SODEMAN'S

PATHOLOGIC PHYSIOLOGY
MECHANISMS OF DISEASE

WILLIAM A. SODEMAN, JR., M.D., F.A.C.P.

Deputy Dean for Academic Affairs,
Professor and Chairman, Department of Comprehensive Medicine,
University of South Florida College of Medicine,
Tampa, Florida

THOMAS M. SODEMAN, M.D., F.C.A.P., F.A.C.P.

Professor and Chairman, Department of Pathology,
Texas Tech University Health Sciences Center School of Medicine,
Lubbock, Texas

SEVENTH EDITION

1985

W. B. SAUNDERS COMPANY

Philadelphia • London • Toronto • Mexico City • Rio de Janeiro • Sydney • Tokyo • Hong Kong

W. B. Saunders Company: West Washington Square
                          Philadelphia, PA 19105

Library of Congress Cataloging in Publication Data

Pathologic physiology.

Sodeman's pathologic physiology.

1. Physiology, Pathological.   I. Sodeman, William A.
   (William Anthony), 1936–   II. Sodeman, Thomas M.
   III. Title. [DNLM: 1. Pathology. QZ 140 S679p]

RB113.P35 1985   616.07   83–7869

ISBN 0–7216–1010–2

Sodeman's PATHOLOGIC PHYSIOLOGY: Mechanisms of Disease   ISBN   0-7216-1010-2

Last digit is the print number: 9   8   7   6   5   4   3   2   1

CONTRIBUTORS

J. A. ABILDSKOV, M.D.

Professor of Medicine and Director, Nora Eccles Harrison Cardiovascular Research and Training Institute, University of Utah School of Medicine; Attending Physician, University of Utah Hospital, Salt Lake City, Utah.

BART BARLOGIE, M.D.

Associate Professor of Medicine, University of Texas Medical School at Houston; Associate Internist/Oncologist, M. D. Anderson Hospital and Tumor Institute; Consultant Professor, Hermann Hospital, Houston, Texas.

RODGER L. BICK, M.D., F.A.C.P.

Clinical Faculty, Hematology/Oncology, UCLA Center for Health Sciences, Los Angeles, California; Associate Professor, Wayne State University School of Medicine, Detroit, Michigan; Chief of Staff, Chief of Hematology/Oncology, and Former Chief of Medicine, San Joaquin Community Hospital; Medical Director, San Joaquin Hematology/Oncology Medical Group, Bakersfield, California.

CHARLES E. BILLINGS, M.D., M.Sc.

Senior Scientist, Ames Research Center, National Aeronautics and Space Administration, Moffett Field, California.

DANE R. BOGGS, M.D.

Professor of Medicine, University of Pittsburgh, School of Medicine, Pittsburgh, Pennsylvania.

GILES G. BOLE, JR., M.D.

Professor of Internal Medicine and Physician-in-Charge, Arthritis Division and Rackham Arthritis Research Unit, University of Michigan Medical School, Ann Arbor, Michigan.

ROBERT J. BOLT, M.D.

Professor, Department of Medicine, University of California, Davis, Davis, California; Attending Physician, University of California Davis Medical Center, Sacramento, California.

GEORGE A. BRAY, M.D.

Professor of Medicine, Professor of Physiology and Biophysics, University of Southern California School of Medicine; Chief, Section of Diabetes and Clinical Nutrition, Los Angeles County-University of Southern California Medical Center, Los Angeles, California.

THOMAS W. BURNS, M.D.

Professor of Medicine and Director, Division of Endocrinology and Metabolism, University of Missouri—Columbia School of Medicine; Attending/Consulting Physician, University of Missouri—Columbia Hospital and Clinics and Harry S. Truman Memorial Veterans Administration Hospital, Columbia, Missouri.

HAROLD E. CARLSON, M.D.

Associate Professor of Internal Medicine, University of Missouri—Columbia School of Medicine; Chief, Endocrinology Section, Harry S. Truman Memorial Veterans Administration Hospital, Columbia, Missouri.

DAVID CENTER, M.D.

Associate Professor of Medicine, Boston University School of Medicine; Associate Professor of Medicine, Pulmonary Medicine Section, Boston University Medical Center, Boston, Massachusetts.

YVONNE E. CUMMINGS, M.D., F.A.C.P.

Associate Professor of Medicine, Division of Nephrology, Department of Internal Medicine, University of South Florida College of Medicine; Attending and Consulting Nephrologist, Tampa General Hospital; Consulting Nephrologist, James A. Haley Veterans Administration Hospital, University Community Hospital, and Memorial Hospital of Tampa, Tampa, Florida.

HAROLD T. DODGE, M.D.

Professor of Medicine, University of Washington School of Medicine; Attending Cardiologist, University Hospital, Seattle, Washington.

LEONARD S. DREIFUS, M.D.

Professor of Medicine, Jefferson Medical College of Thomas Jefferson University; Chief, Cardiovascular Division, Lankenau Hospital, Philadelphia, Pennsylvania.

LOUIS J. ELSAS, II, M.D.

Professor of Pediatrics; Associate Professor, Biochemistry; and Director, Division of Medical Genetics, Emory University School of Medicine; Attending Physician, Emory University Hospital, Grady Memorial Hospital, and Henrietta Egleston Hospital for Children, Atlanta, Georgia.

EDMUND B. FLINK, M.D., Ph.D.

Professor of Medicine, West Virginia University School of Medicine; Attending Physician, West Virginia University Hospital, Morgantown, West Virginia.

RAY W. GIFFORD, JR., M.D.

Chairman, Department of Hypertension/Nephrology, Cleveland Clinic Foundation, Cleveland, Ohio.

ARTHUR C. GUYTON, M.D.

Professor and Chairman, Department of Physiology and Biophysics, University of Mississippi Medical Center, Jackson, Mississippi.

W. PROCTOR HARVEY, M.D.

Professor of Medicine, Division of Cardiology, Georgetown University Medical Center, Washington, D.C.

FRANK L. IBER, M.D.

Professor of Medicine, Division of Gaastroenterology, University of Maryland School of Medicine; Professor of Medicine, Baltimore Veterans Administration Medical Centers, Baltimore, Maryland.

J. WARD KENNEDY, M.D.

Professor of Medicine and Director, Division of Cardiology, University of Washington School of Medicine; Chief of Cardiology, University Hospital, Seattle, Washington.

DAVID M. KLACHKO, M.D.

Professor of Medicine, University of Missouri—Columbia School of Medicine; Attending/Consulting Physician, University of Missouri—Columbia Hospital and Clinics; Attending/Consulting Physician, Harry S. Truman Memorial Veterans Administration Hospital, Columbia, Missouri.

PATRICIA S. LATHAM, M.D.

Assistant Professor of Medicine and Pathology, University of Maryland School of Medicine and Baltimore Veterans Administration Medical Center, Baltimore, Maryland.

ROBIN McFADDEN, M.D.

Assistant Professor of Medicine, University of Western Ontario Faculty of Medicine; Staff, Pulmonary Medicine Section, St. Joseph's Hospital, London, Ontario, Canada.

JOHN C. MARSH, M.D.

Professor of Medicine and Lecturer in Pharmacology, Yale University School of Medicine; Attending Physi-

cian, Yale–New Haven Hospital; Consultant, West Haven Veterans Administration Hospital, New Haven, Connecticut; Consultant, Uncas on Thames Hospital, Norwich, Connecticut.

DEAN T. MASON, M.D.

Physician-in-Chief, Western Heart Institute, Saint Mary's Hospital and Medical Center; Editor-in-Chief, *Medical Heart Journal,* San Francisco, California.

W. KEITH C. MORGAN, M.D.

Professor of Medicine, University of Western Ontario Faculty of Medicine; Director, Sir Adam Beck Chest Unit, University Hospital, London, Ontario, Canada.

CARLOS E. MOYA, M.D.

Clinical Assistant Professor, University of Kansas College of Health Sciences, Kansas City, Kansas; Associate Pathologist, Department of Pathology, Methodist Medical Center, Saint Joseph, Missouri.

H. JUERGEN NORD, M.D., F.A.C.P.

Associate Professor of Medicine, Division of Digestive Diseases and Nutrition, University of South Florida College of Medicine; Chief, U.S.F. Gastroenterology Service, Tampa General Hospital; Attending Physician, James A. Haley Veterans Administration Medical Center, Tampa, Florida.

WILLIAM W. PARMLEY, M.D.

Professor of Medicine, University of California, San Francisco; Chief of Cardiology, University of California Medical Center, San Francisco, California.

ANANDA S. PRASAD, M.D., Ph.D.

Professor of Medicine, Wayne State University School of Medicine; Director, Division of Hematology, Harper Hospital, Detroit, Michigan; Staff, Veterans Administration Hospital, Allen Park, Michigan.

JEAN H. PRIEST, M.D.

Professor, Pediatrics-Medical Genetics; Associate Professor, Pathology, Emory University School of Medicine; Attending Physician, Grady Memorial Hospital and Emory University Hospital, Atlanta, Georgia.

MARTIN N. RABER, M.D.

Associate Professor of Medicine, Division of Hematology/Oncology, University of Texas Medical School at Houston; Attending Physician, Hermann Hospital; Assistant Internist/Oncologist, M. D. Anderson Hospital and Tumor Institute, Houston, Texas.

CHARLES E. REED, M.D.

Professor of Medicine, Mayo Medical School; Consultant, Internal Medicine and Allergy, Mayo Clinic, Rochester, Minnesota.

DOUGLAS SEATON, M.D., M.R.C.P.

Clinical Tutor, Faculty of Clinical Medicine, University of Cambridge, Cambridge, England; Consultant Physician in Respiratory Medicine, Ipswich Hospital, Ipswich, England.

SHEILA SHAH, M.D.

Clinical Assistant Professor, University of Kansas College of Health Sciences, Kansas City, Kansas; Associate Pathologist, Department of Pathology, Methodist Medical Center, Saint Joseph, Missouri.

DANA L. SHIRES, JR., M.D., F.A.C.P.

Professor of Medicine and Director, Division of Nephrology, Department of Internal Medicine, University of South Florida College of Medicine and Affiliated Hospitals; Director, Kidney Transplant Service and University Renal Service, Tampa General Hospital; Consulting Nephrologist, James A. Haley Veterans Administration Hospital and Memorial Hospital of Tampa, Tampa, Florida.

DAVID B. SKINNER, M.D., D.Sc.(Hon.)

Dallas B. Phemister Professor of Surgery, University of Chicago Pritzker School of Medicine; Chairman, Department of Surgery, University of Chicago Medical Center, Chicago, Illinois.

PHILIP J. SNODGRASS, M.D.

Professor of Medicine, Indiana University School of Medicine; Chief, Medical Service, Veterans Administration Medical Center, Indianapolis, Indiana.

THOMAS M. SODEMAN, M.D., F.C.A.P., F.A.C.P.

Professor and Chairman, Department of Pathology, Texas Tech University Health Sciences Center School of Medicine, Lubbock, Texas.

WILLIAM A. SODEMAN, SR., M.D., M.A.C.P.

Academic Advisor and Clinical Professor of Medicine, The Medical College of Ohio, Toledo, Ohio.

WILLIAM A. SODEMAN, JR., M.D., F.A.C.P.

Deputy Dean for Academic Affairs; Professor and Chairman, Department of Comprehensive Medicine, University of South Florida College of Medicine, Tampa, Florida.

JOHN F. STAPLETON, M.D.

Professor of Medicine and Associate Dean, Georgetown University School of Medicine; Medical Director, Georgetown University Hospital, Washington, D.C.

H. J. C. SWAN, M.D., Ph.D.

Professor of Medicine, UCLA School of Medicine; Director, Department of Cardiology, Cedars-Sinai Medical Center, Los Angeles, California.

MORTON N. SWARTZ, M.D.

Professor of Medicine, Harvard Medical School; Chief, Infectious Disease Unit, Massachusetts General Hospital, Boston, Massachusetts.

ANDOR SZENTIVANYI, M.D.

Dean of the College of Medicine and Deputy Vice President for Medical Affairs, University of South Florida College of Medicine, Tampa, Florida

JUDITH SZENTIVANYI, M.D.

Clinical Assistant Professor, Department of Internal Medicine, University of South Florida College of Medicine, Tampa, Florida.

ROBERT C. TARAZI, M.D.

Vice-Chairman, Research Division; Chairman, Clinical Science Department, Cleveland Clinic Foundation, Cleveland, Ohio.

YOSHIO WATANABE, M.D.

Professor of Medicine and Director, Cardiovascular Institute, Fujita Gakuen University School of Medicine, Toyoake, Aichi, Japan.

DAVID W. WATSON, M.D.

Clinical Associate Professor of Medicine, University of California, Davis, Davis, California; Attending Physician, University of California Davis Medical Center, Sacramento, California.

LOUIS WEINSTEIN, M.D., Ph.D.

Lecturer, Department of Medicine, Harvard Medical School; Senior Consultant in Medicine, Brigham and Women's Hospital, Boston, Massachusetts.

JOAN WIKMAN-COFFELT, M.S., Ph.D.

Research Biochemist, University of California, San Francisco, San Francisco, California.

K. LEMONE YIELDING, M.D.

Chairman and Professor of Anatomy, Professor of Medicine, University of South Alabama College of Medicine, Mobile, Alabama.

PREFACE

Thirty-five years ago the first edition of *Pathologic Physiology* was released. Truman was President, the Korean War began, Tennessee Williams published *The Rose Tattoo,* Charles Schultz began drawing Peanuts, and the Nobel Prize in Medicine went to Hench, Kendall, and Reichstein for their work on cortisone. The available medical texts focused on signs, symptoms, differential diagnosis, and therapy. The pathology texts focused on gross and microscopic characteristics. Each was an encyclopedic assemblage of known facts. *Pathologic Physiology* was to serve as a bridge between the technologically maturing basic sciences and the clinical encyclopedias. Since that time the science of medicine has, with increasing success, illuminated the art in a continuum, which this text has both participated in and recorded.

This edition strives to maintain this continuum. We are indebted to the contributors who made this edition possible. Its successes are theirs, while the defects are the editors' responsibility. We are grateful to Mr. John Hanley, the former president of the W. B. Saunders Company, for his continued support and are particularly indebted to Mr. John Dyson, our editor at the W. B. Saunders Company, for his patient counsel through two editions. Our families have been more than tolerant, for revision of a large text is a thief of family time and its publication a family triumph. Their patience and support should not go unrecognized. Dr. William A. Sodeman, Sr., as editor emeritus, has had an equally unsung, but essential, influence which we acknowledge.

Last, our special thanks to Mrs. Alison Goins, who catalogued each manuscript page, illustration, galley, and page proof.

William A. Sodeman, Jr., M.D.
Thomas Sodeman, M.D.

CONTENTS

Section III
RHEUMATOLOGY, ALLERGY, INFECTIOUS DISEASE,
AND HEMATOLOGY

Section V
TOXIC PHYSICAL AND CHEMICAL AGENTS

Section I

SCIENTIFIC FOUNDATIONS

Metabolic Biochemistry

1

Thomas M. Sodeman

Characterization of the normal state and of the complex changes wrought by disease formulates the goal of biochemical research. Locked in the intricate interlinking pathways toward that goal are the sources of the structural elements of cells, their physiology, and their metabolic regulation. The protoplasm of the cell, contained by the cell wall and holding numerous organelles, consists of a mixture of water, minerals, and organic macromolecules. From these mixtures stem the physiologic characteristics of life. The study of these chemical mixtures in terms of their components, synthesis, storage, interaction, and degradation is the foundation of biochemistry, of which a clear understanding is essential. Most, if not all, of the pathologic processes to be discussed in this text involve either primary defects or secondary alterations in biochemical processes.

The biochemical processes of the body occur at a subcellular level and involve synthesis and catabolism of organic material, regulation of exchange of material, and conversion of chemical energy into usable forms. The chemical composition and ratio of compounds of cells are complex and vary among cell types. Oxygen, carbon, hydrogen, nitrogen, phosphorus, and sulfur contribute most of the structural mass of the cell and provide the elements for its intrinsic chemical physiology. Additional elements—for example, the metals sodium and magnesium—are essential to life. Of known elements, only 19 appear to be absolutely necessary. The task of unraveling the chemical nature of cell function and structure is formidable and is certain to lead to change in the understanding of even the most well-established biochemical mechanisms.

The intent of this chapter is to review biochemical principles that govern biologic processes. It is assumed that basic organic chemical concepts

of covalent bonds, bond angles, and the spatial relationships between atoms are familiar. The chemical and physical properties of biochemical compounds in most situations reflect the nature of the functional groups.

Fundamental groups of alcohols, aldehydes, ketones, amines and carboxylic acids are encountered throughout carbohydrate, lipid, and protein metabolism (Table 1–1). Alcohols are hydroxylated hydrocarbons and alkyl derivatives of water. In polyhydric form they represent sugars and, as cyclic or ring forms, steroids. Aldehydes and ketones are composed of a carbonyl group ($-C=O$) with one or two alkyl groups attached. These organic configurations are also present in the polyhydric alcohols of sugars and other organic compounds. Amines are alkyl derivatives of ammonia and, as will be discussed, are essential elements in proteins. The carboxylic functional group consists of a carbonyl and hydroxyl group on the same atom. Functionally, they form weak acids.

These functional groups and their activity in oxidation, esterification, reduction, and other reaction modes provide many of the characteristics of organic compounds.

EQUILIBRIUM

Equilibrium is the process in which a forward reaction is equal to the reverse reaction. Although there is no net change in reactants and products, turnover is occurring on either side of the reaction through equal change. A better term for the equilibrium in biologic processes is "steady state." This implies that a concentration of a substance can be held constant. The equilibrium, or steady state, is nonproductive in the biologic system with regard to the thermodynamics of the system. No free energy is made available by the system. Biologic studies are more concerned with the initial state, routes, and rate of conversion in which energy changes occur. This is, essentially, the study of the kinetics of the reaction. Isolation of a single reaction in an in-vitro system permits an understanding of interaction of the components and the thermodynamics that occur. In-vivo study is more difficult because the components of a reaction, either reactants or products, are influenced by the complex pathways that yield or utilize them in the continuous biologic system. Under these circumstances, equilibrium becomes less important. The concentrations of many substances are held at rigid levels within the body. This steady state is controlled by reactions producing or utilizing the

TABLE 1–1 FUNCTIONAL GROUPS

Alcohol	$R-CH_2-OH$
Aldehyde	$R-C=O$ $\quad\;\; \mid$ $\quad\;\; H$
Ketone	R $\quad \searrow$ $\qquad C=O$ $\quad \nearrow$ R
Amines	$R-NH_2$
Carboxylic acid	$R-COOH$

components. Feedback mechanisms that control enzymes and enzyme substrate induction represent some of the controls that assure availability of reactants and energy necessary for biologic processes. All chemical reactions to some degree are reversible; however, in biochemical pathways, the products of a reaction are usually utilized in the next step. This forces the reaction one way, resulting in irreversibility and nonequilibrium of reaction.

The reaction kinetics and steady state can be expressed mathematically, and the influence of component concentrations, temperature, and pressure can be analyzed to determine the dynamics of the reaction and interacting systems. The environmental demands on in-vivo reactions are difficult to comprehend at the subcellular level. For this reason, reaction characteristics are more commonly thought of in terms of the changing concentrations of intermediates and the effects these may have in regulation of distant but indirectly coupled reactions. A pathologic state may be derived from or result in the inability of regulatory influences to compensate for changes in biochemical interactions. Changes in the immediate kinetics of a reaction or distal reactions can result in the development of new steady states with accumulations or depletions of pathway components. Such effects can be seen in storage diseases, the inability to maintain sufficient glucose levels, and the failure of normal trigger mechanisms to initiate the coagulation cascade in the absence or depression of key factors.

THERMODYNAMICS

Thermodynamics is the study of quantitative changes in energy as biologic reactions pass to equilibrium. It is not concerned with processes at equilibrium, as that is a terminal state in which free energy is zero. The energy produced within a system may take the form of thermal, osmotic, mechanical, chemical, or electrical energy. Transformation of energy from one form to another may be completed in biologic systems.

In the biologic system, energy is primarily obtained by chemical linkage to oxidative reactions. The energy of a system can be considered in two parts. Entropic energy is that energy required internally by the system to maintain its molecular configuration. Enthalpic energy is the energy available externally for work (free energy). In the conversion of glucose in the presence of oxygen to yield carbon dioxide and water, 673,000 cal/mole of free energy are produced that may be transferred by chemical means to reactions requiring energy. In a reaction process, some energy is lost as heat and may not be utilized in chemical reactions.

The difference in energy states of a substrate versus the product is a measure of the extent to which a reaction will proceed. Exergonic reactions (i.e., those that yield energy) may proceed spontaneously. Whether an exergonic reaction will spontaneously occur depends on the energy of activation of the reactants. Each molecule has an average level of energy that maintains its molecular configuration. For a reaction to occur spontaneously, a critical energy level or barrier must be reached so that bonding or exchange may occur between elements. When two atomic orbits merge, a more stable configuration occurs that will require less energy. Enzymes, through the formation of an enzyme-reactant complex, reduce the energy of activation and thus accelerate a reaction. Endergonic reactions, however, require large amounts of energy to proceed.

The energy requirement of reactions plays an important role in determining the availability of products and, therefore, in controlling subsequent reactions. In biologic systems, there is both compartmentalization and linkage of reactions to ensure the efficient availability of reaction products and energy necessary to activate, or drive, a reaction. Energy is usually supplied by chemical means and under strictly controlled mechanisms. The energy released in a reaction may contribute to further activation of the initial substrate or may provide energy for closely associated reactions. The product of the reaction may be sufficiently activated to reduce the energy requirements for the next step.

In the metabolic process, the mechanism of free energy transfer relies heavily on intermediate energy absorbers, for example, the nucleotide *adenosine triphosphate (ATP)*. The advantage of energy absorbers lies in their universal activity, which permits energy transfer in a wide variety of reactions. Throughout the biochemical pathways, ATP has an essential role in providing energy to endergonic processes. ATP is composed of a purine, a ribose, and three phosphate groups. It carries a central position in relation to other organophosphates in its ability to yield and accept high-energy phosphate. ATP has the stability necessary to function as an energy storehouse. The source for the high-energy bond is provided in the respiratory chain oxidation in mitochondria, in the catabolism of substrates (as in the Embden-Meyerhof pathway of glycolysis), and in high-energy storage depots, such as creatine phosphate in muscle. Upon hydrolysis ATP liberates 8.8 cal/mole of free energy. Three factors are involved in this release: (1) a change in resonance energy, (2) ionization-released energy, and (3) relief of electrostatic repulses. The prime reservoir of energy is in the body's macromolecules, which, through metabolic processes, provide high-energy phosphates. Lipids are particularly effective in this process and provide the added advantage of osmotic stability in the cell.

TABLE 1–2 ENZYME CLASSIFICATION

Oxidoreductases
Transferases
Hydrolases
Lyases
Isomerases
Ligases

ENZYMES

Enzymes are protein biocatalysts that reduce the necessary chemical energy for activation of a reaction. They are not consumed, and, therefore, only small quantities are required. In contrast to catalysts, they tend to be reaction-specific. Six functional classes of enzymes have been established and are outlined in Table 1–2.

Almost all biochemical reactions are enzyme-catalyzed. Many enzymes require nonprotein cofactors or coenzymes in their reactions. Coenzymes are important in transferring groups between reactants and, unlike enzymes, are not re-formed in the reaction. B-vitamins are a common structural part of coenzymes.

The three-dimensional structure of enzymes plays an important role in their function and stability. An enzyme, a relatively large molecule in comparison with the substrate, combines with a substrate, altering the enzyme configuration to bring functional or catalytic groups into place.

Enzyme aggregates resulting from association of subunits form a series of multiple molecular forms with similar enzymatic activity but structural differences. One form may dominate over others in a tissue. Clinically, multiple molecular forms are expressed in isoenzymes of dehydrogenases, phosphatases, transaminases, and proteolytic enzymes.

Measurements of circulating enzymes have become routine in the practice of medicine as an indicator of cellular damage or genetic defects. Because of the small quantities present, enzymes are measured by their activity. This has given rise to a number of arbitrary units. Many of the enzymes in plasma have no physiologic function in the blood but represent release from cells and normal cellular degradation. Other enzymes exist in proenzyme forms, for example, coagulation factors and lipoprotein lipase, which, upon activation, play critical roles in the body's homeostatic processes.

METABOLIC REGULATION

The regulation of metabolic processes is particularly controlled by enzyme activity. Control may be based on the amount of enzyme synthesized, enzyme inhibition, activation, degradation, and covalent modification of protein structure.

Regulatory mechanisms also include the availability of substrates or cofactors, transport systems, and compartmentalization of reactions. Compartmentalization permits localization of reaction and independence from potentially influencing processes. It provides an orderly sequence for controlled enzymatic processes linking reactants and assures energy transfer. Compartmentalization does pose problems when reactants must be moved from one compartment to another. Translocation may require a converting process to change a metabolite to a permeable state or form for passage across a membrane and then similar processes for reconversion. Such a process would require two forms of enzymes physically separated.

Metabolic processes tend to maintain a steady state within cells despite short-term changes within the environment. Chemical processes must occur at the right time and rate to meet the coordinated processes in a cell. Enzymes play a key role in this regulation. Many factors are involved in enzyme control. Among those not yet mentioned is control of synthesis by substrate induction, by product repression or feedback repression, by regulated enzyme degradation, and by hormonal and dietary influences. Secondary enzyme activation provides one method of regulation. In this process, a proenzyme is converted to an active form by a second enzyme. This provides a mechanism for concentrating an enzyme at an appropriate site ready for its physiologic demand. Examples can be seen in the coagulation process and in digestive enzymes. Knowledge of these regulatory processes is limited, but they are important in understanding the pathologic physiology of disease and the possible approaches to therapy. The ability to control enzymes may in the future open new avenues for therapeutics.

BIOLOGIC OXIDATION

Free energy in the cell ultimately lies in the oxidative reaction. In biologic systems, this mostly involves the transfer of hydrogen and formation of water. The loss of electrons is known as *chemical oxidation;* a gain in electrons is called *reduction.* The energy released in biologic oxidation may be chemically conserved in high-energy phosphates. This process of coupling of oxidation to high-energy carriers is referred to as *oxidative phosphorylation.* When a coenzyme (e.g., ATP or NAD) is reduced, a mechanism for reoxidation and regeneration, the respiratory chain, is available in the cell. This system provides an assemblage of enzymes in coupled reactions that can transport electrons and provide high-energy bonds. It is compartmentalized in the mitochondria. These high-energy bonds provide a mechanism for storing energy formed in biologic oxidation.

The energy from oxidation of fatty acids, amino acids, and carbohydrates is made available in the mitochondria through the respiratory chain. Numerous enzymes are involved in the oxidative process. Among these are oxidases, aerobic and anaerobic dehydrogenases, hydroperoxidases, and oxygenases. The respiratory chain transports reducing equivalents, hydrogen or electrons, for reaction with oxygen to form water. The order is arranged sequentially, with increasing tendency for free-energy exchange or redox potential. The main mitochondrial chain (Fig. 1–1) is initiated by a NAD-linked dehydrogenase system and proceeds through flavoprotein and cytochrome systems to molecular oxygen. Metabolic pathways feed reducing equivalents (NAD or $FADH_2$) into the system. The terminal cytochrome system possesses many elements, starting with coenzyme Q, which links flavoprotein to cytochrome, and extending through cytochromes C_1, C, A, and A_3. The respiratory chain provides three sites at which energy change is sufficient to permit coupling with ADP to form ATP. Each mole of NADH that enters the chain produces three moles of high-energy phosphate, and each mole of $FADH_2$ yields two moles of this high-energy product. The control of the respiratory process depends on the availability of substrate, ADP, and oxygen.

High-energy bonds are not produced solely in the respiratory chain. Substrate phosphorylation involving the production of high-energy bonds during metabolic oxidation sequences of glucose, lipids, and amino acids will be reviewed later in this chapter during specific discussions. Mechanisms are available to transfer to the mitochondria the NADH produced by glycolysis in the cytosol with substrate-pair translocation systems.

The impact of both mitochondrial and substrate phosphorylation is provision of energy. With oxidation of glucose in the glycolytic process and citric acid cycle, six high-energy phosphate bonds are produced and two are used. These represent phosphorylation at the substrate level. Linkage with the respiratory chain, with reoxidation of reduced coenzymes, yields 34 high-energy bonds per cycle of glucose. Through these processes it is possible to account for 46 per cent of the free energy of glucose metabolism. Under anaerobic conditions, two high-energy phosphate bonds are produced.

CARBOHYDRATE METABOLISM

CARBOHYDRATE STRUCTURE

Carbohydrates may be defined as aldehyde or ketone derivatives or polyhydric alcohols and are divided into four major groups. Monosaccharides, including trioses, tetroses, pentoses, hexoses, and heptoses, are physiologically important carbohydrates. The hexose sugars glucose, fructose, galactose, and mannose are common dietary components and provide a major energy source. D-ribose, a pentose sugar, is an essential component of nucleic acid. Disaccharides such as sucrose, maltose, and lactose are composed of two monosaccharides united by a glycosidic linkage and are common elements of the daily diet. Polysaccharides occur in the forms of starches, glycogen, and dextrins. Polysaccharides in the form of glycosaminoglycans (mucopolysaccharides) and glycoproteins (mucoproteins) are important structural components of the body. Glycoproteins are elements of blood groups and certain hormones.

GLYCOLYSIS

This process, the Embden-Meyerhof pathway, is a complex sequence in which glucose and other carbohydrates are metabolized to pyruvate or lactate. It is an extramitochondrial function, occurring in the cytosols of cells. A schematic outline of the glycolytic process is included in Figure 1–2. In step 1, glucose is phosphorylated to glucose 6-phosphate by hexokinase or, in the liver, by glucokinase. The reaction is irreversible and is associated with an extensive heat loss. Glucose 6-phosphate is a major pivotal compound in carbohydrate metabolism. Processes involving synthesis and degradation of glycogen, from either glucose or citric acid components, and entry into the hexose monophosphate shunt involve this critical component. Step 3 involves an irreversible phosphorylation reaction that is followed by a splitting of the hexose molecule into two triose phosphate molecules. These trioses are interconvertible. The glycolysis pathway continues with oxidation of glyceraldehyde 3-phosphate and the

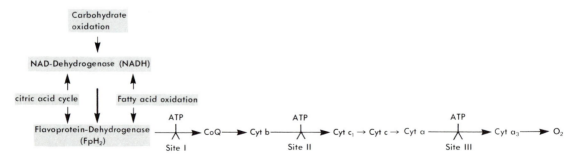

Figure 1–1 Mitochondrial respiratory chain for transport of reducing equivalents.

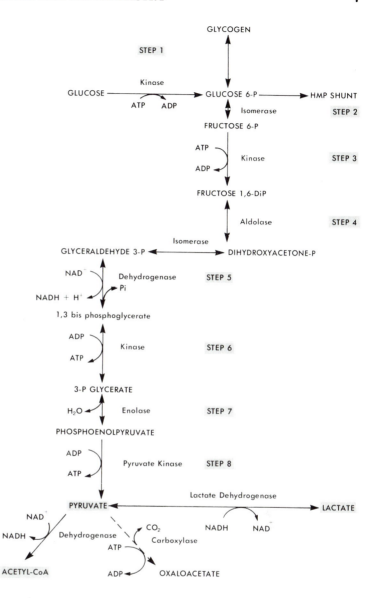

Figure 1–2 Embden-Meyerhof pathway for glycolysis is located in the cytosol and catalyzes the conversion of carbohydrates to pyruvate and lactate.

addition of an inorganic phosphate in a NAD-dependent step. At steps 6 and 8, high energy phosphate bonds are produced. In the latter step, the conversion of phosphoenolpyruvate to pyruvate under the influence of pyruvate kinase, a third irreversible point occurs in the glycolytic pathway.

The outcome from this point depends on the availability of oxygen. Under hypoxic situations, the NADH produced in step 5 is available for conversion of pyruvate to lactate. Under aerobic conditions, the NADH is utilized in the mitochondrial respiratory chain and pyruvate is utilized in the citric acid cycle. Pyruvate enters the mitochondria via a transport system where, under the influence of a pyruvate dehydrogenase enzyme complex, it is converted irreversibly to acetyl-CoA. This complex involves thiamine pyrophosphate, lipoic acid, transacetylase, and two dehydrogen-

ases. $FADH_2$ is produced in the reaction, to be oxidized later by NAD. The process is regulated by ATP, which acts through cyclic AMP (cAMP) to activate a phosphatase that dephosphorylates and activates the enzyme complex.

In addition to supplying acetyl-CoA in the mitochondria, pyruvate supplements the citric acid cycle intermediate, oxaloacetate. This is achieved by pyruvate carboxylase in the presence of ATP and CO_2 in an irreversible reaction. The process is regulated by acetyl-CoA.

HEXOSE MONOPHOSPHATE SHUNT

An alternate pathway for oxidation of glucose 6-phosphate is provided in the hexose monophosphate shunt (HMP), or pentose phosphate shunt

(Fig. 1–3). This process occurs, like glycolysis, in the cytosol. Isolation of the shunt enzymes has demonstrated high levels in liver, red blood cells, and adipose tissue and low activity in skeletal muscle. Through a series of enzyme reactions, glucose 6-phosphate undergoes dehydrogenation and decarboxylation to ribulose 5-phosphate and CO_2. Two NADP-dependent reactions are involved in accepting electrons. If three molecules of glucose 6-phosphate are metabolized in the HMP shunt, three pentoses are formed. By being rearranged through transketolase and aldolase reactions, one molecule of glyceraldehyde 3-phosphate and two molecules of glucose 6-phosphate can be re-formed for final oxidation.

What, then, is the point of the alternate pathway? It appears to be a major source of NADPH. In the red blood cell, approximately 10 per cent of glucose 6-phosphate enters the shunt. The NADPH produced is linked by glutathione enzymes with peroxidase, which provides a mechanism for preventing accumulations of H_2O_2 that would cause oxidative denaturation of hemoglobin. In adipose tissue, NADPH is necessary for the synthesis of fatty acids and steroids. The pentose phosphate shunt also provides sugars for nucleotide and nucleic acid synthesis in the form of ribose 5-phosphate.

GLYCOGENESIS

This process consists of the synthesis of glycogen. It may occur in all tissues but is most prominent in liver and skeletal muscle. The steps include the phosphorylation of glucose to glucose 6-phosphate and then conversion to glucose 1-phosphate by a mutase enzyme. The glucose 1-phosphate then enters a cycle reacting with uridine triphosphate (UTP) and, under the influence of glycogen synthetase, is linked in a 1,4-glycosidic bond with a glucose residue. Through a series of successive linkages, a glycogen molecule is enlarged with branches occurring every 6 to 12 glucose residues. Control of glycogenesis is through the enzyme glycogen synthetase I, which is activated by synthetase phosphatase under the influence of glucose or insulin. Inactivation of glycogen synthetase is influenced by ATP. Adenylate cyclase is stimulated to form 3'5'-cyclic AMP from ATP. This reaction, initiated by epinephrine, norepinephrine, or glucagon, increases cAMP, which activates a protein kinase that converts glycogen synthetase to its inactive form.

GLYCOGENOLYSIS

This process consists of the breakdown of glycogen and is initiated by the action of the enzyme phosphorylase. The phosphorylase enzyme breaks the 1,4 linkage to yield glucose 1-phosphate. Once in the form of glucose 1-phosphate, enzymes exist to convert it in liver or kidney, but not muscle, to free glucose.

Separate distinct forms of phosphorylase exist in muscle and liver cells. In muscle, phosphorylase *a* activity is controlled in part by hormones through the basic cAMP sequence, similar to that described for inactivation of glycogen synthetase. In this process, cAMP activates an enzyme that condenses the inactive dimer, phosphorylase *b,* to the tetramer active form, phosphorylase *a.* Simple muscle contraction is also known to stimulate phosphorylase *a* independent of cAMP. Liver phosphorylase also exists in two forms in the cell. However, it is not influenced by cAMP but controlled by a specific phosphatase.

GLUCONEOGENESIS

In addition to glycogenolysis, the process of gluconeogenesis can provide glucose in dietary

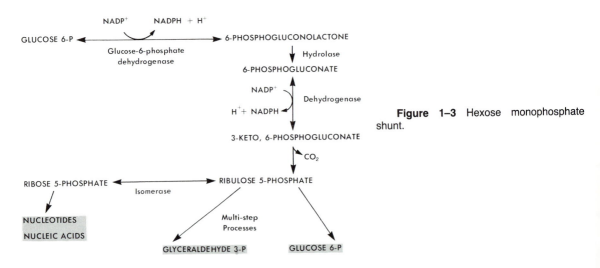

Figure 1–3 Hexose monophosphate shunt.

carbohydrate restriction. In essence, the process is a reversal of glycolytic processes and involves the conversion of noncarbohydrates to glucose. As it is a reversal, gluconeogenesis activities are counterproductive to glycolytic processes.

Three irreversible steps occur in glycolysis that must be overcome to reverse the Embden-Meyerhof pathway. The first irreversible reaction is the conversion of phosphoenolpyruvate to pyruvate. This is accomplished by entry of pyruvate into the mitochondria, where it can be converted to oxaloacetate by pyruvate carboxylase. The mitochondria are not permeable to oxaloacetate. They are, however, permeable to malate, which can be formed by reduction of oxaloacetate. Malate can be translocated by the dicarboxylate transport system to the cytosol for reaction with NAD and reduction to oxaloacetate. Under the influence of carboxykinase, oxaloacetate is converted to the glycolytic intermediate, phosphoenolpyruvate. A high-energy GTP is necessary for this reaction.

The irreversible glycolytic reaction between fructose 1,6-bisphosphate and fructose 6-phosphate and the phosphorylation of glucose to glucose 6-phosphate are handled through enzymatic processes distinct from those in the glycolytic pathway. The enzymes for reversal of glycolysis are present in liver and kidney but not in skeletal muscle.

Glucogenic amino acids, after transamination or deamination, provide members of the citric acid cycle or pyruvate that can be converted to glucose by gluconeogenesis. Similarly, lactate formed via activation of pyruvate and glycerol by glycerokinase to glycerol 3-phosphate enters the gluconeogenesis pathway. Gluconeogenesis in liver and kidney can then meet the body's needs for glucose in carbohydrate starvation once glycogen stores are exhausted.

ALTERNATE CARBOHYDRATE METABOLISM

Glucose can be converted to glucuronic acid with intermediate formation of uridine diphosphoglucuronic acid. The latter is an important conjugant for hormones, drugs, and bilirubin. Glucuronic acid can be metabolized to xylulose and enter the pentose phosphate shunt.

Fructose, through multiple pathways, may enter at several steps in the glycolytic pathway for conversion to glucose. In humans, a great deal of the fructose formed as a product of sucrose digestion is converted in the gastrointestinal wall to glucose. In the liver, it may be stored as glycogen. Fructose may also be metabolized by adipose tissue. Galactose formed by intestinal hydrolysis of lactose may be converted to glucose in the liver through a series of enzyme steps.

LIPIDS

Lipids are a heterogeneous group that, because of their high-energy value, form an important dietary constituent. A classification of lipids is given in Table 1–3. The cornerstone of the lipid molecule is fatty acid. Natural fatty acids usually contain an even number of carbon atoms and may be saturated (no double bonds) or unsaturated (one or more double bonds). Common saturated fatty acids encountered in nature are acetic, palmitic, lignoceric, and butyric. Common unsaturated fatty acids are oleic, palmitoleic, linoleic, and arachidonic acids and prostaglandins.

FATTY ACID OXIDATION

Triacylglycerols are esters of fatty acids and the alcohol glycerol. The fatty acids at the three ester positions may vary, giving rise to a mixed acylglycerol. Less commonly, they will all be of the same type. Hydrolysis of triacylglycerols occurs mostly in adipose tissue with the release of the fatty acid, which forms a complex with albumin in plasma. Glycerol, depending on the tissue availability of glycerokinase, may be reutilized or diffused out of the tissue for use elsewhere. Fatty acids circulating in plasma can be removed and undergo β-oxidation to acetyl-CoA through a series of enzyme reactions in the mitochondria. To enter the mitochondria, fatty acids must first be converted to an acyl-CoA form by the action of thiokinase and ATP in microsomes or on the mitochondrial surface. This is the only step in β-oxidation of fatty acids that requires ATP. For long-chain fatty acids, a carnitine and its enzyme associated with the mitochondrial membrane are essential to penetration of the acyl-CoA form through the mitochondrial wall. Activation of short-chain fatty acids may occur directly within mitochondria, avoiding the carnitine step. Once in the mitochondria, acyl-CoA undergoes a series of dehydrogenase steps to remove two hydrogen atoms. The reduced coenzymes ($FADH_2$ and NADH) may enter the respiratory chain and provide ATP. The final enzymatic step in oxidation splits a two-carbon molecule of acetyl-CoA from the fatty acid

TABLE 1–3 GENERAL CLASSIFICATION OF LIPIDS

Simple Lipids
  Fats—fatty acid esters with glycerol
  Waxes—fatty acid esters with higher alcohols

Compound Lipids
  Phospholipids
  Glycolipids
  Aminolipids

Derived Lipids
  Hydrolysis products of other lipids

chain. In the citric acid cycle, the acetyl-CoA can be further oxidized to CO_2 and water. Beta-oxidation yields considerably more energy than the oxidation of glucose. Fatty acids with odd numbers of carbon atoms yield the three-carbon propionyl-CoA on β-oxidation. This may be converted to succinyl-CoA and enter the citric acid cycle.

FATTY ACID SYNTHESIS

Two pathways are available for fatty acid synthesis. The mitochondrial system involves a reversal, with modifications, of β-oxidation. This system functions under anaerobic conditions and requires ATP, NADH, and NADPH. It adds acetyl-CoA units to existing long-chain fatty acids.

The principal site of fatty acid synthesis is the extramitochondrial system, which consists of a multienzyme functional unit that combines with acetyl-CoA to form acyl units. The initial steps involve a condensation of acetyl-CoA with malonyl-CoA, followed by reduction, dehydration, reduction, and the ultimate transfer of the saturated unit to the outer part of the enzyme complex. Malonyl-CoA is formed from acetyl-CoA in a separate reaction. Within this enzyme unit, the molecules are passed along as the reactions proceed. NADPH, derived primarily from the HMP shunt, acts as the hydrogen donor in both reductions. ATP, Mn^+, and HCO_3^- are also required. The process is repeated, adding acyl radicals until the 16-carbon unit of palmitate is formed. The acetyl-CoA used in both the mitochondrial and extramitochondrial systems is derived from carbohydrate and amino acid oxidation or by β-oxidation. The inability to transfer acetyl-CoA out of the mitochondria for fatty acid synthesis in the extramitochondrial system is overcome by transferring acetyl-CoA as a citrate with cleavage by ATP-citrate lyase in the cytosol to acetyl-CoA and oxaloacetate. Pyruvate may participate in fatty acid synthesis by providing acetyl-CoA in the mitochondria which may then be transferred out as citrate. The oxaloacetate formed may be converted to malate and provide NADPH, it may be utilized for glucose formation, or it may be transported into the mitochondria to function in the citric acid cycle. The main site for elongation of existing long-chain fatty acids is a microsomal system.

LIPID METABOLISM

Nutritionally, lipid may be considered essential or nonessential. The three essential long-chain unsaturated fatty acids that are of metabolic significance and that therefore must be supplied in the diet are linoleic, linolenic, and arachidonic acids. These essential fatty acids are important elements in the structural integrity of the cell and its organelles. The nonessential unsaturated fatty acids can be formed from the corresponding saturated fatty acid forms.

The level of free fatty acids (FFA) in plasma, resulting from lipolysis in adipose tissue, strongly influences metabolism in the liver and skeletal muscle.

TRIACYLGLYCEROL (TRIGLYCERIDES)

Triacylglycerols are synthesized in many tissues. The fatty acid portions of the molecule are provided by the synthesis pathways that have already been discussed. In the liver, kidney, intestines, and lactating mammary glands, glycerol can be provided by the action of glycerokinase, which, in the presence of ATP, forms glycerol 3-phosphate. In those tissues low in glycerokinase (adipose tissue and muscle), the glycerol 3-phosphate is derived from the Embden-Meyerhof pathway.

In triacylglycerol formation, fatty acids are activated to acyl-CoA by thiokinase, ATP, and CoA. The acyl-CoA and glycerol 3-phosphate combine in the presence of a transferase to form a diacylglycerol phosphate. Following a phosphohydrolase reaction, which removes the phosphate, a final acyl-CoA is added to form triacylglycerol.

Degradation of the molecule results from hydrolysis with the release of FFA and glycerol. This reaction depends on lipase (not lipoprotein lipase) and is not a simple reversal of synthesis. The fatty acid released upon hydrolysis may be reconverted into triacylglycerol or oxidized by β-oxidation for entry into the citric acid cycle. Depending on the availability of glycerokinase in tissue, glycerol may be reused or diffused into the plasma for transport to tissues with active glycerokinase.

Glucose availability in adipose tissue plays a key role in the level of FFA in plasma. By providing increased levels of glycerol 3-phosphate, glucose stimulates esterification with fatty acids and decreases the flow of fatty acids into the plasma pool. Glucose in adipose tissue may also be oxidized via the citric acid cycle or the HMP shunt, or it may be converted to long-chain fatty acids. When carbohydrates are plentiful, adipose tissue tends to emphasize energy production and conversion to endogenous fatty acids for synthesis of acylglyerol. As carbohydrates are restricted more glucose is conserved for glycerol 3-phosphate formation and esterification with free fatty acids; less glucose is diverted to energy production. However, lipolysis may exceed the rate of esterification despite the greater proportion of glucose being directed to glycerol 3-phosphate and plasma FFA increase. Energy is derived from oxidation of fatty acids rather than from glucose.

The activity of lipase is influenced by adrenocorticotropic hormone (ACTH), melanocyte-stimulating hormone (MSH), thyroid-stimulating hormone (TSH), growth hormone (GH), epinephrine, and glucagon, all of which have a fat mobilization effect. This is thought to occur by activation of cAMP, which converts inactive lipase to an active form through a protein kinase. Insulin and prostaglandins inhibit lipase by decreasing cAMP synthesis. In addition, insulin stimulates lipogenesis. Most of the studies of glucose and hormone effects on lipid metabolism have been carried out in experimental animals. The extent to which they will hold true in humans is still not clear. Certainly, insulin has clinically demonstrated a corrective effect on fat metabolism in diabetics.

PHOSPHOLIPIDS

The phospholipid groups are defined in Table 1–4. In addition to fatty acids and alcohol, phosphoric acid residue and other compounds, such as nitrogenous bases, are contained by phospholipids. A schematic diagram of their synthesis is presented in Figure 1–4. Phospholipids are synthesized from monoacylglycerol or intermediates of triacylglycerol. In the synthesis of lecithins or cephalins, the nitrogenous bases choline and ethanolamine are converted to active form by ATP and cytidine triphosphate. The phosphorylated base is then transferred to intermediate acylglycerol to form the appropriate phospholipid. Similarly, through transferase activity, inositol is added to acylglycerol molecules to form lipositol.

Cardiolipins are formed from an intermediate of lipositol by reaction with glycerol 3-phosphate. Phosphatidylserine is formed from phosphatidylethanolamine (cephalins) by direct reaction with serine. A plasmalogenic diacylglycerol is formed from dihydroxyacetone phosphate of the glycolytic pathway through the action of a transferase,

TABLE 1–4 PHOSPHOLIPIDS

Phosphatidic acid	(cardiolipid)
Phosphatidylcholine	(lecithin)
Phosphatidylethanolamine	(cephalin)
Phosphatidylinositol	(lipositol)
Phosphatidylserine	(cephalin-like)
Lysophospholipids	(lysolecithins)
Plasmalogens	—
Sphingomyelin	—

NADPH-dependent reductase, and acyl-CoA. The sphingomyelins are phospholipids that contain a complex amino alcohol, sphingol, in place of glycerol. Sphingosine is formed from palmitol-CoA and serine through a series of enzyme reactions followed by reaction with choline and acyl-CoA. Cerebrosides contain the sphingosine fatty acid combination with a galactose moiety. These may further react with activated sulfate to yield sulfatides. An alternate pathway for sphingomyelin synthesis is the formation of ceramide, a sphingosine-acyl derivative, followed by addition of choline. Ceramide may also react with galactose and N-acetylneuraminic acid to form a ganglioside.

These numerous phospholipids play a vital role in the structural integrity of cells and biochemical pathways of many tissues, the details of which are beyond the scope of this review. Their clinical importance lies in inherited enzyme deficiencies that are associated primarily with accumulation. In the case of sulfatides, accumulations result in metachromatic leukodystrophy, sphingomyelin in Niemann-Pick disease, and gangliosides in Tay-Sachs disease. Under normal circumstances, degradation involves the enzymatic hydrolysis into individual components with turnover at their own rates.

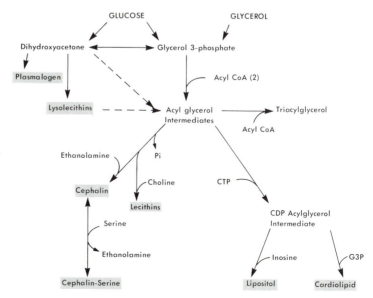

Figure 1–4 Biosynthesis of phospholipids.

PROSTAGLANDINS

The prostaglandins are a series of 20-carbon (eicosanoic) acids derived from fatty acids. The basic structure, prostanoic acid, consists of two carbon chains bonded at the middle by a five-member ring. Variations in double bonds and functional groups give rise to 14 compounds divided into four divisions: A, B, E, and F. The prostaglandins exhibit hormone-like activity and appear to have potential therapeutic uses.

CHOLESTEROL

Steroids have a similar cyclic nucleus that resembles three phenanthrene rings to which a cyclopentane is added. The positions within the steroid nucleus have been internationally defined (Fig. 1–5). Cholesterol is based on this steroid nucleus. Most of cholesterol is synthesized in the body. Dietary cholesterol, however, does affect the production and plasma levels. Cholesterol synthesis involves the microsomal and cytosol fraction of the cell and occurs in such tissues as liver, adrenal cortex, intestine, and aorta. Synthesis can be divided into three basic phases (Fig. 1–6).

The first phase is the formation of mevalonate, which uses a pathway involving condensation of acetyl-CoA molecules into a six-carbon structure. Reduction by NADPH yields mevalonate.

Phase two initially involves phosphorylation of mevalonate, followed by a series of steps involving decarboxylation, condensation of molecules, and a final reduction with the elimination of a pyrophosphate. The end product is squalene, a 30-carbon unit.

The third phase of cholesterol synthesis involves the closure of squalene to form lanosterol, which has the familiar ring-form structure of cholesterol. This phase appears to occur with squalene attached to a carrier protein. Through a series of changes to the side chains and steroid nucleus involving the loss of three methyl groups, cholesterol is formed. Cholesterol on the protein carrier may then be converted to bile acids or steroid hormones. Cholesterol is incorporated into very low density lipoprotein (VLDL) and low density lipoprotein (LDL) for transport in plasma. More than 75 per cent of cholesterol is transported by LDL.

Control of synthesis occurs early in the pathway through a feedback inhibition by cholesterol on the reductive enzyme forming mevalonate. Inhibition by cAMP has also been reported. In tissue cultures, it has been demonstrated that LDL is bound by a receptor on the cell surface. Incorporation by endocytosis into cell lysosomes is followed by splitting off of the cholesterol ester and by hydrolysis to free cholesterol. Free cholesterol inhibits HMG · CoA reductase to slow cholesterol synthesis. Approximately one half the cholesterol eliminated from the body is excreted in feces after conversion to bile acids. The rest is lost as neutral steroids derived from cholesterol in the intestinal mucosa and converted to neutral steroids by bacteria in the lower intestine. Reabsorption of bile acids in the lower ileum provides a feedback inhibition of metabolism of cholesterol in the liver.

PLASMA LIPIDS

Dietary cholesterol is absorbed from the intestine, following which 80 to 90 per cent undergoes esterification with long-chain fatty acids. The esterified cholesterol is incorporated into chylomicrons and VLDL and transported via the lymphatics to plasma. Exogenous cholesterol will suppress endogenous production in liver but cannot eliminate it. Intestinal cholesterol synthesis is little affected by dietary cholesterol, since it seems to be controlled by bile acids. In a similar fashion, cholesterol causes feedback inhibition of its own synthesis. Equilibration of dietary cholesterol with plasma cholesterol takes several days.

Fatty acids in plasma are derived from lipolysis in adipose tissue and from the action of lipoprotein lipase on chylomicrons and VLDL. Carried by albumin, FFA are rapidly removed from circulation by tissues to be utilized in lipid synthesis pathways or to provide energy. In the fasting state, 25 to 50 per cent of energy is derived after β-oxidation of fatty acids and oxidation in the citric acid cycle.

Four major lipid-protein fractions are found in plasma: chylomicrons, VLDL, LDL, and HDL (Table 1–5). One or more apoproteins may be

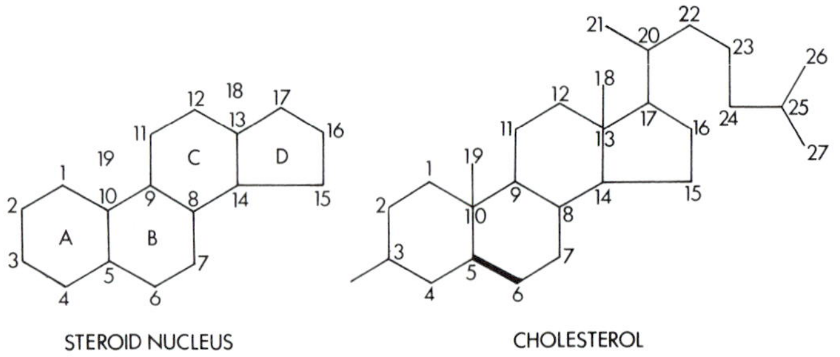

STEROID NUCLEUS   CHOLESTEROL

Figure 1–5 The steroid nucleus with standardized numbering for carbon atoms. The similarity of cholesterol can be seen.

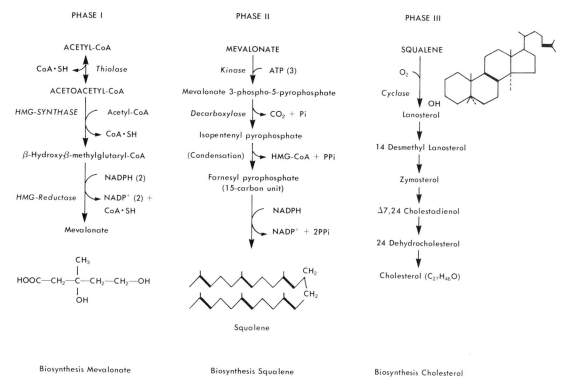

PHASE I

ACETYL-CoA

CoA·SH Thiolase

ACETOACETYL-CoA

HMG-SYNTHASE Acetyl-CoA

CoA·SH

β-Hydroxyβ-methylglutaryl-CoA

NADPH (2)

HMG-Reductase NADP⁺ (2) + CoA·SH

Mevalonate

$$HOOC-CH_2-\underset{\underset{OH}{|}}{\overset{\overset{CH_3}{|}}{C}}-CH_2-CH_2-OH$$

PHASE II

MEVALONATE

Kinase ATP (3)

Mevalonate 3-phospho-5-pyrophosphate

Decarboxylase CO_2 + Pi

Isopentenyl pyrophosphate

(Condensation) HMG-CoA + PPi

Farnesyl pyrophosphate
(15-carbon unit)

NADPH

NADP⁺ + 2PPi

Squalene

PHASE III

SQUALENE

O_2

Cyclase

OH

Lanosterol

14 Desmethyl Lanosterol

Zymosterol

Δ7,24 Cholestadienol

24 Dehydrocholesterol

Cholesterol ($C_{27}H_{46}O$)

Biosynthesis Mevalonate

Biosynthesis Squalene

Biosynthesis Cholesterol

Figure 1–6 Biosynthesis of cholesterol involves three phases: first, the development of mevalonate; second, the condensation to squalene; and third, the ring closure and modification to cholesterol.

associated with the lipids. The apoproteins are grouped into four divisions: apo-A, apo-B, apo-C, and arginine-rich. The apoproteins associated with the lipoprotein fractions are indicated in Table 1–5. A, B, C, and arginine-rich apoproteins contain carbohydrate components and represent glycoproteins. Elements of cholesterol, triacylglycerols, and phospholipids are present in each lipoprotein group; however, one or more of these constituents may be more abundant than the other members. In Table 1–5, the dominant lipid component of each lipoprotein is listed.

Chylomicrons are formed in the gastrointestinal cell by incorporation of the apoprotein B synthesized by ribosomes with triacylglycerol, phospholipid, and cholesterol synthesized in the endoplasmic reticulum. Some portion of the VLDL

TABLE 1–5 LIPOPROTEINS

Lipoprotein	Apoprotein	Major Lipid
Chylomicron	B, CI II III	T
VLDL	B, CI II III Arg-rich	T
LDL	B	C
HDL	AI II, CI II III Arg-rich	P, C

T = triacylglycerol
C = cholesterol
P = phospholipid

is also formed in the intestinal tract, although most is derived from the liver by incorporation of apoprotein and lipid in a fashion similar to that of chylomicrons in the intestine. Release from the cell in both processes is by reverse pinocytosis. The level of chylomicrons and, to a lesser extent, VLDL fluctuates with dietary levels of triacylglycerol. Apoprotein C is added to the chylomicrons and VLDL by transfer from HDL in the plasma.

Chylomicrons are rapidly cleared from plasma at the tissue interface by the action of lipase. About 80 per cent are removed by tissues other than liver. In fact, lipoprotein lipase, essential in clearing chylomicrons from plasma, is not found in significant quantities in hepatic tissue. The liver appears more important in processing lipoprotein remnants. Both phospholipids and apoprotein CII are essential to lipoprotein lipase activity. In the extrahepatic tissue, the triacylglycerol is hydrolyzed, and fatty acids are released for endogenous use or into plasma. The apoprotein C on the chylomicron is transferred to HDL to be reused. A smaller, residual molecule on apoprotein B composed primarily of cholesterol and some triacylglycerol is taken up in the liver and further broken down. It has been suggested that a part of this remnant may form LDL. Most VLDL is produced in the liver as a transport vehicle for endogenously produced triacylglycerol. The VLDL produced in the liver, as well as that from the gastrointestinal tract, undergoes a degradation process similar to that of chylomicrons in extra-hepatic tissues and the liver. In this case, the hepatic-processed remnant is the major source of body LDL. Evidence suggests that degradation of LDL occurs in fibroblasts. HDL is formed in the liver and intestine. Hepatic HDL is coated before release with the apoprotein C, whereas intestinal HDL acquires its apoprotein C by transfer from hepatic HDL.

The lipoproteins of endogenous sources are primarily hepatic in origin. Under normal circumstances, triacylglycerol is rapidly released from the liver. Carbohydrates encourage hepatic fatty acid and triacylglycerol synthesis. Increased levels of free fatty acids are found in the plasma of patients on carbohydrate-restricted or high-fat diets.

KETONES

Acetoacetate, β-hydroxybutyrate, and acetone represent a group of compounds known as *ketone bodies*. They are formed by mitochondrial enzymes in the liver under conditions involving a high rate of fatty acid oxidation. Acetoacetyl-CoA is the initial molecule in ketogenesis and is formed either as a final two-carbon element in β-oxidation or as a product of the condensation of two acetyl-CoA molecules. Acetoacetyl-CoA condenses with acetyl-CoA to form an intermediate that is enzymatically attracted to yield β-hydroxy-β-methyl-glutaryl-CoA and free acetoacetate. The carbons of the original acetyl-CoA are found in the aceto-acetate molecule. β-hydroxybutyrate is formed by the action of an NADH-specific dehydrogenase

enzyme on acetoacetyl-CoA. Acetoacetic and β-hydroxybutyric acids are moderately strong acids that, in excessive amounts, deplete alkali reserves, resulting in clinical ketoacidosis.

Acetoacetate can be taken up in extrahepatic tissue and reactivated to acetoacetyl-CoA. Reactivation cannot occur in the liver. It can then be split by thiolase to acetyl-CoA and oxidized in the citric acid cycle. β-hydroxybutyrate can be reactivated by thiokinase and converted by dehydrogenation to acetoacetyl-CoA to be split and processed in the citric acid cycle. Acetone is formed spontaneously by decarboxylation of acetoacetic acid. Degradation is thought to occur by reversal of decarboxylase. Extrahepatic tissues utilize ketone bodies as energy substrates. They will be oxidized in preference to glucose and fatty acids. At approximately 70 mg/dl the oxidation pathway becomes saturated, and further increases in ketones cause a rise in blood and urinary concentrations. In severely diabetic rats, studies suggest that ketonemia may also be increased by reduced catabolism as well as by increased production.

CITRIC ACID CYCLE

The citric acid cycle, also known as Krebs' cycle, or the tricarboxylic acid cycle, is an essential biochemical sequence providing the final pathway in carbohydrate, lipid, and amino acid oxidation (Fig. 1–7). It is an energy production system that, through a series of mitochondrial reactions, generates high-energy phosphate directly and through coupling with the respiratory chain.

Acetyl residues in an activated state associated with coenzyme A condense with a four-carbon

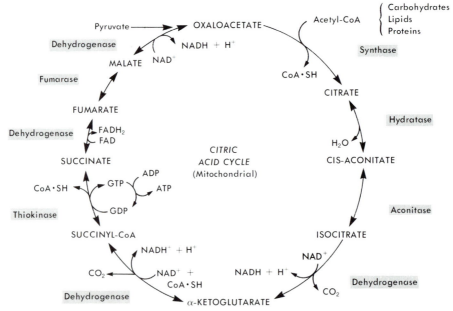

Figure 1–7 The citric acid cycle (Kreb's cycle) provides a pathway for oxidation of carbohydrates, protein, and lipids.

molecule, oxaloacetate, and water in an essentially irreversible mode to form a six-carbon citrate molecule. The coenzyme bond is hydrolyzed in this process, and CoA is split away. Citrate then reacts with an iron-containing enzyme and, by dehydration and rehydration, forms isocitrate. Isocitrate undergoes a dehydrogenation with an NAD-dependent enzyme to form oxalosuccinate, which converts to α-ketoglutarate on decarboxylation. The next reaction involves the irreversible oxidative decarboxylation in a series of steps associated with thiamine diphosphate, lipoate, NAD^+, FAD, and CoA similar to the process of converting pyruvate to acetyl-CoA. This process yields succinyl-CoA and a reduction of NAD to NADH. Succinyl-CoA is converted to succinate by splitting off CoA in the presence of inorganic phosphate. In this step, a high-energy phosphate (GPT) is produced that can be transferred to ADP, forming ATP. Succinate, in the presence of flavoprotein-specific dehydrogenase, is converted to fumarate. Water is added to fumarate to yield malate, which is converted to oxaloacetate by malate dehydrogenase. In this step, a third molecule of NADH is produced. Two carbon atoms are lost in one turn of the cycle, neither from the initial acetyl-CoA. Following a second revolution of the cycle, the initial two entry carbons will be lost as CO_2. The three molecules of NADH and one of $FADH_2$ produced by one turn of the citric acid cycle can be transferred to the respiratory chain. NADH will yield three high-energy phosphates, and $FADH_2$ will yield two. Including the high-energy bond produced in the cycle, a total of 12 phosphate bonds are formed.

The citric acid cycle provides a focal point for glucogenesis and fatty acid synthesis in the liver and kidney. In fatty acid synthesis, acetyl-CoA is transported out of the mitochondria after conversion to citrate and then is reconverted in the cytosol to acetyl-CoA for incorporation into fatty acids. Transamination and deamination of amino acids yield intermediates of the citric acid cycle or pyruvate. These may be converted to oxaloacetate, which may gain access via malate to the cytosol and give rise to glucose by gluconeogenesis. Pyruvate may also give rise to acetyl-CoA for oxidation in the citric acid cycle or conversion to fatty acids.

AMINO ACIDS

Amino acids are the basic building blocks of proteins and are responsible for determining many of the properties of proteins. The general structural formula for amino acids is as follows:

$$\begin{array}{c} NH_2 \\ | \\ R-C-COOH \\ | \\ H \end{array}$$

With the exception of two amino acids, those in proteins have the amino and carboxyl groups attached to the same alpha carbon. At pH 7.4, the amino group exists in a conjugated acid form ($R-NH_3^+$), and the carboxyl group appears in its conjugated base form ($R-COO^-$).

Only 20 of the many amino acids available in nature are involved in the protein structure. These 20 amino acids can be classified into subdivisions based on the charge or lack of charge of their R group. These subdivisions consist of the nonpolar, or hydrophobic, R groups, uncharged (neutral) polar R groups, positively charged R groups, and negatively charged R groups (Table 1–6). They

TABLE 1–6 AMINO ACIDS

Classification	Names (trivial/symbolic/systematic)	
Nonpolar hydrophobic	Alanine (Ala)	2-Aminopropionic acid
	Leucine (Leu)	2-Amino-4-methylpentanoic acid
	Isoleucine (Ile)	2-Amino-3-methylpentanoic acid
	Phenylalanine (Phe)	2-Amino-3-phenylpropionic acid
	Valine (Val)	2-Amino-3-methylbutanoic acid
	Proline (Pro)	2-Pyrrolidine-carboxylic acid
	Methionine (Met)	2-Amino-4-(methylthio) butyric acid
	Tryptophan (Trp)	2-Amino-3-indolepropionic acid
Neutral polarity	Serine (Ser)	2-Amino-3-hydroxypropionic acid
	Threonine (Thr)	2-Amino-3-hydroxybutyric acid
	Tyrosine (Tyr)	2-Amino-3-(p-hydroxyphenyl)propionic acid
	Asparagine (Agn)	2-Amino-succinamic acid
	Glutamine (Gln)	2-Aminoglutaramic acid
	Cysteine (Cys)	2-Amino-3-mercaptopropionic acid
	Glycine (Gly)	Aminoacetic acid
Positively charged	Lysine (Lys)	2,6-Diaminohexanoic acid
	Arginine (Arg)	2-Amino-5-guanidinovaleric acid
	Histidine (His)	2-Amino-1H-imidazole-4-propionic acid
Negatively charged	Aspartic acid (Asp)	Aminosuccinic acid
	Glutamic acid (Glu)	2-Aminoglutaric acid

may also be grouped on the basis of side chain molecular structure. Amino acids, with the exception of glycine, are optically active and may occur in levorotatory or dextrorotatory forms. In proteins, the levorotatory form is encountered. The characteristics of amino acids are due to the reactions of the functional side chain groups and the carboxyl and amino groups.

AMINO ACID CATABOLISM

Amino acids are versatile molecules that, upon catabolism, give rise to nitrogen, which can be converted to various nitrogenous products, and to carbon components, which may enter several pathways. Thirteen of the amino acids are glycogenic. An additional five amino acids may be converted to either carbohydrates or ketones. One amino acid is solely ketogenic (Table 1–7).

In Figure 1–8 the entry points of the various amino acids into the citric acid cycle, the glycolysis pathway, and ketones are indicated. Eleven of the amino acids form acetyl-CoA—either directly, via pyruvate, or indirectly, via acetoacetyl-CoA. Twelve amino acids are converted to citric acid cycle intermediates: five as α-ketoglutarate, three as succinyl-CoA, two as oxaloacetate, and two as fumarate. The carbon skeletons of certain amino acids can enter the citric acid cycle directly; others require extensive modification or cleavage for en-

TABLE 1–7 AMINO ACID CONVERTIBILITY

Glycogenic	Glycogenic-Ketogenic	Ketogenic
Alanine	Lysine	Leucine
Arginine	Tryptophan	
Cystine	Isoleucine	
Aspartate	Phenylalanine	
Glutamate	Tyrosine	
Glycine		
Histidine		
Hydroxyproline		
Methionine		
Proline		
Serine		
Threonine		
Valine		

try into the cycle. Those amino acids that form pyruvate have an option: by conversion to acetyl-CoA, to undergo complete oxidation in the citric acid cycle or, by conversion to oxaloacetic acid, to give rise to glucose.

Glycogenic amino acids, after removal of the amino group by transaminase or oxidative deamination reactions, provide a carbon skeleton that can be metabolized to citric acid cycle intermediates in the liver or kidney. All of them eventually form oxaloacetate in the mitochondrial citric acid cycle and are transported as malate or citrate to the cytosol for reconversion to oxaloacetate. Ox-

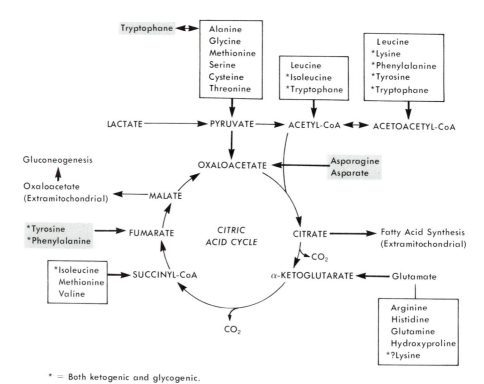

* = Both ketogenic and glycogenic.

Figure 1–8 Route for amino acid metabolism.

aloacetate in the cytosol is converted by decarboxylation, with GTP supplying high-energy phosphate, to phosphoenolpyruvate, an intermediate in the glycolytic pathway. By modified reversal of glycolysis, glucose or glycogen may be formed.

Five amino acids listed in Table 1–7 are both glycogenic and ketogenic. This combined activity is derived from the fact that lysine, isoleucine, phenylalanine, and tyrosine are converted upon degradation to ketogenic acetyl-CoA or acetoacetyl-CoA and intermediate products of the citric acid cycle. Tryptophan can be converted to ketogenic by-products or directly to alanine, which is glycogenic.

Leucine yields neither pyruvate nor citric acid cycle intermediates during catabolism and therefore is not glucogenic. It is converted directly into acetyl-CoA. There is no metabolic pathway by which carbons of acetyl-CoA can give rise to new glucose. The carbons can, however, be incorporated into the glucose molecule. The acetyl-CoA can combine with oxaloacetate in the citric acid cycle to form citrate. During excessive production of amino acids, there is a large input into the citric acid cycle of intermediates, which increases the citrate concentration in the mitochondria. Transported from mitochondria to cytosol, citrate may be cleaved into oxaloacetate and acetyl-CoA. The acetyl-CoA is immediately available for fatty acid synthesis and the oxaloacetate is available for gluconeogenesis.

In catabolism of the amino acids, the amino group may be removed by amino transferases or transaminases and transferred to an alpha carbon of an α-keto acid. This yields an amino form of keto acid and the α-keto analogue of the amino acid (Fig. 1–9). Two common transaminases use α-ketoglutarate or pyruvate as the keto acid. When α-ketoglutarate is used, glutamate is produced. When pyruvate is used, alanine is formed. Glutamate and alanine may then serve as amino group donors for oxidative deamination to nitrogenous products or amino acid production. Transaminases all have a pyridoxal phosphate prosthetic group and are found in the mitochondria and cytosols of cells. They can act on most amino acids, and the reactions are reversible. These reactions are important for the concentration of cytoplasmic amino groups, primarily by formation of glutamate, which can then be transported into the mitochondria and undergo oxidative deamination. Most of the concentration of amino groups is centered around glutamate, which, through the action of glutamate dehydrogenase and the coenzyme NAD^+ or $NADP^+$, yields α-ketoglutarate and ammonia (NH_3) (Fig. 1–9). This reaction may occur in both the cytoplasm and the mitochondria and may accept amino groups from most amino acids. In the mitochondria, the reduced coenzyme may enter the respiratory chain.

UREA SYNTHESIS

Both ammonia produced endogenously from transamination and deamination in tissue and that formed by intestinal bacteria are toxic and must be eliminated from the body or modified. Intestinal ammonia is rapidly removed by the liver and may be reused for amino acid synthesis along with endogenous ammonia by reversal of deamination. The remainder is excreted as urea or uric acid. Only trace levels of ammonia are found in blood.

Besides reversal of deamination, ammonia may react with glutamic acid in an ATP-dependent step to form glutamine. This is a major pathway in brain tissue for removal of ammonia. The glutamine formed in tissue may be transported to the kidney and converted back to ammonia, where it plays a major role in acid-base balance, or to the liver, where glutamine may be hydrolyzed to yield ammonia for conversion to urea. Most ammonia is transported to the liver as glutamine.

The production of urea involves a cyclic pathway. Beginning in the mitochondria, ammonia condenses irreversibly with carbon dioxide in the presence of two ATP molecules to form carbamoyl phosphate (Fig. 1–10). In the next step, a carba-

$$\text{moyl group } (-\overset{\overset{\text{O}}{\|}}{\text{C}}-\text{NH}_2)$$ is donated to ornithine, forming citrulline, which diffuses into the cytosol. At this point, the second amino group is added. It is derived from aspartate and involves a condensation of aspartate and a carbamoyl group of citrulline to form argininosuccinate. ATP is again required in the reaction. The aspartate is formed by the action of aspartate transaminase on glutamate. Next, fumaric acid is cleaved from the argininosuccinate, forming arginine. The last step involves hydrolysis with cleavage of the guanidino group of arginine, re-forming ornithine and releas-

$$\text{ing urea } (\overset{\overset{\text{NH}_2}{|}}{\underset{\underset{\text{NH}_2}{|}}{\text{C}=\text{O}}}). \text{ Urea formed in the liver is the}$$

major pathway of nitrogen excretion in humans. It accounts for 95 per cent of the nitrogen elimi-

Figure 1–9 Generalized examples of the processes of transamination, deamination, and urea formation.

(1) α amino acid + α-Ketoglutarate $\underset{}{\overset{\text{transaminase}}{\rightleftharpoons}}$ α-keto acid + Glutamate

(2) Glutamate + NAD^+ $\underset{}{\overset{\text{Deaminase}}{\rightleftharpoons}}$ NADH + α Ketoglutarate + NH_3

(3) NH_3 + CO_2 + ATP + Ornithine cycle $\longrightarrow$ Urea + ornithine cycle

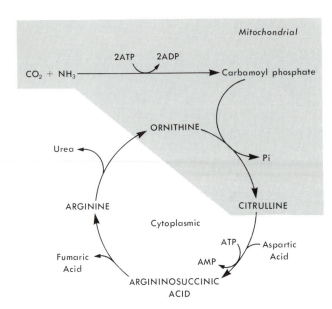

Figure 1–10 Urea synthesis.

nated by the kidney. The cycle costs three moles of ATP, ammonia, CO_2 and aspartate. Three of the amino acids involved do not occur in proteins; these are ornithine, citrulline, and argininosuccinate.

BIOSYNTHESIS OF AMINO ACIDS

As is the case with lipids, some but not all amino acids can be synthesized by humans. Thus, those that cannot be synthesized are called *nutritionally essential amino acids* (Table 1–8). Ammonium ions serve as the nitrogen source for their synthesis. A series of multienzyme steps, many of which are complex, are required for the synthesis of nutritionally essential amino acids by bacteria or plants. These synthesis pathways differ, except for a few common points, from the degradation pathways. The biosynthetic pathways for nutritionally nonessential amino acids are relatively short. They involve three basic methods: (1) synthesis from intermediates of glycolysis, as occurs in formation of serine and glycine, (2) the utilization of citric acid cycle intermediates, as occurs in the formation of alanine, glutamate, and aspartate, and (3) the utilization of other amino acids (Table 1–9). Regulation of synthesis is generally accomplished through feedback inhibition or enzyme synthesis repression.

TABLE 1–8 NUTRITIONALLY ESSENTIAL AMINO ACIDS

Arginine	Methionine
Histidine	Phenylalanine
Isoleucine	Threonine
Leucine	Tryptophan
Lysine	Valine

Amino acids or portions of their structure contribute to synthesis of many other products, including hormones, coenzymes, porphyrins, vitamins, and pigments. The details of these many reactions are beyond the scope of this limited review; however, several examples of specific byproducts will be listed. Glycine contributes both the alpha carbon and nitrogen atoms in the synthesis of porphyrins in hemoglobin. Methionine is a common precursor of methylated molecules. Cysteine is involved in coenzyme A synthesis. Serine is an important fraction of some phospholipids. Tryptophan is the precursor of serotonin; tyrosine is the precursor of melanin, epinephrine, and norepinephrine. Arginine, glycine, and methionine are precursors of creatine, an important storehouse of energy in muscle. Creatinine, the anhydrous form of creatine, is formed by the irreversible nonenzymatic removal of water with the loss of phosphate.

PROTEINS

Proteins are formed by a series of amino acids that are linked by a covalent peptide bond (Fig. 1–11). In the simplest terms, the peptide bond is formed by reaction of an alpha amino group and alpha carboxyl group of separate amino acids with the loss of one mole of water. The uniqueness of each protein lies in the arrangement of its amino acids. This explanation of peptide bond formation is not sufficient in terms of cellular events. In the cell, this reaction occurs on the ribosome and involves several forms of ribonucleic acid. Genetic information that establishes a protein's amino acid sequence is stored in the DNA nucleotide sequence. This information is transcribed and appears in the cytoplasm on messenger RNA

TABLE 1–9 NUTRITIONALLY NONESSENTIAL AMINO ACID SYNTHESIS

	Intermediate	Enzyme	Amino Acid
Citric acid	Oxaloacetate/glutamate	Transaminase	Aspartic acid
	α-Ketoglutarate	Dehydrogenase	Glutamic acid
	Pyruvate/glutamate	Transaminase	Alanine
Glycolysis	3-Phosphoglycerate/glutamate	Transaminase	Serine
	Pyruvate/glyoxylate	Transaminase	Glycine
	$CO_2 + NH_3$	Synthetase	Glycine
Amino Acid	Serine	Transferase	Glycine
	Glutamic acid	Kinase/dehydrogenase	Proline
	Proline (protein bound)	Oxygenase	Hydroxyproline
	Methionine/serine	Transulfuration	Cysteine
	Phenylalanine	Oxygenase	Tyrosine
	Glutamic acid	Synthetase	Glutamine
	Aspartic acid	Synthetase	Asparagine

(mRNA). The cell possesses the mechanism to translate information of mRNA into the sequence of amino acids. It does this through an adapter molecule, transfer RNA (tRNA), that recognizes the specific nucleotide sequence as well as the counterpart amino acid. The process occurs on the ribosome. Since 20 amino acids are involved in protein formation, a similar number of distinct codes are available to identify them. These codes are carried by the nucleotides in mRNA and consist of a three-nucleotide codon providing the potential for 64 individual codes. Three of the 64 are "nonsense codons," which provide a signal to terminate the amino acid polymer. As there are 61 codons left for 20 amino acids, some amino acids have more than one codon. A single tRNA molecule possesses the proper anticodon for a given codon or codons in mRNA needed to recognize and provide an amino acid. Each amino acid added to the peptide chain requires its own tRNA. The tRNA differ from each other in their nucleotide sequences. The recognition by tRNA of its specific amino acid occurs through reaction with the enzyme, aminoacyl-tRNA synthetases. The synthetase enzymes are highly specific for a particular amino acid and tRNA. The reaction between the amino acid and enzyme occurs in the cytoplasm and requires ATP conversion to AMP. The end product is an aminoacyl-AMP-enzyme complex or activated amino acid. This amino acid–enzyme complex then recognizes its specific tRNA and attaches the amino acid at the 3′-hydroxy-adenosyl terminus by an ester linkage. Once attached,

the amino acid plays no role in the recognition of the steps to follow.

Transfer RNA can be thought of as a simple cross. At the top, the amino acid is bonded at the ACC terminus; to the left, the thymidine-pseudouridine-cytidine loop binds to the ribosome surface; the base represents the nucleotide anticodon; and to the right there is a dihydrouracil loop. The ribosome contains two nucleoprotein subunits—a 60S unit and a 40S unit. The mRNA binds to the 40S ribosome under the influence of a protein initiation factor 3 (IF-3). Aminoacyl-tRNA interacts with GTP and initiation factor 2 (IF-2) to form a complex that, in the presence of initiation factor 1 (IF-1), attaches the tRNA to the 40S ribosome. The initiation factors are released and the 40S ribosome particle merges with the 60S unit, hydrolyzing GTP and forming the 80S unit on which there are two binding sites for tRNA. The aminoacyl-tRNA entered initially at the P site, leaving the second site, or A site, free. The next step involves the formation of a peptide bond and elongation of the peptide unit. The second amino acid in an activated state is carried by its tRNA to the A site, where it reacts with an elongation factor (EF-1) and GTP to form a complex. At this time, EF-1 and GTP are released. The amino acid at site A carries out a nucleophilic attachment on the esterified carboxyl group of the amino acid–tRNA at site P under the influence of a transferase. The aminoacyl residue is transferred from the P site tRNA to A site tRNA to form a dipeptide. The tRNA at site P is then discharged,

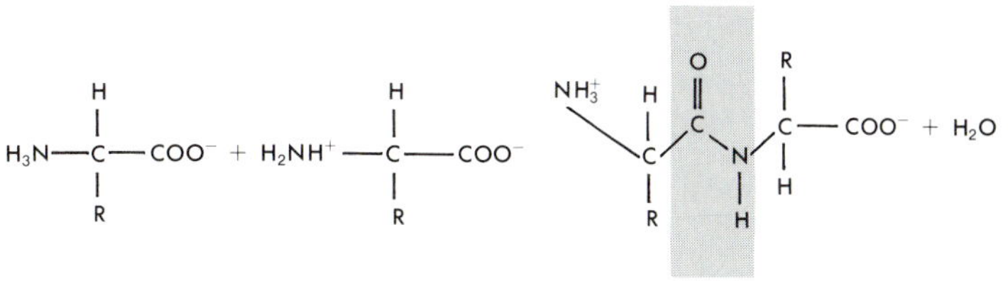

Figure 1–11 Simple formation of the peptide bond.

$$H_3N-\overset{\overset{\displaystyle H}{|}}{\underset{\underset{\displaystyle R}{|}}{C}}-COO^- + H_2NH^+-\overset{\overset{\displaystyle H}{|}}{\underset{\underset{\displaystyle R}{|}}{C}}-COO^- \longrightarrow \overset{NH_3^+}{\underset{\underset{\displaystyle R}{|}}{C}}\overset{\overset{\displaystyle O}{\parallel}}{C}\overset{H}{\underset{\underset{\displaystyle H}{|}}{N}}\overset{\overset{\displaystyle R}{|}}{\underset{\underset{\displaystyle H}{|}}{C}}-COO^- + H_2O$$

and, by the action of EF-2 and GTP, the tRNA at site A is relocated to the P site. Site A is then free for another amino acid–tRNA.

The initiation of the peptide chain begins when the amino acid methionine is brought into the ribosome as N-formylmethionyl-tRNA. Termination of the peptide chain is signaled by a nonsense codon on mRNA appearing at site A. As there is no tRNA that recognizes this, the peptide chain is complete. A releasing factor and enzyme then hydrolyze the bond between the peptide chain and tRNA at the P site. Once the protein is released, the ribosome dissociates to its subunits.

Considerable energy is used in peptide formation. The equivalent of four ATP molecules is required to activate the amino acids, and three GTP molecules are needed for attachment to the ribosome and translocation.

Simple proteins yield amino acids upon hydrolysis; conjugated proteins yield not only amino acids but also organic components referred to as *prosthetic groups*.

Each protein has a characteristic three-dimensional shape, or conformation, that permits classification. The *primary structure* of a protein refers to the basic sequence of covalently linked amino acids. The *secondary structure* refers to the recurring arrangement along one dimension of the polypeptide chain. This is formed by disulfide or hydrogen bonds. Hydrogen bonds are formed by nitrogen and carboxyl oxygen of separate peptides sharing a hydrogen atom. A common secondary conformation is the alpha helix, which consists of a coiled backbone of peptide units. This permits maximal intrachain hydrogen bonding between coils of the helix. The helix has approximately 3.6 amino acids per turn, with hydrogen bonds between every fourth amino acid. The *tertiary structure* refers to the manner in which polypeptide chains bend and fold in three dimensions to form globular proteins. Weak associations, or bonds, are responsible for stabilizing this conformation. These are hydrogen bonds between peptide R groups, hydrophobic interactions between nonpolar R groups, and ionic bonds between oppositely charged side chains. The *quaternary structure* refers to the configuration that develops when individual polypeptide chains group about each other.

The basic properties of the polypeptide are due to the nature of the R side chains, the size of the amino acid polymer, its three-dimensional structure, and associated organic or inorganic molecules. The forces maintaining the conformation of proteins can be interrupted by strong acids or bases, heat, heavy metal, and organic solvents. This process is referred to as *denaturation*.

Proteins may be classified by several methods. Common classifications group proteins as fibrous or globular and as simple or conjugated as well as by their relative solubility and antigenic properties. Examples of fibrous proteins are keratin, collagen, and elastin. In the clinical setting, solubility is used to separate proteins into albumin and globulins. More important are the collected ionic properties of the amino acids in proteins, which permit electrophoretic separation into numerous fractions. For clinical purposes, these are grouped into five classes: albumin, $alpha_1$ globulins, $alpha_2$ globulins, beta globulins, and gamma globulins. Albumin consists of a single polypeptide chain in a globular form. It functions as a nonspecific transport and provides considerable osmotic pressure. The major $alpha_1$ globulins are glycoproteins and high-density lipoproteins; the main $alpha_2$ globulins are haptoglobin, ceruloplasmin, prothrombin, glycoproteins, and VLDL. The major beta globulins are transferrin and LDL. The gamma globulins represent the immunoglobulins.

Proteins in the body are constantly broken down and resynthesized. This turnover is measured by the half-life of proteins, which is approximately 80 days for the average body protein. The average, weight-stable man degrades and synthesizes 400 gm of protein a day. Most of the nitrogen metabolized in the body is contained in protein.

Although this discussion of polypeptide chains has referred primarily to protein, physiologically active free peptides exist. Two common ones are glutathione and bradykinin. In some cases, free peptides represent by-products of protein degradation.

PURINE AND PYRIMIDINE METABOLISM

Figure 1–12 shows the nitrogenous heterocyclic structures of purine and pyrimidine. In humans, there are three major pyrimidines—cytosine, thymine, and uracil—and two major purines—adenine and guanine. Humans can meet their need for these bases by endogenous synthesis and therefore need not rely on dietary sources.

Nucleotides are composed of a purine or pyrimidine base, to which a sugar is attached at N_1 or N_9 position. Free purine and pyrimidines and their nucleosides occur only in trace amounts in cells. Nucleotides are nucleosides phosphorylated on the hydroxyl groups of the sugar. These occur in significant amounts in cells. The pentose sugars incorporated in nucleosides are usually D-ribose or 2-deoxyribose bonded by an *N*-glycosidic bond. For

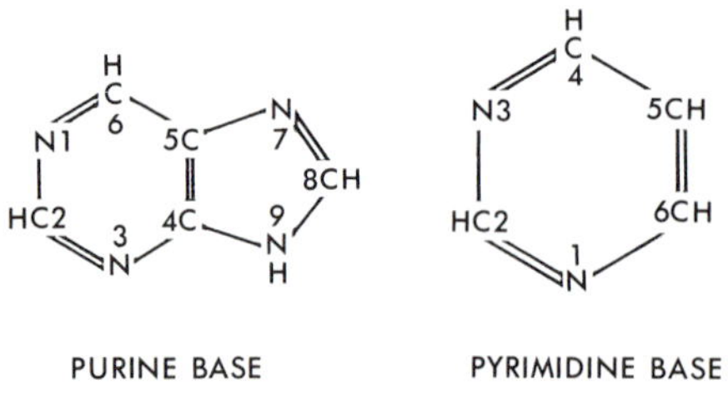

PURINE BASE   PYRIMIDINE BASE

Figure 1–12 Structure of purine and pyrimidine bases, numbered by international system.

example, adenine and a D-ribose sugar together yield adenine ribonucleoside or adenosine; when they are phosphorylated, the product is adenosine monophosphate or adenylate. The abbreviations A, G, C, T, and U may be used to designate a nucleoside base. The prefix "D" is added to the nucleoside to indicate a deoxyribose sugar.

The synthesis pathway for purine in the cytosol is complex and involves the assemblage of the molecule from amino acids and carbon donors. Synthesis involves the phosphorylation of ribose 5-phosphate and ATP to 1-pyrophosphorylribosyl-5-phosphate (PRPP). Glutamine then adds nitrogen (N-9), which is followed by the addition of glycine to form N-7 and carbons 5 and 4 (C-5,4). This step requires ATP. Tetrahydrofolate carrier adds a formyl group at C-8. A second glutamine adds a nitrogen (N-3), again requiring ATP. Under the influence of a third ATP, the imidazole ring is closed, to be followed by a carboxylation reaction adding C-6 from CO_2. Aspartate provides N-1, and formyl-tetrafolate provides C-2, completing the basic inosine monophosphate molecule. This molecule is then converted by amination or by oxidation and amination to guanosine monophosphate (GMP) or adenosine monophosphate (AMP). The monophosphates can be converted to diphosphates or triphosphates by transfer of high-energy groups.

Control of the purine synthesis is primarily directed by the availability of ribose 5-phosphate. Synthesis of ribose 5-phosphate depends on the availability of its substrate and feedback inhibition of the synthesis enzymes by purine. Salvage pathways are available in the body to convert free purine to nucleoside or to phosphorylate nucleotide to limit the loss of purine and to supply tissues that are incapable of purine synthesis. These salvage pathways also involve the interconversion of IMP, GMP, and deoxyribonucleotides to nucleosides.

Catabolism of purine involves conversion to uric acid. The purine nucleoside is acted upon by a phosphorylase to yield the free base guanine or hypoxanthine. Both of these may be converted to xanthine, which, under the influence of xanthine oxidase, yields uric acid (Fig. 1–13).

The pyrimidine nucleotide synthesis requires PRPP, glutamine, CO_2, and aspartate. Thymidine also requires a tetrahydrofolate derivative. Unlike purine, the pyrimidine nucleus is formed separately from the PRPP and added later. Synthesis begins in the cytosol, with the carbamoyl phosphate of glutamine providing N-1 and CO_2 providing C-2. The step is ATP-dependent. The carbamoyl phosphate condenses with aspartate, which provides C-4, C-5, C-6, and N-3. Upon the loss of water a ring structure is formed. Through a series of reductase, transferase, and decarboxylase steps, the molecule is altered, and ribose 5-phosphate is added to form uridine monophosphate (UMP). This molecule may undergo further phosphorylation and amination by glutamine to cytidine triphosphate, or a methyl group can be donated by tetrahydrofolate to form thymidine monophosphate (TMP). Synthesis is controlled by feedback repression and derepression mechanisms. Purine and pyrimidine are synthesized in a coordinated manner.

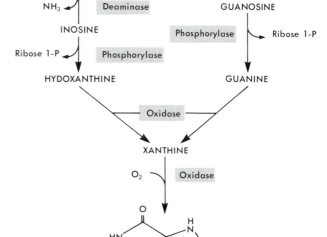

Figure 1–13 Formation of uric acid from purine nucleosides.

Catabolism of pyrimidine occurs mainly in the liver, beginning with the hydrolysis and removal of the ribose-phosphate. Following an NADPH-dependent oxidation and hydration, the ring is broken. In the final step, uracil and cytosine form alanine, CO_2, and NH_3, and thymine forms isobutyric acid, CO_2, and NH_3. Salvage mechanisms are not available for the free pyrimidine bases but are available for the conversion of nucleosides to nucleotides.

The structure and metabolism of nucleic acids are discussed in Chapter 2 and will not be introduced here except to express the fact that the chemical nature of DNA consists of monomeric units of nucleotides linked by a $3'5'$-phosphodiester bridge.

METABOLIC REGULATION

The numerous energy-producing pathways thus far discussed are strictly controlled to provide the necessary continuous flow of energy for cells. These pathways require a constant supply of substrates, enzymes, and cofactors that must be met by the complex transport systems and interconnecting sequences. Factors must be available at the appropriate time and concentration to meet the individual tissue needs and to assure an orderly metabolic process under a variety of nutritional states.

Some reactants in a metabolic pathway reach a steady state; others are at constant nonequilibrium. Unless controlled, the nonequilibrious reactions would rapidly deplete substrates and force equilibrium changes in earlier steady-state substrates. Control of pathways can best be exercised at the nonequilibrium steps. Such control is possible by limiting the enzyme concentration in the reaction, by providing enzyme regulation through feedback or forward control, by controlling the availability of cofactors, and by hormone influence as inducers or repressors of enzyme synthesis.

Obviously, changes in substrate concentration and end-product removal also provide regulatory activity. Clearly, the blood levels of carbohydrates, fatty acids, and amino acids influence the metabolic processes in tissues. Changes in dietary components can indirectly affect metabolic pathways through hormonal mechanisms. Glucocorticoids, glucagon, and epinephrine, for example, function as inducers of glucogenic enzymes, whereas insulin suppresses these enzymes but stimulates glycogenesis, the HMP shunt, and lipogenesis. Since these hormones are responsive to blood glucose, indirect control occurs.

The major organs of the body are capable of carrying out the essential metabolic sequences of glycolysis, citric acid cycle, and lipid and protein processes. Individual characteristics of tissue do exist. For example, the liver is the major absorber from the gastrointestinal tract and plays a significant role in the metabolite distribution. Two thirds of the glucose molecules resulting from digestion are phosphorylated in the liver; the rest circulate to other tissues. Other carbohydrates are totally processed in the liver. Amino acids absorbed by the gastrointestinal tract enter the liver and, like glucose, have several options. They may pass to other tissues for protein synthesis, or they may provide amino acids for protein synthesis in the liver. Amino acids, when in excess, may provide energy, glucose, fatty acids, or other elements, such as porphyrins. The liver also plays the only role in urea formation. Lipids enter the liver from the gastrointestinal tract via either the portal tract or the systemic circulation. The glycerol fraction of lipids is capable of providing glucose, fatty acid fraction, lipoproteins, energy, cholesterol, and ketones.

Adipose tissue utilizes both blood glucose and fatty acids for energy and synthesis. It provides a storehouse for energy in the synthesis of lipids. Similarly, skeletal muscle utilizes both blood glucose and fatty acids to provide energy. Much of the glucose used is stored as glycogen, which provides energy by metabolism to pyruvate or lactate. In muscle, carbohydrates supply less energy than do lipids.

Blood glucose levels are rigidly regulated. Glucose uptake in liver and extrahepatic tissue is related to the concentration in blood. At normal blood glucose levels, the liver produces glucose; at higher levels, production ceases, and a net uptake occurs in liver and extrahepatic tissues. Insulin plays a central regulatory role in this process. It increases uptake by extrahepatic tissues and probably also by hepatic tissue. It appears to increase transport across the cell membranes in addition to stimulating pathway elements. As indicated earlier in this chapter, glucocorticoids lead to gluconeogenesis, resulting in increased protein catabolism and, thus, amino acid uptake in the liver. In addition, insulin inhibits utilization of amino acids in extrahepatic tissue. Growth hormone decreases glucose uptake in muscle and mobilizes fatty acids from adipose tissue. The resultant hyperglycemia stimulates insulin. Adrenocorticotropic hormone (ACTH) can directly enhance the release of fatty acids from adipose tissue, but exerts its primary effect through glucocorticoids. Epinephrine stimulates glycogen breakdown through its activity on hepatic and muscle phosphorylase. Glucagon, stimulated by hypoglycemia, activates phosphorylase in a manner similar to epinephrine, causing glycogenolysis. It also stimulates gluconeogenesis by its effects on proteins.

In carbohydrate restriction, blood glucose levels are maintained by glycogenolysis. As glucagon levels rise, insulin falls and lipolysis increases, causing fat mobilization. Fatty acids impair oxidation of gluconeogenesis and phosphofructokinase. Fatty acids increasingly provide energy for the body. If endogenous gluconeogenesis falls behind glucose utilization, fat mobilization further increases. Under these circumstances, glycerol provides an important source of glucose.

Lipogenesis is the conversion of glucose and intermediates to fat. In a diet high in carbohydrates, lipogenesis is stimulated and fatty acid oxidation is spared in preference to esterification. In high-fat or carbohydrate-restricted diets, the reverse occurs, and FFA levels rise in plasma. The rate-limiting step in lipogenesis appears at the acetyl-CoA carboxylase step by feedback inhibition of acyl-CoA. In effect, if acyl-CoA is not being utilized, further fatty acid synthesis is inhibited. Insulin stimulates lipogenesis by increasing cellular glucose uptake, the production of glycerol 3-phosphate, and the availability of NADPH produced via the HMP shunt. It also inhibits lipolysis by depression of cAMP. The reverse occurs in insulin deficiency. The increased acetyl-CoA may result in increases in cholesterol. Glucocorticoids, ACTH, and epinephrine all increase lipolysis.

Acetyl-CoA is not glucogenic as are certain amino acids, lactate, and glycerol. It is true that acetyl-CoA from β-oxidation may enter the citric acid cycle and that its carbons may end up in glucose or glycogen molecules. However, there is no net conversion to glucose, since the molecule of acetyl-CoA incorporated into the cycle requires one molecule of oxaloacetate. No net change occurs. Similarly, there is no net conversion of fatty acids to amino acids. However, the reverse reaction may occur, with glucogenic amino acids yielding fatty acids by the formation of either pyruvate or acetyl-CoA. Although fatty acids cannot increase glucose, glycerol released upon hydrolysis of triacylglycerols is readily converted to glucose in the liver and kidney, where there are high levels of glycerokinase. In the presence of ATP, glycerol 3-phosphate is produced for gluconeogenesis.

Lactate is formed by glucose oxidation in skeletal muscle under anaerobic conditions. It is also formed in erythrocytes, which lack a citric acid cycle. In the Cori cycle, lactate formed in the skeletal muscle is transported to the kidney or liver, converted to pyruvate, and, by gluconeogenesis, processed to glucose.

REFERENCES

Devlin, T. M.: Textbook of Biochemistry with Clinical Correlations. New York, John Wiley and Sons, 1982.
Dickens, F., Randle, P. J., and Whelan, W. J.: Carbohydrate Metabolism and its Disorders. Vols. 1 and 2. New York, Academic Press, 1968.
Dickerson, R. E., and Geis, I.: The Structure and Action of Proteins. New York, Harper and Row, 1969.
Dixon, M., and Webb, E. C.: Enzymes. 2nd ed. New York, Academic Press, 1964.
Harper, H. A., Rodwell, V. W., and Mayes, P. A.: Review of Physiologic Chemistry. 18th ed. Los Altos, Lange Medical Publications, 1981.
Lehninger, A. L.: Biochemistry. 2nd ed. New York, Worth Publishers, 1975.
Mallette, M. F., Clagett, C. O., Phillips, A. T., and McCarl, R. L.: Introductory Biochemistry. Baltimore, The Williams & Wilkins Co., 1971.
Montgomery, R., Dryer, R. L., Conway, T. W., and Spector, A. A.: Biochemistry: A Case-Oriented Approach. 2nd ed. St. Louis, The C. V. Mosby Company, 1977.
Newsholme, E. A., and Start, C.: Regulation in Metabolism. New York, John Wiley and Sons, 1973.
Stryer, L.: Biochemistry. 2nd ed. San Francisco, W. N. Freeman and Company, 1981.

2

Molecular Biology

K. Lemone Yielding

GENERAL INTRODUCTION

Our present understanding of the chemistry of biologic processes has made it possible to approach human diseases and their management in terms of molecular derangements. For some years, interest in "molecular" disease was concerned with the description of examples of genetically determined molecular defects such as hemoglobinopathies, enzyme deficiencies, storage diseases, and the like. Now, however, the whole array of biologic processes involved in human diseases and their treatment should come into focus. These include all aspects of the function of the human organism as well as those for the variety of parasites that impose their effects.

Molecular biology represents the molecular approach to all biologic processes, not only in the descriptive sense but also with a major emphasis on the nature of the information contained in molecules and how this information is translated into biologic action. This emphasis on information has culminated in the powerful new genetic engineering technologies (see further on) that have already impacted on a wide spectrum of biologic problems. Human health management will profit immediately in three major ways: (1) the generation of highly specific and pure biologicals for treating disease; (2) the direct modification of the informational content and thus of the function of diseased cells; and (3) the elucidation of specific disease mechanisms. The power of these technologies in generating new information is most exciting in terms of solving human health problems. In addition to the traditional interest in inherited diseases, the major area of challenge to be met by the approaches of molecular biology include (1) development and organization; (2) aging and degenerative disease; (3) neoplastic disease and other uncontrolled growth phenomena; (4) adaptive and recovery processes; (5) host-parasite relationships; (6) environmentally provoked diseases and environmental risk assessment; and (7) explanation of the functions of the nervous system, including behavior.

This chapter will summarize the basic principles and our current data base for considering diseases as problems in molecular biology.

Molecular biology is based on two simple premises: (1) Biologic processes can be explained in chemical terms, and, in fact, knowledge of molecular structure can provide the basis for understanding function; and (2) the reality of evolutionary design in biologic systems means that knowledge of complex systems in humans or other

higher organisms can be gained through study of simple organisms (and vice versa). The power of both premises is well illustrated by the substantial advances that have been reported. The progress in our understanding based on structure information is especially impressive in the area of nucleic acids and information transfer. Undeniably, the description of the principles underlying DNA and RNA structure and their study in simple organisms has led to extensive understanding of biologic function. In fact, one of the remarkable achievements of modern science has been the ability to isolate, purify, amplify, and use the nucleic acid (gene) units responsible for specific biologic functions. Thus, genetic engineering, long a dream of the modern molecular biologists, has become a reality. It seems that soon this remarkable achievement will be extended to a wide spectrum of human problems. Understanding nucleic acid structure-function relationships has perhaps resulted in such success partially because of the structural simplicity of these macromolecules. Not only are the monomer repeating units of nucleic acids limited to a select few members but also the two-dimensional structure (sequence) of these polymers dictates the biologic function. Tertiary and quaternary structure, still not fully understood, certainly contribute important features of regulation, organization, and stability, but they apparently do not determine qualitatively the expression of biologic activity.

Structure analysis has not yet revealed the details of function for all classes of biomolecules because of the complexity of their three-dimensional structure and the complexity of their potential interactions in the cell. Progress continues at an impressive rate, however, to confirm the principle that function can be rationalized by knowledge of structure. This first premise carried into the study of disease would mean both that one could explain diseases by identifying and studying relevant abnormal molecules and their deficient or aberrant functions and that therapy should consist of appropriate molecular adjustments.

A major problem is in detecting primary and secondary events in view of the molecular *cascading* seen in biologic systems. Studies of inherited diseases have emphasized the principle of cascading and the distinction between primary and secondary molecular changes in disease, since a single primary molecular defect attributed to a single mutant gene can lead to complex diseases. Genetic diseases, therefore, have provided means for understanding disease mechanisms in all organ systems and thus represent nature's "laboratory" for the study of molecular disease mechanisms. Therapy, too, is complicated by the occurrence of both primary and secondary drug effects, which are subject to the same cascading phenomenon described for disease perturbations. An increased understanding of biologic process coupled with identification of molecular drug targets should accelerate the development of new therapeutic approaches. Diseases provide the "natural" experiment for studying functional consequences of specific molecule changes and thus warrant exhaustive study. Human disease studies have identified a variety of important biochemical concepts that have been tested and extended in simpler systems. Thus, new knowledge obtained with methods in molecular biology can often be generated conveniently and even uniquely in human experiments. The emphasis on molecular details must not cause one to lose sight of the fact, however, that the study of disease demands the integrated application of all disciplines within the medical and biologic sciences.

CHEMICAL PRINCIPLES AND BIOLOGIC SYSTEMS

Biology offers no exception to the full application of fundamental chemical and physical principles. A full description of a biologic process must include thermodynamics and kinetics of the process as well as details of molecular structures involved.

Thermodynamics is the consideration or delineation of all forms of energy in a system. All differences between an initial and final state can be summarized by the expression ΔG (change in "free energy") = ΔH (change in enthalpy) − $T\Delta S$ (change in entropy as a function of temperature). Thus, any possibility for spontaneous change requires a decrease in free energy of the system through an increase in entropy (paraphrased as "disorder") or a decrease in enthalpy ("heat" or "available" energy) or both. *Entropy* is an especially important term in biology because of the extensive (and energetically expensive) ordering of biomolecules in the face of the tendency of all systems of matter to become less ordered. Thus, cells must "live uphill in a downhill world." It is clear that biologic systems cannot be completely "closed," since they must utilize energy from without to maintain their order as well as to achieve energetic events, which must be expressed in terms of positive changes in enthalpy (or measurable energy).

Two very important principles operate. First, biologic systems and subsystems are tightly compartmentalized and highly organized, with stringent preservation of order and function. Second, biologic subsystems are tightly *coupled*. Thus, deg-

radative reactions in one system serve to energize and maintain other systems. This coupling is achieved through highly specific transfer of molecules between compartments and the generation and reaction of so-called "high-energy" molecules that react with appropriate molecular partners to provide reactions that are highly favored energetically. Thus, even if free energy changes in one compartment are unfavorable, they will be coupled chemically with other favorable reactions.

KINETICS

Thermodynamics concerns only initial and final states. *Kinetics* is the study and description of both the route and the rate, and thus is concerned with the rate details of molecular changes. The assignment of equilibrium conditions is based on the thermodynamics of the total system, but even at equilibrium molecular transformations are still occurring. Only *net* change is zero because the "forward" reaction(s) is equal to the "reverse" reaction(s) as dictated by the thermodynamics of the "initial" versus the "final" state(s). In biologic systems, dynamic "steady state" is a much more important concept than simple equilibrium. "Steady state" exists when *concentration(s)* remain constant with time ($dc/dT = 0$). This may be so because the sum of all processes that remove reactants is equal to all the processes that generate reactants.

Most biologic components may be considered within pseudo–steady state systems, since chemical concentrations are maintained so rigorously. The maintenance of these steady states in the face of continual fluctuations in the environment understandably demands the most sensitive and effective regulatory mechanisms. Recognition of biosystems as examples of steady state focuses attention on the importance of these control mechanisms and emphasizes the role of molecular "turnover" and "degradation" as well as rates of formation in the determination of the functioning concentration of any biocomponent. Systematic fluctuations are also important and characteristic of biologic systems, especially those as complex as a human. With each perturbation, there follows an "approach to steady state," the characteristics of which are dictated by the equilibrium and kinetic parameters of the systems involved as well as the intensity and duration of the perturbation. It is also very interesting that many systems go through a continual "oscillation" process of change back and forth between such approaches to steady state. Several examples are diurnal fluctuations of hormonal levels and body temperature, postabsorptive changes in metabolic activities, ion and metabolite distributions in nerve conduction and muscle contraction, menstrual cycling, and regulation of body temperature following perturbations.

The intricate "cascading" and "interlocking" of biologic reaction sequences are widely evident and are the basis for the amplification of single molecular defects into complex disease states. They also account for "distant" adjustment in steady-state concentrations through shifts in rates of precursor formation or product removal. The time required to achieve steady state in a reaction sequence depends on the individual rate constants of the contributing reactions and the volume or quantity ("pool size") of reactants involved. Thus, perturbation can result in a rapid appearance of shifts in concentration of small quantities of intermediates whose turnover is rapid, but it may cause delayed and prolonged changes in the case of slow reactions. Thus, the rapidity of appearance of "disease" can be rationalized on kinetic grounds. The rapidity of change also dictates the type of regulatory mechanism that may be required. With a rapid oscillation, an immediate kinetic *stimulation* or *inhibition* of enzymes or of molecular transport may provide immediate compensation for the perturbation. Slower or prolonged changes in steady state may provoke or require readjustment in *concentrations* of such enzyme catalysts or transport mechanisms. Some aspects of biologic function do not achieve steady state in the strictest sense. Environmental insults, for example, may result in damage that cannot be compensated completely—despite all homeostatic mechanisms—with resultant progressive changes. These changes may be very slow or very rapid, depending on the kinetics of the systems involved.

Biologic systems are also complicated by the kinetics of cell division. For example, a sequence involving slow molecular turnover may not achieve steady state in a cell population that is dividing rapidly. Thus, without any differences in the natures or controls of any chemical processes, reactants may differ considerably in concentration between dividing and nondividing cells owing to the differences in extent to which steady state is approached. Such non–steady state may provide an important regulatory distinction between such cells.

The study of chemical kinetics, therefore, must not ignore the importance of cell kinetics and the changes that occur during the cell cycle. This point is particularly significant when one is considering the response of cell populations to drugs and environmental insults. The kinetic distinctions between cells make it possible to exert control over specific cell populations (e.g., cancer cells), even if no qualitative distinctions can be made on the basis of their chemical processes.

The *rate-limiting steps* for formation and removal of bioconstituents are important to assign because they define vulnerability to perturbations and provide insight into disease as well as therapeutic manipulations. When one is looking at any change in steady state concentration, the following questions should be asked: (1) How critical is control of concentration, and is it primary or secondary to the biologic event in question? (2) What are *contributing processes and pathways*? (Where does it come from and where does it go?) (3) What are *rate-limiting steps*? (4) Over what *volume* are perturbations distributed? (What is the "pool" size?) This determines the magnitude of a significant perturbation and the abruptness of change. (5) Over what *time course* does the perturbation appear? (6) How is the perturbation propagated? (7) Where is control normally exerted?

Catalysis is of extreme importance in biologic systems because reactions must proceed at useful rates, efficient foci for regulation must be available, and chemical product selection must be precise. Enzyme mechanisms, kinetics, and regulation therefore play central roles in the chemical reactions of cells. The unique structures of the catalytic binding sites (on enzymes) that account for catalysis in biologic systems are largely unknown. When these are elucidated, an extraordinary potential will be unleashed for manipulation of biologic processes both through design of highly specific and effective inhibitors and inactivators and through the construction of artificial and replaceable catalysts.

The branching and cascading of chemical pathways provide a high level of complexity in biosystems so that consideration of a reaction in isolation is often meaningless. Thus, the concept of changes in steady state of an individual component must include all its secondary effects on other systems. The "concentration-response curve" is often complex owing to the interaction of multiple components at a control point. Therefore, many examples of complex, cooperative, and high-order response curves are seen in biologic systems.

Kinetics in biosystems must therefore concentrate on several important issues: both chemical and cell kinetics; the concepts of steady state and coupling; the importance of rate limiting steps; pool sizes; enzyme catalysis and regulation; and the occurrence of complex dose-response curves.

MOLECULAR COMPONENTS AND PROCESSES

GENERAL PRINCIPLES

Molecules are the basis for biologic processes. They provide information, structure, energy sources, energy transduction mechanisms, and waste disposal as well as a general milieu in which the cell must survive. The uniqueness of living systems is their high degree of complex order, which in turn must depend on a very complex and complete information system. This information system must be extraordinarily precise and must include self-replication and self-assembly mechanisms. All these features depend on specific molecular properties and can be described in such fundamental terms. In this brief discussion, four major points will be considered:

1. The very high degree of order in biomolecules has a strong dependence on the structural state of water (which constitutes most of the cell). Water, therefore, plays a dominant role in the determination of the cell's molecular properties. Water exists in a highly ordered state owing to its polarizability and resulting self-interactions by hydrogen bonding. Even at cell temperatures, water is, in large part, composed of orderly arrays of molecules in a lattice-like arrangement, as seen in ice. This lattice may be either disrupted or stabilized by the insertion of nonwater molecules, with substantial changes in entropy. Since the cellular concentration of water is better than 50 M, these changes in entropy can represent a major driving force to accomplish seemingly unfavorable reactions. The enthalpy of interactions between solute and water is also important to consider, especially in the case of charged or polarizable molecules, but entropy changes are often the dominant factor in rationalizing the state of biomolecules. This is particularly true with respect to macromolecular structure, in which individual moieties could be either inserted into the surrounding water layer or folded in a manner that excludes water. Water, therefore, determines whether or not biologic arrangements and biologic reactions can occur. In simple terms, the extreme ordering of some biologic molecules can occur because such ordering leads to an increase in disorder of the surrounding water molecules.

2. Weak chemical interactions play large roles in biosystems. These weak interactions include hydrogen bonding; various charge phenomena, including "salt" and dipole bonding; and nonpolar or hydrophobic interactions. Although each is of low energy, their combined totals of energy make them substantial factors in structure determination and serve to stabilize flexible macromolecules into useful shapes, to provide rapidly reversible responses of biomolecules to environmental changes, to generate specialized compartments or domains within cells, to provide for transport systems and molecular movement, and to generate the information-exchange mechanisms on which all life depends. Specialized domains within the covalent macromolecular structure provide the "binding sites" for such weak interactions, with much of their binding energy resulting from water as the cell solvent.

3. Biologic systems function as complex information systems by virtue of their molecular composition. Informational content can be rationalized rather easily when it is recognized that all atoms and molecules are subject to highly specific interactions and are, in that sense, informational. Simple ions have a specific size, charge density, hydration shell, and other features that dictate the potential for interactions. Thus, it is not surprising that an ion such as calcium can play such a dominant role in determining or activating such a variety of cellular mechanisms. Covalent molecules are highly specific in a three-dimensional sense and are, therefore, informational in a very specific way. The directed nature of covalent bonding and resulting three-dimensional specificity provide for the very important molecular templating, which is the basis for recognition and transmission. Sequential arrangements of molecular information bits in macromolecules, the complexity of temporal staging of information, and the interaction between two macromolecules of unique sequence all provide an extremely high order of discrimination. Each small molecule assumes a favored conformation that is based on its own structure in concert with its solvent domain and the influence of specific interactions with other molecules. In the case of a macromolecule, the total three-dimensional structure, although extremely complex, still depends on the state of each of its repeating units. Thus, when a change or interaction occurs, there is not only involvement of the individual reactants but also, possibly, production of rather distant changes in macromolecular conformation and reactivity. It is particularly intriguing to consider the details of the transduction of informational interactions either into a cascade of informational exchange, into messenger function, or into an energetic event. The conformational discriminations of molecules provide the basis for all these events. Thus, the individual information bits in biologic systems are arranged into a hierarchy: template interactions between small molecules based on three-dimensional molecular considerations and the directed nature of covalent bonds; more complex interactions resulting from arrangement of these information bits into a temporal framework within macromolecules; and interactions between such macromolecular arrangements and other macromolecules or small molecules to provide receptor-response loops.

4. Chemical reactivity in cells is tightly controlled through the operation of transfer reactions. Highly reactive chemical groups are transferred from donor to recipient in a controlled fashion that involves sequential steps of decreasing energy rather than the single burst of an exothermic reaction. It is especially interesting from the standpoint of chemical damage that the distribution of oxidative potential involves molecular species that can cause great biologic harm. Thus, the coupling sequences are also accompanied by a variety of scavengers that normally protect the cell against assault by such agents as superoxide radicals, peroxide, singlet oxygen, and hydroxide radicals. These mechanisms may represent important factors in the balance between cell destruction and cell preservation. Through the intervention of transfer reactions, the chemical energy of oxidative reactions is used constructively to maintain cell processes and to promote reactions that may be unfavorable energetically. Any breakdown of

this tight coupling, of course, is destructive to the cell. The whole of intermediary metabolism is concerned with the processes by which this type of control and tight coupling is accomplished and regulated.

STRUCTURES OF MACROMOLECULES

Macromolecules play central roles in biologic systems. A remarkable feature of all macromolecules is their sequential covalent synthesis from a limited number of small precursors and their self-assembly or aggregation into very large structures. With each class of macromolecules the precursors are essentially the same for all life forms, with minor variations in structure that permit discrimination between organisms and between specific functions within the same organism.

Macromolecules serve a variety of functions within living systems, including information storage and retrieval; structural integrity; formation of barriers to interface with the environment and to divide cell compartments; storage of chemical energy; and a variety of effector roles such as catalysis, energy transduction (chemical, thermal, and mechanical), and molecular transpositions to provide secretion and transport. Their three-dimensional structures are derived from the unique secondary and tertiary weak binding of these assembled building blocks, driven energetically by their interactions with each other and, especially, with solvent. The tendency toward self-assembly is often strong, accounting for the aggregation and assembly into supramolecular structures (organelles, membranes, enzyme complexes, etc.). The self-assembly process is the spontaneous result of these molecular interactions and often can be demonstrated in isolated systems. Macromolecular defects may derive from fundamental precursor and assembly problems, from details of minor structural variations, or from the excesses and deficiencies that result purely from kinetic alterations in either formation or turnover.

Table 2-1 presents a summary of the major classes of macromolecules in biologic systems. Each macromolecule is composed of characteristic repeating units arranged in some unique primary sequence. Each possesses some secondary structural feature that derives from the nature of the intramolecular ordering around this primary sequence, and each is characterized by a characteristic set of tertiary and quarternary interactions between the primary bits of information, or repeating units, and between these units and other macromolecules or small molecules. The tertiary and quaternary interactions of these macromolecules are dictated by the primary structure in concert with interactions with the medium and are unique for the individual molecule under a given set of conditions. For each molecule, the biologic properties depend, of course, on these three-dimensional structural characteristics as well as their primary chemical reactive property. Some macromolecules are characterized by their chemical inertness or stability; others are distinguished by their dynamic reactive properties.

Unique binding sites for small molecules on macromolecules provide effector functions essential to the chemical processes of cells as well as the direct communication link between the environment and cell effector functions. Thus, macromolecules represent the receptors at which drugs and other biologically effective signals interact (usually reversibly and often weakly) to provoke substantial biologic consequences.

The major classes of macromolecules—nucleic acids, proteins, carbohydrates, and lipids—will be discussed chiefly in terms of their roles in information storage, transfer, and utilization; structure formation; and effector functions. As already emphasized, all molecules are informational in nature, but nucleic acids represent the primary information system of the cell. Proteins play a major role in determining the structural properties of the cell, and although all constituent molecules are an integral part of the cell structure, carbohydrates and lipids contribute particularly to the structure of membrane barriers and to the intercellular matrix. Proteins play the major role in effector functions and primary communication with the environment. The important structural roles of complex polysaccharides and lipids and their participation in regulation and recognition must also be noted. All these macromolecular constituents interact in forming the cell mass and dictating total cell function.

The detailed study of each set of macromolecules provides a unique challenge to the modern investigator. In each instance, studies involve several approaches. First, primary structure analysis by destructive sequence determination is well advanced and, in principle, solvable for any protein. This has resulted from (1) the ability to cleave massive proteins into unique smaller units by selective backbone hydrolysis using enzymes, and (2) the ability to hydrolyze the backbone chemically by sequential cleavage from the end of the molecule, with identification of each repeating unit. The technology is fully automated and widely available. The limited availability of pure material somewhat restricts successful practice of the procedures, but microtechniques have drastically reduced the quantity of material required.

Proteins are classically separated and purified according to their physical properties. Their unique receptor (ligand binding) and antigenic properties provide an even more powerful means of purification through use of such specific binding materials attached to an insoluble matrix material. Thus, adsorptive columns can be used to remove pure proteins from impure mixtures. This method can be especially powerful when quantities of an appropriate and pure (monoclonal) antibody

TABLE 2-1 MACROMOLECULES IN BIOLOGIC SYSTEMS

	DNA	RNA	Proteins	Glycogen	Mucopolysaccharides (Glycosoaminoglycans)	Hetero-Oligosaccharides
Primary Structure Repeat (Backbone)	Deoxyribose polyphosphate ester of purine and pyrimidine glycosides.	Ribose polyphosphate ester of purine and pyrimidine glycosides.	Peptide bond.	Repeating glycoside of glucose (glucosylglucose).	Disaccharide repeating unit composed of an amino sugar and a uronic acid in glycosidic linkage. All but hyaluronic acid also have O- and N-sulfate groups.	Glycoside residues attached through glycoside linkage to secreted polypeptides, cell wall lipids, and structure and secretory proteins.
Type of Structure	Linear, nonbranching.	Linear, nonbranching.	Linear with complex 3-D constraints.	Linear and branched.	Linear chains, variable in length linked covalently to a polypeptide core.	Often highly branched.
Type of Secondary and Tertiary Interactions	Template interactions are key to biologic role; these complementary self-interactions (intra- and inter-chain ring stacking and H-bonding of purines and pyrimidines) provide highly ordered helical structures that are packed into manageable cellular units by specific binding to proteins.	Same potential as DNA, but less extensive.	H-bonding of peptide unit; noncovalent interactions between side chains (H-bonding, hydrophobic, charge); covalent bonds between side chains spontaneously (s) or enzymically. Supramolecular aggregation is common.	Minimal	Extensive hydrophilic and electrostatic interactions.	May be highly specific (e.g., antigenic templating).
Synthesis and Assembly	Templated sequential addition of primary repeat with occasional postsynthetic modification (e.g., methylation) of specific bases. Segmental repair or segmental resynthesis also occurs.	Same as DNA with more extensive postsynthetic modification by degradation of chain termini and end addition and by removal and splicing of internal sectors.	Templated sequential addition of amino acids. Postsynthetic modifications include segmental hydrolysis, addition of nonpeptide moieties, oxidation and reduction, and condensation.	Sequential addition of glucose units to growing chain; transfer of chain sectors within growing chain to form branch points (enzyme rather than template directed).	Sequential addition and modification in situ of monosaccharide units—directed by specificity of enzymes (not templated).	Sequential addition dictated by specific enzymes and growing chain termini.
Precursors Required in Addition to Enzymes	Deoxypurine and pyrimidine nucleotides. Deoxyribose moiety and thymine are unique to DNA.	Ribose, purine, and pyrimidine nucleotides (uracil is unique to RNA).	Amino acids, tRNA, mRNA, and ribosomes; residues for postsynthetic modification.	UDP glucose.	Polypeptide chain; UDP monosaccharide unit; phosphoadenosine phosphosulfate.	Growing chain termini and appropriate activated glycoside residue.
Size	Immense.	Small to very large.	Small to very large.	Variable and heterogeneous.	Extremely variable; aggregates in excess of 10^6 mol. wt.	Highly variable.
Functions	Primary information storage and transcription.	Information transfer and translation.	Protean—structural, effector, transport, barrier, buffer, regulatory, receptor.	Storage.	Constitute "ground substance" and modulate the solvation and reaction environment of all tissues.	Lubricant; membrane integrity, recognition processes (e.g., antigen-antibody, peptide hormones); regulation of molecular turnover.
Turnover	Primary stability is essential to life; limited segmental turnover occurs through damage and repair.	Some are very stable (e.g., ribosomal RNA), whereas some species turn over rapidly.	From very stable to very labile. Related to inherent (thermodynamic) stability. Final degradation of backbone is largely nonspecific.	Rapid, tightly regulated.	Requires action of specific hydrolytic enzymes to control appropriate concentrations; otherwise, molecules are very stable.	Requires specific hydrolytic enzymes.

have been produced to serve as the reagent. Primary sequence analysis is also well advanced for nucleic acids and is, in fact, now easier and less expensive than for proteins. Despite the fact that each gene of interest is composed of at least three times as many repeating units as the corresponding gene product, the primary structure of any gene is within easy grasp of the modern molecular biologist. This, in combination with the variety of experimental strategies available with nucleic acids, is a powerful approach to the study of biologic function. The templating properties of nucleic acids can be used for their isolation. For example, the appropriate RNA transcript can be used to form a complementary complex with a unique DNA sequence and separate it from a mixture of sequences, all of which have the same physical properties. Furthermore, a small amount of pure DNA (or RNA) can be amplified into whatever quantity is required for study based on the nucleic acid technology now available.

Effective sequence analysis for complex polysaccharides is assisted by advanced chromatographic and mass spectroscopic techniques and through the availability of specific glycosidases with which the terminal sugar at each successive hydrolytic step can be identified and hydrolyzed.

These important analyses may present the most formidable challenge, since the macromolecules of interest may be present on cells in very small amounts and no techniques are available to construct large amounts in vitro. However, there has been considerable progress in the potential for isolation through the development of monoclonal antibodies (see further on), which can now be used to harvest the macromolecules from large quantities of tissues. This is an area of study that promises to shed much light on cell-cell interactions and organization, host parasite relationships, and susceptibility to a variety of diseases. The clinical observation that specific cell surface markers that function ostensibly as "self antigens," or recognition mechanisms, appear to correlate with the frequency of diseases (e.g., ankylosing spondylitis, acquired immune deficiency) suggests that important insights into disease mechanisms will result from elucidation of the structure and function of this important class of macromolecules.

The study of primary sequences in situ within macromolecules is also of considerable value in identifying structure-function relationships in macromolecules. The complementary nature of polynucleotides makes it quite practical to identify short informational sequences within the macromolecule simply by the construction of an appropriate complementary probe. It is entirely practical, for example, to identify a gene by the complementary binding of an isolated messenger molecule. The added technology of synthesizing DNA sequences from messenger molecules by means of reverse transcriptase followed by amplification through cloning permits study of these

sequences in different genetic surroundings (see further on). The major approach to the identification of unique sequences within a large protein molecule has involved the use of the specific antibodies. This is complicated, however, by the fact that these unique sequences are often involved in extensive tertiary structure of the protein, which may considerably modify the ability of an antibody to bind. Moreover, antibody specificity is directed at tertiary as well as primary structure.

Identification of specific binding sites responsible for biologic properties (e.g., enzyme substrate site, antigen combining site, drug "receptor" site, etc.) is a problem of sequence identity as well as of surface topography, and it is complicated by the fact that moieties that are adjacent in the folded, active configuration of a macromolecule may be quite distant from each other in the primary sequence. Furthermore, most site-binding is reversible and may involve quite low concentrations of ligand and receptor. Identification of these moieties can be approached by chemical ablation or perturbation of the macromolecular structure, modification of ligand structure, affinity labeling, and the powerful technique of photoaffinity labeling. Physical studies of the complexes in situ and the use of appropriate model compounds also have proved valuable. Reversible structure perturbations also provide a valuable approach to the study of macromolecular structure and function. This is particularly interesting from the viewpoint of studying mechanisms of biologic regulation, since regulation is effected through reversible perturbations in structure (and function). High-resolution electron microscopy has also made it possible to view directly specific macromolecules within cellular structures and thus to achieve an increased understanding of molecular structure. This technology now appears to be useful in the study of all major classes of macromolecules, particularly when combined with the use of specific tagged antibodies as probes.

One of the most intriguing approaches to the study of biomolecular structure and function has been the construction of model compounds of precursor molecules with modeling of the biologic processes for which these molecules are responsible. The construction, for example, of the lipid bilayer membrane and the insertion of model peptides that serve as either channels or transport carriers has provided a very incisive approach to the understanding of membrane function. The construction of sequences of collagen and elastin has also been used in studies of mechanisms for tissue calcification and offers promise for solution of this intriguing and important biologic problem. The construction of unique protein sequence and topographic models represents a complex and challenging synthetic problem for the chemist.

The "genetic experiment" (provided by either nature or the investigator) has been especially useful in the study of macromolecular structure and function. The study of the structures and function of mutant gene products has long been a major source of progress in understanding structure-function relationships and the nature of biologic regulation. Previously, the major genetic experiment was limited to spontaneous or induced mutations, which are random in nature and often complex in expression. Breakthroughs in plasmid technology now make it possible to clone DNA sequences within a lower organism so that quantities of a gene can be constructed for use in appropriate biologic studies. The whole technology of the construction of these genes and their potential insertion into other cells, of course, has created a tremendous amount of interest and even controversy, but in terms of the medical sciences, it represents one of the major advances in our capacity to study, understand, and modify disease processes (see further on).

Thus, macromolecules can be studied by the specific approaches of destructive analysis, analysis in situ—either the nondestructive sort or that achieved through perturbation effects—and the appropriate construction of models for the study of specific structure-function relationships.

NUCLEIC ACIDS

The roles of nucleic acids in providing the stable storage form for information in cells as well as the templating mechanisms for information read-out (transcription, translation, replication, reverse transcription, repair) are well known and need not be discussed in great detail here. These macromolecules, in providing two-dimensional copies of all the information in an organism to be translated into both time-dependent events and three-dimensional structures, are necessarily immense and present special problems in environmental vulnerability and stability, fidelity of copying and translation, cellular packaging, and mechanisms for precise regulation. These problems are solved through special structural features and cellular processes, which will be summarized briefly.

The nucleic acids illustrate one of the basic premises of molecular biology, namely, that knowledge of molecular structure can lead to an understanding of function. The double-helical structure of DNA proposed by Watson and Crick led to confirmation of the two-dimensional read-out nature of cellular information storage and retrieval, to an understanding of the stable nature of and replicative mechanism for the information system, and to a precise understanding of the chemical nature of genetic variability and mutations. Nucleic acids have both sequence specificity and three-dimensional specificity and provide the basis not only of the primary information system but also for the interaction of regulators so that biologic expression can be modulated. DNA is the

most stable of the nucleic acids and usually represents the stable master copy of information within the cell; RNA is an intermediate expression or vector of information (messenger) and also provides a read-out mechanism for translation. There are, however, exceptions to this generalization in that some viruses consist of RNA rather than DNA.

The structures of RNA and DNA are diagrammed in Figure 2–1. The basic backbone of nucleic acids is a monotonous repeating unit of a sugar phosphate ester that provides stability and whose polyanionic nature assures an extended structure of the polymer for ease in reading and modulation. The information bits consist of unique sequential arrangements of purine and pyrimidine bases, attached by glycosidic bond to the backbone, that provide a reading mechanism through the "templating" action of specific intramolecular interactions of weak hydrogen bonding and ring-stacking. The specific reactive properties of the bases also account for modifications known to impair or change function. For example, the bases are susceptible to modification by alkylating drugs, formation of various adducts, simple chemical cleavage of the glycosidic bond, or modification by absorption of radiant energy. Their specific functions and interactions may also be disrupted by binding of various aromatic heterocyclic drugs that show avidity for ordered sequences of purines and pyrimidines. This is particularly true for binding to the "core" of purine and pyrimidine base pairs in double-stranded DNA.

In addition to their common features, DNA and RNA also show several important differences. First, there is a single copy of DNA made for each chromosome at each cell replication, whereas RNA may be synthesized in multiple copies. Second, DNA is much larger than RNA and thus represents a larger "target" for various insults. Both these factors combine with the critical role of DNA to make the cell particularly vulnerable to DNA damage. Third, the deoxysugar and thymine are unique to DNA and represent specific loci where DNA synthesis can be regulated—a point of considerable importance to chemotherapy. At the same time, the deoxysugar makes the DNA backbone more stable chemically by protecting it against alkaline hydrolysis. Its double helical structure also lends stability and provides a complementary strand for use in replication and repair. The large target size of DNA also accounts for the major lethal effects of ionizing radiation, whereas UV irradiation kills cells largely because of the efficient and specific capture of radiant energy by the pyrimidines in DNA, with formation of dimers and consequent disruption of its information role.

The packaging of nucleic acids into three-dimensional structures serves primary functional and regulatory roles as well as solving cell logistic problems in handling such large molecules. The

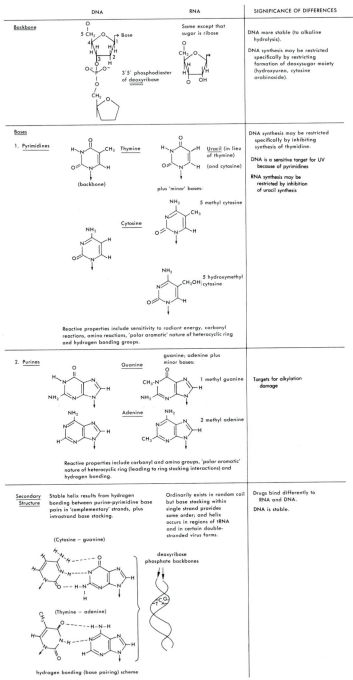

Figure 2–1 Diagram of primary and secondary aspects of DNA and RNA structure (with abbreviated structural formulas, emphasis on three-dimensional arrangement).

nature of "packaging" is related directly to the molecular details of function. For DNA and mRNA reading, sequential access to each of the information bits is required, and extensive three-dimensional structuring probably is not concerned with primary function. The highly structured state of DNA is more likely involved with determining which sequences will be expressed, when, and at what rates. DNA is packaged in a highly ordered fashion around basic protein "cores" interspersed with regions of extended DNA structure. In addition, a large number of acidic proteins as well as RNA molecules are associated with DNA to form cellular chromatin. In cell division of higher eukaryotes, DNA replication is followed by a highly ordered sequence of events in which a contractile protein (spindle protein) segregates the replicated number of chromosomes into their respective daughter cells. Although the different classes of nucleic acid–associated proteins do not contribute directly to the nature of the information provided by the nucleic acids, they are highly important adjuncts to the organization, integrity, and orderly and appropriate expression of such information. The cellular "structuring" of DNA, therefore, involves the binding of a variety of proteins and RNA. Ribosomal RNA is also packaged with a number of specific proteins to serve its biologic function. Transfer RNA, in contrast, assumes specific three-dimensional configurations by virtue of intramolecular interactions dictated by its primary structure and the presence of specific modified bases that are produced post-transcriptionally, to provide specific recognition sites for the enzymes concerned with amino acid activation and for interaction with ribosomal units and with mRNA for translation. Thus, although nucleic acid information is basically two-dimensional in nature, three-dimensional structural considerations are of great importance within the total context of biologic function and regulation. It is apparent that additional information will be forthcoming on the details of secondary structure and their roles in biologic function. It is interesting that despite the long-standing interest in DNA helical structure, an additional configuration, zDNA, was only recently described as an important dynamic variant that may be associated with specific regulatory consequences in DNA function.

The structure of nucleic acids results in a number of types of predictable interactions with other molecules, as shown in Table 2–2. The backbone provides a repetitious, charged, hydrophilic domain for electrostatic binding. The purine and pyrimidine bases contribute a variety of reactive sites (amino and carbonyl groups, heterocyclic rings) and participate in ring-stacking interactions and hydrogen bonding. The highly ordered hydrophobic core of helical DNA is especially suited for hydrophobic and ring-stacking interactions. Thus, DNA, for example, can participate in interactions ranging from electrostatic to hydrophobic and can

react covalently as well. Strong binding of specific ligands often involves two or more of these interaction modes to provide highly cooperative and specific attachment. In addition to a primary mode of covalent reaction, a ligand that is bound noncovalently can be activated in situ to cause covalent damage (e.g., by light activation in the case of furocoumarins or acridines or by oxidation in the case of bleomycin). In the cell, accessibility is determined by the structural state of the polynucleotide, that is, to what extent available sites are blocked by "natural" ligand binding or by complex "packaging." It is highly interesting that binding of ligands within intact cells may exhibit specificities that are much more stringent than in-vitro studies. For example, in the case of ethidium, there appears to be highly selective binding to kinetoplast DNA correlated with its antiparasitic action. The biologic consequences are difficult to predict quantitatively, therefore, because of this variability in binding, the compensatory mechanisms that a cell may employ, and the additional selective factors operating within intact cells. The interactions of ligands with nucleic acids and their consequences represent a challenging topic for study in relation to therapeutic actions and for understanding toxic effects of drugs and environmental chemicals. The reversible nature of much of such binding and the small numbers of bound molecules required for effects have made such studies difficult. The strategy of photoaffinity labeling, in which the small numbers of effector ligands can be fixed covalently by photoactivation in situ, has provided an exciting approach to this problem.

Because the information responsible for a cell's characteristics is encoded in the sequence of DNA, it follows simply that a qualitative change in a DNA locus by removal, addition, or change in a nucleotide base information bit can result in a mutation or change in cell properties. Since the total of an organism's properties depends also on the dynamic interplay of all its systems, normal information expression also requires correct quantitative balance between the different elements of expression, particularly in highly complex organisms that go through a precisely timed sequence of differentiation and cell cycling. When the genetic load is disrupted by a change in chromosomal number, gross errors in differentiation occur (e.g., the various human abnormalities associated with the occurrence of extra chromosomes; see Chapter 3). It is also noteworthy that changes in the information content of the cell can result from the imposition of external genetic material, such as that resulting from virus infections that may simply disrupt cell functions or may cause heritable changes in cell properties such as neoplastic transformation. The steps involved in information storage and processing in nucleic acids are summarized in Table 2–3. These processes are especially pertinent to biologic regulation and can be exploited to explain disease processes or used for

TABLE 2–2 INTERACTIONS OF CHEMICAL AGENTS WITH NUCLEIC ACIDS

Type of Interaction	Drug	Nucleic Acid Structural Site(s) Involved	Effects on DNA Properties and Function	Clinical Use
Covalent	Alkylating agents nitrogen mustard, such antibiotics as mitomycin, etc.	Adds to N-7 position of guanine	Inhibits cell replication; also mutagenic	Cytotoxic agent
	Certain reactive aromatic hydrocarbons (e.g., fluroenyl-acetamide)	Adds to N-8 position of guanine	Mutagenic, carcinogenic	
	Hydrazine and hydroxylamine	Reacts with C=O groups	Mutagenic	
	Nitrous acid	Reacts with NH_2 groups	Mutagenic	
Noncovalent	Polyamines (spermine, spermidine)	Backbone (PO_4)	Stabilizes	
	Basic proteins (histones)	Backbone (PO_4)	Stabilizes	
	Acidic proteins	Specific base sequences	Regulation of structure and function	
	Ions	Backbone, and polar groups of bases	Backbone binding stabilizes, base binding disrupts DNA helix	
	Hydrocarbons	Stacks with purine bases	Mutagenic, carcinogenic	
	Heterocyclic drugs and antibiotics			
	1. Actinomycin	Ring-stacking (intercalation) and charge interaction with backbone (minor groove)	Inhibits RNA synthesis, and to a lesser extent DNA synthesis	Cytotoxic (anticancer)
	2. Streptomycin	Ribosomal RNA	Inhibits protein synthesis	Antibiotic
	3. Aminoquinoline antimalarial drugs	Ring-stacking and charge interaction with backbone	Stabilizes DNA helix, inhibits DNA synthesis and repair; inhibits RNA synthesis poorly	Antiparasitic
	4. Acridines (including quinacrine)	Ring-stacking and charge interaction with backbone	Same spectrum of action as aminoquinolines	Antiparasitic Anticancer
	5. Furocoumarins	?	Photosensitivity	Vitiligo therapy
	6. Adriamycin	Ring-stacking (intercalation)	Inhibits replication	Cytotoxic (anticancer)
	7. Ethidium	Ring-stacking (intercalation)	Inhibits replication	Antiparasitic
	8. Bleomycin	Binding to bases with secondary covalent binding	Inhibits replication	Anticancer
	9. Berenil	Binds to outside of helix	Inhibits replication and transcription	Antiparasitic
	10. Anthracenedione	Base-stacking	Inhibits replication	Anticancer
	11. Elliplicine	Base-stacking	Inhibits replication	Anticancer; antiparasitic
	12. *cis*-Platinum	Base-stacking	Inhibits replication	Anticancer

TABLE 2–3 INFORMATION STORAGE AND PROCESSING

Processes	Steps Required	Enzyme (and possible sites for regulation)

DNA Synthesis	1. Precursor synthesis
	  a. Synthesis of purines and pyrimidines (thymine uniquely)
	  b. Formation of nucleoside
	  c. Phosphorylation to form nucleotides
	  d. Reduction of ribonucleotides to deoxyribonucleotides
	2. Synthesis (formation of polydexoyribose PO₄ backbone in *templated* sequential replicative process to form new duplex)
	3. Superhelical structure formation (winding) and condensation with proteins and packaging into chromosomes
	4. Deployment of contractile protein (spindle) to segregate chromosomes into daughter cells
		1. Enzymes for precursor synthesis (thymidylate synthetase and kinase and ribonucleotide reductase are unique to DNA)
		2. Replicases (template and primer requiring polymerases to form information sequences)
		3. Ligases—to join short segments into total sequences and to restore nicks.
		4. Enzymes acting on secondary and tertiary structure—"unwinding" and "winding" enzymes
		5. Nucleases—"editing" removal of mismatched bases in replication; nicking actions to provide DNA access for normal functions and repair; DNA turnover (cell death) and foreign DNA; "restriction"
		6. Modification enzymes—methylation of specific bases as control points for expression and in control of restriction DNAases
		7. Spindle protein formation attachment and contraction

DNA Repair	1. Recognition of damage (surveillance) 2. Removal and synthesis and/or exchange of limited DNA sequences	1. Specific endonucleases 2. Exonucleases 3. Polymerases 4. Ligases 5. Recombinational enzymes
RNA Synthesis (Transcription)	1. Precursor synthesis (same as for DNA except uracil in lieu of thymine and ribonucleotides are not reduced) 2. Synthesis—templated sequential polymerization with release of RNA product and restoration of DNA duplex. 3. Processing of RNA transcript and transposition to site of function. (Internal sequences are spliced out, 5' end is "capped" with 5'→5' pyrophosphate linked and methylated base, and poly-A tail is added to 3' end)	1. Enzymes of precursor biosynthesis pathways 2. Transcriptase (including factors for initiation which may include enzymes "unwinding" of "rewinding" of DNA template) 3. RNAases and polyadenylating enzymes (processing of mRNA)

Peptide Synthesis (Translation)	1. Formation and assembly of constituents of translation complex
	  a. Template (messenger) transcription
	  b. Formation of ribosomes
	    1) Transcription of unique RNA (ribosomal)
	    2) Synthesis of specific proteins
	    3) Ordered aggregation (assembly)
	  c. Transcription of specific tRNA molecules
	    1) Synthesis
	    2) Modification of specific nucleotides
	    3) Folding into specific 3D structure
	  d. Activation of amino acids (attachment to appropriate tRNA molecules)
	2. Sequential (templated) formation of peptide backbone
	3. Assembly (spontaneous) of secondary and tertiary structure
		1. All enzymes for RNA transcription (above)
		2. Amino acid activating enzymes
		3. tRNA modification enzymes
		4. Peptide synthetase
		5. Transcriptase

Modification of Translation Products (Protein)	1. Synthesis or absorption of various nonprotein moieties 2. Attachment of chemical groups to specific protein side chains 3. Modification of translated primary structure (oxidation, reduction, hydroxylation of side chains; hydrolytic removal of sections of primary sequence)	1. Biosynthetic enzymes for nonprotein moieties 2. Specific transferases for attaching nonprotein moieties. 3. Hydroxylases, oxidoreductases for amino acid side chains. 4. Proteases (specific)
Reverse Transcription	Precursor synthesis (deoxyribonucleotides) Templated (RNA) synthesis of DNA	Reverse transcriptase
Discriminating Protein Regulatory and Effector Functions (Binding, Catalysis, etc.)	1. All steps for specific protein synthesis and modification 2. Signals reception (small molecule binding) 3. Protein response (conformational change) 4. Effector function (catalysis, transport, regulation)	1. All enzymes for protein synthesis and modification 2. All enzymes for synthesis and modification of signal molecule

therapeutic applications. Sites for regulation are also indicated in Table 2–3.

DNA replication is a tightly controlled and precisely ordered process in which each strand of double helical DNA serves as a template for the synthesis of a new DNA strand for distribution to daughter cells. For the complex eukaryotic cell, replication is initiated at specific starting points, and each replicating unit (replicon) is copied on a precise time schedule in which chromosomal organization is maintained. Each parent strand with its complementary newly synthesized daughter strand is packaged into a new chromosome, and these are segregated into the daughter cells by a precise process of mitosis or meiosis in which each genetic locus is preserved. There can be exchange of information segments between identical sectors of chromosomes (crossing over) during both meiosis and mitosis, which serves to give a random assortment of differences in genetic markers carried on different members of a pair of chromosomes. Mitosis and meiosis differ only in the number of chromosomal doublings and the final distribution of chromosomal copies. For mitosis, a simple doubling occurs, with daughter cells identical with the parents in chromosomal number. Meiosis produces cells (terminal germ cells) with half the parent number of chromosomes through final segregation of single chromosomal copies into daughter cells during a reductive division. It is significant that final chromosomal segregation for diploid organisms such as the human produces a cell with no redundancy of information and thus no opportunity to recover information lost during the division processes. For either mitosis or meiosis, failure to segregate chromosomes correctly (nondisjunction) can result in disruption in chromosomal number and size, with resultant impairment of biologic function.

Lack of precision and appropriate control of DNA replication and the attendant cell processes of mitosis and meiosis are obviously detrimental and provide the basis for disease. For example, the growth of neoplastic tissues, the proliferation of pannus in the joints in rheumatoid arthritis, keloid formation, and psoriasis may all represent excessive or inappropriate cell proliferation. Conversely, depression of the bone marrow and immune suppression and ulceration of the intestinal mucosa consequent to the administration of a variety of toxic drugs or in the course of irradiation are examples of inadequate replication and proliferation of cells. Furthermore, disruptions in chromosomal size and number, presumably from nondisjunction or unequal exchange of chromosomal segments, have devastating effects on human development. Replicative processes and chromosomal integrity also provide important targets for damage by a variety of environmental hazards.

An understanding of the specific structures and processes involved in replication also provides the rational basis for regulation. Thus, limitation of the synthesis of thymidine by folic acid antagonists and certain fraudulent nucleotides or inhibition of reductive formation of deoxyribose nucleotides by hydroxyurea or cytosine arabinoside restricts replication at the precursor level. The process of DNA copying by the DNA polymerase can be interfered with by a variety of drugs and antibiotics that interact with the DNA template, such as daunomycin and adriamycin, bleomycin, ethidium bromide, various antimalarials, mitomycin, nitrogen mustard and other alkylating agents, and to some extent actinomycin D. Subsequent to DNA synthesis, the segregation process for the newly synthesized DNA in mitosis can be blocked by the administration of specific mitotic inhibitors such as vincristine and colchicine that interact with the specialized contractile proteins responsible for mitotic segregation of chromosomes. At the present time it is not clear what the signal is in a cell for the start of DNA synthesis and cell division, and no exploitation of this mechanism has been possible for therapeutic purposes. However, cells can be stimulated to divide in vitro by the administration of certain agents such as phytohemagglutinin and pokeweed mitogen, illustrating the potential for regulation of this process.

The central information role of DNA is protected by several important homeostatic mechanisms. First, an "editing" process operates during replication to excise mismatched bases in the new strand through a nuclease action that accompanies the polymerase. Even more interesting are the mechanisms that operate to restore the fidelity of information within preformed DNA. The best understood mechanism is that of excision repair, or *repair synthesis,* in which modified single-stranded segments of DNA are excised and resynthesized complementary to the intact strand. This process is called into action following a variety of environmental insults, including UV or ionizing irradiation, chemical modification of bases, and thermal damage. The actions of a number of specific enzymes have been identified that recognize specific modifications and introduce a break in the damaged DNA strand. The actual excision, resynthesis, and rejoining processes appear to be common to multiple types of damage but are subdivided into "long-gap" and "short-gap" processes ranging from only a few to as many as 2000 bases. Because the information is intact in the complementary strand, these processes can be accomplished with high fidelity. Repair can also be accomplished following replication. New strand synthesis opposite the damaged site either is interrupted to result in a single strand gap or results in errors either during replication or in the daughter cell. Repair of the damaged region can also be accomplished after replication by a recombinational process to retrieve information from another chromosome. Damage at a locus involving both DNA strands either is not repairable or must involve an error-prone process, since neither strand has a complete information copy. Hence, the potent effects of neutron irradiation, which introduces double strand breaks, or multifunctional alkylating agents can be rationalized partly on the grounds of lack of repair.

It has also been recognized that persistence of unrepaired lesions can serve to provoke an error-prone inducible "repair" process, a finding that stresses the importance of regulation in this important system. DNA repair processes (and their regulation) appear to represent, therefore, important homeostatic mechanisms by which the cell preserves the integrity of its basic information system. The possibility also exists that this is the means by which the cell can undergo biologic variations by modification of limited regions of DNA without the necessity for undergoing cell division. Predictably, disease can result from defects in these repair mechanisms because the stability of the information systems for somatic cells may be compromised. Such stability is particularly pertinent to cancer and aging, and it is significant that several repair defects have been identified in human cells in association with increased cancer susceptibility. Human repair defects are summarized in Table 2–4. The identification and study of such "genetic experiments of nature" constitute a powerful approach that will provide invaluable clues to the details and the biologic roles of the DNA repair systems.

Thus, xeroderma pigmentosum, Fanconi's anemia, ataxia telangiectasia, and Down's syndrome are all associated with increased risk of malignancy and have been shown to be defective in repair mechanisms. In addition, it has been reported that the increased aging associated with progeria may also be correlated with a defect in cellular DNA repair. In the case of xeroderma pigmentosum, it has also been shown that the disease can actually be caused by more than one defect, since investigators using isolated cells in in-vitro experiments have identified more than one complementation group. Repair systems may also be exploitable therapeutically for modifying the sensitivity of cancer cells to irradiation and alkylating agents, since such therapy works by introducing repairable lesions into cellular DNA.

The orderly read-out of stored information in the cell occurs through the processes of transcription (synthesis of a messenger RNA) followed by translation of this messenger into protein structure. Transcription represents the appropriate and timely templating of the information strand of the helical DNA into a single strand of messenger RNA, which is the vector for cytoplasmic expression. Studies with model systems in simple organisms have revealed that transcription is a tightly controlled process in which messenger RNA is made appropriate to the needs of the cell. For each gene, transcription must start at a precise initiation point and continue in a sequential fashion to the end of the gene. The details of the control of this process in cells, particularly mammalian cells, are not yet worked out, but it is clear that the initiation process involves both negative and positive control factors and that more than one gene may be controlled coordinately, possibly because a single large messenger is transcribed for several genes (polycistronic messengers). Transcription may be repressed by the binding of some recognition molecule to the initiation region on DNA, so that it cannot occur unless an appropriate signal in the form of a small molecule interacts with this repressor to impede its binding. This permits small molecules to turn on transcription. In a similar fashion, small molecules may serve to turn off transcription if the DNA binding repressor binds more tightly in response to the small molecular signal. These processes of induction and repression are illustrated in Figure 2–2 and are essential to the understanding of enzyme induction and enzyme repression, both of which offer potential for exploitation in therapy. The control of virus infection and expression is also effected through such mechanisms.

When RNA is transcribed, not only is the unique messenger sequence synthesized but also additional RNA at each end of the messenger and

TABLE 2–4 HUMAN DEFECTS IN DNA REPAIR

Xeroderma pigmentosum	In most cases, there is decreased excision of UV photoproducts; variants are deficient in postreplicative repair	Extreme UV sensitivity with high frequency of cancer in UV exposed areas; severe variants have CNS defects.
Ataxia telangiectasia; Bloom's syndrome	Decreased excision repair of ionizing radiation damage; increased radiation sensitivity; decreased chromosomal stability (Bloom's syndrome also sensitive to UV)	Increased cancer susceptibility; immunodeficiency; cerebellar ataxia telangiectasia
Fanconi's anemia	Decreased excision repair following UV and ionizing radiation	Increased cancer susceptibility
Progeria	Cultured cells show decreased capacity to rejoin x-ray strand breaks	Premature aging

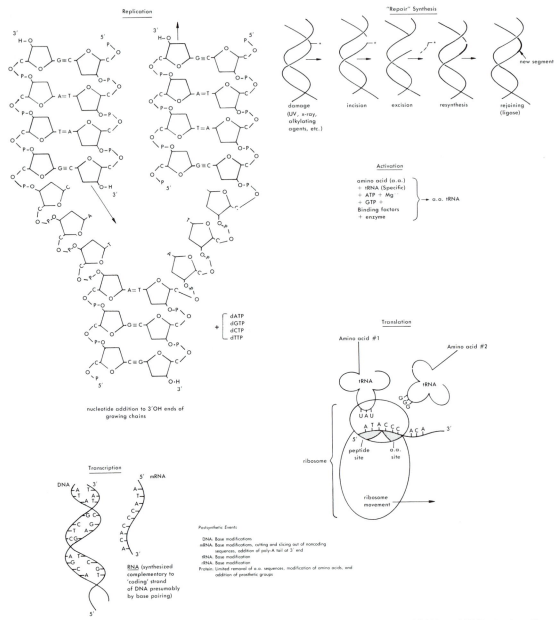

Figure 2–2 Diagrammatic sketch (with abbreviated chemical formula) to follow fate of DNA and RNA structure through replication, repair, transcription, and translation.

long, "noncoding" internal sequences are included. These sequences, therefore, must be processed or eliminated before the message is translated by the cytoplasmic machinery. Furthermore, the ends of the final message are prepared by capping of the 5′ end with a pyrophosphate-linked 5′ nucleotide and specific-base methylation and by attachment of a poly-A "tail" to the 3′ end. These steps of post-transcriptional messenger RNA processing have received considerable emphasis. The roles of the excess RNA synthesized have not been established, but the cell obviously makes a large investment

in energy in order to synthesize these polynucleotide sequences and then to process them following the initial step of transcription.

Transcription offers several potential sites for regulation (and therapeutic manipulation). First, limitation in the unique RNA precursors required for transcription can be accomplished by metabolic blockade or by use of fraudulent nucleotides that compete for incorporation. Second, induction and repression may be accomplished either by the use of the appropriate small molecular signal, usually a product for the gene action in question or a related system, or by the use of fraudulent small molecules that serve to mimic their action. Third, the templating function of DNA may be interfered with by the binding of specific agents, such as actinomycin D, that bind to the DNA template and prevent copying. Fourth, the action of the RNA polymerase itself may be blocked (in bacteria) by such agents as the antibiotic rifamycin. Fifth, the processes by which the very large precursor messenger RNA is modified to provide the final messenger may also be subject to regulation, although the mechanisms involved have not been elucidated.

Translation is the process of converting the linear information sequence in the mRNA transcript into a protein molecule that in turn provides a three-dimensional biologic structure. The molecular structures involved directly in this complex process are RNA derived from processing of the initial mRNA transcript; ribosomes, composed of RNA and a large number of specific proteins; and "charged" transfer RNA, from which all the correct amino acids are transferred sequentially into the growing peptide chain, based on the complementarity between a coding triplet in each tRNA and a triplet sequence within the mRNA. This complex sequence of events depends on a number of processes characteristic of the cascading nature of biologic events, providing multiple points for potential regulation. mRNA must be synthesized (in the appropriate amount and at the right time), processed to remove the noncoding sequences, transported out along the endoplasmic reticulum, and attached to ribosomes. Ribosomes are assembled in the cell from specific species of RNA (rRNA) and a large number of specific proteins, thus requiring transcription of rRNA, the appropriate mRNAs, and the complete processes concerned with translation as well as the proper cell milieu for self-assembly. The availability of tRNAs, charged with appropriate amino acids, requires tRNA transcription, processing, and correct formation of three-dimensional structure; availability of an amino acid pool; action of a series of specific "amino acid–activating" enzymes that act to place the correct amino acid on each tRNA for subsequent transfer to the new protein. Finally, the peptide transfer reaction itself, which occurs on the ribosome, requires simultaneously specific three-dimensional interactions between the ribosome, each tRNA, the growing peptide chain, and the enzyme or enzymes that catalyze the transfer reaction. Thus, translation may be interrupted through changes in any of the structures or processes involved, and it is not surprising that a variety of antibiotics, such as streptomycin, chloramphenicol, puromycin, and cycloheximide, inhibit translation.

The action of interferon is particularly intriguing. These specific proteins are synthesized by mammalian cells in response to the presence of virus nucleic acids, and they appear to interfere specifically with the process of translation of virus messengers without interfering with host messenger. Since interferon production is host-specific but not virus-specific, it can be stimulated in host cells by the administration of synthetic polynucleotides as well as virus nucleic acids, and it thus represents a potential means of controlling virus infections. The role of hormones and various other biologic regulators in modifying the process of translation is also under intensive investigation.

Post-translational events are also important to the process of formation of biologically active proteins. In addition to resulting from the spontaneous folding into tertiary structure (described further on), covalent modification occurs through addition of nonprotein moieties onto amino acid side chains (including nucleotide, PO_4, carbohydrate, lipids, and various prosthetic groups); hydroxylation; ester formation; oxidation (reduction) of side chains; cross-linking between side chains; and proteolysis with removal of amino acid sequences from the primary structure. All these processes produce specific structural changes that relate to biologic function and must be considered as potential regulation (and disease) loci.

Information storage and processing in nucleic acids are important keys to the understanding and control of human diseases. It is especially significant that most of our current knowledge has been acquired during the brief period ranging from the 1950s to the present.

PROTEINS

Proteins constitute the work molecules for biologic systems. They provide structural integrity and specificity, appropriate solution properties and barrier functions (buffers and the like), and specific effector roles, such as transport, energy transduction, and catalysis and regulation. They are, in the strictest sense, informational molecules in that their unique three-dimensional structures provide the basis for all their discriminating interactions and functions. Proteins are especially well suited for biologic diversity because of the endless number of structures that can be generated from sequences of the 20 amino acids available. The most important insight into protein structure and function is the recognition that the primary covalent sequence of amino acids dictates the most favorable secondary structure (hydrogen bonding between peptide bonds in the chain) and tertiary structure (interactions between amino acid side chains) based on the lowest (and most favorable) free energy state of the protein and its surrounding medium. Because of this important governing thermodynamic principle, the read-out of two-dimensional information encoded in nucleic acids into a two-dimensional protein sequence is transformed into a unique three-dimensional structure. Furthermore, the association of protein into aggregates (quaternary structure) or other more complicated macrostructures, such as virus coats, ribosomes, membranes, and others, can also occur spontaneously according to the same governing principle. Current technology has made it quite feasible to learn the primary sequence of any protein so that the structure-function relationships can be established.

Individual amino acids in a protein chain may be viewed as serving two types of roles. First, they determine the unique reactivity required for the discriminating functions of proteins; second, they provide the structural basis for interacting with the environment and determining three-dimensional protein structure and stability. Therefore, modifying a protein (e.g., by genetic "error") may interfere with its functional and regulatory capacity or change its structural stability or both. Defects in red blood cells provide excellent examples of these different defects. Sickle hemoglobin, because of a single amino acid change (glutamate → valine), shows a tertiary structure lability, so that, although it can still bind O_2, its tertiary structure in the deoxygenated state is so distorted that it forces gross deformity of the red blood cells. A variety of other hemoglobin defects, in contrast, have a decreased capacity to bind O_2. Certain mutants for glucose-6-PO_4 dehydrogenase in the red cells show substantial changes in catalytic properties. This also illustrates an excellent example of the seemingly remote biologic effects that may result from an enzyme deficiency due to perturbation of interrelated steady state systems. The ultimate result of this enzyme deficiency is fragility of red blood cells, apparently because the decreased reduction of NADP by glucose-6-PO_4 restricts availability of reduced glutathione for reduction of methemoglobin. Pyruvate kinase deficiency associated with hemolytic anemias appears to result from a defect in enzyme stability that is expressed as the cell ages. It may well be that some instances of apparent complete enzyme absence may instead represent a highly labile although potentially active enzyme, a point of considerable therapeutic interest.

Certain toxic effects also may be explained on the basis of modifications of protein structure, in terms of either functional capacity or structural integrity. Thus, amino acid–specific reagents, such as heavy metals and thiols that react with -SH groups in proteins or reactive organophosphates that react with "active" serines in enzyme catalytic sites, would be expected to have extensive biologic consequences. Modification of the protein environment can also be important in biologic systems. Cryoglobulins, for example, precipitate as the temperature is lowered because of the change in water structure, which in turn promotes protein aggregation. Another physical effect on proteins results from their natural tendency to unfold at interfaces owing to their content of both hydrophobic and hydrophilic groups. This is an important concept to consider, for example, in the construction of heart-lung machines and prosthetic heart valves or arteries and during the infusion of chemical agents into the blood in order to prevent denaturation of blood elements and resulting toxic effects.

Protein secondary structure results from all the backbone rotations around the peptide bond, stabilized by hydrogen bonding between peptide units. When rotation is free and intrachain hydrogen bonding is neither impeded by extremely bulky side chains nor made impossible by the occurrence of an amino acid in the sequence, a regular helix results. The pitch of this helix is dictated by the nature and size of each side chain. Nonhelical regions may be stabilized in folded configurations (so-called "pleated sheet") that may be interspersed between helical regions in a large polypeptide. The regularity of a helical region results in a high degree of cooperativity in its structure stability. Furthermore, the sequential occurrence of repeated sequences within a polypeptide can extend such cooperative stability and a high order of structure over an immense molecule (e.g., collagen, elastin). Although the classic helix and pleated sheet account for most protein secondary structure, much attention is now directed at certain "nonclassic" configurations of peptides, involving especially repeated sequences of polypeptides to generate unique biologic functions, such as ion channels, ion carriers, elastomeric properties, calcification, and so forth. It is particularly exciting that modeling of biologic functions of proteins can now be done both through theoretic calculations and through chemical synthesis of appropriate polypeptide sequences—now made possible through advanced protein technology.

Protein tertiary structure results from all the interactions of the side chains, which generate the final three-dimensional structure. The role of water structure is a most important consideration, since the so-called "hydrophobic" interactions of the amino acid side chains are the most important quantitatively in protein tertiary structure. Such interactions derive their stability from the fact that removal of hydrophobic groups from solution results in a considerable increase in entropy of the water structure stability; thus, protein denaturation and renaturation depend on both thermodynamic and kinetic considerations. The protein, once formed, may be extremely stable even when the surrounding medium is changed, because the energy of activation for a structural transition is high owing to the combined effects of its many weak interactions or because of the imposition of covalent restraints in the form of the covalent disulfide bonds. Conversely, a protein may become quite labile or refuse to renature if it is transported into an environment different from the site of synthesis or if its structure is modified following synthesis. A good example of the latter mechanism of post-translational modification is insulin. Proteolytic removal of a portion of the backbone of the precursor, proinsulin, prior to secretion removes its ability to renature following denaturation. Such proteolysis, in addition to providing biologically active structures at the time and site of need, also provides a limitation on their stability and turnover. This theme of prohormone → hormone transition is repeated many times for protein hormones. Other pertinent examples are clotting factors, the complement system, digestive enzymes, and various kinins. In contrast, some of the effector and regulatory roles of proteins would require that structure transitions be rather freely reversible in the course of their function.

Quaternary structure is a special, although not separable, aspect of protein tertiary structure that serves to generate higher order structures through aggregation of individual protein molecules. This may result simply in multichain proteins (e.g., hemoglobin, gammaglobulin, a variety of enzymes, collagen) or in aggregates between proteins and other molecules. Not only is such aggregation critical to the formation of functional complexes and supramolecular structures, but also provoked changes in these structures are a powerful mechanism for biologic regulation.

Protein tertiary structures provide specific domains for discriminating interactions with other molecules so that proteins may serve their various effector roles and may interact with specific molecular signals from the environment. Moreover, the transitions that occur in tertiary structure provide basic mechanisms for effector roles and for responses to the binding of molecular signals.

Nonprotein moieties in proteins also deserve special consideration, since they impart important properties and functions for structural and effector proteins. The covalent attachment of carbohydrate (via serine, threonine, and arginine covalent bonds) provides special binding properties, such as immunologic specificity, cell recognition, and, perhaps, aspects of cell communication related to regulation. The process of attachment of carbohydrate to proteins in the Golgi apparatus may also serve an important secretory role. Transport lipoproteins have attracted clinical attention since the recognition of specific diseases, such as Tangier disease, in which abnormal lipid deposits in tissues result from deficient transport (for review, see Chapter 23). Lung surfactant is a lipoprotein that normally maintains the unique properties of the gas exchange surfaces of the lung and may provide major insight into understanding and treating lung disease. Lung surfactant appears to be deficient in hyaline membrane disease of the newborn and is a critical target for study in a variety of pulmonary diffusion difficulties (see Chapter 16). Lipoproteins also serve a variety of other functions, such as the construction of membranes and cell organelles, and the lipid and the protein moieties provide extensive means of varying structure. The discovery of the many effects of prostaglandins

has emphasized how potent lipid-protein interactions may also be in regulating biologic systems. A variety of specific small prosthetic molecules, such as heme, pyridoxal, nucleotides, metals, and even PO_4, also provide regulatory and functional properties for catalytic and carrier proteins and illustrate one of the ways minor dietary substances can influence biologic function.

The description and management of diseases in terms of deficiencies or abnormalities of proteins provide an interesting challenge to medical science, the approach to which will require thorough understanding of protein structure and function.

Specific Functional Classes of Proteins

A complete description of all classes of proteins is not feasible within this chapter. However, a brief classification will be useful to focus our attention on specific discussions of disease mechanisms that will follow in later chapters.

Enzymes. Enzymes must serve three structural roles. First, structure must provide highly specific domains for recognition and binding of substrates and coenzymes. This is a demanding information role for this class of protein molecules that accounts for the specificity and selectivity for all the chemical reactions that make up a biologic system. Since such substrate or catalytic sites may be made up by the precise three-dimensional positioning of a few amino acid side chains from different (even distant) parts of the primary sequence, the entire amino acid structure of the protein participates in their generation. The complete description of a catalytic site is a demanding problem that requires, therefore, complete knowledge of three-dimensional structure and the identification of substrate molecule in situ. Although a variety of techniques are available for tentative identification of participating amino acid residues, only x-ray crystallography at present can solve the complete structure.

Second, enzyme structure must provide the chemical mechanisms for the extraordinary efficiency of enzyme catalysis. The understanding of enzyme mechanisms and their structural bases is a demanding and unsolved problem in molecular biology that could ultimately serve as the basis for generating molecular substitutes for deficient enzymes.

Third, enzyme structure must provide for all the discriminating interactions (communication) between enzymes and their environment and for the appropriate response patterns to these environmental signals. The binding sites for such regulatory molecules, or signals, termed *allosteric sites*, are analogous to the substrate sites in their structure and specificity, and reversible changes in enzyme conformation structure provoked by their binding provide the response mechanisms.

In many instances, the regulatory binding sites may be provided by separate protein subunits that are aggregated with the catalytic subunit to provide a coordinated regulatory and effector complex. Coordination of enzyme function also results from specific aggregates of enzymes that are responsible for sequential or interdependent functions. Isoenzymes (isozymes) are minor structural variants of the same protein that occur in different cell types or at specific stages of differentiation resulting from differential expression of redundant genes that are not identical. The fact that active enzymes (and other proteins) are often assembled from subunits amplifies this variability because the final active molecule can be composed of either or both structural forms of each subunit. For example, lactic dehydrogenase is composed of four identical chains that exist in two structural forms. The tetrameric enzyme exists either in pure form or as the predictable mixtures of the three hybrid aggregates, depending on the relative tissue concentrations of the different chains. The biologic functions of isoenzymes are still a matter for study, but their description is often useful diagnostically because it permits identification of the cell type of origin of, for example, an abnormal enzyme level in blood.

The consequences of a single genetic defect in enzyme structure may be expressed principally in terms of substrate binding, catalytic action, regulation, or stability or through changes in all these properties due to the interdependence of protein structure and function.

Other Proteins with Special Binding Domains. Most protein functions depend on specialized binding properties exemplified by enzymes. The differences that exist between groups of proteins can be described in terms of the fates of the protein and its bound ligand or ligands. With enzymes, the primary substrates are modified chemically, and the protein molecule is reusable. With transport proteins, the ligand is released unchanged either through some environmentally provoked nondestructive change in transport protein conformation or through shifts in concentration gradients so that the transport process can be repeated. Thus, protein (peptides) can serve to translocate other molecules through reversible binding processes. A special binding and transport mechanism for peptides has also been defined through the generation of specific transmembrane ion channels through which specific ions can move. The gating for such movement results simply from reversible shifts in peptide conformation. In the case of proteins responsible for host defense (e.g., antibodies, complement, inflammation peptides, clotting factors, etc.) irreversible changes are provoked by ligand binding providing host protection by removal of the ligand or by generation of a new molecular structure from the binding protein. Protein hormones are a special class of binding proteins that bind specific target molecules in cells

and cell surfaces to signal appropriate metabolic processes. Peptides and polypeptides with hormonal action vary in size from the tripeptide hypothalamic releasing factors to thyroglobulin (MW~ 600,000), which serves as the storage form from which active thyroid hormone is released. Hormone receptors for nonprotein hormones are also highly specific receptor proteins that serve to bind hormones in target cells and promote their interactions with their ultimate targets (see also Chapter 4).

The role of peptides and proteins in pharmacologic action also deserves special mention. It has been recognized for many years that many drug actions depend on specific receptors presumed to be protein in nature. The identity of such receptors and how they serve as effectors are central to the final understanding of drug action. Pharmacologically active peptides are especially intriguing. The extraordinary potencies of certain exogenous peptide toxins have long been recognized and provide mechanisms for a number of important disease processes (e.g., tetanus, botulism and "food poisoning," diphtheria, mushroom poisoning, etc.). Such peptide toxins have also been used as probes for studying mechanisms of drug action. The recognition of endogenous peptides with pharmacologic actions has added a new dimension to studies of drug actions in the central nervous system, suggesting that such phenomena as sleep, pain perception, emotional level, and so forth may be controlled by peptide regulators. These and other specialized peptides that serve as neurotransmitters or neuromodulators have provoked intensive studies. In the strictest sense, these agents may be "hormones," since they may be synthesized in one site and serve to modulate activity of other cells. Even structural proteins have specialized binding domains that lead to stable structural aggregates that provide structure and barrier functions against the environment and may serve specific roles in such processes as calcification.

These brief comments illustrate that the specific three-dimensional binding sites provided by protein structures play a central role in the success of biologic systems. The high specificity of the binding processes meets the demanding informational needs of living systems, and the structural changes in the protein or the bound ligand or both serve the large variety of effector roles required. The protein molecule may act, therefore, as a signal or as a transducer of a molecular signal into some biologic response.

Structural Proteins

Collagens, the most abundant proteins in the body, provide the fibrous network that supports all cellular and supracellular structures. Collagen fibers are built up by aggregation of collagen molecules, each of which is composed of a rigid supercoil of three α-chain molecules tightly wound together. The remarkable ordering, strength, and stability of collagen, as well as its biologic variations, can be related to its unique structural features. The different types of collagen are provided by five types of α-chains that differ either in primary gene sequence or from post-translational modification. All α-chains are homologous in the sense that they are composed of repeating tripeptides with the formula -x-y-Gly-, in which 42 per cent of x and y residues are proline + hydroxyproline, and 22 per cent are alanine. The repeating tripeptide structure assures the long range regularity required for fiber assembly and stability.

The biosynthesis of collagen and the assembly of fibers for unique functions require at least eight sequential processes of post-translational modification. The mRNA for each type of α-chain codes for a procollagen molecule that has additional unique sequences at both the initial and terminal ends of the chain. After translation, there is hydroxylation of prolyl and lysyl residues followed by addition of sugar moieties to specific hydroxylysyl groups. Chain association and disulfide bonding then occur, followed by the highly ordered process of triple helix formation and secretion from the cell. The secreted procollagen molecules are then converted into collagen by proteolytic cleavage followed by aggregation into fibers. Fibers are then stabilized to provide the tensile strength by enzymic formation of intra- and interfiber crosslinks through oxidation and condensation of lysine side chains.

This highly ordered sequence of events offers several opportunities for genetic defects and for pharmacologic and toxic intervention. Defects in the genes for α-chain formation lead to specific excesses or deficiencies of collagen types (Ehlers-Danlos type IV; osteogenesis imperfecta). Changes in post-translational mechanisms result in hydroxylysine deficiency (Ehlers-Danlos type VI); deficiencies in proteolysis of procollagen to collagen (Ehlers-Danlos type VII); or deficient cross-linking due to lysyl oxidase deficiency (Ehlers-Danlos type V) or unknown or secondary mechanism (Marfan's syndrome, homocystinuria, Menkes' kinky hair syndrome). The roles of post-translational changes in collagen structure in aging and degeneration are also of great interest. Structural stability provided by collagen molecules can now be discussed in terms of molecular properties. The additional roles of collagen in such processes as calcification, ion sequestering, and transport are also problems of current interest.

Elastin is a fibrous extracellular protein of remarkable properties that imparts the normal elastic and resilient character exhibited by tissues. The precursor of all fibrous elastin, tropoelastin, has a molecular weight of 72,000, and four amino acids, alanine, glycine, proline, and valine, account for 80 per cent of all its 850 amino acids. There are some 38 lysine residues from which specific cross-links are formed to yield stable elastomeric fibers. The complete structure has not been determined, but the partial sequence is characterized by repeating runs of sequential polypeptides, which may account for long-range order in the fiber and the resulting elastomeric properties. The assignment of specific defects in elastin and its post-translational processing and stability to specific disease mechanisms must await more detailed structural knowledge. The importance of maintaining tissue elastic properties is self-evident. In addition, the fact that elastin can serve as a matrix for calcification is highly relevant to formation of atherosclerotic plaques as well as normal calcified tissues.

Keratin is a mixture of structure proteins that provide the "barrier" functions of cornified skin, hair, and nails. The "low-sulfur" component is wound into superhelices to form fibrils that are imbedded in an amorphous matrix. These proteins must then collectively account for the extraordinary properties of the integumental system. Not only do they provide a potent barrier by virtue of their own structure, but they also provide a matrix for deployment of the complex lipids and other skin components that may serve an effector or protective role.

Membrane proteins are of great interest in terms of membrane stability as well as dynamic functions. Basement membranes are collagenous in nature. Cell membranes contain both integral (structural) and peripheral (adherent) proteins that account for specific properties. Integral proteins are characterized by one or more of two unique structural properties. First, they are amphipathic, that is, they are composed of both hydrophobic and hydrophilic domains to facilitate interaction with both the lipid membrane and the aqueous environment. Second, they often have essential nonprotein substituents. For example, glycophorin of red cell membranes is composed of 60 per cent carbohydrate residues. The proteolipid of myelin is extremely rich in fatty acids, probably bound by ester linkages. These nonprotein moieties serve unique functional roles and are responsible for immunologic specificity and cell recognition. A cancer cell presumably is different, either qualitatively or quantitatively, since it displays altered antigenicity as well as loss of contact or density inhibition. Integral membrane proteins apparently have lateral mobility, but they are oriented across the membrane in a highly organized manner. "Peripheral," or adherent, membrane proteins have highly specific interaction sites for membrane attachment and also account for specific properties. Some of these proteins attach reversibly to account for regulation (e.g., peptide hormones). Both integral and peripheral proteins may also serve such effector roles as catalysis and transport.

Although *nuclear proteins* usually are thought of specifically in terms of their information role, they may also be classified as structural proteins. Quantitatively, basic proteins (histones) are the major class and provide the core around which the polyanionic DNA is wound into a stable and organized package. Part of the nuclear "package" is also composed of acidic proteins, which also may serve more specific regulatory and catalytic roles in genetic expression. The nuclear proteins are also important determinants for interactions of drugs and hormones owing to the imposed constraints on DNA structure and availability and to the provision of specific protein receptors.

COMPLEX CARBOHYDRATES

Complex carbohydrates serve important structural and functional roles. The intercellular matrix and surface properties of all tissues are maintained by the acid mucopolysaccharides. This is a group of related heteropolysaccharides containing acidic monosaccharides, usually glucuronic acid, alternating with an acetylated amino sugar. In addition, either or both substituents may be sulfated. These occur as free polysaccharides or in combination with specific proteins to form mucins or mucoproteins. The synthesis of these large molecules from regular repeating units depends on repetitive enzyme processes: sequential coupling of the appropriate precursors, addition of sulfates to sulfated mucopolysaccharides, attachment to protein moieties in the case of mucins, and formation of noncovalent aggregates. There is considerable microheterogeneity in size, ratios of repeating units, extent of modification (sulfation), and loci and extent of protein attachment, since synthesis and secretion depend on these several independently functioning enzyme steps rather than on a template or messenger process. Degradation and turnover for mucopolysaccharides apparently constitute the important control for limiting the amounts of mucopolysaccharides in tissues. This is a critical issue because of the extraordinary stability of these repetitive polymers. In contrast to proteins, which denature readily in the environment and can be degraded by any of a number of peptidases with wide specificity, mucopolysaccharides are stable in solution and require an arsenal of some 40 highly specific hydrolytic enzymes (contained mostly in lysomes) for their stepwise degradation. Thus, deficiencies of these lysosomal hydrolases result in tissue accumulations of their substrates, often referred to as "storage" diseases (see Chapter 3).

LIPIDS

In addition to serving as the storage and transport forms for metabolic fuel, lipids provide structural components for membranes and cell surfaces and are concerned with cell recognition devices at cell surfaces. The molecular details of the latter two classes of functions and the chemical structures required are complex issues of great current interest. A complex lipid consists of long-chain fatty acids esterified (or in ether linkage) to a backbone of glycerol, glycerol phosphate, or sphingosine. Both glycerol phosphate and sphingosine, in turn, may be attached to various additional head groups with large differences in polarity and size. These include simple and modified carbohydrate residues, ethanolamine, choline, and amino acids. Thus, the fatty acids provide a variable nonpolar structure, and the head groups provide extensive ranges of specificity for polar interactions and three-dimensional recognition sites. These structures are ideally suited for construction of membranes, therefore, and for dictating specific interactions at cell surfaces.

The simple lipids, which include sterols, carotenes, and prostaglandins as important members, are also important biologically and are characterized by their abilities to interact with a nonpolar environment. Owing to the unique specificities of their interactions and their high affinities for membranous structures, they can be extremely potent biologically, as evidenced by effects of prostaglandins and steroid hormones. For some actions (e.g., steroid hormones), biologic action involves not only cell membrane penetration but also attachment to specific cytoplasmic receptors, with transport into the nucleus. This combination of an external ligand (signal) with an internal receptor to form a complex intracellular effector molecule is an interesting principle in regulatory biology. It permits a relatively simple signal to interact with an extensive and specific target within the cell.

ASSEMBLY OF COMPLEX BIOLOGIC STRUCTURES

The state of knowledge about macromolecules combined with the current sophistication of electron microscopy provides promising background information on such complex structures as cell membranes, cell organelles, and parasites. The principle of "self-assembly" demonstrated for tertiary and quaternary structure of proteins, based on the structures of the component molecules, also operates for more complex systems, as shown by the in-vitro reassembly of previously disrupted virus capsules, ribosomes, bacterial flagellae, and membrane components of animal cells.

MEMBRANES

The discriminating barrier, transport, communication, and regulatory functions of biologic membranes are essential to living cells, and the structural basis for these functions is under intensive investigation. Membranes do not appear to be simple barriers but complex aggregates of macromolecules that show structural variability, depending on functional requirements. Thus, a myelin sheath, although similar to the plasma membrane of a liver cell, will also display distinct chemical differences. The concept that a membrane in any site is a dynamic complex of individually synthesized macromolecules is important to the question of assembly, stability, turnover, and function, and the structures of the individual component molecules are of critical interest. The lipid bilayer has served as a useful experimental model for the structural features of a membrane, particularly because molecules may be intruded into its structure and serve there as the "catalytic," or "carrier," units. For example, one can demonstrate simple models for ion transport by both carrier and channel mechanisms using peptide antibiotics that bind specific ions. A wide variety of genetic defects in amino acid, sugar phosphate, and ion transport result from specific defects in membrane function. Similarly, membranes are clearly important end organs for the action of specific drugs and hormones as well as for acute toxic diseases and more chronic processes such as demyelination or chronic renal disease. Unfortunately, our knowledge of membrane structure still does not allow mechanistic discussions, but this will be an area of active discovery in the next few years. Genetic diseases may again serve as important study systems for identifying the biochemical basis for function in much the same way as in intermediary metabolism.

CELL ORGANELLES

A detailed discussion of organelles is beyond the scope of this chapter, but a few cogent points should be made about ribosomes, mitochondria, and lysosomes as examples of the potential of the molecular approach.

Ribosomes, complex aggregates of RNA and specific proteins, are the site of protein synthesis as outlined previously and therefore are rate-limiting for many biologic processes. They display self-assembly from experimentally disrupted molecular components and are the site of action of several antibiotics and other drugs. Abnormal, or "mutant," ribosomes occur in microorganisms but probably preclude survival in higher forms, although the possibility that they may provide disease mechanisms cannot be excluded. In animal cells, the endoplasmic reticulum to which the ribosomes are attached is also a major concentration of a variety of enzymes that serve such varied functions as drug metabolism and detoxification.

Mitochondria are complex organelles with extensive responsibility for metabolic and energy support of the cell. They consist of membranous structures into which a variety of catalytic and structural macromolecules are incorporated. In addition, mitochondria contain DNA and can account for the phenomenon of cytoplasmic inheritance, since they carry the information for synthesizing some of their own components. Mitochondria apparently are self-replicating structures, but there is a complex interplay between them and the nucleus, since some of their components are also dictated by nuclear DNA and are synthesized in the cytoplasm. Their structure and self-assembly are further complicated by the fact that their stability varies considerably from tissue to tissue (half-life of 3 days in liver and 30 days in brain); moreover, their various components show different turnover rates. At least one disease appears to represent a defect in mitochondrial morphogenesis (central core myopathy), and experimentally the resistance of malaria to certain chemotherapeutic agents seems to bear an inverse relationship to frequency of mitochondrial bodies in the parasites.

Lysosomes are of special interest as examples of the important role of compartmentalization of biologic function. These organelles contain a rather extensive variety of degradative enzymes and represent potential "suicide packages." On release, these enzymes are involved in digestion of phagocytosed or pinocytosed material, self-resorption in the event of cell death, and maintenance of the normal steady-state concentrations of a variety of tissue components. "Storage diseases" result from deficiencies of lysosomal function, and tissue disruption can occur from excessive lysosomal activation, as might occur as a consequence of chemical toxicity.

MOLECULAR BASIS FOR BIOLOGIC REGULATION

One of the most remarkable features of a living system is the precision with which its numerous chemical processes are integrated and regulated appropriately in response to signals from the environment. To this end, both simple and direct mechanisms exist as well as rather extensive and complex systems such as the endocrine glands. An understanding of the structure and function of macromolecules and cell organelles is the basis for the following discussion of these control phenomena in terms of molecular interactions. The result of perturbing a particular biochemical process depends on the nature of the process, what its role is in each system involved, whether it plays the rate-limiting role, and whether there are other compensating or amplifying mechanisms involved. It is also clearly important to determine whether the perturbation is temporary or chronic. Several general principles may be articulated. First, the regulatory loops that govern biologic processes are driven by molecular signals. This implies, of course, that they must have a specific signal molecule whose steady state concentration and flux vary according to biologic conditions. Second, signal molecules are "received" by binding to macromolecular receptor molecules whose complex structures provide a highly specific discrimination of these changes in concentration. Third, there must be a highly efficient transduction and amplification process to translate the signal into biologic action. This principle supports the prediction that the final target for signal action will be at the nucleic acid, protein, or membrane level to change effector action. Fourth, signal selectivity and cell distribution and specificity are often determined by binding of the initial signal molecule to a highly discriminating macromolecular receptor that then becomes the effective signal (e.g., hormone-receptor complexes). Fifth, through the intervention of specific intermediate targets, multiple types of signals may operate through the generation of a final common messenger of signal action. Sixth, amplification of signal may result from transduction of this whole complex system into fluctuations in the concentrations of some simple ion or molecule that then affects many other targets.

REGULATION OF NUCLEIC ACID–DIRECTED PROCESS

Control of nucleic acid structure and function provides the overall control of biologic function. Regulatory interaction with these macromolecules, which have already been outlined, can result from a variety of chemical agents. In addition to the direct binding of small molecules (e.g., hormones, drugs) to nucleic acids, specificity is amplified by the occurrence of specific receptor proteins that bind regulatory molecules and then interact with specific sites in DNA as receptor-ligand complexes to initiate, stimulate, or inhibit nucleic acid processes. Thus, the specificity and effectiveness of nucleic acid regulation depend in large part on the discriminating binding of proteins. The discoveries that many genes have large "noncoding" internal sequences and that they are organized with long intergene sequences that are also "noncoding" suggest that many potential sites are available for such regulatory interactions.

REGULATION OF MEMBRANE FUNCTION

The compartmentalization of cellular function dictates membrane functions as important regulatory loci. The descriptions of the molecular details of membrane transport and barrier functions are unfolding rapidly and will provide the basis for understanding such regulations. Specific ionophores that can direct transport of specific ions as well as the gating mechanisms for ion channels have already been recognized and have great potential for regulatory intervention. Furthermore, identification of specific membrane binding sites provides a molecular basis for regulation and cell communication that can be exploited for both basic biologic understanding and, potentially, therapeutic manipulation.

REGULATION OF PROTEIN FUNCTION

The effector roles of proteins plus the precise discrimination provided by protein binding sites make this class of macromolecules ideal for monitoring small molecular "signals" from the environment. The strength of such molecular signals (extent of binding) depends simply on their concentration in the milieu. The simplest type of regulation is through competition at the functional site (e.g., at the catalytic site of an enzyme or transport site of a membrane) by fraudulent "substrates." Methotrexate, an analogue of folic acid and a powerful inhibitor of dihydrofolate reductase, a rate-limiting enzyme for thymine (and therefore DNA) synthesis, is an example of such a competitive inhibitor that binds even tighter than the normal substrate. The search for useful competitive inhibitors is a straightforward process based simply on knowledge of substrate structure. For example, allopurinol was developed as a xanthine oxidase competitive inhibitor so that uric acid production could be reduced in gout. By blocking terminal formation of the highly insoluble uric acid, the much more soluble and excretable hypoxanthine becomes the terminal product. Fraudulent substrates also may be metabolized. For example, ingested glycols are oxidized to highly insoluble oxalic acid by alcohol dehydrogenase with castastrophic results because the normal substrate is not available to saturate the enzyme. Similarly, drugs may compete at receptor sites for a natural "regulator" and either produce blockade of normal function or may themselves provoke a response. Table 2–5 lists several examples of well-known competitive inhibitors that have relevance to clinical medicine.

Many proteins also have specific sites, other than the effector or functional sites, that serve as sensors for monitoring the environment through binding a variety of specific regulatory substances. The consequence of such binding is a change in tertiary structure, with resulting change in functional properties. A regulator can thus serve to stimulate or inhibit a reaction, and it need not bear any structural similarity to the substrate for the protein. This provides the molecular mechanism for appropriate regulation of a system by end product (feedback inhibition), cross-linked control between collateral systems, and hormonal and drug control. It also represents another type of macromolecular defect that could lead to disease, namely, defective regulator binding sites with resulting inadequate or inappropriate control. This regulation by binding at nonsubstrate sites has been discussed extensively as "allosteric" regulation. The additional fact that the enzymes thus regulated are usually composed of subunits also

TABLE 2–5 EXAMPLES OF COMPETITIVE INHIBITORS

Drug	Enzyme or Receptor	Reaction or Natural Substrate Inhibited	Examples of Clinical Use
Neostigmine	Acetylcholinesterase	Acetylcholine	Myasthenia gravis; glaucoma
Atropine	Parasympathetic nerve endings (cholinergic endings)	Acetylcholine	Parasympathetic blockade
Guanethidine	Adrenergic endings	Catecholamines	Hypertension
Methyldopa	Dopa decarboxylase	Dopa, $5 - OH$ tryptophan	Hypertension
Ganglionic blocking drugs	Ganglionic receptor	Acetylcholine	Hypertension
Neuromuscular blocking agents (curare, succinyl-choline, etc.)	Neuromuscular junction	Acetylcholine	Anesthesia (muscle relaxation), spastic disorder
Antihistamine	"Histamine receptors"	Histamine	Allergy
Isocarboxazid (Marplan) Nialamide (Niamid) Phenelzine sulfate (Nardil) Tranylcypromine (Parnate)	Monoamine oxidase	Epinephrine, norepinephrine, dopa	Depressive disorders
Tetraethylthiuram disulfide (Antabuse)	Aldehyde dehydrogenase	NAD, acetaldehyde	Alcoholism
Ethanol	Alcohol dehydrogenase	Methanol→formaldehyde and glycol→oxalic acid by alcohol dehydrogenase	Methanol and glycol poisoning
Clomiphene	Estrogen receptor site	Estradiol	Infertility
Allopurinol	Xanthine oxidase	Xanthine, hypoxanthine	Gout

tends to promote cooperative binding of the regulator and substrate molecules, with the result that the system may be very sensitive to small concentration changes over a critical range. This type of regulation, then, results from the detection of small environmental changes through the discrimination of binding by proteins and consequent changes in the three-dimensional structure on which their functional properties depend.

Therapeutically, allosteric regulation offers extensive potential for exploitation. For example, fraudulent feedback inhibitors can be employed to turn off metabolic pathways (as with certain nucleic acid precursors in cancer therapy), or abortive inhibitors can be used that bind but do not inhibit and therefore release a system from normal inhibition.

The simplest type of protein regulation involves detection by the enzyme or other effector molecule of changes in concentration of a small molecular signal. There are also secondary or remote mechanisms involved in regulation. For example, some proteins are modified covalently by specific enzymes to produce more stable changes in structure and function, with the primary regulatory signal operating on the modifying enzyme. Such covalent modifications include limited proteolysis, phosphorylation, glycosylation, thio- and carboxyester formation, and amide formation. The concept of a so-called "secondary messenger" in regulatory processes has also become quite important, although the choice of terms leads to some confusion with the "messenger" role of RNA. This concept, so beautifully established with cyclic AMP, interposes an additional, strictly regulatory enzyme between the environmental signal and the target enzyme or enzymes, with the resulting regulatory enzyme product serving as the final enzyme stimulator or inhibitor. Thus, adenyl cyclase is stimulated or inhibited by a variety of drugs or metabolic products in its catalysis of cyclic AMP production. The levels of the cyclic AMP, in turn, are responsible for the regulation of an extensive array of biologic processes, with consequent amplification and orchestration of the environmental stimulus into function. It is particularly interesting that this mechanism has already been used to rationalize the defect in regulation of the kidney tubule in pseudohypoparathyroidism. A thorough understanding of such secondary regulation mechanisms is of great importance both for understanding diseases and for therapy. It is interesting that calcium has also been proposed as a "second messenger" because its effects are so dramatic and widespread following signal-provoked changes in concentration.

Protein structure may also be modified in less specific ways by changes in the solvent environment. For example, the sickling of red blood cells due to hemoglobin S can be antagonized by urea, which is thought to modify protein structure by increasing solubility of hydrophobic groups through changes in water structure.

Although function is the major consideration

in the aforementioned types of regulation, the influence of such changes on the structural stability of proteins is also very important.

REGULATION OF THE CONCENTRATION OF PROTEINS

The steady-state concentration of a protein or other macromolecule is the sum of all the processes involved in formation and breakdown. Regulation, then, depends on which step is rate-limiting.

Enzyme induction, or environmentally stimulated increase in enzyme level, and enzyme repression, a converse decrease in level, were first elucidated in bacteria and are outstanding examples of mechanistic biology. The models for these processes, as illustrated in Figure 2–3, show transcription to be the rate-limiting process and assume protein stability to be relatively unimportant in these short-lived organisms. Classically, enzymes are induced by substrate and repressed by

end products, so that function is linked to metabolic need. In higher organisms, control signals such as hormones must also be included, and most importantly, all aspects of synthesis and breakdown must be considered. Thus, in addition to transcriptional control, translation, and assembly of final tertiary and quaternary structure (including any covalent modifications or additions of nonprotein moieties), protein stability and consequent turnover are important. Each potential control point provides a locus for malfunction, and each offers a possible site for therapeutic manipulation. It is also clear that regulation may be imposed through secondary effects much in the same way as allosteric regulation (secondary messenger, etc.).

There has been considerable speculation about whether inherited deficiency diseases might become treatable based on gene transfer by plasmids. In fact, much less drastic methods may be applicable if the defect is not a complete deletion of the gene but one of depressed level, since correction

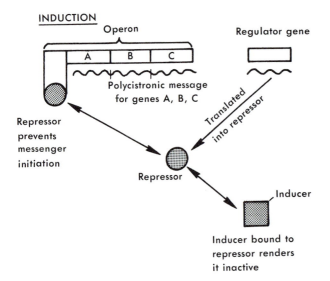

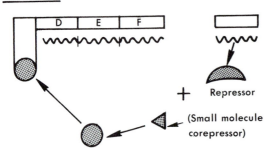

Figure 2–3 Model scheme for induction and repression of protein synthesis operating at the level of RNA transcription.

might be achieved through alterations in the regulation machinery or structure of the macromolecule.

Several diseases are already explicable on the basis of faulty control of protein levels. For example, delta-aminolevulinic acid synthetase is excessive in porphyria, and chemical induction by drugs such as barbiturates results in disease exacerbation. Thalassemia appears to result in depressed (and unbalanced) levels of one of the two types of hemoglobin chains that normally must be available in equal amounts for normal assembly of the protein. Polycythemia results from overactivity of erythropoiesis.

The ability of drugs to perturb steady-state levels of enzymes by interacting at any of the control points is important therapeutically in explaining drug toxicity and for developing insight into such regulatory effects. The ability of barbiturates to induce glucuronyl transferase and mixed-function oxidases has found application in treatment of both congenital jaundice in Crigler-Najjar syndrome and physiologic jaundice of the newborn. It is also well known that tolerance to drugs may be induced through the mechanism of increasing levels of metabolizing enzymes and that "cross tolerance" may be observed (e.g., the tolerance to alcohol evoked by barbiturates and vice versa).

Therapeutic approaches based on regulation of macromolecular levels are limited chiefly by our lack of information about specific disease defects and about mechanisms for producing the appropriate perturbations. Our knowledge about both these points is increasing rapidly, however, and it is clear that this type of thinking will dominate therapeutics. Cancer chemotherapy illustrates how regulatory principles can be applied when the chemical objective is clear and many of the mechanisms are known. Because the problem is one of uncontrolled cell growth, therapy is aimed at preventing cell proliferation and viability, both of which are ultimately dependent on DNA-directed processes. A summary of current chemotherapy reveals that DNA synthesis is inhibited by limitation of precursors, by fraudulent feedback inhibition, by competitive inhibition, and by interference with the DNA template through simple or covalent drug binding and the destructive effects of radiation. The ultimate aim of chemotherapy, to spare normal cells, of course, can be realized only through sufficient knowledge of regulation in both populations of cells.

GENETIC ENGINEERING IN MEDICAL SCIENCES

"Genetic engineering" in medical sciences has three practical goals: (1) the elucidation of fundamental biologic and disease mechanisms, (2) the specific intervention into disease mechanisms, and (3) the efficient creation of very pure biologic products that are important to humans. Other goals, such as manipulation of the environment (e.g., toxic waste product disposal) and increased agricultural development, also have profound health implications. Genetic engineering, simply stated, consists of producing specific biologic products or functions through the insertion, transfer, or amplification of natural or synthetic genetic elements or through the molecular control of the expression of specific genetic elements that are present within the cell. There has been very visible progress in the former, but the specific regulation of existing genes and gene products has been more elusive.

There have been two remarkably successful approaches to gene insertion that have moved "genetic engineering" away from sheer speculation and into the practical arena. Both approaches selectively exploit the information system to generate specific biologic functions through transfer of genetic information into a new setting. The first approach, that of *cell fusion,* simply merges a cell that is producing a specific protein of interest with another (malignant) cell that has been released from stringent control by virtue of the malignant state. The hybrid cell still grows without restraint but produces proteins dictated by its new information source. The new hybrid cells, hybridomas, are selected by their production of new proteins and are propagated in culture and as a tumor in animals as pure clones. Since selected protein is produced in large amounts, it can usually be purified rather successfully from the other proteins that are produced. The key to the success of this approach is the selection of new clones that are large overproducers of the desired protein. The technology emphasized here is cell biology with manipulation, selection, and propagation of cell clones in vitro; selected expansion and growth in animal hosts; and, finally, purification of the gene product. The key to success has been the use of malignant cells to provide recipient cells that are not restrained by the regulatory processes that govern normal cells. This new technology has been especially successful in producing and studying antibody-producing cells and has thus been highly useful in studying the bases for antibody diversification and for producing single, isolated antibody species for use in a wide spectrum of biologic problems. This method is of great practical importance for the design of diagnostic tests for medical practice. Even more impressive is the versatility provided to generate powerful reagents for use in medical research for detection and separation of unique molecules. Figure 2–4 outlines the steps in the generation of a monoclonal antibody.

The second major approach to "genetic engineering," that of *gene insertion,* involves splicing the desired sequences into the genome of simple bacteriophages and plasmids and amplifying and purifying them in the respective bacterial host

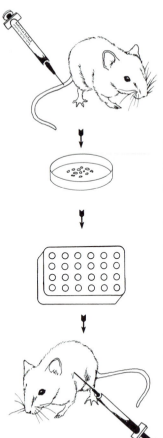

STEPS

Immunization of mouse

Spleen cells removed and fused *in vitro* with mouse myeloma cells

Cells plated in soft agar and screened with antigen for selection of antibody–producing clones

Selected clones expanded and grown in mouse hosts as an ascitic tumor

Ascites fluid collected for isolation of antibody.

Figure 2–4 Generation of monoclonal antibodies.

cells. The desired gene products can then be produced in quantity in these simple "foreign" cells in absolute purity from any other protein produced by cells representing the original source of the gene. Furthermore, production in the new host cell is released from the kinetic restraints of the original host cell because the structural genes can be transferred without the regulatory genes. The completion of the gene transfer cycle would then be the successful transfer of a purified gene back into cells of the original host line that are deficient in the specific gene product. Even this has been accomplished in model systems and will, no doubt, soon be accomplished in humans. This new gene-cloning technology is a direct consequence of the systematic exploitation of the knowledge generated by the molecular approach to biology and results directly from several breakthroughs. Table 2–6 shows significant events in the development of this technology. The sequence of this list does not necessarily correspond to the chronology of discovery.

The general strategies for cloning a gene fragment are shown in Figure 2–5. As illustrated, the fragment may be prepared from a larger DNA sequence by cleavage with a restriction endonu-

clease that recognizes a specific sequence and generates a fragment with *single-stranded regions* at the left and right ends. Since these ends are complementary to other such fragments, they are described as "sticky." Nicking of the plasmid vector with the same endonuclease, therefore, leads to complementary binding of the alien gene fragment to the cut ends. It is then attached with a DNA ligase enzyme to restore covalent continuity of the plasmid. Successful insertion, therefore, requires an appropriate restriction nuclease site in both the plasmid and the gene to be cloned. Alternatively, a restriction enzyme may be used that does not generate single-stranded regions, or the single-stranded regions can be trimmed from the ends of the nicked plasmid or filled in with a polymerase. A blunt-ended fragment of any terminal sequence can then be ligated to the ends. Blunt-end ligation may also be used to attach appropriate restriction sites at the ends of DNA fragments to permit insertion *and retrieval-specific plasmid sites*. The hybrid plasmids are then cloned and amplified by growth in host bacteria. Successful cloning, of course, requires a sensitive method of selecting those clones that are producing the desired gene product. The gene sequence to be

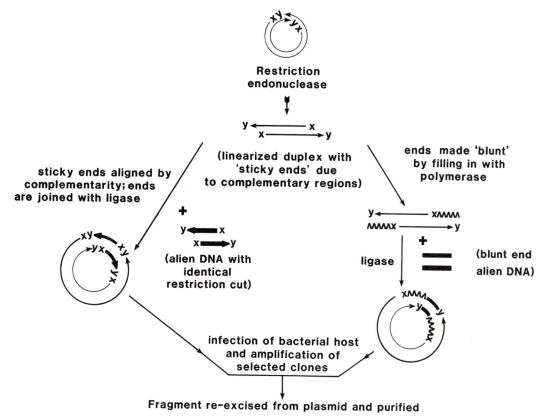

Figure 2–5 Cloning gene fragments in bacterial plasmid.

cloned may be derived directly from the DNA genome, although purification and isolation may be formidable problems. Alternatively, purified messenger RNA can be copied with the reverse transcriptase to yield the complementary DNA sequence, which is then copied with a DNA polymerase to give double-stranded DNA for insertion into the plasmid. The gene cloned will differ, of course, from the parent gene because the processed messenger RNA will not contain the complements for synthesizing any of the intervening sequences that were present in the parent copy DNA. This is a great convenience, however, since the new bacterial host cells are not able to provide all the required processing mechanisms anyway. Another method of generating a cloning fragment is chemical synthesis of the appropriate sequence based on knowledge of the amino acid sequence of the gene product.

It is not surprising that genetic engineering has created such widespread excitement. Already, the approach to production of specific vaccines has been revolutionized, since absolutely pure antigens can be prepared in quantity. Not only can the major antigen components involved in the antibody response be given in isolation but also minor components that may have even greater

potential for generating effective host response can be amplified and studied. The ability to produce human peptide hormones for replacement therapy is also a major advance in therapy. Similarly, the generation of other specialized products (e.g., blood clotting factors, transport proteins, and host defense proteins) offers high potential for therapeutic application. Not only can cloning technology provide extremely pure gene products but also the gene sequences themselves provide tools for both research and diagnosis. For example, prenatal diagnosis of genetic defects with synthetic DNA or DNA probes for identification of genes in situ is a most exciting possibility. The ultimate goal of correcting an inherited defect by insertion of the missing or defective gene seems, indeed, to be a realistic goal!

COMMENTS ON THE MOLECULAR BASIS FOR DISEASE

In order to understand the consequence of molecular derangements in terms of disease, it is clearly essential to define the role or roles of the molecule involved. For example, an enzyme deficit (or toxic damage) could result in a deficiency state

TABLE 2–6 HIGHLIGHTS IN DEVELOPMENT OF GENE CLONING TECHNOLOGY

1. Establishment of a working model for DNA structure and the concept of templating by nucleic acids.
2. Identification of DNA-directed DNA synthesis (DNA → DNA) (replication).
3. Identification of DNA-directed RNA synthesis and establishment of the messenger concept (transcription).
4. Description of RNA-directed protein synthesis (translation).
5. Synthesis of nucleic acids of known sequence (synthetic genes).
6. Elucidation of the nature and specific details of the genetic code (gene structure can be deduced from protein structure).
7. Demonstration that a viral genome can be integrated into and replicated with the host genome.
8. Successful fusion of eukaryotic cells with expression of genes from both parent cells.
9. Identification of RNA-directed DNA-sequence (reverse-transcriptase) DNA gene can be made from its RNA transcript.
10. Identification of site-specific DNA-"cutting" enzymes (restriction endonucleases).
11. Identification of DNA-splicing enzymes.
12. Demonstration that DNA from different sources could be spliced successfully.
13. Generation of successful cloning vectors biochemically through insertion of alien DNA.
14. Successful replication of inserted genes in a simple bacterial host.
15. Refinement of selection techniques.

in the case of a synthetic enzyme, an excess of some cell component if it is a degradative enzyme, seemingly remote or widespread effects if it is a regulatory enzyme, or no expression of disease if compensating regulatory mechanisms are called into play or if there is no current demand for the particular biologic role performed. Thus, a pseudocholine esterase deficiency is not expressed unless the individual is given the appropriate toxic drug; Hurler's and Hunter's syndromes result from defects in normal mucopolysaccharide degradation and turnover, and patients with McArdle's syndrome cannot synthesize glycogen normally. Certain other defects prevent normal cross-linking of metabolic pathways; for example, in galactosemia, galactose cannot be converted to glucose. The disturbance, however, results from accumulation of the substrate rather than from a metabolic deficiency. Diseases also result from excesses, as pointed out in the example of acute intermittent porphyria. In all instances, there may also be far-reaching consequences of a defect resulting from the secondary regulatory roles served by enzyme products. An excellent example of this is the adrenogenital syndrome, in which the molecular defect is hydroxylation of the 11-position of the steroid nucleus to form active adrenal corticoids. Individuals with this disease not only show severe adrenal insufficiency but also are severely masculinized because the normal hydroxysteroid product is not present to regulate (inhibit) early steps in steroid biogenesis, and overproduction of androgens results.

It is also interesting to consider the kinetics of disease development and recovery in terms of perturbation of steady-state concentrations of molecules. Whereas some alterations are manifested immediately owing to rapid achievement of new steady states, others develop slowly, even over the course of many years, either through cumulative defects (e.g., arteriscleroses) or through slow achievement of a new steady state owing to low rates of synthesis and turnover.

Medical Genetics

Louis J. Elsas II
and Jean H. Priest

INTRODUCTION

The field of medical genetics has increased understanding of the pathologic physiology of inherited human disease and our ability to predict and prevent these disease processes. Cellular engineering, mass screening, environmental engineering, genetic counseling, and prenatal diagnosis are some clinical realities that have developed through the application of this body of information. The relatively new field of molecular genetics has introduced recombinant DNA, DNA fragment analysis, and genetic engineering, which provide still higher levels of resolution and application.

The mechanisms and recurrence risks for pathologic processes caused by the interaction of multiple genes and the environment provide accurate figures and alternatives to families seeking counseling for such common anomalies and diseases as cleft palate, pyloric stenosis, spina bifida, hypertension, early onset heart disease, and duodenal ulcer. Other diseases caused by a single mutant gene of large effect conform to mendelian patterns of inheritance. Pedigree analysis provides information about recurrence risks and genetic mechanisms for subsequent offspring and may lead to an understanding of the molecular mechanisms that produce the disease. Testing lipid phenotypes in pedigrees from a large population of early onset heart disease led to the identification of three genes that were found to account for 54 per cent of all myocardial infarctions occurring before 60 years of age.

The chromosome is now recognized as the nuclear structure responsible for the physical transmission of genetic information. Abnormalities in chromosome structure or number are associated with numerous clinical syndromes. Techniques in which extended banding and various staining procedures are used now make possible the identification of individual chromosomes and their subparts. Translocations, deletions, and inversions can now be confirmed and related to abnormal phenotypes. With combinations of pedigree analysis, biochemical analysis, cell fusion, chromosome analysis, and in-situ hybridization with cDNA over 500 human genes have been localized to specific chromosomes.

Progress has been made in characterizing catalytic and structural proteins and relating their function and variation to genetic control. Garrod's assumption that an abnormal gene product resulted in impaired cellular metabolism and produced an "inborn error of metabolism" has been verified and extended in many disorders.

The molecular concepts derived from microbial systems by Watson and Crick for the biochemical transmission of genetic information through deoxyribonucleic acid (DNA), by Jacob and Monod for the regulation of gene expression, and by Nirenberg for the translation of triplet codons in nucleic acids to specific amino acids in a peptide chain have found application in human disease. Single amino acid changes occur in sickle hemoglobin and can be explained by a single base pair substitution (point mutation) in the DNA triplet codon. These and other observations in genetic regulation and variation of hemoglobin chain synthesis and structure provide direct evidence that the genetic concepts derived from microbial systems apply to humans. The genetic axiom "one gene—one enzyme" now extends to "one gene—one polypeptide." With the new resolution provided by molecular biology, it is now recognized that nuclear processing of the mRNA plays a major role in gene expression in humans. Thus, many mutations of the intervening, nonstructural components of the beta globin gene result in absent or reduced beta globin production (thalassemia). In one disorder of the urea cycle, citrullinemia, abnormal processing of the gene for argininosuccinic acid synthetase results in absent or CRM-negative enzyme production.

The "inborn errors of metabolism" include defects of structural proteins, subunits of functioning proteins, transport proteins, proteins involved with coenzyme function, and proteins involved in the repair of DNA itself. In fact, impaired expression of genes caused by abnormalities at transcription, mRNA processing, translation, and post-translational control now are exemplified in humans by significant pathology. Therapeutic maneuvers being studied or used to treat this group of disorders include replacement of target enzymes, deficient enzyme products, or coenzymes; addition of inducers or feedback inhibitors; restriction of toxic precursors or by-products; and replacement of the deficient genes themselves.

The disciplines of population genetics, biochemical genetics, molecular genetics, and cytogenetics unite in studying, defining, counseling, and treating inherited pathologic processes.

This chapter will review basic mendelian genetics as a necessary prerequisite to the principles of human genetics. Three general categories of genetic disorders will then be discussed: (1) dis-

53

eases caused by multiple genes and the environ-ment; (2) diseases associated with chromosomal abnormalities; and (3) diseases caused by single genes of large effect. All genetic diseases cannot be discussed in this chapter, and examples are used arbitrarily to illustrate a category of a pre-sumed pathophysiologic mechanism.

MENDELIAN INHERITANCE

MENDEL'S EXPERIMENTS

Although Rabbi Simon ben Gamaliel (Talmud of Maimonides, 100 A.D.) excused brothers of "bleeders" from circumcision, it was not until 1900 that Mendel's laws of 1860 were accepted and a formal study of patterns of inheritance in humans begun. In 1978, 2811 traits were catalogued in patterns conforming to mendelian inheritance. All these diseases are caused by single genes of large effect.

It is important to begin our discussion of pathologic physiology with Mendel's principles of inheritance. Mendel's observations were made while he was experimenting with *Pisum sativum,* or garden pea plant, between 1856 and 1865. He selected 34 varieties of true-breeding plants and studied *discontinuous characters* such as the length of the stem, the position of the flowers relative to the stem, the seed color, and the coat texture. Since the flower could fertilize itself and be protected from outside artifact, Mendel could cross hybrids derived from true breeders and thus make quantitative calculations of those disparate characteristics that appeared in subsequent gen-erations. In one such experiment, Mendel found that the texture of the seed coat was either wrin-kled or smooth. When he crossed true-breeding plants containing wrinkled seeds with plants con-taining smooth seeds, he found that in the F_1 generation only smooth-coated seeds were present. When he self-fertilized these smooth-seeded (F_1) plants, he found 25 per cent (¼) true-breeding smooth plants, 25 per cent (¼) true-breeding wrin-kled plants, and 50 per cent (2/4) smooth, impure breeders, which, when self-fertilized, reproduced the same 1:2:1 ratio (see diagram).

Mendel recognized that the wrinkled coat was transmitted from the F_1 to the F_2 generation in an unchanged state, although it was not phenotypi-cally evident in the F_1 hybrid plant. To explain the disappearance of this hereditary trait in the F_1 hybrid and its predictable recurrence, he rec-ognized that the physical expression (phenotype) differed from the genetic constitution (genotype), which must be composed of two transmissible characters (genes). Mendel's *first law* stated that a unit of genetic information (gene) was transmis-sible unchanged from generation to generation. His *second law* stated that alternate forms of the gene (later called an *allele*) must segregate during gamete formation and recombine independently in the offspring to provide this 1:2:1 ratio. From the phenotypic expression of these discontinuous traits, the concepts of dominance and recessivity were derived. In the F_1 hybrid derived from two pure-breeding strains, that allele which is ex-pressed is dominant (smooth, S). The unexpressed allele is recessive (wrinkled, w). The genotypes to this experiment can now be written:

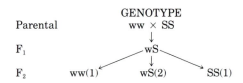

                                   GENOTYPE
    Parental   ww × SS
                                       ↓
    F₁   wS
                                       ↓
    F₂   ww(1)   wS(2)   SS(1)

To test the relationship of transmission be-tween two different discontinuous traits, Mendel designed another set of experiments. He compared the textures of the seeds with their internal color. If he crossed true-breeding plants having smooth seeds and yellow interiors with plants having wrinkled seeds and green interiors, all the F_1 hybrids were smooth and yellow. When this hybrid was self-fertilized, he found a ratio of 9 smooth-yellow seeds, 3 smooth-green, 3 wrinkled-yellow, and 1 wrinkled-green out of a total of 16. These ratios (9/16; 3/16; 1/16) were the product of the probability that either trait would appear inde-pendent of the other. Thus, for the two dominant traits (smooth seeds with yellow interiors), there was a 3/4 × 3/4 probability, or 9/16. For the recessive traits (wrinkled seeds with green inte-

PHENOTYPE

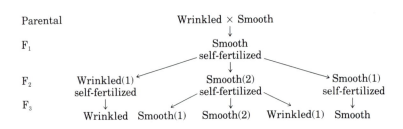

    Parental   Wrinkled × Smooth
                                              ↓
    F₁   Smooth
                                       self-fertilized
                                              ↓
    F₂   Wrinkled(1)   Smooth(2)   Smooth(1)
                  self-fertilized   self-fertilized   self-fertilized
    F₃   ↓   ↓   ↓
                Wrinkled Smooth(1)   Smooth(2) Wrinkled(1)   Smooth

rior), the probability was 1/4 × 1/4, or 1/16. Mendel recognized that the texture of the seed and the color of its interior were independent traits that were not allelic. Thus, his *third law* stated that nonallelic traits do not segregate but assort randomly and recombine with a probability representing the product of their independent probabilities.

Because the botanists of Mendel's time were observing continuous rather than discontinuous traits, his concepts of a unit of inheritance lay dormant until 1900, when they were rediscovered independently by several different geneticists. By 1902, his observations had been applied in a pedigree analysis of humans to explain the patterns of recurrence of brachydactyly. It should be remembered that the concepts of dominance and recessivity were derived from phenotypes. Today, pedigree analyses based on mendelian concepts are used to predict recurrence risks and to offer insights into the abnormal genetic mechanisms producing disease, even when the mechanisms of pathogenesis are unknown.

AUTOSOMAL DOMINANT INHERITANCE

This pattern of inheritance is the most common mode of monogenic transmission in humans, although recessive traits are becoming more prevalent as new metabolic disorders are discovered through modern screening techniques. Most autosomal dominant traits exhibit distinct phenotypic abnormalities, making them relatively easy to detect. From mendelian concepts, one can predict the pedigree pattern for expression of a single dominant gene.

Consider the mating A in Figure 3–1. The heterozygote is affected and, by definition, expresses the dominant trait. If such a parent mates with a homozygous normal, each offspring has a 1/2, or 50 per cent, risk of being an affected heterozygote or homozygous normal. In mating B, two affected heterozygotes mate. Their alleles segregate during gamete formation and recombine randomly. Each offspring has a 1/4, or 25 per cent risk, of being a homozygous normal; a 1/2, or 50 per cent, risk of being an affected heterozygote; and a 1/4, or 25 per cent, risk of being a seriously (lethally?) affected homozygote. Seventy-five per cent (3/4) of the offspring from this mating could be affected by the dominant trait. A schematic pedigree representing an autosomal dominant pattern of inheritance is indicated in Figure 3–2. Since the heterozygote expresses this trait, there is parent-to-offspring transmission, and a vertical pattern of abnormal individuals is produced. Since the mutant gene is located on an autosome, there is an approximately equal distribution of males and females. On the average, 50 per cent of a patient's offspring are affected.

Important in genetic counseling is the fact that each individual pregnancy involves a genetic risk for the given disorder independent of the risk associated with any previous pregnancy. In autosomal dominant patterns of inheritance, if an individual does not express a dominant trait, he cannot transmit it to subsequent generations. This reassuring fact must be tempered against the difficulty of differentiating the disease from other

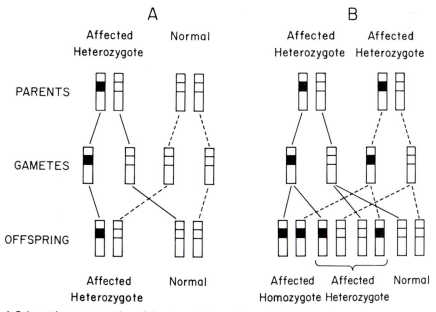

Figure 3–1 Schematic representation of the transmission of an autosomal dominant phenotype. *A* and *B* represent separate matings.

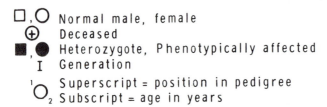

LEGEND:

□ ,○ Normal male, female
 ⊕   Deceased
■ ,● Heterozygote, Phenotypically affected
 I   Generation
 ¹○   Superscript = position in pedigree
 ○₂   Subscript = age in years

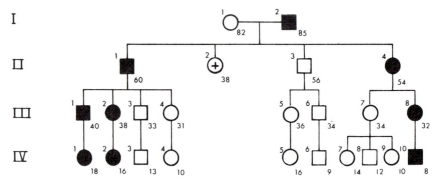

Figure 3–2 Pedigree conforming to an autosomal dominant pattern of inheritance.

similar diseases, the age at which the abnormal phenotype is expressed, and the spectrum of expression. For example, the fact that a child of a patient with familial colonic polyposis (an autosomal dominant trait) does not demonstrate polyps by sigmoidoscopy at age 5 years does not mean that polyps will not occur later in life or that they are not present in regions beyond the view of the sigmoidoscope.

In 1982, 1827 autosomal dominant traits were catalogued, including acute intermittent porphyria, Huntington's chorea, hemorrhagic telangiectasia, Marfan's syndrome, hypertrophic subaortic stenosis, polycystic kidney disease, neurofibromatosis, hereditary nephritis with deafness, familial polyposis, brachydactyly, tuberous sclerosis, and others. Despite our current lack of knowledge regarding the basic defect in many of these disorders, the dominant pattern of inheritance suggests several mechanisms for their expression and molecular control. In a dominant trait the heterozygote expresses the mutant allele. Thus, the mutant gene product could interfere with the function of the normal gene product by producing an abnormal subunit in a protein complex, rendering the complete complex less effective. Examples of this concept are dysfibrinogenemia and abnormalities in structural proteins such as collagen in Marfan's syndrome or in the structural membrane proteins of erythrocytes in hereditary spherocytosis. Dominant mutant alleles might produce proteins that interfere with the regulation of gene expression (repression or feedback control), as in lack of heme in acute intermittent porphyria. The mutant enzyme might overconsume limited substrates, as in

G6PD Hektoen. These concepts will be considered in more detail later when inherited metabolic disorders are discussed.

AUTOSOMAL RECESSIVE INHERITANCE

From the scheme represented in Figure 3–3, one can predict the pattern of inheritance for an autosomal recessive trait. In mating A, a normal homozygote mates with a phenotypically normal carrier of an autosomal recessive trait. In accordance with mendelian principles, the heterozygote does not express the trait. The offspring of such a mating are all phenotypically normal, although, on the average, 50 per cent (1/2) are heterozygotes. Mating B in Figure 3–3 is the more common situation requiring genetic counseling for an autosomal recessive trait. Here, two phenotypically normal parents carry an autosomal recessive mutation and produce an affected child. A recurrence of this phenomenon can be predicted from Mendel's hybridization experiments. On the average, a 1:2:1 ratio of homozygous normal:heterozygous:homozygous abnormal is expected and produces the classic ratio of 3 phenotypic normals to 1 affected. Remember that *each* new offspring of this mating has this risk (25 per cent, or 1/4), independent of previous results. A schematic pedigree conforming to these predictions is outlined in Figure 3–4.

Several differences from the autosomal dominant pedigree outlined in Figure 3–2 are obvious. There is no parent-to-offspring transmission of the phenotypic trait, but siblings are affected, and a

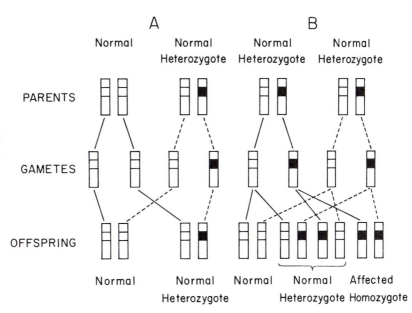

Figure 3–3 Schematic representation of the transmission of an autosomal recessive trait. *A* and *B* represent separate matings.

horizontal pattern as compared with the vertical pattern of dominant inheritance is produced. Twenty-five per cent rather than 50 per cent recurrence in siblings is seen. Since recessive traits are rare in the population, consanguineous matings are more likely to produce the affected homozygote. Subjects III-3 and III-4 are first cousins, and their consanguineous mating is indicated by the horizontal double bar.

In recessive traits with identifiable biochemical abnormalities heterozygotes can be detected by appropriate studies, although they are phenotypically normal under normal environmental conditions. High-risk populations such as adult Jews of eastern European origin are screened for the asymptomatic heterozygous Tay-Sachs disease genotype. The partially closed symbols in Figure 3–4 represent phenotypically normal heterozygotes detectable by biochemical tests. Unlike the situation for the dominant traits, a phenotypically

LEGEND:

□,○ Normal male, female
■ Homozygous abnormal, Phenotypically affected
◪ Heterozygote (detectable), Phenotypically normal
+ Deceased
○—◪ Consanguineous mating
I Generation
¹○₂ Superscript = position in pedigree
     Subscript = age in years

Figure 3–4 Pedigree conforming to an autosomal recessive pattern of inheritance.

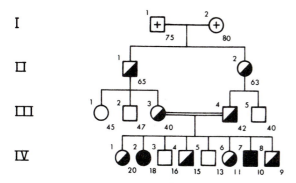

unaffected member in this pedigree cannot be assured that he has no greater risk than the general population for transmitting the disorder. The risk of having an affected offspring is based on the product of the probability that the unaffected member carries the mutant gene, that he will mate with a carrier, and that both mutant genes will be transmitted to the offspring. If heterozygotes can be detected by biochemical means, more precise information can be given. Suppose patient IV-1 in Figure 3–4 seeks counseling regarding recurrence risks and is found by biochemical testing to carry the mutant gene for Tay-Sachs disease. Her mate is then tested. If he carries the mutation, the risk of producing a phenotypi-cally affected child is 25 per cent ($1/2 \times 1/2 = 1/4$). If her mate is normal, all their children will be unaffected, although each has a 50 per cent risk of being a carrier. Since these recessive traits are located on autosomes, males and females are affected equally.

In 1982, 1298 human diseases were classified as autosomal recessive traits. Most of the inborn errors of metabolism are included in this category.

X-LINKED INHERITANCE

In both the previous patterns of inheritance, the mutant gene was located on one of the 22

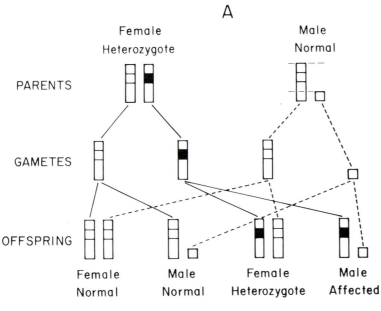

Figure 3–5 *A,* Schematic representation of X-linked transmission: maternal heterozygote. *B,* Schematic representation of the critical mating in X-linked transmission: paternal hemizygote.

human autosomes. Let us now consider a mutation residing on the X chromosome. In Figure 3–5A, a female carrying an X-linked mutation marries a normal male. The expectations of such a mating are that 50 per cent of the female offspring and 50 per cent of the male offspring will inherit the maternal X chromosome containing the mutant gene. If the mutant allele is recessive to the normal allele, the carrier female will not express the trait, but the male, who has only one X chromosome, is hemizygous for the trait and has no normal allele. He, therefore, would express the disorder. The prediction is that half the sons will be affected and the other half will be unaffected and unable to transmit the mutation. Half the daughters will be heterozygotes and carry the mutation and half will be homozygous normal, but all will be phenotypically normal.

Let us turn now to the critical mating (Fig. 3–5B). The mutation is located on the X chromosome of an affected male; all his daughters will inherit this X chromosome containing the mutation, but none of his sons can inherit this disorder because they must all receive his Y chromosome. The pattern of inheritance for an X-linked trait is illustrated by the pedigree in Figure 3–6. Heterozygotes for X-linked traits are indicated by a symbol with a darkened inner circle. If the trait is recessive, only hemizygous males are affected phenotypically. Since maternal uncles of affected

males are commonly affected, an oblique pattern of inheritance is seen. Subject II-1 is an affected male and does not transmit the trait to any of his sons. Both his daughters are carriers and the trait reappears in his grandson, subject IV-2. On the average, half the sons of a carrier female are affected and half the daughters are carriers. A homozygous affected female may appear in a pedigree for an X-linked recessive trait if a hemizygous affected father marries a heterozygous carrier female or, rarely, if the X chromosome containing the normal allele is inactivated during lyonization, leaving only cells with the mutant X chromosome (see discussion of the Lyon hypothesis). In 1982, 243 human diseases were catalogued as X-linked traits.

If the X-linked trait depicted in Figure 3–6 were familial hypophosphatemic rickets, heterozygous females would have abnormally low tubular reabsorption of phosphate and perhaps rickets. This is a dominant X-linked trait. If the trait is rare, twice as many females are affected as males, presumably because there is twice the risk for a female to inherit the mutant X chromosome. If the trait is common, as in Xg blood groups, the ratio of females to males is less than 2:1 (see discussion of the Hardy-Weinberg law). Direct parent-to-offspring transmission is seen. The progeny of subject II-1 provide a critical test of this hypothesis. In this situation, neither of his sons (III-1, III-3) but

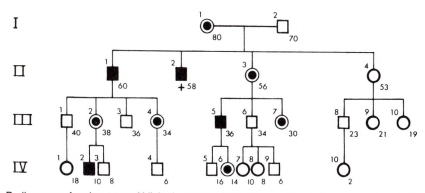

LEGEND:

☐ Normal male
○ Normal female
◉ Heterozygous female, Phenotypically normal or abnormal
■ Hemizygous male, Phenotypically abnormal
+ Deceased
I Generation
Superscript = position in pedigree
Subscript = age in years

Figure 3–6 Pedigree conforming to an X-linked pattern of inheritance. If a heterozygous female is phenotypically normal, the trait is recessive, as in hemophilia A. If she is phenotypically affected, the trait is dominant, as in familial hypophosphatemic rickets.

both his daughters (III-2, III-4) are affected. If such a critical mating were not present, an X-linked dominant trait might be mistaken for an autosomal dominant. Prediction and prevention in this disease are critical. Treatment with oral phosphates and vitamin D should be instituted before weight-bearing age to preserve normal bone growth. An accurate pedigree analysis is therefore essential to prediction, early diagnosis, and prevention.

Y-LINKED INHERITANCE

If a discontinuous trait were located on the Y chromosome, only males would express it. Female descendants could neither inherit nor transmit this trait. Many phenotypic traits were thought inherited by this mechanism, but variable expression in females effectively ruled out this mode of inheritance. At present, genes transmitting a peculiar form of "hairy ears" in males, the H-Y antigen or "testis determining factor" or both are thought to be located on the Y chromosome.

MITOCHONDRIAL INHERITANCE

In the aforementioned patterns of human inheritance, expressed genes are located on DNA located in the cell's nucleus. The mitochondria also contain DNA, and their genetic code in humans is almost completely known. If a mutation were present in the mitochondrial DNA, it would be transmitted from an affected female to all her offspring. However, an affected male would *not* transmit the trait. Why mitochondrial genes are transmitted by maternal inheritance patterns is not clear. Perhaps the mitochondria of spermatozoa are either worn out or recognized as foreign antigens by the fertilized ovum. Whatever the mechanism, the zygote inherits its mitochondrial DNA only from the mother. With cDNA probes and restriction endonuclease maps for mitochondrial DNA fragments, this pattern of transmission has been confirmed in humans. At present, one heritable disease has been associated with maternal transmission, Leber's optic atrophy. This disease is being actively investigated with the assistance of mitochondrial cDNA probes.

There are many problems in analyzing pedigrees for "mendelizing phenotypes." Mendelian inheritance may be simulated by environmental mechanisms. Women with phenylketonuria may produce retarded children with microcephaly and other congenital anomalies even though the children are genotypically heterozygotes for PKU. The retardation presumably is caused by the effect of high concentrations of phenylalanine on the developing fetus. Phenocopies may be produced by intrauterine infections. Rubella virus may produce a syndrome of deafness and chorioretinal degeneration simulating Usher syndrome, an autosomal recessive trait. Environmentally caused diseases may masquerade as mendelian traits. At least one instance is known of a mother affected by the rubella syndrome who produced a child with a similar syndrome. Recessive traits that usually are not clinically manifest in the heterozygous state may produce disease under unusual stressful circumstances: When heterozygotes for sickle cell hemoglobin (AS) are subjected to lowered atmospheric pressure, such as in nonpressurized aircraft flights, a "sickle crisis" may occur. Similarly, if the genetic determinant used in a pedigree analysis of sickle cell disease is erythrocyte sickling upon in-vitro exposure to sodium metabisulfite, a dominant rather than recessive pattern of inheritance would emerge. Despite these semantic problems, pedigree analysis and mendelian classification aid in establishing a probable genetic cause, in predicting high-risk individuals, and in suggesting basic genetic mechanisms. The problems raised by phenotypic expression will be solved by more precise information concerning the mutant gene product.

THE HARDY-WEINBERG LAW: FREQUENCY OF GENES IN A POPULATION

In 1908, an English mathematician, Hardy, and a German physician, Weinberg, independently developed a mathematical formulation for determining the frequency of genotypes in a population. This formula is known as the *Hardy-Weinberg law*, which is quite simply the binomial expansion, stating that given two alleles, p and q, $p + q = 1$. Therefore, for a population at equilibrium where mutation rates are small, where mating is random, and where selection is minimal

$$p^2 + 2pq + q^2 = (p + q)^2 \text{ and}$$

p^2 = frequency of homozygotes for the p allele

$2pq$ = frequency of heterozygotes for p and q alleles

q^2 = frequency of homozygotes for the q allele

From this relationship, one can see that heterozygotes for rare autosomal recessive traits are relatively common. For instance, phenylketonuria may occur in only one of every 10,000 live births. Therefore

$$q^2 = 1/10,000$$

$$q = 1/100$$

Since $p + q = 1$

then $p = 1 - 1/100 = 99/100$

The frequency of heterozygotes in the population is given by the following expression:

$$2pq = 2 \times \frac{99}{100} \times \frac{1}{100}$$

which is approximately

1/50, or 2 per cent

Thus 2 per cent of the population carry the gene for PKU, even though the disease occurs in only 0.01 per cent. The relatively high frequency of heterozygotes also enables one to see why saving homozygous affected individuals and enabling them to reproduce will not alter the gene frequency perceptibly in several centuries.

The Hardy-Weinberg law also enables one to understand why females are affected by X-linked dominant traits twice as often as males. Affected males can have only one genotype, since they are hemizygous. In the Hardy-Weinberg equation, their population frequency is seen by the expression "q." Females who are affected may be either heterozygous (2pq) or homozygous (q^2). Thus, the ratio of the frequency of females to males expressing an X-linked dominant trait is

$$\frac{\text{female}}{\text{male}} = \frac{(2pq + q^2)}{q}$$

If the disorder is rare, the frequency of a homozygous affected female (q^2) is negligible and the expression becomes

$$\frac{\text{female}}{\text{male}} = \frac{2pq}{q}$$

where p is nearly one and the female/male ratio is 2/1. If the trait is common, q^2 cannot be ignored, and this ratio becomes smaller.

MULTIFACTORIAL GENETIC DISORDERS

Although Mendel conducted hybridization studies using discontinuous traits, he also made some observations on traits that blended into a continuum between the parental phenotypes. He recognized that when purple-petaled and white-petaled plants were crossed, an intermediate mauve color was found in the hybrid. When this F_1 hybrid was self-fertilized, a range of color from purple to white was produced in the progeny. These observations seemed to contradict the concept of single-gene effects, but Mendel suggested that flower petal color was determined by more than a single gene and that the expressed color resulted from a blending of these genes. Such common conditions as diabetes, schizophrenia, cleft palate, extremes in intelligence quotient and height, club foot, spina bifida, and pyloric stenosis recur in populations and families with frequencies suggesting some genetic influences. Falconer interpreted these observations in the following manner: (1) There are both heritable and environmental influences acting on the final phenotypic expression; (2) the hereditary component is polygenic and represents a continuum of genetic expression within the population; and (3) the small affected fraction of the population exceeds a threshold liability produced by both a larger number of "risk genes" and the environmental influences to produce the disease (Fig. 3–7). These hypotheses meet certain predicted conditions:

1. If these traits are not monogenic in causation, they will not conform to a mendelian pattern of recessive or dominant inheritance. Therefore, if one looked at the recurrence in first-degree relatives, one would *not* expect to find either a 25 per cent recurrence (autosomal recessive) or a 50 per cent recurrence (autosomal dominant) but rather some other calculable increased risk compared with the general population. There should be a marked reduction in its recurrence from the first-degree relatives to the second-degree relatives but still some definable increased risk relative with the general population. These findings contrast sharply with those for either recessive or dominant

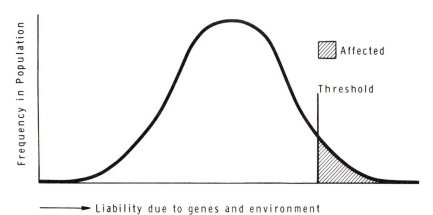

Figure 3–7 Multifactorial inheritance. The continuous distribution of liability to develop a multifactorial disease is determined by many genes and the environment. A threshold of liability indicates the limit beyond which disease is expressed.

inheritance. For mendelian recessive traits, one would expect no increased risk to second-degree relatives, barring consanguinity.

2. A second condition tests the recurrence of traits in monozygous and dizygous twins. In either recessive or dominant monogenic traits, the phenotype must be present in both monozygotic twins (100 per cent concordance). In these forms of inheritance, the recurrence rates in dizygous twins are the same as in first-degree relatives. In a multifactorial trait, one would expect an increased incidence in monozygous twins but not 100 per cent concordance because of different nongenetic influences. The increased incidence found in dizygous twins should reflect this environmental effect. The recurrence rate found in first-degree relatives should be the same in dizygous twins.

3. One might expect that the more severe the disease expression, the greater the recurrence, since more "risk genes" must be present.

4. One might also expect that, if the disease is more frequent in one sex, then the sex with the lower incidence figure would have a higher threshold and would require more "risk genes" to manifest disease.

5. Finally, one might anticipate that in families in which more than a single sibling is affected, the recurrence risks for a third affected offspring would be greater, since, again, more of the "risk genes" must be present in the parents and the probability of liability gene transmission is increased.

Carter's data for cleft lip with or without cleft palate satisfy these criteria. Other known familial causes of cleft lip and palate were excluded, namely, lower lip mucous pits (as seen in Van der Woude syndrome, an autosomal dominant trait; trisomy 13; orofaciodigital syndrome; and so on). Table 3–1 gives the combined data from four different studies in populations with cleft lip. The general incidence of cleft lip is 0.1 per cent. Monozygous twins were both affected in 40 per cent of cases, whereas in dizygous twins both were affected in only 4 per cent. Neither of these values would be consistent with a monogenic disorder. The first-degree relatives had a 40-fold increased frequency over the general population. The second-degree relatives had a ninefold increase, and the third-degree relatives had a fourfold increase. When a more severe form of the disease was present, such as bilateral cleft lip with cleft palate, a higher recurrence risk figure for first-degree relatives was found (6 per cent). When the milder form of the disease, unilateral cleft lip without cleft palate, was present, a lower recurrence risk of 2.5 per cent was found. When two siblings were affected, the recurrence risk for a third affected individual within that family rose to 12 per cent. These data can be explained on the basis of a liability with continuous distribution produced by multiple genes and the environment, with a threshold beyond which the disease is manifest (Fig. 3–7).

Several other relatively common human disorders conform to a multifactorial mode of inheritance (Table 3–2). In some instances, the environmental influences are greater than the heritable component. For example, Carter reminds us that Laplanders and the American Indians swaddle their infants with legs extended and adducted. In both these groups, the incidence of dislocation of the hip is higher than the negligible incidence in certain Asiatic groups such as the Chinese, whose infants are held on a back sling with hips flexed and abducted. The incidence in a population in which neither of these environmental extremes is present is approximately 0.2 per cent. At least two genetic factors (acetabular dysgenesis and familial joint laxity) and at least two environmental factors (breech position at birth and swaddling) have been

TABLE 3–1 MULTIFACTORIAL INHERITANCE OF CLEFT LIP WITH OR WITHOUT CLEFT PALATE

Condition	Incidence in General Population (Per Cent)	Relatives Affected (Per Cent)					
		Monozygous Twin	First Degree		Second Degree		Third Degree
			(Siblings)	(Children)	(Aunts and Uncles)	(Nephews and Nieces)	(First Cousins)
Overall recurrence risk for cleft lip ± cleft palate	0.1	40 (400X)	4.4 ± 0.7 (40X)	3.3 ± 1.2	0.7 ± 0.1 (9X)	1.1 ± 0.5	0.4 ± 0.1 (4X)
Bilateral cleft lip + palate	--	--	6.0		--		--
Unilateral cleft lip + palate	--	--	2.5		--		--
Two affected siblings	--	--	12.0		--		--

Blanks (--) indicate insufficient data.
Numbers in parentheses followed by X (400X) indicate the increased risk relative to the general population.
(Data from Carter, C. O.: Hosp. Pract. 5:45, 1970.)

TABLE 3–2 MULTIFACTORIAL INHERITANCE—EMPIRICAL DATA FROM FAMILIES WITH CONGENITAL MALFORMATIONS

Condition	Incidence in General Population (Per Cent)	Increased Risk Relative to General Population			
		Relatives			
		Monozygous Twin	First Degree	Second Degree	Third Degree
Dislocation of hip (females)	0.2	200X	25X	3X	2X
Pyloric stenosis (males)	0.5	80X	10X (Males)	5X	1.8X
Pyloric stenosis (females)	0.1	--	200X (Males)	20X	1.8X
Spina bifida cystica	0.2	--	10X	--	--
Talipes equinovarus	0.1	300X	25X	5X	2X
Ankylosing spondylitis (males)	0.02	--	35X	10X	3X
Early-onset ischemic heart disease (males)	0.15	--	6X	--	--

Blanks (--) indicate insufficient data.
Numbers in parentheses followed by X (200X) indicate the increased risk relative to the general population.
(Data compiled from Carter, C. O.: Hosp. Pract. 5:45, 1970, and Falconer, D. S.: Ann. Hum. Genet. 29:51, 1965.)

described that adversely affect the incidence and recurrence risk figures for dislocation of the hip. A 25-fold increase over the incidence in the general population is found in first-degree relatives of patients with congenital dislocation of the hip. There is only a threefold and twofold increased risk to second- and third-degree relatives, respectively. In pyloric stenosis, a sex predilection has been demonstrated. Although pyloric stenosis occurs more commonly in males than in females (0.5 vs. 0.1 per cent), the recurrence risk to the sons of affected fathers is ten times the general population risk. In keeping with the postulates for a multifactorial mode of inheritance, the female may require more "risk genes" before manifesting the trait if, perhaps, hormonal influences protect her. If an increased number of "risk genes" are required for her to express the disease, a recurrence risk should be higher in her hormonally unprotected male offspring. Sons of females with pyloric stenosis have a 200-fold increased incidence relative to the general population. Carter has determined that in the London area, the incidence of spina bifida cystica is approximately 0.2 per cent. The recurrence is 2 per cent in families in which one member has been affected. After two children in a family are affected, the risk rises to 12.5 per cent.

These kinds of data are useful in relating recurrence risk figures to families, but the concept of a continuous distribution and "multifactorial" disease should not inhibit attempts to find specific causes within these heterogeneous groups. The "continuous" expression of an enzyme function in population studies may be related to multiple genotypes in that population. Harris clearly demonstrated the continuous distribution of serum cholinesterase (pseudocholinesterase) activity if serum hydrolytic activity alone were the genetic determinant (Fig. 3–8A). Only a small portion of the population (closed squares) was functionally defective and no mendelian pattern was deline-

ated. When other characteristics of the gene products were examined, such as resistance to dibucaine, three phenotypes become evident: "usual," "intermediate," and "atypical" (Fig. 3–8B). This trimodal distribution then suggested mendelian rather than multifactorial inheritance in which "usual" was homozygous normal, "intermediate" was heterozygous, and "atypical" was homozygous abnormal. The discriminant, "dibucaine resistance," resolved the genetic control mechanism for this enzyme function into a mendelian pattern. Since this earlier description, other parameters of resistance, inheritance, and separation of isozymes have demonstrated at least two loci for pseudocholinesterase activity and 10 genotypes to account for the continuous polygenic distribution in the population. Environmental factors such as liver disease, general nutrition, and renal glomerular integrity contribute further to the "multifactorial" pattern of enzyme activity originally found.

CYTOGENETICS

Another mechanism of human disease results from chromosomal abnormalities of two general types. There may be a numerical variation from the normal number, or the normal number may be present but gross structural abnormalities of individual chromosomes may exist. Chromosomal aberrations have been known to occur in plants and animals for a long time, but only since the late 1950s have human cytogenetic techniques advanced sufficiently to demonstrate that such aberrations occur in humans as well.

THE CHROMOSOMES

In humans, the normal chromosome number, 46, was definitively established by 1956. There are

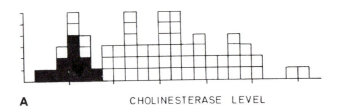

A   CHOLINESTERASE LEVEL

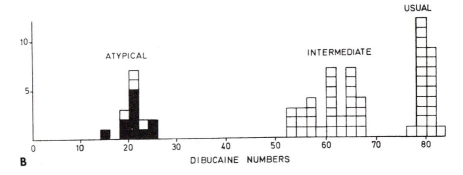

B   DIBUCAINE NUMBERS

Figure 3–8 *A,* Continuous distribution of serum cholinesterase (pseudocholinesterase) activity. Each square represents one individual. Suxamethonium-sensitive individuals are marked in black. *B,* Distribution of dibucaine numbers (percent inhibition) on identical serum specimens. Discrimination of three phenotypes is evident. (From Harris, H., et al.: Acta Genet. Stat. Med. *10*:1, 1960.)

22 pairs of autosomes, which are identical in both sexes, and one pair of sex chromosomes. The latter two chromosomes have a similar appearance in the female, XX, but are dissimilar in the male, one being like the X chromosome of the female and the other, Y, being smaller. The chromosomes appear in metaphase as double structures known as the *chromatids,* which lie adjacent to each other and are connected at a constriction called the *centromere.* An analysis of the chromosomes has permitted their classification based on length and shape, with the latter being determined by position of the centromere. A chromosome is called *metacentric* when its centromere is approximately in the middle, the chromatid arms being about equal in length. The centromere may be toward one end, making the arms on opposite sides of the centromere of unequal length. *Acrocentric* chromosomes are those with the centromere very close to one end. Satellites can be present on acrocentric chromosomes (Fig. 3–9). These are DNA-staining regions on the distal short arm that are separated from it by a secondary constriction (nonstaining

area) now known to contain genes for 18S and 28S ribosomal RNA. Active transcription is indicated by positive silver staining in these secondary constrictions, referred to as *nucleolus organizer regions* (NORs).

The autosomes are divided into seven groups, A to G, depending on their length and position of the centromere. They are numbered from 1 to 22, primarily in order of decreasing length (Table 3–3). The X chromosome by length is placed between chromosomes 7 and 8, but without banding the X cannot be differentiated from other larger members of the C group. The Y is small and acrocentric and usually cannot be differentiated easily from those in group G. The earlier techniques made it possible to group chromosomes in a satisfactory way, but only within groups A and E was it possible to separate individual pairs (Fig. 3–10).

During the early 1970s, newer banding techniques increased the cytogeneticist's ability to distinguish individual chromosomes. Q-banding (quinacrine banding) is produced by quinacrine stain and fluorescence microscopy. G-banding

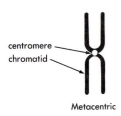

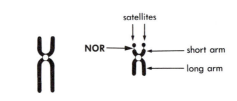

Figure 3–9 Types of human metaphase chromosomes.

TABLE 3-3 MORPHOLOGIC CHARACTERISTICS OF HUMAN METAPHASE CHROMOSOMES

Group	Chromosome Number	Characteristics
A	1, 2, 3	#1 is longest, metacentric #2 is 2nd longest, submetacentric #3 is 3rd longest, metacentric
B	4, 5	Relatively long chromosomes; more submetacentric
C	6 to 12, and X	Medium length, metacentric and submetacentric; X is one of the longer chromosomes in this group
D	13 to 15	Acrocentric chromosomes; longer than G group; have satellites
E	16 to 18	Smaller than above groups: #16 is metacentric #17 and #18 are submetacentric #18 is shorter than #17
F	19, 20	Four small metacentric chromosomes that look like the letter X.
G	21, 22, Y	Short acrocentrics; have satellites; Y is similar but may be slightly longer; long arms closer together and with secondary constriction and no satellites

(Data compiled from references cited under CHROMOSOMAL GENETICS—General in references.)

(Giemsa banding) is produced by various pretreatments, usually trypsin, of chromosomes on slides, followed by a stain, usually Giemsa. R-banding (reverse banding) comes out the other way around—nonstaining bands by Q- and G-banding techniques are positively stained by the R-banding technique (Fig. 3–11). Note that since the ends of most chromosomes do not stain by Q- and G-banding but do stain by R-banding, the latter is useful to detect small terminal deletions or translocations. However, Q- and G-banding techniques are the two that are used most commonly for diagnosis of the chromosome abnormalities discussed later in this chapter. The X-chromosome is easily identified by its characteristic banding pattern; the Y chromosome is identified by bright fluorescence on long arms after Q-banding.

Another technique, called *C-banding (centromere banding),* stains the centromere regions of all human chromosomes except the Y; it shows positive C-banding on the long arms. The chromosome regions stained by this technique are thought to contain DNA with highly repeating base sequences. This type of DNA has been equated with genetic inactivity, and therefore variations in size of C-banded chromosome regions occur in normal individuals and are termed *C-band polymorphisms.* Q-band polymorphisms also occur normally, particularly in the regions of acrocentric chromosome short arms and satellites. Both types of polymorphisms show mendelian inheritance; in any chromosome pair heterozygous for the polymorphism, one member is identifed as *paternal* and one as *maternal* by morphologic

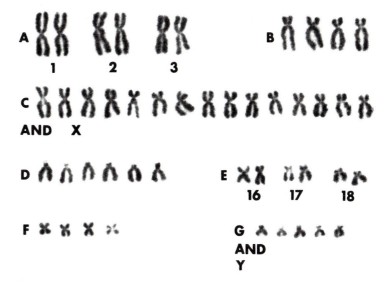

Figure 3–10 Normal male karyotype, shown by standard staining techniques. Forty-six chromosomes are arranged in seven groups (A to G). Note that the X chromosome cannot be differentiated from the C group; the Y is similar to the others of the G group, unless, as a normal variation, it is slightly longer. Normally, the Y has no satellites and does not have an NOR region on the short arm. Only pairs 1, 2, 3, 16, 17, and 18 can be identified within the groups.

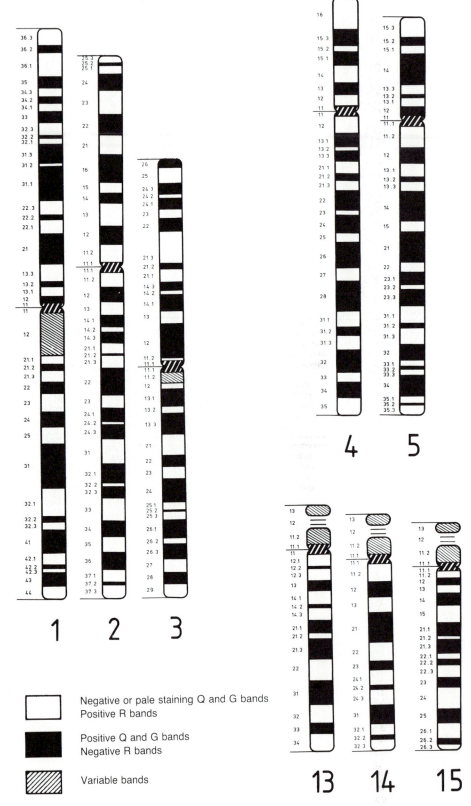

Negative or pale staining Q and G bands
Positive R bands

Positive Q and G bands
Negative R bands

Variable bands

Legend and illustration continued on opposite page

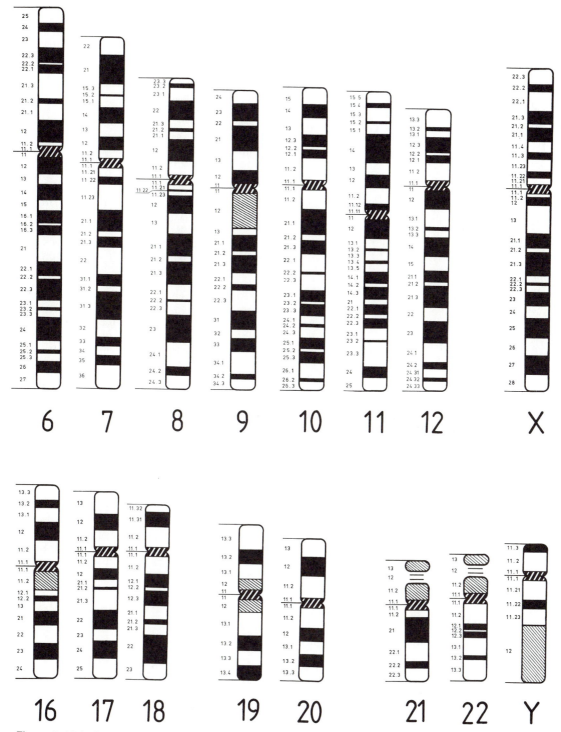

Figure 3–11 A diagrammatic representation of chromosome bands based on the patterns observed in different cells stained with the Q-, G-, or R-band technique, illustrating a haploid karyotype of approximately 550 bands. At least this degree of resolution should be achieved routinely for diagnosis of structural defects in human chromosomal disease states. Regions and bands are numbered consecutively from the centromere outward along each chromosome arm. A band is a part of a chromosome clearly distinguishable from adjacent parts by virtue of its lighter or darker staining intensity. Bands are grouped into regions. Four items are required to designate a particular band: (1) chromosome number, (2) arm symbol (p for short arm and q for long arm), (3) region number, and (4) band number within that region. (Modified from An International System for Human Cytogenetic Nomenclature. High Resolution Banding (1981). Report of the standing committee on Human Cytogenetic Nomenclature. Birth Defects Original Article Series. Vol XVII, No. 5, 1981, March of Dimes Birth Defects Foundation, White Plains, N.Y.; and from Cytogenetics and Cell Genetics Vol. 31, No. 1, 1981, S. Karger AG, Basel.)

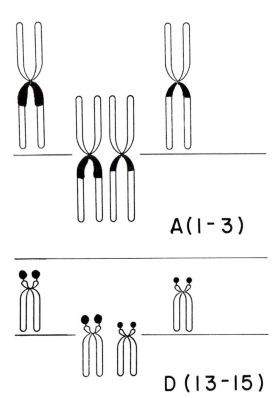

A (I - 3)

D (I3 - I5)

Figure 3–12 *Upper panel,* C-band polymorphism for the A group chromosome 1 is illustrated. To the left is one parental chromosome 1 with a longer C-band; to the right is one chromosome 1 with a shorter C-band from the other parent. In the upper middle is the heterozygous pair 1 in the child, one identifiable member from each parent.

Lower panel, Q-band polymorphism for a D group chromosome is illustrated. To the left is one parental D chromosome (say, chromosome 13) with a large satellite. To the right is a D (13) from the parent, with a smaller satellite. In the lower middle is the heterozygous D (13) pair in the child, one identifiable member from each parent.

study. This important principle is illustrated in more detail in Figure 3–12. Normal variation in length of the Y chromosome occurs in the Q-banded region of its long arm. Each son has his father's Y with respect to this length characteristic.

High-resolution banding is now used to identify more bands on longer metaphase chromosomes. This detailed morphology is accomplished by (1) treating the cells with an agent such as actinomycin D that binds to DNA and maintains a greater degree of extension at metaphase, or (2) synchronizing and harvesting for chromosome studies in early metaphase. The reasons that chromosomes band are not completely understood. As a general rule, G- and Q-positive bands replicate later and are thought to contain less active DNA; R-positive bands replicate earlier and are more active genetically.

MITOSIS AND MEIOSIS

The many cells of the body are derived from division of preceding cells; hence, it is essential that we review briefly mitosis, meiosis, and the cell cycle. The nondividing state of a cell is termed *interphase.* During a portion of this time, termed the *S period* (S), semiconservative DNA replication occurs and chromatids are doubled. The time after mitosis (M) and before S is termed G_1, for gap-1; the time after synthesis of DNA and before the next mitosis is termed G_2 for gap-2 (Fig. 3–13). RNA and protein synthesis occur during all of interphase. The doubled chromatids do not separate until next mitosis.

During interphase the chromosomes are extended; however, as the cell enters prophase of mitosis, they condense and become discrete. In *metaphase,* the next stage, chromosomes are independently oriented (not paired) on the equatorial plate. Duplicated chromatids are held together at the centromere, which is also the attachment point of the chromosome to some of the spindle fibers. During the next stage, *anaphase,* the doubled chromatids move apart, pulled by spindle fibers to each pole of the dividing cell. Each chromatid is now called a chromosome. During *telophase* the nuclear membrane forms about each set of chromosomes, and the cell divides into two daughter cells. Thus, a newly formed cell nucleus contains the same number and kinds of chromosomes as the cell it came from. This paired number of chromosomes in each cell is called *diploid.*

During formation of germ cells, a modification of the process just described occurs called *meiosis.* The chromosomes, instead of remaining independent as in mitosis, line up in pairs during metaphase of the first meiotic division, termed *meiosis I.* One of each pair goes to each daughter cell, giving rise to the haploid number. In *meiosis II,* chromatids separate, as in a mitotic division, and

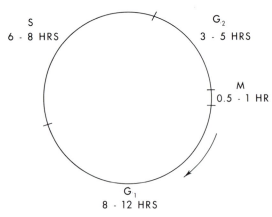

Figure 3–13 Diagram of the cell cycle of most cultured mammalian diploid cells. The approximate length of each part of the cycle is indicated in hours. Direction of progression is indicated by the arrow. Terminology is explained in the text.

the haploid number is again distributed to each daughter cell. Reduction of the diploid number of chromosomes to haploid is essential in sexual reproduction, since fertilization will again join two haploid sets from father and mother to reestablish the diploid.

CHROMOSOMAL ABNORMALITIES

The normal diploid number of chromosomes in humans is 46 in all the somatic cells. In gametes, however, the haploid number is 23 and includes one of each pair. One could suspect that a variation in chromosome number or gross structure would add or subtract many genes from the individual cell and lead to an abnormality. One must bear in mind, however, that some structural changes may occur as normal variations in humans without any significant phenotypic expression. Gross chromosomal abnormalities are associated with a number of clinical disorders. The relationship of chromosomal abnormalities to the disease state in terms of the precise pathophysiologic mechanisms is not known.

Before considering specific syndromes associated with chromosomal abnormalities, it is necessary to review a cytogenetic shorthand, first standardized in 1971 and now in common usage. A brief synopsis of this is presented, incorporating only the common terms or terms used in this chapter. (Table 3–4 summarizes some nomenclature symbols.) The karyotype is written by noting total number of chromosomes followed by the sex chromosomes. For example, 46,XY is the normal male and 46,XX is the normal female karyotype.

In considering numerical aberrations, 45,X indicates a total number of 45 chromosomes with only one X; 47,XXY indicates a total of 47, two X chromosomes and a Y; 47,XX,+18 indicates a female with 47 chromosomes due to trisomy of number 18; and 45,XY,−C indicates a male with 45 chromosomes, the missing one being of the C group.

Chromosomal mosaics are shown by separating the several cell lines by a diagonal slash. For example, 45X/46,XY indicates a chromosome mosaic with two cell lines: One has 45 chromosomes and a single X; the other is normal with 46 chromosomes and XY. The mosaic karyotype, 46,XY/47,XY,+21 indicates a mosaic with one normal male cell line and another with one additional number 21.

In defining structural abnormalities, the short arm of a chromosome is designated with a small "p"; the long arm with a "q." A minus sign (−) after a symbol is used to designate decrease in chromosome material. Therefore, 46,XY,5p− indicates a male with 46 chromosomes, but chromosome 5 has a deletion of the short arm. The karyotype 46,XX,22q− shows a female with normal chromosome number, but a deletion of the

TABLE 3–4 NOMENCLATURE SYMBOLS

A–G	the chromosome groups
1–22	the autosome numbers
X, Y	the sex chromosomes
diagonal (/)	separates cell lines in describing mosaicism
plus sign (+) or minus sign (−)	when placed immediately before the autosome number or group letter designation indicates that the particular whole chromosome is extra or missing; when placed immediately after the arm, structural or other designation indicates an increase or decrease in length
(?)	questionable identification of chromosome or structure
(*)	chromosome or structure explained in text or footnote
:	break—no reunion, as in terminal deletion
::	break and join
→	from-to
ace	acentric
cen	centromere
del	deletion
dic	dicentric
dup	duplication
end	endoreduplication
h	secondary constriction or negatively staining region
i	isochromosome
inv	inversion
inv (p−q+) or inv (p+q−)	pericentric inversion
mar	marker chromosome, unknown origin
mat	maternal origin
mos	mosaic
p	short arm of chromosome
pat	paternal origin
q	long arm of chromosome
r	ring chromosome
rcp	reciprocal translocation
rec	recombinant chromosome
s	satellite
t	translocation
ter	terminal or end
pter	end of short arm
qter	end of long arm
tri	tricentric
repeated symbols	duplication of chromosome structure

long arm of chromosome 22. A plus sign (+) after a symbol is used to designate increase in chromosome material. Therefore, 13p+ indicates increase in length of the short arm of chromosome 13. An isochromosome for X long arm is designated 46,X,i(Xq) in an individual who also has one normal X. A ring X chromosome is written 46,X,r(X) in an individual who also has one normal X.

Translocations are indicated by the letter "t" followed by parentheses that include the chromosomes involved. One type of translocation is used as an example and is designated 45,XX, −14, −21, +t(14q21q); the individual is a female with 45 chromosomes. One chromosome 14 and one 21 are missing. The long arms of these two chromosomes are united in a translocation (t).

The location of any given break point in a chromosomal rearrangement is specified by the band in which that break has occurred. A translocation involving switch of pieces between two different chromosomes (referred to as *reciprocal*) is noted as 46,XY,t(2;5)(q21;q31) when chromosomes 2 and 5 in a male individual break in the long arms at q21 and q31, the region and band number of chromosomes 2 and 5, respectively.

Chromosomal abnormalities may lead to a number of consequences. First, they have been associated with fetal loss, since spontaneously aborted fetuses have a variety of chromosomal defects. The incidence can be as high as 50 per cent in the first trimester, falls to as high as 15

TABLE 3–5 CLASSIFICATION OF CHROMOSOMAL ABNORMALITIES

1. Numerical
    A. Polyploidy
    B. Aneuploidy
        (1) Autosomal
        (2) Sex chromosomal
2. Structural
    A. Translocations
    B. Deletions
    C. Isochromosomes
    D. Ring chromosomes
    E. Inversions

per cent in the second trimester, and is about 1 to 2 per cent in the last trimester of pregnancy. Second, various types of congenital malformation syndromes, most of them associated with mental retardation, result from chromosomal abnormal-

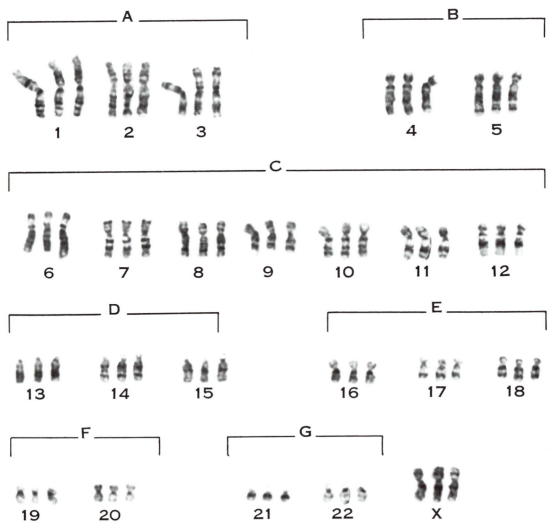

Figure 3–14 A karyotype of a spontaneously aborted fetus, 69,XXX. All autosomes are present in triplicate; the sex chromosomes consist of three X chromosomes.

ity. Surveys of newborn infants report the incidence of viable major chromosome defects to be about 5 per 1000 consecutive births, equally distributed between sex chromosome and autosomal abnormalities. Third, neoplasia is associated with aneuploidy, as will be discussed later in this chapter. Chromosomal abnormalities can be classified into two major groups, numerical and structural (Table 3–5), although these groups overlap to some extent.

NUMERICAL ABNORMALITIES OF THE CHROMOSOMES

Polyploidy

This term refers to the number of chromosomes in multiples of the haploid number, 23. As mentioned previously, the diploid state (46 chromosomes) is normal for somatic cells. Triploidy is a form of polyploidy in which 69 chromosomes are present, three of each chromosome instead of the normal pair (Fig. 3–14). Triploidy is considered to be abnormal because it is found in spontaneously aborted fetuses and, rarely, in liveborn infants. In either case, it is associated with severe congenital malformations. In tetraploidy (92 chromosomes), four of each individual chromosome are present. Tetraploidy occurs normally in some tissues such as liver and is frequently seen, along with diploidy, in culture of amniotic fluid for prenatal chromosomal diagnosis. In this latter situation at birth, infants are phenotypically normal, and the tetraploidy is thought to arise in trophoblast, an extraembryonic tissue. True diploid-tetraploid mosaicism or tetraploidy in the entire individual is associated with severe congenital defects and fetal loss.

Aneuploid States

Aneuploidy is an increase or decrease in the normal (euploid) number of chromosomes that does not involve a full haploid set. The aneuploid state may involve autosomes or sex chromosomes or, sometimes, both. In *trisomy*, a form of aneuploidy in which 47 chromosomes are present, one chromosome of a pair is present three times instead of two. Clearly described congenital malformation syndromes are associated with complete autosomal trisomies, as summarized in Table 3–6.

In *monosomy*, only one chromosome is present in a particular chromosome pair instead of two. Only a few viable cases of full autosomal monosomy are reported, for G group or number 21 chromosome. Monosomy for the X chromosome is well known, however, and is the basis for Turner syndrome. Other aneuploid states may occur that are more complex; some involve trisomy of two chromosomal pairs, producing a karyotype with 48

TABLE 3–6 THE FULL TRISOMY SYNDROMES

Trisomic Chromosome	Brief Clinical Description
8	General dysmorphy of bones; abnormalities of vertebrae and iliac bones; brachymesophalangy; syndactyly; club foot; limitation of joint movement; macrocephaly; mental retardation.
13	Sloping forehead; colobomas; microphthalmia or anophthalmia; arrhinencephaly; cleft lip and palate; cardiac defects; polydactyly; prominent heels; flexion of fingers; apneic spells; seizures; hemangiomas; retarded development.
18	Prominent occiput; small head; small palpebral fissures; flat nasal bridge; small mandible; short sternum; flexed fingers; syndactyly; retarded development; small hypothenar muscles; renal abnormality; rockerbottom feet; hypertonia.
21	Small head; slanting palpebral fissures; epicanthal folds; speckling of iris; flat nasal bridge; large tongue; short neck; cardiac defects; short stature; broad, short hands; incurved fifth finger; single flexion crease in fifth finger; palmar single transverse lines; gap between toes 1 and 2; plantar furrow; hypotonia; hyperextensible joints; frequent infections; mental retardation.
22	Small head; antimongoloid slant of eyes; preauricular skin tags; small chin; cardiac defects; finger-like thumbs; hypotonicity; retarded development; characteristic facies.

chromosomes. An example is the combination of both Down syndrome and Klinefelter syndrome in the same individual (48,XXY,+21).

Nondisjunction

During nuclear division, chromosomes or chromatids normally separate, or disjoin, from each other. Meiotic nondisjunction (failure of disjunction) can occur in the gonads of chromosomally normal males or females (Fig. 3–15), resulting in trisomic offspring after fertilization. If the chromosomes of a pair do not separate in meiosis I, one daughter cell will contain both members. Recall that in some individuals these two members can be distinguished by their polymorphisms, or normal variations in morphology. Therefore, a misdivision in meiosis I is characterized by the presence of two different-looking members of the pair, as shown at the left in Figure 3–15. If the

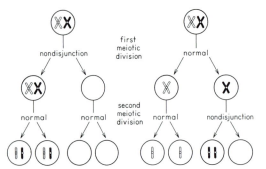

Figure 3–15 Nondisjunction occurring at the first and second meiotic divisions. Nondisjunction at meiosis I produces gametes containing both members of the pair of chromosomes concerned or neither member. Nondisjunction at meiosis II produces gametes containing (or lacking) two identical chromosomes, both derived from the same member of the pair. (From Thompson, J. S., and Thompson, M. W.: Genetics in Medicine. 3rd ed. Philadelphia, W. B. Saunders Co., 1980.)

meiotic I division is normal but nondisjunction occurs in meiosis II, only one type of polymorphic chromosome for any given pair will be present in duplicate, since chromatids of the same chromosome fail to separate in meiosis II (shown at the right in Figure 3–15). This morphologic distinction between a meiotic I and II nondisjunctional error can be used to pinpoint the error in an individual case of trisomy.

Factors leading to the production of nondisjunction are not completely understood. In Down syndrome, incidence of the condition increases with advancing age of the mother. Similar mater-

nal age effect is also noted in other forms of autosomal trisomy. A possible explanation for these observations is that at birth the female already has a lifetime's supply of oocytes. They have entered prophase of meiosis I and remain arrested prior to metaphase of meiosis I until ovulation many years later. The longer this time, the greater the opportunity for damage from infection, drugs, or other environmental factors. The delay in completion of first (reductional) division of meiosis I is greater in older than in younger women. Therefore, a meiotic I error might be predicted in an older woman who produces a trisomic child. Figure 3–16 illustrates proof of meiosis I error in such a situation. The chromosome polymorphisms have been quantitated by a technique using densitometry to record differences in Q-banding along chromosomes 21 from a child with Down syndrome (upper), father (middle), and older mother (lower). These are strip chart recorder tracings that record differences in intensity of fluorescence on the Y coordinate and differences in length of the chromosome on the X coordinate. In chromosome 21, the polymorphic area is in the region of the short arm, which on these tracings is to the left. In this analysis, the problem is to assign or match up the three trisomic chromosomes of the child at the top with the parental chromosomes below. It is fairly easy to see—and computer analysis has proved—that the child has three different-looking chromosomes number 21, two of which are from the mother and one of which is from the father. If you refer again to Figure 3–15 you will note that this situation is found in a meiotic I error. Since this error is in the older

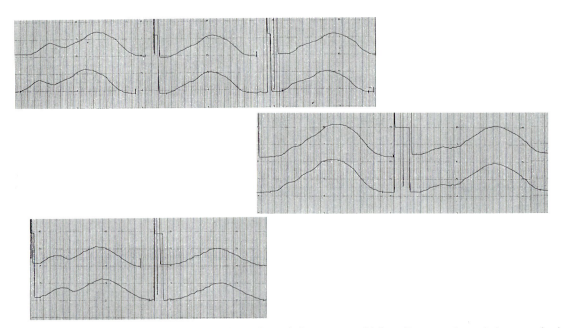

Figure 3–16 Densitometric strip chart recorder tracings of chromosomes 21 from Down syndrome index case *(top)*, father *(middle)*, and mother *(below)*. See text for details.

mother and not the father, our initial prediction is upheld in this example.

Autosomal Aneuploidy

Trisomy 21 and Down Syndrome. In 1959, Lejeune and his colleagues were the first to find that patients with Down syndrome had an extra chromosome belonging to group G. This additional chromosome is now accepted as number 21 on the basis of its characteristic banding pattern. Trisomy for the proximal part of subband 21q22 (Fig. 3–11) is responsible for the clinical syndrome. Production of an enzyme, superoxide dismutase (soluble), is also mapped to the same region on chromosome 21. Activity of this enzyme in trisomy 21 is dose related (i.e., is 1.5 times the level found in diploid individuals) and gene dosage also occurs at the transcriptional level. However, the relationship to clinical symptoms in Down syndrome is not understood. Mapping of human chromosomes and the significance of this important area of study for the understanding of chromosomal disease will be discussed again later.

In the past, a majority of cases of Down syndrome were age-dependent, associated with advancing age of the mother. Maternal meiotic nondisjunction is postulated to be a cause of these trisomic conditions. Exceptions to maternal age–dependence were soon studied in more detail. Some had the following characteristics: (1) There was a familial occurrence; (2) mothers were younger; (3) affected children had 46 instead of 47 chromosomes, but one was abnormal; (4) one clinically normal parent, more frequently but not exclusively the mother, had 45 chromosomes and one of these was the same unusual chromosome. It became apparent from study of this parent that the abnormal chromosome was a translocation of chromosome 21 to a D chromosome, usually number 14; in addition, the parent was missing a separate 21 and a separate number 14, making the total chromosome complement "balanced." The affected child had the 14/21 translocation, one separate 14 and two separate 21s producing clinical symptoms identical with those of trisomy 21. Figure 3–17 illustrates segregation of the involved chromosomes in meiosis of a 14/21 balanced carrier mother. If an ovum receives both a separate 21 and the 14/21 translocation, fertilization by a normal haploid sperm would result in a zygote with translocation Down syndrome.

Another form of Down syndrome is due to translocation of one chromosome 21 to another 21. In this situation, a balanced 21/21 carrier who transmits the translocation in meiosis could produce only offspring with Down syndrome after fertilization by a normal haploid gamete. Carrier state for translocation of 21 to other chromosomes is also reported as a cause of Down syndrome in offspring.

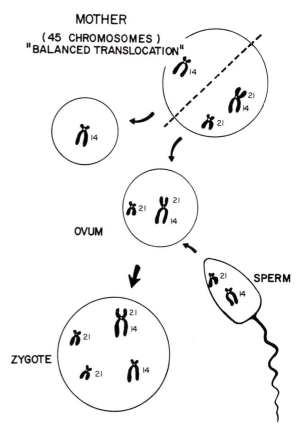

Figure 3–17 The mechanism for production of a 14/21 translocation Down syndrome (see text for detailed explanation). It should be noted that only the split of the primary oocyte producing Down syndrome of the translocation type is shown. Other splits of the oocyte would result in viable offspring with normal chromosomes or with the "balanced" carrier state.

Translocation accounts for only about 5 per cent of cases of Down syndrome followed after birth. Somewhat under 5 per cent are mosaics for 46/47, + 21 and have milder clinical symptoms. The remainder are 47, + 21 trisomics, either dependent or independent of maternal age. Now most genetic clinics are reporting an incidence of about 85 per cent maternal age–independent Down syndrome among cases ascertained by clinical symptoms after birth. Thus, by far the greatest number of individuals with clinical Down syndrome have trisomy 21 for reasons still unknown. Stratification of father's age by mother's reveals some paternal age association for trisomy 21, particularly when paternal age exceeds maternal age by at least 10 years. Penrose has postulated an autosomal recessive inheritance for trisomy 21, but many individual pedigrees do not support this hypothesis. Maternal irradiation, delayed fertilization, and infection are other postulated cases. Reproduction of an individual who is already trisomic is referred to as *secondary (inevitable) nondisjunction* and is known to result in trisomy in offspring. It is possible that a reservoir of undetected 46/47, + 21 mosaics in the general population could serve as a continuing source of trisomic Down syndrome.

Other Autosomal Trisomy Syndromes. Lejeune and coworkers also described a syndrome from full trisomy of chromosome 8. The clinical features are summarized in Table 3–6. Patau and others reported patients with retarded development and a very striking constellation of severe congenital malformations usually incompatible with life; the cause was trisomy of chromosome 13 (Table 3–6). As in the situation of Down syndrome, the clinical picture can also be produced by translocation of a chromosome 13 to another chromosome, most frequently another member of the D group. A slightly more common type of congenital malformation was described by Edwards and coworkers. In this form, there is trisomy of chromosome 18, the smallest member of the E group. Babies who reach term with this condition have characteristic clinical symptoms (Table 3–6). Another syndrome of congenital defects has now been established by banding analysis to be due to trisomy 22.

Sex Chromosomal Aneuploidy

Determination of Sex. The primitive gonad is bipotential and can develop into either an ovary or a testis, depending on the type of sex chromosomes (Fig. 3–18). The search for a testicular organizing substance has led to study of the *H-Y antigen,* a term describing those antigens found only on male cells that induce the formation of serum antibodies. There is now evidence that serologic expression of H-Y antigen maps to the short arm of the Y chromosome. This antigen can apparently direct testicular organization. Therefore, in humans the Y chromosome is male-determining and promotes testicular development from the medullary portion of the primitive gonad. In the presence of two X chromosomes, the cortex of the primitive gonad develops into an ovary. Importance of the Y chromosome is emphasized by the fact that an XXY individual is a male despite the presence of two X chromosomes. In fact, XXXY and XXXXY individuals are also phenotypic males despite the additional X chromosomes. However, a 45,X individual is phenotypically female, but one with failure of ovarian differentiation, and has Turner syndrome. The suggestion is that a second X chromosome is necessary for the primitive gonad to develop into a normal ovary.

Sex Chromatin. In 1949, some years before modern techniques of human chromosome analysis were developed, Barr and coworkers discovered a condensed chromatin mass in cell nuclei of females. A similar body was not present in cell nuclei of males. Female sex chromatin (Barr body; X body) usually appears as a planoconvex condensation of chromatin about 1μ in diameter along the nuclear membrane (Fig. 3–19, top). In 1970, bright fluorescence on the Y chromosome long arm was shown to give a bright spot in interphase, the male sex chromatin (Y body) (Fig. 3–20*A* and Fig. 3–21*A*). Quinacrine stain and fluorescence microscopy are required for its examination. Studies of female and male sex chromatin are very useful in screening for the number of X or Y chromosomes, respectively, present in an individual. In clinical practice, smears of the buccal mucosa are readily available, and these are usually studied.

An X body is seen in at least 15 to 20 per cent of readable buccal smear nuclei of the normal female. Its presence indicates two X chromosomes in the cell, one of which is "inactivated" or condensed to form the female sex chromatin. An X body is not seen in normal males (XY) or in patients with classic Turner syndrome (45,X). The XXX female has cells with two X bodies, and the XXXX individual has cells with three X bodies (Fig. 3–19, middle and bottom). Thus the rule follows: The number of X chromosomes is 1 + n, when n is the number of X bodies.

Condensed chromatin of the X body is associated not only with genetic inactivity and greater condensation of chromosomal DNA but also with late onset and completion of DNA replication within S period of the cell cycle. If tritiated thymidine is supplied to cells late in the S period, late-replicating X chromosomes will incorporate preferentially the tritium label. They will appear heavily labeled with exposed silver grains in photographic emulsion applied over metaphases on microscopic slides, a technique called *autoradiography* (Fig. 3–19). In more recent studies, 5-bromodeoxyuridine (BrdU) is added to cultured cells and, where it is incorporated into chromosomes in place of thymidine, stain by Giemsa or other chromatin dyes is decreased. Thus, late replicating regions along metaphase chromosomes can be

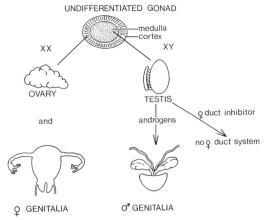

UNDIFFERENTIATED GONAD

medulla
cortex

XX — OVARY — and

XY — TESTIS — androgens

♀ duct inhibitor

no ♀ duct system

♀ GENITALIA   ♂ GENITALIA

Figure 3–18 Development of the gonads and genital ducts. (From Thompson, J. S., and Thompson, M. W.: Genetics in Medicine. 3rd ed. Philadelphia, W. B. Saunders Co., 1980.)

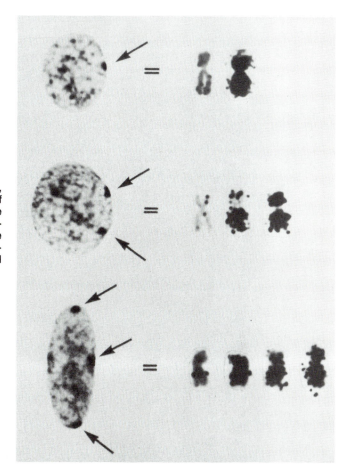

Figure 3–19 Three cell nuclei from XX, XXX, and XXXX individuals are shown. The number of X bodies is designated by the arrows. Alongside each nucleus are the X chromosomes from metaphases after labeling with tritiated thymidine. Note that all X chromosomes in excess of one are late-labeling. (Photograph courtesy of Professor Paul E. Polani.)

identified by differential stain. In fact, replication sequencing in general can be studied by the BrdU incorporation technique, a method referred to as *replication banding*.

A Y body (male sex chromatin) is seen in at least 50 per cent of readable buccal smear nuclei of normal males. Its presence indicates one Y chromosome in the cell; individuals with 47,XYY have two Y bodies (Figs. 3–20 and 3–21). Thus, the rule follows: The number of Y chromosomes is n, where n is the number of Y bodies. Variation in size of the fluorescent segment on the Y chromosome occurs normally and accounts for the overall variability in length of the Y. Rarely, the limits of normal variation are such that no fluorescent spot is seen in interphase in a normal XY individual with a small Y. Perhaps more commonly a heteromorphic region on an autosome can produce a brightly fluorescent region in interphase, resulting in a false "Y-like" body. These situations merely point out that sex chromatin analysis is only a screening procedure for chromosomal sex. Chromosome analysis is the definitive way to identify genetic sex.

Lyon Hypothesis. Observations on female sex chromatin along with other biologic studies on the genetics of mice led Mary Lyon to hypothesize that only one X chromosome is active in each cell during interphase. The second X chromosome, if we may use an analogy from sports, "takes to the sidelines" as an inactive condensed chromatin body. Furthermore, any additional X chromosome also becomes inactive and appears as an X body. This helps explain why additional X chromosomes do not have the same devastating effects that the presence of extra autosomes have in Down syndrome and the other autosomal trisomies.

Basic features of the Lyon hypothesis are that (1) in the female, one X chromosome is genetically inactive and forms the Barr body; (2) the decision about whether maternally derived (X^M) or paternally derived (X^P) chromosome is inactive is made early in embryonic life and is random in each cell; and (3) all cells subsequently have the same inactive X chromosome, either X^M or X^P. Therefore, these cells and all their descendants have the same active X chromosome, X^M or X^P.

The Lyon hypothesis clarifies some confusing

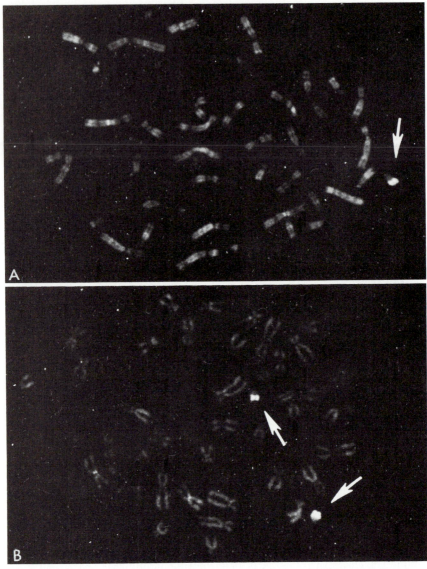

Figure 3–20 Metaphase chromosomes stained with quinacrine mustard. *A,* Photomicrograph showing the Y chromosome in a normal male, 46,XY. *B,* Photomicrograph illustrating two fluorescent Y chromosomes in a male with 47,XYY.

clinical and biologic problems pertaining to quantitative gene expression. Why does the male with only one X chromosome have the same amount of gene product for genes carried on the X chromosome as a female who has two X chromosomes? The level of glucose-6-phosphate dehydrogenase (G6PD), an enzyme with wide tissue distribution in the body, is controlled by an X-linked gene and is equivalent in normal males and females. Levels of X-linked coagulation Factor VIII (antihemophilic globulin) are also equivalent in normal men and women. The mechanism for this "dosage compensation" can be understood in light of the Lyon hypothesis if one of the two X chromosomes of the female is inactive in any particular cell.

Occasionally, a female heterozygous for the hemophilia trait has a bleeding disorder manifested by reduced circulating Factor VIII. Why is this X-linked recessive trait expressed? The Lyon hypothesis provides one explanation. Since inactivation of one X chromosome is initially a random event, by chance alone more X chromosomes containing the normal allele the Factor VIII could be inactivated; most cells, then, would express the mutant allele.

Turner Syndrome (Gonadal Dysgenesis). This syndrome is a form of primary hypogonadism in phenotypic females who have gonadal dysplasia, amenorrhea, short stature, and lack of secondary sex characteristics. A variety of congenital defects,

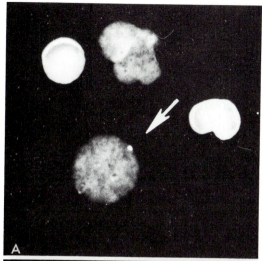

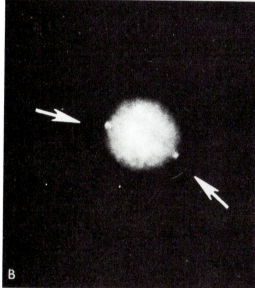

Figure 3–21 Peripheral blood lymphocytes stained with quinacrine mustard. *A,* Photomicrograph demonstrating a single Y body *(arrow). B,* Photomicrograph showing two Y bodies *(arrows)* in a patient with 47,XYY chromosomes.

is believed to account for only a small fraction of the total number of conceptions with the 45,X karyotype. Studies show that this karyotype occurs frequently in spontaneously aborted fetuses. The frequency with which it is found suggests that most of such conceptuses are aborted, and only less than 10 per cent survive to be born and show Turner syndrome.

Interesting associations with Turner syndrome are the clinical accompaniment of Hashimoto's thyroiditis and the even more frequent finding of circulating antibodies to thyroglobulin. These associations may be more common in patients with isochromosome X, described in the next paragraph. The question is raised whether development of antibodies is the consequence of the chromosomal abnormality or whether the reverse might be true. A high incidence of thyroid antibodies has been found in families of these patients, suggesting that the tendency to autoantibody formation in parents might be related to chromosomal abnormalities of the children.

In contrast to the majority of patients with Turner syndrome, a minority were found to be X-chromatin positive, with a normal number of chromosomes. In some of these patients, all the 44 autosomes were normal, as would be expected, and a single normal-appearing X chromosome was present. The other X was a structurally abnormal isochromosome. This chromosome is believed to arise as a result of misdivision through the centromere (as illustrated in Figure 3–22). In this situation, an isochromosome composed of two X long arms shows a characteristic banding pattern, since both arms are mirror images of each other. Isochromosomes for the X short arm apparently do not survive; banding studies do not confirm their existence. It is clear, however, that X chromosomes can break in different places, forming partial isochromosomes, X duplications, or X-X translocations. (Structural abnormalities of chromosomes are described again in the next section.) In the decision as to which X chromosome makes an X body at the time of inactivation, an abnormal X usually becomes the inactive one. X long arm isochromosomes are longer than a normal X and produce a morphologically larger Barr body.

Instances of Turner syndrome with one normal X and a deleted X have been described. The deleted X is termed *Xp-* or *Xq-,* depending on the site of deletion. A ring X, termed *r(X),* is usually considered a form of X deletion, since intact opposite ends of chromosomes do not normally form rings. Therefore, the existence of terminal deletions is assumed but often is difficult to prove, even with banding. Deleted X chromosomes form morphologically smaller X bodies.

Turner mosaics are described with reasonable frequency. Among these are 45,X/46,XX; 45,X/46,XY; 45,X/47,XXX; 45,X/47,XYY; and some with three cell lines, as 45,X/46,XX/47,XXX. The number of Barr bodies per cell and the percentage

including webbing of the neck and coarctation of the aorta, may accompany this syndrome. Nipples are widely spaced on the chest, and pigmented nevi are frequently present on the skin. Lymphedema has been described in the early weeks of life, especially on the feet and lower extremities. The syndrome is accompanied by high gonadotropin secretion in urine and low urinary estrogens, as would be expected in primary gonadal failure. Many of these individuals are X-body negative, and cytogenic studies have shown that their karyotype is 45,X. The incidence of this karyotype in surveys of newborns is about one per 10,000 females.

The number of patients with Turner syndrome

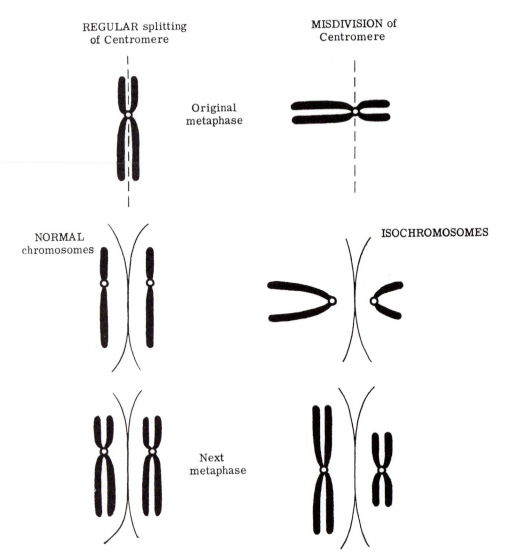

REGULAR splitting of Centromere

MISDIVISION of Centromere

Original metaphase

NORMAL chromosomes

ISOCHROMOSOMES

Next metaphase

Figure 3–22 The mechanism for production of an isochromosome. (From Hamerton, J. L. [ed.]: Chromosomes in Medicine. London, William Heinemann Medical Books, Ltd., 1962.)

of X-body positive cells in buccal smear may be useful in screening for these mosaics. All forms of Turner syndrome other than 45,X may be termed *Turner variants*. They have varying degrees of involvement with features of the syndrome, although gonadal dysgenesis and short stature usually are present. The exact role of the X chromosome in determining stature is not presently settled. Turner variants with a cell line containing a Y chromosome are at risk for gonadal tumors, and therefore the cytogenetic diagnosis is critical for their management.

Originally, it was felt that 45,X Turner syndrome had its origin in meiotic nondisjunction (Fig. 3–23), but another explanation for occurrence of the chromosomal abnormalities found in Turner syndrome has its basis in the relative frequency of mosaic types. This hypothesis suggests that nondisjunction occurs soon after formation of the zygote rather than before. If one X in a cell division of a 46,XX line fails to enter a daughter cell, subsequent cell development could be 45,X/46,XX; if chromatids of one X in a 46,XX cell separate but move to the same daughter cell, subsequently cells should be 45,X/47,XXX or 45,X/46,XX/ 47,XXX; if the Y in a 46,XY cell is not included in a daughter cell, the result would be 45,X or 45,X/46,XY; and so forth. Mosaicism need not necessarily occur if one cell line is lost, particularly if the abnormal cell division occurs very early in the development of the zygote. Absence of a clear maternal-age effect associated with Turner syndrome gives support for the idea that some cases are due to somatic nondisjunction.

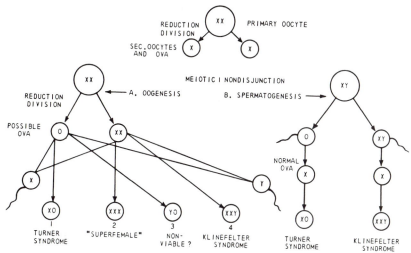

Figure 3–23 Meiotic division and nondisjunction. In normal meiotic division of a primary oocyte, each of the secondary oocytes and ova contains one X chromosome *(upper figure)*. For simplification, the polar bodies are ignored. The same process in spermatogenesis leads to X- or Y-containing sperm. *A,* In meiotic I nondisjunction involving oogenesis, an ovum with no X chromosomes and another with both X chromosomes are shown. In each instance, the result of fertilization by an X-containing sperm and the result of fertilization by a Y-containing sperm are depicted. The possible combinations could lead to Turner syndrome, an XXX "super-female," or Klinefelter syndrome. The YO offspring has not yet been shown for humans. Meiotic nondisjunction is shown occurring in spermatogenesis. Each possible sperm is shown fertilizing a normal ovum.

Multiple-X Females. The normal female has two X chromosomes, but females with more than two X chromosomes have been described. The triple-X female (47,XXX) has two X bodies (Fig. 3–19, middle). Although the first patient with this disorder had amenorrhea and gonadal dysgenesis, no consistent clinical picture has subsequently been defined. Some are fertile and produce clinically normal children. Renal malformations occur with some regularity.

Tetra-X females (48,XXXX) with three X bodies (Fig. 3–19, bottom) and penta-X females (49,XXXXX) with four X bodies have also been described.

Klinefelter Syndrome. This syndrome is a form of primary hypogonadism and infertility in the male. The condition was described in 1942 in phenotypic males who had small, firm testes, azoospermia, and elevated levels of gonadotropin in urine. Gynecomastia occurs in 40 to 50 per cent of the cases. Its association with some degree of mental retardation is evident because of the increased incidence of Klinefelter syndrome in some institutions for the mentally retarded. In the mid 1950s it was first discovered that a number of individuals with the Klinefelter phenotype were X-chromatin positive. Soon after the application of cytogenetic techniques, it was found that these patients had a karyotype of 47,XXY. Now it can be shown that both X and Y bodies are present in the same cell. The incidence of this karyotype in surveys of newborns is about one per 1000 males.

It does not appear to be a usual cause of spontaneous abortion. Several mosaic varieties of Klinefelter syndrome such as 46,XY/47,XXY and 46,XX/47,XXY have been described. The syndrome in some of these patients is incomplete.

One origin of the abnormal karyotype is nondisjunction in meiosis (Fig. 3–23). Pedigree studies using color vision and other X-linked genes as markers indicate maternal or paternal origin for the nondisjunction. Another theoretic mechanism is mitotic nondisjunction.

Additional varieties of Klinefelter syndrome have 48,XXXY and 49,XXXXY chromosomes. The clinical picture of hypogonadism is present, but there may be a greater degree of mental retardation. The 49,XXXXY patients may have several additional features, including radioulnar synostosis and more severe hypogonadism, with hypoplasia of the penis and scrotum.

XYY Individuals. In 1965, a syndrome was described in males with two Y chromosomes. These men were tall, showed antisocial aggressive behavior, and were incarcerated because of crimes of a violent nature. More recent studies have shown that the incidence of this karyotype is not as infrequent as was originally thought. In surveys of newborn infants, the incidence is about one per 1000 males. As these individuals are followed to adulthood, they do not manifest the aggressive behavior problems noted in the biased earlier studies of cases ascertained because of placement in penal institutions.

STRUCTURAL ABNORMALITIES OF THE CHROMOSOMES

Although total number may be normal, the chromosomes may be abnormal in structure (Table 3–5). Structurally abnormal chromosomes have already been considered in connection with Turner syndrome, since structural abnormalities of the X (isochromosome, deletion, ring, translocation) can produce some clinical features resembling complete absence of an X. Structural abnormalities of autosomes, with or without change in total number, can produce clinical features of full or partial trisomies or monosomies or deletion syndromes.

Translocations

If a separated chromosomal fragment becomes attached to another chromosome, it is said to be translocated. Sometimes parts of two different chromosomes exchange places with each other, producing a reciprocal translocation (Fig. 3–24). If the translocated pieces are large enough, the chromosomes involved will be morphologically altered and can be recognized as abnormal. If, however, the translocated pieces are very small, they may be difficult to recognize under the microscope. Small but clinically significant translocations may be undetected for this reason. Translocations can be balanced or unbalanced genetically, examples being the 14/21 and 21/21 translocations already discussed in connection with Down syndrome. Recall that total chromosome number can also be changed by this type of translocation, usually referred to as *centric fusion,* or *Robertsonian translocation.*

Deletions

A number of syndromes associated with the deletion of a piece of chromosome have now been reported (Table 3–7). A well-characterized one is 5p- syndrome, or cri du chat syndrome, first described by Lejeune and others in 1963. The major feature of this disorder is a characteristic mewing cry like that of a cat. The peculiar cry results from abnormal development of the larynx, and this feature is lost as the infant grows older. Some cases are due to translocation, and under these circumstances one parent may be a carrier.

A brief summary of the clinical findings in other deletion syndromes is presented in Table 3–7. Note the overlap between different syndromes as well as characteristic features.

Inversions

Inversions can result from two breaks along the course of a chromosome and realignment after a 180-degree reversal of the order of the chromosome. If the breaks are on the same side of the centromere, a paracentric inversion occurs and the realignment does not change the shape of the chromosome. If the breaks occur on opposite sides of the centromere, a pericentric inversion occurs; if the segments are unequal in size, the position of the centromere may be altered.

Pericentric inversions of chromosome 9 are estimated to occur in about 1 per cent of the normal population in heterozygous form. Although such inversions theoretically could result in unequal crossing-over during meiosis, infertility, fetal loss, and recombinant offspring are probably not in-

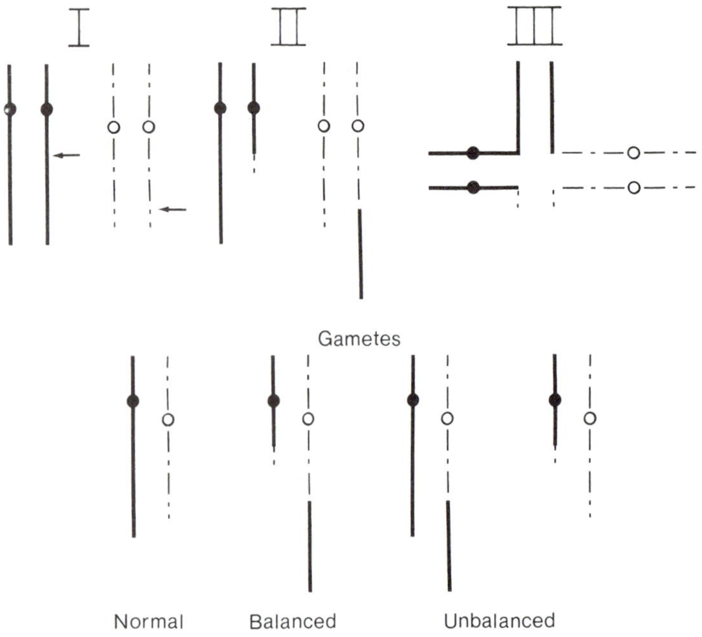

Gametes

Normal   Balanced   Unbalanced

Figure 3–24 Reciprocal translocation and its consequences. Origin by breakage of two nonhomologous chromosomes (I) and reconstitution with the broken ends interchanged (II) are shown. At meiosis, a cross-shaped figure is formed (III) in order for pairing of homologous regions to occur. Gametes formed by this translocation heterozygote are normal and balanced (diagonal separations in part III of diagram) and unbalanced (upper from lower separation in part III of diagram). It is also possible, although less common, for segregation to occur such that both homologous centromeres pass to one gamete (left from right separation in part III of diagram), again producing unbalanced gametes. Normal or balanced gametes result in phenotypically normal offspring, but unbalanced gametes result in zygotes that are partially trisomic and partially monosomic and consequently develop abnormally. (From Thompson, J. S., and Thompson, M. W.: Genetics in Medicine. 3rd ed. Philadelphia, W. B. Saunders Co., 1980.)

TABLE 3–7 THE DELETION SYNDROMES

Chromosome Deletion	Characteristic Clinical Findings
4p-	Midline scalp defect; colobomas; ptosis of eye lids; preauricular dimple or sinus; beaked nose; cleft palate; carplike mouth; hypospadias (males); small birth weight; sacral dimple or sinus; oblique nail striations; severe psychomotor retardation; seizures; delayed bone maturation.
5p-	Small head; hypertelorism; narrow ear canals; high palate; heart disease; hypotonia; cry like a cat; poor muscular development.
13q-	Microcephaly; arrhinencephaly; colobomas; microphthalmia; micrognathia; congenital heart disease; imperforate anus; hypospadias, bifid scrotum; hand and foot anomalies; psychomotor retardation.
18q-	Small head, asymmetric face; hypertelorism; hearing loss, narrow ear canals; maxillary hypoplasia; high palate; heart and renal malformations; failure to thrive; proximally placed thumbs; abnormal toe implantation; hypotonia; mental retardation.
21q-	Antimongoloid slant of eyes; prominent nasal bridge; micrognathia; skeletal malformations; growth retardation; psychomotor retardation; hypertonia.
22q-	Epicanthal folds; microcephaly; high palate; syndactyly of toes; psychomotor retardation; hypotonia.

creased in inversion 9 heterozygotes. Inversions in other chromosomes occur in normal individuals but may result in unbalanced progeny. During evolution, inversions may serve to preserve certain chromosome sequences, since crossing-over produces decreased viability.

CHROMOSOMES AND NEOPLASIA

Leukemia and Lymphomas

In 1961, Nowell and Hungerford reported the association of a G-group chromosomal abnormality with chronic myelogenous leukemia. One chromosome had lost almost half of the distal long arm. This finding was believed to be a deletion, although translocation involving another larger chromosome could not be ruled out. The abnormality was called a *Ph¹ chromosome*, or *Philadelphia chromosome*, after the place of first report. Subsequently, a reciprocal translocation that usually involves chromosomes 22 and 9 was shown (Fig. 3–25). Consistent chromosome exchanges are now regularly observed in specific human leuke-

mias and lymphomas. Concordance between the chromosome location of certain human cellular oncogenes (normal genes homologous to sequences in viruses known to produce cancer) and the breakpoints involved in these chromosome rearrangements is becoming evident. As an example, a translocation common in Burkitt's lymphoma moves the *c-myc* cellular oncogene on chromosome 8 to the locus for the immunoglobulin heavy-chain gene on 14. Removal of normal control could accompany the rearrangement and be a part of the neoplastic process.

Solid Tumors

High-resolution banding tells us that an interstitial deletion in the proximal long arm of chromosome 13 is associated with bilateral retinoblastoma and that an interstitial deletion in the short arm of chromosome 11 is associated with aniridia–Wilms' tumor syndrome. The cellular oncogene for *c-ras* is located at the site of the deletion in chromosome 11. The deletion or, possibly, other mechanisms could remove normal control. These two deletions just mentioned are interesting in that they can be observed in peripheral blood and are not confined to tumor tissue.

Chromosome Breakage Syndromes

Several inherited diseases associated with chromosomal breaks have stimulated a great deal of interest, particularly since they are also associated with leukemia, lymphoma, or solid tumor formation. Bloom syndrome is a rare autosomal recessive disorder characterized by sun-sensitive telangiectatic skin, erythema, low birth weight, stunted growth, and increased chromosome breakage. There are also chromosome rearrangements, some consisting of quadriradial figures (pairing of somatic chromosomes) that are thought to represent cytologic evidence for somatic crossing-over. Leukemia is the more common neoplasm in this disorder.

Fanconi anemia is another disease associated with autosomal recessive inheritance and chromosome breakage, as well as pancytopenia, skin pigmentation, congenital malformations of the skeleton, hypogonadism, and increased risk of leukemia.

Ataxia-telangiectasia (Louis-Bar syndrome) is also associated with chromosomal instability and neoplasia. In this disorder there are progressive cerebellar ataxia, multiple telangiectasia of skin and eye, and recurrent sinopulmonary infections. The inheritance is autosomal recessive.

In the three genetic disorders just mentioned, chromosomal instability has been documented by direct cytogenic observation in individuals homozygous or heterozygous for the responsible genes.

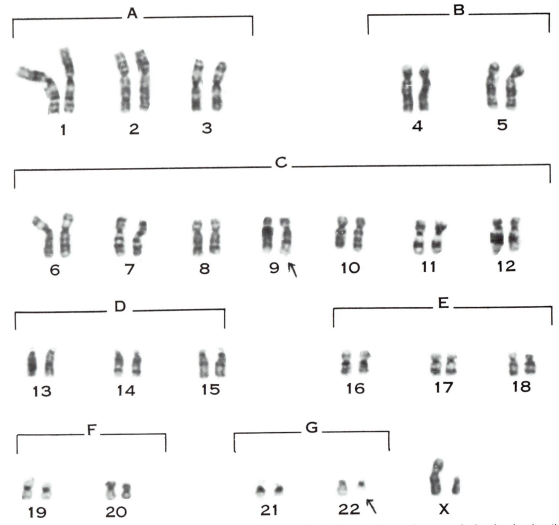

Figure 3–25 Photomicrograph of a metaphase from a patient with chronic myelogenous leukemia showing the translocation between chromosomes 9 and 22 *(arrows)*.

In a fourth genetic disorder, xeroderma pigmentosum, chromosome breaks and rearrangements are less obvious but nevertheless appear to be present, particularly in skin cultures at later subcultures. The inheritance is autosomal recessive, and affected individuals are prone to multiple skin cancers in areas exposed to sunlight. Cultured cells from affected individuals are shown to be defective in DNA repair.

In the disorders just discussed, the critical question is whether a cell with chromosomal rearrangements could become the start of a malignant cell line.

CHROMOSOME MAPPING

The goal of human gene mapping is to determine chromosomal location of all known specific genes. In general terms, the accomplishments of this endeavor would provide a better understanding of how genes function and would be a prerequisite for genetic engineering. The classic method of mapping human genes has been to follow the pattern of inheritance of individual single gene traits through many generations of a family to learn what traits are linked or associated with one another on a single chromosome. Sometimes the exact chromosome could be identified, particularly if it was an X, and in a few cases the linear order of genes and some estimate of their distance apart could be determined by this method.

Newer cytogenetic techniques have permitted identification of chromosome polymorphisms, and these could in turn be used as markers to locate genes coding for specific traits or enzymes. Another method, deletion mapping, has been useful to some extent because if part of a chromosome is absent, products of the missing genes will also be absent.

Nevertheless, family studies in human populations are extremely difficult because families are relatively small, generation time is long, and controlled breeding is not possible. The technique of somatic cell hybridization has greatly increased our ability to map chromosomes, such that each chromosome now has assignments and some chromosomes have many. This method allows fusion of two genetically different parent cells.

The experience to date with chromosomes in hybrid cells, particularly human–other animal cell crosses, shows that there is preferential loss of human chromosomes. If the loss of particular human chromosomes can be correlated with absence of specific gene functions, a step is taken toward gene localization. This problem can be approached statistically, as shown in Table 3–8. In this example, the expression of an enzyme (peptidase A) is correlated with presence of human chromosome 18. Different hybrid cell cultures were each grown, or cloned, from single mouse-human hybrid cells, and each cloned culture was analyzed for presence (+) or absence (−) of peptidase A activity and of particular human chromosomes. Concordant cloned cultures show presence or absence of chromosome and enzyme expression, respectively, whereas discordant cultures show presence of one and absence of the other. Ideally, all clones are concordant and none discordant if enzyme expression is correlated with a particular chromosome. In this example, for chromosome 18 there are 27 concordant and one discordant, the closest fit in this data set. The discordant clone was classified as enzyme (−) and chromosome 18 (+), but in the particular culture only a small percentage of cells were chromosome (+) in spite of cloning, and the enzyme activity was difficult to measure. (Experiments are rarely if ever perfect!)

Results of human chromosome mapping can be summarized by locating symbols for the gene products on the chromosome diagrams presented in Figure 3–11. If exact chromosome location is known, the symbol is placed next to the appropriate band and region. This approach is limited to the kinds of gene products that can be measured in hybrid cell cultures.

MOLECULAR BASIS FOR INHERITANCE

The basic unit of inheritance first postulated by Mendel must have at least three properties: (1) It must control a specific function in the organism; (2) it must replicate and transmit this function from one generation to the next; and (3) it must mutate and produce variations in this function. The basic unit of inheritance should be present in all cells of the organism. The physical basis for these properties is satisfied by the chromosome. Reduction division seen during meiosis and gamete formation, recombination during zygote formation, chromosome replication preceding mitosis, and phenotypic aberrations associated with abnormal chromosomes satisfy these requirements.

Watson and Crick, in 1953, first pointed out that deoxyribonucleic acid (DNA) was a biochemical contained in bacteria and in the cell nucleus of mammals that satisfied requirements for the basic unit of inheritance at a molecular level. The double-helical model, with its base pairs oriented internally and joined by noncovalent bonds, provides a molecular method of replication. Each strand can unwind, separate, and serve as a template for replication of a new thread derived from substrates in the cell. A single strand of DNA permits only the insertion of that base complementary to it on the new strand of DNA as it grows alongside the original strand. This semiconservative model for replication of the DNA molecule was confirmed by Meselson and Stahl in 1958 (Fig. 3–26). The original parent molecule of DNA dissociates, and each strand directs the synthesis of a new strand complementary to itself. Thus, the first generation daughter molecules contain one original and one newly synthesized helical strand. In the second generation, half the molecules are composed of two new strands and half contain an

TABLE 3–8 CORRELATION OF PEPTIDASE A EXPRESSION WITH PRESENCE OF HUMAN CHROMOSOMES

Human Chromosome	Number of Concordant Clones* +/+ or −/−	Number of Discordant Clones* +/− or −/+
1	21	7
2	19	9
3	21	7
4	14	14
5	18	10
6	16	12
7	19	9
8	16	12
9	17	11
10	23	5
11	20	8
12	15	13
13	20	8
14	—	—
15	—	—
16	18	10
17	19	9
18	27	1
19	15	13
20	17	11
21	18	10
22	13	15
X	22	6
Y	17	11

*Presence (+) or absence (−) of enzyme activity is placed to the left of diagonal line (/) and presence (+) or absence (−) of human chromosome to the right.

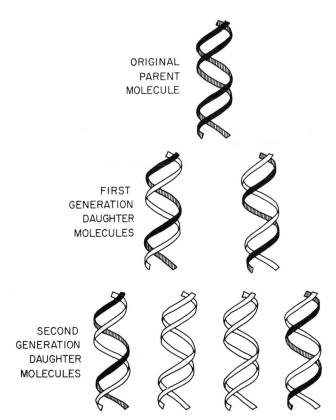

ORIGINAL
PARENT
MOLECULE

FIRST
GENERATION
DAUGHTER
MOLECULES

SECOND
GENERATION
DAUGHTER
MOLECULES

Figure 3–26 Model for semiconservative DNA replication. Solid, black helical strands represent original DNA molecules; open, white strands represent freshly synthesized DNA. In the first generation, there is a 1:1 ratio of old to freshly synthesized strands. In the second generation, only 2 of 8, or one fourth, are original strands. (From Meselson, M., and Stahl, F. W.: Proc. Natl. Acad. Sci. U.S.A. *44*:671, 1958.)

original and a newly formed strand. In microbial systems, purified DNA polymerase can use a primer single strand of DNA and replicate by matching one of the four deoxyribose triphosphates (GTP, ATP, CTP, or TTP) with the complementary base on the primer strand. The chain grows by adding appropriate bases at the 3′ hydroxy group and releasing pyrophosphate. DNA replication in chromosomes of higher organisms is more complex. Several points along the chromosome may replicate at the same time. Because mutants for DNA replication in eukaryotes have been difficult to obtain, the detailed enzymology of DNA replication in humans has not yet been worked out. Helix-destabilizing proteins and a DNA helicase produce a fork. DNA polymerase then proceeds in either continuous or short series along the leading and lagging parent strands. RNA primers are made and used to start new DNA molecules. These replicated strands are finished by DNA ligase, which seals the 3′ end to the 5′ end of the previous fragment. A major difference in eukaryotic DNA replication is that it is not bare DNA but chromatin that is replicated. Chromatin is composed of tightly bound histone proteins that coil into nucleosomes of some 200 base-pair-interval disks. Nucleotide spacing of replication DNA is shorter and the speed of replication is slower for eukaryotic DNA than for prokaryotic DNA.

The double-helix model provides several possibilities for error or mutation. For instance, the base might exist in its tautomeric form and, during replication, pair with a new base not complementary to the original strand. This erroneous base would then direct the insertion of a new base complementary to itself in the second and subsequent generations. Mutations are produced also by chemicals that are structurally similar to the bases. Bromodeoxyuridine is structurally similar to thymine but pairs with guanine rather than adenine. If this pyrimidine analog were incorporated into the DNA strand, guanine would replace adenine in subsequently formed strands. Many other mutagenic agents are known, such as acridine dyes, nitrogen mustards, nitrous acid, and ultraviolet light. Ultraviolet light increases the incidence of interaction between bases on the same strand. These dimers (thymine-thymine) are excised in one process (dark repair). With the other DNA strand as a template, new bases are then inserted. Abnormalities in this repair mechanism are reflected in humans by the disease xeroderma pigmentosum. In this autosomal recessive trait, an endonuclease necessary to initiate repair is defective, and thymine-thymine dimers are not excised at a normal rate.

The DNA molecule can replicate and undergo variation. How does it relate to the organ or cell function? It is known from studies of bacteria and from examples in mammalian systems that the amino acid sequence of a polypeptide chain is determined by the sequence of bases on a single strand of DNA. The basic model for transcription and translation is briefly summarized in Figure 3–27.

There are three classes of ribonucleic acid (RNA) that enable DNA to direct the synthesis of polypeptides. Messenger RNA (mRNA) is formed upon a template of single-stranded DNA. It is a single-stranded nucleic acid similar to DNA but contains ribose rather than deoxyribose and uracil (U) instead of thymine (T). Messenger RNA associates with a second class of stable RNA, ribosomal RNA in the cytoplasm. Amino acids in the cytoplasm are activated by "activating enzymes" and "recognized" by a third class of RNA, soluble (transfer) RNA (sRNA). Soluble RNA has an additional recognition site that binds to complementary base on the mRNA strand. Each amino acid has a specific sRNA that attaches to its carboxy end and to the mRNA-ribosomal complex at the complementary site on the mRNA template. The sequence of amino acids is determined by the mRNA strand, and the amino acids are covalently bound at their carboxy terminal. The length of this peptide is determined by punctuation marks in the genetic code.

Various control mechanisms between DNA and its expression as a polypeptide chain have been postulated from microbial systems. The operon model of Jacob and Monod is indicated in Figure 3–28. In their negative control hypothesis, a repressor protein prevents the structural genes from producing mRNA by binding to a site on the DNA molecule called an *operator*. In the presence of an inducer, the repressor protein is inactivated and does not bind to the operator, and the structural genes in the operon are transcribed. There is indirect evidence for the existence of these working models of DNA regulation in mammalian cells, although no operon per se has been defined.

Eukaryotic DNA has several distinctive regions that do not code for protein but that are important in control of transcription to, and subsequent processing of, messenger RNA. Recognition sites include promoter regions, terminator regions, ribosomal recognition sites for mRNA binding, and control genes. Of current interest are *intervening sequences,* or *introns,* large regions of DNA nucleotides that are transcribed but not translated (Fig. 3–28). These sequences may contain mutations that do not allow for proper processing of messenger RNA and prevent proper gene expression. Examples in humans are those "leaky," or β^+, thalassemias in which splicing of introns is impaired owing to a mutation with subsequent reduction in the *rate* of mature mRNA production and consequent production of β-globin chains. Human DNA is also characterized by sequences of *pseudogenes*. These resemble active genes but are neither transcribed nor translated. In various studies, when complementary ^{32}P-labeled DNA for the human enzyme argininosuccinic acid synthase was hybridized to the human karyotype, it was found that many chromosomes contained DNA that hybridized but that was not expressed. The eukaryotic mRNA differs in several ways from prokaryotic mRNA. It is more stable because of 5′ capping with 7-methylguanylate with its methylated riboses (CAP) and polyadenylation at the 3′ terminus. It is also complexed with proteins that may protect and prolong half-life. This stability is important because it enables splicing of intervening sequences (introns) and joining of exons that eventually will be exported from the nucleus and translated to protein. Export through nuclear membrane and binding to ribosomes for translation must be protected from phosphatases

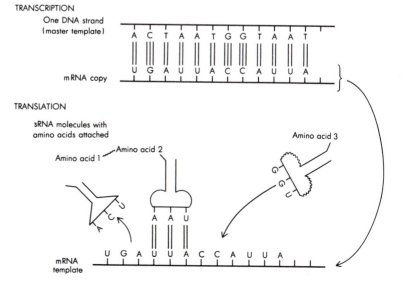

Figure 3–27 A model for the transcription and translation of DNA into proteins. (From Hartman, P. E., and Suskind, S. R.: Gene Action. Foundations of Modern Genetics Series. Englewood Cliffs, Prentice-Hall, Inc., 1965.)

TRANSCRIPTION

One DNA strand (master template)

A C T A A T G G T A A T

U G A U U A C C A U U A

mRNA copy

TRANSLATION

sRNA molecules with amino acids attached

Amino acid 1

Amino acid 2

Amino acid 3

A A U

U G A U U A C C A U U A

mRNA template

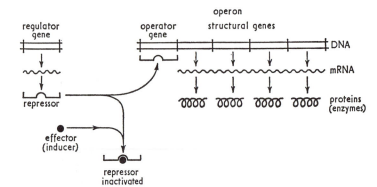

Figure 3–28 The operon model for the negative regulation of mRNA synthesis. Normally, a regulator gene produces a repressor protein that binds to an operator portion of DNA, preventing other genes in the operon from transcribing mRNA. An inducer inactivates the repressor protein, allowing expression of structural genes. (From Davidson, N. J.: The Biochemistry of the Nucleic Acis, 5th ed. New York, Methuen and Co., 1965.)

and exonucleases (Fig. 3–29). The mature eukaryotic message is usually monocistronic as compared with operons or polycistronic messages of bacteria. Thus, "one gene–one polypeptide chain" still applies as a genetic axiom in humans, but the mechanisms involved in the intermediary processes are complex and important in the pathogenesis of human disease.

Regulatory mechanisms exist not only at these processing steps for messenger RNA but also at levels of nuclear membrane transport and translation of mRNA into peptides. The newly synthesized peptide chains also undergo complex modifications with glycosylation and interaction of the peptides with others to form functioning proteins.

A precise definition of the mRNA code for specific amino acids became possible following the discovery by Nirenberg that polyphenylalanine is formed when an artificial mRNA, polyuridylic acid, is added to bacterial ribosomes. The genetic code described in microbial systems functions in higher organisms, including humans. The essential features of the genetic code are that each amino acid is dictated by a sequence of three bases (triplet codons). These triplet codons are arranged in a linear fashion and do not overlap, so that one group of three specifies one amino acid, the next group of three specifies a second amino acid, and so on. The four bases of an mRNA strand (UCAG) can occur in 64 different triplet sequences. Sixty-one triplet combinations are known to specify one of the 20 amino acids. Most of the amino acids have more than one code word, and therefore the genetic code is said to be degenerate. Thus, the process of gene expression in mammalian cells proposes a sequence of events by which single strands of nuclear DNA transcribe their triplet codons to pre-mRNA, which is processed and spliced to mature mRNA, which proceeds through the nuclear membrane and associates with cyto-

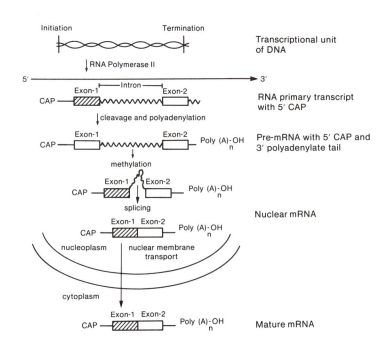

Figure 3–29 Schematic representation of processing of eukaryotic messenger RNA.

plasmic ribosomal complexes. Specific "activated" amino acids bound to tRNA are then added in a linear fashion to form polypeptide chains. A large amount of post-translational change occurs in mammalian polypeptides. In fact, the addition of oligosaccharides is responsible for subcellular localization. *I-cell disease* in humans results from impaired phosphorylation of oligosaccharides on newly synthesized acid hydrolases. They are not directed to lysosomes but instead leak out into the extracellular spaces. Glycosylation and helical formation of collagen are necessary to promote extracellular transport, and defects in these post-translational controls produce *Ehlers-Danlos syndrome, type VI.*

HEMOGLOBIN VARIANTS: A HUMAN MODEL OF MOLECULAR DISEASE

The first direct evidence that gene mutations result in altered human proteins came from observations regarding sickle cell anemia. This disease occurs in a small percentage (1 to 2 per cent) of black populations. It is expressed by severe anemia, infarctions of various organs such as the kidney and lungs, susceptibility to bone infections, and death, frequently in the second decade of life. Erythrocytes subjected to low oxygen tensions became elongated, filamentous, and sickle-shaped. Sickling of the erythrocytes can be demonstrated in 8 per cent of the black population of the United States, and this may occur in the absence of disease. Individuals with sickling are said to have sickle trait. Neel suggested that individuals with the sickle trait were heterozygous and those expressing disease were homozygous for an abnormal gene producing sickle hemoglobin S. Family studies further supported this hypothesis. In 1949, Pauling and coworkers demonstrated that normal hemoglobin and hemoglobin S differed in their electrophoretic properties. Red cells from normal individuals contained only hemoglobin A, but cells from patients with sickle cell trait contained both hemoglobin A and hemoglobin S. A third abnormal hemoglobin, hemoglobin C, was discovered by Itano and Neel. In family studies, this hemoglobin was also determined by a single gene, and heterozygotes for this gene had both hemoglobin A and hemoglobin C in their red blood cells. Homozygotes for the mutant C gene formed only hemoglobin C but clinically had only a mild anemia. That the two mutations were allelic became evident when patients with both mutant hemoglobins were found (double heterozygotes). Since the two hemoglobins were readily differentiated by electrophoresis, pedigree analysis of the two mutations (hemoglobin C and hemoglobin S) could be made. When one parent was a double heterozygote (SC) and the other was normal (AA), offspring were produced with either hemoglobin C trait (AC) or sickle cell trait (AS). No offspring were doubly heterozygous (SC) or homozygous normal (AA). Thus, hemoglobin S, C, and A segregated during meiosis and were presumably alleles.

A molecular basis for these pedigrees became evident when the structure of the variant hemoglobins was determined. Normal hemoglobin A was found to contain four polypeptide chains, two alpha (α_2) and two beta (β_2) chains, each with a characteristic amino acid sequence. The α-chain contained 141 amino acids, the β-chain 146 amino acids, and their precise sequences have been established. The nature of the difference between hemoglobin A and hemoglobin S was determined by Ingram in 1957 when he found that one amino acid in the β-polypeptide chain at position 6 was occupied by glutamic acid in hemoglobin A and by valine in hemoglobin S. This position was subsequently found to be occupied by a lysine residue in hemoglobin C (Table 3–9). In all three of these β-polypeptide chains, the sequence of the other

TABLE 3–9 MUTANT CODONS AND THEIR IDENTIFICATION BY ANALYSIS OF DNA FRAGMENTS PRODUCED BY RESTRICTION ENDONUCLEASES

Variant β-Globin	Amino Acid Sequence at Positions	DNA Sequence at Positions	Size (Kb) of DNA Fragments Produced by:	
			Mst II*	Dde I†
	__ 5 __ 6 __ 7 __	__ 5 __ 6 __ 7 __		
A	__ Pro __ Glu __ Glu __	__ CCT __ GAG __ GAG __	1.15, 0.20	0.17, 0.20
S	__ Pro __ Val __ Glu__	__ CCT __ GTG __ GAG __	1.35	0.37
C	__ Pro __ Lys __ Glu __	__ CCT __ **AAG** __ GAG__	1.15, 0.20	0.17, 0.20

*Mst II recognizes and excises at __/CCTNAGG⌐__ .
†Dde I recognizes and excises at __/CTNAG⌐__ .
"N" represents any nucleotide.

145 amino acids was identical. Thus, the mutations were occurring not only at the same locus but also at the same amino acid position of the chain. In molecular terms, the gene is defined as that sequence of DNA that produces a functional polypeptide chain. The mutations for S and C hemoglobin occur within the gene at identical codon sites (point mutations) and are homoallelic.

There are now powerful methods of diagnosing these types of mutations at the DNA level. By using ^{32}P-labeled complementary DNA probes and cutting up these probes and DNA from patients, one can create maps of DNA fragments to diagnose human diseases at the DNA or gene level (Fig. 3–30 and Table 3–9). Again, the prototypes for this approach have been the hemoglobinopathies. As outlined in Table 3–9, single amino acid substitutions at position 6 of the β-globin chain are caused by single base substitutions. Two restriction endonucleases, Dde I and Mst II, recognize nucleotide sequences that are altered in the sickle globin chain mutation and cause the enzyme to skip over this site. Thus, when the DNA fragments are analyzed by in-situ hybridization after electrophoresis, one large DNA fragment is produced rather than two smaller ones (Fig. 3–30 and Table 3–9). This approach is very important for such diagnostic needs as prenatal monitoring because the sequence of nucleotides in DNA is present even if the gene is not expressed as β-globin. Therefore, a fetus making only 3 to 5 per cent of its hemoglobin from β-chains can be diagnosed from a few micrograms of cellular DNA with these techniques. The limitations of these methods are evident in Figure 3–30 and Table 3–9. The two restriction enzymes do not differentiate the first nucleotide codon in position 6 of the β-globin gene. Therefore, the gene for C-globin chains, which is produced by a mutation of G→A at this position, is not differentiated from a normal A-globin chain.

In most situations at present, the structure-function relationships between normal hemoglobin A, hemoglobin S, and hemoglobin C provide the

best insight into how a single base substitution can result in the expression of a systemic disease. Perutz and Mitchison observed that deoxygenated sickle cell hemoglobin is less soluble in aqueous solutions than deoxygenated normal hemoglobin. These observations suggested a molecular mechanism for the sickling phenomenon. Murayama demonstrated that substitution of valine for glutamic acid at position 6 in the two β-chains of tetrameric hemoglobins allowed intermolecular hydrophobic bonding and molecular stacking between hemoglobin molecules. Perutz and Lehmann suggested that position 6 of the β-polypeptide chain of hemoglobin occupies the surface of the tertiary structure and that normally the polar group (glutamic acid) adheres to a complementary site on its neighboring hemoglobin molecule. In the absence of this polar group, linear aggregates of hemoglobin S occur. In homozygotes for sickle cell disease, the intracellular concentration of hemoglobin S is high and leads to intermolecular stacking. Deoxygenated red blood cells sickle in the venous circulation, increase blood viscosity, impede the circulation of the venous capillaries, block smaller blood vessels, and form thrombi, leading to tissue infarction. The sickled red cells are not able to withstand the stresses of the circulation and have a shorter survival time, leading to hemolytic anemia. A pathologic structural-functional relationship is also seen in patients homozygous for hemoglobin C. These patients have only mild hemolysis as compared with the severe fatal disease produced by hemoglobin S. Substitution of another polar amino acid, lysine, in position 6 of the β-chain (hemoglobin C) does not produce intermolecular stacking and high viscosity, although a tendency to gel is observed under reduced oxygen tension. It is still not clear how a lysine substitution produces this functional defect in hemoglobin C.

Over 100 different variants of the α- and β-chains of hemoglobin have been identified. The functional expression of these mutant gene prod-

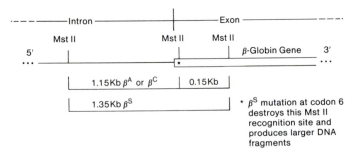

Mst II DNA Pattern	Possible Genotypes
1.35/1.35	SS
1.35/1.15	SA, or SC
1.15/1.15	AA, CC or CA

Figure 3–30 Restriction endonuclease mapping of DNA fragments for the diagnosis of hemoglobinopathies.

ucts depends on the charge and location of the amino acid substitution, the resultant conformational change in the tetrameric hemoglobin molecule, and the interaction of these polypeptides with their four prosthetic heme groups. The *thalassemias* represent a group of chronic hemolytic anemias caused by a reduction in the rate of α- or β-chain synthesis. As already discussed, mutations in introns and deletions of genes are now recognized as the molecular mechanisms for this group of disorders rather than mutations in exons or the structural gene. Homozygotes for β-chain thalassemia manifest severe hemolytic anemia from birth and have a deficiency of normal β-chain production and consequently of normal tetrameric hemoglobin A ($\alpha_2\beta_2$). There is excess production of other normal polypeptide chains, δ or γ. The resultant red cells contain increased amounts of both hemoglobin F ($\alpha_2\gamma_2$) and A₂ ($\alpha_2\delta_2$), are deformed, and are subject to increased hemolysis.

INHERITED METABOLIC DISORDERS

PROTEINS AS MUTANT GENE PRODUCTS

Few mutant proteins other than the hemoglobin peptide chains have had adequate analysis of amino acid sequence to demonstrate single amino acid substitutions. Most inherited metabolic diseases of humans are characterized by the functional derangement imposed on the organism by its mutant gene products. A. E. Garrod first introduced the term "inborn error of metabolism" and described four diseases: alkaptonuria, albinism, cystinuria, and pentosuria, which conformed to mendelian patterns of inheritance and presumably resulted from a block in a major metabolic pathway. He noted that when protein or other precursors of homogentisic acid were administered orally to patients with alkaptonuria, the urinary excretion of homogentisic acid increased. He theorized that this "block-in-reaction sequence" was under genetic control, since pedigree analyses were consistent with an autosomal recessive mode of inheritance. The enzyme defect in alkaptonuria was not discovered until 50 years later, when homogentisic acid oxidase activity was found missing in the liver and kidneys of patients affected with alkaptonuria. Garrod's concepts have been extended from the "one gene—one enzyme" to "one gene—one polypeptide" or "one cistron—one functional polypeptide."

Variations in human proteins do not usually produce a functional impairment. A number of normally functioning protein variants, including hemoglobins, phosphoglucomutase, lactate dehydrogenase, red cell acid phosphatase, and haptoglobin, have been discovered during routine electrophoretic surveys in various normal populations. The vast array of "structural" gene loci in normal individuals was reviewed in detail by Harris. Using electrophoretic surveys, he described the considerable protein polymorphism present in normal populations. He classified the genetic control of these multiple molecular forms into three categories: (1) There may be several gene loci coding for structurally distinct polypeptide chains of a complex protein; (2) there may be only one gene locus but many different alleles at this locus; and (3) there may be secondary "post-translational" modifications of the basic protein. When the mutant gene product results in functional derangement, an inborn error of metabolism exists. The functional defect may be expressed by many different pathogenic mechanisms. The protein prior to mutation may transport substrates across the plasma membrane, catalyze a reaction in a metabolic pathway, interact with other proteins to affect hemostasis, provide active coenzymes from precursor vitamins, excise thymine dimers from normal DNA, and so on. The severity of the clinical pathologic condition produced will depend on the degree of alteration and the metabolic role of the mutant gene product.

The discussion of inherited pathologic physiology will be subdivided into categories according to the metabolic role played by the mutant gene product in the intact organism (Table 3–10). These categories include diseases caused by defective proteins that normally would (1) catalyze plasma membrane transport; (2) catalyze major metabolic pathways with disease caused by accumulation of toxic precursors; (3) catalyze a major pathway with disease caused by overproduction of toxic by-products from a minor pathway; (4) catalyze a needed product in the pathway with disease caused by a deficiency of this product; (5) catalyze products in the major pathway that act as feedback inhibitors

TABLE 3–10 CLASSIFICATION OF INHERITED METABOLIC DISORDERS BY PROTEIN FUNCTIONS THAT ARE DISRUPTED BY MUTATION

Proteins Act As Follows:

1. Catalyze plasma membrane transport.
2. Catalyze major cellular metabolic pathways:
    a. Disease is caused by accumulation of toxic precursors;
    b. Disease is caused by toxic by-products from a normally minor pathway;
    c. Disease is caused by deficiency of end product;
    d. Disease is caused by overproduced intermediates through loss of feedback control.
3. Circulate in blood and provide and maintain various functions (clotting; metal transport; immunity; oxygen transport).
4. Produce or bind coenzymes involved in specific enzymatic reactions.
5. Catalyze the removal of potentially toxic pharmacologic or environmental agents.
6. Maintain structural integrity of organs (collagen, membrane proteins).

and cause disease by overproduction of products; (6) circulate in the blood and have many different functions (clotting, metal binding, immunity, oxygen transport; (7) catalyze the production of specific coenzymes involved in a major pathway; (8) catalyze the removal of potentially toxic pharmacologic or environmental agents and (9) maintain structural integrity of organs and cells (Table 3–10).

INHERITED DISORDERS CAUSED BY DEFECTIVE MEMBRANE TRANSPORT

The jejunal epithelium and the proximal renal tubular epithelium have cells that are differentiated for the transport of essential substrates from outside the cell to its interior. This transport step shares several characteristics with enzymes, such as saturation, steric specificity, energy dependence, competitive and noncompetitive inhibition, and concentrative ability. Direct evidence for the existence of substrate-specific permeases has been obtained from microbial systems. In humans, evidence for their existence is obtained from pedigree analysis of inherited diseases in which this transport function is defective and can be studied. Most of these inherited transport defects have been defined in the intestine or kidney. Table 3–11 lists some inborn errors of membrane transport, the tissues affected, substrates malabsorbed, and the proposed mode of inheritance.

Garrod first recognized the familial occurrence of cystine stone formation, which he ascribed to a block in metabolic reaction sequence. In 1951, Dent and Rose suggested that cystinuria was caused by an error in the renal tubular transport mechanism for cystine, arginine, ornithine, and lysine. These four dibasic amino acids were found in excess in the urine of affected patients. An autosomal recessive mode of inheritance was confirmed by Harris. Rosenberg defined three different forms of cystinuria. Types I, II, and III were distinguished by comparing, in a pedigree analysis, differences in dibasic amino acid transport across the gut in homozygous affected individuals, and in heterozygotes. Variations in urinary excretion of the dibasic amino acids were found. These three genetically distinct types of cystinuria were subsequently demonstrated to be allelic. Type II-III double heterozygotes expressed the clinical phenotype and produced offspring who were either type II or type III heterozygotes, but none was normal or clinically affected. Disease is caused by malabsorption of cystine in the proximal renal tubule. When the urine contains more than 30 mg of cystine per 100 ml, cystine crystallizes and forms stones. Cystinuric homozygotes and double heterozygotes excrete over 600 mg of cystinine in 24 hours. Cystinuria is the most common cause of bladder calculi at birth and may account for 5 per cent of all nephrolithiasis. It is most commonly expressed during the third and fourth decades of life. The urine from members of an affected family should be screened for asymptomatic stone formation. Cystine is more soluble in dilute urine and in an alkaline pH. Stone formation may be decreased by maintaining water diuresis and a

TABLE 3–11 SOME DISEASES CAUSED BY PLASMA MEMBRANE TRANSPORT MUTATIONS

Disease	Tissues Affected	Malabsorbed Substrate	Mode of Inheritance	Clinical Expression
Cystinuria	Kidney ± gut	Cystine ± lysine, arginine, ornithine	Autosomal Recessive	Renal lithiasis (cystine)
Hartnup disease	Gut + kidney	Neutral amino acids	Autosomal Recessive	Nicotinic acid deficiency (pellagra)
Blue diaper syndrome	Gut	Tryptophan	Autosomal Recessive	Hypercalcemia
Methionine malabsorption	Gut	Methionine	Autosomal Recessive(?)	Mental retardation, white hair, failure to thrive
Glucose-galactose malabsorption	Gut + kidney	Glucose and galactose	Autosomal Recessive	Refractory diarrhea
Renal glycosuria	Kidney	Glucose	Autosomal Recessive	Benign glycosuria
Hypophosphatemic rickets	Kidney	Phosphate	X-linked Dominant	Rickets
Congenital chloridorrhea	Gut	Chloride	Autosomal Recessive	Diarrhea, alkalosis
Hereditary spherocytosis	Erythrocyte	Sodium	Autosomal Recessive	Hemolytic anemia
B_{12} malabsorption	Ileum	B_{12}	Autosomal Recessive	Juvenile pernicious anemia

urinary pH above 7.5. Renal stones once formed may be dissolved by the administration of D-penicillamine (β,β-dimethylcysteine), which forms soluble penicillamine-cystine disulfides.

Renal stone formation is but one of many clinical manifestations produced by heritable defects in membrane transport permeases. In Hartnup disease, malabsorption of the neutral amino acids by the intestinal mucosa may have no ill effects. However, if the defect is severe and enough tryptophan is malabsorbed, intracellular nicotinamide deficiency may result. The disease is then expressed as a pellagra-like syndrome with ataxia, sun-sensitive rashes, and dementia. Treatment consists of administration of the deficient vitamin, niacin. In familial glucose-galactose malabsorption, severe osmotic diarrhea occurs in infants from the inability of their jejunal mucosa to transport glucose and other sterically similar monosaccharides. Direct evidence for the genetic control of intestinal glucose transport was obtained by invitro studies of jejunal biopsy material. As seen in Figure 3–31, epithelial cells from an affected homozygote were unable to accumulate glucose over a 60-minute incubation period, whereas cells from her clinically normal brother and normal controls concentrated glucose to levels 15 times that in the extracellular space. Biopsies from both parents demonstrated partial impairment of this transport function. These data indicate that the proband is homozygous for the glucose transport mutation, that her brother is homozygous for the normal allele, and that both parents and her half-sister are heterozygotes, each carrying one mutant and one normal allele. The osmotic diarrhea induced by ingested glucose is prevented by substituting fructose as the dietary carbohydrate source. This monosaccharide has a different steric configuration and membrane transport requirements. In familial glucose-galactose malabsorption, the defect is absence of intestinal glucose transport along with a partial glucose transport defect in the kidney. In *renal glycosuria*, the kidney tubule is unable to reabsorb glucose, but this genetic defect is not expressed by the intestine. In one family, renal glucose transport was quantitated with invivo titration techniques, and an autosomal recessive mode of inheritance was defined (Fig. 3–32). Heterogeneity for renal glucose transport is evidenced by the different types of abnormal curves found in other families with familial glycosuria. In contrast to glucose-galactose malabsorption, renal glucose malabsorption produces no ill effects unless iatrogenic disease arises from a misdiagnosis of diabetes mellitus.

Defective accumulation of phosphate, vitamins, sodium, and chloride may result from other heritable membrane transport mutations. The changes resulting from these defects vary. In familial hypophosphatemic rickets, the best genetic determinant of this X-linked dominant trait is defective phosphate reabsorption by the proximal renal tubule. If this is the initiating event, it is postulated that hypophosphatemia results, hydroxylation of cholecalciferol (vitamin D) is impaired, calcium absorption is reduced, and bone resorption occurs to maintain normal serum phosphate levels. In addition, shortened lower body segments, rickets in children, and osteomalacia in adults may result. In congenital chloridorrhea, adults may manifest malabsorption of chloride by the colon, resulting in watery diarrhea, hypochloremia, and decreased renal chloride filtration. Bicarbonate is reabsorbed in the absence of tubular chloride to maintain a normal electropotential gradient. Increased bicarbonate reabsorption by

Figure 3–31 Jejunal mucosa from the affected proband is unable to accumulate glucose, whereas cells from her brother and from normal controls concentrate to levels 15 times more than that in the extracellular space. Both parents and a half-sister accumulate intermediate amounts of glucose, indicating a partial transport defect and identifying them as heterozygotes for the mutant gene. Distribution ratio is calculated from the ratio of counts per minute per milliliter of intracellular space to counts per minute per milliliter of extracellular space (CPM/ml ICF:CPM/ml ECF).

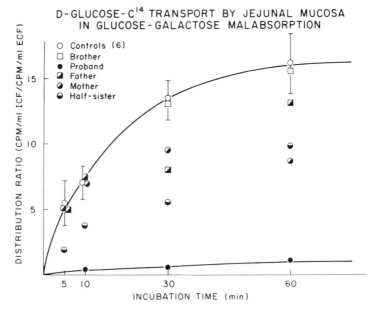

D-GLUCOSE-C^{14} TRANSPORT BY JEJUNAL MUCOSA IN GLUCOSE-GALACTOSE MALABSORPTION

○ Controls (6)
□ Brother
● Proband
◪ Father
◖ Mother
◕ Half-sister

DISTRIBUTION RATIO (CPM/ml ICF/CPM/ml ECF)

INCUBATION TIME (min)

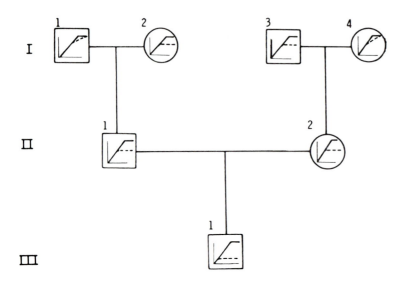

Figure 3–32 Autosomal recessive inheritance of renal glycosuria. The results of renal glucose titration are inscribed within the pedigree symbols. Broken lines (---) represent observed deviation from the theoretic curve (—). The proband (III-1) expresses severe type A glycosuria, and his parents (II-1, II-2) and grandparents I-2- and I-3 have milder forms. Grandparents I-1 and I-4 have normal curves.

the kidney tubule results in continued metabolic alkalosis. In hereditary spherocytosis, impaired erythrocyte membrane permeability to sodium results in a shortened survival of the erythrocyte and hemolytic anemia. This condition is inherited as an autosomal dominant trait with parent-to-offspring transmission. Several observations concerning membrane proteins, specifically spectrin dimer association, give credence to the theory that structural protein defect is a cause of cellular sensitivity to osmotic gradients. In vitamin B_{12} malabsorption, juvenile pernicious anemia results. This autosomal recessive trait is seen in children with normal gastric acid secretion in whom intrinsic factor can be demonstrated but in whom vitamin B_{12} cannot be transported across the intestinal epithelial cell.

INHERITED DISORDERS RESULTING FROM PRECURSOR ACCUMULATION

The most commonly described inborn error of metabolism results from a metabolic block in a major pathway and the accumulation of toxic precursors. One such disease is alkaptonuria, a defect in homogentisic acid oxidase activity. This enzyme normally catalyzes the conversion of homogentisic acid to maleylacetoacetic acid in the oxidative catabolic pathways of tyrosine (Fig. 3–33). Virtual absence of this enzyme in kidney and liver results in the accumulation of homogentisic acid in tissues and excretion into the urine. Homogentisic acid accumulation in cartilaginous tissue is associated with premature arthritis and provides this tissue with the characteristic dark tinge caused by oxidation of homogentisic acid. The disease is not usually manifest until after 30 years of age, and whether tissue deposition could be delayed or prevented with restricted phenylalanine and tyrosine intake is unknown.

Various storage diseases have been delineated in which glycogen, sphingolipids, cystine, or mucopolysaccharides are found in excess in tissues and subcellular organelles. The deposition of these compounds presumably results from a block in their normal metabolic pathway. The precise mechanisms by which intracellular storage of these compounds produces clinical manifestations are being clarified.

In classic galactosemia, a defect in galactose-1-phosphate uridyl transferase results in accumulation of the hexose monophosphate, galactose-1-phosphate and its precursor galactose. Because different errors exist in this catabolic pathway, the pathogenesis of disease in this disorder is somewhat better understood. Galactose-1-phosphate accumulates in liver, kidney, and brain, and produces cirrhosis, renal tubular malabsorption, and mental retardation. The molecular mechanism by which galactose-1-phosphate accumulation interferes with normal cellular function is not clear, although the hexosemonophosphate has been postulated to be a "phosphate sink" preventing adequate production of ATP and other physiologically necessary high-energy phosphate bonds. In another defect in galactose utilization, galactokinase deficiency, galactose is accumulated in the blood and tissues, but galactose-1-phosphate is normal or reduced. In this disorder, cataracts are manifest without impairment of kidney, liver, or brain. Cataract formation in both classic galactose-1-phosphate uridyl transferase deficiency and galactokinase deficiency presumably results from excessive accumulation of galactose and conversion in the lens by aldose reductase in the presence of triphosphopyridine nucleotide to galactitol. This poorly effluxed alcohol is trapped in the lens, creates an osmotic gradient, and produces degeneration of lens fibers. The pathologic condition created by both enzyme defects can be ameliorated if detected early and if dietary restriction of nonessential galactose-containing sugars is instituted.

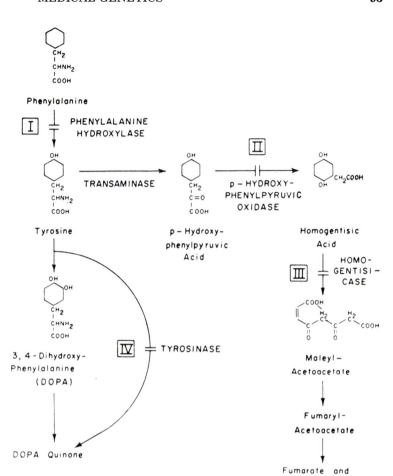

Figure 3–33 The normal metabolic pathway for phenylalanine. *I,* The deficiency of phenylalanine hydroxylase results in phenylketonuria. *II* and *III,* Deficiencies of these enzymes that lead to tyrosinosis and alkaptonuria. *IV,* Deficiency of the enzyme tyrosinase results in albinism. (From Hsia, D.Y.: Inborn Errors of Metabolism. Chicago, Year Book Medical Publishers, Inc., 1959.)

Maple syrup urine disease, or branched-chain ketoaciduria, results from defective decarboxylation of the branched-chain α-keto acids. The reaction sequence is indicated in Figure 3–34. Isoleucine, leucine, and valine, the branched-chain amino acids, are reversibly transaminated to their branched-chain α-keto acid derivatives, α-keto-β-methyl valeric, α-keto isocaproic, and α-keto isovaleric acids. Subsequent decarboxylation of all three of these organic acids to their coenzyme-A derivates is blocked in maple syrup urine disease. The α-keto acids and their branched-chain amino acid precursors accumulate in tissue and blood and are excreted in the urine. Racemers of these branched-chain α-keto acids impart a fragant odor of maple syrup to the patient's urine. The enzyme defect is expressed in leukocytes isolated from the peripheral blood and in fibroblasts cultured from patient's skin. Analogous to α-ketoglutarate decarboxylation, three different enzyme proteins are involved in branched-chain α-keto acid decarboxylation: (1) a thiamine-dependent α-keto acid decarboxylase, (2) a lipoyl-containing transacylase, and (3) a flavoprotein, lipoamide oxidoreductase. Four soluble co-factors are involved in the overall reaction: (1) thiamine pyrophosphate (TPP), (2)

reduced coenzyme A (CoASH), (3) Mg^{++}, and (4) oxidized nicotinamide adenine dinucleotide (NAD^+). The complex of these three enzymes and four cofactors that decarboxylate α-ketoisocaproic acid, α-keto-β-methyl valeric acid, and α-ketoisovaleric acid resides in the inner mitochondrial membrane.

Because phenotypic expression of the acute phase of maple syrup urine disease is ameliorated by restriction of the intake of leucine, isoleucine, and valine, the mechanism of pathogenesis involves toxic effects on brain of excess branched-chain amino acids or their α-keto acid derivatives or both. "Deficiency of end product" has not been implicated. The ultimate production of acetoacetyl CoA, acetyl CoA, and succinyl CoA as well as TPNH-reducing equivalents from catabolism of the branched-chain amino acids may be diminished, but the relative contribution of these essential compounds is small. The severity of clinical expression in the untreated disease is directly related to the concentration and duration of precursor accumulation, to the degree of impaired enzyme function, and to the age of the developing brain at which insult occurs. With dietary restriction in the neonatal period to maintain concentra-

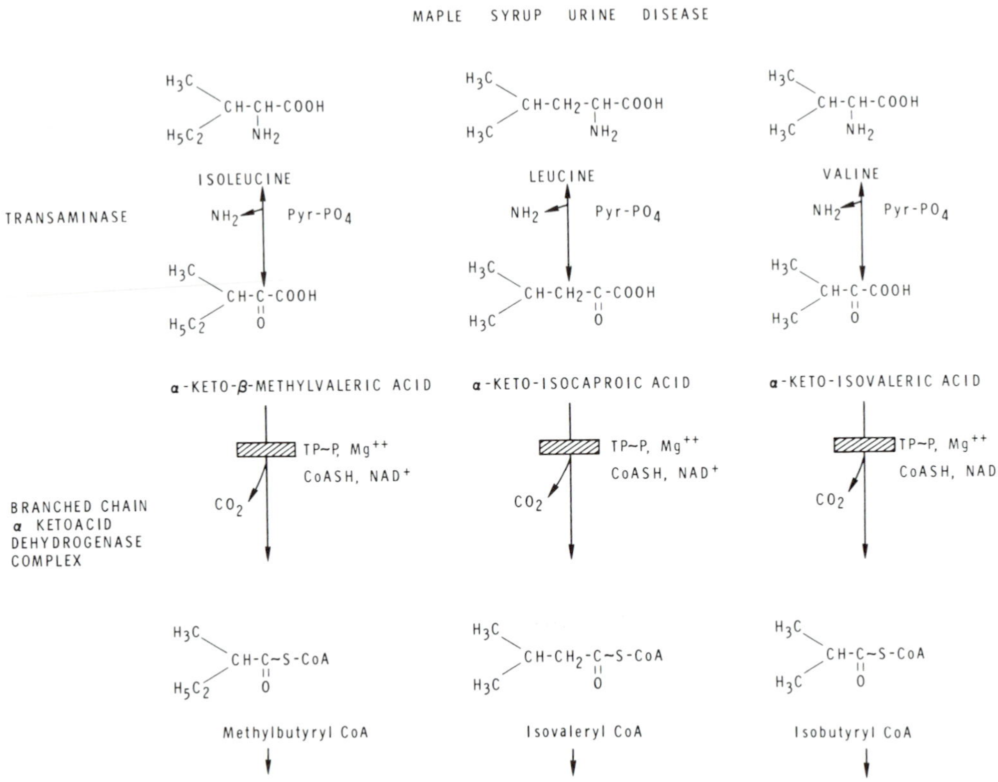

MAPLE   SYRUP   URINE   DISEASE

Figure 3–34 Catabolic pathway for branched-chain amino acids. Bar ▨▨▨ represents block in maple syrup urine disease. TPP, CoASH, Mg^{++} and NAD^+ are soluble cofactors involved in the oxidative decarboxylation of α-keto acids.

tions of leucine below 300 μM, patients can be prevented from expressing irreversible clinical manifestations. In the "classic" form of this disease, mutations produce less than 2 per cent of normal enzyme activity, and the prevention of acute central nervous system depression is difficult unless immediate screening, retrieval, diagnosis, and treatment are implemented within the first week of life. Maternal enzyme protects against the accumulation of branched-chain amino acids in the fetus. In the "intermediate" forms of this disorder, there is 2 to 10 per cent enzyme activity and expression of the acute toxic effect of accumulated branched-chain α-keto acids if protein loading is sufficient. In the "intermittent" form, there is 10 to 20 per cent of normal enzyme activity and often no clinical expression unless the patient is stressed by infections or excessive protein ingestion. If these "intermittent" episodes are frequent in early childhood, mild mental retardation may persist. "Thiamine-responsive" forms have been described, and this response is usually related to stabilization of the enzyme complex by thiamine.

There are two major pathologic consequences to the brain in untreated maple syrup urine disease. In the *acute toxic phase,* usually expressed by neonates with the classic form of the disease, there may be apnea and coma without any appar-

ent specific pathology. Hypoglycemia and hypoalaninemia reflect impaired glucose-alanine homeostasis. There are two general theories concerning the mechanisms of pathogenesis: (1) neurotransmitters are displaced, and (2) energy sources for the brain are suddenly removed. Plasma branched-chain α-keto acids are usually above 1.0 mM during these acute attacks. Since leucine transport across the blood-brain barrier has a K_m in the 0.1 mM range, one can assume equal or greater concentrations of branched-chain amino acids in intracellular brain cells. In most reported studies, the precursor amino acid did not inhibit enzymes producing neurotransmitters. However, very large concentrations of branched-chain α-keto acids, particularly α-ketoisocaproic acid, inhibited important enzymes for brain mitochondrial energy production. The reported K_i's (1.4 to 4.5 mM) were within the range reported in the blood of untreated newborns who died during the acute toxic phase of maple syrup urine disease. There is less direct evidence for the mechanisms of pathogenesis in more chronic situations. Here blood concentrations of branched-chain amino acids may have been abnormal only briefly during infancy, yet mental retardation and spastic paralysis persist. In situations of this type in which diet restriction is the method of treatment, the gross histology and content of lipid, proteolipid, and cerebrosides are normal. In untreated cases, however, brain tissue is characterized by decreased lipids, proteolipids, and cerebrosides. Chronically elevated branched-chain amino acids are potential hazards to the formation of myelin proteolipids. For instance, the condensation of palmitoyl CoA with serine in the production of sphingosine is critical in myelin formation, and if branched-chain amino acids were present in excess, this reaction would be impaired by lowering of serine pools. Critical stable myelin could be altered in early infancy by elevated branched-chain amino acids or α-keto acids and produce permanent neurologic damage.

INHERITED DISEASES CAUSED BY PRODUCTS OF MINOR PATHWAYS

The precursor in the metabolic block of a major pathway may not be the immediate cause of the disease. Instead, by-products of an alternate minor pathway may be the cause. The activity of such a pathway is normally minimal but is enhanced by abnormal precursor accumulation. For example, cataracts in *galactosemia* are not caused by galactose or galactose-1-phosphate; rather, the increased concentration of galactose in lens fibers results in excessive amounts of nondiffusible galactitol produced as a result of an alternate pathway through aldose reductase.

A second example is *phenylketonuria*. A deficiency in phenylalanine hydroxylase results in the accumulation of phenylalanine. It is, however, the deaminated by-product of phenylalanine, phenylpyruvic acid, that produces the characteristic ferric chloride reaction in the urine and metabolic acidosis. Because a moderate elevation of phenylalanine alone is not toxic, these by-products in high concentrations may interfere with central nervous system processes. Although mental retardation and demyelination are irreversible consequences of the untreated disease, the basis for their pathogenesis remains an enigma. An inhibitory effect of phenylalanine has been recognized on tyrosine hydroxylase and tryptophan hydroxylase. This produces a decrease in L-dopa and serotonin in brain and transient effects on performance.

A third example is *hyperoxaluria,* which is characterized by the excretion of large amounts of oxalic acid, nephrolithiasis, nephrocalcinosis, and early renal failure. The stones are formed from calcium oxalate, a nonessential end product of glycine degradation. This disorder is caused by excessive biosynthesis of oxalic acid, which is formed from glycine through the irreversible oxidation of glyoxylic acid. Two causes of excessive accumulation of glyoxylic acid and its insoluble by-product, oxalic acid, have been postulated. In type I, a defect in the soluble enzyme glycolic acid α-ketoglutarate carboligase blocks conversion of glyoxylic acid to α-OH-β-ketoadipate (one of six

alternate routes for glyoxylic acid) and results in accumulation of glyoxylic acid and conversion to oxalic acid. In type II, Williams and Smith described excessive D-glyceric aciduria as well as hyperoxaluria and found deficient D-glyceric acid oxidase in the leukocytes of affected patients and of the mother but not of the father. These authors postulated that a deficiency in this enzyme reduces conversion of glyoxylic acid to glycolic acid. Both types lead primarily to excesses of glyoxylic acid by blocking normal dissimilation and secondarily to increased biosynthesis of oxalic acid normally present but in smaller amounts. These examples, then, represent inborn errors of metabolism, the manifestations of which are caused not by the precursor in the metabolic block but by the overproduction of by-products from the accumulating precursor.

INHERITED DISEASES CAUSED BY DEFICIENCIES OF END PRODUCT

A pathologic condition may result from a mutant gene product that reduces the intracellular concentration of essential end products in its pathway. *Albinism* represents a group of disorders caused by impaired production of melanoprotein from tyrosine. A specialized cell, the melanocyte, is the source of pigment in hair, skin, and eyes. Hydroxylation of L-tyrosine to 3,4-dihydroxyphenylalanine (DOPA) and its subsequent oxidation to dopa-quinone utilize the same enzyme, tyrosinase (Fig. 3–33). Nonenzymatic reactions then occur in the melanocyte, resulting in polymerization of dopa-quinone derivatives and reaction with a specialized protein to form melanoprotein. Melanocytes are present in albinism but do not contain melanin. Many different clinical forms of albinism exist with different genetic patterns of inheritance. Classic oculocutaneous albinism (type I) is expressed as diffuse hypopigmentation of the hair, skin, fundus oculi, and iris. It is inherited as an autosomal recessive trait. Melanocytes are present but are presumably deficient in tyrosinase. The disease expression therefore is due to a deficiency of the end product, melanin, which normally acts as a sunscreen and protects cells from light energy. In albinism, instead of tanning, affected individuals burn on exposure to light. Exposed skin has an increased tendency to develop malignant melanomas. Photophobia, nystagmus, and visual impairment result from melanin deficiency in the eye.

Defective formation of thyroid hormone represents another group of inborn errors of metabolism in which deficiency of the product of the enzyme pathway results in expression of disease. Several different enzymatic defects have been described that produce a deficiency of functioning thyroid hormone. These include (1) an iodide transport defect, (2) iodide organification defects,

(3) a defect in the coupling of iodotyrosyl to form thyroxine, (4) failure to synthesize normal thyroglobulin, and (5) failure to dehalogenate organic iodide. Mental retardation or cretinism is caused by a deficiency in the end product, thyroid hormone.

Congenital adrenal hyperplasia results from an inherited, relative or absolute loss in one of the enzymes that produce normal hormonal steroids from cholesterol. When this block in the normal biosynthetic pathway results in insufficient production of salt-retaining mineralocorticoids and anti-inflammatory glucocorticoids, persistent loss of sodium in the urine, vomiting, dehydration, hypotension, shock, or sudden death may occur. At least five different enzyme deficiencies in this pathway have been described, including those of 21-hydroxylase, 11-hydroxylase, 3 β-hydroxysteroid dehydrogenase, 17-hydroxylase, and 18-hydroxylase. Salt-wasting may occur in all except the 11-hydroxylase deficiency, in which salt-retaining hormones 11-deoxycortisol and 11-deoxycorticosterone are formed in excess and protect the organism against deficient aldosterone production. An autosomal recessive pattern of inheritance is presumed for these disorders.

INHERITED DISEASES CAUSED BY LOSS OF FEEDBACK INHIBITION

In the preceding section, it was shown that deficiency of essential end products in the major metabolic pathway produces abnormalities directly. In the pathogenesis of some heritable disorders, loss of regulation in a metabolic pathway produces the disease state. The failure to synthesize thyroxine results in mental retardation. The total phenotype is due not only to deficient hormone but also to loss of feedback inhibition of hypothalamic thyrotropin releasing factor, excess secretion of TSH, and the formation of excessive thyroid parenchyma. The goiter expressed in familial hypothyroidism results from the loss of end-product inhibition of TSH regulatory control mechanisms.

In the adrenogenital syndrome, particularly in 11-hydroxylase deficiency, the end-product deficiency may not in itself produce the entire syndrome. A precursor, 11-deoxycorticosterone, is accumulated in one group (the 11-hydroxylase deficiencies), conserves renal sodium, and may even produce hypertension. However, another pathologic process in this disorder is masculinization. Normally, cortisol and corticosterone regulate hypothalamic-pituitary ACTH secretion by acting as depressants on corticotropin-releasing factor. Corticotropin-releasing factor acts to stimulate synthesis and release of ACTH. When cortisol production is reduced, as in 21-hydroxylase deficiency, this negative feedback control is lost, more ACTH is produced, and excessive androgenic steroids in the pathway are formed. Levels of

ACTH, 17-ketosteroids, and potent androgens such as testosterone are elevated in plasma and tissues. This pathologic process occurs during intrauterine development and may cause clitoromegaly or ambiguous genitalia in the female infant, macrogenitosomia in the male, and virilization with epiphyseal closure in both. The whole process is reversed by providing exogenous cortisol in physiologic amounts, returning feedback inhibition to the hypothalamic-pituitary-ACTH axis.

One of the most important advances in genetics is the understanding of early-onset coronary heart disease and its relationship to regulation of cholesterol biosynthesis. In a combined biochemical and genetic analysis in 500 survivors of myocardial infarction, Goldstein, Motulsky, and Brown found that over half had a monogenic trait producing one of three plasma lipid phenotypes: familial hypercholesterolemia, familial hypertriglyceridemia, or combined hyperlipidemia. Ten per cent had familial hypercholesterolemia; in the general population, one per 500 persons is affected by this autosomal dominant trait. Subsequent studies using cultured skin fibroblasts, lymphocytes, and cultured aortic smooth muscle cells from homozygous and heterozygous patients with familial hypercholesterolemia demonstrated at least three genetically distinct defects in low-density lipoprotein-cholesterol (LDL-cholesterol) binding and pinocytosis by plasma membrane (Fig. 3–35). The extracellular complex of LDL-cholesterol protects the cell from overaccumulation of cholesterol and its esters. After incorporation through pinocytosis into lysosomes, free cholesterol is released and suppresses the rate-limiting enzyme in cholesterol biosynthesis, hydroxymethyl glutaryl CoA reductase (HMGCoA reductase). Thus, phenotypically affected heterozygotes with partially reduced membrane-binding functions have increased intracellular cholesterol esters and a two- to threefold increase in plasma cholesterol levels. These abnormalities are associated with atherosclerosis and myocardial infarctions between the ages of 35 and 45 years. Homozygously affected individuals occur in the population rarely, with an estimated frequency of one in 1,000,000. By comparison, they have little or no LDL-cholesterol binding and/or invagination, a sixfold or greater elevation in plasma cholesterol, and myocardial infarctions between the ages of 5 and 15 years. Since heterozygotes express early-onset heart disease, familial hypercholesterolemia is an autosomal dominant trait.

In *acute intermittent porphyria,* partial impairment of an enzyme in the heme biosynthetic pathway results in loss of feedback regulation of δ-aminolevulinic acid synthetase. Acute intermittent porphyria is characterized by hepatic overproduction of porphyrin precursors, δ-aminolevulinic acid and porphobilinogen. Increased activity of hepatic δ-aminolevulinic acid synthetase has been described in patients affected with this order.

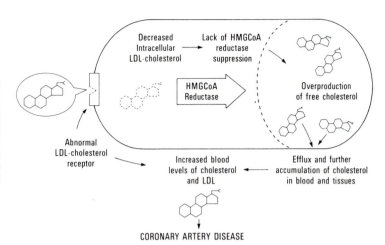

Figure 3–35 Schematic model in familial hypercholesterolemia. Pathogenesis of early-onset heart disease results from genetically determined impairment in the number and function of plasma membrane low-density lipoprotein (LDL)–cholesterol binding sites. Heterozygotes have partial impairment with adult onset of disease expression, whereas affected children who are homozygous lack binding sites and express coronary disease before puberty.

Family studies in 600 patients from Sweden described direct parent-to-offspring transmission, with both sexes equally affected. This indicates an autosomal dominant pattern of inheritance. Meyer and Marver demonstrated a primary partial impairment of the enzyme uroporphyrinogen I synthase. In linkage studies, this enzyme has been localized to the long arm of chromosome 11. Acute intermittent porphyria is characterized by intermittent episodes of severe abdominal pain, psychoses, and paralysis.

Photosensitivity is not present, nor is there excessive excretion of preformed porphyrins. A number of factors are known to provoke acute attacks in patients with this disorder, including steroids, barbiturates, infections, female sex hormones, and starvation. All these agents increase binding proteins for heme production and further reduce available free heme to act as negative control in the biosynthesis of δ-aminolevulinic acid synthetase. During attacks, the urine contains excessive amounts of porphobilinogen, which on standing in an acid pH will polymerize to form porphyrins and other dark reddish pigments. Acute clinical episodes, increased enzyme activity, and excessive production of porphobilinogen are not quantitatively correlated. Other hepatic porphyrias, hereditary coproporphyria, and variegate porphyria also are inherited in an autosomal dominant pattern, have excess porphyrin production, and are caused by enzyme impairment distal to uroporphyrinogen synthase in the heme biosynthetic pathway.

In an inborn error of pyrimidine biosynthesis, *orotic aciduria*, a single rare mutant gene produces a deficiency of two enzyme functions: orotic acid phosphoribosyl transferase (O-PRT) and orotidine-5'-phosphate decarboxylase (ODC). This block results in the accumulation and excretion of a relatively insoluble pyrimidine nucleotide precursor, orotic acid, and reduced synthesis of its mononucleotide product, uridylic acid. Orotic acid is found in the urine of affected children and produces needle-shaped crystals and obstructive urinary-tract symptoms when affected individuals become dehydrated. Children also manifest megaloblastic anemia and psychomotor retardation, presumably caused by "pyrimidine deficiency." A deficiency of this end product, uridylic acid (uridine-5'-monophosphate), results in overproduction of orotic acid, since it acts as a feedback inhibitor of carbamyl phosphate synthetase and aspartate transcarbamylase, initial enzymes in the biosynthetic pathway of uridylic acid production. If the feedback inhibitor uridine is provided by uridine replacement, reduction in the rate of orotic acid overproduction is seen in patients and in cells cultured from their skin. Uridine replacement also improves the anemia and growth retardation.

Another inborn error of nucleotide feedback control is exemplified by defects in purine biosynthesis. The enzyme hypoxanthine-guanine-phosphoribosyltransferase (HGPRTase) acts to catalyze the formation of the mononucleotides inosinic and guanylic acid from hypoxanthine and guanine using phosphoribosyl pyrophosphate (PRPP). Defects in this enzyme result in reduced feedback inhibition of the de-novo synthesis of uric acid, increased cellular concentrations of PRPP, and marked overproduction of uric acid. Patients affected with complete HGPRTase deficiency have severe mental retardation, chorea, spasticity, and a bizarre compulsion to practice self-mutilation. They also exhibit hyperuricemia, urinary uric acid stones, and clinical gout. The gene is located on the X chromosome. Female heterozygotes demonstrate mosaicism for HGPRTase activity in fibroblasts cultured from their skin. Approximately half their cells are unable to incorporate tritiated hypoxanthine into nucleic acids (HGPRTase deficient), whereas the other half have normal enzyme activity. These observations support the Lyon hypothesis for early random and continued X-inactivation. The mechanism by which HGPRTase deficiency interrupts normal brain biochemistry and function is unknown. Two possibilities exist:

(1) an important purine nucleotide is deficient, or (2) an abnormal purine intermediate is overproduced. Neither of these possibilities is confirmed, but uric acid is clearly overproduced, and this aspect of the disease can be classified as an inherited defect resulting in loss of feedback control of de-novo purine biosynthesis.

INHERITED DISEASE ASSOCIATED WITH DEFICIENT OR ABNORMAL CIRCULATING PROTEINS

A wide variety of genetically controlled proteins circulate in the blood. In some, changes in concentration, structure, or function may have no effect on the organism as a whole; in others, such changes may have distinctly deleterious results. Perhaps the best known of this group are disorders of immunoglobulin production. In fact, the field of immunogenetics encompasses not only the control of immunoglobulins but also the complete immune reaction, which includes circulating complement, various regulatory enzymes, leukocytes, and lymphocytes. These concepts are discussed in a later chapter. Reduction in the concentration of thyroxine-binding globulin, a protein controlled by a locus on the X chromosome, reduces the serum protein–bound iodide but does not alter metabolic function. Dominantly inherited variants of the iron-binding protein, transferrin, have been described, but none of these structural mutations has a known effect on iron metabolism. However, a recessively inherited atransferrinemia has been described in which there is a transferrin deficiency with a refractory hypochromic anemia. In Wilson's disease, reduction in circulating ceruloplasmin, a polyamine oxidase that is induced by and binds 95 per cent of serum copper, is associated with copper deposition in almost all tissues of the body. The deposition of copper in liver, brain, eyes, and kidney results in cirrhosis, extrapyramidal tract degeneration, pathognomonic corneal Kayser-Fleischer rings, and renal tubular dysfunction. Removal of copper from these organs with chelating agents such as penicillamine will prevent impairment and in some instances improve organ function. Although reduction in circulating ceruloplasmin remains the best genetic determinant of affected homozygotes, approximately 2 to 3 per cent of patients with phenotypic Wilson's disease have chemically and functionally normal ceruloplasmin. The basic mutant gene product and the relationship between tissue copper and reduced levels of ceruloplasmin remain unsolved.

The hemostatic mechanism in humans is provided by several different factors under genetic control. In classic hemophilia A, an X-linked recessive trait, hemizygous males have diminished functional antihemophilic globulin (Factor VIII, AHG). Vascular hemophilia, or Von Willebrand disease, is an autosomal dominant trait in which there is also a deficiency of Factor VIII. It is interesting that the more serious coagulation defect (classic hemophilia A) more commonly has detectable immunologic AHG that is hemostatically defective, whereas "vascular" hemophilia A (Von Willebrand disease) has no immunoreactive material but the disease is characterized by a less severe defect in hemostasis. Hemophilia B, or Christmas disease, is a defect in Factor IX (plasma thromboplastin component), and, as with Factor VIII, deficiency is transmitted in an X-linked recessive pattern. Studies in families in which classic hemophilia A and hemophilia B were segregating showed that the two disorders were clearly nonallelic.

Several families have been reported with hemostatic defects expressed as mild prolongation of blood and plasma coagulation times and by the presence of abnormal fibrinogens. These dysfibrinogenemias are inherited in an autosomal dominant pattern when prolonged prothrombin time is used as the genetic determinant. Several different abnormal fibrinogens have been described. Ratnoff and Bennett tabulated these variants. Most abnormal fibrinogens are immunologically distinct. Affected individuals have two populations of fibrinogen, normal and mutant. Mammen and coworkers suggested that a substitution of a strongly basic amino acid (arginine) for serine in fibrinogen-Detroit changed the conformational site for active polymerization and resulted in interference with the clotting properties of the normal fibrinogen, which was also present. Another disorder, congenital afibrinogenemia, has been described. In this disorder, there is absent coagulation of blood in the affected individuals, and parents have mild coagulation defects. This disorder is inherited as an autosomal recessive trait. The dominant pattern of inheritance in dysfibrinogenemia and the expressed coagulation defects in "afibrinogenemic" heterozygotes indicate that in both disorders the mutant gene product (fibrinogen) is altered, so that it interferes with the product of its normal allele and results in phenotypic expression.

Congenital abetalipoproteinemia is an autosomal recessive disease characterized by the absence of circulating low-density lipoprotein. This disease is expressed by abnormal red blood cell structure (acanthocytes), steatorrhea, diffuse central nervous system abnormalities (cerebellar, posterior column, peripheral nerve), and engorgement of upper intestinal absorptive cells with triglycerides when fat is present in the diet. The genetic effect is now known to be a block in either the secretion or the synthesis of apoprotein B, which is a component of both LDL and VLDL. Patients affected by this disease have reduced plasma cholesterol, all of which is bound to high-density lipoprotein (HDL). HDL-cholesterol is not taken up by normal fibroblasts, and fails to suppress HMG CoA-reductase or stimulate cholesteryl ester formation (Fig. 3–35). The pathologic processes in red cell membranes and central nervous system may reflect a deficiency of these membranal sterols.

INBORN ERRORS CAUSED BY REDUCED COENZYME BINDING OR PRODUCTION

Renewed interest in cofactor interaction with enzymes has resulted from the immediate therapeutic effects of administering supraphysiologic doses of vitamins whose coenzyme products augment defective enzyme pathways. Rosenberg defined the "vitamin-dependent inborn errors" as genetic disturbances leading to specific biochemical abnormalities, affecting one reaction catalyzed by a vitamin and responding only to pharmacologic amounts of that vitamin. This definition thus clearly differentiates vitamin dependency from vitamin deficiency, which affects many pathways, responds to physiologic amounts of the vitamin, and is acquired. Frimpter first demonstrated decreased cystathionase activity in the liver from patients with *cystathioninuria*. When liver homogenates were incubated with its coenzyme, pyridoxal phosphate, activity was markedly increased. He also showed that cystathionine excretion in patients was lowered significantly by the administration of large amounts of vitamin B_6. Vitamin B_6 is phosphorylated to pyridoxal-5' phosphate or pyridoxamine-5'-phosphate by specific kinases requiring adenosine triphosphate. These phosphorylated compounds act as coenzymes for a large number of apoenzymes that regulate the catabolic pathways for fatty acids, amino acids, and glycogen. Since cystathionase activity alone was impaired in cystathioninuria, a vitamin deficiency was unlikely. Frimpter's work suggested that the mutation in cystathioninuria altered that portion of the specific apoenzyme that bound its active coenzyme, pyridoxal phosphate. Other inborn errors of metabolism demonstrating vitamin B_6 dependency include infantile convulsions, pyridoxine-responsive anemia, xanthurenic aciduria, and homocystinuria. In homocystinuria, B_6 apparently stabilizes the mutant cystathionine synthase and increases its biologic half-life (Step 4, Fig. 3–36).

Four different disorders involved in conversion of B_{12} to its active cofactors have been described. In humans, examples have been demonstrated through studies of vitamin B_{12}–responsive *methylmalonic aciduria*. This disorder arises from impairment in the conversion of methylmalonyl CoA to succinyl CoA. The reaction is catalyzed by the enzyme methylmalonyl CoA-mutase and its coenzyme 5'-deoxyadenosylcobalamin, a vitamin B_{12} derivative. Metabolic ketoacidosis accompanied by coma and shock was a common finding during the early weeks of life in six patients described. Other findings included hypotonia, hepatomegaly, osteoporosis, neutropenia, and thrombocytopenia. The appearance of long-chained ketones, including butanone and hexanone in the urine, intermittent hyperglycinemia and glycinuria, and the excretion of large amounts of the unusual organic acid methylmalonic acid, characterized the biochemical phenotype. In vitro biochemical studies revealed that peripheral blood leukocytes and cultured skin fibroblasts from affected patients were unable to convert methylmalonic acid to succinic acid. Normal levels of tissue and plasma vitamin B_{12} were found. When 1-mg doses of hydroxycobalamin are given to children with this disease, methylmalonic acid excretion falls and white blood cell utilization of methylmalonate rises. If fibroblasts are grown in tissue culture media containing physiologic concentrations of vitamin B_{12}, very low intracellular concentrations of the active coenzyme 5'-deoxyadenosylcobalamin are produced. However, when the cells are grown in medium with 10,000-fold increases of vitamin B_{12}, 5'-deoxyadenosylcobalamin rises to normal levels. Methylmalonate CoA mutase activity and its ability to bind coenzyme are normal in fibroblast homogenates, indicating that the apoenzyme is normal and has a normal affinity for its coenzyme. A primary genetic defect occurs in the production of the coenzyme 5'-deoxyadenosylcobalamin from its precursor, vitamin B_{12} (Step 2, Fig. 3–36). With cell fusion and complementation techniques, at least four genetically different B_{12}-responsive forms of methylmalonic aciduria have been defined in the transport and conversion of B_{12} to its active cofactors.

In these metabolic disorders, defects occur in the binding or the production of coenzymes in-

Figure 3–36 Inborn errors of metabolism expressing vitamin dependency could arise from any of the four mechanisms represented. (Adapted from Rosenberg, L. E.: N. Engl. J. Med. 281:145, 1969, with permission of author.)

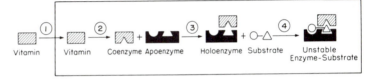

Vitamin → Vitamin → Coenzyme + Apoenzyme → Holoenzyme + Substrate → Unstable Enzyme-Substrate

1. Defective Transport of Vitamin into Cell
2. Defective Conversion of Vitamin to Coenzyme
3. Defective Formation of Holoenzyme
4. Unstable Enzyme-Substrate Complex Resulting in shortened biologic half-life

volved in the major catalytic reaction. Several vitamin dependency syndromes have been evaluated at the molecular level, with the following mechanisms defined: (1) The vitamin may not be transported into a specialized cell; (2) it may fail to convert to its active coenzyme; (3) it may not be bound to its apoenzyme to form a holoenzyme; and (4) vitamins or their coenzyme products may stabilize normal or mutant enzyme complexes in supraphysiologic concentrations. This latter mechanism producing vitamin responsivity has been postulated in thiamine-responsive maple syrup urine disease and pyridoxine-responsive homocystinuria. Therapeutic importance of this type of pathologic physiology is evident. In certain instances, administration of high concentrations of the precursor vitamin may augment the defective coenzyme or enzyme pathway and provide the individual with some protection against the toxic precursor or deficient product resulting from the altered pathway. In several cases, fetuses with B_{12}-responsive methylmalonic aciduria or biotin-responsive multiple carboxylase deficiency were diagnosed prepartum, and they and their mothers were treated with massive doses of B_{12} or biotin. The children at birth were prevented from developing acidemia.

DISEASES CAUSED BY ENZYMES REGULATING DRUG METABOLISM

Some inherited disorders are not expressed until the organism is stressed by the administration of certain drugs. Such a disorder might arise if a mutant gene product did not remove a potentially toxic drug. A well-known example of this disorder is deficiency of *serum cholinesterase*. As described previously, this enzyme hydrolyzes choline esters, notably the muscle relaxant succinyldicholine. Different types of mutant gene products can be analyzed in pedigrees by their resistance to inhibitors. A silent allele has also been described that results in the complete loss of enzyme activity in the homozygous condition. Immunochemical studies suggest that this "silent allele" produces a true absence of the total enzyme protein, whereas other mutant alleles produce products that differ only in their kinetic properties for the binding of cholinesterase and various inhibitors. The abnormal enzymes, however, have similar immunochemical properties, electrophoretic mobilities, and molecular size. Pedigree analyses suggest 10 different phenotypes from three alleles at one locus (E_1). A second locus (E_2) has been described for this protein when examined by starch gel electrophoresis. The E_2 locus is characterized by an isozyme with a fifth subunit (C_5) that is seen in approximately 10 per cent of European people. The functional attributes of this electrophoretic variation are as yet unknown. Individuals who are homozygous for an atypical allele or doubly het-

erozygous for the atypical silent allele are unable to hydrolyze succinyldicholine, a drug used to induce transient muscular paralysis during surgery. Normally, it is removed in minutes, but in affected individuals the drug persists in its pharmacologically active form for a prolonged period of time.

The use of a pedigree and biochemical analysis in the diagnosis and prevention of this disorder in a family is illustrated in Figure 3–37 (compare with Figure 3–8). The 19-year-old proband (III-1) is a healthy football player who had a molar tooth extracted. During surgery, succinyldicholine was administered, and the patient remained paralyzed for 6 hours. A family history indicated that his mother had a similar respiratory arrest 4 years earlier following hysterectomy. Serum from the mother (II-2), proband, and siblings (III-2, III-3) demonstrated reduced hydrolytic activity as well as resistance to dibucaine and fluoride, consistent with the homozygous atypical genotype (AA). This initial family history evaluation suggested direct parent-to-child transmission of an autosomal dominant trait, which was contrary to the usual recessive mode of inheritance for serum cholinesterase deficiency. Serum from the clinically normal father (II-1) showed normal enzyme activity but increased resistance to dibucaine and fluoride, suggesting that the father was heterozygous (AU). This finding provided evidence for an autosomal recessive mode of inheritance. The mother and siblings were advised to avoid succinyldicholine in the future. The normals and heterozygotes were reassured that they were not sensitive.

Identification of another group of inborn errors caused by drug administration resulted from the observations of Hockwald that American blacks develop an acute hemolytic anemia after receiving synthetic antimalarial drugs such as primaquine. This abnormal hemolytic response to the drug was caused by a deficiency of the enzyme glucose-6-phosphate dehydrogenase (G6PD), which normally catalyzes the oxidation of glucose-6-phosphate to 6-phosphogluconate with reduction of the coenzyme NADP to NADPH. This is the first step in the oxidation of glucose via the pentose shunt pathway, which serves to maintain the intracellular concentration of reduced coenzyme NADPH and glutathione. It is postulated that the interaction of primaquine with mutant G6PD results in failure to maintain reduced NADPH, diminution of reduced glutathione, fragility of red cell membrane, and hemolysis. Other drugs can produce these hemolytic crises; these include the sulfonamides, antimalarials, and fava beans (favism). Different mutant G6PD proteins occur in black, Mediterranean, and Middle Eastern populations. They are all X-linked recessive traits. Of 21 variants described, six are associated with hemolytic disease and presumably have specific properties that render red blood cells unstable. Female heterozygotes may be sensitive to these drugs, de-

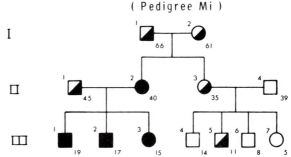

PSEUDOCHOLINESTERASE DEFICIENCY

(Pedigree Mi)

Figure 3–37 An example of combined pedigree and biochemical analysis in a family with pseudocholinesterase deficiency. Members represented by closed symbols are sensitive to succinyldicholine. "A" is atypical and "U" is the usual allele. Dibucaine and fluoride numbers indicate per cent inhibition of hydrolytic activity. (Assays were performed through the courtesy of B. N. LaDu, M.D., Ph.D.)

Patient	Activity*	Dibucaine Number	Fluoride Number	Probable Genotype
I-1	0.573	61.3	48.9	UA
I-2	0.700	64.0	51.5	UA
II-1	0.849	60.7	47.7	UA
II-2	0.421	20.8	23.0	AA
II-3	0.550	57.7	45.0	UA
II-4	1.140	83.0	60.5	UU
III-1	0.394	18.8	26.6	AA
III-2	0.391	12.4	23.2	AA
III-3	0.418	9.8	17.3	AA
III-4	1.054	81.2	64.6	UU
III-5	0.922	59.0	52.0	UA
III-6	1.070	80.3	63.8	UU
III-7	1.140	78.8	62.8	UU
(Normal)	(0.6-1.2)	(77-83)	(57-68)	(UU)

*μmoles benzoylcholine hydrolyzed / min / ml

pending on lyonization effects and the quantitative impairment in G6PD.

Another inherited disease produced by drugs was found after isoniazid (INH) was introduced for tuberculosis therapy. Initial studies revealed two distinct groups of individuals with different rates of removal of INH from the plasma. Evans demonstrated that 6 hours after a 40 mg per kg dose, a group of subjects known as "slow inactivators" had plasma INH concentrations above 4 μg per ml, whereas the "rapid inactivators" had levels below 3 μg per ml. In the urine of the rapid inactivators, the proportion of the drug in an acetylated form was greater than that in the urine of the slow inactivators, who excreted the drug unchanged. Acetylation of INH occurs in the liver as a consequence of the enzyme acetylcoenzyme A transferase. The activity of this enzyme is much greater in the livers of rapid inactivators than in the livers of slow inactivators. This enzyme is also concerned with the acetylation of drugs such as sulfamethazine and sulfadiazine. This pathologic physiology has some significance in the use of the drug for the treatment of tuberculosis. Slow inactivators of INH are more likely to develop peripheral neuropathy after prolonged administration,

but this rare complication of INH treatment can be prevented by the simultaneous administration of pyridoxine. Rapid inactivators may require higher doses to provide adequate circulating levels of the unacetylated active form. It is presumed from pedigree analyses that slow inactivators are homozygous for a "slow allele" and that rapid inactivators are either heterozygous or homozygous for the "rapid allele."

All the aforementioned examples of genetically determined enzyme defects are related to the metabolism of drugs and re-emphasize the interrelationships of genetic and environmental factors in the pathogenesis of disease. Since the underlying genetic differences are brought out by drugs, these and several conditions of a similar nature have been called *pharmacogenetic disorders*. Wider application of this concept would include the effects of life styles on genetically susceptible individuals. Thus, persons heterozygous for α-1-antitrypsin deficiency would develop emphysema if exposed to dust or cigarette smoke. Persons who have decreased negative feedback control for arylhydrocarbon hydroxylase may develop lung cancer if exposed to carcinogenic hydrocarbons. Individuals with high levels of pepsinogen may be prone to duodenal ulcer. The broader term now used for the interplay of genetic susceptibility and the environment is *ecogenetics*.

DISEASES CAUSED BY ABNORMAL STRUCTURAL PROTEINS THAT MAINTAIN STRUCTURAL INTEGRITY OF ORGANS

Collagen is a protein that constitutes the principal structural element of vertebrate connective tissue. Collagen fibers are formed by a series of metabolic processes, as outlined in Figure 3–38. At least five genetically distinct collagen α-chains are translated, hydroxylated, assembled into a triple helix, glycosylated, cleaved, extruded into the extracellular space, and cross-linked by several processes. These functions are catalyzed by several enzymes, including prolyl and lysyl hydroxylases, monosaccharide transferases, procollagen peptidase, and lysyl oxidase. The presence of hydroxylysine and hydroxyproline in the finished product is unique to this protein.

Abnormalities in collagen have been proposed as the causes of many human disorders. A partial list includes pseudoxanthoma elasticum, Marfan syndrome, cutis laxis, osteogenesis imperfecta, Ehlers-Danlos syndrome, chondrodystrophy, and interstitial nephritis. All these diseases are heterogeneous, but recent advances have provided

evidence for specific defects in a group of disorders clinically classified as Ehlers-Danlos syndrome. The composite clinical disorder is characterized by joint laxity, retinal detachment, small cornea, vertebral anomalies, abnormal atrophic scar formation, and hyperextensible, friable skin. At least seven subtypes have been defined on the basis of genetic and phenotypic differences. The first to be defined and evaluated at biochemical and genetic levels is type VI, characterized by hydroxylysine-deficient collagen and impaired lysyl hydroxylase in cultured skin fibroblasts (Figure 3–39). This enzymatic defect has been found partially impaired in skin cultured from both parents, confirming an autosomal recessive pattern of inheritance. Studies on collagen lysyl hydroxylase, a microsomal oxygenase, indicate that vitamin C is a principal physiologic reductant. The patient identified in Figure 3–39 responded to 4 gm per day of vitamin C with increased urinary hydroxylysine production, increase in corneal size, decrease in bleeding time, and improved muscle tone.

Collagen is the most obvious protein involved in maintaining structural integrity of organs. However, several proteins are involved in maintaining cellular structure. For instance, intermolecular stacking of hemoglobin S produces the sickling phenomenon of sickle cell anemia; abnormal spectrin may produce the spherocytes of hereditary spherocytic anemia; and the absence of β-

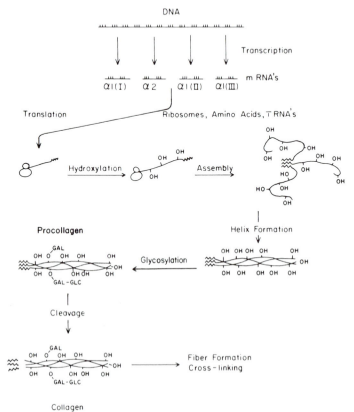

Figure 3–38 Collagen biosynthetic pathway. Processes of transcription, translation, hydroxylation of lysyl and prolyl residues, assembly, and glycosylation occur within cells. Procollagen cleavage and extrusion from the cell occur in association with cell membranes. Fiber formation and cross-linking occur extracellularly. Formation of monomeric collagen is depicted. (From Miller, E. J., and Matukas, V. J.: Fed. Proc. *33*:1197, 1974.)

Ehlers Danlos Syndrome (TYPE VI)

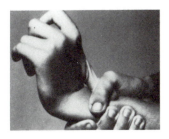

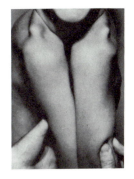

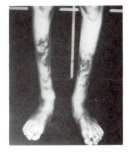

Skin Hydroxylysine (Residues/1000)		HOLYS HOPRO
Patient (JDH)	0.5	0.011
Controls (25)	5.1 ± 0.7	0.061 ± 0.009

Figure 3–39 Hyperflexibility of finger and shoulder joints and abnormally friable skin with scorbutic scar formation in an 8-year-old boy with hydroxylysine-deficient collagen. The patient's cultured skin fibroblasts had less than 10 per cent of normal collagen lysyl hydroxylase activity.

lipoprotein causes the increased sphingomyelin-to-lecithin ratio seen in acanthocytic red cells of patients with abetalipoproteinemia.

APPLICATIONS TO MANAGEMENT OF INHERITED DISEASE

Knowledge in the field of human genetics has grown rapidly, and our concern as physicians has been to find applications for this knowledge. Table 3–12 represents a composite of both factual and speculative approaches to the management of inherited diseases. These therapeutic approaches have been categorized according to the level of recognition of the pathogenic mechanisms. Thus, if what we recognize at present is an abnormal phenotype (as in Down syndrome, muscular dystrophy, and spina bifida), therapeutic approaches are limited to genetic counseling regarding the recurrence risks and to rehabilitation of the patient. In some instances the clinical phenotype may be expressed in cultured fetal cells or in amniotic fluid, and more precise counseling such as antenatal diagnosis can be offered. There are over 200 different disorders currently monitorable by these techniques—some only through indirectly associated findings such as increased amniotic fluid α-fetoprotein in fetuses with open neural tube anomalies or hereditary nephrosis. Another example is diagnosis of a male fetus in the case of X-linked recessive disorders, where the mother is a known or at-risk carrier of an incurable disorder such as Duchenne pseudohypertrophic muscular dystrophy. In many other disorders, specific enzyme defects are demonstrable in cultured amniotic fluid cells and provide more precise criteria for the probable phenotype of the fetus. Genetic counseling will become more precise as techniques of antenatal diagnosis improve. At this level of recognition, treatment of the affected individual must be considered. Sonography has become so sensitive that hydronephrosis due to posterior valve syndrome in the male has been treated surgically before birth. Another example is the reproductive-age female with phenylketonuria. Control of her blood phenylalanine to normal levels during conception and pregnancy may prevent the otherwise absolute risk to her offspring of having microcephaly and mental retardation as a result of elevated maternal phenylalanine.

Many inborn errors of metabolism are revealed by the presence of abnormal concentrations of potentially toxic precursors in an impaired reaction sequence and can be treated before the disease is clinically manifest. The best example of this is the statewide screening of newborn infants for elevated blood phenylalanine levels to diagnose phenylketonuria. Treatment of this group of disorders involves a form of environmental engineering in which the potentially toxic precursor, phenylalanine, is restricted in the diet to prevent manifestations of the clinical phenotype. The sequelae of many other disorders, such as hypothyroidism, galactosemia, maple syrup urine disease, and homocystinuria, are similarly preventable through mass screening (nonselective) of all newborns. Early retrieval, diagnosis, and treatment

TABLE 3–12 THERAPY OF INHERITED DISEASE

Level of Recognition	Treatment

1. Clinical phenotype	1. Genetic counseling
	   a. Antenatal diagnosis
	   b. Rehabilitation

2. Impaired reaction sequence
   a. Toxic precursor
   b. Deficient product
   c. Deficient coenzyme
   d. Sensitivity to environment
	2. Environmental engineering
	   a. Restriction
	   b. Replacement
	   c. Vitamin administration
	   d. Exposure prevention

3. Defective gene product
   a. Enzyme
   b. Structural protein
   c. Regulation
	3. Cellular engineering
	   a. Replacement; bone marrow transplant
	   b. Prevention of structural changes
	   c. Provision of inducer, repressor, or feedback inhibitor

4. Mutant DNA	4. Genetic engineering
	   a. Transformation
	   b. Transduction

before the third week of life are also prerequisites in such a preventive program. In other conditions, such as Hartnup disease, the pellagra-like symptoms are preventable by the administration of the deficient end product, nicotinic acid. In vitamin dependency syndromes such as vitamin-responsive methylmalonic aciduria, the administration of massive amounts of the vitamin precursor will increase the deficient coenzyme and ameliorate the blocked reaction sequence and clinical problems attendant to the untreated condition. Such approaches during the third trimester of pregnancy have prevented newborn manifestations of methylmalonic acidemia by treating the mother with several milligrams of B_{12} per day. Environmental engineering may also be provided in circumstances in which an individual has a mutant gene product reflected only under stressful environmental conditions. The group of pharmacogenetic disorders is a good example of this situation in which patients are sensitive to the administration of primaquine (G6PD deficiency) or succinyldicholine (pseudocholinesterase deficiency). Prediction and prevention can be effected through pedigree analysis and chemical evaluation of "high-risk" members. Speculation in this area grows as we analyze the complex alleles of circulating blood proteins such as the α_1-antitrypsin. Fagerhol has pointed out that functional defects in antitrypsin activity and protein phenotypes may be associated with increased susceptibility to pulmonary disease, cirrhosis, and clotting disorders. As more knowledge is collected relating the structural and functional defects of this group of proteins and as populations are screened for their protein genotype, physicians may offer specific suggestions concerning the best type of environment in which an individual should live. For instance, a presymptomatic patient with α_1-anti-

trypsin deficiency and a protein genotype of ZZ (deficient) or MZ (40 per cent activity) may be advised to live in a rural rather than an urban area to retard the development of lung disease resulting from the polluted environment. Patients from families in which high serum group I pepsinogen is linked to duodenal ulcer may develop life styles amenable to preventing ulcer disease. Similarly, children in families with high blood levels of LDL and cholesterol may be treated with compactin to bypass the LDL-cholesterol receptor, suppress HMG CoA-reductase, reduce cholesterol biosynthesis, and prevent atherosclerosis. Compactin and its analogue, merinolin, are compounds isolated from mold.

In some of the inborn errors alluded to previously, the defective gene product has been defined as a functional or regulatory impairment of cell metabolism. At this level of recognition, therapy can be considered in terms of cellular engineering in which the objective is the replacement of a defective enzyme. This concept is not novel, since we all recognize the value of insulin or antihemophilic globulin in inherited disorders such as diabetes mellitus or hemophilia A. However, the administration of specific enzymes involved in intracellular function remains at present in the area of research. Purified enzymes can be enclosed in semipermeable inert nylon microspherules to protect the enzyme from immune host response. Catalase has been injected intravenously to revert the abnormal biochemical phenotype in acatalasemic mice, and urease has raised the blood ammonia in dogs. If the enzyme is lysosomal or cytoplasmic, its eventual deposition in the reticuloendothelial cells may provide function to the organism in which this enzyme is deficient. Glucocerebrosidase enclosed in liposomes or autologous red blood cell ghosts has alleviated organomegaly in Gaucher's disease. In some of the mucopolysaccharidoses, bone marrow transplants have produced macrophages that provide functioning enzymes. In other instances, the defective gene product may be a structural protein whose molecular structure is recognized. The administration of cyanate and carbamyl phosphate to patients with sickle cell disease is a form of cellular engineering aimed at correcting the molecular aggregation of sickle hemoglobin and is under study. In some disorders, the defective enzyme function may be inducible. Thus, in hepatic glucuronyl transferase deficiency, sodium phenobarbital has enhanced this enzymatic pathway and the perinatal utilization of bilirubin. Steroid hormones may also be effective inducers of some enzymes. In one patient with type III glycogen storage disease, a double enzyme deficiency involving amylo-1,6-glucosidase and glucose-6-phosphatase was described. A fourfold increase in glucose-6-phosphatase activity occurred upon administration of triamcinolone. Repression of an overactive pathway may also become a form of genetic engineering. In orotic aciduria, the administration of uridine represses the initial step of this pathway and reduces the formation of insoluble orotic acid.

Transplantation has become a reality in several heritable disorders. Kidney transplants in Fabry disease have provided ceramide trihexosidase, and reduced deposition of ceramide trihexoses in other organs. Thymus transplants in DiGeorge syndrome and marrow transplants in disorders of immune response have literally cured disease.

Finally, the most intriguing aspect of therapy in inherited human disease involves approaches to gene regulation. The base analogue, 5-azacytidine, induces hypomethylation of DNA and thereby "turns on" fetal hemoglobin genes in patients suffering from thalassemia and sickle cell anemia. Thus, γ-globin chains replace the missing or defective β-globin chains and prolong erythrocyte half-life. Although many of the fundamental genetic and regulatory processes of mammalian cells remain unknown, recombinant DNA technology has demonstrated science's ability to introduce new functional genes into mammalian cells. Although these developments do not provide practical genetic engineering, it is now clear that science has provided means by which genes can be transferred and inserted into mammalian cells. These basic tools will provide answers to many questions concerning gene function and a new approach to treating inherited disorders.

GLOSSARY OF GENETIC TERMS

Acrocentric—Chromosomes with the centromere close to one end.

Alleles—Alternate forms of a gene.

Aneuploid (aneuploidy)—Deviation from the basic diploid number or from exact multiples of the basic (haploid) number in a chromosome series.

Arm (chromosome)—The portion located on either side of the centromere of a metaphase chromosome.

Autosome—Any non–sex chromosomes (22 pairs in humans).

Balanced translocation—Rearrangement of chromosomal material, without genetic effect.

Break (chromosome)—Interruption in staining of the chromosome arm, with displacement in the alignment of the portions on either side of the interruption.

Cell cycle (cell life cycle)—The cycle in the life of a cell that includes progression through mitosis (M) and interphase.

Centromere (also kinetochore or primary constriction)—A nonstaining area on a chromosome, separating the chromosome arms; the point of attachment of the chromosome to the mitotic spindle.

Chromatid—One of two structurally distinguishable (by light microscopy) longitudinal subunits of a metaphase chromosome.

Chromatin—Areas of a cell nucleus that stain with a DNA stain. (See also *Sex chromatin*.)

Cis—Two genes on the same chromosome are cis to each other or coupled.

Cistron—The gene considered on a functional basis as defined by the cis-trans complementation test. Two mutants in the same cistron do not complement; two mutants in different cistrons do.

Codon—A triplet of three bases in a strand of DNA that codes for a specific amino acid.

Complementation—Interaction of two cytoplasmic products to produce a normal phenotype.

Crossing-over—The exchange of genetic material between members of a pair of homologous chromosomes that leads to the formation of recombinants.

Deletion (chromosome)—Absence of part of a chromosome.

Diploid—Possessing two genomes. In humans, somatic cells normally contain the diploid number of chromosomes: 46 (2n).

Discontinuous traits—Two clearly different phenotypes that do not blend with one another.

Dominant—The phenotype expressed in the F_1 heterozygote resulting from a cross between two true-breeding strains. The dominant allele determines the phenotype expressed by a heterozygote.

Endoreduplication (endopolyploidy)—The result of a partial mitosis involving doubling of chromosome number without division of nucleus or cytoplasm.

End-product repression—Repression of synthesis of the messenger RNA from the operon for an anabolic (synthetic) pathway caused by the accumulation of an end product of the pathway.

Episome—A piece of DNA that can either remain separate from the rest of the genome or become integrated into it. A type of plasmid.

F_1—The first filial generation (the progeny) of a cross between two individuals.

Fragment (chromosome)—A portion of a chromosome without a centromere.

Feedback inhibition—Inhibition of an enzyme in an anabolic pathway by an allosteric effect of an end product or derivative of the end product in this pathway.

Frameshift mutation—A mutation arising from the insertion or deletion of a nucleotide pair.

Gap (chromosome)—Interruption in staining of a chromosome arm, without disturbance of alignment of the portions on either side of the interruption.

Gene—(a) Classic mendelian definition: The fundamental biologic unit of heredity transmitted from generation to generation unchanged;
   (b) Molecular definition: Unit of function of a cistron. One gene codes for one polypeptide chain.

Genome—One copy of each allele.

Genotype—The genetic constitution of an individual.

Haploid—A haploid cell contains one copy of a genome. The normal mammalian gamete contains only one member of each chromosome pair and is therefore haploid. In humans, the haploid chromosome number (n) is 23.

Hemizygote—An individual possessing only one allele at a given locus. Since human males have only one X chromosome, they are said to be hemizygous with respect to X-linked genes.

Heterochromatin (heterochromatization; heterochromatic)—Nuclear areas that stain "differently" with DNA stains.

Heterogeneity—One phenotypic effect produced by a number of different genetic mechanisms or genes.

Heterokaryon—Cell with two or more genomes of different types.

Heterozygote—An individual who has two different alleles for a given gene.

Homozygote—An individual possessing a pair of identical alleles for a given gene.

Hyperdiploidy (hypodiploidy)—More (or less) than the diploid number of chromosomes. A form of aneuploidy.

Isochromosome—A chromosome consisting of identical arms on either side of the centromere.

Karyotype—A systematized arrangement of chromosomes.

Linkage—Association of genes on one chromosome.

Locus—A cluster of genes located in a linkage group.

Map distance (genetic distance)—The distance between two genes equal to the number of progeny recombinant for them divided by the total number of progeny.

Meiosis—That form of cell division in the formation of gametes producing the haploid chromosome number (n) from a diploid cell (2n).

Metacentric—Chromosomes with the centromere located in the center, making the two arms on either side of it equal in length.

Missense mutation—A change in a gene resulting in the incorporation of an incorrect amino acid into its product.

Monosomic (monosomy)—One chromosome pair contains 1 instead of 2 chromosomes.

Monozygotic—Twins derived from a single fertilized ovum (identical twins).

Mosaic—An individual or tissue with at least two cell lines, differing in genotype or karyotype, derived from a single zygote.

Mutant—An altered gene, or an individual bearing such an altered gene.

Mutation—An alteration in genetic material that is transmitted from one generation to the next.

Nonsense mutation—A change in a gene resulting in the formation of one of the "stop" codons in place of a codon for a particular amino acid and leading to formation of a partial protein that is terminated at the site of the mutation.

Operon—A genetic unit consisting of an operator and the cistrons whose actions it controls.

Phenocopy—An individual whose appearance is produced by an environmental effect but whose phenotype is similar to one produced by a genetic effect.

Phenotype—The physical constitution of an individual. This includes physical, biochemical, and physiologic makeup of an individual as determined by his genotype and the environment in which he develops.

Pleiotropy—Multiple phenotypic effects produced by a single genetic mechanism or gene (gene pair).

Point mutation—A change in a single base pair.

Polyploidy—The designation for the occurrence of chromosome numbers in multiples of the basic haploid number (n), other than the diploid number (2n), for example, triploidy (3n) and tetraploidy (4n).

Proband—Same as *propositus*.

Propositus—Also called *index case,* or *proband*; the family member who first draws attention to a pedigree of a particular trait.

Protein polymorphism—The occurrence of two or more different forms of the same protein.

Recessive—That phenotype which is *not* expressed in the F_1 heterozygote resulting from a cross between two true breeding strains. In classic genetics, this term can be used only when the F_1 heterozygote is phenotypically identical with that of one of the homozygotes. In human genetics, "recessive" refers to a gene that is expressed only when homozygous.

Recombination—The formation of new combinations of linked genes by crossing-over between them.

Ring (chromosome)—Attachment of opposite ends of a chromosome to form a ring.

Satellite—DNA-staining structure on the distal end of a chromosome arm and separated from it by a secondary constriction.

Secondary constriction—A nonstaining area on a chromosome arm.

Segregation—The separation of alleles and chromosomes during meiosis.

Sex chromatin, female (Barr body, X body)—A characteristic area in the interphase nucleus composed of X-chromosome material that stains heavily with a DNA stain.

Sex chromatin, male (Y body)—A characteristic area in the interphase nucleus composed of Y-chromosome material that fluoresces brightly.

Sex chromosomes—XX in human female; XY in human male: 1 pair is normally present in each individual.

Silent allele—An allele that has no detectable product, presumably produced by a nonsense mutant.

Somatic—Pertaining to cells other than germ cells.

Tetraploid—The quadruple basic number in a chromosome series (4n).

Trans—Two genes on different chromosomes are trans to each other, or in repulsion.

Transcription, RNA—The process by which new RNA is made from a DNA template.

Transduction—A form of recombination in bacteria in which a bacteriophage serves as the DNA vector.

Transformation—The form of recombination in bacteria in which naked DNA serves as the vector.

Translation—The process by which genetic information contained in DNA is carried by mRNA from the nucleus to the cytoplasm and directs amino acid sequences in the synthesis of proteins.

Translocation—The transfer of a piece of one chromosome to another chromosome.

Triploid—The triple basic number in a chromosome series (3n).

Trisomy—The state of having one extra chromosome per cell. Instead of the usual two chromosomes in a homologous pair, there are now three.

X-linked—Genes on the X chromosome or traits determined by such genes are X-linked.

REFERENCES

GENERAL GENETICS

Bergsma, D. (Ed.): Birth Defects. Atlas and Compendium. 2nd ed. The National Foundation. Baltimore, The Williams and Wilkins Co., 1979.

Carter, C. O.: Genetics of common disorders. Br. Med. Bull. 25:52, 1969.

Carter, C. O.: Multifactorial genetic disease. Hosp. Pract. 5:45, 1970.

Carter, C. O., David, P. A., and Laurence, K. M.: A family study of major central nervous system malformations in South Wales. J. Med. Genet. 5:81, 1968.

Carter, C. O., and Evans, K. A.: Inheritance of congenital pyloric stenosis. J. Med. Genet. 6:233, 1969.

Cavalli-Sforza, L. L., and Bodmer, W. F.: The Genetics of Human Populations. San Francisco, W. H. Freeman and Company, 1971.

Edwards, J. H.: The simulation of mendelism. Acta Genet. (Basel) 10:63, 1960.

Falconer, D. S.: The inheritance of liability to certain diseases, estimated from the incidence among relatives. Ann. Hum. Genet. 29:51, 1965.

Haws, D. V., and McKusick, V. A.: Farabee's brachydactylous kindred revisited. Bull. Johns Hopkins Hosp. 113:20, 1963.

Lubs, H. A., and dela Cruz, F. (Eds.): Genetic Counseling. New York, Raven Press, 1977.

McKusick, V. A.: Human Genetics. Englewood Cliffs, New Jersey, Prentice-Hall, Inc., 1964.

McKusick, V. A.: Mendelian Inheritance in Man: Catalogs of Autosomal Dominant, Autosomal Recessive, and X-linked Phenotypes. 6th ed. Baltimore, Johns Hopkins University Press, 1983.

McKusick, V. A., and Claiborne, R. (Eds.): Medical Genetics. New York, HP Publishing Co., Inc., 1973.

Mange, A. P., and Mange, E. J.: Genetics: Human Aspects. Philadelphia, Saunders College, 1980.

Mendel, G.: Versuche über Pflanzenhybriden. Leipzig, Engelmann, 1901. Translated in J. Heredity, 42:1, 1951.

Milunski, A. (Ed.): Genetic Disorders and the Fetus. New York, Plenum Press, 1979.

Riccardi, V. M.: The Genetic Approach to Human Disease. New York, Oxford University Press, 1977.

Simpson, J. L., Golbus, M. S., Martin, A. O., and Sarto, G. E.: Genetics in Obstetrics and Gynecology. New York, Grune & Stratton, 1982.

Smith, D. W.: Recognizable Patterns of Human Malformation. Genetic, Embryologic and Clinical Aspects. 3rd ed. Philadelphia, W. B. Saunders Co., 1982.

Thompson, J. S., and Thompson, M. W.: Genetics in Medicine, 3rd ed. Philadelphia, W. B. Saunders Co., 1980.

Vogel, F., and Motulsky, A. G.: Human Genetics. New York, Springer-Verlag, 1979.

CHROMOSOMAL GENETICS

General

An international system for human cytogenetic nomenclature (1978). Cytogenet. Cell Genet. 21:313, 1978.

An international system for human cytogenetic nomenclature—high-resolution banding (1981). Cytogenet. Cell Genet. 31:1, 1981. Or Birth Defects: Original Article Series XVII:5. New York, March of Dimes Birth Defects Foundation, 1981.

Borgaonkar, D. S.: Chromosomal Variation in Man: A Catalog of Chromosomal Variants and Anomalies. 3rd ed. New York, Alan R. Liss, Inc., 1980.

DuPraw, E. J.: DNA and Chromosomes. New York, Holt, Rinehart and Winston, Inc., 1970, Ch. 9.

Ford, E. H. R.: Human Chromosomes. New York, Academic Press, 1973.

Hamerton, J. L., Canning, N., Ray, M., and Smith, S.: A cytogenetic survey of 14,069 newborn infants. I. Incidence of chromosome abnormalities. Clin. Genet. 8:223, 1975.

Makino, S.: Human Chromosomes. Tokyo, Igaku Shoin Ltd., 1975.

Ohno, S., Klinger, H. P., and Atkin, N. B.: Human oögenesis. Cytogenetics 1:42, 1962.

Paris Conference (1971): Standardization in Human Cytogenet-

ics. Birth Defects. Original Article Series VIII:7. New York, The National Foundation, 1972. Or Paris Conference (1971): Standardization in human cytogenetics. Cytogenetics 11:313, 1972.

Paris Conference (1971), Supplement (1975): Standardization in Human Cytogenetics. Birth Defects: Original Article Series XI:9. New York, The National Foundation, 1975.

Priest, J. H.: Medical Cytogenetics and Cell Culture. 2nd ed. Philadelphia, Lea and Febiger, 1977.

Schwarzacher, H. G., Wolf, U., and Passarge, E. (Eds.): Methods in Human Cytogenetics. New York, Springer-Verlag, Inc., 1974.

Therman, E.: Human Chromosomes. New York, Springer-Verlag, 1980.

Yunis, J. J. (Ed.): Human Chromosome Methodology. New York, Academic Press, 1974.

Chromosome Banding

Arrighi, F. E., and Hsu, T. C.: Localization of heterochromatin in human chromosomes. Cytogenetics 10:81, 1971.

Bobrow, M., Pearson, P. L., Pike, M. C., and El-Alfi, O. S.: Length variation in the quinacrine-binding segment of human Y chromosomes of different sizes. Cytogenetics 10:190, 1971.

Caspersson, T., Lomakka, G., and Zech, L.: The 24 fluorescence patterns of the human metaphase chromosomes—distinguishing characters and variability. Hereditas 67:89, 1971.

Craig-Holmes, A. P., Moore, F. B., and Shaw, M. W.: Polymorphism of human C-band heterochromatin. I. Frequency of variants. Am. J. Hum. Genet. 25:181, 1973.

Dutrillaux, B., and Lejeune, J.: Cytogénétique humaine.—Sur une nouvelle Technique d'Analyse du Caryotype humain. C. R. Acad. Sci. (Paris) 272:2638, 1971.

Seabright, M.: A rapid banding technique for human chromosomes. Lancet 2:971, 1971.

Sex Chromatin

Barr, M. L., Bertram, L. F., and Lindsay, H. A.: The morphology of the nerve cell nucleus, according to sex. Anat. Rec. 107:283, 1950.

Goad, W. B., Robinson, A., and Puck, T. T.: Incidence of aneuploidy in a human population. Am. J. Hum. Genet. 28:62, 1976.

Lyon, M. F.: Sex chromatin and gene action in the mammalian X-chromosome. Am. J. Hum. Genet. 14:135, 1962.

Mittwoch, U.: Sex Chromatin. J. Med. Genet. 1:50, 1964.

Pearson, P. L., Bobrow, M., and Vosa, C. G.: Technique for identifying Y chromosomes in human interphase nuclei. Nature 226:78, 1970.

Priest, J. H.: Medical Cytogenetics and Cell Culture. Sex Chromatin. 2nd ed. Philadelphia, Lea & Febiger, 1977, Ch. 10.

Congenital Defect Syndromes

Allderdice, P. W., Davis, J. G., Miller, O. J., et al.: The 13q-deletion syndrome. Am. J. Hum. Genet. 21:499, 1969.

Becker, K. L., Hoppman, D. L., Albert, A., et al.: Klinefelter's syndrome. Arch. Int. Med. 118:314, 1966.

Beratis, N. G., Kardon, N. B., Hsu, L. Y. F., et al.: Parental mosaicism in trisomy 18. Pediatrics 50:908, 1972.

Borgaonkar, D. S., Mules, E., and Char, F.: Do the 48, XXYY males have a characteristic phenotype? Chem. Genet. 1:272, 1970.

Caldwell, P. D., and Smith, D. W.: The XXY (Klinefelter's) syndrome in childhood: detection and treatment. J. Pediatr. 80:250, 1972.

de Grouchy, J.: Chromosome 18: a topologic approach. J. Pediatr. 66:414, 1965.

Edwards, J. H., Harnden, D. G., Cameron, A. H., et al.: A new trisomic syndrome. Lancet 1:787, 1960.

Ford, C. E., Jones, K. W., Polani, P. E., et al.: A sex-chromosome anomaly in a case of gonadal dysgenesis (Turner's syndrome). Lancet 1:711, 1959.

Grace, E., Drennan, J., Colver, D., and Gordon, R. R.: The 13q-syndrome. J. Med. Genet. 8:351, 1971.

Hsu, L. Y. F., Shapiro, L. R., Gertner, M., et al.: Trisomy 22: a clinical entity. J. Pediatr. 79:12, 1971.

Jacobs, P. A., Baikie, A. G., Court Brown, W. M., et al.: Evidence for the existence of the human "super female." Lancet 2:423, 1959.

Jacobs, P. A., and Strong, J. A.: A case of human intersexuality having a possible XXY sex-determining mechanism. Nature 183:302, 1959.

Klinefelter, H. F., Reifenstein, E. C., and Albright, F.: Syndrome characterized by gynecomastia, aspermatogenesis without A-Leydigism, and increased excretion of follicle-stimulating hormone. J. Clin. Endocrinol. 2:615, 1942.

Lejeune, J., Gautier, M., and Turpin, R.: Étude des chromosomes somatiques de neuf enfants mongoliens. C. R. Acad. Sci. (Paris) 248:1721, 1959.

Lejeune, J., Lafourcad, J., Berger, R., et al.: Trois Cas de Deletion Partielle des Bras Courts d'un Chromosome 5. C. R. Acad. Sci. (D). (Paris) 257:3098, 1963.

Patau, K., Smith, D., Therman, E., et al.: Multiple congenital anomalies caused by an extra autosome. Lancet 1:790, 1960.

Penrose, L. S., and Smith, G. F.: Down's Anomaly. Boston, Little, Brown & Co., 1966.

Polani, P. E., Hunter, W. F., and Lennox, B.: Chromosomal sex in Turner's syndrome with coarctation of the aorta. Lancet 2:120, 1954.

Shepard, T. H.: Catalog of Teratogenic Agents. 4th ed. Baltimore, The Johns Hopkins University Press, 1983.

Sinet, P.-M., Couturier, J., Dutrillaux, B., et al.: Trisomie 21 et superoxyde dismutase-1 (IPO-A). Exp. Cell Res. 97:47, 1976.

Smith, D. W., Patau, K., Therman, E., et al.: The D₁ trisomy syndrome. J. Pediatr. 63:326, 1963.

Tuncbilek, E., Halicioglu, C., and Say, B.: Trisomy-8 syndrome. Humangenetik 23:23, 1974.

Turner, H. H.: A syndrome of infantilism, congenital webbed neck, and cubitus valgus. Endocrinology 23:566, 1938.

Chromosomes and Neoplasia

de Klein, A., van Kessel, A. G., Grosveld, G., et al.: A cellular oncogene is translocated to the Philadelphia chromosome in chronic myelogenous leukaemia. Nature 300:765, 1982.

Nowell, P. C., and Hungerford, D. A.: Chromosome studies in human leukemia. II. Chronic granulocytic leukemia. J. Natl. Cancer Inst. 27:1031, 1961.

Rowley, J. D.: Identification of the constant chromosome regions involved in human hematologic malignant disease. Science 216:749, 1982.

Yunis, J. J., Oken, M. M., Kaplan, M. E., et al.: Distinctive chromosomal abnormalities in histologic subtypes of non-Hodgkin's lymphoma. N. Engl. J. Med. 307:1231, 1982.

Chromosome Mapping

Human Gene Mapping 6 (1981). Cytogenet. Cell Genet. 32:1, 1982.

McKusick, V. A.: The mapping of human chromosomes. Sci. Am. 224:104, 1971.

Pardue, M. L., and Gall, J. G.: Molecular hybridization of radioactive DNA to the DNA of cytological preparations. Proc. Natl. Acad. Sci. U.S.A. 64:600, 1969.

Ruddle, F. H., and Kucherlapati, R. S.: Hybrid cells and human genes. Sci. Am. 231:36, 1974.

Shows, T. B., and Sakaguchi, A. Y.: Gene transfer and gene mapping in mammalian cells in culture. In Vitro 16:55, 1980.

MOLECULAR BASIS FOR INHERITANCE

Alberts, B., Bray, D., Lewis, J., et al.: Molecular Biology of the Cell. New York, Garland Publishing Co., 1983.

Cleaver, J. E.: Defective repair replication of DNA in xeroderma pigmentosum. Nature 218:652, 1968.

Crick, F. H. C.: The genetic code. Proc. Roy. Soc. B 167:331, 1967.

Hartman, P. E., and Suskind, S. R.: Gene Action. 2nd ed. Englewood Cliffs, New Jersey, Prentice-Hall, Inc., 1969.

Ingram, V. M., and Stretton, A. O.: Genetic basis of the thalassaemia diseases. Nature 184:1903, 1959.

Ingram, V. M.: Gene mutations in human haemoglobin: the chemical difference between normal and sickle cell haemoglobin. Nature 180:326, 1957.

Itano, H. A., and Neel, J. V.: A new inherited abnormality of human hemoglobin. Proc. Natl. Acad. Sci. U.S.A. 36:613, 1950.

Jacob, F., and Monod, J.: Genetic regulatory mechanisms in the synthesis of proteins. J. Mol. Biol. 3:318, 1961.

Jacob, F., and Monod, J.: On regulation of gene activity. Cold Spring Harbor Symp. Quant. Biol. 26:193, 1961.

Kornberg, A.: Enzymatic synthesis of DNA. New York, John Wiley and Sons, Inc., 1962.

Meselson, M., and Stahl, F. W.: The replication of DNA in Escherichia coli. Proc. Natl. Acad. Sci. U.S.A. 44:671, 1958.

Murayama, M.: Structure of sickle cell hemoglobin and molecular mechanism of the sickling phenomenon. Clin. Chem. 14:578, 1968.

Neel, J. V.: The inheritance of sickle cell anemia. Science 110:64, 1949.

Neel, J. V.: The inheritance of sickling phenomenon with particular reference to sickle cell disease. Blood 6:389, 1951.

Nirenberg, M. W., and Matthaei, J. H.: The dependence of cell-free protein synthesis in E. coli upon naturally occurring or synthetic polyribonucleotides. Proc. Natl. Acad. Sci. (Wash.) 47:1588, 1961.

Pauling, L., Itano, H. A., Singer, S. J., and Wells, I. C.: Sickle cell anemia, molecular disease. Science 110:543, 1949.

Perutz, M. F., and Lehmann, H.: Molecular pathology of human haemoglobin. Nature 219:902, 1968.

Perutz, M. F., and Mitchison, J. M.: State of haemoglobin in sickle-cell anaemia. Nature 166:677, 1950.

Ptashne, M.: Specific binding of the λ-phage repressor to λ-DNA. Nature 214:232, 1967.

Watson, J. D.: The Double Helix. New York, Atheneum Publishers, 1968.

Watson, J. D.: Molecular Biology of the Gene. 3rd edition. Menlo Park, Cal., W. A. Benjamin, Inc., 1976.

Watson, J. D., and Crick, F. H. C.: Genetical implications of the structure of deoxyribose nucleic acid. Nature (London) 171:964, 1953.

Weatherall, D. J.: Genetics of the thalassaemias. Br. Med. Bull. 25:24, 1969.

Woese, C. R.: The present status of the genetic code. Progr. Nucleic Acid Res. Molec. Biol. 7:107, 1967.

INHERITED METABOLIC DISORDERS
General References

Bondy, P. K., and Rosenberg, L. E. (Eds.): Metabolic Control and Disease. 8th ed. Philadelphia, W. B. Saunders Co., 1980.

Gardner, L. I.: Endocrine and Genetic Diseases of Childhood. 2nd ed. Philadelphia, W. B. Saunders Co., 1975.

Garrod, A. E.: Inborn errors of metabolism (Croonian Lectures). Lancet 2:1, 73, 142, 214, 1908.

Harris, H.: The Principles of Human Biochemical Genetics, 3rd ed. New York, American Elsevier Publishing Co., Inc., 1980.

Nyhan, W. L. (Ed.): Heritable Disorders of Amino Acid Metabolism. New York, John Wiley and Sons, 1974.

Stanbury, J. B., Wyngaarden, J. B., and Frederickson, D. S., et al. (Eds.): The Metabolic Basis of Inherited Disease. 5th ed. New York, McGraw-Hill Book Co., 1983.

Membrane Transport

Bolis, L., Hoffman, J. F., and Leaf, A.: Membranes and Disease. New York, Raven Press, 1976.

Christensen, H. N.: Biological Transport. 2nd ed. Reading, Mass., W. A. Benjamin, 1975.

Crane, R. K.: Intestinal absorption of sugars. Physiol. Rev. 40:789, 1960.

Dent, C. E., and Rose, G. A.: Amino acid metabolism in cystinuria. Q. J. Med. 20:205, 1951.

Elsas, L. J., Busse, D., and Rosenberg, L. E.: Autosomal recessive inheritance of renal glycosuria. Metabolism 20:968, 1971.

Elsas, L. J., Hillman, R. E., Patterson, J. H., and Rosenberg, L. E.: Renal and intestinal hexose transport in familial glucose-galactose malabsorption. J. Clin. Invest. 49:576, 1970.

Elsas, L. J., and Rosenberg, L. E.: Famial renal glycosuria: a genetic reappraisal of hexose transport by kidney and intestine. J. Clin. Invest. 48:1845, 1969.

Evanson, J. M., and Stanbury, S. W.: Congenital chloridorrhea or so-called congenital alkalosis in diarrhea. Gut 6:29, 1965.

Goldberg, L. S., and Fudenberg, H. H.: Familial selective malabsorption of vitamin B_{12}. Re-evaluation of an in vivo intrinsic-factor inhibitor. N. Engl. J. Med. 279:405, 1968.

Jacob, H. S., and Jandl, J. H.: Increased cell membrane permeability in the pathogenesis of hereditary spherocytosis. J. Clin. Invest. 43:1704, 1964.

Milne, M. D., Crawford, M. A., Girao, C. B., and Loughridge, L. W.: The metabolic disorder in Hartnup disease. Q. J. Med. 29:407, 1960.

Pardee, A. B.: Crystallization of a sulfate-binding protein (permease) from Salmonella typhimurium. Science 156:1627, 1967.

Rosenberg, L. E., Downing, S., Durant, J. L., and Segal, S.: Cystinuria: biochemical evidence for three genetically distinct diseases. J. Clin. Invest. 45:365, 1966.

Rosenberg, L. E.: Genetic Heterogeneity in Cystinuria. In Nyhan, W. L. (Ed.): Amino-Acid Metabolism and Genetic Variations. New York, McGraw-Hill Book Co., Inc., 1968.

Scriver, C. R., and Hechtman, P.: Human Genetics of Membrane Transport with Emphasis on Amino Acids. In Harris, H., and Hirschhorn, K. (Eds.): Advances in Human Genetics. New York, Plenum Press, 1970, pp. 211–274.

Shepard, R., Anderson, V. E.: and Eaton, J. W. (Eds.): Membranes and Genetic Disease. Progress in Clinical and Biological Research. Vol. 97. New York, A. R. Liss, Inc., 1982.

Winters, R. W., Graham, J. B., Williams, T. F., et al.: A genetic study of familial hypophosphatemia and vitamin D resistant rickets with a review of the literature. Medicine 37:97, 1958.

Wolfe, L. C., John, V. M., Falcone, J. C., et al.: A genetic defect in the binding of protein 4.1 to spectrin in a kindred with hereditary spherocytosis. N. Engl. J. Med. 307:1367, 1982.

Major Metabolic Pathways

Bongiovanni, A. M.: The adrenogenital syndrome with deficiency of 3 beta-hydroxysteroid dehydrogenase. J. Clin. Invest. 41:2086, 1962.

Childs, B., Grumbach, M. M., and Van Wyk, J. J.: Virilizing adrenal hyperplasia: a genetic and hormonal study. J. Clin. Invest. 35:213, 1956.

Dancis, J, Hutzler, J., and Cox, R. P.: Enzyme defect in skin fibroblasts in intermittent branched-chain ketonuria and in maple syrup urine disease. Biochem. Med. 2:407, 1969.

Dancis, J., Hutzler, J., and Rokkones, T.: Intermittent branched-chain ketonuria, variant of maple-syrup-urine disease. N. Engl. J. Med. 276:84, 1967.

Elsas, L. J., and Danner, O. J.: The role of thiamin in maple syrup urine disease. Ann. N.Y. Acad. Sci. 378:404, 1982.

Fujimoto, W. Y., and Seegmiller, J. E.: Hypoxanthine-guanine phosphoribosyltransferase deficiency: activity in normal, mutant, and heterozygote-cultured human skin fibroblasts. Proc. Natl. Acad. Sci. U.S.A. 65:577, 1970.

Gabrilove, J. L., Sharma, D. L., and Dorfman, R. I.: Adrenocortical 11 beta-hydroxylase deficiency and virilism first manifest in the adult woman. N. Engl. J. Med. 272:1189, 1965.

Goldstein, J. L., and Brown, M. S.: Lipoprotein receptors: genetic defense against atherosclerosis. Clin. Res. 30:417, 1982.

Griffin, R. F., and Elsas, L. J.: Classic Phenylketonuria: diagnosis through heterozygote detection. J. Pediatr. 86:512, 1975.

Hsia, D. Y.: Galactosemia. Springfield, Ill., Charles C Thomas, 1969.

Kinoshita, J. H., Futterman, S., Satoh, K., and Merola, L. O.: Factors affecting the formation of sugar alcohols in ocular lens. Biochem. Biophys. Acta. 74:340, 1963.

Koch, J., Stokstad, E. L., Williams, H. E., and Smith, L. H.: Deficiency of 2-oxo-glutarate: glyoxylate carboligase activity in primary hyperoxaluria. Proc. Natl. Acad. Sci. U.S.A. 57:1123, 1967.

LaDu, B. N., Zannoni, V. G., Laster, L., and Seegmiller, J. E.: The nature of the defect in tyrosine metabolism in alcaptonuria. J. Biol. Chem. 230:251,.1958.

Menkes, J. H., Hurst, P. L., and Craig, J. M.: New syndrome: progressive infantile cerebral dysfunction associated with an unusual urinary substance. Pediatrics 14:462, 1954.

Menkes, J. H.: Maple syrup disease: investigations into the metabolic defect. Neurology 9:826, 1959.

Meyer, U. A., and Marver, H. S.: Intermittent acute porphyria: clinical demonstration of a genetic defect in porphobilinogen metabolism. Clin. Res. 19:398, 1971.

Meyer, U. A., and Schmid, R.: Intermittent acute porphyria: the enzymatic defect in brain dysfunction in metabolic disorders, F. Plum (Ed.). Research Publication, Assoc. Nerv. Ment. Dis. 53:211, 1974.

Motulsky, A. G.: Current concepts in genetics: the genetic hyperlipidemias. N. Engl. J. Med. 294:823, 1976.

O'Brien, W. M., LaDu, B. N., and Bunim, J. J.: Biochemical, pathologic and clinical aspects of alcaptonuria, ochronosis and ochronotic arthropathy. Review of world literature (1584–1962). Am. J. Med. 34:813, 1963.

Rosenbloom, F. M., Henderson, J. F., Caldwell, I. C., et al.: Biochemical bases of accelerated purine biosynthesis de novo in human fibroblasts lacking hypoxanthine-guanine phosphoribosyl-transferase. J. Biol. Chem. 243:1166, 1968.

Tschudy, D. P., Perlroth, M. G., Marver, H. S., et al.: Acute intermittent porphyria: the first "over-production disease" localized to a specific enzyme. Proc. Natl. Acad. Sci. U.S.A. 53:841, 1965.

Williams, H. E., and Smith, L. J., Jr.: L-glyceric aciduria. A new genetic variant of primary hyperoxaluria. N. Engl. J. Med. 278:233, 1968.

Circulating Proteins

Beck, E. A., Charache, P., and Jackson, D. P.: A new inherited coagulation disorder caused by an abnormal fibrinogen (fibrinogen Baltimore). Nature 208:143, 1965.

Elsas, L. J., Hayslett, J. P., Spargo, B. H., et al.: Wilson's disease with reversible renal tubular dysfunction. Ann. Intern. Med. 75:427, 1971.

Fagerhol, M. K., and Laurell, C.-B.: The Pi system: inherited variants of serum $alpha_1$-antitrypsin. In Steinberg, A. G., and Bearn, A. G. (Eds.): Progress in Medical Genetics. 7th ed. New York, Grune & Stratton, 1970.

Forman, W. B., Ratnoff, O. D., and Boyer, M. H.: An inherited qualitative abnormality in plasma fibrinogen: fibrinogen Cleveland. J. Lab. Clin. Med. 72:455, 1968.

Harris, H.: Genes and isozymes. Proc. Roy. Soc. Lond. 174:1, 1969.

Hirschhorn, R.: Adenosine deaminase deficiency and immunodeficiencies. Fed. Proc. 36:2166, 1977.

Holtzman, N. A., Naughton, M. A., Iber, F. L., and Gaumnitz, B. M.: Ceruloplasmin in Wilson's disease. J. Clin. Invest. 46:993, 1967.

Levy, R. I., Fredrickson, D. S., and Laster, L.: The lipoproteins and lipid transport in abetalipoproteinemia. J. Clin. Invest. 45:531, 1966.

Mammen, E. F., Prasad, A. S., Barnhart, M. I., and Au, C. C.: Congenital dysfibrinogenemia: fibrinogen Detroit. J. Clin. Invest. 48:235, 1969.

Ratnoff, O. D., and Bennett, B.: The genetics of hereditary disorders of blood coagulation. Science 179:1291, 1973.

Stites, D. P., Hershgold, E. J., Perlman, J. D., and Fudenberg, H. H.: Factor VIII detection by hemagglutination inhibition: hemophilia A and Von Willebrand's Disease. Science 171:196, 1971.

Coenzyme Function

Danner, D. J., Lemmon, S. K., and Elsas, L. J.: Substrate specificity and stabilization by thiamine pyrophosphate of rat liver branched chain α-ketoacid dehydrogenase. Biochem. Med. 19:27, 1978.

Danner, D. J., Wheeler, F. B., Lemmon, S. K., and Elsas, L. J.: In vivo and in vitro response of human branched chain α-ketoacid dehydrogenase to thiamine and thiamine pyrophosphate. Pediatr. Res. 12:235, 1978.

Elsas, L. J., Danner, D. J., and Rogers, B. L.: Effect of thiamine on normal and mutant human branched chain alpha-ketoacid dehydrogenase. In Gubler, L. J., Fujiwara, M., and Dreyfus, P. (Eds.): Thiamine. New York, John Wiley and Sons, 1974, pp. 335–353.

Elsas, L. J., Miller, R. L., and Priest, R. E.: Inherited human collagen lysyl hydroxylase deficiency: ascorbic acid response. J. Pediatr. *92*:378, 1978.

Elsas, L. J., Pask, B. A., Wheeler, F. B., et al.: Cofactor resistant maple syrup urine disease. Metabolism *21*:929, 1972.

Erbe, R. W.: Inborn errors of folate metabolism. N. Engl. J. Med. *293*:753, 807, 1975.

Fernhoff, P. M., Danner, D. J., and Elsas, L. J.: Vitamin responsive disorders. *In* Garry, P. J. (Ed.): Human Nutrition: Clinical and Biochemical Aspects. Washington, D.C., Am. Assoc. Clin. Chem., 1982.

Frimpter, G. W.: Cystathioninuria: nature of the defect. Science *149*:1095, 1965.

Longhi, R. L., Fleisher, L. D., Tallan, H. H., and Gaull, G. E.: Cystathioninine beta-synthase deficiency: a qualitative abnormality of the deficient enzyme modified by vitamin B₆ therapy. Pediatr. Res. *11*:100, 1977.

Mahoney, M. J., and Rosenberg, L. E.: Inherited defects of B₁₂ metabolism. Am. J. Med. *48*:584, 1970.

Morrow, G., and Barness, L. A.: Combined vitamin responsiveness in homocystinuria. J. Pediatr. *81*:946, 1972.

Rosenberg, L. E.: Inherited amino-acidopathies demonstrating vitamin dependency. N. Engl. J. Med. *281*:145, 1969.

Rosenberg, L. E.: Vitamin responsiveness inherited diseases affecting the nervous system. *In* Plum, F. (Ed.): Brain Dysfunction in Metabolic Disorders. New York, Raven Press, 1974.

Rosenberg, L. E.: Vitamin-responsive inherited metabolic disorders. Adv. Hum. Genet. *6*:1, 1976.

Scriver, C. R.: Vitamin responsive inborn errors of metabolism. Metabolism *22*:1319, 1973.

Scriver, C. R., Clow, C. L., MacKenzie, S., and Delvin, E.: Thiamine-responsive maple syrup urine disease. Lancet *1*:310, 1971.

Pharmacogenetics

Bell, J. C., and Riemensnider, D. K.: Use of serum microbiologic assay technique for estimating patterns of isoniazid metabolism. Am. Rev. Tuberc. *75*:995, 1957.

Evans, D. A., Manley, K. A., and McKusick, V. A.: Genetic control of isoniazid metabolism in man. Br. Med. J. *2*:485, 1960.

Harris, H., Robson, E. B., Glenn-Bott, A. M., and Thornton, J. A.: Evidence for non-allelism between genes affecting human serum cholinesterase. Nature *200*:1185, 1963.

Hockwald, R. S., Arnold, J., Clayman, C. B., and Alving, A. S.: Status of primaquine: toxicity of primaquinine in Negroes: report to Council on Pharmacy and Chemistry. J.A.M.A. *149*:1568, 1952.

Jenne, J. W.: Partial purification and properties of the isoniazid transacetylase in human liver. Its relationship to the acetylation of P-aminosalicylic acid. J. Clin. Invest. *44*:1992, 1965.

Kirkman, H. N.: Glucose-6 phosphate dehydrogenase variants and drug-induced hemolysis. Ann. N.Y. Acad. Sci. *151*:753, 1968.

Structural Proteins

Jacob, H. S., Ruby, A., Overland, E. S., and Mazia, D.: Abnormal membrane protein of red blood cells in hereditary spherocytosis. J. Clin. Invest. *50*:1800, 1977.

McKusick, V. A.: Heritable Disorders of Connective Tissue. 4th ed. St. Louis, C. V. Mosby Co., 1972.

Miller, M. J., and Matukas, V. J.: Biosynthesis of collagen. Fed. Proc. *33*:1197, 1974.

Pinnell, S. R., Krane, S. M., Kenzora, J. E., and Glimcher, M. J.: A heritable disorder of connective tissue. Hydroxylysine-deficient collagen disease. N. Engl. J. Med. *286*:1013, 1972.

MANAGEMENT OF INHERITED DISEASE

Acosta, P. B., and Elsas, L. J.: Dietary Management of Inherited Metabolic Disease: Phenylketonuria, Galactosemia, Tyrosinemia, Homocystinuria, Maple Syrup Urine Disease. Atlanta, ACELMU Publishers, 1976.

Boyer, S. H., Siggers, D. C., and Krueger, L. J.: Caveat to protein replacement therapy for genetic disease: immunological implications of accurate molecular diagnosis. Lancet *2*:654, 1973.

Brady, R. O., Gal, A. E., and Pentcher, P. G.: Evolution of enzyme replacement therapy for lipid storage disease. Life Sci. *15*:1235, 1974.

Brock, D. J. H.: Biochemical and cytological methods in the diagnosis of neural tube defects. Progr. Med. Genet. *2*:1, 1977.

Buckley, R. H., Whisnant, J. K., Schiff, R. I., et al.: Correction of severe combined immunodeficiency by fetal liver cells. N. Eng. J. Med. *294*:1076, 1976.

Cerami, A., and Manning, J. M.: Potassium cyanate as an inhibitor of the sickling erythrocytes in vitro. Proc. Natl. Acad. Sci. *68*:1180, 1971.

Chang, J. C., and Kan, Y. W.: A sensitive new test for sickle-cell anemia. N. Eng. J. Med. *307*:30, 1982.

Childs, B., and Simopoulous, A. P. (Chairpersons): Genetic Screening Programs, Principles, and Research. Assembly of Life Sciences, National Research Council, Washington, D.C., 1975.

Cohen, S. N.: Gene manipulation. N. Eng. J. Med. *294*:883, 1976.

Desnick, R. J., Thorpe, S. R., and Fiddler, M. D.: Toward enzyme therapy for lysosomal storage diseases. Physiol. Rev. *56*:57, 1976.

Desnick, R. J.: Prospects for enzyme therapy in the lysosomal storage diseases of Ashkenazi Jews. *In* Goodman, R. M., and Motulsky, A. G. (Eds.): Genetic Diseases Among Ashkenazi Jews. New York, Raven Press, 1979.

Fratantoni, J. C., Neufeld, E. F., Uhlendorf, B. W., and Jacobson, C. B.: Intrauterine diagnosis of the Hurler and Hunter syndromes. N. Engl. J. Med. *280*:686, 1969.

Gillette, P. N., Petersen, C. M., Lu, Y. S., and Cerami, A.: Sodium cyanate as a potential treatment for sickle-cell disease. N. Engl. J. Med. *290*:654, 1974.

Howell, R. R.: Genetic disease: the present status of treatment. Hosp. Pract. *7*:75, 1972.

Hug, G., and Schubert, W. K.: Lysosomes in type II glycogenosis. Changes during administration of extract from *Aspergillus niger*. J. Cell. Biol. *35*:C1, 1967.

Huntley, C. C., and Stevenson, R. E.: Maternal phenylketonuria. Course of two pregnancies. Obstet. Gynecol. *34*:694, 1969.

Kerr, G. R., Chamove, A. S., Harlow, H. F., and Waisman, H. A.: "Fetal PKU": the effect of maternal hyperphenylalaninemia during pregnancy in the rhesus monkey (*Macaca mulatta*). Pediatrics *42*:27, 1968.

Kraus, L. M., and Kraus, A. P.: Carbamyl phosphate mediated inhibition of the sickling of erythrocytes in vitro. Biochem. Biophys. Res. Comm. *44*:1381, 1971.

Lauer, R. M., Mascarinas, T., Racela, A. S., and Diehl, A. M.: Administration of a mixture of fungal glucosidases to a patient with type II glycogenosis (Pompe's disease). Pediatrics *42*:672, 1968.

Ley, T. J., DeSimone, J., Anagnou, N. P., et al.: 5-Azacytidine selectively increases λ globin synthesis in a patient with β⁺ thalassemia. N. Engl. J. Med. *307*:1469, 1982.

Lubs, H. A., and Lubs, M. L.: Genetic disorders. *In* Burrow, G. N., and Ferris, T. S. (Eds): Complications During Pregnancy. Philadelphia, W. B. Saunders Co., 1975.

Mabuchi, H., Haba, T., Tatami, R., et al.: Effects of an inhibitor of 3-hydroxy-3 methylglutaryl Coenzyme A reductase on serum lipoproteins and ubiquinone-10 levels in patients with familial hypercholesterolemia. N. Engl. J. Med. *305*:478, 1981.

Marion, J. P., Danner, D. J., Ballou, W., et al.: Testing for the Tay-Sachs gene in the Atlanta Jewish population. South. Med. J. *70*:833, 1977.

Merril, C. R., Geier, M. R., and Petricciani, J. C.: Bacterial virus gene expression in human cells. Nature *233*:398, 1971.

Milunsky, A., Littlefield, J. W., Kanfer, J. N., et al.: Prenatal genetic diagnosis (three parts). N. Engl. J. Med. *283*:1370, 1441, 1498, 1970.

Moses, S. W., Levin, S., Chayoth, R., and Steinitz, K.: Enzyme induction in a case of glycogen storage disease. Pediatrics *38*:111, 1966.

Mulligan, R. C., and Berg, P.: Expression of bacterial gene in mammalian cells. Science *209*:1422, 1980.

Nadler, H. L., and Gerbie, A. B.: The role of amniocentesis in the intrauterine detection of genetic disorders. N. Engl. J. Med. 282:596, 1970.

Nalbandian, R. M. (Ed.): Molecular Aspects of Sickle Cell Hemoglobin. Springfield, Ill., Charles C Thomas, 1971.

Philippart, M., Franklin, S. S., and Gordon, A.: Reversal of an inborn sphingolipidosis (Fabry's disease) by kidney transplantation. Ann. Int. Med. 77:195, 1972.

Rabovsky, D.: Molecular biology: gene insertion into mammalian cells. Science 174:933, 1971.

Schimke, R. T., and Doyle, D.: Control of enzyme levels in animal tissues. Ann. Rev. Biochem. 39:929, 1970.

Schwartz, A. G., Cook, P. R., and Harris, H.: Correction of a genetic defect in a mammalian cell. Nature (New Biol.) 230:5, 1971.

Scriver, C. R.: Treatment of inherited disease: realized and potential. Med. Clin. North Am. 53:941, 1969.

Watson, C. J., Bossenmaier, I., Cardinal, R., and Petryka, Z. J.: Repression by hematin of porphyrin biosynthesis in congenital erythropoietic porphyria. Proc. Natl. Acad. Sci. U.S.A. 71:278, 1974.

Yaffe, S. J., Levy, G., Matsuzawa, T., and Baliah, T.: Enhancement of glucuronide-conjugating capacity in a hyperbilirubinemic infant due to apparent enzyme induction by phenobarbital. N. Engl. J. Med. 275:1461, 1966.

Cellular and Molecular Foundations of Immunity, Immunologic Inflammation, and Hypersensitivity*

4

Component Parts and Their Relation to Neurohumoral Control Mechanisms

Andor Szentivanyi, M.D., and Judith Szentivanyi, M.D.

Human life and development are marked by encounters with an infinite range of potentially injurious and destructive agents and stimuli. Of the various defense systems that establish and sustain homeostasis against injurious agents and stimuli, those that will be emphasized in this chapter involve (1) elements that manage first encounters (the inflammatory response), and (2) elements that utilize experience upon re-encounters (the specific immune response). These systems, or defense functions, are anatomically inter-related and physiologically interdependent. Each is in continuous interplay with elements of the internal milieu of the host as well as with elements of the host's environment, and, therefore, closely linked with neurohumoral defense mechanisms.

Regardless of the purpose for which the inflammatory response is set in action, the first encounter is a more or less stereotyped reaction. Cells of predictable type are drawn into the injured area and proceed, for instance, to engulf the foreign material by phagocytosis. Vascular occlusion, fibrin barriers, and other aspects of the inflammatory response serve to localize infection or other injury and initiate repair.

The functions of the immune defense system are the properties of cells distributed throughout the body. They include (1) free or circulating cells of the blood, lymph, and intravascular spaces; (2) similar cells collected into units that allow for close interaction with lymph or circulating blood (lymph nodes, spleen, liver, and bone marrow); and (3) a source or control organ for the system (the thymus gland). Constant interchange of cells between the units provides for rapid dissemination of information to each unit. These systems are, therefore, dynamic, changing constantly in struc-

ture and functional capacity in response to stimuli. Defects in genetic endowment, injuries to cell lines, and factors that alter the rate or quality of accumulation of the memory store of immunologic experience alter the normal developmental patterns and result in clinical disorders, including immunologically based hypersensitive manifestations.

In this chapter, we emphasize and sequentially discuss the cells involved in immunity and immunologic inflammatory reactions (including reactions of hypersensitivity), the effector molecules stored or synthesized and released by these cells, the target cells on which these molecules act, the amplification systems (i.e., complement and kinin systems), and the biochemical controlling mechanisms that modulate the functioning of these various cell types, including their intracellular messenger systems (i.e., cyclic nucleotides).

THE CELLS STORING OR SYNTHESIZING THE EFFECTOR MOLECULES (CHEMICAL MEDIATORS) OF IMMUNOLOGIC INFLAMMATORY RESPONSES AND THEIR INTERRELATIONSHIPS

These cells seem to represent a continuous spectrum of related or unrelated cell types, specialized in the production and storage of various mediators in variable proportions (i.e., of cells that might have a common developmental origin), with differentiation being determined by the specific requirements of the local neurohumoral regulation.

Accounting only for those mediators for which the cell type has been identified, this arbitrary spectrum of mediator-storing, synthesizing, and transporting cells includes neutrophil leukocytes

---

*This chapter incorporates portions of Chapters 4 and 5 of the previous edition, prepared by Robert M. Nakamura and Ernest S. Tucker, III.

(SRS-A*, ECF-A†, enzymes, vascular permeability factors, kinin-generating substances, a complement-activating factor, histamine-releasers, and a neutrophil inhibitory factor [NIF]); basophilic leukocytes (histamine, SRS-A, ECF-A, NCF‡ and PAF§); murine basophilic leukocytes (histamine, SRS-A, ECF-A, PAF, and serotonin); eosinophilic leukocytes (histamine, PAF, and possibly SRS-A); mast cells (histamine, SRS-A, ECF-A, NCF, and PAF); murine mast cells (histamine, SRS-A, ECF-A, PAF, NCF, and serotonin); "chromaffin-positive" mast cells (dopamine in ruminants; in other mammals possibly norepinephrine); enterochromaffin cells (serotonin); chromaffin cells (catecholamines); platelets (depending on species—histamine, serotonin, catecholamines, and prostaglandins); neurosecretory cells (histamine, serotonin, catecholamines, acetylcholine, and prostaglandins); and nerve cells (potentially all amine-mediators as well as prostaglandins and kinins).

Many of these cell types possess different embryologic, morphologic, physicochemical, and general biologic characteristics. Nevertheless, in passing from one member of the mediator-containing cell spectrum to another, obvious transitions can be seen in all these characteristics. Furthermore, when one surveys their properties and their probable physiologic function in the higher organism, certain cohesive features become apparent that set them apart from other body constituents as a distinct, single class of cells that could be included in a generalized concept of neurosecretion.

NEUTROPHILIC LEUKOCYTES

A comparative analysis of this spectrum might be properly introduced with the neutrophilic leukocytes. These cells tend to be fairly uniform in size, with cytoplasm and granules similar to those of stabs. The nucleus is coarsely clumped and segmented into two to five, most frequently three, lobes that are connected by thin chromatin strands.

Neutrophils possess large numbers of cytoplasmic granules. They appear to be of two main types:

1. *Azurophil granules* (also called *primary* granules because they appear first in cellular development). These are large, dense granules that contain various lysosomal hydrolases (such as acid phosphatase) and cationic proteins as well as peroxidase (called *myeloperoxidase*) and an antibacterial substance called *lysozyme.*

2. *Specific* (or *secondary*) *granules*. These are smaller and less dense and contain alkaline phos-

phatase, lysozyme, and lactoferrin (an antibacterial, iron-binding protein) but no lysosomal hydrolases and no peroxidase.

In addition to enzymes, the preformed neutrophil effector molecules include vascular permeability factors, kinin-generating materials, a complement-activating factor generating C5a, and histamine releasers such as cationic proteins. A neutrophil inhibitory factor (NIF), which inhibits motility and responsiveness to chemotactic stimuli but permits phagocytosis, also can be produced by neutrophils. Several substances, including pyrogen, are not preformed but synthesized and released on neutrophil activation. It has also been shown that the calcium ionophore A23187 induces synthesis and secretion of a molecule with properties essentially identical with those of SRS-A. In addition, both the calcium ionophore and phagocytic stimuli induce synthesis and secretion of an eosinophil chemotactic factor similar to ECF-A in molecular size and biologic properties. Thus, neutrophils elaborate some of the same chemical mediators that basophilic leukocytes and mast cells produce during immediate hypersensitivity reactions (see Chapter 5).

BASOPHILIC LEUKOCYTES AND MAST CELLS

Basophilic leukocytes and mast cells contain most of the histamine in adult (though not in fetal) mammalian tissues. They also contain an agent that is chemotactic for homologous eosinophils (ECF-A) and a substance that elicits secretion of histamine and serotonin from platelets (PAF*). Unlike these mediators, SRS-A is not stored within these cells, but elaborated by them during the process of secretion of the other mediators.

For phylogenetic and morphologic reasons, it is customary to distinguish between tissue mast cells and blood mast cells or basophilic leukocytes—commonly referred to as *basophils*. In lower organisms, the tissue mast cells are believed to be intimately related to the basophilic leukocytes and may originate from these basophils, through direct transformation, and from cells of the fixed mesenchyme. With the evolution of the bone marrow, however, partition occurs in the production of these two cell types. The tissue mast cells continue to arise from mesenchymal cells at the sites of former hematopoietic centers, whereas the basophils are formed from basophilic promyelocytes or myelocytes. Their separate origin and habitat in the higher organism are complemented by morphologic differences. In contrast to the tissue mast cell, the basophil is smaller in size, in general more rounded in shape, and has a relatively scanty

---

*Slow-reacting substances of anaphylaxis.
†Eosinophil chemotactic factor of anaphylaxis.
‡Neutrophil chemotactic factor.
§Platelet-activating factor.

---

*This substance, which can be immunologically released from basophilic leukocytes, has yet to be elicited from tissue mast cells.

cytoplasm and a segmented nucleus—characteristics that are retained even by the extravasated basophils. There also appear to be some functional differences between these cell types. Cholinergic and alpha-adrenergic receptors have been described on human lung mast cells but not on basophils. Another difference is that C3a may trigger mediator release from skin mast cells but is less effective on basophils. Cell-mediated inflammatory infiltrates that include basophils—such as cutaneous basophil hypersensitivity, or CBH (see Chapter 5)—indicate that basophils respond to chemotactic stimuli, whereas mast cells do not, although in rodents increased numbers of mast cells are found in certain pathologic states (i.e., in the gastrointestinal tract during parasitic infection). Without adding less well-established and rather insignificant further examples of dissimilarities, we will allow these considerations to serve as the basis of the view that tissue mast cells and basophils belong to separate cell systems.

Despite this view, there are several reasons to consider mast cells and basophils at least as clearly interrelated cell systems representing a functional unit. As already mentioned, direct transformation from one cell to the other is believed to occur in lower organisms. Although evidence indicates that subpopulations of monocytes, macrophages, and lymphocytes also express Fc receptors for IgE antibody, of all mammalian cells only basophils and mast cells exhibit an extraordinary binding affinity for this antibody (see later discussions). The granules of both the basophils and the tissue mast cells give the same metachromatic* reaction and show the same lamellar stratification. Practically all workers up to the present have found histochemical reactions similar in principle, a fact that is in harmony with the identity of the active agents (histamine, SRS-A, ECF-A, heparin and its precursors, etc.) stored or synthesized or both by the two cell types. The basic identity of the active agents is especially significant, since the physiologic importance of the two cell systems is likely to be related to the nature of the active agents that they contain. Both cells show a similar susceptibility to immunologic, osmotic, or chemical release of their active constituents, and in a number of species there is a certain degree of reciprocity between the two kinds of cells, suggesting a compensatory relationship and indicating that they subserve the same physiologic function. Thus, the present chapter will regard the basophils as freely circulating counterparts of a "portion" of the tissue mast cell system. This

reference to the functional heterogeneity of the so-called tissue mast cells will be explained further on, but first—in conjunction with the basophils—the problem of the eosinophilic leukocytes will be discussed.

EOSINOPHILIC LEUKOCYTES

Among other reasons, the eosinophilic leukocytes are included in this discussion because their increase in blood and tissues is a characteristic of hypersensitivity diseases in humans.

Most modern workers agree that the eosinophil is a cell *sui generis,* generically and functionally different from the basophil. It is also widely held that the bone marrow serves as the only source of eosinophil. However, the old concept that the eosinophils may develop outside the bone marrow by heteroplasia of mesenchymal cells or through an "ubiquitous heteroplasia" involving also nonmesodermal precursors (e.g., the epithelial lining of the intestinal crypts) has again gained adherents. Regardless of whether eosinophils can develop outside the marrow or not, the youngest cell among the eosinophilic series is the promyelocyte, which has a "mixed" (i.e., partly basophilic, partly eosinophilic) granulation. The same can be seen in patients with chronic myelocytic leukemia, in which basophilic granules are not infrequently reported in eosinophils. Likewise, observations in the rat's genital tract connective tissue indicate that tissue eosinophils can serve as precursors of tissue mast cells. These cells also exhibit a similarity in their responses to certain neuroendocrine stimuli.

Another reason for discussing the eosinophil among the mediator-containing cells lies in the evidence that has accumulated to indicate that eosinophils may carry histamine, at least in some species and under certain conditions. When such evidence was at first presented, it was rapidly challenged by workers who could not find any constant correlation between the number of eosinophils and the level of histamine in the peripheral blood. In light of subsequent studies, however, these contradictions may be resolved by existence of species differences, by the technical inadequacy of the earlier works in enumerating the different white cells of the blood, and by the unaccountable fact that eosinophils in the blood may be increased without any concomitant elevation in histamine concentration (i.e., eosinophils may contain quite different concentrations of histamine under different conditions).

In healthy humans, the basophils carry about 50 per cent of the total blood histamine, and the eosinophils have about 30 per cent, but the ratio of histamine-load between the respective individual cells is as high as 6:1. Thus, the amount carried by each individual eosinophil is far less and also much more variable than that associated

---

*Metachromasia refers to the strong affinity of the granular material for basic dyes and to the property of altering the original color of the dye. The metachromatic shift in the absorbency spectrum is now known to depend on the stacking of multiple cationic dye molecules on an anionic polymer with a sufficiently high-charge density; the polyanion responsible for the metachromatic staining is the highly electronegative sulphated mucopolysaccharide, heparin.

with each basophil. Sometimes, the eosinophils of humans contain no histamine. To illustrate, eosinophilia could be mentioned, when such a break in the normal relationship to histamine often occurs. Conversely, in human chronic myelocytic leukemia, the basophils are poorer and the eosinophils are richer than normal in histamine.

These issues have been investigated in other species as well. In the dog, all or nearly all of the histamine in blood is carried by eosinophils, but again the amount associated with each individual cell is variable and sometimes negligible. In the guinea pig, however, the eosinophils carry either very little or no histamine at all. The same seems to apply to the eosinophils of oxen.

Perhaps the most revealing feature of the foregoing is the variability of the amount of histamine that is tied to the eosinophils compared with the histamine-load of basophils, which seems much more fixed. This may suggest that the eosinophils are facultative histamine carriers rather than storage cells and serve only to transport histamine, which has been elaborated elsewhere, and that they do this possibly in conjunction with the detoxification and disposal of histamine. Indeed, evidence has been accumulating to support such a view. Thus, local aggregation of eosinophils can be linked not only with their accumulation in areas in which mast cell granules and ECF-A are being released but also with the presence of free histamine in the tissues. Furthermore, histaminase destroys histamine; it is activated by phosphate ions and, in the presence of gaseous oxygen, catalyzes the destruction of histamine, forming hydrogen peroxide. Eosinophils contain a peroxidase that, in the presence of hydrogen peroxide, catalyzes the oxidation of various substances. The detoxification of histamine, therefore, may be accomplished by histaminase in the granules or by some other substance present in the cell that participates at a further stage in histamine breakdown. Direct antihistaminic effects of eosinophils could also be conceived via other specific products of these cells. For instance, extracts of the buffy coat of horse blood injected into guinea pigs selectively lowers the sensitivity to histamine. When the antihistamine effect of such extracts on the bronchi of guinea pigs in vivo is analyzed, a definite correlation is found between the potency of the extracts and eosinophil counts, suggesting that the active principle is derived from the eosinophils. This is supported by the successful extraction of substances with antihistaminic properties from the isolated granules of blood eosinophils. Finally, eosinophils seem to figure prominently in the inactivation not only of histamine but also of SRS-A and PAF. In the presence of halide ions, eosinophil peroxidase can inactivate SRS-A, and eosinophil phospholipase D can inactivate PAF.

At the same time, eosinophils are capable of synthesizing SRS-A—leukotrienes C4 and D4 (LTC4 and LTD4)—and their migration is modulated by complement- and lymphocyte-derived products in addition to the other inflammatory mediators mentioned earlier. Eosinophils also kill antibody-coated parasites and may act synergistically with mast cells in destroying ticks.

HETEROGENEITY OF MAST CELLS

Since their conclusive description by Ehrlich, it has been common practice to refer to those connective tissue elements that avidly bind dyes of the thiazine group and exhibit granular metachromasia as *mast cells*. It appears, however, that the body cells known as mast cells represent a heterogeneous collection of cells that have nothing more in common than that they contain the material that has the property of staining metachromatically.

Thus, mast cells are pleomorphic, with their shape and finer structure varying among different species and also in different parts of the same species. There are not only pertinent morphologic dissimilarities but also differences among and within species in tinctorial reactions in response to histamine liberators, with regard to biochemical composition, and, possibly, with respect to other structural and functional parameters.

Evidence has been presented that tissue mast cells represent at least two morphologically distinct cellular types. One is the so-called *fibroblastic type,* an elongated eel-like structure with a long, pale-staining nucleus and usually bipolar cytoplasmic protrusions that contain bluish-red granules. These granules have a homogeneous structureless internal architecture. The other kind of mast cell is the oval type, a circumscribed mass containing granules composed of subgranular structures in the form of clusters of rolled scrolls, with a finely particulate substance filling the spaces between and within these scroll-like bodies. It seems that the oval type cell, with its coarse and complex granules, is the more classic form of tissue mast cell, perhaps the "typical" mast cell, whereas the fibroblastic type, with its rather simple granule, is probably identical with those cells that were independently described by several groups of workers as *chromaffin cells,* or *chromaffin-positive mast cells.*

Chromaffin-Positive Mast Cells. Designation of these mast cells as *chromaffin cells* rests on the findings described in the subsequent paragraphs.

The granules of these cells give the *chromaffin reaction,* that histochemical characteristic so typical of the adrenal medulla (see further on). They are argentaffin, reduce ferric-ferricyanide, and show a yellow autofluorescence when viewed under near ultraviolet light. In the skin, some correlation has been found between the amount of chromaffin substance contained by these cells on one hand and the vascular tone as well as the catechol content of different cutaneous regions on the other.

Chemically and structurally, the centrally located electron-dense body of the chromaffin granules resembles those granules described for the head cells of the adrenal medulla much more than the granules of the mast cells. In the human skin, these chromaffin-positive mast cells have been frequently encountered in close connection with unmyelinated nerve fibers. The cells rest on these neural elements, but sometimes the nerve fibers may even penetrate the chromaffin-positive mast cells. In either case, it can be demonstrated that the cell membrane of the chromaffin cell is in contact with the cell membrane of the nerve fiber itself or that of the Schwann cell. This, taken together with the fact that these chromaffin-positive mast cells were also shown to be in close contact with smooth muscle cells of small arteries and veins, might indicate that this cell-type is able to release its active constituent or constituents into the smooth muscle cell by impulses propagated through the nerve fiber. Thus, the anatomic relationship is highly reminiscent of that existing between the terminal of an autonomic postganglionic fiber and its effector cell. In mammals, the classic chromaffin cells are also in close anatomic contact with adrenergic nerve fibers, although the latter are conventionally regarded as preganglionic fibers.

These chromaffin-positive mast cells are found most richly in the walls of the blood vessels of the cutis; they are also described, however, as being present in the lung, liver, uterus, urinary bladder, heart, nerves, and striated muscle. In fact, the only tissue so far in which such cells cannot be demonstrated is the placenta. The conspicuous absence of this type of mast cell in the aneural placenta may be a reflection of its genuine relationship to neural structures.

Chromaffin-positive mast cells having relations similar to the autonomic nerves of the cutis, and presenting many similarities to those already mentioned, have also been described in the albino guinea pig by other workers, who called these cells *neurohumoral cells*. On the basis of their histochemical reactions, these neurohumoral cells are believed to contain norepinephrine. The term *neurohumoral* relates to the assumption that these cells have a secretory function, since the granules when stained by the chromhematoxylin-phloxin method appear to be wandering out of the cells into the tubelike extensions, as observed in the supraoptic and paraventricular neurosecretory cells of the hypothalamus and in those of the pineal gland. It is of great significance that such morphologic and histochemical similarities can be shown to exist between these chromaffin-positive mast cells and typical neurosecretory cells, which were found to contain high concentrations of histamine, serotonin, catecholamines, acetylcholine, and prostaglandins.

Tissue mast cells whose granules give a positive chromaffin reaction have also been identified in the liver capsule and gut of the ox, cow, and sheep. In the gastrointestinal mucosa of ruminants, these cells are found in close proximity to the serotonin-storing enterochromaffin cells (see further on). They give positive argentaffin* and Schmorl† reactions in dichromate-fixed material. The fact that the Schmorl reaction is more intense in tissues fixed in formol-dichromate than in formalin-fixed material is consistent with the presence of a catecholamine-like rather than a serotonin-like compound, as are the negative indophenol and alkaline diazonium reactions. Also, the fluorescence produced by these catecholamine-containing mast cells and that produced by the serotonin-containing enterochromaffin cells of the gut contrast strongly, with the former having a silvery-white color and the latter a golden-yellow hue when the tissue is fixed in formol–calcium chloride. The catecholamine that is contained by these cells is probably dopamine, since the cells are located in regions that, when extracted, yield large quantities of dopamine. Thus, the histochemical reactions of these cells are typical only of catecholamine-containing elements, and similar reactions would be expected if these cells possessed epinephrine or norepinephrine or both instead of dopamine.

Because of distinctive morphologic and histochemical differences, the two major types of mast cells (i.e., the chromaffin-positive *fibroblastic type* and the more classic *oval type*) were at first believed to be two unrelated cell types that had only one property in common: granular metachromasia. Further observations, however, have revealed intermediate forms. Cells have been found that contain granules of both types. It may be, therefore, that the two cells are simply variants of the same type, in which case intermediate forms might be expected.

Murine Mast Cells. Before leaving the question of mast cell heterogeneity, the mast cells of rats and mice should be separately mentioned. Justification for this lies in the fact that rats and mice seem unique among the species in possessing demonstrable quantities of serotonin along with histamine in their mast cells. The possibility that some of these cells contain only serotonin and that others contain only histamine is ruled out by the simultaneous occurrence and persistence of both amines in cultures of mast cells that had begun as single cells. Although the possibility remains that the mast cells of some species other than rat and mouse produce and contain serotonin, perhaps in quantities much smaller than those encountered in these two species, or produce this chemical without retaining it, there is not yet unequivocal evidence that this is true.

---

*The *argentaffin reaction* refers to the dark granulation caused by the reduction of ammoniacal silver solutions by catecholamines or serotonin to metallic silver.

†The *Schmorl reaction* refers to the blue coloration of the granular material produced by ferric-ferricyanide solutions.

ENTEROCHROMAFFIN CELLS

The principal storage cell of serotonin is the enterochromaffin cell. The term *enterochromaffin* was coined by Erspamer for cells of the gastrointestinal mucosa whose granules show chromaffin and argentaffin reactions, couple with diazonium salts, and fluoresce after fixation with formaldehyde. Although they are chromaffin, their chromaffinity is different from that shown by the classic chromaffin cells (i.e., the adrenal medullary cells) in that it occurs, and strongly, after formalin fixation. Also, whereas serotonin-containing granules readily couple with alkaline-diazonium compounds, with the reaction leading to the formation of highly colored complexes, catecholamine-containing granules do not; furthermore, only serotonin-containing granules give a positive indophenol reaction and a strongly positive Schmorl reaction in formol-fixed material.

Attention was at first called to a specific relationship between enterochromaffin cells and serotonin by the fact that this amine was shown to be present in the gastrointestinal mucosa of all the animals, birds, reptiles, and amphibians examined and also in the gastrointestinal extracts of species of Elasmobranchii, Chondrostei, and Ascidiacea. In all these species, the gastrointestinal serotonin is localized in the enterochromaffin cells, which are pyramidal cells squeezed in between the cells of the mucosa, with their bases on the basement membrane. Today, these cells are considered to constitute a diffuse system serving specifically for the production of serotonin, which is stored in the enterochromaffin granules.

The developmental history of the enterochromaffin cells is not a settled problem. They may be of local origin from the endoderm or from the neural ectoderm, be it directly from the neural crest or from placodes. However, analogy to the classic chromaffin cells in general suggests a nervous origin, and they certainly seem to be intimately related to the terminal fibers of the submucous nerve plexus. It may be added that serotonin is also contained by a large network of serotoninergic neurons in the brain.

CHROMAFFIN CELLS

The main catecholamine store of the mammalian body is the chromaffin tissue, including the adrenal medullae, paraganglia, and various other extra-adrenal chromaffin cells. The term *chromaffin* refers to the brownish darkening effect of potassium bichromate and of chromic acid on these cells, which causes the formation of a pigmented granularity in their cytoplasm. Chromic acid and bichromate induce this coloration by oxidizing the catecholamines; the oxidized products then condense to form insoluble colored polymers that resemble melanin. The precursors of these cells are derived from the neural crest of the embryo as primordial sympathetic ganglion cells. Only after migrating outside the nervous system do some of the ganglion cells become further differentiated as adrenal medullary cells and, to a lesser extent, as paraganglia (including the organs of Zuckerkandl) or as the chromaffin elements of the carotid body as well as those of the homologous structures related to the great vessels of the thorax. However, extra-adrenal chromaffin cells may occur in any part of the more central adrenergic nervous system, including all parts of the paravertebral chain and the prevertebral sympathetic plexuses. Any sympathetic ganglion may contain chromaffin elements, and isolated cells or discrete bodies may accompany any of the intra-abdominal or thoracic adrenergic nerve fibers.

To date, four catecholamines have been positively identified in the mammalian body: epinephrine, norepinephrine, dopamine, and N-methyl epinephrine. They are unevenly distributed among the various storage cells. In the adrenal medulla, for instance, two types of cells have been demonstrated containing predominantly or exclusively either epinephrine or norepinephrine. The evidence for separate epinephrine-storing versus norepinephrine-storing cells in the medulla rests on (1) differential staining reactions, (2) differential fluorescence, (3) selective susceptibility of the two cell types to the same catecholamine-releasing stimuli, (4) differences in enzymic activities, (5) selective hyperplasia of one or the other cell type following certain stimuli, (6) the survival of the two cell types retaining their original distinct characteristics following transplantation, (7) observations made on isolated granular portions of medullary homogenates showing the existence of separate populations of granules containing predominantly either epinephrine or norepinephrine, and (8) electron-microscopic studies indicating the presence of morphologically different chromaffin granules in adjacent medullary cells.

Distribution patterns of the two cell types are remarkably similar and constant in individual animals of the same species. Conversely, species differences in medullary distribution of the two cell types are well illustrated in the greatly varying relative proportions of the two catecholamines in the medullary tissue of different species. Of the total catecholamines in the adrenal medulla, for instance, average values for norepinephrine are about 20 per cent in humans, 4.5 per cent in rabbits, 11 per cent in guinea pigs, 45 per cent in cats, and 70 per cent in hens. Dopamine and N-methyl epinephrine are also present in the adrenal medulla but usually only in trace amounts. Nevertheless, in some mammals they may show a relatively high value, accounting for 2 per cent of the total catecholamine content.

In contrast to the adrenal medullary cells, the extra-adrenal chromaffin cells, widely scattered throughout the body, contain almost exclusively dopamine. This is evidenced by the fact that there are some organs with a catecholamine content of which 94 to 100 per cent is dopamine. This is true for lung, liver, jejunum, and colon. The possibility that this dopamine is located in the innervating adrenergic neurons of the respective organs is likely in view of the following facts:

1. In the jejunum, more than 80 per cent of the dopamine is located in the mucous membrane, which is very poorly, if at all, innervated.

2. A considerable portion of this dopamine is granular bound, as contrasted with the dopamine of the noradrenergic neurons, which is found exclusively in the cytoplasm.

3. In general, noradrenergic neurons contain a catecholamine mixture of about 50 per cent norepinephrine and 50 per cent dopamine, but never predominantly or exclusively dopamine.

4. In ruminants, it was shown that in these dopamine-rich organs, there indeed exists a special kind of chromaffin cell, the aforementioned dopamine-containing chromaffin-positive mast cell.

Little information is available on the catechol composition of the various other extramedullary chromaffin cells. Among these, the paraganglia certainly contain catecholamines, in some cases (organs of Zuckerkandl) both norepinephrine and epinephrine, whereas chromaffin cells associated with the terminals of postganglionic adrenergic neurons probably contain only epinephrine.

In the spectrum of the mediator-containing storage cells, the gap between mast cells and chromaffin cells appears to be bridged in a rather continuous manner by various chromaffin-positive and serotonin-containing mast cells as well as enterochromaffin cells. Likewise, the transition between chromaffin cells and classic nerve cells appears to be even more continuous because of the existence of the so-called *neurosecretory cells*, which are also qualified members of the mediator-containing cell spectrum. That the arbitrary interpolation of the neurosecretory cell between chromaffin cells and nerve cells as their natural connecting link is indeed justified will be evident from the following discussion.

Consider, for instance, the most representative chromaffin cell, the adrenal medullary cell, which is derived from the embryonic sympathetic ganglia. This ganglionic ancestry is further exemplified by the unusual anatomic relationship of these cells to their innervating autonomic fibers. The latter, reaching the adrenal gland via the lesser splanchnic nerve and through direct branches from the lumbar sympathetic trunk, terminate among the medullary chromaffin cells without the interposition of postganglionic neurons. Both cholinesterase activity and the synaptic vesicles, the characteristic storage organelles of the cholinergic neurotransmitter (acetylcholine), are confined to the presynaptic terminals of the splanchnic fibers, whereas the catecholamine-containing storage granules are localized postsynap-

tically in the medullary chromaffin cells. This arrangement is consistent with the concept that the nerve fibers represent the preganglionic cholinergic innervation of the chromaffin cells, with the limiting membrane of the latter standing for the postganglionic membrane, whereas the cells themselves substitute for the terminals of the postganglionic adrenergic neurons. The commonly shared characteristics of electrophysiologic properties and sensitivity to various ganglion blocking agents further testify to the specific relationship between their limiting membrane and the postganglionic adrenergic membrane. This is well illustrated by the excellent agreement between the sensitivity of both membranes to methonium compounds of various chain lengths; in both cases, decamethonium ($^{C}10$) is ineffective, and hexamethonium ($^{C}6$) is the most potent.

The medullary chromaffin cells, therefore, may be regarded as the embryologic, anatomic, and functional analogues of the adrenergic ganglion cells. Nevertheless, the medullary chromaffin cells are not nerve cells in that they possess neither axons nor dendrites, and they liberate their secretions directly at the surface of the cell body and thence into the circulation instead of at the distal end of an axon in the vicinity of the target cell. With respect to these three differences, the chromaffin cells resemble endocrine cells more than nerve cells. There are, however, cells that defy classification as either nervous or endocrine, combining most of the typical structural and functional features of both elements in one single cell type: the aforementioned neurosecretory cells.

NEUROSECRETORY CELLS

Neurosecretory cells possess most of the ordinary features of nerve cells, including synaptic excitability, impulse conduction, Nissl bodies in their cytoplasm, and a neuroectodermal origin. However, although they receive nervous impulses that serve as their specific activating stimuli and these impulses are propagated through their axons in the usual manner, the impulses are not passed on to other neurons or effector cells. Instead, the propagated nerve impulse serves only to release the hormonal material from its storing cytoplasmic granule at the nerve terminal, which is produced in the perikaryon of the cell and passed along the axon to the terminal. Thus, the main function of the neurosecretory cells consists of the production and release of hormones or other active substances into the blood either to act on distant target cells (as in the case of some neurohypophyseal or pineal hormones) or to stimulate the cells of another gland (adenohypophysis).

Although neurosecretory cells occur widely throughout the vertebrate and invertebrate phyla, the most comprehensive and integrated view of the structure-function relationships of neurosecretory systems and their target cells is available in mammals (especially for those located in the hypothalamus and pineal gland), for which there is a considerable background of anatomic and experimental information.

Therefore, these hypothalamic and pineal formations will serve here for the illustration of a neurosecretory cell. First, we shall mention the neurosecretory cell groups in the ventral anterior hypothalamus of humans and other vertebrates, namely, the supraoptic and paraventricular nuclei, which are part of a hypothalamoneurohypophyseal neurosecretory system. The cell bodies, or perikarya, of these neurosecretory cells form closely packed cellular condensations in the aforementioned nuclei, and the axonic processes run downward through the hypophyseal stalk into the posterior lobe of the pituitary, where they end as typical nerve terminals.

In these neurosecretory cells, the hormonal materials enclosed in cytoplasmic granules are mainly elaborated in the perikarya of the supraoptic and paraventricular neurons and transported by axoplasmic flow from the hypothalamus via the supraopticohypophyseal tract into the posterior pituitary, where they are stored and released. It is possible, however, that secretory granules are also formed along the axon and that they undergo a progressive increase in size and volume during the axoplasmic streaming. In other words, it might be that the axonal transport of the hormone-containing granules is supplemented with that of a progressive synthesis of the hormonal material along the axon until a quantal, or maturation, size of the granule is reached.

These features are complemented by the presence of typical synaptic vesicles in the terminals of the supraopticohypophyseal neurons. Since the synaptic vesicles represent the most constant and specific component of synaptic endings in general, and since they are the storage organelles of acetylcholine and other synaptic mediators, it is difficult to link their presence with anything but the release of the hormones lodged in the neighboring membrane-bound particles. This implies that the electrical events that have been recorded in single neurons do not act directly in the release of the granular material but by way of acetylcholine, a neurotransmitter that is also stored in the same terminals. This arrangement is consistent with our current concepts of neuronal activity and impulse transmission in general.

In the hypothalamus, there are neurosecretory systems other than the supraopticoparaventriculoneurohypophyseal complex (e.g., in the nucleus lateralis tuberis, the nucleus periventricularis infundibularis, and the area periventricularis posterior). These and other hypothalamic neurosecretory cells, such as those in the anterior part of the median eminence and those in the mamillary and posterior tuberal regions, evidently formulate materials that control the output of pituitary trophic hormones (e.g., corticotropin-releasing factor), whereas others produce trophic hormones that act on peripherally located glands. Furthermore, neurosecretory material can be traced from the hypothalamus along pathways other than the supraopticohypophyseal tract (i.e., to the septum, the habenula, and the midbrain). These observations are suggestive of a general neurosecretory function of practically all the representative nuclear groupings of the hypothalamus, for which there is further evidence in the production or storage or both of effector molecules such as epinephrine, norepinephrine, dopamine, acetylcholine, histamine, serotonin, prostaglandins, and the like in the very same areas.

The only other comparable area in the brain in which such concentration of these mediators has been shown to occur is the pineal gland, the specific cell type of which is the pinealocyte, a typical neurosecretory cell. Earlier histologic studies demonstrated that the pineal gland consists of a single type of cell, originally called *parenchymal*, and that these parenchymal cells arise from the same source as the nerve cells or the neuroglia but seem to represent a specific cell type with a characteristic neurosecretory structure and function. Electron-microscopic observations have confirmed these conclusions, and the term *pinealocyte*, proposed for the designation of this specific cell type, will be used in this discussion.

Pinealocytes have long processes that extend for considerable distances and end in bulblike swellings in the interlobular connective tissue. In the center of the lobules, these processes radiate in all directions from the cells, whereas toward the periphery of the lobules, the cells tend to become polarized in one or two processes. The secretory material is concentrated in the processes of the pinealocytes in the perivascular spaces. Under the electron microscope, it can be seen that the two types of vesicles, one containing light homogeneous material and the other containing heterogeneous material that encloses a dark osmium granule, are the main components of the processes.

Norepinephrine and serotonin (and possibly histamine), which occur in high concentrations in this tissue, are stored in those vesicles containing the dense osmium granules. However, it is not known whether the specific hormonal product of pinealocytes, the melatonin, is stored in the dense or in the light vesicles. It is, however, important that melatonin (5-methoxy-*N*-acetyl tryptamine) is derived from serotonin by N-acetylation and O-methylation and that the two enzymes involved in these chemical transformations are exclusively found in the pineal gland.

The neurosecretory cells logically lead us to the next major mediator-storing cell system, the nervous system, the structural and functional units of which are the nerve cells, or neurons.

NERVE CELLS (NEURONS)

The nervous system is a highly cellular entity, the structural units of which are its cells, known as *nerve cells*, or neurons. The protoplasm of the neuron may be extended into several processes. These processes are not intercellular substance but prolongations of the cytoplasm of the cell. The term *nerve cell* is often used to designate the body of the cell immediately surrounding the nucleus, and the processes are called *nerve fibers*. This is a misleading usage of these terms, since it implies that the fiber is not part of the cell. It is more appropriate to call the part of the cell surrounding the nucleus the *perikaryon*, or *cell body*.

In most cases, one process of each neuron serves to convey impulses away from the perikaryon. This process is called the axon.* The remaining processes, which are called *dendrites*, receive impulses and convey them to the perikaryon.

Perikaryon. As just mentioned, the mass of cytoplasm that surrounds the nucleus is called the *cell body*, or *perikaryon*. This cytoplasm contains organelles and inclusions typically encountered in most mammalian cells, albeit in different arrangements and concentrations. Notable among them are the nucleus, mitochondria, Golgi formations, pigment, fat droplets, microtubules, Nissl bodies, and neurofibrils. The latter two most typify nerve cells.

The perikaryon also contains primary lysosomes. Neuronal lysosomes are probably engaged in the degradation of unsaturated lipids and the detoxification of end products of cellular activity. Fat bodies of various sizes containing a yellow pigment may also be demonstrated in some perikarya, although not in the processes. It is now generally accepted that the yellowish-brown pigment granules, also referred to as *lipofuscin granules*, represent secondary lysosomes.

The Neuronal Processes. Each axon originates from the axon *hillock*, a cone-shaped elevation of the perikaryon, and ends as *telodendria*, an arborization of delicate branching nerve terminations. The surface of the axon is covered by the cell membrane, the *axolemma*. The cytoplasm of the axon, called *axoplasm*, is continuous with that of the perikaryon, and there is evidence for a continuous discharge of neuronal cell products into the axon and a flow of axoplasm to the very terminations. Neurotubules and neurofilaments serve as directional guides for the cytoplasmic transport of cellular ingredients from the perikaryon to more distal parts of the cell. In addition, axons and dendrites also exhibit structures called *neurofibrils*, which are aggregates of submicroscopic neurotubules and neurofilaments.

Nerve Endings. As the axon approaches the site of its termination, it exhibits structural features not found more proximally. Thus, the preterminal part of the axon is expanded to form a terminal button, or *end-bulb*, and beadlike swellings occur along the axon. In both these structures, the most striking feature is the occurrence of large numbers of microvesicles, which have been dubbed *synaptic vesicles*. They can be subdivided into three categories: (1) small granulated vesicles, (2) large granulated vesicles, and (3) clear vesicles.

The small granulated vesicles average 300 to 500 Å in diameter and have a dense core that contains norepinephrine. The large granulated vesicles average 800 to 1000 Å in diameter and are synthesized in the perikaryon and transported along the axon. They represent storage sites for norepinephrine and are assumed to be precursor structures of the small granulated vesicles. The clear vesicles of parasympathetic nerves contain acetylcholine as do similar vesicles in the synaptic termination of motor end-plates. It is presently not known whether the clear vesicles of adrenergic nerve endings are acetylcholine-containing organelles or membranous "ghosts" representing the final stage of a continuous transition from large to small granulated vesicles.

Functional Interpretations from Cytology. If we were to try to infer the functions of a neuron from the foregoing cellular machinery, we would be entitled to the following assumptions. Despite wide variations in cell shape, size, and volume, most nerve cells possess large amounts of unattached ribosomes, presumably for the synthesis of intracellular materials such as enzymes and structural macromolecules. However, the cell body is also filled with varying quantities of rough endoplasmic reticulum and smooth endoplasmic reticulum indicative of cells that package synthetic material for transcellular secretion. Thus, we anticipate the neuron to be a dynamic secretory cell with broad synthetic capabilities.

Although organelles with such synthesizing capabilities characterize both the dendrite and perikaryon cytoplasm, they are not found within the axon. This indicates that the perikaryon synthesizes all the required macromolecules for the axon and that a process of somatofugal transport carries them from the perikaryon down the axon. Regardless of the rate at which macromolecules can be transported down the axon, certain actions of the nerve terminal, such as the release of transmitters, occur at rates that still exceed the amount arriving from the perikaryon. In these cases, the nerve terminals have acquired the necessary enzymes in order to synthesize the neurotransmitters de novo from amino acids present in the extracellular fluid spaces. Nerve terminals are specialized functionally in yet another way that helps decrease their need for transmitter synthesis: Almost all neurochemical types of nerve terminals except those releasing acetylcholine are

---

*Although this definition of *axon* is true for most neurons, it is not accurate for the peripheral process of the sensory neuron, which conducts impulses toward the perikaryon and is, nonetheless, called an axon.

able to reaccumulate actively the transmitters that they release.*

PLATELETS

Platelets are small (2 to 4 μm diameter), anucleated, circulating, granule-containing cells derived from bone marrow megakaryocytes. They interact with damaged endothelium, participate in hemostasis and coagulation, and are also active in immunologic inflammatory reactions in that they adhere to immune complexes and release the mediators stored in their granules.

In the blood, serotonin is contained in platelets; virtually none is found in platelet-free plasma if this has been prepared in such a way as to avoid platelet damage. The serotonin content of platelets of different species varies considerably. In humans, 10^8 platelets contain about 60 ng of serotonin, whereas in the same number of rabbit platelets, which are slightly smaller in size, there is about 15 times as much. A similar species variation is shown by histamine, which is also contained by platelets of some species, especially by those of rabbits. Epinephrine and norepinephrine are also among the amine constituents of platelets. Their presence in platelets presumably represents catecholamines that have been taken up from the plasma; the same may apply for the source of their serotonin and/or histamine contents. In fact, the main reason for placing the discussion of platelets following that of the neuron relates to the striking resemblance between their respective catecholamine re-uptake functions, because of which the platelet has been considered a circulating cellular equivalent of the postganglionic adrenergic neuron. This parallelism together with other interrelationships among the storage cells of the chemical mediators will be discussed later.

THYMIC EPITHELIAL CELLS AND HASSALL's CORPUSCLES

Usually, the thymus is composed of two lobes that are covered by a fibrous capsule. This capsule gives off numerous trabeculae that subdivide each lobe into many lobules. The lobules are composed of a cortex and medulla. Most of the thymic epithelial cells are within the medulla, and a few are found as a thin layer in the subcapsular cortex. The Hassall's corpuscles are oval bodies consisting of concentrically arranged squamous-appearing cells that are found only in the medulla.

The thymic epithelial cells arise from the neural crest, migrate to the thymus gland, and secrete immunomodulatory hormones that are responsible for the terminal differentiation of T-

lymphocytes (see later). These epithelial cells, therefore, are both developmentally and functionally highly reminiscent of the earlier described neurosecretory cells. Although the origin of Hassall's corpuscles is not known, they also participate in the production of immunomodulatory peptides. Collectively, therefore, they represent a hormonal secretory cell system, enclosed in one organ that is a major controlling source of the operation of the immune response (see further on).

LYMPHOCYTES AND MONONUCLEAR CELLS

Lymphocytes are mononuclear cells whose cytoplasm contains no specific-staining granules. They arise from a maturation sequence that is simpler than that of granulocytes: lymphoblast—prolymphocyte—lymphocyte. Maturation as viewed histochemically consists of progressive intensification of chromatin staining and coarsening of its texture as cell and nucleus become smaller. Mature lymphocytes are rich in free ribosomes and contain a few mitochondria, a small Golgi, and a few lysosomes.

Lymphocytes can be functionally subdivided into T cells (thymus-derived, or thymus-dependent lymphocytes) and B cells (bone-marrow–derived, or bursal-equivalent cells, i.e., antibody-secreting plasma cells and their precursors). T-lymphocytes contain at least four functional subclasses: helper cells, suppressor cells, lymphokine-producing cells, and cytolytically active cells. Cell-mediated immune, or delayed-hypersensitivity (DH), reactions are probably mediated by lymphokine-producing lymphocytes, which can attract and activate macrophages. Cytolytically active T cells are induced during graft rejection and viral infections. These "killer" T cells are directed against, and kill, the foreign graft cell surface antigens and virally altered cell surface antigens, respectively.

Another mononuclear cell is the monocyte. This cell has a lobulated nucleus with reticular chromatin strands. Although sometimes it is difficult to distinguish a monocyte from an atypical large lymphocyte, the two cell types show clearly different histochemical characteristics. Monocytes arise in the bone marrow, sojourn in the blood for about 24 to 36 hours, and then enter the tissues, where they may persist for long periods of time. They are precursors of tissue macrophages, which are differentiated mononuclear phagocytes that reside in the tissues. Transformation of monocyte to macrophage is accompanied by fundamental changes in cell structure and metabolism. As they develop into macrophages, the cells become large, with an increase in mitochondria and a growing dependence for energy on tricarboxylic acid cycle activity (unlike their monocytic precursors, which depend primarily on glycolysis). Macrophages characteristically contain large numbers of heter-

---

*In the case of the cholinergic synapse, choline is taken up by the presynaptic terminal.

ogeneous dense granules. These granules contain acid hydrolases and are probably "secondary lysosomes" resulting from the fusion of the primary lysosomes with phagocytic vacuoles. Another typical feature of macrophages is the presence of abundant small pinocytic ("drinking") vesicles.

Although macrophages are present in all tissues (in connective tissue they are called *histiocytes* and in serous cavities *pleural* and *peritoneal macrophages*), they are especially dense in "filter" organs—liver (Kupffer cells), lung (alveolar macrophages), spleen and lymph nodes (free and fixed macrophages)—where, perched on endothelial cells and reticulum fibers, they constitute a sentry network. These cells of the network were grouped by Aschoff into what he termed the *reticuloendothelial system*. Today, it is realized that this term is inappropriate and should be replaced by *mononuclear phagocyte system*.

Mononuclear phagocytes (monocytes and macrophages), like neutrophils, can ingest and kill bacteria (particularly pyogenic bacteria) during all phases of their life cycle. Macrophages, especially those previously activated by antigens, are more efficient in killing and ingesting bacteria than monocytes. Because of their long life, macrophages are also responsible for the digestion of bacteria killed by neutrophils. They are actively pinocytotic and possibly play a role in normal serum protein catabolism. They also clear and digest senescent blood cells. They have important biosynthetic capacities and produce large quantities of lysozyme as well as proteins of the complement and fibrinolytic systems and a group of presently incompletely defined substances termed *monokines*. Macrophages in various specific locations may have properties unique to their site (i.e., alveolar macrophages show greater rates of oxygen consumption than do peritoneal macrophages) and as yet undetermined local functions.

Macrophages together with lymphocytes are involved in immune responses that include programming lymphocytes for antibody formation and containment, if not killing, of "facultative" intracellular parasites, viruses, protozoa, certain fungi, and mycobacteria. These activities lead us to the discussion of one of the most important homeostatic defense mechanisms—the immune response.

OPERATION OF THE IMMUNE RESPONSE: CELLULAR DYNAMICS AND ORGANIZATIONAL CHARACTERISTICS

Immunology has become the "Rosetta stone" of modern medicine. It has helped explain and demystify many puzzling diseases. The importance of the immune response in protecting and preserving a normal state of health is well known. By contrast, the role of the immune response and immune reactions in the pathogenesis of disease is now increasingly apparent. Indeed, because of these conflicting biologic and pathologic activities, immunologic responses and reactions sometimes appear as enigmas.

Our present knowledge of the intricacy and complexity of the immune response has been growing greatly since the beginning of the twentieth century. Since the 1970s, there have been giant steps in this accumulation of knowledge. We are rapidly approaching a point at which the biochemical and cellular details of the immune response will be so well known that we will be able to "map" an individual's potential for immune reactivity to a wide range of chemical and biologic factors. Also, we should soon be able to understand how the protective aspects of the immune response become subverted to those that are damaging and destructive.

Immunology today can be likened to a large octopus with tentacles that extend into many areas of biology and medicine. At the center of the discipline, there is a body of facts and observations, theories and hypotheses, that can be considered the current "dogma" of the science. In this chapter and in Chapter 5, this body of knowledge is presented with an emphasis on the main points and principles that have now been well confirmed and that are basic to a critical understanding of immunology. We will occasionally digress from our central discussion in order to highlight or emphasize a point of information and to show its application to a specific problem in the clinic or the laboratory.

Embryologists and developmental biologists have shown the evolution of adaptive systems from the simple to complex multicellular organisms. It has been observed that the phenomenon of enzyme induction in bacteria is similar to the induction of antibody in a higher organism. In the bacterium, adaptive enzyme induction occurs when there is a limitation of available substrate material for energy metabolism or other vital functions. This substrate limitation induces a genetic activation that leads to the formation of a specific group of proteins possessing enzymatic activity that will allow the bacterium to metabolize and assimilate the substrate. In the case of an antibody response, we will see later that there is also a genetic activation followed by elaboration of the specific antibody protein that reacts with the initiating antigen. In this context, the immune response appears to be an adaptive response predetermined by the genetic makeup of the organism. As an adaptive mechanism, it is an important determinant of the organism's ability to survive and prosper. Without the ability to mount an immune response, an organism would readily succumb to any of a variety of lethal factors.

In higher organisms such as vertebrates, the immune response is of great complexity and diversity. However, in lower organisms, such as the primitive unicellular and multicellular forms, one does not encounter the specifically reactive cells and molecules that characterize the immune response in higher animals. At the primitive level, reaction of the organism to hazardous factors occurs by less specific means. Commonly, the organism simply moves away to avoid a noxious agent. At other times, an offending material may be phagocytosed and digested, and thus its potentially harmful effect is inactivated. In the higher organisms, such nonspecific forms of protection persist, but they are enhanced by more specific and potent humoral and cellular components of the immune response. The complexity, diversity, and specificity of the immune response afford a greater margin of protection. Those reactions of higher organisms that correspond to primitive forms are due to the biochemical and cellular factors of the general inflammatory response.

The inflammatory response is notably augmented by the immune response. This augmentation occurs because of specific antibody and reactive lymphocytes that amplify host mediator systems to destroy or inactivate pathogenic factors. It provides considerable protection for the host but, as mentioned, also can lead to damage of the host's tissues. The conditions of health operate to maintain a delicate balance between these potentially opposing forces. This interplay has been explored extensively, and we now understand many intricacies of its operation.

A CONVENIENT MODEL OF THE IMMUNE SYSTEM

One can best understand the structure and function of the immune system by referring to a simplified model. The model that has been selected is one of a simple servomechanism. Self-regulating, or homeostatic, systems are characteristic of many biologic systems. They are readily understood in our modern world of cybernetics and computers, which causes us to think in terms of servoregulated systems.

The specific model we will follow is illustrated in Figure 4–1. It has the following components: an input signal, a central unit for processing the signal, an output produced by the central unit, and a feedback loop that links the output to the input signal. We can find many examples of analogous mechanical systems, such as thermostatically controlled central heating systems and computer-controlled machines and devices. In biologic systems, examples are equally numerous, such as the simple neurogenic reflex arc and the control mechanisms that regulate respiratory and cardiovascular activity.

In our model, each of the immune components is identified by analogy with those of the servoregulatory system. The stimulating antigen, immunogen, is identified as the input signal or stimulus. The lymphatic tissues and cells are

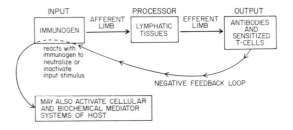

A MODEL OF THE IMMUNE SYSTEM DEPICTING INTERRELATIONS OF THE MAJOR COMPONENTS

Figure 4–1

designated as the central processor. Antibodies and specifically reactive T-lymphocytes are the output of the lymphatic tissues. A feedback loop is created by reactivity of the antibodies and reactive T-lymphocytes with the immunogen. The feedback effect is negative, since the result of antibody or reactive T-lymphocyte combining with immunogen is to neutralize or inactivate, thus diminishing its input to the system.

The pathway, or direction, followed by the input signal, or immunogen, to the lymphatic tissues (central processing apparatus) is called the *afferent limb*; the pathway of the output signal of antibody and reactive T-lymphocytes from the lymphatic tissues is designated the *efferent limb*.

By frequently referring to the model throughout the following discussions, the reader will be able to maintain a perspective for understanding the general way in which the immune system operates. Each upcoming section will provide important details about the major components of the immune system. At the conclusion, the reader should be able to arrange the information in such a way that the functional interrelationships of the components are apparent.

IMMUNOGENS, ANTIGENS, AND ALLERGENS

In our model, the input signal is known as the *stimulating antigen*, or *immunogen*. In earlier literature, the term *antigen* was used as an all-inclusive one to indicate any substance that could elicit an immune response as well as react with the antibody or lymphocytes produced. Various studies have necessitated a redefinition of terms that will allow researchers to clarify those substances that elicit an immune response. The term *immunogen* is now the preferred name for a substance or material that will stimulate an immune response in a sensitive and immunocompetent host. Immunogen is considered the special class of antigens denoting those that are capable of immune stimulation. Those immunogens that give rise to hypersensitivity through the specific stimulation of IgE antibody production are called *al-*

lergens. Other types of antigen may exhibit reactivity with antibodies or sensitized lymphocytes but do not produce a stimulatory effect.

To be considered an immunogen, an antigen must be shown to elicit an immune response in some animal. The immune response may occur either as antibody production or as proliferation of specifically reactive T-lymphocytes. It is now known that each of the different populations of cells leading to production of antibody or sensitized lymphocytes reacts only with specific sites on the entire immunogen. These reactive sites on the immunogen molecule are called *determinants*. As illustrated in Figure 4–2, a single immunogen molecule may possess many different antigenic determinants along its molecular structure. Each of these determinants possesses a specific chemical composition and physical configuration that impart a unique molecular configuration to the determinant. As will be mentioned again later, each of these different determinants reacts with a different B- or T-lymphocyte within the tissues of a responsive animal. The ability of a particular B- or T-lymphocyte to react with a specific immunogenic determinant is regulated by the genome of the animal through the production of specific recognition molecules on the surface membranes of the lymphocytes.

The terms now used to denote the structure of immunogenic determinants are *carrier determinant* and *haptenic determinant*. These are used to designate two general classes of such molecular configurations found along the surface of immunogens. Carrier determinants are the structural areas that occur along the integral part of the molecule and depend on the folding and arrangement of the polymeric chains that constitute the macromolecule. By contrast, haptenic determinants are chemical groupings that usually project from the integral structure of the molecule and exist as discrete and sharply defined chemical groupings, such as side chains or groups that have been chemically linked at particular points along the molecular surface. The illustrations of these determinants as shown in Figure 4–2 will aid the reader in understanding the differences between these two types of structures. Thinking of the haptenic determinants as spines that project from a leaf of a cactus and the carrier determinants as folds of the leaf itself may also help one to comprehend the differences.

It is apparent that naturally occurring immunogens and antigens possess a variety of determinants, so that the total immune response to an immunogen is quite varied and diverse. Indeed, we find that there are individual and separate antibodies as well as populations of reactive T-lymphocytes formed in response to each different determinant. Stated in another way, we find in the blood of an animal who had developed an immune response that there are different populations of antibodies and sensitized T-lymphocytes,

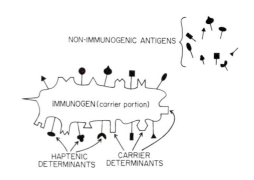

DIAGRAM ILLUSTRATING DIFFERENCE BETWEEN AN IMMUNOGEN AND NON-IMMUNOGENIC ANTIGENS

Figure 4–2

each reactive with a different individual antigenic determinant. This explains the considerable heterogeneity of the immune response to an immunogen and the great diversity and heterogeneity apparent when one compares the immune response with similar immunogens in different animals.

Antigens that function as immunogens have certain physical and chemical characteristics. One of these is the overall three-dimensional size and shape of the molecule, which is best expressed in terms of molecular weight. In general, macromolecules of small size—that is, with molecular weights less than 6000 daltons—usually do not behave as immunogens. Those ranging in size from 6000 to 30,000 daltons are often poor immunogens and require the use of adjuvants.* Larger macromolecules, especially those above the molecular weight range of 35,000 to 40,000 daltons, are usually good immunogens.

The chemical structure of the molecule is also important; for example, nonpolar lipid molecules are poor immunogens compared with those having molecular polarity. The route of administration affects the degree of response to a particular immunogen. An immunogen that is administered and then becomes sequestered or trapped does not have access to lymphocytes; consequently, it will not stimulate a response. Selection of the responding animal is also important because genetic factors determine the responses different animals give to the same immunogen. Instances frequently occur in which a given animal or species is unresponsive to a particular immunogen, whereas another may produce a marked response. Some molecules can be made immunogenic by being chemically linked or coupled to a larger macromolecule. In such instances, the coupled chemical becomes the haptenic determinant, and the substrate macromolecule provides the carrier determinants.

Another consideration that is important in establishing whether a substance is an immuno-

---

*An *immunologic adjuvant* may be defined as a compound capable of aiding or potentiating an immune response.

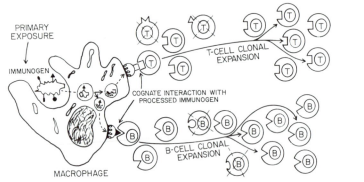

Figure 4–3

SCHEMATIC ILLUSTRATION OF EVENTS IN THE PRIMARY IMMUNE
RESPONSE SHOWING STIMULATION OF VIRGIN T AND B LYMPHOCYTES
BY REACTION WITH PROCESSED IMMUNOGEN

gen concerns whether it can cause the cross-linking of specific receptors on lymphocyte membrane
surfaces at the time of initial recognition contact.
As we will note again in a later section, such cross-
linking activates enzyme systems in the cell, leading to blast transformation and subsequent cell
multiplication. Some immunogens have similar
repeating haptenic determinants that are closely
spaced and that produce cross-linking on direct
contact with the recognition lymphocyte. However,
most immunogens require a type of modification,
called *processing*, before they are able to react
effectively with the receptors on lymphocytes. This
processing occurs within monocytes and histiocytes. The sequence of events in processing (Fig.
4–3) begins with phagocytosis of the antigen, followed by intracellular breakdown of the immunogenic molecule into smaller antigenic determinants that are then coupled with a material from
the cell similar to ribonucleic acid (RNA). The
processed antigen then moves to the cell surface,
where contact with recognition lymphocytes occurs. Processed antigen is thus put in a form that
is reactive with the lymphocyte receptors. Contact
with the receptors causes the activation sequence
leading to lymphocyte proliferation and differentiation.

The reaction of recognition lymphocytes with
the processed antigen is now known to be more
complex than a simple one-to-one stoichiometric
relationship between antigen and responding lymphocyte. In the past few years, it has been discovered that there are populations of lymphocytes
that provide a helper function to augment production of antibody or sensitized lymphocytes and
others that exhibit a suppressor effect. These
helper and suppressor cells arise from subpopulations of T-lymphocytes and are relatively specific
in their reactivity with individual immunogens.
More recently, they have been found to secrete
soluble factors that appear to be the active substances that evolve either a helper or a suppressor
effect, depending on the cell of origin. These cells

will be discussed later; we mention them here in
order to emphasize the complexity of immunogen
initiation of the immune response.

The studies that have shown the action of
helper and suppressor cells have also demonstrated that, in general, B cells recognize and react
with haptenic determinants of an immunogen,
whereas T cells preferentially react with the carrier determinants (Fig. 4–4). Experiments with
immunogens of varied haptenic and carrier determinants have also shown that in many instances
in which T- or B-cell reaction occurs with a haptenic determinant, the subsequent differentiation
to a plasma cell with production of antibody or
differentiation of specifically reactive T-lymphocytes does not occur in the absence of a concomitant helper T-cell reaction with the carrier determinants.

DEVELOPMENT AND MATURATION OF LYMPHOID TISSUES

The immune response to an immunogen depends on normally developed and functioning lymphocytic cells that possess the genetically determined receptors for reacting with the particular
immunogen. Thus, normal immune functions (immunocompetence and immunoresponsiveness) depend on the full development and maturation of
lymphoid tissues. Investigations in experimental
embryology have shown that the earliest appearance of specific cells destined to become the mature
lymphocytic tissues occurs during the first trimester in the primitive yolk sac. Later, during the
second and third trimesters, these primitive cells
are found in the fetal liver and spleen. Finally,
they accumulate in the marrow of the long bones.
These are primitive stem cells that not only give
rise to immature lymphocytes but also produce
other important cell lines of the blood, including
erythrocytic, myelocytic, and megakaryocytic cell
types (Fig. 4–5).

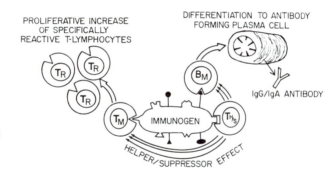

Figure 4–4

SCHEMATIC ILLUSTRATION OF EVENTS IN THE SECONDARY IMMUNE
RESPONSE SHOWING DIFFERENTIAL STIMULATION OF T AND B
MEMORY CELLS AND HELPER AND SUPPRESSOR T-LYMPHOCYTES

Production of primitive lymphocytes from these stem cell foci appears to occur as the result of certain stimuli of normal differentiation and development that have not yet been identified and whose specific mode of action is still undefined. These primitive lymphocytes then undergo further differentiation, which causes them to segregate into two major types. One type has a high affinity for localization in the thymus. After release from the marrow foci of primitive stem cells, the lymphocytes enter the circulation and "home" to the thymus through a mechanism of specific attraction not yet fully understood. These cells are designated *primitive*, or *immature* T-lymphocytes because of this affinity for thymic localization.

Another type of immature lymphocyte moves from the stem cell foci to other areas in the bone marrow in humans and many other vertebrates. In the chicken, these cells localize preferentially in a structure of the hind gut known as the *bursa of Fabricius*. These immature lymphocytes are referred to as *B cells,* or *bursal-equivalent cells,* because of their tendency to localize in the bone marrow foci in the human and other vertebrates or the bursal structure in the chicken.

The immature T- and B-lymphocytes undergo a period of maturation and differentiation in the tissues in which they have homed. After they become mature cells, they emerge and enter the circulation, disseminating throughout the body to populate the peripheral lymphatic tissues, which include the lymph nodes, lymphoepithelial tissues, spleen, and the recirculating pool of lymphocytes in blood and lymphatic channels (Fig. 4–5). The cell surfaces of mature T- and B-lymphocytes have specific recognition molecules that enable them to react with specific immunogens.

The majority of these T- and B-lymphocytes show a pattern of constant recirculation through the lymphatics and the peripheral blood, so there is a continuing change of the cell population at all times. In the lymphatics, specifically the lymph nodes and spleen, there is a preferential accumulation of the different cell types in specific anatomic areas. The B-lymphocytes accumulate in the cortical areas of lymph nodes and tend to recircu-

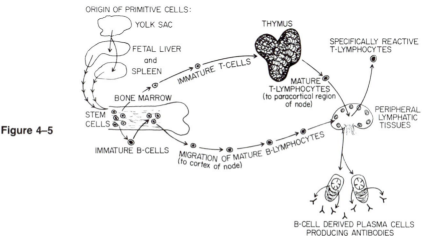

Figure 4–5

SEQUENCE OF DEVELOPMENTAL MATURATION OF LYMPHATIC TISSUES

late about the cortical sinuses, whereas T-lympho-cytes predominate in the paracortical zones of lymph nodes. In the spleen, the small pencillar arteries found in the center of the lymphatic ag-gregates are surrounded by a cuff of cells that are predominantly T-lymphocytes. The B-lymphocytes tend to cluster eccentric to this zone and occasion-ally show follicle formation. The T- and B-lympho-cytes in the circulating blood re-enter the lymph nodes across specialized vascular structures known as the *postcapillary venules* (Fig. 4–6). These ven-ules possess a type of endothelial cell that exhibits a high profile and is called *high endothelium.* Postcapillary high endothelial venules predomi-nate in the junctional zone between the cortex and paracortex of the lymph nodes. By traversing these structures, the T- and B-lymphocytes can rapidly re-enter the lymph nodes from the circulation and circulate through the sinuses of the node, exiting along the medullary sinuses into draining lym-phatic channels. They then enter subsequent nodes in the chain and eventually return to the blood by way of drainage through the thoracic duct.

The next chapter, which deals with the patho-physiology of immunologic and related diseases, will emphasize that failure of development and normal maturation of the lymphocytes at any point in the sequence can lead to a deficit of immune function. Some defects may be partial and selec-tive, causing only minor impairment. Others may be of critical importance to survival. Defects that often lead to a lethal outcome are those associated with a significant impairment of T-lymphocyte function, either alone or in combination with a B-lymphocyte deficiency.

The events of differentiation and maturation of T- and B-lymphocytes are not as well known in the human as in some experimental animals. There is a strong presumption, however, that the sequence of events is similar. In the mouse, im-mature T-lymphocytes possess varied membrane receptors for different biochemical factors. These

include thymic hormone receptors, beta-adrenergic receptors, and others. When maturation is com-plete, the T-lymphocyte has lost many of these receptors and emerges with fewer receptors for biologic factors, but it has newly formed receptors for immunogen that develop during maturation. A similar change in membrane receptors is thought to occur in the maturation of B-lymphocytes.

Mature T- and B-lymphocytes have specific recognition molecules on their cell membranes that bind to specific immunogenic determinants. These molecules are different in T- and B-lympho-cytes and vary in specificity among individual lymphocytes of either T or B type. An individual lymphocyte carries recognition molecules only for a specific individual determinant, usually one quite different from the specificity of its neighbors. This high degree of selectivity and specificity has been of great interest to geneticists because it appears to represent almost complete genetic (al-lelic) exclusion within each individual lymphocyte. Each lymphocyte appears to be programmed with a specific membrane receptor to respond only to certain determinant structures; the vast remain-der of genetic information in each cell appears to be suppressed or excluded by mechanisms not yet understood.

It has been established that the genes that determine the ability of an animal to respond to various immunogens are contained within the gene complex known as the *histocompatibility gene loci.* In the mouse, these genes are located in the H2 region; in the human, the histocompatibility loci are designated by the abbreviation HLA (hu-man leukocyte antigens). In the human and the mouse, there are different regions along these genetic loci that determine an individual's capac-ities for an immune response; these regions are specifically known as the *immune response genes,* or *IR genes.* Within the IR genes are specific loci that code for recognition of individual immuno-genic determinants. As already indicated, only a

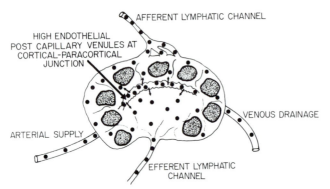

AFFERENT LYMPHATIC CHANNEL

HIGH ENDOTHELIAL
POST CAPILLARY VENULES AT
CORTICAL-PARACORTICAL
JUNCTION

ARTERIAL SUPPLY

VENOUS DRAINAGE

EFFERENT LYMPHATIC
CHANNEL

Figure 4–6

DIAGRAM OF LYMPH NODE CIRCULATION SHOWING LOCATION OF HIGH ENDOTHELIAL POST CAPILLARY VENULES WHERE LYMPHOCYTES TRANSIT DIRECTLY INTO NODE FROM BLOOD CIRCULATION

single locus becomes expressed in the form of a membrane receptor for each individual lymphocyte of either T or B type. When the mechanisms of this selective allelic exclusion become understood, a significant advance in understanding gene function will have been made.

The identification and chemical structure of the specific receptors on membranes of T- and B-lymphocytes have attracted considerable interest. It has been clearly determined that the receptor molecules on mature B-lymphocytes are identical with the particular immunoglobulin that the cell will form after differentiating to a plasma cell. Immunoglobulins are the specific antibody products of the immune response by B-lymphocytes. Their chemistry and structure will be covered in more detail later, but it should be pointed out here that there are five major classes of immunoglobulins identified by letters of the alphabet preceded by the prefix Ig—thus, the designations IgG, IgM, IgA, IgD, and IgE. Each of the immunoglobulin classes is made by a different B-lymphocyte, and each individual immunoglobulin made will vary with the stimulating immunogen.

It has been found that those B-lymphocytes that have not reached full maturity exhibit a change in the type of immunoglobulin receptor on the cell surface, which shifts initially from IgM to IgD and continues changing until the lymphocytes reach final maturity, at which stage the immunoglobulin receptor is identical with the type and specificity that the B-lymphocyte will secrete on stimulation. For example, a B-lymphocyte that will ultimately secrete immunoglobulin of IgG type in response to a bacterial antigen may at first be found to possess a receptor of the IgM type, which then shifts to IgD and finally to IgG. It should be emphasized, however, that at any point in this maturation sequence, should antigen contact occur, the cell will be stimulated to proliferation with secretion of the specific IgG immunoglobulin as genetically determined. There is some experimental evidence favoring the view that less mature cells possessing IgM and IgD receptors function as latent cells in the initial primary response and as memory cells in the secondary immune response. These responses will be discussed in more detail later.

The membrane receptors on T cells are not immunoglobulins, but they do possess a similar high degree of specificity for the immunogen. As with B cells, T cells also exhibit a wide range of receptor specificities from cell to cell, each having different reactivity with a different immunogen. The receptors on T-lymphocytes appear to be genetically determined in the same way as the immunoglobulin receptors on B cells. Experimental studies aimed at identification of the chemical structure of the T-cell receptor have shown the receptor to occur in close physical association with the HLA antigens on the cell surfaces. This close surface association corresponds to the close relationships of the loci within the genome. Aside from data indicating that the T-cell receptor is a glycoprotein, there is as yet no information as to its structural configuration. Presumably the amino acid sequence varies considerably in order to accommodate a wide range of cellular reactivity with different immunogenic molecules.

The membrane and intracellular biochemical events that occur following immunogen contact with the lymphocyte receptors lead to a marked change in cellular activity. In B-lymphocytes, the binding of antigen results in a phenomenon called *capping*, which results in movement of the antigen to concentrate in one area on the cell membrane. Following this, the B cell exhibits increased synthetic metabolic activity accompanied by cellular enlargement and increase in nuclear size, a change that is described as *blast transformation*. Soon after blast transformation occurs, the cells enter the mitotic cycle and undergo division. This leads to an increase in the number of specific lymphocytes identical with the original. This proliferative increase is called *clonal expansion* (Fig. 4–3). T cells undergo a similar increase in numbers as a consequence of immunogen stimulation.

As T- and B-lymphocytes increase in numbers following the first exposure to immunogen, some of them continue differentiation into specialized effector cells; others remain as memory cells that will respond to subsequent immunogen exposure. Some B-lymphocytes continue differentiation to form plasma cells, which manufacture and secrete antibody. T cells, however, differentiate to form subclasses of reactive cells. Some T cells become either helper or suppressor cells; others become antigen-reactive sensitized cells. Some of these latter cells can directly fix to antigens on tissue cells and cause death; some respond to antigen by the production of soluble factors, known as *lymphokines*, that promote cellular infiltrative reactions in tissue. The type of T-lymphocyte that kills on direct contact with tissue is called a *killer* (K) *T-lymphocyte*. These will be discussed in detail in Chapter 5.

CHARACTERISTICS OF THE IMMUNE RESPONSE

Attention is now directed to the sequence of events that constitute the steps in the immune response from initial immunogen exposure to production of antibody or reactive lymphocytes. It was previously emphasized that both T- and B-lymphocytes are in constant recirculation through the lymphatic tissues, lymph, and blood. Many studies have shown that the lymphocytes in the peripheral blood are approximately 80 per cent T-lymphocytes, whereas approximately 15 to 20 per cent are B cells. The total number of lymphocytes circulating each day has been estimated at 10 to 12 times the number found in the blood at any given time. T-lymphocytes also circulate through the extravascular interstitial tissue of organs such as skin, kidney, ovary, uterus, testis, and others; B-lymphocytes do not. As mentioned earlier, both T- and B-lymphocytes re-enter lymph nodes directly from the blood via the high endothelial postcapillary venules near the junction of cortex and paracortex in the lymph node (Fig. 4–6).

Immunogen exposure may occur in a variety of ways. It can result from ingestion and absorption across the gastrointestinal tract, from inhalation and absorption along the mucosa of the respiratory tract, from infection, or from direct inoculation by injection or a penetrating wound. Some antigens may be absorbed directly across the skin barrier. Following entry of antigen into the tissues or circulation, nonspecific inflammatory and cellular reactions occur, leading to clearance, degradation, or sequestration of the antigens in the tissues. Phagocytic cells, especially polymorphonuclear leukocytes, tissue macrophages, and cells of the mononuclear phagocyte system, are the main participants in this phagocytic encounter with immunogen. The majority of antigens may be effectively eliminated by this first encounter. It is during this reaction that the antigen becomes "processed," as was discussed previously (Fig. 4–3).

The processed antigen is released to the surface of the phagocyte (macrophage), where contact with recognition lymphocytes occurs (Fig. 4–3). Some processed antigen is also released into the circulation and may randomly contact and interact with specific recognition lymphocytes either in the circulation or in the lymphatic tissues. Lymphocytes that react on this first exposure to immunogen follow the proliferative sequence of events already described and may differentiate further to give rise to a limited amount of antibody production, formation of specifically reactive T cells, or production of abundant memory cells. The responding cell may be either T or B type or both, depending on the immunogen characteristics and recognition by virgin lymphocytes. The antibody response from the first encounter is mainly of the IgM class and is formed in a much smaller quantity than that produced following subsequent immunogen exposure. This initial antibody production does not appear to depend on T-helper cells. There is evidence that it is of IgM type because those receptors or recognition lymphocytes are more easily cross-linked by direct contact with small antigenic determinants and do not require facilitation by T-helper cells.

All the events that occur on the first encounter with antigen are described together as the *primary immune response*, which usually requires a period of 4 to 7 days to become fully developed following antigen exposure. The actual tissue sites of the cellular reaction are determined by the point of antigen contact. T cells traversing the tissues may encounter either native or processed immunogens at their site of entry; B-lymphocytes and other T-lymphocytes encounter antigen in regional lymph nodes after drainage from the site of entry. This contact in the local lymph nodes leads to cellular reactivity and proliferation. The sequence of changes observed in such a stimulated lymph node reflect those cellular events of proliferation and differentiation. In the early phase, the lymph node appears hypercellular and exhibits a change that has been called *sinus plugging*. All the sinuses within the paracortical region initially appear engorged with cells, followed by engorgement of the cortical zone and the medullary sinuses. Later, as the cell engorgement declines in the paracortex, hyperplasia of follicles appears in the cortical area. Cells in the paracortex during this engorgement are quite large and deeply basophilic, with prominent large nuclei characteristic of the blast transformation preceding the proliferative increase in cells. At this time, the lymph node becomes grossly enlarged and may become tender because of pressure and stretching on the surrounding tissues. After 5 to 7 days, plasma cells can be found in the medullary sinuses accompanied by immature cells that appear to be blast forms of plasma cells. Increases in antibody concentration can be detected in the draining lymph as well as in the peripheral circulation. The plasma cells do not leave the node but remain in the sinuses and secrete antibody into the lymph fluid leaving the node. In the spleen, similar cellular responses occur in the malpighian follicles, where the lymphocytes are arranged in clusters. The increase in lymphocytes may, in addition to the activation and enlargement of the histiocytes along splenic sinusoids, cause splenic enlargement. Such enlargement is commonly encountered when there is massive intravascular antigenic exposure, as occurs with sepsis.

After the first encounter and response to immunogen, an individual is said to be sensitized and possesses a certain level of specific antibody to the initiating immunogen as well as a certain population of reactive T-lymphocytes. There are also increased numbers of recognition lymphocytes of either T or B type or both, depending on the nature of the primary reaction. The individual is thus in a condition of heightened responsiveness and will have increased reactivity on subsequent exposure to the same or similar immunogen. The overall effect of the first exposure is an increase in the numbers of specific recognition lymphocytes, which thereby raises the potential level of immune response even to a small dose of the immunogen encountered at a later time.

The *secondary immune response* occurs in a sensitized individual. It has also been called the *anamnestic response*, a term derived from the Greek word meaning *to recall* or *recollect*. In the secondary response, the biochemical and cellular changes parallel those of the primary response but occur faster and in much greater quantity. There are also some qualitative differences, however, with regard to the classes of antibody formed. In the secondary response, IgG is the major class of antibody, whereas in the primary response IgM predominated. Also, the important role of helper and suppressor cells in the regulation of the secondary immune response is becoming understood. In experimental studies, it has been shown that some animals that fail to respond to a particular immunogen do so because of the effects of suppressor cells. In other instances, it has been shown that failure of response is due to lack of a T-helper cell effect. The studies demonstrating these points have also shown that T cells principally react with the carrier determinants of an antigen, whereas B cells react with the haptenic determinants (Fig. 4–4). In animals sensitized to the haptenic determinants but not to the carrier determinants, an effective secondary immune response fails to develop. It has been further shown that the carrier effect could be substituted by a phenomenon called the *allogeneic effect*. These studies have been carried out by cell transfer experiments of lymphocytes from an allogeneic donor strain to the sensitized animal. The allogeneic cells appear to exhibit an augmentation of B-cell response similar to that of the carrier-specific T-helper cells. Thus, the term *allogeneic effect* refers to a form of general immunopotentiation in which specific stimulation of T cells results in the release of subcellular factors active in the regulation of the immune response.

The cellular and tissue changes of the secondary response are similar to those of the primary response, but even greater cellular proliferation and engorgement of lymph nodes with marked hyperplastic activity in follicles of the cortex are found. The medullary sinuses of the nodes become engorged with large blast cells as well as abundant plasma cells synthesizing and secreting antibody. Because of the marked cellularity, lymph nodes become enlarged and tender.

The secondary immune response is also reflected in the increase of peripheral lymphocyte count and specific antibody in the circulation. These are the products of the immune response, and their measurement can provide pertinent clinical information regarding the immunocompetence and immunoresponsiveness of an individual. The ability to produce a substantial secondary immune response indicates immunocompetence and normal functioning of the entire immune system, since both T- and B-lymphocytes participate in that response.

SPECIFICALLY REACTIVE T CELLS

Formation of increased numbers of T cells specifically reactive for certain immunogens and antigens parallels those cellular events described in antibody production. The specifically reactive T cells can be thought of as analogous to specific antibody. The sites for interaction (binding) with antigen are cell membrane receptors, in contrast with the structural binding sites in molecules of antibody. The chemical composition and structure of such antigen binding sites in T cells are not the same as those of immunoglobulins.

Two major classes of specifically reactive T cells have now been described, although the pace of current investigative work suggests that others will no doubt be discovered and described in the near future. Those currently in central focus are called *regulatory T cells* (helper or suppressor) and *effector T cells*. The latter are distinguished by a response on contact with antigen, causing either synthesis and release of biologically active factors (lymphokines) or cell death on contact with cell-linked antigens. Regulatory T cells function by helping or suppressing B-cell antibody response or T-cell effector response. Some of the points made earlier regarding the primary immune response should be re-emphasized for T cells. It was noted that clonal proliferation ensues following the initial interaction of immunogen and virgin recognition T- and B-lymphocytes. It was emphasized that recognition T-lymphocytes generally recognize and react with the carrier determinants of an immunogen. Clonal expansion of T-lymphocytes yields a greater number of specifically reactive cells. The individual thus has a greater capacity for response on subsequent exposure to immunogen. This is the same state of affairs observed with B-cell clonal expansion.

Regulatory activity by T-lymphocytes was initially discovered through some animal experiments already mentioned. Such regulatory T cells in humans have been observed in in-vitro test systems, and they parallel the experimental animal findings. There is now agreement that such cells are important in the immune response in humans, although, as in the animal studies, the details of the mechanisms of regulation are not fully known. Most recently, it has been shown that there are soluble factors formed by both helper and suppressor T cells that are specifically reactive with antigen and closely associated with histocompatibility antigens of the cell membranes. Earlier studies indicated a necessity for close proximity of the regulatory T cells to the specifically responding effector T cell or responding B cell in order to achieve an effect, whether it was helper or suppressor. Regulatory T cells have been observed to affect activities of both T cells and B cells, as emphasized in Figure 4–4.

In experimental studies, the sensitivity of suppressor cells to low doses of irradiation and cytotoxic agents, such as cyclophosphamide, has been noted and applied in experiments on suppressor cell function. This point has not been clearly confirmed in humans, but there is strong suspicion that a similar sensitivity may exist. Also, it has been shown that some T-lymphocyte regulatory cells have receptors for an Fc structure of IgG and that others have receptors for the Fc of IgM. Those with Fc gamma (IgG) receptors appear to have a helper function; those with Fc mu (IgM) have been associated with suppressor activity.

Effector T cells are key participants in immunologic reactions known under such various labels as *delayed hypersensitivity, cell-mediated immunity, tuberculin-type hypersensitivity,* and *cellular hypersensitivity*. All these terms designate the sequence of events following interaction of antigen and specifically reactive T cells that commonly lead to lymphocytic infiltrates and granuloma formation in tissues. Many experimental studies conducted by various investigators since the 1960s have clarified the basic mechanisms of T-cell tissue reactions. There are two principal pathogenic sequences, and either may destroy the antigen or damage the tissue in which the reaction takes place. One reaction sequence occurs when an effector T-lymphocyte migrating through the tissue reacts with antigen. Following contact with antigen, intense biochemical activity occurs in the cell, resulting in protein and nucleic acid synthesis and later leading to cell division. Before division, however, there is a secretory phase, with the production of numerous biochemical substances that are secreted into the local tissue from the cytoplasm of the activated lymphocyte or lymphocytes. These substances, called *lymphokines*, have been found in both experimental and clinical studies to exhibit a wide range of biologic activities. They principally have an effect on other cells, producing activation, chemotaxis, or inhibitory changes. These effects on cells cause the succession of events of monocyte/macrophage recruitment (chemotaxis) into tissue, followed by phagocytosis of antigen with formation and release of digestive enzymes that destroy antigen and produce tissue necrosis.

The other principal mode of T-cell effector activity is cell killing. It occurs when the reactive antigen is part of, or closely linked to, a cell membrane in close association with histocompatibility antigens. In this sequence the corresponding T-lymphocyte reacts with the specific surface antigen and thereby comes in close contact with the cell, inducing a biochemical effect that causes death of the antigen-bearing cell. This killing is presumed to be due to a cytotoxic factor from the T-lymphocyte. Such a cell is called a *killer (K) T-cell*. These K-cell reactions will be covered in more detail in Chapter 5.

IMMUNOLOGIC MEMORY

The concept of memory in the immune system implies a capacity for recall recognition of an immunogen due to previous exposure. This capacity resides in recognition lymphocytes, which arise from the clonal expansion following an initial exposure to the immunogen. It is now recognized that the phenomenon of immunologic memory is a direct function of the increased numbers of recognition lymphocytes formed following the first immunogen exposure. During the primary response, the clonal proliferation of stimulated T- or B-lymphocytes produces progeny with reactivity identical with the original. This substantially increases the numbers of reactive cells with respect to the original population. Some of the progeny continue differentiation to form plasma cells and specific antibody or form populations of effector and regulatory T-lymphocytes. Most of the progeny do not undergo further differentiation but exist as copies of the original recognition lymphocytes within the tissues and circulating lymphocyte pool. Because of this increase in recognition cells, subsequent exposure to the immunogen causes a much greater response, as measured by serum-antibody production or numbers of specifically reactive T-lymphocytes. They appear to have developed more quickly and in greater quantity. This rapidity, however, is more apparent than real because the increased numbers of recognition cells react in greater numbers to form the differentiated cell types that produce antibody and reactive lymphocytes. The quantity and apparent speed of the response are a function of the sensitivity of the assay systems used to detect antibody and reactive cells. Current data do not show that the time interval between immunogen exposure and cellular response is substantially different for individual lymphocytes in either the primary or secondary immune responses. The phenomenon of immunologic memory thus is mainly quantitative. It provides the important condition of increased numbers of reactive cells. This augments the immune response necessary to assure host protection against the many hazardous factors with which we constantly come into contact. Primary immunization and booster stimulation in medical practice provide the needed increase in reactive cells that give a potent anamnestic host response when infection or exposure to toxins or other dangerous biologic materials occurs.

THE EFFECTOR MOLECULES OF IMMUNE, INFLAMMATORY, AND HYPERSENSITIVITY RESPONSES

This section describes the immunoglobulins and the nature of the other effector molecules stored, synthesized, and released by the preceding catalogue of cells, and the humoral amplification (i.e., complement, kinin, coagulation, and fibrinolytic) and messenger systems (i.e., cyclic nucleotides) that are connected with immune, inflammatory, and hypersensitivity responses.

IMMUNOGLOBULINS

Referring to the earlier described arbitrary model of the immune system, one should note that antibody is one of the major products of the immune response. Antibodies are immunoglobulins. In humans and other higher vertebrates, immunoglobulins are designated by an alphabetic letter according to their particular class. They were first identified among the gamma globulins in electrophoretic studies by Tiselius and Kabat in the 1930s. Little was known about their molecular structure or their physical, chemical, and biologic characteristics until the work undertaken during the 1950s. Today there is considerable information about the immunoglobulins of humans and many other species.

As already mentioned, in humans and other higher animals there are five different classes of immunoglobulins. These have been separated according to their chemical structure and designated by the prefix *Ig* followed by the letter of the alphabet denoting the class (i.e., IgG, IgA, IgM, IgE, and IgD). The alphabetic class designation derives from the Greek letters assigned to the larger polypeptide chains, known as *heavy (H) chains*, which make up part of the structure of each immunoglobulin. For example, it was determined that those molecules designated *IgG* all possess H chains whose amino acid composition and antigenicity are similar. These chains are designated as gamma (γ) for IgG; mu (μ) for IgM; alpha (α) for IgA; epsilon (ε) for IgE; and delta (δ) for IgD.

The basic structure of immunoglobulins has been determined by Porter and Edelman and other investigators in work undertaken since the 1960s. The basic unit of immunoglobulin structure is epitomized by that of immunoglobulin IgG. Each molecule of IgG has been shown to contain four polypeptide chains: two identical longer chains known as *heavy (H) chains* and two identical shorter polypeptide chains called *light (L) chains*. They are held together in a three-dimensional configuration by inter- and intrachain disulfide

bonds. Each of the polypeptide chains, heavy and light, has been shown to exhibit a constant region and a variable region in each molecule. The constant regions of the heavy chains are the same for all molecules of a given immunoglobulin class made by a single individual (isotypes). The constant region of the light chains is the same for either of two classes of light chain molecules, designated either kappa (κ) or lambda (λ), in a given individual. The variable regions of both heavy and light chains differ among immunoglobulins in a single individual. These variable regions contribute to the structure of the antigen-binding site on the antibody molecule. It appears that the variability is directly related to the specificity for antigen-binding.

A schematic illustration of the structure of IgG is provided in Figure 4–7. The aforementioned constant and variable regions and the general location of the interchain disulfide bonds are shown. The molecule is also divided into other major parts, represented in the diagram as the Fab portion and the Fc portion. The Fab portion contains those parts of heavy and light chains structurally arranged to form the two antigen-binding sites, hence the term *fragment antigen binding (Fab)*. The Fc portion of the molecule is composed of the two segments of each heavy chain, including the interchain disulfide bond. As indicated in the diagram, the proteolytic enzyme, pepsin, will cleave the immunoglobulin molecule just above the inter–H-chain disulfide bond to yield peptide fragments from the Fc region and a divalent fragment, the $F(ab')_2$ fragment. Papain, by contrast, cleaves the molecule below that disulfide bond, yielding intact Fc fragment and univalent Fab fragments.

The Fc portion of the immunoglobulin molecule accounts for biologic activities other than antigen-binding. These include complement-fixing

Figure 4–7

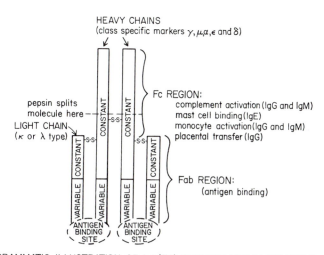

DIAGRAMMATIC ILLUSTRATION OF IgG(7S) IMMUNOGLOBULIN MOLECULE SHOWING MAJOR STRUCTURAL COMPONENTS AND REACTIVE SITES (IgA, IgE and IgD have similar structure)

activity (exhibited by IgM and IgG), specific transfer across the placental barrier (IgG), specific attachment to the cell membranes of basophils and mast cells (IgE), and fixation to cell membrane receptors of lymphocytes, monocytes, and macrophages (IgG and IgE). The significance of these different biologic activities will become apparent in the discussions of immunologic tissue injury in Chapter 5.

All immunoglobulins have a basic unit of structure similar to IgG and exhibit similar physical and chemical characteristics. As noted earlier, their amino-acid composition causes them to be relatively basic when compared with other serum proteins. They migrate with the gamma and slow beta globulin fractions on electrophoresis. Each basic unit possesses two sites for antigen-binding and thus is considered bivalent. The molecular weight of the intact molecule of IgG is approximately 150,000 daltons. This results in a sedimentation coefficient of 7S in the ultracentrifuge on density gradient analysis. Each of the H chains has a molecular weight of approximately 50,000 daltons; each L chain is approximately 24,000 daltons. The immunoglobulins IgG, IgE, and IgD typically exhibit the four-chain, 7S structure, whereas IgA and IgM occur as polymers of the 7S units, thus exhibiting larger size and higher sedimentation coefficients. IgA may occur as a monomer similar to the IgG basic unit but also occurs as a dimer and trimer with sedimentation coefficients ranging up to 13S. IgM normally occurs as a pentamer composed of five 7S units linked together by a disulfide glycopeptide chain known as the J chain. IgM has a high sedimentation coefficient of 19S. The J chain also provides the link for IgA polymeric forms. The J chain is synthesized by all plasma cells, even those that do not produce polymeric forms of immunoglobulin. The polymeric forms of IgA and IgM are schematically illustrated in Figure 4–8. Because of their large size with increased numbers of antigen-binding sites, they are of higher valence than the 7S molecules. Because of this, they are much more efficient in binding antigen in reactions such as agglutination and immune complex formation.

It was mentioned that immunoglobulins are produced by plasma cells that differentiate from immunogen-stimulated B-lymphocytes. The class and specificity of the immunoglobulin produced by each individual plasma cell differ according to the stimulating immunogen that selectively reacts with the immunoglobulin receptors present on the surface of the particular virgin, or recognition, B-lymphocyte. The marked degree of diversity in immunoglobulin response arises from the diverse recognition lymphocytes in a given individual. Antibodies will be produced to the many different determinants of a single immunogen, which will usually be of different classes and subclasses as well as have varying antigen reactivities. Because of such heterogeneity, there will be a wide range of antibody reactivity in a given antiserum for the

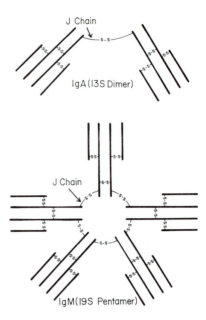

POLYMERIC STRUCTURES OF IMMUNOGLOBULINS IgA AND IgM

Figure 4–8

different determinants. Some of the antibodies will have a high affinity for, and bind strongly to, some of the antigen determinants; others will be of low affinity and will bind weakly. In general, larger immunogens with an abundance of heterogeneous determinants elicit an extremely heterogeneous antibody response, whereas a more homogeneous response occurs to immunogens of uniform composition. Indeed, a highly purified immunogen of uniform structure with determinants of identical or closely similar arrangement may produce an antibody response restricted to a single class of immunoglobulin with a limited range of reactivity. Commonly, however, most immunogens are quite heterogeneous and result in a polymorphic response.

In humans and other vertebrates, the relative concentration of immunoglobulins in the circulation shows IgG to predominate, with average serum values in the human adult measuring approximately 1200 mg/dl, whereas IgM values are about 125 mg/dl, IgA values are around 210 mg/dl, and IgE values are between 40 and 100 ng/dl. IgD is usually present in trace quantities. The finding of normal levels of serum immunoglobulins generally indicates a normal state of immunocompetence and immunoresponsiveness.

LYMPHOKINES, MONOKINES, AND CYTOKINES

As the preceding section may imply, the antibody has been the focal effector molecule of immunologic thinking and investigation since the

1930s. Even in the era of modern immunology, the antibody molecule continued to dominate concepts that sought to explain the functioning of the immune system. Only in the 1970s did researchers develop an awareness and growing appreciation that lymphocytic and monocytic products other than immunoglobulins are largely responsible for a complex array of cell cooperative activities. We now know that these *lymphokine* and *monokine* activities have an essential role in the communication of immunocompetent and accessory cells and, consequently, in the regulation of the immune system.

At this early point in the development of this field, it is not possible to state with any certainty the types, numbers, range, and sequence of activities in biochemical or enzymatic cascades by which this growing spectrum of effector molecules fits precisely into the multicellular network that constitutes the immune system. Therefore, the discussion that follows will have to be severely limited to a brief account of some of the best known of these effector molecules.

Furthermore, it is to be added that many of these agents, such as lymphotoxins, growth inhibitory factors, interferons, and colony-stimulating factors, are produced by a wide variety of normal, damaged, or infected cells (fibroblasts, keratinocytes, Langerhans' cells, tumor cells, etc.). In the broader sense, these substances are *cytokines*. They can properly be regarded as lymphokines or monokines only when produced by stimulated lymphocytes or activated macrophages; in these instances, the lymphocytes and macrophages play the role of focusing and intensifying a phylogenetically ancient, traditional, nonspecific inflammatory mechanism at the site of a specific response.

Effector Molecules of Activated Lymphocytes

This range of substances includes effector molecules that affect (1) macrophages, (2) polymorphonuclear leukocytes, (3) lymphocytes, and (4) other cell types.

Products of Activated Lymphocytes Affecting Macrophages. The first of the lymphokines to be described was the *macrophage migration inhibitory factor (MIF)*. Human MIF has a molecular weight of 23,000 to 55,000; on electrophoresis it migrates with the albumin; it is heat-stable and sensitive to chymotrypsin and neuraminidase; and its buoyant density indicates that it is a glycoprotein. Several studies demonstrate that MIF is heterogeneous, and, although there are various hypotheses, it is not yet known how MIF influences macrophage migration. Another lymphokine, originally called *macrophage activation factor (MAF)*, is a macromolecule either very similar to or identical with MIF. Both pH3-MIF and pH5-MIF are capable of causing in-vitro macrophage activation that is essentially identical with that produced by

MAF. The changes observed include increased adherence to culture vessel, increased oxidation of glucose through the hexose monophosphate shunt together with increased levels of lactate dehydrogenase in cytoplasm, increased incorporation of glucosamine into membrane components, and increased ruffled membrane activity. Likewise, an enhanced bacteriostasis, phagocytosis, pinocytosis, tumoricidal and membrane adenylate cyclase activities, and the appearance of increased numbers of cytoplasmic granules may be observable. By contrast, MAF, as MIF, produces a decrease in electron-dense surface material and reduced levels of certain lysosomal enzymes (acid phosphatase, cathepsin-D, and B-glucuronidase). At present, it is not known how the inhibition of macrophage migration is related to the late activation of these cells, especially if the two activities reside in the same lymphokine molecule. This refers to the as yet undetermined difference in time needed for the development of these two activities: Inhibition of migration of macrophages may be observed within 24 hours, whereas activation of macrophages takes several days to occur. A possible explanation for this difference may lie in the observation that inhibition of macrophage migration is a reversible process (i.e., cells initially inhibited may again migrate and actually at a higher rate than usual). In other words, the initial MIF effect on a macrophage may change its surface properties so that it becomes more sticky. Later on, as the full complement of the aforementioned metabolic changes occur with the resultant macrophage activation, the overall functional capacity of the cell is enhanced.

Antigen- and mitogen-activated lymphocytes also elaborate a chemotactic substance that selectively attracts macrophages or monocytes. This *macrophage chemotactic factor (MCF)*, like MIF, is heterogeneous, as indicated by isoelectric focusing showing peak activities with a pI of 10.1 and 5.6. Production of MCF is antigen-specific, and it is heat-stable at 56°C, with a molecular weight of 12,000 to 25,000 in humans. On electrophoresis, MCF migrates in the part of the gel associated with albumin, and its buoyant density is similar to that of pure protein.

Products of Activated Lymphocytes Affecting Polymorphonuclear Leukocytes. Polymorphonuclear leukocytes are inhibited in their migration by a soluble material called *leukocyte inhibitory factor (LIF)*. LIF, which is produced by sensitized lymphocytes exposed to specific antigen or stimulation by concanavalin A, inhibits polymorphonuclear migration, but not that of macrophages. Physicochemically, it appears to be a protease with an approximate molecular weight of 68,000, stability to heat at 56°C, a charge similar to that of albumin, and resistance to neuraminidase but not to chymotrypsin. Separately from LIF, there are chemotactic factors for neutrophils, basophils, and eosinophils produced by sensitized lymphocytes. They are similar in molecular weight, ranging from 24,000 to 55,000, and it is presently unclear whether these factors are all distinct molecular entities or the same substance with chemotactic activity for multiple cell types. Nevertheless, there is some evidence for the existence of two factors that affect the directed movement of eosinophils. One of these requires the interaction of the substance with specific antigen-antibody complexes in order to generate chemotactic activity, whereas the other is active in the absence of antigen-antibody complexes.

Another agent that has been described specifically affects the basophil leukocytes. This factor, called *histamine releasing factor (HRF)*, is produced by sensitized human lymphocytes in response to antigen and nonspecifically by mitogens or viral agents. It has the capacity to induce histamine release from human basophils in a noncytotoxic manner, it is nondialyzable, it is heatstable, and it has a molecular weight of 12,000.

Products of Immunologically Activated Lymphocytes Affecting Nonsensitized Lymphocytes.

Activation by specific antigen results in the release of a substance from sensitized lymphocytes that has mitogenic activity for nonsensitized lymphocytes. This factor is known by the designation *lymphocyte mitogenic factor (LMF)*. This material induces normal lymphocytes to undergo blast transformation and cell multiplication.

LMF is a nondialyzable macromolecule that is heat-stable and resistant to RNase and DNase as well as treatment with proteolytic enzymes. It has a molecular weight of approximately 20,000 to 30,000.

In this category, there are some other factors released on stimulation by specific antigen from lymphocytes that modulate antibody production. These factors have not been well characterized, and it is not known whether they are the same factor acting at a different concentration or several distinct molecular entities. In any case, a material has been described in the mouse that triggers B cells to make IgM class antibody to sheep red cells, and some other soluble factors have been reported that also increase IgG and IgE antibody production. In humans, an effector substance released by activated lymphocytes induces B cells to proliferate, lose their C3 receptors, and increase their protein synthesis, and it stimulates production of IgG antibody to specific antigens. Conversely, there are also factors capable of suppressing antibody production. Both the enhancing and the antibody-suppressing factors appear to be nondialyzable, heat-stable macromolecules with molecular weights of 25,000 to 55,000.

Sensitized lymphocytes also contain a substance that is released by either disruption of the cells or stimulation of them with a specific antigen. This material was first described by Lawrence and named by him *transfer factor* because in human beings it was possible to transfer delayed-type hypersensitivity (DH) to previously unreactive recipients with extracts of these sensitized cells obtained from skin test–positive donors. Transfer factor (TF) has a molecular weight of less than 4000, and although several laboratories have been successful in partially purifying the active agent, so far no one has produced a homogeneous preparation. Nevertheless, the essential functional components of the molecule appear to be a peptide, a purine base, ribose, and a phosphodiester group.

TF can specifically transfer DH without preparing the host to make antibody against the same antigen. The mechanism by which this is accomplished is not known, but there are two current hypotheses that may be mentioned. One suggestion is that TF enhances antigen sensitivity by potentially responsive T cells. In this view, the cytoplasmic membranes of the T cells possess receptors for antigenic determinants and for specific TFs. Activation of the cell with antigen stimulates release of the membrane-associated TF as well as other lymphokines. TF in turn interacts with membrane-receptors on other cells that are potentially reactive to the antigen and renders them more responsive. This cascade effect expands the number of responding cells and thereby provides for clonal expansion, which is a requirement for transfer. A second suggested mechanism involves facilitation of antigen-processing and presentation to T cells. Such an effect could occur if TF acted on macrophages or other accessory cells and facilitated cell cooperation, but it would not be antigen-specific. This could explain some of the "nonspecific" effects of TF, such as amplification of DNA synthesis by antigen- and mitogen-stimulated cells in vitro.

Effector Molecules Acting on Cell Types Other Than Lymphocytes.

Additional products of activated lymphocytes include cytotoxic factors (i.e., lymphotoxins that can kill bystander cells or tumor cells); growth inhibitory factors, which prevent the proliferation or cloning of their cells; a group of vertebrate glycoproteins with broad antiviral activity called *interferons*; factors capable of activating the clotting sequence; effector molecules that increase vascular permeability; colony-stimulating factors; and an agent that activates osteoclasts to solubilize bone.

Thus, sensitized human lymphocytes, in response to specific antigens or mitogens, release an effector molecule or molecules that have cytotoxic effects on certain target cells. Such material or materials are generally referred to as *lymphotoxin (LT)*. The physicochemical properties of human lymphotoxin are heterogeneous, and there are at least three distinguishable molecular species, known as α-LT, β-LT, and δ-LT. Of these, the best characterized so far is α-LT, with a molecular weight of 75,000 to 100,000, an isoelectric point of 6.8 to 8.0, and stability to heat at 56°C, to storage at 4°C, and to treatment with DNase, RNase, and neuraminidase. On polyacrylamide gel electrophoresis, it appears to be an $\alpha_2{}'\beta$-globulin. As to its mechanism of action, it is believed that the lymphocyte, having been activated by intimate contact with target cell membranes, is induced to synthesize LT, which binds to the target cell membrane, where it effects target cell lysis. Disruption, or physical dislodgment, of target cell membrane then promotes the lymphocyte's release from the target cell and subsequent cessation of LT secretion.

Some activities also have been described that, rather than causing lysis, inhibit the growth pattern of target cells, specifically involving inhibition of proliferation and inhibition of cloning. It is presently unclear whether the effects of lysis and the foregoing growth inhibitions reflect the activities of three separate macromolecules or of one and the same effector molecule that can exert different effects on different cells, depending upon its concentration in its immediate microenvironment.

As stated earlier, another category of lymphokines, the interferons, represent a group of vertebrate glycoproteins first described by Isaacs and Lindenmann as soluble factors interfering with viral multiplication. Interferons are heterogeneous in terms of both their cellular origin and their mode of induction. Their most recent classification, based on their antigenicities and molecular structures, defines the three antigenic types and numerous subtype interferons: (1) the antigenic type α, formerly called *human leukocyte* and *lymphoblastoid*; (2) type β, fibroblast interferon; and (3) type δ, for the type II, immune, or T-type interferons. One places the designation of the animal species from which the interferon is derived in front of the type designation, using the standard abbreviation 1FN for interferon (e.g., human = Hu1FN-α or Hu1FN-β). Subtypings based on molecular weights are parenthetically indicated—for example, Hu1FN-α(21K), and numerical subtypes refer to sequence heterogeneities such as Hu1FN-α and Hu1FN-β$_2$.

All three interferon types are found in human and animal systems both in vivo and in vitro. On the basis of the sequencing of several of the interferons and their genes, α-interferons are a heterogeneous group of proteins. Similar heterogeneities are expected to be found in ongoing investigations among β- and δ-interferons. The three types of interferons are established to be distinct not only antigenically but also with respect to several other properties (e.g., molecular weights, stabilities, cross-species activities, and biologic activities).

Extensive work on α- and β-interferons as purely antiviral agents has also revealed several nonantiviral activities. Their first primary effect on interferon-pretreated cells is a better response to the inducers, with production of higher levels of interferon. Many other nonantiviral properties are now known to be induced by α- and β-interferons, including inhibition of nonviral agents

(bacteria, protozoans), cellular multiplication and inhibition, toxicity enhancement, increased or depressed cellular synthetic activities, and cell surface alterations. In addition, α- and β-interferons have become noted for their immunomodulatory actions, such as enhancement of immunocytolysis (either cell-mediated or antibody-dependent), promotion of phagocytosis, macrophage activation, inhibition of delayed-type hypersensitivity and graft-versus-host reactions, and effects on humoral antibody production. Several of these assorted activities have now been documented as being induced by either very highly purified or even pure interferon preparations, suggesting that interferons are pleiotypic biologic response modifiers.

Essentially the same properties are possessed by δ-interferon preparations, except that this type of interferon appears to have a much higher antitumor activity than the other types in general and a more potent influence on the antitumor activity of macrophages in particular. With respect to immunomodulatory activities, δ-interferon has both immunosuppressive and immunoenhancing properties. In a comparison between β- and δ-interferon, it was shown that the immunosuppressive activity of β-interferon appears to produce an effect on β-lymphocytes, whereas the immunoenhancing property of δ-interferon appears to produce an effect on T-lymphocytes.

Of the various factors capable of activating the blood-clotting sequence, the "procoagulant factor," or "tissue factor," produced by lymphocytes and monocytes is to be mentioned here. Mononuclear cells, stimulated by antigen or mitogen, produce a procoagulant material that, when incubated with Factor VIII–deficient plasma, is able to correct the prolonged clotting time. This substance is antigenically distinct from Factor VIII and has been identified as "tissue factor." Because of the technical difficulties produced by its lability, it has not yet been well characterized, and its pathophysiologic importance also has yet to be determined. Nevertheless, it is intriguing to consider its possible relation to certain manifestations characterized by both lymphocytic infiltration and pathologic thrombosis, such as rejection of a transplanted kidney and the delayed-hypersensitivity skin test.

A vasoactive substance that increases vascular permeability, called *lymph node permeability factor (LNPF)*, could be extracted from lymph nodes of immunized animals but could also be obtained in equal amounts from nonimmune animals. The fact that it is released without an immunologic stimulus and is found in numerous nonlymphoid tissues suggests that it may not play a primary role in the delayed hypersensitivity reaction as it was originally believed. It may, however, serve as one of the many secondary mediators of the inflammatory process per se through its release subsequent to cell or tissue injury.

Another category of effector molecules included in this section involves the *colony stimulating factors (CSF)*, which are a group of soluble factors that in tissue culture stimulate the differentiation of immature bone-marrow precursor cells into granulocytes and macrophages. They were so named because they were the only macromolecular requirement, besides components in fetal calf serum, for the formation of colonies of granulocytes or macrophages or both by hematopoietic cells cultured in semisolid medium. Although blood monocytes and tissue macrophages appear to be major sources of these agents, it is now established that lymphocytes may also actively produce them during immunologic reactions. Colony-stimulating factors are heat-stable glycoproteins with molecular weights in the range of 40,000 to 60,000.

Osteoclast-activating factor (OAF) is an effector molecule produced by lymphocytes in vitro following antigenic or mitogenic stimulation. It is capable of forming osteoclasts in bone and activating these cells. OAF has a molecular weight of 13,000 to 25,000, is heat-labile, is inactivated by proteolytic enzymes, and can be differentiated from all other established bone-resorbing substance. The nature of its role in immunobiology is unclear at the present time.

MACROPHAGE-DERIVED EFFECTOR MOLECULES

Phagocytosis by macrophages has been studied since the late 1800s, but it is only since the 1970s that the importance of macrophages as secretory cells has been recognized. Over 50 secretion products of macrophages have been identified so far. Some of the secretion products of the macrophage influence the inflammatory process at its many steps. Lysosome and complement components are secreted constitutively by macrophages in all states of stimulation. Secretion of other products such as arachidonic metabolites, acid hydrolases, and neutral proteinases is triggered and regulated by engagement of specific receptors, by endocytosis, or by exposure of macrophages to membrane-active drugs, including tumor pronators, ionophores, and endotoxin. Activated lymphocytes, tissue pH oxygen tension, and various other factors are also operative in the regulation of macrophage secretion, which in turn controls the role of macrophages in the inflammatory process.

In this section, we address the macrophage not in its role as the professional phagocyte but rather in the context of the initiation of immune responses induced by mitogens or specific antigens. Such roles of the macrophage may be divided into two functional categories: (1) antigen- or mitogen-binding, -processing, and -presentation; and (2) synthesis and secretion of a class of effector molecules, the monokines, that act in conjunction with

antigen or mitogen to initiate and modulate both T- and B-lymphocyte–mediated immune responses.

As the chemical purification and characterization of these essentially lymphostimulatory factors proceeded, it became increasingly evident that many or most of the properties originally attributed to these factors by various bioassays in fact reside in one and the same effector molecule. Thus, a consensus was reached at the Second International Lymphokine workshop in 1979 with regard to the definition of the most extensively studied monokine, *lymphocyte activating factor (LAF)*. On the basis of a number of independent and collaborative studies, it was concluded that LAF is the molecular entity responsible for the biologic activities associated with the terms *mitogenic protein (MP)*, *helper peaks-1 (HP-1)*, *T-cell–replacing factor III (TRF-III)*, *T-cell–replacing factor Mø (TRF$_M$)*, *B-cell–activating factor (BAF)*, and *B-cell–differentiation factor (BDF)*. In order to free the terminology from the constraints associated with definitions by single bioassays, investigators accepted a revised term for LAF, *interleukin-1 (IL1)* ("between leukocytes").

Macrophages stimulated with antigen, endotoxin, and other phagocytic stimulants release IL1. Human IL1 has been purified to homogeneity and identified as a glycoprotein with a molecular weight of 15,000. Studies are currently under way to determine its precise molecular structure. This IL1 has been demonstrated to fulfill most of the requirements for macrophages in a competent immune and inflammatory response in general. Thus, IL1 stimulates T-lymphocytes, fibroblasts, and synovial cells; regulates B-lymphocyte differentiation; controls the growth of bone marrow cells; and effects the generation of cytotoxic T-lymphocytes. Furthermore, IL1 stimulates the release of acute phase reactants by hepatocytes, induces the release of prostaglandin and collagenase from synovial cells, and increases the numbers of circulating neutrophils. There is also conclusive evidence that IL1 is identical with "endogenous pyrogen," the elusive macrophage-derived fever-producing factor.

Nevertheless, IL1 cannot replace the functional properties of antigen-processing and antigen-presentation performed by macrophages. Likewise, IL1 cannot substitute for histocompatibility antigens found on the surface of macrophages, and the aforementioned properties of IL1 may be due to its ability to initiate the release of a lymphokine, termed interleukin 2 (IL2) (previously known as T-cell growth factor) from helper T-lymphocytes.

Two major species of IL2 have been purified that are separable by charge (pI 4.3 and 4.9) and size (molecular weights of 25,000 and 21,000, respectively). Differences between them appear to be due to glycosylation, and an inverse relationship of size to charge in these different molecular forms is also determinable. Various studies on a human T lymphoma cell line showed that the major species of IL2 secreted by these cells has a pI of 7.75 and a molecular weight of 13,500. Both IL1 and IL2 are glycoproteins and exhibit a number of common biologic properties, including the enhancement of thymocyte mitogenic response to phytohemagglutinin and concanavalin A as well as the stimulation of antigen-dependent, cell-mediated, and humoral immune responses. However, IL2 can be readily distinguished from IL1 by its ability to initiate and maintain T-lymphocytes in continuous culture. Finally, most recent studies have identified another glycoprotein of 41,000 daltons, termed *interleukin 3* (IL3), that appears to promote hematopoietic progenitor cell proliferation and differentiation.

The functional relationship between IL1 and IL2 in the context of macrophage and I-cell interactions in the expression and regulation of immunity may be stated as follows. Activation of helper and delayed-hypersensitivity (DH) reactive T cells by antigen requires two signals, each of which is mediated by the macrophage. The first signal requires the presentation of antigen in a manner suitable for recognition by T cells. The second signal is associated with the synthesis of IL1 by macrophage and is necessary for full T-cell activation to proceed.

The precise events involved in the ability of macrophages to present antigen to T cells are not completely understood. Nevertheless, activation of helper and DH-reactive T cells requires that they recognize antigen in conjunction with self-Ia determinants. Therefore, display of Ia determinants by macrophages constitutes a minimal requirement for their antigen-presenting capabilities.

The second signal required for activation of helper and DH-reactive T cells involves the synthesis and release of IL1 by the macrophage. IL1 exerts its effect by stimulating the production of IL2 by T cells, and it is IL2 that then acts in concert with the first signal mediated by antigen plus Ia to allow full T-cell activation to proceed. It is unclear whether the T cells that are sensitive to the action of IL2 actually synthesize IL2. To date, only malignant T-cell lines have been shown to be capable of both synthesizing and responding to IL2.

In any case, the sequence in which the two signals act upon reactive T cells to induce their activation appears to be as follows. First, T cells interact with antigen presented in conjunction with Ia, resulting in an increase in the expression of receptors for IL2. Second, synthesis of IL1 by macrophages induces synthesis of IL2 by T cells, and it is the action of IL2 that then allows full T-cell activation to proceed. An obvious missing link in these interactions is represented by the signal that induced IL1 production by macrophages. It is possible that no signal is required and that synthesis of sufficient amounts of IL1 is a constitutive function of macrophages and other accessory cells.

THYMOSINS AND OTHER THYMIC HORMONES

As repeatedly stated earlier, it is now recognized that the thymus is responsible for the normal maturation of many different functional subclasses of T-lymphocytes (e.g., helper, suppressor, and cytotoxic effector cells). The thymus exerts its influence by the release of various effector molecules both within its own microenvironment and at distant target tissue sites (e.g., peripheral lymphoid tissues) via these molecules secreted into the blood. In this sense, the thymus-derived effector molecules behave like hormones, and the thymus itself acts as an endocrine organ. These immunomodulatory hormones are produced by the medullary thymic epithelial cells and the Hassall's corpuscles.

A number of laboratories have succeeded in isolating and purifying factors with thymic hormone—like activity from both the thymus tissue and serum. Several of these effector molecules, such as thymosin fraction 5, thymic humoral factor, and thymic Factor X, have been reported to restore immunocompetence in patients with a wide range of primary and secondary immunodeficiency disorders (see Chapter 5).

Preparations of these thymic products are in various stages of chemical and biologic characterization and include thymosin fraction 5, thymopoietin I and II (TP), thymic humoral factor (THF), facteur thymique serique (FTS), and thymic Factor X (TFX).

Thymosin fraction 5 has been found to contain a number of active peptides with molecular weights ranging from 1000 to 15,000. Several of the thymosin peptides (α_1, β_3, and β_4) have now been purified to homogeneity and sequenced. Two of them (thymosin α_1, molecular weight of 3108; thymosin β_4, molecular weight of 4982) have been synthesized. As far as their role in T-cell maturation is concerned, thymosin β_3 and β_4 promote early stem cell differentiation to the prothymocyte stage. Thymosin α_1 supports both early and late steps of T-cell differentiation. Thymosin α_7 is associated with the generation of functionally mature suppressor T cells and thymosin α_1 with the generation of helper T cells.

The recognition of thymopoietin (initially named *thymin*) resulted from experimental studies related to the human disease *myasthenia gravis*. This disease is characterized by a deficit in neuromuscular transmission and by thymic malfunction. On the basis of a biologic assay measuring impairment of neuromuscular transmission, researchers first isolated thymopoietin by following its capacity to induce blockage, as is seen in patients with myasthenia gravis. Subsequently, two factors were identified on the basis of their ability to induce the differentiation of bone marrow cells into mature T cells in vitro, and the peptides have been designated *thymopoietin I* and *thymopoietin II*. Since they are immunologically cross-reactive and have indistinguishable biologic activities, they appear to be closely related polypeptides, which is also reflected by the fact that thymopoietins I and II differ by only two amino acid residues. Thus, the two thymopoietins probably represent isohormonal variation. Thymopoietin II has a molecular weight of 5562 daltons, and the synthesis of its entire chain of 49 amino acids has been accomplished. Some of the most important biologic properties of the thymopoietins include (1) induction of differentiation of prothymocytes to thymocytes, as detected by cell surface markers, and functional characteristics (i.e., responsiveness to T cell mitogens); (2) enhancement of lymphoid cell transcription and translation of DNA; (3) inhibition of early-stage and induction of late-stage B-cell differentiation; and (4) induction of complement receptors on human granulocytes.

Thymic humoral factor (THF) was discovered through the demonstration that thymic tissue in millipore chambers implanted into neonatally thymectomized mice led to the restoration of specific immunologic competence in these animals. Purification of the THF to homogeneity has been achieved, and, based on leucine as unity, the minimal molecular weight is 3220. Since many of the extensive biologic data reported for THF have been obtained with the earlier, relatively impure thymic extract and have not been reassessed with homogeneous THF, the biologic properties of this agent will not be discussed here.

When thymic fragments taken from myasthenia gravis patients are transplanted into selected individuals with leukemia and Hodgkin's disease, manifestations of immunologic enhancements appear in the recipients a short time after the thymic transplant. The active agent responsible for this thymic effect is a protein with a molecular weight of approximately 4200, named *thymic Factor X (TFX)*. Comparisons of amino acid composition of TFX, thymosin α_1, the thymopoietins, and THF show no evident similarities. In the absence of sequence analysis of TFX, the data available cannot as yet contribute to clarification of the question regarding its possible chemical relationship to the other putative thymic hormones.

TFX increases rosette formation by lymphocytes as well as the intracellular concentration of cAMP and protein kinase of lymphocytes in patients with chronic lymphocytic leukemia. It also restores the azathioprine sensitivity of spleen rosette-forming cells from adult thymectomized mice. In case of in-vivo treatment with TFX, this thymic hormone increases the number of blood lymphocytes and their response to mitogens.

In the course of studies assessing the immunologic status and the relative likelihood of kidney rejection in patients with renal transplants, another thymic hormone–like activity has been detected in the sera of these patients. Subsequently, the active agent has been isolated directly from serum and termed *facteur thymique serique (FTS)*. The agent has a molecular weight of 847 and has been characterized as a nonapeptide with the following amino acid composition: Glu-Ala-Lys-Ser-Glu-Gly-Gly-Ser-Asn. Synthesis of the molecule has been achieved, and the synthetic and natural FTS show comparable biologic activities. Some of the more significant of the latter include (1) restoration of responsiveness of adult thymectomized animals to mitogens and of their capacity to generate cytotoxic lymphoid cells to restrain the growth of virus-induced sarcoma; (2) inhibition of antibody production to thymus-independent antigen and of the development of contact sensitivity; (3) delay of allogeneic skin graft rejection through the generation of suppressor T cells and prevention of appearance of autoimmune hemolytic anemia and Sjögren syndrome in animal models; and (4) transformation of cortisone-sensitive thymocytes into cortisone-resistant thymocytes.

In closing this section, it is to be added that many other less well-defined thymic factors have been described. At the time of this writing, their chemical and biologic characterization, however, has not progressed to the point that they could be included here.

THE EFFECTOR MOLECULES OF IMMUNOLOGIC AND HYPERSENSITIVE INFLAMMATORY RESPONSES GENERATED BY ANTIGEN-ANTIBODY INTERACTIONS

This section describes the individual components of immunologic or hypersensitive inflammatory responses, which are initiated by interaction of antigen with antibody. The interaction, if on the surface of a basophil, mast cell, lymphocyte, or any of the other components of the spectrum of cells described earlier, may trigger the release of effector molecules (mediators). Activation of the amplification systems (kinin or complement) by antigen-antibody interaction or a secondary mechanism also induces the generation of biologically active mediators. Both the primary and secondary mediators induce pathophysiologic changes by mechanisms that include contraction of vascular and other smooth muscle, chemotaxis of inflammatory cells, and either activation or inhibition of secretion from inflammatory cells.

Many questions remain to be answered concerning the concept of release of biologically active substances as the responsible mediators of the clinical manifestations of immunologic and hypersensitive inflammatory responses. Thus, there is much disagreement regarding the relative importance of any one of the known chemical mediators of such reactivities in general and in individual reactions in particular.

It would seem that there are no two instances (even representing the same type of manifestation) that would be strictly comparable, and in the final analysis the relative significance of a given mediator will depend on a multitude of various determining factors. Schematically, the following circumstances or factors seem to determine the relative significance of a mediator and, thus, the nature of the response at any one time:

1. The physicochemical and biologic character and the quantities of immunologic reactants participating in the event.
2. Susceptibility of the local mediator—or its precursor—to store cells to the immunologic or inflammatory injury.
3. Types and relative amounts of active mediators present in the area of injury.
4. The local occurrence of mediators in a pre-existing store or the presence of precursors or substrates that can give rise to the active principles.
5. Local availability of appropriate enzymes or other mechanisms required for such an activation.
6. Relative efficiency of the primarily released mediator to mobilize another active agent.
7. Factors such as diffusibility, rate of inactivation of the mediator, and the proximity of the target cells to the site of release or activation.
8. The functional state of these target cells and that of their mediator-specific receptors.
9. Relative potency of the primarily released mediator to sensitize the target cells to the action of the secondarily mobilized agent.
10. The persistence of the manifestation: The number of active agents entering into the reaction is increasing with the time, and the relative significance of any of these is varying with the stage the reaction has reached.

With these qualifications in mind, one can determine that the currently established chemical mediators of immunologic and hypersensitive inflammatory reactions include amines, peptides, lipid substances, Hageman factor pathway enzymes, other enzymes, (mast cell granules), and proteoglycans.

In the first group, we find the physiologically and pharmacologically familiar and chemically defined amine mediators such as histamine, serotonin, catecholamines, and acetylcholine.*

The second group includes bradykinin, a nonapeptide whose amino acid sequence is H-Arg-Pro-Pro-Gly-Phe-Ser-Pro-Phe-Art-OH, and the "eosinophil chemotactic factors of anaphylaxis" (ECF-A). As mentioned previously, several cells that participate in the organization of inflammatory, immune, or hypersensitivity responses can synthesize these factors, release them, or both. In some tissues, such as lung, ECF-A activity is contained in two tetrapeptides, Val-Gly-Ser-Glu and Ala-Gly-Ser-Glu. However, in other tissues or cells, no

information is so far available on the precise amino acid sequence of these tetrapeptides.

The first established member of the third group is the "slow-reacting substance of anaphylaxis" (SRS-A), which has been shown to consist of two leukotrienes, which are cysteine-containing products of the lipoxygenase pathway of arachidonic acid metabolism. Chemically, the first one is 5-hydroxy-6-S-glutathionyl-7, 9, 11, 14-eicosatetraenoic acid (LTC_4), and the second one is 5-hydroxy-6-sulfidocysteinyl-glycine-7, 9, 11, 14-eicosatetraenoic acid (LTD_4). A third biologically active leukotriene (LTE_4) can be formed by metabolic removal of glycine from LTD_4. Other important mediators in this group are the prostaglandins, which are also derived from arachidonic acids but through the cyclo-oxygenase enzyme pathway. Activation of the cyclo-oxygenase pathway results in the formation of endoperoxides, which are then metabolized further to thromboxanes or prostaglandins. Chemically, the prostaglandins are 20-carbon unsaturated carboxylic acids with a cyclopentane ring. Of the family, the E_1, E_2, D_2, I_2, F_2, F_{2a} classes and thromboxane A_2 and B_2 have so far been proved as authentic mediators of hypersensitivity responses, although they are synthesized and released by a variety of nonimmunologic inflammatory and other stimuli. A final group of mediators of the third category, which (1) are produced by basophils, mast cells, and neutrophils; (2) are released by immunologic and other stimuli; and (3) activate platelets to aggregate and release mediators, are called *platelet activating factors*, or *PAF*. The structure of human PAF has not yet been defined, but rabbit PAF has been purified and identified as two closely related phospholipids (1-0-hexadecyl/octadecyl-2-acetyl-sn-glyceryl-3-phosphorylcholine).

The fourth category of mediators involves several high molecular weight, Hageman factor pathway–associated proteolytic enzymes that were originally described as *arginine esterases*. There are at least three enzymatic activities associated with Hagemen factor pathways in immunologic reactions: (1) kinin-generating (i.e., kallikrein-like); (2) prekallikrein-activating; and (3) Hageman factor–cleaving and –activating. The original kinin-generating activity associated with basophils has been called *BK-A*, or *basophil kallikrein of anaphylaxis*.

The fifth category of mediators includes a number of enzymes that are found in recast cell granules such as chymotrypsin (rodents), trypsin (humans), superoxide dismutase, peroxidase, carboxypeptidase A, exoglycosidases, and arylsulfatases. These enzymes contribute to the tissue destruction accompanying late-phase hypersensitivity reactions or participate in antiparasitic infection responses. Finally, the last group of effector molecules involves the family of proteoglycans, which are chemically high–molecular weight, sulfated acid mucopolysaccharides that are preformed and stored in the granular storage sites of mast

*It is convenient to refer to acetylcholine herein as an amine.

cells and other storage cells and are released by the antigen-antibody interaction.

Collectively, the various groups of these effector molecules produce an increase in blood flow, capillary permeability, constriction of smooth muscles, secretion of mucous glands, and anticoagulation. These are the component features of the anaphylactic and/or acute allergic inflammation.

THE PHARMACOLOGICALLY ACTIVE EFFECTOR MOLECULES OF IMMEDIATE HYPERSENSITIVITIES AS THE NATURAL CHEMICAL ORGANIZERS OF NEUROHUMORAL CONTROL

Of all the various groups of pharmacologically active effector molecules described in the preceding section, special mention should be made of the catecholamines, since all the other mediators release, or are capable of releasing, these amines. They are, therefore, at least potential participants in immediate hypersensitivities of both the nonatopic and atopic varieties. Although in this capacity—in contrast with the other mediators—they usually have no untoward effect, under certain conditions (i.e., atopy) their entry into the reaction may be harmful. Of further importance is the fact that in many tissues of most species, the catecholamines are the principal natural antagonists of both the primary and secondary mediators and thus play a major role in determining the nature of ultimate reactivity of the effector cells to these substances released by immune or other mechanisms.

The discovery that a major group of hypersensitivities is mediated by pharmacologically active substances was a revolutionary advance in the history of allergy. It supplied the long-awaited explanation for the elusive fact that the symptoms of immediate hypersensitivities are wholly unrelated to the physicochemical or biologic properties of the offending antigen. As various naturally occurring pharmacologically active agents were shown to mediate hypersensitivity responses, neurophysiologic research proceeded to demonstrate that impulse transmission from one neuron to another is accomplished through chemical transmitter substances. These two parallel processes of chemical identification ultimately converged in the common recognition that many, if not most, of the pharmacologic mediators of hypersensitivity reactions also are the physiologic (chemical) transmitters (or, in a broader sense, chemical organizers) of neural integration.

Emergence of Pharmacologic Mediation in Allergy

Histamine became the first compound to be suspected as a possible mediator as early as 1911

by Sir Henry Dale; by 1919, Dale was capable of concluding that histamine was the long-sought "anaphylatoxin" that had been hypothesized from work on guinea pig anaphylaxis. This was complemented by the description and experimental analysis of the "triple response" by Sir Thomas Lewis. As early as 1927, Lewis recognized that this response, which occurs after injury to the skin by physical, thermal, or chemical agents, is similar to the reaction resulting from intradermal injection of histamine and to the phenomenon of human urticaria. In the succeeding two decades, as the result of a series of investigations by various workers, histamine gained wide acceptance as a mediator of certain hypersensitive manifestations.

The immune release of acetylcholine was demonstrated subsequently in animal anaphylaxis and later in some human allergic reactions. In the mid-1950s, a third amine mediator, serotonin, was implicated in animal anaphylaxis. By that time, it was established that these three amines release or are capable of releasing their principal amine antagonists, the catecholamines, and that the latter can similarly mobilize each of the preceding three agents. This led to the realization of the conspicuous fact that *the entire class of naturally occurring, physiologically important biogenic-amines participates, either primarily or secondarily, in the pharmacologic mediation of the allergic response.*

The dawn of the antihistaminic era broke in the 1930s, and the availability of antihistamines unmasked the existence of still another mediator, SRS-A. The appreciation that neither histamine nor highly purified SRS-A is chemotactic for homologous eosinophils led to the discovery of ECF-A, a third mast cell–connected mediator of immediate hypersensitivities. Similarly, the use of antihistamines and other specific antagonists as analytic tools cleared the way for the recognition that still other mediators, such as bradykinin and the prostaglandins, are released by antigen-antibody reactions.

Emergence of Chemical Transmission in Neurophysiology

In 1921, Otto Loewi presented the first evidence that transmission of the nerve impulse at the junctional gaps of the autonomic nervous system is accomplished by humoral substances. These substances were designated *Vagusstoffe* and *Acceleransstoffe,* corresponding respectively to the substances released from vagal and sympathetic terminals. Vagusstoffe later was shown to be identical with acetylcholine, and Acceleransstoffe was found to be the same as norepinephrine.

Peripheral Nervous System. From these works, the emerging picture of chemical transmission in the autonomic nervous system or in the efferent peripheral nervous system in general can be divided into two classes, cholinergic (release acetylcholine from their terminals) and adrenergic (release norepinephrine from their nerve endings). Derived from the "two-unit" organizational principle of the mammalian nervous system, the term *cholinergic* implies transmission from the first to the second neuron through acetylcholine, whereas the term *adrenergic* implies transmission through norepinephrine.

In addition, a network of nonadrenergic and noncholinergic inhibitory neurons represents a third neural component of the autonomic nervous system. ATP has been postulated to be the inhibitory transmitter released from these neurons, and since the effect of stimulation of these nerves on smooth muscle can be reproduced by exogenous purine nucleotides and nucleosides, these neurons have been termed *purinergic*. Existence of this system has been shown most satisfactorily in the gastrointestinal tract, but presence of purinergic inhibitory nerves also has been postulated in the lung and trachea, the blood vessels, and the urogenital system.

Central Nervous System. In the central nervous system, this "two-unit" arrangement as a basic structural principle is preserved, and the mechanism by which a nerve impulse is transmitted across the junctional gap between one neuron and the next is fundamentally the same. Thus, central transmitters are liberated in the same way from synaptic vesicles or cytoplasmic storage granules in the presynaptic terminals and act in the same manner as transmitters at peripheral junctions. Furthermore, synaptic regions of both central and peripheral neurons are electrically inexcitable. These considerations led to the conclusion that transmission of the nerve impulse must be mediated chemically at all central as well as peripheral junctions.

There is strong evidence that acetylcholine serves as a major transmitter in the central nervous system. However, not all central neurons transmit impulses by liberation of acetylcholine, and the three catecholamines (epinephrine, norepinephrine, and dopamine), histamine, serotonin, and the prostaglandins also have been implicated in central transmission or in some form of modulation of the nerve impulse in the central nervous system. In the peripheral nervous system, tryptaminergic neurons (in which serotonin functions as a neurotransmitter) has been demonstrated in invertebrates, and evidence is accumulating that histamine, the prostaglandins, and the plasma kinins exert an important modulatory influence on autonomic control.

THE RECEPTOR AS THE PHARMACOLOGICALLY SPECIFIC EFFECTOR-CELL COMPONENT OF MEDIATOR ACTION

The pharmacologic mediators elicit their characteristic effect through the activation of certain cells that are specific effectors. These cells, called *effector cells,* are further defined as cells that are endowed with receptive substances *(receptors)* possessing sites with a steric configuration complementary to the mediator in question. The released or administered mediator combines with the complementary receptor site, thereby initiating a chain of biochemical reactions that culminates in the observable biologic response. From the standpoint of specificity of action, the strategically important component of the effector cell is the receptor. Most receptors have not been isolated and purified, and despite irrefutable evidence for their existence, their properties are thus still largely conjectural.

The Adrenergic Receptors

The receptor concept implies two distinct functions: (1) recognition of specific pharmacologically active molecules, such as catecholamines; and (2) stimulation of biologic processes (e.g., through changes in ion permeability) or of enzyme activity.

Pharmacologic Classification of Adrenergic Receptors. Because the exact nature of the various adrenergic receptors has not been known, receptors conventionally have been described by the effector response resulting from their activation or by the absence of this response resulting from their selective blockade or by both. Classified on this basis, there are two principal types of adrenergic receptors, termed, for convenience, *alpha* and *beta* by Ahlquist. Over the years, this dualistic receptor classification has been validated and extended. Thus, at least two major types of beta receptors have been delineated. One type, termed *beta₁-receptors,* has relatively high affinity for norepinephrine, which is generally equipotent with epinephrine and a third to a quarter as potent as isoproterenol. A second type, termed *beta₂-receptors,* is found in vascular, bronchial, and uterine smooth muscle, and also appears to mediate the metabolic effects of catecholamines in skeletal muscle and liver. Beta₂-receptors have much higher affinity for isoproterenol than norepinephrine (about 100 times). A further subclassification of receptor types has been directed toward alpha₁-receptors in that the classic alpha-receptors on effector sites are now referred to as *alpha₁-receptors.* This is in contrast with alpha-receptors on postganglionic adrenergic nerve endings, which are called *alpha₂-receptors.*

Physiologic- and Adenylate Cyclase–Coupled Beta-Adrenergic Receptors. The enzyme *adenylate cyclase* has been shown to be stimulated by catecholamines in virtually all tissues in which beta-receptors can be demonstrated by pharmacologic means. Therefore, an immediate question of major importance concerns how closely the properties of beta-adrenergic receptors linked to adenylate cyclase resemble those of beta-receptors delineated by classic pharmacologic techniques in more intact preparations. This question may now be answered by stating that the adenylate cyclase–coupled beta-adrenergic receptors display specificity and other characteristics identical with those of beta-adrenergic receptors defined by pharmacologic experiments.

Investigators have overcome earlier technical difficulties involved in direct identification of beta-adrenergic receptors by ligand-binding studies by using high–specific activity, high-affinity, beta-adrenergic antagonists to label receptors in adenylate cyclase–containing membrane fractions. Beta-adrenergic receptor–binding sites labeled with $(-)-[''H]$-alprenolol* possess all the essential characteristics to be expected of beta-receptors. These include (1) rapid and reversible kinetics of binding; (2) strict specificity, stereospecificity, and affinity appropriate to the adenylate cyclase–coupled beta-adrenergic receptors; and (3) saturability.

The ability to examine directly the binding interaction of the ligands with the beta-adrenergic receptor has made it possible for one to assess the nature of the receptors and their relationship with the adenylate cyclase enzyme. Thus, the beta-adrenergic receptors are probably lipoproteins. They appear to be located in membrane fractions close to the catalytic unit of adenylate cyclase, although a variety of characteristics indicate that the binding sites are distinct from the adenylate cyclase enzyme.

Furthermore, at least two factors influence the extent of enzyme stimulation produced by a given level of beta-receptor occupancy: (1) membrane phospholipids, and (2) guanyl nucleotides. The manner in which these substances modulate signal transfer from receptor to enzyme distal to receptor-binding remains unclear. Similarly, although the receptors seem localized to cell membranes, attempts to prove their accessibility at the cell surface with a variety of immobilized catecholamine derivatives have so far been frustrated by the chemical instability of the derivatives.

Biochemical Consequences of Adrenergic Stimulation. Little is known about the biochemical consequences of alpha-adrenergic stimulation. By contrast, much more is known about the events that occur subsequent to beta-receptor occupancy, at least in the most extensively studied system—the epinephrine- and glucagon-induced regulation of glycogen breakdown and synthesis in liver and muscle.

The adrenergic receptor, when occupied by a catecholamine, indirectly activates the enzyme called *adenylate cyclase*. This activation involves a component of the cell membrane, sometimes referred to as *guanyl nucleotide–binding protein*. The activation of adenylate cyclase is modulated by several substances, the chief of which is *guanosine triphosphate (GTP)*, a chemical analogue of ATP and also the chemical precursor of *3′,5′-guanosine monophosphate,* or *cyclic GMP* (which is discussed later). By some mechanism of unknown nature, GTP sensitizes the receptor—guanyl nucleotide–binding protein—adenylate cyclase system to catecholamine action.

Adenylate cyclase (formerly called *adenyl cyclase*) has been detected in nearly every mammalian cell in which it has been sought and is also present in cells of many lower organisms. With the single exception of the soluble adenylate cyclase from *Brevibacterium liquefaciens,* the enzyme has been found to be associated with the cell membrane. In the case of certain types of muscles, adenylate cyclase appears to be bound to the membranes of the sarcoplasmic reticulum. However, it can be argued that the transverse tubular segments of this reticulum are extensions of the cell membrane. To date, in spite of major efforts, the enzyme has defied all attempts of researchers to isolate it in a highly purified form.

In the presence of magnesium ions, the adrenergically activated adenylate cyclase catalyzes the formation of a cyclic nucleotide from ATP and 1 mole of pyrophosphate per mole of ATP utilized. This cyclic* nucleotide, adenosine 3′,5′-monophosphate (cyclic AMP), is a mononucleotide of adenylic acid, with the phosphate group diesterified at carbons 3′ and 5′ of the ribose moiety.

Cyclic AMP then functions as an intracellular mediator, a "second messenger" of catecholamine or hormonal action, by modifying enzyme activities and permeability barriers. This is accomplished through the activation of a class of enzymes known as *protein kinases*. These enzymes consist of two types of subunits, one catalytic and the other regulatory. When the catalytic and regulatory subunits are complexed, the enzymes are inactive. Activation occurs when cyclic AMP complexes with regulatory subunits, allowing the catalytic subunits to perform their function, which is the phosphorylation of many different proteins. It is believed that these phosphorylations stimulate a cascade of biochemical reactions that produce the intracellular alterations of metabolic, genetic, electrochemical, and mechanical activities that may be regulated by cyclic AMP. Conversely, protein kinase is inactivated when the enzyme's regulatory subunits recombine with its catalytic subunits. This occurs when the concentration of cyclic AMP is no longer high enough to provide for complex formation with the regulatory subunit.

---

*The term $(-)-[''H]$-alprenolol refers to the labeled material obtained by catalytic reduction of $(-)-$alprenolol with tritium. By mass spectroscopy, this material is in fact *di*- [''H]-hydroalprenolol. The biologic activity of nonradioactive dihydroalprenolol, *di*-[''H]-hydroalprenolol, and alprenolol are identical, as shown by competitive-binding and adenylate-cyclase experiments.

---

*The phosphate group is attached not to a single position on the ribose group (as is the case with ordinary varieties of AMP) but at two different points, the 3′ and 5′ positions, producing a ring that accounts for the term *cyclic*.

Regulation of the intracellular concentration of cyclic AMP is a function shared with adenylate cyclase by one or more specific cyclic adenosine-3′,5′-monophosphate phosphodiesterases. This enzyme hydrolyzes the 3′-phosphate ester bond of cyclic AMP to yield 5′-AMP. It requires a divalent cation for catalytic activity (usually Mg + +), seems to be ubiquitous, and may exist in the cell in a soluble or a particulate form or both. The enzyme has been purified by a number of investigators, and its characteristics have been reported in detail.

Cholinergic Receptors

As with the adrenergic receptors, the exact nature of cholinergic receptors is now known, and they too are described by the effector response resulting from their activation.

Pharmacologic Classification of Cholinergic Receptors. There are at least three types of cholinergic receptors: (1) atropine-sensitive (muscarinic); (2) tetraethylammonium-sensitive (nicotinic); and (3) curare-sensitive (nicotinic). They correspond to the cholinergic receptor of the postganglionic cholinergic, synaptic, and neuromuscular (striated muscle) junctions, respectively. Nevertheless, the possibility that acetylcholine has only one receptor has not been excluded. Thus, the apparent differences in susceptibility to various cholinergic blocking agents may reflect not qualitative but quantitative differences that rest on nonreceptor factors such as those controlling the accessibility of acetylcholine or that of its blocking agent to the receptor site.

The Cholinergic Receptor Protein. From extensive studies on purified receptors from fish electric organs, it has been adduced that the cholinergic receptors are proteins, but not enzymes, and have a molecular weight of 42,000. The receptor is most probably a lipoprotein with four subunits, and in its membrane environment it is positioned in proximity to the enzyme *acetylcholinesterase*.

Cholinergic Activity and Cyclic GMP. Under a variety of experimental conditions, cholinergic stimulation leads to the intracellular accumulation of cyclic 3′,5′-guanosine monophosphate (cyclic GMP). This substance is similar to cyclic AMP except that the purine base guanine replaces the adenine ring of the latter. Besides cAMP, cGMP is the only cyclic nucleotide that is known with certainty to occur in nature. It has been detected in all mammalian tissues investigated so far, and, in most tissues, its levels are generally at least tenfold lower than those of cyclic AMP. A specific enzyme system, guanylate cyclase, catalyzes the synthesis of cyclic GMP from guanosine triphosphate (GTP), and hormones or other agents that activate adenylate cyclase do not stimulate (in physiologic concentrations) guanylate cyclase.

The two cyclic nucleotides, cAMP and cGMP, have been shown to exert opposing effects, with a reciprocal counterregulatory interplay similar to that of the adrenergic and cholinergic divisions of the autonomic nervous system. It is possible, therefore, that cyclic GMP will prove to be a biochemical intermediate of cholinergic action.

THE SIGNIFICANCE OF THE CYCLIC NUCLEOTIDE SYSTEM IN IMMUNOLOGIC PROCESSES

Following the discovery of the cyclic nucleotide system by Earl Sutherland, these agents have been gradually identified as key intermediates in the response of cells to exogenous stimuli: Essentially all nucleated mammalian cells contain cAMP, and the cyclic nucleotide has been implicated as a regulatory agent in virtually every organ and tissue. In view of the diversity of intracellular processes now known to the affected by cAMP, its involvement in immune processes would have to be strongly suspected. The very nature of the immune response with its requirements for specific cellular recognition, for cellular proliferation and differentiation, for short-range communication between cells, and for secretion of antibody and nonspecific mediators makes this involvement all the more likely. Our review will consider areas of involvement of cAMP in immune processes in terms of what is now known.

A full appreciation of the significance of these considerations requires a closer definition both of the general role of cyclic AMP in cell function and of the primary biologic mission of the lymphocyte. A generalized interpretation of all of the available evidence indicates that cyclic AMP participates in those biologic processes that involve the promotion of preprogrammed events consistent with the differentiated phenotype (i.e., the functions for which that cell type is developed—e.g., for the liver, glucose production from glycogen; for the adrenal gland, steroid production; for fat tissue, lipolysis). As for the lymphocyte, its mature circulating form is a resting cell (restricted "G_1,"), the biology of which, among other responses, is dominated by clonal proliferation on exposure to antigen. The lymphocyte thus appears to be an exception among cells in that its dominant response seems to be antagonized rather than promoted by cyclic AMP. In fact, cAMP apparently participates as an inhibitory regulator of the functions of virtually every cell involved in the expression of the immune response, including the B- and T-lymphocytes and their subpopulations, macrophages, polymorphonuclear and basophilic leukocytes, mast cells, and platelets. The illuminating lawfulness of this unusual biologic paradox seems to suggest that, in the effector cells that participate in the organization of an immune or immunologically mediated inflammatory response, the cellular regulatory role of cyclic AMP may represent a highly specific key function.

In terms of mechanism and site of action, the effects of the cyclic nucleotides may be on the afferent area of the immune response arc (e.g., the sensitization phase) or on the efferent, effector phase. Often it is difficult to be certain which phase is involved, and frequently both are. Moreover, the specific site of action within the phase may be difficult to ascertain.

Cyclic Nucleotides and the Sensitization Phase

All cells of the immune network contain both cAMP and cGMP and possess the enzymes catalyzing their synthesis as well as their destruction, providing the same possibilities for regulation of cellular function inherent in other cells.

Intracellular levels of cyclic AMP in human peripheral lymphocytes can be increased up to several-fold by beta-adrenergic agents, E-series prostaglandins, and various glucocorticoids. Parallel with their cyclic AMP–increasing effects, these agents all inhibit the proliferation of lymphocytes. This antiproliferative effect of beta-adrenergically–induced cAMP accumulation in lymphocytes correlates well with extensive similar observations on nonlymphocytic normal as well as transformed cells in tissue culture and other preparations, indicating that cyclic AMP is an inhibitor of cell proliferation in a variety of cell systems.

In addition to the antiproliferative effect exhibited by catecholamines acting through beta-adrenergic receptors, there exists a proliferation-augmenting action resulting from an alpha-adrenergic mechanism. Analysis of this mechanism has shown that alpha-adrenergic stimulation increases lymphocytic glucose uptake and use as well as glycogen accumulation and that norepinephrine acting through this alpha-adrenergic mechanism directly stimulates adenosine triphosphatases (ATPases) in lymphocytic plasma membranes. The relationship of cyclic nucleotides to these transport-linked enzymes remains unclear at this time, and, although such action of norepinephrine has been linked to cyclic GMP in vas deferens and in platelets, this association has not yet been reported in lymphocytes, nor has a direct link of cyclic GMP to membrane ATPases been established.

Agents that increase cyclic GMP in lymphocytes, such as acetylcholine, also augment proliferation of these cells. This action of acetylcholine involves an atropine-sensitive muscarinic receptor mechanism. To date, it has not been possible to show that acetylcholine exerts any positive influence on calcium influx or transport of nutrients into lymphocytes, indicating that the proliferation-promoting action of acetylcholine may be directly linked to cyclic GMP phosphodiesterase by imidazole, which also augments mitogen-induced human lymphocyte proliferation.

Another naturally occurring substance shown to act on lymphocytes is insulin. The latter was found to increase glucose uptake in lymphocytes and to augment lymphocyte proliferation in response to mitogenic and allogeneic stimulation. The mechanism of this insulin action on lymphocytes has not been studied in detail, but it has been shown in other cells that insulin inhibits intracellular accumulation of cyclic AMP through inhibition of adenylate cyclase or stimulation of cAMP phosphodiesterase or both. Insulin action also has been linked to cyclic GMP accumulation in fibroblasts, fat cells, and liver cells, and at least one laboratory found twofold to threefold increases in cGMP in lymphocytes following exposure to insulin.

For all the complexities involved in the regulation of lymphocyte proliferation by cyclic nucleotides, including the many controversial aspects, other texts should be consulted. For our purposes, it will suffice to state that alpha-adrenergic, beta-adrenergic, and cholinergic mechanisms as well as their biochemical correlates, the cyclic nucleotides, could conceivably have a major controlling influence on the proliferation of lymphocytes. This control appears to be bidirectional inasmuch as cholinergic and alpha-adrenergic influences enhance lymphocyte proliferation, whereas beta-adrenergic effects inhibit it. The bidirectional character of this regulation, however, may be more apparent than real, since we have no evidence for a regulatory role of acetylcholine outside the synaptic, or junctional, clefts. Therefore, the established presence of a muscarinic acetylcholine receptor on lymphocytes may or may not have physiologic significance. Thus, it is possible that autonomic regulation of lymphocyte replication is essentially adrenergic in character. This possibility received important support from observations made on the effects of chemical or surgical sympathectomy on lymphopoiesis in anterior eye chamber thymic explants. The significance of this point lies in the fact that the main impetus in the induction of the immune response consists of the replication of cells selected by the antigen from a large number of pre-existing clones of lymphocytes. Replication is needed to generate the necessary mass of cells with specificity for antigen and thereby to convert a pre-existing capability into the quantitative reality of antibody production. Any specific or nonspecific effect on this highly critical replication step would, therefore, be expected to have immunomodulatory potential.

Cyclic Nucleotides and the Effector Phase

Amphetamine, phenylethylamine, tyramine, and other substances that induce sympathomimetic activity indirectly through the endogenous release of catecholamines are capable of liberating histamine. The same can be accomplished by the exogenous administration of catechol-amines and of their specific blocking agents. Al-though nonimmunologic histamine release is elic-ited by all these agents, they render sensitized mast cells incapable of responding to antigen chal-lenge with histamine release.

Analysis of these seemingly contradictory findings suggests that (1) adrenergic agents inter-fere with binding or release of histamine because of their catecholamine-like intrinsic activity; and (2) they operate on a cellular system that is anti-gen-activated and thus central to the mechanism of the allergic reaction.

The first conclusion is supported by residual agonistic activity of the blocking agents employed, since the only common feature of these directly acting adrenergic compounds is their basic cate-cholamine structure. The second conclusion is based on the observation that methylxanthines also inhibit immunologic release of histamine. Thus, when ragweed antigen was made to interact in vitro with IgE antibody on the surface of leu-kocytes from ragweed-sensitive human donors, both methylxanthines and catecholamines inhib-ited histamine release. The significance of these findings is evidenced by the fact that methylxan-thines are competitive inhibitors of the specific phosphodiesterase that inactivates cyclic 3′, 5′-AMP, and thereby they may induce "adrenergic action" by increasing the intracellular concentra-tion of the compound. Indeed, catecholamines and methylxanthines were found to act synergistically in inhibiting histamine release, and the phospho-diesterase-inhibitory potencies of the various methylxanthines correlated well with their inhib-itory effects on histamine release. Of further sig-nificance is the fact that the methylxanthines and catecholamines were shown to inhibit only if added to the cells when antigen was present. They had no effect if removed from the environment of the sensitized cells before antigen exposure. The aden-ylate cyclase system therefore must be considered a critical regulatory system in allergic histamine release.

Besides beta-adrenergic agents, prostaglan-dins of the E series, prostacyclin, adenosine, and histamine (i.e., substances that interact with cell membrane receptors that activate adenylate cy-clase) also inhibit allergic release of histamine or of other pharmacologic mediators of immediate hypersensitivity. Inhibition of allergic mediator release by these agents is generally paralleled by an increase in the intracellular concentration of cyclic AMP in the respective cell preparations. Furthermore, since the release-inhibitory activi-ties of these agents are blocked by their specific antagonists, it is presumed that these agents in-crease cyclic AMP by acting on receptors linked to adenylate cyclase. The mechanism by which cAMP blocks mediator release is not known, but current evidence suggests that cyclic AMP acts early in the release process, that it is linked to the oblig-atory inward flux of calcium, and that it is related

to microtubule function. There are, however, ex-ceptions when changes in cyclic nucleotide levels do not correlate with inhibition of immunologic mediator release. The nature of such dissociation between cyclic AMP elevation and inhibition is unclear but may be explained if there are func-tionally separate intracellular cAMP pools and if a product of the lipoxygenase or some other path-way can selectively block a biochemical sequence linking adenylate cyclase activation to inhibition of mediator release.

The effect of changes in intracellular cyclic GMP levels on allergic mediator release has been less extensively studied. In lung tissue, alpha-adrenergic and cholinergic stimulation increases cyclic GMP levels, and such effects as well as extracellular cyclic GMP derivatives potentiate antigen-induced mediator release. However, cyclic GMP does not enhance release from rat mast cells and has minimal or no effect on immunologic mediator release from basophils. Furthermore, it is not known whether cGMP-induced enhancement of pulmonary mediator release is a direct effect of alpha-adrenergic or cholinergic agents on the mast cells or whether it reflects their actions on other cell types. Nevertheless, in this context it may be added that pertussis or pharmacologically estab-lished beta-adrenergic blockade has been reported to cause peritoneal mast cell degranulation in rats and mice, whereas beta-adrenergic stimulation protects these cells against propranolol-induced degranulation. As judged by the PCA reaction in guinea pigs, propranolol has the same enhancing effect on immunologic mediator release.

The role of the adenylate cyclase–linked beta-adrenergic receptor system in the constitutional basis of diseases of atopic allergy will be discussed in Chapter 5.

THE COMPLEMENT SYSTEM

The complement system consists of a series of serum glycoproteins that possess many effector functions. Two distinct routes exist for complement activation: the classical and the alternative path-ways. Since both pathways result in sequential activation of components (i.e., for several reactions in these pathways, the product of one step is the enzyme that catalyzes the next step), the amount of activated component can be markedly amplified in each succeeding step. The intermediate products of the complement pathway possess several types of biologic activity, including chemotaxis of cells, activation of cells for mediator release, and smooth muscle contraction. Activation of the entire com-plement sequence results in cell lysis.

The steps in the activation of the complement system initiated by immune reactions are called the *classical pathway of complement activation* (Fig. 4–9). The classical complement pathway will be contrasted with the *alternative pathway,* which involves nonimmune activation of the complement and serum properdin systems (Fig. 4–10).

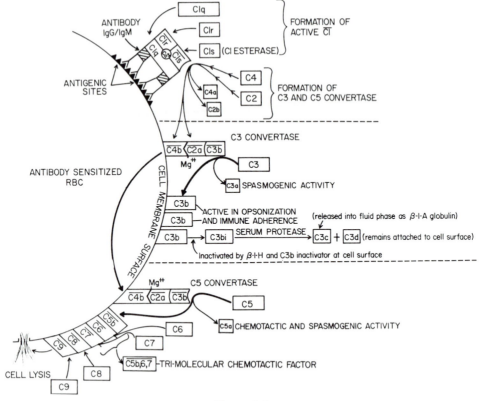

Figure 4-9

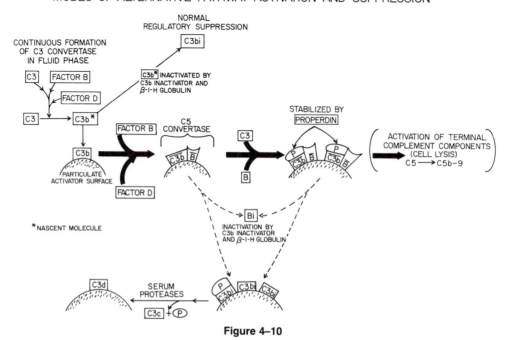

Figure 4-10

In the classical pathway, the immune complex formed must be of a certain physical size that provides a macromolecular surface upon which the activation (fixation) of the components can occur. A system usually employed for complement assays consists of sheep erythrocytes sensitized with an IgM rabbit antibody (hemolysin), to which is added a source of complement, usually human serum. The immune reactants "fix" along the cell membrane, which provides the structural surface upon which activation occurs. As a result of binding to antigen, there is a steric change in the antibody molecules that exposes hidden structural sites in the Fc portion of the molecules to which the initial reacting component of complement, C1q, attaches. It has been shown that binding of a single molecule of IgM, because of its polymeric structure, or of two closely adjacent molecules of IgG will provide the binding site of C1q. Following the attachment of C1q, the remainder of all the 11 proteins that constitute the nine components of the complement system become sequentially activated. At different steps in the activation sequence, molecular fragments are generated that exhibit a variety of biologic activities. These play a major role as mediators of the tissue effects of these reactions.

Following binding of C1q, activation of C1r and C1s occurs, which, in the presence of calcium, forms a trimolecular complex designated the *activated C1 complex*. The esterase activity of C1 shows a specific substrate affinity for components C2 and C4. Both these components are cleaved by C1 esterase, with each yielding two fragments, designated *a* and *b*. The 4b fragment combines with the 2a fragment in the presence of magnesium and binds to other sites on the cell membrane. This enzymatic complex is called *C3 convertase (C4b2a)*. It has enzymatic activity that cleaves C3, yielding fragments C3b and a small peptide fragment, C3a. The C3b fragment may then bind to specific receptors at other sites on the cell membrane, where it shows biologic activities such as immune adherence and opsonization for phagocytosis.

The residual C3b molecules remain with the C4b2a complex to form a trimolecular enzyme called *C5 convertase (C4b2a3b)*, which has high substrate affinity for complement component C5. C3b is also a link between the classical and alternative pathways of complement activation. As we will see later, it also participates in activation of the alternative pathway sequence. The C3a fragment is released into the fluid phase and exhibits an activity described as *spasmogenic*. This term refers to the molecule's pharmacologic activity of causing smooth muscle contraction through the release of granule factors from basophils and mast cells. Previously, this fragment was thought to have chemotactic activity, but more modern studies have shown that sort of activity only with the C5a cleavage fragment, which is produced later in the activation sequence.

The trimolecular C5 convertase (C4b2a3b) cleaves C5 into a and b fragments. The C5a fragment is released into the fluid phase, and it shows both chemotactic and spasmogenic activities, as previously mentioned. The C5b fragment attaches to the cell membrane, providing a point for subsequent attachment to the remainder of the terminal components of the complement system, C6, C7, C8, and C9. This terminal assembly leads to cell membrane disequilibrium, resulting in hemolysis, or breakdown, of the lipoprotein membrane. As a transient product, the trimolecular complex (C5b, 6, 7) may dissociate from the cell surface into the fluid phase as another factor chemotactic for neutrophils and monocytes.

Activation of the alternative pathway is illustrated in Figure 4–10 and can be contrasted with that of the classical pathway. It now appears that there is an ongoing activation of the alternative pathway by the association of complement C3, properdin factor B (C3 proactivator), and properdin factor D (C3 proactivator convertase). This complex produces enzymatic cleavage of C3, yielding a continuous low-level production of C3b. The C3b generated in this manner is a nascent molecule with a short life, since it normally is inactivated by the C3b inactivator enhanced by beta-1-H globulin in the blood. However, in the presence of certain types of surfaces known as *activator surfaces*, the nascent C3b molecule becomes bound to the activator surface and is protected from inactivation. On the activator surface, further reaction with factors B and D yields an enzymatic complex composed of C3b and activated factor B (C3b, B) along the surface. This enzymatic complex possesses C5-cleaving activity and is called the *C5 convertase of the alternative pathway*. As shown in Figure 4–10, this convertase can be stabilized by the molecule, properdin. It acts as the trigger molecule for activating the terminal complement components, just as in the classical pathway, leading to cell lysis, or disruption, of the lipoprotein membrane surface of the activator.

The extent of activation of the alternative pathway is limited by the access of C3b inactivator and beta-1-H globulin on C3b molecules at the surface. On certain surfaces, the integrity of the C3b, B complex is protected because of restrictions due to the cell surface properties. In other instances in which there is no cell surface restriction, the inactivators rapidly cleave C3b and B to inactive molecules, which in turn are further cleaved by serum proteases to inactive polypeptides. In contrast to earlier studies in which it seemed that a specific activator triggered activation of the alternative pathway, it now appears that the alternative pathway is continuously activated at a low level and is normally under regulatory suppression by C3b inactivator and beta-1-H globulin. Augmentation occurs in the presence of a particular activator surface that binds and protects the C3b from the serum inactivators. Surfaces that behave as particulate activators include bacterial cell walls, polysaccharides, aggregated immunoglobulins, and rabbit erythrocytes. Sheep erythrocytes, lacking the restrictive surface properties, are poor activator surfaces for the alternative pathway.

Activation of the classical complement pathway by immune complexes results in the immunopathologic features of the Arthus phenomenon, serum sickness, and a variety of immune complex diseases. These are discussed in Chapter 5. Conversely, complement is not directly involved in atopic or nonatopic manifestations of immediate hypersensitivities, although there is some suggestive evidence that under certain circumstances histamine release may be activated by some complement components.

REFERENCES

Austen, K. F.: Tissue mast cells in immediate hypersensitivity. In Dixon, F. J., and Fisher, D. W., (Eds.): The Biology of Immunologic Disease. Sunderland, Mass., Sinauer Associates, Inc., 1983, pp. 223–234.

Bach, F. H., Bonavida, B., Vitetta, E. S., and Fox, C. F. (Eds.): T and B Lymphocytes: Recognition and Function. New York, Academic Press, 1979.

Barrett, J. F.: Textbook of Immunology. 4th ed. St. Louis, The C. V. Mosby Co., 1983.

Bloom, F. E. (Ed.): Peptides: Integrators of Cell and Tissue Function. New York, Raven Press, 1980.

Bona, C. A.: Idiotypes and Lymphocytes. New York, Academic Press, 1981.

Bona, C. A., and Kohler, H. (Eds.): Immune networks. Ann. N.Y. Acad. Sci. Vol. 418, 240–248, 1983.

deGaetano, G., and Garattini, S. (Eds.): Platelets: A Multidisciplinary Approach. New York, Raven Press, 1978.

Friedman, H., Klein, T. W., and Szentivanyi, A. (Eds.): Immunomodulation by Bacteria and Their Products. New York, Plenum Press, 1981.

Fudenberg, H. H., Pink, J. R. L., Wang, A., and Douglas, S. D.: Basic immunogenetics. New York, Oxford University Press, 1978.

Fujii, S., Moriya, H., and Suzuki, T. (Eds.): Kinins—II: Biochemistry, Pathophysiology, and Clinical Aspects. New York, Plenum Press, 1978.

Fujii, S., Moriya, H., and Suzuki, T. (Eds.): Kinins—II: Systemic Proteases and Cellular Function. New York, Plenum Press, 1978.

Ganellin, C. R., and Parsons, M. E. (Eds.): Pharmacology of Histamine Receptors. Bristol, Wright PSC, 1982.

Gross, F., and Vogel, H. G. (Eds.): Enzymatic Release of Vasoactive Peptides. New York, Raven Press, 1980.

Haberland, G. L., and Hamberg, U. (Eds.): Current Concepts in Kinin Research. Oxford, Pergamon Press, 1979.

Hadden, J. W., Chedid, L., Dukor, P., et al. (Eds.): Advances in Immunopharmacology 2. Proceedings of the Second International Conference on Immunopharmacology, July 1982, Washington, USA. Oxford, Pergamon Press, 1983.

Hadden, J. W., and Stewart, W. E., II (Eds.): The Lymphokines: Biochemistry and Biological Activity. Clifton, N.J., Humana Press, 1981.

Jacobs, S., and Cuatrecasas, P. (Eds.): Membrane Receptors—Methods for Purification and Characterization. Receptors and Recognition, Series B, vol. 11. London, Chapman and Hall, 1981.

Kalsner, S. (Ed.): Trends in Autonomic Pharmacology. Vol. 1. Baltimore, Urban & Schwarzenberg, 1979.

Kalsner, S. (Ed.): Trends in Autonomic Pharmacology. Vol. 2. Baltimore, Urban & Schwarzenberg, 1982.

Karnovsky, M. L., and Bolis, L. (Eds.): Phagocytosis—Past and Future. New York, Academic Press, 1982.

Kelsall, M. A., and Crabb, E. D.: Lymphocytes and Mast Cells. Baltimore, Williams and Wilkins, 1959.

Khan, A., and Hill, N. O. (Eds.): Human Lymphokines: The Biological Immune Response Modifiers. New York, Academic Press, 1982.

Klein, R. L., Lagercrantz, H., and Zimmermann, H. (Eds.): Neurotransmitter vesicles. New York, Academic Press, 1982.

Mahmoud, A. A. F., and Austen, K. F. (Eds.): The Eosinophil in Health and Disease. New York, Grune & Stratton, 1980.

McGhee, J. R., and Mestecky, J. (Eds.): The Secretory Immune System. Proceedings of the Conference on the Secretory Immune System, May 4–7, 1982, The New York Academy of Sciences. Ann. N.Y. Acad. Sci. Vol. 409, 461–498, 1982.

Merigan, T. C., and Friedman, R. M. (Eds.): Interferons. New York, Academic Press, 1982.

Mizel, S. B. (Ed.): Lymphokines in Antibody and Cytotoxic Responses. Vol. 6. Lymphokines: A Form for Immunoregulatory Cell Products. New York, Academic Press, 1982.

Movat, H. Z. (Ed.): Inflammation, Immunity and Hypersensitivity: Cellular and Molecular Mechanisms. 2nd ed. Hagerstown, Md., Harper & Row, 1979.

Nowotny, A.: Basic Exercises in Immunochemistry. 2nd ed. Berlin, Springer-Verlag, 1979.

Pick, E. (Ed.): Lymphokines. Vol. 7. New York, Academic Press, 1982.

Plaut, M., and Lichtenstein, L. M.: Cellular and chemical basis of the allergic inflammatory response: component parts and control mechanisms. In Middleton, E., Jr., Reed, C. E., and Ellis, E. (Eds.): Allergy: Principles and Practice. 2nd ed. Vol. 1. St. Louis, The C. V. Mosby Co., 1983, pp. 119–146.

Stewart, W. E., II: The Interferon System. 2nd ed. Vienna, Springer-Verlag, 1981.

Szentivanyi, A., Krzanowski, J. J., and Polson, J. B.: The autonomic nervous system: structure and function. In Middleton, E., Jr., Reed, C. E., and Ellis, E. (Eds.): Allergy, Principles and Practice. 2nd ed. Vol. 1. St. Louis, The C. V. Mosby Co., 1983, p. 303–331.

Szentivanyi, A., Middleton, E., Jr., Williams, J. F., and Friedman, H.: Effect of microbial agents on the immune network and associated pharmacologic reactivities. In Middleton, E., Jr., Reed, C. E., and Ellis, E. (Eds.): Allergy, Principles and Practice. 2nd ed. Vol. 1. St. Louis, The C. V. Mosby Co., 1983, pp. 211–236.

Unanue, E. R., and Rosenthal, A. S. (Eds.): Macrophage Regulation and Immunity. Proceedings of the Conference, Regulatory Role of Macrophages in Immunity. Mar. 12–14, 1979, Augusta, Mich. New York, Academic Press, 1980.

Weir, D. M. (Ed.): Handbook of Experimental Immunology. 3rd ed. Vol. 1: Immunochemistry. Oxford, Blackwell Scientific Publications, 1978.

Williams, L. T., and Lefkowitz, R. J.: Receptor Binding Studies in Adrenergic Pharmacology. New York, Raven Press, 1978.

Williams, R. C., Jr. (Ed.): Lymphocytes and Their Interactions: Recent Observations. Kroc Foundation Series, No. 4. New York, Raven Press, 1975.

Yamamura, Y., and Kotani, S. (Eds.): Immunomodulation by microbial products and related synthetic compounds. Proceedings of an international symposium. Osaka. July 27–29, 1981. Amsterdam, Excerpta Medica, 1982.

The Pathophysiology of Immunologic and Related Diseases*

5

Andor Szentivanyi, M.D., and Judith Szentivanyi, M.D.

This chapter describes the pathophysiologic mechanisms of immunologic and related disorders in four sections. In the first section, the immunodeficiency diseases are presented as they may involve some, many, or all major components of the immune system, including lymphocytes, phagocytic cells, and the complement proteins, regardless of whether the defective function is genetically determined or acquired. This is followed by an analysis of the immunobiology and immunopathology of cancer in the second section.

The third section considers, within the conceptual framework of autoimmunity, the established patterns of autoimmune reactions encountered in human disease, and the last section discusses the principal pathways of immunologic tissue injuries.

IMMUNODEFICIENCY DISEASES

Current understanding of the pathogenesis of immunodeficiencies originated with the discovery in chickens and mice that immunologic functions were mediated by two developmentally independent but functionally interacting cell types. These are T cells originating in the thymus and B cells developing within the avian bursa of Fabricius or the mammalian bone marrow. Good and his associates in 1967 were the first to recognize the pathogenic significance of these observations in human immunodeficiencies and lymphoid malignancies. Application of these concepts in subsequent years has largely depended on the development of the means to identify, enumerate, and study the functions of lymphocytes from humans and experimental animals in vitro.

Four major aspects of the immune system are involved in the defense against various viral, bacterial, and other microbial infections. These systems consist of (1) B-cell, or antibody-mediated, immunity; (2) T-cell, or cell-mediated, immunity; (3) phagocytic mechanisms; and (4) the complement system. Each of these systems can act independently or in conjunction with one or more of the others. The immunodeficiency disorders can be classified under five major categories (Table 5–1): (1) antibody, or B-cell, deficiency diseases; (2) cellular, or T-cell, immunodeficiency diseases; (3) combined B- and T-cell immunodeficiency diseases; (4) diseases with a phagocytic dysfunction; and (5) complement abnormalities and immune deficiency diseases.

TABLE 5–1 CLASSIFICATION OF PRIMARY IMMUNODEFICIENCY DISORDERS

I. B-Cell (Antibody) Immunodeficiency Diseases
 X-linked congenital hypogammaglobulinemia
 X-linked immunodeficiency of IgG and IgA with hyper IgM
 Common variable immunodeficiency
 Selective IgA deficiency
 Selective IgM deficiency
 Selective deficiency of IgG subclasses

II. T-Cell (Cellular) Immunodeficiency Diseases
 Congenital thymic hypoplasia
 Chronic mucocutaneous candidiasis

III. Combined B-Cell and T-Cell Immunodeficiency Diseases
 Severe combined immunodeficiency diseases
 Cellular and antibody immunodeficiency with abnormal immunoglobulin synthesis (Nezelof's syndrome)
 Wiskott-Aldrich syndrome (immunodeficiency with eczema and thrombocytopenia)
 Immunodeficiency with short-limbed dwarfism
 Immunodeficiency with enzyme deficiency
  (a) Adenosine diaminase deficiency
  (b) Nucleoside phosphorylase deficiency

IV. Phagocytic Dysfunction
 Chronic granulomatous disease
 Glucose-6-phosphate dehydrogenase deficiency
 Myeloperoxidase deficiency
 Chediak-Higashi syndrome
 Job's syndrome
 Tuftsin deficiency

V. Complement Abnormalities and Immunodeficiency Diseases
 C1q, C1r, C1s deficiency
 C2 deficiency
 C3 deficiency
 C5 dysfunction

(Modified from Ammann, A. J., and Fudenberg, H. H. *In* Fudenberg, H. H., et al. (Eds.): Basic and Clinical Immunology. Los Altos, CA, Lange Medical Publications, 1976, p. 334.)

*This chapter incorporates portions of Chapters 4 and 5 of the previous edition, prepared by Ernest S. Tucker, III, and Robert M. Nakamura.

TABLE 5–2 EXAMPLES OF SECONDARY IMMUNODEFICIENCY SYNDROMES

I. T-Cell (Cellular) Immunodeficiency
   Malignant diseases such as Hodgkin's disease and chronic infections (e.g., leprosy, sarcoidosis)
   Aging
   Intestinal lymphangiectasis (obstruction of lymph flow)

II. B-Cell (Antibody) Immunodeficiency
   Lymphomas (decreased antibody synthesis)
   Nephrotic syndrome (increased loss and catabolism of immunoglobulins)
   Multiple myeloma, macroglobulinemia (increased abnormal and defective immunoglobulins and decreased synthesis of normal immunoglobulins and antibody)

The immunodeficiency diseases may be categorized into those that are *primary,* resulting from a failure of proper development of the humoral or cellular immune system or both. Often excluded from the primary group of immunodeficiency diseases are hypercatabolic disorders and disorders of the complement system. The *secondary,* or acquired, immunodeficiency diseases may occur in patients in association with a variety of diseases and include immunodeficiency states associated with intestinal lymphangiectasia, protein-losing enteropathy, X-irradiation, immunosuppressive and cytotoxic drugs, lymphoreticular malignancies, and so forth. Some examples of secondary immunodeficiency syndromes are listed in Table 5–2.

PRIMARY IMMUNODEFICIENCY DISEASES

Despite the impressive amount of information gained of the functional derangements and cellular abnormalities in the various primary immunodeficiency disorders as of the end of 1983, the fundamental biologic errors, with only two exceptions, remain unknown for all of them. These exceptions involve two defects accompanied by purine salvage pathway enzyme deficiencies (see later). In many other immunodeficiencies, the genetic errors must, by definition, be located on the X chromosome. Not one of the primary immunodeficiencies appears to reflect defects involving HLA-linked immune response genes on chromosome 6. Furthermore, since trace amounts of immunoglobulins of all five isotypes are usually present in the sera of even the most severely agammaglobulinemic patient, it is also unlikely that these deficiencies are due to deletions of genes encoding for immunoglobulin heavy chains. This does not, however, exclude the possibility of regulating genetic defects.

Primary B-Cell Immunodeficiency Diseases

The stem cell differentiates and gives rise to a population of precursor B cells, which can be found in the marrow and spleen. The cells acquire an ability to express surface immunoglobulin. Fully mature B cells can synthesize immunoglobulin and express it on the surface; they differentiate into cells capable of secreting antibody in response to an antigenic stimulation. The B cells and T cells are identified by certain surface markers, as listed in Table 5–3. The classic B cell is identified by surface Ig and Fc and complement receptors. The mature, small B-lymphocyte is itself only a precursor for the plasma cells that appear on antigenic stimulation (Fig. 5–1). The deficient humoral immune system can result from the failure of these terminal stages of differentiation despite the presence of normal-appearing small B-lymphocytes.

Deficient T-helper function also can decrease and compromise the humoral response. Production of IgA, IgG, and IgE appears to require T-helper function. IgM production is less dependent on T-cell help. The development of mature T cells is due to the precursor lymphoid cells, which mature under the influence of the thymus. Prethymic cells may migrate to the intact thymus gland and differentiate into an immunocompetent T cell under the influence of thymic hormones. The thymus plays a definite role in the normal maturation of the T cells.

There are four types of primary panhypogammaglobulinemia involving all classes of immunoglobulins (including IgG, IgA, IgM, IgD, and IgE), which will be discussed subsequently.

Transient Hypogammaglobulinemia of Infancy. This is a relatively benign condition. Babies

TABLE 5–3 LYMPHOCYTE SURFACE MARKERS

Surface Marker	T Cell	B Cell
1. Rosettes with sheep erythrocyte (E)	+	−
2. Antithymocyte heteroantisera	+	−
3. Easily detectable surface immunoglobulin	−	+
4. Anti–B-cell heteroantisera	−	+
5. Complement receptors (EAC rosettes)	−	+
6. IgG Fc receptor		
a. IgG coated erythrocyte rosettes	±	+
b. Aggregated IgG	−	+

MATURATION OF B-CELLS

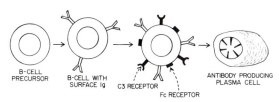

Figure 5–1

are born with mostly maternal gamma globulins that have passed through the placenta. The adopted maternal gamma globulin is naturally catabolized during the first 6 months of life, and normally the infant's own immunogobulin system becomes competent. Some children may have a prolonged physiologic depression of the initiation of gamma globulin synthesis that may last 2 or 3 years. The number of B-lymphocytes with surface immunoglobulin or complement receptors remains normal. The affected child is susceptible to bacterial respiratory infections and bronchitis. In children between 1.5 and 2.5 years of age, immunoglobulin production usually becomes normal. These patients have an excellent prognosis and rarely require treatment. With any low levels of IgG, treatment with immune serum globulin may be indicated. This disorder should be distinguished from the more serious immunoglobulin defects with a poor prognosis.

X-Linked Hypogammaglobulinemia. This syndrome was first recognized by Bruton in 1952 and is characterized by a deficiency of B-lymphocytes that results in failure of production of immunoglobulin of all classes. This is a pure B-cell deficiency in which normal cellular immunity is present with a very low concentration of circulating immunoglobulins. This disorder is X-linked, and usually only males are affected. The serum concentration of IgG is usually below 100 mg/dl, and IgA, IgM, and IgD are commonly undetectable. The immunoglobulin-producing B cells usually are absent in the bone marrow, blood, lymphoid tissue, and mucosal tissue. The lymph nodes show a paucity of germinal centers and plasma cells.

During the first few months of life, the infants are protected by the placental transfer of the maternal IgG antibody. After the maternal placentally transferred IgG has been catabolized, these patients are susceptible to severe recurrent infections with common bacteria, including pharyngitis, otitis media, pneumonia secondary to streptococci, *Staphylococcus aureus, Hemophilus influenzae,* and *Neisseria meningitidis.* The diagnosis usually is made by demonstration of panhypogammaglobulinemia, diminished number of circulating surface-bearing immunoglobulin-containing B cells, and family history of other males with the disease in the mother's family.

Sex-Linked Hypogammaglobulinemia With Normal or Increased IgM. In this disorder, IgG and IgA are deficient, whereas IgM levels are normal to increased. B cells bearing IgM type antibodies can be demonstrated. The thymus-dependent system is normal, and the immunologic abnormalities indicate an arrest in the development of B cells from the IgM- to the IgG-producing cells. Most of the cases of this sex-linked recessive disorder are males. There is also a high incidence of neutropenia, thrombocytopenia, hemolytic anemia, and B-cell lymphomas.

An acquired form of this abnormality may be a consequence of congenital rubella infection, transcobalamin II deficiency, and hypogammaglobulinemia. Transcobalamin II deficiency has been found to be associated with a panhypogammaglobulinemia and is a transport protein involved in vitamin B_{12} metabolism. This disease is inherited as an autosomal recessive trait. Megaloblastic anemia, granulocytopenia, and thrombocytopenia can be found. B- and T-cells are demonstrated by their surface markers, although antibody production is low to absent.

Common Variable, Unclassifiable Immunodeficiency. This is the most common type of panhypogammaglobulinemia in which both sexes are affected. In this disease, the degree of immunoglobulin deficiency is less marked than in the X-linked form. The clinical onset is usually delayed until late childhood or adulthood. There is a great variation in the time of onset, clinical manifestation, and the degree of disordered T-cell cellular immunity. There has also been a high associated incidence of other immunologic abnormalities, such as systemic lupus erythematosus, hemolytic anemia, and thrombocytopenic purpura. The following four different types of defects have been identified in these common variable immunodeficient patients:

1. B cells are absent.

2. B cells are present in a resting state with decreased antibody production. The B cells are unresponsive to T-cell mitogenic signal in the presence of antigen.

3. B cells are present, and these cells are responsive to the T-cell signal in the presence of antigen. IgE is synthesized but not secreted. In this case, there is a defect with failure of glycosylation of the heavy chain of the immunoglobulin, which suggests that the secretion defect is due to a failure of incorporation of carbohydrate into the immunoglobulin molecule.

4. Normal B cells that are suppressed by humoral factors or suppressor T cells are present. Experiments have indicated that T cells from some patients with common variable immunodeficiency actually suppressed normal lymphocyte synthesis of Ig after pokeweed mitogen stimulation in culture. Since T cells are involved in modulating the terminal differentiation of B cells to immunoglobulin-secreting cells, some patients with common

variable immunodeficiency probably have an abnormality of T-cell regulators that is responsible for perpetuating hypogammaglobulinemia.

Selective Immunoglobulin Deficiency Disorders

There are six possible combinations of the deficits of the three major immunoglobulins. In addition, subclass deficiencies of IgG have been found.

Selective Deficiency of IgA. Selective deficiency of serum IgA is the most common primary immunodeficiency in humans, and the incidence is four to seven in 1000 patients. Autosomal dominant and recessive inheritance have been reported. Serum IgA levels are usually below 5 to 10 mg/dl. The IgA-producing cells are decreased, and secretory IgA and the external secretions are low to absent. Free secretory component is usually found. In many cases, the IgM levels in the external secretion in IgM-producing cells, and external secretory sites are increased. The defect appears to be at the level of the terminal differentiation of B cells to plasma cells.

IgA deficiency is a result of a variety of genetic defects and can be produced by a congenital rubella virus, cytomegalovirus, or *Toxoplasma gondii* infection. The selective IgA deficiency has a striking association with autoimmune diseases, nontropical sprue, or ataxia telangiectasia.

In approximately 80 per cent of cases, ataxia telangiectasia is associated with an IgA deficiency. Recently, a deficiency of secretory component has been described in a patient with chronic intestinal candidiasis. The serum levels of IgA were normal, but neither IgA nor secretory component could be demonstrated in external secretions. Patients with a serum IgA deficiency who receive blood transfusions can develop an anaphylactoid reaction, since IgA is often recognized as a foreign protein in transfused blood.

Selective IgM Deficiency. The selective IgM deficiency is the second most common selective immunodeficiency disorder. In most cases, the IgM serum levels are below 20 mg/dl. Many of these patients have recurrent infections with septicemia, meningitis, gastrointestinal disorders, atrophic skin diseases, and lymphoreticular malignancies. Because IgM has a short half-life, replacement therapy to raise IgM level is difficult.

IgG Subclass Deficiency. Selective deficiencies of different combinations of IgG1, IgG2, IgG3, and IgG4 have been reported. Total IgG level in these cases may be normal or slightly decreased. Diagnosis is usually indicated by a restricted heterogeneity of the electrophoretic mobility of the IgG or the lack of antibody production against certain antigens. It requires the quantitative measurement of IgG subclasses.

Primary T-Cell Disorders

Very few pure T-cell cellular disorders are seen. The majority of the T-cell immunodeficiency disorders are associated with some aberration in the humoral immune system to form antibodies. This is in concert with the observation that most antigens such as proteins and haptens require both the T cells and B cells for normal antibody production. Thus, a complete absence of T-cells will result in a defect of antibody production to all T-cell–dependent antigens. Many of the immunodeficiencies may initially be classified primarily as a T-cell or B-cell defect. However, when followed for a prolonged time, the immunodeficiency becomes severe and may eventuate in combined T- and B-cell deficiency. The patients with a T-cell immunodeficiency are susceptible to a variety of infectious agents, such as viruses, bacteria, and protozoa, which usually result in intracellular types of infections.

Congenital Thymic Aplasia (DiGeorge's Syndrome). The diagnosis of congenital thymic aplasia, or DiGeorge's syndrome, usually is made shortly after birth, since these patients present with congenital heart disease and hypoparathyroidism. Clinically, the patient shows hypocalcemia, which appears within 24 hours after birth and is frequently associated with tetany.

DiGeorge's syndrome results from interference with normal embryonic development at approximately 12 weeks' gestation. The thymus and parathyroid glands develop from the epithelial evaginations of the third and fourth pharyngeal pouches. In many patients with DiGeorge's syndrome, the thymus is not completely absent but is hypoplastic or in an abnormal location. The terms "complete" and "partial" DiGeorge's syndrome are used to describe various degrees of immunodeficiency found in such patients. The complete absence of the thymus could result in a definite defect in the humoral antibody system, whereas the patient with a partial thymus gland would show primary manifestations of a T-cell deficiency. The peripheral lymphocyte count is low, and the number of circulating T cells is low or absent at the time of birth. The studies of B-cell immunity are difficult to interpret, since IgG in fetal serum at birth represents maternal transfer of gamma globulin. IgM and IgA are normally present in very small amounts in newborns.

The congenital heart disease associated with DiGeorge's syndrome may require immediate corrective surgery. Calcium is administered to correct the hypocalcemia, and vitamin D and parathyroid hormone are used to treat hypoparathyroidism. Fetal thymus transplant at less than 14 weeks' gestation is the treatment of choice to correct the T-cell abnormality. The fetal thymus transplant has been successfully used in cases of DiGeorge's syndrome, with rapid reconstitution of T-cell immunity. The mechanism of reconstitution of T-cell immunity with the fetal transplant may be due to a humoral factor within the thymus, since one patient with DiGeorge's syndrome has been reconstituted with implantation of fetal thymus in a millipore chamber.

Fresh blood transfusions with live leukocytes should not be given to patients with a T-cell immune defect because of a possible graft-versus-host reaction. The blood products should first be irradiated (3000 R).

Chronic Mucocutaneous Candidiasis With and Without Endocrinopathy. The majority of these patients have only minor defects in T-cell immunity. They usually have a chronic *Candida* infection of the skin and mucous membranes associated with idiopathic endocrinopathy. The etiology of the disease is not well defined. There may be a basic autoimmune disorder associated with the T-cell defect. A wide variety of endocrine abnormalities have been seen, including hypoparathyroidism, Addison's disease, and diabetes. The total lymphocyte count and lymphocyte response to phytohemagglutinin and other mitogens and the total number of T cells are normal. Delayed-hypersensitivity skin tests to a variety of antigens are normal, but the hallmark of the disease is an absent delayed-hypersensitivity skin test response to *Candida* antigen in the presence of severe *Candida* infection. B-cell immunity is intact in patients with chronic mucocutaneous candidiasis, and immunoglobulin levels usually are normal to elevated.

Primary T- and B-Cell Disorders

Severe Combined Immunodeficiency. There are two major forms of severe combined immunodeficiency disease. Each is inherited in a distinctive pattern. The X-linked recessive form was previously termed *X-linked lymphopenic agammaglobulinemia*. The autosomal recessive form was initially termed the *Swiss type of autosomal recessive lymphopenic agammaglobulinemia*. Both disorders are characterized by a complete absence of T- and B-cell immunity, and the patients rarely survive beyond 1 year of age because of poor resistance to infections. The etiology of severe combined immunodeficiency disease is not known. It is commonly believed that the disorder is a result of a defect in the stem cell differentiation with absence of normal development of immunocompetent T cells and B cells. However, some evidence suggests that there may be other etiologic factors. Patients with deficiency of the enzyme adenosine deaminase have demonstrated laboratory and clinical manifestations of a severe combined T- and B-cell immunodeficiency.

The majority of patients with severe combined T- and B-cell immunodeficiency become symptomatic before 6 months of age with recurrent respiratory infections, *Candida* infections of the skin

and mouth, and diarrhea. There are a certain number of infants with mild combined immunodeficiency disease who appear quite normal at 6 to 9 months of age and who may not demonstrate an increased incidence of infection. Patients suspected of having such an immunodeficiency should never be immunized with live attenuated viral vaccine, since there is complication of paralytic polio or fatal encephalitis following immunization with live polio, live measles, or mumps vaccine. *Pneumocystis carinii* and progressive vaccinia are frequent complications.

The T-cell abnormalities are present at birth with lymphopenia. Other findings are a decreased number of T cells, absence of peripheral blood lymphocyte response to PHA and allogeneic cells, and absent thymus shadow. Adenosine deaminase deficiency may be seen in individuals with severe combined immunodeficiency, although the majority of this group of patients have normal enzyme levels. Studies of B-cell immunity are abnormal, with an absence of antibody response following immunization. Biopsy of lymph node and skin will show depletion of T- and B-dependent areas. Biopsy of colonic mucosa will demonstrate an absence of plasma cells.

Cellular Immunodeficiency With Abnormal Immunoglobulin Synthesis (Nezelof's Syndrome). Patients with this disorder demonstrate the following features: (1) susceptibility to viral, bacterial, fungal, and protozoal infections; (2) abnormally depressed T-cell function; and (3) a varying degree of antibody immunodeficiency with various levels of specific immunoglobulins. The disease is sporadic, has no genetic pattern, and is found in both males and females.

The primary defect is a T-cell deficiency, and the B-cell abnormalities are the result of failure of normal T- and B-cell interaction. As already discussed, a complete absence of T cells will result in B-cell abnormalities with defective antibody production to many antigens.

The immunologic defect in these cases has been treated with fetal thymus transplantation and transfer factor, and thymosin has been used with partial success in the reconstitution of T-cell immunity.

Wiskott-Aldrich Syndrome. Patients with Wiskott-Aldrich syndrome show thrombocytopenia, which may be present at birth. The disorder is inherited and sex-linked recessive. The primary defect may be in the macrophages, although the patients demonstrate T- and B-cell abnormalities. The macrophages and immune lymphocytes are unable to process polysaccharide antigen normally. The consequence is an inability to form antibody against polysaccharide-containing organisms such as *Hemophilus influenzae*, pneumococcus, and coliform bacillus. As patients become older, they manifest a gradual loss of both T- and B-cell functions.

The patients show complications of thrombo-

cytopenia with bleeding, ecchymosis, and petechiae. Anemia is frequently present, and a
Coombs'-positive hemolytic anemia may be seen.
Infants with Wiskott-Aldrich syndrome may be
protected during the first 5 to 6 months of life by
maternal antibody. Subsequently, they experience
recurrent viral and bacterial infections, with
eczema of the skin. These patients have a higher
incidence of lymphoreticular malignancies than
does the normal control population.

Studies of the T-cell function during early
infancy may be normal. Varying degrees of T- and
B-cell dysfunction may be seen with progression
of the disease. The patient shows an absence of
blood group IgM isoagglutinins, and no antibody
response is seen following immunization with a
polysaccharide antigen such as typhoid. Often,
there is a normal to elevated level of serum IgG,
decreased serum IgM, and elevated IgA and IgE
levels.

**Immunodeficiency With Ataxia Telangiecta-
sia.** By 4 years of age, patients with ataxia telangiectasia usually develop characteristic symptoms
of ataxia, telangiectasia, and recurrent sinopulmonary infections. Telangiectasia, usually present
by 2 years of age, is seen on the bulbar conjunctiva,
on the ears, and over the bridge of the nose. This
disorder is inherited as an autosomal recessive.
The disease may involve a primary immunologic
defect with secondary involvement of other organs
resulting from a viral or autoimmune disease.

About 80 per cent of patients with ataxia
telangiectasia lack both serum and secretory IgA.
In a majority of the cases, both IgA and IgE may
be absent. Antibody to IgA may develop in these
patients, similar to the situation seen in selective
serum IgA immunodeficiency. In these patients,
circulating IgA–bearing lymphocytes are present.
Cell-mediated immunity is usually impaired, and
the thymus gland is hypoplastic. There is lymphopenia, with depressed response of T cells to mitogen and allogeneic cells.

The immune defects in ataxia telangiectasia
resemble those of the congenitally nude mouse
with selective IgA deficiency. In these nude mice,
the IgA deficiency and the T-cell defect were corrected with thymic allografts. Thus, the primary
T-cell defect in ataxia telangiectasia could result
in IgA and IgG deficiency by failure to facilitate
normal development or suppression of B-cell maturation.

**Immunodeficiency With Short-Limbed Dwarf-
ism.** This immunodeficiency exists as three distinct syndromes. The most severe form (type I) is
associated with severe combined immunodeficiency disease. Type II is associated with cellular
immunodeficiency, and type III is associated with
antibody immunodeficiency. The severity of the
immunologic defects varies in each disorder. All
three show similar skeletal abnormalities, and
these disorders appear to be inherited in an autosomal manner. In short-limbed dwarfism associ-

ated with severe combined immunodeficiency, the
patients become ill in infancy with viral, bacterial,
fungal, or protozoal infections. Patients with short-
limbed dwarfism and cellular immunodeficiency
are susceptible to recurrent respiratory tract infections.

Individuals with short-limbed dwarfism and
antibody deficiency remain well for 5 to 6 months
of life and then experience recurrent bacterial
infections following a course similar to that of
patients with congenital hypogammaglobulinemia.

Immunodeficiency With Enzyme Deficiency.
Two forms of enzyme deficiency exist in association
with immunodeficiency. The first to be discovered
was adenosine deaminase deficiency, which is associated with both T- and B-cell immunodeficiency.
The second was nucleoside phosphorylase, which
is associated with a T-cell immunodeficiency.
Adenosine deaminase and nucleoside phosphorylase are enzymes necessary for the catabolism of
the purine adenosine. Adenosine deaminase catalyzes the conversion of adenosine to inosine, and
nucleoside phosphorylase catalyzes the conversion
of inosine to hypoxanthine. The exact mechanism
by which a deficiency of the enzyme results in the
immune defect is not known. It is postulated that
the immunodeficiency is the result of pyrimidine
starvation secondary to accumulation of adenine
nucleotides. Other possibilities are that elevated
adenosine results in altered immune function and
that accumulated adenosine suppresses lymphocyte functions. The mode of inheritance of these
enzyme defects is autosomal recessive. The carrier
state can be shown in both sexes by decreased
adenosine deaminase or nucleoside phosphorylase
activity.

The degrees of immunodeficiency may be variable. Patients with adenosine deaminase deficiency may have severe combined immunodeficiency or partial defects in T- and B-cell immunity
or in B- or T-cell immunity alone. These patients
usually become symptomatic after the first 6 or 12
months.

The diagnosis of immunodeficiency with enzyme deficiency may be best established by enzyme
assays of red cells. White blood cells and tissue
are also deficient in the enzyme. An intrauterine
diagnosis of adenosine deaminase has been made
with the use of cultured amniotic cells. Patients
with nucleoside phosphorylase deficiency are unable to form uric acid. One may make a rapid
diagnosis of immunodeficiency with nucleoside
phosphorylase by measuring the serum or urine
uric acid, which is extremely low.

Disorders of the Complement System

There are a few significant defects in the
complement system that may lead to a state of
susceptibility to infection. The genetically deter-

mined abnormalities of the complement system have been described and can be classified into the following categories:

1. Defects in inhibitors that result in spontaneous consumption of complement components.

2. Synthesis of defective complement molecules.

3. Absence of a complement component.

Hereditary angioedema is caused by defective synthesis of C1 esterase inhibitor. In normal persons, the C1 esterase inhibitor blocks the activity of C1s and therefore is capable of suppressing the progression of the complement sequence beyond C1. Patients with hereditary angioedema suffer from episodic triggering of the complement system and develop angioedematous reactions in tissues, particularly those of the upper respiratory tract. Recurrent attacks of edema usually involve the skin, gastrointestinal tract, and respiratory mucosa, and involvement of the larynx can be very serious. Hereditary angioedema may exist in two genetic variants. In one type, there is an absence of the C1 esterase inhibitor; the other variety may involve the formation of a nonfunctional C1 esterase molecule.

Patients with C3 deficiency may have repeated infections with pyogenic bacteria. The C3 deficiency leads to an absence of complement-mediated immunoadherence and opsonization as well as defective activation of the latter components of complement. C3 deficiency may occur in different ways, such as failure of synthesis of C3 and absence of C3 inactivator leading to hypercatabolism of C3. Patients with a defect in C3 catabolism as a result of abnormal activity of C3 inactivator may suffer from recurrent pyogenic infections. Treatment consists of replacement of C3 with normal plasma.

Familial C5 dysfunction has been described in patients with Leiner's syndrome who suffer from generalized seborrheic dermatitis, severe diarrhea, and recurrent bacterial infections, usually of the gram-negative variety. Autosomal recessive C2 deficiency may be associated with diseases such as systemic lupus erythematosus. In these individuals, the biologic functions of the complement system may be impaired.

Phagocytic Disorders

Phagocytic disorders can be divided into extrinsic and intrinsic defects. The extrinsic disorders may be secondary to (1) deficiency of antibody and complement factors; (2) suppression of the phagocytic cells by immunosuppressive agents; (3) interference with phagocytic function by corticosteroids; and (4) suppression of circulating neutrophils by autoantibodies.

Intrinsic phagocytic disorders are related to enzymatic deficiencies within the metabolic pathway necessary for killing the bacteria. They include chronic granulomatous disease with a deficiency of NADPH or NADH oxidase, myeloperoxidase deficiency, and glucose-6-phosphate dehydrogenase deficiency.

Chronic Granulomatous Disease (CGD). The major immunologic features include (1) susceptibility to infection with unusual organisms of low virulence such as *Staphylococcus albus* and *Serratia marcescens*; (2) a sex-linked inheritance, with several female variants; (3) onset of symptoms occurs by 2 years of age, with pneumonia, draining lymphadenitis, and splenomegaly; and (4) confirmation of diagnosis by quantitative nitroblue tetrazolium test and quantitative killing curve of bacteria.

The chronic granulomatous disease is inherited as a sex-linked disorder, with manifestations appearing in the first 2 years of life. A rare female variant of this disease has been described. The enzymatic deficiency in chronic granulomatous disease is felt to be either NADH or NADPH oxidase. In the female variant, glutathione peroxidase is believed to be deficient. With the enzymatic deficiency, the intracellular metabolism of the neutrophils and monocytes is abnormal, and there are decreased oxygen consumption and decreased utilization of glucose by the hexose monophosphate shunt, with decreased production of hydrogen peroxide as well as diminished iodinization of bacteria and decreased superoxide anion production. The net result is decreased intracellular killing of certain bacteria and fungi. These individuals are susceptible to the so-called organisms that have low virulence for normal individuals; such organisms have a catalase enzyme and will destroy the hydrogen peroxide that may be present in the cell.

The recommended test for diagnosis of chronic granulomatous disease is the quantitative nitroblue tetrazolium (NBT) test. This test is based on the fact that normal leukocytes reduce the NBT dye at a normal rate during in vitro phagocytosis of particles such as latex. The leukocytes of patients with CGD show no nitroblue tetrazolium dye reduction, whereas carriers may have normal or reduced nitroblue tetrazolium reduction noted mainly in the polymorphs and the monocytes. Patients with CGD are unable to kill certain bacteria at a normal rate. The peripheral white count usually is elevated, even if the patient does not have active infection. Cell immunity is normal, and complement factors may be elevated. There are two variants of the disease. One is the female variant of chronic granulomatous disease associated with deficient glutathione peroxidase; the other is associated with a deficient glucose-6-phosphate dehydrogenase.

Chediak-Higashi Syndrome. This disease is a multisystem autosomal recessive disorder. The symptoms include recurrent bacterial infection with a variety of organisms, hepatosplenomegaly, partial albinism, central nervous system abnormalities, and a high incidence of lymphoreticular malignancy.

The characteristic abnormality is a giant cytoplasmic granular inclusion in white blood cells and platelets that is observed on routine peripheral blood smears. There may be an abnormal neutrophil chemotaxis with abnormal intracellular killing of organisms, which also include streptococci and pneumococci as well as organisms found in chronic granulomatous disease. The killing defect consists of delayed killing time. Oxygen consumption, hydrogen peroxide formation, and hexose monophosphate shunt activity are normal.

Job's Syndrome. Job's syndrome was originally described as a disease of recurrent "cold" staphylococcal abscesses of the skin, lymph nodes, or subcutaneous tissue. Most of these patients do not have abnormal immunologic tests. There have been reports that Job's syndrome may be a variant of chronic granulomatous disease.

Tuftsin Deficiency. This disorder has been reported as a familial deficiency of a phagocytosis-stimulating tetrapeptide (Thr-Lys-Pro-Arg), which is cleaved from a parent immunoglobulin (termed *leukokinin*) molecule in the spleen. It was discovered at Tufts University by Najjar, who named it *tuftsin*. Tuftsin also appears to be absent in patients who have been splenectomized. Local and severe systemic infections occur. Microorganisms include *Candida, Staphylococcus aureus,* and *Streptococcus pneumoniae.*

SECONDARY IMMUNE DEFICIENCY DISEASES

Depressed immune functions occur quite frequently as a consequence of various disease states. The secondary immunodeficiencies are frequently observed in certain infections, malignant conditions (especially those involving the lymphoid system), loss of proteins from the body, drug therapy, aging, and debilitating diseases. The secondary immunodeficiency may affect both the humoral and cellular immune systems. Examples of certain disorders primarily associated with a T- or B-cell defect are shown in Table 5–2. In many cases, both the T- and B-cell systems may be suppressed to a variable degree.

In certain infections such as rubella, there may be a decrease in the immune function. Many lymphoproliferative disorders are accompanied by a secondary immunodeficiency state. This includes multiple myeloma, Waldenstrom's macroglobulinemia, and other lymphoproliferative diseases. These disorders have often been called *monoclonal gammopathies* because excessive amounts of monoclonal types of immunoglobulins are produced. Patients with multiple myeloma frequently suffer recurrent infections and have an unusual susceptibility to various bacterial and fungal infections. The antibody synthesis against exogenously administered antigen is markedly decreased. Patients with Hodgkin's disease develop a progressive immunodeficiency of the cellular immune system, but their humoral immune functions appear essentially normal. It has been discovered that there is a serum factor involved that may be a beta lipoprotein that acts as an immunosuppressive factor. Patients who have active chronic hepatitis B infections have also been known to possess a serum factor that suppresses cellular immune function.

Patients with chronic lymphocytic leukemia develop deficiency of both T- and B-cell immune systems. Both immune systems are essentially normal in acute lymphocytic leukemia. In the latter phases of these lymphoreticular malignant conditions, defective host defense mechanisms allow recurrent infections.

Patients with nephrotic syndrome have low serum levels of albumin and gamma globulin because excessive amounts of these proteins are lost in the urine. Protein losses from the intestinal tract during certain acute and chronic diseases of the bowel may lead to hypogammaglobulinemia and intestinal lymphangiectasia. Both serum proteins and lymphocytes are lost in the stool.

The Acquired Immunodeficiency Syndrome (AIDS)

This disorder, first noted in male homosexuals, is a new, highly lethal epidemic immunodeficiency disease of obscure pathogenesis primarily affecting the T-cell system. At least four major groups of individuals appear to be at risk for AIDS: homosexual men, abusers of intravenous drugs with no history of homosexuality, Haitian immigrants who are not homosexuals and who do not abuse drugs, and hemophiliacs.

Patients with this syndrome present with life-threatening opportunistic infections or Kaposi's sarcoma or both. The immunologic abnormalities found in AIDS are those of a severe and profound cellular immunodeficiency. These include an absence of delayed hypersensitivity; an absolute lymphopenia caused by an absolute deficiency of helper T-cells (T4+ cells); reversal of the usual ratio of phenotypic T-helper to T-suppressor blood cells; depressed lymphocyte responses to mitogens; and an impaired natural killer (NK) cell function in vitro. In contrast, hypergammaglobulinemia is the rule, and antibody titers to a wide range of antigens are often very high; nevertheless, there is some evidence for a B-cell defect as well. Complement components are normal. Elevated interferon and thymosin levels have been reported in most of these patients.

Because AIDS apparently represents a profound progressive and irreversible loss of cell-mediated immunity, several laboratories initiated extensive studies of the thymus gland in the early

1980s. In the aggregate, these studies reveal an essential destruction of the Hassall's corpuscles and marked alterations in the appearance of the thymic epithelial cells. Most of the latter become spindled, have pyknotic nuclei, and appear to be inactive. It is to be recalled here that the thymic epithelial cells produce thymosin α_1, thymosin β_3 and β_4, thymopoietin, thymulin, and most probably other biologically active peptides. Hassall's corpuscles elaborate thymosin α_7. As stated in Chapter 4, these thymic hormones have a profound regulatory role in the terminal differentiation of T cells.

Despite the epidemiologic data suggesting a transmissible, possibly viral, agent as the cause of the immune alterations in AIDS, so far no specific agent has been linked etiologically to the disease. Cytomegalovirus hepatitis and herpesviruses, which were initially thought to be the leading candidates, are no longer considered the causes of this disease. A most recent hypothesis is that AIDS may be caused by a human retrovirus related to the human T-cell leukemia virus (HTLV). This is supported by the following considerations: (1) HTLV is a lymphotrophic retrovirus that preferentially infects helper T cells; (2) another retrovirus, the feline leukemia virus, causes thymic atrophy, lymphopenia, and profound immunosuppression; (3) HTLV has been isolated from peripheral blood lymphocytes of several patients with AIDS; and (4) antibodies specifically reactive with internal structural proteins of HTLV have been found more frequently in the sera of patients with AIDS than in normal sera.

Emergence of HTLV as an etiologic agent also raises the possibility that AIDS is an immune complex–mediated thymic dysfunction. Indeed, the histopathologic changes formed in the thymus glands of patients with AIDS are consistent with an organ-specific immune-complex attack on Hassall's corpuscles and thymic epithelial cells. In accord with this is the finding that HTLV contains an internal structural protein (p19) that strongly cross-reacts with the epithelial cells of the thymus. Also, some of the abnormal laboratory values found in AIDS patients reflect an autoimmune process. Often, there are very great elevations of the immunoglobulins, especially polyclonal IgG, and circulating immune complexes are frequently found. As discussed before, differentiation of circulating T-lymphocytes is thymus-dependent, and there are significant changes in these cells in AIDS. Elevations of β_2-microglobulins as well as thymosin α_1 may reflect cellular death of lymphocytes and thymic epithelial cells, respectively. When normal thymus is incubated with serum from AIDS patients and then with FITC–goat antihuman globulin, the Hassall's corpuscles are fluorescent, a finding not seen with normal sera or with those from other autoimmune syndromes. These observations form the basis of the postulate that AIDS may represent an organ-specific immune complex attack by polyclonal immunoglobulins directed against the thymic epithelial cells and Hassall's corpuscles.

DIAGNOSIS AND LABORATORY EVALUATION OF IMMUNODEFICIENCY DISORDERS

The Clinical Manifestations of the Immunodeficient Patient. Recurrent infection is the hallmark of the immunodeficient patient. The following types of infection may suggest an immunologic defect:

1. Recurrent infection caused by bacteria of high grade virulence.
2. Those caused by low-grade virulence or unusual organisms.
3. Those caused by fungi and unusual reactions to vaccines.

The nature of the immune deficiency determines the spectrum of infections that may be encountered. The primary T-cell deficiencies demonstrate an unusual susceptibility to intracellular infections, which may be caused by viruses, fungi, and certain bacteria such as *Mycobacterium tuberculosis*. B-cell deficiencies allow infections by organisms that are largely disposed by opsonization (e.g., pneumococci, staphylococci, and streptococci).

In the evaluation of patients suspected of immunodeficiency diseases, one should obtain a detailed history. Some of the important points to be investigated are as follows:

1. History of allergy and tests completed in past.
2. Prior surgery, particularly tonsillectomy and adenoidectomy as well as appendectomy. Results of pathologic examination on excised tissue may help in the assessment of the immune system.
3. Radiation therapy to the thymus or nasopharynx.
4. Sites of infections and organisms recovered; age at onset of infections.
5. Previous immunizations and reactions.
6. Prior gamma globulin treatment.
7. Family history of collagen diseases, endocrine disorders, tumor, or early death.

Evaluation of the T-cell Deficiency. Generally, a T-cell deficiency is indicated by increased susceptibility to infection by fungi, viruses, atypical acid-fast organisms, and some of the so-called "lower-grade" pathogens. Various organisms that are involved include *Candida albicans*, vaccinia and mumps virus, *Mycoplasma*, and *Pneumocystis carinii*. *Pneumocystis carinii* is frequently involved and produces pulmonary lesions in patients with a combined B- and T-cell deficiency. In these patients, the pneumonia shows characteristic accumulations of foamy, pink-staining exudate containing many *Pneumocystis* organisms. The

following tests are used for the evaluation of the
T-cell system:

1. Absolute lymphocyte count.
2. Delayed type skin reaction.
3. Lymphocyte stimulation test.
4. Migration inhibitory factor test.
5. Examination of circulating lymphocytes for
T-cell markers.
6. Radiologic evidence of normal lymphoid
tissues.

Skin tests for delayed hypersensitivity to common antigens may be of little help in young children who have not had the opportunity to develop a cell-mediated immune reaction to the antigens. However, a negative skin test to *Candida* antigens in children suffering from infection with this fungus has a diagnostic usefulness. Morphologic analysis of the small lymphocytes in the peripheral blood and the deep cortical areas of biopsy lymph nodes provides some information about the adequacy of the T-cell system.

Evaluation of the B-cell System. The deficiency of the B-cell system is generally indicated with frequent bouts of infections with pathogenic organisms causing otitis media, pneumonia, meningitis, and other infections. Such organisms include pneumococcus, *Streptococcus, Hemophilus, Meningococcus,* and hepatitis virus. A variety of immunologic tests are available for quantitation of the immunoglobulin levels. The antibody tests for humoral immunity can be divided into two groups: (1) tests for the presence of immunoglobulin and existing antibodies to common antigens; and (2) tests for antibody formation following active immunization. The immunoglobulin levels can be quantitated by various techniques, including radial immunodiffusion, immunofluorescence, and other immunoprecipitin techniques. There should be some caution in the evaluation of immunoglobulin levels in adult sera, as they may vary greatly among individuals. The measurements may not be reliable in the case of quantitation of various monoclonal gamma globulins owing to the nature of the specificity of the antisera and the various standards used. Absence or low serum levels of one or more immunoglobulins may have three possible causes:

1. Absence or decreased number of B cells in circulation of lymphoid tissue.
2. A defect in the immunoglobulin secretion by B cells.
3. An increased rate of immunoglobulin catabolism.

Tests that can be carried out to distinguish between the various possibilities involve the immunofluorescent staining of the membrane of the various lymphocytes to analyze the B-cell population in the circulation as well as in the lymph nodes. In addition, one can look for the presence of germinal centers and plasma cells in the lymph nodes.

Tests for T-cell Function

ABSOLUTE LYMPHOCYTE COUNT. The count in normal children usually is above 2000/mm³ during the first 4 years of life. The lymphocyte count during maturation is an average of 2500, with a lower limit of 1000/mm³. Normal infants should show a count greater than 1500 small lymphocytes per millimeter.

DELAYED-TYPE SKIN REACTIONS. Five different antigens may be employed: *Trichophyton, Candida,* streptokinase-streptodornase, mumps, and purified protein derivative (PPD). Most normal persons show a positive response to one or more antigens. The most consistently positive antigen is *Candida,* which shows a positive delayed skin reaction in 80 to 95 per cent of normal persons 7 months of age or older. If skin reactions to the aforementioned delayed-hypersensitivity antigens are negative, sensitivity tests to 2,4-dinitrochlorobenzene may be indicated.

LYMPHOCYTE STIMULATION TEST. This test is an in-vitro test useful in the diagnosis of thymic dysplasia in infants whose absolute lymphocyte count appears within the normal range. In this test, a pure lymphocyte fraction obtained from peripheral blood is cultured with phytohemagglutinin (PHA). Lymphocytes from normal persons will show 50 per cent or more conversion to blast forms, whereas cells from individuals with thymic abnormalities demonstrate little or no transformation of lymphocytes in culture.

MIGRATION INHIBITORY FACTOR TEST. The sensitized thymus-derived T-lymphocytes in the presence of antigen release a number of factors, one of which inhibits the migration of macrophages from capillary tubes. Production of the migration inhibitory factor (MIF) is a good in-vitro indicator of the presence of cell-mediated immunity.

EXAMINATION OF CIRCULATING LYMPHOCYTES FOR T-CELL MARKERS (Table 5–3). Human T-lymphocytes have a surface receptor for sheep erythrocytes that provides a reliable marker for the identification of T cells. This reaction is temperature-dependent, requiring reduced temperature and prolonged incubation at 4°C. E-rosette formation requires viable lymphocytes and has been shown to be dependent on a surface receptor.

The method of enumerating peripheral E rosettes involves isolating lymphocytes on a Ficoll-Hypaque gradient to remove human erythrocytes and adding an excess ratio of sheep erythrocytes to lymphocytes, then incubating the cells overnight at 4°C and resuspending and counting cells with more than three or more adherent red cells/lymphocytes. The percentage of peripheral blood lymphocytes that form E rosettes in normal adults varies between 65 and 78 per cent.

Antithymocyte serum, the antisera to T cells, has been developed by immunization of animals with human thymus cells and human or monkey thymus cell suspensions. Extensive absorption with erythrocytes, immunoglobulin, and B cells, such as B-cell chronic lymphatic leukemia or cultured B-cell lines and human fetal embryonic liver cells, is required to render such antisera specific for human T cells. If the absorbed antiserum is used in immunofluorescence tests, approximately 80 per cent of peripheral blood lymphocytes are identified as T cells. Various studies have demonstrated a subpopulation of T cells with a surface receptor for the Fc portion of the IgG. This group of T cells with Fc receptors may represent T-helper cells.

RADIOLOGIC EVIDENCE OF NORMAL LYMPHOID TISSUE OF THYMUS AND PHARYNX.

LYMPH NODE BIOPSY. A depletion of paracortical lymphoid cells indicates a T-cell defect.

Tests for B-cell Function

The various tests for B-cell function could be presented in two groups: (1) tests for presence of immunoglobulins and existing antibodies to common antigens, and (2) tests for antibody formation following active immunization.

TESTS FOR PRESENCE OF IMMUNOGLOBULINS AND EXISTING ANTIBODIES TO COMMON ANTIGENS.

Schick Test. If an individual has been previously immunized with diphtheria toxoid and his humoral immune system is normal, the Schick test will be negative. A positive Schick test in such cases is presumptive evidence of IgG deficiency.

A and B Isohemagglutinins. Isohemagglutinins are present normally after about 1 year of age and are primarily of the IgM class. The absence of isohemagglutinins is presumptive evidence of IgM deficiency. The isoagglutinin titer in the first 2 years of life is low.

Immunoelectrophoresis. This test is used to determine qualitative levels of immunoglobulins IgG, IgM, and IgA. The sera of newborns show a normal absence of IgM and IgA.

Quantitative and Immunoglobulin Determinations. IgG concentration of 200 mg/dl is considered the lower adult threshold value. IgA deficiency shows less than 5 mg/dl of serum.

Quantitation of IgG Subclasses. Patients with normal levels of immunoglobulins may have a history of recurrent pyogenic infection that is associated with selective IgG subclass deficiencies.

Rectal Mucosal Biopsy Examination. A biopsy may be taken for routine histology and immunofluorescent localization of IgG, IgM, and IgA immunoglobulins. Infants over 1 month of age will have many plasma cells in the lamina propria of the rectal mucosa. This is a good screening test for evidence of antibody production in suspected humoral immune deficiency cases.

Circulating B-Lymphocytes for Surface Immunoglobulins (Table 5–3). The presence of easily detectable surface immunoglobulin as determined by vital staining with immunofluorescent antisera of IgG heavy chain determinants has been applied to identify B cells. So that some of the problems related to Fc receptors are avoided, reagents using

Fab and (Fab')₂ digest of antisera are employed. Careful attention to temperature during the staining procedure is observed, and incubation of cells at 37°C and washing before staining with immunofluorescent conjugates have been reported to facilitate detection of lymphocytes with stable surface Ig. The dominant surface Ig determinants on B cells in normal individuals are IgM and IgD. Many B cells carry both these determinants. The significance of the strong representation of IgD, besides its minor contribution to serum Ig, has suggested that it may be important in the clonal maturation of B cells or in triggering further events affecting B-cell response. The number of circulating B cells with easily detectable surface Ig in peripheral blood of normal adults has ranged from 8 to 15 per cent.

B cells have a surface receptor for the third component of complement and have been utilized as a means of detecting B cells in suspension. The most widely applied method demonstrates complement receptors using sheep erythrocytes sensitized with purified IgM antibodies and reacted with complement. These EAC cells can then be demonstrated to adhere to B-lymphocytes to form rosettes through the complement surface receptor. Peripheral blood lymphocytes in normal individuals with EAC receptors also have surface Ig markers. Many B cells have receptors for the Fc portion of the IgG and may be identified by use of IgG-coated erythrocytes or fluorescent-tagged aggregated IgG. Such a receptor is also present on monocytes and some T-cells. Since some B cells apparently lack Fc receptor, application of this technique as a lymphocyte marker probe is limited. The identification of a population of lymphoid cells that have Fc IgG receptor but lack other B- and T-cell markers has raised the question concerning whether there may be a third population of lymphoid cells. The cell responsible for lymphoid cell-mediated antibody-dependent cytotoxicity has been shown to have Fc receptors without other identifying surface markers.

TESTS FOR ANTIBODY FORMATION FOLLOWING ACTIVE IMMUNIZATION.

Diptheria, Pertussis, and Tetanus (DPT) Vaccination. A standard dose is given weekly for 3 successive weeks. Following immunization with diphtheria toxoid, one can administer a Schick test. A positive Schick test is seen in agammaglobulinemia.

Active Immunization with Typhoid Vaccine. Typhoid immunization can be given once a week for 3 weeks. Typhoid O and H agglutinins can be easily determined in the clinical laboratory. The anti-H titer after three injections will be 160 or greater, and patients with an antibody deficiency may have a titer of less than 1:5.

THE IMMUNOLOGY OF CANCER

At various points in the preceding section, we have repeatedly referred to observations indicating an important relationship between some impairment of the immune status and the occurrence of cancer. It is appropriate, therefore, that in the sequential order of this chapter the immunology of cancer follows the presentation of diseases of immunodeficiency.

Cancer can be defined as a disease that can be triggered and influenced by a wide variety of factors such as viruses, genes, and chemical and physical agents. The factors involved in a particular tumor may be single or multiple.

The objectives of tumor immunology are to explore the complex immunologic interrelationship between the host and the tumor and to manipulate this relationship for the purpose of diagnosis, prevention, and treatment of cancer.

TUMOR ANTIGENS

It is well established that the existence of specific antigens on tumors induced by chemical, physical, or viral agents may elicit an immunologic response in the host. Antigens associated with the tumor that can be qualitatively, quantitatively, or temporally different from normal cells are called *tumor-associated antigens (TAA)*. Antigens present in tumor cells but absent in normal cells have been called *tumor-specific antigens (TSA)*. Antigens that are able to induce an immune response or resistance to tumor growth in the autochthonous host have been called *tumor-specific transplantation antigens (TSTA)*. The majority of the tumors, including those induced by chemical carcinogens and viruses as well as spontaneously arising tumors, carry antigens that elicit an immune response in the host.

During carcinogenesis, there is often a retrogressive dedifferentiation, normally repressed in the mature normal cell, that leads to increased expression of the genetic information. This process leads to increased formation of fetal or embryonic components of the cell. With the advent of sensitive immunologic assay methods, there has been increasing evidence that extremely small amounts of fetal antigens may be present in normal adult persons. With development of a tumor, there is a reversion of the cell to the embryonic form, and the fetal antigens are formed in increasing amounts. Therefore, the quantitative measurement of fetal antigens is useful—practically diagnostic—in the characterization of certain tumors that produce large quantities of these antigens. The embryonic or fetal antigens are more correctly referred to as *tumor-associated phase-specific antigens (TAPSA)*, since such antigens are found in high concentration in fetal and tumor tissues and in very low concentration in normal adult tissues.

The tumor cells, when compared with their normal counterparts, may show the following features:

1. Deletion of normal surface cell antigens.

2. Membrane alteration with changes in composition and immunochemical reactivity.

3. Formation of tumor-specific antigens (TSA).

4. Retrogressive dedifferentiation with formation of tumor-associated phase-specific antigens (TAPSA) or fetal antigens.

Deletion of Normal Surface Cell Antigens

An early loss of the blood group antigens A, B, and H has been shown in many human epithelial cancers, such as squamous cell carcinoma of the cervix, head, and neck. Tests for the presence or absence of A, B, and H antigens on histologic sections of tumor have been used for early immunologic diagnosis of carcinoma. The exact mechanism leading to deletion of normal surface antigens in tumor cells is unknown. One postulated mechanism is that the cell surface may combine with the carcinogen to form a neoantigen, leading to antibody production; the resulting autoantibody causes the deletion of the surface antigen.

Membrane Alterations of Tumor Cells

When compared with their normal counterparts, the surface membranes of tumor cells demonstrate many physicochemical and immunochemical differences. Surface membrane changes in tumor cells definitely involve a difference in the distribution and density of normal membrane macromolecules. Tumor cells are more susceptible than normal cells to agglutination by plant agglutinins, such as concanavalin A and wheat germ agglutinins. In addition, there are alterations in the lipid and glycoprotein composition of tumor cell membranes.

Tumor-Specific Antigens (TSA) and Tumor-Specific Transplantation Antigens (TSTA)

Tumors may be induced experimentally by chemical or physical agents and viruses. Individually distinct antigens are expressed in tumors induced by chemical or physical agents, so cross-immunization is rarely possible, even in the presence of tumors of similar morphology induced by the same carcinogen. In contrast to the virus-induced tumor, each new tumor has unique properties of its own antigenic specificity. However, tumors induced by the same virus in different species may display identical tumor antigens, which are related and specific for the virus-induced tumor. Individually specific neoantigens may be shown in several tumors of one host induced by the same carcinogen. The absence of immunologic cross-reactivity in certain tumor antigens induced by chemical carcinogens such as methylcholanthrene has been proved. The neoantigens of chemically induced tumors are best demonstrated by in-vitro serologic techniques such as immunodiffusion and immunofluorescence.

There are two major categories of tumor-associated antigens in virus-induced neoplasms: (1) the virus-specific antigens; and (2) the newly formed antigens that were not present in normal cells before neoplastic transformation. Virus-induced tumors have been shown to have individually specific antigens in addition to the common antigens coded by the virus. Antigens belonging in the second category may arise as a product of specific interaction of the viral genome with the host genome, resulting in uncovering of normal or pre-existing cell products such as fetal embryonic antigens.

Two categories of tumor antigens have been distinguished: (1) those that form part of the cell surface; and (2) those that do not. Those that do not form a part of the cell surface are exemplified by certain virus-related antigens of the DNA viruses. They may be products of viral genes, although not incorporated into virus particles, and may continue to be produced within tumor cells that no longer release infectious virus. The group-specific antigens of RNA oncogenic viruses provide another example; in this case, the antigens are components of the virus particle and are not known to play any part in the rejection of tumor cells. The group-specific antigens are located intracellularly and elicit an immune response that can be demonstrated serologically. The antigens responsible for rejection reactions and relevant to immunotherapy are at the cell surface, where they make the cell vulnerable to attack by humoral and cellular immune responses. These cell-surface antigens are called *TSTA* because the usual techniques for their demonstration involve transplantation of tumor cells from one host organism to another. There is a common belief that a distinction could be made between chemically induced tumors and virus-induced tumors, since chemically induced tumors possess unique TSTA and virus-induced tumors share a TSTA common to all tumors. This difference is relative rather than absolute, and thus individually distinct TSTA may be a characteristic of tumors generally. This feature of individually distinct TSTA is often overlooked in virus-induced tumors with a virus-related cross-reacting antigen.

One of the best examples for the existence of a human tumor virus is the Epstein-Barr virus (EBV), which is a DNA virus. EBV is closely associated with infectious mononucleosis, Burkitt's lymphoma, and nasopharyngeal carcinoma, and it is believed to be the etiologic agent in infectious mononucleosis. Current evidence has been obtained for the presence of the EBV genome in tumor biopsies of Burkitt's lymphoma and nasopharyngeal carcinoma. However, the EBV genome has not been found in a variety of other lymphoproliferative diseases.

There is some indirect evidence that cervical carcinoma may result from herpes simplex virus type II infection. Preliminary studies for herpes simplex viral genome in cervical cancer biopsies with nucleic acid hybridization have produced both positive and negative results.

RNA tumor viruses have been demonstrated in association with mouse mammary carcinoma, mouse leukemia, and mammary carcinoma in Rhesus monkeys. The hypothesis for the viral etiology of human breast cancer stems from the various studies of mouse mammary cancer. The evidence for etiologic association of an RNA tumor virus in human breast cancer is still incomplete. A recognizable virus has not been isolated from human breast cancer tissue, and the virus-like particles that have been isolated from human milk have not been shown to have biologic tumor-inducing activity.

There are experimental data to support the concept that RNA viruses may be involved in the pathogenesis of human leukemia. However, there is no convincing evidence that viral particles seen with the electron microscope are regularly present in leukemic cells. In addition, the virus-like particles have been noted in normal patients.

Phase-Specific Fetal Antigens Associated with Human Tumors

Trace amounts of fetal antigens and the probable regression of gene activity at a given phase in the adult differentiated cell can be detected in normal adult tissue. Many of the fetal antigens that can be considered as phase-specific gene products appear in malignant tumors in larger amounts than in normal tissue. The tumor cells can arise from either (1) a transformation of normal cells, with a retrogressive dedifferentiation of phase-specific gene products; or (2) undifferentiated cell populations that express significant amounts of the fetal phase-specific gene product.

Table 5–4 lists some of the more common fetal and placental antigens associated with human tumors. The fetal antigens that can be transported across the cell membranes are significant, since immunologic tests for the quantitation of such antigens are useful as tumor markers. Alpha-fetoprotein (AFP) has a high binding affinity to estrogen and may play a role in hormonal regulation. There is some evidence that AFP has immunoregulatory properties with a suppressive effect on antibody synthesis. This phenomenon has been demonstrated in vitro to a T-cell–dependent antigen in both the primary and secondary antibody response. The exact physiologic role for most of the other fetal proteins is not well known. However, certain fetal proteins such as carcinoembryonic antigen (CEA) and AFP are tumor mark-

TABLE 5–4 FETAL AND PLACENTAL ANTIGENS ASSOCIATED WITH HUMAN TUMORS

Antigen	Fetal Tissue of Origin	Principal Type of Tumors
I. Fetal Antigens		
1. Alpha-fetoprotein (AFP)	Liver	Hepatomas, teratomas
2. Carcinoembryonic antigen (CEA) and subspecies CEA-S	GI tract	GI tract and variety of other tumors
3. α_2H-ferroprotein	Liver	Leukemia, Hodgkin's disease
4. Fetal sulfoglycoprotein	GI tract	Stomach cancer
5. β-oncofetal antigen	Fetal organs	All types of carcinoma
6. γ-fetoprotein (γFP)	GI tract, spleen, thymus	Many different tumors
7. Pancreatic oncofetal antigen	Pancreas	Pancreatic tumors
II. Placental Antigens		
1. Human chorionic gonadotropin (HCG)	Trophoblasts	Choriocarcinoma, teratocarcinoma
2. Placental alkaline phosphatase	Placenta	Various tumors

ers, and assays for the antigens are useful to monitor the tumor growth, as discussed subsequently.

THE IMMUNE RESPONSE TO TUMOR

It is generally accepted that cell-mediated and humoral immune responses play a major role in host-tumor relationships. Histologic evidence of immune response to the tumor is indicated by infiltration of several types of mononuclear inflammatory cells, including lymphocytes and histiocytes, and increased cellularity of the regional lymph nodes. The ability of the host to distinguish the tumor-associated antigens as well as foreign antigens and to respond to them forms the basis of the classic immunologic surveillance theory of host defense against neoplasia. Immune cells play a significant role in these host defense mechanisms against neoplasia.

The cell-mediated immune mechanisms play a significant role in tumor rejection responses. The tumor-specific immune responses can be monitored in vitro by employing a cytotoxicity test that demonstrates the cytotoxic or cytostatic effects of sensitized lymphocytes by determining their capacity to inhibit the growth of tumor cells in culture. In-vitro studies have shown that immunocompetent cells can destroy tumor cells. At least

four distinct reactions against tumor cells have been described. They are discussed subsequently.

Lysis of Tumor Cells by Activated T Cells (Fig. 5–2). The contact of a sensitized T-lymphocyte with a target cell results in selective destruction and increased permeability of the plasma membrane of the target cells.

Lysis of Tumor Cells in the Presence of Antibody and Complement (Fig. 5–3). This is the classic reaction of lysis of cells with antibody and complement. The binding of complement components requires suitable aggregation of surface-bound immunoglobulin; such aggregation requires close apposition of several molecules of the membrane tumor antigens.

Antibody-Dependent Cellular Cytotoxicity (ADCC) of Tumor Cell. ADCC is mediated by nonimmune and nonspecific effector cells that lack T- or B-cell markers. The effector cells are called K, or killer cells. They initiate lysis of the tumor cells bound with sensitizing antibody to specific tumor antigens. The cytotoxicity is mediated by nonimmune mononuclear cells attacking antibody-sensitized target cells through the Fc receptors (Fig. 5–4). Free immune complexes can inhibit the K cell function, presumably by binding to the Fc receptors. There may be competition for these receptors between free immune complexes and target-bound antibodies. Very low dilutions of

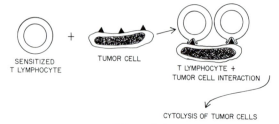

LYSIS OF TUMOR CELLS BY ACTIVATED T CELLS

Figure 5–2

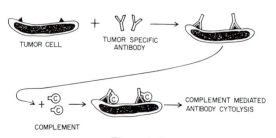

LYSIS OF TUMOR CELLS BY ANTIBODY AND COMPLEMENT

Figure 5–3

ANTIBODY DEPENDENT CELLULAR CYTOTOXICITY OF TUMOR CELLS

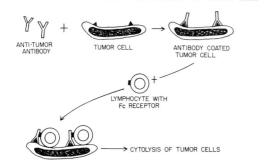

Figure 5–4

antiserum insufficient to induce complement-dependent lysis may still be effective in inducing ADCC. There is evidence to demonstrate that the effector cells are neither T cells nor the classic B cells.

Lysis of Tumor Cells by Armed Macrophages. Peritoneal macrophages can become specifically cytotoxic after incubation with either immune lymphoid cells or cell-free supernatant from cultures consisting of sensitized lymphocytes and specific macrophage arming factor (SMAF) (Fig. 5–5). The SMAF is believed to be smaller than the intact immunoglobulin and has a specific recognition site for the target cells. The type of lymphocyte involved in the generation of SMAF has not been definitely characterized. This phenomenon has been primarily demonstrated in experiments with mice.

IMMUNE SURVEILLANCE, IMMUNODEFICIENCY, AND CANCER

Immune surveillance is the mechanism whereby the host mounts an immune response against antigens expressed by the tumor. By somatic mutation or other equivalent processes, the immune system is able to recognize and eliminate foreign patterns of antigens arising in the body. The concept of immune surveillance suggests that a mutant cell that is potentially responsible for neoplastic transformation develops neoantigens and elicits an immunologic host response. The immunologic response monitored against this antigen is sufficient so that a clone of immunocompetent cells can appear and eliminate the abnormal mutants.

It is generally accepted that some form of an immune surveillance mechanism occurs continuously, but there is considerable controversy as to whether the surveillance mechanism requires immunologic rejection rather than elimination by nonimmunologic mechanisms. The evidence for an immune surveillance system is as follows:

1. After renal transplantation, patients taking immunosuppressive drugs develop an increased incidence of tumor.

2. Stimulation of immune reactivity by specific immunization or nonspecific methods causes a decreased incidence of tumor after infection with certain oncogenic viruses.

3. There is increased incidence of both lymphoreticular and solid tumors in patients with immunodeficiency diseases.

The increased incidence of cancer with old age has been cited as an example of the association of human malignancy with impaired immunologic status and thus as evidence supporting the concept of immunosurveillance. Observed exceptions to the increased incidence of cancer with old age are germ cell tumors of the testes, which occur mostly in young men, and nodular sclerosing Hodgkin's disease, which is seen mostly in young women.

It is well established that the incidence of malignancy is greatly increased in patients with congenital immunodeficiency diseases in comparison with the general population. The incidence of cancer is roughly 10 per cent for patients with Wiskott-Aldrich syndrome, common variable immunodeficiency, or ataxia telangiectasia, and it is

LYSIS OF TUMOR CELLS BY MACROPHAGES AND SPECIFIC MACROPHAGE ARMING FACTOR

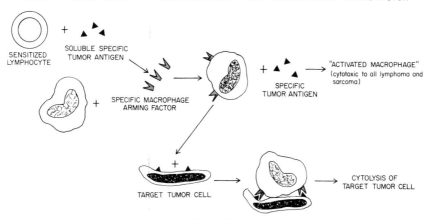

Figure 5–5

about 5 per cent for patients with Bruton-type agammaglobulinemia or severe combined immunodeficiency.

If the concept of immunosurveillance is valid, one would predict an excess of cancer in patients with impaired immunity secondary to other diseases. In patients with respiratory sarcoidosis and lepromatous leprosy, a depressed T-lymphocyte function has been demonstrated, although there is no evidence that leprosy is associated with increased risk of malignancy. However, the risk of developing cancer in patients with respiratory sarcoidosis was found to be greater than in the general population.

Recipients of renal transplants constitute the largest group of patients receiving immunosuppressive drugs over a prolonged period. Renal transplant patients showed an increased incidence of lymphoma 35 times that of the general population, and the tumors were mostly reticulum cell sarcomas. Risk of skin cancer was four times higher than normal, and the risk of other types of cancer was slightly higher than expected. It has been postulated that herpesvirus infection in a setting of prolonged antigenic stimulation may be responsible for the increased incidence of lymphoid malignancy and epithelial tumors of the skin, lip, and cervix in patients on immunosuppressive therapy. It is well known that the majority of transplant recipients showed evidence of infections with herpesvirus, especially cytomegalovirus. The evidence for herpesvirus etiology for other cancers is weaker than it is for the EBV and Burkitt's lymphoma; however, serologic evidence points to the association of the EBV with nasopharyngeal carcinoma and herpes simplex type II with cervical carcinoma. It is of interest that cervical carcinoma is among the few nonlymphoid malignancies occurring with greater frequency among transplant patients than in the general population.

The immune surveillance theory has been challenged with the observation that malignancies in individuals with immunodeficiency are usually in the lymphoreticular system. Schwartz has proposed that the defect in immunity does not involve a failure of surveillance against neoplastic cells but that the disordered immune system in immunodeficient patients is unable to terminate the lymphoproliferative response to antigenic stimulation and the subsequent formation of lymphoreticular tumors.

In transplant patients, the majority of the tumors (60 per cent) were reported to be of lymphoid origin, and the frequency was even higher in patients who were congenitally T-cell–deficient. This is *not* consistent with the immune surveillance concept, which states that neoplastic cells should appear spontaneously in the body and be rejected by the immune system. There is no increased incidence of mammary carcinoma, which is a common tumor, in immunodeficient patients. Skin, lip, and cervical cancers are the only epithelial tumors that show a slightly increased incidence in transplant patients. It is suspected that these epithelial tumors are of viral origin. Thus, patients with defective T-cell systems are more susceptible to virus infections and virus-related tumors.

MECHANISMS OF TUMOR ESCAPE AND IMMUNOLOGIC ENHANCEMENT

There are numerous factors that can facilitate the escape of tumor cells from the immune surveillance mechanism. Some of the important considerations are as follows:

1. Modulation of the cell-surface antigenic structure with alteration of the host immune response.

2. Rapid turnover of antigenic cell-surface antigens with release of large amounts of free tumor-associated antigens and immune complexes.

3. Production of tumor cell-specific antibody and host tissue enzymes that inactivate suppressor lymphoid cells.

4. Rapid growth of the malignant cells, with formation of a large tumor mass.

5. Development of a varying tumor cell population that is less immunogenic to the host.

6. Appearance of suppressor cells that dampen host immune response against the tumor cells.

7. Immunosuppressive agents responsible for neoplastic transformation.

8. Immune deficiencies in the host.

Many serum factors, including antigen-antibody complexes, antigens, and antibody capable of blocking the cytotoxic effect of sensitized cells, can provide important escape mechanisms. The nature of blocking serum factors and the mechanism of blocking have been only partially elucidated. Blocking may occur by binding of serum factors to antigens, thus preventing cellular recognition by specific lymphoid effector cells. The degree of blocking produced by immune complexes is critically related to their physical configuration. The most effective complexes are small and soluble because large complexes are readily removed from the circulation by the reticuloendothelial cells. Small complexes with a molecular weight of less than 1,000,000 are stable and are potent inhibitors of effector cells in antibody-dependent cytotoxicity.

Proposed mechanisms for the ability of serum factors to suppress host immune response against neoplastic cells have been categorized as afferent, central, or efferent inhibition, depending on which portion of the immune system is blocked.

Afferent Blockade. Antibodies or antibody parts of immune complexes bind to antigenic determinants on the tumor and mask the antigenic sites, thus preventing recognition by the host immune cells.

Efferent Blockade. The antigenic sites of the tumor are masked by antibody or immune complexes or both, which prevents recognition and destruction of the tumor cells by immune effector cells. Soluble antigens and antigen-antibody complexes may bind to recognition sites of the immune effector cells and interfere with the ability of these cells to recognize the target tumor cells.

Central Blockade. Tolerogenic soluble serum factors or suppressor cells or both could induce a state of tolerance and prevent a tumor-destructive immune response.

The afferent blockade is an important mechanism for enhancing tumor growth in vivo. The effector mechanism is a plausible explanation for blocking in vitro with the use of hyperimmune antisera. Enhancement is often achieved with a single injection of antiserum, yet the binding of antibody to tumor cells is a transient phenomenon. The masking hypothesis is difficult to explain with the observation that very small quantities of antiserum are sufficient to induce enhancement. It seems more plausible that enhancement may be the result of an effector cell inhibition or central blockade.

IMMUNOLOGIC EVALUATION AND DIAGNOSIS OF CANCER

There are several approaches to the immunodiagnosis of cancer, as shown in Table 5–5. A popular approach is the detection of tumor-associated antigens. Several of the various assays may seem promising, although the usefulness, sensitivity, and specificity of most of the assays remain to be determined.

The tumor-associated antigens may be found in larger quantities in tumor cells than in normal cells. To be useful for immunodiagnosis, the tumor antigens should be common to a variety of tumors, at least of the same histologic type, and appear and persist in circulation or in biologic fluids. Common antigens in tumors have been identified and classified in the following categories:

Virus-Induced or Associated. Tumors induced by the same virus may share some of the same common tumor-associated antigens even when they differ in morphologic appearance.

Fetal or Embryonic Antigens. Such antigens are present on normal fetal cells and in a variety of tumors, regardless of etiology.

Tissue Antigens. Normal tissue antigens may be expressed in larger amounts in tumor cells, and

TABLE 5–5 IMMUNODIAGNOSIS OF CANCER

I. Detection of tumor-associated antigens on tumor cells and in plasma and biologic fluids
II. Immune competence of cancer patients
III. Immune response to tumor-associated antigens
 A. Humoral immunity
 B. Cell-mediated immunity

some of these may be specific for the organ from which the tumor is derived.

Assays for Tumor-Associated Antigens

Circulating antigens potentially useful for immunodiagnosis of cancer may be divided into categories of fetal antigens, hormones, and miscellaneous. A useful test would have the features of a high specificity with high sensitivity, with a definite quantitative difference from normal to benign cases. Currently, many of the tumor cell markers are useful for following patients known to have tumor, but they have not been proved useful for early detection of cancer patients prior to metastatic lesions.

The fetal and placental antigens suggested for possible diagnostic application are listed in Table 5–4. CEA is present in nonmalignant adult tissue and normal plasma. The use of serum CEA assays to differentiate between patients with tumors and patients with benign disease depends on relative concentrates of CEA in tumor tissue versus other nontumor tissues and the destruction of the barrier to leakage of CEA into the plasma. Many of the studies of patients with benign gastrointestinal disease and cancer patients with localized disease have demonstrated a large percentage of false-positives, and many patients with localized GI cancer do not have elevated CEA values. More recently, a subspecies assay for CEA, called CEA-S, has been developed. The assay for CEA-S detected a higher proportion of patients with GI cancer and demonstrated a very low incidence of false-positive and false-negative results in noncancer patients. Currently, CEA and CEA-S assays are most useful in monitoring patients with cancer known to produce CEA substances to indicate prognosis.

Alpha-fetoprotein (AFP) has been found to be present in small amounts in normal serum. Serum AFP assays are useful in the differential diagnosis and serve to monitor patients with hepatoma, choriocarcinoma, and testicular tumors. More recently, serum and amniotic fluid AFP assays have been useful for the detection of neural tube defects of the fetus during pregnancy.

Investigations of the various other tumors associated with fetal antigens are currently under way; however, their practical usefulness has not been sufficiently documented.

Certain hormones have been reported to be useful as tumor markers. Human chorionic gonadotropin (HCG) and human placental lactogen (HPL) may be ectopically produced by a small proportion of tumors arising in areas outside the reproductive tract. HCG assays have been useful in monitoring choriocarcinoma and certain testicular tumors known to produce HCG. Pro-ACTH (adrenocortical trophic hormone) may be useful in the diagnosis of lung cancer, and a high percentage of patients with lung cancer have demonstrated elevated serum ACTH in preliminary studies.

Tests for Immune Competence in Immunodiagnosis of Cancer

There is a correlation between general immunocompetence and the level of specific tumor immunity with extent of disease and prognosis in patients in a wide variety of malignancies. The changes in levels of general immunocompetence and specific tumor immunity will parallel the changes in the clinical status of the patient with cancer. In almost every type of human cancer tested, patients who have a poor, depressed immune competence have a worse prognosis than patients demonstrating a normal immune system.

Immunocompetence declines markedly with advancing disease, and the patient becomes more immunodeficient. Progressive tumor growth with resulting immunodeficiency has been observed in Hodgkin's disease, leukemia, lymphomas, and a wide variety of solid epithelial tumors, such as carcinomas of the breast, lung, colon, head, and neck. In Hodgkin's disease, there is often a depressed cell-mediated immune reaction; in chronic lymphocytic leukemia, humoral antibody response is impaired, whereas the cell-mediated immunity is slightly depressed. Cell-mediated immunity and inflammation may be markedly suppressed in various solid tumors, whereas the antibody response is only mildly impaired.

The depression of the immune competence of cancer patients may be useful diagnostically. In the normal or benign disease population, decreased immune competence may have diagnostic implications. It has been demonstrated that immune functions that are impaired in cancer patients include delayed hypersensitivity responses, peripheral blood lymphocyte counts, lymphocyte blastogenic responses, T-lymphocyte levels, B-lymphocyte levels, serum immunoglobulin levels, complement levels, primary and secondary antibody responses, specific antitumor levels, in-vivo delayed hypersensitivity to tumor antigens, and in-vitro lymphocyte cytotoxicity to target cells.

Immune response and various nonimmunologic host defense mechanisms can be evaluated in cancer patients by a variety of techniques, as enumerated in Table 5–6. Cellular immunity can be evaluated in many ways; for example, the delayed hypersensitivity skin test; measurement of the lymphocyte blastogenic response to mitogens or antigens; and the production of migration inhibitory factor. Measurements as simple as lymphocyte and monocyte counts in the peripheral blood may be useful and may correlate with prognosis.

One can quantitate humoral immunity by measuring immunoglobulin levels, isoantibody titers, complement levels, primary antibody response to antigens (e.g., typhoid or keyhole limpet hemocyanin), and secondary response to antigens (e.g., tetanus and diphtheria).

Immune Response to Tumor-Associated Antigens

There have been several human studies involving immune response to specific tumor-associated antigens. The tests for delayed hypersensitivity reactions to extracts of tumors have been done in a manner similar to the tests for the common bacterial-fungal antigens. Routine hypersensitivity skin test reactions have been observed in patients with leukemia, colon cancer, breast carcinoma, carcinoma of the lung, and cancer of the cervix. Skin test reactivity to leukemia-associated antigens has been shown to correlate with

---

TABLE 5–6 ASSAYS FOR IMMUNE COMPETENCE IN TUMOR PATIENTS

I. Cellular Immunity
1. Skin tests for delayed hypersensitivity
   a. Tests for previous sensitization with recall antigens (e.g., *Candida,* streptokinase–streptodornase, trichophytin, mumps)
   b. Primary sensitization (e.g., dinitrochlorobenzene)
2. Quantitation for circulating T- and B-lymphocytes
   a. E-rosette assay for T-lymphocytes
   b. Immunofluorescent assays for B-lymphocytes
3. Lymphocyte function
   a. Total WBC and total lymphocyte count
   b. Response to mitogens, PHA, Con A, and pokeweed
   c. Production of lymphokines
4. Macrophage function

II. Humoral Immunity
1. Quantitative immunoglobulins
2. Isoantibody levels (blood group isoagglutinins)
3. Serum complement level
4. Primary antibody response to typhoid, keyhole limpet hemocyanin
5. Secondary antibody response to antigens such as tetanus and diphtheria

the clinical status of the patient. In general, delayed hypersensitivity skin tests to the specific tumor-associated antigens correlate with the clinical state and are useful for monitoring response to therapy. Because of the possible hazard of inoculation of cancer antigen into patients who do not have cancer, the potential usefulness of such skin tests for cancer screening and diagnosis is limited.

Cell-mediated cytotoxicity assays may have a possible application in immunodiagnosis. The lymphocytes removed from patients with cancer can exhibit in-vitro growth of the tumor cells or may demonstrate cytotoxic inhibition of the cultured tumor cells. Such assays are performed primarily in the larger diagnostic cancer centers, primarily on a clinical investigation basis.

Leukocyte migration inhibition assays have been performed with the use of patient cells reacted with the extract of the tumor tissue. Reactivity to common tumor-associated antigens has been observed by this method in patients with breast cancer, malignant melanoma, lymphoma, and leukemia. Further, the leukocyte migration assay has been reported to show good correlation with delayed-hypersensitivity skin test reactions.

Potential fruitful approaches that remain to be developed are useful tests for the detection of antibodies to tumor-associated antigens. Antibodies to common tumor antigens have been described in melanoma and osteosarcoma. The specificity of the reactions in melanoma and osteosarcoma must be studied further. This approach is very sensitive and can be useful for the early diagnosis of cancer.

IMMUNOTHERAPY

There are many problems associated with current methods of immunotherapy. The human tumor antigens have not been well defined in terms of location (e.g., cytoplasm or surface), immunogenicity, cross-reactivity with normal tissue antigens, and interaction with host immune surveillance systems. The approaches to enhance the normal immune system to combat and contain the growth of cancer have been (1) increasing cell-mediated immunity; (2) augmenting antibody-mediated immunity; and (3) stimulating the general immunocompetence with use of specific and nonspecific reagents.

There are seven major approaches to immunotherapy listed in Table 5–7.

Active Nonspecific Immunotherapy

This mode of therapy usually involves use of adjuvants such as BCG or *Corynebacterium parvum* to increase the general immunocompetence with augmentation of cell-mediated and humoral response. These nonspecific adjuvant reagents may have one or more of the following immunologic effects: (1) increase in general immunocompetence; (2) augmentation of cell-mediated or humoral responses; (3) expansion of T-lymphocyte population and activation of the macrophages; or (4) enhancement of the reticuloendothelial system. This approach has been used in the therapy of many tumors, such as melanoma, leukemia, colon cancer, lung carcinoma, and breast carcinoma, with variable degrees of success.

Immunorestoration

Certain agents such as levamisole and thymosin have been used to restore cell-mediated responsiveness. Levamisole is a chemical agent that probably acts through a cyclic nucleotide or prostaglandin system in lymphocytes and helps restore cell-mediated responsiveness in sensitized hosts.

In patients who are immunodeficient and immunosuppressed, the administration of thymic hormones has been shown to increase the percentage of peripheral circulating E-rosette T-cell types of lymphocytes. The possibility of thymic factors that can augment cell-mediated response of cancer patients has been shown to enhance in-

TABLE 5–7 APPROACHES TO IMMUNOTHERAPY OF CANCER

Approach	Mechanism of Action
1. Active-nonspecific	Increase general immunocompetence
	Activate macrophages
2. Immunorestorative	Restore immunocompetence
3. Active-specific	Increase specific cell-mediated–humoral antitumor immunity
4. Adoptive	Transfer tumor immunity from immune cells
5. Passive	Transfer humoral tumor-specific antibodies, cytotoxic, deblocking, opsonizing, antibody-dependent cellular cytotoxicity or drug- or isotope-transporting antibody
6. Local	Locally active macrophages kill tumor cells by bystander effect of delayed hypersensitivity; induce specific tumor immunity
7. Combination of above	

(Modified from Hersh, E. M. et al.: Immunotherapy of cancer. *In* Becker, F. F., ed.: Cancer, A Comprehensive Treatise, Vol. 6, p. 425. New York, Plenum Press, 1977.)

vitro cell function. Preliminary results have demonstrated some clinical improvement in tumor patients; however, further studies are needed to determine the true therapeutic benefits.

Active Specific Immunotherapy

This mode of therapy includes immunization with tumor cells or antigens. The tumor cells may be modified with virus or chemicals prior to immunization to enhance specific cell-mediated and humoral immunity in the host. Specific stimulation of immunity has been attempted by the following:

Unmodified Cancer Cells or Cell Surface Antigens as Immunogens. Allogeneic cancer cells as immunogens have been used in the immunotherapy of human leukemia. The human leukemia cells were irradiated to prevent cell division and injected periodically into recipients previously induced into remission of acute lymphocytic leukemia by chemotherapy. Concurrent with the tumor vaccine, BCG was administered. The immunotherapy with both irradiated allogeneic cells and BCG was synergistic, whereas either modality alone was ineffective.

Treatment of Cancer Cells with Neuraminidase. This is based on the hypothesis that enzymatic removal of sialic acid residues from cancer cell membranes increases their immunogenicity and facilitates immunospecific rejection. The efficacy of this treatment has not been established.

Virus-modified Cancer Cells. Virus infections of cells may produce strongly immunogenic viral antigens on the cell surface that enhance the immunogenicity of weak tumor-specific antigens. The immune response is not directed to the virus alone because rejection of subsequent tumor challenge is tumor-specific. These studies have been extended to humans with malignant disease on a limited basis. No therapeutic benefits have been noted in patients with osteogenic sarcoma given influenza virus-infected autologous or allogeneic tumor cells.

Chemically Modified Membranes on Cancer Cells. Chemicals can be coupled to tumor cell membranes and enhance the cell-mediated cytotoxicity in experimental animal tumor models. Most of the experimental work has been in animal models using substances such as 2,4-dinitrophenol. This approach is still in the early stages of clinical experimentation for treatment of human tumors.

Adoptive Immunotherapy

This mode of therapy utilizes transfer of cells or cell products from a specifically immunocompetent donor to a tumor-bearing recipient. The therapy may involve transfer of T-lymphocytes, transfer factor, or immune RNA extracted from sensitized lymphocytes.

Transfusion of Normal T-Lymphocytes. Often in cancer patients, the T-lymphocytes are depressed primarily or secondarily, and the therapeutic infusion of normal T cells will initiate or augment an antitumor response. One major obstacle of adoptive immunotherapy is the histocompatibility antigen difference. Without HLA matching, the donor cells will survive, and a severe graft-versus-host reaction may occur in an immunosuppressed recipient.

Transfusion of Sensitized T-Lymphocytes. The transfusion of allogeneic sensitized T-lymphocytes in the form of leukocyte transfusion was one of the first methods used in immunotherapy of human cancer. The donors and recipients should be matched with respect to the ABO blood group and HLA antigens. This mode of therapy has been only partially successful in humans.

Treatment with Transfer Factor. Transfer factor has been used to activate the immune response in cancer patients and other immunodeficient diseases. The small molecular weight transfer factor derived from sensitized T-lymphocytes can program recipient lymphocytes to develop certain aspects of specific cellular immunity, such as T-cell–mediated cytotoxicity. Transfer factor therapy has been used in cases of human malignant melanomas, resulting in prolongation of life span and an interval of time for clinical recurrence of the tumor.

Transfer of Immune RNA. RNA is extracted from sensitized donor immune lymphocytes and injected into the recipient host. Experimental studies have shown that immunotherapy with immune RNA is more effective in inhibiting tumor growth if administered at a period when there is small tumor mass with growth in the early stages. This mode of therapy is not very effective when immune RNA is given to an animal with a well-established growing tumor. This approach in humans is still in the early stages of clinical investigation, and the mechanism of action and beneficial effects have yet to be determined.

Passive Immunotherapy

This refers to transfer of antitumor antibodies from an immune donor to a recipient host with tumor. The use of tumor-specific antibodies has been applied with some success in experimental animal models. However, studies of immunotherapy with antibodies in humans have not been adequately tested. Most of the reported human studies have not been very successful. There has been hesitation on the part of oncologists, since it is possible to enhance the growth of the tumor by administration of tumor antibodies by blocking specific cell-mediated immunity.

A better approach currently being used is to couple certain cytotoxic agents (e.g., organic chemicals and radioactive substances) to specific antibodies and to employ such reagents to kill tumor cells selectively.

Local Immunotherapy

This method refers to the injection of active-nonspecific or adoptive immunotherapeutic reagents directly into the tumor in order to induce local killing and enhance specific tumor immunity of the general host immune system.

Combinations of the aforementioned modes of immunotherapy have been used with variable results. In general, one can summarize by stating that immunotherapy by itself has not been found to be very effective in most cases, although it has demonstrated some benefit when administered in conjunction with cancer chemotherapy.

DISEASES OF AUTOIMMUNITY

In this section, it will be seen that the different forms of autoimmune disease correlate with the type of immune response in a given disorder. Some autoimmune diseases exhibit both T-cell–dependent and antibody-dependent injury, but others are not associated with a clearly defined pathogenesis. We are now much closer to an understanding of the autoimmune phenomenon than before, but we still lack the needed information to define with assurance all the factors in the developmental mechanism of autoimmunity. The discussion will indicate that the puzzle is not how we develop an immune response to our own tissues as antigens but rather how we develop and normally maintain a state of unresponsiveness. Key answers will no doubt be forthcoming from current and future research.

DEFINITIONS OF AUTOIMMUNITY

Autoimmunity can be defined as a failure of an organism to recognize its own tissue and includes any immune response to the host's own tissue, whether it is humoral (e.g., circulating autoantibodies) or cellular (e.g., delayed hypersensitivity). Autoimmunity is a concept that may explain the pathogenesis of a number of diseases and is a major immunologic phenomenon in clinical medicine.

The body is endowed with mechanisms to distinguish self from nonself. However, as will be discussed, there are many pathways for the breakdown of the control mechanisms underlying self-recognition. Such breakdowns result in an autoimmune response. Autoantibodies that react with the tissue antigens of the host may or may not cause tissue injury and produce disease. The term *autoimmune disease* has been generally assigned to those conditions in which an immune mechanism of injury has contributed to the pathogenesis of

the disease. In certain of the diseases, such as organ-specific autoimmune thyroiditis, the autoimmune response is the major factor in initiating the tissue injury. However, there are many other diseases in which the immunologic response is notably secondary to the initial tissue injury. Detection of autoantibodies may be of equal value in the diagnosis of the latter group of diseases. Autoimmunity may play a role in a wide range of clinical situations, including aging, response to viral and other microbial infections, organ-specific immunologic diseases, and generalized systemic immunologic diseases such as systemic lupus erythematosus.

The term *autoallergic* is often used interchangeably with the word *autoimmune*. The term *allergy* was originated by von Pirquet in 1906 to describe an altered reaction to repeated injections of heterologous gamma globulin to diphtheria toxin. Thus, allergy is often used to mean harmful altered reactions secondary to immune mechanisms. Today, the term *allergy* is most commonly applied to diseases characterized by hypersensitivity reaction, such as hay fever and asthma, which are mediated by cytophilic IgE antibodies. Hypersensitivity has been used to describe immune reactions similar to allergy and also to describe nonimmunologic reactions, such as nonimmune hypersensitivity to drugs.

Autoimmunity that is observed in clinical and experimental circumstances can be defined as an apparent termination of the natural unresponsive state to self. Immunologic tolerance is the result of an active physiologic process and is not simply the lack of immune response. There are two types of immunologic tolerance: One results in a central unresponsive state characterized by an irreversible loss of competent lymphocytes; the other is a peripheral inhibition in which competent cells are present but suppressed. A definition of *unresponsiveness* is the inability to make a detectable immune response to an antigenic challenge, as distinguished from so-called *tolerance*, which is a term commonly used in transplantation immunology in addition to nonimmunologic events to describe endurance without ill effects of substances such as endotoxins and drugs. However, for the purposes of this section, the terms *unresponsiveness* and *tolerance* will be used interchangeably, since the discussion will be confined to immune mechanisms.

CONCEPT OF UNRESPONSIVE STATE OR TOLERANCE AND RELATION TO AUTOIMMUNITY

Currently, it is believed that a person becomes unresponsive to his own tissue antigens during fetal development and that the natural unresponsive state develops as a result of direct contact between the self-constituents and receptor sites on the surface of lymphocytes reactive to these antigens. This is a phenomenon that was first predicted by Burnet, who developed the clonal selection theory, which proposed that the contact of antibody-forming cells with their respective antigens during fetal or early postnatal life led to destruction or inactivation with elimination of the corresponding clones. Since then, many investigators have artificially induced an unresponsive state to a wide variety of antigens during the newborn period when an immature immune system was present.

The mode of induction of the natural unresponsive state is probably by two mechanisms: (1) The clones are immunocompetent cells capable of reacting to self antigens and are eliminated by a mechanism of the clonal theory of Burnet; and (2) antigen-producing cells are made unresponsive by early exposure to self antigen. The clonal selection theory was not easily reconciled with the observations on the experimental induction of autoimmunity. Weigle and coworkers showed that injections of cross-reacting thyroglobulins of other species in the absence of adjuvant elicited formation of autoantibodies against thyroglobulin and experimental thyroiditis. It became clear that the T cells and B cells interact in the production of autoantibodies and that the mechanisms of induction of the unresponsive state at the cellular level of the T cells and B cells are different.

In the cellular aspects of unresponsiveness, the cells involved are macrophages, B cells, T cells, and antibody-producing B cells from the bone marrow. The evidence for direct cooperation between the T- and B-lymphocytes is well confirmed. When specific antigen-sensitive cells interact for production of antibodies, specifically reactive T cells and B cells must both interact. Although macrophages play a major role in the establishment of the unresponsiveness, they appear to be nonspecific and under genetic control.

Both T- and B-lymphocytes can become unresponsive or tolerant. However, the kinetics of tolerance in these two lymphocyte populations differ greatly. Many autoantigens, such as thyroglobulin, protein hormones, and solubilized membrane antigens, circulate in limited concentrations in the body fluids. With limited concentrations of these self components, the unresponsive state is maintained only in the T cells, not in the B cells. The natural unresponsive state is maintained to antigens such as native thyroglobulin because of the lack of T-helper cell signal, and autoantibody production is *not* initiated (Fig. 5–6).

In other studies, it has been found that high doses of antigen can induce unresponsiveness in both T- and B-lymphocytes. This has been demonstrated experimentally with injection of human gamma globulin in mice. Experiments in mice have shown that thymocytes become tolerant to human gamma globulin within 24 hours of exposure and that this tolerance lasts for 100 days. By contrast, B-cell tolerance requires an induction period of 15 to 21 days. The long latent period

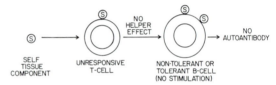

NATURAL UNRESPONSIVE STATE

Figure 5–6

between exposure and tolerance to human gamma globulin in mice may indicate a relative resistance of the bone marrow cells to tolerance or a requirement for thymic cell–bone marrow interaction before tolerance can be induced. Even with high doses of antigen, the unresponsive state of B-lymphocytes is often incomplete, and some antibody of low affinity can still be formed. In the case of thyroglobulin and the involvement in thyroiditis, only the T-lymphocytes may be tolerant, leaving B-lymphocytes able to respond to autoantigens suitably presented to them with T-lymphocyte help. Mechanisms allowing the requirement for specific T-lymphocytes responding to autoantigens to be bypassed are discussed later in this section. Tolerance to autoantigen based on the selective unresponsiveness of T-lymphocytes can be easily bypassed by various viral and microbial infections and other events.

In contrast to the situation observed in the unresponsive state to thyroglobulin and thyroiditis, neither T cells nor B cells appear to be unresponsive to basic protein, and specific antigen-binding cells to basic protein have been detected in both T- and B-cell populations. By deleting either the T- or B-cells from these populations as specifically bound basic proteins, researchers have demonstrated that T-cells, not antibody, are responsible for induction of experimental allergic encephalitis.

Several studies have demonstrated the existence of antireceptor or anti-idiotypic antibodies, which may arise as a result of various T-cell bypass mechanisms described further on. These antibodies may block the expression of an immune response and produce a tolerance-like situation to self antigen. When an animal makes an immune response to a given antigen, autoantibodies directed to the antibody made as the result of the antigenic stimulus also may be produced. The idiotypic determinants characteristic of a given antibody may also be present on lymphocytes with receptor for the antigen. Thus, the autoantibody to the idiotype may block or suppress the immune response to a given antigen, and the loss of the control mechanism could lead to expression of an autoimmune response to self antigens.

GENETIC FACTORS IN AUTOIMMUNITY

The genetic basis of immunologic regulation is an important area of research today. A group of genes located within the major histocompatibility locus (MHC) play important roles in immunologic regulation. The differences and susceptibility to various viruses and the intensity of the cellular immune response of graft-versus-host reaction is also controlled within the cluster of genes located within the major histocompatibility region.

Genetically determined cell surface antigens termed *Ia* are important immunologic factors involved in antigen recognition, cellular interaction, and cellular cooperation. Much evidence suggests that genes associated with the major histocompatibility locus in humans (HLA) may be important in the immune regulation and in the pathogenesis of autoimmunity. Many autoimmune disorders have been found to be associated with a particular HLA haplotype. The majority of the associations are with the second locus genes, and this may be close to the human immune response (Ir) genes. The association of HLA antigens has been found to be marked in cases of ankylosing spondylitis, in which as many as 90 per cent of patients are found to possess HLA-B27 antigens. It should be noted that the association does not imply that the disease is caused by possession of the HLA-B27 antigen. Certain autoimmune diseases, particularly the organ-specific disorders, such as idiopathic Addison's disease, Graves' disease, chronic active hepatitis, and Sjögren's syndrome, occur more frequently in individuals who have HLA-B8. Other diseases, such as multiple sclerosis and rheumatoid arthritis, appear to be associated with lymphocyte-defined genetic loci whose products on the cell membranes are responsible for mixed lymphocyte reactivity.

Autoimmunity and autoimmune diseases are frequently associated with genetic and viral factors that interact with the immune system and influence regulation. Genetically determined lymphocyte membranes in humans determine the magnitude of response and mixed lymphocyte reactions and may be closely associated in the development of autoimmunity. Although the exact mechanisms by which genetic factors and autoimmunity are related are unclear, it is likely that the immune response (Ir) genes, lymphocytic surface antigen, and possible receptors for specific viruses are involved. Viruses and other infectious agents are often associated with autoimmunity. Many virus buds from cell surfaces can incorporate normal membrane constituents as part of their viral envelope. Such combinations of viral and host tissue antigens may become immunogenic and give rise to autoimmune responses.

GENERAL THEORIES AND MECHANISMS OF AUTOIMMUNITY

Autoimmunity arises when there is a disordered regulation and interaction of T cells and B cells in response to antigenic stimulation. The T- and B-cell interaction may be imbalanced as a consequence of genetic, viral, and environmental mechanisms acting singly or in combination. A central mechanism in this concept involves a disturbance of the delicate balance between the suppressor and helper activity of regulatory T cells. Either an excess of T-cell activity or a deficiency of suppressor activity could lead to development of autoimmunity. The autoimmune state could probably arise by several mechanisms: (1) a bypass of either T-cell specificity or the need for T cells in the presence of competent B cells; (2) a stimulation of competent T cells or B cells or both in case of sequestered self antigens; and (3) a loss of suppressor activity preventing autoantibody to self antigens. Depending on the disease, any one or a combination of these possibilities may play a role involving a host of mediators in the autoimmune state and may result from a humoral response, a cellular response, or a combination of both.

T-Cell Bypass Mechanism of Autoimmunity

Most autoantigens, such as thyroglobulin, protein hormones, and soluble membrane antigen, circulate in very low doses. Prolonged exposure to these would produce selective tolerance in T-lymphocytes, leaving B-lymphocytes able to bind autoantigens and to be stimulated by autoantigens presented to them with appropriate T-lymphocyte help. Under such circumstance, the requirements for T-lymphocytes responding to autoantigenic determinants can be bypassed (Fig. 5–7).

In Figure 5–7, one can note that in the normal state the T cell is tolerant and the B cell is competent; no autoantibody is formed because the absence of the T-cell helper signals the presence of the autoantigen. However, the autoantigens will form immunogenic units with antigens that are able to initiate the T-cell helper signal to stimulate

T-CELL BYPASS MECHANISM OF AUTOIMMUNITY

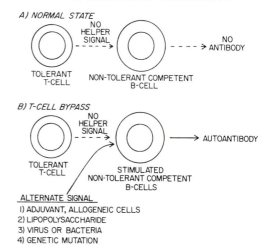

Figure 5–7

TABLE 5–8 TYPES OF REACTIONS INVOLVING BYPASS OF T-CELL SPECIFICITY IN THE PRESENCE
OF COMPETENT B CELLS

1. Binding of foreign haptens as drugs to host tissue.
2. Infections by viruses and bacteria that alter host autoantigens.
3. Exposure to altered or cross-reacting antigens (i.e., enzyme degradation and viral and bacterial infections).
4. Stimulation of competent B cells by bacterial lipopolysaccharide (LPS).
5. Nonspecific stimulation of helper T-cell activity with adjuvant.
6. Graft-versus-host reaction (nonspecific stimulation of helper T-cell activity with allogeneic cells).

the existing immunocompetent B cell. Among the helper determinants are viruses, bacteria, and drugs. Any procedure that nonspecifically activates lymphocytes, such as adjuvants or graft-versus-host reaction with allogeneic cells, can stimulate production of autoantibodies by the bypass of T-cell specificity.

The types of autoimmune reactions involving bypass of T-cell specificity in the presence of competent B cells are listed in Table 5–8.

Autoimmunity Following Administration of Drugs. Some autoimmune manifestations following drug administration are remarkably specific. Thus, in patients treated with alpha-methyldopa, Coombs'-positive autoimmune hemolytic anemias are not uncommon. Often, the autoantigen in the body is IgG-directed against the E antigen of the Rh series. The production of antinuclear factors in a syndrome like systemic lupus erythematosus is relatively frequent in patients treated with procainamide and hydralazine. There often is a coupling of drug or metabolite to an autoantigen that initiates a host T-lymphocyte reaction against the antigenic determinants of the drug; subsequently, autoantibodies are formed through a T-cell helper effect (Fig. 5–8). In some patients, following administration of hydantoin, there is generalized lymphoid hyperplasia and plasmacytosis with production of a variety of antibodies with specificity for erythrocytes. In such cases, it is believed that hydantoin derivatives become attached to the surface of lymphoid cells and modify their major histocompatibility antigen complex in such a way that autologous T-lymphocyte recognizes them as foreign and reacts to them. There is also another situation in which nitrofurantoin treatment can result in a wide variety of autoantibodies, including some with specificity for human albumin. A lupus-like syndrome with pulmonary reactions has

been described in patients treated with nitrofurantoin.

Virus Infections. Virus infections can elicit autoantibody formation by two mechanisms. First, the viral antigens and autoantigens may become associated to form immunogenic units. Viral antigens stimulating host T-lymphocytes could then function as helper determinants, thereby stimulating B-lymphocyte responses to autoantigens. Second, some viruses such as the Epstein-Barr virus (EBV) stimulate proliferation of the B-lymphocyte cell line with autoantibody production. There are two ways in which viral and host antigens can form immunogenic units. Host antigens can be incorporated in the envelopes of some viruses, and viral antigens can appear on the surfaces of infected host cells (Fig. 5–9). The viral antigens also may form complexes with and modify histocompatibility antigens or other membrane constituents such as the contractile protein, actin. The modified viral antigens could stimulate T-cell helper effect and elicit autoantibody formation (Fig. 5–10).

In humans, infection with viruses such as influenza, measles, varicella, and herpes simplex has often resulted in autoimmune manifestations such as platelet and red cell autoantibodies. The development of cold autoagglutinins after *Mycoplasma pneumoniae* infection probably occurs by a

AUTOIMMUNITY FOLLOWING ADMINISTRATION OF DRUG HAPTEN

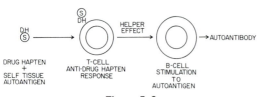

DRUG HAPTEN
+
SELF TISSUE
AUTOANTIGEN

T-CELL
ANTI-DRUG HAPTEN
RESPONSE

B-CELL
STIMULATION
TO
AUTOANTIGEN

Figure 5–8

INTERACTION OF VIRUS, VIRAL ANTIGENS AND SELF-TISSUE
ANTIGENS TO FORM IMMUNOGENIC UNITS

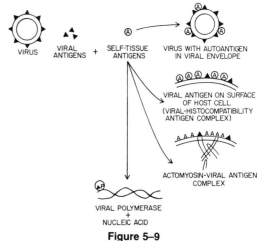

Figure 5–9

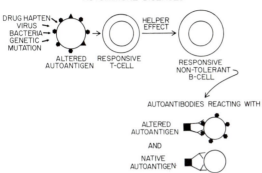

AUTOANTIBODY FORMATION IN CERTAIN ORGAN SPECIFIC
AUTOIMMUNE DISEASES

Figure 5–10

T-cell bypass mechanism. Following infectious mononucleosis, many patients' sera often react against several autoantigens. These include autoantibodies against nuclei, lymphocytes, erythrocytes, and smooth muscle. In addition, cross-reactive heterophile antibodies may be noted following infectious mononucleosis and other infections. The autoantibody is produced by a mechanism similar to that observed in altered self component with virus or bacteria.

There has been much speculation about the possible involvement of an oncornavirus in the pathogenesis of human systemic lupus erythematosus.

Degradation and Alteration of Autoantigens. Tissue damage with alteration of host antigens may play a role in eliciting autoimmune reactions. Partial degradation can expose antigenic determinants that are not available in the native molecules, and these can react with T-lymphocytes to induce autoimmunity. Many bacterial, viral, and parasitic infections are associated with transient positive tests for antiglobulin of the rheumatoid factor type, and among the underlying mechanisms is either partial degradation or alteration of immunoglobulin.

Adjuvant and Bacterial Infections. Immunologic adjuvants are nonspecific B-lymphocyte stimulators, such as lipopolysaccharide and purified protein derivatives (Fig. 5–11). These immunologic adjuvants may induce autoimmune responses. It is possible that diseases such as pertussis and other bacterial infections involving liberation of products with adjuvant activities could produce polyclonal lymphocyte activation and autoimmunity. In rheumatic fever, there is cross-reaction of some determinants of the organism with the host tissue. Other determinants of the same molecule or complexes could be recognized by host T-lymphocytes and function as helper determinants. Antibody to cardiolipin and cold autoantibodies to erythrocytes in syphilis and antibody to myocardial antigens in rheumatic fever can result from chronic infections or repeated injections of bacteria.

Graft-Versus-Host Reaction (Allogeneic Cells). The primary event in graft-versus-host reaction (GVH) is the response of donor T-lymphocytes to the major histocompatibility complex on lymphoid and hematopoietic cells of the recipient. A major effect is the stimulation of lymphoid tissue in the recipient, with development of lymphoreticular hyperplasia with germinal center enlargement and plasmacytosis. There is proliferation of recipient B-lymphocytes under the influence of a donor T-lymphocyte signal (Fig. 5–11).

In a normal person, autoantibody formation does not occur because T-lymphocytes are unable to react to autoantigens. However, when lymphocytes are nonspecifically stimulated, as in the graft-versus-host reaction, there is an allogeneic effect leading to the production of antibodies that normally requires T-lymphocyte help (Fig. 5–11). In this mechanism, the need for carrier-specific T-lymphocytes in the immune response can be bypassed; hence, the graft-versus-host reaction results in the formation of autoantibodies. This mechanism has been shown to result in autoantibodies in various experimental animal models of such conditions as glomerulonephritis and Coombs'-positive autoimmune hemolytic anemia.

Autoimmune Thyroiditis and Organ-Specific Autoimmune Diseases. The classic example of the mechanism of T-cell specificity bypass mechanism is thyroiditis. Overwhelming evidence in studies of experimental thyroiditis as well as human thyroiditis has shown that the major factor in initiating tissue injury is the humoral autoantibody response.

It was previously thought that thyroglobulin was a sequestered antigen; however, various experiments subsequently showed that thyroglobulin was a semisequestered antigen present in the circulation in very small amounts after birth and that it was able to equilibrate between the intra- and extravascular compartments. In these organs, which are frequently associated with autoimmune diseases, it is felt that extremely low concentrations of self antigen, such as thyroglobulin, are in circulation and that these concentrations are sufficient to maintain tolerance only at the level of the T cells, not at the level of the B or bone marrow cells. This is not a completely healthy condition, since the unresponsiveness at the thymus level is adequate to inhibit any antibody response; however, it superimposes upon this a situation such as virus transformation or genetic

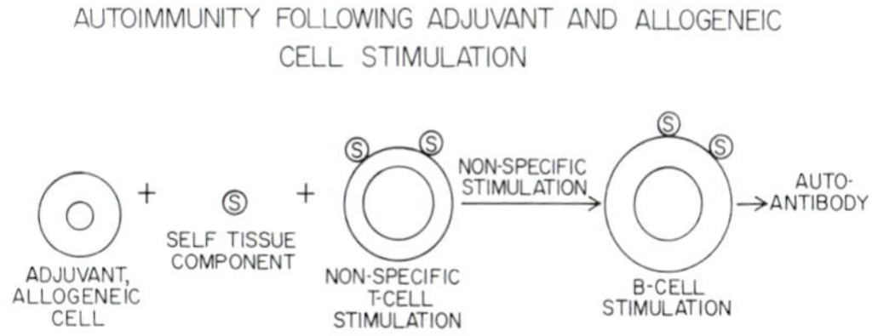

AUTOIMMUNITY FOLLOWING ADJUVANT AND ALLOGENEIC
CELL STIMULATION

Figure 5–11

mutation. This permits the thymus cells to react with the altered portion, the self antigen. The interaction takes place with the immunocompetent bone marrow cells, and the autoimmune process is initiated (Fig. 5–10).

The mechanism involved in thyroiditis may operate in the organ-specific diseases (e.g., primary adrenal gland atrophy, parathyroid hypoplasia, and primary ovarian atrophy). These organs release extremely small concentrations of self antigens during the development of the natural unresponsive state, and tolerance is developed at the T-cell level and not at the B-cell level.

Sequestered Antigen Release Mechanism of Autoimmunity

It was formerly believed that many autoantigens are secluded from immunocompetent cells in the body; however, many antigens formerly thought to be secluded, such as thyroglobulin protein hormones, now are known to circulate in small amounts—approximately 100 ng/ml in the case of thyroglobulin. Cell membrane constituents such as major histocompatibility antigens are likewise known to circulate in low quantities. However, there may well be segregation of some antigens in normal persons. An example is the ocular lens, which is segregated from blood vessels and lymphatics; its constituents do not normally elicit immune responses. The basic protein of myelin probably is effectively secluded from immunocompetent cells. In normal human adults, neither T cells nor B cells appear to be tolerant to basic protein, and specific binding cells to basic protein can be detected in both T cells and B cells. This can explain the observation that T cells and the cellular (delayed-sensitivity) mechanism constitute the primary mechanism of injury in experimental allergic encephalitis (Fig. 5–12).

Loss of Suppressor Cell Activity in Autoimmunity

Several investigators have hypothesized that T cells are involved in controlling B cells by suppressing B-cell–dependent synthesis of autoan-

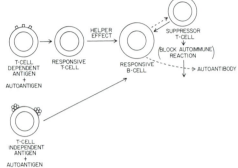

SUPPRESSOR T-CELLS IN THE PREVENTION OF AUTOIMMUNE REACTIONS

Figure 5–13

tibody. As shown in Figure 5–13, the T-lymphocytes can inhibit autoimmune responses and provide a general mechanism for preventing or delaying them. Evidence has accumulated that the population of T-lymphocytes with suppressor and helper effects is distinct. The major evidence for suppressor control is that antibody is made at a fairly steady rate that is not influenced by injecting more antigen; injection of antilymphocyte serum causes a large temporary rise in the number of antibody-secreting cells, and tolerance to many self-components may be maintained by active suppressor mechanisms.

With a loss of suppressor cell activity due to aging, immune deficiency syndromes (i.e., thymic hypoplasia), or other disease mechanisms, the self-reactive B cells are permitted to proliferate, with resultant production of autoantibody and auto-reactive lymphocytes (Fig. 5–14).

Experimental evidence to support the concept of loss of suppressor T-cell activity in development of autoimmune reactions is as follows:

1. Following early thymectomy, a strain of leghorn chickens developed a form of autoimmune thyroiditis more severe than that which occurs spontaneously.

2. Spleen cells from old New Zealand Black mice (NZB), when transplanted to young NZB mice depleted of T cells by antilymphocyte serum, will induce a persistent Coombs'-positive hemolytic anemia.

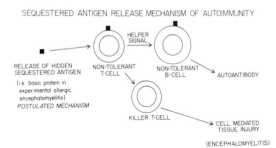

SEQUESTERED ANTIGEN RELEASE MECHANISM OF AUTOIMMUNITY

Figure 5–12

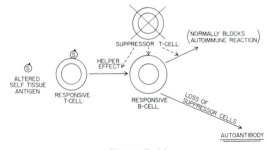

LOSS OF SUPPRESSOR CELL ACTIVITY IN AUTOIMMUNITY

Figure 5–14

Summary of Mechanisms of Autoimmunity

It is apparent that numerous mechanisms may initiate an autoimmune response. The autoimmune reaction is the result of disruption of the normal pathways of interaction of T cells and B cells with autoantigens. Autoimmunity may arise whenever there is a state of immunologic imbalance in which B-cell activity is excessive and suppressor T-cell activity is diminished. This imbalance may occur as a consequence of genetic, viral, and environmental mechanisms acting singly or in combination. Manipulation of autoantigens in a way to stimulate helper T-cell functions, such as the use of adjuvants, immunogenic carriers, or cross-reactive antigens, also induces the autoimmune phenomenon. Furthermore, the decrease in normal suppressor cell activity caused by aging, cancer, or other disease mechanisms, may permit self-reactive cells to proliferate, resulting in the production of autoantibody and autoreactive lymphocytes.

CLASSIFICATION OF HUMAN AUTOIMMUNE DISEASES

The autoimmune disorders can be broadly separated into three main groups: (1) organ-specific diseases, (2) non–organ-specific diseases, and (3) diseases with non–organ-specific autoantibodies but with lesions restricted to one or only a few organs (Table 5–9).

Organ-Specific Autoimmune Disease. These disorders are characterized by chronic inflammatory changes in a specific organ. The autoantibodies in this group of diseases exhibit specificity for antigens of the diseased organ. Such autoantibodies may demonstrate species specificity, and familial clustering of diseases within this group occurs with remarkable frequency. Examples of this group are (1) Hashimoto's autoimmune thyroiditis, (2) primary hypothyroidism, (3) thyrotoxicosis (Graves' disease), (4) chronic atrophic gastritis, (5) primary adrenal atrophy, (6) post–rabies vaccination encephalomyelitis, and (7) autoimmune hemolytic anemia.

The pathogenic mechanism in autoimmune thyroiditis probably involves a bypass of T-cell specificity to initiate production of autoantibodies. It has been postulated that a deficiency in T cells may be the key factor in initiating the whole process, and ultimately all categories of cells may be involved.

In thyrotoxicosis, there is human thyroid-stimulating immunoglobulin, which is probably an anti-TSH receptor with a thyroid-stimulating activity that acts longer than TSH. These antibodies can be either human-specific or cross-reactive with other species, and they closely mimic TSH. The thyroid-stimulating antibodies initiate the transduction process, which results in stimulation of adenyl cyclase with increased thyroid hormone release.

Non–Organ-Specific Autoimmune Diseases. These diseases are characterized by widespread pathologic change in many different organs and tissues throughout the body. Furthermore, the associated serum autoantibodies often lack organ and species specificity, and experimental lesions are not readily produced; however, similar diseases arise spontaneously in certain inbred animal strains. Examples of this group are (1) systemic lupus erythematosus, (2) rheumatoid arthritis, and (3) various other connective tissue disorders, such as progressive systemic sclerosis (scleroderma).

In the group of non–organ-specific autoimmune diseases, the primary mechanism of injury is by immune complexes. In systemic lupus erythematosus, the pathogenic complex is the DNA–anti-DNA complex. The factors involved in production of anti-DNA antibody are probably complex, with an abnormal imbalance and interaction of viral, genetic, and immunologic factors.

Disorders with Non–Organ-Specific Autoantibodies and with Lesions Restricted to One or Few Organs. By definition, these diseases combine the features of both organ-specific and non–organ-specific categories. Examples of this group are (1) primary biliary cirrhosis, and (2) chronic aggressive hepatitis.

The autoimmune liver disorders are characterized by the production of non–organ-specific and non–species-specific antibodies, such as antimitochondrial and anti–smooth muscle cell antibodies. The relationships of these antibodies to immune injury and the lesion are unknown. The levels of the antibodies do not correlate with the severity or duration of the disease. There is evidence that the mechanisms of immunologic injury in liver disorders involve primarily a cellular immune mechanism operating via the suppressor cell and cytotoxic affector cell functions. In addition, there are humoral immunoregulatory factors that modulate the cellular functions of the immune system in the pathogenesis of the immunologic liver disorders.

CLINICAL OBSERVATIONS THAT INDICATE AUTOIMMUNE PATHOGENESIS

Autoimmune disorders are frequently associated with malignancies, immune deficiency syndromes, and aging. Possible autoimmune pathogenesis in a given disease is indicated when one observes (1) the existence of autoantibodies; (2) amyloid deposits of denatured gamma globulin; (3) hypergammaglobulinemia with elevation of various immunoglobulins; (4) vasculitis, serositis, and glomerulonephritis, which suggest an immune complex disease; and (5) existence of other diseases, such as endocrinopathies, known to be associated with autoimmune disorders.

TABLE 5–9 ANTIBODIES IN VARIOUS AUTOIMMUNE DISEASES

Diseases	Antigen Involved	Methods for Detection of Antibody
Organ-Specific, Endocrine		
Autoimmune thyroiditis, primary myxedema, thyrotoxicosis	Thyroglobulin	Immunofluorescent test (IFT) (indirect)–methanol-fixed human thyroid
		Passive hemagglutination
		Latex agglutination
	Cytoplasmic microsome	IFT (indirect)–unfixed human hyperplastic thyroid tissue
		Passive hemagglutination
		Complement fixation
Thyrotoxicosis	Thyroid cell surface antigen	Bioassay–mouse thyroid stimulation in vivo
		Radioimmunoassay with inhibition of TSH on human thyroid tissue receptor
Addison's disease	Adrenal cell cytoplasm	IFT (indirect) on unfixed human adrenal cortex
Parathyroid	Parathyroid cytoplasmic antigen	IFT (indirect) human parathyroid gland
Early-onset diabetes	Islet cell	IFT on human or guinea pig pancreas
Non–Organ-Specific Diseases		
Lupus erythematosus	Nuclear antigens	
Dermatomyositis		
Periarteritis nodosa		
Scleroderma		
Rheumatoid arthritis	Altered gamma globulin	Latex agglutination (rheumatoid factor)
		Rose test, sheep cell agglutination
	Rheumatoid arthritis precipitin	Immunodiffusion
Sjögren's syndrome		
Polymyositis		
Other collagen diseases		
"Autoimmune" liver diseases		
Alimentary Tract Diseases		
Atrophic gastritis	Parietal cell microsomes	IFT (indirect)–human or mouse gastric mucosa substrate
Pernicious anemia	Intrinsic factor	Radioactive vitamin B_{12}–binding assay
Sjögren's syndrome	Salivary duct cells	IFT (indirect)–unfixed human salivary gland
Ulcerative colitis	Colon, lipopoly-saccharide	IFT (indirect)–human or rat colon
Celiac disease	Reticulin	IFT (indirect)–rat kidney, liver
Crohn's disease	Reticulin	IFT (indirect)–rat kidney, liver
Liver Diseases		
Chronic aggressive hepatitis	Smooth muscle (actin)	IFT (indirect)–rat gastric mucosa, human cervical tissue
	Liver/kidney microsomal	IFT (indirect)–rat kidney and liver
Primary biliary cirrhosis	Mitochondrial	IFT (indirect)–rat kidney, unfixed
Other		
Myasthenia gravis	Skeletal or heart muscle	IFT (indirect)–rat skeletal muscle and calf thymus
	Acetylcholine receptor	Radioimmunoassay
Goodpasture's syndrome	Glomerular and lung basement membrane	IFT (direct)–biopsy of patient's kidney
		IFT (indirect)–patients serum on human kidney substrate
		Radioimmunoassay on serum
Pemphigus vulgaris	Prickle cell desmosomes	IFT (direct and indirect)–human skin
		Peroxidase-labeled antibody
Bullous pemphigoid	Epithelial basement membrane	IFT (direct and indirect)–human skin
		Peroxidase-labeled antibody
Cicatricial pemphigoid	Epithelial basement membrane	IFT (direct) on biopsy of mucous membrane–indirect on human skin
Dermatitis herpetiformis	Reticulin	IFT (indirect)–rat kidney, liver
Autoimmune hemolytic anemia	Red cell	Coombs' antiglobulin test (direct and indirect)
Central nervous system demyelinating diseases (i.e., multiple sclerosis)	Myelin	IFT (indirect)–mammalian spinal cord

(From Nakamura, R. M., and Tucker, E. S.: *In* Henry, J. B. [Ed.]: Clinical Diagnosis by Laboratory Methods. 16th ed. Philadelphia, W. B. Saunders Company, 1978, Chap. 35.)

GENERAL LABORATORY TESTS

The most commonly used tests for the diagnosis of autoimmune disorders involve the detection of circulating antibodies. Tests for cellular sensitivity are done in the larger centers, primarily on an investigative basis.

Immunofluorescence, enzyme-labeled antibody, and radioimmunoassay methods utilize primary antigen-antibody binding reactions and, because of their high sensitivity, are preferred for the detection of circulating and tissue-bound antibodies and antigens.

Tests that involve secondary antigen-antibody preparations, such as complement fixation, agglutination, and precipitation in agar gel, may not be as sensitive as immunofluorescence or radioimmunoassay in some circumstances, but they may be technically more suitable for the identification of certain autoantibodies.

The indirect immunofluorescence test (IFT) and the more recently developed peroxidase-labeled antibody method are the most widely used immunohistochemical procedures for the detection of serum autoantibodies in the clinical laboratory. Both methods can be used to demonstrate (1) autoimmune antibodies in serum; (2) tissue localization and fixation of autoantibody; and (3) deposition of antigen-antibody complexes in kidney, vessels, and other tissues.

In addition to tissue autoantibody detection, numerous other methods have proved useful in the evaluation of patients with suspected autoimmune disorders. These include various assays for cell-mediated immunity that have potential usefulness in studying patients with autoimmune thyroiditis, certain liver diseases, and rheumatoid arthritis. Still other, less cumbersome methods are frequently employed, such as (1) rheumatoid factors; (2) immune complexes in serum or joint fluid; (3) quantitation of serum immunoglobulins; (4) immunoelectrophoresis of serum and other body fluids; (5) cryoglobulins; (6) complement assays; and (7) biopsy of kidney, vessel, or joint for immunofluorescence localization of antibody and immune complexes.

Interpretation of Serum Autoantibody Levels. In general, the level of antibody is high in patients with autoimmune disorders and low in apparently healthy persons. A very high titer of autoantibody is significant, but a low or absent titer of autoantibody does not rule out the possibility of an autoimmune disorder. For example, in severe thyroiditis, at the height of the disease the gland may act as an immunoadsorbent and remove circulating antibody. In addition, thyroglobulin may be released into the circulation during the acute stage, neutralizing circulating autoantibody. Therefore, the level, or titer, of a given antibody must be interpreted in relation to the stage or treatment of a particular disease.

When adults are tested for rheumatoid factor and the antibodies to nuclear, parietal cell, thyroglobulin, thyroid epithelial cell, reticulin, mitochondrial, and smooth muscle, the incidence of autoantibodies in the general adult population to one or more antigens at a level of 1:10 titer or greater varies from approximately 21 to 27 per cent, with a higher incidence in females. The incidence of certain autoantibodies increases with advancing age. In one study, 50 per cent of subjects over 60 years of age demonstrated low titers of one or more autoantibodies.

The antinuclear, antiparietal cell, and antithyroid antibodies are age- and sex-dependent, with an increasing incidence in females and older persons. However, the incidences of smooth muscle antibody and rheumatoid factor do not correlate with age and sex. The incidences of smooth muscle antibody and rheumatoid factor are similar in males and females.

AUTOIMMUNITY AND NEOPLASIA

Autoimmune reactions to damaged or altered tissue may facilitate malignant degeneration with adoptive loss of cellular components. Human cancer and autoimmunity may be related, since (1) certain autoimmune diseases may be considered precancerous and are associated with a higher incidence of cancer than occurs in the control population; and (2) the host immune response to the invading cancer may initiate immunologic injury with formation of nonmetastatic distant lesions.

There may be a step-by-step developmental sequence from normal immunologic regulation through autoimmunity and benign lymphoproliferation, leading ultimately to lymphoid neoplasia. Considerable evidence from studies in humans and animals suggests that autoimmunity, monoclonal immunoglobulin production, and malignant lymphocytic and plasma cell proliferation may be related events. There is a clear association between autoimmunity and the lymphoma that occurs in Sjögren's syndrome. Sjögren's syndrome represents a lymphocytic attack on the salivary and lacrimal glands, and the disease is associated with rheumatoid arthritis in almost 50 per cent of cases. Sjögren's syndrome often is benign, leading to progressive oral and ocular dryness. However, some patients exhibit an aggressive course, demonstrating lymphocytic infiltrates with lymphadenopathy. The term *pseudolymphoma* has been applied to this condition, and some patients with this abnormality develop malignant lymphomas without necessarily passing through the pseudolymphoma state. The lymphomas are often highly undifferentiated and may be associated with hypogammaglobulinemia and loss of antibodies.

A pathologic entity termed *immunoblastic lymphadenopathy* has been described, a lesion that has been confused with Hodgkin's disease. The lymph node shows immunoblastic proliferation in the B-lymphocyte plasma cell series, with proliferation of small vessels and deposits of amorphous interstitial material. The cellular proliferation is considered benign; however, the clinical course is associated with a poor prognosis. Many of the patients show hypersensitivity reaction to drugs, and this entity supports the concept that there is uncontrolled immunoblastic proliferation following an antigenic stimulus, and a true neoplasm may develop.

IMMUNE MECHANISMS IN TISSUE DAMAGE

Advances in knowledge of the immune response and immune reactivity achieved since the early 1960s have been accompanied by a more complete understanding of the different pathways of immune tissue injury. In the section that follows, these varied pathogenic mechanisms will be examined.

The different types of immune reactivities were briefly described in the context of the discussions of various sections of Chapter 4. Antibodies and effector T-lymphocytes were noted to participate in essentially different pathogenic sequences, all of which lead to a common effect of direct neutralization or inactivation of antigen or indirect inactivation due to cellular and biochemical mediating mechanisms. During the course of extensive experiments in animals, each of the major mechanisms of immune injury has been studied and each step in the pathogenic sequences has been defined.

Based on this new understanding, the various types of immunopathologic processes have been subdivided by the classification by Coombs and Gell into the following four basic types:

Type I: Immediate hypersensitivities
Type II: Cytotoxic tissue injury
Type III: Immune complex tissue injury
Type IV: Cell-mediated immune tissue injuries

As we shall see later, this classification is oversimplified because of the complex interrelationships that exist between the several events that constitute an inflammatory response. Nevertheless, this view represents the closest approximation of the various basic patterns of immune tissue injury, and the classification does not depend on the host species or on the method of antigen exposure. Another valuable feature of the classification is its integrated emphasis on the important central point that in these various patterns of immune injury the tissue damage results from the immune activation of cellular and biochemical mediator systems of the host. The combination of the immune reactants produces only minimal direct effects, but as a trigger mechanism it sets the destructive factors into play.

Type I Reactions (Immediate Hypersensitivities)

The term *immediate hypersensitivity* denotes an immunologic sensitivity to antigens that manifests itself by tissue reactions occurring within minutes after the antigen combines with its appropriate antibody. Such a reaction may occur in any member of a species (nonatopic immediate hypersensitivity) or only in certain predisposed or hyperreactive members (atopic immediate hypersensitivity).

The prototype of the nonatopic immediate hypersensitivity is local or generalized anaphylaxis, whereas manifestations of atopic immediate hypersensitivity include bronchial asthma, hay fever, allergic rhinitis, chronic urticaria, and atopic dermatitis.

Nonatopic Immediate Hypersensitivities

The term *anaphylaxis* was coined to represent the prototype of this group of manifestations under the following historical circumstances. In 1890, von Behring discovered the prophylactic use of antiserum against diphtheria toxin. In a search for other prophylactic antisera, Portier and Richet noted an immediate shocklike reaction in a sensitive dog to a sea anemone toxin; they called this harmful reaction *antiphylaxis,* or *anaphylaxis,* to denote the antithesis of the helpful *prophylaxis.* For the purpose of this discussion, anaphylaxis is defined as a manifestation of immediate hypersensitivity resulting from the in-vivo interaction of cellular sites with antigen and specific antibody.

Terminology. *"Generalized anaphylaxis"* refers to a shocklike state occurring within minutes following an appropriate antigen-antibody reaction. Upon the first exposure of an animal to an antigen, a cytotropic antibody may form that sensitizes mast cells, basophils, and other cells, storing and/or synthesizing pharmacologically active effector molecules in tissues and in blood. After a second exposure to the antigen, the animal so sensitized reacts with the explosive release of the foregoing effector molecules, which results in the hemodynamic, bronchial, and cutaneous manifestations of shock. In this particular example, furthermore, we are referring to *active* anaphylaxis, since the final clinical manifestation is dependent on the active production of cytotropic antibodies by the test animal. If, however, the test animal is the recipient of cytotropic antibodies produced by a donor animal, the condition of the test animal resulting from exposure to the antigen is called *passive* anaphylaxis.

Another term, *local anaphylaxis,* is used for describing the anaphylactic response of a specific target organ (e.g., the bronchial tree, gastrointestinal tract, nasal mucosa, or skin). Under experimental conditions, such a reactivity may be induced by passive sensitization of the tissue in question with antibody-containing serum obtained from a sensitized donor; subsequent intravenous or local administration of the corresponding antigen will then result in a local anaphylactic reaction. An illustrative example of this kind of reactivity is the so-called *passive cutaneous anaphylaxis (PCA)*, in which an animal is injected intracutaneously with serum from a sensitive animal of the same or another species. After a certain latent period, required for the cutaneous fixation of the antibody, the antigen is administered intravenously along with Evans blue dye, which will react with the skin-fixed antibody, causing the release of histamine from cutaneous mast cells. The histamine release results in local vasodilation and leakage of albumin, to which the blue dye is attached, producing a blue spot. The latter indicates that an anaphylactic reaction has taken place in the skin.

For experimental purposes, several in-vitro tissue models of anaphylaxis have been developed. Of these, the earliest model is the Schultz-Dale test, which uses isolated smooth muscle from a sensitized animal (e.g., ileum, uterus, and tracheal ring). Frequently employed alternative models include finely chopped lung slices, skin fragments, peritoneal mast cells, and circulating basophils obtained from actively or passively sensitized tissues.

General Characteristics of the Anaphylactic Pattern of Immunologic Tissue Injury. The sequence of biochemical and cellular events in anaphylactic tissue injury is much better understood than it was in the 1970s. Initially, the immunoresponsive host becomes sensitized by developing a significant cytotropic antibody response on exposure to the stimulating immunogen. Theoretically, any immunogen should be able to elicit anaphylaxis in a properly sensitized host. These may be proteins, chemical haptens such as drugs attached to proteins, carbohydrates, or, occasionally, nucleic acids. Cellular antigens such as red cells or bacteria usually cause weak and inconsistent sensitization.

Cytotropic antibodies—primarily the IgG and IgE classes, but, in special circumstances, IgA and IgM—may also be involved in anaphylactic sensitization. Nevertheless, homocytotropic antibodies (i.e., antibodies that will sensitize an animal of the same species) are cardinal in such reactions, and these are of the IgE class in all species so far examined. In general, 10 to 14 days are required after immunization before IgG antibodies result in active anaphylactic sensitization, whereas IgE sensitization may occur earlier. Passive sensitization has a latent period (the time needed for the antibody to attach to the cells storing or synthesizing the pharmacologically active effector molecules) of 3 to 6 hours for IgG antibodies, and it is short-lived because the IgG molecules become detached from these cells within 12 to 24 hours. However, passive sensitization with IgE antibody, although it may occur within 6 hours, becomes strong by 24 to 72 hours. Consequently, anaphylactic reactions occurring after 48 to 72 hours are practically exclusively due to IgE antibodies, since IgG antibodies are already detached from the target cells and, therefore, do not participate in such a reaction. IgE antibodies remain fixed to the target basophils, mast cells, and so forth for about 6 weeks in humans.

Following the initiation of antibody production, the cytotropic antibodies (primarily IgE) that are formed disseminate throughout the circulation to become almost selectively and uniquely attached to the cell membranes of basophils in the circulation and mast cells in the tissues. The attachment occurs through a structural area in the Fc part of the antibody molecule to a specific receptor on the basophil or mast cell membrane. Although some evidence indicates that subpopulations of monocytes, macrophages, and lymphocytes also express Fc receptors for IgE antibody, of all mammalian cells only basophils and mast cells exhibit an extraordinary binding affinity for this antibody. There is a relative abundance of these IgE molecules bound along the membrane, and they are located close to each other physically. When the IgE becomes attached, the cells are said to be sensitized, and the individual is now in a sensitive state for reactivity on subsequent exposure to the antigen (Fig. 5–15).

A second, or subsequent, exposure can occur via many routes, such as inhalation, ingestion, or injection. The immunogen (antigen, allergen) must move across membrane and tissue barriers in order to come to the surface of the sensitized cells. When this close encounter occurs with an immunogen of sufficient size to react with the immunogen-binding sites of two closely adjacent IgE molecules, it produces a "bridging" effect. In this molecular interaction, one immunogen molecule combines with two antibody molecules to form a bridge. This bridging brings together two IgE receptor molecules, which results in distortion of the cell membrane, triggering an enzymatic cascade that causes the release of pharmacologically active effector molecules responsible for the clinical symptomatology of anaphylaxis. The optimal ration of antigen to antibody for elicitation of anaphylaxis is slight to moderate antigen excess. So-called *toxic complexes* of composition Ag_3Ab_2 or Ag_5Ab_3 best trigger anaphylactic reactions. These are small complexes that best bridge surface receptors in the combining site of sensitizing antibodies. Complexes of Ag_2Ab_1 formed in extreme antigen excess do not trigger anaphylaxis. Such complexes are unable to bridge antibodies because both combining sites on each antibody molecule are attached to two different antigen molecules. Large amounts of antibody are complexed by relatively few antigens in zones of antibody excess or at the optimal

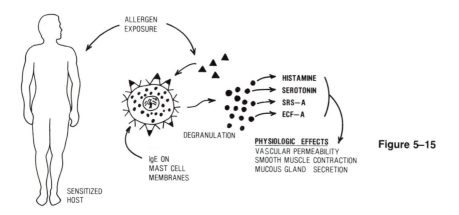

Figure 5–15

PATHOGENIC EVENTS IN ANAPHYLAXIS

proportions for precipitation. These are usually insufficient for triggering anaphylactic reactions, but in these zones minimal anaphylaxis may occur.

As already stated, the bridging effect of the antigen-antibody interaction results in the release of stored (preformed) and newly formed pharmacologically active effector molecules. These agents (described in detail in Chapter 4) include amines, peptides, lipid substances, Hageman factor pathway and other enzymes, and proteoglycans. Collectively, they produce an increase in blood flow, capillary permeability, constriction of smooth muscles, and secretion of mucous glands. These varied effects account for the sudden tissue changes characteristic of local and systemic anaphylactic reaction (Fig. 5–15).

The particular tissue site of the reaction depends on the portal of entry (route of exposure) of the antigen. Antigens that are inhaled make contact with mast cells by crossing the mucous membranes of the nose, the sinuses, and the lower respiratory tract. The local effects in these tissues are characterized by a marked increase in mucus secretion, with congestion and edema of the mucous membranes. The effect on bronchi and bronchiolar smooth muscle causes constriction with impairment of air flow, severely restricting pulmonary exchange and usually associated with the sudden onset of wheezing respirations.

Ingestion of antigens in food substances or oral medications can cause local and diffuse reactions in the gastrointestinal tract. Such exposure may produce symptoms of acute onset, commonly in the form of intestinal hypermotility, dyspepsia, colicky pain, and a sensation of fullness and bloating. These symptoms occur because of local release of pharmacologically active effector molecules by the immune reaction along the submucosa of the gastrointestinal tract. Antigens may also be absorbed into the circulation from the gastrointestinal tract and disseminate throughout the body, resulting in generalized systemic reactions or localized reactions in the skin and viscera or both.

In the skin, the acute reactions can present as edematous papules or larger urticarial lesions. Acute systemic reactions can occur following the injection of an antigen, such as a drug or vaccine, in individuals with marked sensitivity. The condition of acute anaphylaxis can lead to shock, respiratory insufficiency, and death unless there is immediate treatment. Such profound systemic reaction is due to the massive intravascular release of effector molecules from the circulating basophils.

Atopic Immediate Hypersensitivities (Diseases of Atopic Allergy)

As stated earlier, manifestations of atopic immediate hypersensitivity include bronchial asthma, hay fever, allergic rhinitis, certain forms of chronic urticaria, and atopic dermatitis. These diseases are discussed in detail in Chapter 18, and, therefore, the discussions that follow will be confined to the problems of the constitutional basis of atopic immediate hypersensitivities or disease of atopic allergy.

Only a minority of the population shows some form of atopic disease in spite of the fact that, by and large, identical conditions of antigen exposure must be presumed to exist for all members of the population. The nature of the constitutional basis of atopy, that is, of the underlying determinant for the development of atopic disease, is as yet unexplained.

Many theories of the constitutional basis of atopy have been proposed since Coca and Cooke's original definition. Only two general ideas, however, have survived: (1) the perception of atopy as a primary disorder of the immune system with sequelae in the various effector tissues; and (2) a concept of atopy as a primary autonomic imbalance, essentially beta-adrenergic in character, with sequelae in effector cells *including* those engaged in the production of antibodies. The autonomic imbalance is perceived *as caused not by some disorder of the autonomic nervous system itself but by a defective functioning of its effector cells.*

These two concepts are not mutually exclusive. In fact, they may be interdependent. Although the immune features of atopic disease can be understood within the framework of a basic adrenergic disorder of various effector cells, many, if not most, of the nonimmune features of atopic conditions are not readily explicable on the basis of the primary immune abnormality.

The Original Concept of Atopy. At the time when the first concepts of atopy were being developed, it had long been known that hay fever and asthma often occurred together in the same individual and that both conditions showed a marked familial tendency. Similarly, it had been recognized that acute and chronic urticaria as well as gastrointestinal manifestations of idiosyncrasy to a specific food were more common in patients with these diseases than in the general population, and a relation to infantile eczema (Besnier's prurigo, neurodermatitis) also was observed. Eczema was found to occur more frequently in the children of patients with hay fever or asthma, and individuals who had eczema in infancy showed an unusual incidence of hay fever and asthma later in life.

These diseases were, therefore, considered together by Cooke and Vander Veer as a special group of diseases of human sensitization with a hereditary background, and these authors concluded that such "sensitized individuals transmit to their offspring not their own specific sensitization, but an unusual capacity for developing bioplastic reactivities to any foreign proteins." With further progress in determining additional characteristics of "human sensitization" in contrast to those of experimental anaphylaxis in laboratory animals, Coca and Cooke concluded that a clear distinction must be made between two types of hypersensitivity manifestations: (1) the *anaphylactic* type of allergic response to abnormal substances, and (2) the *atopic* type of response to substances that are generally innocuous. As they stated:

"This latter sub-group evidently needs a special term by which it may be conveniently designated and this need is satisfactorily met with the word atopy, which was kindly suggested by Professor Edward D. Perry of Columbia University. The Greek word ἀτοπία from which the term was derived, was used in the sense of a strange disease. However, it is not, on that account, necessary to include under the term all strange diseases; the use of the term can be restricted to the hay fever and asthma group."

To these, Wise and Sulzberger then added neurodermatitis under the new designation of "atopic dermatitis." Based on the close association of this condition with other atopic manifestations, Wise and Sulzberger concluded that the skin lesions of this disorder were the cutaneous analog of hay fever and asthma and suggested that the name *atopic dermatitis* replace *disseminated neurodermatitis.*

Several characteristics of the atopic state emerged from these early concepts: Atopy was felt to be a hereditary manifestation, subject to a dominant gene, a peculiarly human disorder with a reacting serum element different from classic antibodies and reminiscent of the Wasserman reagin (hence the name, *atopic reagin*). Atopic antibodies, furthermore, seemed to occur only in humans, many times without any demonstrable prior exposure to incitant substances and induced by agents that often appeared to be nonantigenic (*atopens* of Grove and Coca).

Over the years, most of these postulated differences between atopy and anaphylaxis were gradually eliminated. Thus, antibody essentially identical with atopic reagin was found by Ishizaka in various animal species. Moreover, atopic disease was shown by Patterson to occur in animals. Some of the other distinctions between anaphylaxis and atopy also were amenable to various alternative explanations, indicating that these conditions may not be separated by wide and irreconcilable differences as it was believed by the originators of the concept of atopy. Nevertheless, some differences remained, and other important new differences emerged, making it imperative that a concept of atopy be reformulated.

The Reformulated Concept of Atopy. Since the 1960s, it has become increasingly evident that in addition to some of the remaining immunologic differences between anaphylaxis and atopic allergy, there are critically important nonimmune differences between the immediate hypersensitivities of the atopic and nonatopic. Thus, it appears that in anaphylaxis we are dealing with a normal (physiologic) antibody response to an unnatural exposure to antigen, whereas in atopic allergy an "abnormal" antibody response to natural antigenic exposure seems to be involved. Anaphylactic reactivity of the sensitized individual depends on the release of an amount of pharmacologically active effector molecules sufficient to be toxic for most members of the same species. *In contrast, individuals with atopic disease possess a quantitatively and qualitatively abnormal reactivity to otherwise nontoxic concentrations of endogenously released or exogenously administered pharmacologic mediators.* Furthermore, the quantitative change consistently is in the direction of a decreased response when beta-adrenergic agents are the agonists and consistently in the direction of an increased response when any one of the other pharmacologically active effector molecules is involved.

Another essential difference between the atopic and nonatopic varieties of immediate hypersensitivities is the major contributory role played by infection in atopy, whereas infection has not been shown to be causally related to anaphylactic allergy—anaphylaxis, the Arthus reaction, or serum sickness. Moreover, *atopic conditions can be precipitated by a number of totally unrelated stimuli,* whereas anaphylaxis can be brought about only by the specific antigen. Finally, the latter conditions may be produced artificially, but *atopic disease, with its spontaneous pattern of familial occurrence, cannot be induced at will.* Acute human pulmonary anaphylaxis, which can include asthmatic features, for example, has never been reported to lead to the development of bronchial asthma or other atopic disease.

In the reformulation of the original concept of atopy by Szentivanyi, *the essential difference between immediate hypersensitivities of the nonatopic and atopic varieties is that the former conditions are mediated by normal immune and pharmacologic mechanisms, whereas atopy is based on abnormal immune and pharmacologic mechanisms. This difference between anaphylaxis and atopy is regarded as fundamental. In this view, furthermore, it is the altered pharmacologic reactivity that is considered as the uniformly present, single atopic characteristic of pathognomonic significance.*

Development of the Beta-Adrenergic Approach to the Study of the Constitutional Basis of Atopy.
Authentic atopy cannot be produced at will in animals or humans—neither induced directly nor transferred passively. In addition to animal models of anaphylaxis, there are a number of experimental models simulating human atopy as well as isolated systems suitable for studying segmented areas of atopic reactivity. As such, they are useful for the analysis of some of the individual events (i.e., mediator release) in the human reaction. Nevertheless, these in-vivo and in-vitro models are anaphylactic variants and represent immunologically and pharmacologically normal reactivities. Therefore, they cannot be used for the study of the constitutional abnormality in atopy.

The two experimental models for the study of the constitutional basis of atopy

The search for a laboratory model was guided by the premise that, if it is to be meaningful, the model must be able to imitate not only the immunologic but also the pharmacologic abnormality of the atopic state. As discussed in Chapter 4, the latter is manifested against substances that, in mammalian physiology, serve as the natural chemical organizers of autonomic action. It seemed likely, therefore, that an abnormal reactivity to these agents could be most effectively produced through some alteration of normal autonomic regulation significant enough to result in an autonomic imbalance.

The Hypothalamically "Imbalanced" Anaphylactic Guinea Pig.
The first attempts to establish a more meaningful experimental counterpart of

the atopic state were made by Filipp and Szentivanyi in the years from 1952 to 1958 during studies of hypothalamically "imbalanced" anaphylactic guinea pigs. Briefly, by electrolytic removal of one hypothalamic division or electric stimulation of the antagonistic division, it was possible to alter profoundly the anaphylactic reactivity of guinea pigs both immunologically and pharmacologically. From both the immunologic and pharmacologic standpoints, the conditions so produced more closely approximated those of the human atopic state than does anaphylaxis. Nevertheless, it was felt that the artificiality of such surgically induced hypothalamic imbalance is far removed from the natural setting (involving various inherited or acquired factors or both) that may surround the development of an atopic state. In their efforts to discover a more accurate representation of those naturally occurring conditions—some of which (i.e., infection) may conceivably serve as a developmental background for atopy—some researchers found that the *Bordetella pertussis*–induced hypersensitive state served as a more appropriate model.

The *Bordetella Pertussis*–induced Hypersensitive State of Mice and Rats.
Injection of live or killed *Bordetella pertussis* organisms into certain strains of mice and rats modifies the normal responses of these animals to a number of various stimuli. The possible applicability of the results of these investigations to atopy is implied by the following principal features of the *B. pertussis*–induced altered responsiveness: (1) hypersensitivity to endogenously released or exogenously administered histamine, serotonin, bradykinin, slow-reacting substance A, some prostaglandins, and, at least in two strains, to acetylcholine; (2) hypersensitivity to less specific stimuli, such as cold, changes in atmospheric pressure, and respiratory irritants; (3) in contrast with these increased sensitivities, a reduced beta-adrenergic sensitivity to catecholamines and, concerning some metabolic parameters, a reversal of normal beta-adrenergic activity; (4) enhanced antibody formation in general (adjuvant activity) and facilitated production in the quantity of antibodies of the IgE class; and (5) presence of a marked eosinophilia.

According to Szentivanyi and Fishel, the major advance in these experiments that has paved the way for a meaningful analogy to atopic disorders has been the finding that hypersensitivity of the pertussis-sensitized mouse to pharmacologic mediators may be due to an acquired autonomic imbalance caused primarily by a reduced functioning of the beta-receptors or of some of the reactions between receptor activation and adrenergic end response. In particular, the deprivation of the normal beta-adrenergic inhibition of peripheral (extrahepatic) uptake of glucose appears to be instrumental in the production of the hypersensitivity to the various pharmacologic mediators. In addition, this increased rate of entry of glucose may well be the biochemical explanation for the pertussis-induced alterations of the immune response.

Principal tenets of the beta-adrenergic theory of atopic disorder

The previously discussed considerations and conclusions of the two consecutive series of animal experiments have culminated in the postulation of the beta-adrenergic theory of atopic disorders reported by Szentivanyi. *This theory regards these disorders (i.e., perennial and seasonal alleric rhinitis, bronchial asthma, and atopic dermatitis) not as* immunologic diseases *but as unique patterns of altered reactivities to a broad spectrum of immunologic, psychic, infectious, chemical, and physical stimuli. This view gives to the antigen-antibody interaction the same role as that of a broad category of nonspecific stimuli that function only to trigger the same defective homeostatic mechanism in the various effector cells of the biochemical reaction sequence of immediate hypersensitivities.*

Activation of the same defective mechanism by such a broad spectrum of unrelated stimuli is believed to be made possible by the unusual character of the pharmacologic mediators as a biologically distinct class of natural substances. As discussed in Chapter 4, these mediators, when viewed from the standpoint of their probable physiologic function, are the chemical organizers of autonomic action, that is, of homeostatic control. Consequently, regardless of the immunologic or nonimmunologic nature of the triggering event, its chemical realization would be expected to be brought about by essentially the same mediators.

Homeostatic adjustment to these influences requires, among other things, mobilization of the adrenergic neurotransmitters and their balanced (uninhibited) interaction with their effector systems. The theory postulates that *the constitutional basis of atopy lies in the reduced functioning of the beta-adrenergic effector system, irrespective of what the triggering event may chemically be in a particular case (e.g., immunologic, infectious, or psychic). In this situation, the adrenergic neurotransmitters are released in the face of a relatively unresponsive beta-adrenergic effector system, and the resultant autonomic imbalance deprives the effector tissues of their normal counterregulatory adjustment. This constellation of mediators and effectors then leads to a unique pattern of quantitatively and qualitatively altered reactivity to the chemical organizers of autonomic action, mostly in response to trivial trauma.*

The most critical component of this malfunctioning effector system is the adenylate cyclase–coupled beta-adrenergic receptor, or, more specifically, the receptor–transducer–adenylate cyclase complex. It follows, therefore, that the fundamental abnormality common to all atopic persons may lie in an inherited or acquired lesion that causes defective functioning of this complex. This reduced responsiveness to catecholamines could reflect alterations at any of a number of sites, including (1) changes in the affinity of catecholamines and their receptor sites; (2) decreases in the concentration of beta receptors; (3) "interconversion" of adrenergic receptors from beta to alpha; (4) alterations in the efficiency of coupling of activated receptors to the catalytic units of adenylate cyclase; and (5) reductions in the concentration of adenylate cyclase. Alternatively, the postulated lesion may occur at a point beyond the cAMP generation step in the biochemical sequence leading to the adrenergic end response; in a cAMP-related pathway; in a complementary interacting or modulating system such as that provided by the prostaglandins; or in an intracellular messenger system with counterregulatory potential, such as that connected with cyclic GMP. Nevertheless, *the currently available evidence seems to favor the possibility that the postulated lesion lies at an early point of the adrenergic reaction sequence, involving either a reduction in beta-receptor concentration or mechanisms similar to those that may occur in receptor interconversions.*

Progression of the disease process from a subclinical to a clinical form conceivably requires the operation of a preparatory and a triggering factor. The preparatory factor involves the postulated abnormality, and it may be familial (presumably hereditary) or acquired in nature; however, in either case, it must set the stage for the development of a functional imbalance. The triggering event must be appropriate to result in an increase in the rate of firing of adrenergic neurons, in the release of catecholamines from extraneuronal stores, or in any conceivable mediator constellations suitable to make the latent abnormality clinically manifest. However, the preparatory and triggering factors need not be separate or unrelated entities. Infection (probably viral), for example, could serve in both capacities.

With the exception of nonnucleated erythrocytes, the adenylate cyclase system has been found to be present in all animal cells examined to date. Its ubiquitous character suggests, therefore, that *the ultimate clinical manifestation of the fundamentally same atopic abnormality will be determined by the type of cell primarily involved, that is, by the effector cell system that primarily harbors the postulated abnormality* (cells of bronchial tissue versus those of nasal mucosa and skin and the circulating cells of blood).

Evolution of research strategy in the experimental analysis of the beta-adrenergic theory

In the experimental analysis of this theory, both chronologically and in research strategy, four phases can be distinguished. In the wake of the early presentations of the theory (1962 to 1972), manifestations of reduced asthmatic responsiveness to catecholamines as measured by various systemic parameters of beta-adrenergic reactivity were found. These studies showed less rise in blood sugar, free fatty acids, lactate, pyruvate, pulse rate, and urinary and plasma cAMP levels as well as a reduced eosinopenic response following beta-adrenergic stimulation in asthmatic patients. Reduction in adrenergic responsiveness correlated well with the severity of the disease and with the degree of pharmacologic hypersensitivity, as judged by exposure to acetylcholine.

Although these results were highly compatible with the beta-adrenergic theory, their interpretation was handicapped by the limitations of in-vivo studies involving complex homeostatic regulations. It was, therefore, of importance that in the second phase of the experimental analysis of the beta-adrenergic theory (1972 to 1975), the same pattern of reduced beta-adrenergic responsiveness was demonstrable in in-vitro preparations of isolated cells derived from asthmatic individuals. In such studies, leukocytes and lymphocytes from asthmatic donors exhibited a reduced cAMP response to beta-adrenergic agonists but an intact response to prostaglandin E_1, suggesting that the biochemical defect may in fact be at the level of the beta-adrenoceptor.

However, as the continuing analysis of the beta-adrenergic approach to atopy entered its third phase (1975 to 1978), several methodologic and theoretical problems emerged, casting doubt on the validity of interpretation of the foregoing findings on leukocytes and lymphocytes as well as on the supportive value of these findings for the de facto existence of the postulated beta-adrenergic abnormality. These problems are connected with the develoment of the radioligand-binding methodology.

Specifically, emergence of this technology in the study of adrenoceptors has resulted in an array of new problems in current research on atopic disease. These include (1) the similarities and differences between agonist-induced desensitization and manifestations of beta-adrenergic subsensitivity in diseases of atopic allergy and some related conditions; (2) discovery of the reciprocal changes in alpha- and beta-adrenergic reactivities as well as in their respective receptor concentrations and, if indeed there are such reciprocal changes, their nature; and (3) consideration of the various developmental mechanisms that may be operative in the induction of beta-adrenergic subsensitivities in atopic disease.

The first study of physiologically relevant beta-adrenoceptors in human lymphocytes using the beta-specific radioligand [³H]dihydroalprenolol ([³H]DHA) was conducted in 1976. By 1980, a reduction in the numbers of beta-receptors was demonstrated in lymphocytes of asthmatic patients. The first question that could be raised by these findings concerns whether the reduced numbers of lymphocytic beta-receptors in bronchial asthma are due to an authentic beta-adrenergic abnormality inherent in the atopic constitution itself or to quantitative shifts in lymphocyte subpopulations possessing different numbers of beta-receptors in their membranes.

Researchers addressed this question in later studies by comparing B- and T-lymphocytes obtained from the same population of peripheral blood lymphocytes to determine whether differences existed in the concentration or affinity of beta-adrenoceptors on their membranes or their beta-adrenergically responsive intracellular cAMP levels. No significant difference was found in the respective numbers of beta-adrenoceptors or in the dissociation constants for [³H]DHA between B cells and T cells. Cyclic AMP accumulations in whole lymphocytes were also comparable, although a tendency toward lower basal and stimulated levels in the T cells was evident. These findings, together with additional observations discussed subsequently, appear to indicate that reductions in numbers of lymphocytic beta-adrenoceptors in bronchial asthma are not likely to be caused by possible differences in the proportions of circulating B- and T-lymphocytes.

In subsequent studies, the degree of reduction in lymphocytic beta-receptor numbers correlated well with disease severity and airway obstruction among patients. Those asthmatic patients with more severe disease and greater airway obstruction showed lower numbers of lymphocytic beta-receptors. Nevertheless, it remained unclear whether this correlation could have been entirely accounted for by differences in drug treatment. Theophylline preparations were predominantly used, and administration of beta-adrenergic agonists was limited. Likewise, the decrease in the numbers of beta-receptors was as apparent in asthmatic patients who received no adrenergic bronchodilators as in those who did receive such drugs. In any case, these studies raised the question concerning whether manifestations of beta-adrenergic subsensitivities in asthma may be due to the disease itself or to adrenergic medication taken by the patients.

Although drug-induced beta-adrenergic desensitization may clearly cause decreasd beta-adrenergic reactivity or contribute in many situations to the overall beta-adrenergic subsensitivity, beta-adrenergic subsensitivity appears to be a fundamental characteristic of atopy for the following reasons:

1. Decreased beta-adrenergic responses to catecholamines by no means represent a consistent feature of adrenergic therapy.

2. There are findings to indicate that adrenoceptor susceptibility to agonist desensitization varies with the receptor subtype as well as with the tissue involved and that some adrenoceptors may not be subject to down-regulation.

3. Beta-adrenergic subsensitivity in asthma can be shown to occur also during periods without symptoms or medication or under circumstances in which prior or concurrent medication can be only one contributing factor to defective beta-adrenergic function.

4. In fact, there is evidence to suggest that atopic asthmatic and nonasthmatic atopic subjects may not develop beta-adrenergic subsensitivity as readily as do normal individuals.

5. Beta-adrenergic subsensitivity is also demonstrable in atopic conditions (atopic dermatitis) in which adrenergic medication has never been involved.

6. Most importantly, because of methodologic developments, different patterns of drug-induced, versus disease-induced, beta-adrenergic subsensitivities may now be recognized in lung tissue, lymphocytes, and adipocytes in atopic asthma.

In the aggregate, these findings indicate that, depending on the selectivity of the agonist used, drug-induced beta-adrenergic subsensitivity results in a reduction in the number of the relatively affected beta-receptors, whereas in beta-adrenergic subsensitivity induced by the atopic state, some other mechanism or mechanisms are involved that result in a concurrent rise in the numbers of alpha-adrenoceptors.

Inverse changes in lymphocytic beta-receptor–binding can also be shown in asthmatic subjects when the effects of guanine nucleotides on $beta_2$-agonist–binding are studied. The normal effect of guanosine triphosphate (GTP) and its synthetic analogue, 5-guanylyl-imido-diphosphate (Gpp(NH)p), is a reduction in the apparent affinity of agonists in competing for beta-adrenergic binding sites. This was originally shown in studies on the binding of the beta-agonist [³H]hydroxybenzyl-isoproterenol ([³H]HBI) to frog erythrocyte membranes. In these experiments, after a steady-state level of [³H]HBI binding to frog erythrocyte membranes was attained, Gpp(NH)p was added to the incubation, resulting in a very rapid dissociation of a large portion of the bound [³H]HBI. Other nucleotides have a similar effect on agonist binding in the following order of potency: GTP > guanosine-5'-diphosphate > ATP = guanosine-5'-monophosphate. It is to be noted that this aspect of agonist binding contrasts markedly with the binding of a radioligand *antagonist,* such as [³H]DHA, which is not affected by the addition of guanine nucleotide to the incubation mixture.

When this experimental design was used for the study of the binding of [³H]HBI to lymphocytic membranes in the presence and absence of the guanine nucleotide, it was found that Gpp(NH)p caused a substantial *decrease* in [³H]HBI-binding in patients without airways disease and in those with nonreversibly obstructed airways disease but an increase in reversibly obstructed airways disease (asthma). At present, the nature of such a reversal in the normal effect of Gpp(NH)p is un-clear, but it raises the possibility of some biochemical membrane disorder that possibly involves multiple receptor abnormalities.

Under these circumstances, it is important to mention some of the results of studies designed to determine whether there is any change in cholinergic (muscarinic) receptor numbers in lymphocytic and lung membranes of patients with airways disease and atopic dermatitis. With the use of [³H]quinuclidinyl benzilate ([³H]QNB), a stereospecific radioligand for muscarinic cholinergic receptors, it was shown that there were (1) a significant reduction in the number of cholinergic receptors in the lung preparations of asthmatic patients; and (2) no difference in the number of receptors in lymphocytic membranes derived from the groups with nonreversibly obstructed airways disease (asthma) or atopic dermatitis. Thus, what is seen is a dichotomy between lymphocytes and lung with respect to the cholinergic receptor in the face of a completely identical pattern of behavior in the lymphocytes and lung specimens with regard to adrenoceptors.

Several interpretations could be offered for the phenomenon, but the most directly applicable one is that the adrenergic abnormality, although contributory to the leading tissue manifestations of atopic allergy, is connected primarily with the constitutional basis of atopy and not with the bronchial pathology of obstruction. An even more complicated question concerns how one can possibly find a reduction in the number of muscarinic cholinergic receptors in lung membranes derived from patients with reversible obstruction (asthma) when these patients show an exquisite bronchial hyperreactivity to cholinergic agents. At present, one can offer only two possible interpretations. One is that the bronchial hyperreactivity to cholinergic agents in asthma is not mediated through cholinergic mechanisms but is basically caused by the adrenergic abnormality that is also responsible for the atopic feature of the disease. An attractive second possibility is that the reduction in muscarinic receptor numbers is caused by a heightened vagus activity, resulting in a cholinergic downturn and ultimately producing a pharmacologic "denervation supersensitivity" to cholinergic agents.

In addition to these findings concerning adrenergic and cholinergic receptors, evidence is accumlating that manifestations of an imbalance between the two histamine receptor systems (H_1 and H_2 receptors) are present in various animal models of allergic reactions. These changes in the relative relationships of the two histamine receptor systems are highly reminiscent of the observations described earlier in that in most adrenoceptor measurements obtained in asthma, the change in the relative proportions of the two main adrenoceptor types appeared to occur in a mutually reciprocal manner—that is, a decrease in one receptor type was associated with a concurrent increase in the other receptor type. As stated earlier, the significance of these reciprocal changes is seen in the fact that they may be demonstrable in beta-adrenergic subsensitivities of some manifestation of human atopic diseases or in some of their animal models but not in beta-adrenergic subsensitivity produced by agonist desensitization. In case of the latter, depending on the agonist's selectivity or the lack of it, we find either a reduction in the number of all adrenoceptor types or a selective reduction in one type of adrenoceptor corresponding to the selectivity of the agonist. The critical point is that a selective reduction in the number of one adrenoceptor type is not matched by a concurrent rise in the number of another adrenoceptor type in case of agonist desensitization.

The nature of the reciprocal counterregulatory changes in numbers and reactivities of adrenoceptor types

Since adrenoceptors are no longer imaginary entities but morphologic realities, the question that provides the framework for discussion of the foregoing reciprocal changes could be stated as follows: Are adrenoceptor subtypes real in the physiologic sense, or do they become apparent only when certain chemicals are applied to them?

Three different arguments are apparent:

1. There is only one kind of adrenoceptor. It responds best to epinephrine. This adrenoceptor also responds to the two other natural catecholamines (dopamine, norepinephrine), and any apparent differences are due to the association of the receptor with different cells (e.g., smooth muscle, exocrine gland, or other effector cells).

2. There are two or more adrenoceptor subtypes because norepinephrine (adrenergic neurohormone, or neurotransmitter) and epinephrine (metabolic hormone) have different functions.

3. All adrenoceptors and their subtypes are different, depending on the cell membrane on which they are located.

The "Interconversion" Controversy. In the pattern of receptor behavior, the mutually reciprocal changes between functionally antagonistic adrenoceptors in atopic disease and in some of its animal models appear to be consistent enough to be reminiscent of the phenomenon of receptor "interconversion."

EVIDENCE SUPPORTING THE CONCEPT OF RECEPTOR INTERCONVERSION. The existence of such a phenomenon was originally suggested by Kunos and Szentivanyi on the basis of the finding that the beta-receptors of the frog heart could be converted to alpha-receptors by cold. This and subsequent observations were interpreted to indicate that alpha- and beta-receptors may represent different conformations of a metabolically controlled single receptor rather than separate and independent molecular entities.

The original observation on the effect of temperature shifting the balance of the adrenoceptors of the frog heart has been extended to include similar "shifts" under a number of conditions associated with low metabolic activity, including hibernation in frogs, low ambient temperatures, low rates of contraction, hypoxia, muscarinic cholinergic stimulation, some metabolic inhibitors, myocardial ischemia, adrenalectomy, and hypothyroidism.

Conversely, beta-directed shifts in adrenoceptor balance appear to be operative in insulin-deficient or insulin-deprived conditions such as human and alloxan diabetes. In human diabetes, some of the noradrenergic reactions of blood vessels normally sensitive only to alpha-adrenergic antagonists can be inhibited by beta-blocking agents. This beta-sensitive noradrenergic constriction, found previously in alloxan-diabetic rabbits, now appears to be an inherent characteristic of various diabetic vascular reactions, regardless of whether the diabetes has been induced by alloxan or has developed spontaneously.

Likewise, in experiments measuring alpha- and beta-receptor concentrations with [³H]dihydrocryocryptine ([³H]DHE) and [³H]DHA in myocardial homogenates of hypothyroid rats, an increase in the number of [³H]DHA-binding sites and a matching decrease in the [³H]DHE-binding sites, without changes in binding affinity, were found after a 6-day treatment with 0.5 mg kg^{-1} T_3. In another laboratory, similar changes were found as early as 2 days after treatment of hypophysectomized rats with 0.2 mg kg^{-1} T_4. The latter treatment schedule does not lead to cardiac hypertrophy but is sufficient to reverse completely the shift from beta- to alpha-type force and rate responses of atria, which develop over several weeks after hypophysectomy. In myocardial homogenates from these rats, the density of beta-receptors, identified as high-affinity [³H]DHA-binding, increased from 27.5 ± 2.7 (H_x) to 45.5 ± 5.7 fmol mg^{-1} protein ($H_x + T_4$), whereas the density of alpha-receptors, identified as prazosin-suppressible binding of [³H]WB-4101, decreased from 38.7 ± 3.1 (H_x) to 18.7 ± 2.5 fmol mg^{-1} protein ($H_x + T_4$). These observations demonstrate that reciprocal changes in alpha- and beta-receptor reactivities in the rat heart are associated with similar reciprocal changes in receptor numbers. It is pertinent to add that although thyroid hormones are known to induce the synthesis of a number of cell components, their effect on alpha- and beta-receptors may be a rapid and direct one that does not necessarily involve altered turnover of receptor protein. For instance, hypothyroidism in dogs changes the erythropoietic action of catecholamines from a beta$_2$- to an alpha-type response, and incubation of culture bone marrow cells from hypothyroid dogs with 100 mM T_4 for as little as 30 minutes reverses the response pattern from alpha-type response to beta-type response. There are many more examples of reciprocal changes in alpha- and beta-receptor responses in various other tissues and of factors other than thyroid state or temperature that can produce similar alterations.

EVIDENCE AGAINST THE CONCEPT OF RECEPTOR INTERCONVERSION. The information that has been interpreted by various workers as having provided evidence against the concept of receptor interconversion can be classed into two categories.

The first involves data obtained primarily through traditional physiopharmacologic analysis or radioligand binding studies from 1975 through 1979. The data and their interpretation developed in these publications are limited to suggesting that in one of the many conditions associated with reciprocal changes in alpha- and beta-receptor numbers or reactivities or both, such changes may not be detected under certain experimental conditions or may be attributed to nonspecific drug effects. None of these studies was undertaken in patients with atopic disease or in their animal models.

Since 1979, a more significantly important category of information has been developed; this involves detailed structural analysis of beta- and alpha-adrenoceptors provided by a number of new technical approaches, including target-size analysis radiation inactivation, receptor affinity probes, and immunologic studies wih monoclonal and antireceptor autoantibodies. Taken together, these structural studies indicate that alpha- and beta-receptors have distinct molecular identities.

The two significant questions about the reciprocal adrenoceptor changes

The critical questions that may be raised by the foregoing observations are as follows:

1. Are there, in fact, valid examples of reciprocal changes in alpha- and beta-receptor reactivities and in their respective concentrations?

2. If there are such examples, what is their mechanism?

The Validity of Examples of Reciprocal Adrenoceptor Changes. As was discussed earlier, there is substantial evidence to suggest that indeed there are valid examples of reciprocal changes in alpha- and beta-receptor reactivities as well as in their respective concentrations. Nevertheless, additional work is required to determine the ultimate validity of these observations and their physiologic and pathologic significance, especially in studies that were carried out by radioligand binding techniques.

Thus, the cells used to study adrenoceptors, primarily blood cells, often represent a mixture of several distinct populations, resulting in conflicting observations. For instance, the number of beta-receptors on PMNs seems to be normal in subjects with asthma unless they receive adrenergic ago-

nists. In sharp contrast, lymphocytes of asthmatic patients show a significant decrease in radioligand binding to beta-receptors, independent of agonist therapy. The same disparity in beta-receptor behavior between PMNs and lymphocytes can be shown to exist in patients with atopic dermatitis. Finally, in an article in which PMNs and lymphocytes were studied simultaneously in asthmatic patients for the first time in the literature, it was found that the patients not receiving drugs showed a significant reduction in beta-receptor concentration in lymphocytic membranes but not in PMN membranes. This consistent disparity in receptor behavior between PMNs and lymphocytes appears to be of pathognomonic significance for human asthma and atopic dermatitis.

Although studies to date have not indicated any difference in beta-receptor numbers or affinities for agonists or antagonists between B and T cells, there is some indication that different mononuclear cell types (T cells, B cells, null cells, and monocytes) do not accumulate the same amount of cAMP when stimulated with isoproterenol, and the results vary with the method used to separate the cells. It is possible that future studies emphasizing less perturbing methods to separate these various cell populations (i.e., centrifugal elutriation) will eliminate these variations in cAMP concentrations.

Another concern that has been raised in connection with lymphocytic alpha-receptors concerns the possibility that the [³H]DHE-binding in such studies represented alpha-receptors on platelets that may have contaminated the cell preparations. Although such a possibility cannot be entirely ruled out at present, it seems highly unlikely in view of the following considerations. In several experiments in which subtype-specific radioligands were used for the purpose of analyzing adrenoceptor subtype behavior in what appears to be two different subsets of asthmatic subjects, it was found that (1) lymphocytic alpha-adrenoceptors consist of both alpha$_1$- and alpha$_2$-subtypes, (2) the alpha-directed reciprocal shifts in lymphocytes of asthmatic patients are primarily confined to alpha$_2$-receptors, and (3) the adrenergic abnormality is not present in individuals with asymptomatic triad asthma (i.e., in patients whose asthma is combined with hypersensitivity to aspirin and presence of nasal polyps). This latter group therefore may represent patients with a type of asthma that is without the atopic abnormality or that is based on a different pathogenesis. This possibility is further supported by the findings on adipocytes obtained from the same patients and showing the same alpha$_2$-directed reciprocal shift that has been found on lymphocytes, indicating the same adrenoceptor subtype behavior in a cell preparation in which no contamination with platelets is possible. Since no adrenoceptor shift similar to that in lymphocytes could be demonstrated in adipocytes obtained from patients with triad asthma, these findings lend additional support to the notion that this subset of asthma may have a different pathogenetic background.

The Mechanisms of the Reciprocal Adrenoceptor Changes. In the conceptual framework of the interconversion hypothesis, two major mechanisms have been suggested.

According to one speculation, alpha- and beta-receptors may represent allosteric configurations of the same structure. Furthermore, since allosteric enzymes can be influenced by compounds unrelated to the specific substrate, allosteric adrenergic receptors could be appropriately influenced by the postulated modulator substance that has reportedly altered the balance of alpha- and beta-adrenergic vascular responses in skeletal muscle or by hormones.

The second approach focuses on the physical state of membrane lipids, which is known to be temperature-dependent and which can profoundly influence many membrane-associated processes. Indeed, there is evidence that membrane lipids have an essential role in the coupling between beta-adrenergic binding sites and adenylate cyclase, and discontinuities in the Arrhenius plots of catechol-activated adenylate cyclases were found at temperatures similar to the critical temperature for changes in adrenergic receptor properties. Binding of GTP to a regulatory site, which has already been implicated in the catecholamine-induced activation of adenylate cyclase, was proposed to be the temperature-sensitive event, since GTP analogues abolished the break in the Arrhenius plot.

However, in view of the earlier described structural differences between adrenoceptors, the reciprocal changes between receptors under various physiologic and pathologic conditions appear to suggest a functional rather than a morphologic relationship between these receptor entities. Nevertheless, many of the aforementioned findings may in fact be compatible with an actual interconversion of alpha- and beta-receptors at the same time that they are equally compatible with separate but functionally coupled receptor molecules. It is also possible that the mechanism of similar reciprocal changes in receptor responses under different conditions varies. Some of the later findings on the molecular characteristics of alpha- and beta-receptors may suggest that the two binding sites reside on different macromolecules or on different subunits of the same macromolecule and do not exclude a possible functional coupling of the two in the intact membrane.

We shall not be able to reach definitive conclusions on the nature of these reciprocal receptor changes until a new technology emerges that will enable us to study adrenoceptors in vivo in their natural membrane environment. Most investigators study adrenoceptors on cell fragments ("membranes") suspended in a nonphysiologic buffer with the virtual removal of the entire internal cell milieu. At this point, the receptors are "binding sites" and not biologically functioning receptors. Although such studies conducted with broken cells are informative in many ways, results obtained in this manner cannot lead to full understanding of how receptors are regulated in vivo.

It appears that such a new technology for the noninvasive in-vivo study of adrenoceptors on internal organs of patients is in fact in development. The first paper on the visualization of beta-receptor occupancy in the intact animal with nuclear-isotope scanning has already appeared in the literature. The two other highly promising technical approaches to such studies involved nuclear magnetic resonance and positron-emission tomography. Nuclear magnetic resonance is a technique that uses magnetic fields and electromagnetic energy. These magnetic fields interact with the basic unit of human matter, the atom, yielding biochemical data and images that allow investigation of molecular mechanisms in vivo. Positron-emission tomography is a technique that allows visualization of basic biologic processes through the images produced. Radioisotopes, positron-emitting substances made with a cyclotron, are added to natural body components (carbohydrates, water, protein, etc.). These radioactive substances are traced and imaged as they engage in fundamental biologic reactions. Thus, we are not far from making "beta-receptor scans" an integral part of our future receptor studies and, it is hoped, from clarifying the mechanisms involved in the contribution of the reciprocal adrenoceptor changes to the development of some forms of beta-adrenergic subsensitivity.

Developmental mechanisms of beta-adrenergic subsensitivity in asthma

An acute asthmatic episode may be seen as the dramatic culmination of an internal struggle for homeostasis. Initiated by a remarkable range of environmental or internal factors, the struggle probably begins at the site of an inherited or acquired intrinsic defect or imbalance at the molecular level. Then, regardless of the initiating agent or event, the physiologic "dominoes"—otherwise normal homeostatic responses—begin to fall along the characteristic asthma pathway.

In returning to the apparent central feature of the atopic abnormality (the intrinsic defect) that is the beta-adrenergic subsensitivity of the effector cells that participate in the cellular organization of the atopic response, the question may be raised of how such an abnormality could develop. At present, at least three major developmental mechanisms can be envisaged. The abnormality may be (1) acquired by a functional regulatory shift caused by hormonal changes, infection, allergic tissue injury, or other event; (2) genetically determined; or (3) caused by autoimmune disease. In case of a given atopic disorder, one, two, or all three of these major mechanisms may be operative.

As to the possibility of inheritance, it has been demonstrated in histamine-sensitive and histamine-insensitive strains of guinea pigs that the in-vivo histamine-induced reduction in lung compliance in the guinea pig is inversely related to its in-vitro tracheal threshold sensitivity to beta-adrenergic activation. It has been known also since the beginning of the twentieth century that broad ranges of differing autonomic reactivities can occur in humans in both health and disease. Thus, genetically determined differences in adrenergic reactivities are known to exist.

Considerations of an autonomic imbalance caused by a beta-adrenergic deficit have consistently emphasized that infections of both bacterial and viral varieties may produce the same type of damage in autonomic effector cells that has been described for the histamine-sensitizing factor of *Bordetella pertussis* and endotoxin of gram-negative bacteria. Endotoxin sensitization of human bronchial smooth muscle to alpha-adrenergic activation has, in fact, been reported previously. In these studies, phenylepinephrine-induced contractions were enhanced two to 10 times in normal lungs and 1000 times in lungs from a patient with chronic bronchitis, and endotoxin also caused a decrease in cAMP of the tissue. More recently, it was found that endotoxin produces a significant alpha-directed shift in adrenoceptor number.

Killed influenza virus vaccine, which has no local inflammatory activity, increases the sensitivity of asthmatic patients to aerosolized methacholine. During several reported viral respiratory infections that provoked an attack of asthma, the responsiveness of peripheral lymphocytes and granulocytes to beta-adrenergic activation was shown to be reduced more than usual. This additional reduction in beta-adrenergic reactivity during upper respiratory infections was also shown to apply to both the cAMP-synthesizing and the lysosomal enzyme–releasing properties of granulocytes. Also, it has been repeatedly observed that patients who have chronic bronchitis, with no previous history of asthma, may experience frank asthmatic attacks during therapy with a beta-adrenergic blocking agent instituted for some unrelated reason. Observations of cAMP-mediated changes in adrenoceptor specificities after virus transformation of a cultured cell line are also available.

All hormonal agents that have been studied so far (i.e., corticosteroids, thyroid hormones, insulin, and estrogen) are capable of producing an alpha- or beta-oriented shift in adrenoceptor numbers. Of these, the most extensively studied are the glucocorticoids, which can also produce an increase in beta- and a decrease in alpha-adrenoceptor numbers.

Finally, the adrenergic abnormality may be due to autoimmune mechanisms. Several workers have noted that autoantibodies to beta$_2$-adrenoceptors can be identified in the plasma of some atopic subjects. Although these antibodies appear to be heterogeneous, they share the ability to affect binding of ^{125}I-labeled protein A to calf lung membranes, to inhibit binding of beta-adrenergic radioligand to calf lung beta$_2$-adrenergic receptors, and to precipitate solubilized calf lung beta-adrenergic receptors in an indirect immunoprecipitation assay. The presence of autoantibodies to beta$_2$-adrenoceptors in these subjects correlates with a reduced beta$_2$- and an increased alpha-adrenergic responsiveness.

These findings will have to be interpreted against a background of new information on autoantibodies in some other conditions in which their presence may alter hormone and neurotransmitter receptor densities, thereby contributing to the development of these diseases. For example, muscle weakness and fatigue in myasthenia gravis are due to antibodies directed at nicotinic acetylcholine receptors at the neuromuscular end-plates, whose function is markedly impaired. The hyperthyroid state in Graves' disease is currently being attributed to the presence of circulating autoantibodies to the thyrotropin receptor, and the severe insulin resistance in type B insulin-resistant diabetes has been ascribed to autoantibodies to the insulin receptor. Thus, we may be witnessing the emergence of a new group of conditions that are receptor diseases, and atopic allergy or some subsets of it may ultimately be recognized as legitimate members of this group.

TYPE II REACTIONS (CYTOTOXIC TISSUE INJURY)

Type II reactions are cytotoxic and involve the combination of IgG or IgM antibodies with antigenic determinants on a cell membrane. A free antigen or hapten also may be adsorbed to a tissue component or cell membrane, and antibody subsequently combines with this adsorbed antigen. Complement fixation frequently occurs in this situation and leads to cell damage. The usual sequelae of attachment of circulating antibody to either a tissue antigen or membrane-adsorbed antigen are, therefore, as follows: (1) cell lysis or cell inactivation with activation of complement; (2) phagocytosis of the target cells with or without activation of complement; and (3) lysis or inactivation in the presence of effector killer cells.

Complement-Dependent Antibody Lysis

The target for the cytotoxic reaction may be either a formed blood element or a specific cell type within a particular tissue. This form of injury follows immune reactions of antigen and antibody in which the antibody is of the IgG or IgM class. These are the only two classes of immunoglobulins that activate the complement system as immune reactants. Immune complexes formed by IgG, IgA, and IgD do not exhibit complement-activating effects, and, indeed, among the four subclasses of IgG, only subclasses IgG1 and IgG3 exhibit substantial complement activation.

The conditions of sensitivity in complement-dependent disorders are that the individual has been exposed to the antigen previously and has produced an antibody response of IgM or IgG or both. Subsequent exposure to the reactive antigen then results in immune complex formation, which initiates activation of the complement system. The antigens in this form of hypersensitivity are often derived from infections with microorganisms (e.g., bacteria, fungi, and viruses); from injections or inoculations in the course of immunization or blood transfusion; or from drug therapy.

The steps in the activation of the complement system, initiated by such immune reactions and called the *classical pathway of complement activation,* are described in Chapter 4. The so-called *alternative complement pathway* is also discussed in the preceding chapter. This pathway involves nonimmune activation of the complement and the serum properdin systems.

Red cell lysis is an illustrative example of type II cytotoxic reaction, involving the lysis of red blood cells by a complement-dependent antibody–lysing process or phenomenon that classically occurs during transfusions with grossly incompatible blood. Platelets, polymorphonuclear leukocytes, and lymphocytes can also be lysed by similar mechanisms under certain conditions.

One can produce type II reactions in any tissue by inducing heterologous antibodies to different tissue components. Some of these tissue reactions have been studied extensively in lower species and are of great importance in humans, especially in the kidney and skin. In humans, deposition of antibodies in a linear pattern along the human glomerular basement membranes occurs in three groups of diseases:

1. Abnormalities related to renal transplantation. In earlier years of renal transplantation, people were treated with antilymphocyte antisera. Today, these antisera are known to have contained antibodies against glomerular basement membranes that deposited along the glomerular basement membrane of the transplanted kidney. This situation is analogous to classic nephrotoxic serum nephritis.

2. Goodpasture's syndrome, in which there is deposition of antibodies directed against glomerular and pulmonary basement membranes, accounting for the symptoms of hematuria, renal failure, and recurrent hemoptysis.

3. Several other diseases, such as scleroderma, diabetic glomerulonephritis, systemic lupus ery-

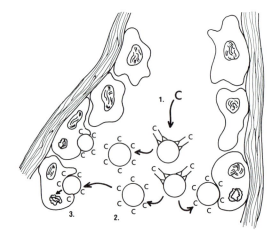

PATHOGENIC SEQUENCE IN COMPLEMENT DEPENDENT CYTOTOXICITY
1. COMPLEMENT ACTIVATION BY ANTIGEN—ANTIBODY REACTIONS ON ERYTHROCYTE SURFACE
2. COMPLEMENT (C3b) ON CELL SURFACE
3. PHAGOCYTOSIS AND INTRACELLULAR DESTRUCTION OF ERYTHROCYTE FACILITATED BY COMPLEMENT (C3b) ON CELL SURFACES

Figure 5–16

thematosus, malignant hypertension, polyarteritis nodosa, and toxemia of pregnancy.

In these situations, the primary disease leads to renal damage, which in turn sensitizes the patient to glomerular basement membrane. In the skin, type II reactions caused by linear deposition of antibody against the basement membrane at the dermal-epidermal junction occur in pemphigoid disorders.

Another type of complement-dependent cell destruction occurs as a result of immune adherence. In this situation, there is immune activation of complement along a cell surface that generates abundant C3b, and C3b molecules attach to the cell surface. They act as specific receptors that facilitate rapid phagocytic clearance of the coated cells from the circulation by immune adherence. This causes the C3b-covered cells to attach to receptors on reticuloendothelial cells (Fig. 5–16). Phagocytosis occurs and is followed by intracellular destruction of the engulfed cell or particle. When the cells affected are erythrocytes, chronic severe reactions of this type can lead to profound anemia and are incorrectly termed *hemolytic. Phagocytic anemia* would be a more appropriate diagnostic term. If leukocytes or platelets are the target cells, they are cleared from the circulation in a similar manner. Commonly, these reactions are due to an immune reaction with antigens intrinsic to or linked to the cell surface.

Antibody-Mediated Killer Cell Toxicity

Another mechanism of antibody-dependent cell injury has been described. It is called *antibody-*

dependent cytotoxicity, or *natural killer (K)–cell destruction.* The sequence of events in this form of tissue injury is illustrated in Figure 5–17. It can be seen that a target cell that possesses antigens along the cell surface, either as part of the cell membrane or linked to the cell membrane, can bind antibody through the Fab region along the surface. Following this, the small mononuclear (natural killer) cells of the circulation that have a receptor site for the Fc portion of IgG come close to the antibody-coated target cell and contact the cell by receptor-binding with the Fc portion of the antibody molecules. This cell contact is then followed by release of a biochemical factor that kills the target cell, which undergoes fragmentation and dissolution. In this reaction, the specificity derives from the antigen-antibody reaction, whereas the killer cell (K cell) effect is essentially nonspecific. It is attracted to the target antigens by reaction of its Fc receptor with the antibody molecule bound to cell antigens. This mechanism of destruction appears to be due to release of a biochemical factor via an energy- and calcium-dependent reaction contingent upon microtubule function in the K cell.

As a mode of tissue injury, these K-cell reactions appear to be of importance in conditions in which cells develop virus-associated, drug-induced, or tumor-associated antigens closely linked to HLA antigens on the cell membranes. It also promises to provide the basis for an important therapeutic approach to the specific immunologic treatment of neoplasms.

TYPE III REACTIONS (IMMUNE COMPLEX TISSUE INJURY)

Type III reactions are characterized by localization of antigen-antibody complexes in tissues and an associated inflammatory response. Typical manifestations of this group are the Arthus phenomenon, serum sickness, and immune complex diseases.

The Arthus Phenomenon

The Arthus phenomenon was described in 1903 by Nicolas-Maurice Arthus in experimental animals as a local necrotic lesion resulting from a local antigen-antibody reaction. In its classic form, following the intradermal injection of antigen into a sensitized rabbit, the area shows local swelling and erythema in 1 to 2 hours, which increases to a maximum within 3 to 6 hours and disappears within 10 to 12 hours. Originally, the Arthus phenomenon was believed to be a local variant of systemic anaphylaxis, but now it is regarded as a prototype of an inflammatory lesion due to immune complex disease, as described further on.

One human clinical example of an Arthus reaction is hypersensitivity pneumonitis, or extrinsic allergic alveolitis, which is caused by inhalation of organic dusts.

Serum Sickness

In the early decades of the twentieth century, patients frequently developed serum sickness after treatment with horse serum as an antiserum to diphtheria, tetanus, or other organisms. It is seen today only in underdeveloped countries in which alternative methods of active immunization may not be available. In developed countries today, it occurs only as a reaction to drugs such as penicillin or consequent to renal allotransplantation in patients who receive heterologous antilymphocyte serum.

Like the Arthus phenomenon, serum sickness was for a long time regarded as a manifestation of

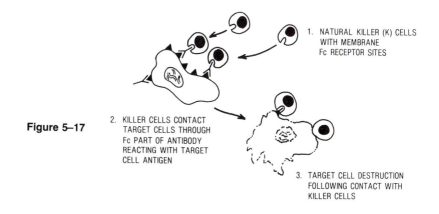

Figure 5–17

1. NATURAL KILLER (K) CELLS WITH MEMBRANE Fc RECEPTOR SITES

2. KILLER CELLS CONTACT TARGET CELLS THROUGH Fc PART OF ANTIBODY REACTING WITH TARGET CELL ANTIGEN

3. TARGET CELL DESTRUCTION FOLLOWING CONTACT WITH KILLER CELLS

MECHANISM OF ANTIBODY DEPENDENT KILLER (K) CELL DESTRUCTION OF TARGET CELL immediate hypersensitivity, but now we know that its key pathogenetic feature is the formation of antigen-antibody complexes in the bloodstream and their subsequent deposition throughout the body.

Immune Complex Diseases

Disorders associated with significant clinical features secondary to formation and deposition of immune complexes are now collectively termed *immune complex diseases*.

The critical pathologic feature of these diseases is that formation of the immune complex is followed by entrapment of the complex in the tissue. This provides the focus for development of the lesion. Complement activation occurs on the immune complex in the tissue, yielding chemotactic factors that specifically attract the neutrophils. Once in the tissue, the neutrophils release destructive hydrolytic enzymes from their lysosomal granules. The degradative action of these enzymes produces the necrotic destructive lesion at the site of immune complex localization. This pathogenic sequence of immune complex injury is illustrated in Figure 5–18.

Some examples of disseminated immune complex disease in humans include systemic lupus erythematosus, various forms of acute and chronic glomerulonephritis, polyarteritis nodosa, Hashimoto's thyroiditis, rheumatoid arthritis, dermatitis herpetiformis, Crohn's disease, and disorders associated with a variety of infectious and neoplastic diseases.

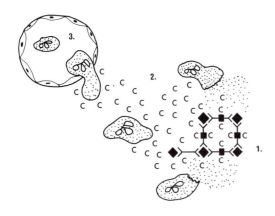

IMMUNE COMMUNE COMPLEX TISSUE INJURY
PATHOGENIC SEQUENCE:

1. COMPLEMENT ACTIVATION BY ANTIGEN—ANTIBODY COMPLEX LODGED IN TISSUE
2. COMPLEMENT CHEMOTAXIS OF NEUTROPHILS INTO TISSUE SITE OF IMMUNE REACTION WITH RELEASE OF DESTRUCTIVE LYSOSOMAL ENZYMES
3. MIGRATION OF NEUTROPHIL FROM BLOOD VESSEL DUE TO CHEMOATTRACTION

Figure 5–18

TYPE IV REACTIONS (CELL-MEDIATED IMMUNE TISSUE INJURIES)

Cell-mediated immune reactions occur as the result of the interactions between actively sensitized lymphocytes and specific antigens. They are mediated by the release of lymphokines or by direct cytotoxicity or by both. Historically, the classic lesion of a cell-mediated immune reaction is the delayed–skin-hypersensitivity reaction (i.e., the tuberculin reaction). Mechanistically, discussion of cell-mediated reactions can be most effectively arranged around (1) the T-cell–dependent reaction, leading to granulomatous injury, and (2) the T-lymphocyte–cytotoxicity reactions.

T-Cell Reactions

Granulomatous injury

The forms of immune injury so far discussed have involved reactions of antigen with antibody, a product of B cells. We will now consider those reactions that depend on T-lymphocyte activation and response. T cells in these reactions serve as both reacting cells and effector cells.

In the type of T-cell–dependent reaction resulting in the formation of a granuloma, the T cell reacts with the stimulating antigen through specific receptors on the cell surface. Consequent to this contact, the T-lymphocyte is stimulated to increased metabolic activity and exhibits nuclear enlargement with cytoplasmic basophilia, a change described as *blast formation*. Along with the increased metabolic activity, there is production of many soluble biochemical factors that cause certain physiologic and biologic effects (Fig. 5–19).

These factors, the lymphokines (extensively discussed in Chapter 4), are the primary mediators of this reaction sequence. The activities of the lymphokines include stimulation and activation of blood monocytes, which cause transformation of the monocytes to macrophages; a chemotactic effect on monocytes to attract them specifically into tissue; and a migration inhibition effect that limits motility of monocytes and macrophages once they have arrived at the tissue site. These lymphokines mediate the cellular events that produce a characteristic histopathologic lesion known as a *granuloma*. This sequence of events is illustrated in Figure 5–19. It shows diagrammatically the initial contact of effector T-lymphocyte with antigen, followed by synthesis and release of lymphokines, then by recruitment of monocytes from the circulation due to the chemotactic effect of the lymphokines, and finally transformation of monocytes into macrophages, with increased activity in cytoplasmic digestive vacuoles. Often, the individual macrophages cluster and fuse around a central site of antigen concentration, which may show focal necrotic change due to leakage of proteolytic en-

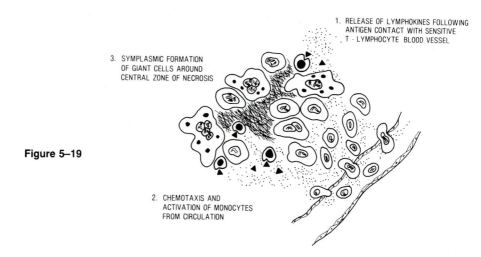

Figure 5–19

1. RELEASE OF LYMPHOKINES FOLLOWING ANTIGEN CONTACT WITH SENSITIVE T - LYMPHOCYTE BLOOD VESSEL

3. SYMPLASMIC FORMATION OF GIANT CELLS AROUND CENTRAL ZONE OF NECROSIS

2. CHEMOTAXIS AND ACTIVATION OF MONOCYTES FROM CIRCULATION

EVENTS IN THE DEVELOPMENT OF T—LYMPHOCYTE DEPENDENT HYPERSENSITIVITY GRANULOMATOUS LESION

zymes. These events give rise to the typical appearance of a granuloma, with multinucleate giant cells surrounding a central area of necrotic change bounded by a mantle of mononuclear cells. Such a necrotic or cellular granuloma is a characteristic lesion of delayed-hypersensitivity reactions. It is often observed in certain infectious diseases in which there is antigen persistence with marked T-cell reactivity, as in tuberculosis and in fungal and viral infections.

T-Lymphocyte cytotoxicity reaction

A variant of immune injury produced by T-lymphocytes in a role as effector cells is called *cytotoxic,* or killer (K)-cell–infiltrative, reactions. This type occurs as a result of contact by the effector lymphocyte with histocompatibility-linked antigens on the surface of target cells. The se-

quence of events is illustrated in Figure 5–20. Cell contact of the T-lymphocyte produces killing through a mechanism similar to that already discussed under antibody-dependent natural killer–cell cytotoxicity. The principal difference in the mechanism is that the T-cell contacts the antigen directly, rather than through antibody linkage as in the antibody-dependent form of injury. The killing effect appears to be due to release of a biochemical factor from the T-lymphocyte. It is energy-dependent and related to the integrity of microtubule function of the killer T cell. Close contact with the target cell appears necessary to initiate the killing reaction. Some examples of such tissue reactions in human disease are the acute phase of homograft rejection, autoimmune tissue lesions, viral infections, and some forms of dermatitis.

The granulomatous and cytotoxic forms of T-cell reactivity can occur together, although one

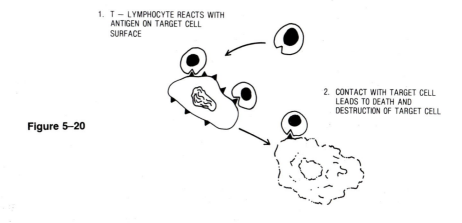

Figure 5–20

1. T — LYMPHOCYTE REACTS WITH ANTIGEN ON TARGET CELL SURFACE

2. CONTACT WITH TARGET CELL LEADS TO DEATH AND DESTRUCTION OF TARGET CELL

EVENTS IN CYTOTOXIC T—LYMPHOCYTE REACTION

usually predominates as the primary form of the reaction. The site of lesions in these immunologic diseases as well as others depends on the localization of the immune reactants. This is usually determined by the portal of entry of the antigen, which often induces a local tissue reaction limited to the entry site or which also enters the circulation and becomes widely disseminated, with lesions throughout the body. The potential for dissemination of the reaction gives many variations of clinical patterns in immunologic disease. These patterns may vary considerably, even though there is a final common sequence of injury.

SUMMARY OF MECHANISMS IN TISSUE DAMAGE

The four types of immune mechanisms have been discussed as separate, distinct entities. In reality, however, an immune reaction may involve a mixture of these various mechanisms. Thus, we see a combination of type II and type III reactions in virus infections. Penicillin may produce an acute fatal type I anaphylaxis, a type II reaction with hemolytic anemia, a type III reaction clinically resembling serum sickness, or a type IV delayed-hypersensitivity reaction.

REFERENCES

Askenase, P. W.: Effector and regulatory mechanisms in delayed-type hypersensitivity. In Middleton, E., Jr., Reed, C. E., and Ellis, E. (Eds.): Allergy: Principles and Practice. 2nd ed. Vol. 1. St. Louis, The C. V. Mosby Co., 1983, pp. 147–165.

Bach, F. H., Bonavida, B., Vitetta, E. S., and Fox, C. F. (Eds.): T and B Lymphocytes: Recognition and Function. New York, Academic Press, 1979.

Barrett, D. J., et al.: Clinical and immunologic spectrum of the DiGeorge syndrome. J. Clin. Lab. Immunol. 6:1, 1981.

Barrett, J. F.: Textbook of Immunology. 4th ed. St. Louis, The C. V. Mosby Co., 1983.

Benacerraf, B.: Role of MHC gene products in immune regulation. Science 212:1229, 1981.

Bergsma, D. (Ed.): Immunologic Deficiency Diseases in Man. Birth Defects Original Article Series, Vol. IV, No. 1, Feb. 1968.

Bierman, C. W., and Pearlman, D. S. (Eds.): Allergic Diseases of Infancy, Childhood and Adolescence. Philadelphia, W. B. Saunders Co., 1980.

Bridges, B. A., and Harnden, D. G.: Untangling ataxia-telangiectasia. Nature 289:222, 1981.

Chandra, R. K.: Immunodeficiency in undernutrition and overnutrition. Nutr. Rev. 39:225, 1981.

Ciba Foundation Symposium 15 (new series): Corneal Graft Failure. Amsterdam, Associated Scientific Publishers, 1972.

Cochran, A. J.: Man, Cancer and Immunity. New York, Academic Press, 1978.

Cohen, M. S., et al.: Fungal infection in chronic granulomatous disease. Am. J. Med. 71:59, 1981.

Cowan, M. D., and Ammann, A. J.: Immunodeficiency associated with inherited metabolic disorders. Clin. Haematol. 10:139, 1981.

Dausset, J., and Svejgaard, A. (Eds.): HLA and Disease. Baltimore, Williams & Wilkins Co., 1977.

deWeck, A. L., and Blumenthal, M. N. (Eds.): HLA and Allergy. Monographs in Allergy. Vol. 11. Basel, S. Karger, 1977.

Dixon, F. J.: Murine SLE models and autoimmune disease. In Dixon, F. J., and Fisher, D. W. (Eds.): The Biology of Immunologic Disease. Sunderland, Mass., Sinauer Associates, Inc., 1983, pp. 235–245.

Ferrone, S., Curtoni, E. S., and Gorini, S. (Eds.): HLA Antigens in Clinical Medicine and Biology. New York, Garland STPM Press, 1979.

Friedman, H., Klein, T. W., and Szentivanyi, A. (Eds.): Immunomodulation by Bacteria and Their Products. New York, Plenum Press, 1981.

Goodman, M. G., and Weigle, W. O.: Role of polyclonal B-cell activation in self/non-self discrimination. Immunol. Today 2:54, 1981.

Hadden, J. W., Chedid, L., Dukor, P., et al.: (Eds.): Advances in Immunopharmacology 2. Proceedings of the Second International Conference on Immunopharmacology, July 1982, Washington, USA. Oxford, Pergamon Press, 1983.

Haliotis, T., et al.: Chediak-Higashi gene in humans. 1. Impairment of natural killer function. J. Exp. Med. 151:1039, 1980.

Hanna, C. (Ed.): Symposium on Suppression of Graft Rejection with Emphasis on the Cornea. Nov. 5–6, 1965; Little Rock, Ark. (Available from Williams & Wilkins Co., Baltimore, Md.)

Hay, J. B. (Ed.): Animal Models of Immunologic Process. London, Academic Press, 1982.

Heberman, R. B. (Ed.): NK Cells and Other Natural Effector Cells. New York, Academic Press, 1982.

Heberman, R. B., and Friedman, H. (Eds.): The Reticuloendothelial System: A Comprehensive Treatise: Vol. 5. Cancer. New York, Plenum Press, 1983.

Inman, R. D., and Day, N. K.: Immunologic and clinical aspects of immune complex disease. Am. J. Med. 70:1097, 1981.

Jacobs, S., and Cuatrecasas, P. (Eds.): Membrane Receptors—Methods for Purification and Characterization. Receptors and Recognition, Series B, Vol. 11. London, Chapman and Hall, 1981.

Kalsner, S. (Ed.): Trends in Autonomic Pharmacology. Vol. 1. Baltimore, Urban & Schwarzenberg, 1979.

Kalsner, S. (Ed.): Trends in Autonomic Pharmacology. Vol. 2. Baltimore, Urban & Schwarzenberg, 1982.

Karnovsky, M. L., and Bolis, L. (Eds.): Phagocytosis—Past and Future. New York, Academic Press, 1982.

Klein, T., Specter, S., Friedman, H., and Szentivanyi, A. (Eds.): Biological Response Modifiers in Human Oncology and Immunology. New York, Plenum Press, 1983.

Kohler, P. F.: Immune complexes and allergic diseases. In Middleton, E., Jr., Reed, C. E., and Ellis, E. (Eds.): Allergy: Principles and Practice. 2nd ed. Vol. 1. St. Louis, The C. V. Mosby Co., 1983, pp. 167–199.

Lindstrom, J.: Autoimmune response to acetylcholine receptors in myasthenia gravis and its animal model. Adv. Immunol. 27:1, 1979.

McGhee, J. R., and Mestecky, J. (Eds.): The Secretory Immune System. Proceedings of the Conference on the Secretory Immune System, May 4–7, 1982, at The New York Academy of Sciences. Ann. N.Y. Acad. Sci., Vol. 409.

Middleton, E., Jr., Reed, C. E., and Ellis, E. (Eds.): Allergy: Principles and Practice. 2nd ed. Vol. 1. St. Louis, The C. V. Mosby Co., 1983.

Mizel, S. B. (Ed.): Lymphokines in Antibody and Cytotoxic Responses. Vol. 6. Lymphokines: A Forum for Immunoregulatory Cell Products. New York, Academic Press, 1982.

Morley, J. (Ed.): Bronchial Hyperreactivity. London, Academic Press, 1982.

Muller-Eberhard, H. J.: Complement abnormalities in human disease. In Dixon, F. J., and Fisher, D. W. (Eds.): The Biology of Immunologic Disease. Sunderland, Mass., Sinauer Associates, Inc., 1983, pp. 167–176.

Ochs, H.: Intravenous immunoglobulin therapy of patients with primary immunodeficiency syndromes. In Immunoglobulins: Characteristics and Uses of Intravenous Preparations. U.S. Department of Health and Human Services, 1981, pp. 9–14.

Oettgen, H. F.: Immunologic aspects of cancer. In Dixon, F. J., and Fisher, D. W. (Eds.): The Biology of Immunologic Disease. Sunderland, Mass., Sinauer Associates, Inc., 1983, pp. 187–195.

Oxelius, V. A., et al.: IgG subclass deficiency in selective IgA deficiency. N. Engl. J. Med. *305*:1476, 1981.

Panwa, S. G., Pahwa, R. N., and Good, R. A.: Heterogeneity of B lymphocyte differentiation in severe combined immunodeficiency disease. J. Clin. Invest. *66*:543, 1980.

Parkman, R., et al.: Complete correction of the Wiskott-Aldrich syndrome by allogeneic bone marrow transplantation. N. Engl. J. Med. *298*:921, 1978.

Peterson, B. H., et al.: *Neisseria meningitidis* and *Neisseria gonorrhoeae* bacteremia associated with C6, C7, or C8 deficiency. Ann. Intern. Med. *90*:917, 1979.

Sell, S. (Ed.): Cancer Markers: Developmental and Diagnostic Significance. Clifton, N.J., Humana Press, 1980.

Siegal, F. P.: Cellular differentiation markers in lymphoproliferative diseases. *In* Dixon, F. J., and Fisher, D. W. (Eds.): The Biology of Immunologic Disease. Sunderland, Mass., Sinauer Associates, Inc., 1983, pp. 197–208.

Siegel, R. I., et al.: Deficiency of T helper cells in transient hypogammaglobulinemia of infancy. N. Engl. J. Med. *305*:1307, 1981.

Stobo, J. F.: Autoimmune antireceptor diseases. *In* Dixon, F. J., and Fisher, D. W. (Eds.): The Biology of Immunologic Disease. Sunderland, Mass., Sinauer Associates, Inc., 1983, pp. 275–282.

Szentivanyi, A., and Friedman, H. (Eds.): Viruses, Immunity and Immunodeficiency. New York, Plenum Press (in press).

Szentivanyi, A., Middleton, E., Jr., Williams, J. F., and Friedman, H.: Effect of microbial agents on the immune network and associated pharmacologic reactivities. *In* Middleton, E.,

Jr., Reed, C. E., and Ellis, E. (Eds.): Allergy: Principles and Practice. 2nd ed. Vol. 1. St. Louis, The C. V. Mosby Co., 1983, pp. 211–236.

Szentivanyi, A., Polson, J. B., and Szentivanyi, J.: Manifestations and mechanisms of adrenergic subsensitivity in asthma. *In* Weiss, E. B., and Segal, M. S. (Eds.): Bronchial Asthma: Mechanisms and Therapeutics. 2nd ed. Boston, Little, Brown and Co., 1984.

Szentivanyi, A., and Williams, J. F.: The constitutional basis of atopic disease. *In* Bierman, C. W., and Pearlman, D. W. (Eds.): Allergic Diseases of Infancy, Childhood and Adolescence. Philadelphia, W. B. Saunders Co., 1981, pp. 173–210.

Trentin, J. J. (Ed.): Cross-Reacting Antigens and Neoantigens (with Implications for Autoimmunity and Cancer Immunity). Baltimore, The Williams & Wilkins Co., 1967.

Twomey, J. J. (Ed.): The pathophysiology of human immunologic disorders. Baltimore, Urban & Schwarzenberg, 1982.

Waters, H. (Ed.): The Handbook of Cancer Immunology. Vols. 1–9, New York, Garland STPM Press, 1978–1981.

Weigle, W. O.: Analysis of autoimmunity through experimental models of thyroiditis and allergic encephalomyelitis. Adv. Immunol. *30*:159, 1980.

Williams, L. T., and Lefkowitz, R. J.: Receptor Binding Studies in Adrenergic Pharmacology. New York, Raven Press, 1978.

Williams, R. C., Jr. (Ed.): Lymphocytes and Their Interactions: Recent Observations. Kroc Foundation Series, No. 4, New York, Raven Press, 1975.

Yamamura, Y., and Kotani, S. (Eds.): Immunomodulation by Microbial Products and Related Synthetic Compounds. Proceedings of an International Symposium, Osaka, July 27–29, 1981. Amsterdam, Excerpta Medica, 1982.

Section II

CARDIORENAL AND RESPIRATORY SYSTEMS

Integrated Dynamics of the Circulation and Body Fluids

6

Arthur C. Guyton

It would be pointless to review in this chapter all the details of hemodynamics, such as the interrelationships between pressure, resistance, and flow, or the problems of blood viscosity, or the differences between streamline and nonstreamline blood flow, because these are found in every textbook of medical physiology. However, although the integrative aspects of hemodynamics are extremely important to the clinician, they are rarely written about. It is these aspects that will be covered in this chapter.

BASIC PHILOSOPHY OF THE CIRCULATORY SYSTEM

The purpose of the circulatory system is to provide transport for nutrients, excreta, and other substances to and from the cells. To do this there are two major groups of hemodynamic systems. One of these is geared to provide a continuous pressure level in the arterial tree, and the other is organized to control blood flow in each individual section of the circulation in accord with local needs. It will be the aim of this chapter to show how the different circulatory mechanisms operate together to provide continuous automatic function of the circulation and how dysfunction can lead to circulatory inadequacy.

BASIC FACTORS IN OVERALL CIRCULATORY FUNCTION AND REGULATION

Figure 6–1 depicts the basic factors in overall function of the circulation and also shows their interrelationships. First, let us describe the six factors located around the periphery of the diagram in blocks 1 through 6, beginning with arterial pressure. (1) When the arterial pressure increases, this causes the renal output of water and electrolytes to increase also. (2) Increased loss of water and electrolytes from the kidneys reduces the extracellular fluid volume. (3) This reduction of extracellular fluid volume causes a similar decrease in blood volume. (4) The decrease in blood volume decreases the mean circulatory filling pressure (the tightness with which the circulation is filled with blood). (5) Decreasing this factor decreases venous return and cardiac output. (6) The

decrease in cardiac output obviously decreases arterial pressure.

Thus, one sees that an initial increase in arterial pressure causes a series of events that in turn tend to reduce the arterial pressure back toward normal. Conversely, a decrease in arterial pressure will cause exactly opposite effects, this time raising the diminished pressure back toward normal.

As one studies this circuit of Figure 6–1 (blocks 1 through 6), he sees that it is a negative feedback hemodynamic mechanism that tends always to return the functional variables of the circulation toward their normal levels. It is negative feedback loops such as this one that provide most control functions in the body. This specific hemodynamic negative feedback loop of Figure 6–1 is the most basic control loop of the circulatory system. Furthermore, complete understanding of this mechanism can help explain many clinical circulatory abnormalities, as we shall see in subsequent pages.

Effects of Water and Electrolyte Intake. The two inside blocks of Figure 6–1 also deserve special mention. Block 7 shows that one's intake of water and electrolytes also plays a major role in overall control of the circulation, obviously counterbalancing renal output of water and electrolytes.

Effect of Total Peripheral Resistance and Autoregulation. Total peripheral resistance (block 8) has two very significant effects on circulatory regulation: (1) An increase in total peripheral resistance tends to increase arterial pressure, but (2) an increase in total peripheral resistance also tends to decrease venous return and cardiac output. The second of these two effects is often forgotten; many times its effect of reducing arterial pressure is more potent than the direct effect of the resistance to increase arterial pressure. For instance, when the total peripheral resistance increases because of venous constriction, the tendency to decrease cardiac output is much greater than the tendency to increase arterial pressure. Therefore, in this instance, the arterial pressure actually decreases instead of increasing because of the greatly decreased cardiac output. This interplay between the positive and negative effects of total peripheral resistance on pressure is mentioned here merely to illustrate one of the falsities that has crept into much understanding of circulatory hemodynamics, namely, a widespread impression that total peripheral resistance and

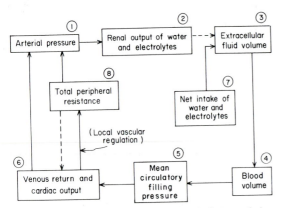

Figure 6–1 The major hemodynamic factors of circulatory function and their interrelationships.

arterial pressure are always directly related to each other.

It is also noted in block 8 that an increase in cardiac output can increase total peripheral resistance, as illustrated by the dark arrow leading from block 6 to block 8. This effect is frequently overlooked in schemes of circulatory function. It results from the ability of tissues to control their own local blood flows, which will be discussed later in this chapter. When the cardiac output becomes too great, the blood flow through the tissues is also excessive, and local vascular reactions in the tissues attempt to return their flow to normal. As a result, the local blood vessels constrict, thereby increasing total peripheral resistance. Conversely, whenever the cardiac output falls too low and blood flow in the tissues diminishes, the local vasculature dilates. This effect of cardiac output on vascular resistance is called *autoregulation*, the result of which is a tendency for the total peripheral resistance to change in the same direction as the change in cardiac output. The effect, however, is not an instantaneous one. A small part of it occurs within the first minute or so, still more within the next hour, and much more over a period of days and weeks, as will be discussed later in this chapter in relation to local blood flow regulation.

With this rapid introduction to the major functional factors in circulatory control, now let us turn to one of the more specific circulatory functions.

LOCAL BLOOD FLOW AND ITS REGULATION

Every clinician is familiar with the ability of local tissues to protect their own blood flows. For instance, if a femoral artery suddenly becomes occluded, within 60 to 90 seconds collateral blood vessels open to supply blood to the leg. Then, during the next several weeks to several months, the collaterals become progressively larger, until

finally blood flow can be almost as adequate as before, particularly in very young persons.

Exactly the opposite effects occur when blood flow to the tissues becomes too great. Some degree of acute constriction of the blood vessels occurs within the first minute or so, and this is followed gradually over days, weeks, and months by actual decrease in vascular dimensions.

MECHANISMS OF LOCAL BLOOD FLOW REGULATION: ROLE OF OXYGEN

Different tissues have different mechanisms for control of local blood flow, depending on their special local needs. However, the majority of the tissues control local blood flow in relation to their need for oxygen. This is particularly true of all types of muscle—skeletal, cardiac, and smooth—which together make up approximately one half the body. Diminished oxygen delivery causes up to a fourfold increase in blood flow within seconds to minutes; then, additional vasodilatation occurs during the ensuing half hour to hour.

In some tissues, this effect of oxygen lack to control local blood flow is overshadowed by other more potent local factors for controlling blood flow. For instance, in the brain the factor that plays the most potent role is usually carbon dioxide; any increase in carbon dioxide level causes increased blood flow, thereby providing increased removal of the excess carbon dioxide from the brain tissue. However, when the brain becomes moderately or extremely hypoxic, vasodilatation occurs because of function of the hypoxia mechanism in exactly the same way as it occurs in muscle.

Possible Vasodilator Substances Released in Response to Oxygen Deficiency. The basic mechanism by which decreased oxygen delivery to the tissues causes vasodilatation is still unknown. Some research workers believe that diminished oxygen in the tissues causes some humoral vasodilator factor to be released into the tissue fluids and that this in turn actively dilates the local vessels. The substance that has received widest attention in recent years has been *adenosine*, one of the breakdown products of adenosine triphosphate, which is released in small quantities into the tissue fluid in hypoxic states. Other possible vasodilator substances that have been suggested include potassium, osmotic substances of any nature, adenosine triphosphate, carbon dioxide, lactic acid, and histamine. All these in sufficient quantities can indeed cause vasodilatation, but to date none of them has been absolutely proved to be *the* major cause of the dilatation that occurs in hypoxia.

Possible Vasodilatation Caused by Oxygen Deficiency Per Se. More recently, experiments have shown that the vasodilating effect of tissue hypoxia could result from simple decrease of oxygen itself in the tissues rather than from the presence of vasodilator substances. Absence of oxygen prevents formation of significant quantities of ATP and other high-energy compounds in the smooth muscle cells of the vascular walls, so the strength of contraction of these cells is diminished in exactly the same way that the strength of contraction of skeletal muscle is diminished in hypoxia. Obviously, this could easily cause local vasodilatation when too little oxygen is available to the tissues.

Long-term Changes in Blood Vessels During Prolonged Ischemia or Hypoxia. In animals kept for months at high altitudes, the actual sizes and numbers of vessels in the tissues increase, causing a phenomenon called "increased vascularity." Furthermore, return of these animals to normal altitudes causes the vascularity to return toward normal. Essentially the same effects occur when the tissues are made ischemic because of large artery obstruction. Unfortunately, the causes of these changes in vascularity are not yet known, but the vascularity changes themselves help maintain proper delivery of oxygen and other nutrients to the tissues.

Other Normal and Pathologic Factors in Local Blood Flow Regulation. In the skin, local blood flow is controlled almost entirely by the body temperature control mechanism, acting mainly by means of nervous constriction or dilatation of the skin vessels.

In the kidneys, blood flow is controlled primarily by the renal excretory loads, especially by the presence of excess sodium and other electrolytes in the plasma; also, some of the end products of metabolism such as urea help control renal blood flow. Only when the kidneys become extremely hypoxic does the hypoxia mechanism play any significant role in renal blood flow regulation.

Finally, any pathologic state that causes a direct shunt from the arteries to the veins increases the local blood flow and contributes to the overall control of the circulation. Thus, either minute pathologic arteriovenous fistulae or major A-V fistulae will increase blood flow.

Local Blood Flow Regulation During Increased Tissue Activity. The local blood flow regulating mechanisms also respond to increased cellular activity. For example, Figure 6–2 shows the effect of progressive increase in work output during exercise on both oxygen consumption and cardiac output, illustrating that as tissue metabolism increases (indicated by increasing oxygen consumption), blood flow through the entire body also increases (indicated by the increasing cardiac output). Other conditions in which increased tissue activity causes vascular dilatation include (1) increased metabolism of the tissues caused by thyrotoxicosis, (2) increased tissue activity caused by excessive catecholamines, and (3) increased metabolism caused by fever. Therefore, the increased local blood flows and increased cardiac outputs observed in these conditions can all be ascribed to the increased activities in the local tissue cells themselves.

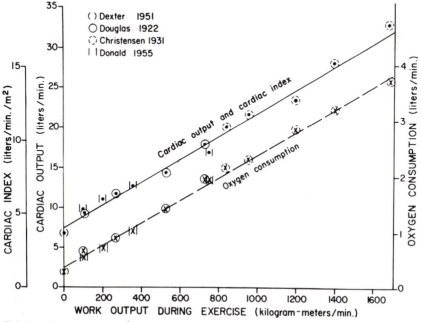

Figure 6–2 Relationship between cardiac output and work output *(solid curve)* and between oxygen consumption and work output *(dashed curve)* during exercise. (Reprinted from Guyton, A. C., et al.: Circulatory Physiology: Cardiac Output and Its Regulation. 2nd ed. Philadelphia, W. B. Saunders Co., 1973.)

CARDIAC OUTPUT: HEMODYNAMIC FACTORS AND ITS REGULATION

When one thinks of cardiac output regulation, he almost immediately thinks of the heart, but under normal conditions 90 to 95 per cent of cardiac output regulation is determined by peripheral circulatory factors, and not more than 5 to 10 per cent by the heart itself. However, when the heart becomes diseased and is unable to provide adequate pumping capacity, the limiting factor in cardiac output regulation then becomes the heart.

ROLE OF THE HEART IN CARDIAC OUTPUT REGULATION

Even under resting conditions, the normal human heart is capable of pumping between 10 and 15 liters of blood per minute, although it actually pumps only 5 to 6 liters. The simple reason for this difference is that only this smaller amount of blood flows into the heart from the veins, and, however much pumping capacity the heart may have, it can never pump more blood than flows into it. The normal heart merely keeps the input veins pumped almost dry, which can be illustrated by injecting a contrast medium into any of the peripheral veins and noting the slitlike character of the veins where they pass through the abdomen or neck.

Effect of the Nervous System on Heart Pumping Capacity. In dog studies, maximal sympathetic stimulation of the heart can increase its pumping capacity about 70 to 100 per cent. However, maximal vagal stimulation can stop the heart for a few seconds until the ventricles begin to beat at a very slow rate, driven by a ventricular pacemaker. After the ventricles have thus "escaped" from the vagal stimulation, the maximum pumping capacity of the heart is reduced to about 50 per cent of normal. Therefore, the total range of nervous control of heart pumping is probably between −50 per cent and +100 per cent.

Effect of Cardiac Hypertrophy on Heart Pumping Capacity. In athletes who train for endurance, the maximum cardiac output can be increased 50 to 100 per cent by the training procedure. At least part of this effect is caused by cardiac hypertrophy. Likewise, from study of certain disease conditions (e.g., left-to-right shunts) in which the heart must pump greatly increased amounts of blood indefinitely, one can also conclude that heart hypertrophy can increase heart pumping capacity as much as 100 per cent.

Cardiac Reserve. The difference between heart pumping capacity and the actual amount of blood pumped by the heart under resting conditions is called the "cardiac reserve." Thus, if the heart of a well-trained athlete is capable of pumping 30 liters per minute but under resting conditions pumps only 5 liters, the cardiac reserve is 25 liters. Expressing this as a percentage, which is the usual method, one can determine that this person has a cardiac reserve of 500 per cent above normal. The more asthenic person, however, rarely has a cardiac reserve greater than 250 to 350 per cent.

ROLE OF PERIPHERAL CIRCULATION IN CARDIAC OUTPUT CONTROL

If the peripheral blood vessels were rigid tubes, the peripheral circulation would play essentially no role in cardiac output regulation because whenever the heart would pump increased quantities of blood into a peripheral vessel an equal amount of blood would be returned instantaneously to the input side of the heart. However, the fact that the peripheral vessels are highly distensible prevents this instantaneous increase in venous return. Instead, the extra blood pumped by the heart at first simply distends the arterial tree. Then it is allowed to flow through the small tissue vessels into the veins and, finally, back to the heart only at the will of the tissues. Consequently, it is frequently said that cardiac output is controlled by venous return and that venous return is controlled by the tissues. This means simply that whatever amount of blood is allowed to flow through the small vessels of the tissues into the veins and thence into the heart is also the amount of blood that the heart pumps.

Cardiac Output Regulation as the Sum of Local Blood Flow Regulations. The factors that control local blood flow in the peripheral circulation change from minute to minute in accord with the needs of the tissues, as already discussed, and there is simultaneous alteration of venous return and cardiac output. Therefore, another way of looking at normal cardiac output regulation is simply to state that it is the sum of all the local blood flow regulations. If return of blood to the heart from any single tissue increases, cardiac output increases by approximately a similar increment.

This principle is illustrated very forcefully when one studies the effects of an arteriovenous fistula on circulatory function, as illustrated in Figure 6–3. This figure shows an instantaneous increase in cardiac output resulting from opening the fistula. The primary effect is to allow direct flow of blood from the arteries into the veins, and the surge of blood returning to the heart instantaneously increases the cardiac output. Within another few seconds, the nervous reflexes further compensate for the fistula by causing blood reservoirs to constrict throughout the body, thereby making still more blood available to be pumped by the heart. Then, during the next several days, renal retention of water and salt (for reasons discussed earlier in this chapter in relation to Figure 6–1) causes the blood volume to increase,

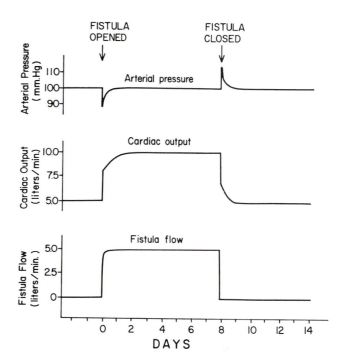

Figure 6–3 Effect of suddenly opening and suddenly closing an A-V fistula, showing changes in fistual flow, cardiac output, and arterial pressure.

making even more blood available to the heart. Thus, within 2 to 3 days, there is full compensation to opening the A-V fistula, and *the cardiac output is increased by an amount exactly equal to the fistula flow*, if the heart does not go into failure.

Role of Blood Volume and "Mean Circulatory Filling Pressure" in Cardiac Output Regulation. Another noncardiac factor that normally plays a supporting role, and under certain abnormal conditions plays the major role, in cardiac output regulation is the blood volume and its ability to fill the circulatory system, as measured by the "mean circulatory filling pressure." When the blood volume is increased, the quantity of blood in each vessel in the body also tends to increase. Therefore, the pressure in each vessel becomes slightly greater than normal. The algebraic sum of these pressures, weighted in proportion to the capacitances of the respective vascular segments, is the mean circulatory filling pressure. Unfortunately, this has never been measured in the human being, but it is probably near that observed in the dog, 7 mm Hg. This is also the average pressure in the peripheral circulation that tends to push blood toward the venous input side of the heart. Both mathematically and experimentally, it has been demonstrated that if all other factors remain constant, venous return increases directly in proportion to an increase in mean circulatory filling pressure. However, the right atrial pressure exerts a back pressure to reduce flow of blood into the heart. Putting both these factors together, one finds that *return of blood to the heart is directly proportional to the mean circulatory filling pressure minus the right atrial pressure*.

EFFECT OF VASCULAR CAPACITY ON FILLING PRESSURE. The capacity of the circulatory system itself is another factor that helps determine the mean circulatory filling pressure. Obviously, the greater the capacity, the greater must be the blood volume to create the same degree of filling pressure. Furthermore, the capacity of the circulatory system can be changed by nervous stimulation, hormonal effects, fever, and so forth. Some of these factors will be discussed later in the chapter in relation to blood volume regulation, but it is very clear that the tightness with which the circulatory system is filled with blood is determined by the ratio of the blood volume to the capacity of the system itself. Therefore, with regard to control of the circulation, one needs to think in terms of mean circulatory filling pressure and not in terms of blood volume itself.

Role of Mean Circulatory Filling Pressure in Circulatory Shock and in Heart Failure. There are two very important applications of the concept of circulatory filling pressure to clinical medicine—one to help explain circulatory shock and the other to explain one of the compensations in congestive heart failure. In circulatory shock, the blood volume is usually greatly decreased, but shock can also result from excessive dilatation of the vasculature, which simply increases the capacity of the system. That is, either decreased blood volume or increased vascular capacity decreases the mean circulatory filling pressure below its normal value and correspondingly can reduce venous return and cardiac output. In the early stages of some types of shock (e.g., hemorrhagic), the pumping capacity of the heart actually increases far above normal because of reflex nervous stimulation of the heart. Yet, despite this, the venous return is still too low, and the cardiac output cannot rise above the venous return; hence, the patient is in circulatory shock despite massive pumping effort by the heart. Thus, the concept of mean circulatory filling pressure is an extremely important one in understanding abnormal control of the circulation in circulatory shock.

In congestive heart failure, the primary abnormality occurs in the heart itself, but even a very weak heart often delivers normal blood volume if it is constantly primed with excessive amounts of blood entering the right atrium. In severe congestive heart failure, the kidneys function very poorly, causing diminished urinary output and consequent increase in extracellular fluid volume and blood volume. As a result, the mean circulatory filling pressure sometimes rises to as high as 20 to 30 mm Hg, which is three to four times the normal value. This excessive pressure plays a significant role in pushing extra quantities of blood toward the heart, often compensating completely for the weak heart, so that cardiac output is normal. This is an example in which one hemodynamic factor, an increase in blood volume and mean circulatory filling pressure, opposes another factor, decreased pumping ability of the heart, to afford almost normal delivery of blood to the tissues despite a severe abnormality in the circulation. Unfortunately, however, there often comes the time when the heart becomes so weak that, whatever the increase in blood volume and mean circulatory pressure, the heart still cannot pump enough blood to supply the tissues adequately. Therefore, kidney function never returns to normal, and fluid continues to be retained indefinitely. This obviously leads to the state of *decompensation.*

QUANTITATIVE METHOD FOR ASSESSING RESPECTIVE ROLES OF THE HEART AND PERIPHERAL CIRCULATION IN CARDIAC OUTPUT REGULATION

Figure 6–4 demonstrates graphically the relative roles of the heart and of the peripheral circulation in cardiac output regulation. Note first the curve labeled "cardiac output curve." This illustrates the effect of increasing right atrial pressure on cardiac output, showing that as the pressure rises from about −4 mm Hg to +6 mm Hg, the cardiac output rises from zero to a plateau level of about 13 liters per minute.

The curve labeled "venous return curve" shows the effect on venous return of increasing right atrial pressure. As the right atrial pressure rises to approach approximately 7 mm Hg (the mean circulatory filling pressure), the venous return falls toward zero.

Now, let us see what happens when the two

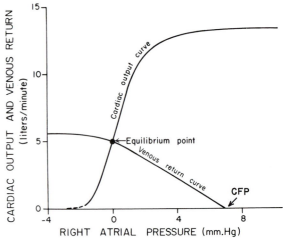

Figure 6–4 Interrelationship between cardiac output and venous return, showing (1) that the ability of the heart to pump blood can be expressed by *cardiac output curves,* (2) that the ability of blood to flow into the heart can be expressed by *venous return curves,* and (3) that the actual operating conditions of the circulation are expressed by the equilibrium point at which the two curves cross. The point labeled "CFP" represents the mean circulatory filling pressure of the system. (Modified from Guyton, A. C., et al.: Circulatory Physiology: Cardiac Output and Its Regulation. 2nd ed. Philadelphia, W. B. Saunders Co., 1973.)

curves interact with each other. First, let us assume that the right atrial pressure is 7 mm Hg. At this pressure, the cardiac output is 13 liters per minute and venous return is zero. Therefore, blood will be pumped rapidly out of the right atrium, and the right atrial pressure will decrease. Venous return will increase upward along the venous return curve, whereas cardiac output will decrease downward along the cardiac output curve. As long as there is greater cardiac output than venous return, the blood volume in the heart will be decreasing and the right atrial pressure will be falling. But when the right atrial pressure reaches that point at which the two curves cross each other, venous return and cardiac output become equal, and the right atrial pressure also becomes stable. Therefore, this point is called an "equilibrium point," depicting the steady-state operational condition of the circulation. In Figure 6–4, which represents the normal condition of the circulation, the equilibrium point shows a cardiac output of approximately 5 liters per minute and a right atrial pressure of approximately 0 mm Hg (with reference to atmospheric pressure).

Analysis of Sequential Events Following Acute Heart Failure. We can now use the principle of equating venous return and cardiac output curves to analyze the sequence of events following an acute heart attack. In Figure 6–5, the two dark curves represent the same normal curves as those in Figure 6–4. Immediately after the heart attack, assuming that it occurs within seconds, the pe-

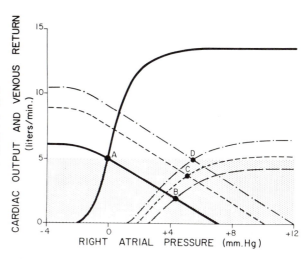

Figure 6–5 Use of cardiac output and venous return curves to analyze changes in cardiac output and right atrial pressure following acute onset of cardiac failure, showing complete cardiac output compensation at equilibrium point D after a week or more of recovery. (Reprinted from Guyton, A. C., et al.: Circulatory Physiology: Cardiac Output and Its Regulation. 2nd ed. Philadelphia, W. B. Saunders Co., 1973.)

ripheral circulation has not yet been changed at all. However, the strength of the heart has been reduced to a level represented by the long-dashed curve in the figure. This equates with the normal venous return curve at point B, showing that instantaneously the cardiac output falls to 2 liters per minute while the right atrial pressure rises to 4 mm Hg. At this low cardiac output, the person is likely to faint and is certain to become very weak.

EFFECT OF CIRCULATORY REFLEXES. Within seconds, the cardiovascular reflexes become active, and they change both the venous return curve and the cardiac output curve to the small-dashed curves. The venous return curve is changed because sympathetic stimulation tightens the blood vessels around the blood, thereby increasing the mean circulatory filling pressure and in turn promoting greater tendency for blood to flow from the peripheral vessels to the heart. The cardiac function curve is increased because sympathetic stimulation increases the strength of contraction of the undamaged portions of the heart. These sympathetic reflexes begin to act within 2 to 3 seconds and reach full development in 30 seconds to 1 minute. Therefore, the cardiac output rises by the end of this time from point B to the new equilibrium point, C, which represents a cardiac output of 3.5 liters per minute and an atrial pressure of 5.5 mm Hg.

EFFECT OF HEART RECOVERY AND FLUID RETENTION. During the next week, the strength of the heart improves because of (1) increase in collateral circulation to the ischemic areas of the heart, (2) some degree of hypertrophy of the undamaged heart muscle, and (3) stiffening of the infarcted portion of the myocardium to reduce aneurysmal bulging of this area. The low cardiac output causes simultaneous retention of water and salt by the kidneys for a variety of different reasons, thereby increasing the mean circulatory filling pressure even more and further elevating the venous return

curve. Therefore, the respective venous return and cardiac output curves become those represented by the dot-dashes, and the new equilibrium point becomes point D in Figure 6–5. By this time, the cardiac output has returned to normal, and renal output of water and salt is again in balance with the intake of water and salt. However, in the meantime, the body has accumulated fluid, the blood volume has increased a small amount, and the right atrial pressure has now risen to 6 mm Hg. Yet, despite the fact that the pumping capacity of the heart is only one half normal, the cardiac output has returned essentially to normal. This demonstrates again the importance of the peripheral circulatory system in long-range control of cardiac output.

CARDIAC OUTPUT IN ABNORMAL STATES

Figure 6–6 illustrates the effects of different abnormal states on cardiac output. One can readily understand most of the different factors that decrease the cardiac output in such states as myocardial infarction, hemorrhagic shock, traumatic shock, valvular heart disease, and cardiac shock. However, the factors that increase the cardiac output above normal are not so readily understood.

High Output States. Each one of the high output states illustrated in Figure 6–6 is associated with reduced total peripheral resistance. For instance, in beriberi the total peripheral resistance is often reduced to as low as 50 per cent of normal, and in patients with A-V shunts the total peripheral resistance occasionally is reduced to as low as 30 to 40 per cent of normal. In anemia, blood viscosity is greatly reduced, and diminished delivery of oxygen to the tissues causes vasodilatation; thus, two different effects decrease the total peripheral resistance. In pulmonary disease, diminished delivery of oxygen to the tissues can dilate

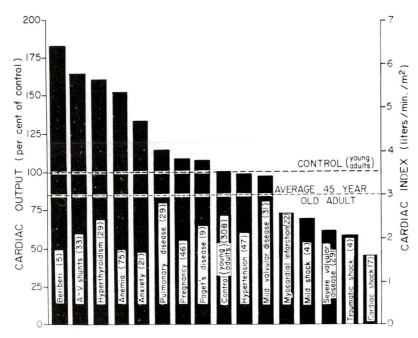

Figure 6–6 Cardiac output in different pathologic conditions. The figures in parentheses represent the number of patients from which the average values were obtained. Constructed from data in National Academy of Sciences: Handbook of Circulation. Philadelphia, W. B. Saunders Co., 1959.)

the peripheral vessels, and increased metabolism because of extra respiratory effort dilates the blood vessels in the respiratory muscles; both these effects reduce the total peripheral resistance. Finally, in both pregnancy and Paget's disease, increased vascular shunting decreases total peripheral resistance.

Thus, in none of these high cardiac output conditions can one ascribe the high output to excess pumping capacity of the heart. Instead, one finds the total peripheral resistance to be decreased and the cause of the increased cardiac output to be increased venous return. Indeed, in many of these conditions, the pumping capacity of the heart is actually reduced rather than increased.

One might suspect hyperthyroidism and anxiety to be exceptions to this rule because the heart becomes hyperactive in both these states. However, increasing heart activity by pacing it with a pacemaker at a high rate in a normal resting person or in an animal does not significantly alter cardiac output, even though this procedure does indeed increase the pumping capacity of the heart itself up to heart rates of about 150 beats per minute. Therefore, at present, there is no proven condition in which higher than normal cardiac output is caused by increased pumping capacity of the heart itself. The increased pumping capacity merely *increases the cardiac reserve*, not the cardiac output.

Low Output Caused by Cardiac Insufficiency. The above principles illustrate once again that as long as the heart has unused cardiac reserve, the cardiac output is controlled almost entirely by factors in the peripheral circulation. However,

when the cardiac reserve approaches zero, and particularly when the cardiac pumping capacity actually falls below the needs of the body's tissues, the heart does then become the limiting factor in the control of cardiac output. This is illustrated in Figure 6–6 by the cardiac outputs in patients with myocardial infarction, severe valvular heart disease, and cardiac shock. All these conditions impose limits on the amount of blood that the heart can pump. In these conditions, the peripheral tissues lose their ability to control their own local blood flows because the heart does not supply enough blood flow to allow this luxury. Therefore, the flows in the respective tissues will no longer be distributed according to the needs of the tissues. As a consequence, one would expect some tissues to deteriorate more than others. The most notably affected organs are often the kidneys, degeneration of which can cause death of the person even if all the other tissues do survive.

VENOUS PRESSURE: ITS REGULATION AND ITS ABNORMALITIES

Venous pressure regulation is inextricably tied to the regulation of cardiac output, which one can see by referring to both Figures 6–4 and 6–5. At the same time that venous return interacts with the cardiac pumping capacity to determine cardiac output, it also determines right atrial pressure, which is also central venous pressure. In general, increased pumping capacity of the heart is associated with reduced central venous pressure, whereas diminished pumping capacity is associated with elevated central venous pressure. Also, any peripheral circulatory factor that increases venous return is associated with increased central venous pressure, and any factor that reduces venous return is associated with diminished central venous pressure. However, when factors affect both the heart and the peripheral circulation at the same time, the central venous pressure is then determined by a balance between the two respective factors; the only way to determine this balance accurately is by using some quantitative method, such as the graphic method illustrated in Figures 6–4 and 6–5.

Mean Circulatory Filling Pressure as the Upper Limit of Central Venous Pressure. Referring again to Figure 6–4, one will note that as the right atrial pressure rises to approach the mean circulatory filling pressure, venous return approaches zero. Therefore, the upper limit to which the central venous pressure can rise is the mean circulatory filling pressure. The normal value for this filling pressure in the dog (it has never been measured in human beings) is 7 mm Hg. However, when the venous return and cardiac output fall below normal, nervous reflexes can increase the filling pressure up to levels as high as 18 to 20 mm Hg. Therefore, if the normal heart is weakened slowly enough for the reflexes to develop completely, cardiac output will decrease to zero only when the right atrial pressure rises to a maximum value of 18 to 20 mm Hg.

In pathologic conditions that cause retention of body fluids and consequent increase in blood volume, the mean circulatory filling pressure, even without reflex stimulation, can be as high as 20 to 30 mm Hg—in congestive failure, for instance. Therefore, progressive deterioration of the heart over a period of weeks or months can cause the central venous pressure to rise to maximum values of 20 to 30 mm Hg or perhaps even higher for minutes at a time because of superimposed action of sympathetic reflexes.

Peripheral Venous Pressure Versus Central Venous Pressure. Unfortunately, the peripheral venous pressure does not always correlate well with central venous pressure. The reason for this is that veins are frequently compressed in their courses to the heart, and the pressure beyond each compression point must rise enough to overcome the compression before the blood vessel will open to allow blood flow. The peripheral venous pressure, therefore, is more often a measure of the degree of venous compression than a measure of the central venous pressure. For this reason, to obtain meaningful venous pressure measurements, one must usually pass a catheter into a central vein. The tip of this catheter need not pass all the way into the right atrium, however, because the negative intrathoracic pressure keeps the central veins widely open so that central venous pressure measured anywhere inside the thoracic cavity will be within 1 mm Hg of the right atrial pressure itself.

When the central venous pressure rises above 6 to 10 mm Hg, the pressure in many or most of the peripheral veins then becomes great enough to overcome external compression on the veins. When this happens, the peripheral veins also remain filled essentially all the time, and the resistance between the peripheral veins and the central veins becomes very slight. Therefore, now, the pressure measured in the peripheral veins becomes nearly equal to the pressure in the central veins (except for hydrostatic pressure difference). Furthermore, pressure waves generated in the right atrium as a result of cardiac pumping are now transmitted with ease backward along the veins. This accounts for the obvious pulsation of the veins in the neck in congestive heart failure.

Hydrostatic Reference Level for Measuring Venous Pressure at the Tricuspid Valve. Extremely minute changes in central venous pressure can have marked effects on the output of the heart, which can be understood by referring again to the cardiac output curve in Figure 6–4. In this figure, an increase in right atrial pressure from 0 to 1 mm Hg is shown to increase the cardiac output approximately 30 per cent. Therefore, all central venous pressures must be measured at a very exact hydrostatic pressure level to be meaningful. Different reference levels have been suggested, such as one third the thickness of the chest behind the sternum, 10 cm anterior to the back, and so forth. However, physiologic studies have shown that there is one point in the heart at which the central venous pressure changes less than 1 mm Hg, regardless of the position of the animal. This is the very midpoint of the tricuspid valve. A basic physiologic reason for the constancy of pressure at this point is the following: Whenever the pressure at the tricuspid valve rises above its normal control value, the right ventricle fills more than normally and automatically pumps the increased quantity of blood out of the right ventricle; this obviously decreases the tricuspid pressure back toward normal. Conversely, decreased pressure at the tricuspid valve decreases the filling of the ventricle so that less blood is pumped; therefore, the pressure rises once again to its normal control value at the tricuspid valve level.

Thus, a physiologic hydrostatic reference point for measurement of venous pressure is the midpoint of the tricuspid valve. However, if the venous pressure is always measured with the patient in precisely the same position from one time to another and from one patient to another, any of the hydrostatic reference points—such as 10 cm in front of the patient's back—will usually serve adequately except for very thick or very thin persons. One of the most unforgivable mistakes, however, is to refer the measured pressure to the level of the catheter tip when the pressure is measured by a transducer at the external catheter end because it makes no significant difference where the tip of the catheter lies in the central veins; the hydrostatic column of blood inside the veins beyond the tip of the catheter compensates almost completely for changes in position of the catheter tip, still making it essential that the pressure be measured in relation to the level of the tricuspid valve.

ARTERIAL PRESSURE AND HEMODYNAMIC FACTORS IN ITS REGULATION

Fortunately, our bodies possess a large number of arterial pressure control mechanisms, no one of which can regulate arterial pressure under all conditions, although the total consortium of these mechanisms performs admirably. Eight of the best known arterial pressure control systems are described in the following sections. The first three of these are strictly nervous reflex controls—the baroreceptor reflex, the chemoreceptor reflex, and the central nervous system ischemic response. These all react within seconds and therefore are the principal controllers of arterial pressure from second to second or from minute to minute. The other mechanisms are slower to function, but, because of their very great feedback gains, they are the principal long-term pressure controllers. Especially important is the *renal–body fluid pressure* regulating mechanism, which has enough gain to override the other control mechanisms over periods of weeks and months.

The Baroreceptor Reflex. An increase in arterial pressure stretches the *baroreceptors* (also called "pressoreceptors") located in the carotid sinuses, in the arch of the aorta, and, to a much lesser extent, in other large central arteries. Signals from these are transmitted to the brain stem and thence back to the peripheral blood vessels to dilate them and also to the heart to decrease its pumping activity; both these effects reduce the arterial pressure back toward normal.

The Chemoreceptor Reflex. A decrease in arterial pressure decreases blood flow to the *chemoreceptors* in the carotid and aortic bodies. The decreased flow reduces the available oxygen to the chemoreceptors and also enhances the buildup of carbon dioxide in these receptors. Both these effects stimulate the chemoreceptors, causing them also to transmit signals by way of the brain stem to the blood vessels and heart, this time raising the arterial pressure back toward normal.

The Central Nervous System Ischemic Response. When the arterial pressure is reduced below approximately 60 mm Hg, the brain stem becomes ischemic and elicits the so-called "central nervous system ischemic response." This sends powerful signals through the sympathetic nerves to the blood vessels to cause vasoconstriction and to the heart to enhance its pumping activity, thus bringing the arterial pressure back up to a level that will prevent brain ischemia.

Stress Relaxation. When the arterial pressure rises above normal because of an acute increase in blood volume, such as immediately following massive blood infusion, the pressure frequently is increased in all or most of the other vessels of the circulation as well as in the arteries. The smooth muscle cells of all the vessels gradually become stretched, a phenomenon called "stress relaxation." This increases the capacity of the vascular tree, thereby decreasing the mean circulatory filling pressure, decreasing cardiac output, and decreasing arterial pressure back toward normal. Conversely, when the pressures in all the respective vessels fall acutely to a level below normal, the blood vessels slowly contract around the blood and return the pressure back upward toward normal.

The Capillary-Fluid Shift Mechanism. Increase in arterial pressure is frequently accompanied by an increase in capillary pressure, especially after an acute increase in blood volume. When this occurs, excess fluid begins to filter from the capillaries into the tissue spaces, thereby reducing the blood volume, reducing cardiac output, and reducing arterial pressure back toward normal. This effect also operates in the opposite direction when the capillary pressure falls below normal.

The Renin-Angiotensin-Vasoconstrictor Mechanism. Decrease in arterial pressure below normal causes the kidneys to release renin. The renin in turn enzymatically splits angiotensin from renin substrate in the plasma proteins. The angiotensin then causes peripheral vasoconstriction. The vasoconstriction results in increased total peripheral resistance and thereby returns the arterial pressure back upward toward normal.

The Aldosterone Pressure Regulating Mechanism. Decrease in arterial pressure increases aldosterone secretion. This occurs to some extent because angiotensin stimulates the adrenal cortex, but most of the effect probably occurs because of other not yet understood effects of decreased arterial pressure acting either directly or indirectly on the adrenal glands. The increased aldosterone in turn causes renal retention of salt, which then has several indirect effects to cause the kidneys also to retain water. The increased water and salt increase the extracellular fluid volume, which increases blood volume, which increases cardiac output, which in turn increases arterial pressure back toward normal.

The Renal–Body Fluid Pressure Regulating Mechanism. A decrease in arterial pressure has a direct effect on the kidneys to reduce renal output of water and salt. This results primarily from (1) decreased glomerular filtration rate caused by decreased glomerular pressure, and (2) increased tubular reabsorption caused by reduced peritubular capillary pressure. The result is retention of water and salt in the body and consequent progressive increase in extracellular fluid volume and blood volume as the person ingests additional quantites of water and salt. The increase in blood volume increases cardiac output and thereby returns the arterial pressure toward normal. This mechanism is the important hydrodynamic feedback control system illustrated at the outset of this chapter in Figure 6–1.

INTERACTION OF DIFFERENT PRESSURE CONTROL SYSTEMS—THE CONCEPT OF FEEDBACK GAIN

The greatest problem in understanding arterial pressure regulation has been to understand how all the different pressure regulating mechanisms interact with one another and under what conditions different mechanisms are important. To understand this, it is first necessary to explain the concept of feedback gain in control systems.

Let us assume that the normal arterial pressure is 100 mm Hg and that some abnormal factor suddenly increases this pressure to 180 mm Hg. The baroreceptors become stretched, and within seconds the baroreceptor reflex returns the arterial pressure to about 110 mm Hg. Thus, 70 mm Hg compensation occurs, and there is still 10 mm Hg abnormality. The ratio of these two values, 70/10, is a mathematical measure of the ability of the control system to control arterial pressure; this ratio is also an expression of the feedback gain of the system. In this case, the feedback gain is 70 divided by 10, or a gain factor of 7.

Another example, this one involving the renal–blood volume pressure control mechanism is as follows: If the arterial pressure is increased above its control value by sudden closure of a large

arteriovenous fistula, the kidneys begin to excrete more than the net intake of water and salt. Consequently, the body fluid volumes decrease, cardiac output decreases, and arterial pressure returns to normal. Furthermore, the arterial pressure will not stop falling until urinary output of water and salt returns exactly to equal the intake, which means that the arterial pressure must return all the way to its control value, not merely to a limited degree. Therefore, the correction is some finite value, and the final abnormality is zero. A finite value divided by zero is infinity. Therefore, the renal–body fluid feedback mechanism for control of arterial pressure has a feedback gain of infinity when allowed enough time to respond fully.

In a similar manner, we can derive at least estimated gains for the eight well-known arterial pressure control mechanisms. The values for these are approximately the following when each is operating under optimal conditions:

CNS ischemic response	11.0
Baroreceptor reflex	7.0
Chemoreceptor reflex	4.0
Stress relaxation mechanism	2.8
Capillary-fluid shift mechanism	2.5
Renin-angiotensin vasoconstrictor mechanism	1.6
Aldosterone, body fluid pressure control mechanism	1.0
Renal–body fluid pressure control mechanism	∞

Response Time Courses of Respective Arterial Pressure Control Mechanisms. Figure 6–7 illustrates approximate response time courses of the different pressure control mechanisms. Note that the time scale is approximately a logarithmic one, beginning with seconds and then extending

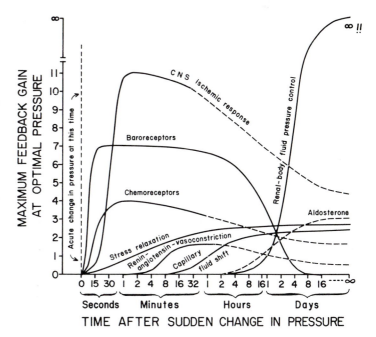

Figure 6–7 Response time courses of the major arterial blood pressure regulating mechanisms. This figure also shows approximate feedback gains of these mechanisms at different times after their responses have been initiated. Note especially the infinite gain that occurs in the renal–body fluid pressure control mechanism at infinite time. (Reprinted from Guyton, A. C.: Circulatory Physiology III: Arterial Pressure and Hypertension. Philadelphia, W. B. Saunders Co., 1980.)

MAXIMUM FEEDBACK GAIN AT OPTIMAL PRESSURE

Acute change in pressure at this time

CNS Ischemic response

Renal-body fluid pressure control

Baroreceptors

Chemoreceptors

Stress relaxation

Renin-angiotensin-vasoconstriction

Capillary fluid shift

Aldosterone

Seconds   Minutes   Hours   Days

TIME AFTER SUDDEN CHANGE IN PRESSURE

to minutes, hours, and days. The three nervous feedback mechanisms—the baroreceptor, the chemoreceptor, and the CNS ischemic effect—all begin to act within seconds and reach full gains within 30 seconds to a minute. Therefore, these are the mechanisms that are most important for control of arterial pressure from second to second or from minute to minute. They are the mechanisms that prevent sudden death following rapid bleeding and that prevent fainting when a person stands up. Each of the three nervous pressure control mechanisms operates in a different pressure range. The baroreceptors function most effectively at pressures between 80 and 180 mm Hg, the chemoreceptors between 40 and 100 mm Hg, and the CNS ischemic response mainly below 60 mm Hg. The extreme gain of the CNS ischemic response at very low pressure causes it to resist strongly any final decrease of pressure below about 30 mm Hg. It stimulates the sympathetic nervous system to its maximum, causing a very forceful heart beat and the highest possible degree of sympathetic constriction of the peripheral vessels. Therefore, this mechanism is frequently called the "last-ditch stand" against final circulatory collapse.

At least three non-nervous pressure control mechanisms begin to operate within minutes and continue to operate for perhaps hours or days. These are the stress relaxation mechanism, the renin-angiotensin-vasoconstrictor mechanism, and the capillary-fluid shift mechanism. None of them has a major amount of gain, but when added to the gains of the other mechanisms they play very significant roles in maintaining normal arterial pressure temporarily in such conditions as slow bleeding, dehydration, and loss of the nervous controls of the circulation.

Finally come the long-term controls of arterial pressure, which are based primarily on retention of water and salt by the kidneys. The aldosterone mechanism has a finite gain, whereas the direct renal–body fluid pressure control mechanism has infinite gain if given adequate time to come to full equilibrium, which in practice is several weeks. Because of this infinite gain, the renal–body fluid pressure control mechanism is the one that under long-term conditions dominates arterial pressure control for reasons that will be discussed in more detail in the following section.

IMPORTANCE OF INFINITE GAIN IN THE RENAL–BODY FLUID PRESSURE CONTROL MECHANISM AND ITS SIGNIFICANCE IN LONG-TERM ARTERIAL PRESSURE REGULATION

When two or more control systems attempt to control the same factor at the same time, the contribution of each of the systems toward the final level of control is determined by the ratio of

their gains. Note in Figure 6–7 that, at infinity time, the renal–body fluid pressure control system has infinite gain, whereas all the others have finite gains. Therefore, the ratio of the renal–body fluid pressure control system gain to all the others is infinity divided by some finite value, which is still infinity. Consequently, the long-term arterial pressure level calculates to be determined entirely by the renal–body fluid pressure control system. Let us explain this mechanism more fully.

Renal output of water and electrolytes is highly dependent upon arterial pressure. This effect is illustrated in Figure 6–8 by the curve labeled "normal renal output curve." This curve was determined in dogs by infusing sodium chloride solution at increasing rates for several days to several weeks while also recording the effect on mean arterial pressure and on urinary output. As illustrated, a very slight increase in arterial pressure is associated with a tremendous increase in renal output of both water and salt. Conversely, a very slight decrease in arterial pressure is associated with a marked decrease in output. Only part of the increase in urinary output is caused by the rise in pressure itself. However, other simultaneous effects also increase the output, which is the cause of the extremely steep curve in Figure 6–8. For instance, during fluid loading, the rate of secretion of renin by the kidneys decreases, and this greatly increases the excretion of both salt and water. Likewise, fluid loading is usually associated with a decrease in aldosterone, which also allows increased urinary output. Finally, fluid

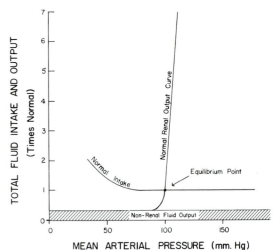

Figure 6–8 Relationship between mean arterial pressure and (1) normal fluid intake (curve labeled "normal intake") and (2) normal fluid output (curve labeled "normal renal output curve"). The point at which these two curves cross, called the "equilibrium point," depicts the pressure at which the arterial pressure will stablize in the long-term, steady-state condition. (Reprinted from Guyton, A. C.: Circulatory Physiology III: Arterial Pressure and Hypertension. Philadelphia, W. B. Saunders Co., 1980.)

loading is often associated with decreased sympathetic activity, this also acting to increase urinary output.

Even though we do not know all the causes of the extreme steepness of the curve depicting the relationship between urinary output and arterial pressure, one can readily understand its importance for long-term control of arterial pressure. That is, whenever the arterial pressure rises above normal, this is generally associated with a tremendous increase in urinary output, which in turn causes the pressure to fall back toward normal. Conversely, a decrease in arterial pressure causes fluid retention, which also increases the pressure back toward normal.

Equilibration between Fluid Intake and Fluid Output. Also shown in Figure 6–8 is a curve labeled "normal intake" showing that at normal arterial pressures the intake of water and salt by a normal person remains essentially constant. Only when the pressure is very low is this not true, presumably because ischemia of the thirst center in the brain causes some increase in fluid intake.

It is axiomatic that the rate of fluid intake must over an extended period of time equal the rate of fluid output. This occurs where the two curves in Figure 6–8 cross each other at the point labeled *equilibrium point.* If ever the arterial pressure rises too high, one can expect that the urinary output will also become excessive. As a consequence, the rate of fluid loss from the body becomes greater than fluid intake. Over an extended period of time, this will cause the arterial pressure to fall and also cause the renal output of fluid to decrease until total fluid output again equals fluid intake. When this has been achieved, the arterial pressure becomes stabilized. Conversely, if the pressure falls too low, the fluid intake becomes greater than the output; the body fluids build up until the intake and output again become equal and the pressure stabilizes.

If one will think for a few moments about the meaning of the diagram in Figure 6–8, he will see that the renal–body fluid pressure control mechanism has the capability of stabilizing the arterial pressure to a very precise level. This is the result of the infinite gain feature of this control mechanism. That is, this system continues to modify the fluid volume until the precise pressure point is reached, which is what is meant by "infinite gain."

Effect of Changes in Renal Function or Fluid Intake on the Arterial Pressure Level. Figure 6–9 illustrates two fluid intake curves representing two levels of fluid intake (consisting of approximately isotonic water and salt solution) and four different renal output curves, each representing a different state of kidney function. The normal renal output curve and the normal intake curve cross each other at point A. Therefore, the arterial pressure normally will stabilize only at point A. At any other point, there will be either a negative

or positive fluid balance that will continue until the pressure returns to point A.

To the far right in the figure is a renal output curve labeled "bilateral renal artery constriction." This is the curve recorded when both renal arteries are constricted, and it is also the curve recorded in rats that have spontaneous hypertension. Note that this output curve crosses the intake curve at point D. Therefore, as long as the kidneys operate in this state and the intake of fluid is normal, the only steady-state arterial pressure level that can be achieved is that represented by point D, or a level of approximately 155 mm Hg. At any other pressure level, there will be either a positive or negative fluid balance that will continue until the pressure returns to this level.

Now, note the curve labeled "vasoconstrictor." When a vasoconstrictor substance circulates in the body, it constricts not only the arterioles in the limbs, splanchnic areas, and so forth; it constricts the renal arterioles as well. As a consequence, the renal output curve decreases to the one shown in the figure. This curve crosses the normal intake curve at point C. Therefore, the arterial pressure over any extended period of time will stabilize at point C.

Finally, note the curve labeled "30% renal mass." This curve crosses the normal intake curve at a pressure slightly greater than 100 mm Hg. In other words, as long as the intake of fluid remains normal, the arterial pressure will hardly be changed from normal, even though 70 per cent of the kidney mass has been removed. In fact, animal experiments show that simple removal of kidney mass will rarely raise the arterial pressure more than 10 mm Hg as long as fluid and salt intake remain normal. Instead, the animal always goes into uremia before a significant rise in pressure occurs. However, if the animal is simultaneously loaded with a high intake of water and salt, the arterial pressure does rise markedly. This is illustrated by point B in Figure 6–9, where the high intake curve crosses the low renal mass curve, showing an arterial pressure of approximately 140 mm Hg. Thus, when there is decreased renal mass, the arterial pressure is determined to a great extent by the rate of water and salt intake. In a normal animal, however, the intake of water and salt has very little effect on the arterial pressure. This can be understood by noting the point at which the high intake curve crosses the normal renal output curve; this crossing point occurs at an arterial pressure level of approximately 105 mm Hg, which represents hardly any rise in arterial pressure.

In summary, the level at which the arterial pressure stabilizes is determined by the point at which the fluid output curve crosses the intake curve. At any other pressure level, there will be either a positive or negative fluid balance that will continue until the pressure returns to the stable level dictated by the point at which the two curves cross. However, if ever either of these two curves itself changes, then the pressure also will change accordingly.

Determinants of the Long-term Level of Arterial Pressure. From the previous discussion one sees that there are only two basic factors that in the long run determine the arterial pressure level. These are the fluid intake curve and the renal output curve, as illustrated in Figures 6–8 and 6–9. However, one will understand that anything that affects the shape or quantitative level of either of these two curves can also affect the long-term level of arterial pressure. Since the intake of fluid (and salt) remains relatively constant from one person to another and from day to day, the arterial pressure level is most often determined by the characteristics of the output curve. Most clinicians already know the different factors that can shift this curve to high pressure levels, but let us list a few of these:

1. Certain types of kidney disease, especially pathologic constriction of the renal vasculature. Also, thickening of the glomerular membrane, which tends to decrease the rate of glomerular filtration, will elevate the long-term arterial pressure level.

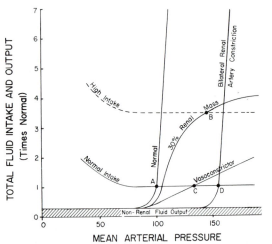

Figure 6–9 Fluid intake and fluid output curves under different conditions. The long-term level at which the arterial pressure will stabilize is determined by (1) the fluid intake curve under which the subject is operating and (2) the fluid output curve under which the subject is operating. Point A depicts the arterial pressure under normal conditions. Point B depicts the arterial pressure when the renal mass has been reduced to only 30 per cent of normal and there is also a high level of fluid intake. Point C depicts the long-term arterial pressure level when the animal or person is under the long-term influence of a vasoconstrictor substance and there is a simultaneous normal fluid intake. Point D depicts the long-term arterial pressure level when there is a normal fluid intake and simultaneous constriction of both renal arteries. (Reprinted from Guyton, A. C.: Circulatory Physiology III: Arterial Pressure and Hypertension. Philadelphia, W. B. Saunders Co., 1980.)

2. Excessive reabsorption of electrolytes and fluid by the tubules. This occurs especially in the presence of excess steroids.

3. Constriction of the renal vasculature as a result of circulating hormones. Hypertension of this type is illustrated by the hypertension that occurs in patients with pheochromocytomas and in patients with reninomas. In the first instance, the catecholamines cause marked constriction, especially of the afferent arterioles of the kidneys. In the second instance, the renin causes formation of angiotensin II, which in turn constricts the arterioles of the kidneys and also increases salt and water reabsorption by the renal tubules.

4. Sympathetic stimulation of the kidneys, which constricts the renal arterioles and results in a tendency toward diminished formation of glomerular filtrate.

5. Changes in electrolyte intake, which in turn alter the urinary volume output by the kidneys.

In summary, any factor that alters the shape or quantitative level of either the fluid intake curve or the fluid output curve depicted in Figures 6–8 and 6–9 is a determinant of the long-term arterial pressure level.

Lack of Correlation in Many Instances of Arterial Pressure with Cardiac Output, Total Peripheral Resistance, and Blood Volume. For years, investigators have argued the importance of total peripheral resistance, cardiac output, blood volume, and extracellular fluid volume in the regulation of the long-term level of arterial pressure. However, one will note that none of these factors has a direct effect on either the normal fluid intake curve or the normal renal output curve illustrated in Figures 6–8 and 6–9. Therefore, no one of these four factors is a *primary* determinant of the long-term steady-state level of arterial pressure. For example, a change in cardiac output obviously can cause a temporary change in arterial pressure. But if this altered arterial pressure then causes the fluid output to become unequal to the fluid intake, the total peripheral resistance, blood volume, and/or cardiac output will automatically be altered as needed until the level of arterial pressure that will once again bring intake and output into balance is achieved.

Therefore, total peripheral resistance, blood volume, and cardiac output are all *dependent variables* in the system.

It is extremely important to understand the difference between the *determinants* of the long-term arterial pressure level and the dependent variables because a change in a determinant will always of necessity alter the long-term pressure. However, a change in one of the dependent variables will simply throw the system out of balance temporarily, but the system will automatically readjust the dependent variables until the arterial pressure comes back exactly to where it was. Therefore, it is essentially fruitless to argue whether or not one of the dependent variables correlates with arterial pressure. For instance, in the type of hypertension that occurs immediately after a massive transfusion, the total peripheral resistance is at first greatly reduced, whereas cardiac output is greatly elevated. However, in hypertension caused by a pheochromocytoma, the total peripheral resistance is greatly increased, whereas the cardiac output is often reduced. Thus, these factors are nothing more than manipulated pawns in the regulation of arterial pressure.

Role of Blood Flow Autoregulation in Both Arterial Pressure Regulation and Hypertension.

Much has been written in the last 20 years about the relationship of "autoregulation" to arterial pressure control and hypertension. Also, a number of investigators working in the field of hypertension have spoken frequently of the "autoregulation theory of hypertension" and have ascribed this theory partly to the author of this chapter and partly to a few other research workers. However, there really is no such thing as an "autoregulation theory of hypertension." That is, autoregulation never causes hypertension. Yet, autoregulation does almost certainly account for the following three extremely important findings in many persons with hypertension: (1) the very high total peripheral resistance, (2) the normal or nearly normal cardiac output, and (3) the normal or nearly normal extracellular fluid volume and blood volume. Therefore, let us explain the role of autoregulation in arterial pressure control and hypertension.

First, it should be recognized that the term "autoregulation" applies to autoregulation of *blood flow*, not of pressure. A good definition of autoregulation is that the rate of blood flow through each tissue is automatically controlled by local tissue factors in such a way that changing the arterial pressure will not significantly change the blood flow, except transiently.

Second, if there were no such mechanism as autoregulation—that is, if the blood vessels were all rigid tubes—all the renal–body fluid pressure mechanisms discussed in the previous sections of this chapter would still be entirely operative. That is, if the arterial pressure becomes too low to cause normal output of water and salt, the arterial pressure will rise until the kidney begins to excrete the same amount of water and salt that is ingested. Furthermore, whether or not the autoregulation mechanism is present makes no difference in the final pressure level that will be attained. Thus, blood flow autoregulation does not enter into the determination of the arterial pressure level.

Third, no proved vasoconstrictor factor, such as a circulating hormone or increased sympathetic stimulation, has yet been found in essential hypertension. In fact, even the plasma concentration of renin is normal or below normal in most essential hypertensive patients. Also, 40 years ago thousands of patients were sympathectomized for hypertension, and in a very well-studied group of 2500 patients, the decrease in blood pressure caused by sympathectomy lasted for only a few weeks or months, even though the sympathetic nerves did not grow back. What is it, then, that increases the total peripheral resistance in essential hypertension in the probable absence of either a generalized circulating vasoconstrictor substance or increased sympathetic stimulation?

Fourth, pure volume-loading hypertension has been produced in many dogs by removing most of the kidney mass and then infusing large amounts of saline for weeks or months. At the onset of this hypertension, both the blood volume and the cardiac output increase greatly, whereas the total peripheral resistance actually falls below normal. Thus, the initial onset of this type of hypertension is caused by increased blood volume and increased cardiac output, not by increased total peripheral resistance. During the next 2 weeks, the total peripheral resistance rises to a very high level, whereas both the cardiac output and blood volume return to levels not significantly greater than normal. Therefore, even this pure volume-loading hypertension, once it has reached its chronic state, is a *high-resistance hypertension*, not a high–blood-volume/high–cardiac-output hypertension. Furthermore, the high resistance that occurs in this hypertension develops *after* the hypertension has developed, not at the time that the hypertension appears.

Fifth, in a few types of hypertension, vasoconstrictor substances are found in the blood—for instance, in those types of hypertension in which the kidneys secrete large quantities of renin. In these types, the total peripheral resistance may be elevated from the very start. If too much renin is secreted and excessive vasoconstriction occurs, it is possible for the blood-flow autoregulation mechanism actually to work in the backwards direction to decrease the undue vascular resistance caused by the renin—otherwise, the tissues of the body might well become so ischemic that they would be destroyed.

Now, using the aforementioned facts, let us find what the role of autoregulation is in arterial pressure regulation. By all means, autoregulation refers to autoregulation of blood flow, not autoregulation of pressure. That is, if the blood flow becomes too great anywhere in the body, within each individual tissue is a local feedback mechanism to decrease this flow back toward the normal value. Conversely, if the flow falls below normal, the autoregulation mechanism operates in exactly the opposite direction, to increase the flow back toward normal. This mechanism serves to maintain an appropriate rate of blood flow to each tissue according to its needs. In the volume-loading hypertension experiment referred to previously, the increase in volume initially increased the cardiac output and caused hypertension, but, at the same time, it also increased the blood flow to excessive levels. Because the blood flow autoregulation mechanism is always functioning, it would tend, over a period of time, to constrict the local arterioles and return the tissue blood flows to either normal or very nearly normal. Therefore, the cardiac output also would return to nearly normal, but the arteriolar constriction that decreases the flow would greatly increase the total peripheral resistance at the same time. Also, as the arterioles constrict, this would decrease the capillary pressure, allowing any excess fluid that had transuded into the tissue spaces to be reabsorbed into the circulation. Finally, the rising arterial pressure would increase the renal output of water and salt. The combination of these effects would return the fluid volume almost to the normal level. The consequence of this whole sequence would be a *volume-loading hypertension* in which the total peripheral resistance was greatly elevated while the cardiac output and blood volume were so near to normal that usual measuring techniques might not be able to distinguish elevations at all.

If there were superimposed generalized vasoconstrictor factors such as renin or increased sympathetic stimulation, these could readily take the place of the autoregulation phenomenon in causing the increased resistance in hypertension, but they are not necessary because autoregulation itself can increase the resistance if they are not present.

In summary, autoregulation never causes hypertension. It probably does account for the increased total peripheral resistance, the normal cardiac output, and the normal blood volume in many instances of hypertension. In fact, in essential hypertension, in which no generalized vasoconstrictor factor has yet been proved, it is very likely that autoregulation is responsible for the high total peripheral resistance and the normal cardiac output and blood volume in these patients.

CAPILLARIES AND CAPILLARY EXCHANGE

The body has roughly 10 billion capillaries, and their total cross-sectional area is a thousand or more times the total cross-sectional area of the aorta. It is rare that any cell of the body lies more than 30 to 50 microns from the nearest capillary. These facts bespeak the functions of the capillaries, namely, to deliver nutrients or humoral agents to the cells and to remove excreta from the cells.

The principal means of capillary exchange of both water and nutrients between the blood and the interstitial fluid is the process of *diffusion*. In fact, diffusion is so great through the capillary walls that water molecules diffuse in each direction many times as rapidly as the blood itself flows in the capillaries. Therefore, there is constant mixing of most of the constituents of the interstitial fluids with those of the blood.

DYNAMIC EQUILIBRIUM AT THE CAPILLARY MEMBRANES

Figure 6–10 illustrates a capillary in juxtaposition to its surrounding tissues. It also shows colloid osmotic pressures and hydrostatic pressures on each side of the capillary membrane. It is the dynamic equilibrium at this capillary membrane that prevents excessive quantities of fluid from filtering through the capillary membranes into the interstitial spaces. This can be explained as follows.

Since plasma proteins leak through the capillary membrane to only a slight extent, their concentration in the blood remains relatively high, causing a normal plasma colloid osmotic pressure of about 28 mm Hg in the human being. The plasma protein that does leak into the interstitial spaces creates an average interstitial fluid colloid osmotic pressure of about 5 mm Hg, varying from as little as 1 to 2 mm Hg in some tissues with only slightly porous capillary membranes, such as in the brain, to as high as 20 to 25 mm Hg in tissues with extremely porous membranes, as in the liver. The colloid osmotic pressure of the plasma is so much greater than that of the interstitial fluid that it creates a continual net force for movement of fluid from the interstitial spaces into the capillaries. In Figure 6–10 this difference between the two colloid osmotic pressures is shown to be 28 minus 5, or 23 mm Hg, that is, a *net* colloid osmotic absorptive pressure of this amount.

The average capillary pressure, as measured in several different ways, averages about 17 mm Hg. This value is considerably lower than the 25 mm Hg so often taught in the past. This hydrostatic pressure tends to force fluid outward through the capillary membrane. Yet, when it competes with the 23 mm Hg colloid osmotic absorptive pressure attempting to move fluid inward, one finds 6 mm Hg more absorptive pressure than hydrostatic pressure tending to force fluid outward. Therefore, under normal circumstances, there is a net absorptive capability of the capillaries, which can create a *negative* pressure (less than atmospheric pressure) in the interstitial spaces averaging about −6 mm Hg. Studying Figure 6–10 again, one can note that there is a hydrostatic pressure of −6.5 mm Hg in the tissue spaces rather than the theoretic value of −6. The extra 0.5 mm Hg is caused by the pumping action of the lymphatics, which causes a minute trickle of fluid to flow from the tissue spaces into the lymph vessel and thereby creates slightly more negative pressure in the interstitial spaces than can theoretically be accounted for by the colloid osmotic and hydrostatic forces at the capillary membrane.

If we now add separately the colloid osmotic and the hydrostatic forces on the two sides of the membrane, we find a colloid osmotic pressure difference of 23.0 mm Hg (28 minus 5) attempting to cause absorption and a hydrostatic difference of

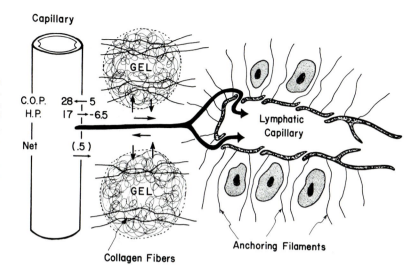

Figure 6–10 Capillary, tissue fluid, and lymph vessel relationships, illustrating dynamics at the capillary membrane, net outflow of fluid from the capillaries into the lymph vessels, and diffusional exchange of fluid and dissolved substances within the free fluid of the interstitial spaces and between the free fluid and the gel fluid.

23.5 mm Hg (17 minus −6.5) attempting to force fluid outward from the capillaries. Summing these values shows that there is a net *filtration pressure* averaging about 0.5 mm Hg at the capillary membrane. This 0.5 mm Hg represents a continual state of nonequilibrium at the membrane, and it causes net filtration of fluid out of the capillaries into the tissue spaces, thereby providing the small trickle of fluid that flows into the lymph vessels. The lymph vessels in turn transport the fluid back into the circulation, so that a steady state develops, with neither loss of fluid out of the circulation nor gain of fluid.

LYMPHATIC DRAINAGE FROM THE TISSUES

In a sense, the lymphatic system is older than the venous system because at lower phylogenic levels of animalhood whole blood is discharged directly from small blood vessels into the tissue spaces; the blood cells, along with other tissue fluid constituents, are then drained into lymphatic vessels that pump the mixture back toward the heart. In higher species of animals, some of these early vessels have remained relatively unchanged and have become the lymph vessels; others have changed into a less porous tubular system that comprises the capillaries and veins. The lymph vessels still perform the same function that they did in the lower animals, namely, they drain any excess fluid, cells, and debris that collect in the interstitial spaces.

DETERMINANTS OF LYMPH FLOW

The rate of lymph flow is determined by four major factors: (1) pumping action of the lymph vessels themselves, (2) pumping effect of tissue

motion, (3) pumping action at the tips of the terminal lymphatic capillaries, and (4) the pressure of fluid in the tissue spaces.

Lymphatic Valves and Pumping Action of the Lymph Vessels. The lymph vessels undergo continual rhythmic contraction, this occurring in all lymph vessels from the lymph capillaries up to the thoracic duct itself. Also, all lymph vessels larger than the lymph capillaries have valves that are all oriented toward the point of discharge from the lymphatic system into the circulation at the junctures of the jugular and subclavian veins. Because of this orientation of the valves, contraction of a section of a lymph vessel will propel fluid toward the circulation but never backward toward the tissues. Combining this valve function with the natural rhythmic contraction of lymph vessels, some of the larger lymph vessels can pump against a pressure head as great as 20 to 40 mm Hg.

Lymphatic Pumping Caused by Tissue Motion. Obviously, any tissue motion that compresses the lymph vessels from the outside can also compress fluid from one lymph vessel segment to another, but only in the direction that the valves are oriented. Therefore, tissue motion provides another propelling force that causes flow in the lymph vessels.

The Terminal Lymphatic Capillary Pump. Lymphatic contraction or compression also causes lymphatic pumping at the very tips of the lymphatic capillaries in some animals and perhaps also in humans; this can be understood by referring again to Figure 6–10. The endothelial cells lining the lymphatic capillary are shown in this figure to overlap each other. At the point of overlap, the cells are not attached to each other, but instead their inner edges can flap to the interior. Therefore, if the pressure outside the capillary is greater than that inside, fluid can push the flaps open and move to the interior. On the other hand, if the capillary is compressed or if it contracts so that the pressure inside becomes greater than that on the outside, any attempt of the fluid to escape from the capillary will close the flaps. Thus, the junctures between the endothelial cells are actually valves, allowing fluid to move into the lymphatic capillary but not in the outward direction.

Other structures important to terminal lymphatic pumping are the *anchoring filaments*. These are shown attached to the outside surfaces of the endothelial cells. They extend into the surrounding tissues, where they are held tightly between the cells by the hyaluronic acid gel that fills the intercellular space. When the tissues are compressed, the cells compress the lymphatic capillary and cause fluid to move away from the capillary toward the larger lymphatics. Then, when the tissues recoil because of the tissue turgor, the anchoring filaments pull the lymphatic capillary to an open position. Experiments indicate that this creates a negative pressure inside the capillary and causes fluid to flow from the surrounding tissue areas into the lymphatic capillary. Once filled, another cycle of compression of the capillary will again force fluid into the larger lymph vessels. Thus, tissue motion of any type creates actual sucking at the very tips of the terminal lymphatic capillaries, and it is this sucking action that keeps the trickle of fluid flowing from the tissue spaces into the lymphatic system and from there back into the blood circulation.

Motion pictures have shown that, at least in some animals, even the terminal lymphatic capillaries undergo rhythmic contraction several times a minute, presumably caused by myofibrillae in the cytoplasm of the endothelial cells themselves. Obviously, this contraction also aids in the suction pump action of the terminal lymphatic capillaries. It is still a question whether this rhythmic motion is strong enough to be of significant value in comparison with the tissue motion itself.

Effect of Interstitial Fluid Pressure on Lymph Flow. Though the large lymph vessels can pump against a pressure head up to 20 to 40 mm Hg, the suction pump at the tips of the lymphatic capillaries seems to be a relatively weak one, having in most tissues a suction limit of about -7 mm Hg. In other words, if the interstitial fluid pressure falls below -7 mm Hg, lymph flow becomes essentially zero, despite full pumping by the terminal suction pump.

When the interstitial fluid pressure rises above -7 mm Hg, the lymphatic suction pump begins to function, and the rate of lymph flow increases almost linearly until the interstitial fluid pressure rises to slightly more than atmospheric pressure. The normal rate of lymph flow from a typical peripheral tissue at a normal interstitial fluid pressure of approximately -6.5 mm Hg is about 0.1 ml of lymph per 100 gm of tissue per hour, illustrating the extremely slow trickle of fluid that normally flows in the lymphatics. However, when the interstitial fluid pressure rises to approach 0 mm Hg (atmospheric pressure level), lymph flow increases 10- to 50-fold, now delivering as much as 1 to 5 ml per 100 gm of tissue per hour.

INTERSTITIAL FLUID DYNAMICS AND EDEMA

There is a very common misbelief that the interstitial spaces are large, baggy chambers filled with freely mobile fluid. Even though the interstitial fluid spaces do represent about one sixth of the total tissue by volume, this concept is still far from the truth. Instead, the interstitial compartment is highly structured, filled primarily with two types of structural elements: (1) collagen fibers and (2) a gel matrix composed mainly of hyaluronic acid. The amount of freely mobile fluid in normal tissue spaces is probably a fraction of 1 per cent.

Figure 6–10 illustrates two gel masses lying between a blood capillary and a lymphatic capillary and also surrounded by tissue cells. Actually, this diagram is very much out of proportion because it shows a large free fluid space between the two gel bodies, whereas in normal tissues this space is nothing more than minute sluices along the cell surfaces. This figure also shows two types of fluid mobility that occur within the interstitial spaces. The large curved arrows show a net trickle of fluid from the capillary through the tissue free fluid sluice and thence into the lymphatic capillary. The small arrows illustrate diffusion of substances into and out of the blood capillary and also back and forth between the free fluid space and the gel. Thus, continual dynamic equilibria exist between the different fluid compartments of the tissues.

Interstitial Pressures—Interstitial Fluid Pressure, Solid Tissue Pressure, and Total Tissue Pressure. In an earlier section of this chapter we pointed out that the normal *interstitial fluid pressure* in the free fluid of the interstitial spaces is about -6.5 mm Hg, which is caused by the terminal lymphatic suction mechanism and by a tendency for the colloid osmotic pressure of the plasma to cause absorption of fluid from the tissue spaces through the capillary walls.

However, another type of pressure also occurs in the interstitial spaces. This is pressure exerted by the solid elements of the tissues and is called *solid tissue pressure*. When fluid is removed from the free fluid spaces by capillary osmosis or by lymphatic pumping, the decreased pressure in the free fluid immediately sucks fluid from the gel into the free fluid, and this fluid also is removed. Therefore, suction occurs in the entire interstitial space. In consequence, the walls of the interstitial spaces crowd toward each other—only to be held apart by the positive solid tissue pressure exerted by the solid structures in the spaces.

The solid structures in the interstitial spaces that exert solid tissue pressure are mainly the collagen fibers and the reticulum of the hyaluronic acid gel. At present, we do not know how much of the solid tissue pressure is caused by the gel and how much by the collagen and other fibers. However, the sum of these pressures must be great enough to oppose the negative suction effect of the interstitial fluid pressure, and it must also be great enough to overcome any other compressional forces that exist on the tissues, such as pressure exerted by a blood pressure cuff, pressure caused by turgor of the skin, pressure caused by compression points on the surface of the body, and so forth. When the skin and other tissues exert zero turgor and there is no compression from outside the body, the algebraically averaged solid tissue pressure must exactly equal the negative interstitial fluid pressure. If the fluid pressure is −6.5, then the solid tissue pressure must be 6.5. If we assume that skin elasticity causes the skin to press against the tissue with a pressure of another 2 mm Hg, the solid tissue pressure would be 8.5 mm Hg.

Finally, one can sum the interstitial fluid pressure and the solid tissue pressure to determine still another quality, the *total tissue pressure,* which is the pressure acting on any surface in a tissue by the combined effects of both the fluid and the solid elements. Assuming an average interstitial fluid pressure of −6.5 mm Hg and a solid tissue pressure of 8.5 mm Hg, one can calculate that the total tissue pressure would be 2.0 mm Hg.

Significance of the Different Types of Tissue Pressure. Because the aforementioned three types of tissue pressure all exist in the tissue spaces and because different methods for measuring tissue pressure measure different pressures, major confusion has developed regarding the true tissue pressure and its significance. However, if the reader follows the logic of the previous discussion, he can readily see that each of the different types of tissue pressure has its own peculiar significance, as follows:

Interstitial fluid pressure is the pressure that promotes fluid movement (1) from one part of a tissue to another part, (2) through the pores of a capillary membrane, or (3) from the tissue spaces into the lymphatics. In other words, interstitial fluid pressure relates to the fluids themselves and the forces that cause their mobility in the tissues.

Solid tissue pressure is pressure caused by contact points between solid elements of the tissues. Therefore, the greater the solid tissue pressure, the greater will be the forces exerted by these contact pressure points and, therefore, the greater will be the distortional forces caused in the tissues. It is solid tissue pressure that causes the shapes of cells to be irregular, causes at least part of the folding of the fibers in the tissue spaces, and distorts such structures as capillaries, and so forth.

Summation of interstitial fluid pressure and solid tissue pressure, which together equal total tissue pressure, can be accomplished by any structure that is capable of combining forces over a spatial domain. For instance, if fluid is compressing a capillary at one point and a fiber is compressing the capillary at a slightly different point, the elastic coefficient of the capillary membrane allows it to summate these two compressional forces even though they are not acting at precisely the same point. This is also true of cell membranes and of any other solid surface in a tissue. Therefore, total tissue pressure can act on any solid surface in a tissue. One of the most important of these solid surfaces is the blood vessels. Thus, the compressional force of the tissues against the blood vessels is equal to the total tissue pressure and is not equal to either the interstitial fluid pressure or the solid tissue pressure alone except when one of these is zero.

If we recognize, in accord with a discussion in the previous section, that interstitial fluid pressure, solid tissue pressure, and total tissue pressure usually are very different from each other, the importance of distinguishing them becomes clear. In clinical medicine, the two that are especially important are the interstitial fluid pressure, which is related primarily to the problem of interstitial fluid edema, and total tissue pressure, which is related primarily to the problem of blood vessel collapse.

Measurement of the Different Types of Tissue Pressure. MEASUREMENT OF TOTAL TISSUE PRESSURE. Methods are now available for measuring both interstitial fluid pressure and total tissue pressure. From these two values one can calculate the algebraically averaged solid tissue pressure.

The time-honored method for measuring tissue pressure has been to insert a minute needle into the tissue, then to inject about 1 μl of fluid at the tip of the needle, and, finally, to measure the pressure in this minute bolus of injected fluid using an extremely low compliance pressure measuring device. When pressure is measured in this manner, it gives a value of 1 to 3 mm Hg in most soft tissues, which is equal to the total tissue pressure. One might ask why this method measures total tissue pressure rather than interstitial fluid pressure, particularly since fluid is at the tip of the needle. The answer to this is that the fluid injected into the tissue temporarily displaces the solid tissue elements, so that the solid tissue pressure at this point is temporarily zero. Therefore, until the small bolus of fluid is absorbed, the pressure measured is the total tissue pressure, not the interstitial fluid pressure.

MEASUREMENT OF INTERSTITIAL FLUID PRESSURE. To measure interstitial fluid pressure, one must insert into the tissue some device that can remain there long enough for the fluid in the interstitial spaces to come to equilibrium with the fluid in the device. The method that has been used most successfully thus far has been to implant a small, hollow, but porous capsule, 1.0 to 2.0 cm in diameter, in the tissue. Over a period of days, the fluid inside the capsule comes to equilibrium with the fluid in the surrounding spaces. When pressure is measured inside this capsule, it is found to average about −6.5 mm Hg in most subcutaneous tissue. However, negativity is not present in tissues with tight capsules (e.g., the kidneys, which have pressures of about +6 mm Hg).

Unfortunately, the implanted capsule method cannot be used in clinical patients, although it has been applied in a few instances in human beings. A newer method has been developed that gives an indication of the interstitial fluid pressure but probably does not measure its true value in most instances. This is a wick method in which a small wick of cotton protruding from the tip of a 1-mm Teflon tube is inserted into the tissue and allowed to come to equilibrium for about ½ hour. A low displacement manometer connected to the Teflon tube then records a pressure of about −1 to −3 mm Hg, a less negative pressure than that usually measured with the perforated capsule. However, the fact that this method does measure a negative pressure demonstrates that other methods besides the porous capsule method can also be used for measuring negative interstitial fluid pressure. Furthermore, the wick method can be applied to the human being, although the problem of bleeding around the inserted wick is likely to nullify the validity of the pressure measurements. Those who have employed this method thus far in human beings have used it primarily for determining *changes* in interstitial fluid pressure rather than for measuring true value of the pressure.

REGULATION OF INTERSTITIAL FLUID PRESSURE

The interstitial fluid pressure is reasonably constant most of the time and remains at a subatmospheric pressure level in essentially all external soft tissues. This regulation of the interstitial fluid pressure is achieved in the following way. If the pressure becomes too great, lymph flow increases. The lymph flow in turn drains some of the excess fluid from the interstitial spaces and reduces the pressure. Even more important, however, the increased lymph drainage carries increased quantities of protein away from the interstitial spaces, thereby reducing the interstitial fluid colloid osmotic pressure. When this happens, the still high colloid osmotic pressure of the plasma then causes osmotic reabsorption of additional fluid from the interstitial spaces directly into the blood through the capillary walls. This second effect normally accounts for 90 per cent or more of the reabsorption of excess fluid from the usual tissue space, whereas the lymphatic drainage mechanism accounts for less than 10 per cent of this activity. In severe edematous states, however, the lymphatic drainage mechanism becomes progressively more important, sometimes outdoing the osmosis mechanism because of the extreme rates of lymph flow that occur at high interstitial fluid pressures.

REGULATION OF INTERSTITIAL FLUID VOLUME

Obviously, the regulation of interstitial fluid volume is also closely related to the regulation of interstitial fluid pressure, because whenever the interstitial fluid volume increases the tissue spaces expand, and, correspondingly, the interstitial fluid pressure increases. The same sequence as that described previously for interstitial fluid pressure regulation ensues once more: namely, increased pressure increases lymph flow, decreases tissue fluid colloid osmotic pressure, increases capillary osmotic absorption of fluid from the tissue spaces, and thereby returns interstitial fluid volume toward normal. Therefore, all these factors operate together in a simple but extremely important basic control system to keep the interstitial fluid pressure, protein concentration, and fluid volume all normally regulated to very exact levels.

PHYSIOLOGIC BASIS OF EDEMA

Positive Interstitial Fluid Pressure as Cause of Edema. In several thousand measurements of interstitial fluid pressure using the perforated capsule technique and encompassing both nonedematous and edematous tissues, investigators have found that loose areolar subcutaneous tissues will invariably be edematous if the interstitial fluid pressure is positive—that is, above atmospheric pressure; however, the tissues will be nonedematous if the pressure is negative (less than atmospheric pressure). Therefore, whether or not edema exists in these tissues seems to be determined by a simple factor: whether the interstitial fluid pressure is above atmospheric pressure or less than atmospheric pressure.

The Normally "Dry" State of the Interstitial "Free" Fluid Compartment. The fluid in the interstitial fluid compartment exists in two states: (1) a "free" state in which the fluid flows freely; and (2) a "gel" or "nonmobile" state. Figure 6–11 illustrates the approximate volumes of interstitial fluid in both these states at the different interstitial fluid pressures. At a normal pressure of −6.5 mm Hg, there is essentially zero free fluid, as shown in the figure, whereas there are approximately 12 liters of nonmobile gel fluid in the adult human being.

Thus, in the normal interstitial fluid spaces, the interstitial fluid volume is regulated to essentially zero free fluid. Furthermore, whenever any significant amount of free fluid begins to develop in the tissues, the lymphatic and capillary osmotic mechanisms normally return this free fluid to the circulatory system almost immediately. Thus, in effect, the mechanisms for regulating interstitial fluid volume normally maintain an almost completely "dry" state in the *free* fluid portion of the interstitial spaces. The fluid that does exist in the interstitial spaces is almost entirely that fluid which is bound in the form of a gel.

Character of the Interstitial Fluids in Edema—Pitting Edema. Note also in Figure 6–11 the changes in both free fluid and nonmobile fluid volumes when the interstitial fluid pressure rises. The nonmobile fluid volume increases about 30 per cent as the interstitial fluid pressure rises from −6.5 mm Hg up to zero. This is caused by the natural tendency of the gel reticulum to expand and thereby to pull fluid into the gel. However, when the free interstitial fluid pressure rises above zero, the gel has by then expanded to its limit, so that thereafter the nonmobile gel fluid volume does not increase further. Instead, above the critical level of zero pressure the free interstitial fluid volume increases drastically, a change that constitutes the state of frank edema.

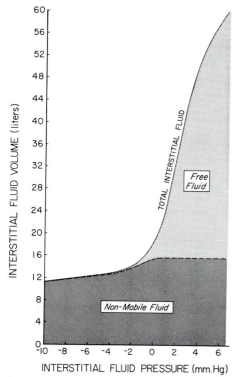

Figure 6–11 Changes in total interstitial fluid volume, free fluid volume, and nonmobile fluid volume (gel fluid) in the tissue spaces as the interstitial fluid pressure rises from a negative value of −10 up to a positive value of 7 mm Hg. Note the rapid appearance of free fluid in the interstitial spaces as the interstitial fluid pressure crosses from the subatmospheric pressure range into the supra-atmospheric pressure range. (Reprinted from Guyton, A. C., Granger, H. J., and Taylor, A. E.: Physiol. Rev. *51:*527, 1971.)

The large increase in *free* fluid volume as the interstitial fluid pressure rises above atmospheric pressure accounts for the pitting phenomenon that can be demonstrated in most forms of extracellular fluid edema. Free fluid is highly mobile in the tissue spaces, whereas the gel fluid is almost completely nonmobile. Therefore, in the normal state of the interstitial spaces, pitting does not occur. However, when vast amounts of free fluid develop, the fluid can be made to flow freely from one sector of the tissues to another. Thus, pressure with a finger on an edematous area will move fluid from the point of compression, and a pit will remain for a few seconds to a minute or more after the finger is removed—that is, until the fluid has time to flow back into the pitted area.

The high mobility of free fluid in edema also explains several other clinical phenomena, such as the continual weeping of wounds in edematous tissues and the difficulty for wounds to heal in edematous tissues. It explains, too, at least part of the dependent nature of edema. For instance, if a person has generalized edema, fluid can actually flow through the tissues from the top side of the body to the low side, such as from one breast to the other in a patient lying on her side. Obviously, another cause of dependent edema is high pressure in the dependent capillaries.

Role of Gel in the Interstitial Spaces. Although very little research has been performed on the functional importance of gel in interstitial spaces, the gel probably has at least three very valuable functions:

1. The gel prevents dependent edema in the normal person. Measurements of fluid flow in free fluid versus those of fluid flow through hyaluronic gel have shown a difference of several hundred thousandfold. In other words, the fact that the tissue spaces normally are filled with gel and not with free fluid prevents the fluid from flowing from the upper parts of the body to the lower parts. Since one sixth of the human body is composed of interstitial fluid, it is apparent that if the fluid were not in a gel state, both legs would almost certainly be perpetually edematous.

2. The nonmobile nature of the gel prevents spread of infection in the tissues. Indeed, some bacteria, such as streptococci, are extremely pathogenic simply because they secrete hyaluronidase to dissolve the gel and allow movement of the local fluids with consequent spread of the bacteria.

3. The gel probably is important to keep the formed elements of the tissues separated at appropriate distances from each other. Since most nutrients are transported from the capillaries to the cells and most excreta from the cells to the capillaries by the process of diffusion, it is essential that appropriate avenues be maintained for adequate diffusion through the spaces. If the cells should be crowded completely upon each other, enough space between cells would not be available for the diffusion process, and one would expect

outlying cells to be deficient in certain nutrients. For instance, glucose will not diffuse through cells because it becomes trapped inside cells. Therefore, it is essential that glucose diffuse *between* cells if it is to reach those cells far removed from the capillaries. Fortunately, such substances diffuse in tissue gel almost as rapidly as in free fluid. However, the diffusion process operates most efficiently for short distances of diffusion. Therefore, it is important that the mechanism for controlling interstitial fluid volume maintain the volume only at a certain level—not too little, not too much. This is accomplished by the mechanism that maintains the tissue fluid compartment normally dry of free fluid and limits the volume to the gel fluid.

Tissue Nutrition in Edema. One of the major problems in edema is nutrition of the tissue cells because expansion of the tissue spaces increases the distances required for diffusion. Every physician becomes cognizant of this when treating varicose ulcers of the leg, since it is very difficult if not impossible for these to heal in a continuously edematous leg. Also, nutrition of essentially any tissue of the body can be compromised at least to some extent by edema. Indeed, functional measurements in the heart have even shown that an edematous myocardium has considerably decreased pumping capability.

Role of Capillary and Lymphatic Dynamics in Causation of Edema. The roles of the capillaries and the lymphatics in causing edema are so well known that they require only passing mention here. There are basically four dynamic abnormalities that can cause edema: (1) high capillary pressure, (2) low plasma colloid osmotic pressure, (3) increased permeability of the capillaries, and (4) blockage of the lymphatics. All these tend to increase the interstitial fluid pressure, and when this pressure rises above the atmospheric pressure level, edema occurs. Increased permeability of the capillaries increases the tendency for edema mainly because of leakage of plasma protein through the very porous capillary walls. This in turn causes buildup of protein in the interstitial spaces as well as loss of protein from the blood, thus causing greatly enhanced tissue colloid osmotic pressure as well as reduced plasma colloid osmotic pressure.

SAFETY FACTORS AGAINST EDEMA

Fortunately, the human being has tremendous capability for resisting the development of edema. For instance, the capillary pressure in a typical tissue must rise from the normal level of about 17 mm Hg to about 34 mm Hg—that is, to two times the normal pressure—before edema will appear, or the colloid osmotic pressure of the plasma must fall from the normal level of 28 mm Hg to below 10 mm Hg before edema will occur. From the previous discussion of interstitial fluid dynamics

of edema, one can readily understand how these tremendous safety factors come about.

Basically, edema cannot occur until the interstitial fluid pressure rises above atmospheric pressure, and there are three different mechanisms that come into play to prevent this from occurring. These are the following:

1. The normal negative interstitial fluid pressure of approximately −6.5 mm Hg must be lost before edema can occur. Therefore, the aforementioned mechanisms for maintenance of the normal negative interstitial fluid pressure constitute the first safety factor.

2. When the interstitial fluid pressure begins to rise, lymph flow increases rapidly, increasing an average of 20- to 25-fold by the time the interstitial pressure rises from its normally negative value to the level of atmospheric pressure. This greatly enhanced lymph flow constitutes a second safety factor against edema. Approximately 7 mm Hg excess filtration pressure is required across the capillary membrane to form the amount of lymph that can be carried away by this high level of lymph flow.

3. When the lymph flow increases, the rapid movement of fluid through the interstitial spaces toward the lymph vessels washes protein out of the interstitial spaces. This decreases the colloid osmotic pressure in the interstitial fluid from the normal value of about 5 mm Hg to approximately 1 mm Hg. Therefore, the plasma colloid osmotic pressure becomes 4 mm Hg more effective for absorbing fluid from the tissue spaces. This adds another 4 mm Hg of safety factor.

Adding the aforementioned safety factors, 6.5 + 7.0 + 4.0, one finds a total safety factor of approximately 17.5 mm Hg. This explains the necessity for the colloid osmotic pressure to decrease from the normal value of 28 to 10 mm Hg before edema will occur. It also explains the doubling of capillary pressure required before edema occurs, an increase from 17 to 34 mm Hg, or a safety factor of 17 mm Hg. Finally, experiments have also shown that edema can be caused in a normal arm exposed to an external vacuum greater than 18 mm Hg but cannot be caused by a vacuum less than 18 mm Hg.

There obviously is a clinical state one might call "pre-edema," which means a condition in which much of the safety factor has been dissipated even though the edema state itself has not yet been reached.

BLOOD VOLUME AND ITS REGULATION

Hemodynamic Factors. The basic hemodynamic mechanisms for blood volume regulation can be understood by combining the discussions from previous sections of this chapter. First, referring again to Figure 6–1, one notes that an increase in blood volume increases cardiac output, which increases arterial pressure, which increases urinary output, which decreases extracellular fluid volume, which finally returns the blood volume to normal. Thus, this is a purely hydrodynamic mechanism in which the kidneys are made to eliminate fluid until the volume returns to its normal level. All steps of this mechanism have been proved in individual physiologic experiments. Illustrative of this mechanism is the following experiment that we have run a number of times: In animals with normal hormonal systems and with the nervous system completely destroyed, infusion of several hundred milliliters of saline causes approximately a tenfold increase in urinary output within less than 1 minute. This increase continues, but with progressive decrement, for an hour or more until the urinary output gradually dwindles back to its control value. In the meantime, essentially all the excess saline infused is recovered in the urine.

Hormonal Factors. Two different hormones have been especially implicated in blood volume regulation: antidiuretic hormone and aldosterone. However, when either of these two hormones is infused for as long as a month into an animal at rates several times as high as the normal secretory rate, it is rare that the blood volume will change more than a few per cent, and the extracellular fluid volume also usually will change no more than 5 to 15 per cent.

This brings up the question of what these two hormones actually control if it is not volume. Studies have demonstrated that ADH is mainly concerned with control of the sodium concentration in the extracellular fluid and aldosterone with control of potassium concentration. When both the thirst and ADH mechanisms are blocked, sodium concentration varies very widely depending on the intake of salt or water or both. Also, when excess quantities of ADH are secreted, the sodium concentration decreases markedly. The mechanism of this effect is the following: The ADH causes an initial retention of water by the kidneys, but this in turn sets into play a number of different effects, including a slight rise in arterial pressure, that cause a secondary increase in urinary output containing large amounts of salt. Consequently, the sodium concentration of the extracellular fluids decreases, whereas the water content of the body increases slightly.

In the case of aldosterone, it has been taught so frequently that aldosterone controls body sodium that it is difficult to understand why aldosterone actually is far more effective in the control of extracellular fluid potassium than in the control of extracellular fluid sodium. Aldosterone does indeed cause excessive renal tubular reabsorption of sodium; it also causes excessive secretion of potassium. When excessive amounts of sodium begin to appear in the extracellular fluid, the ADH and thirst mechanisms automatically increase the body water as well and therefore bring the sodium

concentration back to the normal level. As a result, aldosterone usually fails to affect sodium concentration measurably. Therefore, the major effect of aldosterone on the extracellular fluid is on the potassium concentration rather than on sodium concentration.

Nervous Factors. Dilatation of the atria of the heart initiates potent nervous vasodilating reflexes to the kidneys and also transmits signals to the neurohypophysis to diminish the secretion of antidiuretic hormone. Both these effects increase the output of urine. Therefore, it is frequently said that the atrial receptors are "volume receptors" that detect increases in blood volume and in turn help to rectify the abnormality. However, this mechanism seems to be important in volume regulation only transiently, because the high atrial pressures occurring in heart failure do not cause continued excessive urinary output, as the mechanism would suggest.

RELATIONSHIP BETWEEN BLOOD VOLUME REGULATION AND INTERSTITIAL FLUID VOLUME REGULATION

Retention of fluid by the kidneys does not mean that the fluid will remain in the blood, because extracellular fluid is partitioned between the plasma compartment of the blood and the two interstitial fluid compartments, the free fluid compartment and the gel compartment. Under normal circumstances, in the absence of edema, the free fluid compartment volume of the interstitial spaces is essentially zero, and it is only the gel compartment with which we are concerned. When extra amounts of fluid are available, the tendency for the gel to swell causes it to absorb moderate amounts of the extra fluid. However, in dehydration states fluid is pulled out of the gel and returned to the circulation either by capillary osmosis or through the lymphatics. Therefore, there is a dynamic equilibrium between the plasma volume and the interstitial gel volume.

Measurements have shown that infusion of a balanced electrolyte solution into the circulatory system of a nonedematous person will cause approximately two thirds of the fluid to enter the gel compartment of the tissue spaces and the remainder to stay in the blood. Therefore, in the pre-edema state, retention of water and salt by the kidneys increases both blood volume and interstitial fluid volume. Conversely, dehydration decreases both of these; indeed, severe dehydration can cause circulatory shock.

Increase in Tissue Compliance in Edema. An entirely different effect occurs once the edema stage is reached, that is, once the interstitial fluid pressure rises above atmospheric pressure level. Referring again to Figure 6–11, one notes that the total interstitial fluid volume now increases extremely rapidly with very little additional rise in the interstitial fluid pressure. This contrasts with the marked rise in pressure that occurs with only a small volume increase in nonedematous tissues. The reason for this difference is that the normal tissue spaces are in a compacted state, and the volume cannot change without simultaneous marked changes in the negative pressure that causes the compaction. However, once the interstitial fluid pressure rises into the positive pressure range, the compaction of the tissues has been relieved. Now, the only major restraining force is the skin, and measurements show that the skin exerts less than one twenty fifth as much restraining force on changes in the interstitial fluid volume as do the elastic forces of tissue compaction. To express this another way, in the negative interstitial fluid pressure range, the compliance of the tissue space is slight, whereas in the positive interstitial fluid pressure range the looseness of the skin and other tissue elements allows the compliance to increase 25-fold.

Therefore, once the interstitial pressure rises to a positive value, tremendous quantities of free fluid begin to collect in the very loose tissue spaces, and this fluid collects despite extremely little additional rise in interstitial fluid pressure.

Safety Valve Function of the Interstitial Fluid Spaces for Excesses of Blood Volume. The significance of edema to the circulatory system probably has escaped most physiologists and clinicians alike. The ability for tremendous quantities of fluid to collect rapidly in tissue spaces when the blood volume rises above a certain critical level is actually an important safety valve for the circulatory system. Were it not for this, it would be difficult to infuse more than 2 to 3 liters of electrolyte solution into a normal patient without killing him, which one can demonstrate any time he wishes by simply infusing several liters of fluid intravenously at a rate that is too rapid, all of it within 1 minute, for the fluid to transude out of the capillaries into the interstitial spaces. Pressures throughout the system rise to extreme values and can cause rupture of vessels, arrhythmias of the heart, and typical signs of acute cardiac failure.

Therefore, the edema mechanism is an important safety valve for blood volume control in the human being. Furthermore, this "safety valve" opens at a very exact capillary pressure level—at exactly that capillary pressure at which the total safety factor against edema has been dissipated.

SIGNIFICANCE OF BLOOD VOLUME MEASUREMENTS AND OF MEAN CIRCULATORY FILLING PRESSURE

Because it is very easy to measure blood volume by injecting any type of indicator material that will stay in the circulatory system and then measuring the degree of dilution of the indicator, blood volume measurements are frequently made; however, they are rarely of great significance. The reason for this is elementary: Blood volume is automatically adjusted to fit the capacity of the circulatory system itself, and even such conditions as varicose veins can change both the capacity of the circulatory system and the blood volume markedly. Likewise, a state of vasoconstriction, as occurs in patients with pheochromocytomas, can greatly reduce the capacity of the circulation; vasodilatation, as caused by block of the sympathetic nervous system, can increase the capacity of the system.

The tightness with which blood volume fills the circulatory system is measured by the mean circulatory filling pressure, and this can change as a result of a variation in either blood volume or circulatory capacity. From our earlier discussion of cardiac output regulation, it is clear that it is not blood volume per se that affects venous return and cardiac output but, instead, the mean circulatory filling pressure. Therefore, alteration of the mean circulatory filling pressure, whether it be caused by a change in blood volume or a change in capacity of the system, has essentially the same effect on the circulation.

Consequently, the factor that needs to be measured, so far as the dynamics of the circulation are concerned, is not blood volume but, instead, mean circulatory filling pressure. In animal experiments, in which it is possible to stop the heart and to bring pressures to equilibrium throughout the system, it is possible to measure this pressure, the normal value for which is 7 mm Hg. In human beings, this measurement has never been achieved. In the meantime, one can understand why blood volume measurements are much less useful in explaining hemodynamic function of the circulation than are such functional measurements as arterial pressure and cardiac output.

PULMONARY CIRCULATION

Many, but not all, of the hemodynamic principles that apply to the systemic circulation also apply to the pulmonary circulation. For instance, the pulmonary system is a low-pressure system with a mean pulmonary arterial pressure of only 13 mm Hg and systolic and diastolic pressures of 22 mm Hg and 8 mm Hg, respectively. For this reason, the pulmonary system has correspondingly thinner arterial and arteriolar vasculature, as well as less smooth muscle in the vessel walls. This is very fortunate because the pulmonary vasculature receives the same stroke volume output from the right heart that the entire systemic arterial tree receives from the the left heart. The high degree of distensibility of the pulmonary arteries, despite their short length, is of major advantage in allowing the pulmonary vascular tree to absorb the large thrust of blood with each heart beat. Also, because of very low pulmonary vascular resistance from the arteries to the veins—only about one tenth that of the systemic circulation—there is marked runoff of blood from the pulmonary arteries to the left atrium even before systole is complete, which decreases the quantity of blood that must be accommodated in the pulmonary arterial tree. These two factors acting together cause the pulmonary arterial pulse pressure to be only about 14 mm Hg, in contrast to 40 mm Hg in the aorta.

Effect of Alveolar Hypoxia on Local Vascular Resistance. There are three important exceptions to the usual rule that blood flow is distributed almost equally to all alveoli. The first of these exceptions occurs when some alveoli are ventilated to a lesser extent than others. If the poorly ventilated alveoli were perfused with blood to the same extent as the other alveoli, the oxygen levels in the poorly ventilated alveoli would become depressed, thereby creating hypoxia also in the blood leaving these alveoli. However, the direct effect of hypoxia on the local vasculature is vasoconstriction; this reduces the perfusion of the affected alveoli and thereby shunts blood flow to other alveoli that are better ventilated. Unfortunately, however, this mechanism is a weak one — that is, it does not have a very high feedback gain. Therefore, it is not as important a mechanism as one might wish it to be to control distribution of blood flow to the respective alveoli.

Pulmonary physiologists have also pointed out that hypoxia occurring in widespread areas of alveoli at the same time—for instance, as often occurs in emphysema—can sometimes cause enough vasoconstriction of the total pulmonary vasculature to elevate pulmonary arterial pressure significantly. Occasionally, the rise in pulmonary arterial pressure is enough to cause right heart failure with corresponding reduction in cardiac output. Oxygen therapy often helps relieve this condition, presumably by decreasing the pulmonary vascular resistance.

Effect of Atelectasis on Local Blood Flow. The second condition in which unequal distribution of alveolar blood flow occurs to a significant extent is atelectasis. When a bronchus is blocked, the alveoli beyond the block begin to collapse within minutes, and whole segments of the lung can become collapsed over a period of hours. The mechanical collapse of the alveoli causes the solid tissues between the alveoli to close tightly around the local blood vessels, in some cases actually kinking the vessels. As a result, in total atelectasis as much as 75 per cent of blood flow is usually shunted to the normal lung tissue. This is actually a very fortunate effect because it helps ensure that essentially all the blood flow passing through the lungs will flow in juxtaposition to ventilated alveoli and will bypass the nonventilated alveoli.

Effect of Hydrostatic Pressure on Local Blood Flow in the Lung. Still a third hemodynamic factor that causes nonuniform blood flow in the pulmonary circulation is the different hydrostatic levels of the different parts of the lung. When a person is in a standing position, the apex of his lung lies as much as 10 to 15 cm above the midlevel of the heart, which means that the pulmonary arterial pressures are only barely high enough to pump blood through the apical vessels. Indeed, only the systolic pressure is high enough, so that blood flows through the apical vessels in spurts synchronized with cardiac systole. At the base of the lung, however, located some 10 cm below the level of the heart, the pulmonary vessels are subjected not only to normal pulmonary vascular pressure but also to an additional 7 mm Hg hydrostatic pressure. Therefore, both the diastolic and systolic pressures are considerably elevated in the base of the lung, and the blood flows through this region continuously throughout systole and diastole. This difference creates another problem, namely, that in the standing, quiet state the base of the lung is overperfused, whereas the apex is underperfused. This effect is partially compensated by the fact that the base of the lung is, for mechanical reasons, ventilated to a greater extent than is the apex. Fortunately, during exercise, when the fullest functional capacity of the lungs is needed, the pulmonary pressures rise throughout the lungs, and all portions reach almost optimal ventilation-perfusion ratios.

PULMONARY EDEMA

Capillary dynamics in the lungs obey almost exactly the same principles as those discussed earlier for the systemic circulation, but a few differences are important.

Normal Mechanism for Keeping the Alveoli "Dry." To keep the alveoli in their normal "dry" state — that is, filled with air rather than with fluid — the pulmonary interstitial fluid pressure is almost certainly negative in the same way that it is in peripheral tissues. Indirect measurements indicate this pressure to be about −8 mm Hg. Negative pressure in the interstitial spaces of the lungs obviously would keep the alveolar membrane pulled tightly against the capillaries. It would also provide an absorptive force for causing absorption of any stray fluid that might occur in the alveoli, thus returning the alveoli to their normal dry state.

If, however, the interstitial fluid pressure of the lungs should ever rise into the positive range, one would expect pulmonary edema to result in the same way that edema results in peripheral tissues.

Safety Factor Against Pulmonary Edema. The safety factor against edema in the lungs is greater than in systemic tissues. The pulmonary capillary pressure must be increased acutely to approximately 30 mm Hg, or to about 2 mm Hg greater than the colloid osmotic pressure of the blood, before pulmonary edema will ensue. Since the normal pulmonary capillary pressure in the human being is probably about 7 mm Hg, the safety factor against pulmonary edema can be calculated to be approximately 23 mm Hg, compared with 18 mm Hg in the systemic circulation. An acute increase in pulmonary capillary pressure above 30 mm Hg will cause rapid fluid transudation into the lungs (based on studies in dogs), and when the pressure is raised acutely to 50 mm Hg it can cause lethal pulmonary edema in as little as one half hour.

Role of Lymphatics in Chronic Pulmonary Edema. In chronic pulmonary edema, still another safety factor occurs. Even a few weeks of greatly elevated left atrial pressure causes marked overgrowth of the pulmonary lymphatics, increasing their lymph-carrying capacity sometimes as much as tenfold. Therefore, one would expect that pulmonary capillary pressure would then have to rise much higher than the 30 mm Hg required in acute conditions before pulmonary edema would occur. This corresponds to the finding in many catheter laboratories that patients with chronic mitral stenosis frequently have chronic elevations of pulmonary capillary pressure in the 35 to 45 mm Hg pressure range without evident pulmonary edema.

Alveolar Flooding in Pulmonary Edema. Another primary difference between pulmonary edema and systemic edema is that the limiting boundary of the pulmonary interstitial spaces, the alveolar membrane, is a very thin, weak, one–cell layer membrane. Therefore, in contrast to the skin on the surface of the body, the alveolar membrane cannot withstand significant amounts of positive pressure in the interstitial spaces of the lungs. Evidence at present indicates that these alveolar membranes begin to break when the interstitial fluid pressure rises even a fraction of a mm Hg into the positive pressure range. When this happens, fluid in the interstitial spaces of the lungs simply flows immediately into the alveoli. Therefore, only very mild pulmonary edema can be confined to the interstitial spaces; if this edema develops to any significant extent, a major share of the edema fluid immediately flows through the broken alveolar membranes into the alveoli themselves, which accounts for the alveolar flooding that occurs in most instances of pulmonary edema.

ARTERIAL PULSATION

The clinically important features of arterial pulsation are so well understood by most clinicians that they deserve little comment. However, it is important to review a few simple principles.

Arterial Elasticity and Net Stroke Volume as Determinants of Arterial Pulse Pressure. The basic determinants of arterial pulse pressure are twofold: (1) the elasticity of the arteries; and (2) the *net* stroke volume output of the heart, which is defined as the stroke volume of the heart minus the volume runoff through the small vessels during the period of systole. In other words, the greater the net gain of blood volume in the arterial tree between the beginning of systole and the end of systole, the greater also will be the arterial pulse pressure. Also, the higher the volume elasticity coefficient of the arterial vessels — that is, the less the compliance — the greater will be the pulse pressure.

Obviously, a large number of other factors can affect one or both of these two basic determinants of the pulse pressure. These include the presence or absence of arteriosclerosis, the degree of active vasoconstriction or vasodilatation of the arterial tree, and the sizes of the arteries themselves, all of which affect the volume elasticity coefficient of the arterial system. Factors that can affect the net stroke volume output include cardiac output, heart rate, and degree of peripheral vasodilatation. That is, stroke volume output is equal to cardiac output divided by heart rate, and net stroke volume output is stroke volume diminished by the amount of blood runoff during systole.

Diminished Peripheral Pulsation. The clinical habit of feeling the peripheral pulse can be a highly valuable art, even to the extent that a few clinicians in the past reputedly could estimate arterial pressure quite accurately by feeling the radial artery, although in general this method is no longer practiced by clinicians. Only two features of the peripheral arterial pulse are now usually noted by the clinician—the pulse frequency pattern and the intensity of pulsation.

The significance of diminished intensity of the peripheral pulse is illustrated in Figure 6–12, which shows a recorded arterial pulse curve from the dorsalis pedis artery before and after stimulation of the sympathetic nerves. Note that the pulse pressure diminished markedly following the vasoconstriction and that the mean pressure level also diminished. This figure demonstrates that there is a high degree of correlation between the intensity of peripheral arterial pulsation and tissue perfusion. Consequently, the clinical dictum that diminished pulsation means diminished tissue perfusion is indeed a well-founded one, although, of course, this also has its exceptions, especially when collateral vessels have taken over the function of a normally pulsatile artery.

Some physiologists have claimed that arterial pulsation *per se* plays a significant role in helping maintain peripheral perfusion. However, this is still a very doubtful concept and has been both supported and denied by different investigators. The only value of peripheral arterial pulsation that has thus far been proved beyond doubt is its capability, in at least some instances, to promote lymph flow. In a completely pulseless tissue, lymph flow has been found in animals to be greatly diminished, particularly when the animal is under

Figure 6–12 Pressure contour in the dorsalis pedis artery recorded first under normal conditions and second during stimulation of the sympathetic nerves supplying the femoral artery. (Modified from Alexander, R. S., and Kantrowitz, A.: Surgery 33:42, 1953.)

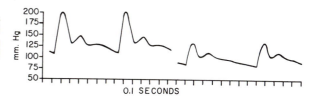

the influence of anesthesia, such as sodium pentobarbital, that can block lymph vessel vasomotion.

The Hemodynamic Anomaly of Pulsus Alternans. Pulsus alternans is a condition in which the arterial pulse alternates — usually every other heart beat: first strong, then weak, then strong, and continuing in this alternating pattern. Thus far, it has never been satisfactorily explained. It is mentioned here because several basic studies of circulatory hemodynamics have offered a possible explanation. One of these was a computer study in which the systemic circulation and the pulmonary circulation were simulated mathematically to operate in a complete circuit. In performing different experiments with the simulation, several conditions were found in which typical pulsus alternans occurred. One of these was abnormality of ventricular response to changes in atrial pressure. When the computer was programmed so that a very minute change in atrial pressure would cause marked change in ventricular output, the left ventricle would first pump an extremely large quantity of blood into the systemic circulation

during one heart beat, but during the next heart beat the right ventricle would pump an extremely large quantity into the lungs, the blood volume oscillating back and forth between the pulmonary circulation and the systemic circulation, It was also possible to cause oscillation of the blood volume between the central circulation of the chest region and the more peripheral circulation. Furthermore, the system frequently would be working completely normally and would then be thrown into pulsus alternans by some transient event that occurred in the simulated circulation. This is completely in accord with typical findings in the clinical catheter laboratory, when a sudden event related to the catheterization procedure itself often can cause pulsus alternans in the patient.

This phenomenon and its possible explanation have been discussed here because, if the explanation is correct, the phenomenon is strictly a hemodynamic problem resulting from resonance within the mechanical system itself, not too unlike the resonance that occurs in the pipe of a pipe organ, with pressure waves reflecting back and forth from one end of the pipe to the other.

REFERENCES

Berne, R. M., and Rubio, R.: Coronary circulation. *In* Berne, R. M., et al. (Eds.): Handbook of Physiology. Sec 2. Vol. I. Baltimore, Williams & Wilkins, 1979, p. 873.

Bevan, J. A., et al. (Eds.): Vascular Neuroeffector Mechanisms. New York, Raven Press, 1980.

Coleman, T. G., and Guyton, A. C.: Hypertension caused by salt loading in the dog. III. Onset transients of cardiac output and other circulatory variables. Circ. Res. 25:153, 1969.

Fishman, A. P.: Hypoxia in the pulmonary circulation. Circ. Res 38:221, 1976.

Genest, J., et al.: Hypertension. New York, McGraw-Hill Book Co., 1977.

Gibbs, C. L.: Cardiac energetics. Physiol. Rev., 58:174, 1978.

Goetz, K. L., et al.: Atrial receptors and renal function. Physiol. Rev., 55:157, 1975.

Granger, H. J., and Guyton, A. C.: Autoregulation of the total systemic circulation following destruction of the central nervous system in the dog. Circ. Res., 25:379, 1969.

Green, J. F.: Determinants of systemic blood flow. International Review of Physiology: Cardiovascular Physiology III. Vol. 18. Baltimore, University Park Press, 1979, p. 33.

Gregg, D. E.: Coronary Circulation in Health and Disease. Philadelphia, Lea and Febiger, 1950.

Guyton, A. C.: Arterial Pressure and Hypertension. Philadelphia, W. B. Saunders Co., 1980.

Guyton, A. C., Coleman, T. G., Cowley, A. W., Jr., et al.: A systems analysis approach to understanding long-range arterial blood pressure control and hypertension. Circ. Res. 35:159, 1974.

Guyton, A. C., Jones, C. E., and Coleman, T. G. (Eds.): Circulatory Physiology: Cardiac Output and Its Regulation. 2nd ed. Philadelphia, W. B. Saunders Co., 1973.

Guyton, A. C., Taylor, A. E., and Granger, H. J. (Eds.): Circulatory Physiology II. Dynamics and Control of the Body Fluids. Philadelphia, W. B. Saunders Co., 1975.

Guyton, A. C., et al.: Integration and control of circulatory function. Int. Rev. Physiol., 9:341, 1976.

Hughes, J. M. B.: Pulmonary circulatory and fluid balance Int. Rev. Physiol. 14:135, 1977.

Keatinge, W. R., and Harman, M. C.: Local Mechanisms Controlling Blood Vessels. New York, Academic Press, 1979.

Manning, R. D., Jr., et al.: Essential role of mean circulatory filling pressure in salt-induced hypertension. Am. J. Physiol., 236:R40, 1979.

Oberg, B.: Overall cardiovascular regulation. Annu. Rev. Physiol., 38:537, 1976.

Parker, J. C., et al.: Pulmonary transcapillary exchange and pulmonary edema. International Review of Physiology: Cardiovascular Physiology III. Vol. 18. Baltimore, University Park Press, 1979. p. 261.

Rapaport, E. (Ed.): Current Controversies in Cardiovascular Disease. Philadelphia, W. B. Saunders Co., 1980.

Schaper, W. (Ed.): The Pathophysiology of Myocardial Perfusion. New York. Elsevier/North-Holland. 1979.

Sparks, H. V., Jr., and Belloni, F. L.: The peripheral circulation: Local regulation. Annu. Rev. Physiol., 40:67, 1978.

Vander, A. J.: Control of renin release. Physiol. Rev., 47:359, 1967.

Wenger, N. K. (Ed.): Exercise and the Heart. Philadelphia. F. A. Davis Co., 1978.

Willis, J. (Ed.): The Heart: Update, New York, McGraw-Hill, 1979.

7 Systemic Arterial Pressure*

Robert C. Tarazi and Ray W. Gifford, Jr.

The pressure in arteries and veins was first measured in 1733 by Stephen Hales, who inserted a cannula into an artery and a vein of a mare and noted the rise of the blood column in a tube. The arterial column rose approximately 8 feet, whereas the venous column rose only 12 inches. Since that time, tubes have been successfully inserted into various segments of the circulation of conscious unrestrained subjects and the pressure determined by sensitive manometers with high frequency of response. Thus, a map could be drawn of pressure variations along the circulatory circuit and of its fluctuations with different phases of the cardiac cycle (Fig. 7–1). The marked drop of pressure observed at the systemic arteriolar level led to a subdivision of the circulation into a "high-pressure" (resistance) segment and a "low-pressure" (capacitance) segment. The first is thought to be mainly concerned with flow distribution and regulation, and the second with priming of the cardiac pump and control of its output and, possibly, with regulation of intravascular volume. Important as these subdivisions are, the essential unity of the circulation must not be forgotten. A greater transmission of pressure from arteries to capillaries (as by arteriolar vasodilatation) may increase capillary ultrafiltration and reduce intravascular volume while concomitantly increasing venous return. Conversely, venoconstriction may, under certain conditions, relocate blood to the cardiopulmonary area, enhance cardiac output, and thus influence arterial pressure. Blood pressure in capillaries, veins, and the lesser circulation is discussed elsewhere in this text and will be referred to here only insofar as it influences systemic arterial pressure.

Left ventricular contraction provides a phasic output of energy for the circulation; during systole, the intraventricular pressure rises from an average of 8 mm Hg to about 120 mm Hg under normal conditions. Blood is ejected into the aorta when the intraventricular pressure forces open the semilunar valves; during that portion of the cycle, systolic pressure is practically equal in the ventricle and aorta. At the end of systole, the heart muscle relaxes, and as intraventricular pressure falls steeply, the semilunar valve is closed. While blood is running from the arterioles into capillaries and veins, the large arteries, which had absorbed part of the energy of systole, now recoil on the diminishing volume of blood left by ventricular ejection, so that arterial pressure falls gradually during diastole. Thus, the arterial pressure pulse results from the ejection of a small volume of blood into a partly filled container of limited distensibility. This ejection at first distends only the proximal portion of the aorta, but the pressure wave generated is then rapidly transmitted to the rest of the arterial tree, with a velocity inversely proportional to the distensibility of the vessels involved. Since compliance of the arterial tree is less far out from the central aorta, the pulse wave velocity increases the farther it travels. When the wave reaches the main branching sites, but especially the precapillary resistance barrier, it is reflected back. Summation of the advancing waves with reflected waves may alter pulse tracings to a greater or lesser extent, depending on the particular artery considered, the speed of wave transmission, and the degree of peripheral vasoconstriction at that time. Particularly obvious is the peaking of pulse waves in the femoral arteries, when the size of the wave often becomes greater than in more central vessels, possibly resulting in phasic backflow. Conditions stiffening arterial walls such as hypertension or sclerosis will also increase pulse wave velocity.

Pulse wave velocity must not be confused with the velocity of blood flow. The actual volume of blood yielded by the heart will have moved only a few centimeters by the time the pressure wave has reached the distal ends of the arterial system. Blood movement can be likened to the result of pushing a series of billiard balls: Applying force on a ball at one end displaces another at the other end. As total surface area of the vasculature increases with repeated branching of the vessels, blood flow velocity decreases; concurrently, the pulse wave velocity increases. This explains why the velocity of the pressure pulse is approximately 15 times that of blood flow in the aorta but may be as great as 100 times the velocity of blood flow in the distal arteries.

DETERMINATION OF ARTERIAL PRESSURE AND DEFINITION OF TERMS

Arterial pressure can be determined either directly (intra-arterial insertion of a needle or tube

---

*Many concepts and mechanisms described in this chapter are related to general concepts discussed in Chapter 6.

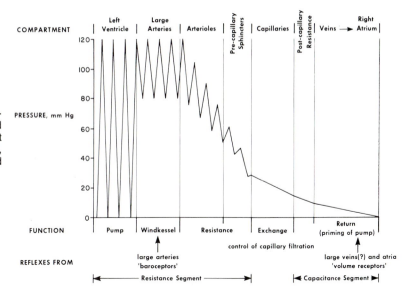

Figure 7–1 Functional subdivisions of the systemic circulation and pressure variations in its different segments. (After Folkow, B., and Neil, E.: Circulation. New York, Oxford University Press, 1971.)

connected to a manometer) or indirectly, usually by auscultation over an artery to which pressure is applied proximally (sphygmomanometry). The choice of method will depend on purpose; the accuracy of determinations does not depend on the method used as much as on the attention given to seemingly minor but really quite important details.

DIRECT METHOD

The pressure determined in this way depends on the type of manometer to which the intra-

arterial cannula is connected. The older U-tube mercury manometer has so much inertia that it cannot rise and fall rapidly and therefore simply oscillates around a mean level of pressure. To record faithfully rapidly changing pressures, manometers with higher frequency responses are currently used with optimal damping to ensure a uniform output throughout the range of frequencies expected. The records obtained are illustrated in Figure 7–2. The difference between the highest (systolic) and lowest (diastolic) pressure of a cycle is called the "pulse pressure" (PP). An integrated mean for the pressure developed throughout a whole cardiac cycle can either be recorded by

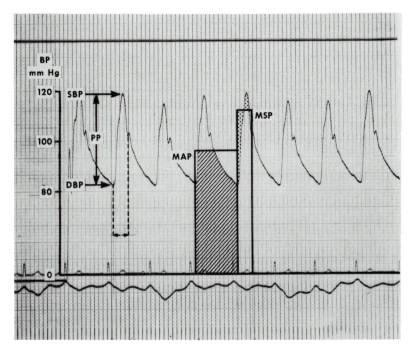

Figure 7–2 The line defining mean arterial pressure (MAP) can be drawn so that the area added (blank) is equivalent to the area subtracted (blank) from the whole cardiac cycle. Similarly, mean systolic pressure (MSP) can be estimated by adding an area (stippled) equivalent to that subtracted (stippled) from the ventricular ejection period only (from onset of pulse to incisure).

electronically damping the response of the recording system or be determined by planimetry. The *mean arterial pressure* (MAP) thus obtained reflects the average pressure pushing blood through the systemic circulation and is therefore used to calculate peripheral resistance (see later discussion); it is not equal to the arithmetic mean of the systolic and diastolic pressures but depends in part on the heart rate and relative duration of systole and diastole. A close approximation is obtained as follows:

$$MAP = DBP + \tfrac{1}{3} PP.$$

The *mean systolic pressure* (MSP) is determined by integrating the area under the systolic part of the cycle; again, the following calculation yields a close approximation in most conditions:

$$MSP = DBP + 0.8 PP.$$

Its main use is in calculations of cardiac work and tension-time indices; it is closely related to myocardial oxygen consumption, since pressure work is more costly to the heart than volume work.

INDIRECT METHOD

The instrument universally used is the sphygmomanometer; the arterial pressure is usually measured in humans at the brachial artery with the subject seated or lying down, with the arm slightly flexed and at heart level. Time should be allowed for recovery from recent exercise or excitement; clothing should not constrict the arm, and the patient should be put as much at ease as possible. A cloth-covered rubber bag is placed firmly and snugly around the upper arm, with its lower edge about an inch above the antecubital space. The bag should be 20 per cent wider than the diameter of the limb on which it is to be used (12 to 14 cm for the average adult but wider for obese patients) and should be long enough (25 to 30 cm) to encircle the limb almost completely. There should be no bulging or displacement of the bag when inflated. The air pressure inside the bag is determined by a mercury manometer or by an aneroid manometer calibrated against a mercury manometer. While the brachial or radial pulse is palpated, the bag is inflated to a pressure 30 mm Hg higher than that required to obliterate the pulse. The pressure is then gradually reduced at a rate approximately 2 to 3 mm Hg per second while a stethoscope, which is applied firmly but with as little pressure as possible over the previously palpated brachial artery, is employed. As the pressure in the bag falls, a series of sounds—the Korotkoff sounds—are heard as follows:

Phase I: A clear, sharp, snapping sound appears suddenly and grows louder.

Phase II: Sound is softened and becomes prolonged into a murmur.

Phase III: Sound again becomes crisper and increases in intensity.

Phase IV: Distinct abrupt muffling of the sound.

Phase V: Sounds disappear.

It is universally agreed that the first appearance of vascular sounds (phase I) indicates the breakthrough of the pulse wave and gives the systolic pressure. In contrast, the best index of diastolic pressure is still a subject of controversy. The American Heart Association recommended phase IV in 1967 but then chose phase V in 1969. Part of the controversy is due to individual differences regarding ease or dependability in recognition of "muffling" as opposed to "disappearance" of a sound. Numerous studies have shown that phase V corresponds more closely to the direct intra-arterial diastolic pressure; however, this may be only an empiric coincidence. There is no logical connection in the laws of physics between phase V and diastolic pressure, whereas the abrupt muffling of the arterial sound (phase IV) signals that blood flow is no longer impeded during diastole by the cuff pressure. In practice, there is usually little difference between the two phases, but they may become widely separated when arterial flow is increased. In such cases it is best to note both phases, so that blood pressure is recorded as, for example, 128/88/76. The first figure represents the systolic (phase I); the second, the diastolic (phase IV); and the third, phase V pressure.

Sometimes, particularly in some hypertensive patients, the usual sounds heard over the brachial artery when the cuff pressure is high disappear as the pressure is reduced and then reappear at a lower level. This early, temporary disappearance of sound is called the *auscultatory gap* and occurs during the latter part of phase I and phase II. Because this gap may cover a range of 40 mm Hg, one can seriously underestimate the systolic pressure or overestimate the diastolic pressure, unless its presence is excluded by first palpating for disappearance of the radial pulse as the cuff pressure is raised.

When all sounds have disappeared, the cuff should be deflated rapidly and completely. Before further determinations are made, 1 to 2 minutes should elapse for the release of blood trapped in the veins.

An important sign to be looked for actively, especially in patients with some indication of cardiac dysfunction, is *pulsus alternans*. One detects this by noting that after the first sounds are heard and as pressure is reduced, their rate suddenly doubles, strong sounds alternating with weak sounds. It is an important sign of left ventricular failure and should be carefully distinguished from arrhythmia (irregular intervals between sounds) or respiratory variations of arterial pressure. The degree of alternans (interval between phase I and level of doubling of the sounds) and the heart rate at the moment should be carefully noted. The wider the alternans and the slower the heart rate at the time, the more seriously must this sign be viewed; minor degrees of alteration are not uncommon with marked tachycardia.

Blood pressure can also be determined during sphygmomanometry in three other ways. The first, the *palpatory,* involves palpating the radial pulse and noting the pressure at which it returns, after it has been obliterated by elevation of the pressure in the cuff above the pressure in the brachial artery. This method is not used extensively for several reasons. In the first place, only the systolic pressure can be determined, and, in general, it is inaccurate, being too low by approximately 5 to 10 mm Hg. However, the method is useful, in part at least, in ascertaining from the absence of the radial pulse that the brachial pulse is exceeded, a point that cannot always be settled by the auscultatory method.

The second is the *oscillometric.* In the Pachon oscillometer, two rubber bags are contained in the cuff, and the pressure in these bags is transmitted to a recording manometer. The mechanism is so arranged that when the column of blood reaches the lower cuff, the pulsation is reversed on the record. The entrance of the column of blood into the artery under the second cuff and the reversal of the record signal the systolic pressure. As the pressure is further reduced, the oscillations become greater and greater until they suddenly diminish markedly in size. This point is commonly taken as the diastolic pressure, but the precise point on the record at which the change occurs is not always evident.

The third method depends on a Doppler effect and is gaining in importance and popularity, especially in pediatric practice and for patients with peripheral vascular disease. A narrow ultrasonic beam is directed toward any peripheral artery; when pressure in the sphygmomanometer cuff exceeds the systolic level, the artery collapses. Then, as pressure within the cuff is gradually lowered, the empty artery begins to receive blood flow intermittently and then continuously. The effects of these variations on ultrasonography can be recognized by auscultation or recorded after suitable amplification.

Slight differences in pressure between both arms are not uncommon on repeated determinations; however, meaningful comparisons can be made only by simultaneous determinations of blood pressure on both sides. Care must be taken to utilize cuffs appropriate to each arm's size; significant differences are reproducible and usually greater than 10 mm Hg. They usually are due to some obstruction in arterial supply to the arm with the lower pressure.

The blood pressure may be taken in other parts of the body, particularly in the leg. When this is done, the patient rests in the horizontal position and the cuff is placed around the thigh, the sound being elicited over the artery in the popliteal space by application of the diaphragm of the stethoscope there. A special wide "thigh-cuff" should be used, wrapped firmly, but not tightly, with the compression bag over the posterior aspect of the midthigh. The systolic pressure thus recorded in the thigh is higher by 10 to 40 mm Hg than that in the arm, but the diastolic is essentially the same. This difference is mainly spurious (uncomfortable position, difficulty of proper compression), although a minor part may be related to the effect of reflected pulse waves. It is accentuated in aortic insufficiency (Hill's sign), but more importantly it disappears or becomes reversed (arm pressure > thigh pressure) in coarctation of the aorta or obstruction at the aortic bifurcation and sometimes in abdominal aortic aneurysms.

CORRELATION BETWEEN DIRECT AND INDIRECT METHODS

Cuff readings are closely related to direct measurements, although levels are on the average 5 mm Hg too low for the systolic and 8 mm Hg too high for the diastolic (taken as phase IV). Actually, the disappearance of sounds (phase V) often coincides with diastolic pressure measured directly but it is less easy to define in some cases than phase IV and admits of wider variations. One of the most important factors affecting the accuracy of indirect recordings is the size of cuff used and its proper application to ensure adequate and even compression of the artery. The smaller the cuff in relation to the arm circumference, the higher the recorded pressure and the greater the error.

In both methods, the relation of the arm and manometer to the "heart level" is crucial; lowering or raising the arm from that level will increase or reduce recorded pressure because of hydrostatic factors involved, hence the importance of keeping the arm level with the fourth intercostal space whenever blood pressure is determined while the subject is sitting or standing.

AMBULATORY BLOOD PRESSURE MONITORING

There are several methods of ambulatory blood pressure monitoring. Continuous intra-arterial pressures can be monitored and recorded through an indwelling needle in the radial artery (Oxford-Medilog system). Indirect, patient-operated ambulatory recorders (Remler) have been available for several years. The most recent development is a fully automatic system that measures and records blood pressure every 7.5 to 30 minutes (Del Mar Avionics). With both the Oxford intra-arterial device and the Del Mar Avionics system, it is possible to measure blood pressure during sleep, which the patient-operated Remler apparatus cannot do.

Although ambulatory blood pressure monitoring is a valuable research tool, it has few clinical applications at this time. The casual blood pressure determination has been the basis for all studies on the natural history of hypertension as well as the effects of treatment. Whether ambulatory blood pressure monitoring can provide information not available from casual and home blood pressure determinations (which are much less expensive and not as cumbersome) in making clinical decisions regarding the necessity for and effectiveness of treatment is conjectural and will ultimately depend on establishing a whole new set of data based on the prognostic implications of ambulatory versus casual and home blood pressure averages.

BASIC FACTORS DETERMINING ARTERIAL PRESSURE

PRESSURE, FLOW, AND RESISTANCE

Blood flow through vessels depends on two factors—the pressure head driving it and the resistance it meets. The relationship between these factors is defined by some basic hydrodynamic laws developed by Newton, Hagen, Poiseuille, and others. Translated into clinical terms, these laws have become essential to the understanding of arterial pressure variations in health and disease.

As just stated, the flow of any liquid along a tube is associated with a pressure gradient along that tube dependent on the rate of flow and on the resistance it meets. Because resistance (R) cannot be measured directly, it is calculated as the ratio of the pressure gradient (ΔP) to the rate of flow (F):

$$R = \Delta P/F \qquad (1)$$

The rate of flow of liquids within cylindrical vessels can be mathematically deduced from Newton's principles on laminar movement of fluids. If the liquid is of uniform viscosity and its flow streamlined and nonpulsatile, then

$$F = \frac{\Delta P \times r^4}{l \times v} \times \frac{\pi}{8} \qquad (2)$$

(r = radius of vessel, l = its length, and v = the fluid viscosity; $\frac{\pi}{8}$ is a constant, arising from calculus derivations).

Strictly speaking, these conditions are not met in the circulation, but despite the obvious differences, this fundamental law (Poiseuille) is largely valid for hemodynamic studies. The calculations

derived from it are very useful in assessing the relative parts played by blood flow and peripheral resistance in changes of arterial pressure. The clinical equivalents of F, ΔP, and R (formula 1) in the systemic circulation are cardiac output (CO), mean arterial pressure (MAP), and total peripheral resistance (TPR), respectively. Cardiac output and mean arterial pressure are determined directly and TPR is calculated as their ratio.* Rearranging the terms in (1) leads to the basic equation describing the relationship of arterial pressure, cardiac output, and peripheral resistance

$$MAP = CO \times TPR \qquad (3)$$

It is important to realize the approximations and simplifications involved in this formula and the consequent reservations involved in its application to the intact organism. An example of simplification is the use of MAP as the equivalent of ΔP: The marked difference between systemic arterial and central venous pressure as well as the relatively small fluctuations of the latter allows its disregard in calculations of resistance in the systemic circulation. This simplification naturally is not possible for the pulmonary circulation; in calculations of pulmonary vascular resistance, the pulmonary wedge pressure or left atrial pressure must be subtracted from the mean pulmonary arterial pressure.

The main reservation relates to the understanding and evaluation of changes in total peripheral resistance; the simplicity of this formula must not lure one into simplistic interpretations of that calculated value. The first caveat: Total peripheral resistance is the composite of the vascular resistance of each organ. Resistances to flow obey the same laws as electric resistances for combinations of series and of parallel arrangements. Therefore, a change in TPR does not necessarily indicate that similar quantitative or even similar directional changes are occurring in all individual vascular territories. The second caveat concerns the relationship of ΔTPR to vasoconstriction and dilatation. Calculating according to the usual physiologic limits of blood viscosity and assuming a constant vascular length in the same individual, one can determine that variations in resistance will usually result from active, passive, or structural changes of vessel diameter. Since the radius is magnified to the fourth power in equation

---

*Resistance can be calculated from either cardiac output or from cardiac index (CI = CO/body surface area); since cardiac output is related to body size but MAP is not, the latter approach is preferable. In either case, resistance can be expressed in arbitrary units, PRU (peripheral resistance units) = $\left(\frac{mm\ Hg}{L/mm/m^2}\right)$ or in fundamental units of force. For the latter, pressure in mm Hg is converted to dynes/cm^2 (1 mm Hg = 1333 dynes/cm^2) and flow to cm^3/sec (1 L = 1000/60 cm^3/sec); the calculated resistance is then expressed in dynes sec/cm^5. This can be achieved practically by multiplying PRU by 80.

2, flow and pressure are markedly affected by relatively small changes in vessel size. One is strongly tempted to translate immediately ΔTPR into an index of peripheral arteriolar vasoconstriction. Although this may frequently be correct, one must not fail to recognize the important role that large and small arteriovenous shunts, precapillary sphincters, passive arterial variations, structural changes, and collateral vessels may sometimes play in these changes.

FACTORS DETERMINING PULSE PRESSURE

Aside from forces regulating the average level of arterial pressure, a number of factors determine the width of pulsations around the mean. This discussion concerns those factors affecting central pulse pressure rather than the local variations already mentioned, resulting from reflected waves and altered distensibility of various peripheral portions of the arterial tree.

The aorta and its main branches take up a relatively large volume of blood under pressure during systolic ejection; during diastole, the pressure energy thus stored is gradually used to press blood onward. This "Windkessel function" helps transform an intermittent input to a more even outflow (Wiggers). Determination of pulse pressure will therefore relate mainly to quantity of blood ejected per beat (stroke volume) and to compliance of the aorta and large vessels; to a lesser degree, pulse pressure will be determined by speed of ejection of blood. The aortic wall is not a perfectly elastic material and its viscous components imply that the more rapidly blood is ejected, the greater its resistance to stretch and therefore the larger the rise in pulse pressure.

Obviously, the larger the stroke volume, the wider the pulse pressure; the causes of increased stroke volume are usually evident (aortic insufficiency, complete heart block, various high output states). In contrast, conditions associated with diminished aortic compliance are not often clinically evident but are suspected on the basis of the resultant systolic hypertension and wide pulse pressure. The effects of altered compliance can be readily appreciated from the physical definition of the term:

Vascular compliance (or volume distensibility) =

$$\frac{\text{Increase in volume } (\Delta V)}{\text{Increase in pressure } (\Delta P)}$$

Translated into clinical terms,

$$\text{Aortic compliance} = \frac{\text{Stroke volume}}{\text{Pulse pressure}}$$

from which follow:

(a) Stroke volume =
Pulse pressure × Aortic compliance

(b) Pulse pressure = $\dfrac{\text{Stroke volume}}{\text{Aortic compliance}}$

If compliance were constant, stroke volume could be deduced from pulse pressure, and cardiac output could then be calculated by multiplying pulse pressure by heart rate. Unfortunately, variables are too great for useful interpretations of the formula.

It is readily seen that decrease in compliance will result in wider pulse pressure per each milliliter of blood ejected. Compliance decreases slightly as arterial pressure increases or with sympathetic stimulation; it is markedly reduced by loss or fragmentation of aortic elastic and muscular tissue, as occurs with age or extensive atheromatous involvement with secondary medial fibrosis or intimal calcification. Reduction of aortic distensibility per se leads to a slight decline in diastolic and a marked rise in systolic pressures (isolated systolic hypertension). Diastolic hypertension cannot therefore be ascribed to reduced aortic compliance alone. The wide pulse pressure found in many subjects with diastolic hypertension poses a special problem. In experimental models, with aortic distensibility held constant, increasing peripheral resistance will be associated with declining pulse pressure. Inordinate rise of systolic pressure in patients with diastolic hypertension therefore reflects either a large stroke volume or, more frequently, a secondary loss of large vessel distensibility.

EFFECT OF AGE AND ENVIRONMENTAL FACTORS ON ARTERIAL BLOOD PRESSURE

Definition of a "normal" arterial blood pressure is so closely linked to the concept of hypertension that it is better to discuss it later in that section. For now, it is sufficient to point out the often wide variations in both systolic and diastolic pressures encountered from moment to moment in the same subject. Most are related to such obvious causes as body movement, position, pain, emotional stress, and the like. Under ordinary conditions, blood pressure measured even after a few minutes' rest in the doctor's office (casual pressure) is markedly higher than that recorded under basal conditions. Smirk defined "basal pressure" as the one recorded in the morning 10 to 12 hours postprandially; after an additional half hour rest in a warm room, repeated recordings are obtained over 30 to 45 minutes to the lowest attainable levels in a monotonous, silent environment. Home blood pressures recorded by the patient himself or by a lay relative often approximate basal levels. The difference (casual minus basal) is called "supplemental pressure." Although the basal pressure might statistically be more closely related to the clinical consequences of hypertension, it has found little clinical acceptance. Most epidemiologic and clinical experience has been derived from studies of casual pressure.

Age, Sex, and Body Build. Until adulthood is reached, the age factor may make a remarkable difference (Fig. 7–3); subsequent changes with age vary in different populations and from subject to subject. In some, pressure does not rise with age; in others, the rate of rise is quite marked. Studies in Wales suggest that the rate of rise, in Western populations at least, correlates with the initial level of blood pressure. Young men tend to have higher pressures than young women, but between ages 35 and 45 the curves for systolic pressure cross, and women's pressures subsequently rise more steeply with age than men's. There is no evidence that menopause is associated with a unique hypertension. Obese subjects tend to have higher blood pressure that cannot be accounted for by a systematic error due to increased arm circumference.

Posture and Exercise. With standing, pulse pressure narrows as the systolic drops slightly and the diastolic rises by about 5 mm Hg, so that mean arterial pressure does not vary by more than ±5 to 10 mm Hg. Changes in arterial pressure with dynamic exercise (cycling, walking) are proportional to the severity of exercise; this pressure may reach 200/100 when exercise becomes strenuous. Static exercise (e.g., sustained contraction of forearm muscles) is associated with an abrupt

reflex rise in pressure proportional to the muscular tension developed.

Variations With Daily Activities. The extent of these variations as recorded by automatic recorders is quite impressive, averaging in one study 24 mm Hg (range 15 to 40) for systolic and 14 mm Hg (5 to 20) for diastolic in normotensive subjects. Arterial pressure falls profoundly during sleep but is most unstable in REM (rapid eye movement) sleep. Relation of pressure variations to nocturnal cardiovascular accidents is still conjectural.

SOME ASPECTS OF ARTERIAL PRESSURE REGULATION

Arterial blood pressure is only one aspect in a highly integrated cardiovascular control system. Accordingly, to understand its disturbances one should consider the cardiovascular system as a whole, including not only cardiac performance and peripheral resistance but also the indirect effect of capacitance vessels on blood flow and the ways in which hemodynamic functions can be modified by sympathetic neural activity and hormonal factors. Control of circulatory pressure must be closely associated with control of the volume distending the circulation, and arterial pressure reflects, in part, this relationship between container (blood vessels) and content (blood volume). Hence, the mechanisms regulating the size and distribution

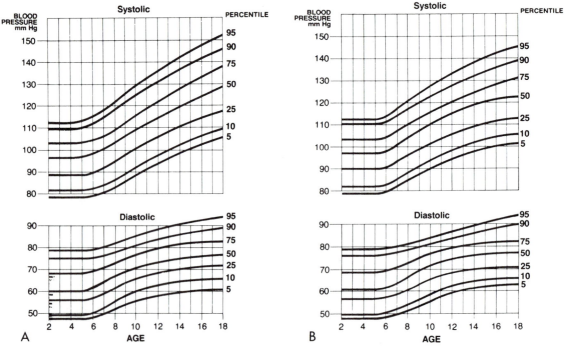

Figure 7–3 *A,* Percentiles of blood pressure measurement in boys (right arm, seated). *B,* Percentiles of blood pressure measurements in girls (right arm, seated). (Reprinted with permission from Report of the Task Force on Blood Pressure Control in Children. Pediatrics 59:803, 1977.)

of extracellular fluids must be considered along with factors controlling hemodynamic functions. The reader is referred to the 1983 references for Tarazi.

HEMODYNAMIC ASPECTS

Physical bases of mean arterial and pulse pressure have already been discussed. Arterial pressure can be regulated by variations of either cardiac output or peripheral resistance or both.

Interrelationship Between Output and Resistance. In acute studies, cardiac response to changes in peripheral resistance is to increase output for a decrease in peripheral resistance and to decrease output for an increase in resistance. Thus, any effect on pressure is at least attenuated. This relationship underlines the importance of peripheral factors in determining cardiac output (given normal myocardial contractility) by controlling the flow of blood from arteries to veins. Conversely, primary changes in output lead to reciprocal changes in peripheral resistance, tending to maintain pressure constant. This relationship is probably mediated principally through baroreceptor reflexes (see later discussion).

Chronic changes in blood flow unrelated to local needs of tissues have been associated with a different type of long-term readjustment. In such cases, a persistent inappropriate increase of cardiac output is thought to induce a progressive constriction of local vessels over a period of days or months until finally blood flow through the tissues returns to near normal. Return of output to normal is associated with increased peripheral resistance (Fig. 7–4). This sequence of events has been termed "total body autoregulation"; the term is an extrapolation to the whole organism from a phenomenon first described in local isolated circulation. Local regulation of blood flow to the needs of the tissues depends on (1) concentration of local metabolites, and (2) myogenic response of vessel wall to stretch (Bayliss mechanism).

The total circulation is affected by these local tissue factors but also by multifaceted neural, humoral, and structural influences. Whether extrapolation of the term "autoregulation" to that situation is justified has been hotly debated (see also Chapter 7). Obviously, the term means different things to different investigators; for some, development of collateral vessels is a phenomenon of long-term flow regulation. Whatever its exact mechanism, the concept supposes that regulation of flow to the needs of the tissues has been disassociated from and has superseded pressure regulation. As regards regional circulations (renal, cerebral, etc.), maintenance of blood flow despite pressure variations (within limits) has been well established. For the systemic circulation as a whole, the term "autoregulation" has been invoked to both describe and explain the transition of a

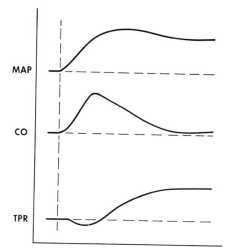

Figure 7–4 Diagrammatic illustration of the results of a sustained increase in cardiac output (CO) unrelated to peripheral demands; as output rises, mean arterial pressure (MAP) increases while total peripheral resistance (TPR) remains unchanged or even decreases slightly. Within a few weeks, however, TPR increases and cardiac output returns toward normal; MAP remains elevated because of the persistent increase in resistance.

"high flow–normal or low resistance" pattern to a "normal flow–high resistance" situation.

This concept is particularly important in relation to current theories regarding hypertension. The transition from high output to high resistance has been described in many experimental hypertensions; the present debate centers on whether it is an obligatory step in the initiation and evolution of most forms of hypertension. In many situations, in both humans and animals, it has been shown that a high output hypertension can persist for a long time without apparent secondary rise of TPR. More important, prevention of the initial rise in cardiac output did not in many instances prevent the development of increased resistance and hypertension. Thus, even when present, the evolution from a high output to a high resistance state may not necessarily mean "autoregulation"; it may depend on many factors including neural or humoral mechanisms as well as the effects of structural changes on resistance vessels and cardiac performance.

Blood Vessels and Arterial Blood Pressure. All systemic vessels—arteries, veins, and capillaries—participate in their own way in arterial blood pressure regulation. The following classification of blood vessels is based on the functional characteristics of each segment (Folkow and Neil, 1971):

1. "Windkessel" vessels (aorta and its large branches) damp the pulsatile output from the left ventricle and help steady the blood flow to the periphery; their main effect is on pulse pressure.

2. Resistance vessels (small arteries and arterioles) furnish most of total resistance to flow and regulate the distribution of cardiac output.

Their high intrinsic (myogenic) tone is continuously modified by physical, chemical, and neural influences. As flow is proportional to the fourth power of the radius, seemingly minor changes in diameter may exert a powerful influence on blood pressure (Poiseuille's law).

3. Exchange vessels (capillaries) are guarded by precapillary sphincters and postcapillary resistance vessels (venules and small veins). Diffusion, filtration, and reabsorption occur through the capillary walls, but the capillaries themselves have no active influence on this exchange. The net fluid transfer between plasma and interstitial fluid, given normal plasma oncotic pressure, depends on the ratio of precapillary to postcapillary resistance, which is controlled by sphincters and resistance vessels at either end of the capillaries. Changes in this ratio affect primarily blood volume and indirectly arterial pressure. A fall in pressure at the arteriolar end will favor intravascular shift of fluid and thus help to some degree in restoring arterial pressure. Conversely, venoconstriction will favor capillary filtration and reduction of plasma volume.

4. Capacitance vessels (veins) add little to peripheral resistance but accommodate the larger portion of blood volume and thus play an important role in circulatory regulation. They are well supplied by sympathetic nerves and may react differently from resistance vessels to nervous and humoral stimuli. To ascribe a role to veins in regulation of arterial pressure may seem paradoxical, but cardiac output depends on venous return. Venoconstriction resulting from sympathetic stimulation will not significantly alter peripheral resistance but will lead to decreased venous capacity. This will enhance a translocation of blood out of systemic veins into the cardiopulmonary area, raise cardiac output, and thus help prevent or correct falls in arterial pressure due to blood loss or excessive peripheral pooling.

INTRAVASCULAR VOLUME AND ARTERIAL PRESSURE

The vascular circuit just described is obviously not a homogeneous system; each of its subdivisions has its own pressure/volume characteristics. The arterial segment has limited distensibility and is maintained at high pressure and low volume; it is thought to contain about 20 per cent of the total blood volume. Although the capillary bed is of considerable length, it contains only 5 per cent of the total blood volume. Capillary pressure is determined by the balance of constriction between precapillary arterioles and postcapillary venules. The venous side of the circulation is a low-pressure, highly distensible compartment that contains about 75 per cent of the intravascular volume.

Both the arterial and venous compartments are importantly affected by sympathetic vasomotor outflow, but, characteristically, these effects are different. Neural influences alter arterial capacity and volume only slightly, but small changes in that segment will affect arterial pressure directly. In contrast, sympathetic vasomotor activity plays a large role in determining venous capacity, but the contribution of veins to total peripheral resistance is small. More important is their control of venous return and influence on cardiac output. In that respect and within certain limits, the distribution of intravascular volume may be more important than its magnitude; thus, it is possible to have, on the one hand, a large blood volume, venous pooling, low central blood volume, and low cardiac output or, on the other, a small blood volume, diminished venous capacity, a disproportionately high central blood volume, and a normal or even increased cardiac output.

The potential of vascular adaptability is such that changes in blood volume are not normally reflected to any important degree in arterial pressure variations unless the change is acute or excessive (hemorrhage). Conditions marked by hypervolemia (polycythemia vera) are not necessarily associated with hypertension. This efficacy of adaptation implies that important disturbances in regulation may lead to only subtle changes in pressure/volume relationships. However, arterial pressure becomes quite sensitive to blood volume changes when neural reflexes are interfered with. A small blood loss that would normally be well tolerated may lead to profound hypotension if suffered by a patient treated with neural blocking agents. Conversely, fluid retention and plasma volume expansion will nullify an initial good response to hypotensive agents that interfere with neural regulatory mechanisms, whether centrally (e.g., clonidine, methyldopa), peripherally (reserpine, guanethidine), or by alpha-adrenergic blockade (prazosin).

Factors regulating blood volume are beyond the scope of this discussion; they include renal excretory mechanisms, balance between interstitial and intravascular components of extracellular fluid volume, and neurohumoral control mechanisms (see appropriate sections).

PRINCIPLES OF VASCULAR CONTROL

The inherent myogenic activity of vessel walls is responsible for a *basal vascular tone* that is locally regulated by the vasodilator action of tissue metabolites. Superimposed on this, neurogenic mechanisms exert a "remote" control to adjust the circulation to the requirements of the body as a whole. Various circulating hormones add their excitatory or inhibitory influences.

Vascular innervation is not restricted to arteries; all vessels except capillaries are innervated.

Arterioles are supplied by two sets of nerves—sympathetic vasoconstrictors (alpha-adrenergic) and other vasodilator fibers. Sympathetic nerve fibers reach the vessels either from plexuses along their walls or through somatic nerve trunks. This distribution is important, for stripping the greater vessels of their nerve supply will not affect the smaller vessels. The more important neural influence on the arterial side is vasoconstriction; similarly, the overriding effect of sympathetic stimulation on veins is alpha-adrenergic vasoconstriction. Thus, the main effects of sympathetic stimulation are increases in resistance and enhancement of venous return.

Vasodilator fibers are less widespread and not tonically active. Beta-adrenergic receptors are found in arteries and probably in veins; their functional importance is debated. Cholinergic sympathetic vasodilator nerves supply only the larger resistance vessels of skeletal muscle and are activated mainly when the animal is alerted (defense reaction); as most other regions are vasoconstricted, the muscles may thus be provided with near maximum blood supply. Parasympathetic vasodilator nerves supply some specialized tissues such as salivary glands and external genitalia.

Hormonal influences include circulating epinephrine (from adrenal medulla), which stimulates both alpha- and beta-receptors, so that it usually causes a redistribution of blood flow; myocardium, muscle, and liver receive more blood at the expense of other circuits (kidney, skin, gastrointestinal tract) that are vasoconstricted. Angiotensin is discussed later. Many other "vasoactive agents" are known (prostaglandins, histamine, serotonin, vasopressin); specialized reviews should be consulted for details of their effects. Particular note, however, should be made of prostaglandins, a ubiquitous series of compounds synthesized in a variety of tissues from essential unsaturated fatty acids, predominantly arachidonic acid. The work of some investigators has led to growing awareness of the importance of these acids as local hormones, meaning that they are involved principally in the modulation of regional circulation in the tissues in which they are formed.

The "prostaglandin system" has proved particularly important in helping achieve the delicate balance needed between vasoconstrictor and vasodilator factors. Intensive work by Vane, Oates, McGiff and others has led to more precise definition of the products of arachidonic acid metabolism. Release of this 20-carbon unsaturated fatty acid is the first step in the synthesis of prostaglandins and thromboxanes; this release can be stimulated by kinins and angiotensins. Conversely, the prostaglandins produced from arachidonic acid can inhibit or augment the action of these vasoactive hormones. This represents one of the many delicate balances between vasoconstrictor and vasodilator agents that can modulate blood flow according to tissue needs.

After arachidonic acid is released from tissue stores, it is transformed into cyclic endoperoxides by a cyclo-oxygenase present in most cells; these endoperoxides are acted upon by different enzymes to form either prostaglandins or thromboxanes. The final products formed vary with the type of tissue, the physiologic state, and the presence of injury or disease (McGiff, 1979). Thromboxane A_2 is a vasoconstrictive agent that stimulates platelet aggregation, whereas prostacyclin (PGI_2) is a vasodilator that inhibits platelet aggregation; here is obviously another mechanism by which blood flow and patency of vessels can be modulated. Thromboxanes are produced mostly by platelets, although they can also be produced in vessel walls; the major source of circulating prostacyclins is the lung, but prostacyclin can also be synthesized in vascular walls. The capacity for prostacyclin synthesis varies greatly among vessels and is markedly influenced by age and hormonal background. Anti-inflammatory agents such as indomethacin and aspirin can inhibit the synthesis of prostaglandin and thromboxanes, thus interfering to various degrees according to the agent and dose used with platelet aggregation, vasoconstriction, or vasodilation (Fig. 7–5).

As regards blood pressure regulation, the development of hypertension may reflect stimulation of vasopressor mechanisms, but it may also be due to failure of a vasodilator system such as prostaglandins. This balance between the renin-angiotensin system, adrenergic influences, and local prostacyclin production has been particularly studied in the kidney. Prevention of prostaglandin synthesis with indomethacin intensifies and prolongs the renal vasoconstrictive effects of angiotensin II (Fig. 7–6).

Finally, it is important to remember, especially in the context of blood pressure regulation, that salt-water equilibrium profoundly affects the activity and responsiveness of smooth muscles. Changes in sodium gradient across cell membrane may enhance constriction (if intracellular sodium is increased) or relaxation (if sodium is depleted). The effects of intracellular sodium (Na_i) on vascular smooth muscle have been variously attributed to alterations in depolarization of the cell membrane, increase in intracellular calcium, and even enhanced protein synthesis and early vascular hypertrophy. Increase in intracellular calcium can be linked to increased Na_i through different types of Na-Ca exchange mechanisms; the net result would be enhancement of both vascular smooth muscle tone and cardiac performance. The hypertension associated with volume-expanded states has been tentatively attributed to increase in a "natriuretic factor" induced by volume expansion, the net result of which would be to depress the Na/K pump and increase intracellular calcium concentration. Much remains to be explored in this field. The role of other ions, such as potassium and magnesium, has been studied extensively in vitro and in vivo. In actual practice, however, the situ-

[Eicosatrienoic acid] Arachidonic acid [Eicosapentaenoic acid]

$$\downarrow$$

Cyclic endoperoxides $(PGG_2 \rightarrow PGH_2)$

Prostacyclin $(PGI_2)^*$	Prostaglandin E_2	Thromboxane A_2^{**}
$\downarrow$		$\downarrow$
6-keto $PGF_{1\alpha}$	Prostaglandin $F_{2\alpha}$	Thromboxane B_2

Predominant effect	*Inhibit platelet aggregation *Vasodilatation	E_2: vasodilatation $F_{2\alpha}$: venoconstriction	**Accelerates platelet aggregation **Vasoconstriction

Figure 7–5 Simplified scheme of prostaglandin synthesis and actions. The hydrolysis products 6-keto $PGF_{1\alpha}$ and thromboxane B_2 have little biologic activity. Eicosatrienoic acid and eicosapentaenoic acid give rise to products having one and three double bonds, respectively. Interestingly, the number of double bonds in the side chains usually does not fundamentally alter the biologic properties of prostaglandins, but thromboxanes A_1 and A_3 have been reported to be unable to induce platelet aggregation. (Modified with permission from McGiff, J. C.: Prostaglandins in circulatory disorders. *Triangle* 18:101, 1979.)

ation is more complex than can be discerned through controlled experiments. Salt and water equilibrium involves changes in volume (intra- and extravascular) as well as in ion gradients. Changes in serum electrolytes usually involve more than one; Haddy has pointed out the synergistic effect of some common combinations. Thus,

a reduction in serum potassium would enhance the effect of a simultaneous rise in serum calcium to increase myocardial contractility and induce vasoconstriction. A practical example is the frequent production of this particular combination by hemodialysis; its effect on arterial pressure is counterbalanced by the simultaneous loss of fluid

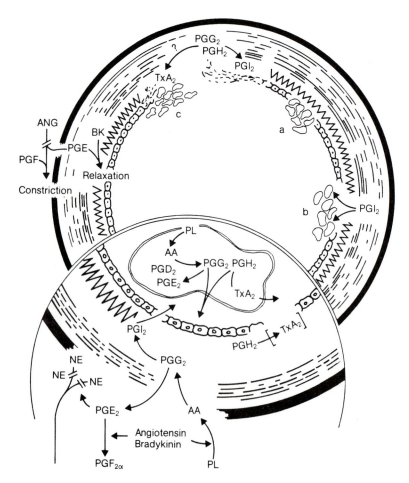

Figure 7–6 Schema of the cross section of a blood vessel with enlargement of the vascular wall showing possible platelet–endothelial surface interactions. Thromboxane (TxA_2) generated by platelets is related to aggregation and subsequent deposition of platelets at the blood-endothelial interface (a), which can be prevented by prostacyclin (PGI_2) synthesized by the vascular wall (b). TxA_2 may be formed by diseased blood vessels (c). PGE_2, also formed by blood vessels, blunts the vasoconstrictor action of angiotensin (ANG) and augments the vasodilator action of bradykinin (BK), whereas $PGF_{2\alpha}$ may augment angiotensin-induced vasoconstriction. In the enlargement, arachidonic acid (AA) can be released from tissue stores—e.g., phospholipids (PL)—in response to either angiotensin or bradykinin, which can also accelerate enzymatic conversion of PGE_2 to $PGF_{2\alpha}$. PGE_2 but not $PGF_{2\alpha}$ can inhibit release of norepinephrine (NE) from nerve endings in the vascular wall. (Reprinted with permission from McGiff, J. C.: Prostaglandins in circulatory disorders. *Triangle* 18:101, 1979.)

and modulated by the humoral and neurogenic responses to hypovolemia. Thus, even in relatively simple situations, the control of arterial pressure remains a multifactorial process.

NEURAL REFLEXES AND "CENTRAL" REACTIONS

Neural circulatory reflexes act mainly to stabilize arterial pressure at the levels set for a particular subject. They help buffer the impact of stimuli by raising arterial pressure when it is lowered or decreasing it when it rises. When neural activity is impaired by drugs or disease, arterial pressure may fluctuate widely between hypertension in the supine position and hypotension with fainting on standing.

Like all neural reflexes, they involve an afferent and an efferent limb joined through a center (the vasomotor center). They are activated by sensory receptors in different parts of the circulation; the most important are located in the carotid sinus and aortic arch. These stretch receptors are sensitive to expansion or deformation of the arterial wall and respond more to a pulsatile than to an equivalent steady pressure (the term *baroreceptor* is inaccurate because they do not respond to pressure per se). Fibers from the carotid sinus travel cephalad in the glossopharyngeal nerve; those from the aortic arch employ the vagus. The carotid sinus reflex is normally the more powerful, possibly because it guards the blood supply to the central nervous system. But other sensitive vascular areas (e.g., the mesenteric) can also induce compensatory blood pressure responses in anesthetized animals with cut sinus nerves and vagi (Heymans).

The stretch receptors are activated when arterial pressure rises and the consequent impulses inhibit the tonic activity of the vasomotor center. This latter term is applied to a group of neurons located in the upper medulla and lower pons that normally maintain a slow rate of firing to essentially all sympathetic vasoconstrictor fibers. Baroreceptor impulses normally exert an inhibitory influence on the center; when blood pressure tends to fall, their activity is reduced, and the vasomotor center is thus liberated. The consequent increase in sympathetic discharge helps restore pressure to normal. The vasomotor center influences the heart as well as the peripheral vessels, so that increase or reduction of cardiac activity (chronotropic and inotropic) parallels the increase or decrease in vasoconstrictor impulses. Efferent impulses travel along the two components of the autonomic system—sympathetic and parasympathetic. Of these, the sympathetic is of greater importance because of its wider distribution to the peripheral vasculature and in the heart, going to both atria and both ventricles. Vagal fibers supply mainly the sinoatrial and atrioventricular nodes and the atria; there is evidence, however, of some parasympathetic influence on ventricular function as well.

These reflexes play a major role in circulatory adjustments to postural changes (see discussion of hypotension). Both sides of the reflex are demonstrated in responses to the Valsalva maneuver (a sustained increase in intrathoracic pressure obtained by blowing against some resistance for 20 to 30 seconds). During the period of straining, venous return is sharply curtailed and cardiac output decreased, so that systolic pressure falls. Resultant reflex sympathetic stimulation increases heart rate and limits fall in diastolic pressure. When straining is suddenly stopped, blood rushes into the thorax and the resurgent cardiac output is thrust into an arterial system whose outflow resistance has been increased. This results in a brief overshoot of arterial pressure; the opposite reflex readjustment then leads to bradycardia and a decline of pressure to prestrain levels.

These sequential variations with the Valsalva maneuvers usually are classified into four phases (Fig. 7–7): Phase 1 is a brief rise in pressure with onset of straining; phase 2 is the reduction in pulse pressure and increase in heart rate; phase 3 is a further drop in pressure as straining is suddenly stopped and the resultant increased pulmonary vascular capacity momentarily reduces return to the left ventricle further; phase 4 refers to the overshoot in arterial pressure and reflex bradycardia. These responses, however, depend not only on the integrity of neural reflexes but also on the degree of volemia and on cardiac compensation. In heart failure, blood pressure actually rises during straining, and phase 4 is abolished ("square-wave" response).

The effectiveness of this system in controlling excessive pressure fluctuations immediately raises the question of its inability to prevent hypertension. This failure is related to the fact that the receptors eventually adapt to whatever pressure level they are exposed to if this pressure is maintained long enough (Fig. 7–8). This resetting of baroreceptors not only prevents the reflex from functioning as a long-term control system but also may act in reverse, increasing the difficulties of initiating antihypertensive therapy.

Apart from reflexes originating in the "high-pressure" circuit, there are also thoracic sensory endings beginning in the "low-pressure" segment, the fibers from which are vagal in location. They respond to shifts in blood volume or rather to distention in vessel walls related to such shifts. Some experiments suggest that vagal fibers originating in the cardiopulmonary region exert, like the carotid and aortic baroreceptors, a tonic inhibition of the vasomotor center. Further, vagal afferents from the cardiopulmonary region also play an important role in blood volume regulation. Stimulation of cardiac receptors, especially in the left atrium, leads to increased excretion of water

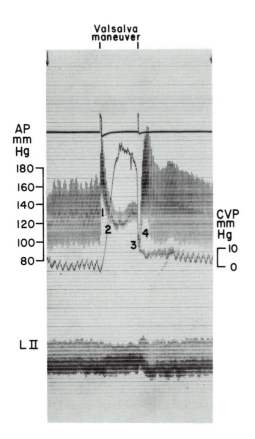

Figure 7–7 Response to a Valsalva maneuver performed for 20 seconds. From above downward are shown (a) signal indicating beginning and end of straining; (b) arterial pressure (AP) showing four phases: *1,* initial rise with onset of straining; *2,* the fall in pulse pressure as venous return is temporarily diminished; *3,* a further fall in pressure with the first deep breaths on cessation of strain; and *4,* the pressure overshoot as an increased left ventricular output is now thrown in a constricted vascular bed; (c) central venous pressure (CVP) tracing showing the marked increase during straining; (d) electrocardiogram (lead II), which shows the slowing in heart rate with phase 4 after its increase during phase 2.

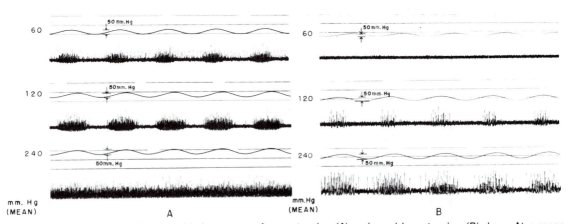

Figure 7–8 Neurogram from carotid sinus nerve of normotensive *(A)* and renal hypertensive *(B)* dogs. At a mean arterial pressure of 60 mm Hg, nerve activity was clearly present in the normotensive dog but absent in the hypertensive animal. At 240 mm Hg MAP, firing was continuous in *A* but still intermittent in *B*, suggesting that the normal range of baroreceptor response had been shifted upward in the hypertensive animal. (After McCubbin, J., et al.: Baroreceptor function in chronic renal hypertension. Circ. Res. *4*:205, 1965, by permission of The American Heart Association, Inc.)

and sodium related in various degrees to renal vasodilatation as well as to reduction of ADH, inhibition of renin release, and possibly stimulation of a blood-borne diuretic agent. Translated into clinical terms, left atrial and pulmonary congestion should lead to reduction of plasma volume; conversely, a drop in cardiopulmonary volume leads to vasoconstriction and to retention of water and salt.

Reflexes mediated through vagal afferents are *usually* depressor. In contrast, reflexes carried from the heart and large vessels through sympathetic afferents are usually pressor. These sympathetic cardiac afferents can lead to reflex increases in myocardial contractility, heart rate, and peripheral resistance. They may be important in some types of paroxysmal hypertension.

Of less importance for arterial pressure control are chemoreceptor reflexes. They are not very effective in the normal pressure range, but in hypertensive states diminished arterial oxygen concentration excites the carotid and aortic bodies, thus reflexly elevating arterial pressure.

It is evident that there are many inputs to the central nervous system. Reflexes of opposing nature may be evoked simultaneously. Reflexes from somatic afferents during isometric exercise may override the carotid baroceptor reflexes and lead to tachycardia despite the increase in arterial pressure. However, the reflex vasoconstrictor response to that type of exercise is enhanced by reducing the input from cardiopulmonary (low pressure) receptors. Review of the 1976 report by Mancia and coworkers suggests that the carotid sinus reflex dominates when the carotid sinus, cardiopulmonary, and carotid chemoreflexes interact. The cardiopulmonary receptors appear to become more effective in pressure regulation only when input from the carotid baroreceptors is decreased or when chemoreceptors are activated. The net effect of these many reflexes depends on central integration of this information; moreover, the activity of the higher centers themselves can modulate this interaction of reflexes. Sjostrand has shown that the balance between vasodilator and vasoconstrictive reflexes induced by standing up or by volume depletion could be tipped toward hypotension under the influence of emotional stimuli or anesthesia.

"Central Reactions." In contrast to the feedback system of baroreceptor reflex, these reactions do not serve to control arterial pressure. The circulatory response to hypothalamic stimulation is a marked blood pressure rise with profound inotropic and chronotropic excitation of the heart. It represents a full mobilization of the organism for fight or flight. It is mentioned here because its frequent repetition or its possible evolution into a conditioned reflex, has been proposed as a possible cause for hypertension. Conversely, the "playing dead" reaction (profound bradycardia, hypotension, and fainting occurring in some animals when cornered) may be analogous in some cases of emotional fainting in patients. In these conditions, the muscle cholinergic vasodilator system is markedly activated.

THE KIDNEY AND BLOOD PRESSURE REGULATION

There are two aspects of the close relationship existing between systemic arterial pressure levels and renal function. The first relates to the excretory function of the kidney; diminished excretion of salt and water in the face of maintained intake leads to hypervolemia and hypertension to achieve greater filtration and a new equilibrium between intake and output.

The second mechanism is related to a more "active" process, a renal pressor system capable of raising pressure directly when activated. Although these two mechanisms are often associated, they can also be dissociated in both clinical and experimental situations. This is discussed at greater length under Mechanisms in Hypertension; at this point only the *renal pressor system* will be described.

The importance of this system with regard to hypertension is that its end product, angiotensin II, is the most potent pressor substance known and also a stimulator of aldosterone. The system itself is really two enzyme systems in series (Fig. 7–9). In the first section, a proteolytic enzyme of renal origin called *renin* reacts with a circulating alpha-2-globulin (renin substrate or angiotensinogen) to release to decapeptide angiotensin I. This serves as substrate for converting enzyme that, by releasing two amino acids, produces the octapeptide, angiotensin II; the converting enzyme is present in plasma and tissues, and there is evidence to suggest that in some species the major conversion of angiotensin I to II occurs in the lung. Angiotensin II is inactivated by plasma and tissue angiotensinases. Renin not only is active in circulating blood but is also stored in arterial walls; the importance of this local storage and possible later activation has not yet been determined. Still under investigation too is a phospholipid renin inhibitor system dependent on a renal phospholipase and a circulating phospholipid inhibitor.

Angiotensin I has no direct effect on arterial pressure, whereas only nanograms of angiotensin II can produce substantial elevations. Information currently available suggests that the plasma concentration of angiotensin II is usually less than 100 pg per ml. Because of difficulties in measuring circulating angiotensin, current information concerning the renal pressor system comes from studies of plasma renin activity (PRA); it should be emphasized that the methods widely used provide an estimate of the activity of renin but do not measure it directly.

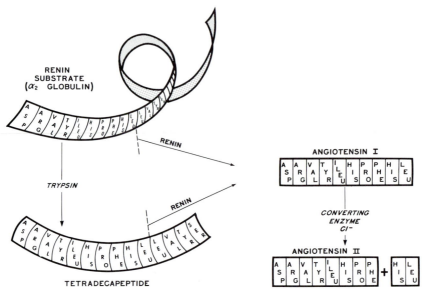

Figure 7–9 Renin-angiotensin system . The normal amino acid sequence of angiotensin II is essential to its biologic action; recently, analogs obtained by substitution of some amino acids have been shown to block, through competitive inhibition, various effects of the octapeptide. They are therefore very useful tools for investigation (? treatment) of some types of hypertension. (After F. M. Bumpus. *In* Page, I. H., and McCubbin, J.: Renal Hypertension. Chicago, Year Book Medical Publishers, 1969.)

Source of Renin—The Juxtaglomerular Apparatus.

Renin comes from the kidney—hence the term "renal pressor system." It is formed and stored in the juxtaglomerular (JG) apparatus, or complex, at the vascular pole of the glomerulus. At this point, the macula densa portion of the distal tubule is in close proximity to the afferent and efferent arterioles. The JG complex is composed of granular cells in the afferent arterioles, the macula densa and the polkissen, a group of cells in the triangle formed by the afferent and efferent arteriole and the distal tubule. The complex is richly innervated by sympathetic nerve fibers.

Renin seems to be primarily located in the granular cells of the afferent arteriole; experimentally, there is a close relationship between the granularity of these cells and their renal renin content. The role of the macula densa in renin production has not yet been exactly defined. However, its cells are in close contact with JG cells and their cytologic characteristics are distinct from those of other cells in the distal tubule, suggesting a difference in function at this site. The strategic location of the JG apparatus between an arteriole and a tubule seems particularly suited to a system apparently related to both arterial pressure and sodium excretion.

It was first assumed that the factor stimulating *renin release* was renal ischemia, but this was later disproved, since release could be stimulated by alterations in sodium balance that do not produce ischemia and by reductions in perfusion pressure too small to decrease renal blood flow signif-

icantly. Two concepts regarding the mechanism of renin release were then developed, the intrarenal baroreceptor hypothesis and the macula densa theory. According to the first, the renal afferent arterioles and JG cells respond to changes in stretch that could be secondary to changes in intravascular volume or in arterial pressure. For others, the macula densa is a primary sensing element responding to changes in the sodium load reaching it. Neither theory can explain all experimental observations, and it seems possible that both types of receptor exist and that they influence each other. In addition to these intrarenal mechanisms, sympathetic nerves and circulating humoral agents may play important modifying roles.

A common denominator for the many stimuli that affect renin release is "effective blood volume"; this term is a conceptual expression of the degree of filling of the vascular system. It is of course related to the actual total blood volume but not dependent on it alone. It is influenced as well by the distribution of that volume as well as by the tone of the vessels that contain it; its apparent correlates in clinical situations also include the level of serum sodium. Rapid reduction of intravascular volume increases PRA, as does the complex chronic effect of low-sodium diets or diuretic treatment. Conversely, plasma volume expansion turns off the stimulus for renin release and reduces PRA. So predictable are these responses that dietary sodium restriction and intravenous sodium chloride infusion are used as standard tests of the renal pressor system. These maneuvers alter blood volume (and extracellular fluid volume) and sodium balance; under normal conditions both stimuli act in the same direction on renin release. Under experimental conditions the two stimuli can be dissociated, and it would seem that changes in intravascular volume predominate over changes in serum sodium in determining PRA. That is not to say that serum sodium plays no role in influencing renin release. On the contrary, this has been clearly shown in animal experiments utilizing renal perfusion techniques with which it is possible to vary sodium concentration of the perfusate without varying that of the whole body. In these studies, hyponatremia increased renin release and hypernatremia diminished it. It has been suggested that diuretic drugs increase PRA not only because they decrease plasma volume but also because they diminish sodium transport by macula densa cells. In this connection, changes in serum potassium must be taken into account in the interpretation of renin data. Hypokalemia may stimulate and hyperkalemia may inhibit PRA, independent of associated alterations in either aldosterone secretion or sodium balance.

Although it is not essential to renin release, the sympathetic nervous system may alter it directly or indirectly. The role of arterial baroreceptors in the control of renin release is debatable; however, cardiopulmonary receptors appear to exert a tonic restraint on renin release by reflex inhibition of sympathetic outflow to the kidney. Conditions associated with rise in PRA are usually those associated with increased sympathetic activity (upright posture, hypovolemia). Both alpha- and beta-adrenergic blocking drugs have been shown to diminish PRA. In addition to manipulations of sodium intake, upright posture is frequently used as a clinical test of renin release. Patients with idiopathic orthostatic hypotension sometimes fail to show the expected increase of PRA with standing.

Pressor Effects of the Renin-Angiotensin System. Although angiotensin II is the most powerful vasoconstrictor agent, its direct effect on resistance vessels might not be its most important contribution to arterial pressure regulation except in special cases. Possibly of greater significance for circulatory control are its effects on aldosterone secretion and sympathetic functions.

Infusions of even small subpressor doses of angiotensin lead to a marked increase in aldosterone secretion. The resultant fluid retention and increase in sodium stores set the stage for blood pressure elevation, water retention by increasing extracellular fluid volume, and sodium retention by increasing vascular responsiveness to vasoconstrictor agents.

Angiotensin has major effects on sympathetic nervous activity. It enhances activity through a direct stimulatory action on the vasomotor center; the area postrema is one place in which blood-brain barrier against angiotensin breaks down. Peripherally, it enhances sympathetic nerve effects by diminishing neuronal norepinephrine uptake, thus allowing a greater concentration of the neurohormone to reach vascular receptor sites. Angiotensin is also a potent stimulus for catecholamine release from the adrenal medulla. Thus, it is obvious that no matter how potent a vasoconstrictor angiotensin may be in its own right, it has the potential to affect arterial pressure in many other ways. Its effects on nerve function suggest that angiotensin may eventually prove to be an important modulator of neural activity.

Renal Pressor System and Hypertension. It is obvious by now that "renin" has emerged as a very complex system as regards both its control mechanisms and the extent of its effects. Assessment of its participation in hypertension is therefore *not* easy. It has been attempted along two lines, both of which are applicable to humans; their value and limitations for investigation, diagnosis, and therapy must therefore be clearly outlined. The first consists of determination of plasma renin activity (PRA) or, less frequently, of one or the other of its components (renin concentration or angiotensin II). Valuable as they are, estimates of peripheral plasma renin activity (PRA) cannot be expected to define all disturbances of this system. A normal PRA does not rule out the possibility of important minor variations in circulating angiotensin II. Conversely, an elevated PRA can be found in normotensive states such as hepatic cirrhosis or the nephrotic syndrome, showing that there is more to any hypertension than the renal pressure system. The number of factors affecting renin release make it clear that reported levels of renin activity cannot, therefore, be interpreted out of context. They can be evaluated correctly only in relation to clinical setting, posture of patient at the time of sampling, level of arterial pressure, sodium balance (24-hour urinary sodium), serum electrolytes, and some estimate of intravascular volume.

The second approach is to determine the effect on arterial pressure of interference at different points with the renin-angiotensin cascade (Table 7–1).

Thus, beta-adrenergic blockers have been used to reduce renin release; inhibitors of the converting enzyme diminish or prevent the formation of angiotensin II while angiotensin antagonists compete with it for binding to end-organ receptors. This approach is useful in that it attempts to define more or less directly the functional importance of the renin system. However, each agent used has other actions besides its effect on "renin" and may elicit counteractions that cloud the picture. Beta blockade has important hemodynamic and possible central nervous system effects; converting enzyme inhibition leads to increased bradykinin levels because that same converting enzyme is responsible for bradykinin degradation. Angiotensin antagonists come closer to the goal but some have significant agonist effects and all do not interfere equally with all actions of angiotensin.

The renal pressor system has been implicated

TABLE 7–1 AGENTS INTERFERING WITH THE RENAL PRESSOR SYSTEM

Renin Cascade	Interference			
	Agent	Action	"Caveats"	
Angiotensinogen (1) Renin	(1) β-blockers	Interfere with renin release	Hemodynamic and CNS effects	
Angiotensin I (2) CE	(2) Converting enzyme (CE) inhibitors	Competitive antagonism of CE	Increased bradykinin	
Angiotensin II (3) end organs (3) Angiotensin III	(3) Angiotensin antagonists	Competitive inhibition	(a) Agonist effect (b) Unequal action on different receptors	
Inactive fragments				

in malignant hypertension, renovascular hypertension, and the hypertension induced by oral contraceptives. In most other hypertensions, there is no clear evidence of its participation. In primary aldosteronism, aldosterone alone is increased, whereas PRA is suppressed. Animal studies have suggested that excess renin may cause vascular injury; the lesions are those of arteriolar necrosis and might be related to changes seen in accelerated hypertension. There is no evidence to date that "renin" is related to the common atherosclerotic complications of hypertension.

Each type of hypertension is discussed separately, so we will refer here only to that related to the use of oral contraceptives. The estrogen component of these agents increases renin substrate, and although renin itself is not necessarily increased, more angiotensin is formed, and circulating angiotensin is usually increased. Hypertension, however, occurs only in a few of the women so treated; its exact nature has not yet been determined, nor has its relationship to possible genetic predisposition, association with sympathetic disturbance, or dependence on fluid retention. Clinical studies with blockers of the renal pressor system might give some of the answers needed. Practically, however, when treatment is discontinued, the components of the renal pressor system return to normal levels and the hypertension disappears.

HYPERTENSION*

Hypertension means elevated arterial pressure, either systolic or diastolic or both, as is often the case. In the past, diastolic elevation was con-

*See also Chapters 6 and 14.

sidered the hallmark of hypertension, whereas systolic blood pressure was thought to be more variable and its elevation inconsequential. More recent evidence has shown both assumptions to be false; diastolic pressure levels vary as much as the systolic, and systolic hypertension is associated with increased morbidity and mortality. The close relation between mean systolic pressure and myocardial oxygen requirements shows that systolic hypertension is not hemodynamically insignificant; it imposes a costly load on the heart and seems as closely related to cardiac hypertrophy as diastolic hypertension, if not more so. The basic mechanisms of systolic hypertension have been reviewed, and this discussion will deal with what is called "diastolic hypertension," although systolic pressure is elevated as well.

Hypertension by itself is not a diagnosis. It is the result of a number of diseases and disturbances — some serious and progressive, others transient — and it can be classified in many ways. The following is modified from Pickering:

1. By kind
   a. Systolic hypertension
   b. Diastolic hypertension
2. By degree
   a. Nonmalignant
   b. Malignant
3. By cause
   a. Primary or unexplained — essential hypertension
   b. Secondary hypertension

A list of causes is given in Table 7–2.

DEFINITION OF HYPERTENSION

To speak of elevated arterial pressure begs the question of what constitutes "normal" pressure

TABLE 7–2 AN ETIOLOGIC CLASSIFICATION OF HYPERTENSION

I. *Arterial Hypertension (elevation of systolic and diastolic blood pressures)*
 A. Essential hypertension
  1. Labile (intermittent)
  2. Established ("fixed")
 B. Renal hypertension
  1. Kidney disease
   a. Glomerulonephritis
   b. Chronic pyelonephritis
   c. Congenital polycystic kidneys
   d. Obstructive uropathy
   e. Diabetic glomerulosclerosis
   f. Interstitial nephritis due to analgesics, gout, hypercalcemia
   g. Connective tissue diseases, periarteritis nodosa, scleroderma, lupus erythematosus
   h. Renal tumor
   i. Renal amyloidosis
   j. Radiation nephritis
   k. Hereditary nephritis
  2. Renal arterial disease
   a. Fibrous dysplasias
   b. Atherosclerotic disease
   c. Embolic obstruction
   d. Traumatic arterial dissection or occlusion
  3. Compression of kidney
   a. Perinephritis
   b. Perirenal hematoma, usually posttraumatic
 C. Endocrine hypertension
  1. Catecholamine excess: pheochromocytoma
  2. "Steroid" hypertension
   a. Mineralocorticoid excess
    (1) Primary aldosteronism
    (2) Functional enzymatic block leading to adrenal hyperplasia (e.g., 11-hydroxylase deficiency in adrenogenital syndrome, 17-hydroxylase deficiency, androgen-induced hydroxylase deficiency in masculinizing tumors)
    (3) Iatrogenic: excess DOC or fluorinated steroid administration
   b. Glucocorticoid excess—various causes of Cushing syndrome (adrenal, pituitary, ectopic ACTH syndromes, ovarian tumors)
  3. Oral contraceptives
  4. Condition associated with hypertension
   a. Acromegaly
   b. Thyroid disorders
    (1) Myxedema
    (2) Thyrotoxicosis, usually a cause of systolic, not diastolic, hypertension
 D. Neurogenic hypertension
  1. Anxiety states (?)
  2. Intracranial disease
   a. Increased intracranial pressure
   b. Encephalitis
   c. Diencephalic syndrome
   d. Lead encephalopathy
  3. Disturbances in vasomotor center
   a. Bulbar poliomyelitis
   b. Disturbances in vascular supply
  4. Spinal cord and peripheral nerves
   a. Transection of the cord, transverse myelitis
   b. Polyneuritis
   c. Porphyria
 E. Hypertension of coarctation of the aorta
 F. Hypertension of toxemia of pregnancy
  1. Pre-eclampsia
  2. Eclampsia
II. *Systolic Hypertension*
 A. Caused mainly by an increased stroke output of the left ventricle
  1. Complete heart block
  2. Aortic regurgitation
  3. Patent ductus arteriosus
  4. Thyrotoxicosis
  5. Arteriovenous fistula
  6. Paget's disease of bone
 B. Caused mainly by a decreased distensibility of the aorta
  1. Arteriosclerosis of aorta
  2. Coarctation of aorta

levels. Mathematical limits can be defined by population surveys (means, standard deviations), but the absence of a demonstrable cause for deviation from the norm in the vast majority of cases has led to a re-examination of basic concepts regarding the nature of hypertension. Put simply, the question concerns whether there is a natural dividing line between normal and raised arterial pressure, or whether hypertension is a purely quantitative alteration of a biophysical measurement (pressure). In the first case, hypertension would be a specific disease leading to pressure elevation; in the second, it would be a simple quantitative deviation from normal with no specific point at which the disease can be said to begin.

The controversy is not yet completely settled. According to one school of thought (Platt et al.), hypertension is a specific disease entity. Two groups exist — those whose pressures do and those whose pressures do not increase with age — and the difference between them is determined by monogenic inheritance. Pickering and co-workers have argued very strongly that arterial pressure is a biophysical characteristic, like height, whose frequency distribution curves show no natural subdivision into separate groups and which is governed by a graded multifactorial or polygenic inheritance. Arguments are based on complicated statistical analysis of population surveys but also fundamentally, we think, on the persistent failure to uncover the "fault" that would explain essential hypertension.

A very important benefit of these discussions has been the attention drawn to the quantitative aspects of hypertension. Whatever its basic nature, there is no doubt about the importance of the actual level of pressure. Perhaps in no other disease does the quantitative deviation of a single variable so influence the course and complications of the disorder. Studies by life insurance companies have shown an impressive relationship between mortality and blood pressure levels extending over the whole range of arterial pressures, with no sudden break at any point. Aside from specific characteristics of diseases associated with hypertension, high blood pressure has consequences of its own. Many are closely related to the level of pressure itself and are prevented or reversed by adequate pressure control. These would include left ventricular failure, hypertensive encephalopathy, and the malignant phase. Fibrinoid necrosis can occur in any form of hypertension, with the possible exception of aortic coarctation, if the pressure is high enough. The relationship with pressure is less clear-cut for other complications; atherosclerotic complications are more frequent in hypertensive patients but may develop in normotensive subjects. In this case the duration of hypertension may be more important than its level. Nevertheless, most controlled clinical trials of antihypertensive therapy have shown that the incidence of strokes can be reduced by control of arterial pressure, and the study of the Hypertension Detection and Follow-up Program (HDFP) has shown that the incidence of myocardial infarction may also be decreased when blood pressure is controlled.

GENERAL PATHOPHYSIOLOGIC ASPECTS IN HYPERTENSION

The number of unrelated diseases associated with hypertension indicates that there must be a variety of factors that produce a chronic rise of blood pressure. These are called "pressor mechanisms." In a sense, this term is a misnomer because, with the exception of pheochromocytoma, the physiologic abnormalities associated with hypertension have not been shown to be causal. Although these abnormalities represent distinct aberrations of a number of cardiovascular control systems, the degrees to which they participate in arterial pressure elevation are not known. There is a real difference between recognizing the "cause" of a particular hypertension and describing its mechanism.

Hypertension is a disease of regulation; the mosaic theory proposed by Page in 1949 stressed the multifactorial response of the body to environmental influences. A disturbance of one factor will lead to automatic involvement of others, so that a whole new set of relationships may be established, often making it very difficult to decide which came first.

Some of these secondary alterations may be responsible for what might be termed *postcausal* hypertension, meaning persistence of hypertension even after removal of its primary cause. This can be shown experimentally in hypertension produced by renal arterial constriction. Removal of the ischemic kidney will reduce blood pressure only if performed within a certain time after the provoking maneuver; if nephrectomy is delayed, hypertension will not be relieved. A clinical counterpart of this situation might be surmised when removal of apparently primary causes (e.g., adrenocortical tumor, pheochromocytoma, renal arterial stenosis) fails to relieve the patient of his hypertension. It is, however, very difficult in humans to ascertain whether one is not dealing with the coexistence of two separate causes for the hypertensive disease (e.g., renal arterial stenosis in a patient with essential hypertension).

Of the possible factors helping perpetuate hypertension, the following three are of particular interest:

1. The vulnerability of the renal vessels to increased pressure loads, leading to development of arteriolar nephrosclerosis.

2. The structural adaptation of vessel walls to hypertension; the thickened wall amplifies the luminal reduction produced by even normal stimuli.

3. Resetting of baroreceptors: The fact that carotid sinus reflexes are active in hypertensive patients led to questioning why they did not prevent hypertension. McCubbin and coworkers showed in dogs with chronic renal hypertension that there is a shifting upward in response of baroreceptors, that is, an adaptation resetting the reflex to operate normally at higher pressure levels (Fig. 7–8). Once developed, this resetting may well for a time counter attempts at reducing arterial pressure.

SECONDARY HYPERTENSION

The mechanisms responsible for a secondary hypertension are not completely known in all cases. The following is a summary of some of the main types. A certain degree of overlapping is unavoidable, and this section should be read along with that on essential hypertension.

Renal Hypertension*

One of the important results of various studies has been the differentiation of hypertensive states associated with renal disease into two types—one related, at least initially, to activation of some pressor mechanism, and the other related to loss of renal substance and possibly of an antipressor effect. The first is exemplified by unilateral renal arterial stenosis and the second by the anephric state. In a schematic form that admits of many exceptions, the first type is characterized in man by elevated plasma renin activity (especially in recent hypertension), low plasma volume, and in-

*See also Chapter 14.

dices of increased neurogenic activity. The second type is marked by a positive correlation between blood volume and arterial pressure and very low or absent circulating renin; neurogenic activity fluctuates inversely with the degree of volemia. Patients with bilateral renal disease show varying mixtures of these two extremes, with either the "renal" or "renoprival" element predominating according to the type or stage of the lesion (Fig. 7–10).

Renovascular Hypertension. A large body of knowledge has been accumulated concerning this type of hypertension since the classic experiments of Goldblatt in dogs. Essential to proper evaluation of experimental studies is the realization of the extent of differences that may result from variation in techniques, timing of observations, and animal species used. More relevant perhaps to clinical situations is the extent of interference with the kidneys. Clipping of one renal artery is different from bilateral clipping; again, unilateral narrowing of a renal artery leaving the contralateral kidney intact differs in hemodynamic and humoral results from unilateral clipping with contralateral nephrectomy. Essential to the difference is the degree of fluid retention associated with bilateral maneuvers; the greater the retention, the lower the PRA and the smaller the response to angiotensin antagonists. This interaction of volume factors with the renal pressor system does not negate the role of either.

Studies in humans have shown not only that cardiac output was elevated in many patients with renovascular hypertension but also that this increase alone was not responsible for the maintenance of their hypertension. Total peripheral resistance was raised in patients with both normal and elevated outputs; successful surgical repair or nephrectomy was associated with reduction in resistance more often than with reduction in output. This common participation of varying degrees of increased output and resistance in the mainte-

nance of renovascular hypertension in humans corresponds to experimental studies in rats and dogs. Although the early rise of arterial pressure following clipping of renal arteries or cellophane wrapping of the kidney is primarily due to increased cardiac output, later stages are characterized by a delayed rise in peripheral resistance with a return of output toward normal. The change in hemodynamic pattern with time has been related to autoregulatory mechanisms discussed earlier in this chapter.

The increase of output and initiation of hypertension following renal arterial clipping have been related to fluid retention consequent on the reduction in renal perfusion pressure. However, no change in blood volume was noted in the initial stages of perinephritic hypertension in dogs when cardiac output was rising; indeed, in both humans and dogs with chronic renovascular hypertension plasma volume is slightly reduced. The combination of lower intravascular volume and increased cardiac output suggested an increased tone of the capacitance vessels shifting blood toward the heart. This is presumably related to enhanced sympathetic activity by angiotensin, since the latter has little, if any, direct effect on veins. Simultaneous stimulation of arterioles directly or indirectly (Fig. 7–11) helps set the stage for increased peripheral resistance. Once established, hypertension may be perpetuated by the development of secondary factors obscuring the initial disturbance (see later discussion).

It is generally agreed that the renal pressor system plays an important role in the early stages of renovascular hypertension; its participation in the chronic stage is much more debatable. This is probably because of the number of factors involved in any hypertension of sufficient duration. Doubts regarding the role of "renin" in this condition are based in part on the normal PRA in long-term renal arterial clip experiments. However, a normal PRA does not negate the possibility that angioten-

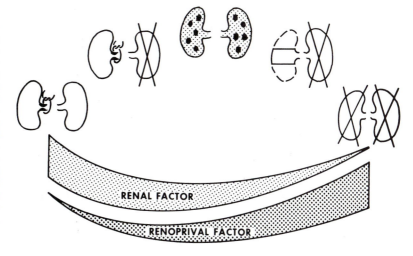

Figure 7–10 Renal and renoprival mechanisms in various types of "renal" hypertension. At one extreme is the renal mechanism activated by critical narrowing of one renal artery, the other remaining intact; at the other, removal of both kidneys leads to a renoprival volume-dependent state. In between these two extremes, both renal and renoprival factors participate in different combinations in the development of hypertension, depending on amount of renal tissue lost and on impairment of circulation through the remainder. (Modified from Tarazi, R. C., et al.: Pathol. Biol. 16:547, 1968.)

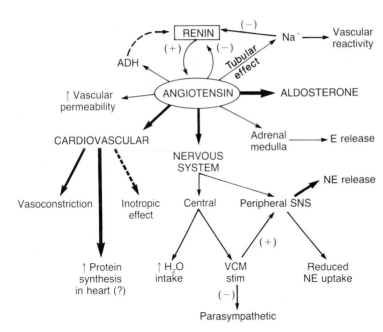

Figure 7–11 Multiple effects of angiotensin. Angiotensin is much more than a simple vasoconstrictive agent; it can stimulate adrenergic mechanisms through both central and peripheral effects. Its vascular effects are further potentiated by its stimulation of aldosterone synthesis and consequent increased sodium reabsorption.

sin II may be marginally increased; further, the effects of the renal pressor system may be amplified by any degree of fluid retention. As regards clinical situations, it is important to recall that conclusions from animal studies might not apply unreservedly to humans.

Control of hypertension has been achieved in some patients by unilateral nephrectomy or surgical correction of long-standing renal arterial stenosis. In deciding which patients will respond to these measures, one may find PRA determinations or assessment of BP response to angiotensin antagonists to be useful if properly evaluated (see previous discussion); however, these methods have not proved very reliable in predicting the outcome of corrective surgery for renovascular hypertension. Peripheral plasma renin activity is not infrequently elevated in patients with renal arterial stenosis and seems to be directly related to the height of diastolic arterial pressure. This is important to remember, since these patients in a hospital setting often have mild labile hypertension, and a finding of normal PRA does not mean that the hypertension is nonrenal. Because peripheral PRA is inconsistently elevated in renovascular hypertensive subjects, measurements in renal venous blood have been advocated. Results have been correct in a majority of instances; they are based on the likelihood that in unilateral renal arterial stenosis the affected kidney will produce, either spontaneously or in response to adequate stimulation, more renin than the unaffected kidney.

Hypertension and Renal Parenchymal Disease. This type of hypertension is so often complicated by the features attendant on diminished kidney function that acceptable studies of its mechanism in humans have been very difficult to obtain. Furthermore, the time course of renal

decompensation can be compressed into a few days or extended over several years, so that hypertensive mechanisms may be quite different from one case to the other. Whether the diseased kidneys are still present or have been removed is another important factor; in some instances, the characteristics of hypertension are radically altered by bilateral nephrectomy, even though the removed organs had practically no excretory function left.

The dependence of arterial pressure on volume expansion characterizes the hypertension associated with loss of renal tissue. In contrast with the slight plasma volume contraction seen in essential and renovascular hypertension is the direct correlation between arterial pressure and intravascular volume found in many patients with renal parenchymal disease (Fig. 7–12). In each patient, however, the hypertensive features will depend on the individual proportion of the renal and renoprival elements outlined earlier.

The hypertension of acute glomerulonephritis has been related to hypervolemia with consequent circulatory congestion, high ventricular filling pressure, and increased cardiac output, the total peripheral resistance remaining inappropriately normal in the face of increased blood flow.

In patients with end-stage kidney disease, two varieties of hypertension may be seen. The first and more common is volume-dependent. The height of the arterial pressure is related to the degree of volemia and can be controlled by diuretics (if still effective) or by dialysis; PRA is not elevated. The second type involves patients who do not respond well to dehydration or the usual vasodilators; their hypertension seems to depend on continued activation of the renal pressor system and is markedly reduced (or made easier to manage) by nephrectomy.

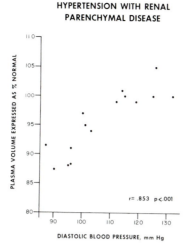

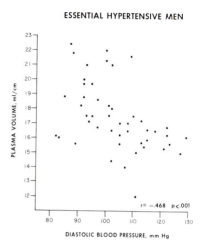

Figure 7–12 Contrasting relationship of intravascular volume and arterial pressure in essential hypertensive men and patients with renal parenchymal disease. (After Tarazi, R. C., et al.: Arch Intern. Med. *125*:835, 1970. Copyright 1970, American Medical Association.)

Hemodynamic findings in the hypertension of renal parenchymal disease are quite variable because of the number of complicating factors present, such as degree of anemia, fluid balance, myocardial status, and so on. However, when conditions are strictly controlled, the increase in pressure is found to depend on an absolute or relative increase in total peripheral resistance. It differs from essential hypertension in the absence of a preferential redistribution of blood flow to the muscles. Brod and colleagues, who reported these findings, interpret them as a definite qualitative difference from the "patterns of persistent stress or preparedness to exercise characteristic of essential hypertension."

Coarctation of the Aorta

The hypertension associated with coarctation of the aorta is an experiment of nature of considerable hemodynamic interest. It has demonstrated that the body can adjust peripheral resistance differently in organs above and below the coarctation so as to provide all of them with a normal blood flow. Unfortunately, the mechanism of this precise adjustment has not yet been determined, although it offers the best possible example for autoregulation of blood flow.

Although the renal arteries usually are below the aortic constriction, there is no unequivocal evidence for activation of a renal pressor mechanism. The hypertension is probably related to the mechanical obstruction. Cardiac output in coarctation is usually increased; the ejection of a large stroke volume into an aorta with decreased capacity and relatively limited runoff accounts for the large pressure found in vessels above the area of constriction. As output and rate of ejection are increased with exercise, so is the systolic blood pressure, often to alarming levels, even in patients who have near normal blood pressure at rest. By

diminishing this increase of cardiac output with intravenous propranolol, blood pressure rise with exercise is attenuated despite the significant increase in total peripheral resistance induced by the drug.

The importance of adaptive changes to hypertension can be seen in the occasional complications that follow surgical repair. When the obstruction is removed, vessels below the coarctation are suddenly exposed to higher pressures than they are used to; concomitantly, baroreceptor reflexes are activated by the drop of pressure in their area. The result may be a hypertensive crisis with arteriolar necrosis in the mesenteric vessels.

Pheochromocytoma

Most interesting and unusual is the hypertensive state associated with pheochromocytoma, a tumor of the medullary portion of the adrenal gland. It is one of the rare types in which the actual pressor mechanism is known. The tumors contain large amounts of epinephrine and norepinephrine in varying proportions. Hypertension may be persistent but is often paroxysmal. Symptoms result from release of the hormones from the tumor, causing sudden rapid rises in blood pressure, tachycardia, anxiety, headache, perspiration, nausea, and epigastric and precordial pain. All symptoms do not always appear, but it would be a most unusual patient who would not have at least one or two. Norepinephrine produces no tachycardia and does not affect the cardiac output. Epinephrine does both and produces hypermetabolism and hyperglycemia as well. Variations in the clinical picture depend in large part on these variables, but there are exceptions. The only definitive means of making the diagnosis are biochemical tests showing increased catecholamine secretion or excretion; these include determination of plasma or urinary catecholamines, urinary vanillylmandelic acid (VMA), and metanephrines either during a hypertensive period or following a provocative test. Intravenous glucagon (1 or 2 mg) may bring on an attack and incites both a blood pressure response and an increase in the plasma catecholamines as reliably as histamine does. The clonidine suppression test is predicated on the principle that a centrally acting adrenergic inhibiting agent will reduce the increased plasma catecholamines that are due to neural stimulation, whereas high levels produced by an adrenal tumor are not altered. The blood pressure response to orally administered clonidine in patients with essential hypertension does not differ from that in patients with pheochromocytoma.

However, three hours after oral administration of 0.3 mg of clonidine, plasma catecholamines will be reduced by at least 50 per cent in patients with essential hypertension but will not be suppressed in patients with pheochromocytoma. Alpha-adrenergic blocking agents (e.g., phentolamine, dibenzyline, and prazosin) will reduce elevated pressure that is due to pheochromocytoma. Phentolamine can be given by intravenous bolus to control acute hypertensive episodes in patients with pheochromocytoma; dibenzyline or prazosin is preferred for oral therapy in medical management if tumors are inoperable. Beta-adrenergic blockers may be needed to control tachycardia or ventricular irritability induced by excess catecholamines. Since beta blockade would leave alpha-mediated vasoconstriction unopposed, beta blockers should be given only under cover of alpha-adrenergic blocking agents.

Primary Aldosteronism (Conn's Disease)

The frequency of this condition as a cause of hypertension is not known. It is certainly a more frequent cause than is pheochromocytoma; however, it is less common than autopsy findings of small adrenocortical nodules might suggest. It results from autonomous hypersecretion of aldosterone by small single or multiple tumors of the adrenal cortex zona glomerulosa; sometimes only bilateral hyperplasia is found, with no strictly defined tumor (see Chapter 34). Its importance stems from the possibility of specific therapy or surgical cure for this type of hypertension.

The diagnosis is suggested by the presence of hypokalemia and inappropriate kaliuresis (>30.0 mEq daily urinary potassium excretion with a serum potassium <3.5 mEq/L) in a hypertensive patient with no history of recent diuretic therapy; the clinical picture is otherwise very similar to that of essential hypertension. The specific endocrine derangement is indicated by (1) low plasma renin activity that cannot be stimulated by low sodium intake (thus excluding secondary aldosteronism), and (2) more specifically, increased aldosterone excretion that cannot be suppressed by high sodium intake (thus reflecting the abnormality in regulation). Adrenal venography has been recommended for localization of the lesion; more recently, CT sector scanning and radioactive isotopes that are concentrated in the adrenal cortex have been introduced to avoid some of the hazards of venography.

The metabolic abnormalities in primary aldosteronism are better understood than the mechanism of its hypertension. Increased aldosterone excretion leads to sodium and water retention; stimulation of potassium-for-sodium exchange in the distal tubule leads to hypokalemia from excessive potassium loss in the urine. Increase in extracellular sodium and relative expansion of plasma volume probably account for the suppression of plasma renin activity, since administration of spironolactone can stimulate it. The classic hemodynamic pattern of this hypertension includes hypervolemia, increased cardiac output, and an elevated total peripheral resistance. But this can be modified by excessive rises in blood pressure or by coincident essential hypertension; in such cases, plasma volume and cardiac output may be reduced to low normal levels.

There are other causes of hypertension due to *mineralocorticoid excess*, all sharing the same pattern of suppressed plasma renin activity and easily induced hypokalemia (Fig. 7–13). Some result from excess administration of sodium-retaining steroids or steroid-like substances (e.g., licorice) and simply require discontinuing the drug or readjusting its dose. Others are due to enzymatic blocks (congenital or acquired) in hydroxylation of adrenal steroids at the 11 or 17 position. These blocks interfere with the production of cortisol and hence with its negative feedback control over ACTH production. The resultant excessive ACTH drive leads to adrenal hypersecretion of mineralocorticoids and consequent hypertension. Treatment consists of ACTH suppression by dexamethasone. Still other cases result from disordered hormonal production by adrenal and extra-adrenal tumors.

ESSENTIAL HYPERTENSION

By far the commonest type, essential hypertension remains a diagnosis by exclusion, reached only after the various causes of elevated arterial pressure are ruled out. It is characterized by a strong hereditary element and a long natural course, so that in early phases the subject appears normal except for the high blood pressure.

All the mechanisms discussed earlier have been at one time or another linked with essential hypertension. It is obviously very difficult in slowly developing asymptomatic processes to differentiate primary factors from secondary reactions. At this time, no animal model exists for essential hypertension; the relation of genetic

SIMPLIFIED SCHEME OF MINERALOCORTICOID HYPERTENSIONS

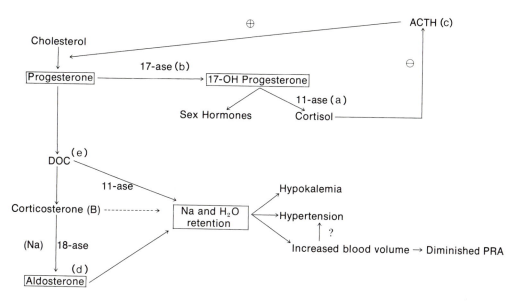

Key:
⊕ Positive stimulus
⊖ Negative feedback
11-ase, 17-ase = 11 beta- or 17 alpha-hydroxylase
PRA = plasma renin activity

(a) 11 beta-hydroxylase deficiency leads to decreased cortisol; the increased ACTH drive leads to hypertension secondary to DOC excess and to accumulation of 17-OH products increasing androgenic hormones.
(b) 17 alpha-hydroxylase deficiency leads to decreased cortisol and therefore to increased ACTH drive, but sex hormones are usually absent owing to lack of 17-hydroxylation; hypertension is related to increased DOC and corticosterone as sodium retention decreases their conversion to aldosterone.
(c) Combined DOC, corticosterone, and aldosterone excess occurs in adrenocortical tumors, especially if malignant, and in disordered ACTH drive (ectopic); cortisol is also usually increased in these cases.
(d) In primary aldosteronism, only aldosterone is increased.
(e) Iatrogenic hypertension usually results from excess DOC or fluorinated cortisol derivatives with unrestricted salt intake.

Figure 7–13

strains of spontaneously hypertensive rats to the human disease is still conjectural. Another difficulty is the lack of homogeneity resulting from lack of precision in diagnosis; there are probably different subgroups still included, for want of a better definition, in the general category of "essential, or idiopathic, hypertension."

Hemodynamic Characteristics

The main development in this area concerns the relationship between fixed and labile essential hypertension. Well-established essential hypertension is associated with a normal cardiac output and elevated peripheral resistance. The elevated resistance seems to be uniformly distributed in practically all vascular territories except in the kidney, where it may be more intense, and in the skeletal muscular system, where it is slightly less marked. This pattern was likened by Brod to a constant preparedness for exercise or response to

unspecified stress. Within this general framework a certain gradation has been described wherein a progressive reduction of resting cardiac output occurred with development of progressive cardiac involvement in the course of the disease. Even before cardiac decompensation occurred, cardiac output was reduced (and total peripheral resistance further increased) in hypertensive patients with definite left ventricular hypertrophy (Tarazi).

Contrasting with the aforementioned findings, an increasing number of studies from laboratories in the United States and Europe have established that a large proportion of patients with intermittent, usually mild elevations of arterial pressure (borderline hypertension) have increased cardiac output and normal, near normal, or subnormal values of total peripheral resistance. The suggestion is that this pattern of "increased output-normal resistance" is the beginning phase leading to increased resistance and fixed hypertension. Longitudinal studies by Lund-Johansen and Ohm have indeed shown a transition from high to normal cardiac output in untreated borderline hypertensives followed over 20 years. However, although a normal or low cardiac output is most frequent among established essential hypertensives and a high output is common in borderline hypertension, exceptions *do* occur in both conditions. It is still possible, therefore, that in some patients a high output may represent a qualitatively different hemodynamic type of the disease.

The reason for the increased output in borderline hypertension is not clear; oxygen consumption is normal for that level of output in contrast with other high output states. Resting heart rate, although slightly faster than normal, is not faster than that in other forms of hypertension. This finding reawakened interest in the old suggestion that an "augmented force" of the heart beat could play a role in the genesis of hypertension, but an increase in output might also represent a normal cardiac response to constriction of the capacitance vessels and central redistribution of blood. Similarities with hemodynamic findings in renovascular hypertension are obvious; however, the mechanisms involved in essential hypertension are still purely conjectural.

In these considerations of increased output, it must be remembered that in the final analysis, hypertension is the result of failure of the peripheral circulation to adapt to systemic flow. Indeed, some abnormality in peripheral circulatory adjustment is demonstrable even in patients with "normal total peripheral resistance." Although correctly said to be "within normal range," their resistance is abnormally high for their cardiac output, as is shown by comparison with normotensive subjects with equivalent levels of output. The abnormality is clearly revealed during muscular exercise.

In the absence of cardiac failure, response to dynamic exercise in hypertensive patients is much the same as in normal subjects. Cardiac output increases proportionally to oxygen uptake, and peripheral resistance falls. This fall is never to normal levels, so that blood pressure remains high; although the heart responded normally, the extent of reduction in peripheral resistance was not commensurate with the rise in output, especially in young subjects. The anomaly of peripheral reactions in hypertension is also shown in the pattern of response to stressful interviews. In these studies, the resultant increase of blood pressure was due to increased cardiac output in 80 per cent of normal subjects, whereas most hypertensive patients responded by an increase in total peripheral resistance.

Neurogenic Factors

The obvious effects of emotional factors on arterial pressure have led to many assumptions regarding the role of *psychogenic factors* in essential hypertension. It has been suggested that frequent psychogenic rises in blood pressure may culminate in fixed hypertension. The corticohypothalamic "defense reaction" not only may be activated by manifest threats but also is said to occur whenever "alertness" is raised. Repeated increases in arterial pressure would lead to structural adaptation (hypertrophy) of the arterioles, which in turn would amplify the vasoconstrictive effects of even normal nerve traffic or circulating substances. Various alterations found in essential hypertension — namely, altered regional blood flow, modest increase in basal heart rate, and decrease in plasma volume — have been likened to the pattern of "preparedness to exercise."

Despite its attractiveness, this hypothesis still remains to be proved, since there is no firm evidence that psychogenic stimuli result in chronic sustained hypertension. These stimuli are difficult to quantitate, and nerve traffic, although measurable in some superficial nerves in humans, cannot be adequately quantitated nor taken to represent precisely the overall level of sympathetic activity in various organs. Studies showing excessive pressure rise in hypertensive patients in response to stressful experiences do not differentiate between increased sympathetic outflow from vasomotor centers and increased vascular responsiveness to normal outflow. The problem is complicated by the possible influence of such poorly defined factors as personality traits. Pavlov noted that it is easier to produce a neurotic state in "sanguine" than in "melancholic" dogs. Promising studies are being conducted in the area of conditioned blood pressure control and the effects of reticular formation on baroreceptor activity.

The hypertension produced in laboratory animals by sinoaortic denervation does not bear any real resemblance to essential hypertension. It is accompanied by wide swings of blood pressure and marked tachycardia; the pressure falls to normal levels when the animal is quiet or asleep and is usually sensitive to neural blocking agents. Apart from rare cases of polyneuritis involving the ninth cranial nerve, disturbances of the baroreceptor mechanism probably do not have a causative role in essential hypertension. Secondary resetting of their threshold and/or diminished sensitivity of the reflex due to functional or structural changes in the carotid arteries might theoretically play a minor role in its maintenance.

The striking antihypertensive effectiveness of drugs that suppress adrenergic functions is still one of the main evidences that neural factors operate in some way to maintain hypertension. A clinically applicable way to estimate their importance is to determine the immediate pressure response to an intravenous injection of a ganglion blocker. In various studies, the pressure reduction obtained in essential hypertensive subjects correlated significantly with preinjection diastolic pressure and total peripheral resistance. Again, the higher the pressure and the resistance, the smaller the plasma volume, so that intravascular volume was inversely related to sympathetic activity. At present, there is no way of knowing whether intravascular volume is decreased because increased sympathetic tone has reduced vascular capacity or whether increased sympathetic outflow is a compensatory response to a reduced plasma volume.

An important aspect developed over the past decade is the close and reciprocal interaction between the renal pressor and sympathetic nervous systems. The potentiating action of angiotensin on the cardiovascular effects of the sympathetic nervous system has already been discussed. However, sympathetic hyperactivity may help trigger the renin-angiotensin system by restricting blood flow to the kidney (a part of the "defense reaction"). Thus, whether a neurogenic or a hormonal factor is the initial event, both may interreact to maintain a more sustained neurohumoral drive on the cardiovascular system (Folkow and Neil). The clinical relevance of these relationships is underlined by the experience that renovascular hypertension can be effectively treated by drugs that suppress adrenergic activity.

Extracellular Fluid and Blood Volume

There now seems little question that plasma volume is quite regularly altered in various forms of hypertension. It is reduced in essential hypertension in relation to the level of diastolic pressure and peripheral resistance, so that the higher the resistance, the lower the volume. Since extracellular fluid volume is usually normal in this condition, the reduction in plasma volume probably reflects a subtle abnormality in the distribution of fluid between its intravascular and interstitial compartments. Hypertension accompanying renal arterial disease or pheochromocytoma is also characterized by reduced plasma volume.

In contrast, plasma volume is modestly expanded in primary aldosteronism, although not as consistently as is usually suggested. The more striking abnormality is the positive correlation between total blood volume and arterial pressure found in patients with renal parenchymal disease (see Renal Hypertension). Finally, a subgroup of essential hypertension has been described with plasma volume either expanded or inappropriately normal for height of diastolic pressure. This group possibly represents the same type of hypertension as is being tentatively described by various investigators as having increased extracellular fluid volume, increased exchangeable sodium, and hyporeninemia with no evidence of primary aldosteronism.

The clinical relevance of volume studies is not limited to diagnostic considerations. As indicated previously, pressure responsiveness to ganglion

blockers is inversely related to degree of volemia, hence the greater sensitivity of patients with low plasma volume (spontaneous or diuretic-induced) to neural blocking drugs. Conversely, pressure response to these drugs is attenuated or lost when hypervolemia develops, as it often does during their administration. The increase in plasma volume during treatment results from diminished tone of capacitance vessels with resultant transfer of fluid from the interstitial to the intravascular compartment and is accentuated by actual fluid retention. This "false tolerance" to the neural blocking drugs is reversed and pressure control is restored by adequate volume depletion with diuretics.

Renal Pressor System

At present, there is no indication of any gross abnormality of this system in nonmalignant essential hypertension. Plasma renin levels are usually within normal range but can occasionally be quite low and unresponsive to the usual stimuli used to increase circulating renin. Laragh and coworkers have classified essential hypertensive subjects into low-, normal-, and high-renin categories, suggesting that the first type of patient depends more on volume factors and the latter two on renin mechanisms. An attractive hypothesis links these observations with those on volume factors in the following scheme. Essential hypertension could be viewed as being of two subtypes: one with normal to high PRA, contracted plasma volume, and probably increased sympathetic drive; the second with low PRA, expanded plasma volume, and particular responsiveness to diuretic therapy. However, it is not yet clear whether this subdivision describes different subtypes or only extremes at either end of a graded spectrum of variations. Exceptions do occur; levels of PRA are influenced by age, and long-term studies are needed to determine whether some of these differences are not simply time-dependent. It is important to note that the renin angiotensin system does not necessarily represent the central factor in this concept; its variations, like those of plasma volume and cardiac output, may be only a reflection of different levels of sympathetic activity. This is another illustration of the difficulty in deciding which of the many possible pressor mechanisms is the prime mover in hypertension.

In the majority of subjects with essential hypertension, aldosterone secretion correlates normally with urinary sodium excretion. In some, however, discrepancies between levels of plasma renin activity and aldosterone excretion have been described, especially under the stimulus of sodium deprivation. The role of this hormonal imbalance is still not clear.

Malignant hypertension—of whatever origin—is associated with marked secondary aldosteronism: high plasma renin activity, hyponatremia, hypokalemia, and great rises of aldosterone excretion. Activation of the renin-angiotensin system in this condition has been viewed as partly responsible for the intensification of the vascular disease and of hyponatremia.

Summary. This review of pathophysiologic mechanisms in essential hypertension has revealed multifactorial disturbances. Any of the numerous changes that occur in hypertension cannot be considered alone; the complexity of relationships and the practical impossibility of differentiating primary from secondary factors explain the failure of finding a "single" cause of essential hypertension.

Alterations with Antihypertensive Therapy

Recent developments have led to concerted efforts for control of hypertension; this is often achieved by drug therapy that introduces marked alterations in mechanisms regulating arterial pressure. Better understanding of these alterations will help accurate evaluation of problems in the increasing number of treated hypertensive subjects.

Attempts at lowering arterial pressure set in motion a number of counter-reactions; further, all antihypertensive drugs in common use have one or more actions that tend to thwart their own effectiveness. Thus, sympatholytics as well as vasodilators can cause fluid retention and plasma volume expansion. During treatment with beta blockers, peripheral resistance can increase and thus limit the reduction in blood pressure. Conversely, treatment with many vasodilators reduces peripheral resistance but reflexly increases cardiac output. Both diuretic agents and vasodilators increase plasma renin activity, which may antagonize their antihypertensive effects, although this has not been established. Thus, hypertension remains a multifactorial problem not only in its initiation and in its maintenance but also in its response to therapy.

The clinical implications of these observations are twofold: (1) Studies of the physiologic characteristic of any hypertension may be misleading if made while patients are on antihypertensive therapy or too soon after it is stopped. (2) Antihypertensive agents sometimes fail simply because one pressor mechanism has been substituted for another. Most patients with moderate or severe hypertension will require a combination of drugs; the choice must be based on a consideration of the mechanisms involved and balanced in order to minimize the counteractions anticipated from each of its components.

HYPOTENSION

GENERAL CONSIDERATIONS AND DEFINITION OF TERMS

Low systemic arterial pressure impairs tissue perfusion; however, the pressure level at which blood flow is critically diminished will vary, depending on the extent and rate of reduction in blood pressure, local condition of the vessels, and adequacy of compensating mechanisms. Hence, a numerical definition of hypotension raises the same problems of "normalcy" as a numerical definition of hypertension. Some normal subjects have arterial pressures below 90/60 mm Hg with no apparent cause and no sign of ill-effect. The brain can apparently be adequately perfused, even in the upright position, by systolic pressures as low as 60 mm Hg or less. The symptoms of diminished vitality, easy fatigue, and dizziness that have been sometimes loosely ascribed to hypotension (systolic below 100 mm Hg) are just as frequently found in normotensive as in hypotensive patients.

A low arterial pressure level by itself is not necessarily a pathologic finding; in fact, chronic "hypotension" in the absence of associated disease may be a favorable condition because of the diminished cardiovascular load. Pathologic hypotension is the level at which blood flow to vital organs (brain, heart, kidneys) is impaired. Obviously, perfusion will be more easily impaired by acute hypotension than by a chronic reduction in arterial pressure that may allow time for more effective compensatory adjustments of blood flow. The effects of hypotension may be subdivided into (1) those resulting directly from impaired organ perfusion (e.g., fainting due to cerebral ischemia) and (2) those due to activation of compensatory mechanisms (e.g., sweating and tachycardia from sympathetic stimulation secondary to decreased baroreceptor activity). The resulting clinical picture will therefore vary markedly with the cause of hypotension, its time course, the pattern of blood flow alteration, the activation of compensatory mechanisms or their failure, and any pre- or coexisting disease.

Postural Hypotension. This is characterized by a marked fall in arterial pressure with dizziness and possibly syncope when the patient is standing but a quite adequate circulation and pressure when the individual is lying down (Fig. 7–14).

Although acute hypotension (postural, cardiac, or reflex) is one of the commonest causes of syncope, the two terms are not synonymous. *Syncope* refers to a sudden, transient loss of consciousness; it is indeed very frequently due to hypotension and impaired cerebral perfusion but might in other instances result from biochemical derangements such as hypoglycemia or reflect cerebral dysfunction as in the cerebral type of carotid sinus syndrome. Most fainting spells (vasovagal attacks

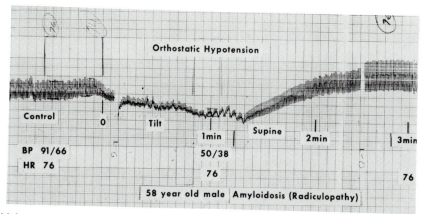

Figure 7-14 Intra-arterial pressure record of a patient with postural hypotension due to loss of sympathetic nerve function. Note the rapid (as opposed to sudden) reduction in pressure from the beginning of head-up tilt and the unchanged heart rate despite the fall in pressure. As soon as the patient is returned to the horizontal position, arterial pressure begins to rise to even hypertensive levels; this tilt-back overshoot occurs following head-up tilt in patients with organic or drug-induced sympathetic dysfunction and has been related to liberation of catecholamines.

or vasodepressor syncope) occur when the subject is standing and are associated with a fall in arterial pressure. They differ from "postural hypotension" in that they may occur when the subject is in the supine position, an extraprovocative factor is usually present (emotional disturbance, sight of blood, pain, hot weather), and signs of vagal activity (slowing pulse, nausea) are evident. Whereas all symptoms associated with postural hypotension quickly disappear as soon as the patient lies or falls down, the vasovagal disturbance clears much more slowly. Vasodepressor syncope is characterized by a sudden reduction in peripheral vascular resistance (Fig. 7-15), venoconstriction rather than dilatation, and little change in cardiac output. There is no evidence for excessive plasma volume contraction.

Shock. Despite its lack of precision, this term does evoke an impressive and readily recognizable picture and will certainly continue to be used clinically. It describes a condition of marked weakness; a variable degree of mental torpor with weak, rapid, thready pulse, cold clammy skin, and unobtainable or very low arterial pressure by usual method of examination. Many of these signs may not necessarily be found; arterial pressure may occasionally be relatively normal, especially if the patient was previously hypertensive. In some cases central pressure obtained by arterial cannulation may be high while brachial pressure is clinically unobtainable owing to marked peripheral vasoconstriction. Mentation may be unexpectedly clear if peripheral and renal vasoconstriction are intense enough to secure adequate cerebral blood flow. Instead of being cold and clammy, the skin may be dry and hot in cases of bacteremic shock. However, despite these variations, the picture is usually readily recognizable; the basic fault is a gross impairment of tissue perfusion due to marked reduction in cardiac output. The subject is much too extensive to be covered in this chapter; it is important, however, to underline its differences from other types of hypotension and to realize that in any hypotension, the body suffers not from the fall in arterial pressure per se but from the reduced blood flow that hypotension produces or signifies.

Chronic Hypotension. Chronic hypotension with vague or nonspecific symptoms may be asso-

Figure 7-15 Semidiagrammatic illustration of hemodynamic events in vasodepressor syncope and in orthostatic hypotension due to loss of sympathetic activity. In the former, the drop in blood pressure occurs suddenly after a normal response to tilt (simulated in this case by lower body negative pressure, LBNP); heart rate and total peripheral resistance increase before they suddenly drop. In contrast, arterial pressure is gradually reduced to hypotensive levels in patients with sympathetic paralysis (see Fig. 7-14), with no change in either TPR or heart rate. Note also the post-tilt overshoot of the arterial pressure.

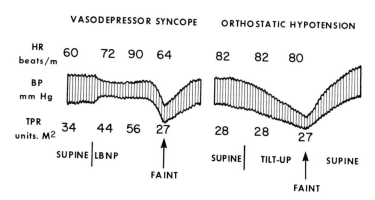

ciated with a variety of diseases such as aortic stenosis, adrenocortical insufficiency, malabsorption syndrome, severe cardiac failure, and constrictive pericarditis. The clinical picture is dominated by the primary disease of which hypotension is only a sign. Some of these conditions may be associated with postural hypotension also. In contrast with such secondary forms of hypotension, an idiopathic, chronically low arterial pressure is not really a pathologic condition. Indeed, statistical studies would suggest enhanced longevity for apparently healthy people with idiopathic hypotension.

PATHOPHYSIOLOGY OF POSTURAL HYPOTENSION

Adjustment to Postural Changes. The pressure in a column of fluid depends on its specific gravity and the vertical distance from the point of measurement to the reference level; hence, the pressure at the bottom of the U tube will obviously be higher than that at the top. However, the pressure head required to drive fluid through a system of horizontal tubes will not be altered by the addition to that system of an unyielding U tube dipping below the line of flow. Similarly, if blood vessels were rigid tubes, standing up would not affect arterial or venous blood pressure at the heart's level and cardiac output would not change. The intravascular pressures in the feet would be markedly increased by an amount equal to their distance below the phlebostatic or zero point, but the arteriovenous gradient would not be altered, since arterial and venous pressures would be affected to the same extent.

Vessels, however, are not rigid, impermeable tubes. As we stand, the pull of gravity pools blood in distensible veins below the heart and plasma is lost to interstitial fluid as capillary pressure and ultrafiltration increase. Diminished venous return reduces cardiac output and unless compensatory mechanisms perform adequately the subsequent fall in arterial pressure will result in impaired cerebral perfusion and loss of consciousness. Fortunately, adjustment mechanisms normally are quite effective and arterial pressure is maintained (see Chapter 6). Even with passive head-up tilt, which exaggerates the effect of gravity by minimizing the support derived from contraction of the lower limb muscles, mean arterial pressure varies only by ±10 mm Hg.

This stability is due to an almost instantaneous reflex increase in sympathetic vasomotor outflow (see Neural Reflexes). Obviously, vasoconstriction must occur in the resistance vessels to offset the effect of reduction in output and in the capacitance vessels to diminish pooling and help hasten venous return. As part of this sympathetic stimulation, heart rate increases slightly. The same reflexes are involved in bleeding or when mechanical factors hinder venous return (e.g., recumbency in late pregnancy).

Associated with this increased sympathetic activity, catecholamine concentration is increased in plasma and urine. The increase in epinephrine is due to reflex sympathetic stimulation of the adrenal medulla, and the increase in norepinephrine is mostly due to increased activity of the sympathetic vasomotor nerves. Other hormones are also involved in the response to upright posture; renin and aldosterone secretion are increased, and there is even some evidence that antidiuretic hormone may be released, probably in response to reduced tension on intrathoracic volume receptors. Plasma renin activity is elevated within a few minutes of upright tilt, but its rise lags behind the reflex increase in pulse rate and diastolic blood pressure. Renin release is markedly affected by sympathetic nerve activity and circulating catecholamines and may be impaired in some patients with autonomic nerve disease or during treatment with adrenergic blocking drugs; however, increased catecholamine production is not an indispensable prerequisite for adequate stimulation of renin and aldosterone in the upright posture.

Whatever the reflex effects on resistance vessels, the capillary vessels in the feet during standing must still contend with a pressure exceeding 100 mm Hg, far above the maximum colloid osmotic pressure of plasma proteins. Plasma loss by diffusion could thus be enormous; this is prevented by contraction of precapillary sphincters, thus effectively shutting off filtration from a large number of dependent capillary beds. In addition, counterpressures develop in dependent areas to prevent overdistention of veins and help balance some of the rise in capillary pressure. Intramuscular tissue pressure increases with muscular contraction. Lower limb veins are compressed when leg and thigh muscles contract, and blood is pushed upward; as the muscles relax, backward flow of blood is prevented by intravenous valves. By interrupting the column of blood in the veins at different points, valves also prevent transmission of the full weight of that column to small dependent venules. Thus, "muscular pumping" helps lower both venous pressure and effective capillary filtering pressure; when this is interfered with, the incidence of fainting is increased. This may happen in normal subjects standing motionless at attention, or in those tilted passively and then supported in the upright position, or in patients with incompetent venous valves and dilated varicose veins.

Cerebral Circulation. The oxygen requirements of the central nervous system are fairly constant, and cerebral blood flow must therefore be kept constant if consciousness and life are to be preserved. The cerebral vessels are remarkably unresponsive to the usual neural and hormonal stimuli; the constancy of flow is secured by local autoregulatory mechanisms dependent on local production of carbon dioxide and local oxygen needs. Arterial P_{CO_2} is the most powerful regulator of cerebral flow; doubling P_{CO_2} approximately doubles cerebral flow, whereas a decrease in oxygen saturation to about 75 per cent increases flow approximately 40 per cent. However, the vasodilator effect of oxygen deficiency increases at very low saturations. This close adaptation of cerebral flow to neuronal metabolic needs ensures an impressively constant flow over wide ranges of arterial pressure down to quite low levels (50 to 60 mm Hg mean pressure). Thus, whenever widespread, sympathetic vasoconstriction develops (shock, hemorrhage, or upright posture), the cerebral vasculature is not materially affected by it, but blood is redistributed toward the brain (and heart) from other constricted vascular beds. Moreover, since cerebral vessels and cerebrospinal fluid are enclosed within a rigid cavity, variations in cerebrospinal fluid or extravascular pressure with standing parallel very closely the variations in intravascular pressure, thus increasing the stability of the cerebral circulation. The stability of cerebral flow despite marked fluctuations in arterial pressure may explain why antihypertensive therapy is very rarely associated with cerebral damage, even when transient hypotension develops. As soon as blood pressure is increased beyond a minimal level (as by lying down), cerebral blood flow is rapidly restored to near normal.

Pathophysiologic Classification. Orthostatic hypotension is characterized by a fall of at least 20 mm Hg in both systolic and diastolic pressure on assumption of the standing position; in severe cases, the patient cannot even stand up, since simple sitting leads to severe reduction in blood pressure. Severe hypotension may also develop in positions other than standing; women in late pregnancy may faint when lying on their backs, and patients with atrial myxoma or pedunculated intra-atrial thrombus may faint on sitting up. These type of postural hypotension are due to impaired ventricular filling and diminished cardiac output.

Orthostatic hypotension is the commonest form of postural hypotension; the blood pressure in the supine position may be reduced, normal, or even elevated. The patient may feel and look quite normal when lying down, or some circulatory disorder may be apparent (e.g., rapid pulse and low arterial pressure as in hemorrhage or adrenocortical insufficiency). However, whatever the cause of the orthostatic fall in pressure, the clinical picture on standing is common to all (Table 7–3). The patient feels dizzy, weak, and faint; ataxia, blurring of vision, or occasionally some dysarthria develops, and unless he lies down promptly, he may become unconscious. All symptoms, including syncope, clear up rapidly with the patient in the supine position.

Postural hypotension may have different causes (Table 7–4) that can essentially be linked to either of two basic mechanisms. In the first group, cardiac output is so reduced that despite reflex sympathetic stimulation, arterial pressure falls (sympathicotonic type). The second group is characterized by failure of the barostatic mechanism at some point along the reflex arc; hence, there are no or inappropriately few signs of sympathetic activity. Reflexes may be interfered with by disease or simply slowed by such factors as aging, prolonged recumbency, physical exhaustion, and starvation. The commonest cause of orthostatic hypotension, however, is inhibition of sympathetic reflexes by drugs that interfere with ganglionic transmission or with norepinephrine liberation at the nerve endings or that block alpha-adrenergic receptors (Table 7–4). The effects of bed rest on sympathetic activity are particularly important to note, since even short periods of inactivity may aggravate orthostatic hypotension due to other causes. By the same token, repeated head-up tilting may reduce the postural fall in pressure produced by some neurologic lesions. To these two major mechanisms, a hemodynamic disturbance and a failure of adequate autonomic response, one may add a third, namely, the activation of vasodilator reflexes as in vasovagal attacks and the pacemaker syndrome (Tarazi and Fouad).

Clinical differentiation of various types is not always easy. When present, signs of associated disease or history of drug intake give helpful clues, but determination of the mechanism involved and localization of the lesion require a stepwise, reasoned approach. Causes listed in group I are usually readily differentiated from those in group II-B by the intensity of sympathetic activity in the first group and its relative absence in the second (Table 7–4). Clinical signs of increased sympathetic drive include pallor, sweating, and tachycardia; hemodynamic studies may document the simultaneous increase in peripheral resistance, diminution in forearm blood flow, and venoconstriction. The absence of these signs despite the fall in arterial pressure characterizes neurogenic hypotension (Table 7–4). However, although the absence of tachycardia during hypotension indicates an inadequate neural response, its presence does not necessarily exclude a neurogenic lesion. Thus, heart rate may increase in early idiopathic hypotension before cardiac nerves are involved or in hypotension due to lumbar sympathectomy. The same remarks apply to pallor and sweating. Failure of peripheral resistance to increase is particularly significant. The picture in vasodepressor syncope is quite different; here the pulse actually slows and peripheral resistance suddenly falls as the patient faints (Fig. 7–15).

LOCALIZATION OF DEFECT IN THE BARORECEPTOR ARC (GROUP II-B). Lesions in the efferent limb will be characterized by loss of pressure responses to all reflex pressor maneuvers, whatever the origin of the reflex—baroreceptor as in the Valsalva maneuver, pain as in cold pressor test, or psycho-

TABLE 7–3 HEMODYNAMIC RESPONSES IN ORTHOSTATIC HYPOTENSION

	Normal	Oligemia or Diminished Venous Return	Idiopathic Orthostatic Hypotension	
			Early	*Advanced*
1. Standing Up				
Blood pressure	Little change: mean arterial pressure varies by <10 mm Hg	Reduction in both systolic and diastolic pressures, sometimes quite marked		
Heart rate	Increased by about 15%	Marked increase	Slight increase	No change
Cardiac output	Reduced, usually 10 to 20%	Reduced to varying degree	Reduced, usually >25%	Reduced >25%
Total peripheral resistance	Increased by 15 to 20%	Marked increase	Slight increase may occur	No increase
2. Phenylephrine				
Blood pressure	Increased, depending on dose	Normal response	Response > normal because of denervation hypersensitivity	
Heart rate	Slowed with blood pressure rise	Normal response	Response may be normal	No change despite rise in blood pressure
3. Valsalva Maneuver Overshoot (Phase IV)	Rise in diastolic pressure averages 25 to 35% of control	Normal or increased	Absent	Absent, and return from phase III may be quite slow

TABLE 7–4 POSTURAL HYPOTENSION

I. *Diminished Cardiac Output*
  A. Interference with venous return and cardiac filling at the muscular, venous, or cardiac level:
    1. Poor muscular pumping mechanism
      a. Muscular atrophy
      b. Poor postural adjustment in young asthenic persons standing at strict attention
      c. Passive tilting
    2. Venous disease
      a. Incompetent valves
      b. Varicose veins
      c. Obstruction (e.g., late pregnancy)
    3. Cardiac: tamponade, constrictive pericarditis, atrial myxoma, ball valve thrombus
  B. Absolute or relative depletion of intravascular volume
    1. Relative: due to dilatation of capacitance vessels by drugs (e.g., nitrites) or disease (e.g., venous angiomatosis)
    2. Absolute
      a. Hemorrhage, internal or external
      b. Excessive loss of fluid by diuresis, vomiting, diarrhea
      c. Increased capillary permeability with loss of fluid in interstitial spaces
      d. Urinary salt wasting due to selective hypoaldosteronism
  C. Diminished myocardial performance*
    1. Myocarditis, severe coronary arterial disease
    2. Postural arrhythmias with excessively slow or extremely rapid heart rate
    3. Outlet obstruction as in aortic or pulmonary stenosis (usually leads to exercise rather than orthostatic hypotension)

II. *Impaired Peripheral Resistance*
  A. Arteriolar
    1. Disease: relatively rare (e.g., amyloidosis), and then usually associated with neural involvement as well
    2. Arteriolar vasodilators as nitrites or nitroprusside
  B. Neurologic dysfunction
    1. Lesion in afferent limb: Tabes dorsalis, rarely in polyneuritis
    2. Lesion in central nervous system
      a. Some forms of chronic idiopathic hypotension; possible relation to Shy-Drager syndrome
      b. Parkinsonism either isolated or part of a more extensive degenerative disease
      c. Cerebral arteriosclerosis
      d. Syringomyelia, various myelopathies, Wernicke's syndrome, tumors
      e. Drugs (e.g., meprobamate)
    3. Lesion in efferent sympathetic limb (parasympathetic may be affected but is not responsible for hypotension)
      a. Some forms of chronic idiopathic hypotension
      b. Polyneuritis (e.g., diabetes, porphyria)
      c. Myelopathies
      d. Iatrogenic
        (1) Postsympathectomy
        (2) Neural blocking drugs
          (a) Ganglion blocking agents adrenergic blockers
          (b) Monoamine oxidase inhibitors
          (c) L-Dopa

III. *Undetermined or Mixed Mechanisms*
  A. Adrenocortical insufficiency: possibly related to cardiac dysfunction and aggravated by fluid loss; reactions of resistance and capacitance vessels said to be normal
  B. Diabetic acidosis
  C. Pheochromocytoma (distinctly uncommon)

*Note: Cardiac failure as such as is *not* a cause of orthostatic hypotension; in fact, patients in congestive failure tolerate head-up tilt very well, possibly because of their hypervolemia.

logic as in stressful mental arithmetic. These stimuli will not raise blood pressure as they normally should because the final common neural pathway is not functioning. However, arteriolar responsiveness to norepinephrine infusion will be intact or indeed exaggerated (denervation hypersensitivity) in contrast with the impaired responsiveness found in purely arteriolar lesions. Similarly, loss of reflex sweating (warming contralateral limb) despite the presence of responsive sweat glands suggests an efferent or central sympathetic defect. In many but not all cases of efferent limb dysfunction, the cardiac nerves (sympathetic and parasympathetic) are involved; if the heart is functionally denervated, its rate will be higher than expected and fixed, unresponsive to atropine injections, carotid sinus stimulation, or increase in arterial pressure by phenylephrine. If neural involvement is not far advanced (early idiopathic postural hypotension) or is localized (as following lumbar sympathectomy), demonstration of reflex cardiac slowing will indicate that afferent nerves, medullary centers, and parasympathetic efferent nerves are intact.

Pathophysiologic localization of central lesions is more difficult; reflex pressor responses are also interfered with. Some help may be derived from the presence of other neural signs (rigidity, parkinsonism, nystagmus, alterations of deep reflexes, etc.), but especially from demonstration of intact peripheral sympathetic innervation. One can most readily achieve this by showing increased toe or finger blood flow with local anesthesia of the corresponding nerves. Lesions of afferent baroreceptor nerves may be suspected when orthostatic reflexes are absent (hypotension and unchanged heart rate during head-up tilt), in contrast with normal pressor responses to cold stimulus and mental arithmetic, normal peripheral blood flow response to nerve blockade, and intact vagal supply to the heart (increased rate following atropine injection). The loss of baroreceptor sensitivity may be demonstrated by absence of reflex bradycardia when blood pressure is raised and lack of pressor response to maneuvers lowering arterial pressure.

IDIOPATHIC ORTHOSTATIC HYPOTENSION

This syndrome affects men more frequently than women; it is a slowly progressive condition marked by obvious neural autonomic involvement (postural hypotension, loss of sweating, fixed heart rate), subtle neurologic signs (pupillary abnormalities, generalized hyperreflexia, disturbed bladder regulation), and usually intact sensation and mental faculties. Association with parkinsonism is particularly frequent and may be very disabling. In many instances, the disease may represent variants of the syndrome described by Shy and Drager but not all forms are necessarily related to

the same pathologic alterations. Some may be due to involvement of sympathetic nerves and others to degeneration of preganglionic spinal neurons. The initial description of the syndrome by Bradbury and Eggleston stressed the triad of postural hypotension gradually increased in severity, anhydrosis slowly spreading to involve most of the body surface, and impotence. Plasma and urinary catecholamines are usually decreased. Responses of the renin-angiotensin-aldosterone system were impaired in some patients and reported as normal in others. In our experience, abnormalities in PRA were not helpful in localization of the lesion. Plasma volume is often contracted, and because of reduced sympathetic support cardiac performance becomes overly dependent on changes in preload.

CEREBROVASCULAR DISEASE AND HYPOTENSION

A sudden fall in systemic blood pressure can cause focal neurologic impairment, especially in patients with atherosclerotic narrowing or occlusion of intracranial vessels or of the carotid or vertebral arteries. However, cerebrovascular disease may itself cause hypotension and fainting, so that determination of which event came first may be very difficult. The question is particularly relevant in antihypertensive therapy; it is our opinion that hypotension has been grossly overrated as a cause of strokes. Though hypotensive episodes were very frequent in the heroic days of ganglion blocking therapy, the incidence of permanent neurologic damage was not particularly increased. This impression is supported by the rarity of cerebral infarction in patients with idiopathic orthostatic hypotension, many of whom are elderly and subject to frequent hypotensive spells.

Postural hypotension is more common in patients with cerebrovascular disease than in normal controls. Central interference with the baroreceptor reflex may be one cause; pressor response to the Valsalva maneuver is often blunted and may be completely absent in elderly patients with cerebral atherosclerosis. Patients may easily faint while coughing or when straining at stool or during micturition, possibly because of reflex failure of vasoconstriction in the face of diminished venous return rather than because of laryngeal or vesical reflexes. However, anatomic interference with baroreceptor arc may not be the only factor. A study of such patients showed that they often have barely adequate reflexes to cope with mild stress; they can maintain an adequate systemic blood pressure and orthostatic responses unless an additional factor such as a sedative drug or prolonged rest is added. Recumbency even for relatively short periods such as a night's rest reduces sympathetic activity; hypotension is therefore aggravated in the early morning hours. Prolonged recumbency adds the additional stress of blood volume contraction.

REFERENCES

Beevers, D. B., Bloxham, C. A., Backhouse, C. I., Lim, C. C., and Watson, R. D. S.: The Remler M2000 semi-automatic blood pressure recorder. Br. Heart J. *42*:366, 1979.

Bergenwald, L., Freyschuss, U., and Sjostrand, T.: The mechanism of orthostatic and haemorrhagic fainting. Scand. J. Clin. Lab. Invest. *37*:209, 1977.

Bevan, A. I., Honour, A. J., and Scott, F. H.: Direct arterial pressure recording in unrestricted man. Clin. Sci. *36*:329, 1969.

Friedman, S. M., and Friedman, C. L.: Cell permeability, sodium transport, and the hypertensive process in the rat. Circ. Res. *39*:433, 1976.

Folkow, B., and Neil, E.: Circulation. New York, Oxford University Press, 1971.

Folkow, B.: Physiological aspects of primary hypertension. Physiol. Rev. *62*:347, 1982.

Genest, J., Kuchel, O., Hamet, P., and Cantin, M. (Eds.): Hypertension. 2nd ed. New York, McGraw-Hill Book Co., 1983.

Haddy, F. J., Pamnani, M. B., and Clough, D. L.: Humoral factors and the sodium-potassium pump in volume-expanded hypertension. Life Sci. *24*:2105, 1979.

Hypertension Detection and Follow-Up Program Cooperative Group: Five-year findings of the hypertension detection and follow-up program. 1. Reduction in mortality of persons with high blood pressure, including mild hypertension. J.A.M.A., *242*:2562, 1979.

Laragh, J. H.: Vasoconstriction-volume analysis for understanding and treating hypertension: The use of renin and aldosterone profiles. Am. J. Med. *55*:261, 1973.

Lund-Johansen, P., and Ohm, O. J.: Haemodynamic long-term effects of beta-receptor blocking agents in hypertension: a comparison between alprenolol, atenolol, metoprolol and timolol. Clin. Sci. Mol. Med. *51*:481S, 1976.

Mancia, B., Lorenz, R. R., and Shepherd, J. T.: Reflex control of circulation by heart and lungs. *In* Guyton, A. C., and Cowley, A. W. (Eds.): Cardiovascular Physiology II. Vol. 9. Baltimore, University Park Press, 1976, pp. 111–144.

McGiff, J. C.: Prostaglandins in circulatory disorders. Triangle *18*:101, 1979.

Pickering, T. G., Harshfield, G. A., Kleinert, H. D., Blank, S., and Laragh, J. H.: Blood pressure during normal daily activities, sleep and exercise. J.A.M.A. *247*:992, 1982.

Platt, R.: The nature of essential hypertension. *In* Bock, K. D., and Cottier, P. T. (Eds.): Essential Hypertension. Berlin, Springer Verlag, 1960, p. 39.

Sjostrand, T.: Regulation of blood volume. Scand. J. Clin. Lab. Invest. *36*:209, 1976.

Tarazi, R. C., and Fouad, F. M.: Circulatory dynamics in chronic autonomic insufficiency. *In* Bannister, R. (Ed.): Autonomic Failure. London, Oxford University Press, 1983.

Tarazi, R. C.: Hemodynamics of hypertension. *In* Genest, J., Kuchel, O., and Hamet, P. (Eds.): Hypertension: Physiopathology and Treatment. New York, McGraw-Hill Book Co., 1983, pp. 15–42.

Mechanisms of Cardiac Contraction: Structural, Biochemical, and Functional Relations in the Normal and Diseased Heart

8

Joan Wikman-Coffelt and Dean T. Mason

The clinician has appreciated for many years that major improvements in the understanding and management of heart disease attend advances in knowledge of the fundamental mechanisms making up and governing contraction of cardiac muscle in normal and pathologic states. Although a complete detailed elucidation of the contractile process is not yet available and controversy remains concerning certain of its aspects, intensive investigation undertaken since the 1960s has provided a considerable body of new information that has permitted formulation of the events involved in myocardial contraction in health and disease. These advances have been stimulated by contributions from members of several disciplines, including the clinical investigator, physiologist, pharmacologist, biochemist, and anatomist, through the development of a multiplicity of improved techniques and their application to experimental biologic systems and to patients.

The purpose here is to present the status of this field and the progress that has taken place, particularly at the level of the myocardial cell, in enhancing the clinical understanding of the mechanisms and regulation of contraction of the normal and diseased heart. The discussion that follows is intended to provide an overall integrated conceptual view of the various principal characteristics of the myocardium relating to the complex phenomenon of cardiac contraction. Attention is focused on the subcellular organizational structure of heart muscle and the biochemical processes that control the energy system within the myocardium. Proceeding from this anatomic and metabolic background, the mechanism linking electrical excitation of heart muscle with activation of its contractile machinery is considered, and the molecular biochemical basis of the contractile process itself is analyzed. Finally, the function of the normal and failing heart is assessed in terms of its muscle mechanical properties. Emphasis will be placed on the clinical meaning of the events constituting cardiac contraction in order to trans-

late important basic concepts into improved principles and practical information applicable to evaluation and care of the patient with cardiovascular disease.

MYOCARDIAL ULTRASTRUCTURE

Sophisticated delineation of the microanatomic features of heart muscle has now become possible with the recent development and utilization of modern methods in the examination of cardiac morphology. These studies have shown clearly that there is a definite relationship between the fine spatial architecture of heart muscle (Fig. 8–1) and the contractile mechanism of the functioning ventricle. Thus, a subcellular structural basis has been established for myocardial mechanical activity and cardiac pump performance in which the fundamental individual contractile component is recognized to be the *sarcomere*.

MYOCARDIAL CELL AND MYOFIBRILS

The gross musculature of the ventricles is traditionally described as being encircled by superficial, middle, and deep muscle bundles that arise and insert at the fibrous skeleton of the valve annuli. Spiral bundles represent a transitional continuum with outer and inner fibers at right angles to those in the midwall. Under the light microscope, the muscle bundles are composed of individual branching striated muscle cells, or fibers, approximately 50 μ long and 15 μ wide, oriented in the same direction within a given bundle (Fig. 8–2). In turn, the muscle fiber contains multiple parallel rows of longitudinal *myofibrils* that traverse the entire length of the cell. Each myofibril consists of several of the basic contractile units, sarcomeres, which are joined serially, end to end, in a single line (Fig. 8–2*B*).

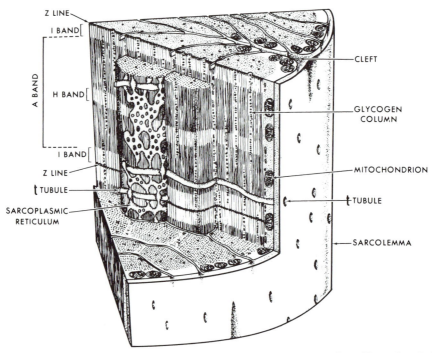

Figure 8–1 Three-dimensional cross-sectional view of a single myocardial cell, or fiber. (Reproduced with permission from Wikman-Coffelt, J., et al.: *In* Mason, D. T. [Ed.]: Congestive Heart Failure. New York, Yorke Medical Books, 1976.)

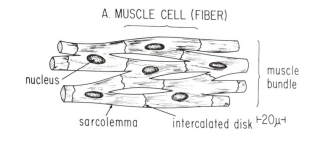

A. MUSCLE CELL (FIBER)

nucleus

muscle bundle

sarcolemma   intercalated disk ⊢20μ⊣

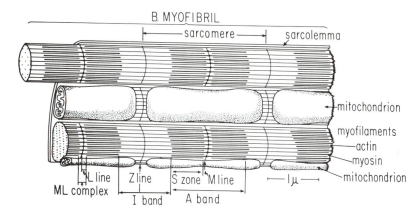

B. MYOFIBRIL

sarcomere   sarcolemma

mitochondrion

myofilaments
actin
myosin
mitochondrion

L line   Z line   S zone   M line   ⊢1μ⊣
ML complex
I band   A band

D. SARCOMERE & MYOFILAMENT
(RELAXED)

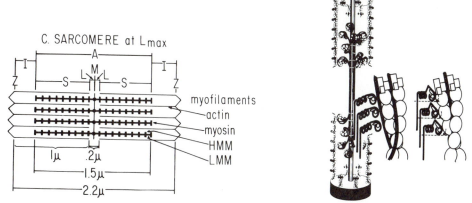

C. SARCOMERE at L$_{max}$

myofilaments
actin
myosin
HMM
LMM

1μ   .2μ
1.5μ
2.2μ

Figure 8–2 *A,* Myocardial structure viewed under light microscope showing syncytium of cells, or fibers. Since the intercalated disks (derivatives of the cell's superficial sarcolemma-transtubular membrane system) represent true cell-to-cell junctions, the myocardium constitutes a functional but not a true anatomic syncytium. *B,* Ultrastructure of longitudinal section of an individual fiber schematized from electron microscope demonstrating parallel myofibrils composed of serially connected sarcomeres in register with sarcomeres of adjacent fibrils. Horizontal rows of mitochondria are situated throughout the cell. *C,* Diagrammatic representation of a sarcomere at L$_{max}$ (resting length at which active tension becomes maximal) showing overlapping arrangement of thick (myosin) and thin (actin) myofilaments. *D,* A sarcomere with three myosin heads protruding and showing their position in relation to the thin filaments in the relaxed state. Following depression of troponin via calcium binding, myosin binds to actin, and contraction commences. S = S zone (area of actin-myosin overlap); HMM = heavy meromyosin; LMM = light meromysin.

SARCOMERE AND MYOFILAMENTS

Further delineation of myocardial morphology, or ultrastructure, requires the resolution and magnification powers of the electron microscope (Fig. 8–3). The sarcomeres themselves are composed of specific arrangements of two sets of overlapping *myofilaments* of contractile proteins: *thick filaments* of myosin molecules and *thin filaments* of actin molecules (Fig. 8–2C). It is the biochemical and biophysical interactions that occur at precise sites between these strands of actin and myosin aggregates that ultimately produce contraction with generation of force and shortening of heart muscle. Within an individual myocardial cell, the sarcomere bodies of neighboring myofibrils lie next to each other with their ends adjacent, so that the banded organization of contractile proteins inside the sarcomere imparts a cross-striated appearance to the muscle fiber.

The relative densities of the cross-bands identify the location of the contractile proteins within the sarcomere (Figs. 8–2C and 8–3). The myosin filaments are indicated by the broad dark *A band* of constant length (1.5 μ in the center portion of the sarcomere); the stationary myosin units are held to each other by linkages at the midpoint of their filaments, shown by the dark M line. Surrounding the myosin units are the sliding actin filaments of constant length (1.0 μ) attached at either end of the sarcomere at the dark Z line, which also connects adjacent sarcomeres at this point. The Z bands and intercalated disks have an important generative function in the production of new sarcomeres (Legato). From the light *I band* of variable dimension, the actin filaments run centrally to be largely covered by the fixed myosin framework. Under physiologic conditions, overall sarcomere length (Z to Z distance) varies during the cardiac cycle between 1.5 and 2.2 μ, depending on the degree of end-diastolic fiber stretch and the extent of shortening during contraction. Immediately lateral on both sides of the M line is a thin light L line. In acutely overstretched skeletal muscle and to a lesser degree in myocardium, a pathologic wide H zone appears, indicating partial

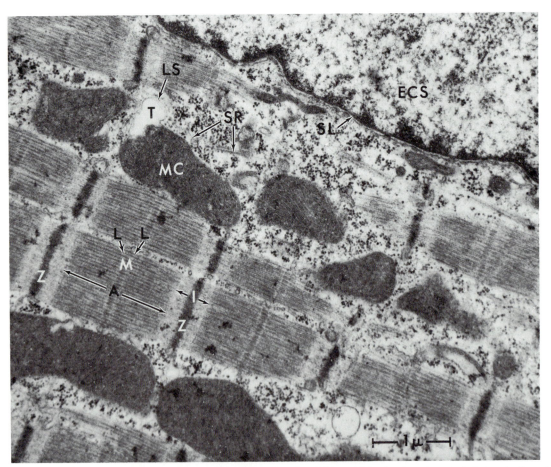

Figure 8–3 Electron micrograph of longitudinal section of canine right ventricle showing characteristic bands (A and I) and lines (Z, M, and L) of sarcomere substructure. Individual sarcomeres are delineated by dark Z lines. MC = mitochondrion; SL = sarcolemma; T = sarcotubule; LS = lateral sac of sarcoplasmic reticulum (SR); ECS = extracellular space.

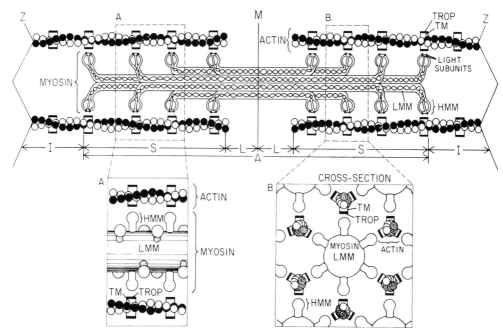

Figure 8–4 Diagrammatic representation of the contractile proteins of heart muscle during relaxation indicating the relative longitudinal configurations and positions of actin and myosin filaments and modulatory proteins, tropomyosin (TM) and troponin (TROP), as viewed by electron microscopy. Each thick filament is composed of horizontal aggregations of myosin molecules with long shafts (light meromyosin: LMM) and cross-bridge heads (heavy meromyosin: HMM) containing light subunits regulating myosin ATPase activity that interact with myosin-binding sites on actin of the thin filament during contraction. Insets *A* (horizontal view) and *B* (cross section) indicate three-dimensional orientation of actin-myosin relationships within the S zone, demonstrating hexagonal lattice of six thin filaments arranged around each thick filament and each thin filament surrounded by three thick filaments.

disengagement of the thick and thin filaments. In contrast, slippage and malalignment of myofibrils appear to be the principal morphologic alterations in chronic excessive dilation of the ventricle. Alterations in molecular composition and physical structure of the contractile proteins and myofilaments themselves are not found in heart failure.

CONTRACTILE PROTEINS: THIN FILAMENTS

Concerning the two primary contractile proteins of the sarcomere, the *actin* and *myosin* chains possess distinct structural and functional properties (Fig. 8–4). The thin filament is principally constituted by two helical chains of globular actin molecules (Figs. 8–4 and 8–5). As observed in cross-section of the sarcomere, each thin filament is surrounded by three thick filaments, and each thick filament is encompassed by six thin filaments (Fig. 8–4*B*). Although actin enhances the enzymatic action of myosin ATPase to more active actomyosin ATPase, there is no enzymatic participation of actin itself in the contractile mechanism. Instead, the physiologic role of actin is its ability to combine reversibly at specific binding sites on the thin filament with the myosin cross-bridges, one myosin head attaching to each active actin

site. Thus, according to the sliding filament theory of contraction offered by Huxley, formation of cross-bridges between active sites of actin and myosin causes inward movement of the thin filament centrally along the fixed thick filament

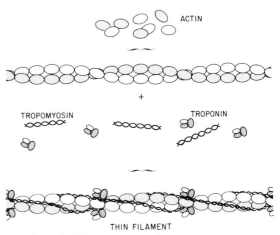

Figure 8–5 Representation of the components of a thin filament. *A*, Depolymerized globular actin. *B*, Polymerized fibrous actin, tropomysin, and troponin. *C*, The reconstituted thin filament composed of fibrous actin with tropomyosin alongside the actin grooves and troponin at each turn of the double helix of actin.

framework. In this contractile process, the lengths of the two filaments remain unchanged while the sarcomere shortens.

In addition to the two primary contractile proteins, actin and myosin, two regulatory proteins, *tropomyosin* and *troponin,* are located along the thin actin filament (Fig. 8–4). Tropomyosin and troponin are not contractile proteins as such but rather they serve a regulatory role in the contractile mechanism of inhibiting or activating the actin-myosin interaction. Tropomyosin molecules lie in elongated chains longitudinally along the paired actin strands of the thin filament. Troponin is attached at regular intervals to tropomyosin, coinciding with the grooves of the actin double helix. During relaxation of cardiac muscles, troponin in consort with tropomyosin prevents cross-bridge reaction between actin and myosin. As demonstrated by Ebashi, troponin contains the receptor protein for the specific binding of calcium in the contractile system. Although calcium is considered in the broad sense as the activator of mechanical contraction, this action actually functions as the specific inactivator of the troponin-tropomyosin complex's inhibition of actin-myosin linkage formation. Two further protein subcomponents complete the troponin structure (Fig. 8–6): a tropomyosin-binding protein and an actin-myosin interaction inhibitor.

For further clarification, the assembly of proteins (actin, tropomyosin, and troponin) that constitute the thin filament is depicted in Figure 8–5. During polymerization, depolymerized globular actin (Fig. 8–5A) is converted to the fibrous form, resulting in a double helix with seven actin molecules to a turn (Fig. 8–5B). Conversion of depolymerized actin to polymerized actin occurs with the addition of ATP and calcium. As also shown in Figure 8–5B, tropomyosin is a long linear molecule composed of two subunits with a double helical conformation. The reconstituted polymerized thin filament is represented in Figure 8–5C. Troponin is a globular molecule, affixed near the end of each tropomyosin molecule, consisting of three subunits termed *troponin I, C, and T* (Fig. 8–6). As indicated, the reaction between actin and myosin is controlled by troponin and tropomyosin. During contraction, actin is *turned on* and reacts with myosin. In contrast, during relaxation actin is *turned off,* thus repulsing myosin with the result that no interaction takes place; a single tropomyosin molecule traverses seven actin molecules, thereby masking the actin sites for interaction with myosin. *Troponin I,* like tropomyosin, has the ability to regulate the interaction between actin and myosin. *Troponin T* serves to bind the troponin complex to tropomyosin. *Troponin C* binds available Ca^{++} for initiation of contraction and deactivates the inhibitory action of troponin I. Thus, troponin C-Ca^{++} becomes a derepressor, exerting a conformational change that forces tropomyosin into the helical groove of actin, thereby exposing the actin sites for interaction with myosin. Recent evidence indicates that phosphorylation of troponin I plays an important role in the contraction process, since this subunit is phosphorylated by myocardial *cyclic AMP-dependent protein kinase.* Phosphorylation of troponin I, activated by isoproterenol, decreases the calcium sensitivity of actomyosin by reducing the affinity of troponin C for calcium. A cross-talk exists between cAMP and calcium. Since cAMP increases the influx of calcium, it would concurrently decrease the calcium sensitivity of troponin and thus help conserve energy by allowing for an increase in rate of contraction and relaxation without correspondingly causing an increase in the number of cross-bridges formed.

CONTRACTILE PROTEINS: THICK FILAMENTS

The thick filament is composed of staggered parallel clusters of a few hundred myosin molecules (Fig. 8–4), each characterized by an elongated rodlike core of interwoven paired helical coils *(light meromyosin)* with globular lateral endings, or heads *(heavy meromyosin).* The globular projection contains the principal functional component of myosin: the cross-bridge of the thick filament that interacts with actin of the thin filament to produce contraction (Fig. 8–4). Further, each globular cross-bridge is paired with light myosin subunits at their termination. These light subunits *(light chains)* of heavy meromyosin are thought to influence the level of enzyme activity of *myosin adenosine triphosphatase* (ATPase)

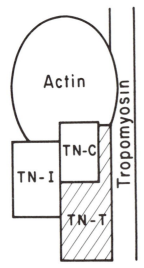

Figure 8–6 Representation of the three subunits of troponin (TN) showing their relation to the other proteins of the thin filament. (Reproduced with permission from Wikman-Coffelt, J., et al.: *In* Mason, D. T. [Ed.]: Congestive Heart Failure. New York, Yorke Medical Books, 1976.)

in the remaining portion of the heavy meromyosin *(heavy chains),* as well as to influence the intensity of the actin-myosin linkage itself (i.e., stroke work). Myosin ATPase splits the terminal phosphate bond off ATP and thereby liberates the energy for the contractile process. The rate of both ATP splitting and stroke work is decreased with a decrease in pH. One can then assume that the velocity and tension of muscle shortening in the heart is decreased with acidity, as occurs in ischemia.

The ultrastructure of interdigitating thick and thin filaments is illustrated in Figure 8–7 as they appear in longitudinal section. Three thick and four thin filaments are shown, tropomyosin is in the groove of the double helix of actin molecules, and troponin is located at every seventh actin molecule. The thick filaments are composed of bundles of myosin molecules, each consisting of a central strand with lateral terminating heads that spiral outward from the core of the cylinder. These

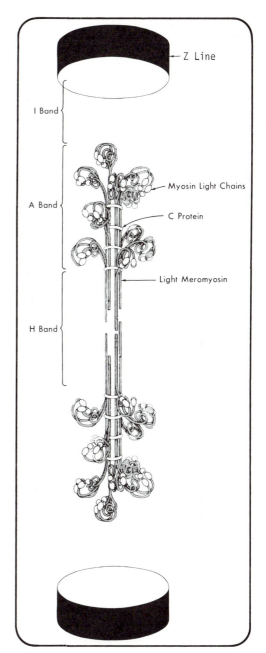

Figure 8–8 Three-dimensional view of a single thick filament containing several pairs of myosin molecules. (Reproduced with permission from Wikman-Coffelt, J., et al.: *In* Mason, D. T. [Ed.]: Congestive Heart Failure. New York, Yorke Medical Books, 1976.)

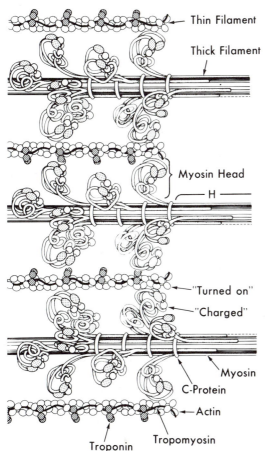

Figure 8–7 Diagrammatic representation of alternating myofilaments in longitudinal view in a portion of a lateral section of thick filaments. H = midzone ML band of the thick filaments. (Reproduced with permission from Wikman-Coffelt, J., et al.: *In* Mason, D. T. [Ed.]: Congestive Heart Failure. New York, Yorke Medical Books, 1976.)

myosin molecules are grouped sequentially so that the myosin heads spiral along both A band sections of the filament. The myosin heads establish cross-bridge contact with actin, and enzymatic activity in the myosin heads takes place. Figure 8–8 provides a three-dimensional view of a single thick filament with several pairs of myosin aggregates.

The manner by which the nature and nomenclature of the myosin fragments of the whole myosin oligomere have been established is represented in Figure 8–9. The proteolytic enzyme trypsin hydrolyzes whole myosin at the *hinge region* (M bridge) to produce two fragment pairs, light meromyosin and heavy meromyosin. Heavy meromyosin is separated by papain digestion into its two components: *heavy meromyosins S_1 and S_2* (Fig. 8–9). Figure 8–10 delineates the configuration of one (220,000 molecular weight) of the two heavy chains constituting whole myosin. The *myosin head* (heavy meromyosin S_1) contains two light chains wrapped within this segment, and it is specifically this heavy chain S_1 component in which the ATPase activity of myosin and the site of myosin that forms the cross-bridge with actin are contained. Heavy chain S_2 meromyosin forms a tight helix, whereas meromyosin S_1 is elliptically shaped (Fig. 8–10). Light meromyosin constitutes the backbone of the thick filaments. Movement of the heavy meromyosin S_1 head, by changing the degree of its *head angle* (Fig. 8–10), results in pushing the thin filaments together during contraction. This is diagrammatically summarized in Figure 8–11.

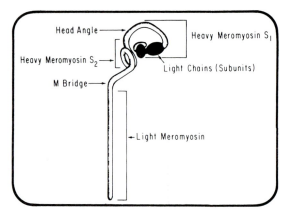

Figure 8–10 Representation of the configuration of one of the two heavy chains of whole myosin. The myosin heavy chain is composed of light meromyosin and heavy meromyosin (HMM). The M bridge is between light and heavy meromyosin, and the head angle is between heavy meromyosins S_1 and S_2. In addition, two myosin light chains are bound within the heavy chain myosin head (HMM S_1). (Reproduced with permission from Wikman-Coffelt, J., et al.: *In* Mason, D. T. [Ed.]: Congestive Heart Failure. New York, Yorke Medical Books, 1976.)

SUPERFICIAL MEMBRANE SYSTEM

In addition to the sarcomere contractile apparatus that occupies approximately one half the myocardial fiber, there are other important specialized subcellular constituents. The individual myocardial fibers are covered by the *sarcolemma*

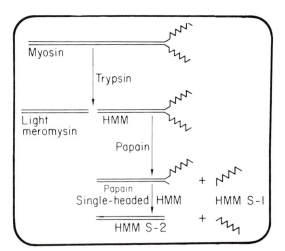

Figure 8–9 Separation of the components of whole myosin by cleavage with proteolytic enzymes. Trypsin produces the two major fragments: light meromyosin and heavy meromyosin (HMM). Papain digestion results in division of heavy meromyosin into its S_2 and S_1 fragments. (Reproduced with permission from Wikman-Coffelt, J., et al.: *In* Mason, D. T. [Ed.]: Congestive Heart Failure. New York, Yorke Medical Books, 1976.)

membrane, of which the *intercalated disks* and *transverse tubular system* are derivatives of major significance (Figs. 8–1, 8–3, and 8–12). The intercalated disks are situated at intercellular junctions between the terminal sarcomeres of the cell, thereby locking fibers together at their ends. In the ventricular myocardium, deep invaginations at frequent intervals of the sarcolemma from the fiber surface vertically into the interior of each cell constitute the complex transtubular network, or T system. The intercalated disks and transverse tubular membranes provide pathways for rapid transmission of the depolarizing impulses that electrically excite adjacent fibers and the intracellular membrane sarcomere contractile system. In addition to contributing a vehicle for excitation, the transtubular system provides a comprehensive extension of the extracellular space throughout the cell so that transmembrane cation transport of sodium, potassium, and calcium accompanying depolarization, repolarization, excitation-contraction coupling, and relaxation occurs quickly and synchronously within myocardial fibers. Furthermore, the T system furnishes a conduit for ready entry and egress of metabolites and other substances between the interstitial medium and the sarcoplasm, and access is afforded to cardiovascular drugs, such as digitalis and antiarrhythmic agents, for their action on intracellular membranes and related enzyme systems in the vicinity of the contractile apparatus within the entire fiber, even if the drugs do not actually cross the membrane in clinically meaningful doses.

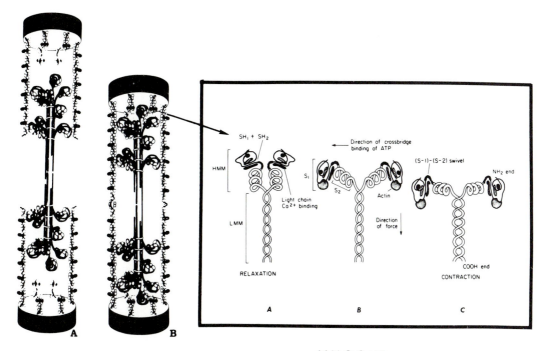

SARCOMERE

MYOSIN

Figure 8–11 A sarcomere in the relaxed *(A)* and contracted *(B)* state (left panel). The inset (right panel) shows the conformation of myosin during relaxation *(A)*, during the binding of actin *(B)*, and during contraction *(C)*. (Reproduced with permission from Wikman-Coffelt, J., et al.: Am. Heart J. *103*:935, 1982.)

SARCOPLASMIC RETICULUM

An extensive intracellular tubular membrane system, the *sarcoplasmic reticulum* (Figs. 8–1, 8–3, and 8–12), complements the transtubular T system structurally and functionally in support of the process of excitation-contraction coupling and mechanical relaxation. The T-tubular system is in contact with the extracellular environment and runs a vertical pathway through the width of the sarcomere I bands. The sarcoplasmic reticulum is entirely within the cell, and its general orientation is at right angles to the T system, so that the sarcotubular structure courses longitudinally in the A band region (actin-myosin cross-bridge area) along the rows of sarcomeres with multiple branching interconnections. *Lateral sac* cuff modifications *(terminal cisternae)* of the narrow sar-

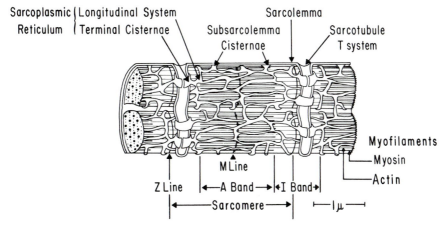

Figure 8–12 Longitudinal diagram of myocardial ultrastructure reconstructed from electron micrographs showing relationships between the superficial (sarcolemma and wide T system) and intracellular (sarcoplasmic reticulum) membranes of the cardiac fiber.

coplasmic reticulum (longitudinal L system) occur at its point of contact with the wider T system in the lateral I band on one side of the Z line. The sarcotubular lateral sacs store calcium; the intracellular transport of calcium from this area is important in linking membrane excitation with troponin of the contractile apparatus. Also, lateral sacs abut the intercalated disks and sarcolemma to provide each of the specialized membranes with a complete system for excitation-contraction coupling. An interesting exception is the Purkinje cell, which has no transverse tubular system. Perhaps dissimilarities in the electrical and contractile responses of different types of cardiac cells to pharmacologic agents are, in part, the result of variations in the extent and nature of development of the transtubular network and inherent modifications in the characteristics of the superficial membranes.

MITOCHONDRIA

The final myocardial substructure to be considered is the *mitochondrion,* which contains the aerobic biochemical systems of the fiber (Figs. 8–1, 8–3, and 8–12). The mitochondria, located between the myofibrils, are abundant in accordance with the heart's high requirement for oxygen, and they constitute nearly 30 per cent of the myocardial cell. The mitochondria, situated near the A bands and thus myosin ATPase, are the metabolic power plants in which oxygen and appropriate substrates are utilized to produce ATP, the final direct energy source for myocardial contraction and other biochemical reactions. In the cytoplasm or sarcoplasm, glycogen granules are stored and the process of anaerobic glycolysis is operative. Morphologically, the mitochondrion is surrounded by a membrane from which there are numerous cristae infoldings on which the process of oxidative phosphorylation takes place. In addition, the mitochondrial membranes are capable of accumulating calcium, which might serve as an internal buffer against abnormal rises of sarcoplasmic calcium during diastole and perhaps might represent a mechanism influencing myocardial compliance or a source of activator calcium.

MYOCARDIAL METABOLISM

The principal biochemical processes that relate to the ultimate contractile function of the ventricle include those involved in regulation of energy metabolism, contractile machinery of the sarcomere, the muscle relaxing system, electrical and transport activity of the membranes, and protein synthesis within the fiber. It is emphasized that these chemical mechanisms are interrelated, and alterations in any one of them may influence activity in the other pathways. For conceptual

purposes, the sequence of reactions important in myocardial energy metabolism is substrate availability and energy production, storage, and utilization.

ENERGETICS

Normal heart muscle is uniquely dependent on *aerobic* metabolism for its energy supply. To satisfy this need, the myocardium requires the delivery of a continuous supply of large quantities of oxygen via the coronary circulation. The oxygen demand of the heart is considerably greater than for other organs, and, since myocardial oxygen extraction is nearly maximal at body rest, increases in oxygen need are primarily accomplished by elevations of coronary blood flow. *Myocardial oxygen consumption* of the ventricle is principally determined by three hemodynamic-related variables: (1) intramyocardial systolic tension (primarily governed by systolic pressure and ventricular volume); (2) contractility; and (3) heart rate (Fig. 8–13). In addition to these three major determinants, external work or ventricular shortening *(Fenn effect),* energy of activation-relaxation, and basal diastolic energy requirements contribute to a relatively minor degree to overall myocardial oxygen requirements (Fig. 8–13). In considering the effects of an intervention on myocardial oxygen consumption, such as with the administration of digitalis or nitroglycerin, one must appreciate that the final result quantitatively is dependent on the entire hemodynamic functional status of the heart, an interplay among the more important factors regulating oxygen utilization, and the summation of their individual actions.

Oxidative Phosphorylation. Since ATP is the immediate energy source for the contractile apparatus and biochemical reactions elsewhere in the cell, myocardial energy metabolism is normally directed toward aerobic production of ATP in the mitochondria by substrate oxidation (dehydrogenation of citric acid intermediates requiring nicotinamide adenine dinucleotide), with discharge of carbon dioxide in the *Krebs cycle,* consequent transport of hydrogen and its electrons through the respiratory chain of flavoproteins and cytochromes (resulting in oxygen consumption and making of water), and *oxidative phosphorylation,* in which inorganic phosphate acquires a high-energy bond and combines with adenosine diphosphate (ADP) to form ATP (Fig. 8–14). Schwartz has shown depressed mitochondrial energy production in the severely failing myocardium, whereas respiratory function in the mitochondria is increased in the hypertrophied heart prior to failure. Although abnormalities in mitochondrial energy metabolism may contribute to myocardial dysfunction in heart failure, these biochemical aberrations generally are not considered causative of failure due to chronic hemodynamic overload.

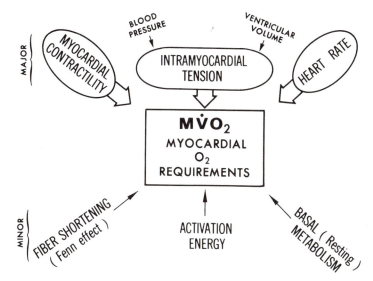

Figure 8–13 Major and minor determinants of myocardial oxygen consumption (MV̇O₂).

The predominant substrate fuel for myocardial ATP synthesis consists of the circulating *free fatty acids,* consumption of which accounts for the majority of oxygen extracted by the heart. Concerning other primary substrates, normally *blood glucose* is used preferentially in the postprandial state. Circulating lactate is also an important fuel, particularly when its blood concentration is evaluated by prolonged skeletal muscle exercise. Blood pyruvate, like glucose, lactate, and free fatty acids, is readily taken up by the myocardium in proportion to its arterial blood concentration. Blood-borne ketone bodies and even amino acids may serve as substrates in certain abnormal conditions. Conversion of the substrate fuels into acetyl-coenzyme A is necessary for their entry into the citric acid cycle for aerobic ATP production. Concerning blood glucose as substrate in myocardial energy systems, after the substance is transported across the sarcolemma-transtubular membranes and metabolized to glucose-6-phosphate under the influence of insulin, it may be stored as glycogen or undergo an aerobic glycolysis to pyruvate in the sarcoplasm. In normal conditions, pyruvate is oxidized to acetyl-coenzyme A and undergoes aerobic metabolism in the citric acid cycle within the mitochondria.

Lactate acts as a relief valve for excess NADH. Oxidation of NADH in the mitochondria leads to ATP production, as shown in Figure 8–15. Two NADHs are produced per glycosyl unit. They are transported into the mitochondria via the citric acid cycle; if this transport is slow, as in the glucose-perfused heart, NADH accumulates and can have a feedback inhibition on glycolysis. In order to prevent accumulation, it is oxidized via lactic dehydrogenase as pyruvate is converted to lactate (Fig. 8–16). In the glucose-perfused heart, in which glucose is the only substrate, one can observe cyclical changes in the pyruvate:lactate and ATP:ADP ratios that are due to this slow transport of NADH into mitochondria.

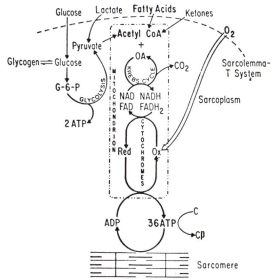

Figure 8–14 Metabolic pathways for energy (ATP) production shown diagrammatically within the cardiac cell. NAD = nicotinamide adenine dinucleotide; FAD = flavin adenine dinucleotide; NADH = reduced NAD; FADH₂ = reduced FAD; Ox = oxidation; Red = reduction; CP = creatine phosphate; C = creatine; G-6-P = glucose-6-phosphate. See text for further explanation.

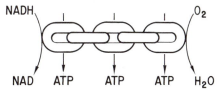

Figure 8–15 Diagrammatic representation of the electron transport chain showing the oxidation of NADH and the reduction of oxygen to water. The by-product is ATP.

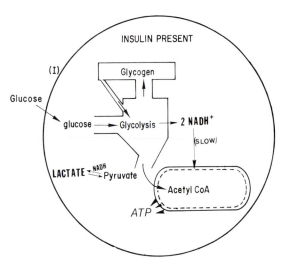

Figure 8–16 Diagrammatic depiction of the glycolytic mill in a muscle fiber. Lactic dehydrogenase uses NADH in the conversion of pyruvate to lactate.

Anaerobic Glycolysis. The importance of *anaerobic glycolysis* as a source of energy varies with the state of oxygenation of the myocardium. Normally, glycolysis is of considerably less significance, since this entire process results in only two ATP molecules for each molecule of glucose, whereas each glucose molecule provides 36 molecules of ATP in the aerobic pathways (Fig. 8–14). When myocardial oxygen delivery falls, there is increased glycolysis, although this is an ineffective process alone for maintaining energy supply, and ATP levels decline. Also, less pyruvate enters the citric acid cycle during enhanced glycolytic metabolism in myocardial hypoxia. Consequently, in the heart relatively deprived of oxygen, pyruvate is reduced to *lactate*.

Oxidative phosphorylation acts as a proton "sink" for all the H^+ produced during contraction. One H^+ is produced per each ATP hydrolyzed by myosin. With a decrease in oxidative phosphorylation, the H^+ sink is lost and intracellular acidity builds up. There is an equilibrium of H^+ during glycolysis; lactate cannot ionize at a physiologic pH. A shift in metabolism occurs with a decrease in oxidative phosphorylation such that a conducive pH is eventually reached, promoting extracellular transport of undesirable by-products. One such product is lactate.

The hypoxic myocardium may produce more lactate than it consumes, with the result that coronary sinus blood will contain more lactate than systemic arterial blood. In contrast, lactate concentration is greater in arterial blood than in the coronary venous effluent in the normally metabolizing heart owing to myocardial lactate extraction for aerobic synthesis of ATP. By selective catheterization of the coronary sinus, Gorlin has shown that detection of abnormal myocardial lac-

tate metabolism or balance provides a useful biochemical means for the objective identification of myocardial ischemia in patients with coronary artery disease. Furthermore, when the abnormality is not present at rest in patients with angina pectoris, it can often be revealed by increasing the mechanical and metabolic activity of the heart by the performance of exercise, by increasing heart rate with a pacemaker catheter, or by administration of isoproterenol.

Creatine Phosphate. In regard to myocardial energy storage, *creatine phosphate* functions as a limited reservoir of high-energy phosphate to maintain ATP. Thus, following the cleavage of ATP by myofibrillar ATPase to ADP and inorganic phosphate in the contraction reaction and by the additional myocardial ATPases in other biochemical processes requiring energy utilization, ADP is replenished with a high-energy phosphate from creatine phosphate or by oxidative phosphorylation to re-form ATP.

The buffering action of phosphocreatine is depicted in Figure 8–17. The forward action of phosphocreatine to ATP utilizes an H^+. With the increase in intracellular acidity, the reaction increases in the forward direction. As a result, in ischemia phosphocreatine is depleted before ATP. In some types of heart failure, phosphocreatine is decreased more than ATP; whereas in cardiomyopathy in hamsters, ATP is decreased to a greater extent than phosphocreatine. This may be due to a deficiency in nucleotides in the heart failure state. Along with the decrease in high-energy phosphates, there is an increase in the end products, ADP and inorganic phosphate. The accumulation of end products may decrease the free energy of ATP hydrolysis to a point at which the calcium pump may be hindered. Such a decrease in the free energy of ATP hydrolysis in heart failure has been associated with a decrease in contractility. However, along with the decrease in high energy phosphates and the increase in end products there is a shift in metabolism and an increase in intracellular acidity. Acidity, however, is known to decrease actin-activated myosin ATPase activity

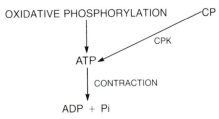

Figure 8–17 Phosphocreatine buffers ATP via creatine kinase. ATP is resynthesized mainly through either oxidative phosphorylation or phosphocreatine. Both forms of replenishing ATP utilize protons, thus balancing the hydrogen ions produced during contraction and maintaining the pH in equilibrium.

and thereby affect cardiac performance. Thus, it may not be possible to separate intracellular acidity from a decrease in high-energy phosphates. The two may be interrelated and work concurrently to cause a decrease in contractility.

PROTEIN SYNTHESIS

The mechanisms of protein synthesis in the heart are generally the same as those in other organs. Protein synthesis in the myocardium provides a continuously operative system for renewal of fiber structure and enzymatic machinery, as well as a rapidly responsive compensatory mechanism for ventricular hypertrophy induced by cardiac mechanical stress. ATP is consumed in the process of protein synthesis, which consists of the stages of (1) *replication* in the nucleus (DNA-controlled synthesis of DNA by *DNA polymerase*); (2) *transcription* in the nucleus, in which nucleoli are centers of RNA activity (RNA synthesis by *RNA polymerase* on the chromosomal template); and (3) *translation,* involving three types of RNA in the sarcoplasm (formation of specific proteins on ribosomal RNA, directed by messenger RNA containing the genetic code, from amino acids carried by transfer RNA).

Excessive intramyocardial tension appears to be the transducer that couples mechanical systolic overload with increased protein synthesis. Increased muscle mass resulting from chronic elevation of hemodynamic burden is due to hypertrophy rather than hyperplasia of myocardial fibers, although there is some proliferation of connective tissue cells. Activation of all stages of protein synthesis occurs rapidly after hemodynamic stress, with increases in DNA in connective tissue cells and elevation of RNA synthesis and incorporation of amino acids into proteins in myocardial cells. For example, even the creation of acute mild pulmonary stenosis in dogs is a potent stimulus

for RNA and protein synthesis within 24 hours after pulmonary banding, resulting in substantially increased weight of the hypertrophied right ventricle with correspondingly increased myosin content.

Transcription. Transcription is the process by which genetic information, stored in nuclear DNA, is transferred to RNA. The result is the formation of nucleotide polymers containing triplet codons corresponding to those found in DNA. The regulation of the transcription system involving a repressor is depicted in Figure 8–18. In the transcription process of gene control, a regulatory gene directs the synthesis of a specific protein; the repressor binds to a metabolite or hormone and serves as the regulatory signal. This binding can either activate or inactivate the repressor, depending on whether the system is repressive or inductive. The repressor in its active state binds the genetic operator and prevents production of messenger RNA from the associated structural gene. In contrast, in an inductive system, the operator remains repressed until the regulatory metabolite complexes with and prevents function of the repressor. With this model of gene control applied to the myosin system via the transcription process, the cell possesses the ability to respond rapidly to new environmental stress, such as excessive ventricular hemodynamic burden leading to myocardial hypertrophy. Further, the rapid elevation in RNA synthesis that occurs (for example, in the right ventricle with pulmonary stenosis) may be aided by the availability of an additional factor that acts as an inducer at the transcriptional level.

Translation. Translation is the cellular process through which information that has been transcribed to RNA is utilized to produce proteins (Fig. 8–19). Protein synthesis takes place on cellular particles called *ribosomes* that travel along the instruction tape of messenger RNA reading the genetic message. The process of translation is divided into three stages: (1) initiation; (2) elon-

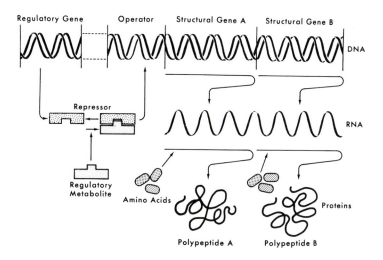

Figure 8–18 Diagram of two genes under one operator constituting a genome and the regulatory gene codes for the repressor, which in turn has the ability to repress or induce transcription of the genome, depending on the presence of certain metabolites in the system. (Reproduced with permission from Wikman-Coffelt, J., et al.: *In* Mason, D. T. [Ed.]: Congestive Heart Failure. New York, Yorke Medical Books, 1976.)

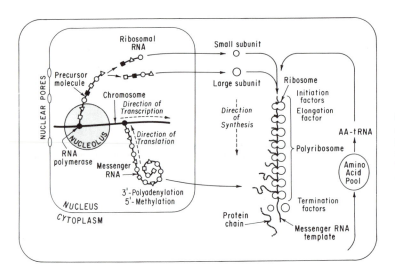

Figure 8–19 Diagram of transcription in the cytoplasm. The transcription of ribosomal RNA is restricted to the nucleolus. The two ribosomal RNA molecules (28S and 18S RNA) are derived from the larger parent precursor molecule, which separates into the two.

gation; and (3) termination. Before the sequence of translation is discussed, it is beneficial to examine the three different types of RNA involved in the process and the respective role of each type of RNA.

Ribosomal RNA (rRNA) is one of the three major types of RNA manufactured during the process of transcription. This type of RNA is transcribed from genes located on chromosomes found in the nucleolus. Initially, a precursor RNA molecule is formed and later cleaved to form an 18S and a 28S RNA subunit. The 28S subunit combines with several types of proteins, moves out of the nucleus, and eventually forms the 60S component of the ribosomes. Likewise, the 18S subunit combines with protein, as well as with a smaller 5S RNA molecule, and thus forms the 40S component of the ribosome. The many different proteins that compose the ribosome are in equilibrium with a pool of free ribosomal proteins in the cytoplasm of the cell. The turnover rate varies for each of these proteins.

Messenger RNA (mRNA) is the second of the three types of RNA made in the nucleus and transported to the cytoplasm for production of a protein such as myosin. The mRNA molecules for myosin heavy chains have been purified. It appears that both mRNA and its carrier protein are complexed to the smaller ribosomal subunits when they reach the cytoplasm (Fig. 8–19). When mRNA was purified from the cytoplasm of various cells, it was found to be characterized by its long stretches of polyadenylic acid, one of the four nucleotides constituting RNA. Unlike rRNA and tRNA (discussed subsequently), mRNA has little tertiary structure and is thus very susceptible to ribonuclease cleavage.

Transfer RNA (tRNA) is the third type of RNA molecule. It is the smallest of the three. Several tRNA varieties have been sequenced, and it has been found that the molecule has an over-

all clover-leaf configuration, with about 80 per cent of its nucleotides paired. Each amino acid has specific tRNA varieties to which it binds. Further, each amino acid also has a specific aminoacyl-tRNA synthetase enzyme that is responsible for mediating this binding reaction. Certain regions of these individual tRNA molecules contain the anticodon that can match up with the corresponding mRNA codon. This system provides the capacity for accurate recognition between amino acid and code of the mRNA to ensure the proper placement of each amino acid in precise sequences in the formation of a specific polypeptide chain.

Specific Protein Synthesis. Protein synthesis is initiated by the complexing of mRNA to the 40S particle of the ribosome. This event is followed by the combination of the 40S particle with the associated mRNA to the larger 60S subunit of the ribosome. To begin translation of the mRNA tape, various soluble initiation factors are required. Certain of these factors, along with guanosine 5'-triphosphate (GTP) and the correct concentration of magnesium (Mg^{++}) and ammonium (NH_4^+) ions, provide the condition for the binding of the first tRNA-associated amino acid to the initiating codon of the mRNA.

The complete ribosome contains two binding sites for tRNA. One site, located on the 40S ribosomal subunit, is designated the *aminoacyl-tRNA binding site*; the other site on the subunit is referred to as the *peptidyl-tRNA binding site*. The specific tRNA associated with amino acid formylmethionine is required for the initiation of translation. It appears that the structure of this molecule enables it to move directly from the aminoacyl site to the peptidyl site on the ribosome, despite the fact that it has only one amino acid bound to it. This translocation reaction allows the binding of a new tRNA and associated amino acid to the recently vacated 30S site of the ribosome. It is believed that the hydrolysis of GTP provides the energy needed in this translocation reaction. Two soluble factors, aminoacyl transferase I and II, along with sulfhydryl compounds and Mg^{++} and NH_4^+, also play a role in this translocation.

The peptide bond formation necessary to bind the two separate amino acids is catalyzed by peptidyl synthetase, located in the 60S ribosomal subunit, and does not require soluble initiation factors or GTP. By continuing the cycle of tRNA binding, peptide bond formation, and translocation, it is possible to form peptides containing specific amino acid sequences governed by the code provided by the mRNA (Fig. 8–20).

Protein synthesis is concluded when the ribosome reads a terminator codon located on the mRNA. The terminator codon, in conjunction with certain releasing factors, dissociates the ribosome into its original 40S and 60S subunits and provides for the release of the protein and mRNA. Interestingly, it is possible for several ribosomes to read a single mRNA molecule at the same time. In this situation, the group of ribosomes is referred to as a *polyribosome*.

Myosin Synthesis. Increase in myosin synthesis is accompanied by augmentation of myosin ATPase activity in certain situations, such as in the stressed ventricle in the presence of mild pulmonary or mild aortic stenosis. At the same time, in these specific hemodynamic situations, the proportion of myosin heavy chains to myosin light chains is increased. In other studies, it has been shown that myosin heavy chains have a turnover rate that is twice that of myosin light chains. A phenomenon such as the disparate turnover rates of light and heavy chains of myosin may be the result of regulation at the level of translation or transcription.

It is possible that a type of regulation at the translation level described for hemoglobin occurs in myosin synthesis: a selective translation of α or β chains, depending on the presence of messenger-specific translational factors. The greater turnover rate of myosin heavy chains may be due to greater affinity of availability of translational factors for the messenger for myosin heavy chains.

Conversely, the greater synthesis of myosin heavy chains in comparison with that of light chains may be due to control at the transcriptional level. As shown in Figure 8–18, each of the myosin chains may be under different genetic control, so that an activator of one gene would not necessarily be a potent activator of other genes. Gene amplification, which constitutes multiple copies of certain genome sequences, occurs in mammalian tissues. The possibility exists that there is redundance of genes for myosin chains. Gene duplication facilitates speedy transcription when certain molecules are in great demand, such as occurs with ribosomes. This allows for several simultaneous transcriptions of the same type of molecule. Thus, it is speculated that there may be various degrees of gene duplication of the myosin chains (Fig. 8–18), with each of the light and heavy chains having its code in a separate genome controlled by its own operator.

As shown by Meerson, Rabinowitz and Nair, and others, activation of all stages of protein synthesis occurs rapidly following acute stress, with increased DNA in connective tissue cells and elevations of RNA and incorporation of amino acids into proteins in myocardial cells. With chronic hemodynamic overload, however, there is some diminution of these processes.

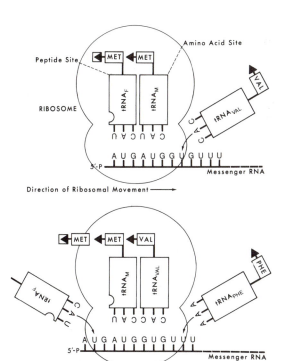

Figure 8–20 Diagram of translation occurring on the messenger RNA complexed to the ribosome. The process of translation begins at the 5′ end of the messenger RNA. The transfer RNA molecules are shuttling amino acids to the peptide site to form the growing peptide chain. (Reproduced with permission from Wikman-Coffelt, J., et al.: *In* Mason, D. T. [Ed.]: Congestive Heart Failure. New York, Yorke Medical Books, 1976.)

CYCLIC AMP (cAMP)

Another important biochemical system in heart muscle is that involved with the intracellular regulatory substance, cyclic AMP (*adenosine monophosphate*), discovered by Sutherland. Cyclic AMP is synthesized in the sarcoplasm from ATP by stimulation of the enzyme adenylate cyclase of the plasma sarcolemma and transtubular membranes. The activity of adenylate cyclase is enhanced by beta-adrenergic receptor stimulation located also in the plasma membranes. It has been suggested that the positive inotropic action of several cardiovascular agents is mediated by activation of this process leading to increased cAMP formation: catecholamines by stimulation of the beta receptor, and glucagon, thyroid hormone, and tolbutamide by direct action on adenylate cyclase. Furthermore, the increased contractility produced by aminophylline has been attributed to the drug's ability to inhibit phosphodiesterase, an intracellular enzyme that inactivates cAMP. The mechanism through which cAMP increases myocardial glycogenolysis has been established (cyclic nucleotide stimulation of protein kinase causes phosphorylation of phosphorylase kinase from ATP, which in turn activates the phosphorylase enzyme, degrading glycogen). Concerning the significance of cAMP in the modulation of cardiac contraction, evidence suggests that myocardial cAMP-dependent protein kinase phosphorylates protein components in sarcoplasmic reticulum governing calcium transport and in troponin itself, thereby influencing the effects of calcium in the contractile reaction. Cyclic AMP is essential to contraction. It plays both a regulatory and a modulatory role in the cardiac cycle. The influx of calcium with membrane depolarization may increase intracellular cAMP levels, perhaps through calcium activation of calmodulin. Thus, cAMP increases with depolarization but is rapidly degraded; by the end of peak systole, the cAMP values are returned to levels similar to those seen in the resting phase. Oscillations of cAMP with the cardiac cycle are shown in Figure 8–21. Cyclic AMP modulates the slow calcium channels. Levels of free calcium appear to regulate cAMP concentrations, and levels of cAMP regulate calcium concentrations. This cross-talk between calcium and cAMP appears to occur not only at the level of message transmission but also at the level of the response to calcium or cAMP-dependent protein phosphorylation. Immediately following an increased workload on the heart, there is an augmentation of cAMP, whereas in heart failure there appears to be a deficiency of cAMP. Concerning the heart failure state, adenylate cyclase activity is not altered, but its stimulation by certain cardiovascular agents may be impaired.

NOREPINEPHRINE

Examination of the biosynthesis of *myocardial norepinephrine* is important in the consideration of mechanisms governing mechanical performance of heart muscle, since this hormone is the neurotransmitter directly linking cardiac sympathetic activity with beta receptor stimulation, resulting in elevated contractility and heart rate. The sympathetic nervous system normally exerts a major regulatory role in the augmentation of cardiovascular function in response to increased metabolic demands of the peripheral tissues, such as during physical exercise. The rich sympathetic innervation of heart muscle permits the heart to produce the majority of its own norepinephrine requirements. In the terminals of sympathetic nerves, norepinephrine is synthesized through a series of steps from tyrosine, in which *tyrosine hydroxylase* is the rate-limiting enzyme. The neurotransmitter is stored in the nerve ending in granules that protect it from enzymatic destruction by monoamine oxidase in the neuronal cytoplasm. In response to sympathetic impulses, norepinephrine is released to activate myocardial beta receptors. Importantly, in the failing heart the activity of

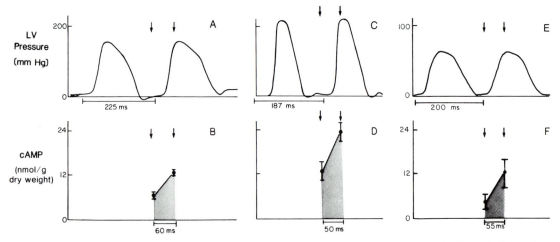

Figure 8–21 Pressure tracings *(A, C,* and *E)* and corresponding myocardial cAMP values *(B, D,* and *F)* are shown. Rat hearts were perfused for 20 min and then freeze-clamped at points in the cardiac cycle as indicated by the arrows (i.e., at the end of diastole 10 msec prior to stimulation and at peak force). In *A* and *B,* rat hearts were perfused with 2.5 mM calcium. In *C* and *D,* rat hearts were perfused with 3.5 mM free calcium and 10^{-8} M isoproterenol. In *E* and *F,* rat hearts were perfused with 0.8 mM free calcium. (Reproduced with permission from Wikman-Coffelt, J., et al.: Biochem. Biophys. Res. Commun. *111*:450, 1983.)

tyrosine hydroxylase is markedly reduced, thus resulting in severe decrease of myocardial norepinephrine. The depression of norepinephrine appears to be the result of disturbed metabolic function in the neuron rather than actual loss of neural tissue. While this defect deprives the dysfunctioning ventricle of an adaptive mechanism for increasing its contractility, the depletion of myocardial norepinephrine is not responsible for the intrinsic weakness of the failing muscle. In heart failure, there is supersensitivity of myocardial beta receptors to circulating norepinephrine, and blood levels of this hormone are elevated because of its increased synthesis in the peripheral vasculature and the adrenal medulla; thus, this supporting mechanism is restored, in part, to the failing heart.

It is apparent that a number of highly important biochemical processes are operative in the intact ventricle. Their complete integrity of function and proper integration are essential to normal mechanical and hemodynamic performance of the heart. Although aberrations have been identified in certain of these systems in the failing myocardium, the current view is that abnormalities in myocardial energy metabolism, protein synthesis, AMP reactions, and norepinephrine production may contribute by encroaching on compensatory mechanisms but do not play the primary causative role in the onset of congestive heart failure induced by chronic hemodynamic overload. A more promising probability is that the biochemical defect or constellation of abnormalities resides in the mechanism of excitation-contraction coupling and the function of the contractile proteins.

EXCITATION-CONTRACTION COUPLING AND THE CONTRACTILE PROCESS

ELECTRICAL EXCITATION

The electrical event constituting excitation of the myocardial fiber involves *depolarization* of the cell by rapid ingress of sodium into the sarcoplasm (*phase 0 spike* of the *action potential*) (Fig. 8–22), followed by egress extracellularly of an equal amount of potassium (repolarization of the action potential). Depolarization and repolarization do not require ATP energy. Instead, the rapid Na^+ influx constituting complete phase 0 depolarization is a passive process that appears to be governed by activated Na^+ carriers (electrostatically controlled fast membrane channels or pores). The rate of rise of the spike action potential determines *conduction velocity;* relative to the surface EKG, phase 0 depolarization in the ventricles is denoted by the QRS complex, in the atria by the P wave, and collectively by the P–R interval in the sinoatrial node and the atrioventricular node.

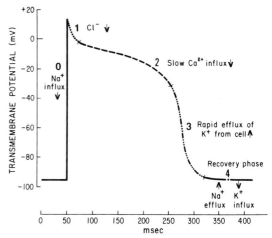

Figure 8–22 Diagram of ventricular muscle fiber action potential correlating phasic voltage changes with flux of cations in and out of the cell during the cardiac cycle.

The relationship of a wave of depolarization to a pressure tracing in the rat heart is shown in Figure 8–23A. Free calcium as demonstrated by aequorin measurements, as described by Wier, is shown in Figure 8–23B. In Figure 8–23C, the increase in cAMP in relation to a pressure tracing and the wave of depolarization is shown.

Although the *repolarization* period is signified by three stages (phases 1, 2, and 3), the mechanism is accomplished most quickly during *phase 3* by rapid K^+ efflux from the fiber (Fig. 8–22). More germane to the present discussion of the subcel-

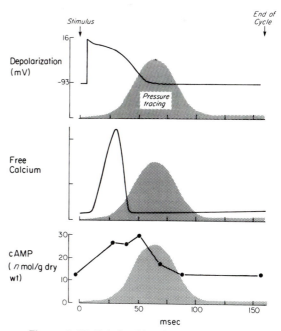

Figure 8–23 Relationship of depolarization, calcium influx, and cyclical changes in cAMP with an intraventricular pressure tracing.

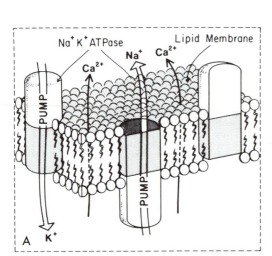

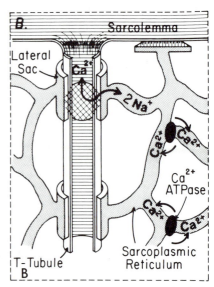

Figure 8–24 *A,* Diagram of the transtubular cell membrane composed of phospholipids interspersed with the Na^+ – K^+ ATPase pump proteins operative during diastole (phase 4) establishing the increased extracellular Na^+ and increased intracellular K^+ gradients. *B,* The transtubular cell membrane proteins mediating the Na^+ – Ca^{++} exchange system are shown associated with the sarcoplasmic reticulum. The T-tubules mediate such exchange between the sarcoplasmic reticulum and the extracellular space during phases 2 (Ca^{++} entrance) and 4 (Ca^{++} exit) of the electrophysiologic cycle.

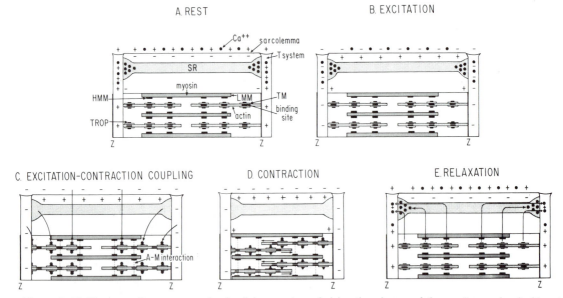

Figure 8–25 Diagrammatic sequence of subcellular events underlying the phases of the cardiac cycle. *A,* At rest, extracellular calcium (solid dots) is concentrated in the interstitial medium around the sarcolemma and in the T system, and intracellular calcium (solid dots) is sequestered in the lateral sacs of the sarcoplasmic reticulum (SR). *B,* With electrical excitation, complete depolarization of the fiber occurs by rapid influx of sodium during phase O of the spike action potential, resulting in positive intracellular voltage. *C,* Excitation-contraction coupling is triggered by excitation, resulting in release of intracellular calcium from the SR and entry of extracellular calcium during phase 2 of the action potential, with delivery of calcium (arrows) to troponin of the contractile apparatus within the sarcomeres. Calcium binding to troponin derepresses troponin (TROP)-tropomyosin (TM) inhibition of myosin linkage with specific binding site on actin. Thereby, actin-myosin (A-M) interaction initiates contraction. *D,* The process of contraction occurs through sequential making and breaking of A-M interconnections, with consequent sliding of actin centrally (arrows) along the fixed myosin filaments, producing force development and sarcomeric shortening. *E,* Relaxation occurs with removal of calcium by SR (arrows), with calcium returned extracellularly and sequestered in SR lateral sacs. Repolarization takes place by potassium efflux with re-establishment of negative intracellular voltage that, in diastole, is maintained with sodium extrusion and potassium return by sarcolemma–T membrane pump ATPase activity.

lular events involved in cardiac contraction, gradual inward Ca^{++} current occurs via slow calcium channels during the *phase 2* action potential plateau (Fig. 8–22), resulting in Ca^{++} movement into the cell, which is important in the process of excitation-contraction coupling. Simultaneous relatively slow egress of K^+ appears to take place during phase 2. The entire repolarization period constitutes the action potential *duration* that governs the *refractory period* of heart muscle and is represented for the ventricles on the surface EKG by the Q–T interval.

During diastole, following repolarization, the *phase 4* recovery portion of the electrophysiologic cycle ensues in which the depolarization-entered Na^+ leaves the cell and the repolarization-egress K^+ returns into the fiber (Fig. 8–22). These cation exchanges during mechanical relaxation require the active energy-utilizing transport mechanism of the *transtubular Na^+-K^+ATPase pump* (Fig. 8–24A). Phase 2 Ca^{++} is removed from the fiber during the resting period by a sarcolemma Na^+-Ca^{++} exchange transport system (Fig. 8–24B). Schwartz and Langer have proposed the sarcolemma-transtubular membrane sodium-potassium pump ATPase enzyme as the pharmacologic receptor for *digitalis,* and the increased calcium influx responsible for the positive inotropic effect of the glycoside may result from the drug's interference with this enzyme pump. There appears to be reduction of membrane sodium-potassium ATPase activity in heart failure.

MECHANICAL ACTIVATION

When the stimulating impulse from the cardiac pacemaker arrives at the surface of the myocardial cell (Fig. 8–25A) an orderly sequence of events is initiated in which *calcium* movement is the chief component linking electrical excitation of the fiber with *mechanical activation* of the contractile machinery in the sarcomere. Excitation of the individual cell proceeds as the depolarization wave spreads throughout the entire fiber along the sarcolemma and its interior transtubular membrane system (Fig. 8–25B). When the depolarizing current in the transtubular system reaches the intimately apposed cisternae calcium depots of the sarcoplasmic reticulum, ionic calcium release is triggered from the lateral sacs into the sarcoplasm (Fig. 8–25C). Together with an apparently smaller but crucial quantity of ionic calcium influx across the sarcolemma-transtubular membrane occurring during phase 2 of the transmembrane action potential, this discharged calcium immediately diffuses to the sarcomeres, where it binds to the specific troponin C calcium-receptor protein (Fig. 8–6) on the thin myofilaments in the overlap region (A band) between the thick and thin filaments (Fig. 8–7).

Mechanical activation is then achieved by the binding of activator-calcium to troponin C, which overcomes the troponin I-tropomyosin complex inhibition of actin and myosin interaction, with the result that actin-myosin electrostatic cross-bridges are formed. Delineation of the precise mechanism of activation involved is shown in Figure 8–26. Thus Ca^{++} binding to troponin C produces structural alteration of the troponin C protein, which is transmitted through troponin I to tropomyosin, so that tropomyosin moves deeper into the groove of the double helix of actin molecules. In this manner, these configurational changes of the troponin-tropomyosin complex free the actin-binding sites to link directly with the myosin heads, thereby allowing actomyosin ATPase activity to occur with initiation of the active state of the contractile process. The temporal course of the entire *excitation-contraction coupling* process takes place relatively quickly, as indicated clinically by the average 0.06-second delay between the beginning of the scaler electrocardiographic QRS complex and the onset of isovolumic ventricular contraction.

CONTRACTILE MECHANISM

The onset of contraction takes place with development of force and contractile element shortening by the *cyclic interaction* of *actin-myosin linkages* pulling the thin filaments along the immobile thick filaments towards the center of the sarcomeres. It is believed that the electrostatic links are next broken as myosin binds another ATP. Thus, a repetitive sequence of making and breaking cross-linkages is established as the actin filament slides past the myosin filament during the entire course of ventricular contraction. For shortening of the sarcomere to occur, each actin-myosin cross-bridge must perform sequentially as shown in Figure 8–27. It is thus necessary for the myosin head to attach to actin, swivel, detach, and then reattach to the next actin-binding site at a point farther laterally on the thin filament. The result is a rowing motion of the myosin heads pulling the thin filaments together centrally and causing their overlap with decreasing distance between Z lines, thereby producing sarcomere, myofilament, muscle fiber, and ultimately ventricular shortening.

The structural features of whole myosin, relationships of myosin heavy chains within the thick filament, and the movement of a myosin heavy chain during contraction are shown in Figure 8–28. Both the light meromyosin backbone (tail region) and the proximal lateral heavy meromyosin S_2 portion form a tight helix; the terminal lateral myosin head extension, heavy meromyosin S_2, is elliptically shaped (Fig. 8–28A). The thick filament is formed by myosin molecules stacked in series, joined only by the light meromyosin tail portions, with the M bridge being the hinge region

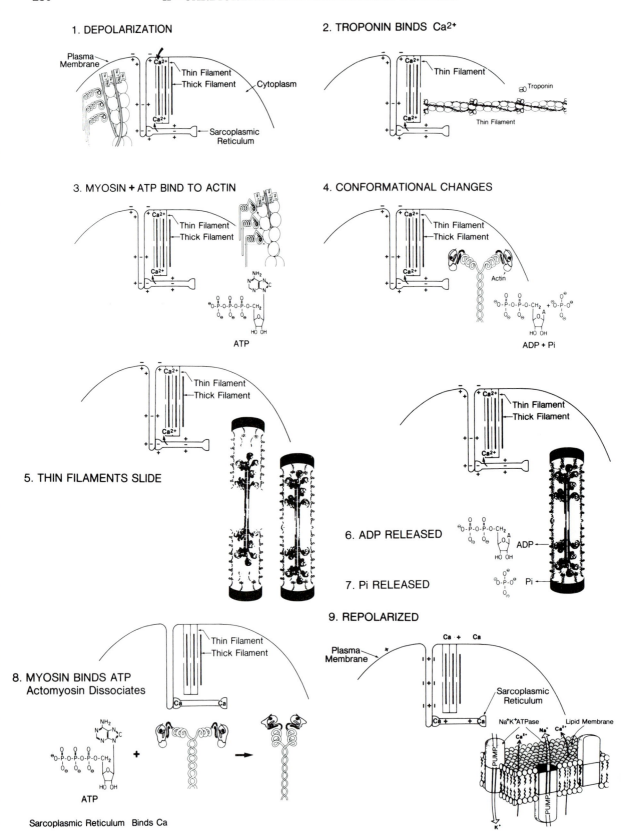

Figure 8–26 *See legend on opposite page.*

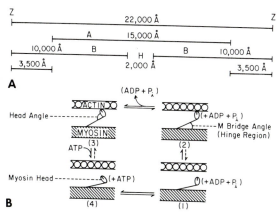

A

B

Figure 8–27 Panel *A* shows the spacing of the myofibrillar proteins within the resting sarcomere. A = thick filament; B = two thin filaments; H = central H zone; Z = two Z lines. Panel *B* shows the sequence of the process of activation of myosin. Diagrammed are the configurational changes that occur in heavy meromyosin due to the binding of ATP and cation to the myosin head with hydrolysis of ATP by myosin ATPase, resulting in subsequent sliding of the actin filaments. Frames 2 through 4 represent progressive phases of the active state, and the resting state is shown in frame 1.

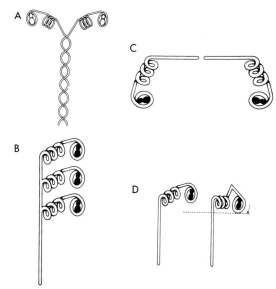

Figure 8–28 *A*, Whole myosin molecule showing the two different types of light chains in the myosin heads associated with the remainder of myosin: the heavy chains constituting heavy meromyosins S_1 and S_2 and light meromyosin. *B*, Serial stacking of the myosin heavy chains in which the tail region (light meromyosin) of one myosin heavy chain complexes with the tail regions of the adjacent myosin heavy chains. *C*, Tail-to-tail repulsion of two myosin heavy chains at the sarcomere center H zone. The right side of *D* delineates the movement of the head angle of a single myosin head (arrow) to the distance indicated by the horizontal broken line and lightening of the heavy meromyosin S_2 coil during the active state; the left side of *D* represents the myosin chain configuration in the resting state.

of the single-spaced heavy meromyosin spiraling outward (Fig. 8–28*B*); the midportion of the thick filament is without heavy meromyosin (Fig. 8–28*C*). With binding of ATP and cation to the myosin head in the active state, the bridge angle increases and the heavy meromyosin S_2 coil tightens to bring the myosin head in contact with actin; with ATP hydrolysis by myosin ATPase in the myosin head, the head angle (junction between meromyosins S_1 and S_2) increases so that inward swivel of the myosin head occurs, thus propelling the actin filament toward the center of the sarcomere (Fig. 8–28*D*).

Figure 8–29*A* is a three-dimensional model of a sarcomere in the relaxed state in which the thick filament is shown with two of the six thin filaments that surround it. On contraction, the thin filaments move centrally, thereby closing the area of the H band (Fig. 8–29*B*). Thus, this sequence in Figure 8–29 *A* and *B* demonstrates the systolic movement of the thin filaments, bringing the Z lines attached to the distal end of the thin fila-

ments closer together after a sequence of ATP hydrolytic cycles takes place in the myosin heads during the active state. The Z lines are the terminal ends of the sarcomere and thus demarcate the zone of contact between the sarcomeres in series. From these observations, it is apparent that when the sarcomeres shorten during contraction, the whole cardiac fiber in turn shortens. The proteins that compose the Z lines are bound tightly to the outer ends of the fibrous actin molecules.

The decrease in distance between the Z lines of a single sarcomere upon contraction results in the partial or total disappearance of the I bands,

Figure 8–26 Diagrammatic sequence of the molecular events of the modulator and contractile proteins constituting excitation-contraction coupling. During the resting state at the time of depolarization, the troponin-tropomyosin complex blocks myosin head contact with actin *(1)*. With greater calcium delivered to troponin C, troponin C–calcium binding overcomes troponin I–tropomyosin interaction *(2)*. Thus, the troponin-tropomyosin conformational change allows for the active sites of the actin molecule to become exposed to the myosin heads. Myosin-ATP or myosin-ADP binds to actin *(3)*. If the myosin-ATP binds, ATP is rapidly hydrolyzed by actomyosin *(4)*. Following hydrolysis, myosin goes through several conformational changes as the end products (ADP + Pi) are transferred to different positions in the oligomer *(5)*. The conformational changes result in shortening of the sarcomere *(5)*. The end products are released *(6 and 7)*. If the sarcoplasmic reticulum binds calcium, cycling stops and myosin goes into the relaxed state *(8)*. During relaxation, repolarization takes place *(9)*.

depending on the degree of shortening. Shortening may terminate when myosin is in contact with the Z lines (Fig. 8–27B). However, systolic shortening may terminate before myosin reaches the Z lines,

or, conversely, contraction may continue to the extreme extent of compressing the thick filaments into a wavy pattern and causing the thin filaments to slip past one another in the H band region.

MECHANICAL RELAXATION

The phase of the excitation-contraction activating coupling process in which calcium is delivered to the contractile apparatus does not require ATP energy. The contractile reaction involving myosin ATPase utilizes the great majority of total myocardial energy, which varies according to the muscle-loading conditions and contractile state. Following development of the fully active contractile state, the active process of relaxation ensues, with calcium departing from the sarcomere and rapidly binding to the sarcoplasmic reticulum (Fig. 8–25E). The cation is then pumped back into the lateral sacs by *sarcotubular calcium pump ATPase* (relaxing factor) (Fig. 8–24B), the total energy needed for relaxation being relatively small.

Concerning calcium dynamics, essentially no sarcoplasmic calcium is present during diastole, and the quantity of available calcium stored intracellularly is insufficient in itself to activate subsequent systole. Myocardial cells are not able to contract in a calcium-free external medium, and, unlike skeletal muscle, cardiac muscle requires some extracellular calcium for contraction. The total amount of calcium provided to the sarcoplasm from internal and external sources is normally sufficient to activate all myosin molecules of the thick filament, with contraction taking place when a critical threshold of sarcoplasmic calcium concentration is reached. The greater the rate and quantity of calcium delivered to troponin, the faster the rate and number of activated interactions between actin and myosin, with a consequently more rapid rate of tension development, greater maximum tension, and increased contractility.

MYOSIN ATPase ACTIVITY

One of the most intriguing aspects of contractile protein performance relates to the elucidation of the molecular alterations of myosin determining the degree of myosin ATPase activity, since increased rate of myosin ATPase hydrolysis of ATP during the active state stimulates the intensity of actin-myosin linkages and thereby correlates directly with a greater degree of cardiac contractility. In this regard, the function of the two myosin light chains contained within the coil of a single myosin head, meromyosin S_2 (Fig. 8–10), is of particular importance. Previously, the concept was entertained that both light subunits simply suppressed the activity of myosin ATPase within the head of the myosin heavy chains. Various heavy and light chain dissociation and reassociation

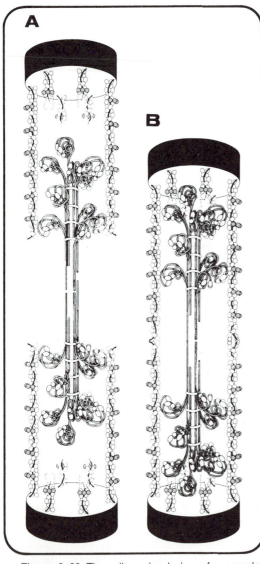

Figure 8–29 Three-dimensional view of a complete thick filament surrounded at each of its ends by six thin filaments, two of which are shown in full length. The lateral limits of the sarcomere are shown by the disc-like Z lines to which the lateral ends of the thin filaments are attached. In A, the sarcomere is in the relaxed state with the central ends of the thin filaments extending only up to the beginning of the central H zone. In B (active state of complete contraction), the central ends of the actin filaments from both sides of the sarcomere are in contact, thereby entirely closing the H zone. In addition, the movement of the thin filaments towards the middle of the sarcomere during systole decreases the distance between the two Z lines; this process underlies cardiac muscle shortening during contraction. (Reproduced with permission from Wikman-Coffelt, al.: *In* Mason, D. T. [Ed.]: Congestive Heart Failure. New York, Yorke Medical Books, 1976.)

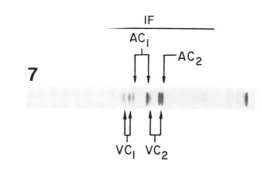

Figure 8-30 Two-dimensional electrophoresis of atrial and ventricular myosin light chains. The combined light chains were electrophoresed in the first dimension (top) with 2 per cent ampholines composed of 1.6 per cent of pH range 4 to 6 and 0.4 per cent pH range 3 to 10, and then electrophoresed through a gradient of polyacrylamide (5 to 20 per cent) containing a detergent, sodium dodecylsulfate. This showed for the first time that atrial and ventricular myosins were isozymes. VC = ventricular light chains; AC = atrial light chains. (Reproduced with permission from Long et al.: Biochem. Biophys. Res. Commun. 76:626, 1977.)

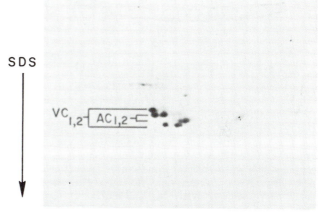

studies have shown that the function of the myosin light chains is considerably more complex, with each light subunit possessing quite different properties. These two light chains are designated C_1 (28,000 molecular weight) and C_2 (18,000 MW). The larger light chain (C_1) is variable in structure among different species; the smaller light chain (C_2) binds calcium, becoming more firmly attached to the myosin head with such Ca^{++} binding, and the C_2 light subunit spans the distance from the actin linkage site to the hinge angle of heavy meromyosin S_2 (Fig. 8–10).

Importantly, concerning canine myosin light chains, the immunologic properties of electrophoresis (Fig. 8–30) and the degree of Ca^{++}-stimulated myosin ATPase function differ markedly between atrial and ventricular myocardium. Furthermore, among different animal species, ventricular myosin light chains evaluated by radioimmunoassay against antimyosin ventricular light chains are immunologically distinct (Fig. 8–31), and the levels of ventricular myocardial ATPase activity (Fig. 8–32) vary considerably. In general, the smaller animals (rat, guinea pig, cat, rabbit) with greater basal metabolic rate normally demonstrate higher ventricular myosin ATPase activity at greater optimal pH than larger species (dog, sheep, human) (Fig. 8–32).

The light chains play a subtle role in modify-

ing regulated actomyosin ATPase activity. In the absence of the regulatory proteins, the light chains from atrial and ventricular myosins can be completely cross-hybridized and shown not to affect actin-activated myosin ATPase activity. However, in the presence of the regulatory proteins, the calcium sensitivity is modified by the presence and type of myosin light chain.

The myosins between the atria and ventricle exist as isozymes. Such isomyosins are enzymes with related function but demonstrate modifications in structure and activity. A shift in isomyosins, as can occur in the ventricles subject to an increased workload, can cause either an increase or a decrease in the force and velocity of muscle shortening and possibly the degree of oxygen consumption. At least in the rat, rabbit, and hamster, and possibly the dog, there are three isomyosins: V1, V2, and V3. From temperature-sensitive measurements of papillary muscles it was shown that there was a greater liberation of heat per unit tension in muscles containing V1 than in those containing V3. Myosin with the slow ATPase activity (V3) has a longer cross-bridge on-time and thus is able to generate more tension per ATP utilized than is myosin with the fast ATPase activity (V1). There is an inverse relationship between the economy of tension development and actin-activated myosin ATPase activity. At low

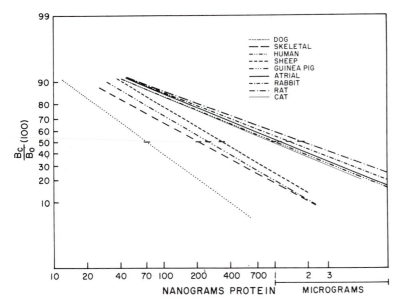

Figure 8–31 Homologous radioimmunoassay of myosin against antimyosin of ventricular light chains from different animal species, demonstrating limited species cross-reactivity and disparate antigenic sites of cardiac myosin light chains among the various species. Concerning the smaller versus the larger animals, considerable differences in the immunologic and structural properties of the ventricular light chains were observed.

calcium concentrations, it is possible that muscles that contain mainly V3 myosin will require less ATP per unit tension and thus consume less oxygen. A shift towards isomyosin V3 is a compensatory mechanism occurring in advanced hypertension and heart failure that is beneficial for conserving energy. With the induction of isomyosin V1 there is a faster pumping force that allows for better systemic circulation, whereas with V3 the benefit is economy of ATP utilization per unit tension.

As mentioned previously, greater concentrations of Ca^{++} delivered to the contractile proteins during the active state increase both the number and maximum turnover rate of actin-myosin cross-bridge formation, thus elevating both contractile force and contractility. Influencing these phenomena are apparently both Ca^{++} binding and phosphorylation of troponin and myosin, as well as interrelationships between myosin ATPase activity and cross-bridge linkage. Elevation of myosin ATPase activity increases both the number and

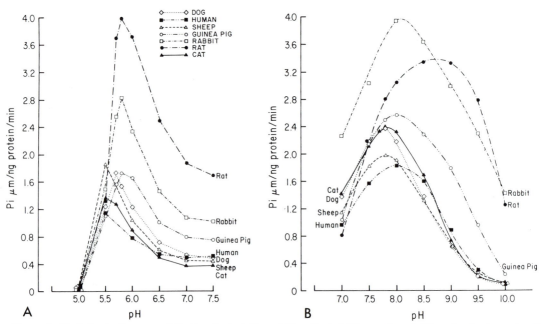

Figure 8–32 Optimal pH curves of Ca^{++}-activated *(A)* and K^+-activated *(B)* myosins of different animal species. The smaller animals demonstrated greater myosin ATPase activity and higher optimal pH values than the larger animal species.

intensity of actin-myosin connections, depending on the number of available Ca^{++}-turned-on actin molecules. Phosphorylation of troponin I decreases calcium sensitivity of troponin $C\text{-}Ca^{++}$ derepressor activity. This derepressor activity of troponin C is regained in the presence of elevated Ca^{++} concentrations, whereas in consort there is increased phosphorylation of myosin light chain $C_2\text{-}Ca^{++}$ binding affinity. In addition, myosin light chains may play a role in enhancing Ca^{++} sensitivity of troponin C. Furthermore, Ca^{++} binding of myosin heavy chains may enhance myosin ATPase activity. With purified enzyme systems, acute changes in myosin ATPase activity have not been demonstrated; instead, all changes in myosin ATPase activity seen experimentally have been produced by animal preparations of chronic ventricular hemodynamic overload or have occurred in animals with chronic primary contractility disturbance.

CARDIAC HYPERTROPHY AND FAILURE

Although the induction of ventricular hypertrophy may result from different factors (including pressure overload, volume overload, hormonal influences, exercise, hypoxia, and primary disturbances of contractility), development of hypertrophy caused by all these conditions is characterized by a common initial mechanism of protein synthesis. The stress engendered by these stimuli causes activation of the genetic apparatus of the myocardial cell, resulting in enhancement of nucleic acid and protein synthesis as well as induction of new genetic expressions. Thus, myocardial cellular hypertrophy results from these biochemical sequences, thereby providing prolonged adaptation for the heart.

Ventricular pressure or volume overload leads to *increased wall tension* and stretch of muscle fibers, thus resulting in increased end-diastolic sarcomere length, which in turn activates the growth process of myocardial cellular hypertrophy. Present evidence suggests that this genetic activation mechanism appears to be preceded by changes in *tissue PO_2* and *PCO_2* and an alteration in the *phosphorylation potential* secondary to the increased workload demand. Elevation of myocardial norepinephrine induced by tension and muscle stretch may also play a role in the activation of the early ventricular hypertrophy process. Therefore, the common final pathway in the hypertrophy process may be mediated via norepinephrine released from sympathetic nerve endings in the myocardium by increased wall tension. This neurotransmitter may, in turn, trigger the biochemical process of hypertrophy; thus, *norepinephrine* has been considered a myocardial cellular hypertrophy hormone and perhaps the hypertrophying factor itself. The increased levels of norepinephrine may thereby elicit rises in *cAMP*, thus in-

creasing *RNA polymerase* activity, resulting in elevated *protein synthesis* and thus myocardial hypertrophy. In this regard, RNA polymerase has been shown to increase during early stages of cardiac hypertrophy; this enzyme is activated by cAMP, which in turn leads to increases in RNA; as the result, protein content is augmented.

Since an increase in muscle mass accompanies hypertrophy, ventricular systolic stress is lessened. In this manner, the hypertrophy process compensates for an excessive hemodynamic load by producing more sarcomeres and, in some types of hypertrophy, improves cardiac function to normal. A new principle described herein is the concept of physiologic versus pathologic ventricular hypertrophy in response to disparate settings. *Physiologic hypertrophy* is signified by normal or augmented contractile state with concomitant levels of myosin ATPase activity, in contrast to *pathologic hypertrophy,* characterized by depressed contractility and diminished myosin ATPase function.

Biochemical and mechanical alterations of cardiac performance, myosin ATPase activity and contractility, respectively, which distinguish physiologic from pathologic ventricular hypertrophy, are dependent on at least four principal variables: (1) *degree of stress;* (2) *duration of stress;* (3) *nature of inciting stimulus;* and (4) *species, age, and health* of the animal studied. *Hyperthyroidism* affords a useful experimental model of physiologic hypertrophy in which left ventricular weight is considerably increased, as well as myosin ATPase activity and hemodynamic and mechanical indices of contractility. Concerning experimental examples of *chronic hemodynamic overload* in dogs, mild right or left ventricular outflow obstruction causes sustained increases in myosin ATPase and inotropic function for several weeks in the stress-hypertrophied ventricle prior to eventual depression of such activity (Fig. 8–33). In contrast, severe canine pulmonary or aortic stenosis results in the immediate progressive declines in myosin ATPase activity and contractility in the stressed hypertrophied ventricle (Fig. 8–33). Thus, differential responses of physiologic versus pathologic hypertrophy in the stressed ventricle are produced by chronic right or left ventricular pressure overloading, the type of hypertrophy being dependent on the severity and duration of the hemodynamic burden.

The primary disorder or combination of abnormalities responsible for *depressed contractile state* of the hypertrophied ventricle with the development of heart failure appears to result from defective *excitation-contraction coupling,* a shift in metabolism, and/or dysfunction of the *contractile proteins.*

Enhancement of the rate and quantity of calcium influx from external sources (e.g., digitalis) appears to be an important mechanism for increasing myocardial contractility. Negative inotropic drugs diminish this calcium influx, and Briggs has shown their reduction of sarcotubular calcium

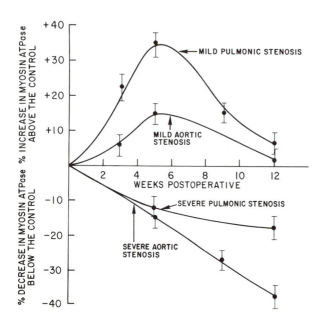

Figure 8–33 Comparison of disparate canine myosin ATPase function (K$^+$-activated enzymatic V$_{max}$ values) from hemodynamically stressed ventricles under different degrees and durations of right and left ventricular outflow obstruction.

pump ATPase. Concerning depressed contractility in heart failure, there may be abnormal transport of calcium by the sarcoplasmic reticulum, as evidenced by its impairment of calcium uptake, binding, release, and pump ATPase activity and demonstrated by Schwartz, Gertz, Chidsey, and others. Chidsey has suggested a maldistribution of myocardial intracellular calcium in chronic hemodynamic overload in which depressed sarcoplasmic function leads to increased mitochondrial sequestration of calcium, with total intracellular calcium being unaltered. In the final phase of ischemic heart disease, exhaustion of ATP supply for myosin ATPase leads to the development of irreversible ventricular contracture, whereas decreased contractility in the earlier stage of ischemia due to disturbed excitation-contraction coupling may be reversible with reperfusion of the myocardium with oxygenated blood.

In regard to dysfunction of the contractile proteins in heart failure, attention has been focused on abnormal energy utilization. Thus, the activity of myofibrillar ATPase is reduced in the failing myocardium, as demonstrated by Alpert, Sonnenblick, Luchi, and others. Diminished activity of this enzyme in heart failure reduces the velocity of interaction between actin-myosin linkages and thereby influences the contractile state. The failing heart does not appear to be inefficient in its conversion of chemical energy to mechanical work. Additional considerations are that dysfunction of hypertrophied muscle may be related to (1) a shift towards isomyosin V3, (2) a calcium overload leading to a decrease in oxidative phosphorylation, and thus (3) a loss in the proton sink, causing intracellular acidity. Intracellular acidity, a shift towards isomyosin V3, and a decrease in

the free energy of ATP hydrolysis due to the decrease in oxidative phosphorylation will all concurrently cause a decrease in contractility. With a decrease in intracellular pH, the conformation of myosin is altered, causing a shift in its three-dimensional configuration and thus lowering its ATPase activity. With intracellular acidity, the flux of calcium as well as protein phosphorylation increases. Phosphorylation of troponin and myosin lowers their calcium sensitivity, whereas phosphorylation of phospholamban, an important calcium-binding protein in the sarcoplasmic reticulum and perhaps also present in the sarcolemma, increases its calcium sensitivity. The net result is a requirement for more calcium by the myofibrillar proteins and membranes to attain similar contractility and a faster calcium pumping rate. Finally, the decrease in contractility during heart failure is due to the decrease in intracellular pH, the low energy reserve, and the shift towards isomyosin V3, the isomyosin with low ATPase activity.

A postulated mechanism whereby contractility is depressed in heart failure is summarized in Figure 8–34. This series of mechanisms has been demonstrated in the cardiomyopathic Syrian hamster as it develops heart failure. Through a possible membrane defect or an oversized heart, oxidative phosphorylation is diminished. Thus, oxidation of NADH is decreased; accumulation of NADH has a feedback inhibition on glyceraldehyde-3-phosphate dehydrogenase, thereby lowering glycolysis. The oxidation of NADH is partially alleviated by conversion of pyruvate to lactate via lactic dehydrogenase, thus utilizing NADH. Norepinephrine and cAMP are lowered, and the Kreb's cycle is depressed. As a result, the transport of NADH into the mitochondria via the Kreb's cycle is re-

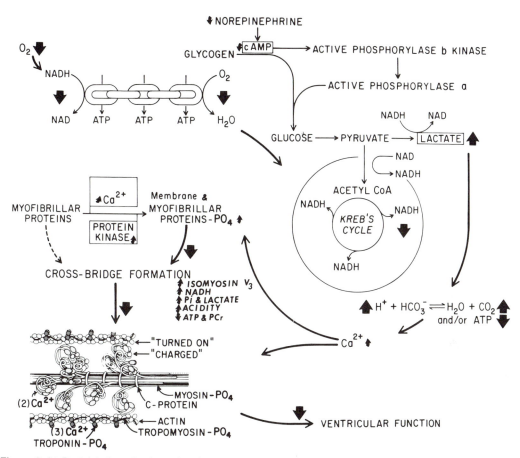

Figure 8–34 Postulated mechanism whereby myocardial contractility is depressed in chronic hemodynamic overload. Reduction in oxidative phosphorylation is followed by an accumulation of NADH, an increase in lactate, and an increase in hydrogen ions. With an increase in intracellular acidity there is a corresponding increase in intracellular calcium. Phosphorylation of myofibrillar proteins increases in order to lower the calcium sensitivity and conserve energy utilization. Phosphorylation of membrane protein increases so that the efflux and binding of calcium ions are increased. The lower pH alters the conformation of myosin and thus decreases contractility.

duced, causing a further increase in cytosolic NADH levels. With the depressed proton sink due to the decrease in oxidative phosphorylation, the pH decreases until it reaches a conducive steady state for efflux of end products. The intracellular acidity causes an increase in the calcium flux. Calcium-activated calmodulin-mediated protein phosphorylation increases, as described by Cheung. With myofibrillar protein phosphorylation, more calcium is required to activate cross-bridge interaction. With calcium-activated phosphorylation of phospholamban, a calcium ATPase protein of the membranes, there is an increased rate in the calcium binding. The decrease in pH causes a shift in the conformation of myosin, decreasing its interaction with actin. The shift towards isomyosin V3 results in a slower rate of

ATPase activity, thus decreasing the velocity of muscle shortening and thereby conserving energy. All the mechanisms of heart failure are conducive to a decrease in oxygen consumption, ATP utilization, and a decrease in contractility, as observed in the cardiomyopathic Syrian hamster.

Finally, it is likely that in circumstances in which there is divergence of results and views concerning the causative, contributory, or coincidental nature of certain biochemical abnormalities in the pathogenesis of depressed mechanical function and contractility in the failing myocardium, these dissimilarities reflect basic differences in the types of heart failure studied: acute or chronic, mild or severe, experimental or human, idiopathic, drug-induced, ischemic, or volume or pressure overload.

REFERENCES

MYOCARDIAL ULTRASTRUCTURE

Braunwald, E., Chidsey, C. A., Pool, P. E., et al.: Congestive heart failure: biochemical and physiological considerations. Ann. Intern. Med. *64*:4, 1966.

Braunwald, E., Ross, J., Jr., and Sonnenblick, E. H. *In* Braunwald, E., et al. (Eds.): Mechanisms of Contraction of the Normal and Failing Heart. Boston, Little, Brown and Co., 1976.

Carney, J. A., and Brown, A. L., Jr.: Human cardiac myosin: electron microscopic observations. Circ. Res. *17*:336, 1965.

Cole, H. A., and Perry, S. V.: The phosphorylation of troponin I from cardiac muscle. Biochem. J. *149*:525, 1975.

Davies, R. E.: Molecular theory of muscle contraction: calcium-dependent contractions with hydrogen bond formation plus ATP-dependent extensions of part of myosin-actin cross-bridges. Nature (London) *199*:1068, 1963.

Ebashi, S., and Endo, M.: Calcium ion and muscle contraction. *In* Butler, J. A. V., and Noble, N. (Eds.): Progress in Biophysics and Molecular Biology. New York, Pergamon Press, 1968, p. 123.

Grant, R. P.: Notes on the muscular architecture of the left ventricle. Circulation *32*:301, 1965.

Hanson, J., and Lowy, J.: Molecular basis of contractility in muscle. Br. M. Bull *21*:264, 1965.

Haugaard, N., Haugaard, E. S., Lee, N. H., and Horn, R. S.: Possible role of mitochondria in regulation of cardiac contractility. Fed. Proc. *28*:1657, 1969.

Huxley, H. E.: Structural arrangements and contraction mechanism in striated muscle. Proc. Roy. Soc. London (Biol.) *160*:442, 1964.

Katz, A. M.: Contractile proteins of the heart. Physiol. Rev. *50*:63, 1970.

Katz, A. M.: Physiology of the Heart. New York, Raven Press, 1977.

Legato, M. J.: Sarcomerogenesis in human myocardium. J. Mol. Cell. Cardiol. *1*:425, 1970.

Mope, L., McClellan, G. B., and Winegrad, S.: Calcium sensitivity of the contractile system and phosphorylation of troponin in hyperpermeable cardiac cells. J. Gen. Physiol. *72*:737, 1978.

Potter, J. D., Piascki, T., Wisler, P. L., et al.: Calcium-dependent regulation of brain and cardiac adenylate cyclase. Ann. N.Y. Acad. Sci. *356*:220, 231, 1980.

Ross, J., Jr., Sonnenblick, E. H., Taylor, R. R., et al.: Diastolic geometry and sarcomere lengths in the chronically dilated canine left ventricle. Circ. Res. *28*:49, 1971.

Solaro, R. J., Holroyde, T. H., Crouch, S., et al.: Myofilament protein phosphorylation in striated muscle. *In* Rosen, O. M., and Krebs, E. G. (Eds.): Protein Phosphorylation, Eighth Cold Spring Harbor Conference on Cell Proliferation. New York, Cold Spring Harbor, 1981.

Spiro, D., and Sonnenblick, E. H.: Structural conditions in the hypertrophied and failure heart. *In* Mason, D. T. (Ed.): Congestive Heart Failure. New York, Yorke Medical Books, 1976, pp. 13–24.

Srivastava, S., Muhlrad, A., and Wikman-Coffelt, J.: Influence of myosin heavy chains on the Ca^{2+}-binding properties of light chain LC2. Biochem. J. *193*:925, 1981.

Wikman-Coffelt, J., Fenner, C., Salel, A. F., et al. *In* Mason, D. T. (Ed.): Congestive Heart Failure. New York, Yorke Medical Books, 1976, pp. 53–75.

Wikman-Coffelt, J., Parmley, W. W., and Mason, D. T.: Relation of myosin isozymes to the heart as a pump. Am. Heart J. *103*:934, 1982.

Wilkinson, J. M., Perry, S. V., Cole, H. A., and Trayer, I. P.: The regulatory proteins of the myofibril. Separation and biological activity of the components of inhibitory-factor preparations. Biochem. J. *127*:215, 1972.

MYOCARDIAL METABOLISM

Alpert, N. R., Hamrell, B. B., and Halpren, W.: Mechanical and biochemical correlates of cardiac hypertrophy. Circ. Res. *35*(Suppl. 2):71, 1974.

Braunwald, E.: Control of myocardial oxygen consumption: physiologic and clinical correlations. Am. J. Cardiol. *27*:416, 1971.

Cheung, W. Y.: Calmodulin. Sci. Am. *246*:62, 1982.

Chidsey, C. A., Braunwald, E., Morrow, A. G., and Mason, D. T.: Myocardial norepinephrine concentration in man: effects of reserpine and of congestive heart failure. N. Engl. J. Med. *269*:653, 1963.

Cohen, L. S., Elliott, W. C., Rolett, E. L., and Gorlin, R.: Hemodynamic studies during angina pectoris. Circulation *31*:409, 1965.

Coleman, H. N., Sonnenblick, E. H., and Braunwald, E.: Myocardial oxygen consumption associated with external work: the Fenn effect. Am. J. Physiol. *217*:291, 1969.

Cooper, G., Gunning, J. F., Harrison, C. E., and Coleman, H. N.: Contractile and energetic behavior of hypertrophied and failing myocardium. *In* Mason, D. T. (Ed.): Congestive Heart Failure. New York, Yorke Medical Books, 1976, pp. 97–110.

Covell, J. W., Braunwald, E., Ross, J., and Sonnenblick, E. H.: Studies on digitalis. XVI. Effects on myocardial oxygen consumption. J. Clin. Invest. *45*:1535, 1966.

Covell, J., W., Chidsey, C. A., and Braunwald, E.: Reduction of the cardiac response to postganglionic sympathetic nerve stimulation in experimental heart failure. Circ. Res. *19*:51, 1966.

Epstein, S. E., Skelton, C. L., Levey, G. S., and Entman, M.: Adenyl cyclase and myocardial contractility. Ann. Intern. Med. *72*:561, 1970.

Hochachka, P. W., and Mommsen, T. P.: Protons and Anaerobiosis. Science *219*:1391, 1983.

Kammermeier, H., Schmidt, P., and Jungling, E.: Free energy change of ATP hydrolysis: a causal factor of early hypoxic failure of the myocardium. J. Mol. Cell. Cardiol. *14*:267, 1982.

Katz, A. N.: Effects of ischemia on the contractile process of heart muscle. *In* Mason, D. T. (Ed.): Congestive Heart Failure. New York, Yorke Medical Books, 1976, pp. 77–84.

Kobayashi, K., and Neely, J. R.: Control of maximum rates of glycolysis in rat cardiac muscle. Circ. Res. *44*:166, 1979.

Kramer, R. S., Mason, D. T., and Braunwald, E.: Augmented sympathetic neurotransmitter activity in the peripheral vascular bed of patients with congestive heart failure and cardiac norepinephrine depletion. Circulation *38*:629, 1968.

Laks, M. M., Morady, F., Garner, D., and Swann, H. J. C.: Temporal changes in canine right ventricular volume, mass, cell size, and sarcomere length after banding the pulmonary artery. Cardiovasc. Res. *8*:106, 1974.

Lindenmayer, G. E., Sordahl, L. A., Harigaya, S., et al.: Some biochemical studies on subcellular systems isolated from fresh recipient human cardiac tissue obtained during transplantation. Am. J. Cardiol. *27*:277, 1971.

Lindenmayer, G. E., Sordahl, L. A., and Schwartz, A.: Reevaluation of oxidative phosphorylation in cardiac muscle from normal animals and animals in heart failure. Circ. Res. *23*:439, 1968.

Mason, D. T.: Autonomic nervous system and regulation of cardiovascular performance. Anesthesiology *29*:670, 1968.

Mason, D. T.: The Failing Heart. Disease-a-Month Series. Chicago, Year Book Medical Publishers, January, 1977.

Mason, D. T., Zelis, R., and Amsterdam, E. A.: Role of the sympathetic nervous system in congestive heart failure. *In* Bortelli, C., and Zanchetti, Z. (Eds.): Cardiovascular Regulation in Health and Disease. Milan, Cardiovascular Research Institute, 1971, pp. 159–172.

Meerson, F., Alekhina, G. M., Aleksandrov, P. N., and Bazardjan, A. G.: Dynamics of nucleic acid and protein synthesis of the myocardium in compensatory hyperfunction and hypertrophy of the heart. Am. J. Cardiol. *22*:337, 1968.

Meerson, F. and Pomoinitsky, V. D.: The role of high-energy phosphate compounds in the development of cardiac hypertrophy. J. Mol. Cell. Cardiol. *4*:571, 1972.

Morkin, E., and Ashford, R. P.: Myocardial DNA synthesis in experimental cardiac hypertrophy. Am. J. Physiol. *215*:1409, 1968.

Nair, K. G., Cutiletta, A. F., Koide, R., and Rabinowitz, M.: Biochemical correlates of cardiac hypertrophy. Circ. Res. *23*:451, 1968.

Namm, D. H., and Mayer, S. E.: Effects of epinephrine on cardiac cyclic 3',5'-AMP, phosphorylase kinase and phosphorylase. Molec. Pharmacol. 4:61, 1968.

Opie, L. M.: Metabolism of the heart in health and disease, Parts 1 to 3. Am. Heart J. 76:865, 1968; 77:100 and 383, 1969.

Pool, P. E., Covell, J. W., Levitt, M., et al.: Reduction of cardiac tyrosine hydroxylase activity in experimental congestive heart failure. Circ. Res. 20:349, 1967.

Pool, P. E., Spann, J. F., Jr., and Buccino, R. A.: Myocardial high energy phosphate stores in cardiac hypertrophy and heart failure. Circ. Res. 21:365, 1967.

Potter, J. D., Piascki, T., Wisler, P. L., et al.: Calcium-dependent regulation of brain and cardiac adenylate cyclase. Ann. N.Y. Acad. Sci. 356:220, 1980.

Rabinowitz, M., and Zak, R.: Mitochondria and cardiac hypertrophy. Circ. Res. 36:367, 1975.

Rabinowitz, M., Nair, K. G., and Zak, R.: Cellular and subcellular basis of cardiac hypertrophy. Med. Clin. North Am. 54:211, 1970.

Rall, T. W., Sutherland, E. W., and Berthet, J.: The relationship of epinephrine and glucagon to liver phosphorylase. IV. Effect of epinephrine and glucagon on the reactivation of phosphorylase in liver homogenates. J. Biol. Chem. 224:463, 1957.

Rinaldi, M. L., Capony, J. P., and Demaille, J. G.: The cyclic AMP-dependent modulation of cardiac sarcolemmal slow calcium channels. J. Mol. Cell. Cardiol. 14:279, 1982.

Schwartz, A., Sordahl, L. A., Entman, M. L., et al.: Abnormal biochemistry in heart failure. In Mason, D. T. (Ed.): Congestive Heart Failure. New York, Yorke Medical Books, 1976, pp. 25–44.

Sievers, R., Parmley, W. W., and Wikman-Coffelt, J.: Energy levels at systole versus diastole in normal hamster hearts versus myopathic hamster hearts. Submitted for publication.

Sobel, B. E., Henry, P. D., Robison, A., et al.: Depressed adenyl cyclase activity in the failing guinea pig heart. Circ. Res. 24:507, 1969.

Spann, J. F., Jr., Buccino, R. A., Sonnenblick, E. H., and Braunwald, E.: Contractile state of cardiac muscle obtained from cats with experimentally produced ventricular hypertrophy and heart failure. Circ. Res. 21:341, 1967.

Spann, J. F., Jr., Chidsey, C. A., Pool, P. E., and Braunwald, E.: Mechanism of norepinephrine depletion in experimental heart failure produced by aortic constriction in the guinea pig. Circ. Res. 17:312, 1965.

Vogel, J. H. K., and Chidsey, C. A.: Cardiac adrenergic activity in experimental heart failure assessed with beta receptor blockade. Am. J. Cardiol. 24:198, 1969.

Wikman-Coffelt, J., Fenner, C., Coffelt, R. J., et al.: Chronological effects of mild pressure overload on myosin ATPase activity in the canine right ventricle. J. Mol. Cell. Cardiol. 7:219, 1975.

Wikman-Coffelt, J., Fenner, C., McPherson, J., et al.: Alterations of subunit composition and ATPase activity of myosin in early hypertrophied right ventricles of dogs with mild experimental pulmonic stenosis. J. Mol. Cell. Cardiol. 7:513, 1975.

Wikman-Coffelt, J., and Mason, D. T.: Mechanism of decreased contractility in chronic hemodynamic overload. In Mason, D. T. (Ed.): Advances in Heart Disease, I. New York, Grune & Stratton, 1977, pp. 491–504.

Wikman-Coffelt, J., and Mason, D. T.: The contractile proteins of cardiac muscle: myosin function in the normal and hemodynamically overloaded heart. In Mason, D. T. (Ed.): Advances in Heart Disease, II. New York, Grune & Stratton, 1978.

Wikman-Coffelt, J., Parmley, W. W., and Mason, D. T.: The cardiac hypertrophy process: analyses of factors determining pathological vs. physiological development. Circ. Res. 45:697, 1979.

Wikman-Coffelt, J., Salel, A. F., and Mason, D. T.: Differential responses of canine myosin ATPase activity and tissue gases in the pressure overloaded ventricle dependent upon degree of obstruction: mild versus severe pulmonic and aortic stenosis. Recent Adv. Stud. Card. Struct. Metab. 12:367, 1978.

Wikman-Coffelt, J., Sievers, R., Coffelt, R. J., and Parmley, W. W.: Biochemical and mechanical correlates at peak systole in myopathic Syrian hamster. Basic Res. Cardiol. In press.

Wikman-Coffelt, J., Sievers, R., Coffelt, R. J., and Parmley, W. W.: Oscillations of cAMP with the cardiac cycle. Biochem. Biophys. Res. Commun. 111:450, 1983.

Wikman-Coffelt, J., Sievers, R., Coffelt, R. J., and Parmley, W. W.: The cardiac cycle: regulation and energy oscillations. Am. J. Physiol. (Heart & Circ. Physiol.) In press.

Wikman-Coffelt, J., Walsh, R., Fenner, C., et al.: Effects of severe hemodynamic pressure overload on the properties of canine left ventricular myosins. Mechanism by which myosin ATPase activity is lowered during chronic increased hemodynamic stress. J. Mol. Cell. Cardiol. 8:263, 1976.

Wikman-Coffelt, J., Zelis, R., Fenner, C., and Mason, D. T.: Studies on the synthesis and degradation of light and heavy chains of cardiac myosin. J. Biol. Chem. 248:5206, 1973.

Zak, R., Martin, A. F., Reddy, M. K., and Rabinowitz, M.: Control of protein balance in hypertrophied cardiac muscle. Circ. Res. 38(Suppl. 1):146, 1976.

EXCITATION-CONTRACTION COUPLING AND THE CONTRACTILE PROCESS

Banerjee, S. K., Flink, I. L., and Morkin, E.: Enzymatic properties of native and N-ethylmaleimide-modified cardiac myosin from normal and thyrotoxic rabbits. Circ. Res. 39:319, 1976.

Beeler, G. W., Jr., and Reuter, H.: Membrane calcium current in ventricular myocardial fibers. J. Physiol. (London) 207:191, 1970.

Besch, H. R., Allen, J. C., Glick, G., and Schwartz, A.: Correlation between the inotropic action of ouabain and its effects on subcellular enzyme systems from canine myocardium. J. Pharmacol. Exp. Ther. 171:1, 1970.

Chandler, B. M., Sonnenblick, E. H., Spann, J. F., and Pool, P. E.: Association of depressed myofibrillar adenosine triphosphates and reduced contractility in experimental heart failure. Circ. Res. 21:717, 1967.

Conway, G., Heazlitt, R. A., Montag, J., and Mattingly, S. F.: The ATPase activity of cardiac myosin from failing and hypertrophied hearts. J. Mol. Cell. Cardiol. 7:817, 1975.

Draper, M., Taylor, N., and Alpert, N. R.: Alteration in contractile protein in hypertrophied guinea pig hearts. In Alpert, N. R. (Ed.): Cardiac Hypertrophy. New York, Academic Press, 1971, p. 315.

Fabian, F., Mason, D. T., and Wikman-Coffelt, J.: Calcium-binding properties of cardiac and skeletal muscle myosins. F.E.B.S. Letter 81:381, 1977.

Fuchs, F., Gertz, E. W., and Briggs, F. N.: The effect of quinidine on calcium accumulation by isolated sarcoplasmic reticulum of skeletal and cardiac muscle. J. Gen. Physiol. 52:955, 1968.

Gertz, E. W., Hess, M. L., Lain, R. F., and Briggs, F. N.: Activity of the vesicular calcium pump in the spontaneously failing heart lung preparation. Circ. Res. 20:477, 1967.

Harigaya, S., and Schwartz, A.: Rate of calcium binding and uptake in normal animal and failing human cardiac muscle. Circ. Res. 25:781, 1969.

Higuchi, M., Stewart, D., Mason, D. T., et al.: Immunological electrophoretic and kinetic properties of cardiac myosins from various species. Comp. Biochem. Physiol. 60:495, 1978.

Hoffman, B. F., and Cranefield, P. F.: Physiological basis of cardiac arrhythmias. Am. J. Med. 37:670, 1964.

Hollosi, G., Srivastava, S., and Wikman-Coffelt, J.: Cross-hybridization of cardiac myosin isozymes: atrial and ventricular myosins. F.E.B.S. Letter 120:199, 1980.

Huxley, H. E.: Mechanism of muscular contraction: recent structural studies suggest a revealing model for cross-bridge action at variable filament spacing. Science 164:1356, 1969.

Ito, Y., and Chidsey, C. A.: Intracellular calcium and myocardial contractility. IV. Distribution of calcium in the failing heart. J. Mol. Cell. Cardiol. 4:507, 1972.

Langer, G. A., and Serena, S. D.: Effects of strophanthidin upon conduction and ionic exchange in rabbit ventricular myocardium: relation to control of active state. J. Mol. Cell. Cardiol. 1:65, 1970.

Long, L., Fabian, F., Mason, D. T., and Wikman-Coffelt, J.: A new cardiac myosin characterized from the canine atria. Biochem. Biophys. Res. Comm. 76:626, 1977.

Luchi, R. J., Kritcher, E. M., and Thyrum, P. T.: Reduced cardiac myosin adenosine triphosphate activity in dogs with spontaneously occurring heart failure. Circ. Res. 24:513, 1969.

Mason, D. T., Vera, Z., DeMaria, A. N., et al.: Treatment of tachyarrhythmias. *In* Mason, D. T. (Ed.): Cardiac Emergencies. Baltimore, Williams & Wilkins Co., 1978.

Nayler, W. G., and Merrillees, N. C. R.: Cellular exchange of calcium. *In* Harris, P., and Opie, L. H. (Eds.): Calcium and the Heart. New York, Academic Press, 1971, pp. 24–65.

Pool, P. E., Chandler, B. M., Spann, J. F., Jr., et al.: Mechanochemistry of cardiac muscle. IV. Utilization of high-energy phosphates in experimental heart failure in cats. Circ. Res. *24:*313, 1969.

Schwartz, A.: Calcium and the sarcoplasmic reticulum. *In* Harris, P., and Opie, L. H. (Eds.): Calcium and the Heart. New York, Academic Press, 1971, pp. 66–92.

Sordahl, L. A., Wood, W. G., and Schwartz, A.: Production of cardiac hypertrophy and failure in rabbits with Ameroid clips. J. Mol. Cell. Cardiol., *1:*341, 1970.

Sulakhe, P. V., and Dhalla, N. S.: Excitation-contraction coupling in the heart. VII. Calcium accumulation in subcellular particles in congestive heart failure. J. Clin. Invest. *50:*1019, 1971.

Swynghedauw, B., Leger, J. J., and Schwartz, K.: The myosin isozyme hypothesis in chronic heart overloading. J. Mol. Cell. Cardiol. *8:*915, 1975.

Thomas, L. L., and Alpert, N. R.: Functional integrity of the SH_1 in myosin from hypertrophied myocardium. Biochim. Biophys. Acta *481:*680, 1977.

Wier, W. G.: Calcium transients during excitation-contraction coupling in mammalian heart: aequorin signals of canine purkinje fibers. Science *207:*1085, 1980.

Wikman-Coffelt, J., Fenner, C., Walsh, R., et al.: Comparison of mild versus severe pressure overload on the enzymatic activity of myosin in the canine ventricles. Biochem. Med. *14:*139, 1975.

Wikman-Coffelt, J., Walsh, R., Fenner, C., et al.: Activity and molecular changes in left ventricular and right ventricular myosin during right ventricular volume overload. Biochem. Med. *14:*33, 1975.

MYOCARDIAL FUNCTION

Abbott, B. C., and Mommaerts, W. F. H. M.: A study of inotropic mechanisms in the papillary muscle preparation. J. Gen. Physiol. *42:*533, 1959.

Brady, A. J.: Active state in cardiac muscle. Physiol. Rev. *48:*570, 1968.

Braunwald, E., Ross, J., Jr., Gault, J. H., et al.: Assessment of cardiac function. Ann. Intern. Med. *70:*369, 1969.

Brutsaert, D. L., Claes, V. A., and Sonnenblick, E. H.: Velocity of shortening of unloaded heart muscle and the length-tension relation. Circ. Res. *29:*63, 1971.

Bunnell, I. L., Grant, C., and Greene, D. G.: Left ventricular function derived from the pressure-volume diagram. Am. J. Med. *39:*881, 1965.

Capone, R. J., Mason, D. T., Amsterdam, E. A., and Zelis, R.: The effect of mitral regurgitation and ventricular aneurysm on Vmax calculated from pressure-velocity data during "isovolumic" systole. Circulation *43*(Suppl. 2):96, 1971.

Cooper, R. H., O'Rourke, R. A., Karliner, J. S., et al.: Comparison of ultrasound and cineangiographic measurements of the mean rate of circumferential fiber shortening in man. Circulation *46:*914, 1972.

Covell, J. W., Ross, J., Jr., Sonnenblick, E. H., and Braunwald, E.: Comparison of the force-velocity relation and the ventricular function curve as measures of the contractile state of the intact heart. Circ. Res. *19:*364, 1966.

DeMaria, A. N., Bonanno, J. A., Amsterdam, E. A., et al.: Radarkymography. *In* Weissler, A. M. (Ed.): Noninvasive Techniques in Cardiac Evaluation. New York, Grune & Stratton, 1974, pp. 275–300.

DeMaria, A. N., Kamiyama, T., Peng, C. L., et al.: Alterations of ventricular function and myocardial contractility indices induced by ventricular asynchrony. Clin. Res. *21:*414, 1973.

DeMaria, A. N., Neumann, A. L., and Mason, D. T.: Echographic evaluation of cardiac function. *In* Mason, D. T. (Ed.): Congestive Heart Failure. New York, Yorke Medical Books, 1976, pp. 91–224.

Dodge, H. T., and Baxley, W. A.: Left ventricular volume and mass and their significance in heart disease. Am. J. Cardiol. *23:*528, 1969.

Falsetti, H. L., Mates, R. E., Greene, D. G., et al.: Vmax as an index of contractile state in man. Circulation *43:*467, 1971.

Forrester, J. S., Diamond, G., Parmley, W. W., and Swan, H. J. C.: Early increase in left ventricular compliance after myocardial infarction. J. Clin. Invest. *51:*598, 1972.

Frank, M. J., and Levinson, G. E.: An index of the contractile state of the myocardium in man. J. Clin. Invest. *47:*1615, 1968.

Fry, D. L., Griggs, D. M., Jr., and Greenfield, J. C., Jr.: Myocardial mechanics: tension-velocity-length relations of heart muscle. Circ. Res. *14:*73, 1964.

Gaasch, W. H., Battle, W. E., Oboler, A. A., et al.: Left ventricular stress and compliance in man with special reference to normalized ventricular function curves. Circulation *45:*756, 1972.

Gabe, I. T., Gault, J., Ross, J., Jr., et al.: Measurement of instantaneous blood flow velocity and pressure in conscious man with a catheter-tip velocity probe. Circulation *40:*603, 1969.

Gault, J. H., Ross, J., Jr., and Braunwald, E.: Contractile state of the left ventricle in man: instantaneous tension-velocity-length relations in patients with and without disease of the left ventricular myocardium. Circ. Res. *22:*451, 1968.

Gleeson, W. L., and Braunwald, E.: Studies on the first derivative of the ventricular pressure pulse in man. J. Clin. Invest. *41:*80, 1962.

Glick, G., Sonnenblick, E. H., and Braunwald, E.: Myocardial force-velocity relations studied in intact unanesthetized man. J. Clin. Invest. *44:*978, 1965.

Gordon, A. M., Huxley, A. F., and Julian, F. G.: Variation in isometric tension with sarcomere length in vertebrate muscle fibres. J. Physiol. *184:*170, 1966.

Grossman, W., Brooks, H., Meister, S., et al.: New technique for determining instantaneous myocardial force-velocity relation in the intact heart. Circ. Res. *28:*290, 1971.

Grossman, W., Hayes, F., Paraskos, J. A., et al.: Alterations in preload and myocardial mechanics in the dog and in man. Circ. Res. *31:*83, 1972.

Herman, M. V., and Gorlin, R.: Implications of left ventricular asynergy. Am. J. Cardiol. *23:*538, 1969.

Hill, A. V.: The heat of shortening and the dynamic constants of muscle. Proc. Roy. Soc. London (Series B) *126:*136, 1938.

Karliner, J. S., Gault, J. H., Eckberg, D. E., et al.: Mean velocity of fiber shortening. A simplified measure of left ventricular myocardial contractility. Circulation *44:*323, 1971.

Levine, H. J.: Clinical Cardiovascular Physiology. New York, Grune & Stratton, 1976.

Levine, H. J., and Britman, M. A.: Force-velocity relations in intact dog heart. J. Clin. Invest. *43:*1383, 1964.

Levine, H. J., McIntyre, K. M., Lipana, J. G., and Bing, O. H. L.: Force-velocity relations in failing and nonfailing hearts of subjects with aortic stenosis. Am. J. Med. Sci. *259:*79, 1970.

Mason, D. T.: Usefulness and limitations of the rate of rise of intraventricular pressure (dp/dt) in the evaluation of myocardial contractility in man. Am. J. Cardiol. *23:*516, 1969.

Mason, D. T.: Regulation of cardiac performance in clinical heart disease: interactions between contractile state, mechanical abnormalities and ventricular compensatory mechanisms. Am. J. Cardiol. *32:*437, 1973.

Mason, D. T.: Afterload reduction and cardiac performance: physiologic basis of systemic vasodilators as a new approach in treatment of congestive heart failure. Am. J. Med. *65:*106, 1978.

Mason, D. T., and Braunwald, E.: Studies on digitalis. IX. Effects of ouabain on the nonfailing human heart. J. Clin. Invest. *42:*7, 1963.

Mason, D. T., and Braunwald, E.: Hemodynamic techniques in the investigation of cardiovascular function in man. *In* Gordon, B. (Ed.): Clinical Cardiopulmonary Physiology. 3rd ed. New York, Grune and Stratton, 1969, p. 153.

Mason, D. T., Braunwald, E., Covell, J. W., et al.: Assessment of cardiac contractility: the relation between the rate of pressure rise and ventricular pressure during isovolumic systole. Circulation *44:*47, 1971.

Mason, D. T., Miller, R. R., and DeMaria, A. N.: Cardiac catheterization in the clinical assessment of heart disease and ventricular performance. In Mason, D. T. (Ed.): Congestive Heart Failure. New York, Yorke Medical Books, 1976, pp. 225–271.

Mason, D. T., Sonnenblick, E. G., Ross, J., Jr., et al.: Time to peak dp/dt: a useful measurement for evaluating the contractile state of the human heart. Circulation 32(Suppl. 2):145, 1965.

Mason, D. T., Spann, J. F., Jr., and Zelis, R.: Quantification of the contractile state of the intact human heart. Maximal velocity of contractile element shortening determined by the instantaneous relation between the rate of pressure rise and pressure in the left ventricle during isovolumic systole. Am. J. Cardiol 26:248, 1970.

Mason, D. T., Spann, J. F., Jr., Zelis, R., and Amsterdam, E. A.: Alterations of hemodynamics and myocardial mechanics in patients with congestive heart failure: pathophysiologic mechanisms and assessment of cardiac function and ventricular contractility. Prog. Cardiovasc. Dis. 12:507, 1970.

Mason, D. T., and Zelis, R.: Clinical quantification of cardiac contractility by mechanical properties of isovolumic systole. In Besse, P., and Bricaud, H. (Eds.): Left Ventricular Performance in Man. Paris, Expansion Scientifique, 1975, pp. 9–22.

Mason, D. T., Zelis, R., Amsterdam, E. A., and Massumi, R. A.: Clinical determination of left ventricular contractility by hemodynamics and myocardial mechanics. In Yu, P. N., and Goodwin, J. F. (Eds.): Progress in Cardiology. Philadelphia, Lea and Febiger, 1972, pp. 121–154.

Mason, D. T., Spann, J. F., Jr., Zelis, R. and Amsterdam, E.: Comparison of the contractile state of the normal hypertrophied and failing heart in man. In Alpert, N. R. (Ed.): Cardiac Hypertrophy. New York, Academic Press, 1971, pp. 433–444.

McCullagh, W. H., Covell, J. W., and Ross, J., Jr.: Left ventricular dilatation and diastolic compliance changes during chronic volume overloading. Circulation 45:943, 1972.

McDonald, I. G.: Contraction of the hypertrophied left ventricle in man studied by cineradiography of epicardial markers. Am. J. Cardiol. 30:587, 1972.

Mehmel, H. C., Krayenbuehl, H. P., and Wirz, P.: Isovolumic contraction dynamics in man according to two different muscle models. J. Appl. Physiol. 33:409, 1972.

Mirsky, I., Ghista, D., and Sandler, H.: Cardiac Mechanics: Physiological, Clinical, and Mathematical Considerations. New York, John Wiley & Sons, 1974.

Mitchell, J. H., Hefner, L. L., and Monroe, R. G.: Performance of the left ventricle. Am. J. Med. 53:481, 1972.

Parmley, W. W., Chuck, L., and Sonnenblick, E. H.: Relation of Vmax to different models of cardiac muscle. Circ. Res. 30:34, 1972.

Peterson, K. L., Uther, J. B., Shabetai, R., and Braunwald, E.: Instantaneous left ventricular tension-velocity relations obtained with an electromagnetic velocity catheter in the ascending aorta. Clin. Res. 20:173, 1972.

Rackley, C. E., Dodge, H. T., Coble, Y. D., and Hay, R. E.: A method for determining left ventricular mass in man. Circulation 29:666, 1964.

Rackley, C. E., Russell, R. O., Moraski, R. E., et al.: Catheterization evaluation of cardiac function in acute and chronic coronary artery disease. In Mason, D. T. (Ed.): Congestive Heart Failure. New York, Yorke Medical Books, 1976, pp. 273–290.

Ross, J., Jr., Covell, J. W., Sonnenblick, E. H., and Braunwald, E.: Contractile state of the heart characterized by force-velocity relations in variably afterloaded and isovolumic beats. Circ. Res. 18:149, 1966.

Ross, J., Jr., Gault, J. H., Mason, D. T., et al.: Left ventricular performance during muscular exercise in patients with and without cardiac dysfunction. Circulation 34:597, 1966.

Russell, R. O., Jr., Frimer, M., Porter, C. M., et al: Left ventricular power in heart disease. Am. J. Cardiol. 23:136, 1969.

Salel, A. F., Kamiyama, T., Peng, C. L., et al.: Pressure-velocity curves in the evaluation of right ventricular contractility. Circulation 46(Suppl. 2):216, 1972.

Sarnoff, S. J., and Mitchell, J. H.: Control of function of heart. In Hamilton, W. F., and Dow, P. (Eds.): Handbook of Physiology. Vol I, Section 2. Washington, D.C., American Physiological Society, 1962, pp. 489–532.

Siegel, J. H., and Sonnenblick, E. H.: Isometric time-tension relationships as an index of myocardial contractility. Circ. Res. 12:597, 1963.

Sonnenblick, E. H.: Implications of muscle mechanics in the heart. Fed. Proc. 21:975, 1962.

Sonnenblick, E. H.: Instantaneous force-velocity-length determinants in the contraction of heart muscle. Circ. Res. 16:441, 1965.

Sonnenblick, E. H.: Contractility of cardiac muscle. Circ. Res. 27:479, 1970.

Sonnenblick, E. H., Ross, J., Jr., Spotnitz, H. M., et al.: The ultrastructure of the heart in systole and diastole: changes in sarcomere length. Circ. Res. 21:423, 1967.

Taylor, R. R., Ross, J., Jr., Covell, J. W., and Sonnenblick, E. H.: A quantitative analysis of left ventricular myocardial function in the intact, sedated dog. Circ. Res. 21:99, 1967.

Urschel, C. W., Covell, J. W., Sonnenblick, E. H., et al.: Myocardial mechanics in aortic and mitral valvular regurgitation: the concept of instantaneous impedance as a determinant of the performance of the intact heart. J. Clin. Invest. 47:867, 1968.

Urschel, C. W., Henderson, A. H., and Sonnenblick, E. H.: Model dependency of ventricular force-velocity relations: importance of developed pressure. Fed. Proc. 29:719, 1970.

Wolk, M. H., Keefe, J. F., Bing, O. H. L., et al.: Estimation of Vmax in auxotonic systoles from the rate of relative increase of isovolumic pressure: (dp/dt)KP. J. Clin. Invest. 50:1276, 1971.

Yang, S. S., Bentivoglio, L. G., Maranhao, V., and Goldberg, H.: Cardiac Catheterization Data and Hemodynamic Parameters. Philadelphia, F. A. Davis Co., 1972.

Yeatman, L. A., Jr., Parmley, W. W., and Sonnenblick, E. H.: Effect of temperature on series elasticity and contractile element motion in heart muscle. Am. J. Physiol. 217:1030, 1969.

Yeatman, L. A., Jr., Parmley, W. W., Urschel, C. W., and Sonnenblick, E. H.: Dynamics of contractile elements in isometric contractions of cardiac muscle. Am. J. Physiol. 220:534, 1971.

Zelis, R., Amsterdam, E. A., and Mason, D. T.: "Isometric" Vmax as an index of contractility independent of series elastic and fiber shortening: implications concerning pressure-velocity data in myocardial fibrosis, valvular regurgitation, ventricular aneurysm and ventricular septal defect. Circulation 44(Suppl. 2):89, 1971.

9

Cardiac Output, Cardiac Performance, Hypertrophy, Dilatation, Valvular Disease, Ischemic Heart Disease, and Pericardial Disease

Harold T. Dodge and J. Ward Kennedy

CARDIAC OUTPUT

The measurement of cardiac output by what is now known as the Fick principle was first applied in animals at the end of the nineteenth century. Since this method requires sampling of mixed venous blood from the pulmonary artery or right ventricle, its application to humans followed the development of right heart catheterization in the 1940s. The indicator dilution method for determining cardiac output was developed by Stewart in 1897 and by Hamilton in 1929 and became widely applied in the 1950s. Both the direct Fick and indicator dilution methods have become standard techniques in cardiac catheterization laboratories and are now frequently used in intensive and coronary care units for the serial measurement of cardiac output during the course of severe illness. More recently, the development of sensitive thermistor probes has allowed modification of the indicator dilution method to the thermodilution method, in which warm or cool saline instead of a dye is used as an indicator. The development and wide application of angiocardiography have provided another method for measurement of the output of the heart by analysis of the change in volume (stroke volume) of the left ventricle during the cardiac cycle. Quantitative angiocardiographic methods for measuring left ventricular stroke volume and minute output are particularly useful in evaluating ventricular performance in patients with heart disease, as will be discussed later.

In addition to the aforementioned methods for directly measuring cardiac output in humans, there have also been many methods devised to estimate cardiac output indirectly. These include analysis of arterial pulse waves; the ballistocardiogram; systolic time intervals using electrocardiographic, phonocardiographic, and carotid pulse wave data; ultrasonic echocardiography; and, most recently, the development and application of instruments for measuring blood-flow velocity with ultrasound by the Doppler shift principle. Although some of these methods are useful in predicting directional changes in cardiac output during the course of illness, they all appear to be less accurate than the direct Fick and indicator dilution methods.

FICK METHOD

This method depends on a knowledge of the quantity of oxygen entering the system measured as the oxygen consumption as determined from samples of expired air and the difference in oxygen content between venous and arterial blood. Since venous blood from different parts of the body has a variable oxygen content, it must be mixed to obtain a sample that represents total body venous oxygen content. When blood passes through the right ventricle, adequate mixing occurs. The mixed venous sample for Fick cardiac output determination is therefore obtained from the pulmonary artery through a right heart catheter. Occasionally, a right ventricular sampling site is utilized when the pulmonary artery cannot be entered. The arterial sample may be obtained from any convenient peripheral artery in the absence of a right-to-left cardiac shunt. When a shunt is present, the sample must be obtained upstream from the shunt.

The formula for determining cardiac output (CO) is as follows:

$$\text{Cardiac output} = \frac{\text{Oxygen consumption}}{\text{Arteriovenous oxygen difference}}$$

A typical value for oxygen consumption in an average-sized adult male at rest is 240 ml per minute. The normal resting arteriovenous oxygen difference is in the range of 40 ml of O_2 per liter of blood. Substituting into the formula,

$$\text{CO} = \frac{240}{40} = 6.0 \text{ L/minute}$$

Errors in the measurement of oxygen consumption and oxygen content of arterial and venous blood result in a total error of the method of

8 to 10 per cent. In applying the method, the chief limitations are the necessity of right heart catheterization and the cooperation of the patient to obtain a representative sample of expired air that can be used for measuring oxygen consumption.

INDICATOR DILUTION METHOD

The indicator dilution technique is preferred over the direct Fick method in many laboratories because it eliminates the need for right heart catheterization. A known quantity of indicator (I), usually indocyanine green, is injected into the venous circulation and the resultant time-concentration curve is determined by continuous withdrawal of arterial blood through a densitometer.

$$\text{Cardiac output} = \frac{I}{C \cdot t}$$

where C represents the mean concentration of the indicator during the time (t) from the appearance to disappearance of the indicator as determined from the time-concentration curve. The validity of the method depends on two assumptions: (1) that there is complete mixing of indicator prior to sampling, and (2) that the indicator concentration curve with respect to time represents only the first passage of the indicator past the sampling site. Since recirculation of indicator distorts the terminal portion of the primary curve to a greater or lesser extent, depending on the injection and sampling sites and the status of circulatory dynamics, various methods have been developed to separate the primary curve from the recirculation curve. These methods are based on the assumption that the fall of concentration in the primary curve follows an exponential time course that can be determined by relating the logarithm of the concentration to time. The time-concentration curve is plotted on a semilogarithmic graph, and the initial portion of the primary curve is identified and then extrapolated as a straight line to zero. This process eliminates the recirculation component of the curve and thus defines the primary curve. An adequate portion of the primary curve must be obtained to permit this extrapolation. From the primary curve, values for (C) and (t) are determined. Small special-purpose computers are now available to separate the primary and recirculation curves and give immediate cardiac output results.

THERMODILUTION TECHNIQUE

The thermodilution technique is similar to the indicator dilution technique but has the advantage that there is no significant recirculation of the indicator, since the temperature difference of the injectate and the blood is lost into tissue prior to recirculation. In general, there is good agreement between the results of the Fick, indicator dilution, and thermodilution methods for determining cardiac output in humans. The development of a balloon-tipped, flow-directed thermodilution catheter that can be inserted into the pulmonary artery without fluoroscopic control has greatly facilitated the use of the thermodilution cardiac output technique. This method is now widely used as an aid in the care of critically ill cardiac patients.

NORMAL CARDIAC OUTPUT

Since the cardiac output is a fundamental measurement of cardiac function, it has been the subject of extensive study in normal animals and humans at rest and during various stresses and in patients with all types of heart diseases. This subject was well reviewed by Wade and Bishop in 1962. Cardiac output is best expressed in terms of body size, and, in general, body surface area is used instead of body weight. The term *cardiac index* is used to refer to the cardiac output per square meter of body surface area. It is frequently convenient to express the output of the heart per beat as stroke volume or the cardiac index per beat as stroke index. The resting cardiac index in a normal human is approximately 3.3 L per minute per M^2, with a low value of about 2.8 L per minute per M^2. Cardiac output decreases with age at the rate of approximately 25 ml per minute per M^2 per year after early adulthood. With a resting heart rate of 70 beats per minute, the normal stroke index is 46 ml.

REGULATION OF CARDIAC OUTPUT

The cardiac output normally increases under the stimulus of muscular exercise up to five times the resting value, depending somewhat on the age and physical training of the individual. There are many factors that make possible such large changes of flow, some of which will be described subsequently.

The return of venous blood to the right heart is regulated in such a manner that the venous return equals the systemic output of the left ventricle. Venous return to a great extent is regulated by alterations in the tone of the venous capacitance vessels, which contain most of the blood volume. Increases or decreases in venous tone therefore have a marked effect on the filling of the right atrium and ventricle and thereby on the output of the left ventricle. Increases or decreases of circulating blood volume also cause respective changes of venous return and cardiac output if not compensated for by changes in venous tone. Cardiac output may increase for a short time with increases in blood volume as occurs with overtransfusion, but compensatory increased volume of venous capacitance vessels soon reduces the right ventricular filling volume, pressure, and output. In patients with chronic heart failure, circulating blood volume is chronically increased owing to retention of sodium and water by the kidneys, and venous tone is increased. As a result, an increased volume of blood is present in the central circulation, which elevates the filling volume and pressure of the two ventricles to maintain cardiac output through the Frank-Starling mechanism. Accordingly, venous return is a major factor in the control of cardiac output in both health and disease and is determined by the blood volume and the capacity and tone of the venous bed.

AUTONOMIC CONTROL OF CARDIAC OUTPUT

The autonomic nervous system significantly controls cardiac output by acting on heart rate, myocardial contractility, and vasomotor tone. In general, parasympathetic tone is greater than sympathetic tone when an individual is at rest. Maximal stimuli to increase sympathetic tone occur during heavy exercise and under severe psychologic stress. Increased parasympathetic tone occurs with vomiting, occasionally in response to severe pain, and with vigorous carotid sinus massage. Sympathetic nerve stimulation has a positive inotropic and chronotropic effect on the heart, resulting in increased heart rate and increased myocardial contractility, which results in increased force, extent, and velocity of myocardial fiber shortening. This causes an increase in stroke volume, provided that venous return is adequate to maintain filling of the right ventricle. In contrast to this, increased parasympathetic tone decreases the heart rate and has little or no effect on contractility of the ventricles. Peripheral vasculature tone increases with sympathetic stimulation, and this results in increased venous return to the right heart, increased ventricular filling pressure, and increased stroke volume. The effects of increased sympathetic tone (i.e., increased heart rate, increased myocardial contractility, and increased venous return) all combine to increase cardiac output.

PERIPHERAL OXYGEN REQUIREMENT

In general, cardiac output varies according to the requirement of the peripheral tissues for oxygen. Control of regional circulation is maintained so that cardiac output is shunted to the particular organ in need of oxygen. For example, during physical exertion blood flow is preferentially increased to the working muscles and reduced to the splanchnic bed and kidneys. When there is a marked reduction in cardiac output, as in some patients with heart failure, there is reduced blood flow to the skin, muscle, and splanchnic vascular

beds. As the cardiac output drops further, renal and finally cerebral blood flow falls. Regulation of regional blood flow therefore plays an important role in maintaining the tissue oxygen needs of the body during various activities and under many different conditions.

VASCULAR RESISTANCE

The peripheral vasculature of the systemic circulation and, to a lesser extent, of the pulmonary circulation is under autonomic nervous system and hormonal control. The vascular resistance, therefore, will vary according to the hemodynamic state of the patient. Systemic vascular resistance becomes chronically elevated in idiopathic or renal vascular hypertension. In chronic mitral stenosis, pulmonary vascular resistance is chronically elevated. It is frequently important to determine the systemic and/or pulmonary vascular resistance.

The resistance of a vascular bed can be calculated if the flow and pressure drop across the bed are known. For these calculations, mean pressures are utilized, and the values are reported in dynes-second centimeters^{-5} (dsc^{-5}). In order to calculate resistance in dsc^{-5}, one must convert pressure measured in mm Hg into dynes per cm^2 by multiplying by 1332. One converts liters per minute to ml per second by multiplying further by 0.06, obtaining a conversion factor of 80.

Therefore:

$$\text{Resistance in dsc}^{-5} = \frac{\text{Mean pressure (mm Hg)} \times 80}{\text{Flow (L/min)}}$$

Systemic vascular resistance (SVR) is calculated as follows:

$$\text{SVR} = \frac{\text{Mean arterial pressure} \times 80}{\text{Cardiac output (L/min)}}$$

Total pulmonary artery resistance is calculated in a similar manner. In some instances, it is also useful to measure the pulmonary vascular resistance (PVR) in order to separate the components of total pulmonary resistance, which results from the pulmonary vasculature, from that component resulting from left atrial pressure. This is, of course, most useful in evaluating patients with left atrial hypertension, such as occurs with mitral stenosis or left ventricular failure. One determines pulmonary vascular resistance by using the pulmonary flow and the difference between the mean pulmonary artery (Pa mean) and mean left atrial pressure (LA mean).

$$\text{PVR} = \frac{(\text{Pa mean} - \text{LA mean}) \times 80}{\text{Pulmonary flow (L/min)}}$$

Normal values for systemic, total pulmonary, and pulmonary vascular resistance are listed in Table 9–1 as reported by Barratt-Boyes in 1958.

TABLE 9–1 NORMAL VALUES: INTRACARDIAC PRESSURES

	Systolic	Diastolic	Mean
Right atrium	3–7	0–2	0–6
Right ventricle	15–30	0–5	—
Pulmonary artery	15–30	6–12	9–17
Left atrium	—	—	5–12
Left ventricle	100–140	2–12	—
Vascular resistance			
Systemic	1130 ± 178 dsc^{-5}		
Total pulmonary	205 ± 51 dsc^{-5}		
Pulmonary vascular	67 ± 23 dsc^{-5}		

(Adapted from data in Barratt-Boyes, B. G., and Wood, E. H.: J. Lab. Clin. Med. *51*:72, 1958.)

As is apparent from these values, total pulmonary resistance is mostly the result of left atrial pressure, not resistance in the pulmonary vasculature. In other words, about two thirds of right heart pressure work goes into filling the left heart under normal resting conditions.

THERAPEUTIC CONTROL OF CARDIAC OUTPUT

In situations of high or low cardiac output due to disease, the physician often attempts to control the cardiac output with drugs or other maneuvers. In several different circumstances, cardiac output is abnormally high, as in febrile patients, conditions of increased metabolism such as thyrotoxicosis, arteriovenous shunts, severe anemia, and ineffective oxygen-carrying capacity of hemoglobin, as in carbon monoxide poisoning. In all these conditions, cardiac output returns toward normal with correction of the abnormality that caused the elevated output.

In conditions of abnormally low cardiac output, the physician often is faced with a more difficult problem. Low cardiac output due to inadequate venous return as a result of inadequate blood volume is easily treated with transfusion or fluid replacement. Low cardiac output due to bradycardia may be successfully treated with drugs or an artificial pacemaker. When cardiac output is inadequate because of poor myocardial contraction, sympathomimetic drugs or digitalis glycosides may be used to increase myocardial contractile force. At times, venous filling pressure may be artificially elevated above normal levels by the administration of saline or plasma in an attempt to increase cardiac output. Unfortunately, the depressed cardiac output such as occurs in advanced myocardial failure often remains low despite current therapeutic methods.

Work by several investigators has shown that chronic reduction of peripheral vascular resistance or ventricular afterload may be achieved by various arterial and venous dilating drugs, such as sublingual and topical nitroglycerin, sublingual and oral isosorbide dinitrate, oral hydralazine, and nitroglycerin and nitroprusside given by continuous infusion. These vasodilating agents, which are now often referred to as "afterload-reducing drugs," produce increased cardiac output with no increase in cardiac work by reducing systemic vascular resistance. When used in patients with advanced heart failure or cardiogenic shock or both, these agents have been associated with reduced mortality and improved medical management of heart failure.

CARDIAC CATHETERIZATION

The technique of cardiac catheterization merits brief mention in a text of pathologic physiology because much of what is known of altered cardiac function in various disease states has been gained through the use of this technique. Cardiac catheterization was first carried out by Forssmann in 1929 when he passed a catheter transvenously into his own right atrium. André Cournand and colleagues introduced the use of this important technique for the study of normal and pathologic physiology. Today, all chambers of the heart and much of the venous and arterial vasculature are regularly catheterized for purposes of blood sampling, pressure recording, and the injection of radiographic contrast material for angiographic visualization. The usual sites of catheter insertion include the veins of the antecubital fossa, the femoral vein, and the brachial and femoral arteries. Large vessels may be entered safely with the percutaneous Seldinger technique. This method involves needle puncture of the vessel with insertion of a flexible guide wire over which the catheter is inserted. When smaller vessels are entered, a small incision with isolation of the vessel for cannulation is required.

Catheterization of the right atrium, ventricle, and pulmonary artery is performed by advancing a catheter from a large peripheral vein through these chambers under fluoroscopic guidance. The development of a flow-directed balloon-tipped catheter by Swan and Ganz now permits right heart catheterization without fluoroscopy. One catheterizes the large arteries, aorta, and left ventricle in a manner similar to that used in the right heart by passing the catheter retrograde from an insertion site in a large artery—usually the brachial or femoral artery. Specially designed catheters are used to cannulate selectively the left and right coronary arteries for purposes of coronary angiography. The left atrium is the cardiac chamber least accessible to the cardiologist. It is usually catheterized by the transseptal technique in which, with the aid of a long needle, a catheter is passed across the interatrial septum from the right to the left atrium. Occasionally, the left atrium is catheterized retrograde across the mitral valve from the left ventricle. In the hands of an experienced cardiac catheterization team, the risk of death resulting from these procedures is between one and two per 1000 patients.

INTRACARDIAC PRESSURE RECORDINGS

Recording pressure in the various chambers of the heart and the great vessels is often a major goal of cardiac catheterization. This is usually accomplished by attaching a fluid-filled catheter to a pressure transducer. The electrical output of the transducer is amplified, displayed on an oscilloscope, and recorded on paper or on magnetic tape. The system is calibrated, and the zero level of the transducers is set at the level of the midthorax. Normal pressures for the various cardiac chambers are given in Table 9–1. At times, it is more convenient to limit catheterization to the right side of the heart. When this is the case, an estimate of pulmonary venous pressure and left atrial pressure can be obtained by passing an endhole catheter out into a terminal pulmonary artery. When "wedged" in this position, the catheter records the pressure transmitted back across the pulmonary capillary bed from the pulmonary veins. This pressure is termed the *pulmonary wedge (pulmonary capillary) pressure*. The mean pulmonary wedge pressure will generally be within 2 mm Hg of the mean left atrial pressure, unless pulmonary venous obstruction is present.

In the last several years, various types of catheters have been developed that contain a pressure transducer at the distal tip. These catheter tip manometers are capable of recording pressures more accurately in the heart because they are free from the hydraulic damping effects, time delays, and motion artifacts that distort pressures recorded through fluid-filled catheters. These improved pressure-recording systems have allowed the detailed analysis of the rapid pressure changes that occur in the right and left ventricle during early systole and early diastole. The maximum rate of rise of the left ventricular pressure, generally referred to as LV dp/dt, has been used as an index of left ventricular myocardial performance. Catheter tip manometers make it possible to record LV dp/dt with sufficient accuracy to permit their use for evaluating myocardial contractility in humans. Multiple variables influence the LV dp/dt, including heart rate, filling pressure (preload), aortic diastole pressure (afterload), myocardial inotropic state, and left ventricular diastolic volume. Because of these many influences, LV dp/dt is more useful in evaluating changes of myocardial performance in a single patient than in comparing the myocardial performance in one patient with that of another.

Various types of valvular abnormalities due to congenital and rheumatic heart disease can now be treated surgically, so that it has become important to evaluate precisely the severity of valve stenosis or incompetence or both. Congenital aortic, pulmonary, and postrheumatic mitral and aortic valve stenosis are the most common types of valvular stenosis, although the other cardiac valves may become stenotic on either a congenital or rheumatic basis. Cardiac catheterization is required to measure the pressure on each side of a stenotic valve, so that the pressure gradient across the valve can be determined. Figure 9–1 is taken from the simultaneous recording of left ventricular and aortic pressure in a patient with aortic stenosis. The high-fidelity left ventricular pressure was obtained with a catheter tip manometer. The shaded area represents the gradient across the stenotic aortic valve. The mean gradient can be obtained by dividing the shaded area by the duration of the valve gradient. Figure 9–2 is taken from simultaneous pressure recordings in the left atrium and left ventricle in a patient with mitral stenosis. The left ventricular pressure was recorded through a fluid-filled catheter and there is some oscillation in the pressure during diastole, indicating an underdamped pressure manometer system. The diastolic gradient across the mitral valve is represented by the shaded area. In these two examples, large pressure gradients are present across these stenotic valves, but since the pressure gradient is a function of both valve orifice size and flow across the valve, the severity of valvular stenosis is best determined by calculation of the cross-sectional area of the valve. This can be done with the formulas developed by Gorlin and Gorlin. These relate the gradient in pressure across the valve during the period of valve flow and rate of flow across the valve to the area of the valve orifice. Empirical correction factors have been introduced based on surgical and postmortem observations.

The basic formula is as follows:

$$\text{Valve orifice} = \frac{\text{Valve flow}}{(K)\ \sqrt{\text{Pressure gradient}}}$$

In the case of the mitral valve the valve flow is measured per diastolic second, whereas in the calculation of the area of the aortic valve orifice the flow is determined per systolic second. The pressure gradient is the mean difference in pressure across the valve during diastolic filling for mitral stenosis and systolic ejection for aortic stenosis. The K values are 31.0 and 44.5 for the mitral and aortic valves, respectively. When there is no valvular incompetence or intracardiac shunt, the flow across the valve is equal to the cardiac output. When valvular incompetence is also present, the flow across the valve is increased and must be taken into account if an accurate valve area is to be obtained. Usually, the mitral valve orifice is constricted to less than 1.2 cm^2 or the aortic valve to less than 1.0 cm^2 before symptoms develop that are significant enough for the physician to consider surgical correction.

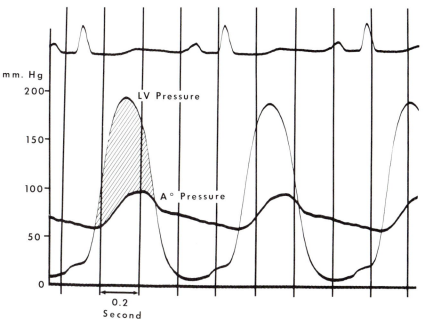

Figure 9–1 Left ventricular and central aortic pressure in a patient with tight valvular aortic stenosis. The shaded area indicates the pressure gradient across the valve during systole.

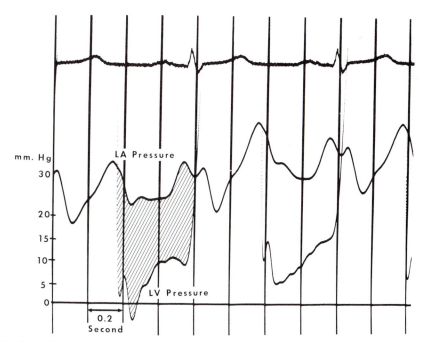

Figure 9–2 Left ventricular and left atrial pressure in a patient with mitral stenosis. Only the lower portion of the left ventricular pressure is seen. The shaded area indicates the pressure gradient across the mitral valve during diastole.

INTRACARDIAC SHUNTS

Cardiac catheterization techniques are used to locate and quantify intracardiac shunts. This is generally done through determination of the oxygen content of blood samples from the appropriate cardiac chambers and great vessels. Frequently, the cardiac catheter will pass through the intracardiac defect or abnormal venous or arterial channel directly, demonstrating its presence. The introduction of a dye, radiopaque contrast media, or hydrogen gas may also be used to detect or demonstrate abnormal blood flow.

LEFT-TO-RIGHT SHUNTS

Abnormal shunting of blood occurs most commonly from the systemic to the venous circulation and is identified by the demonstration of oxygenated blood entering the venous circulation. Conditions in which this occurs include patent ductus arteriosus; aorticopulmonary window; atrial septal defect; ventricular septal defect; and anomalous pulmonary venous drainage to the vena cava, coronary sinus, or right atrium. Occasionally, left-to-right shunts may develop following birth, as with the rupture of a sinus of Valsalva aneurysm into the right heart or the development of a ventricular septal defect following infarction of the interventricular septum. Arteriovenous fistulae may be congenital or acquired and result in a functional arteriovenous shunting of blood.

In general, these defects are easy to recognize at cardiac catheterization by sampling blood from the appropriate sites on the right side of the heart. An increase in oxygen saturation or content occurs at the level of the shunt, thus localizing it anatomically. By comparing the oxygen content of mixed venous blood proximal and distal to the level of the shunt, the volume of the shunt can be calculated utilizing the Fick principle. As shown subsequently, these formulas yield a value for systemic blood flow and pulmonary blood flow. The difference between the two is the shunt flow. The ratio of pulmonary to systemic flow is often used to express the severity of the shunt. For example, if the pulmonary flow is 10 L per minute and the systemic flow is 5 L per minute, the magnitude of the shunt would be 2:1.

In the case of a ventricular septal defect and in the absence of right-to-left shunting, for example,

$$\text{Pulmonary blood flow} = \frac{O_2 \text{ consumption (ml/min)}}{\text{Systemic arterial } O_2 \text{ content} - \text{Pulmonary arterial } O_2 \text{ content}}$$

$$\text{Systemic blood flow} = \frac{O_2 \text{ consumption (ml/min)}}{\text{Systemic arterial } O_2 \text{ content} - \text{Right atrial } O_2 \text{ content}}$$

$$\text{Left-to-right shunt flow} = \text{Pulmonary blood flow} - \text{Systemic blood flow}$$

In the case of an atrial septal defect, the mixed venous O_2 content needs to be obtained from samples taken in the inferior (IVC) and superior (SVC) venae cavae. In this situation,

$$\text{Mixed venous } O_2 \text{ content} = \frac{\text{SVC } O_2 + 2 \text{ IVC } O_2}{3}$$

The 2:1 ratio is employed because of the large blood flow in the IVC relative to that in the SVC. In resting subjects, the oxygen content of IVC blood is higher than that of SVC samples because of the contribution of renal venous blood, which has a relatively high oxygen content.

CYANOTIC HEART DISEASE

The term *cyanotic heart disease* refers to systemic arterial oxygen desaturation due to a cardiovascular abnormality. Cyanosis is generally the result of the shunting of systemic venous blood into the systemic arterial circulation and occurs in such conditions as tetralogy of Fallot, single ventricle, truncus arteriosus, tricuspid atresia, and transposition of the great vessels.

For right-to-left shunting to occur across a patent ductus, ventricular septal defect, or atrial septal defect, the pressure on the right side of the defect must be higher than on the left side at least at some time during the cardiac cycle. Occasionally, right-to-left shunting occurs only during exercise and may be noted by exertional cyanosis. Right-to-left shunting occurs across a patent ductus either because it is located distal to a coarctation of the aorta or because of the presence of pulmonary hypertension of such severity that the total pulmonary resistance is greater than the systemic resistance. In this situation, there may be differential cyanosis, with cyanosis greater in the lower extremities. When right-to-left shunting occurs in patients with ventricular septal defect it is associated with either pulmonary hypertension due to increased pulmonary vascular resistance or pulmonary stenosis of the valvular or infundibular type. Pulmonary stenosis and ventricular septal defect are most often seen as features of the tetralogy of Fallot, the other two features being right ventricular hypertrophy and dextroposition of the aorta with overriding of the interventricular septum, so that the aorta communicates more or less directly with the right ventricular outflow tract. Atrial septal defect is less often associated with a right-to-left shunt. When this occurs, pulmonary hypertension has resulted in right ventricular failure and elevation of right atrial pressure to a level higher than the pressure in the left atrium. In the combination of atrial septal defect and tricuspid stenosis, right-to-left shunting at the atrial level will occur without pulmonary stenosis or right ventricular failure.

The calculation of right-to-left shunt is similar to the calculation of left-to-right shunts except that pulmonary venous blood must be either sampled or assumed to be 98 per cent saturated. If the patient is breathing oxygen, it can be assumed that the sample is fully saturated. Pulmonary blood flow (PBF) is then determined by the following formula:

$$PBF = \frac{O_2 \text{ consumption}}{\text{Pulmonary venous } O_2 - \text{Pulmonary arterial } O_2}$$

The systemic flow is calculated as follows:

$$SF = \frac{O_2 \text{ consumption}}{\text{Systemic arterial } O_2 - \text{Mixed venous } O_2}$$

The mixed venous O_2 should be obtained proximal to the shunt, since a bidirectional shunt may be present. The magnitude of right-to-left shunt is determined by subtracting the pulmonary blood flow from the systemic blood flow. When a bidirectional shunt is present, the effective pulmonary blood flow (Eff Pul BF) must be determined. This is the quantity of blood that picks up oxygen while circulating through the lungs and is determined by the following formula:

$$Eff\ Pul\ BF = \frac{O_2 \text{ consumption}}{\text{Pulmonary venous } O_2 - \text{Mixed venous } O_2}$$

A bidirectional shunt may then be calculated as follows:

Right-to-left shunt =
        Systemic flow − Effective pulmonary flow

Left-to-right shunt =
        Pulmonary flow − Effective pulmonary flow

The validity of flow values determined by these methods depends on rapid and accurate sampling of blood in the various cardiac chambers and vessels concerned. Blood entering the right atrium from the superior vena cava, inferior vena cava, and coronary sinus varies considerably in its O_2 content. The inferior vena cava blood has a high O_2 content owing to a large component of renal venous blood, whereas the coronary venous blood has a very low O_2 content. The atrium does not mix the blood well, so that blood flows in a laminar fashion through the atrium and into the right ventricle. Better mixing occurs here, so that the blood entering the pulmonary artery is usually

relatively homogeneous. The nonmixing of blood in the right atrium and vena cava possibly results in sampling errors and, consequently, in inaccurate shunt flow calculations. Rapid sampling and duplicate measurements can, however, give good estimates of flow that are of value in the clinical evaluation of patients.

Frequently, a left-to-right shunt is associated with pulmonary hypertension. When the pulmonary vascular resistance reaches systemic levels, right-to-left shunting develops and surgical correction of the defect becomes hazardous, if not impossible. In the presence of pulmonary hypertension due to cardiac shunts, great care must be taken in calculating blood flow and pulmonary artery pressure so that accurate pulmonary resistance values can be obtained. In borderline cases it may be useful to measure pulmonary flow and pressure before and during oxygen administration. If pulmonary vascular resistance falls with oxygen administration, surgical correction may be possible, whereas a failure of pulmonary artery pressure to drop suggests that pulmonary vascular resistance is fixed and not due in part to anoxia.

LEFT VENTRICULAR VOLUME AND MASS

There are now four methods of determining left ventricular chamber volumes in humans: (1) indicator dilution, (2) radiographic contrast angiocardiography, (3) isotope angiography, and (4) echocardiography. With the indicator dilution methods, an indicator is injected into the left ventricle and sampled immediately above the aortic valves with a sensor that responds rapidly to changes in the concentration of the indicator. The indicator dilution curves show a steplike decrease in indicator concentration, with the change of concentration per beat being a function of the volume of the left ventricle at end-diastole and the dilution with each stroke (stroke volume). End-diastolic volume (EDV) is computed as follows:

$$EDV = \frac{\text{Stroke volume}}{\left(1 - \dfrac{Cn}{Cn-1}\right)}$$

where stroke volume is determined by the standard indicator dilution method for measuring cardiac output, and $\dfrac{Cn}{Cn-1}$ is the ratio of beat-to-beat changes of concentration of indicator in the aorta. The accuracy of the volume determination depends on complete mixing of indicator in the left ventricle, a concentration of dye in the aorta that is equivalent to that in the ventricle, and a sufficiently high-frequency response of the system for indicator detection to determine accurately indicator concentration and ventricular washout

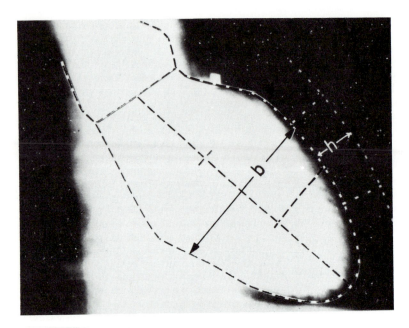

Figure 9–3 Angiocardiogram with the left ventricle and a segment of left ventricular wall outlined. Wall thickness is indicated by *h* and semi-diameter by *b*. (From Dodge, H. T.: Determination of left ventricular mass. Radiol. Clin. North Am. 9:459, 1971.)

as a step function. Various indicators have been used, including dyes, saline, and cold saline with appropriate indicator detection systems. These methods have the advantage of requiring a small volume of indicator that does not in itself cause physiologic changes, and measurements can be repeated frequently. In general, the indicator dilution methods have given larger end-diastolic and residual volumes than the angiocardiographic methods. This difference may be related to uneven mixing of the indicator.

Left ventricular chamber volumes can also be determined from angiocardiograms and cineangiocardiograms taken in biplane as well as single plane projections (Fig. 9–3). The methods most generally used assume that the left ventricle can be represented by an ellipsoid reference figure, with volume computed as

$$V = 4/3 \ \pi \ abc$$

where a equals the major semidiameter, and b and c equal the two minor semidiameters. The differences in methods used for computing volume by various laboratories are due to differences in the methods applied for determining the chamber dimensions. It has been demonstrated that in most

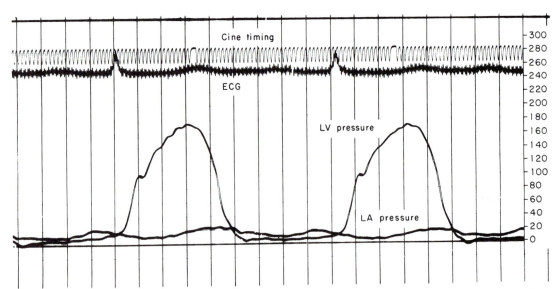

Figure 9–4 Recording of time of cine filming (65 frames per second) with respect to the ECG and left ventricular and atrial pressure in a patient with mitral stenosis.

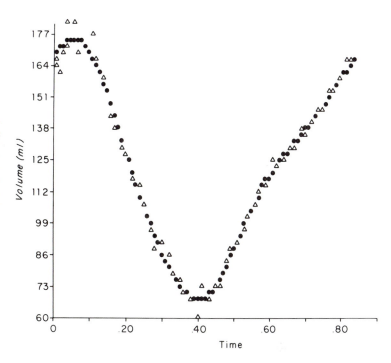

Figure 9–5 Left ventricular volumes computed from cine films taken at 65 frames per second are plotted as triangles with respect to time within the cardiac cycle. From these computed volumes a volume curve has been generated, as shown by the solid circles, through the use of a curve-fitting computer program.

subjects the two minor semidiameters (b and c) are similar. Accordingly, chamber volume can be computed from films taken in a single projection by assuming that b and c are equal, and the formula for computing volume becomes

$$P = 4/3 \ \pi \ ab^2$$

When the time of filming is recorded with the electrocardiogram and left ventricular pressure, as shown in Figure 9–4, the computed volumes can be related to time within the cardiac cycle to construct a left ventricular volume curve as shown in Figure 9–5. From this volume curve, end-diastolic, end-systolic, and stroke volumes can be determined. The portion of the end-diastolic volume ejected with systole $\left(\dfrac{SV}{EDV}\right)$ has been termed the *systolic ejection fraction*. From the slopes of the ejection and filling limbs, respectively, the rates of ventricular ejection and filling, respectively, can be computed. In addition, the angiocardiographic methods provide information on ventricular shape

and dimensions, permit visualization of focal contraction abnormalities as seen in ischemic heart disease, and also provide information on wall thickness. When added to chamber dimensions, the latter has made it possible to compute left ventricular mass as follows:

Vol LV chamber + Wall = $4/3\pi$ (a + h)(b + h)(c + h)

LV mass (gm) = [(Vol chamber + wall) −
Vol chamber] 1.050

where a, b, and c equal chamber semidiameters as previously defined, h equals wall thickness, and 1.050 is the specific gravity of heart muscle. Normal values for left ventricular chamber volumes, ejection fraction, wall thickness, and mass are given in Table 9–2.

With the rapid development of nuclear medicine techniques in cardiology, several methods for determining cardiac chamber volumes and left and right ventricular systolic ejection fractions have become available. The most useful are those uti-

TABLE 9–2 NORMAL VALUES IN ADULTS AND CHILDREN

	End-Diastolic Volume (ml/M²)	Stroke Volume (ml/M²)	End-Systolic Volume (ml/M²)	Ejection Fraction (SV/EDV)	Wall Thickness (mm)	Left Ventricle Mass (gm/M²)
Adults	70±20	45±13	24	0.67±0.08	10.9±2.0	92±16
Children and Infants						
Less than 2 years of age	42±10	28.6	13.4	0.68±0.05		96±11
More than 2 years of age (3 to 16 years)	73±11	44±5	27±7	0.63±0.05		86±11

(From Dodge, H. T.: Determination of left ventricular volume and mass. Radiol. Clin. North Am. *9*:459, 1971.)

lizing a gamma scintillation camera (Anger camera) to record radioactivity in the heart chambers. Activity can be observed following the intravenous bolus injection of the radionuclide as it passes through the right heart, pulmonary circulation, and left heart chambers. This "first pass" technique has the advantage of sequential observation of the four cardiac chambers so that overlapping of the chambers is avoided. With the "first pass" technique, the radioactive material is in the heart for only a short time, so the resolution of the gamma camera images is limited by low radioactivity counting rates. The blood pool method, currently favored by many laboratories, utilizes radioactive agents that are bound to red blood cells or albumin, so that the tracer remains in the intravascular compartment. The patient is monitored by an electrocardiogram, which is linked to the gamma camera so that the radionuclide images of the heart can be timed with the cardiac cycle. In this manner, a high resolution image of the cardiac chambers can be developed over several hundred heart beats for each phase of the cardiac cycle, as illustrated in Figure 9–6. This usually requires 2 to 6 minutes of imaging, during which time the patient must remain in a constant hemodynamic state and at relatively unchanging heart rate.

These radionuclide techniques for imaging the

EJECTION
FRACTION

R-WAVE
SYNCHRONOUS
EQUILIBRIUM
IMAGES

^{99m}Tc-RBC

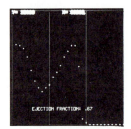

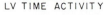

LV TIME ACTIVITY

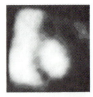

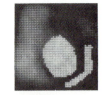

END DIASTOLIC IMAGE   LV AND BKG REGIONS

Figure 9–6 This figure illustrates the technique of isotope angiography for the determination of left ventricular ejection fraction. In the lower left panel is the end-diastolic image of the heart in the left anterior oblique view. In the right lower panel the region of the left ventricle has been identified, and to the right a background region (BKG) from which background radiation levels are determined is visible. Cardiac images are developed by collecting scintillation information in 0.04-second windows over several hundred cardiac cycles by interfacing the gamma camera-computer with the electrocardiogram. In the upper panel, the time activity from the left ventricular region of interest is displayed, and the computed ejection fraction is presented. In this case, the time activity curve is normal, and the ejection fraction is 67 per cent.

cardiac chambers have collectively been termed *isotope angiography*. Advances in technology have been rapid in this field, such that it is likely that several types of standard radiographic contrast angiography can be replaced by this safer, noninvasive method. Like radiographic contrast angiography, isotope angiography requires expensive imaging equipment and subjects the patient to ionizing radiation. Expense and minimal radiation hazard will limit its use.

Echocardiography is a technique that utilizes pulsed high-frequency sound to determine the position and motion of cardiac structures. Like radionuclide techniques, the field of ultrasound has developed rapidly and now has many clinical applications. In cardiology, ultrasound first became clinically useful for the evaluation of mitral valve abnormalities because the anterior leaflet of the mitral valve formed a large, relatively flat surface for the reflection of sound waves. Early use of ultrasonography was also applied for the evaluation of pericardial effusions because the presence of fluid between the posterior left ventricular wall and lung gave an easily recognizable echo-free space. As equipment improved and experience increased, many other structures of the heart have been usefully evaluated by echocardiography, including left atrial and left ventricular chamber dimensions. The change in these dimensions during the various phases of the cardiac cycle has allowed investigators to estimate left ventricular volume, stroke volume, and ejection fraction from echocardiograms. The thickness of the posterior left ventricular wall can also be estimated by echocardiography, so that an estimate of left ventricular muscle mass can also be made if one assumes that wall thickness is uniform in its distribution. Although echocardiographic measurements of left ventricular dimensions are useful, the single probe technique does not provide a view of the long axis of the ventricle, so that the length-area method for calculating volumes described above is not applicable to echocardiographic data. Two-dimensional echocardiography, which is now generally used, provides images of sections of the left ventricle in longitudinal or cross-sectional planes. This technique provides much more quantitative information concerning left ventricular dimensions and function than the original echocardiographic methods. Echocardiography has the great advantage of being entirely noninvasive and almost entirely without hazardous side-effects. Unfortunately, the transmission of ultrasound is very poor through lung tissue. In about one third of older adults, lung tissue between the heart and chest wall prevents a satisfactory echocardiographic examination.

LEFT VENTRICULAR PUMP FUNCTION

The left ventricular end-diastolic volume in the normal adult of average size is in the range of

120 to 130 ml. Approximately two thirds of this end-diastolic volume is ejected with systole. Values for this ejection fraction that are greater than 0.5 are usually accepted as normal (Table 9–2).

In the presence of lesions that place a chronic volume overload on the left ventricle, the ventricle dilates, but the relationship between stroke volume and end-diastolic volume remains much as in the normal; namely, greater than one half the end-diastolic volume is ejected during systole. The left ventricular stroke volume with very severe aortic and/or mitral valve insufficiency may approach, but rarely exceeds, 300 ml. With lesions that place a chronic pressure overload on the left ventricle, as is observed with aortic valvular stenosis, the left ventricle hypertrophies with a thickened wall, but end-diastolic volume and ejection fraction are similar to those observed in normal subjects. This is in contrast to the ventricular dilatation and reduced ejection fraction observed with acute pressure loads. Ventricular hypertrophy very likely provides the mechanism whereby the ventricle with a chronic pressure overload functions at a normal volume and with a normal ejection fraction.

With myocardial disease the left ventricle dilates inappropriately for the stroke volume, so that the residual volume is increased and the ejection fraction reduced. In patients with severe myocardial disease, ejection fractions of less than 0.10 are occasionally observed. Even in the presence of mechanical overloads such as those imposed by valvular heart disease, the relationship of stroke volume and end-diastolic volume as expressed by the ejection fraction has proved to be of value in assessing myocardial function.

The difference between left ventricular stroke volume, as determined by the angiocardiographic method and forward flow, or effective cardiac output per stroke, as measured by the Fick or indicator dilution methods, provides a method for quantifying the volume of regurgitant flow in patients with aortic and/or mitral valve insufficiency and shunt flow in patients with ventricular septal defect. An example of findings in a patient with mitral insufficiency is shown in Figure 9–7. Patients with severe valvular insufficiency may have regurgitant volumes per stroke in the range of 250 ml that may be in excess of 80 per cent of the left ventricular stroke volume. Left ventricular minute outputs in such patients may be as large as 25 to 30 liters per minute.

From the slopes of the ejection and filling limbs of ventricular volume curves the rates of ventricular ejection and filling respectively can be determined. Figure 9–8 shows a curve of ventricular filling and ejection rates calculated from a ventricular volume curve in a patient with ischemic heart disease. The maximum rates of filling and ejection are usually similar, and in the normal resting subject they are in the range of 500 ml per second. With severe aortic and/or mitral valve insufficiency, peak-ejection and filling rates ap-

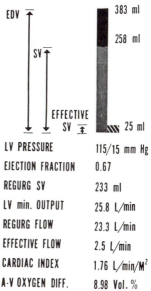

EDV	383 ml
	258 ml
SV	
EFFECTIVE SV	25 ml
LV PRESSURE	115/15 mm Hg
EJECTION FRACTION	0.67
REGURG SV	233 ml
LV min. OUTPUT	25.8 L/min
REGURG FLOW	23.3 L/min
EFFECTIVE FLOW	2.5 L/min
CARDIAC INDEX	1.76 L/min/M²
A-V OXYGEN DIFF.	8.98 Vol. %

Figure 9–7 Left ventricular pressure, volume, and cardiac output data from a patient with severe mitral valve insufficiency. The end-diastolic volume, stroke volume, and effective stroke volume, or forward flow, are as indicated. (Adapted from Dodge, H. T., and Baxley, W. A. *In* Gordon, B. L. [Ed.]: Clinical Cardiopulmonary Physiology. 3rd ed. New York, Grune and Stratton, Inc., 1969. By permission of Grune and Stratton, Inc.)

proach 1500 ml per second. Peak values as low as 200 ml per second are observed in patients with mitral stenosis, aortic stenosis, or severe myocardial disease.

Chronic disease is often associated with altered left ventricular distensibility. Figure 9–9 shows left ventricular end-diastolic pressure-volume relationships of patients with chronic heart disease. End-diastolic volumes of as much as four times normal are observed with filling pressures that are within the normal range. With the increased distensibility, the ventricle functions at a large volume with little or no increase in filling pressure or pulmonary venous pressure. This is important because pulmonary venous hypertension secondary to an elevated ventricular filling pressure is associated with dyspnea. In general, patients with more distensible left ventricles are those with chronic volume overloads or longstanding chronic myocardial disease.

Reduced ventricular distensibility is often observed with thick-walled hypertrophied left ventricles, as occurs with aortic valve stenosis or hypertrophic subvalvular aortic stenosis. Here the filling pressure may be elevated in the presence of a normal ventricular end-diastolic volume. Some patients with ischemic heart disease also have elevated filling pressures with normal end-diastolic volumes.

The functional characteristics of the left ventricle as a pump in performing pressure-volume work can be determined from the ventricular pres-

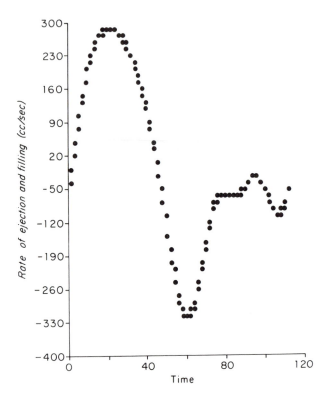

Figure 9–8 Rate of left ventricular ejection and filling with respect to time within the cardiac cycle as determined from the first derivative of a left ventricular volume curve. The positive values are seen during ejection, and negative values occur during ventricular filling. Zero time is the onset of QRS of the EKG.

sure-volume relationships (Fig. 9–10). By relating pressure and volume with respect to time, one can construct a pressure volume curve, with pressure on the vertical axis and volume on the horizontal axis. The height of the curve is determined by the systolic pressure, location on the horizontal axis by the end-diastolic volume, and the excursion along the horizontal axis by the stroke volume. The superior and inferior portions of the curves represent pressure-volume relationships during systole and diastole respectively. The shape of the curve is altered by mechanical defects such as aortic or mitral insufficiency, which shorten or abolish the isovolumic contraction and/or relaxa-

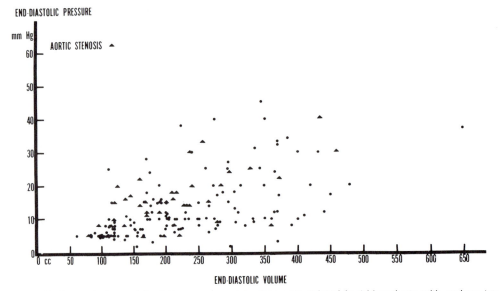

Figure 9–9 Left ventricular end-diastolic pressure and volume are related in 144 patients with various types and durations of heart diseases. Patients with aortic valvular or subaortic stenosis are designated by the triangles. (From Dodge, H. T., and Baxley, W. A.: Hemodynamic aspects of heart failure. Am. J. Cardiol. 22:24, 1968.)

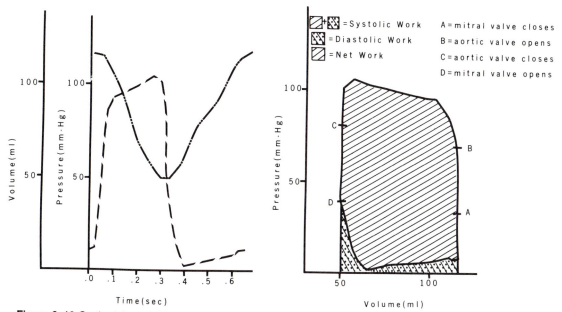

Figure 9–10 On the left are left ventricular pressure and volume curves plotted with respect to time after the QRS of the electrocardiogram. On the right, a pressure-volume curve has been constructed, with work values as indicated by the shaded areas. Mitral valve closure is delayed within the isovolumic contraction period because of an elevated left atrial pressure due to mitral stenosis. The mitral valve opens early in the isovolumic relaxation period, also because of an elevated left atrial pressure from mitral stenosis.

tion period. Differences in locations and shapes of pressure-volume curves as determined from patients with various heart diseases are illustrated in Figure 9–11.

Left ventricular systolic work is determined from the pressure-volume relations during systole and is illustrated by the area beneath the systolic portion of the curve in Figure 9–10, or

$$\text{Systolic work} = \int_{V_d}^{V_s} P d V$$

where V_s and V_d are the end-systolic and end-diastolic volumes, respectively, and P is the ventricular systolic pressure. Systolic stroke work values as much as three to four times normal are observed with severe mitral and aortic valve insufficiency. Values as much as four to five times normal occur when severe valvular insufficiency is associated with ventricular hypertension from aortic stenosis.

The level of work expended in distending the diastolic left ventricle can be determined from the pressure-volume relationships of the left ventricle during diastole. This is illustrated by the area beneath the pressure-volume curve of Figure 9–10, or

$$\text{Diastolic work} = \int_{V_s}^{V_d} P d V$$

where P and V are the pressure and volume, respectively, during diastole. With left ventricular

failure and an elevated left ventricular filling pressure, increased work is performed in distending the diastolic left ventricle. This work is performed by the left atrium and right ventricle and is the physiologic basis for the left atrial dilatation and right ventricular dilatation and hypertrophy observed with chronic left ventricular failure.

The difference between the systolic work and diastolic work values has been termed *net work* and is represented by the area enclosed by the pressure-volume loop shown in Figure 9–10. In considering the left ventricle as a pump, the net work is then the energy delivered as pressure-volume work in systole less the energy expended in distending the left ventricle as pressure-volume work during diastole. With increasing left ventricular failure, net work is decreased relative to systolic and diastolic work. This is illustrated in Figure 9–12, which shows a pressure-volume curve from a patient with a left ventricular end-diastolic volume of 525 ml and pressure of 20 mm Hg. Systolic work is 37.5 gram-meters per stroke. Diastolic work is nearly 30 per cent of this, and net work is only 26.5 gram-meters per stroke.

The most accurate method for computing left ventricular systolic and net work values is from ventricular pressure and volume curves as just described. However, left ventricular stroke work (LVSW) may also be estimated from stroke volume (SV) and left ventricular systolic pressure (LVSP) as follows:

$$\text{LVSW} = \text{SV} (\overline{\text{LVSP}} - \text{LVEDP})$$

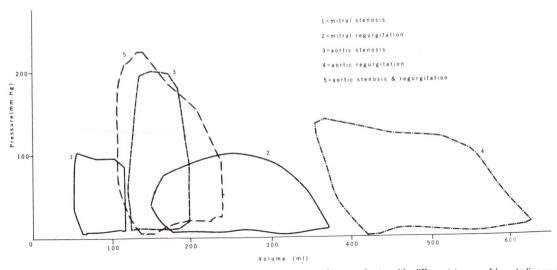

Figure 9–11 Examples of left ventricular pressure-volume curves from patients with different types of heart diseases (mitral stenosis, mitral regurgitation, aortic stenosis, aortic regurgitation, and aortic stenosis and regurgitation). The curve from the patient with mitral stenosis shows well-defined isovolumic contraction and relaxation periods, a normal stroke volume, and relatively normal stroke work. The larger stroke-work values in the other patients can be roughly estimated by comparing the areas beneath the systolic limbs of the pressure-volume curves. The patients with aortic regurgitation, mitral regurgitation, and aortic stenosis and regurgitation have greatly elevated stroke work values with large stroke volumes, as is evident by the excursion of the curves along the horizontal or volume axis. The abnormality in shape and location of these curves is evident. Patients with valvular insufficiency have a shortening or absence of isovolumic contraction and relaxation periods. Patients with aortic valve stenosis have elevated systolic pressures. Patients with large stroke volumes have elevated end-diastolic volumes.

where $\overline{\text{LVSP}}$ equals the mean left ventricular systolic pressure during ejection and LVEDP is left ventricular end-diastolic pressure.

Ventricular power is the rate at which work is performed and can be calculated from the systolic pressure-volume relationships of the left ventricle as $P \times dV/dt$, where P is instantaneous pressure and dV/dt the instantaneous rate of ejection. Peak power values in the range of 500 grammeters per second are observed in normal resting human subjects and values in excess of four times this in patients with severe aortic and/or mitral valve disease.

In chronic heart disease left ventricular hypertrophy is observed as a response to chronic pressure and/or volume overloads and also in association with chronic left ventricular dilatation. In patients with valvular heart disease and as shown in Figure 9–13, where left ventricular weight is related to left ventricular stroke work, the extent of hypertrophy is directly related to the workload. The manner in which the heart hypertrophies differs, however, depending on whether the increased work is a result of a pressure or volume overload. With compensated volume overloads, the wall shows only a small amount of thickening as end-diastolic volume is increased, and the ratio of left ventricular mass to end-diastolic volume is close to 1.0. With pressure overloads, the wall thickness is considerably in-

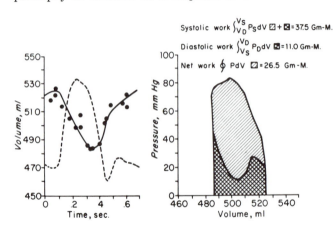

Figure 9–12 Left ventricular pressure, volume, and pressure-volume curves from a patient with ischemic heart disease and left ventricular failure. The various pressure-volume work components are designated and described in the text. (Adapted from Dodge, H. T., and Baxley, W. A.: Hemodynamic aspects of heart failure. Am. J. Cardiol. 22:24, 1968.)

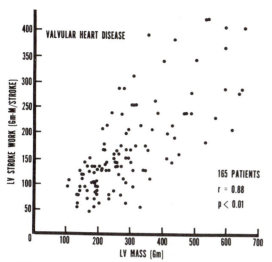

Figure 9–13 Relationship of left ventricular stroke work and mass in 165 patients with valvular heart disease. (From Dodge, H. T., and Baxley, W. A.: Left ventricular volume and mass and their significance in heart disease. Am. J. Cardiol. 23:528, 1969.)

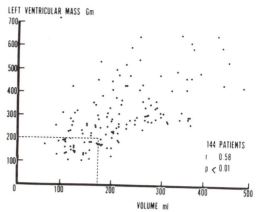

Figure 9–14 Relationship of left ventricular end-diastolic volume and mass in 144 patients with various types of heart diseases. (From Dodge, H. T., and Baxley, W. A.: Hemodynamic aspects of heart failure. Am. J. Cardiol. 22:24, 1968.)

creased, with end-diastolic volume being relatively normal so that the ratio of left ventricular mass to end-diastolic volume is greater than 1.0. It has been shown that in compensated valvular heart disease and with either pressure or volume overloads, the wall thickness is increased in proportion to chamber dimensions and systolic pressure, so that systolic wall stress or force per unit of cross-sectional area of ventricular wall remains relatively normal.

Left ventricular hypertrophy is also observed in the presence of chronic left ventricular dilatation, even when left ventricular stroke work is diminished, as occurs in patients with myocardial disease. In Figure 9–14 left ventricular end-diastolic volume is related to left ventricular mass and, as can be seen, increase in left ventricular weight is roughly proportional to that of volume. Significant ventricular dilatation is regularly associated with ventricular hypertrophy in humans with chronic heart disease. The stimulus to hypertrophy is very likely the increased wall force that occurs with the increased chamber dimensions and reduced wall thickness that accompany ventricular dilatation.

The above observations on increased left ventricular mass in the presence of chronic work overloads and ventricular dilatation are consistent with a growth of myocardium in patients with chronic heart disease. In experimental animals with left ventricular dilatation and hypertrophy from an induced chronic volume overload, maximal sarcomere lengths have been shown to be unchanged from the 2.2 μ observed in the normal left ventricle. This together with the observations of increased myocardial mass in humans with chronic heart disease suggests that growth of new

myocardium and sarcomeres is an important adaptive mechanism in chronic heart disease and that the Frank-Starling mechanism may not be important in these chronic adjustments. There is currently a controversy concerning the contractile state of myocardium that is hypertrophied in response to pressure and volume overloads. Some groups have reported normal and others depressed contractility when expressed per unit of myocardium.

MYOCARDIAL PERFORMANCE

Myocardial performance can be more directly evaluated in the intact heart through an analysis of wall forces and motion. The forces present within the myocardium of the chamber walls are a function of the chamber pressure, dimensions, and wall thickness. A method for computing these forces for the left ventricle is to assume that the ventricle can be represented as a thin-walled ellipsoid of revolution and to apply Laplace's law:

$$\frac{T_1}{R_1} + \frac{T_2}{R_2} = P$$

where T_1 and T_2 are mean wall tensions in the meridional and circumferential directions, respectively, and R_1 and R_2 are the associated principal radii of curvature. P is chamber pressure. Tension is expressed in force per linear cm, if dimensions are expressed in terms of cm, and can be considered as the force acting per cm of slits in the wall placed perpendicular to the principal radii of curvature. The wall forces also can be expressed in terms of stress (σ) or force per unit area (cm²) by dividing tension by wall thickness (h). Laplace's law then becomes

$$\frac{\sigma_1}{R_1} \quad \frac{\sigma_2}{R_2} = \frac{p}{h}$$

where σ_1 and σ_2 equal wall stress in the directions of the principal radii of curvature. Wall stress or force per unit area is expressed in the same units as those used for chamber pressure. The largest wall force values are in the circumferential direction.

Because of the aforementioned relationships between chamber pressure, wall thickness, and wall stress, wall stress increases more rapidly than chamber pressure as chamber dimensions increase and wall thickness decreases, as occurs when the diastolic left ventricle is acutely distended. During systole, chamber dimensions decrease and wall thickness increases so that wall stress decreases relative to chamber pressure. As described previously, in compensated heart disease associated with chronic pressure or volume overloads, wall thickness is increased so that wall stress values are similar to those found in normal subjects. In subjects with left ventricular failure, large wall stress values are frequently present, indicating that myocardial hypertrophy has not been adequate to compensate for the increase in dimensions and decrease of wall thickness as the chamber has dilated.

The relationship of wall stresses in the directions of the principal chamber axes to wall motion expressed in terms of change of these axes during systole has provided a method for expressing myocardial performance of the intact ventricle in terms of force, extent, and velocity of shortening. This has been used to apply knowledge concerning the relationships of force to the extent and velocity of myocardial contraction as determined in in-vitro studies to the intact ventricle of experimental animals and humans.

In-vitro studies of contractile characteristics of myocardium indicate that the myocardial contractile state can be evaluated independently of preload or the Frank-Starling effect from an analysis of myocardial force and velocity of contraction relationships. With this approach to evaluating myocardial contractility, a model to represent the contractile apparatus of the myocardium is assumed. This model consists of a contractile element (CE), a series elastic element (SE), and, for a three-component model, a parallel elastic element. Myocardial contractility is expressed in terms of velocity of contraction of the contractile element (VCE) with respect to force to determine force-VCE relationships. These force-velocity relationships, when extrapolated to zero force, provide a measure of VCE under zero load, which has been termed V_{max}. Some studies indicated that V_{max} is independent of fiber length, or the Frank-Starling effect. However, there is controversy concerning the validity of this concept when applied to isolated heart muscle preparations and even more controversy when applied to evaluate the myocardial contractile state of the intact ventricle of experimental animals and man. For a further discussion of these concepts refer to the section on heart muscle and its dynamics (see Chapter 7).

The preceding studies and concepts are the basis for evaluation of myocardial contractile state of the intact ventricle in experimental animals and humans from high-fidelity ventricular pressure data recorded during the isovolumic contraction period and from studies of ejection phase dynamics. During the isovolumic period, if one assumes no change of cardiac dimensions and wall thickness,

$$\text{VCE} = \frac{(dp/dt)}{(K \times P)}$$

where K is equal to the elastic modulus of the series elastic element and P is the corresponding isovolumic pressure. VCE extrapolated to zero pressure provides a measure of V_{max}, an index of myocardial contractility. If a three-component model with a parallel elastic component is assumed, developed pressure (DP) is substituted for P in the aforementioned equation. DP is computed as P minus the initial or end-diastolic pressure. The expression $(dP/dt)/(K \times DP)$ is said to be less sensitive to changes of preload and to provide a more precise index of myocardial contractile state. These isovolumic indices have proved to be of limited value for evaluation of the status of myocardial performance in individual patients. They have more value when used for assessment of any change in myocardial performance that occurs in response to an intervention or drug in an individual animal or human subject.

Indices of myocardial contractile state as determined from the ventricular ejection phase include the ejection fraction, the velocity of ventricular circumference change (VCF), VCF at peak wall stress which is equivalent to VCE, peak VCE and VCE extrapolated to zero load, or V_{max}. These computations require knowledge of chamber dimensions, pressure, and wall thickness, and instantaneous changes of these parameters during systole. A shortcoming of these ejection phase indices for evaluating a myocardial contractile state is their sensitivity to alterations in preload and afterload. Accordingly, these indices are of limited value for evaluation of the status of myocardial performance when there are marked changes in preload and afterload as in aortic and/or mitral valve insufficiency or in aortic valve stenosis.

Because of the shortcomings of the aforementioned ejection phase indices, the use of end-systolic pressure and volume or wall stress and volume relationships has been reported for assessment of the status of myocardial performance. These indices of myocardial performance are based on studies in the isolated heart by Suga and Sagawa and their coworkers, who demonstrated that under conditions of changing preload or afterload or both there is a linear relationship between end-systolic pressure and volume and that the slope of the line (Ees, or m) and the intercept with the pressure axis at V_o can be used to evaluate myocardial contractile state. With increased contractility, the line defining end-systolic pressure and volume relationship shifts to the left and has a steeper slope. It has also been shown that in intact experimental animals and in humans there is a linear relationship between changes in end-systolic volume and pressure or in end-systolic volume and wall stress, and that these relationships may be used to evaluate the status of myocardial performance. However, there are still a number of problems with the applications of this method of evaluating myocardial performance in humans. First, the method requires repeated measurements of ventricular end-systolic pressure and volume under conditions of induced changes of preload or afterload or both. The methods for inducing preload and afterload changes must not in themselves induce reflex changes in contractility in intact experimental animals and humans. In addition, there is a problem in defining end-systolic pressure and volume, particularly in patients with aortic and/or mitral valve insufficiency. Studies of this technique and methods for resolving the problems concerned with its application are the subject of hemodynamic investigations in a number of laboratories. The reader is referred to the 1981 editorial by Sagawa and to the section on heart muscle and its dynamics for further discussions of the theoretical basis for these concepts and their applications in the evaluation of the myocardial contractile state (see Chapter 7).

HEMODYNAMICS OF HEART FAILURE

Cardiac enlargement, increased ventricular filling pressure, and a low cardiac output at rest, or relative to the demands of some stress such as exercise, are features of heart failure. Basically, the clinical picture of heart failure is the result of a decreased ability of the heart to contract, an increased pressure-volume load, a combination of increased load and depressed contractility, or occasionally interference with venous return to the heart, as occurs with constrictive pericarditis. Figure 9–7 illustrates an example of failure resulting from a large volume overload due to mitral regurgitation. In humans with chronic heart disease and ventricular failure, there is compensation for the decreased myocardial contractility and increased mechanical pressure and volume loads by cardiac dilatation (Frank-Starling mechanism) and by cardiac hypertrophy as previously described. It is often difficult to determine precisely when in the course of chronic heart disease these compensatory mechanisms become inadequate to maintain cardiac output and heart failure develops. In fact, these mechanisms of chamber dilatation and hypertrophy can be viewed as early manifestations of cardiac decompensation, as they represent the initial adjustments of the diseased heart. Because there are limits to the extent of

cardiac dilatation and hypertrophy that occur in disease, once these compensatory mechanisms develop there is a diminished capacity of the heart to adjust to further increases in mechanical loads or further decreases of myocardial contractility.

A fundamental mechanism by which the ventricles maintain stroke volume in response to acute increases of systolic pressure (afterload), volume overload, or depression of contractility is chamber dilatation, which has been termed the *Frank-Starling mechanism*. The increased fiber length that occurs with chamber dilatation is associated with an increased force and extent of contraction. Figure 9–15 shows what have been termed *ventricular function curves*. With normal myocardial function, chamber volume enlargement is associated with increases of stroke work and stroke volume along a theoretically normal curve. With depressed myocardial function, lower stroke volume and stroke work are generated from a given end-diastolic volume, and stroke volume is maintained through ventricular dilatation. A depressed systolic ejection fraction, as is observed in humans with myocardial disease, is a numerical expression of a depressed ventricular function curve, since it indicates inappropriate chamber enlargement with a low stroke volume and large residual volume relative to end-diastolic volume. Drugs that have a positive inotropic effect elevate a depressed ventricular function curve.

With acute increases of ventricular end-diastolic volume there is an eventual leveling off of the ventricular function curves, so that further increases in volume result in no further increase in stroke work or stroke volume. Indeed, under some conditions a descending limb of the function curves has been demonstrated. With ventricular dilatation, ventricular diastolic pressure is increased, and filling pressure is often used as an index of diastolic volume or preload in determining ventricular response to a changing preload. In patients with heart failure due to acute myocardial

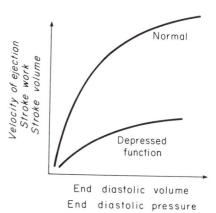

Figure 9–15 Schematic representation of a normal and a depressed ventricular function curve as defined by the relationship of parameters as given on the horizontal and vertical axes.

infarction, it has been shown that little increase or even a fall of stroke volume occurs with elevation of left ventricular end-diastolic pressure beyond 22 to 25 mm Hg.

As described previously, chronic increases of ventricular chamber volume or work load are associated with ventricular hypertrophy. There is a question concerning the role of the Frank-Starling mechanism in the adjustments to chronic increases of ventricular volume and pressure loads, and hypertrophy may be the dominant response to chronic loads.

Measures of ventricular pump performance in addition to stroke volume relative to end-diastolic volume (ejection fraction) can be used in the assessment of myocardial performance in chronic heart disease. These are stroke work, ventricular ejection rate, or peak power. As with stroke volume, none of these parameters has significance in the evaluation of myocardial performance unless the measure is related to ventricular end-diastolic volume. In the presence of myocardial disease, depressed values relative to volume are observed. This is illustrated in Figure 9–16, in which stroke power normalized for end-diastolic volume is related to the ejection fraction.

There is a problem with using stroke work relative to volume to assess myocardial performance in chronic heart disease. As described previously, the adjustment to chronic systolic pressure overload is ventricular hypertrophy rather than dilatation. Accordingly, stroke work relative to chamber volume is high in compensated pressure overload states and decreases with myocardial failure, but it still may be high relative to the stroke work/end-diastolic volume relationships observed in other types of heart disease. As a result, stroke work/end-diastolic volume does not appear to provide a very useful index for evaluating myocardial performance in chronic heart disease.

With ventricular failure, abnormally low values for ventricular performance are also obtained by analysis of ventricular pressure changes during isovolumic contraction (dp/dt) and of wall force and motion relationships. The velocity of circumference change relative to end-diastolic circumference (VCF) is depressed. Derived values for peak VCE, VCE at peak stress, and V_{max} are also depressed.

ISCHEMIC HEART DISEASE

Ischemic heart disease results from an inadequate supply of oxygenated blood to the myocardium. For practical purposes this disease is due to atherosclerotic occlusive disease of the large extramural coronary arteries, although disease of these vessels occasionally results from other pathologic processes such as embolization, fibromuscular disease of the arteries, and arteritis of variable etiology. Atherosclerosis, although usually diffusely distributed in the proximal portions of the coronary arteries, tends to cause localized areas of stenosis or occlusion. The localized distribution of highly stenotic or occlusive lesions results in regional areas of ischemic or infarcted myocardium. Myocardial functional abnormalities are therefore usually of a segmental or regional distribution in patients with ischemic heart disease. When myocardial damage becomes very extensive owing to multiple sites of high-grade stenosis or occlusions of coronary arteries, the entire left ventricle may exhibit reduced contraction. In order to evaluate left ventricular performance in ischemic heart disease it is necessary to study the extent and severity of regional contraction abnormalities.

SELECTIVE CORONARY ARTERIOGRAPHY

Selective coronary arteriography, which was developed by Mason Sones in the late 1950s, is required to define precisely the presence and severity of coronary atherosclerosis. This method is carried out by the insertion of a catheter into the right brachial or a femoral artery and selective cannulation of each coronary orifice. Three to 7 ml of radiographic contrast material are injected over

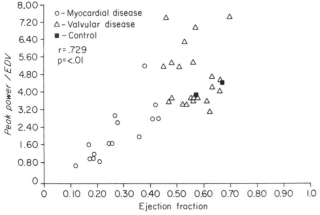

Figure 9–16 A significant correlation is demonstrated for the relationship of left ventricular peak power normalized for end-diastolic volume and ejection fraction in 39 subjects with various types of heart diseases as coded. The subjects indicated as "control" had no demonstrable disease affecting the left ventricle. (From Gensini, G. G. [Ed.]: The Study of the Systemic, Coronary and Myocardial Effects of Nitrates. Springfield, Illinois, Charles C Thomas, 1972.)

1 to 3 seconds, while the image is recorded with a high-gain image intensifier cineangiographic system. High quality cineangiograms of the coronary arteries currently have a resolution of between 75 and 100 line pairs per inch. The right coronary artery is studied in at least two views, and a minimum of three views of the left coronary artery are filmed. Stenosis in these vessels can be easily appreciated and its severity graded relatively accurately. Pharmacologic agents such as nitroglycerin may be given and the studies repeated in order to evaluate the presence of coronary artery spasm. Selective coronary arteriography is also carried out in conjunction with other catheterization techniques in the evaluation of older patients with valvular heart disease, since valvular and coronary heart disease may coexist. Selective coronary arteriography is a safe procedure when carried out by experienced teams. Reports from experienced laboratories indicate that mortality from these procedures rarely occurs, except in very ill patients with disease of the left main coronary artery or with advanced atherosclerosis of all three major coronary arteries. Overall mortality resulting from the procedure is between one and two deaths per thousand studies.

Most angiographers grade lesions by the percentage of greatest diameter narrowing as seen on multiple views of the vessel as compared with nearby segments of normal appearing vessel. Despite many limiting factors, this method of clinically reading coronary arteriograms has been effective in selecting patients for coronary artery surgery. Lesions of greater than 70 per cent stenosis of major proximal coronary vessels are considered to be hemodynamically significant. This statement implies that lesions of this severity limit coronary blood flow and result in myocardial ischemia and angina pectoris. Gould and coworkers have studied the flow and pressure gradients across adjustable coronary occluders on the circumflex coronary arteries of dogs. They have shown that in the resting animal coronary flow is not reduced until an 80 to 85 per cent stenosis is applied. When coronary flow is greatly increased with coronary vasodilating drugs to mimic severe exercise, coronary blood flow is reduced by a stenosis of 40 to 50 per cent. These observations indicate that coronary flow reserve, or the ability to increase coronary flow across a stenosis, begins to be limited with mild coronary stenosis but an actual decrease in resting flow requires severe narrowing of the vessel.

In patients with ischemic heart disease, coronary arterial stenoses are usually multiple, may be located serially along a vessel, and may be connected in parallel through the presence of collateral vessels. Additionally, the hemodynamic effect of a particular atherosclerotic lesion depends not only on the severity of stenosis but also on its length and shape. For example, an irregular lesion that causes increased turbulence of blood flow will have greater pressure loss across it than a smooth lesion that permits more laminar flow. A great deal remains to be learned about the proper physiologic evaluation of coronary atherosclerotic lesions.

Evaluation of regional contraction abnormalities is difficult because it requires that all aspects of the left ventricle, including its apex, free wall, anterior and posterior surfaces, and septum, be visualized and studied. At this time, angiocardiography is the best method available for visualizing the left ventricle and for the detailed evaluation of segmental abnormalities of left ventricular contraction. The evaluation of left ventricular function in patients with ischemic heart disease is best carried out in conjunction with selective coronary arteriography. Indications for study include angina pectoris, symptoms of heart failure, and persistent chest pain following recovery from a myocardial infarction. Occasionally, patients with heart failure of uncertain etiology are also studied in this manner. Left ventricular angiocardiography is carried out in single or biplane views with ciné filming techniques. In most situations, single plane cineangiocardiography is adequate for clinical purposes, although biplane methods are preferable. One method for evaluating ventricular segmental contraction abnormalities is by analysis of end-diastolic and systolic films. This may be carried out by tracing the outline of the opacified chamber. By superimposing systolic and diastolic outlines, the symmetry and extent of contraction can be assessed.

Regional contraction abnormalities can be conveniently divided into five types:

1. *Normal:* The entire ventricular wall moves inward appropriately toward the geometric center of the ventricle. Occasional patients with small volumes and normal ejection fractions have ventricles that appear asymmetric at end-systole owing to distortion of the cavity shape by the papillary muscles.

2. *Borderline abnormal:* The ventricle demonstrates a minor degree of contraction asymmetry involving less than 25 per cent of the wall.

3. *Localized akinesis or hypokinesis:* More than 25 per cent but less than 75 per cent of the ventricular wall has diminished or absent contraction.

4. *Localized dyskinesis:* More than 25 per cent of the ventricular wall demonstrates paradoxic outward motion during systole.

5. *Diffuse akinesis or hypokinesis:* More than 75 per cent of the ventricular surface has diminished or absent contraction.

Selective coronary arteriograms usually demonstrate that the coronary vessels that supply an akinetic or dyskinetic region have severe stenosis or total occlusion. Often, however, severely stenotic or occluded coronary vessels supply areas of myocardium that appear to contract normally. Severe coronary artery disease is not, therefore, necessarily associated with areas of abnormal myocardial contraction, at least in the resting subject. Generally, there has been a good correlation between definite electrocardiographic evidence of myocardial infarction and regional contraction abnormalities as assessed by left ventricular angiocardiography. The opposite, however, is not true. Frequently, a severe myocardial contraction abnormality may be present and the electrocardiogram does not definitely localize an infarct to that region of the heart. Electrocardiography, selective coronary arteriography, and left ventricular angiography are all essential to full evaluation of the patient with ischemic heart disease. Each method yields information not available from the others and together they give a rather complete picture of the left ventricle, its blood supply, electrical integrity, and contractile function.

VENTRICULAR PERFORMANCE IN ISCHEMIC HEART DISEASE

The incidence of significant segmental contraction abnormalities in patients with ischemic heart disease varies with the patient group submitted to angiocardiographic studies. Patients with angina pectoris without a history of electrocardiographic evidence of prior myocardial infarction often have a normal contraction pattern. Not infrequently, however, these patients have a modest reduction in ejection fraction and an elevation of diastolic pressure. Under the stress of tachycardia induced with right atrial pacing, the end-diastolic pressure often becomes abnormally elevated, and abnormal contraction patterns may appear or become more marked. Diastolic pressure rise is especially likely to occur in those in whom pacing induces anginal pain. Exercise in this group of patients is also associated with the development of regional contraction abnormalities, with decreased ejection fraction, and with increased left ventricular end-diastolic pressure and subnormal increase in cardiac output.

The majority of patients who have suffered a myocardial infarction and have associated electrocardiographic evidence of myocardial scar will have a segmental area of abnormal left ventricular contraction. It has been postulated that akinesis of more than 25 per cent of the ventricular myocardium must result in either ventricular dilatation or reduction in stroke volume. This theory rests on estimates of the limits of contractile element shortening that can occur under physiologic conditions. Quantitative assessment of the extent of segmental contraction abnormality in large groups of patients suggests that this theory is essentially correct. When more than 25 to 30 per cent of the left ventricular wall is akinetic or dyskinetic, ventricular dilatation and reduced ejection fraction are usually present. The left ven-

tricular end-diastolic pressure is also elevated in most of these patients. Major contraction abnormalities (type 4 or 5) are nearly always associated with a history of heart failure and a resting ejection fraction below 40 per cent.

Methods are now available that permit more precise analysis of segmental left ventricular performance in patients with coronary artery disease. Such studies are performed from analysis of chamber margins or regional wall thickening from each frame of cineventriculograms taken at 60 frames per second or higher rates. Normal standards for extent and timing of wall motion have been established for these techniques and are used as a basis for determining the frequency and extent of segmental wall motion abnormalities in patients with coronary disease. Such studies have demonstrated that most patients with greater than 70 per cent narrowing of a coronary artery have segmental abnormalities of extent or timing of contraction in the region of the left ventricle supplied by the narrowed coronary artery. These abnormalities often are detected neither by subjective analysis of the ciné films nor by the more common form of analysis of an end-diastolic and an apparent end-systolic film. In fact, the more detailed types of analyses have demonstrated that even in the normal there may be no one ciné film that represents maximum inward contraction for all segments of the ventricle. In patients with ischemic heart disease, abnormalities of timing of wall motion and differences in timing of wall motion of different regions of the left ventricle are very common and often quite marked. Delayed maximum inward motion and, accordingly, relaxation are particularly common. Whether the abnormalities of timing of wall motion are manifestations of myocardial weakness, damage, ischemia, or delayed timing of depolarization is unknown. The asynchronous segmental wall motion and delayed inward motion and relaxation do undoubtedly contribute to the reduced ventricular systolic performance and perhaps to the increased wall stiffness in diastole observed in patients with ischemic heart disease. There are commonly segments with hyperkinesia to compensate for segments that are hypokinetic, so that, although substantial regions of the ventricle are hypokinetic, overall ventricular diastolic volume and ejection fraction may be normal. Figure 9–17 illustrates the application of a technique for analysis of segmental extent and timing of wall motion in a patient with coronary artery disease.

Left ventricular myocardial hypertrophy is frequently present in patients with ischemic heart disease. This appears to be closely related to a history of congestive heart failure and the presence of left ventricular dilatation. There is a close correlation between the increase in left ventricular diastolic volume and the increase in myocardial mass. However, the degree of myocardial hypertrophy relative to diastolic volume is less in is-

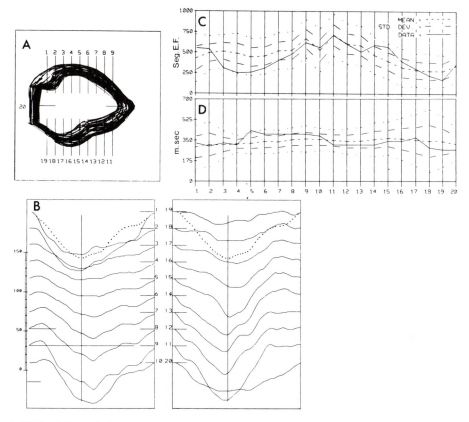

Figure 9–17 The left ventricular chamber margins for systole and diastole of one heart beat have been digitized from a cineventriculogram filmed at 60 frames per second in the anteroposterior projection, stored in computer memory, and played back with the long axes superimposed as shown in *A*. Segmental border motion is determined along each of the numbered hemiaxes, also shown in panel *A,* and displayed with respect to time by the solid line curves in *B*. The chamber volume curve is illustrated by the dotted curves in *B*. In *C* and *D* the segmental ejection fractions (fractional motion toward the long axis) and time from QRS to maximum inward segment motion, respectively, are illustrated by the solid lines and related to normal values. Mean normal values with one and two standard deviations from the mean are designated by the dotted and dashed lines. It is evident that the patient represented here has hypokinesia of segments 3 to 7, hyperkinesia of segments 14 and 15, and delayed time to maximum inward segment motion in segments 5 to 8.

chemic heart disease than in patients with valvular heart disease. This is probably due to the fact that these patients usually do not have an increased volume or pressure load on the left ventricle. In addition, the lesser degree of left ventricular hypertrophy in ischemic heart disease may be related to shorter duration of disease or an expression of inadequate coronary arterial blood supply.

It is of interest that the electrocardiogram is relatively insensitive in detecting the presence of left ventricular hypertrophy in patients with ischemic heart disease. It should be remembered that ventricular hypertrophy as estimated from angiocardiograms or as determined from left ventricular weight at autopsy does not separate normal myocardial tissue from fibrous tissue and scar and is therefore subject to variable error in estimating actual muscle mass, depending on the extent of ischemic damage present. The presence of considerable fibrosis and scarring may account

for the disparity between electrocardiographic and angiocardiographic evidence of ventricular hypertrophy.

MITRAL REGURGITATION IN ISCHEMIC HEART DISEASE

Mild mitral regurgitation is frequently present in patients with ischemic heart disease. It is often intermittent and associated with the presence of congestive heart failure, or it may be present only during episodes of myocardial ischemia. Mitral regurgitation in ischemic heart disease may be the result of papillary muscle dysfunction, dilatation of the mitral annulus secondary to left ventricular dilatation, or papillary muscle rupture.

The two papillary muscles of the left ventricle receive their blood supply from terminal branches of the anterior descending and posterior descending coronary arteries. Since the terminal portions of these muscles are free in the ventricular cavity, they are directly subjected to intercavity pressure. The combination of these two factors may explain why these small muscles are especially vulnerable to ischemia and infarction. The papillary muscles must contract in concert with the ventricle so that the mitral valve is held in a competent position across the mitral orifice throughout systole. Failure of these muscles to contract will result in prolapse of the mitral valve into the left atrium during the later portion of systole, as indicated in Figure 9–18. Clinically, this will result in a mid- or late systolic ejection murmur, which is characteristic of papillary muscle dysfunction. When left ventricular dilatation is extensive, the papillary muscles are pulled down and laterally away from the mitral valve. If the muscles contract with systole in a normal manner, the mitral valve will be held down in the ventricle in an incompetent position throughout systole, as illustrated in Figure 9–18B. This situation will usually result in a blowing pansystolic murmur. This type of regurgitation frequently disappears when treatment for congestive heart failure results in reduction in left ventricular volume. It is of interest that patients with long-standing left ventricular dilatation of any cause often develop mitral regurgitation. At surgical or postmortem examination, some of these patients are found to have a dilated mitral annulus and normal valve leaflets, indicating the mitral incompetence has resulted from enlargement of the mitral annulus secondary to ventricular dilatation. It is not certain how often mitral regurgitation is due to displacement of the papillary muscle by a dilated ventricular cavity and how often annular dilatation plays an important role in the production of valve incompetence.

Quantitative angiocardiographic assessment of patients with ischemic heart disease indicates that in those patients with mitral regurgitation there is evidence of extensive ventricular dilatation, with the left ventricular end-diastolic volume greater than 150 ml per M^2 in the majority of cases. In addition, these patients nearly always have a history of myocardial infarction and congestive heart failure. Left ventricular contraction patterns are also nearly always distinctly abnormal. These findings are not consistent with isolated ischemia or infarction of one or the other papillary muscle but are indicative of more widespread damage of the left ventricular myocardium. A number of studies have been carried out in an attempt to create papillary muscle dysfunction in dogs. One or both papillary muscles have been injected with sclerosing material, and in one study the base of a papillary muscle was ligated. In those animals in which damage was confined to the papillary muscle, mitral regurgitation did not result. When the underlying left ventricular wall was also injured, mitral valve incompetence developed. These animal studies and clinical expe-

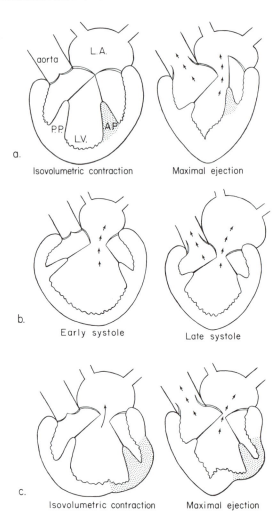

Figure 9–18 The mechanism of mitral regurgitation secondary to ischemia or infarction of the anterior lateral papillary is shown in a. During isovolumic contraction and early systole the mitral valve is competent, but during the maximal ejection period the anterior valve leaflet prolapses into the left atrium and mitral regurgitation results.

The mechanism of mitral regurgitation secondary to left ventricular chamber dilatation is shown in b.

The mechanism of mitral regurgitation that results from infarction of the papillary muscle and the underlying left ventricular wall is shown in c. In this example, the infarcted left ventricular wall is aneurysmal and bulges out during systole. (Adapted from Burch, G. E., DePasquale, N. P., and Phillips, J. H.: Am. Heart J. 75:399, 1968. Copyright 1968, American Medical Association.)

rience in humans suggest that mitral regurgitation in ischemic heart disease is the result of extensive ischemia or infarction of the papillary muscle and the underlying ventricular wall, as seen diagrammatically in Figure 9–18C.

In rare instances, mitral regurgitation develops acutely during the early phase of recovery from myocardial infarction as a result of rupture of a papillary muscle. When the entire muscle body ruptures, the resultant regurgitation is of severe proportions, and pulmonary edema, shock, and death occur rapidly in nearly all instances. Immediate support of the circulation and replacement of the mitral valve is now possible and will undoubtedly result in a few survivals in this group of patients. At times, only one or two heads of the papillary muscle with their attached chordae tendineae rupture. In these instances, the regurgitation that results is less severe, and survival with or without surgical treatment may be possible.

RUPTURE OF THE INTERVENTRICULAR SEPTUM

The development of an interventricular septal defect is an unusual and serious complication of acute myocardial infarction. In most such cases, there is the sudden development of a systolic murmur associated with heart failure and often systemic arterial hypotension. Septal rupture usually occurs during the first 6 days following myocardial infarction in patients who have extensive transmural infarction of the anterior or posterior wall that also involves the interventricular septum. The prognosis in these patients remains poor despite attempts at surgical repair because of the extensive myocardial damage usually present.

VENTRICULAR ANEURYSMS

Angiocardiographic studies have shown that small areas of the left ventricular wall that bulge paradoxically with ventricular systole are common in patients who have had a transmural myocardial infarction. Large ventricular aneurysms that are apparent on simple chest radiographs and fluoroscopy are less common and probably occur in 3 to 10 per cent of patients who survive transmural myocardial infarction. Large ventricular aneurysms have a profound effect on left ventricular dynamics because as they expand with systole they accept a volume load from the contractile portion of the ventricle. However, the volume load is rarely marked and does not approach the levels of volume load observed in patients with moderate or severe aortic or mitral valve insufficiency. Patients with large ventricular aneurysms usually develop congestive heart failure, probably as a result of the loss of a substantial portion of contractile muscle as well as the mechanical effects of the aneurysm. Since most ventricular aneurysms are lined with mural thrombi they are also associated with an increased incidence of systemic embolization. In addition, recurrent ventricular arrhythmias are common in these patients. Surgical resection of large ventricular aneurysms is indicated for heart failure that is resistant to medical treatment and in patients who have had systemic embolization that cannot be controlled with anticoagulants. Occasionally, aneurysms have been resected for recurrent episodes of ventricular tachycardia with apparent success. The risk and success of aneurysm resection depend on the functional capacity of the remaining myocardium.

VALVULAR HEART DISEASE

Diseases of various types affect the cardiac valves and result in valvular stenosis, regurgitation, or a combination of these lesions. Rheumatic endocarditis remains the main cause of chronic valvular deformity and resultant dysfunction, despite the reduction in the incidence of rheumatic fever that has occurred since the introduction of effective antibiotics in Western countries. Rheumatic fever and especially virulent forms of rheumatic valvular disease continue to constitute a major health problem in the developing countries. There has been an increasing appreciation of other etiologic factors responsible for valvular heart disease. It is now known, for example, that many cases of isolated aortic stenosis result from congenital bicuspid malformations of the valve. Many causes of pure mitral regurgitation are also recognized, including congenital abnormalities, dysfunction and rupture of the papillary muscles, rupture of chordae tendineae, mitral annular dilatation, and myxomatous degeneration of the valve leaflets, resulting in prolapse of the mitral valve. Bacterial endocarditis continues to be an important cause of mitral, aortic, and tricuspid valve destruction, although changes in the clinical and bacteriologic picture have resulted from the widespread use of antibiotics.

MITRAL STENOSIS

Mitral stenosis for practical purposes is due to rheumatic heart disease, although a congenital form of the disease and obstruction of the valve orifice due to left atrial myxoma do occur. The valve becomes thickened, and there is fusion of the valve commissures. Calcification of the valve leaflets and mitral annulus is often present. The chordae tendineae are thickened, shortened, and fused to a variable degree. Generally, the valve orifice will be reduced to 1.2 cm^2 or less in cross-sectional area before significant symptoms develop. The major effect of mitral valve obstruction is a chronic increase in left atrial and pulmonary venous pressure. This increased pressure is transmitted back to the pulmonary capillaries and pulmonary artery. There is resultant interstitial edema and marked thickening of the alveolar walls. The small muscular pulmonary arteries and arterioles develop marked muscular hypertrophy and there is reduction in the lumen of these vessels. As one would suspect from these anatomic changes in severe mitral stenosis there may be elevation of pulmonary artery pressure that is greater than can be accounted for by the elevation in pulmonary venous and left atrial pressure, indicating increased resistance across the pulmonary vascular bed. This increased pulmonary vascular resistance may at times rise to systemic levels with resultant severe pulmonary artery hypertension.

The major symptom in mitral stenosis is exertional dyspnea. As the disease advances, dyspnea at rest and marked fatigue develop. Right heart failure and functional tricuspid regurgitation often occur, and peripheral edema and ascites may then become prominent.

The lungs in mitral stenosis become fibrotic and noncompliant. There is abnormal distribution of alveolar perfusion and ventilation that results in functional shunting of blood through the lungs. The upper lobes have increased perfusion, whereas flow to the bases is reduced. This feature of mitral stenosis can often be appreciated on upright chest radiographs.

Despite the marked anatomic changes that occur in the lungs of patients with severe mitral stenosis, pulmonary artery hypertension and increased pulmonary vascular resistance are reversible following surgery that successfully relieves mitral valve obstruction. Studies in patients immediately following mitral valve replacement have shown that the pulmonary artery pressure and calculated pulmonary vascular resistance fall rapidly within the first few days following valve replacement. Studies done several weeks later indicate that further reduction in vascular resistance occurs with time. The reversibility of pulmonary vascular resistance in mitral stenosis contrasts with the irreversible nature of the high pulmonary vascular resistance that develops in some patients with congenital heart disease with left-to-right shunts.

The left atrium in mitral stenosis becomes increased in volume, and the atrial wall becomes hypertrophied. In a study of 25 patients, atrial volume ranged from 44 to 288 ml per M^2, the average volume being more than three times the normal value. Occasional patients have been seen who have giant left atria, but marked left atrial enlargement is usually associated with mitral regurgitation. The maximum volume of the atrium is not linearly related to the severity of mitral stenosis, since other factors such as the duration of disease and the severity of rheumatic involvement of the atrial myocardium are factors in determining atrial volume. As long as sinus rhythm persists, atrial contraction plays an important role in forcing blood through the obstructed mitral orifice into the left ventricle. Unfortunately, the majority of patients with mitral stenosis eventually develop atrial fibrillation. Presumably, this is the result of chronic atrial hypertension and dilatation, although the exact mechanisms are not clear. Atrial fibrillation has three deleterious effects: (1) it reduces left ventricular

filling; (2) it usually results in an increase in heart rate, with resultant decrease in the diastolic portion of the cardiac cycle; and (3) it allows stagnation of blood in the dilated left atrium and its appendage. For cardiac output to be maintained in the face of atrial fibrillation, left atrial pressure must increase to compensate for loss of atrial contraction and reduced diastolic filling time. This increase in atrial pressure may result in the development of left atrial thrombi, which then often embolize with devastating consequences. Control of the heart rate in patients with atrial fibrillation and anticoagulant therapy are, therefore, major therapeutic measures in this disease.

Mitral stenosis is unique among acquired disease of the left side of the heart because it protects rather than stresses the left ventricle. Studies of the left ventricle indicate that in the majority of cases the ventricular volume and mass are normal. In an occasional advanced case, however, actual atrophy of the ventricular myocardium may occur. Despite normal diastolic volume, the left ventricular stroke volume often is reduced. This combination of reduced stroke volume and normal diastolic volume results in a reduced ejection fraction in about one third of patients with mitral stenosis, with half of these having an ejection fraction below 40 per cent. It is not clear at this time whether this reduced ejection fraction is indicative of myocardial dysfunction or whether it is merely an expression of reduced filling volume and pressure (preload).

Right ventricular hypertrophy accompanies the development of pulmonary hypertension in patients with mitral stenosis. Since the right ventricle is unaccustomed to developing high pressures, it often dilates, and functional tricuspid regurgitation frequently occurs. Venous hypertension, congestive hepatomegaly, peripheral edema, and ascites then follow. Sustained pulmonary hypertension occasionally causes dilatation of the pulmonary artery and annulus of the pulmonary valve, with resultant pulmonary valvular insufficiency. Since associated aortic valve insufficiency is commonly present in patients with mitral stenosis, the differentiation of aortic from pulmonary valve insufficiency requires cardiac catheterization and angiocardiography. Both tricuspid and pulmonary valve insufficiency can be expected to become less prominent or disappear entirely following successful mitral valve repair or replacement.

Since mitral stenosis commonly occurs in young women, the disease is often complicated by pregnancy. During pregnancy, there is an increase in both blood volume and cardiac output. Although these changes may be accommodated by patients with other types of heart disease of modest severity, they are poorly tolerated by the patient with mitral stenosis. Not uncommonly, in fact, the first symptoms of heart disease leading to the diagnosis of mitral stenosis occur during pregnancy. Reduction of activity and control of blood volume with low-sodium diet and diuretics are generally successful in bringing these patients through pregnancy and delivery. Occasionally, these measures are not adequate, and mitral commissurotomy is required during the second trimester.

Surgical Considerations. Mitral commissurotomy can be performed with or without the aid of cardiopulmonary bypass. This operation, as it is performed today, is highly successful in the majority of cases in relieving mitral valve obstruction at least temporarily. The operation can be carried out with low mortality in functional class 2 and class 3 patients, but it is associated with a considerably higher mortality in class 4 patients. Most cardiac surgery centers therefore recommend that this operation be performed on patients with mitral stenosis when they become significantly disabled by symptoms of their disease. It is best to operate on patients well before they have developed severe limitation, since the operative mortality increases greatly and the benefits of surgery are reduced. If valve replacement is contemplated because of heavy valve calcification or associated mitral regurgitation or both, surgery should be delayed longer, since operative mortality is greater and long-term results are less favorable with this procedure.

MITRAL REGURGITATION

Mitral regurgitation may occur as a "pure" lesion or may be associated with mitral stenosis. When it is associated with stenosis it is nearly always due to rheumatic heart disease, whereas "pure" mitral regurgitation may be the result of many different diseases.

Pure mitral regurgitation resulting from papillary muscle dysfunction and papillary muscle rupture has been discussed in the section on ischemic heart disease. Other causes of mitral regurgitation are ruptured chordae tendineae, mitral annular dilatation and displacement of the papillary muscle due to ventricular dilatation, dysfunction of the mitral valve apparatus due to endocardial fibrosis, and postrheumatic deformity of the valve. Congenital clefts of the mitral valve occur and are often associated with atrial septal defects of the primum type. Myxomatous degeneration of the valve leaflets also occurs.

In the past, mitral regurgitation was thought to be a benign condition. Although considerable mitral regurgitation may be well tolerated for years, there is no question that it can cause left ventricular failure and death. The hemodynamics of left ventricular ejection are greatly altered in mitral regurgitation. Normally during the isovolumic phase of systole the myocardial fibers develop tension without shortening. When the intracavitary pressure reaches the pressure in the aorta, the aortic valve opens and ejection occurs. In the

presence of mitral regurgitation, the isovolumic phase of systole is greatly shortened, or eliminated, since ejection into the left atrium occurs as soon as left ventricular pressure exceeds left atrial pressure.

Angiographic studies of patients with pure mitral regurgitation have shown that there is left ventricular dilatation that is linearly related to the severity of valvular regurgitation. There is also left ventricular hypertrophy, although this is less than that seen with aortic regurgitation of similar magnitude. The systolic ejection fraction is generally in the normal range in patients with mitral regurgitation of rheumatic etiology, but it is nearly always depressed when regurgitation is due to ischemic heart disease or congestive cardiomyopathy. Chronic mitral regurgitation is frequently present in idiopathic hypertrophic subaortic stenosis, but it is usually mild to moderate and results from displacement of the papillary muscles by the distorted hypertrophied ventricle rather than from disease of the mitral leaflets or annulus. The left ventricle has a normal or increased ejection fraction in contrast to the depressed ejection fraction seen with other types of cardiomyopathy.

The left atrium is always enlarged in patients with chronic mitral regurgitation and is generally larger than in patients with mitral stenosis, as shown in Table 9–3. In a small number of cases, it reaches giant proportions (greater than 300 ml per M^2). The maximum atrial volume is a poor guide to the severity of mitral regurgitation, but the change in atrial volume during the cardiac cycle is increased in mitral regurgitation and has been shown to be related to the severity of regurgitation. The large cyclic change in atrial volume does not depend on atrial contraction, since it occurs passively early in diastole. Only the small increment of atrial emptying that results from atrial contraction is lost when atrial fibrillation develops in these patients.

TABLE 9–3 LEFT ATRIAL VOLUME IN MITRAL VALVE DISEASE

	Number of Cases	Mean	1 SD	Range of Volume
Maximum LA volume (ml/M²)				
Normal	22	35	9	22–50
Mitral stenosis	25	117	57	44–288
Mitral stenosis and regurgitation	27	180	106	84–594
Mitral regurgitation	27	183	116	63–547
LA volume change (ml/M²)				
Normal	22	18	7.4	5–30
Mitral stenosis	25	14	9	1–45
Mitral stenosis and regurgitation	26	23	11	4–50
Mitral regurgitation	27	46	27	12–124

(By permission of the American Heart Association, Inc.)

Pulmonary artery pressure is variable in mitral regurgitation and depends on the severity of valvular regurgitation and, more importantly, on the compliance of the left atrium and the pulmonary venous bed. Most often, left atrial volume is moderately increased and the atrial wall is relatively stiff, so that there is a large systolic pulse pressure, or "V" wave, seen in the left atrial pressure tracing. This large "V" wave plus a variable increase in pulmonary vascular resistance results in elevation of the pulmonary artery and right ventricular pressure. In some cases of chronic mitral regurgitation, however, the left atrium is unusually large and distensible. This large baglike structure absorbs the regurgitant volume from the left ventricle with little increase in pressure. In these circumstances, severe mitral regurgitation may be present with normal pulmonary artery pressure. When mitral regurgitation develops acutely, such as occurs with ruptured chordae tendineae, a small noncompliant left atrium is suddenly subjected to a large pressure and volume load. The left atrial "V" wave may be extremely high (in the range of 60 to 80 mm Hg) and pulmonary artery pressure is likewise greatly elevated. This combination of events often results in the sudden onset of pulmonary edema.

Surgical treatment of pure mitral regurgitation requires cardiopulmonary bypass with open repair of the valve or prosthetic replacement. Valve clefts and fenestrations may be repaired directly or patched with pericardium or fabric. Unfortunately, most patients have severely deformed or thickened valves that cannot be repaired and must be replaced.

COMBINED MITRAL STENOSIS AND REGURGITATION

Rheumatic involvement of the mitral valve frequently distorts the leaflets and supporting structures so that a combination of stenosis and regurgitation results. Scarring is usually severe in these cases, and heavy calcification is frequently present. The symptoms and clinical features will depend on whether stenosis or regurgitation is the dominant hemodynamic lesion.

Abnormalities in atrial and ventricular function and anatomy are generally midway between those seen in either pure stenosis or regurgitation alone. Quantitation of the severity of regurgitation in a series of these patients showed that regurgitation flows of more than 5.0 liters per minute per M^2 occurred only when valve stenosis was absent.

The presence of both stenosis and regurgitation is of therapeutic importance because surgical treatment nearly always requires valve replacement. These patients are usually treated with medical management until they reach functional class 3 status.

Several patients have now been evaluated with quantitative angiographic or echocardiographic techniques before and after clinically successful mitral valve surgery. After surgical treatment for mitral stenosis, there is the expected reduction in left atrial and right heart pressures with increase in resting cardiac output. Left ventricular volume and mass show little change following surgery, since they are usually normal in these patients preoperatively. In patients with mitral regurgitation, successful surgical correction usually results in a reduction in left atrial and right-sided pressures. Left ventricular volume is reduced toward normal, but there is little regression in left ventricular muscle mass. In patients with reduced left ventricular pump function as measured by a low preoperative ejection fraction, there is often a further decline in ejection fraction following surgery. In patients with normal ventricular function prior to surgery, some remain normal, and others have a reduced ejection fraction after surgery. The fall in ejection fraction in some patients after surgery indicates that it is probably due to an increase in left ventricular afterload, which occurs when the mitral valve becomes competent and no longer allows ejection of blood from the left ventricle into the low-pressure left atrium. These studies suggest that patients with mitral regurgitation should be treated surgically prior to the development of left ventricular dysfunction.

AORTIC VALVE DISEASE

Aortic stenosis is most often the result of rheumatic endocarditis and is frequently associated with mitral valve disease. When aortic stenosis occurs as an isolated lesion and there is no history of rheumatic fever, the disease is likely to be the result of a congenital malformation of the valve. It is now known from autopsy studies that bicuspid and other malformations of the aortic valve are common congenital cardiac abnormalities. It is the gradual thickening, fibrosis, and calcification of these abnormal valves that eventually result in isolated calcific aortic stenosis in middle and later life.

Aortic stenosis in its pure form uncomplicated by valvular incompetence presents a systolic pressure load on the left ventricle. This pressure load develops gradually as the valve stenosis becomes more severe and ventricular hypertrophy progresses at a rate adequate to maintain normal cardiac output. Severe aortic valve obstruction may be present for a prolonged period, during which time the patient remains asymptomatic. Eventually, owing to either further valve narrowing or decrease in myocardial performance, the cardiac output cannot increase adequately to meet the demand of exercise. The patient then develops exertional dyspnea and may also experience angina pectoris, lightheadedness, or actual syncope.

Finally, with further deterioration in myocardial function, congestive heart failure develops.

Evaluation of patients who have exertional lightheadedness or syncope has shown that hypotension develops with physical exertion and at that time symptoms appear. This hypotension that occurs with upright exercise is the result of limited ability to increase cardiac output. The available blood flow is preferentially shunted to the low resistance bed of the working leg muscles, with resulting hypotension and cerebral ischemia. The same phenomenon can be observed in patients with tight mitral stenosis, although syncope is uncommon.

Angina pectoris often occurs in patients with aortic stenosis. Since aortic stenosis occurs most commonly in middle-aged men, associated atherosclerotic heart disease may be the cause of the anginal syndrome. When aortic obstruction is severe, however, angina pectoris frequently occurs in the presence of normal coronary arteries. Angina results from inadequate oxygen supply to the myocardium. In aortic stenosis, this is due to a combination of factors, including increased myocardial oxygen consumption resulting from increased pressure work, left ventricular hypertrophy, and reduced coronary artery perfusion pressure. The reduction in coronary perfusion pressure occurs because of low aortic root pressure and elevated left ventricular chamber pressure during systole and to some extent in the later portion of diastole.

When syncope or angina or both are present in a patient with aortic stenosis, there is a high risk of sudden death, which often is associated with physical exertion. It is probable that this is secondary to exertional hypotension resulting in reduced coronary arterial blood flow, myocardial ischemia, and the development of ventricular fibrillation. Patients with tight aortic stenosis and symptoms of angina pectoris or syncope or both require urgent evaluation and surgical correction.

MYOCARDIAL FUNCTION IN AORTIC STENOSIS

Prior to the onset of myocardial failure, the left ventricle responds to a pressure load by hypertrophy without chamber dilatation. The left ventricle in aortic stenosis therefore has normal volume and hypertrophy of the left ventricular myocardium including the wall, trabeculae, and papillary muscles. Ventricular ejection fraction is usually maintained in the normal range. The left ventricular systolic pressure may be as high as 300 mm Hg, although it is usually in the range of 200 mm Hg. This results in a large pressure gradient across the stenotic valve. The aortic pressure is low, has a small pulse pressure, and is slow-rising with an anacrotic notch.

Despite a normal end-diastolic volume and ejection fraction, the filling pressure may be significantly elevated before the onset of congestive heart failure. This is the result of vigorous left atrial contraction ejecting blood into the thick-walled noncompliant left ventricle. The elevation of end-diastolic pressure is, therefore, a poor indication of left ventricular myocardial failure in these patients.

In patients with aortic stenosis who have developed congestive heart failure the left ventricle often shows moderate chamber dilatation, reduced stroke volume, reduced ejection fraction, and marked elevation in left ventricular end-diastolic pressure. As the myocardium progressively weakens, the pressure generated in the chamber is reduced, and the flow and pressure gradient across the valve fall. If only the pressure gradient is measured during cardiac catheterization and the flow and valve orifice are not determined, the severity of valve stenosis may not be fully appreciated.

Treatment of Aortic Stenosis. Once severe aortic stenosis has resulted in significant dyspnea, angina, syncope, or congestive heart failure, surgical replacement of the valve is required.

The evaluation of patients by quantitative angiocardiographic techniques before and after surgery indicates that there is a reduction in left ventricular systolic pressure work, a decrease in end-diastolic pressure, and little change in end-diastolic volume. Patients with a low ejection fraction before surgery usually have an increase in ejection fraction toward normal after surgery. Figure 9–19 illustrates the pressure-volume in a patient with aortic stenosis without myocardial failure before and after successful homograft aortic valve replacement. The difference in the area enclosed by the two loops represents the reduction in pressure-volume work following surgery. The end-diastolic volume is unchanged despite a fall in the diastolic pressure. Studies of left ventricular mass before and 1 year after surgery suggest that myocardial hypertrophy regresses substantially following successful surgical treatment.

AORTIC REGURGITATION

Unlike aortic stenosis, aortic regurgitation is a disease of many causes, rheumatic heart disease being the major one. Other causes include syphilitic aortitis, congenital malformations of the aortic valve (often associated with a high ventricular septal defect), Marfan's syndrome with ascending aortic dissection, aneurysm with aortic annular dilatation, and cusp rupture secondary to chest wall trauma. When bacterial endocarditis involves the aortic valve, severe regurgitation often results. Severe hypertension occasionally causes mild aortic regurgitation that is reversible when the blood pressure is lowered.

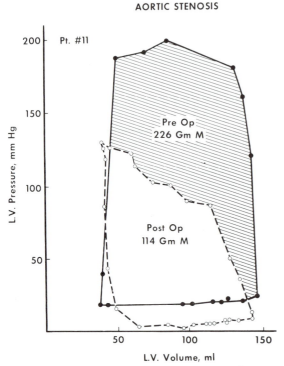

AORTIC STENOSIS

Pt. #11

Pre Op
226 Gm M

Post Op
114 Gm M

Figure 9–19 Left ventricular pressure-volume diagrams constructed from cardiac catheterization and angiocardiographic data acquired before and after successful aortic valve replacement for severe aortic stenosis. The area beneath the systolic portion of each loop represents the pressure-volume systolic stroke work of the left ventricle. Preoperatively, systolic work was 226 gram-meters per beat; following aortic valve replacement, systolic work fell to 114 gram-meters per beat. The shaded area indicates the reduction in work as a result of surgery. (Adapted from Kennedy, J. W., Twiss, R. D., Blackmon, J. R., and Merendino, K. A.: Hemodynamic studies one year after homograft aortic valve replacement. Circulation 37–38 (Suppl. 2):110, 1968. By permission of the American Heart Association, Inc.)

Aortic regurgitation, when severe, places a large volume load on the left ventricle. Since the large stroke volume is ejected into the high-resistance systemic circulation, a component of pressure overload also occurs in this disease in contrast to the pure volume overload seen in mitral regurgitation. The stroke volume is greatly increased, and its forceful ejection from the ventricle results in a wide pulse pressure and often in an elevation in aortic systolic pressure. The leaking aortic valve results in retrograde flow in the aorta during diastole and a fall in aortic diastolic pressure. The impressive peripheral vascular findings in this disease, which include pistol-shot pulses, pulsating capillaries in the nail beds, and systolic head bobbing, are expressions of widened arterial pulse pressure and/or retrograde diastolic flow in large arteries.

Left ventricular enlargement is a major feature of this disease with both hypertrophy of the myocardium and an increased chamber volume. As in mitral regurgitation, the ventricular diastolic volume is increased in direct proportion to the volume of regurgitation, and in extreme cases it may reach nearly 800 ml (Fig. 9–20). The total left ventricular stroke volume is greatly increased, with the forward or systemic stroke volume remaining in the normal range until left ventricular failure develops. Total left ventricular stroke volume, including forward and regurgitant fractions, may reach 300 ml or more, with total output approaching 30 L per minute. This level of ventricular output occasionally seen in these patients at rest is about the same as that achieved by a well-trained healthy young man during maximum exercise. The limits of left ventricular output, therefore, seem to be quite similar in health and in the individual with a compensated left ventricle and severe aortic regurgitation. However, the large minute outputs observed with aortic valve insufficiency are primarily a result of the large stroke volume, whereas the increased outputs observed with exercise are primarily achieved by an increased heart rate. With aortic regurgitation, left ventricular mass may be very large, approaching 1000 gm in severe cases, and averaged 425 gm in 38 cases studied by quantitative angiocardiography. This condition produces the largest left ventricles seen in clinical medicine.

Left ventricular filling pressure depends on the severity of aortic regurgitation, the left ventricular myocardial compliance, and the heart rate. When aortic regurgitation is very severe, the

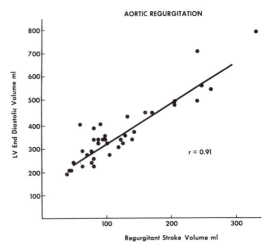

AORTIC REGURGITATION

r = 0.91

Figure 9–20 The relationship between the left ventricular end-diastolic volume and the regurgitant stroke volume in 38 patients with pure aortic regurgitation. There is a linear relationship between the severity of regurgitation and the ventricular end-diastolic volume. (From Kennedy, J. W., Twiss, R. D., Blackmon, J. R., and Dodge, H. T.: Quantitative angiocardiography, III. Relationship of left ventricular pressure, volume and mass in aortic valve disease. Circulation *38*:838, 1968. By permission of The American Heart Association, Inc.)

pressures in the aorta and left ventricle may equilibrate during the end of diastole, usually at a level of 30 to 40 mm Hg. This is most likely to occur if the patient has bradycardia. In Figure 9–21, the left ventricular and aortic pressures are seen in a man with severe aortic regurgitation and sinus bradycardia at a rate of 54 per minute. At end-diastole, the pressure in the aorta is 48 mm Hg and 35 mm Hg in the left ventricle. Following right atrial pacing at a rate of 82 per minute, the end-diastolic pressure in the aorta became normal at 75 mm Hg and fell to 10 mm Hg in the left ventricle. This change in heart rate also resulted in a reduced left ventricular end-diastolic volume and regurgitant flow per beat but no significant change in the volume of aortic regurgitation per minute. This effect of heart rate on ventricular filling pressure accounts for the fact that some patients with aortic regurgitation have dyspnea and angina at rest but have little exercise limitation.

Angina is relatively common in aortic regurgitation, although not as frequent as in aortic stenosis. Left ventricular oxygen consumption is increased in aortic regurgitation because of the associated pressure-volume overload and the ventricular hypertrophy. In addition, the pressure gradient between the aortic root and the intramyocardial and subendocardial coronary vessels is reduced as a result of low aortic diastolic pressure and elevated left ventricular filling pressure. The occurrence of angina pectoris is therefore easily explained in this disease. When aortic regurgitation occurs in middle age, coronary atherosclerosis is also likely to be a contributing factor as a cause

of angina, especially when aortic regurgitation is not severe. Patients with syphilitic aortitis may get calcification and obstruction of one or both of the coronary ostia, which will account for an occasional case of angina in this disease.

When congestive heart failure develops in patients with aortic regurgitation, there is either further dilatation of the ventricle, decrease in the total left ventricular stroke volume, or both, so that the ejection fraction falls, the ventricular filling pressure increases, and pulmonary vascular congestion develops. With marked left ventricular dilatation, functional mitral regurgitation occurs owing to enlargement of the mitral annulus or displacement or excessive lengthening of the papillary muscles. The development of mitral regurgitation results in a further decrease of forward output, and this combination of valvular defects is poorly tolerated.

Bacterial endocarditis of the aortic valve often results in the sudden development of severe aortic regurgitation due to fenestration, tearing, or rupture of one or more valve cusps. The sudden pressure-volume overload imposed on the normal left ventricle is poorly tolerated and there is extreme elevation of ventricular filling pressure and acute dilatation of the chamber. Pulmonary edema may develop suddenly and immediate surgery is often required as a life-saving measure. If the patient survives without surgical treatment, the left ventricle gradually dilates and the myocardium hypertrophies as the left ventricle adjusts to the chronic pressure-volume overload.

Treatment of Aortic Regurgitation. Medical treatment is useful in controlling congestive heart

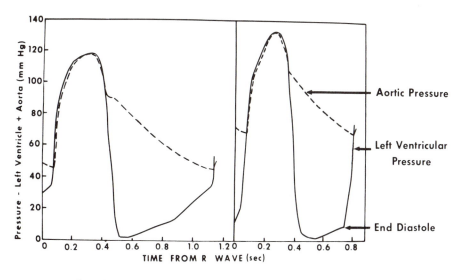

Heart Rate =54   Heart Rate = 82

Figure 9–21 Left ventricular and aortic pressure in a patient with severe aortic regurgitation and sinus bradycardia heart rate 54 (left panel) and during right atrial pacing at heart rate 82 (right panel). With pacing, the aortic pressure during diastole has increased, whereas the left ventricular end-diastolic pressure has decreased to a normal level. (From Judge, T. P., Kennedy, J. W., Bennett, L. J., et al.: The quantitative hemodynamic effects of heart rate in aortic regurgitation. Circulation 44:355, 1971.)

failure. The primary form of treatment is valve replacement. Risk of surgery in aortic regurgitation varies with the cause of the disease, age of the patient, and myocardial function. In patients without myocardial failure the surgical mortality is in the range of 2 to 5 per cent.

Studies of patients before and after successful valve replacement for severe aortic regurgitation indicate that the end-diastolic volume is greatly reduced following surgery, although it may not return completely to normal. The filling pressure and pressure-volume work are also decreased toward normal, and left ventricular hypertrophy regresses but does not become normal. When ventricular function is depressed prior to surgery, as indicated by a low preoperative ejection fraction, it remains abnormal in many patients following surgical correction.

COMBINED AORTIC STENOSIS AND REGURGITATION

The combination of aortic stenosis and regurgitation results from thickened deformed valve leaflets that cannot open or close properly. The disease is most often due to rheumatic endocarditis but also is the frequent result of a congenitally malformed valve. The clinical and hemodynamic pictures depend on whether stenosis or regurgitation is the predominant lesion. Very severe aortic regurgitation does not occur in the presence of significant valve obstruction, so that the marked peripheral vascular signs of aortic regurgitation are less prominent or absent. Surgical treatment is indicated when the patient is disabled by symptoms and valve replacement is nearly always required.

COMBINED AORTIC AND MITRAL VALVE DISEASE

When disease of both the mitral and aortic valves is present, one lesion may alter the effects of the other and the overall hemodynamic picture. The most detrimental combination of valve lesions is aortic stenosis and mitral regurgitation because aortic valve obstruction increases the severity of mitral regurgitation and decreases systemic flow. When both aortic and mitral stenosis occur together, the left ventricle is protected from pressure load by limited filling and may fail to undergo the usual hypertrophy. Because of decreased flow, the murmurs of both lesions will be diminished, particularly that of aortic stenosis, and the diagnosis may be difficult to make at the bedside. Proper surgical treatment requires that obstruction at both valves be relieved.

Tricuspid Valve Disease

In patients with valvular heart disease, tricuspid valve disease is usually associated with mitral valve disease. Tricuspid regurgitation is most often functional and secondary to pulmonary hypertension and right ventricular dilatation. Such functional tricuspid regurgitation usually regresses when mitral valve disease has been adequately treated surgically and there is no residual left ventricular failure to elevate pulmonary vascular pressures. Occasionally, the tricuspid valve is structurally abnormal owing to involvement by the rheumatic process with organic tricuspid stenosis, tricuspid regurgitation, or both. In this situation, the tricuspid valve may require valvuloplasty or replacement. Other types of tricuspid valve disease include congenital tricuspid stenosis and atresia, Ebstein's anomaly of the tricuspid valve, and tricuspid valve insufficiency from endocardial fibrosis of the right heart as occurs in the carcinoid syndrome.

THE CARDIOMYOPATHIES

The term *cardiomyopathy* refers to a group of diseases that involve the myocardium directly. The term *primary myocardial disease* has been used to refer to the subgroup of cardiomyopathies that are idiopathic, and the term *secondary myocardial disease* has been used to designate the group in which causative factors are known. Although there is no uniform agreement on terminology, Fowler has suggested that *cardiomyopathy* is a satisfactory term for this entire group of diseases. Further classification into idiopathic and secondary cardiomyopathy seems sensible and should avoid confusion. A classification from Fowler is given in Table 9–4. The list of secondary cardiomyopathies is long, but the number of cases represented by that group is quite small.

The true incidence of the various cardiomyopathies is not well known because of the tendency to diagnose ischemic heart disease when obvious congenital and rheumatic heart disease are not present. When carefully looked for, various types of cardiomyopathy are frequently recognized. It must be remembered that the specific incidence will vary considerably, depending on the particular population of patients concerned. It is known that idiopathic cardiomyopathy is more frequent among indigent patient populations than in individuals from higher socioeconomic groups. Recent animal experiments suggest that exercise in the face of active myocarditis due to virus infection or Chagas disease is associated with an increase in myocardial damage. Nutritional deficiency has a similar detrimental influence. These studies offer a possible explanation for the higher incidence of these diseases in indigent populations.

TABLE 9–4 CLASSIFICATION OF CARDIOMYOPATHIES

Idiopathic cardiomyopathy
  Nonobstructive cardiomyopathy
    Alcoholic cardiomyopathy
    Postinfectious cardiomyopathy (when infectious
      agent cannot be identified)
    Familial cardiomyopathy
    Peripartal cardiomyopathy
    Cardiomyopathy without identifiable antecedent
      illness
  Obstructive cardiomyopathy
    Familial
    Nonfamilial

Secondary cardiomyopathy
  Myocarditis
    Viral: Coxsackie B, Coxsackie A, echovirus,
      influenza virus, infectious
      mononucleosis
    Rheumatic
    Septic (including bacterial endocarditis)
    Diphtheritic
    Syphilitic
    Chagas disease
    Trichinosis
    Allergic
    Toxic
    Uremic
    Toxoplasmic
  Neuromuscular and neurologic disorders
    Progressive muscular dystrophy;
      pseudohypertrophic and facioscapulohumeral
      muscular dystrophy
    Friedreich's ataxia
    Myotonic muscular dystrophy
  Connective tissue disease: rheumatoid disease,
    dermatomyositis, scleroderma, disseminated
    lupus erythematosus
  Mucopolysaccharidosis (e.g., Hurler syndrome,
    Hunter syndrome)
  Sarcoidosis
  Amyloid disease
  Primary and metastatic tumors
  Metabolic disorders
    Glycogen storage disease
    Nutritional deficiency
      Beriberi
      Kwashiorkor
    Thyrotoxicosis
    Myxedema
    Hemochromatosis
    Nutritional cirrhosis

(From Fowler, N. O.: Progr. Cardiovasc. Dis. *14*:113, 1971. By permission of Grune & Stratton, Inc.)

IDIOPATHIC CARDIOMYOPATHY

There are two general categories of diseases in the idiopathic group—obstructive and nonobstructive. The obstructive cardiomyopathies are very different from the nonobstructive in their hemodynamic manifestations and will be discussed first.

Obstructive Cardiomyopathies. The obstructive cardiomyopathies, known as *idiopathic hypertrophic subaortic stenosis (IHSS),* have been well studied since the classic report of Braunwald and colleagues in the early 1960s. The unusual dynamic character of the obstruction has been defined, and rational methods of medical and surgical treatment have been developed. A familial incidence has been recognized in about 30 per cent of cases, but the etiology remains obscure.

This disease has been recognized from infancy to old age but is usually seen in young adults. It is manifest by palpitations, angina on effort, or postexertional syncope and is associated with a high incidence of sudden death. Symptoms of pulmonary congestion and congestive heart failure develop late in the disease. Physical examination reveals a systolic ejection murmur at the lower left sternal border and an intact aortic second sound. There is an associated murmur of mitral insufficiency in about 50 per cent of cases. The ejection murmur increases in intensity with standing, during the Valsalva maneuver, or following the administration of amyl nitrite or nitroglycerin. The beat following a premature contraction is characterized by an increase in the systolic pressure gradient and in the intensity of the ejection murmur and by a reduced arterial pulse pressure. Treatment with digitalis may cause an increase in the murmur and a worsening of symptoms and is contraindicated in this disease. Hemodynamic studies reveal a pressure gradient between the left ventricular inflow tract and outflow tract. The pressure gradient is increased by the aforementioned drugs and maneuvers and is often decreased by the administration of a beta-blocking drug such as propranolol.

Left ventricular angiocardiography usually reveals generalized left ventricular hypertrophy with marked hypertrophy of the papillary muscles. The basal portion of the interventricular septum is greatly hypertrophied, although this may be difficult to appreciate by angiography. The end-diastolic volume of the left ventricle is usually normal, but the end-systolic volume is smaller than normal, with almost complete obliteration of the apical portion of the ventricle, which may appear as a finger-shaped cavity. Quantitative angiocardiographic evaluation reveals an increased ejection fraction and marked increase in left ventricular mass. The coronary arteries often appear to be unusually large.

Left ventricular end-diastolic pressure is usually elevated and may be extremely high, whereas left ventricular dp/dt is elevated as well. The high filling pressure in combination with an elevated ejection fraction and LV dp/dt suggest that the myocardium is noncompliant but retains normal or has increased contractility.

Surgical exploration reveals a normal aortic valve and localized hypertrophy of the basal portion of the interventricular septum just below the aortic valve. This area of the septum may be fibrotic, and there is often considerable thickening of the endocardium. It appears, therefore, that outflow obstruction develops in this disease because the anterior leaflet of the mitral valve is pulled into apposition with the hypertrophied interventricular septum during systole. The actual site of obstruction is often difficult to visualize by angiography.

Echocardiography has become accepted as a useful noninvasive technique for the diagnosis of IHSS (idiopathic hypertrophic subaortic stenosis). The echocardiogram usually demonstrates asymmetric thickening of the basal portion of the interventricular septum as compared with the thickness of the posterior left ventricular wall in a ratio of ≥1.3:1. In addition, the anterior leaflet of the mitral valve can be shown to move anteriorly toward the septum during systole instead of posteriorly, as in normals. The echo recording often shows the anterior leaflet echoes joining the echoes of the septum, suggesting that at least a portion of the valve contacts the septum during mid- or late systole. This is strong evidence that the outflow obstruction present in IHSS occurs as a result of this phenomenon. Some patients have only asymmetric septal hypertrophy (ASH), without abnormal motion of the mitral valve or other evidence of obstruction. ASH is often found in asymptomatic family members of patients with IHSS, suggesting that ASH may be a genetic marker of the disease.

From the preceding description, it can be appreciated that conditions that reduce end-diastolic volume or increase the contractile state of the left ventricle will tend to increase the subvalvular pressure gradient. These include inotropic drugs such as isoproterenol and digitalis glycosides, reduced venous return to the left heart as induced by postural changes, the Valsalva maneuver or loss of blood volume, and reduced left ventricular afterload as induced with nitroglycerin or amyl nitrite. Beta-blocking drugs are specific for this disease in that they can be shown to reduce or eliminate the outflow obstruction in many of these cases. When severe obstruction is present that does not respond to beta blockade, surgical treatment with excision of the hypertrophied muscle of the outflow tract may be beneficial.

Nonobstructive Cardiomyopathies. The majority of idiopathic cardiomyopathies are of the nonobstructive type. In the United States, they are found most often in patients who consume large amounts of alcohol or in women during the immediate pre- or postpartum periods. Although alcohol administration has been shown to reduce ventricular contractility, the actual etiologic role of alcohol in the production of chronic progressive cardiomyopathy is not known. Peripartum cardiomyopathy is also not well understood, although it is most common in poorly nourished individuals, suggesting the importance of nutritional factors.

In years past, it was thought that most cases of chronic heart disease were either of valvular etiology or due to chronic myocarditis. When the high incidence of ischemic heart disease in Western countries became appreciated, chronic myocarditis became an unusual diagnosis. Although there are well-documented cases of acute viral or bacterial myocarditis having progressed to produce chronic myocardial failure, in general there is complete recovery. In fact, it is extremely unusual to see patients with cardiomyopathy in whom one can obtain a history suggesting an infectious etiology. Therefore, although the concept that chronic cardiomyopathy is due to either prior or continuing low-grade myocarditis is appealing, there is little evidence to support this view.

Most patients with nonobstructive cardiomyopathy present with symptoms and signs of heart failure, but occasionally arrhythmias are the presenting complaint. Chest pain is unusual. The heart is large, and all four chambers are frequently involved. Auscultation reveals a prominent atrial and/or ventricular gallop sound and there may be no murmur. When a murmur is present it is due to functional mitral and/or tricuspid regurgitation.

Cardiac catheterization usually reveals elevated atrial pressures with large "a" waves. The end-diastolic pressure is elevated in both ventricles, and the pulmonary artery pressure is elevated secondary to the elevation of the left heart filling pressure. The cardiac output is low, and the arteriovenous oxygen difference may be greatly elevated. Left ventricular dp/dt is depressed.

Angiocardiography reveals dilated cardiac chambers. The left ventricle has an increased diastolic volume and poor stroke volume, yielding a low ejection fraction, usually below 40 per cent. In severe cases, the ejection fraction may be as low as 10 per cent. The papillary muscles are not prominent, but the left ventricular free wall is generally hypertrophied to a modest degree. Left ventricular mass is elevated and is generally equal to the diastolic volume of the left ventricle, yielding a left ventricular mass to end-diastolic volume ratio of about one.

Occasionally, there is a restrictive hemodynamic pattern seen in these patients with marked elevation in venous pressure and high plateau diastolic pressures seen in all cardiac chambers as is found in constrictive pericarditis. At times, it may be difficult to distinguish this disease from constrictive pericarditis without the aid of pericardial and myocardial biopsy. The restrictive form of the disease is seen most often in patients who either have myocardial infiltration with amyloid or hemochromatosis or have marked thickening and fibrosis of the endocardium. A form of extreme endomyocardial fibrosis is prevalent among natives of Uganda. In this condition, there is dense fibrosis of endocardium and myocardium with involvement of the papillary muscles resulting in mitral regurgitation. The etiology of this disease remains obscure.

SECONDARY CARDIOMYOPATHIES

Cardiomyopathy may be associated with a large number of specific disease entities, as shown in Table 9–4. Myocardial involvement as is seen with most of these diseases has hemodynamic features similar to those observed with the non-obstructive cardiomyopathies described previously. There is loss of myocardial contractile force with ventricular dilatation, high filling pressure, low ejection fraction, and low cardiac output. When there is myocardial infiltration, there is a tendency toward reduced myocardial compliance and a restrictive filling pattern. Exceptions are the cardiomyopathies associated with thyrotoxicosis and beriberi, in which cardiac output is elevated.

Specific cardiomyopathies are associated with certain neuromuscular diseases, including Friedreich's ataxia and the muscular dystrophies. In Friedreich's ataxia there is progressive myocardial fibrosis and obliterative disease of the small coronary arteries that is not due to atherosclerosis. The basis for the relationship between the neuromuscular disease and the cardiomyopathy is not apparent at this time.

Unfortunately, the majority of patients with cardiomyopathy represent difficult therapeutic problems. Cardiomyopathies due to infections and those due to a nutritional or metabolic abnormality may often be treated specifically. Patients with obstructive cardiomyopathy usually respond favorably to therapy with drugs or surgery. The majority of patients with the nonobstructive types of cardiomyopathy will show a favorable clinical response to nonspecific measures such as bed rest, digitalis, diuretics, and unloading therapy. However, these diseases are usually progressive, and response to therapy becomes less satisfactory as the disease progresses. Cardiac transplantation is now considered a useful form of therapy for some of these patients.

PERICARDIAL DISEASE

The pericardium, a fibrous sac surrounding the heart, consists of an outer parietal and inner visceral portion lined by a serous surface and normally contains a small amount of serous fluid. It has been demonstrated to have a function in limiting acute dilatation of the heart, and it possibly serves to isolate the heart from the lungs and to inhibit the spread of infection from the lungs to the heart. These functions do not seem to be very important in that surgical removal of the pericardium is unassociated with abnormalities of heart function, although there may be some increase in the size of the cardiac silhouette on radiographs. Disease of the pericardium is manifest through pain, pericardial effusion, or pericardial constriction of the heart.

Pericardial pain is associated with inflammation or other conditions that irritate the pericardium. The most common cause of pericardial pain is acute pericarditis, but pain also occurs with irritation from leakage of blood into the pericardium, as may be associated with trauma, perforation of the heart, or dissecting aneurysm. The pain is substernal or precordial in location and, in contrast to the pain accompanying myocardial infarction, is accentuated by respiratory movements and occasionally by swallowing. The patient is often more comfortable when sitting and leaning forward. The pain may radiate to the neck, left shoulder, arm, or back. Studies have demonstrated that pain sensation arises from the inferior portion of the parietal pericardium and is transmitted via the phrenic nerves. However, pericardial pain has been relieved by stellate ganglion block, suggesting that at least some pericardial pain fibers travel with the sympathetic nerves.

PERICARDITIS

The most frequent cause of acute pericarditis is so-called *acute idiopathic (nonspecific) pericarditis*. Pericarditis also occurs in association with a large number of other diseases and conditions, including myocardial infarction, postmyocardial infarction, and post-thoracotomy syndrome; specific bacterial, viral, and fungal infections; neoplasms and uremia; certain drug sensitivity reactions; and connective tissue disorders such as rheumatic fever and lupus erythematosus. The pain is often severe and may simulate the pain of myocardial infarction. Inflammatory disease of the pericardium is usually accompanied by systemic signs associated with inflammation, such as fever and leukocytosis. On auscultation, there is usually a pericardial friction rub, which is a scratchy sound, often with three separate components associated with atrial systole, ventricular systole, and ventricular diastole. There are often electrocardiographic changes that are characterized by an S–T current of injury directed downward and to the left in the direction of the cardiac apex, probably a result of diffuse epicardial injury. Over a period of days, and as the S–T subsides, the T wave characteristically becomes abnormal and directed up toward the right shoulder, away from the cardiac apex. Pericarditis is usually associated with pericardial effusion, which is manifest as an increase in the size of the heart on radiographs and occasionally by evidence of pericardial tamponade.

PERICARDIAL EFFUSION

Whether pericardial effusion is associated with pericardial tamponade depends on the rate and volume of fluid accumulation within the pericardium. Acute effusions or bleeding or both of 200 to 300 ml within the pericardium may result in tamponade. When pericardial fluid accumulates slowly, the pericardial sac enlarges, so that more than a liter may be present with no evidence of tamponade.

Large pericardial effusions are usually observed with the more chronic forms of pericarditis, and, in contrast to acute pericarditis, pain is slight or absent. Pericardial effusion is also common in myxedema and congestive heart failure. The pressure-volume characteristics of the pericardium are such that substantial amounts of fluid may accumulate with little increase in pressure. However, a volume is reached at which pressure begins to rise rapidly with further small increases in volume.

On examination, the patient with pericardial effusion characteristically shows an increase in the area of cardiac dullness to percussion with a quiet precordium and distant heart sounds. The cardiac silhouette is enlarged, often with a "waterbottle" configuration. Low voltage is often present on the electrocardiogram.

With pericardial tamponade there is interference with diastolic filling of the heart, resulting in an elevated filling pressure. A characteristic hemodynamic feature of pericardial tamponade is elevation of right and left atrial pressure and the diastolic pressure in the right and left ventricles to similar levels, as is observed in constrictive pericarditis (Fig. 9–22). This feature is often helpful in differentiating pericardial tamponade from left ventricular failure, which is associated with higher filling pressures on the left side of the heart. Dyspnea is usually present, but orthopnea is generally absent unless tamponade is severe. Arterial hypotension also occurs with severe tamponade.

Pulsus paradoxicus is a classic finding in pericardial tamponade and is recognized by a rise and fall of systemic systolic arterial pressure of more than 8 to 10 mm Hg in the recumbent subject during quiet respiration. There have been a number of explanations for this phenomenon. It appears to be related to increased filling of the right heart with reduced filling of the left heart during inspiration. Because in pericardial tamponade there is a restriction of diastolic volume of the entire heart, an increase in diastolic volume of the right ventricle, as occurs during inspiration, must be associated with a reduced diastolic volume of the left heart. An increased pulmonary blood volume is also suggested as contributing to reduced filling of the left ventricle during inspiration. It should be appreciated that pulsus paradoxicus is not a specific finding for pericardial tamponade but also may occur with any condition associated with larger than normal respiratory changes of intrathoracic pressure and with heart failure.

The differentiation of pericardial effusion and tamponade from generalized cardiac enlargement is a rather common clinical problem. Demonstration of pericardial fluid by echocardiography or of a wide margin between the cardiac chamber and the external surface of the cardiac shadow by a radioisotope blood pool scan, by angiocardiography, or by filming following the introduction of carbon dioxide into the venous circulation is often helpful. The demonstration of fluid by pericardiocentesis, of course, establishes the diagnosis of pericardial effusion. Examination of the fluid may also be helpful in establishing an etiologic basis for pericardial effusion and pericarditis.

The treatment for pericardial tamponade is removal of pericardial fluid. This results in prompt relief of symptoms that are due to the tamponade.

CONSTRICTIVE PERICARDITIS

Constrictive pericarditis occurs when pericardial fibrosis and thickening result in restriction of diastolic filling of the heart. In this condition, the

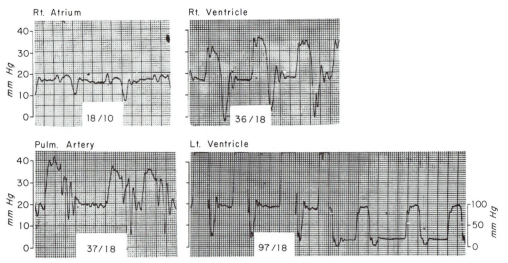

Figure 9–22 Pressures from a patient with constrictive pericarditis. The similarity of pressures during diastole in the right atrium, pulmonary artery, and right and left ventricles is shown. Both right and left ventricular diastolic pressures show a characteristic early diastolic dip followed by a diastolic plateau.

visceral and parietal layers of the pericardium are adherent and may be greatly thickened and densely fibrotic with areas of calcification. Pericardial constriction is known to occur with or following infection of the pericardium with tuberculosis, pyogenic organisms, certain viral diseases, and with acute idiopathic pericarditis. It also occurs with neoplastic involvement of the pericardium, with certain connective tissue disorders such as lupus erythematosus, following radiation therapy, and following hemopericardium from a variety of causes. However, in most patients it is not possible to establish a cause.

The laboratory and clinical findings are consequences of the restricted diastolic filling that results in venous pressure elevation. Because the entire heart is encased in this sac, filling pressures are usually elevated to similar levels on the two sides of the heart, so that right and left atrial, right and left ventricular diastolic, pulmonary wedge, and pulmonary artery diastolic pressures are nearly equal. This is illustrated in Figure 9–22. Other features of the pressure tracings characteristic of constrictive pericarditis are as follows: (1) a rapid fall of ventricular pressure in early diastole resulting in an early diastolic dip followed by a flat diastolic plateau (see right and left ventricular pressures in Figure 9–22); (2) a rapid descent of right atrial pressure with the onset of ventricular filling ("y" descent), which often results in a right atrial pressure curve that has a "w" or "m" configuration. Right ventricular and pulmonary artery systolic pressures are usually only modestly elevated, with the right ventricular diastolic pressure one third or more of the systolic pressure, as shown in Figure 9–22. These pressure findings are not absolutely diagnostic of constrictive pericarditis and occasionally occur with chronic myocardial failure and fibrosis. However, with left ventricular failure the filling pressure is usually higher on the left side of the heart, and right ventricular and pulmonary artery systolic pressures are usually higher than is observed with constrictive pericarditis. Stroke volume is small, but, unless constriction is severe, the cardiac index is only slightly reduced and increases with exercise through an increase in heart rate. The cardiac chamber volumes are characteristically normal or reduced. A thickened wall of the heart due to pericardial thickening can usually be demonstrated by angiocardiography or by positioning a cardiac catheter against the wall of the right atrium at the time of cardiac catheterization, so that the distance from the endocardium to the external surface of the right atrium can be visualized.

Patients with constrictive pericarditis may have an elevated venous pressure for long periods prior to the development of other symptoms or signs such as edema and exertional dyspnea. Edema often appears as ascites and in longstanding cases may be complicated by cardiac cirrhosis of the liver. Weeping of plasma with plasma proteins into the gastrointestinal tract as a result of venous pressure elevation may contribute to hypoproteinemia, which is observed in severe cases of long duration. In spite of an elevated venous pressure and edema, orthopnea is usually absent, and pulmonary edema is unusual.

On examination, patients with constrictive pericarditis have findings associated with an elevated systemic venous pressure and peripheral edema. Pleural effusion is often present. The area of cardiac dullness and the cardiac silhouette are of normal size or only moderately enlarged on radiographs. Heart sounds may be distant, and a pericardial knock sound in early diastole resembling a third heart sound is often present. A paradoxic pulse is occasionally observed. The electrocardiogram commonly has low voltage and flat or abnormally directed T waves. Atrial fibrillation is present in approximately one third of patients. On chest radiographs or fluoroscopic examination, approximately 50 per cent of patients with constrictive pericarditis have pericardial calcification.

In patients with constrictive pericarditis and edema, symptomatic improvement is observed following diuresis induced by one of the diuretic drugs. However, surgical removal of the constricting pericardium is the definitive form of treatment.

REFERENCES

GENERAL

Braunwald, E.: Heart Disease. 2nd ed. Philadelphia, W. B. Saunders Co., 1984.

Grossman, W. (Ed.): Cardiac Catheterization and Angiography. 2nd ed. Philadelphia, Lea and Febiger, 1980.

Hurst, J. W., Logue, R. B., Rackley, C. E., Schlant, R. C., Sonnenblick, E. H., Wallace, A. G., and Wenger, N. K. (Eds.): The Heart, Arteries and Veins. 5th ed. New York, McGraw-Hill Book Co., 1982.

Johnson, R. A., Haber, E., and Austen, W. G. (Eds.): The Practice of Cardiology. The Medical and Surgical Cardiac Units at the Massachusetts General Hospital. Boston, Little, Brown & Co., 1980.

CARDIAC OUTPUT, PRESSURE MEASUREMENTS, AND CARDIAC CATHETERIZATION

Barratt-Boyes, B. G., and Wood, E. H.: Cardiac output and related measurements and pressure values in the right heart and associated vessels, together with an analysis of the hemodynamic response to the inhalation of high oxygen mixtures in healthy subjects. J. Lab. Clin. Med. 51:72, 1958.

Brandfonbrener, M., Landowne, M., and Shock, N. W.: Changes in cardiac output with age. Circulation 12:557, 1955.

Burch, G. E., and DePasquale, N. P.: Cardiac performance in relation to blood volume. Am. J. Cardiol. 14:784, 1964.

Donald, K. W., Bishop, J. M., and Wade, O. L.: Effect of nursing positions on cardiac output of man with a note on the repeatability of measurements of cardiac output by the direct Fick method and with data on subjects with normal cardiovascular system. Clin. Sci. 12:199, 1953.

Dow, P.: Estimations of cardiac output and central blood volume by dye dilution. Physiol. Rev. 36:77, 1956.

Fegler, G.: The reliability of the thermo-dilution method for determination of the cardiac output and the blood flow in central veins. Q. J. Exp. Physiol. 42:254, 1957.

Fry, D. L., Noble, F. W., and Mallos, A. J.: An evaluation of modern pressure recording systems. Circ. Res. 5:40, 1957.

Gorlin, R., and Gorlin, S. G.: Hydraulic formula for calculation of the area of the stenotic mitral valve, other cardiac valves and central circulatory shunts. Am. Heart J. *1*:41, 1951.

Hamilton, W. F., Riley, R. L., Attah, A. M., et al.: Comparison of Fick and dye injection methods of measuring cardiac output in man. Am. J. Physiol. *153*:309, 1948.

Kinsmann, J. M., More, J. W., and Hamilton, W. F.: Studies on the circulation. Injection method; physical and mathematical considerations. Am. J. Physiol. *89*:322, 1929.

Mandel, D.: A Practice of Cardiac Catheterization. Chapter 13. Oxford, Blackwell Scientific Publications, 1968.

Reeves, J. T., Grover, R. F., Filley, G. F., and Blount, S. G., Jr.: Cardiac output in normal resting man. J. Appl. Physiol. *16*:276, 1961.

Samet, P., Bernstein, W. H., and Levine, S.: Transseptal left heart dynamics in 32 normal subjects. Dis. Chest *47*:633, 1965.

Selzer, A., and Sudrann, R. B.: Reliability of the determination of cardiac output in man by means of the Fick principle. Circ. Res. *6*:485, 1958.

Shapiro, G. G., and Kravetz, L. J.: Damped and undamped frequency responses of underdamped catheter manometer systems. Am. Heart J. *80*:226, 1970.

Stewart, G. N.: Researches on the circulation time and on the influences which affect it. J. Physiol. *22*:169, 1887.

Swan, H. J., Marcus, H. S., and Allen, H. N.: Cardiac flow, volumes and pressure. *In* Conn, H. L., and Horwitz, O. (Eds.): Cardiac and Vascular Diseases. Philadelphia, Lea and Febiger, 1971, pp. 54–73.

Swan, H. J. C., Ganz, W., Forrester, J., et al.: Catheterization of the heart in man with the use of a flow-directed balloon-tipped catheter. N. Engl. J. Med. *283*:445, 1970.

Thomassen, B.: Cardiac output in normal subjects under standard basal conditions. The repeatability of measurements by the Fick method. Scand. J. Clin. Lab. Invest. *9*:365, 1957.

Visscher, M. B., and Johnson, J. A.: The Fick principle: analysis of potential errors in its conventional application. J. Appl. Physiol. *5*:635, 1953.

Wade, O. L., and Bishop, J. M.: Cardiac Output and Regional Blood Flow. Philadelphia, F. A. Davis Co., 1962.

Yanof, H. M., Rosen, A. L., McDonald, N. M., and McDonald, D. A.: A critical study of the response of manometers to forced oscillations. Phys. Med. Biol. *8*:407, 1963.

LEFT VENTRICULAR VOLUME, MASS, PUMP FUNCTION, AND MYOCARDIAL PERFORMANCE

Bartle, S. H., and Sanmarco, M. E.: Comparison of angiocardiographic and thermal washout techniques for left ventricular volume measurement. Am. J. Cardiol. *18*:235, 1966.

Borer, J. S., Bacharach, S. L., Green, M. V., et al.: Real time radionuclide cineangiography in the noninvasive evaluation of global and regional left ventricular function at rest and during exercise in patients with coronary artery disease. N. Engl. J. Med. *296*:839, 1977.

Bove, A. A., and Lynch, P. R.: Measurement of canine left ventricular performance by cineradiography of the heart. J. Appl. Physiol. *29*:877, 1970.

Bristow, J. D., Van Zee, B. E., and Judkins, M. P.: Systolic and diastolic abnormalities of the left ventricle in coronary artery disease. Circulation *42*:219, 1970.

Bunnell, I. L., Grant, C., and Greene, D. G.: Left ventricular function derived from the pressure-volume diagram. Am. J. Med. *39*:881, 1965.

Burns, J. W., Covell, J. W., Myers, R., and Ross, J., Jr.: Comparison of directly measured left ventricular wall stress and stress calculated from geometric reference figures. Circ. Res. *28*:611, 1971.

Carabello, B. A., Nolan, S. P., and McGuire, L. B.: Assessments of preoperative left ventricular function in patients with mitral regurgitation; value of the end-systolic wall stress–end-systolic volume ratio. Circulation *64*:1212, 1981.

Davila, J. C., and Sanmarco, M. E.: An analysis of the fit of mathematical models applicable to the measurement of left ventricular volume. Am. J. Cardiol. *18*:31, 1966.

Dodge, H. T.: Determination of left ventricular volume and mass. Radiol. Clin. North Am. *9*:459, 1971.

Dodge, H. T., and Baxley, W. A.: Left ventricular volume and mass and their significance in heart disease. Am. J. Cardiol. *23*:528, 1969.

Dodge, H. T., Hay, R. E., and Sandler, H.: An angiocardiographic method for directly determining left ventricular stroke volume in man. Circ. Res. *11*:739, 1962.

Dodge, H. T., Sandler, H., Ballew, D. W., and Lord, J. D., Jr.: The use of biplane angiocardiography for the measurement of left ventricular volume in man. Am. Heart J. *60*:762, 1960.

Dodge, H. T., Sandler, H., Baxley, W. A., and Hawley, R. R.: Usefulness and limitations of radiographic methods for determining left ventricular volume. Am. J. Cardiol. *18*:10, 1966.

Falsetti, H. J., Mates, R. E., Greene, D. G., and Bunnell, I. L.: V_{max} as an index of contractile state in man. Circulation *43*:323, 1971.

Feigenbaum, H.: Echocardiography. 2nd ed. Philadelphia, Lea and Febiger, 1976.

Gault, J. H., Covell, J. W., Braunwald, E., and Ross, J., Jr.: Left ventricular performance following correction of free aortic regurgitation. Circulation *42*:773, 1970.

Gault, J. H., Ross, J., Jr., and Braunwald, E.: Contractile state of the left ventricle in man. Circ. Res. *22*:451, 1958.

Graham, T. P., Jr., Jarmakani, M. M., Canent, R. V., et al.: Characterization of left heart volumes and mass in normal children and in infants with intrinsic myocardial disease. Circulation *38*:826, 1968.

Graham, T. P., Jr., Jarmakani, M. M., Canent, R. V., Jr., and Morrow, M. N.: Left heart volume estimation in infancy and childhood. Circulation *43*:895, 1971.

Gramiak, R., and Wang, R. C.: Cardiac Ultrasound. St. Louis, C. V. Mosby Co., 1975.

Grant, C., Greene, D. G., and Bunnell, I. L.: Left ventricular enlargement and hypertrophy. Am. J. Med. *39*:895, 1965.

Greene, D. G., Carlisle, R., Grant, C., and Bunnell, I. L.: Estimation of left ventricular volume by one-plane cineangiography. Circulation *35*:61, 1967.

Grossman, W., Braunwald, E., Mann, T., et al.: Contractile state of the left ventricle in man as evaluated from end-systolic pressure-volume relations. Circulation *56*:845, 1977.

Holt, J. P.: Estimation of the residual volume of the ventricle of the dog heart by two indicator dilution techniques. Circ. Res. *4*:187, 1956.

Hood, W. P., Jr., Rackley, C. E., and Rolett, E. L.: Wall stress in the normal and hypertrophied human left ventricle. Am. J. Cardiol. *22*:550, 1968.

Hood, W. P., Jr., Thomson, W. J., Rackley, C. E., and Rolett, E. L.: Comparison of calculations of left ventricular wall stress in man from thin-walled and thick-walled ellipsoidal models. Circ. Res. *24*:575, 1969.

Hugenholtz, P. G., Kaplan, E., and Hull, E.: Determination of left ventricular wall thickness by angiocardiography. Am. Heart J. *78*:513, 1969.

Hugenholtz, P. G., Wagner, H. R., and Sandler, H.: The in-vivo determination of left ventricular volume: comparison of the fiberoptic-indicator dilution and the angiocardiographic methods. Circulation *37*:489, 1968.

Jarmakani, M. M., Graham, T. P., Jr., Canent, R. V., and Capp, M. P.: The effect of corrective surgery on left heart volume and mass in children with ventricular septal defect. Am. J. Cardiol. *27*:254, 1971.

Jarmakani, M. M., Graham, T. P., Jr., Canent, R. V., et al.: Effect of site of shunt on left heart-volume characteristics in children with ventricular septal defect and patent ductus arteriosus. Circulation *40*:411, 1969.

Karliner, J. S., Gault, J. H., Eckberg, D., et al.: Mean velocity of fiber shortening. A simplified measure of left ventricular myocardial contractility. Circulation *44*:323, 1971.

Kasser, I. S., and Kennedy, J. W.: Measurement of left ventricular volumes in man by single plane cineangiocardiography. Invest. Radiol. *4*:83, 1969.

Kennedy, J. W., Baxley, W. A., Figley, M. M., et al.: Quantitative angiocardiography. The normal left ventricle in man. Circulation *34*:272, 1966.

Levine, J. H., McIntyre, K. M., Lipana, J. G., and Bing, O. H. L.: Force velocity relations in failing and nonfailing hearts of subjects with aortic stenosis. Am. J. Med. Sci. *259*:79, 1970.

Mason, D. T., Spann, J. F., Jr., and Zelis, R.: Quantification of the contractile state of the intact left ventricle. Maximal velocity of contractile element shortening determined by the instantaneous relation between the rate of pressure rise and pressure in the left ventricle isovolumic systole. Am. J. Cardiol. *26*:248, 1970.

Mehmel, H. C., Stockins, B., Ruffmann, K., et al.: The linearity of the end-systolic pressure-volume relationship in man and its sensitivity for assessment of left ventricular function. Circulation *63*:1216, 1981.

Mirsky, I.: Left ventricular stresses in the intact human heart. Biophys. J. *9*:189, 1969.

Pouleur, H., Rousseau, M. F., Van Eyll, C., et al.: Assessment of left ventricular contractility from late systolic stress-volume relations. Circulation *65*:1204, 1982.

Rackley, C. E., Dear, H. D., Baxley, W. A., et al.: Left ventricular chamber volume, mass and function in severe coronary artery disease. Circulation *41*:605, 1970.

Rackley, C. E., Dodge, H. T., Coble, Y. D., Jr., and Hay, R. E.: A method for determining left ventricular mass in man. Circulation *29*:666, 1964.

Rapaport, E., Wiegand, B. D., and Bristow, J. D.: Estimation of left ventricular residual volume in the dog by a thermodilution method. Circ. Res. *11*:803, 1962.

Ross, J., Jr., and Sobel, B. E.: Regulation of cardiac contraction. Ann. Rev. Physiol. *34*:47, 1972.

Ross, J., Jr., Sonnenblick, E. H., Taylor, R. R., et al.: Diastolic geometry and sarcomere lengths in the chronically dilated canine left ventricle. Circ. Res. *28*:49, 1971.

Sagawa, K.: Editorial: The end-systolic pressure-volume relation of the ventricle; definition, modifications and clinical use. Circulation *63*:1223, 1981.

Sandler, H., and Dodge, H. T.: Left ventricular tension and stress in man. Circ. Res. *13*:91, 1963.

Sandler, H., and Dodge, H. T.: The use of single plane angiocardiograms for the calculation of left ventricular volume in man. Am. Heart J. *75*:325, 1968.

Sandler, H., Dodge, H. T., Hay, R. E., and Rackley, C. E.: Quantitation of valvular insufficiency in man by angiocardiography. Am. Heart J. *65*:501, 1963.

Schelbert, H. R., Verba, J. W., Johnson, A. D., et al.: Nontraumatic determination of left ventricular ejection fraction by radionuclide angiocardiography. Circulation *51*:902, 1975.

Suga, H. and Sagawa, K.: Instantaneous pressure-volume relationships and their ratio in the excised, supported canine left ventricle. Circ. Res. *35*:117, 1974.

Suga, H., Sagawa, K., and Shoukas, A. A.: Load independence of the instantaneous, pressure-volume ratio of the canine left ventricle and effects of epinephrine and heart rate on the ratio. Circ. Res. *32*:314, 1973.

Swan, H. J. C., and Beck, W.: Ventricular non-mixing as a source of error in the estimation of ventricular volume by the indicator-dilution method. Circ. Res. *8*:989, 1960.

Taylor, R. R., Covell, J. W., and Ross, J., Jr.: Left ventricular function in experimental aorto-caval fistula with circulatory congestion and fluid retention. J. Clin. Invest. *47*:1333, 1968.

Turina, M., Bussmann, W. D., and Krayenbuhl, H. P.: Contractility of the hypertrophied canine heart in chronic volume overload. Cardiovasc. Res. *3*:486, 1969.

Urschel, C. W., Covell, J. W., Sonnenblick, E. H., et al.: Myocardial mechanics in aortic and mitral valvular regurgitation. The concept of instantaneous impedance as a determinant of the performance of the intact heart. J. Clin. Invest. *47*:867, 1968.

HEMODYNAMICS OF HEART FAILURE

Baxley, W. A., Jones, W. B., and Dodge, H. T.: Left ventricular anatomical and functional abnormalities in chronic postinfarction heart failure. Ann. Intern. Med. *74*:499, 1971.

Braunwald, E., Frahm, C. J., and Ross, J., Jr.: Studies on Starling's law of the heart. V. Left ventricular function in man. J. Clin. Invest. *40*:1882, 1961.

Braunwald, E., Ross, J., Jr., and Sonnenblick, E. H.: Mechanism of contraction of the normal and failing heart. N. Engl. J. Med. *277*:794, 853, 910, 962, 1012; 1967.

Chatterjee, K., and Swan, H. J. C.: Vasodilator therapy in acute myocardial infarction. Mod. Concepts Cardiovasc. Dis. *43*:119, 1974.

Cohn, J. N., Khatri, I. M., and Hamosh, P.: Diagnostic and therapeutic value of bedside monitoring of left ventricular pressure. Am. J. Cardiol. *23*:107, 1969.

Cohn, J. W., Mathew, K. J., Franciosa, J. A., and Snow, J. A.: Chronic vasodilator therapy in the management of cardiogenic shock and intractable left ventricular failure. Ann. Int. Med. *81*:777, 1974.

Dodge, H. T., and Baxley, W. A.: Hemodynamic aspects of heart failure. Am. J. Cardiol. *22*:24, 1968.

Patterson, S. W., Piper, H., and Starling, E. H.: The regulation of the heart beat. J. Physiol. *48*:465, 1914.

Rapaport, E., and Scheinman, M.: Rationale and limitations of hemodynamic measurements in patients with acute infarction. Mod. Concepts Cardiovasc. Dis. *38*:55, 1969.

Russell, R. O., Jr., Porter, C. M., Frimer, M., and Dodge, H. T.: Left ventricular power in man. Am. Heart J. *81*:799, 1971.

Russell, R. O., Jr., Rackley, C. E., Pombo, J., et al.: Effects of increasing left ventricular filling pressure in patients with acute myocardial infarction. J. Clin. Invest. *49*:1539, 1970.

Sarnoff, S. J., and Bergland, E.: Ventricular function. I. Starling's law of the heart studied by means of simultaneous right and left ventricular function curves in the dog. Circulation *9*:706, 1954.

ISCHEMIC HEART DISEASE

Barnard, P. M., and Kennedy, J. H.: Postinfarctional ventricular septal defect. Circulation *32*:76, 1965.

Bashour, F. A.: Mitral regurgitation following myocardial infarction. The syndrome of papillary mitral regurgitation. Dis. Chest *48*:113, 1965.

Baxley, W. A., Jones, W. B., and Dodge, H. T.: Left ventricular anatomical and functional abnormalities in chronic postinfarction heart failure. Ann. Intern. Med. *74*:499, 1971.

Bristow, J. D., Bruce, E. V., and Judkins, M. P.: Systolic and diastolic abnormalities of the left ventricle in coronary artery disease. Studies in patients with little or no enlargement of ventricular volume. Circulation *42*:219, 1970.

Burch, G. E., DePasquale, N. P., and Phillips, J. H.: The syndrome of papillary muscle dysfunction. Am. Heart J. *75*:399, 1968.

Daggett, W. M., Burwell, L. R., Lawson, D. W., and Austen, W. G.: Resection of acute ventricular aneurysm and ruptured interventricular septum after myocardial infarction. N. Engl. J. Med. *283*:1507, 1970.

Dumesnil, J. G., Ritman, E. L., Fry, R. L., et al.: Quantitative determinations of regional left ventricular wall dynamics by roentgen videometry. Circulation *50*:700, 1974.

Effler, D. B., Favaloro, R. G., Groves, L. K., and Loop, F. D.: The simple approach to direct coronary artery surgery. J. Thorac. Cardiovasc. Surg. *62*:503, 1971.

Effler, D. B., Groves, L. K., and Favaloro, R.: Surgical repair of ventricularr aneurysm. Dis. Chest *48*:37, 1965.

Falsetti, H. L., Geraci, A. R., Bunnell, I. L., et al.: Function of left ventricle and extent of coronary lesions: failure of correlation in cineangiographic studies. Chest *59*:610, 1971.

Gould, K. L., and Lipscomb, K.: Effects of coronary stenoses on coronary flow reserve and resistance. Am. J. Cardiol. *34*:48, 1974.

Hamilton, G. H., Murray, J. A., and Kennedy, J. W.: Quantitative angiocardiography in ischemic heart disease. The spectrum of abnormal left ventricular function and the role of abnormally contracting segments. Circulation *45*:1065, 1972.

Herman, M. V., Heinle, R. A., Klein, M. D., and Gorlin, R.: Localized disorders in myocardial contraction. N. Engl. J. Med. *277*:222, 1967.

Miller, G. E., Cohn, K. E., Kerth, W. J., et al.: Experimental papillary muscle infarction. J. Thorac. Cardiovasc. Surg. *56*:611, 1968.

Rackley, C. E., Dear, H. D., Baxley, W. A., et al.: Left ventricular chamber volume, mass and function in severe coronary artery disease. Circulation *41*:605, 1970.

Schrinert, G., Falsetti, H. L., Bunnell, I. L., et al.: Excision of akinetic left ventricular wall of intractable heart failure. Ann. Intern. Med. *70*:437, 1969.

Selzer, A., Gerbode, F., and Kerth, W. J. Clinical hemodynamic and surgical considerations of rupture of the ventricular septum after myocardial infarction. Am. Heart J. 78:598, 1969.

Sharma, B., Goodwin, J. F., Raphael, M. J., et al.: Left ventricular angiography on exercise. A new method of assessing left ventricular function in ischemic heart disease. Br. Heart J. 38:49, 1976.

Stewart, D. K., Dodge, H. T., and Frimer, M.: Quantitative analysis of regional myocardial performance in coronary heart disease. In Cardiovascular Imaging and Image Processing: Theory and Practice, 1975. Society of Photo-optical Instrument Engineers, Bellingham, Washington, 72:217, 1976.

Stinson, E. B., Becker, J., and Shumway, N. E.: Successful repair of postinfarction ventricular septal defect and biventricular aneurysm. J. Thorac. Cardiovasc. Surg. 58:20, 1969.

Swithinbank, J. M.: Perforation of the interventricular septum in myocardial infarction. Br. Heart J. 21:562, 1959.

MITRAL VALVE DISEASE

Arvidsson, H.: Angiocardiographic observations in mitral valve disease, with special reference to the volume variations in the left atrium. Acta Radiol., suppl. 158, p. 1, 1958.

Blackmon, J. R., Rowell, L. B., Kennedy, J. W., et al.: Physiologic significance of maximal oxygen intake in "pure" mitral stenosis. Circulation 36:497, 1967.

Braunwald, E.: Mitral regurgitation: physiological, clinical and surgical considerations. N. Engl. J. Med. 281:425, 1969.

Braunwald, E., and Awe, W. C.: Syndrome of severe mitral regurgitation and normal left atrial pressure. Circulation 27:29, 1963.

Braunwald, E., Braunwald, N. S., Ross, J., Jr., and Morrow, A. G.: Effects of mitral valve replacement on the pulmonary vascular dynamics of patients with pulmonary hypertension. N. Engl. J. Med. 273:509, 1965.

Dalen, J. E., Matloff, J. M., Evans, G. L., et al.: Early reduction in pulmonary vascular resistance after mitral valve replacement. N. Engl. J. Med. 227:387, 1967.

DeSanctis, R. W., Dean, D. C., and Bland, E. F.: Extreme left atrial enlargement. Circulation 29:14, 1964.

Ellis, L. B., and Harken, D. E.: Closed valvuloplasty for mitral stenosis. N. Engl. J. Med. 270:643, 1964.

Friedberg, C. K.: Diseases of the Heart. 3rd ed., Chapter 27. Philadelphia, W. B. Saunders Co., 1966.

Friedman, W. F., and Braunwald, E.: Alterations in regional pulmonary blood flow in mitral valve disease studies by radioisotope scanning. Circulation 24:363, 1966.

Gerami, S., Messmer, B. J., Hallman, G. L., and Cooley, D. A.: Open mitral commissurotomy, results of 100 conservative cases. J. Thorac. Cardiovasc. Surg. 62:366, 1971.

Hawley, R. R., Dodge, H. T., and Graham, T. P.: Left atrial volume and volume changes in heart disease. Circulation 34:989, 1966.

Hessel, E. A., Kennedy, J. W., and Merendino, K. A.: A reappraisal of nonprosthetic reconstructive surgery for mitral regurgitation based on an analysis of early and late results. J. Thorac. Cardiovasc. Surg. 52:193, 1966.

Kennedy, J. W., Yarnall, S. R., Murray, J. A., and Figley, M. M.: Quantitative angiocardiography: IV. Relationships of left atrial and ventricular pressure and volume in mitral valve disease. Circulation 41:817, 1970.

Manhas, D. R., Hessel, E. A., Winterscheid, L. C., et al.: Repair of mitral incompetence secondary to ruptured chordae tendineae. Circulation 43:688, 1971.

Merendino, K. A., Thomas, G. I., Jesseph, J. E., et al.: The open correction of rheumatic mitral regurgitation and/or stenosis: with special reference to regurgitation treated by posteromedial annuloplasty utilizing a pump oxygenator. Ann. Surg. 150:5, 1959.

Oleson, K. H.: The natural history of 271 patients with mitral stenosis under medical treatment. Br. Heart J. 27:349, 1962.

Osmundson, P. J., Callahan, J. A., and Edward, J. E.: Ruptured mitral chordae tendineae. Circulation 23:42, 1961.

Roberts, W. C., Braunwald, E., and Morrow, A. G.: Acute severe mitral regurgitation secondary to ruptured chordae tendin-

eae: clinical, hemodynamic and pathologic considerations. Circulation 33:58, 1966.

Row, J. C., Bland, E. F., Sprague, H. B., and White, P. D.: The course of mitral stenosis without surgery. Ann. Intern. Med. 52:741, 1960.

Sanders, C. A., Armstrong, P. W., Willerson, J. T., and Dinsmore, R. E.: Etiology and differential diagnosis of acute mitral regurgitation. Prog. Cardiovasc. Dis. 14:129, 1971.

Sanders, C. A., Scannell, J. G., Hawthorne, J. W., and Austen, W. G.: Severe mitral regurgitation secondary to ruptured chordae tendineae. Circulation 31:506, 1965.

AORTIC VALVE DISEASE

Anderson, F. L., Tsagaris, T. J., Tikoff, G., et al.: Hemodynamic effects of exercise in patients with aortic stenosis. Am. J. Med. 46:872, 1969.

Angell, W. W., Stenson, E. B., Ibur, A. B., and Shumway, W. E.: Multiple valve replacement with fresh aortic homograft. J. Thorac. Cardiovasc. Surg. 56:323, 1968.

Barratt-Boyes, B. G., and Roche, A. H. G.: A review of aortic valve homografts over a six and one-half year period. Ann. Surg. 170:483, 1969.

Duvoisin, G. E., Wallace, R. B., Ellis, F. H., et al.: Late result of cardiac valve replacement. Circulation (suppl. 2) 37–38: 1175, 1968.

Glancy, D. L., and Epstein, S. E.: Differential diagnosis of type and severity of obstruction to left ventricular outflow. Prog. Cardiovasc. Dis. 14:153, 1971.

Judge, T. P., Kennedy, J. W., Bennett, L. J., et al.: The quantitative hemodynamic effects of heart rate in aortic regurgitation. Circulation 44:355, 1971.

Kennedy, J. W., Twiss, R. D., Blackmon, J. R., and Dodge, H. T.: Quantitative angiocardiography. III. Relationships of left ventricular pressure, volume and mass in aortic valve disease. Circulation 38:838, 1968.

Morrow, A. G., Roberts, W. C., Ross, J., et al.: Obstruction to left ventricular outflow. NIH Clinical Staff Conference. Ann. Intern. Med. 69:1285, 1968.

Najafi, H.: Aortic insufficiency. Clinical manifestations and surgical treatment. Am. Heart J. 82:120, 1971.

Roberts, W. C.: The structure of the aortic valve in clinically isolated aortic stenosis. Circulation 42:91, 1970.

Rotman, M., Morris, J. J., Behar, V. S., et al.: Aortic valve disease—comparison of types and their medical and surgical management. Am. J. Med. 51:241, 1971.

Segal, J., Harvey, W. P., and Hufnagel, C.: A clinical study of 100 cases of severe aortic insufficiency. Am. J. Med. 21:200, 1956.

Shean, F. C., Austen, W. G., Buckley, M. J., et al.: Survival after Starr-Edwards aortic valve replacement. Circulation 44:1, 1971.

Spangnuolo, M., Kloth, H., Taranta, D., et al.: Natural history of rheumatic aortic regurgitation: criteria predictive of death, congestive heart failure and angina in young patients. Circulation 44:368, 1971.

Wagner, H. R., Hugenhaltz, P. G., and Sandler, H.: Congenital aortic stenosis, compensating mechanisms in pure pressure overload. Circulation (suppl. 6) 37–38:199, 1968.

THE CARDIOMYOPATHIES

Ablemann, W. H.: Experimental infection with Trypanosoma cruzi (Chagas' disease). A model of acute and chronic myocardiopathy. Ann. N. Y. Acad. Sci. 153:137, 1969.

Adalman, A. G., McLoughlin, M. J., Merquis, Y., et al.: Left ventricular cineangiographic observations in muscular subaortic stenosis. Am. J. Cardiol. 24:689, 1969.

Akbarian, M., Yankopoulos, N. A., and Abelmann, W. H.: Hemodynamic studies in beriberi heart disease. Am. J. Med. 41:197, 1966.

Alexander, C. S.: Idiopathic heart disease. I. Analysis of 100 cases with special reference to chronic alcoholism. Am. J. Med. 41:213, 1966.

Alexander, C. S.: Idiopathic heart disease. II. Electron microscopic examination of myocardial biopsy specimens in alcoholic heart disease. Am. J. Med. 41:229, 1966.

Bashour, F. A., McConnell, T., Skinner, W., and Hanson, M.: Myocardial sarcoidosis. Dis. Chest 53:413, 1968.

Braunwald, E., Lambrew, C.T., Rockoff, S. D., et al.: Idiopathic hypertrophic subaortic stenosis. I. A description of the disease based upon an analysis of 64 patients. Circulation *30*:3, 119; 1964.

Burch, G. E., and DePasquale, N.: Alcoholic cardiomyopathy. A review. Am. J. Cardiol. *23*:723, 1969.

Burch, G. E., and Giles, T. D.: Alcoholic cardiomyopathy. Concept of the disease and its treatment. Am. J. Med. *50*:141, 1971.

Chambers, R. J., Beck, W., and Schrire, V.: Ventricular dynamics in Bantu cardiomyopathy. Am. Heart J. *78*:493, 1969.

Fowler, N. O.: Differential diagnosis of cardiomyopathies. Progr. Cardiovasc. Dis. *14*:133, 1971.

Frank, S., and Braunwald, E.: Idiopathic hypertrophic subaortic stenosis. Clinical analysis of 126 patients with emphasis on natural history. Circulation *37*:759, 1968.

Goodwin, J. F.: Congestive and hypertrophic cardiomyopathies. Lancet *1*:731, 1970.

Hamby, R. I.: Primary myocardial disease. A prospective clinical and hemodynamic evaluation in 100 patients. Medicine *49*:55, 1970.

James, T. N.: Observations on the cardiovascular involvement including the cardiac conduction system in progressive muscular dystrophy. Am. Heart J. *63*:48, 1962.

Lerner, A. M.: Virus myopericarditis. Ann. Intern. Med. *59*:1068, 1968.

Mattingly, T. W.: The clinical and hemodynamic features of primary myocardial disease. Trans. Am. Clin. Climat. Assoc. *70*:132, 1958.

Mitchell, J. A., and Cohen, L. S.: Alcohol and the heart. Current Concepts Cardiov. Dis. *39*:109, 1970.

Perloff, J. K., deLeon, A. C., Jr., and O'Doherty, D.: The cardiomyopathy of progressive muscular dystrophy. Circulation *33*:625, 1966.

Perloff, J. K., Lindgren, K. M., and Groves, B. M.: Uncommon or commonly unrecognized causes of heart failure. Progr. Cardiovasc. Dis. *12*:409, 1970.

Popp, R. L., and Harrison, D. C.: Ultrasound in the diagnosis and evaluation of therapy of idiopathic hypertrophic subaortic stenosis. Circulation *40*:905, 1969.

Shaw, P. M., Gramiak, R., Kramer, D. H., and Yu, P. N.: Determinants of atrial and ventricular gallop sounds in primary myocardial disease. N. Engl. J. Med. *278*:753, 1968.

Wagner, P.: Beriberi heart disease. Physiologic data and difficulties in diagnosis. Am. Heart J. *69*:200, 1965.

PERICARDIAL DISEASE

Berglund, E., Sarnoff, S. J., and Isaacs, J. P.: Ventricular function: role of the pericardium in regulation of cardiovascular hemodynamics. Circ. Res. *3*:133, 1955.

Bradley, E. C.: Acute benign pericarditis. Am. Heart J. *67*:121, 1964.

Capps, J. A.: Pain from the pleura and pericardium. J. Nerv. Ment. Dis. *23*:263, 1943.

Conn, H. L., Jr., and Horwitz, O. (Eds.): Cardiac and Vascular Diseases. Philadelphia, Lea and Febiger, 1971, p. 1326.

Cooley, J. C., Clagett, O. T., and Kirklin, J. W.: Surgical aspects of chronic constrictive pericarditis. A review of 72 operative cases. Ann. Surg. *147*:488, 1958.

Dalton, J. C., Pearson, R. J., and White, P. D.: Constrictive pericarditis. A review and long-term follow-up of 78 cases. Ann. Intern. Med. *45*:445, 1956.

Dressler, W.: The post-myocardial infarction syndrome. Arch. Intern. Med. *103*:28, 1959.

Drusin, L. M.: Post-pericardiotomy syndrome: a six year epidemiologic study. N. Engl. J. Med. *272*:597, 1965.

Effler, D. B.: Chronic constrictive pericarditis treated with pericardiectomy. Am. J. Cardiol. *7*:62, 1961.

Engle, M. A., and Ito, T.: The postpericardiotomy syndrome. Am. J. Cardiol. *7*:73, 1961.

Gimlette, T. M. D.: Constrictive pericarditis. Br. Heart J. *21*:9, 1959.

Guntheroth, W. G., Morgan, B. C., and Mullins, G. H.: Effect of respiration on venous return and stroke volume in cardiac tamponade. Circ. Res. *20*:381, 1967.

Harrison, E. C., Crawford, D. W., and Lau, F. Y. K.: Sequential left ventricular function studies before and after pericardiectomy for constrictive pericarditis. Am. J. Cardiol. *26*:319, 1970.

Harvey, W. P.: Auscultatory findings in disease of the pericardium. Am. J. Cardiol. *7*:15, 1961.

Hurst, J. W., Logue, R. B., Rackley, C. E., Schlant, R. C., Sonnenblick, E. H., Wallace, A. G., and Wenger, N. K. (Eds.): The Heart, Arteries and Veins. 5th ed. New York, McGraw-Hill Book Co., 1982.

McKusich, V. A.: Chronic constrictive pericarditis. Some clinical and laboratory observations. Bull. Johns Hopkins Hosp. *90*:3, 1952.

Portal, R. W., Besterman, E. M. M., Chambers, R. J., et al.: Prognosis after operation for constrictive pericarditis. Br. Med. J. *1*:563, 1966.

Shobetai, R., Fowler, N. O., Fenton, J. C., and Masangkay, M.: Pulsus paradoxus. J. Clin. Invest. *44*:1882, 1965.

Weissbein, A., and Heller, F. N.: A method of treatment for pericardial pain. Circulation *24*:607, 1961.

Wood, P.: Chronic constrictive pericarditis. Am. J. Cardiol. *7*:48, 1961.

Yu, P. N. G., Lovejoy, F. W., Jr., Joos, H. A., et al.: Right auricular and ventricular pressure patterns in constrictive pericarditis. Circulation *7*:102, 1953.

10 Congestive Heart Failure

H. J. C. Swan and William W. Parmley

INTRODUCTION

The general term *congestive heart failure* is used to designate a common series of syndromes seen in the clinical practice of medicine. These syndromes consist of the symptoms and physical signs associated with (1) failure of the left ventricle as a pump, (2) failure of the right ventricle as a pump, (3) pulmonary venous hypertension, and (4) systemic venous hypertension. Although these factors may be present alone or in combination in a given patient and are frequently interrelated from the standpoint of mechanism, it is relevant to separate the general mechanics and consequences of failure of the left ventricle as a pump from those of failure of the right ventricle as a pump. For example, the usual consequences of failure of the left ventricle as a pump are an increase in pulmonary venous pressure with the associated symptoms of dyspnea and the findings of rales in the lung fields or of pleural effusion. However, pulmonary congestion and edema may also be a consequence of alteration of pulmonary capillary permeability by the direct effects of toxic gases or of central nervous system damage. The symptoms associated with failure of the right ventricle usually include ankle edema, abdominal swelling, and right subcostal pain, which may be accompanied by peripheral edema, an enlarged liver, ascites, and increased jugular venous pulsation and pressure. Systemic venous congestion with the symptoms and signs of right heart failure may be due to failure of the right ventricle associated with chronic obstructive lung disease in association with normal left ventricular function or indeed might occur in the absence of primary disease of the heart itself as a consequence of primary pericardial disease with or without effusion.

DEFINITION OF HEART FAILURE

Perhaps it is appropriate to consider initially a rather broad physiologic definition of heart failure rather than the more specific clinical syndromes. Warren and Stead indicated that heart failure is that state that results from the inability of the heart to pump sufficient blood to the body tissues to meet ordinary metabolic demands. Indeed, when the heart is unable to meet the normal resting metabolic needs of the body tissues, ventricular stroke volume is usually profoundly decreased. Minor or moderate depressions of ventricular performance do not usually result in this

alteration because compensating mechanisms become operative. One of the primary compensatory mechanisms available to the body to improve cardiac performance is to increase the heart rate and thus the frequency of emptying of the left ventricle. In the majority of mammalian species in which cardiac output increases under conditions of increased demand, the principal mechanism operates by increasing heart rate with a relatively unchanged level of stroke volume.

Using the current convention for the expression of flow values in the cardiovascular system in terms of body surface area (BSA), one finds that the normal stroke volume in a younger subject averages approximately 60 ml per beat per M^2. At a rate of 60 beats per minute, this results in a cardiac output of 3.6 L per minute per M^2, and during severe exercise at a heart rate of 180 beats per minute, a cardiac index of 10.8 L per minute per M^2 may be achieved in the absence of any changes in stroke volume. Although small changes in stroke volume do occur, this is a secondary mechanism in the control of cardiac output. In patients with seriously reduced cardiac performance, one of the principal hemodynamic alterations is that the left ventricle may eject as little as 20 ml per beat per M^2, or one third of normal stroke volume. However, a sinus tachycardia at a rate of 120 beats per minute will result in a cardiac index of 2.4 L per minute per M^2, which usually is adequate to meet resting metabolic needs.

In addition, partly as a consequence of the reduction in total cardiac output and the associated reduction of renal blood flow, the circulating blood volume increases. This, along with other factors, results in an enhanced filling pressure in the chambers of both right and left ventricles, the "preload reserve." An increased filling pressure results in a larger end-diastolic volume with a greater degree of fiber stretch. Thus, the performance of the heart may be enhanced secondarily for any given level of intrinsic contractile state by a greater fiber stretch—an additional mechanism to improve the function of the heart as a pump. However, as a consequence of the increased left ventricular diastolic pressure, there is increased pressure upstream in the left atrium and therefore in the pulmonary veins and capillaries that is transmitted into the pulmonary arteries. This results in an increase in pulmonary artery systolic, mean, and diastolic pressures. Hence, the right ventricle must do more work and progressively encounters greater difficulty in overcoming its outflow resistance, and a similar process of failure affects the right ventricle with the manifestations of systemic venous congestion. As a result, the common sequence of clinical congestive heart failure is a reduced left ventricular stroke volume accompanied by tachycardia and an increased left ventricular filling pressure, which tend partly to restore cardiac output and hence tissue perfusion but with an increase in myocardial oxygen needs, which are a direct function of both heart rate and left ventricular filling pressure (preload).

However, an important penalty for this compensation is the congestive changes in the lungs with increases in pulmonary arterial pressure and increased systemic venous pressure with congestive changes and edema. As a further generalization, it should be recognized that neither ventricle of the heart in the nonhypertrophied state is able to sustain significant acute increases in afterload.

NORMAL CARDIAC PERFORMANCE

It is necessary to review briefly certain characteristics of cardiac performance in the normal heart for a comparative background. During ventricular contraction, in association with shortening of the myocardial sarcomere, the volume and the shape of both ventricles alter. The principal shortening occurs in the free wall of each cardiac chamber, with lesser degrees of shortening occurring in the ventricular septum and in the base-to-apex dimension. The right and left ventricles differ in their geometric contraction characteristics. The right ventricle ejects its content by approximating the free wall to the right ventricular aspect of the ventricular septum. In contrast, the thicker-walled left ventricle contracts in a more circumferential manner, changing from an ellipsoid configuration during diastole to a narrow truncated cone during systole. This change in ventricular volumes between systole and diastole is the process by means of which blood is expelled from the ventricle. Since ventricular volumes are frequently dramatically altered in patients with heart failure, quantitative emphasis will be placed on the consideration of ventricular volumes and their change. Data pertaining to the accompaniments of normal cardiac function are included in Table 10–1.

LEFT VENTRICULAR EJECTION

The following pertains to the ejection characteristics of the left ventricle. The normal left ventricle has a volume of approximately 90 ml per M^2 at end diastole (EDV). During contraction it ejects approximately two thirds of its content, or 60 ml per M^2, into the aorta—the stroke volume (SV)—and at end systole it contains a residual volume of 30 ml per M^2 (ESV). As a convenient measure of the pumping function of the left ventricle, the ratio of ejected or stroke volume to the

TABLE 10–1 NORMAL VALUES FOR CARDIAC PERFORMANCE AT REST

Cardiac index (L/min/M^2)	3.6
Heart rate (beats/min)	60-90
Stroke index (ml/M^2)	60
Stroke work index (gm-meters/M^2)	60
End-diastolic volume (ml/M^2)	90
End-systolic volume (ml/M^2)	30
Ejection fraction	0.67
LV end-diastolic pressure (mm Hg)	<12
LV max dp/dt (mm Hg/sec)	1500
Segmental wall motion (% inward movement)	
Apical	30%
Anterior	50%
Inferior	40%

end-diastolic volume—the ejection fraction (EF)—may be readily calculated: EF = SV/EDV. Utilizing the foregoing data, the normal ejection fraction is approximately 0.66 and may vary from 0.60 to approximately 0.78. Deviations outside this range usually are abnormal. Note that this expression (EF) of ventricular performance will take into account abnormal valve leakage as well as the magnitude of forward blood flow. Thus, it is possible to describe the performance of the ventricle in patients with valvar incompetence in terms of the magnitude and proportion of volume ejected during ventricular contraction. Since EDV − ESV = total volume ejected, regurgitant volume (RV) is equal to (EDV − ESV) − SV, where SV = forward stroke volume.

The ejection fraction must not be confused with measures of the contractile state of the myocardium. Although it is possible to determine the instantaneous rate of volume change and thus arrive at an interpretation of ventricular function more closely related to the rate of sarcomere shortening, the ejection fraction accounts only for the ability of the heart to discharge its contents without relation to the time course or energetics of that process. The ejection fraction is one practically useful measure of pump function in the description of the heart in normal and abnormal states. Although the contractile state is usually depressed when the EF is reduced, normal values for EF may be found in the presence of a reduced contractile state, particularly when afterload falls.

VENTRICULAR CONTRACTION PATTERNS

Contraction of the ventricular wall is essentially a uniform process in the normal heart. The different elements and regions of the ventricular wall are displaced over a basically similar time course, occurring together for practical purposes over the whole mass of ventricular muscle. Normal end-systolic contraction, expressed as 1 minus the ratio of the end-systolic diameter to end-diastolic diameter for anterior, inferior, and apical segments, is given in Table 10–1. In the presence of certain abnormalities of intraventricular conduction, myocardial disease, or sequential underperfusion of the ventricle, this synchronous contraction may not be maintained. Under such circumstances, specific elements of the myocardium may contract at a time later than the normally contracting myocardium, may not contract at all, and, under certain circumstances, may actually bulge or paradox during contraction of the remainder of the ventricle (Fig. 10–1). Each of these abnormalities of ventricular wall motion is mechanically inefficient and metabolically costly to the ventricle.

In addition to the process of contraction, the cardiac ventricles also are subjected to geometric changes associated with ventricular filling. Following ventricular systole, the sarcomeres of the myocardium lengthen to their resting position, thus markedly reducing the tension in the myocardial wall. This reduction in tension immediately results in passive changes in the internal dimensions of the ventricular cavity, particularly associated with the tendency of connective tissue and supportive elements to return to a position of least energy. This may result in diastolic suction when, following relaxation of the contractile elements, the heart develops a negative intracavity pressure and tends to "suck" blood into its cavity.

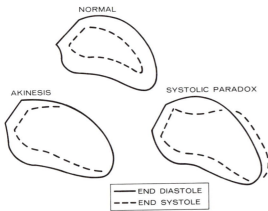

Figure 10–1 Normal and abnormal ventricular contraction patterns. The ventricular contours are shown as they might appear in a cineangiogram obtained in the right anterior-oblique projection. The solid line indicates the contour of the ventricular chamber at end diastole, and the dotted line indicates the position of the ventricular wall at the end systole. Normally, the inward movement of the ventricular wall is uniform, involving all portions of the ventricle to approximately the same degree. In patients with diffuse cardiac disease, there is failure of contraction in all dimensions. In patients with localized cardiac disease, as shown in the two lower figures, there may be failure of movement of the affected portion of the ventricular wall, which is either scarred or stiffened (left). In certain instances the affected area may actually bulge during systole (right), providing not only a failure of contribution to contraction but also a fundamental mechanical disadvantage.

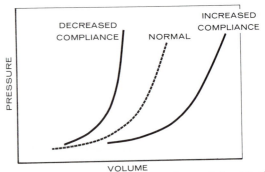

Figure 10–2 Passive pressure-volume relationship of the ventricles. The dotted line in the center indicates the general relationship between pressure and volume. As volume is increased initially, there is only a small rise in pressure. As volume increase continues, the rise in pressure is greater. Each of the solid lines indicates the alteration in pressure-volume relationships in decreased compliance (left) and increased compliance (right). This can be considered as a greater or lesser degree of stiffness of the ventricle in relation to the filling volume. Ventricular compliance is a dynamic phenomenon, and this property can change rapidly.

However, this mechanism plays a small part in filling of the ventricles, which is accomplished from the atria and great veins by reason of a slightly positive pressure within the vascular system relative to that external to the ventricle. The passive pressure-volume curve—representative of ventricular compliance—is concave to its pressure axis, so that blood is accepted in relatively large volumes from a low end-systolic volume, with very little change in filling pressure (Fig. 10–2). However, if filling is prolonged, the pressure will rise at an increasingly rapid level as the stiffer part of the ventricular pressure-volume curve is reached. Little attention has been paid to the passive pressure-volume relationships of the ventricle, yet they are all important in the concepts of heart failure. In normal human cardiac dynamics, the end-systolic volume of 30 ml per M^2 is achieved at a filling pressure of between 0 and 3 mm Hg. Addition of 60 ml per M^2 (equivalent to the succeeding stroke volume) results in an increase in intraventricular pressure to between 8 and 12 mm Hg at end diastole.

Thus, it is possible to describe the complete cardiac cycle in volumetric and pressure terms (Fig. 10–3). If we commence our consideration at the beginning of systole with an end-diastolic pressure of 12 mm Hg and an end-diastolic volume of 90 ml per M^2, the intramyocardial tension rapidly increases until the intraventricular pressure equals that in the aortic root. No net volume change occurs, although a slight distortion of the ventricular wall accompanies the movement of the mitral valve leaflets posterior into the left atrium. When the pressure in the ventricle reaches and exceeds that in the aortic root, ejection commences. In the normal heart, between one half and two

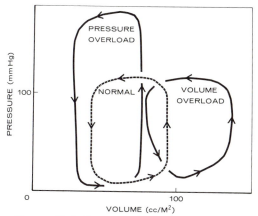

Figure 10–3 Pressure-volume relationships for the normal and abnormal ventricle. The dotted line indicates the normal pressure-volume loop (see text for details). With pressure overload and concentric hypertrophy there may be a reduction in end-diastolic volume. However, greater work is performed in the generation of pressure for ejection of blood from the ventricle. In the presence of volume overload, there is an increase in all dimensions of the ventricle, so that the end-diastolic volume is substantially increased. The volume ejected is also increased, and the end-systolic volume is greater than normal in proportion to the magnitude of volume overload and the degree of compensation of the ventricle.

thirds of the stroke volume is discharged from the ventricle during the first third of systole, whereas the flow into the aorta during the last third of systole is between 10 and 20 per cent of the total. The rates of change of dimension and volume follow a similar time course. For this reason, the normal heart has considerable adaptability at high heart rates, and even with considerable shortening of the duration of ventricular systole is still able to eject a great part of its content. However, when failure of the heart as a pump supervenes, the proportionate ejection of blood from the ventricle is more evenly distributed across the duration of ventricular systole, and the reserve capabilities of the ventricle are thus curtailed.

At the end of ventricular systole, the volume content of the ventricle has been reduced by the stroke volume and has returned to its end-systolic volume of 30 ml per M^2. Following reduction of intramyocardial tension as a result of sarcomere relaxation, the pressure in the ventricle drops to between 0 and 3 mm Hg. At this point, the pressure in the atrium is sufficient to open the atrioventricular valve and allow for the maximal rate of filling of the ventricle, which in the normal heart follows a time course that is similar to that of systole. Thus, approximately half of ventricular filling occurs in the first third of ventricular diastole, with a barely measurable increase in intraventricular pressure. The volume rate of filling of the ventricle is progressively reduced as ventricular pressure rises according to the passive compliance characteristics of the myocardial wall until

end diastole, at which time atrial contraction adds a final increment of stroke volume to the ventricle. When atrial contraction has been completed and the atrioventricular valves have commenced to float into their presystolic position, ventricular systole commences, and the cycle is repeated. The contraction pattern of the free wall of the ventricle is fundamentally uniform, with the greatest degree of shortening in the free wall and the least degree of shortening in the long axis and septal dimensions.

In addition, mechanisms of fundamental importance in the control and modification of normal or abnormal cardiac function include the tripartite relation between function and contractile state and presystolic fiber length—the Frank-Starling relationship (Fig. 10–4). The importance of these factors in the normal heart has already received consideration and will be discussed only in the context of heart failure per se. However, a central theme of critical importance in heart failure is a consideration of the factors that control myocardial oxygen consumption.

MYOCARDIAL OXYGEN CONSUMPTION

Since the report of Evans and Matsuoka in 1915, it has been generally appreciated that myocardial oxygen uptake is directly related to mean arterial pressure but is affected much less by changes in cardiac output. This generalization that pressure-work is much more costly than flow-work has been the framework upon which most of the subsequent studies of oxygen consumption have been performed. Furthermore, this concept has

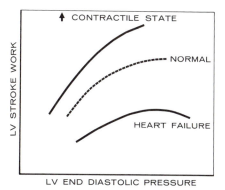

Figure 10–4 The relationship between left ventricular performance and left ventricular filling pressure (Frank-Starling relationship). Normally, an increased end-diastolic pressure is accompanied by a substantive increase in performance (dotted line). In the presence of an enhanced contractile state in the same heart, the levels of performance are proportionately greater. In the presence of heart failure, the performance is less, and when a critical level of diastolic pressure is reached, further increments of pressure are associated with a small reduction in performance.

TABLE 10–2 MYOCARDIAL OXYGEN CONSUMPTION

Major Determinants
    Heart rate
    Tension development
    Contractile state
    Basal
Minor Determinants
    Activation
    Depolarization
    Direct metabolic effect of catecholamines

direct relevance to the pathophysiology of congestive heart failure and its effective therapy.

Fundamental studies in recent years by Sarnoff, Sonnenblick, Braunwald and associates have greatly enhanced our appreciation of the quantitative aspects of myocardial oxygen consumption. The important determinants of myocardial oxygen consumption are listed in Table 10–2 and are divided for convenience into those of major and minor importance. The subsequent discussion will focus on the relative importance of each of these determinants. The oxygen consumption of the beating heart ranges from about 8 to 15 ml per minute per 100 gm myocardium, whereas the oxygen consumption of the noncontracting heart is approximately 2 ml per minute per 100 gm. Thus, the basal requirements for oxygen are approximately 20 per cent of the total needs and are required for the normal metabolic processes in the myocardium that are not associated with contraction.

TENSION-TIME INDEX

The initial observations that pressure-work was a major determinant of oxygen consumption were extended by Sarnoff and associates, who demonstrated under carefully controlled conditions in the dog that there was a close relationship between the product of developed intraventricular pressure and the time for which it was maintained and the measured myocardial oxygen consumption. This concept of a "tension-time index" has been of fundamental importance in relating the alterations in oxygen consumption that occur with changes in intraventricular pressure. Subsequently, the importance of wall tension rather than intraventricular pressure was emphasized. Since wall tension, according to Laplace's law, is a direct function of the radius and intraventricular pressure, wall tension will be increased at the same intraventricular pressure if the heart dilates. Thus, in the enlarged failing heart, wall tension will be increased and myocardial oxygen consumption augmented, although there may be no change in ventricular pressure (Fig. 10–5). This fact further emphasizes the therapeutic importance of reducing the size of the failing heart. This may be accomplished by a reduction of circulating blood volume with diuretics; by increasing venous capacitance with venodilators, which redistributes blood away from the chest; or by inotropic stimulation as with digitalis, which can empty the ventricle more effectively and thus reduce the intraventricular volume.

Despite the obvious importance of the tension-time index as a determinant of myocardial oxygen consumption, it was observed in conscious dogs that myocardial oxygen consumption correlated poorly with the tension-time index during exercise or sympathetic stimulation. Similarly, the administration of inotropic agents, such as isoproterenol, often produced little change or even a decrease in the tension-time index, whereas oxygen consumption was greatly augmented. In a series of studies by Sonnenblick and associates, it became apparent that the velocity of contraction of the myocardium (as an index of the contractile state of the heart) was also a major determinant of myocardial oxygen consumption. Thus, when the tension-time index was maintained relatively constant, oxygen consumption was greatly augmented by changes in contractile state produced by paired electrical stimulation, norepinephrine, or an increase in calcium concentration. At the present time, therefore, it appears that any intervention that increases the contractility of the myocardium will also increase myocardial oxygen consumption.

The minor determinants of myocardial oxygen consumption listed in Table 10–2 are of much less importance. For example, it has been estimated that the depolarization process requires only about 0.04 ml oxygen per minute per 100 gm when the heart is stimulated at a frequency of approxi-

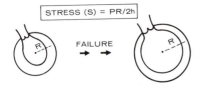

STRESS (S) = PR/2h

FAILURE →→

VENTRICULAR PRESSURE, —————— P : SAME
RADIUS, ———————————— R : INCREASED
WALL THICKNESS, ——————— h : SAME OR DECREASED
WALL STRESS, —————————— S : INCREASED
MYOCARDIAL O₂ CONSUMPTION, MVO₂ : INCREASED

Figure 10–5 Relation of cardiac size to wall stress and to myocardial oxygen consumption. In heart failure, the end-diastolic volume (related to radius) is increased. Even when the wall thickness and internal pressure remain unchanged, the wall stress is increased in accordance with Laplace's law. Hence, the myocardial oxygen consumption is increased.

mately 100 beats per minute. This amounts to approximately 0.5 per cent of the total oxygen consumed by the normal working heart. The direct metabolic effect of catecholamines on the nonbeating heart was determined by administering isoproterenol to the arrested canine heart. The subsequent increase in basal oxygen consumption was relatively minor, on the order of 5 to 10 per cent of that occurring when the same hearts were contracting.

PERFORMANCE OF THE HEART AS A PUMP AND AS A MUSCLE

The performance of the heart *as a pump* is usually designated in terms of pressure and flow. Since the performance of the heart *as a muscle* is generally designated in terms of shortening and wall stress, the relationship between intraventricular pressure and wall stress is of importance. This material is considered extensively in Chapter 9, and the following comments are intended to be used in conjunction with material from that chapter.

VENTRICULAR HYPERTROPHY

Laplace's law is fundamental to the understanding of the pathophysiology of various forms of heart disease. For example, when a heart undergoes hypertrophy secondary to arterial hypertension, the necessity to produce an increased intraventricular pressure is met by thickening of the wall. From Laplace's law, it should be noted that if intraventricular pressure and wall thickness increase proportionately (at a constant radius), wall stress will tend to remain the same. It has been noted in some experimental models of hypertrophy, however, that hypertrophied muscle may actually generate less force per cross-sectional area than normal muscle. If this is the case, wall thickness must increase proportionately more than intraventricular pressure in order to generate the appropriate pressure.

Laplace's law also offers some explanation as to why the left ventricle may hypertrophy, although there is no increase in arterial pressure. When heart failure and cardiac dilatation occur, there is increased wall stress in the free wall of the left ventricle, although there may be no change in intraventricular pressure. This increase in both diastolic and systolic wall stress serves as a stimulus to hypertrophy, without an increase in arterial systolic pressure. Another mandatory consequence of cardiac dilatation is an increase in myocardial oxygen needs. Additionally, there may be nonreversible structural changes in chronic dilatation (e.g., fiber slippage, increased connective tissue content, etc.) that explain the failure of the heart to return to its original size after the causative factors are removed.

For example, in patients with aortic insufficiency who undergo aortic valve replacement, those patients whose hearts return toward normal size also have an improvement in cardiac function, whereas those patients whose hearts remain enlarged (presumably because of irreversible structural changes) have little improvement in cardiac function. Although heart size may increase to enormous proportions following dilatation, there is no concomitant increase in sarcomere length. Instead, sarcomere lengths tend to remain close to their optimal length of 2.2 μ. This presumably can occur both because of the addition of sarcomeres in series and because of fiber slippage, which allows the heart to expand considerably but keeps sarcomeres at a reasonably optimal length. In patients with cardiac dilatation, a beneficial therapeutic intervention generally tends to reduce heart size, with a concomitant reduction in oxygen consumption. This effect is most often produced by salt restriction or diuretics, which reduce intravascular volume; by venodilators, which redistribute blood peripherally; and/or by digitalis, which increases contractile force and allows the heart to empty more completely and return to a smaller size. Reduction of afterload by vasodilator drugs also enhances cardiac emptying and can reduce heart size.

Ross has pointed out that altered cardiac loading conditions can produce failure of the heart even when contractility is normal. Also, favorable or compensated loading conditions can mask the presence of depressed myocardial contractility. Thus, heart failure without myocardial depression may exist as a consequence of sudden aortic or mitral regurgitation afterload mismatch with limited preload reserve. If the mechanical overload develops over a longer time, slow adaption (hypertrophy) occurs to compensate for the overload and thus prevents heart failure. On the contrary, favorable loading conditions (e.g., chronic mitral regurgitation) may mask depressed myocardial contractility. Mild encroachment on the preload reserve with a reduction in afterload will thus allow normal pump function in patients with chronic valvular regurgitation.

Although the most widely used ejection-phase functional index is the ejection fraction, it is afterload-sensitive. End-systolic pressure-volume and end-systolic wall-stress-volume frameworks are particularly useful for the analysis of both mismatch and chronic cardiac adaptation in terms of the pathophysiology of heart failure. A linear relationship has been demonstrated between end-systolic volume and end-systolic pressure that is not afterload-sensitive. Although we can separate the functions of the heart as a pump from those of the heart as a muscle, these relationships are highly complex in health and disease. Also, they are markedly dependent on adaptive mechanisms affecting not only the heart but also the mechanisms of peripheral circulatory control (see Chapter 6). As Guyton has demonstrated (Fig. 6–7), although baroreceptor and chemoreceptor compensatory mechanisms are initially rapid, their sensitivity is reduced at approximately 2 days. Later, control of systemic vessels is mediated by stress relaxation, renin-angiotensin vasoconstriction, and aldosterone. However, at 24 to 48 hours, renal–body fluid adjustments dominate the fundamental mechanisms of systemic arterial vasoconstriction. Thus, interventions that affect autonomic response may be more effective in modulating the vasoconstriction associated with acute heart failure, whereas angiotensin-inhibiting agents, diuretics, and salt and water control become effective at a later time, as in chronic heart failure.

CORONARY CIRCULATION

One organ system deserving particular consideration is the coronary circulation. In the absence of occlusive disease of the epicardial coronary arteries, the coronary circulation is autoregulatory. It appears to function at an abnormally low Po_2 (20 to 23 mm Hg), and there is a very effective extraction of oxygen from the incoming arterial blood. The coronary blood flow varies directly and almost linearly with myocardial oxygen consumption, since there is no reserve available to cardiac muscle by any further widening of the arterial venous oxygen difference. The thermodilution method described by Ganz permits the study of rapid changes in the coronary circulation in humans, and, in particular, the response to acute intervention. In subjects with normal coronary vessels, the mean coronary sinus blood flow was 122 ml per minute—values similar to those reported for other methods. Blood flow in patients with epicardial occlusive coronary artery disease was not different at rest. However, during activity, normal subjects can increase coronary blood flow to a much greater degree. Although drugs, heart rate, and cardiac arrhythmias cause important changes, the highest resting levels and the greatest increases in coronary blood flow have been determined in subjects in whom a pressure load either existed or was imposed on the left ventricle. In heart failure, coronary blood flow is usually normal.

COMMON UNDERLYING MECHANISMS IN CLINICAL CARDIAC FAILURE (Table 10–3)

These mechanisms are considered in detail in Chapter 9. Chronic mechanical overload is compensated by mild ventricular dilation and myocardial hypertrophy. Primary or secondary cardiomyopathy results in a progressive decrease in cardiac muscle and pump performance. In either situation, congestive failure occurs when the ca-

TABLE 10–3 FACTORS IN THE CAUSATION OF HEART FAILURE

A. Increased metabolic (output) demand
　1. Anemia, thyrotoxicosis, fever, beriberi
　2. A-V fistula, Paget's disease, left-to-right shunts
B. Increased left ventricular work
　1. Coarctation of aorta, aortic stenosis, subaortic stenosis
　2. Hypertension: primary, secondary
C. Compromised ventricular contraction
　1. Pericarditis, endomyocardial fibrosis
　2. Cardiomyopathies: infiltrative, idiopathic
D. Coronary artery disease
　1. Ischemia, infarction
　2. Fibrosis, scar, aneurysm
E. Disorders of filling
　1. Mitral, tricuspid stenosis
　2. Pericardial disease, cardiac tamponade
F. Volume overload
　1. Aortic incompetence, mitral incompetence
　2. Transfusion
G. Intrinsic depression of contractile state
　1. Acute myocarditis
　2. Cardiomyopathy
H. Arrhythmias
　1. Tachyarrhythmias—sinus, atrial, nodal, ventricular
　2. Bradyarrhythmias—sinus, partial or complete A-V block

pacity of the heart to discharge a volume of blood against the existing afterload is not sufficient for ordinary metabolic requirements.

BIOCHEMICAL AND MECHANICAL ALTERATIONS IN HEART FAILURE

The myocardium, unlike skeletal muscle, depends almost exclusively on aerobic metabolism and cannot develop any appreciable oxygen debt. Because of its large number of mitochondria, the heart is fundamentally suited to function in an aerobic manner. Normally, the myocardium can adapt itself to a wide number of substrates and is capable of utilizing almost all nutritional substances that come to it via the coronary circulation. These include glucose, pyruvate, lactate, free and esterified fatty acids, acetate, ketone bodies, and amino acids. Thus, in a postprandial state, the myocardium uses primarily glucose, lactate, and pyruvate, with a respiratory quotient approaching 1.0. During fasting conditions, the arterial concentrations of free fatty acids and ketones are much higher, and the heart will utilize these substrates, with a reduction in the respiratory quotient toward 0.8. When glucose is metabolized via the glycolytic and citric acid cycles, 36 of the 38 moles of ATP formed per mole of glucose oxidized are produced as a result of aerobic mitochondrial activity. This emphasizes the importance of aerobic oxidation of glucose in terms of energy production in the form of ATP.

When any portion of myocardium becomes anaerobic, lactate is produced locally, and this has been used, for example, as an indication of ischemia during cardiac catheterization. Normally, uptake of lactate from the arterial blood by the normal myocardium is greater than 10 per cent. With the onset of ischemia, however, tissue lactate is formed as the end product of glycolysis and cannot be metabolized further because of ischemic depression of the citric acid cycle. This results in a level of coronary venous lactate higher than in arterial blood; that is, lactate is produced by the myocardium. Lactate production demonstrated by arteriovenous measurements across the heart is typical of the regional ischemia associated with coronary artery disease.

MECHANICAL FACTORS (Table 10–4)

In several animal models demonstrating heart failure, it has been noted that failing heart muscle has a decreased ability to shorten with a normal velocity. Since the shortening velocity at zero load (Vmax) has been used as an index of contractile state (see Chapter 8), this decrease in velocity of shortening suggests a decrease in the contractile state of the failing muscle. Furthermore, the muscle is unable to develop the same force per unit mass as normal muscle and has a reduced maximum rate of force development.

BIOCHEMICAL FACTORS (Table 10–4)

Numerous studies have been carried out to investigate the potential reasons for these findings. For example, tissue catecholamines are reduced in the failing myocardium, suggesting that there has been an increased excretion rate by augmented sympathetic tone in an attempt to maintain compensation. This is not responsible for

TABLE 10–4 THE FAILING MYOCARDIUM

A. Mechanical alterations
  1. Decrease in force development/cross-sectional area
  2. Decrease in maximum rate of force development
  3. Decrease in velocity of shortening
B. Biochemical alterations
  1. Catecholamines
    a. Reduced tissue content
    b. Reduced synthesis (tyrosine hydroxylase)
  2. Biochemical
    a. Reduced actomyosin-ATPase
    b. Increased hydroxyproline (hypertrophy)
    c. Variable reduction in ATP
    d. Decreased calcium binding by sarcoplasmic reticulum
    e. Decreased adenyl cyclase activity
  3. Exogenous
    a. Increased cortisol, catecholamines, and free fatty acids

the decrease in contractile state, however, since contractile state is not affected by depletion of catecholamines by either reserpinization or denervation. Additional studies in failing heart muscle have revealed a reduction in activity of the enzyme tyrosine hydroxylase, which is in the synthetic pathway of norepinephrine in the myocardium. Thus, there may be not only an increased excretion of norepinephrine but also a decreased rate of synthesis to help account for the depletion of tissue catecholamines. It also has been noted that during the process of hypertrophy there is an increased collagen content of the myocardium, as manifested by an increased hydroxyproline concentration. Whether or not this collagen tissue interferes with the process of contraction is not clear. Even if one corrects contractile measurements for this dilution of normal cardiac tissue by connective tissue, the remaining myocardium still appears to be functioning at a reduced level of contractile state.

ACTOMYOSIN-ATPase

One biochemical alteration of considerable importance in the failing heart is a reduction in actomyosin-ATPase activity. This enzyme is intimately associated with the myosin filament and actin-myosin cross bridges and is responsible for splitting the ATP that provides the energy for contraction. Studies by Barany have demonstrated that actomyosin-ATPase activity in a wide variety of species is closely related to contractile state, as measured by Vmax, the maximal velocity of shortening at zero load. Thus, there is a mechanical-biochemical correlation in failing heart muscle in that both velocity of muscular contraction and baseline actomyosin-ATPase activity are reduced. The reduction in actomyosin-ATPase is the result of the formation of a myosin isozyme (V_3) with reduced enzyme activity. ATP serves as the immediate source of high-energy phosphate bonds for the process of contraction, although creatine phosphate also contains high-energy bonds. In order for this latter energy to be utilized, however, there must be an interchange between creatine phosphate and ADP to form ATP, which is the final source of energy for cardiac contraction. Studies in failing heart muscle have suggested that the levels of ATP are variably reduced in the failing myocardium. A reduction in energy supply does not appear to be the sole reason for a decrease in contractile state.

It has also been noted that there is decreased binding of calcium by the sarcoplasmic reticulum in the failing myocardium. Calcium is the initiator of cardiac contraction by binding with troponin and releasing troponin's inhibition of the interaction of actin and myosin. The reduced ability of the sarcoplasmic reticulum to bind calcium might lead to reduced stores of calcium in the myocardium. Theoretically, this might produce a decreased availability of calcium to the myoplasm and a consequent decrease to contractile state.

In guinea pigs with inherited cardiomyopathy, it has also been noted that adenyl cyclase activity is decreased. This enzyme is intimately associated with the actions of the catecholamines via the beta-adrenergic pathway. Catecholamines, such as norepinephrine, stimulate adenyl cyclase activity and convert ATP to cyclic AMP. Cyclic AMP in turn activates phosphorylase activity and promotes glycogenolysis, making more glucose available for the glycolytic cycle. In addition, cyclic AMP enhances calcium availability to the myofilaments and produces an increase in contractile state. This reduction in adenyl cyclase activity, however, does not appear to be the mechanism responsible for the decrease in contractile state, since the level of this enzyme can vary considerably (depending on the catecholamine content of the myocardium) without affecting basal levels of contraction.

EXOGENOUS FACTORS

Several exogenous factors have important effects on cardiac function during heart failure. An elevation in plasma catecholamines is the most important factor. This catecholamine response is apparently part of the overall response of the body to the stress associated with heart failure and also includes elevations of cortisol and free fatty acids. Of some interest is the potential role of increased levels of catecholamines and free fatty acids in producing arrhythmias in the setting of acute heart failure, particularly acute myocardial infarction. Whether the elevation of these substances is responsible for the arrhythmias observed or merely reflects the serious nature of the underlying heart disease is not yet clear.

In summary, although there are several biochemical alterations of importance in the failing heart, it is not yet known whether these various abnormalities are merely associated with or in some way are responsible for the decreased contractility of the failing heart.

RENAL PHYSIOLOGY IN CONGESTIVE HEART FAILURE*

Renal mechanisms are intimately involved in the retention of fluid and electrolytes and thus the peripheral edema that follows congestive heart failure. The basic response of the kidney to a fall in cardiac output is retention of salt and water. This receptor response apparently has difficulty in discriminating between a true fall in plasma volume, such as might occur with blood loss or fluid

*See also Chapter 14.

depletion, and a fall in effective circulating volume caused by a depression of cardiac function. The stimulus for retention of salt and water, however, will persist until adequate cardiac output is restored. This results in an increase in extracellular fluid volume, in total body water, and in total exchangeable sodium and chloride. Aldosterone secretion and the concentration of antidiuretic hormone also are increased.

Normally, about 98 per cent of the sodium filtered by the glomeruli is reabsorbed by the tubular system. The great bulk of this is reabsorbed in the proximal tubules. A smaller amount is absorbed in the collecting duct and the ascending loop of Henle, whereas the remainder, which is not excreted in the urine, is reabsorbed in the distal tubule by ion exchange with hydrogen or potassium. This mechanism is the principal means for excretion of potassium ion. Under the influence of enhanced aldosterone, total exchangeable potassium in the body may actually be reduced owing to this reabsorption of sodium in the distal tubule.

The rate of sodium excretion is determined by the balance between glomerular filtration and tubular reabsorption. In congestive heart failure, the glomerular filtration rate is commonly reduced to at least one half the normal rate. However, there appears to be increased tubular reabsorption of sodium, suggesting that this latter factor is the most significant cause of sodium accumulation, whereas the fall in glomerular filtration rate is only a contributory factor. Although it is not the exclusive factor, the role of aldosterone in this regard appears to be of primary importance in producing the retention of sodium ions. The sequence of events in this series apparently includes the release of renin from the renal afferent arterioles and juxtaglomerular cells, which transforms angiotensinogen to a decapeptide, angiotensin I. A converting enzyme changes this material to an octapeptide, angiotensin II, which is the immediate factor stimulating the secretion of aldosterone by the zona glomerulosa of the adrenal cortex. Presumably, decreased pressure or volume in the afferent arterioles is the signal mechanism that activates this system. The retention of sodium, therefore, is accompanied by the retention of water and expansion of the circulating blood volume. This in turn leads to filtration of the retained fluid as edema into tissue spaces and occasionally as pleural or peritoneal effusions.

Associated with this retention of fluid is also a decrease in free water clearance. Therefore, patients who have a continued large intake of water will be unable to clear this water through their kidneys and may develop dilutional hyponatremia. Thus, in severe heart failure, it is clear that therapy must include not only a restriction of salt intake but also limited restriction of fluid intake, together with appropriate diuretics. Because of the propensity for potassium loss with increased aldosterone secretion and the administration of certain diuretics such as the thiazides, it is often important to provide oral potassium supplements, particularly in patients who are digitalized. Alternatively, the use of aldosterone antagonists in addition to other diuretics may maintain reasonable potassium balance.

CONTROL OF PERIPHERAL CIRCULATION

In the normal circulation at rest, the total blood flow is divided in a relatively constant proportion among the different organ systems of the body (Table 10–5). Skeletal muscle and the splanchnic and renal beds each receive approximately 20 per cent of the total cardiac output. The cerebral circulation and blood flow through the skin each account for a further 10 per cent of total blood flow. The coronary vascular system receives 4 per cent of the total cardiac output. During activity the cerebral blood flow remains relatively constant. Flow in other segments of the circulation alters in accord with metabolic demand. Thus, during exercise, skeletal muscle blood flow increases promptly and may account for more than 50 per cent of the total cardiac output. At the same time, there is a major increase in skin blood flow, presumably to facilitate the loss of metabolic heat from the body. Although the proportion of blood flow passing to the other circulatory elements is decreased, the absolute level of blood flow is maintained.

In skeletal muscle, the arterioles are under essentially local control. The local vascular resistance is determined by the relative degree of vasodilatation resulting from the production of metabolites in skeletal muscle. When the muscle is relatively inactive, the production of metabolites is low, and the "net" vascular tone remains high.

TABLE 10–5 REGIONAL DISTRIBUTION OF CARDIAC OUTPUT

	Normal		Cardiac Failure	
	Rest	Exercise	Rest	Exercise
Cardiac output (L/min/M²)	3.0	6.0	1.5	2.3
Blood flows (% of cardiac output)				
Muscle	20	50	36	60
Splanchnic	25	12	25	10
Renal	20	9	10	4
Cerebral	12	6	12	12
Coronary	4	4	9	10
Skin	9	15	3	1
Blood flows (absolute values in ml/min/M²)				
Muscle	600	3000	540	1380
Renal	600	540	150	92
Coronary	120	240	135	230

(From Mason, D. T.: Mod. Conc. Cardiovasc. Dis. 36:25, 1967. By permission of The American Heart Association, Inc.)

As metabolic products are formed and their concentration rises, vasodilatation occurs, which has the autoregulatory effect of enhancing the removal of these substances with a tendency to restore the previous level of vasomotor tone. In addition, skeletal muscle is under modest degrees of autonomic control. The circulation in the skin is principally regulated by the autonomic nervous system. Vasodilatation occurs by reason of release of constrictor tone centrally mediated. This appears to be predominantly a heat regulatory mechanism.

HEART FAILURE

In heart failure, however, there is a reduction in total cardiac output at rest, and there is a failure to increase cardiac output proportionate with activity. Hence, there is a redistribution of the absolute magnitude of organ blood flow in this state, which is further accentuated during exercise. In patients with borderline cardiac compensation of heart failure, the coronary blood flow is preserved. In fact, the coronary blood flow may be much greater proportionate to cardiac output in patients with heart failure than in patients with normally compensated circulations. Relatively speaking, there is a diminution in renal blood flow and, to a lesser extent, in splanchnic blood flow. The skeletal muscles retain their usual proportion of blood flow (Table 10–5).

During activity, there is a pronounced alteration in the distribution of blood flow. Cerebral blood flow is maintained, but there is a marked reduction in blood flow to the splanchnic and renal beds. Within the limits of total cardiac output, blood flow to actively exercising skeletal muscle increases. This, however, is strictly limited by the availability of blood flow. In contrast, normal skin blood flow is not increased in heart failure, owing to sustained vasoconstriction. Vascular reactivity is profoundly altered in heart failure. First, there is an increased resting peripheral resistance throughout the organ systems, both collectively and individually. Thus, the balance between the concentration of dilating metabolites and the vascular tone in skeletal muscle is substantially altered so that a greater concentration is necessary to sustain a given level of vasodilatation. This may also be seen in the responses of skeletal muscle and skin to reactive hyperemia. In such instances, the magnitude of dilatation is greatly reduced. In addition, there is an abnormal response to ordinary autonomic reflexes. The vasodilatation in the skin is significantly reduced following heating, and responses to such mechanisms as acute tilting and the Valsalva maneuver are altered. In a normal subject, there is a significant and transient overshoot in arterial blood pressure following the Valsalva maneuver. This overshoot is absent in patients with heart failure, suggesting that the peripheral vascular tone is already high and is not particularly modified during the Valsalva maneuver, nor is stroke volume substantially increased. Heart failure is characterized by an increase in sympathetic vascular tone, which is in direct proportion to the severity of the failure.

Shock. One particular syndrome characterizing the failing heart is worthy of note. In the shock state, peripheral vascular responses may be grossly abnormal. Initially, there is a marked increase in peripheral vascular resistance in such patients, although occasionally reduced peripheral vascular resistance and reflex vasodilation due to stimulation of cardiac receptors have been described. However, in the presence of prolonged and severe hypoxia with resulting lactic acidemia and acidosis, a specific paralysis of peripheral vessels occurs. In the shock syndrome, the ability of skeletal muscle vessels to dilate is almost completely abolished. The reactive hyperemic response is negligible in spite of the fact that presumably high levels of vasodilating substances are present in the resting as well as the exercising muscle.

HEART FAILURE IN ISCHEMIC HEART DISEASE AND ACUTE MYOCARDIAL INFARCTION

Occlusive coronary artery disease is a special disorder of cardiac function that warrants separate consideration from a practical as well as a pathophysiologic standpoint. The processes of atherosclerosis result in the formation of obstructive lesions in the coronary vascular tree that, because of either degree or location, may substantially interfere with the magnitude of coronary blood flow. When the myocardial oxygen demand of the tissue in the distribution of each vessel exceeds the capacity of the restricted arterial bed to supply it with oxygenated blood, ischemic changes result. These changes are usually characterized by the development of chest pain of cardiac origin—angina pectoris—but this is a variable symptom. It is now clear that patients with coronary artery disease and angina pectoris have significant but reversible ventricular dysfunction that is due to ischemia alone. When the degree of ischemia is

extremely severe or the vessel is acutely and completely blocked, major changes occur, both in the structure of the myocardium and in ventricular function. The dynamic nature of this process is shown in Figure 10–6. Patients with acute myocardial infarction are usually classified as (1) being uncomplicated, (2) uncomplicated apart from transient cardiac arrhythmias, (3) exhibiting heart failure of mild degree, (4) exhibiting heart failure of moderate degree, and (5) exhibiting cardiogenic shock. This classification is not always entirely precise, since a true reduction of cardiac performance is not always coincidental with the signs and symptoms of pulmonary venous congestion, which are the usual clinical hallmarks of the diagnosis of heart failure (Fig. 10–7). Thus, the measured values for cardiac performance may show the cardiac output, stroke volume, and stroke work to be normal or even increased in a given patient; may be reduced moderately to levels consistent with normal cardiac performance; or may be reduced profoundly.

Left ventricular filling pressure may be normal, but it is frequently increased. The level of left ventricular filling pressure or pulmonary venous and distending pressure correlates with the presence of increased vascular markings of the lungs on chest radiographs, clinical signs of pulmonary venous congestion, and clinical signs of enhanced filling pressure—third and fourth heart sounds (Fig. 10–8). However, the relationship of cardiac performance to filling pressure is poor, in that patients may have normal cardiac performance with low or high ventricular filling pressures and reduced cardiac performance with low or high ventricular filling pressure.

The time course of changes in these hemodynamics is somewhat variable. Left ventricular filling pressure usually decreases in 2 to 4 days to normal levels, irrespective of whether the cardiac output has been normal or moderately decreased. Pulmonary congesting pressure—pulmonary venous pressure—falls spontaneously without any treatment or with diuretics, which initially act by enhancing venous capacitance and then have a later (½ hour) effect on salt and water excretion.

In myocardial infarction, agents such as digi-

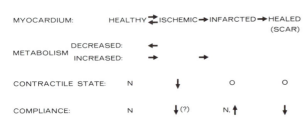

Figure 10–6 Dynamic representation of the changes in the function of myocardium on coronary heart disease. There is a reversible relation between healthy and ischemic myocardium determined by the level of cardiac metabolism. The reaction becomes irreversible when ischemic tissue passes into the infarcted state and undergoes necrosis and healing in the form of fibrosis or scar. The contractile state is reduced to a varying degree (frequently severely) in ischemia and of course is absent in infarcted or scarred myocardium. The compliant state of myocardium may be decreased during ischemia (ventricular stiffening) and may be normal or increased in infarcted myocardium. Following healing, myocardial scars are noncompliant and extremely stiff, with a minimal mechanical disadvantage.

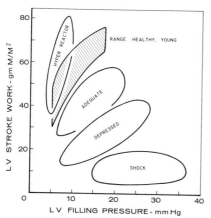

Figure 10–7 Relation of ventricular performance to filling pressure in patients with coronary heart disease and myocardial infarction. A wide spectrum of ventricular response exists. Certain patients may exhibit normal performance characteristics or performance characteristics that are inappropriately enhanced for the sedated, resting individual. Differing degrees of depression of ventricular performance exist that are related dominantly to the magnitude and location of the infarcted-ischemic tissue and the presence of additional mechanical lesions such as mitral valve incompetence. Patients with profound depression of ventricular function usually exhibit the shock state and experience a very high mortality.

talis and the catecholamines do not exhibit a powerful inotropic effect. In patients with normal or increased cardiac output, there is a small increase in cardiac output or stroke work of approximately 10 to 15 per cent. On the contrary, in patients with severe depression of cardiac function, this does not take place. Hence, patients who are severely ill and who require the use of cardiac stimulators do not respond favorably to inotropic agents. This may be due to total failure of the infarcted or ischemic tissue to respond (the normal myocardium is already maximally active). A wide variety of effects appear to result from myocardial infarction (Fig. 10–7). In a small infarct, there are few contractile elements that are rendered inactive. In addition, acute myocardial ischemia or infarction or both appear to mediate strong sympathetic activity. Therefore, certain patients in the ischemic-infarction syndrome exhibit tachycardia or hypertension in the presence of a normal or increased cardiac output. A second group of patients have an infarct of medium size. In this instance more contractile elements have been rendered ineffective and the cardiac output is usually more depressed. However, the diastolic compliant state of the ventricle is variable. In many patients, there is good evidence that the ventricle is stiff and may be exhibiting ischemic contracture. This diastolic stiffness also appears to have a time course similar to that of the change in diastolic filling pressure, so that in 2 to 5 days diastolic pressure has declined and the characteristics of diastolic stiffness have disappeared. The presence

of a loud fourth heart sound in the majority of patients with acute myocardial infarction and the typical configuration of the left ventricular pressure pulse renders an increased diastolic stiffness likely (Fig. 10–8).

If the infarct is large, many contractile elements are rendered nonfunctional, and the ejection fraction (EF) is proportionately reduced (Fig. 10–9). Not infrequently, additional mechanical lesions are present. Of these, perhaps the most important is paradox of the area of the myocardial infarct. If the infarct does not stiffen (decreased ventricular compliance), it distends as intraventricular pressure rises (Fig. 10–10). The work performed by the normally contracting elements is therefore wasted in the distention of the infarct. In addition, mitral insufficiency due to chronic papillary muscle dysfunction or recent dysfunction as a consequence of ventricular dilatation or papillary muscle abnormality can add to the burden of the already disordered ventricle. In the same way as ventricular paradox, mitral insufficiency or intraventricular flow can acutely and profoundly depress cardiac pump function. In this regard, a soft systolic murmur at the apex of the heart in patients with acute myocardial infarction should never be regarded as an innocent, inconsequential sign. It may be evidence of mitral insufficiency of only moderate magnitude but of a degree sufficient to account for a substantial proportion of the reduced cardiac output. In certain instances the mitral insufficiency may be completely silent, with the murmur returning only as cardiac compensation is partly restored.

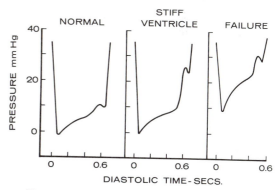

Figure 10–8 Left ventricular diastolic pressure pulses in patients with and without heart disease. In each instance ventricular systole is excluded, and the tracing represents only the events in diastole. Note (left) the early diastolic pressure approaching zero with an "a" wave of approximately 10 mm Hg in magnitude. In acute myocardial infarction, the early diastolic contour of the pressure pulse remains unchanged, but there is an "a" wave of large magnitude, possibly owing to an increased ventricular stiffness and, therefore, a shift to the left of the diastolic pressure-volume relation. In the right panel is a tracing of a patient with chronic congestive heart failure and elevated early diastolic as well as late diastolic and "a" wave pressures.

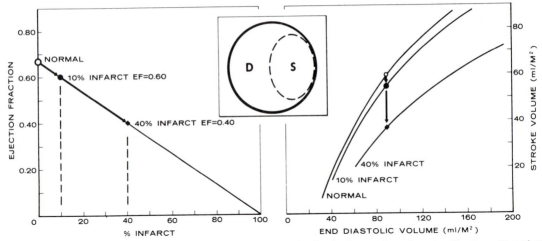

Figure 10–9 Diagrammatic representation of the effect of reduction in the number of contractile elements activated during ventricular systole. In myocardial ischemia or infarction, as the contractile units are rendered nonfunctional the overall performance of the ventricle falls. This is expressed in the left panel as the ejection fraction, or the portion of ventricular content expelled during systole, and on the right panel as isopleths of stroke volume as a function of end-diastolic volume. Note that obligatory reductions in stroke volume must occur as a function of the increasing magnitude of cardiac muscle involved. Further, the ventricle cannot dilate rapidly to compensate for this loss.

The most profound form of depression of cardiac function results in a clinical syndrome known as *shock*. Shock may be associated with a number of causes, including acute infection, acute loss of blood volume, and acute profound destruction of myocardial elements. The reduction of approximately 40 per cent of the contractile elements in the myocardium causes a fall in cardiac performance to the order of magnitude seen in patients in or close to cardiogenic shock. If, however, additional mechanical lesions are present, these effects are additive to the factors depressing the circulatory state and result in a sufficient depression of

cardiac function to cause shock in spite of the presence of an infarct of lesser size.

It has been found that patients exhibiting the shock state do indeed fall into appropriate pathophysiologic groupings. The younger patients with a first infarction who progress rapidly through their illness and die in cardiogenic shock have large myocardial infarcts, usually resulting from an acute anterolateral or anteroseptal infarction consequent on a major occlusion in the left coronary arterial system. These individuals account for approximately 55 per cent of the patients. Another 15 to 20 per cent of patients have an

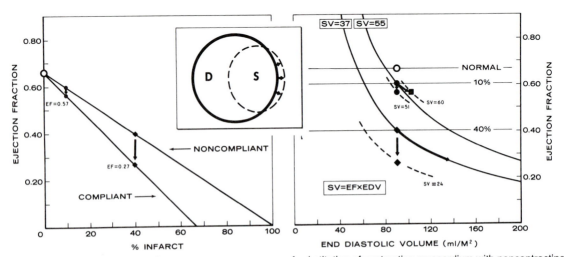

Figure 10–10 Ventricular performance as a consequence of substitution of contracting myocardium with noncontracting but compliant elements. In this instance, the nonfunctional fibers elongate and the ventricle distends as a consequence of the rise in intraventricular pressure occasioned by contraction of the healthy elements. The mechanical disadvantage is evident (compare with Fig. 10–9).

additional definable mechanical lesion such as those already indicated, and the remaining approximately 30 per cent of patients have end-stage heart disease. In this last group, the imposition of new small myocardial infarction upon chronic heart disease is sufficient to depress function so that an adequate performance can no longer be maintained.

SYMPTOMS AND SIGNS OF HEART FAILURE

We shall relate the symptoms and signs of heart failure to the four subsystems previously introduced: the left ventricle, the right ventricle, the pulmonary venous circulation, and the systemic venous circulation.

LEFT VENTRICULAR FAILURE

The principal symptom associated with failure of the left ventricle as a pump consists of those complaints related to reduced organ perfusion (Table 10–6). Easy fatigability and extreme weakness of the musculoskeletal system are characteristic. Dyspnea is principally due to the associated pulmonary venous congestion. The extremities are frequently cool and pale. At times there is forgetfulness, and if the condition is prolonged and severe, there is ultimately evidence of dysfunction in many organ systems, including the gut, kidney, and liver. Severe peripheral cyanosis and indeed gangrene may occur in profound chronic heart failure. The signs include tachycardia, with a heart rate exceeding 100 beats per minute, and a slight reduction in blood pressure. The pulse pressure is usually narrowed. Cardiomegaly may be present owing to the nature of the underlying disease, but the heart size may be normal. The first sound is usually muffled and less distinctive than normal. If diastolic blood pressure is diminished, the second heart sound at the pulmonary

and aortic areas is reduced. Diagnostic physical findings in significant heart failure include the presence of third and fourth heart sounds (Fig. 10–8). These sounds relate to heightened filling pressure in the left ventricle: The former is associated with a rapid filling of an already partially filled ventricle at the beginning of atrial emptying; the latter is associated with an enhanced rate of pressure rise in the ventricle at end diastole. If a murmur is present, it usually is related to the underlying disease but is reduced in intensity. In heart failure, the diastolic murmur of mitral stenosis may be totally absent. In like manner, in acute myocardial infarction a systolic murmur associated with papillary muscle disease may not be apparent but will be detected as cardiac function improves. The apex beat is usually diffuse and rather weak, with or without associated abnormal pulsation. The carotid pulse may be slow in its upstroke, although this is not a consistent finding.

RIGHT VENTRICULAR FAILURE

Right ventricular dysfunction may be associated with dyspnea, as in patients with acute pulmonary embolization. More importantly, there is moderate fatigue, which is not so severe as that associated with comparable degrees of left heart failure. Frequently, a right ventricular lift and an accentuated second heart sound at the pulmonary area may be evidence of the presence of concomitant pulmonary hypertension. Occasionally, a pulmonary diastolic murmur is heard owing to the presence of extremely severe pulmonary hypertension. The second sound of the pulmonary area may also be widely split (Table 10–6).

PULMONARY VENOUS CONGESTION

The principal symptom of pulmonary venous congestion is dyspnea, as occurs following exertion

TABLE 10–6 PRINCIPAL CLINICAL SYMPTOMS AND PHYSICAL SIGNS OF RIGHT AND LEFT HEART FAILURE

	Left Heart Failure	Right Heart Failure
Symptoms	Fatigue, weakness	Weight gain
	Obtundation	Ankle swelling, pigmentation
	Cyanosis	Abdominal distention
	Exertion dyspnea	Subcostal pain
	Cough	Neck pulsations
	Orthopnea, paroxysmal nocturnal dyspnea	Jaundice
	Anorexia	Fatigue, weakness
	Diaphoresis	
Signs	Tachycardia	Edema, acites
	Apex diffuse	Increased second sound (second
	First sound ↓	component) of pulmonary area
	Third and fourth sounds present	Left parasternal lift
	Moist rales, pleural effusion	Increased jugular venous pressure

in patients with a serious degree of heart failure. If the precipitating cause is acute, as with rupture of a cardiac valve, sudden severe shortness of breath may rapidly disable the patient. Orthopnea exists when the patient is unable to lie flat and is due to a high level of pulmonary venous pressure. Paroxysmal nocturnal dyspnea usually is not associated with severe elevation of pulmonary venous pressure but occurs when a patient with more moderate elevations sleeps flat, allowing a slow accumulation of fluid throughout the interstitial spaces of the lungs. When this reaches a critical value, it is necessary for the patient to assume the upright posture, so that redistribution of interstitial and alveolar fluid can allow effective respiration to be restored. Acute pulmonary edema is associated with a very rapid development of severe dyspnea, even with the patient in the upright position. It may be associated with the production of frothy bright red sputum. The patient will (naturally) be extremely apprehensive. On examination, patients with overt heart failure will be found to exhibit an increase in the frequency and depth of breathing. On auscultation of the chest, the findings depend on the degree of pulmonary venous hypertension. Patients with mild heart failure may have relatively few rales at both bases. In patients with acute pulmonary edema, it is possible to identify rales up to the thoracic apex. Unequal distribution of rales in the right and left chest is a frequent finding. Pleural effusion is often an accompaniment and may be so small as to be detectable only on chest radiographs, usually involving the right thoracic cavity. Radiographs of the chest reveal several changes that relate to the severity of the heart failure. In the mildest examples, there are increased vascular markings in the lower lobe pulmonary veins. As the pulmonary congestion becomes more severe, the upper pulmonary veins become more prominent, whereas the lower lobe veins actually appear to become smaller. Hilar congestion and interstitial edema are followed by generalized edema, with a ground-glass appearance across the thorax. Pleural effusions may be noted as just indicated, in the right or left chest cavities or bilaterally.

SYSTEMIC VENOUS CONGESTION

The principal symptoms relate to swelling of the ankles and dependent parts, abdominal swelling, and subcostal pain. The neck veins may be distended and pulsatile. On examination, edema may be identified and abdominal swelling found associated with ascites or a large and tender liver. The liver may pulsate in the presence of tricuspid incompetence. Neck veins are frequently distended with a high venous pressure, so that even with the patient sitting at 45 to 60 degrees from the horizontal, the neck veins remain filled. In the presence of tricuspid incompetence, venous pulsa-

tion characterized by "a" and "v" waves may be identified.

PHYSIOLOGIC PRINCIPLES IN THE THERAPY OF HEART FAILURE

Effective therapy requires an adjustment of the environment or creation of a milieu that will favorably influence the cardiac state. Hence, rational treatment depends on effective measures to reverse altered physiology.

The principles in the management of heart failure are to reduce cardiac demand, improve cardiac performance, maximize the rate and completeness of healing, and reverse associated disorders of organ function and fluid balance. It is not our purpose to discuss the mode of action or practical uses of inotropic or diuretic drugs or other conventional therapeutic modalities or to detail the mechanical benefits consequent on successful surgical treatment of congenital or valvular disease.

ALTERATIONS OF PRELOAD, AFTERLOAD, AND CONTRACTILE STATE

It is convenient to think of the mechanical function of the heart in terms of its three principal determinants: preload, afterload, and contractile state (Table 10–7). *Preload* refers to initial and diastolic fiber length. Thus, changes in preload describe the Starling function curve. In the intact heart, preload is often considered in terms of either end-diastolic pressure or end-diastolic volume.

Since patients with power failure may have either high or low filling pressure, it is important to optimize the filling pressure to the most beneficial place on the Starling curve. Studies in patients with acute myocardial infarction, for example, have shown that a pulmonary capillary wedge pressure of approximately 15 to 18 mm Hg provides the optimal cardiac performance, as measured by stroke volume or stroke work. Higher values of left ventricular filling pressure do not augment stroke volume any further, and lower values of filling pressure may reduce stroke volume by the Starling mechanism. Furthermore, high levels of filling pressure may lead to pulmo-

TABLE 10–7 EFFECTS OF ALTERATIONS IN PRELOAD, AFTERLOAD, AND CONTRACTILE STATE ON STROKE VOLUME

	Preload (LVEDP)	Afterload (Arterial Pressure)	Contractile State
Increase in S.V.	↑	↓	↑
Decrease in S.V.	↓	↑	↓

nary congestion, increased work of breathing, and increased myocardial oxygen consumption due to cardiac dilatation and Laplace's law. These factors emphasize the importance of optimizing the left ventricular filling pressure in patients with cardiac failure.

Afterload refers to the load against which the heart must work. It is convenient to think of afterload as aortic pressure, although in reality the afterload corresponds to wall stress, which is related to pressure by Laplace's law. Of importance is the fact that changes in afterload may affect cardiac performance at a given preload. For example, if afterload is abruptly increased, there will be a corresponding reduction in stroke volume, with subsequent compensatory mechanisms tending to return toward normal. Similarly, if there is a corresponding reduction in afterload, there is an initial increase in stroke volume. This latter fact is the basis for the use of arteriolar vasodilators in the management of patients with either acute or chronic heart failure. Data indicate that there is an excessive rise in systemic vascular resistance in heart failure, which of itself can further reduce cardiac output. Arteriolar vasodilation will lower this elevated resistance and increase cardiac output. Drugs such as nitroprusside reduce arterial pressure and systemic vascular resistance. This therapy is very beneficial in many patients in that it produces an increase in cardiac output and a reduction in left ventricular filling pressure in association with a fall in systemic vascular resistance and arterial pressure. The fall in left ventricular filling pressure is probably due to both venodilation, with a reduction in venous return, and more complete systolic emptying as a result of a reduction in afterload.

Among patients who might especially benefit from a reduction of afterload are those with acute myocardial infarction and a hypertensive reaction. Reduction of blood pressure would markedly reduce oxygen needs of the heart and might limit the size of the infarct by reducing the surrounding ischemic zone. Reduction of the afterload has also been shown to be effective in patients with heart failure associated with severe mitral regurgitation. A fall in afterload reduces the regurgitant fraction and increases forward flow and cardiac output. It should be noted, however, that reduction of afterload also reduces diastolic filling pressure, which is the coronary perfusing pressure. Too great a reduction of arterial pressure, therefore, may be deleterious by reason of a concomitant reduction of coronary blood flow.

The third determinant of mechanical performance, *contractile state*, refers to the ability of the heart to alter its contractile force at a given preload and afterload in response to such factors as intrinsic catecholamine stimulation, circulating catecholamines, and exogenous interventions (e.g., digitalis, norepinephrine, isoproterenol, paired electrical stimulation, etc.). In chronic heart fail-

ure, the use of digitalis to increase contractile force, improve systolic emptying, and reduce heart size is accepted as having beneficial effects on the circulation. In the case of acute power failure due to severe myocardial infarction, however, the potential role of these positive inotropic agents is unclear. The effects of drugs such as digitalis, isoproterenol, and norepinephrine are relatively slight in this setting and may even be deleterious, owing to their propensity to produce arrhythmias and the obligatory increase in myocardial oxygen needs because of the increase in contractile state. The general lack of response to positive inotropic agents in acute power failure following infarction may be related to the fact that much of the myocardium is nonresponsive (infarcted) and therefore unable to increase its contractile state. In addition, the normally responsive myocardium is already maximally stimulated by intrinsic sympathetic tone or circulating catecholamines. Studies of myocardial mechanics have shown that there is a ceiling of contractility; if reached through the use of one agent, this ceiling cannot be exceeded, even though another potent inotropic agent is added. Therefore, the relative lack of response of patients with power failure following myocardial infarction to all inotropic agents may be due to these factors and suggests that these agents may have limited value in this particular setting. Of equal or greater importance may be the correction of such factors as anoxia, arrhythmias, acidosis, and relative hypovolemia.

MECHANICAL CIRCULATORY ASSIST

When one considers the management of cardiac decompensation, it is logical to examine the possibility of adding to the circulating bloodstream energy other than that provided by the contracting left ventricle. With this objective in mind, attention has been paid to the possibility of total or partial circulatory support by artificial mechanical devices.

Total cardiac replacement by an auxiliary heart has been attempted in a few patients. In most of these endeavors, the cardiac chambers themselves have not been removed but have been used in a nonfunctional manner as part of the conduit traversed by blood to an auxiliary ventricle, either in a portion of the arterial system or between the apex of the left ventricle and the aorta. These devices have sustained the circulation for short periods of time. They require the provision of an external power source with an appropriate transcutaneous connection to the working pump. In addition, the technical problems associated with insertion and vascular connections and the formation of thrombi on the surfaces in contact with flowing blood have not yet been satisfactorily resolved. In the relatively short duration of total cardiac function thus far attempted in humans, no limitation seems to be imposed by the strength-durability characteristics of the materials utilized.

An artificial heart powered by an atomic energy source appears to be feasible in the future. Prototype heart pumps have been used for relatively long periods in calves. An atomic power source would allow total implantation, probably within the abdomen, and the problems of radiation shielding and heat dissipation are solvable. It is predicted that such devices will be developed within the next decade with approximately a 10-year life span, determined by the stress-strain characteristics of the pump materials. There is no foreseeable limitation imposed by the energy source.

Temporary circulatory assist implies that fundamental abnormal processes may be reversible if the cardiovascular system is supported for a finite period of time or until more definitive forms of therapy can be undertaken. Circulatory support for hours, or even several days, is now feasible and has been utilized in human patients. However, it has been found that in many instances the degree of myocardial damage that has caused the need for circulatory support is so great as to preclude long-term survival. Hence, many patients must be subjected subsequently to procedures to correct mechanically disadvantageous cardiac lesions or to provide cardiac revascularization by means of aortocoronary artery anastomosis.

The use of the heart-lung bypass machine conventionally employed in cardiovascular surgery has been suggested for the temporary support of the circulation. Although this is feasible for periods of approximately 3 hours, the oxygenators do not allow prolonged total support of the circulation. Apparently, membrane oxygenators more adequately preserve the structure of the formed elements in the blood and do not lead to thrombus formation. With these devices, total circulatory support has been undertaken for 24 to 60 hours in a small number of patients. As an extension of this principle, total support of the circulation utilizing the patient's lung as the oxygenator has been proposed. However, there are significant technical difficulties in recovering the oxygenated blood effectively from the left atrium or in the procedures necessary to totally empty the ventricle.

Mechanical counterpulsation refers to a form of partial mechanical support of the circulation. It is well known that when the heart exhibits failure, it is an extremely poor pressure pump, but it is less disabled than a volume pump. Therefore, reduction of the opening pressure at the aortic valve and a reduction of blood pressure during ventricular systole favor the more complete emptying of the left ventricle. Although this can be accomplished by the reduction of peripheral vascular resistance through administration of dilating drugs, it is done at the expense of coronary perfusion, since a sustained pressure greater than 60 mm Hg is probably needed during diastole to maintain coronary perfusion. Hence, the most favorable circumstance would be a fundamental reversal of the normal sequence of the cardiac cycle, that is, a fall in aortic pressure during ventricular systole and a rise in pressure during ventricular diastole. A number of procedures have been employed to accomplish these ends. Of these, the best known is insertion into the descending thoracic aorta of a sausage-shaped 30-ml balloon that is supported by a rigid catheter. The balloon is connected to a source of compressed helium, which is allowed access to the balloon via a control valve synchronized with the cardiac cycle. Thus, just before or at the time of ventricular systole, the balloon is evacuated of gas, and hence the volume in the aorta is acutely reduced by approximately 30 ml. Consequently, there is a brisk fall in aortic pressure, so that ventricular ejection occurs at a point earlier in the cardiac cycle and at a much lower pressure level. When cardiac ejection is complete and the aortic valve closes, the balloon is reinflated, adding a volume equivalent to 30 ml to the aortic content, thus raising the intra-aortic pressure. These events are indicated diagrammatically in Figure 10–11. Coronary perfusion pressure is increased during ventricular diastole, whereas the stimulus to myocardial oxygen consumption is diminished because isometric contraction is shortened and maximal left ventricular wall tension is decreased.

Usually within 10 to 15 minutes after its initiation, this form of circulatory support can

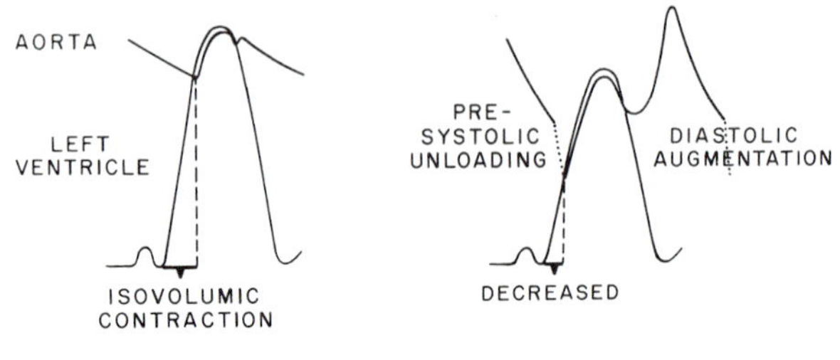

Figure 10–11 The mechanical consequences of counterpulsation. This diagram represents aortic and left ventricular pressure pulses *(left panel)* and the changes consequent upon counterpulsation *(right panel)*. During counterpulsation, the pressure in the aorta during the isometric phase of ventricular contraction suddenly falls. Hence, the aortic valve can open at a lower pressure and early in the cardiac cycle. This may favorably influence the level of myocardial oxygen consumption. Since the aortic capacitance has been increased (see text), the absolute magnitude of pressure generated during ventricular systole is reduced. When the aortic valve closes, aortic pressure is artificially increased by the counterpulsation device, thus providing a higher head of pressure for the maintenance of coronary arterial blood flow.

reverse profound depression of cardiovascular pump function. There is a prompt improvement in cardiac output, reduction in filling pressure, improved organ perfusion, and reversal of metabolic alterations. However, this technique necessitates insertion of the balloon into the vascular system, a precise synchronization of the electrical action of the heart with the inflation and deflation sequences, and an experienced team of clinicians to manage other aspects of patient care.

REFERENCES

Braunwald, E.: The determinants of myocardial oxygen consumption. Thirteenth Bowditch Lecture. Physiologist *12*:65, 1969.

Braunwald, E., Chidsey, C. A., Pool, P. E., et al.: Clinical Staff Conference. Congestive heart failure: biochemical and physiological considerations. Ann. Intern. Med. *64*:904, 1966.

Braunwald, E., Ross, J., and Sonnenblick, E. H.: Mechanisms of contraction of the normal and failing heart. Boston, Little, Brown and Co., 1968.

Chatterjee, K., and Parmley, W. W.: Vasodilators therapy for acute myocardial infarction and chronic congestive heart failure. J. Am. Coll. Cardiol. *1*:133, 1983.

Dodge, H. T., and Baxley, W. A.: Hemodynamic aspects of heart failure. Am. J. Cardiol. *22*:24, 1968.

Ford, L. E.: Heart size. Circ. Res. *39*:297, 1976.

Friedberg, C. K. (Ed.): Congestive Heart Failure. New York, Grune & Stratton, 1970, pp. 1–70, 97–171, 195–288.

Ganz, W., Tamura, K., Marcus, H. S., et al.: Measurement of coronary sinus blood flow by continuous thermodilution in man. Circulation *44*:181, 1971.

Herman, M. V., and Gorlin, R.: Implications of left ventricular asynergy. Am. J. Cardiol. *23*:538, 1969.

Katz, A. M., and Brady, A. J.: Mechanial and biochemical correlates of cardiac contraction (I and II). Modern Conc. Cardiovasc. Dis. *40*:39 and *40*:45, 1971.

Maroko, P. R., Kjekshus, J. K., Sobel, B. E., et al.: Factors influencing infarct size following experimental coronary artery occlusions. Circulation *43*:67, 1971.

Mason, D. T.: Control of peripheral circulation in health and disease. Modern Conc. Cardiovasc. Dis. *36*:25, 1967.

Parmley, W. W., Tyberg, J. V., and Glantz, S.: Cardiac Dynamics. Ann. Rev. Physiol. *39*:277, 1977.

Ross, J., Jr.: Cardiac function and myocardial contractility of perspective. JACC *1*:52, 1983.

Sagawa, K.: The end systolic pressure volume relation of the ventricle: definition, modifications and clinical use. Circulation *63*:1223, 1981.

Spann, J. F., Jr., Mason, D. T., and Zelis, R.: Recent advances in the understanding of congestive heart failure. Modern Conc. Cardiovasc. Dis. *39*:73, 1970.

Swan, H. J. C., Forrester, J. S., Diamond, G., et al.: The hemodynamic basis of shock and acute myocardial infarction: a conceptual model. Circulation *45*:1097, 1972.

11 Heart Sounds, Murmurs, and Precordial Movements*†

John F. Stapleton and W. Proctor Harvey

During each cardiac cycle the heart generates many vibrations that are transmitted through surrounding tissues to the chest wall. These arise from the contractile and expansile movements of the cardiac chambers, from valvular opening and closure, from tissue motion caused by blood flow, and from the bloodstream itself.

Vibrations having low frequency (0 to 30 cycles per second) cause subaudible chest wall pulsations that can be palpated when sufficiently forceful. Vibrations having higher frequency (30 to 500 cycles per second) enter the range of human audibility and can be heard at the chest surface when sufficiently loud. Such audible vibrations are called *heart sounds* when brief and *murmurs* when sustained. Figure 11–1 illustrates the sensitivity of the human ear to cardiovascular sound.

HEART SOUNDS AND MURMURS

The first heart sound (S_1) begins as the ventricles start to contract. Minor vibrations coinciding with the earliest contractile movement may initiate S_1, occurring as early as 0.02 to 0.03 sec after electrocardiographic QRS begins. The first major vibrations then commence 0.06 sec after the onset of QRS (Fig. 11–2), 0.02 to 0.04 sec after rising left ventricular pressure exceeds left atrial pressure. These vibrations begin at the instant the closing mitral leaflets meet—as demonstrated echocardiographically (Fig. 11–3A). Since these initial vibrations of S_1 coincide with mitral closure, the term *mitral component of S_1 or M_1* is applied.

A second set of vibrations begins about 0.03 sec after onset of M_1. This component coincides exactly with tricuspid closure (Fig. 11–3B); hence it is called the *tricuspid component of S_1, or T_1*. A few minor vibrations may follow T_1, completing the first heart sound. These final vibrations coincide with beginning movement of the aortic valve cusps and could derive from this structure. The total first sound lasts 0.04 to 0.10 sec, including the small initial and final oscillations.

The first sound is usually loudest over the cardiac apex, where M_1 predominates and T_1 is

normally absent or faint. At the lower left sternal border, T_1 is often well heard following M_1. Many normal individuals have distinct splitting of S_1 at this area (Figs. 11–4 and 11–5). When T_1 is accentuated, it may be louder than M_1 at the apex. When this occurs, abnormally forceful tricuspid closure is present, as commonly occurs with atrial septal defect. Ebstein's anomaly often causes a singularly loud and late T_1.

At the cardiac base, the normal S_1 consists primarily of M_1 unless T_1 is exaggerated.

The electrocardiographic P–R interval influences the intensity of S_1. Short intervals intensify S_1; long intervals diminish it. When P–R is less than 0.20, the intervals relate inversely to the loudness of S_1. Intervals longer than 0.20 are associated with faint first sounds. When P–R exceeds 0.50 sec, the first sound may recover normal intensity.

The first sound/P–R relationship is explained by the proximity of ventricular systole to atrial systole. The mitral and tricuspid leaflets are opened wide by atrial contraction. When ventricular systole occurs promptly, there is greater leaflet excursion than when ventricular contraction is delayed, allowing the leaflets to float passively together before systole begins. The loudness of S_1 varies directly with the magnitude of leaflet excursion.

Conditions that increase the force of ventricular contraction usually increase the intensity of the first sound. Such conditions include thyrotoxicosis, severe anemia, exercise, excitement, and stimulatory drugs such as epinephrine. Mitral stenosis, by stiffening the mitral leaflets, causes a loud and often high-pitched first sound. Conditions that diminish cardiac function, such as myocardial infarction and myxedema, tend to soften the first sound, irrespective of the P–R interval.

Obesity, left pneumothorax, emphysema, and pericardial or left pleural effusion may also diminish heart sounds owing to intervening tissue, fluid, or air.

Delayed onset of the first sound characterizes mitral stenosis, which impairs leaflet mobility and elevates left atrial pressure. The delay can be detected by measuring the interval between the onset of QRS on the electrocardiogram and the onset of the first major vibrations of the first sound as recorded on a phonocardiogram (normal <0.06). This measurement correlates with the severity of

*Supported in part by U.S. Public Health grants, The Benjamin May Memorial Fund, and Metropolitan Heart Guild.

†We wish to express our appreciation to Mr. Bernard Salb for his assistance in preparing this chapter.

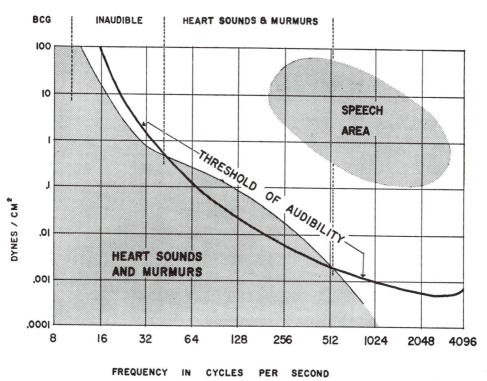

Figure 11–1 Graph illustrating the frequency spectrum of human hearing. Note that only a small component of total cardiac sound can be detected by the human ear. (Reprinted by permission from Butterworth, J. S., Chassin, M. R., and McGrath, R.: Cardiac Auscultation including Audiovisual Principles. 2nd ed. New York, Grune and Stratton, 1960.)

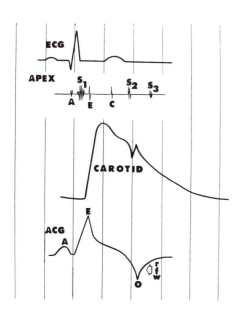

Figure 11–2 Heart sounds heard at the apex correlated with the electrocardiogram *(ECG),* carotid artery pulse tracing *(CAROTID),* and apex cardiogram *(ACG).*

Sound tracing: A = atrial sound or S_4 (left atrial); S_1 = first heart sound; E = aortic ejection sound; C = systolic click; S_2 = second heart sound; S_3 = ventricular filling sound.

Apex cardiogram *(ACG):* E = peak of apical impulse; O = beginning of ventricular rapid filling *(rfw).*

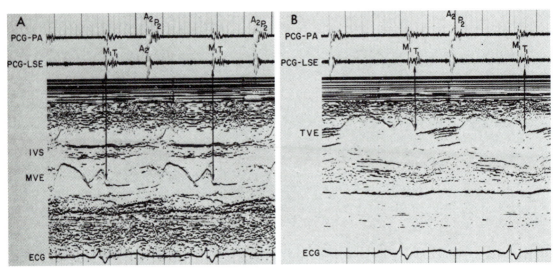

Figure 11-3 Echophonocardiogram from a young woman whose heart was normal except for right bundle branch block. *A*, The C point of the mitral valve echo *(MVE)* occurs at the time of M_1. *B*, The C point of the tricuspid valve echo *(TVE)* is coincident with T_1. *IVS* = interventricular septum. (From Waider, W., and Craige, E.: Am. J. Cardiol. *35*:346, 1975.)

mitral obstruction. Systemic hypertension may also delay the onset of the first heart sound.

When systolic ejection ends, aortic and pulmonary pressures exceed the declining pressures of the relaxing ventricles, causing the aortic and pulmonary valves to shut. The second heart sound (S_2) arises from this process. Normally, it splits into two distinct components, the first arising from aortic valve closure (A_2), the second arising from pulmonary valve closure (P_2).

Echocardiographic tracking of semilunar valve closure reveals this event to precede S_2 slightly, which occurs when the distending cusps close, arresting the rebounding backward surge of blood.

The aortic component (A_2) normally can be heard all over the precordium, being maximal in the aortic area. The pulmonary component (P_2) is usually loudest in the pulmonary area (Fig. 11–6) but often extends to the tricuspid region (Fig. 11–5). Hence, splitting of the second sound is best heard over the pulmonary area and along the mid-left sternal border (Figs. 11–5 and 11–6). Aortic closure usually causes a louder sound than pulmonary closure, even in the pulmonary region; however, in some young individuals P_2 may normally exceed A_2 in the pulmonary region.

The interval between aortic valve closure and A_2 averages 0.01 to 0.015 sec, whereas the interval between pulmonary valve closure and P_2 is longer, ranging from 0.03 to 0.09 sec. The greater distensibility of the pulmonary vascular bed probably accounts for this longer interval. When pulmonary capacity is further increased by inspiration, P_2 occurs even later. At the same time, inspiratory venous inflow lengthens right ventricular systole, delaying pulmonary valve closure, whereas inspi-

ratory increase in pulmonary vascular capacity reduces flow into the left heart, thereby shortening left ventricular systole and causing slightly earlier aortic valve closure. These inspiratory events, leading to earlier A_2 and later P_2, cause audibly widened splitting of the second heart sound in many normal people. Usually, expiration fuses the two components of S_2 (Fig. 11–4).

Inspiratory splitting of S_2 was first described by Potain in 1866 but then forgotten for many years until re-emphasized by Leatham in 1958.

Complete right bundle branch block, by retarding right ventricular depolarization, delays pulmonary valve closure, resulting in wide splitting of the second sound even during expiration; inspiration further widens the split. Conversely, conditions that prolong or delay left ventricular systole may cause A_2 to follow P_2. When this occurs, splitting increases with expiration and narrows with inspiration, a finding called *paradoxic (reversed) splitting of the second sound* (Fig. 11–7). Complete left bundle branch block commonly causes this phenomenon by impeding left ventricular depolarization and so delaying aortic closure. Severe aortic stenosis occasionally prolongs left ventricular ejection sufficiently to cause paradoxic splitting. Right ventricular pacing and right ventricular extrasystoles simulate left bundle branch block by depolarizing the right ventricle before the left, causing reversed splitting of S_2. Other infrequent causes of reversed splitting include patent ductus arteriosus, angina pectoris, myocardial infarction, and, rarely, systemic hypertension.

In uncomplicated atrial septal defect with significant left-to-right shunt, the right and left ventricles share a functionally common atrium and

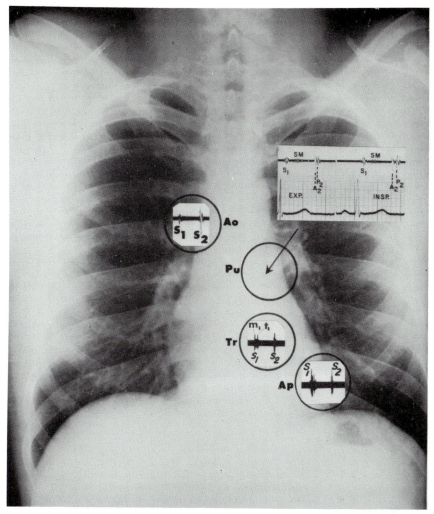

Figure 11–4 Heart sounds as heard over different valve areas. *Ao* = aortic area: Here the first sound *(S₁)* is faint and the second sound *(S₂)* is loud and single. *Pu* = pulmonary area: Here S₁ is reduced and S₂ is loud and split into two components, *A₂* (aortic closure) and *P₂* (pulmonary closure). The split S₂ widens with inspiration and narrows with expiration. *Tr* = tricuspid area: S₁ splits into two components, *M1* (mitral closure) and *T1* (tricuspid closure). *Ap* = apex: S₁ is loud with faint before and after vibrations. S₂ is single and less intense than S₁ at the apex. *SM* = systolic murmur; *INSP* = inspiration; *EXP* = expiration.

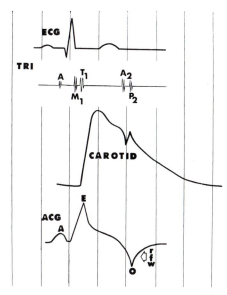

Figure 11– 5 Heart sounds heard over the tricuspid region *(TRI)* correlated with the electrocardiogram *(ECG)*, carotid artery pulse tracing *(CAROTID),* and apex cardiogram *(ACG).*

Sound tracing: *A* = atrial sound or S₄ (right atrial); *M₁* = mitral valve closure sound; *T₁* = tricuspid valve closure sound; *A₂* = aortic valve closure sound; *P₂* = pulmonary valve closure sound.

Apex cardiogram *(ACG): E* = peak of apical impulse; *O* = beginning of ventricular rapid filling *(rfw).*

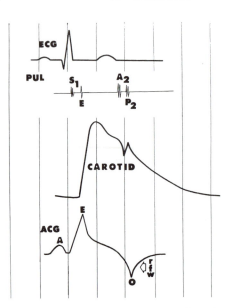

Figure 11–6 Heart sounds heard over the pulmonary area *(PUL)* correlated with the electrocardiogram *(ECG)*, carotid artery pulse tracing *(CAROTID)*, and apex cardiogram *(ACG)*.

Sound tracing: S_1 = first heart sound; E = pulmonary ejection sound; A_2 = aortic valve closure sound; P_2 = pulmonary valve closure sound.

Apex cardiogram (ACG): E = peak of apical impulse; O = beginning of ventricular rapid filling *(rfw)*.

have similar duration of systole. A_2 and P_2 remain clearly separate during both inspiration and expiration, exhibiting little or no respiratory variation (Fig. 11–8). This phenomenon, known as *fixed splitting,* characterizes left-to-right shunting of blood at the atrial level and is a valuable diagnostic sign, although occasional patients with atrial septal defects may present normal splitting of S_2.

Splitting of S_2 is "fixed" and widened in atrial septal defect because P_2 is unduly delayed. Although left and right ventricular systole end together, the copious pulmonary vascular bed takes longer than usual to reverse pulmonary flow and distend the pulmonary cusps. This mechanism explains persistence of "fixed" splitting of S_2 in some patients after surgical closure of atrial defects, since large pulmonary vascular capacity persists.

Pulmonary or systemic hypertension produces forceful closure of the pulmonary or aortic valve. Loud A_2 or P_2 often accompanies aortic or pulmonary hypertension. The accentuated P_2 of pulmonary hypertension is sometimes palpable, if sought. It often occurs early, close to, or fused with A_2, causing a resounding single S_2 over the pulmonary area. This results from the quick reversal of pulmonary blood flow upon valve closure, owing to the high resistance–low capacity vascular bed of severe pulmonary hypertension. Cor pulmonale due to either acute massive pulmonary embolism or chronic lung disease may lengthen right ventricular systole. In these cases, P_2 is both loud and late; the second sound becomes widely split, with accentuation of the delayed pulmonary component. The hyperactive circulation of thyrotoxicosis or severe anemia also intensifies the second sound; however, these disorders also increase the first heart sound, unlike hypertension, which selectively augments the second sound.

Impaired mobility of a semilunar valve will diminish its closure sound. The aortic second sound of calcific aortic stenosis is sometimes faint or even absent, whereas congenital aortic stenosis with its supple valve structure usually generates a normal or increased closure sound. Severe pulmonary stenosis greatly diminishes (and delays) P_2 (Fig. 11–12), whereas mild pulmonary stenosis does so only slightly.

Posterior location of the pulmonary valve, as in certain congenital defects such as transposition of the great vessels, may also diminish or even abolish P_2.

Most children and many young adults have a normal third heart sound (S_3) in early diastole. This sound coincides with the rapid filling phase of left ventricular diastole and is variously known as a *physiologic third sound,* a *ventricular filling sound,* or simply S_3. Its genesis is unclear; it probably derives from sudden deceleration of the

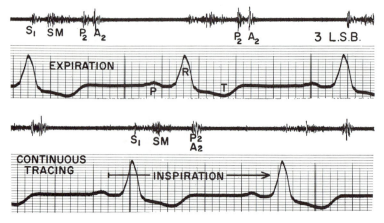

Figure 11–7 Paradoxical splitting of the second sound. The aortic valve closure sound *(A₂)* follows the pulmonary valve closure sound *(P₂)*. Inspiration delays P_2, narrowing the split. Compare with Figure 11–4, which illustrates normal inspiratory separation of A_2 and P_2. S_1 = first heart sound; *SM* = systolic murmur. (Reproduced from Levine, S. A., and Harvey, W. P.: Clinical Auscultation of the Heart. 2d ed. Philadelphia, W. B. Saunders Co., 1959.)

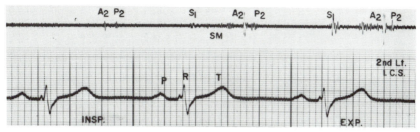

Figure 11–8 Fixed splitting of the second sound. Widely split second sound without significant respiratory variation of the interval between aortic closure *(A₂)* and pulmonary closure *(P₂)*. This finding characterizes most individuals with atrial septal defect. S_1 = first heart sound; *SM* = systolic murmur.

dilating left ventricular wall during early diastolic rapid filling. The third heart sound is low pitched, best heard at the apex, and usually faint, although occasionally this sound is prominent and may have after-vibrations that extend its duration. Although a third sound during left ventricular rapid filling is physiologic during childhood and youth, this sound in middle life and beyond denotes cardiac dysfunction, usually myocardial failure. It is an early and subtle sign of cardiac decompensation, having great diagnostic and prognostic value. Its detection often requires deliberate listening in a quiet room. Occasionally, regurgitant disease of the aortic or mitral valve exaggerates ventricular filling enough to produce a third sound.

Another extra heart sound may occur during atrial systole. This sound, known as the *atrial sound, or fourth heart sound (S₄),* probably arises from sudden deceleration of the left ventricular wall as it dilates during atrial contraction—the same mechanism that creates S₃. Atrial sounds may be heard in apparently healthy individuals, particularly in the older age groups. When atrioventricular block separates atrial from ventricular contraction, atrial sounds frequently become audible. Audible right atrial sounds are never normal.

Left atrial sounds begin about 0.17 sec (range: 0.14 to 0.24) after the onset of the electrocardiographic P, coinciding with the peak of the precordial atrial movement. The sound is low-pitched, apical, and usually faint. Its closeness to the first sound at times may simulate wide splitting of the first sound. Firm stethoscope pressure will frequently eliminate the low frequency atrial sound, but will not abolish M₁ or T₁. When prominent, the sound can be heard medial to the apex, sometimes extending to the sternal border. Right atrial sounds begin about 0.12 sec (range: 0.09 to 0.16) after the onset of P and are low pitched, usually faint, and best heard over the tricuspid area. Right atrial sounds may increase during inspiration. Faint vibrations often can be recorded preceding an audible atrial sound; these vibrations, usually inaudible, probably arise from myocardial contraction.

Atrial sounds are likely to appear whenever there is increased resistance to ventricular filling.

Various myocardial diseases impede ventricular filling by reducing myocardial compliance and thereby cause atrial sounds. Cardiomyopathies frequently cause atrial sounds; the concentric hypertrophy of aortic stenosis and systemic hypertension also stiffens the ventricular wall, leading to vigorous atrial contraction. Atrial sounds regularly accompany these diseases. Acute myocardial infarction often causes high diastolic ventricular filling pressure, low ventricular compliance, and atrioventricular block; hence, atrial sounds appear in most patients with acute myocardial infarction and frequently persist after the acute stage.

When atrial and ventricular diastolic sounds result from heart disease, the term *gallop rhythm* is often applied, because these extra sounds impart the cadence of a cantering horse to the heart rhythm—particularly when the ventricular rate is rapid. Thus, the atrial and ventricular sounds of heart disease are usually called *gallop sounds.* A patient with cardiac failure may have a ventricular (or third sound) gallop, an atrial (or fourth sound) gallop, or both. When tachycardia is present, a diastolic gallop sound may be difficult to classify. When slowing occurs, identification can be made by noting a constant relationship of the ventricular gallop to the second sound and a constant relationship of the atrial gallop to the electrocardiographic P and, usually, to the first sound (Fig. 11–9).

Atrial and ventricular sounds frequently coexist *(quadruple rhythm).* When close together, this combination of sounds may resemble a short, low-pitched rumbling murmur. At times, as in an occasional patient with cardiomyopathy, the rumble is erroneously diagnosed as mitral stenosis. When diastole so shortens that these sounds fuse, a single sound may result, known as a *summation gallop sound.*

Patients with constrictive pericarditis often present an extra sound in early diastole (often designated "pericardial knock") that coincides with sudden arrest of the expanding ventricle as the constricting pericardium abruptly halts diastolic filling.

A third sound often follows closely upon the second sound in mitral stenosis. Known as the

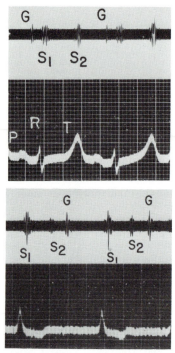

Figure 11–9 Upper panel displays a gallop sound *(G)* related to atrial systole. This sound is known as an "atrial gallop," an "atrial sound," or a "fourth heart sound *(S₄).*" S_1 = first heart sound; S_2 = second heart sound.

Lower panel displays a gallop sound *(G)* related to ventricular rapid filling. This sound is known as a "ventricular filling sound," a "ventricular gallop," or a "third heart sound *(S₃).*" S_1 = first heart sound; S_2 = second heart sound.

opening snap, it probably derives from the suddenly arrested descent (or "checking") of the stiffened mitral valve that occurs as the valve opens in early diastole (Fig. 11–10). This sound signifies the end of isovolumetric relaxation; it is usually high-pitched and best heard at the apex but can transmit widely. It follows the aortic closure sound by 0.06 to 0.12 sec. This measurement, which can be readily made with a phonocardiogram and approximated by careful auscultation, correlates with the severity of mitral obstruction, the shorter A_2-opening snap periods corresponding to higher grades of stenosis. This interval varies with heart rate, since shorter cycle lengths are associated with higher left atrial pressure and earlier mitral valve opening. When mitral stenosis greatly reduces valve mobility, as with dense calcification, the mitral opening snap may become fainter and occasionally disappears.

An opening snap may rarely occur without valvular stenosis when vigorous blood flow causes brisk opening and forceful arrest of the descending leaflets. Atrial septal defect, mitral regurgitation, thyrotoxicosis, and other high-flow conditions occasionally cause opening snaps.

Extra heart sounds also occur during systole. Patients with congenital aortic or pulmonary stenosis often have an early systolic sound that closely follows the first sound. Known as an *aortic or pulmonary ejection sound,* it signifies the end of isovolumetric contraction, coinciding with the maximum excursion of the deformed semilunar valve and the beginning of ejection. Loudness of ejection sounds correlates with the magnitude of valve cusp movement. Aortic ejection sounds are best heard in the aortic area (Fig. 11–12) and at the apex (Fig. 11–2). Pulmonary ejection sounds are best heard in the pulmonary area (Figs. 11–6 and 11–12) and characteristically diminish with inspiration; they are generally faint or absent at the apex. Ejection sounds often occur with pulmonary or systemic hypertension or with abnormal dilatation of the ascending aorta or pulmonary artery; these ejection sounds arise from vigorous opening movement of the semilunar cusps. An aortic ejection sound may be heard over the aortic and apical areas with coarctation of the aorta, and a pulmonary ejection sound is common with idiopathic dilatation of the pulmonary artery. Aortic ejection sounds can occur with thyrotoxicosis and other high-output states.

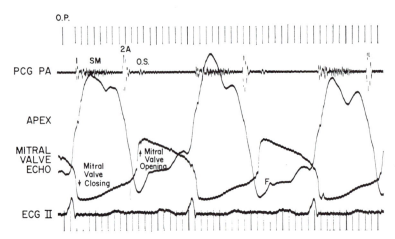

Figure 11–10 The apex cardiogram permits precise timing of the onset of ventricular systole, as signified by the upstroke of the systolic movement. Note that the mitral valve is in a relatively wide open position at the onset of ventricular contraction. *F* = filling wave. (From Fortuin, N. J., and Craige, E.: Br. Heart J. *35*:75, 1973.)

Other sounds may also occur during systolic ejection; such sounds are frequently brief and high-pitched and therefore called "clicks." The "midsystolic click" is a commonly used expression denoting the usual timing of such sounds (Figs. 11–2 and 11–11). A murmur may follow the click, occupying late systole (v.i.). Systolic clicks—with or without a murmur—arise from prolapse of one or both mitral leaflets into the left atrium during systole. This entity is also called "floppy valve syndrome," "billowing valve syndrome," and "Barlow's disease." Angiograms of patients with this finding commonly demonstrate one or both mitral leaflets to be so copious as to prolapse into the left atrium during late systole, permitting regurgitation; the posterior leaflet is most commonly involved. The click coincides with maximum leaflet excursion and probably arises from the suddenly arrested motion of the affected leaflet(s) and chordae tendineae. Clicks may be single or multiple. The standing position may intensify clicks, cause them to occur earlier in systole, or produce clicks not audible during recumbency.

Audible vibrations that persist beyond the brief acoustic impact of a discrete heart sound constitute a heart *murmur;* a murmur is a rapid succession of heart sounds. Most investigators have attributed murmurs to blood flow through irregular or narrowed orifices or through dilated segments of major arteries, through abnormal intracardiac and arteriovenous communications, or backward through incompetent valves. Murmurs also can arise from rapid blood flow through normal structures. The actual genesis of murmur vibrations has not been established with certainty. There are two sources of sound that account for the many varieties of murmurs: the bloodstream itself and solid structures that are caused to vibrate by flowing blood. Murmurs arising from the blood itself are thought to derive from vortex (eddy) formation or from turbulence created as blood flows through different orifices, chambers, and tubes at varying rates. Murmurs arising from solid structures usually represent the vibrations of heart valves or other cardiac or vascular tissue set into motion by the bloodstream.

Murmurs are classified according to timing, location, and loudness. Most murmurs are either systolic or diastolic; murmurs that continue throughout systole and diastole are called *continuous murmurs.* The examiner may categorize loudness according to six grades of intensity. Grade I murmurs are so faint that intent listening is required over several cardiac cycles. Grade II murmurs are also faint but audible immediately upon listening. Grades III and IV represent increasing loudness. Grade VI murmurs are so loud as to be audible through the stethoscope head held just off the chest wall. Grade V murmurs are very loud but cannot be heard off the chest. Grades IV, V, and VI murmurs cause palpable chest wall vibrations, felt by the hand as a gentle, throbbing sensation resembling the purr of a cat. This finding, known as a *thrill,* occurs where the murmur is loudest and represents the tactile counterpart of a loud murmur. The significance of a thrill is that of the underlying murmur.

The examiner localizes the murmur according to the area of maximal intensity. Thus, he may record a grade III apical systolic murmur or a grade II pulmonary diastolic murmur or a grade VI aortic systolic murmur. Many murmurs have

Figure 11–11 Upper left panel displays the holosystolic murmur of severe mitral regurgitation. The murmur *(sm)* extends from the first sound *(S₁)* to the second sound *(S₂)*.

Lower left panel displays the late systolic murmur *(sm)* of mitral regurgitation due to prolapse of posterior mitral leaflet. S_1 = first sound; S_2 = second sound; C = systolic click; sm = systolic murmur.

Vertical panel on right displays the systolic murmur *(SM)* of acute mitral regurgitation due to rupture of chordae tendineae. Note rapid decline of systolic vibrations in late systole *(arrows).* Upper sound tracing recorded in aortic area *(2 i-s);* lower sound tracing recorded over the cardiac apex. S_1 = first heart sound; S_2 = second heart sound.

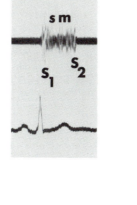

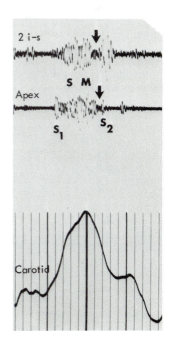

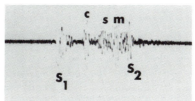

special pitch characteristics that merit description. Thus, diastolic flow across a stenotic mitral valve causes low-pitched vibrations usually described as a *rumble*. A high-pitched murmur is often called a *blow* or *blowing murmur*. Another category, the musical murmur, includes many curious harmonic patterns colorfully labeled "seagull," "cooing dove," "twanging string," and other epithets. The musical tonality derives from a single predominating frequency that usually arises from a vibrating structure within the heart, such as a perforated valve cusp or ruptured chordae tendineae.

Expert auscultation refines timing beyond the simple designation of systolic, diastolic, or continuous. A murmur may extend throughout systole or may be limited to early or late systole. A murmur may steadily intensify (crescendo), may steadily decline (decrescendo), or may have a midway loudness peak. Such variations often have meaning and should be noted. The term *holosystolic* (or *pansystolic*) signifies vibrations that commence with the first heart sound and cease at the second heart sound. A holosystolic murmur invariably indicates systolic regurgitation through the mitral or tricuspid valve or through a ventricular septal defect. Holosystolic murmurs are often called *regurgitant murmurs*. These murmurs are holosystolic because left ventricular pressure exceeds left atrial pressure throughout systole (mitral regurgitation) or because right ventricular pressure exceeds right atrial pressure throughout systole (tricuspid regurgitation) or because left ventricular pressure exceeds right ventricular pressure throughout systole (ventricular septal defect).

The systolic murmur of significant mitral regurgitation is typically a holosystolic murmur, heard best at the cardiac apex (Fig. 11–11). However, this lesion does not always generate a holosystolic murmur. Mild to moderate mitral incompetence often causes a decrescendo systolic murmur that subsides before S_2. The regurgitation of mitral valve prolapse is usually limited to late systole, causing a late systolic murmur. Acute mitral regurgitation causes a murmur that is loud in early and mid systole, decreasing in late systole but remaining holosystolic. The murmur of acute mitral regurgitation diminishes in late systole because the tense left atrial wall of sudden mitral incompetence does not dilate in response to overfilling; instead, mounting left atrial pressure develops during ventricular systole until atrial pressure exceeds the declining pressure of late ventricular systole, thereby reducing regurgitation and its resultant murmur in late systole (Fig. 11–11). This murmur often transmits well to the cardiac base.

The most frequent cause of chronic, pure mitral regurgitation—occurring as a solitary lesion—is mitral valve prolapse. The murmur of prolapse is commonly initiated by one or more systolic clicks as described previously (Fig. 11–11). The Valsalva maneuver or standing posture may move the click(s) earlier and lengthen the murmur or produce it, if previously unheard. Occasionally, mitral valve prolapse produces a holosystolic murmur; such may develop after infective endocarditis or rupture of chordae tendineae or both.

Mitral regurgitation—as an isolated chronic disorder—is seldom due to rheumatic fever. However, mitral regurgitation commonly accompanies rheumatic mitral stenosis or rheumatic aortic valve disease or both. Rheumatic fever residua include fused leaflets and short, thick, fused chordae tendineae that impede normal valve closure. Rheumatic mitral regurgitation may cause a musical murmur that is due to the dominant frequencies generated by the deformed valve.

Left ventricular dilatation of any cause may displace the papillary muscles and dilate the mitral annulus, disrupting normal valve closure. Left atrial enlargement itself may further impede closure by exerting traction on the mitral annulus. Other causes of mitral regurgitation recognized with increasing frequency are papillary muscle dysfunction, ruptured chordae tendineae, calcified mitral annulus fibrosus, myxomatous mitral cusps, bacterial endocarditis, endocardial fibroelastosis, and various congenital anomalies.

The systolic murmur of tricuspid regurgitation is maximal in the fourth left interspace at the lower sternal edge. It may be holosystolic but sometimes fades out in the latter half of systole. It is often faint and easily overlooked. The murmur usually becomes louder during inspiration. This important characteristic results from the increased right ventricular filling caused by inspiration. Respiratory change can be subtle, requiring careful listening. Tricuspid regurgitation may result from leaflet deformity due to rheumatic fever. It is peculiarly common in heroin addicts, resulting from tricuspid bacterial endocarditis in these individuals. Tricuspid regurgitation frequently accompanies severe right ventricular hypertension of any cause, since dilatation of the right ventricle may displace the papillary muscles and/or dilate the tricuspid ring to such an extent that normal valve closure is not possible.

Blood flow across an irregular or stenotic semilunar valve causes a systolic murmur that commences after the first sound, increases to a peak in the middle third of systole, and then declines in late systole, ceasing before closure of the affected pulmonary or aortic valve. Sound tracings reveal a diamond shape; this acoustic pattern has been termed an *ejection murmur*. Such murmurs are often harsh and loud, radiate widely, and may be associated with decreased intensity of A_2 or P_2 when valvular stenosis reduces leaflet mobility (Fig. 11–12).

Murmurs of aortic and pulmonary stenosis are generally loudest at the aortic or pulmonary areas of the chest wall, respectively. Good transmission

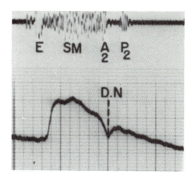

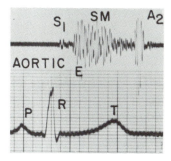

Figure 11-12 Upper panel displays the ejection systolic murmur of pulmonary valve stenosis. Note the pulmonary ejection sound (E), which initiates the diamond-contoured murmur, which subsides before a late and softened pulmonary closure sound (P_2). A_2 = aortic closure sound; SM = systolic murmur; DN = dicrotic incisura.

Lower panel displays the systolic ejection murmur of aortic stenosis. This murmur begins after S_1, has midsystolic peak, and then declines before aortic closure (A_2). E = aortic ejection sound; SM = systolic murmur; S_1 = first heart sound.

to the clavicles and neck characterizes the murmurs of semilunar valve stenosis, although in older patients with aortic stenosis, particularly those with increased anteroposterior chest diameter, the aortic murmur may be loudest at the apex and sometimes has a high-frequency musical quality.

Some ejection murmurs relate to high velocity of blood flow through a normal semilunar valve. Such murmurs are common in conditions such as thyrotoxicosis, pregnancy, fever, excitement, and other states that increase stroke volume. Murmurs like these, which do not arise from structural alteration within the heart, are called *functional murmurs,* in contrast to those arising from anatomic defects, which are called *organic (significant) murmurs.*

Innocent murmurs are those that arise in healthy individuals who have no evidence of increased cardiac output or other circulatory alteration. They are most common in children but are also frequently encountered in the adult. The usual murmur is early to midsystolic, of grade I or II intensity, occasionally grade III. It is most common in the lower, left parasternal region or in the pulmonary area, although also frequently heard over the aortic and apical areas. Innocent murmurs are seldom loudest at the apex. The genesis of these murmurs is not known, although some appear to arise from high-velocity blood flow through the aortic or pulmonic valves.

Most systolic murmurs are innocent; most diastolic murmurs are organic. Abnormal vibrations during diastole usually result from regurgitation through an incompetent aortic or pulmonary valve or from stenosis of the mitral or tricuspid valve. Incompetence of a semilunar valve leads to a high-pitched descrescendo murmur, commencing with A_2 or P_2 and subsiding in mid- or late diastole (Fig. 11-13). Incompetence of the aortic valve results from the leaflet thickening and fusion of rheumatic fever; from dilatation of the aortic valve ring and separation of cusps associated with syphilis or ankylosing (rheumatoid) spondylitis; from cusp perforation or laceration due to bacterial endocarditis or injury; from cusp prolapse due to either dissecting aneurysm or loss of supporting septal tissue with certain ventricular septal defects; or from poor apposition of congenital bicuspid leaflets. All these anatomic deformities permit regurgitation when aortic pressure exceeds ventricular pressure during diastole. This pressure differential is highest in early diastole and declines as aortic pressure declines, hence the decrescendo pattern of murmur intensity.

Pulmonary valve insufficiency most commonly results from marked pulmonary arterial hypertension. Elevated pulmonary artery diastolic pressure may dilate the pulmonary valve ring sufficiently to prevent complete cusp apposition. A high-pitched, usually soft, decrescendo murmur is heard in the pulmonary region. Rarely, congenital deformity of the pulmonary leaflets permits regurgitation. Here the pulmonary artery pressure is normal and the diastolic pressure gradient across the valve is small. The murmur may be similar to that caused by pulmonary hypertension but in some patients it is short, is medium- to low-pitched, and does not commence promptly with P_2 but develops in early diastole, separated from P_2 by a brief pause (Fig. 11-13). It also may increase coincident with inspiration.

The low-pitched apical diastolic murmur or rumble of mitral stenosis is separated from the second sound by a brief interval (0.06 to 0.12 sec) that corresponds to the left ventricular isovolumetric relaxation period. The rumble begins when the mitral valve opens and blood flows through the obstructed orifice at greater than normal velocity. The murmur usually commences with the mitral opening snap sound. As the pressure gradient between atrium and ventricle subsides in mid and late diastole, the rumble diminishes. If atrial systole, by raising left atrial pressure or constricting the mitral orifice, or both, increases the gradient, the murmur will accentuate just

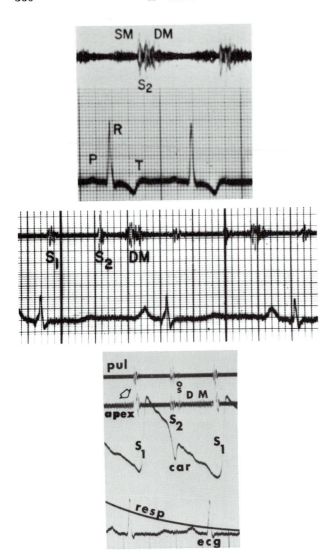

Figure 11–13 Upper panel displays the decrescendo diastolic murmur *(DM)* of aortic regurgitation, which begins at aortic closure *(S₂)* and fades out in late diastole. Most patients with significant aortic regurgitation have a systolic ejection murmur in the aortic region as shown here *(SM).*

Middle panel displays the short, early diastolic murmur *(DM)* of congenital pulmonary regurgitation. Note the brief pause between the second heart sound *(S₂)* and the onset of this diamond-contoured murmur, which subsides quickly as pulmonary artery and right ventricular pressure equalize in middiastole. S_1 = first heart sound. (Reprinted by permission from Collins, N., Braunwald, E., and Morrow, A.: Am. J. Med. *28:*159, 1960.)

Lower panel depicts the rumbling diastolic murmur *(DM)* of mitral stenosis, which begins after opening snap *(OS),* which is present in the pulmonary area *(pul)* as well as at the apex. The murmur accentuates with atrial systole (arrow). *Car* = carotid pulse; *resp* = respiration; *ecg* = electrocardiogram.

before the first sound, creating a crescendo rumble terminating in the exaggerated first sound of mitral stenosis (Fig. 11–13). Although atrial fibrillation abolishes atrial systole, thereby reducing the velocity of presystolic flow, a crescendo presystolic murmur may persist, owing to early systolic contraction of the mitral ring while blood still flows into the ventricle. Sometimes the presystolic rumble disappears altogether with atrial fibrillation. It may also persist, only with shorter cycles.

Tricuspid stenosis causes a diastolic murmur that is similar to the rumble of mitral stenosis but usually subsides earlier in diastole, probably because the gradient across the stenotic tricuspid valve is generally smaller than that across the stenotic mitral valve. This murmur is maximal along the lower left parasternal region. It characteristically accentuates with inspiration. This interesting diagnostic feature relates to increased venous return to the right atrium and greater flow through the tricuspid valve as inspiration lowers intrathoracic pressure, thereby facilitating venous flow into the chest.

One of the most striking cardiac murmurs is that caused by patent ductus arteriosus and other arteriovenous communications. Since arterial pressure exceeds venous pressure throughout the cardiac cycle, such murmurs extend from systole through S_2 into diastole, waxing and waning as pressure gradients and flow velocity wax and wane. The murmur is termed *continuous* and may be high-pitched but often contains loud vibrations of medium and low frequency. When this is so, the murmur has a characteristic musical cadence that has earned the descriptive label of *machinery murmur.* The murmur of patent ductus arteriosus waxes in late systole, peaking at S_2 and declining during diastole. This contour relates to the larger pressure gradient at this time between upper descending aorta and main pulmonary trunk. These

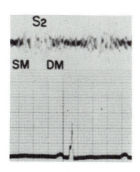

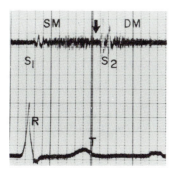

Figure 11–14 Upper panel displays the continuous murmur of patent ductus arteriosus, which persists throughout the cardiac cycle, reaching its peak in late systole and early diastole, forming an envelope about the second sound (*S₂*). SM = systolic component of murmur; *DM* = diastolic component of murmur. Contrast this murmur with the to-and-fro systolic *(SM)* and diastolic *(DM)* murmurs of ventricular septal defect and aortic regurgitation seen in the lower panel. Note declining late systolic vibrations *(arrow)* in contrast to the late systolic crescendo of the continuous murmur.

murmurs must be distinguished from the "to-and-fro" systolic and diastolic murmur of aortic stenosis and regurgitation or of ventricular septal defect and aortic regurgitation that do not envelop S₂ as does the continuous murmur of patent ductus arteriosus (Fig. 11–14).

Pericarditis causes a characteristic rough, scraping sound called a *pericardial friction rub*. The inflamed pericardial and epicardial surfaces move against each other to create this sound. Since the rub relates to movement, it occurs with three major movements of the cardiac cycle—atrial sys-

tole, early ventricular systole, and rapid ventricular diastolic filling. Therefore, the typical friction rub will often have three discrete, high-pitched grating noises corresponding to the cardiac movements described (Fig. 11–15). Frequently, only two components can be heard, as when atrial fibrillation eliminates atrial systole; rarely, only a single rub is present.

The sounds are usually maximal over the lower left parasternal area and often have to be sought intently, with the stethoscope diaphragm pressed firmly against the skin. A typical three-component pericardial friction rub is a highly specific and therefore valuable finding that indicates the presence of some form of pericarditis. A two-component rub is also important evidence of pericardial disease, but a single rubbing sound does not reliably implicate the pericardium, since an occasional cardiac murmur has a similar scratchy or grating quality. The pericarditis is nearly always acute, although chronic pericardial disease, such as a calcified plaque, may rarely account for a pericardial rub.

PRECORDIAL MOVEMENTS

Four major pulsations dominate the precordial movement pattern. These are (1) a brief, small outward thrust coinciding with atrial contraction; (2) a larger, brisk outward movement that starts during isovolumetric contraction and is followed quickly by (3) a steep, inward movement as systolic ejection begins; and (4) an outward movement that develops in early diastole and that corresponds to ventricular filling. This last movement ascends at first rapidly, then more slowly, to a diastolic plateau that precedes the next atrial systole.

Improved recording techniques and hemodynamic correlation have led to better understanding of chest wall motion. The most prevalent method of recording these movements is apex cardiography. According to this technique, a funnel or cup pickup is held to the precordium over the cardiac apex; chest wall displacement causes this device to transmit impulses to a transducer recording system (Fig. 11–16). The pulsations are so inscribed that upward deflections indicate outward

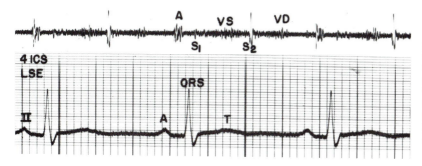

Figure 11–15 The typical pericardial friction rub has three components corresponding to the three major movements of the cardiac cycle: atrial systole *(A)*, ventricular systole *(VS)*, and early diastolic filling *(VD)*. *4ICS/LSE* = fourth intercostal space, left sternal edge. S₁ = first heart sound; S₂ = second heart sound.

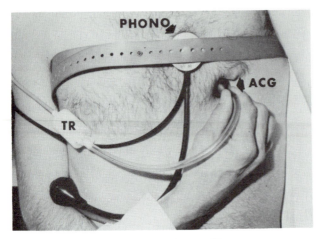

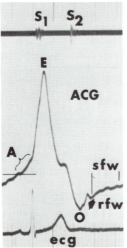

Figure 11–16 The upper panel depicts the recording of an apex cardiogram by means of a funnel that is handheld over the apex and that transmits the increased air pressure caused by displacement to a transducer and graphic recorder. *Phono* = phonocardiographic microphone; *ACG* = apex cardiographic funnel pickup; *TR* = transducer.

The lower panel displays the apex cardiogram *(ACG)* of a healthy young male adult. Note the four major precordial movements: atrial contraction *(A);* early systolic outward thrust peaking at *E;* steep downward deflection following *E,* representing systolic retraction (nadir of the systolic inward movement, labeled *O,* approximates atrioventricular valve opening); outward diastolic movement to the presystolic baseline, commencing at *O,* with the brisk upward deflection of rapid ventricular filling *(rfw)* followed by the more gradual ascending deflection of slow ventricular filling *(sfw).*

movements and downward deflections represent inward movements. The apex cardiograph best records localized impulses, since diffuse pulsations that move the pickup device as a whole do not adequately register. For this reason, recordings usually are made with the patient turned on his left side so as to exaggerate the cardiac apex impulse.

Figure 11–16 depicts a normal apex cardiogram. Note the four major movements just described: a small atrial thrust, labeled *A,* is followed by a steep upward deflection corresponding to beginning ventricular contraction. Systolic ejection starts at *E,* whereupon the tracing descends, at first steeply but then more slowly, leveling off in late systole. The curve descends abruptly again in early diastole to a nadir labeled *O.* At this point, the mitral valve opens and rapid diastolic filling begins, causing a steeply ascending deflection followed by a more gradual ascent during slow ventricular filling until atrial systole starts another cardiac cycle.

Other recording systems are more precise than apex cardiography but seldom used because of the additional time and trouble. Among these are kinetocardiography and displacement cardiography; both these methods use externally supported pickup devices that register movements much as the palpating hand perceives them. Figure 11–17 displays the flexible metal bellows pickup used for kinetocardiography and portrays a normal apical impulse recorded by this means. The four major movements are readily seen, although the contour differs from that of the apex cardiogram.

Displacement cardiography (DCG) is another recording system that produces curves similar to kinetocardiograms. This method records the changing electromagnetic field of the moving heart by means of an oscillator suspended above the precordium.

Aside from these recording methods, there are other techniques, such as impulse cardiography and precordial accelerocardiography, that yield useful information when properly interpreted.

Numerous physiologic studies of intracardiac pressure and flow as well as bidimensional angiocardiography have clarified the cardiac events that cause precordial pulsations. Normally, only the

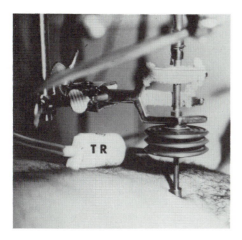

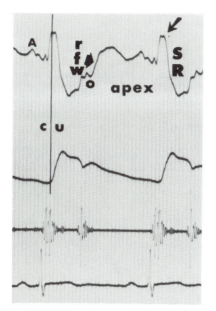

Figure 11–17 The upper panel depicts the recording of a kinetocardiogram with a flexible metal bellows probe held to the chest wall by external support. Air pressure changes within the bellows—as caused by chest wall displacement—are transmitted to a transducer *(TR)* and graphic recorder.

The lower panel displays a normal apex kinetocardiogram recorded with carotid pulse, heart sound, and electrocardiographic tracings. Note the four major movements: atrial *(A)*, apical impulse *(arrow)*, systolic retraction *(SR)*, and early diastolic filling *(rfw)*. *CU* = carotid upstroke; *O* = beginning of ventricular filling.

ventricles contact the chest wall, the right ventricle underlying the lower left parasternal area while the left ventricle relates to the lateral precordium at the cardiac apex. The right ventricle, therefore, is the anterior ventricle that accounts for most of the anterior surface of the heart.

During atrial systole, the ventricles move slightly forward, causing a diffuse outward precordial movement that is not normally palpable but is readily recorded. As systolic contraction begins, a brief outward thrust occurs that can be recorded across the precordium and that is often palpable in the fourth or fifth left intercostal space within 10 cm of the midsternal line. This movement represents the apical impulse or point of maximal impulse (PMI). It corresponds anatomically to the anteroseptal region of the left ventricle above the actual apex. The apex impulse begins during isovolumetric contraction. When the left ventricular base begins to descend, the heart rotates slightly counterclockwise, and the apex thrusts against the chest wall. The impulse rises briskly to a peak that coincides with the onset of left ventricular ejection. At this instant the outward thrust quickly retracts; during the remainder of systole the apex tracing registers sustained retraction. This inward component of the systolic precordial movement sequence is larger and more prolonged than the apical impulse yet is less easily appreciated. Systolic retraction is diffuse; it can be detected sometimes by observing the motion of an unheld stethoscope head resting on the left parasternal precordium during held expiration. As ventricular contraction ceases, the atrioventricular valves open, ventricular rapid filling begins, and the retracted precordium returns to its preatrial systolic baseline—at first swiftly, then more slowly. This movement can usually be recorded but is not normally seen or felt.

Increased left ventricular volume due to hypertrophy or dilatation or both affects the location, amplitude, duration, and area of the apical impulse. Normally, in the supine posture, this impulse occupies an area less than 3 cm in diameter and is confined to one interspace. Increased area often indicates underlying cardiac disease but may represent normal heart action in young, slender individuals, particularly when the anteroposterior chest diameter is narrowed by sternal depression, by straightening of the thoracic spine, or by simple disproportion between the lateral and anteroposterior chest dimensions that places the heart closer than usual to the anterior chest wall.

It is difficult to establish normal values for amplitude of chest wall pulsations. Most recording techniques do not accurately quantitate movements, although some investigators have developed measurable values that are useful when properly interpreted. Every physician must determine for himself what constitutes normal amplitude by palpating many normal patients and developing a "feel" for the average apical impulse. Abnormal amplitude often indicates underlying heart disease but may occur in patients with normal hearts and overactive circulation due to thyrotoxicosis, severe anemia, or other extracardiac causes of high cardiac output. Increased outward excursion of the apical impulse also may occur in young patients with slender chest configuration, especially if anteroposterior diameter is narrow.

Left ventricular hypertrophy and dilatation of any cause can heighten the amplitude and extend the area of apical impulse and may also displace it leftward. Conditions that greatly increase left ventricular diastolic volume such as severe aortic or mitral regurgitation cause the most marked displacement of the apical impulse. Conditions that elevate left ventricular systolic pressure, such as aortic stenosis and hypertension, do not increase total left ventricular volume as much as the regurgitant disorders just cited. Hence, leftward displacement of the apical impulse is found later in pressure overloading than in volume overloading conditions.

The normal apex impulse is a quick, early systolic thrust. Prolongation of this movement is an important and sensitive indication of abnormality. Impulse duration is easily measured on recordings and readily appreciated on palpation, especially if the examiner auscultates at the same time. Abnormally sustained outward movement correlates better with early left ventricular hypertrophy than does any other impulse characteristic and sometimes better than does the electrocardiogram or radiograph. Prolongation of the apical impulse is a more specific abnormality than increased amplitude or area, since there is little overlap with the normal brief impulse. Moreover, the patient with sustained systolic outward movement often has reduced stroke volume and ejection fraction as compared with the patient with abnormally heightened but unsustained apical impulse who usually has normal stroke volume and ejection fraction. Thus, the prolonged apical impulse is not only a more specific but often a more serious finding. Figure 11–18 displays the sustained outward apex movement of a patient with advanced left ventricular hypertrophy and dilatation.

Mitral regurgitation may cause a characteristic precordial movement pattern. Initially, this lesion can cause leftward displacement of a localized pulsation that may evolve, with increasing duration and severity of disease, into a diffuse, systolic impulse, extending from apex to sternum owing to medial rotation of the anterior left ventricular wall. A prominent late systolic outward movement especially characterizes mitral regurgitation. This pulsation is maximal over the lower sternum and left parasternal region and peaks just after the second heart sound (Fig. 11–19). It relates to forward thrust of the ventricles caused by filling of the distended left atrium, which probably impinges on the vertebral column, thereby moving the heart forward. When this movement coexists with the apical impulse of left ventricular hypertrophy, the asynchronous timing of the two movements can be readily appreciated by simultaneous palpation with both hands.

Since the right ventricle underlies the midprecordium, conditions enlarging this ventricle affect chest wall pulsation in this area. Volume overloading conditions such as atrial septal defect cause brisk diffuse early systolic outward movement of the lower left parasternal area, with rapid decline in late systole. Pressure overloading disorders such as pulmonary stenosis give rise to more sustained, diffuse systolic outward movement, often extending from sternum to apex. Mitral stenosis with pulmonary hypertension causes a more medial systolic movement; the maximal thrust is often sternal.

Transmural myocardial infarction frequently causes abnormally sustained systolic outward movement, usually of the midprecordium or apex but occasionally of the sternal or even epigastric areas. This impulse, commonly called a *systolic bulge,* relates to the failure of infarcted myocardium to contract normally. Sometimes this expansile movement derives from an anatomic ventricular aneurysm; more often the bulge correlates with contraction failure of infarcted tissue in the absence of true aneurysm. This movement pattern may characterize old or recent myocardial infarction and may occur transiently during angina pectoris.

Cardiomyopathies can also lead to precordial movement abnormalities that typify enlargement of either ventricle or both. Combined hypertrophy can be suspected when abnormal apical and lower left parasternal systolic outward movements are separated by a zone of quiescence or even systolic retraction.

Atrial systole, when exaggerated, may suffi-

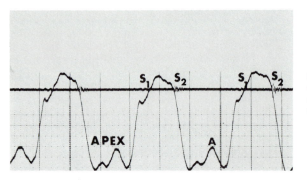

Figure 11–18 Apex impulse tracing (kinetocardiogram) of a patient with severe aortic regurgitation and congestive heart failure. Note the pronounced, sustained outward systolic movement, preceded by a smaller outward thrust corresponding to atrial systole *(A).*

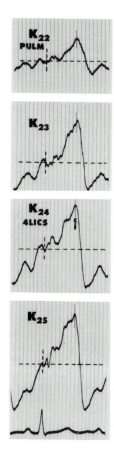

Figure 11–19 Movement tracings (kinetocardiogram) recorded along the left sternal border of a patient with severe mitral regurgitation. A prominent late systolic outward thrust is present from the pulmonary area (*K₂₂*) to the fifth left interspace (*K₂₅*). This results from forward displacement of the ventricles owing to late systolic distention of the dilated left atrium. *CI* = carotid incisura. Vertical dotted line represents peak of the *R* wave of electrocardiogram. Horizontal dotted line represents baseline of kinetocardiogram. (Reprinted by permission from Stapleton, J., and Groves, B.: Am. Heart J. *81*:409, 1971.)

ciently amplify atrial chest wall pulsations so as to render them palpable. This occurs when resistance to ventricular filling is high, as with the concentric hypertrophy of aortic or pulmonary stenosis or of systemic or pulmonary hypertension. The altered myocardial compliance of cardiomyopathies or myocardial infarction also may lead to palpable presystolic impulses. Atrial sounds usually accompany atrial movements. Since atrial hypertrophy often coexists with ventricular hypertrophy, palpable atrial movement is frequently associated with the lifting thrust of ventricular enlargement. The examiner then feels a double or bifid impulse. Such double pulsations are common in clinical practice.

Important pulsations may also occur during diastolic filling. A loud ventricular gallop sound may be associated with a simultaneous brief precordial thrust that corresponds to an exaggerated diastolic rapid filling wave. Thus, the examiner may see, feel, and hear the vibrations of the ventricular gallop phenomenon. Atrial and ventricular rapid filling movements are exaggerated in the left lateral recumbent posture. Palpation in this posture will sometimes detect pulsations not felt with the patient supine.

Constrictive pericarditis and restrictive cardiomyopathy may cause a vigorous, outward impulse in early diastole that is easily mistaken for the movement of ventricular hypertrophy unless the physician carefully times his palpation. This movement corresponds to the sudden arrest of rapid early diastolic filling by restricting pericardium or myocardium.

Careful auscultation and palpation of cardiac vibrations will yield many valuable diagnostic and prognostic clues without patient discomfort and at minimal cost. The examination requires only a few moments of intent observation and knowledge of fundamental normal and abnormal findings. As with other sources of evaluative information, the physician must fit auscultatory and palpatory findings into the total clinical context.

REFERENCES

Adolph, R. J., and Fowler, N. O.: The second heart sound: a screening test for heart disease. Mod. Concepts Cardiovasc. Dis. *39*:91, 1970.

Conn, R. D., and Cole, J. S.: The cardiac apex impulse. Ann. Intern. Med. *75*:185, 1971.

Craige, E., and Millward, D. K.: Diastolic and continuous murmurs. Progr. Cardiovasc. Dis. *14*:38, 1971.

Davie, J. C., Langley, J. O., Dodson, W. H., and Eddleman, E. E.: Clinical and kinetocardiographic studies of paradoxical precordial motion. Am. Heart J. *63*:775, 1962.

Deliyannis, A. A., Gillam, P. M. S., Mounsey, J. P. D., and Steiner, R. E.: The cardiac impulse and the motion of the heart. Br. Heart J. *26*:396, 1964.

Eddleman, E. E., and Thomas, H. D.: The recognition and differentiation of right ventricular pressure and flow loads. Am. J. Cardiol. *4*:652, 1959.

Fortuin, N. J., and Craige, E.: Echocardiographic studies of

genesis of mitral diastolic murmurs. Br. Heart J. *35*:75–81, 1973.

Harvey, W. P., and Stapleton, J. F.: Clinical aspects of gallop rhythm with particular reference to diastolic gallops. Circulation *18*:1017, 1958.

Heintzen, P.: The genesis of the normally split first heart sound. Am. Heart J. *62*:332, 1961.

Leatham, A.: Systolic murmurs. Circulation *17*:601, 1958.

Leatham, A., and Towers, M.: Splitting of the second heart sound. Br. Heart J. *12*:575, 1951.

Levine, S. A., and Harvey, W. P.: Clinical Auscultation of the Heart. 2nd ed. Philadelphia, W. B. Saunders Co., 1958.

McCall, B. W., and Price, J. L.: Movement of the mitral valve cusps in relation to first heart sound and opening snap in patients with mitral stenosis. Br. Heart J. *29*:417, 1967.

McDonald, I. G.: The shape and movements of the human left ventricle during systole. Am. J. Cardiol. *26*:221, 1970.

McKusick, V. A. (Ed.): Symposium on Cardiovascular Sound. Circulation *16*:270, 1957.

Reddy, P. S., Shaver, J. A., and Leonard, J. J.: Cardiac systolic murmurs: pathophysiology and differential diagnosis. Progr. Cardiovasc. Dis. *14*:1, 1971.

Ronan, J. A., Steelman, R. B., DeLeon, A. C., et al.: The clinical diagnosis of acute severe mitral insufficiency. Am. J. Cardiol. *27*:284, 1971.

Stapleton, J. F., and Harvey, W. P.: Systolic Sounds. Am. Heart J. *91*:383–392, 1976.

Sutton, G. C., and Craige, E.: Quantitation of precordial movement. Circulation *35*:476, 1967.

Sutton, G. C., Taylor, A. P., and Craige, E.: Relationship between quantitated precordial movement and left ventricular function. Circulation *61*:179, 1970.

Tantouzas, P., and Shillingford, J.: Impulse cardiogram in early diagnosis of left ventricular dysfunction in hypertension. Br. Heart J. *31*:97, 1969.

Waider, W., and Craige, E.: First heart sound and ejection sounds. Am. J. Cardiol., *35*:346, 1975.

Weitzman, D.: The mechanism and significance of the auricular sound. Br. Heart J. *17*:70, 1955.

The Electrocardiogram **12**

J. A. Abildskov

INTRODUCTION

The electrocardiogram is a record of electrical phenomena that occur in the heart and result in an electrical field distributed throughout the body. The usual electrocardiographic examination for medical diagnostic purposes is carried out with electrodes located at multiple sites on the body surface. When two electrodes are connected by a conductor, current flows in the conductor, and a suitable instrument placed in this current path records evidence of the potential difference between the electrode sites. Such instruments are designated electrocardiographs, and the electrode arrangement constitutes an electrocardiographic lead. The electrocardiograph furnishes records in which deflections are calibrated in terms of voltage on the vertical axis and time is represented on the horizontal axis. The conventional electrocardiogram is thus a Cartesian coordinate graph in which voltage variations are plotted against time, as illustrated in Figure 12–1. Many other displays of the same data are possible, one of which has been designated the "vectorcardiogram," also illustrated in Figure 12–1. In that display, voltage variations from one set of electrodes are plotted against those from another electrode combination rather than against time as in the electrocardiogram. It should be recognized that different displays of data from particular electrode combinations involve the same information from the body surface, but the accessibility of particular items of this information varies with the display. Thus, the relation of voltage to time is clearly evident in the electrocardiogram but not in the vectorcardiogram. In the vectorcardiogram, however, the relation of voltage variations from one set of electrodes to those in another electrode set is precisely indicated. The precision of this relation in the vectorcardiogram when it is recorded from a cathode ray oscilloscope is difficult to achieve even with simultaneously recorded electrocardiographic leads and is impossible to establish with nonsimultaneous leads.

The time-based electrocardiogram is the most commonly employed and widely useful examination of cardiac electrical activity for medical diagnostic purposes. The vectorcardiogram has more limited diagnostic utility and is less often employed, while the many other possible displays of electrical events in the heart are still less frequently used. The discussion that follows will concern the time-based electrocardiogram unless otherwise specified.

As it is used at present, electrocardiographic examination is a major diagnostic method. Certain abnormalities of waveform are the best available clinical evidence of myocardial infarction. Other abnormalities, although often less specific, are useful evidence of a variety of cardiac and extracardiac states ranging from cardiac enlargement and myocardial ischemia to electrolyte and neurologic disorders. The electrocardiogram is the most certain means of identifying the cardiac rhythm at the time of examination and of detecting changes of rhythm when the record is continuously monitored. The ease and almost risk-free nature of electrocardiographic examination enhance its medical usefulness.

The present role of the electrocardiogram in medical diagnosis has been achieved in two ways. One of these has been the empiric correlation of electrocardiographic findings with particular states, the nature of which has been established by other clinical evidence or by pathologic observations. This is the most certain means of establishing the diagnostic utility of particular electrocardiographic findings, and observations for which the diagnostic significance is suspected on other grounds must still be subjected to the actual test of diagnostic success or failure in patients.

The other means by which the diagnostic role of the electrocardiogram has been established is that of defining the physiologic basis of the record in normal and abnormal states. Increasing knowledge of the pertinent physiologic mechanisms has increased the degree to which electrocardiographic findings can be explained in these terms. Such explanation of electrocardiographic findings on the basis of their physiologic mechanism is desirable for teaching purposes. This approach is also likely to be the major means by which further improvements in electrocardiographic diagnoses are achieved, and understanding of the physiologic mechanisms will be the best preparation for the utilization of these improvements.

The material that follows has been organized into seven sections. The first of these describes the *total system* involved in electrocardiography. The various components of the electrocardiographic system are not equally well understood nor are they equally important to diagnostic electrocardiography. This section will therefore specify those components of the total system for which the roles

ELECTROCARDIOGRAM:

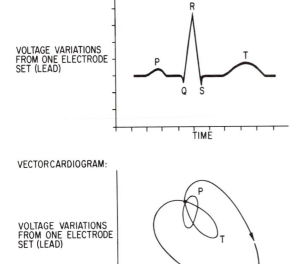

VOLTAGE VARIATIONS
FROM ONE ELECTRODE
SET (LEAD)

VECTORCARDIOGRAM:

VOLTAGE VARIATIONS
FROM ONE ELECTRODE
SET (LEAD)

VOLTAGE VARIATIONS FROM
A SECOND ELECTRODE SET

Figure 12–1 The electrocardiogram and vectorcardiogram. Both records reflect potential differences between electrode combinations. In the electrocardiogram these potential differences are recorded as voltage vs. time. The vectorcardiogram presents voltage variations from one electrode set, constituting a lead, vs. voltage variations from another lead.

are most fully defined and application of which to diagnostic electrocardiography is most important.

The second section presents a brief description of *electrocardiographic leads,* including those that constitute the present routine electrocardiographic examination. This is an extremely complex subject, and detailed consideration is not appropriate in this text. The section will be largely limited to those items that must be appreciated in order for subsequent sections of this text to be understood. These items include description of the electrocardiogram in terms of the electrical axis.

The third section will consider the *cardiac basis of the electrocardiogram* in general terms applicable to both atrial and ventricular muscle and to the specialized conduction system. The description in this section of the relation between cardiac events and the waveform of the body surface electrocardiogram is, in the author's opinion, the most useful approach to employing the electrocardiogram in medical diagnosis available at present.

In the fourth and fifth sections, the relation of cardiac events during *excitation* to electrocardiographic waveform will be specifically applied to *atria* and *ventricles,* and the process of *atrial recovery* will be considered briefly.

Ventricular recovery and its electrocardiographic expressions in the ST-T deflection will be considered in the sixth section. The discussion will emphasize similarities between the cardiac state during recovery and that during excitation and will attempt to elucidate the physiologic basis of the ST-T deflection and QRS complex in the same terms.

The seventh section will concern *pathologic states* and their electrocardiographic manifestations using the same terms employed in previous sections to explain the normal electrocardiogram. The pathologic states considered in this section have been chosen as examples and are only a few of those in which the electrocardiogram has diagnostic utility. Texts of medicine, cardiology, and clinical electrocardiography that describe the diagnostic range of the electrocardiogram are available. The purpose of this text is to describe physiologic mechanisms, and this is done through the use of selected examples of pathologic states.

THE ELECTROCARDIOGRAPHIC SYSTEM

The total system involved in electrocardiography is illustrated in diagrammatic form in Figure 12–2. The major component of the system is the heart, which is the site of origin of events reflected in the electrocardiogram. As the generator of the electrocardiogram, the heart can be considered at the level of intra- and extracellular ion relations in the resting and excited states. The generator can also be considered at the level of the cell membrane across which ion concentration gradients exist and ion movements occur. At still another level, the generator can be considered at the cellular level in terms of the transmembrane action potential. Finally, the generator can be considered at the organ level, at which the gross sequence of electrical events during excitation and recovery can be described.

At present, the most useful level at which to consider the physiologic basis of the body surface electrocardiogram is the gross sequence of electrical events together with certain information from the transmembrane action potential. It is at these various levels that the cardiac basis of the electrocardiogram will be described in the next section.

Extracardiac components of the electrocardiographic system include a complex, three-dimensional conductive medium. This medium consists of tissues with different conductive properties and the geometrically complex and variable boundaries of the body. These portions of the electrocardiographic system undoubtedly influence the body surface electrocardiogram, and the degree and nature of their influence has been and continues to be the subject of intensive study. At present, however, the role of these factors has not been sufficiently well defined that they can be usefully

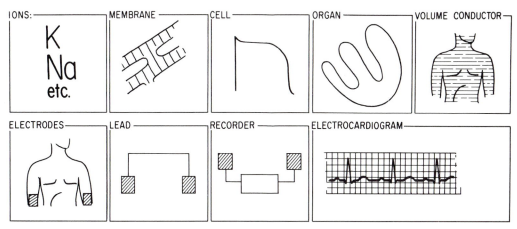

Figure 12–2 The total electrocardiographic system, consisting of ionic gradients across cell membranes, cellular events reflected by the transmembrane action potential, the sequence of electrical events at the organ level, and extracardiac portions of the system, including the conducting medium, recorder, and records.

considered in routine diagnostic electrocardiography. Further definition of the role of nonuniform conductive properties and complex boundary conditions can be expected to refine electrocardiographic diagnosis in the future, however.

The remaining portions of the electrocardiographic system are the electrodes with which potentials on the body surface are sampled, the combinations of electrodes that constitute "leads," and the instruments with which potentials are displayed or recorded or both.

ELECTROCARDIOGRAPHIC LEADS

The combination of a minimum of two electrodes in contact with the body and connected to provide a path for current flow between them constitutes an electrocardiographic lead. The term "lead" is also generally used to refer to the actual electrocardiogram recorded from an electrode combination. The waveform in the electrocardiogram is a description of potential differences at the electrodes constituting the lead as they vary with time. Electrocardiographic examination usually consists of obtaining electrocardiograms from multiple electrode sites. The examination considered to be routine at present includes nine electrode sites with 12 leads consisting of various combinations of these electrodes. Electrodes on the right and left arms and left leg and at six specified sites on the precordium are employed. Leads are designated as "standard," "precordial," and "unipolar" limb leads.

The standard lead designated as I consists of right and left arm electrodes, with the polarity of the recording system so arranged that an upright deflection on the recording occurs when the left arm potential is positive with respect to the right arm. Standard leads II and III consist of electrodes on the right arm and left leg and on the left arm

and left leg, respectively, both arranged to yield an upright deflection when the left leg potential is positive with respect to the arm.

Precordial leads consist of six electrodes at specified sites on the anterior and left lateral thorax, and a central terminal to which right and left arm and left leg electrodes are all connected. These leads are designated "V_1," through "V_6," and each consists of a precordial electrode and the central terminal, with the polarity arranged to result in an upward deflection when the precordial electrode is positive with respect to the central terminal.

The remaining three "unipolar" limb leads consist of electrodes on the arms and the left leg, each of which is combined with a modified central terminal to which the other two limb electrodes are connected. The polarity of these leads is so arranged that an upward deflection results when the single limb electrode is positive with respect to the modified central terminal. Leads recorded with the modified central terminal yield larger deflections than would occur with a terminal to which all three limb electrodes were connected and are known as "augmented leads" and are designated by the symbols "aV_L," "aV_R," and "aV_F" for the three unipolar limb leads. It should be noted that the term "unipolar" lead is a misnomer, since a complete circuit is required to record an electrocardiogram. The term is applied to leads in which one side of the circuit is connected to all three limb electrodes in the case of precordial leads, or to two of these in the case of augmented limb leads. It is applied because potential variations at the central terminal, although neither zero nor negligible, are small, and potential variations at the precordial or limb location of the other electrode are chiefly responsible for the electrocardiographic waveform. Examples of standard, precordial, and unipolar limb leads are shown in Figure 12–3.

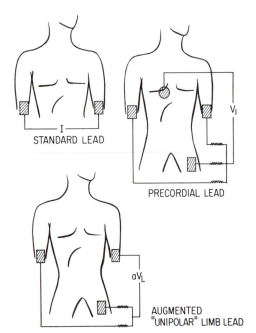

Figure 12–3 Examples of the three varieties of leads employed in the usual 12-lead electrocardiographic examination.

The electrode sites used in the routine 12-lead electrocardiographic examination have been selected according to a combination of technical considerations such as ease and reproducibility of electrode placement; theoretic considerations, including design of the central terminal; empiric evidence of their diagnostic merit; and informed intuition. It is unlikely that they constitute the optimal possible electrocardiographic examination. They do, however, furnish a large amount of diagnostically useful information, and this is the standard by which possible future modifications must be evaluated.

One can appreciate one of the fundamental problems of diagnostic electrocardiography by realizing that a pattern of potential variation due to cardiac electrical events exists at all points on the body surface. This pattern can be defined by recording from extremely large numbers of electrode sites and determining the potential distribution at multiple moments during the cardiac cycle. These patterns constitute virtually all the electrocardiographic information present on the body surface, but sampling from such large numbers of electrodes presents major technical problems. Research is in progress in this area using computer techniques to display the data as isopotential maps at frequent intervals during the cardiac cycle. These studies have definitely demonstrated diagnostically useful information beyond that furnished by the present routine electrocardiographic examination, and this is an extremely promising area for improved electrocardiographic diagnosis

in the future. Improved automated methods may make examinations with large numbers of electrodes practical, or it may be possible to identify limited numbers of electrode sites that furnish all or most of the diagnostic information possible from body surface electrocardiograms. This information will include that provided by leads with selective sensitivity to particular cardiac areas and may make regional cardiac examination by electrocardiography possible. Such examination may permit the identification and quantification of localized hypertrophy; measurement of myocardial infarction and other localized lesion size; and the recognition, localization, and estimation of size and severity of local abnormalities of ventricular repolarization.

Electrode arrangements, or systems, designated as "vectorcardiographic," or "orthogonal" lead systems are in actual clinical use, usually for the purpose of recording vectorcardiograms with the cathode ray oscilloscope or collecting electrocardiographic data for programs of computer analysis. These systems consist of multiple electrodes that in various combinations and with the contribution of individual electrodes weighted by resistor networks yield effects of cardiac electrical activity on three mutually perpendicular axes, namely, horizontal (X), vertical (Y), and anteroposterior (Z) axes. These systems have been designed on the basis of the dimensions and geometry of the human thorax and position of the heart within the thorax. Some of the systems also include qualitative consideration of the nonuniform conductive properties of the body. Evidence has been obtained that the three leads from such electrode systems contain most of the information furnished by the routine 12-lead examination. In addition, there is evidence that the range of normal variability of such leads is less than that of the 12-lead examination. Despite such findings, which suggest that a simpler examination may provide an equal, or nearly equal, amount of diagnostic information with less normal variability and may be more sensitive to abnormalities, these leads are not extensively employed. The major deterrents to their widespread use have probably been the extensive experience and familiarity with 12-lead examination, the relative lack of standards for interpretation of orthogonal leads, and particularly the lack of convincing evidence that their actual diagnostic merit is substantially greater than that of the 12-lead examination now in use.

ELECTRICAL AXIS

Certain features of the electrocardiogram can be conveniently described as the "electrical axis." This description is usually applied to the QRS complex, but there is no inherent reason that it cannot be used to describe other electrocardiographic deflections. In essence, the description consists of relating features in one electrocardiographic lead to those in one or more additional leads. A deflection in one lead can be specified as having a particular amplitude and a positive or negative polarity. As one that can be specified by two terms, this is a scalar quantity, and individual EKG leads are often referred to as "scalar leads." If the relation of one lead to another is known, the magnitude and polarity of electrocardiographic deflections in both may be specified by a single vector quantity that has the additional feature of a specific direction. An example is shown in Figure 12–4. The peak deflection in two leads is illustrated, together with the geometric relation assumed to exist between these leads. The vector shown identifies the deflection in lead I as positive and having an amplitude of four units, whereas that in lead II is also positive and has a magnitude of three units. The term for this vector as usually employed in diagnostic electrocardiography is "electrical axis."

This description of electrocardiographic deflections may be applied to the instantaneous deflection in two simultaneous leads and then constitutes the "instantaneous axis." A number of successive instantaneous axes during the QRS complex would have their termini located on the QRS loop of the vectorcardiogram. One can also plot an axis using the area of deflections. The axis plotted from QRS area in two leads is properly referred to as the "mean electrical axis of the QRS." In actual routine interpretation of electrocardiograms, an approximation of the mean axis is usually employed. The algebraic sum of peak deflections in a lead is determined and used with a similar sum from another lead to determine the vector that identifies these quantities in the leads being considered.

THE CARDIAC BASIS OF THE ELECTROCARDIOGRAM

As stated earlier, the most useful level at which to consider the physiologic basis of the electrocardiogram is the gross sequence of electrical events on the organ level together with certain information provided by the cellular transmembrane action potential. At the gross level, the cardiac state reflected by an electrocardiographic deflection at a given moment is that of a boundary between areas in different electrical states. When the heart is uniformly in the resting state, no such boundaries exist and the isoelectric reference line of the electrocardiogram is established. When excitation is in progress, one or more boundaries exist between excited muscle and that still in the resting state. The varying size and geometry of boundaries during atrial excitation determine the form of the P wave, and those during ventricular excitation determine the QRS complex waveform. After excitation in ventricular muscle, there is a period during which the electrical state changes slowly, as reflected by the plateau of the transmembrane action potential. During this period all ventricular muscle is in the same or nearly same electrical state, and the isoelectric or nearly isoelectric ST segment of the electrocardiogram reflects this condition. As more rapid changes in electrical state occur during the downstroke of the transmembrane action potential, boundaries of potential difference appear between areas in which the stage of recovery differs from that in an adjacent area.

One of the fundamental and most useful relations in electrocardiography is that between a boundary of potential difference in the heart and

Figure 12–4 The electrical axis. In this representation of electrocardiographic features, the geometric relation of the leads must be known or assumed. Here, leads I and II are assumed to form sides of an equilateral triangle. The peak QRS deflection in each is indicated, and these values have been employed to plot a vector. In the portion of the illustration showing this vector, the midpoint of the leads has been superimposed.

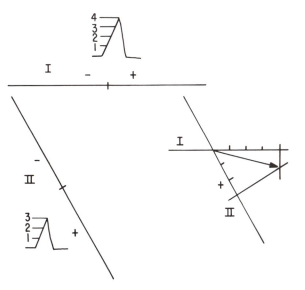

the potential at recording electrodes on the body surface. Potential at a recording electrode is influenced by the distance of the recording electrode from the boundary, the magnitude of potential difference across the boundary, and the geometry of the boundary.

It has also been demonstrated that cardiac fiber orientation influences the extracellular potential field. These influences of anistropy suggest a nonuniform current density at boundaries between cardiac muscle in different electrical states. The influences are such that the equivalent cardiac generator of the electrocardiogram cannot be represented by dipole sources perpendicular to boundaries. This differs from the previously widely accepted theory that assumed a uniform dipole layer perpendicular to boundaries in cardiac muscle. At present, the evidences of nonuniform current density are based on small excitation boundaries that occur shortly after ectopic stimulation. The influences of nonuniform current density both on realistic normal or abnormal activation boundaries spreading through the entire cardiac mass and on repolarization boundaries are not yet known. To the extent that such boundaries are parallel to cardiac fiber direction, a uniform dipole layer perpendicular to boundaries is probably a reasonable approximation of cardiac sources of the electrocardiogram. The success of cardiac generator models that have assumed such sources in explaining major features of the normal and abnormal electrocardiogram suggests that this is at least partially the case. For this reason and because effects of nonuniform current density of realistic cardiac boundaries are not yet adequately defined, this section will be presented in terms of classic uniform dipole layers as the equivalent cardiac generator of the electrocardiogram. Future research concerning effects of cardiac fiber orientation is, however, likely to provide a more detailed and accurate explanation of the cardiac basis of the electrocardiogram.

Figure 12–5 diagrams a closed boundary of potential difference in excitable tissue. If the boundary illustrated is considered to be an excitation front, the magnitude of potential difference across the boundary will be that between excited and resting tissue and will be related to the height of the transmembrane action potential upstroke. Tissue on the excited side of the boundary will have a potential related to the end of the upstroke of the transmembrane action potential, whereas tissue not yet excited will be at resting membrane potential level. The polarity of potential difference will be negative in excited tissue and positive in resting tissue. When the boundary is closed as illustrated, potential differences in all directions are present, and the electrocardiographic effects of one segment of the boundary are canceled by effects of an opposing portion of the boundary. A closed boundary of potential difference will not be expressed by an electrocardiographic deflection,

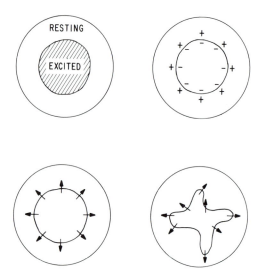

Figure 12–5 Diagrammatic representation of boundaries of potential difference. As described in the text, closed boundaries will not be expressed as electrocardiographic deflections.

regardless of the dimensions of the boundary and regardless of the magnitude of potential difference across the boundary. The foregoing is true of closed boundaries, regardless of their shape, and is true of three-dimensional boundaries as well as those located in a single plane.

It is extremely important that the implications of this relation for diagnostic electrocardiography be appreciated. It should be evident, for example, that the size of electrocardiographic deflections is unlikely to have a simple and direct relation to heart size. It should also be evident that the size of a myocardial infarct or other destructive lesion will not necessarily be proportional to the magnitude of electrocardiographic alterations produced by the lesion. It should further be evident from the relation described that the electrocardiographic effect of a given unclosed boundary will be related to the degree by which it fails to be a closed boundary. A boundary with uncanceled portions is shown in Figure 12–6. The boundary shown can be closed by the line *ab*, and the length of this line will be related to uncanceled portions of the boundary and to the magnitude of electrocardiographic effects of the boundary. In relating boundaries of potential difference to the electrocardiogram, it is convenient to employ vectors as shown in the figure. A vector directed toward the positive side of the boundary, perpendicular to the line closing the boundary and having a magnitude equal or proportional to the closing line, indicates the polarity and magnitude of the electrocardiographic deflection in a particular lead by its projection on the lead axis. If the boundary has spatial form it cannot be closed by a line, and the electrocardiographic effect will be related to the area of the surface necessary to close the boundary.

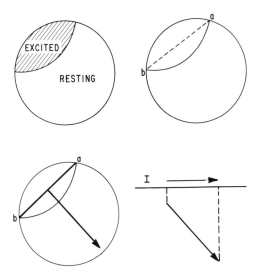

Figure 12–6 Diagrammatic representation of an unclosed boundary of potential difference. The electrocardiographic expression of such a boundary will be related to the quantity necessary to close the boundary. This quantity is the line a-b in the example shown. The electrocardiographic effect of such a boundary is conveniently obtained by constructing a vector perpendicular to the closing line with a magnitude equal or proportional to the line and by projecting the vector on lead axes.

Although the cardiac events responsible for electrocardiographic deflections during excitation and recovery are similar in that both consist of boundaries of potential difference between areas in different electrical states, they differ in significant ways. These differences in the cardiac states of activation and recovery will be introduced here and further explained in a subsequent section. One of the differences between excitation and recovery is the greater time required for the latter process. In individual cells, excitation occurs during the upstroke of the transmembrane action potential and requires only 1 or 2 milliseconds for completion. Recovery as reflected by the transmembrane action potential downstroke begins immediately after excitation, but, because of the special features of cardiac recovery reflected by the plateau of the action potential, excited tissue remains at a potential level near that of the peak upstroke during the normal propagation of excitation. These events make it possible to regard excitation as a moving boundary of potential difference. If sequential boundaries are considered, the electrocardiographic effects of later boundaries can be considered without reference to those of earlier boundaries.

Because of the substantially longer time required for recovery, the potential difference boundaries that exist during that process cannot be related to the electrocardiogram in the same manner as excitation. When potential differences arise between two areas that have reached different stages of recovery, the resulting boundary continues to exist until recovery is complete in both areas. During this time, additional boundaries between other areas that reach different stages of recovery are established and also remain present until recovery is complete in the areas involved. The cardiac state responsible for the ST-T deflection of the electrocardiogram cannot therefore be considered as a moving boundary of potential difference, but must be considered as one in which multiple boundaries coexist. Potential differences across these boundaries vary according to the stage of recovery reached on the two sides of each boundary. The relations between each boundary of potential difference during recovery and an electrocardiographic lead are similar to those occurring during excitation. The electrocardiographic expressions of both are related to the magnitude of potential difference across the boundary, polarity of this difference, and the quantity necessary to close the boundary that defines the uncanceled portion of the boundary.

ATRIAL EXCITATION AND THE P WAVE

Normal cardiac excitation begins in the right atrium, specifically in the specialized tissue constituting the sinoatrial node. This structure is located near the junction of the atrium and superior vena cava. According to James, the human sinoatrial node is approximately $2 \times 5 \times 15$ mm in size and is pierced by a central artery that provides the arterial supply of the node and a large area of surrounding atrial myocardium.

On the cellular level, excitation consists of a sudden increase in membrane permeability to sodium, probably due to inactivation of mechanisms that normally extrude sodium from cells during the resting state. The property of automaticity, or pacemaker activity, normally exhibited by the sinoatrial node consists of slow diastolic depolarization in which the potential difference between interior and exterior of the pacemaking cell declines to a critical point. At the threshold value of membrane potential, the rapid changes of membrane potential characteristic of excitation occur in the pacemaker cell. Propagation of excitation to surrounding cells occurs as a result of local current flow between excited and nonexcited cells. This acts as a depolarizing current in the same manner as current supplied from an external stimulus source.

The property of automaticity is not restricted to the sinoatrial node, and other portions of the specialized conduction system are also capable of pacemaker activity. Normally, however, slow diastolic depolarization occurs at a higher rate in the sinoatrial node than in other sites also capable of pacemaker activity. The normal sequence of atrial excitation during sinus rhythm is determined by the exact pacemaker site within the sinoatrial node and by the atrial properties that determine the velocity of propagation.

In addition to the sinoatrial node, other sites in both right and left atria have been demonstrated to be capable of pacemaker function. It is not yet clear how frequently or under what conditions these areas are likely to initiate the cardiac rhythm, but the wide variability of P waveform may be partially due to such extra sinus node origins of supraventricular rhythm.

In the thin-walled atria, activation sequence in the endocardial-epicardial dimension is not a significant factor in determining P waveform, and atrial activation can be considered a surface phenomenon. It has usually been considered an atrial property that activation spreads with uniform velocity from the pacemaker site. There is, however, both anatomic and functional evidence of specialized preferential conduction paths. Anatomic evidence of three paths containing specialized fibers in direct continuity and extending from the sinoatrial to atrioventricular node and to the left atrium has been reported. Physiologic evidence of such paths, including the effect of localized lesions on P waveform, has also been reported. Conflicting physiologic findings have also been reported, however, ranging from evidence of simple radial spread of excitation with uniform velocity to evidence that excitation spreads in broad areas corresponding to gross anatomic landmarks. These areas are reported to form separate inputs to the AV node but without evidence of narrow, specialized internodal tracts.

Whether atrial excitation is propagated uniformly or via specialized tracts, the physiologic basis of many features of normal and abnormal P waves can be reasonably well explained. Even uniform propagation of excitation would result in geometrically complex boundaries of potential difference in the anatomically complex atria. The location of the sinoatrial node determines some of the major features of atrial excitation sequence and P waveform. The normal pacemaker has a superior and slightly posterior location within the right atrium; thus, the overall direction of atrial excitation is obliged to be leftward, downward, and slightly anterior. This results in upright P waves in leads I, II, and aV_F and usually in all precordial leads. The relation of the overall direction of atrial excitation to the standard leads is illustrated diagrammatically in Figure 12–7. As shown in that figure, the normal P wave amplitude in lead II is likely to be larger than that in lead I, whereas lead III may show isoelectric P waves or waves of either polarity with only minor differences in the geometric relation of atrial excitation to that lead axis.

The relation of sequential boundaries of potential difference during atrial excitation to electrocardiographic leads I and II is illustrated in Figure 12–8. It should be noted that the time of onset of the P deflection differs in this example. The first boundary is so located that it produces no effect in lead I but results in a deflection in lead II. This illustrates that the duration of the P wave in any one lead is not necessarily indicative of the total time required for atrial excitation. Similar considerations apply to other electrocardiographic deflections and the actual duration of the cardiac process that they reflect.

Atrial repolarization results in an electrocardiographic deflection, usually designated the Ta wave, whose peak amplitude is smaller and duration is longer than the P wave. The Ta wave is responsible for the level of the PR segment in relation to the isoelectric interval of the electrocardiogram. The wave also extends into and modifies the form of the QRS complex and the level of the ST segment. Although the Ta deflection has not been extensively studied, it is usually of opposite polarity to the P wave it follows and its area is approximately equal to that of the P wave. At present, the major diagnostic significance of the Ta wave concerns its influence on ST segment level. When large upright P waves are present in a given lead, the Ta deflection can be expected to

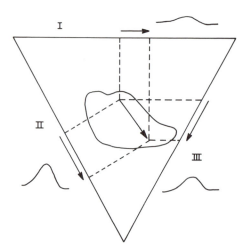

Figure 12–7 Diagrammatic representation of the atria and standard electrocardiographic leads. The average direction of spread of atrial excitation is indicated by the vector, and the usual normal relation of P wave amplitude in the standard leads is shown.

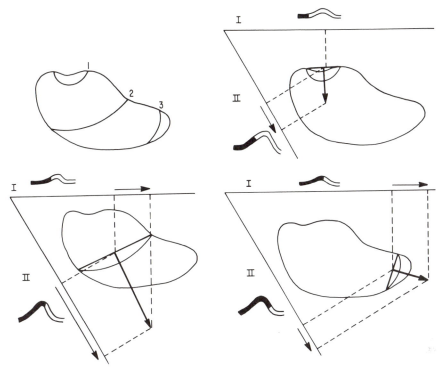

Figure 12–8 Diagrammatic representation of the atria and three sequential excitation boundaries. The electrocardiographic expressions of these boundaries on leads I and II are illustrated.

be proportional and may result in ST segment depression in that lead. Such ST segment depression is not the result of ventricular abnormalities but may be erroneously attributed to these if the effects of atrial repolarization on ST segment level are not appreciated. The Ta wave and its effect on ST segment level are illustrated diagrammatically in Figure 12–9. P wave amplitude and area are often increased with increases in heart rate, and the resulting increase in amplitude and area of the Ta deflection may result in ST segment displacement. Diagnostic errors are therefore especially likely in postexercise electrocardiograms in which ST segment displacement is a frequent manifestation of ischemic heart disease. The tachycardia produced by exercise may result in increased amplitude of the P waves, which are then followed by larger Ta waves superimposed on and displacing the ST segment.

VENTRICULAR EXCITATION AND THE QRS COMPLEX

Normal cardiac excitation originating in the sinoatrial node and spreading through the atria is delivered to the atrioventricular junctional tissues and via these to the specialized intraventricular conduction system. Major components of the junctional and intraventricular conduction system are the atrioventricular node, bundle of His, right and left bundle branches, and the subendocardial Purkinje network. Activation of junctional and intraventricular conduction systems is not expressed as a distinct deflection in the body surface electrocardiogram and normally occurs during the PR segment of that record. Catheter-mounted intracardiac electrodes positioned near portions of the junctional and specialized intraventricular conduction system show evidence of excitation in these structures and are providing valuable data concerning normal cardiac physiology, drug ef-

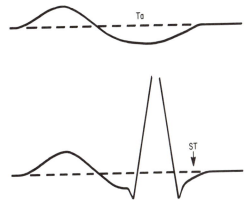

Figure 12–9 Diagrammatic representation of the P and Ta waves and the influence of the latter on ST segment level.

fects, and, in some cases, diagnostically useful information concerning cardiac rhythm.

The QRS complex reflects excitation in ventricular muscle after the process has reached that level via the Purkinje network. The pattern or sequence of ventricular activation has been defined in considerable detail in the hearts of several species, including humans. The time of activation of multiple small areas has been determined, and the major features of the activation sequence so demonstrated account for the principal features of the QRS complex.

Figure 12–10 illustrates diagrammatically some of the major features of ventricular activation order. Excitation of ventricular muscle occurs first on the left side of the interventricular septum in approximately its midportion. The process continues to spread in this area and next appears on the endocardial surfaces of both right and left ventricles near their apices. Excitation then spreads from these three zones from endocardium toward epicardium and from apex toward base in the free ventricular walls and from both right and left, although chiefly from the left, in the interventricular septum. Activation of the thick basal portion of the left ventricular wall and activation of the superior portion of the interventricular septum are the latest events during ventricular excitation.

The relation of boundaries representative of the normal ventricular activation sequence to some leads of the routine electrocardiogram is illustrated diagrammatically in Figure 12–11. As described in previous sections, the electrocardiographic effects of each boundary are related to the quantity necessary to close the boundary and the magnitude of potential difference across the boundary. It is probable that the latter quantity is equal, or nearly so, for all normal activation boundaries, so that the relative size of closing

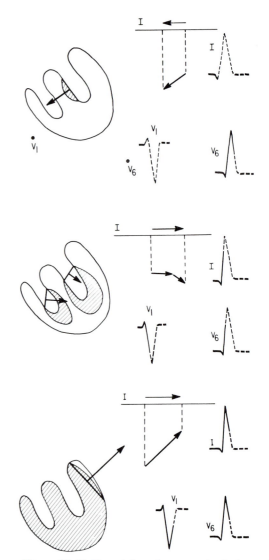

Figure 12–11 The relation of some major features of ventricular activation sequence to electrocardiographic deflections in leads I, V_1, and V_6.

boundaries is directly related to electrocardiographic effects. Early activation in the left side of the interventricular septum results in a boundary of potential difference with the negative side on the left. This is reasonably consistently expressed in the normal electrocardiogram by negative deflections in leads having one electrode on the left (I, aV_L, V_5, and V_6) and polarity so arranged that an upward deflection occurs when the left electrode is positive with respect to the other electrode involved in each lead. Since the negative deflection in these leads is the initial portion of the QRS complex, it constitutes a Q wave. In contrast, precordial lead V_1, in which one electrode is located to the right of the chest midline and has a polarity such that an upward deflection occurs when that electrode is positive with respect to the

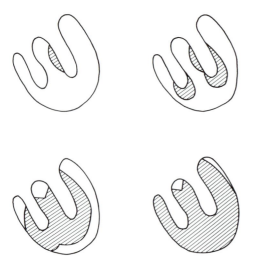

Figure 12–10 Representation of some of the major features of the normal ventricular activation sequence.

central terminal that is the other connection of that lead, reflects early septal activation as an R wave. In a similar fashion, the other boundaries illustrated in Figure 12–11 account for R waves in leads I and V_6 and S waves in V_1 as well as major features of the QRS complex in other leads not illustrated.

Cardiac events responsible for late portions of the QRS complex include activation of the basal portion of the left ventricular wall and of the upper portion of the interventricular septum. The latter event is variable and sometimes occurs in a right-ward direction, resulting in a late negative deflection or S wave in lead I and other leads with an electrode on the left side. Absence of S waves in these leads is a normal variant, however.

One of the informative relations between cardiac events during ventricular excitation and the electrocardiogram is the degree to which the events cancel their electrocardiographic expression. The normal magnitude of this effect provides a useful insight into the diagnostic limits of electrocardiography. A totally closed boundary, as previously described, has no expression in the electrocardiogram and can be said to be 100 per cent canceled. Actual boundaries during ventricular excitation are not usually completely closed, but during much of the normal process the quantity necessary to close boundaries is small in comparison to the boundaries themselves. Theoretic, experimental, and clinical estimates of the degree to which events during normal ventricular excitation cancel their electrocardiographic effects suggest that 70 to 90 per cent of the ventricular mass is excited without contributing to the body surface electrocardiogram. This is illustrated in Figure 12–12 with a boundary characteristic of left ventricular activation during the midportion of the QRS complex. Such considerations indicate that large destructive lesions may have only minor electrocardiographic effects when they involve areas whose excitation is not normally expressed in the electrocardiogram. They further suggest that small lesions appropriately located in areas

whose normal excitation is expressed in the QRS waveform with only a small degree of cancellation may have marked effects on that form.

VENTRICULAR REPOLARIZATION AND THE ST-T DEFLECTION

The cardiac state responsible for the ST-T deflection is similar to that responsible for the QRS complex in certain respects, but there are also important differences. Both excitation and recovery result in states in which boundaries of potential difference exist between cardiac areas in different physiologic states. In the case of excitation, these boundaries are located between areas of excited and resting muscle. During recovery, boundaries are located between areas that have reached different stages of repolarization. If particular excitation and recovery boundaries are considered, their electrocardiographic effects are determined by the same factors. In both cases, the geometry of the boundary and its relation to the electrocardiographic lead under consideration are determinants of the electrocardiographic effect. A closed boundary between areas in different stages of recovery is similar to a closed excitation boundary in having no electrocardiographic expression. The effect of both excitation and recovery boundaries is related to the degree to which they fail to be closed and thereby fail to cancel their electrocardiographic effects.

Both excitation and recovery boundaries produce electrocardiographic effects related to the magnitude of potential difference across the boundary. In the case of excitation boundaries, this value is the potential difference between excited and resting muscle and is related to the height of the transmembrane action potential upstroke. During recovery, the potential difference across a particular boundary is determined by the stage of recovery present on the two sides of the boundary as reflected by the relative height of action potential downstrokes and is always a fraction of the potential difference between excited and resting tissue. Potential differences at any one time during recovery are therefore smaller than the potential difference across activation boundaries. The difference across activation boundaries represents the maximal difference in potential between fully excited and resting muscle, whereas the potential difference at a given moment during recovery is some portion of that between fully excited and resting levels. Another difference in the cardiac states of excitation and recovery is that potential difference across recovery boundaries varies with time in relation to variations in the relative height of transmembrane action potential downstrokes on the two sides of the boundary. In addition, there is a marked difference in the length of time during which activation and recovery boundaries persist. Activation of individ-

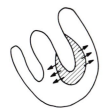 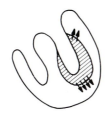

Figure 12–12 Illustration of the cancellation of electrocardiographic effects of portions of a representative boundary during ventricular activation. As shown in the diagram on the left, some portions of the boundary constitute equal and oppositely directed potential differences and cancel each other's electrocardiographic expression. Only those portions of the boundary indicated in the diagram on the right that do not have opposing portions result in electrocardiographic deflections.

ual cells is accomplished during 1 or 2 milliseconds as the action potential upstroke occurs, and individual activation boundaries persist only that length of time. Successive activation boundaries separated by more than that amount of time can be considered individually. The first produces an electrocardiographic effect and then disappears by the time the second boundary comes into existence and produces its electrocardiographic result. This is equivalent to considering activation as a process in which boundaries of potential difference move within cardiac muscle. In contrast, recovery in individual cells requires a considerably longer time, and a given boundary between areas recovering at different rates continues to exist until the repolarization process is complete on both sides of the boundary. During this time, additional boundaries between other cardiac areas with different recovery rates are established. At a given moment during repolarization, the cardiac source of the ST-T deflection may thus be multiple boundaries of potential difference that are widely distributed in ventricular muscle.

To illustrate some of the relations between the cardiac state of recovery and the ST-T deflection, it is helpful to consider a simplified activation sequence and organization of recovery properties. As illustrated in Figure 12–13, ventricular muscle can be considered as two groups of fibers, with all those in each group activated simultaneously and having particular recovery properties. The activation sequence can then be described as excitation of area A, followed by excitation of area B. This sequence of activation is depicted in the figure by the upstrokes of action potentials designated "A" and "B." In the interval between upstrokes A and B, a boundary of potential difference between cardiac areas A and B exists, and the magnitude of potential difference across this boundary is related to the height of the action potential up-

stroke in area A. After area B has also been excited and during the action potential plateau in both areas, there is no potential difference between them. During the downstroke of the action potential, however, potential differences again exist between cardiac areas A and B. At any moment, the magnitude of this difference is a fraction of that between fully excited and resting muscle.

Figure 12–13 can also be used to illustrate the relation of QRS and T wave polarity. An electrocardiographic lead has been arranged so that the potential difference between cardiac areas A and B results in an upward deflection when A is in the excited and B in the resting state. As shown in the figure, that polarity of potential difference is represented by the action potential from area A being located above that from area B. If action potentials are of equal duration, as shown in the figure, the action potential from area A will be completed before that from area B. During the downstroke of these action potentials, the polarity of potential differences between cardiac areas A and B will be opposite that which existed during excitation. This state will result in a T wave of opposite polarity to the QRS deflection.

One of the major features of the normal electrocardiogram is a T wave with the same polarity as the major QRS deflection in most leads and under most circumstances. This suggests that action potentials are of nonuniform duration and is, in fact, compatible with an inverse sequence of activation and of recovery. Actual physiologic data concerning the normal recovery sequence are difficult to obtain and are limited, but those that are available are compatible with such an inverse excitation and recovery sequence in ventricular muscle. Subendocardial muscle is excited early during ventricular excitation but has been demonstrated to have a longer refractory period and longer action potential downstroke than subepicardial muscle. Limited data suggest that an apex to base gradient of recovery properties also exists and apical muscle that is normally excited earlier than that at the ventricular base has the longer recovery time. The physiologic mechanism or mechanisms responsible for these normal variations in recovery properties have not been established. Variations in tension to which fibers are subjected, temperature differences, and other mechanisms have been suspected. Whatever the responsible mechanisms are, the normal recovery properties are such that they tend to equalize actual recovery times following a normal sequence of ventricular excitation. This probably has protective functions in that inequalities of recovery time have been strongly implicated in the mechanism of cardiac arrhythmias.

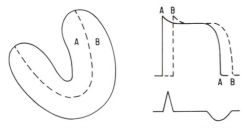

Figure 12–13 Relations between the cardiac state of recovery and the ST-T deflection. In this figure, ventricular muscle is illustrated as two groups of fibers, with an excitation sequence such that fiber group A is excited first. The transmembrane action potentials for fiber groups A and B are shown, and the interval between upstrokes A and B represents the QRS interval. The interval in which action potentials A and B are both at the plateau level represents the ST segment portion of the electrocardiogram, and the onset to completion of rapid downstrokes corresponds to the T wave. Action potentials of the same form and duration for the two fiber groups are shown and, as illustrated, result in QRS and T deflections of opposite polarity.

PATHOLOGIC STATES

The physiologic basis of electrocardiographic abnormalities in certain pathologic states will be considered in this section. The pathologic states to be considered have been selected on the basis of their diagnostic importance and because understanding of the mechanisms by which they modify the electrocardiogram is sufficiently complete to make these mechanisms diagnostically useful.

ATRIAL ENLARGEMENT

The physiologic basis of electrocardiographic features associated with atrial enlargement can be qualitatively appreciated even with simplification of assumptions concerning atrial anatomy and activation order. A diagrammatic representation of the atria and a simple radial excitation spread is illustrated in Figure 12–14, together with P waves in the standard electrocardiographic leads. A representation of left atrial enlargement is also shown and, as illustrated, results in several successive excitation boundaries of nearly equal

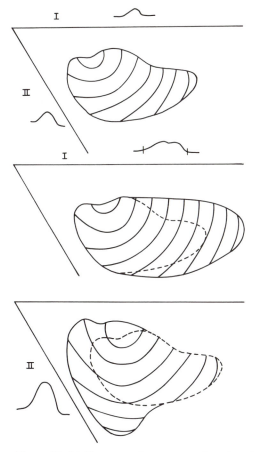

Figure 12–14 Diagrammatic representation of excitation in normal atria and in the states of left and right atrial enlargement. As illustrated, left atrial enlargement results in several successive fronts that are of similar geometry and are so oriented that a flat-topped or notched P wave in lead I results. Right atrial enlargement results in excitation boundaries directed roughly parallel to the axis of standard lead II and results in high P waves in that lead.

length and approximately the same relation to standard electrocardiographic leads. Potential differences across these boundaries are oriented roughly parallel to the left-right axis of the body, so that the most characteristic evidences of left atrial enlargement are likely to occur in lead I. In that lead, the greater time necessary for completion of excitation is evidenced by prolongation of the P wave, and the nearly identical successive boundaries characteristically result in a flat-topped or notched P wave.

Right atrial enlargement is also diagrammatically depicted in Figure 12–14. As illustrated, extension of activation boundaries into the enlarged atrium results in greater potential differences in the vertical axis of the body that are reflected by abnormally high and often peaked P waves in lead II and lead aV_F. Larger than normal P waves often occur in lead I as well but are less characteristic of right atrial enlargement than those in leads II and aV_F.

MYOCARDIAL INFARCTION

Recognition of this frequent and significant lesion is one of the major areas of clinical utility of the electrocardiogram. Positive electrocardiographic findings are the best available evidence of this lesion, and the physiologic mechanisms of these are sufficiently well defined to explain the findings in a useful fashion. Alterations of the waveform of the ventricular complex are the major electrocardiographic manifestations of myocardial infarction, and all portions of this complex, including QRS, ST, and T deflections, may be changed.

The QRS alterations are most specific and provide evidence of the location as well as the presence of infarction. Two major mechanisms operate to alter the QRS complex. One of these is the simple loss of excitable tissue that during its activation contributed to QRS complex waveform prior to infarction. The second mechanism is alteration of the excitation sequence in ventricular muscle not actually involved by the infarct.

The loss of ventricular muscle that during its excitation previously contributed to the form of the QRS complex is the mechanism responsible for the most characteristic and diagnostically useful evidence of the presence and location of myocardial infarction. This mechanism is illustrated in Figure 12–15. Under the heading of "normal" in that figure, an activation boundary is shown on a diagrammatic ventricular section. As illustrated, the uncanceled portion of the boundary results in a positive deflection in lead I. In the diagram headed "infarction," loss of excitable tissue in the lateral left ventricular wall is represented, together with the remaining portion of the excitation boundary previously illustrated. The uncanceled portion of the remaining boundary now results in a negative deflection in lead I. This is the general mechanism by which myocardial infarction results in Q waves

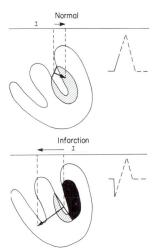

Figure 12–15 The mechanism of alteration of the QRS complex by loss of excitable tissue in myocardial infarction. In the upper diagram a representative excitation boundary in the left ventricle is shown and, as illustrated, is responsible for an upward deflection in lead I. The lower diagram shows part of the same boundary remaining after tissue loss indicated by the solid area. As shown, the remaining portion of the boundary results in a Q wave in lead I.

in leads in which normal ventricular activation is represented by upward deflections. The leads in which Q deflections occur are dependent on the location of infarction. As illustrated, lateral wall infarction may result in Q waves in lead I that are actually the result of activation in ventricular muscle not involved in the infarct. Similarly, lateral wall lesions may produce Q waves in lead aV_L and precordial leads V_5 and V_6. A similar mechanism accounts for Q waves in leads II, III, and aV_F with inferior wall location of infarction and leads V_1 through V_4 with anterior wall infarcts. Posterior wall infarcts are also reflected by QRS alterations in precordial leads V_1 through V_4, but the changes consist of increased amplitude of R waves, since normal activation in the posterior wall is reflected by downward deflections in these leads, and destruction of part of that wall leaves anteriorly directed activation unopposed.

The portion of the QRS complex in which changes due to the loss of excitable tissue occur depends on the location of the infarct with respect to the normal ventricular activation sequence. Abnormally deep or wide Q waves in leads normally containing an R wave reflect an infarct or portion of an infarct involving areas normally activated during early portions of the QRS complex. Subendocardial and intramural lesions or the subendocardial and intramural portions of transmural lesions are thus most likely to produce pathologic Q waves, which are the most definitive electrocardiographic evidence of infarction. Destructive lesions in this location are also more likely to produce marked QRS alterations than similar lesions located in subepicardial areas.

Early activation boundaries in subendocardial and intramural regions surround the ventricular cavities and include portions with potential differences oriented in multiple directions. When tissue loss removes a portion of such a boundary having a particular potential difference direction, portions of the boundary with potential differences in other directions determine QRS form that is often markedly different after infarction. Subepicardial lesions alter activation fronts in which potential differences are largely present in a particular direction. Removal of part of such a boundary can be expected to alter late portions of the QRS complex, but the direction of the boundary before and after such a destructive lesion is likely to be similar. The presence of subepicardial destructive lesions is thus likely to alter the detailed form of the QRS complex, but changes will be small compared to those associated with lesions in other locations. Actual myocardial infarcts are often transmural, or nearly so, but transmural involvement is not a necessity for diagnostically significant alterations of the QRS complex.

It should be clearly recognized that pathologic Q waves do not occur with all infarcts or with all infarct locations. These waves have special diagnostic significance because they represent a marked deviation from normal QRS waveform and do not overlap the range of normal variation of that waveform. Less marked QRS waveform changes may be expected with infarcts of particular size and in particular locations. For example, a lateral wall infarct may reduce the amplitude of R waves in leads I, aV_L, V_5, and V_6 but fail to produce Q waves if the size or location of the lesion is appropriate. Such a QRS waveform may not lie outside the range of normal variation and is less useful diagnostically than the more marked change to a pathologic Q wave.

The second factor that may alter QRS waveform with myocardial infarction is altered excitation sequence in ventricular muscle other than that destroyed by infarction. This mechanism is sometimes called "peri-infarction block," and that term will be employed in this text, although it has also been used with a more limited meaning. Whatever terminology is employed, a destructive myocardial lesion may alter activation sequence in remaining excitable muscle by affecting the spread of excitation in that muscle. Specialized conduction fibers may be interrupted by the lesion, so that areas normally excited via these fibers must be activated by other routes. Even without interruption of specialized fibers, the route of normal activation to a particular area through ventricular muscle may include the area of the destructive lesion, and other paths bypassing the lesion are then taken by the excitation process.

Alterations of the QRS complex by the mechanism of peri-infarction block mainly occur in mid and terminal portions of the complex. In actual diagnostic situations, it is difficult to distinguish such alterations from ones due to tissue loss in areas normally excited during these portions of the QRS complex. Only if the destructive lesion is known to be restricted to areas normally activated during early portions of the QRS complex can alterations of later QRS deflections be attributed to peri-infarction block with certainty. Since this information is not available ante mortem, the QRS alterations due to peri-infarction block are considerably less helpful diagnostically than those due to tissue loss. In addition, QRS alterations by the mechanism of peri-infarction block of necessity involve later portions of the QRS complex, which has a wider range of normal variability than initial deflections, so that changes in the late QRS may not be recognizable unless a preinfarction electrocardiogram is available.

QRS changes due to loss of excitable tissue are likely to be systematic, particularly when areas normally excited during early portions of the ventricular activation process are involved. At this time during the activation process, excitation is spreading in multiple directions, and the localized loss of excitable tissue is likely to leave excitation fronts directed away from the area of the lesion. In a similar manner, there is at least a tendency for QRS alterations due to peri-infarction block to be systematic. In this case, however, the muscle near the destructive lesion is likely to be the area in which activation sequence is most markedly altered, and the spread of excitation into this region is thus directed toward the lesion. These systematic features of QRS alteration by tissue loss and peri-infarction block may be visualized by an electrocardiographic lead containing an R and S wave during normal excitation. Destruction of excitable tissue during early portions of ventricular activation may alter the initial QRS deflection by changing it from an R to a Q deflection, whereas the mechanism of peri-infarction block may alter the terminal QRS in an opposite direction, changing the S wave to an R deflection.

ST segments and T waves are also likely to be altered by acute infarction and to change serially over a period of weeks or months. In old infarction, T wave abnormalities often persist, and ST segment displacement may persist in instances of ventricular aneurysm. The physiologic mechanism of both ST segment displacement and T wave abnormalities includes alteration of the duration and form of intracellular action potentials. An additional mechanism, namely reduced resting membrane potential, is also involved in ST segment displacement during acute infarction. Figure 12–16 illustrates the relation of action potential form to the electrocardiogram at various stages of myocardial infarction. For the purposes of this text, the heart may again be considered as consisting of two populations of cells with different intrinsic recovery properties. The normal state, in which the area activated earliest is represented by the action potential of longest duration, is

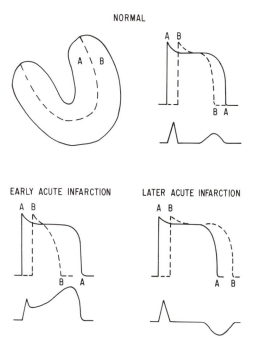

Figure 12–16 The relation of transmembrane action potential alterations by myocardial infarction to ST-T abnormalities. The normal state in which ventricular areas activated early have shorter action potentials and in which QRS and T deflections have the same polarity is illustrated in the upper portion of the figure. Early acute infarction results in reduced action potential duration, and ST displacement due to loss of the action potential plateau and increased T wave amplitude due to shorter action potential duration result. In later stages of infarction, action potential duration in ischemic tissue is prolonged, and T wave inversion occurs, as illustrated in the lower portion of the figure.

illustrated. The area represented by action potential B is excited at a later time but completes the recovery process first. As illustrated, potential differences between these areas during the plateau characteristic of cardiac muscle are small, and the ST segment is nearly isoelectric. The polarity of potential differences between the two areas is the same during excitation and recovery, so that a lead reflecting an upright QRS complex also reflects an upright T wave.

Acute ischemia shortens the duration of the transmembrane action potential and increases the slope of that portion of the record normally represented by a plateau. The mechanism of these action potential changes is not certain, but it is most likely that they are the result of local hyperkalemia due to potassium release from injured cells. As illustrated under the heading of "early acute infarction," such alterations are associated with ST segment displacement and increased amplitude of the T waves but with normal polarity of the latter deflection.

Later in the course of acute infarction, ischemic cells exhibit prolonged recovery time. As illustrated, this produces a state in which the polarities of potential differences during excitation and recovery are different from each other, and the polarities of QRS and T deflections therefore differ, the latter being abnormal. ST segment displacement decreases as cells recover and action potentials exhibit a more nearly normal plateau, or as injured cells become inexcitable.

INTRAVENTRICULAR CONDUCTION DISORDERS

Disorders in the delivery of excitation to ventricular muscle by the intraventricular portion of the specialized conduction system result in abnormal atrioventricular relations or anomalies of the QRS complex waveform. Abnormal atrioventricular relations occur with conduction disorders in the junctional tissues, including the atrioventricular node and bundle of His, or bilaterally in more distal portions of the intraventricular conduction system and range from prolonged conduction time, resulting in a prolonged PR interval in the electrocardiogram, to total failure of conduction, resulting in independent cardiac rhythms in the atria and ventricles, with the electrocardiogram showing unrelated P waves and QRST complexes.

Abnormalities of conduction in the specialized conduction system below the level of bifurcation of the bundle of His into right and left bundle branches result in anomalies of QRS waveform. Some of these abnormalities have considerable diagnostic utility, and they can be recognized only with electrocardiographic examination.

The physiologic basis of the distinctive QRS waveform associated with complete failure of con-

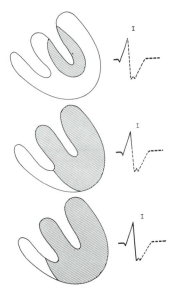

Figure 12–18 Ventricular activation sequence and QRS waveform in lead I in complete right bundle branch block.

duction through the left bundle branch is shown in Figure 12–17. Ventricular excitation reaches ventricular muscle exclusively via the right bundle branch, and its spread through ventricular muscle necessarily occurs in a right-to-left direction. Leads in which one of the electrodes is located on the left side of the body and that result in an upward deflection when that electrode is positive with respect to the other electrode involved in the lead thus show exclusively positive QRS deflections. Leads I, aV_L, V_5, and V_6 of the 12-lead electrocardiogram have this characteristic in left bundle branch block. In addition, most leads will reflect the abnormally long time required for the completion of ventricular activation by prolongation of the QRS complex. Normal ventricular activation delivered via both right and left bundle branches spreads simultaneously in right and left ventricles and determines the normal QRS duration. When bundle branch block is present and activation is delivered only via the functioning branch, an abnormally long time is required for completion of activation in the contralateral ventricle. A QRS duration of 0.12 second or more is usually considered the most useful index of complete bundle branch block.

The physiologic basis of QRS form in right bundle branch block is illustrated in Figure 12–18. As with left bundle branch block, the QRS duration is prolonged. In right bundle branch block, however, excitation occurs normally in the left ventricle. Early left septal activation may therefore give rise to a small Q wave in leads I, aV_L, V_5, and V_6 as in the normal state. This is followed by normal left ventricular activation proceeding leftward in the free left ventricular wall

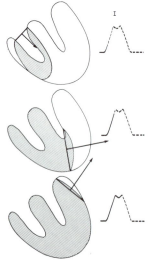

Figure 12–17 Ventricular activation sequence and QRS waveform in lead I in complete left bundle branch block.

and rightward in the interventricular septum. As illustrated, this combination of events gives rise to an R wave in lead I and similarly oriented leads. After completion of left ventricular activation including activation of the interventricular septum, activation of the free right ventricular wall takes place and results in an S wave in leads I, aV_L, V_5, and V_6. This deflection and the prolonged QRS duration constitute characteristic electrocardiographic features of right bundle branch block. Also, the anterior location of the free right ventricular wall results in additional major electrocardiographic evidence of right bundle branch block. The late activation of this structure proceeds anteriorly as well as to the right and results in prominent late R waves in one or more of the precordial leads V_1 through V_3. These deflections are preceded by normal R and S waves in these leads and are therefore known as "R prime waves."

The T waves associated with bundle branch block are influenced by the abnormal ventricular activation sequence as well as by the intrinsic recovery characteristics of ventricular muscle. The gross abnormalities of activation sequence and QRS form in these states also result in gross alterations of T waveform, even if ventricular recovery characteristics are normal. In general, the recovery sequence alterations secondary to activation sequence abnormalities in bundle branch block tend to produce QRS and T complexes of opposite polarity, even if intrinsic recovery properties remain the same. The clinical significance of bundle branch blocks is an appropriate subject for texts of diagnostic electrocardiography and cardiology. As previously mentioned, however, the recognition of these states can be accomplished only by electrocardiographic means.

In addition to block at the level of major right and left bundle branches, other abnormalities of intraventricular conduction exist. Slower than normal conduction can occur under appropriate circumstances at any level in the heart, and in the case of the intraventricular conduction system distal to bifurcation of the bundle of His, such conduction can alter QRS form in fashions that resemble bundle branch block but that are less marked.

Furthermore, conduction defects may occur at sites more distal than the major bundle branches. Evidence has been reported that the left bundle branch consists of two major subdivisions, one of which is distributed to anterosuperior and the other to posteroinferior left ventricular muscle. On the basis of findings to be expected with block of each of these, electrocardiograms can be classified in terms of anterosuperior and posteroinferior left fascicular block. Anatomic evidence for distinct subdivisions of the left bundle is conflicting, but classification of electrocardiograms as evidencing fascicular block is being widely employed. The major criterion proposed for recognition of these entities is the electrical axis of the QRS with anterosuperior fascicular block resulting in left axis deviation and posteroinferior block resulting in right axis deviation. Axis deviation compatible with these entities is often associated with right bundle branch block, and the presence of this conduction defect is compatible with the view that the axis deviation is also the result of a conduction disorder.

13 Arrhythmias—Mechanisms and Pathogenesis

Yoshio Watanabe, Leonard S. Dreifus, and William A. Sodeman, Sr.

A cardiac arrhythmia is any deviation from the normal rhythm of the heart beat, the requirements for "normal" being as follows:

1. The rhythm originates in the sinus (sinoatrial) node. In other words, the sinus node assumes the role of pacemaker of the heart.

2. The frequency of sinoatrial impulse formation is within an optimal range—usually between 60 and 100 per minute in adults.

3. Within this range, the rate must be reasonably regular.

4. Every sinus impulse is transmitted to the ventricles through the normal atrioventricular (AV) conducting system, and with a normal, constant conduction time.

5. Intraventricular conduction is also normal, with the impulse traveling through the His bundle, bundle branches, or fascicles and the peripheral Purkinje network. From this definition, it becomes readily apparent that cardiac arrhythmias include alterations in the site, frequency, or regularity of impulse formation as well as abnormalities in the order, velocity, or regularity of conduction of excitation. Thus, disorders such as first-degree AV block and bundle branch block are included among the cardiac arrhythmias, even though the rhythm is of sinus origin and quite regular.

For clinical purposes, classification of cardiac arrhythmias is usually based on the origin of impulses (supraventricular or ventricular) and their mode of appearance (premature systole, tachycardia, flutter, fibrillation, etc.). From the electrophysiologic standpoint, however, genesis of cardiac arrhythmias is often divided into three categories: (1) disturbances of impulse formation; (2) disturbances of conduction; and (3) a combination of both (Table 13–1).

ABNORMALITIES OF IMPULSE FORMATION

ALTERATIONS IN PHYSIOLOGIC AUTOMATICITY

Physiologic automaticity is a property of the fibers of the specialized conducting system that allows them to generate their own impulses under physiologic conditions. Transmembrane potentials, as recorded with the use of glass microelectrode techniques, usually remain at a constant level (which is negative intracellularly) in the working muscle fibers of the atria and the ventricles when the fibers are not excited. In the fibers of the sinus node, in contrast, the membrane potential becomes gradually less negative during the electrical diastole (phase 4), a phenomenon called *diastolic depolarization.* When the loss of membrane potential reaches a critical level called the *threshold potential,* a rapid reversal of the membrane potential (phase 0 depolarization) ensues, generating a new action potential. These relationships are illustrated in Figures 13–1 and 13–2.

It is apparent from Figure 13–2 that the frequency of impulse formation due to automaticity is determined by the time required for the membrane potential to reach the threshold potential. More specifically, the cycle length is increased and the frequency of discharge is decreased when

TABLE 13–1 ELECTROPHYSIOLOGIC MECHANISMS OF CARDIAC ARRHYTHMIAS

I. Abnormalities of Impulse Formation:
  A. Alterations of physiologic automaticity in the specialized conducting fibers:
    1. Enhanced automaticity
    2. Depressed automaticity
  B. Development of abnormal automaticity in the atrial and ventricular muscle fibers
  C. Other mechanisms of impulse formation:
    1. Oscillations of membrane potential
    2. Delayed afterdepolarization (transient depolarization)
    3. Early afterdepolarization
    4. Local potential differences causing re-excitation of certain fibers, due to either asynchronous repolarization or partial depolarization
II. Disturbances of Conduction of Excitation:
  A. Decremental conduction
  B. Inhomogeneous conduction
  C. Conduction delay and block
  D. Unidirectional block
  E. Reentry
III. Combined Disturbances of Impulse Formation and Conduction:
  A. Parasystole
  B. Ectopic rhythms with exit block
  C. Fibrillation

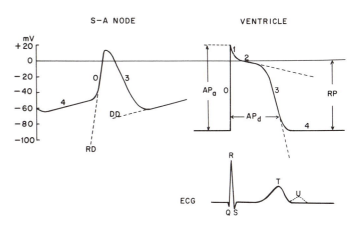

Figure 13–1 Transmembrane action potentials from the sinus node *(left)* and a ventricular muscle fiber *(right)*. The sinus nodal action potential is characterized by a gradual decrease in the resting membrane potential during phase 4 (DD, diastolic depolarization), a less negative membrane potential, small action potential amplitude (APa), slower rate of depolarization during phase 0 (RD), and the lack of phase 2 (plateau) in its repolarization phase. Other abbreviations are RP, membrane resting potential; APd, action potential duration, the time relationships between the ventricular complexes in the electrocardiogram and ventricular action potential as shown with ECG. (Reproduced from Watanabe, Y.: Electrophysiology of cardiac arrhythmias. Clin. Res. *51*:607, 1974.)

either (1) the distance between the maximal diastolic potential (the deepest membrane potential attained at the end of an action potential) and the threshold potential is greater, or (2) the slope of the diastolic depolarization is less steep. This second factor is especially important, and the enhancement and depression of automaticity usually are associated with an increase and decrease in the slope of phase 4 depolarization, respectively. The automaticity in the sinus node is significantly affected by alterations in the autonomic nervous system. For instance, an increase in the vagal tone would make the maximal diastolic potential more negative and farther away from the threshold potential (hyperpolarization) and also decrease the velocity of diastolic depolarization, thus resulting in prolongation of the sinus cycle length (sinus bradycardia). Contrariwise, an increased sympathetic tone will increase the slope of diastolic depolarization and accelerate the sinus mechanism (sinus tachycardia). The respiratory sinus arrhythmia results from phasic alterations in the automaticity of the sinus node due to variations in the autonomic nervous tone associated with respiratory movement. Maneuvers stimulating the vagus

nerve, such as carotid sinus massage, will release acetylcholine in the sinus node region, and a marked suppression of the sinus automaticity may result in sinus arrest. Marked sinus bradycardia, often seen in athletes during rest, is ascribed to the dominance of vagal over sympathetic tone. The frequency of impulse formation in the sinus node is higher in infants and children, often exceeding 100 beats per minute, whereas 60 to 100 beats per minute is considered the normal range for adults. Furthermore, the sinus rate tends to be lower in the aged.

Automatic fibers outside the sinus node are found in the so-called "intra-atrial conducting system," including the bundles of Bachmann, Wenckebach, and Thorel, the AN and NH regions of the AV node, the His bundle, the right and left bundle branches, and the more peripheral Purkinje fibers. Hence, impulse formation can arise from various portions of the AV conducting system. However, the slope of phase 4 depolarization usually is steepest in the fibers of the sinus node, and the loss of membrane potential reaches the threshold level there earlier than in other automatic fibers. This is the reason that the sinus node

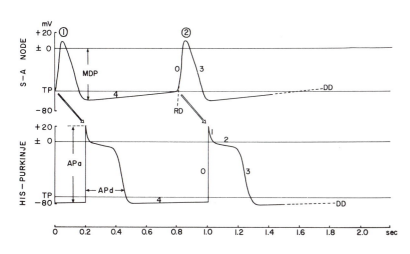

Figure 13–2 Transmembrane potentials of the SA nodal and the His-Purkinje fibers are schematically shown. The slope of diastolic depolarization (Dd) is steeper, and the threshold potential (TP) is attained earlier in the SA nodal fiber than in the His-Purkinje fiber. Thus, the His-Purkinje system is discharged by propagated sinus impulses *(arrows)*. Note the differences in the action potential amplitude (APa), the action potential duration (APd), the rate of phase 0 depolarization (RD), and the time course of repolarization (phases 1, 2, and 3) between the two fiber types. MDP, maximal diastolic potential. (Reproduced with permission from Watanabe, Y., and Dreifus, L. S.: Am. Heart J. *76*:114, 1968.)

becomes the pacemaker of the entire heart under normal conditions. Figure 13–2 shows that the transmembrane potential of the His-Purkinje fibers (bottom diagram) has a slower rate of phase 4 depolarization than that of the sinus node (top diagram); hence, the next sinus impulse will be transmitted to these His-Purkinje fibers and will produce phase 0 depolarization before their own threshold potential is reached. The fibers of the specialized conducting system, other than the sinus node, thus remain as a latent pacemaker. One reason for the lower automatic activity of these subsidiary pacemakers has been attributed to the mechanism of so-called "over-drive suppression." For instance, when the sinus nodal fibers are excited by extrinsic electrical stimuli at a higher frequency, the rate of diastolic depolarization is temporarily decreased, resulting in a decrease in the frequency of impulse formation. The higher the frequency of stimulation and the longer its duration, the more marked the depression of automaticity. Thus, it is possible that other fibers of the specialized conducting system would sustain certain degrees of suppression of their automaticity because of their repetitive depolarization by the sinus impulses.

Several mechanisms related to the genesis of cardiac arrhythmias will be readily apparent from the diagrams in Figure 13–2. First, if the arrival of the sinus impulses to the automatic fibers in other portions of the specialized conducting system is delayed for any reason, the diastolic depolarization in those fibers will proceed uninterrupted, eventually reaching their threshold potential and generating a new impulse. An impulse thus generated usually causes ventricular excitation and prevents a prolonged period of ventricular asystole. This is a physiologic safety mechanism that manifests itself on the electrocardiogram as an escape beat. A series of these escape beats will constitute an escape rhythm. Major causes for such an escape impulse formation include sinus arrhythmia, sinus arrest, and nonconducted atrial

premature systoles (which delay the sinus impulse formation) and sinoatrial (SA) block or AV block (which prevents the transmission of normally formed sinus impulses to the downstream fibers). It is also readily understood that escape beats appear after an interval longer than the cycle length of the basic rhythm. The AV junction usually possesses the next highest order of automatic activity, and escape beats most commonly arise in this area. Less frequently, escape beats may originate in the Purkinje fibers below the bifurcation of the His bundle or within the atrial tissue. When the level of the AV conduction block is located below the bifurcation of the His bundle, the escape impulse formation should naturally arise below the site of block and take the form of idioventricular beats. A rare example of sinus escape beats was previously observed when a slowing of the basic AV junctional rhythm permitted impulse formation in the sinus node, which had a lower intrinsic automaticity than the AV junctional pacemaker.

In the so-called "sick sinus syndrome," the presence of lesions in the AV junctional area is often suggested when failure of escape impulse formation in the AV junction produces long periods of asystole. This indicates depression of subsidiary automatic foci, an insufficient physiologic safety mechanism. There are occasions on which automaticity is depressed in the sinus node and in most portions of the AV conducting system. In these instances, the site of impulse formation may gradually shift from the sinus node to the AV junction and farther down to the intraventricular conducting system, eventually leading to ventricular standstill. Such "downward displacement of the pacemaker" is often seen immediately prior to death in a patient with acute myocardial infarction or other types of organic heart disease. It constitutes the most serious type of arrhythmia caused by depression of physiologic automaticity (Fig. 13–3).

In contrast to the rhythm disorders resulting

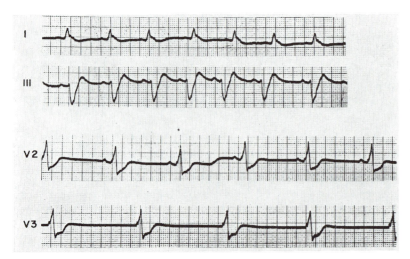

Figure 13–3 An example of so-called "downward displacement of the pacemaker." In leads I and III, sinus rhythm at the rate of 70 per minute with a marked intraventricular conduction disturbance is evident. The sinus rate is decreased to approximately 45 per minute in lead V2, whereas a slow AV junctional or idioventricular rhythm at the rate of 33 per minute without any discernible P waves is visible in V3. Ventricular standstill soon supervened. (Reproduced from Watanabe, Y.: Genesis of cardiac arrhythmias. Intensivmed. Prax. *10*:109, 1973.)

Figure 13–4 *A,* Diagram similar to Figure 13–2 illustrates an accelerated impulse formation in the His-Purkinje system. The sinus node is discharging at a normal rate. However, the His-Purkinje fiber generates its own impulses before a propagated sinus impulse arrives at this region because of an enhanced automaticity (increased phase 4 depolarization). Interference (or collision) of the two independently formed impulses may occur at different levels within the AV transmission system *(arrows)*. *B,* A clinical example of AV junctional tachycardia. The R–R intervals are shorter than the P–P intervals, and AV dissociation is present. (Reproduced with permission from Watanabe, Y.: Genesis of cardiac arrhythmias. Intensivmed. Prax. *10*:109, 1973.)

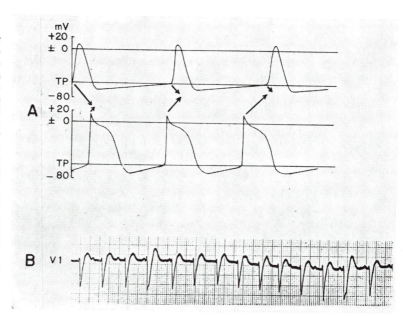

from decreased automaticity, enhanced automaticity in the fibers of the specialized conducting system other than the sinus node may cause a higher rate of impulse formation in these fibers compared with the sinus rhythm. Then, such ectopic impulses (impulses originating outside the sinus node) could control the atria, the ventricles, or both. Ectopic tachycardias resulting from this mechanism would not show sudden onset and offset, and they would probably take the form of nonparoxysmal tachycardia. A diagram illustrating the relationship of enhanced ectopic automaticity and the sinus node and an electrocardiographic example of nonparoxysmal AV junctional tachycardia are shown in Figure 13–4. Depending on the site of enhanced ectopic automaticity, an atrial, AV junctional, or ventricular variety of nonparoxysmal tachycardia will be identified.

It is apparent from the aforementioned observations that changes in the physiologic automaticity in fibers of the AV conducting system can produce various types of cardiac arrhythmia. The automaticity of the His-Purkinje system is enhanced by excessive administration of cardiac glycosides, catecholamines, and hypokalemia, whereas their automaticity can be depressed by hyperkalemia and various antiarrhythmic agents.

DEVELOPMENT OF ABNORMAL AUTOMATICITY

Under certain abnormal conditions, diastolic (phase 4) depolarization and resultant spontaneous impulse formation may be observed in the working muscle fibers of the atria and the ventricles. These ordinarily possess no such ability. Such phenomena can be termed *abnormal automaticity.* A report

by Müller in 1965 showed that when the atrial or ventricular muscle fibers were perfused by a solution containing neither potassium nor calcium, these fibers developed a prominent diastolic depolarization, leading to regular impulse formation. A decrease in the resting membrane potential, or a partial depolarization of the cell membrane, was observed before the development of such automatic impulse formation. Particularly in the atrial muscle fibers, the reduction of the membrane potential reached about -45 mV. Müller explained these findings as a combination of the following two events: (1) loss of membrane potential due to decreased potassium permeability brought about by the lack of potassium ions; and (2) an increased sodium permeability caused by the absence of calcium. Although the results just cited show clearly that even the working myocardial fibers outside the specialized conducting system can develop typical phase 4 depolarization and automatic impulse formation, perfusion of these tissues with potassium- and calcium-free solution is highly unphysiologic and incompatible with life. Therefore, it was considered at that time that the development of such abnormal automaticity could not play a major role in the genesis of clinical cardiac arrhythmias.

It has also been shown that local application of barium chloride ($BaCl_2$) to the working myocardial fibers can produce regular impulse formation due to diastolic depolarization. Partial depolarization of the cell membrane again preceded this type of impulse formation, suggesting the importance of decreased membrane potential levels in the production of abnormal automaticity. However, the presence of barium ions at the high concentrations used in these experiments cannot be expected in the clinical setting.

Partial depolarization of myocardial fibers due to the passage of a depolarizing current to the cell membrane has been shown to produce abnormal automaticity. This indicates that, under certain pathophysiologic conditions in the presence of organic heart diseases, ectopic impulse formation due to such an abnormal automaticity may indeed produce various arrhythmias. For instance, in the presence of myocardial infarction, ischemic ventricular fibers with a reduced membrane potential may develop diastolic depolarization and acquire abnormal automaticity. It is evident that the role of this mechanism in the genesis of clinical arrhythmias requires continuing study.

OSCILLATIONS OF MEMBRANE POTENTIAL AND AFTERDEPOLARIZATIONS

Oscillations of the membrane potential, or so-called "oscillatory afterpotentials," have been observed in several different fiber types under various conditions. In 1959, Matsuda observed in ventricular muscle fibers after the application of aconitine that the completion of repolarization was followed by a decrease in the membrane potential, which produced several small oscillations of the membrane potential not reaching the threshold level. The first of these oscillatory afterpotentials was the largest, and a gradual decrease in their amplitude was followed by their disappearance. When the drug effects were exaggerated, the first afterpotential became greater, reached the threshold potential, and generated a new action potential. The second action potential was again followed by a similar afterpotential, finally resulting in a repetitive discharge at frequencies of 150 to 450 per minute. One criticism of this report noted that such repetitive discharges were produced in Purkinje fibers contained in the preparation.

In any event, it is apparent that abnormal impulse formation at high frequencies may arise in some portions of the ventricle in the presence of this alkaloid. As indicated by the term *afterpotential,* such alterations of the membrane potential are predicated on the presence of an initial action potential. This is the major difference between this mechanism and physiologic or abnormal automaticity, as the latter does not require an initiating beat.

West observed oscillations of the membrane potential in the sinus node of the rabbit heart. When the sinus node preparation was perfused with a solution containing 30 per cent of the normal sodium concentration and 20 µg per liter of isoproterenol, an action potential produced by electrical stimulation was followed by a series of spontaneous discharges of progressively decreasing amplitude leading to subthreshold oscillations. After several (up to 10) small oscillations of 2 to 3 mV, the amplitudes again gradually increased

until, on reaching the threshold potential, a series of spontaneous impulses occurred. The frequency of such subthreshold oscillations of the membrane potential was 200 to 250 per minute, similar to that of the action potentials.

Oscillations of the membrane potential also have been observed in Purkinje fibers under various experimental conditions. For example, Cranefield and others have observed that canine Purkinje fibers superfused with a sodium-free perfusate or with $BaCl_2$ develop phasic variations of the resting membrane potential. A gradual increase in their amplitudes to the threshold potential resulted in the generation of an action potential. This action potential was followed by hyperpolarization of the cell membrane, which, in turn, was followed by depolarization and a spontaneous discharge. Since this type of potential change precedes the development of a spontaneous rhythm, these authors termed it *oscillatory prepotential* in contradistinction to oscillatory afterpotentials. The frequency of these oscillations was about 10 to 20 beats per minute, as was the resultant spontaneous rhythm. In some of the perfused Purkinje fibers, the spontaneous rhythm was terminated by a premature response due to a single electrical stimulus. Subsequent development of subthreshold oscillations was associated with a phenomenon similar to that observed in the sinus node, with initial waning and subsequent waxing until repetitive action potentials were formed. This mechanism of sustained rhythmic activity resulting from a progressive increase in amplitude of the oscillatory potentials may superficially appear similar to the diastolic depolarization in physiologic automaticity. In this experimentally induced mechanism, however, it is said that a rather rapid transition from hyperpolarization to partial depolarization brings about a loss of membrane potential to the threshold level; hence, it requires a preceding action potential.

Although these oscillations of the membrane potential may appear quite important as a mechanism of impulse formation in the myocardium, most of the experimental conditions producing the phenomena are unphysiologic and are not expected to occur clinically. One exception, reported by Vassalle, showed the development of oscillatory prepotentials with subsequent periods of spontaneous impulse formation in Purkinje fibers when the extracellular potassium concentration was lowered from 5.4 to 2.7 mM. Since this degree of hypokalemia can be observed in patients, ectopic impulse formation in the ventricles due to this mechanism may not definitely be ruled out.

Two types of afterdepolarization have been noted and are discussed subsequently:

1. When Purkinje fibers are electrically stimulated in the presence of rather high concentrations of cardiac glycosides, the termination of an action potential is often followed by a transient loss of membrane potential. This is termed either

delayed afterdepolarization or *transient depolarization*. When the frequency of electrical stimulation is relatively low, the degree of depolarization is small and the membrane potential returns to a more negative level. In contrast, stimulation at higher frequencies causes an increase in depolarization sufficient to attain the threshold potential and to generate a new action potential. Usually, only one action potential is formed, and it is followed by a subthreshold transient depolarization. The amplitude of such afterdepolarizations increases when the extracellular calcium concentration is high or the potassium concentration is low. These observations led Ferrier and Moe to suggest that coupled ventricular premature systoles in the form of ventricular bigeminy as an expression of so-called "digitalis arrhythmia" probably result from this mechanism. Clinical observations of aggravation of digitalis arrhythmias by hypercalcemia or hypokalemia may support this contention. It has also been shown that the ionic mechanism producing this delayed afterdepolarization is what is now known to be slow inward currents carried mainly by calcium ions. Indeed, this transient depolarization is abolished by manganese ions, which inhibit such slow inward currents.

2. The second variety is called *early afterdepolarization*. In this process, when ventricular muscle fibers are perfused with aconitine, repolarization is often brought to a halt at a membrane potential level of about -70 mV, at which point partial depolarization resumes. This depolarization may reach the threshold potential and produce several short action potentials in the form of spike discharges. These are finally followed by the completion of phase 3 repolarization and a return to the resting membrane potential level. Rather like the oscillatory afterpotentials described earlier, generation of these abnormal impulses under the influence of aconitine is observed only when the myocardial preparations are electrically stimulated. In other words, aconitine arrhythmias appear to require a preceding beat. Other reports have shown that aconitine produces similar phenomena in Purkinje fibers, whereas veratrine causes an extreme prolongation of phase 2 of repolarization (plateau), from which repetitive spike discharges may arise. These observations suggest the possible role of early afterdepolarizations in the genesis of arrhythmias, although questions can be raised about their clinical significance.

Alternatively, the following mechanism might possibly occur in the clinical setting. In a patient given a moderate amount of ouabain, when the membrane potential in the Purkinje fibers is reduced to -40 to -60 mV by the passage of a depolarizing current, repetitive impulse formation could develop at a frequency higher than that of the original spontaneous rhythm owing to physiologic automaticity. The changes in the transmembrane potential during such sustained rhythmic activity appear similar to enhanced diastolic depolarization. However, this particular type of repetitive discharge occurs at a membrane potential level of -40 to -60 mV, whereas diastolic depolarization in the presence of physiologic automaticity starts at a level of -85 to -90 mV. Furthermore, the maximal rate of depolarization during phase 0, or the upstroke velocity of the action potential, is quite rapid in the latter, whereas it is extremely slow in the former. These two modes of impulse formation thus appear to show qualitative rather than quantitative differences. Transition between the two mechanisms is easily produced by applying either depolarizing or hyperpolarizing currents to the cell membrane. The possibility that this form of abnormal impulse formation may occur in injured Purkinje fibers, especially in the presence of excessive cardiac glycosides, cannot be ruled out.

It must be re-emphasized here that these abnormal mechanisms of impulse formation—abnormal automaticity, oscillations of the membrane potential, and afterdepolarizations—occur in Purkinje fibers as well as ventricular muscle when their transmembrane potential is reduced to a level similar to that found in a normally automatic sinus node. Furthermore, it is now widely accepted that both the sinus nodal action potentials and these abnormal modes of impulse formation depend on ionic currents through the so-called "slow channels" (slow inward currents). Certain investigators have therefore suggested two classifications of mechanisms of impulse formation: (1) those occurring at a membrane potential level of -90 to -70 mV; and (2) those occurring at -60 to -40 mV.

Still another method of classification is to group the physiologic automaticity of the specialized conducting system with abnormal automaticity of the working myocardial fibers and then to contrast them with oscillatory potentials and afterdepolarizations. The former varieties represent true spontaneous impulse formation; the latter are triggered by a preceding action potential.

The classification we have adopted in this chapter is based more on clinical considerations, as automatic activity under physiologic conditions is seen only in the sinus node and other fibers of the specialized conducting system. Other mechanisms of impulse formation appear to occur only under abnormal conditions.

Re-excitation of certain fibers due to local potential differences, as listed in Table 13–1, probably plays a role in the genesis of rhythm disorders, particularly in the initiation and the maintenance of fibrillation. A new term, *reflection,* has been given to this phenomenon by certain investigators, although its differentiation from the so-called "microreentries" and other mechanisms of abnormal impulse formation in partially depolarized fibers may be rather difficult.

Possible clinical implications of these abnormal mechanisms of impulse formation can be suggested. If the rate of impulse formation caused by abnormal automaticity in the working myocardial fibers exceeds that of the sinus rhythm, nonparoxysmal ectopic tachycardias may be produced, whereas oscillatory afterpotentials and the various afterdepolarizations may result in coupled premature systoles. It has further been suggested that paroxysmal ectopic tachycardias, usually ascribed to reentry movements, could be caused by these oscillatory events. The role of these mechanisms in the genesis of digitalis arrhythmias and of either unifocal or multifocal impulse formation in the initiation of cardiac fibrillation perhaps cannot be ruled out.

DISTURBANCES OF CONDUCTION OF EXCITATION

FACTORS CONTROLLING IMPULSE TRANSMISSION

The various factors that control impulse transmission in the myocardium are listed in Table 13–2. Since an extensive review of these problems has previously been published elsewhere, only some of the more important factors will be discussed in this chapter.

The primary determinants of conductivity include (1) effectiveness of impulses produced by depolarization of the upstream fibers; and (2) the excitability of downstream fibers responding to such impulses. With respect to the first factor, it can be generalized that the greater the amplitude and the upstroke velocity of phase 0 of an action potential, the higher its effectiveness as an impulse and the greater its conduction velocity. Smaller action potential amplitudes and decreased rates of phase 0 depolarization will be associated with depressed conductivity. Under physiologic conditions, Purkinje fibers have the most rapid rate of phase 0 depolarization (several hundred volts per second) of all fiber types and also show the highest conduction velocity (3.0 to 3.5 m per second).

In fibers of the atria, ventricles, and the Purkinje system, whose phase 0 depolarization depends on a rapid inflow of sodium ions across the cell membrane (fast sodium channel), a greater (more negative) membrane potential immediately prior to excitation will be associated with both a greater amplitude and a greater rate of rise of the action potential. This is explained by more complete activation of the so-called "sodium carriers" as a function of the transmembrane potential, and this relationship is expressed by membrane responsiveness curves (Fig. 13–5).

The membrane responsiveness curve in a given myocardial fiber should remain constant as long as its physiologic environment is stable, but it can vary with changing conditions. Quinidine,

TABLE 13–2 FACTORS CONTROLLING IMPULSE TRANSMISSION

I. **Primary determinants of conductivity:**
  A. Physiologic factors:
    1. Effectiveness of stimuli produced by depolarization of upstream fibers
    2. Excitability of responding downstream fibers
    3. Temporal fluctuation of 1 or 2
  B. Anatomic factors:
    1. Fiber diameter
    2. Geometric arrangement of fibers

II. **Abnormal conduction phenomena resulting from alterations in the primary determinants of conductivity:**
  A. Decremental conduction
  B. Inhomogeneous conduction
  C. Conduction delay and block
  D. Unidirectional block
  E. Reentry

III. **Abnormal conduction phenomena secondarily affecting conductivity:**
  A. Conduction delay and block:
    1. Effects of conduction delay on the action potential duration (prolongation)
    2. Effects of conduction block on the action potential duration of fibers proximal to the site of propagation failure (shortening)
    3. Effects of conduction block on the action potential duration of fibers distal to the site of propagation failure (prolongation)
    4. Effects of conduction delay or block on excitability of the downstream fibers
    5. Conduction delay or block causing impulse formation in the downstream fibers
  B. Reentry:
    1. Collision of re-entrant impulse with the more slowly advancing, antegrade wave of excitation resulting in cancellation of both wavefronts
    2. Further disorganization of the excitation front (increased inhomogeneity) in subsequent impulse transmission
    3. Reorganization of the excitation front (decreased inhomogeneity) in subsequent impulse transmission

for instance, is known to shift the membrane responsiveness curve downward and to the right. The upstroke velocity of an action potential would then be decreased, even though the level of membrane potential remains unchanged (Fig. 13–5). A shift of this curve upward and to the left will increase the rate of phase 0 depolarization and improve conductivity without any changes in the transmembrane potential. However, various factors that reduce the membrane potential will consequently decrease the rate of depolarization and conduction velocity. Increased extracellular potassium concentrations, myocardial ischemia (hypoxia), and excessive administration of certain antiarrhythmic agents will produce partial depolarization of the cell membrane and depress conduction. Contrariwise, an increase in the resting membrane potential (hyperpolarization) tends to improve conductivity. Certain degrees of hypoka-

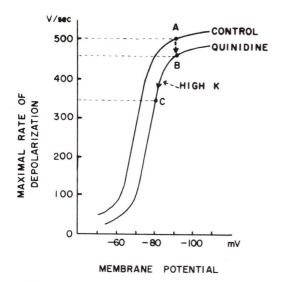

Figure 13–5 Membrane responsiveness curves correlating the level of membrane potential and the maximal rate of depolarization. The shift of the curve downward and to the right by quinidine (A→B) and the effect of a decrease in the membrane potential due to high potassium (B→C) are illustrated.

lemia (e.g., 1.5 mM) may exert such effects on atrial and ventricular muscle fibers.

In fibers of the AV conducting system showing automatic activity, the transmembrane potential will be progressively decreased during electrical diastole because of phase 4 depolarization. Then, action potentials produced by impulses arriving at these fibers later in diastole will show a slower rate of rise and a smaller amplitude of phase 0, and the conduction velocity is decreased. Depres-

sion of conductivity due to this mechanism becomes more marked in the presence of a longer electrical diastole or a greater rate of phase 4 depolarization. Conduction disturbances resulting from this mechanism are often called *phase 4 block* (Fig. 13–6, bottom).

The interval between two impulses may affect conductivity through the change in the membrane potential in a way different from that seen in phase 4 block. This is a sudden shortening of the cycle length of stimulation. In this instance, the wave of excitation arrives at the downstream fibers before the repolarization from a previous excitation is complete. Then, even when these fibers respond with a second action potential, its phase 0 will start from a reduced membrane potential level and show a much slower upstroke velocity. Since this type of conduction disturbance results from encroachment on the phase 3 repolarization by an excitation front, it is often called *phase 3 block* in contrast to the phase 4 block just described (Fig. 13–6, top).

In addition to the levels of membrane potential at the onset of excitation (so-called "take-off potential"), the level of threshold potential may affect the rate of rise of an action potential. It has been shown that a more marked diastolic depolarization is associated with a less negative threshold potential and, hence, with a slower rate of phase 0 depolarization. Conductivity will thus be depressed in those fibers showing distinct phase 4 depolarization. Exit block from an ectopic pacemaker and the so-called "protection block" around a parasystolic focus could possibly be explained by this mechanism, since impulse formation in these ectopic sites results from automatic activity in a group of fibers. The role of slow channels may

Figure 13–6 Schematic diagrams illustrating the mechanisms of phase 3 block *(top)* and phase 4 block *(bottom)*. In phase 3 block, a premature impulse may arrive at certain downstream fibers during their phase 3 of repolarization because of their longer action potential duration compared with the upstream fibers. This will result in a premature action potential with a reduced amplitude and slower upstroke velocity, and conduction may become decremental *(left)*. Still earlier arrival of an impulse may find the downstream fibers refractory, resulting in a complete block *(right)*. In phase 4 block *(bottom diagram)*, impulses arriving later in electrical diastole (phase 4) cause an action potential with decreased amplitude and rate of rise of phase 0 because of the loss of membrane potential due to phase 4 depolarization. Note that depolarization of this fiber immediately after a preceding action potential produces an action potential with a better conductivity *(broken lines)*.

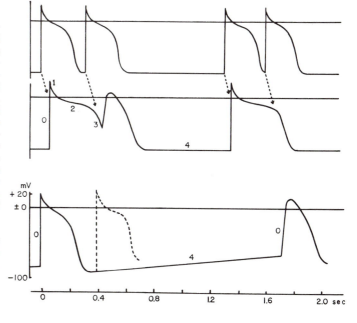

deserve special attention with reference to these phenomena.

Ever since the ionic theory was developed in neurophysiology by Hodgkin and others, it has been postulated that ionic currents similar to those observed in nerve fibers are responsible for the generation of myocardial action potential. However, various experimental data gradually accumulated since the late 1960s have forced a major revision of that concept. It has been demonstrated that the slow channels, in addition to the fast sodium channel, play a major role in the production of cardiac action potentials. This important development in cardiac electrophysiology has been extensively reviewed by several investigators, and a brief discussion here appears in order.

It is now widely accepted that the initial rapid depolarization (phase 0) of the myocardial action potential is produced by a rapid inflow of sodium ions across the cell membrane, exactly as in nerve fibers (fast channel or fast sodium current). The prolonged action potential characteristically seen in myocardial fibers, however, appears to depend on a much slower influx of ions, and these slow inward currents are thought to be carried mainly by calcium and in part by sodium. The electrophysiologic characteristics of these two channels are compared in Table 13–3, which indicates their qualitative rather than quantitative differences. When the membrane potential is significantly decreased (e.g., by partial depolarization), the fast sodium channel is partially inactivated and the phase 0 depolarization becomes dependent mostly on slow inward currents. Slower rate of rise of the action potential and the depression of conduction in these circumstances (so-called "slow responses") are thus explained by a change in the ionic mechanism. This further illustrates the importance of the level of membrane potential in determining conduction of excitation.

It has been pointed out in the previous section that the development of abnormal automaticity or afterdepolarizations in the atrial, ventricular, or Purkinje fibers is observed when these fibers are partially depolarized to a membrane potential level similar to that of sinus nodal fibers. Also, with reference to conduction of excitation, the fibers of the sinus node as well as the AV node appear to act like partially depolarized fibers of the working myocardium and the Purkinje system. In other words, the slowly rising action potentials seen in the sinus node and the N region of the AV node, under physiologic conditions, are now considered to depend on slow inward currents, whereas the role of the fast sodium channel in these fibers is minimal, if any. The ions carrying these slow inward currents in sinus and AV nodal fibers again appear to be mainly calcium, but several experimental studies have shown that the presence of slow sodium current cannot be ruled out.

The various mechanisms that cause alterations of conductivity, as just described, depend mostly on the changes in the membrane potential. They are said to be *voltage-dependent,* except in the case of a shift of membrane responsiveness curve. In contrast, the possibility of *time-dependent* changes in conductivity has been suggested. For instance, in ventricular muscle fibers under the influence of certain drugs, including quinidine and chlorpromazine, partial refractoriness may continue beyond the completion of repolarization. Then, action potentials generated immediately after the end of phase 3 repolarization will show a slower upstroke velocity than those occurring later in electrical diastole, even though the same level of resting membrane potential has been attained. This phenomenon is different from a rightward shift of the membrane responsiveness curve. The rate of phase 0 depolarization varies as a function of time during phase 4 in the former, whereas the rate of rise of action potentials may remain steady at a new lower level throughout electrical diastole in the latter. These time-dependent disturbances in conduction are explained by delayed recovery of the fast sodium channel from its inactivation, compared with the restoration of the resting membrane potential. Nevertheless, it will be understood that the effectiveness of an impulse produced by depolarization of upstream fibers is affected by various factors in a complex manner.

TABLE 13–3 COMPARISON OF FAST CHANNEL AND SLOW CHANNEL

	Fast Channel	Slow Channel
Activation and inactivation	Proceed rapidly; inactivated upon loss of membrane potential	Proceed slowly; activated at lower (less negative) membrane potential levels
Maximal rate of phase 0 depolarization	Usually several hundred volts per second	Usually on the order of 1 to 10 volts per second
Propagation of excitation	Rapid, with high safety factor	Slow, with low safety factor
Ions carrying the current	Sodium	Mainly calcium; partly sodium (and certain other ions?)
Factors that inhibit the channel	Tetrodotoxin	Manganese, lanthanum, verapamil, D 600, etc.; insensitive to tetrodotoxin

The excitability of downstream fibers is the second primary determinant of conductivity. The diastolic threshold of excitation is determined by the minimal strength of stimulus (or the minimal amount of current) required to produce full depolarization of fibers during their phase 4. When this current requirement is greater, the excitability of the fibers is lower, and vice versa. One mechanism for an increased threshold of excitation is increased distance between the membrane resting potential and the threshold potential. If for some reason the diastolic threshold of excitation in a given myocardial tissue is elevated, the strength of stimulus originally sufficient to excite this tissue may now become ineffective (subthreshold stimulation), causing a conduction block.

Generally speaking, the excitability of the myocardium tends to remain constant during electrical diastole, but undergoes a significant change with the onset of electrical systole (action potential). These fibers usually do not respond to a second stimulus from the beginning of phase 0 through phase 2 (plateau), until a certain point in phase 3 of repolarization is reached, regardless of the strength of the currents applied. This is called the *effective refractory period,* and it is followed by a *relative refractory period.* During the latter phase, cellular excitability is less than that during electrical diastole, and fibers respond only to stronger stimuli, producing an action potential with a slower upstroke velocity and a reduced amplitude.

With reference to the excitability of downstream fibers, brief comments are in order on the phenomena of supernormal excitability and the Wedensky effect. Principally in fibers of the specialized conducting system, excitability toward the end of the relative refractory period may transiently become higher than during electrical diastole. This is termed the *supernormal period of excitability.* In this phase, when repolarization has proceeded just beyond the level of the threshold potential but has not reached the resting potential, a small amount of current or a weaker stimulus could possibly decrease the membrane potential to the threshold level and excite these fibers. When the strength of impulses transmitted to a group of myocardial fibers is only slightly below the diastolic threshold, those fibers may respond only during the supernormal period of excitability and produce an action potential. Such phenomena are often observed clinically when the batteries of an electronic pacemaker are depleted.

Conversely, the Wedensky effect represents a transient increase in tissue excitability after a supramaximal impulse. One major difference between the Wedensky effect and supernormal excitability is that the latter has a very brief duration (i.e., less than 50 msec), whereas the Wedensky effect lasts much longer and may affect excitability in several subsequent depolarizations. These two phenomena have often been invoked to

explain the genesis of coupled premature systoles. For instance, an abnormal source of current (such as an injury current between ischemic and nonischemic myocardial fibers) may produce a propagated response only during the supernormal period of excitability and, hence, a premature beat with a fixed time interval from the preceding excitation. If impulses arriving from upstream fibers are barely sufficient to excite an area of conduction disturbance with a lower excitability, propagation of an excitation front may occur only during this period of supernormality, not during electrical diastole. This mechanism may possibly explain one type of supernormal AV conduction. However, the Wedensky effect may explain the observation that, in the presence of high grades of AV block, one successfully conducted beat sometimes is followed by conduction of several subsequent supraventricular impulses. Here, propagation of one excitation front may have increased the excitability of the depressed fibers at the site of the conduction failure.

These two physiologic factors that primarily determine the conductivity in the myocardium may not always remain stable in a given cardiac tissue and could vary depending on conditions. Fluctuations in cardiac hemodynamics, oxygen supply to the myocardium, autonomic nerve tone, or heart rate may cause slight variations in conductivity. Although these subtle changes probably do not have a significant effect on cardiac fibers under the normal physiologic conditions, they may well determine the success or failure of propagation in fibers with reduced conductivity. Certain cases of so-called "Mobitz type II AV block" could possibly be explained by this mechanism.

In addition to these physiologic determinants of conductivity, several anatomic factors must be considered. It is known that conductivity usually is better in fibers with larger diameters, and the high conduction velocity seen in Purkinje fibers can be ascribed in part to their larger diameter. Geometric arrangement of the fibers also appears to play a role in impulse transmission. When a larger fiber strand divides into several smaller ones, conductivity may be decreased because of the division of the wavefront of excitation and a decreased current density. However, summation of several different wavefronts, with appropriate timing, may improve the conductivity in more distal tissue. Indeed, increased amplitude and upstroke velocity of an action potential due to summation have often been demonstrated in the AV node as well as in Purkinje fibers. In a preparation in which two larger pieces of atrial tissue were connected by a small strand of fibers, conduction block tended to develop when the excitation front attempted to invade the larger tissue through the isthmus, whereas propagation from the larger tissue to the smaller strand was well maintained. These observations are in keeping with the aforementioned concepts and have been used to explain the intermittency of conduction through accessory pathways that occurs in the WPW syndrome. It must be pointed out that summation of excitation fronts is more easily demonstrated in the presence of slow responses.

ABNORMAL CONDUCTION PHENOMENA CAUSED BY ALTERATIONS IN THE PRIMARY DETERMINANTS OF CONDUCTIVITY

Changes in the various determinants of conductivity, whether alone or in combination, may produce several abnormal conduction phenomena (Table 13–2):

1. *Decremental conduction* can be defined as a gradual decrease in the effectiveness of stimulus and in the magnitude of response along a pathway of conduction that is anatomically uniform but functionally depressed. Such decremental conduction will develop more easily in the presence of reduced membrane potentials. In a group of partially depolarized fibers, for example, the rate of rise of an action potential will be lower than in more normal cardiac tissue, and its effectiveness as a stimulus will be decreased. When the downstream fibers also have a lower transmembrane potential, their response may be progressively reduced, even to the point of propagation failure. Small action potentials due to slow inward currents may again be important in the development of this phenomenon. In fibers having lower membrane potentials and slower upstroke velocity of the action potential under physiologic conditions (e.g., the N region of the AV node), decremental conduction due to various pathophysiologic factors can be expected more frequently.

2. The next variety of abnormal conduction phenomena, which we have termed *inhomogeneous conduction,* is explained as follows. When depression of conductivity results in a nonuniform decrement at a given portion of the conducting system, the wavefront of excitation becomes fractionated. This fractionation will be associated with a decreased effectiveness of the stimulus compared with the smoother and more organized wavefront that produces synchronous depolarization in adjacent fibers. It can then be suggested that decremental conduction is unlikely to develop in a tissue in which fibers run parallel to one another, forming a compact strand. In sharp contrast, fractionation of the excitation front could be observed more frequently in the AV node, where frequent ramifications and anastomoses of small fibers form a complex network.

This concept of inhomogeneous conduction presupposes that a smooth excitation front with synchronous depolarization of a group of fibers is accompanied by better conductivity and that the opposite also holds true. When impulses from atrial and ventricular tissues attempt to invade

the AV node, their synchronous arrival at the fibers of the N region produce an action potential with greater amplitude and upstroke velocity. It has also been demonstrated that synchronization of two excitation fronts invading AV nodal tissue from two atrial sites causes a successful transmission of the impulse across the AV node, whereas the arrival of only one of the wavefronts or their asynchronous arrival is associated with an intranodal conduction block. The significance of inhomogeneous conduction in determining AV nodal conductivity has thus been established. When this inhomogeneity is markedly exaggerated, transmission of an impulse may be blocked on one side of the AV node while slow but successful conduction occurs on the other side. This phenomenon is called *functional longitudinal dissociation* and is considered to be responsible for reciprocal beating and reciprocal tachycardia (paroxysmal AV junctional tachycardia). The distinction between this mechanism and the more recently advocated mechanism of so-called "dual AV nodal pathways" probably requires more extensive study. Functional longitudinal dissociation has been shown to occur in myocardial tissues other than the AV node (e.g., in the His bundle or peripheral Purkinje fibers). Nevertheless, it may be said that inhomogeneous conduction is a transverse, or parallel, expression of depressed conductivity, whereas decremental conduction is a longitudinal, or series, expression of depressed conduction.

3. The third variety of abnormal conduction phenomena, *conduction delay and block,* can result from any of the previously described mechanisms. However, the most common causes of conduction block, at least in tissues other than the AV node, are probably (a) loss of the membrane potential (due to either partial depolarization or diastolic depolarization) and the resultant appearance of slow responses: and (b) the presence of a refractory tissue (or a tissue with lowered excitability) in the pathway of conduction. The role of conduction delay and block in the genesis of various arrhythmias will be discussed in the next section.

4. *Unidirectional block,* or *unidirectional conduction,* is a special type of conduction block. It was first demonstrated experimentally by Schmitt and Erlanger and is considered responsible for reentry movements. The genesis of this phenomenon is usually attributed to different degrees of decrement, depending on the direction of conduction. We believe that anatomic structures, as illustrated in Figure 13–7, may facilitate the production of unidirectional block. The wavefront of excitation could become irregular and fractionated in one direction, whereas merging and summation of excitation fronts may occur in an opposite direction. We have previously demonstrated unidirectional block within the AV node, and similar phenomena also appear to occur in the Purkinje fibers.

5. *Reentry* is one of the mechanisms most frequently invoked in various cardiac arrhyth-

mias. The requirements for the production of reentry movement include (a) either the presence of two anatomically separated pathways or the existence of functional longitudinal dissociation in the conducting tissue with different degrees of depression of conductivity in those two pathways; and (b) the development of unidirectional block in one of the pathways (Fig. 13–8). One additional factor is a shortened refractory period in those fibers that are to be invaded by the reentrant impulse that allows them to be reexcited after an initial depolarization. Although reentry movement is often classified into macroreentries and microreentries (depending on the size of the reentry circuit), the distinction between these two varieties is far from clear. However, WPW tachycardias, most instances of atrial flutter, and reciprocal movements within the AV junction probably represent macroreentry, whereas microreentry movements may develop in any portion of the myocardium, causing various premature systoles, paroxysmal ectopic tachycardias, and fibrillation. As has been shown in Table 13–2, these several abnormal conduction phenomena will secondarily affect transmission of subsequent impulses in a complex manner. Readers are referred to the original articles for more detailed discussion.

THE ROLE OF CONDUCTION DELAY AND BLOCK IN THE GENESIS OF ARRHYTHMIAS

Conduction delay and block (failure of propagation) can cause numerous varieties of arrhythmia. Their direct expressions in the clinical setting are usually called some kind of "block," for example, sinoatrial (SA) block, atrioventricular (AV) block, exit block from the pacemaker site in the presence of an ectopic rhythm, and intraventricular conduction disturbances (bundle branch block and fascicular block). In these arrhythmias, disturbances of conduction will produce irregularities in the P–P, P–R, or R–R interval or an abnormal prolongation of the P–R or QRS interval. These

usually are identified in electrocardiographic records.

SA block generally becomes of clinical significance only when some of the impulses regularly formed in the sinus node fail to excite the atrial tissue (second degree block). Resultant longer P–P intervals then correspond to simple multiples of a basic sinus cycle length. Two different mechanisms for SA block appear to exist. When a P wave drops out in the presence of certain types of drugs or high extracellular potassium concentrations, the atrial tissue is not depolarized in its entirety because of decrements in atrial conduction. Thus, this condition may be considered intraatrial block (Fig. 13–9). It has been suggested that, under these conditions, sinus impulses may be successfully transmitted to the ventricles without being accompanied by identifiable P waves, a phenomenon termed *sinoventricular conduction*. An increased resistance of the fibers of the intraatrial conducting system (or internodal tracts) greater than that of the working atrial muscle fibers against elevated potassium concentrations or depressant drugs probably could explain such a mechanism. However, transmission of sinus impulses to the surrounding atrial muscle or to the internodal tract may fail at the atrial junction when an organic lesion involves the so-called "perinodal fibers." This second mechanism was simulated by Sano through the creation of small incisions adjacent to the sinus nodal tissue. In the past, first degree SA block (or simple prolongation of the SA conduction time) was considered only a theoretic entity. However, diagnosis of this condition now appears to be possible by measuring the SA conduction time from the difference between the return cycle after an atrial premature systole and the basic sinus cycle.

AV block usually is classified as first, second, or third degree block, depending on the severity of the conduction disturbance. Second degree AV block has been further classified into type 1 (Wenckebach periodicity) and type 2 (Mobitz type II). Precise electrophysiologic mechanisms underlying these two types have not been fully illus-

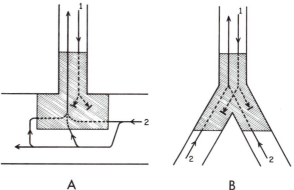

Figure 13–7 Schematic diagrams illustrating possible mechanisms of unidirectional conduction. In *A*, conductivity is depressed at the junction of a small fiber strand and a larger myocardial tissue *(shaded area).* Excitation front invading this area from above *(arrow 1)* is blocked as the action current is "diluted" at this junction, whereas retrograde wavefront of excitation *(arrow 2)* successfully traverses this area because of summation of impulses. Similar relationship exists at the branching portion of a fiber strand *(B).*

A   B

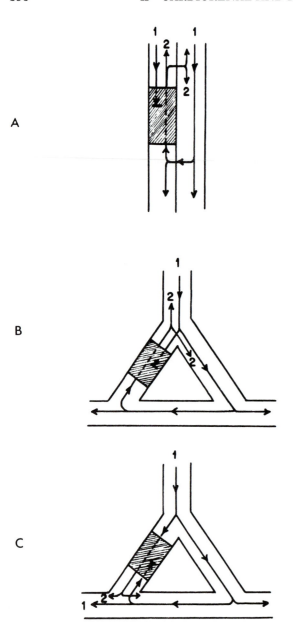

A

B

C

Figure 13–8 Diagrammatic representation of re-entry mechanism. Localized areas of depressed conductivity with the property of unidirectional block *(shaded areas)*, in the presence of either functional longitudinal dissociation *(A)* or two anatomically separate pathways *(B)*, cause re-excitation of the initially depolarized tissue by the impulse traversing these depressed areas in a retrograde fashion *(arrow 2)*. In *C*, an excitation wave traversing the depressed area at a reduced speed may finally emerge from this area *(arrow 2)* to re-excite the distal tissue, which once was depolarized by the same impulse rapidly traveling down a second pathway with a better conductivity *(arrow 1)*. Presence of unidirectional conduction is required in this model also. (Reproduced from Watanabe, Y.: Electrophysiologic knowledge necessary for the understanding of cardiac arrhythmias. Medicina *13*:17, 1976.)

Figure 13–9 An experimental record showing SA, or intra-atrial, block observed in an isolated, perfused rabbit heart. Note the decreased rate of phase 0 depolarization in propagated response in this atrial fiber *(A)* adjacent to the AV node and two successive local responses upon failure of AV transmission. SA, electrogram from the SA nodal region; V, ventricular electrogram. Bottom diagram shows the AV junctional region. CS, ostium of coronary sinus; AVR, fibrous atrioventricular ring; HB, His bundle. (Reproduced from Watanabe, Y., and Dreifus, L. S.: Cardiac Arrhythmias: Electrophysiologic Basis for Clinical Interpretation. New York, Grune & Stratton, 1977.)

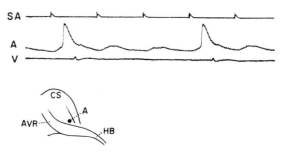

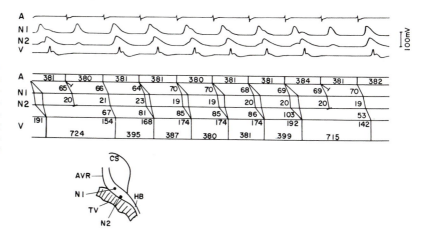

Figure 13–10 Mobitz type 1 block with higher (7:6) conduction ratio. Fibers N1 and N2 are located in the NH region. Note progressive step formation in downstream fiber (N2) and concomitant development of hump in repolarization phase of upstream fiber (N1).

trated, although it has been shown that the former is caused mainly by conduction disturbances within the AV node, whereas the latter in most instances is produced by disorders of His-Purkinje conduction. These observations suggest a propensity toward the development of Wenckebach-type block in the presence of slow responses. Indeed, this type of conduction phenomenon also has been demonstrated in Purkinje fibers and ventricular muscle fibers when their membrane potential was significantly reduced and their conductivity markedly depressed. The possible role of inhomogeneous conduction in the production of Wenckebach phenomenon has been suggested experimentally (Fig. 13–10). It has also been shown that certain instances of Mobitz type II block have resulted from an abnormal premature depolarization of certain portions of the conducting system, which creates a refractory tissue and prevents the transmission of an impulse arriving from the upstream fibers. Such a premature depolarization may be produced by various mechanisms of impulse formation, as discussed earlier, or it possibly may result from reentry movement caused by conduction disturbance. An example of the latter mechanism is shown in Figure 13–11. Disturbances of impulse transmission due to such premature depolarizations constitute one variety of concealed conduction, and they are considered a direct expression of conduction delay and block.

In the case of so-called "protection block" around a parasystolic pacemaker, the presence of a conduction disturbance is not immediately apparent on the electrocardiogram. This is often called *entrance block* in contrast to exit block; it prevents the invasion of a parasystolic pacemaker by other impulses, enabling the pacemaker to maintain its regular impulse formation. Protection block around the parasystolic focus and exit block from the site of ectopic impulse formation will be discussed in greater detail in the following section on the combination of abnormal impulse formation and disturbances of conduction.

Various intraventricular conduction disturbances as another direct expression of abnormal impulse transmission do not reveal themselves as irregularities of the heart beat. However, they may indirectly facilitate the production of various ventricular arrhythmias. In contrast to patients with normal ventricular conduction, those patients with bundle branch or fascicular blocks show a higher incidence of ventricular premature systoles, which tend to originate from the regions of blocked bundles or fascicles. Ventricular tachycardias also appear to arise in areas of conduction disturbance. Although certain reservations must be made before accepting these observations as evidence for reentry movements, the role of conduction disturbances in the genesis of abnormal impulse formation appears to be well established.

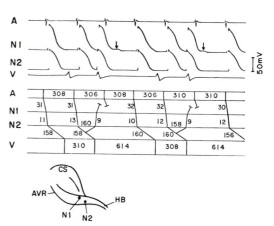

Figure 13–11 Mobitz type 2 block due to concealed re-excitation in AV junction. Fibers N1 and N2 are located in NH region. The third group of action potentials is premature. The action potentials show reversed order of excitation (depolarization of fiber N1 follows that of N2), suggesting retrograde activation of NH fibers. The third atrial impulse is blocked in NH region. (Reproduced from Watanabe, Y., and Dreifus, L. S.: Am. Heart J. *70*:505, 1965.)

SUPERNORMAL CONDUCTION

Supernormal AV conduction has been the focus of great clinical interest, although similar supernormal conduction in the intra-atrial conducting system has also been suggested. Supernormal AV conduction is defined as an apparently paradoxic improvement in the conduction of an impulse when its conductivity is expected to be further depressed from the previous sequence of AV conduction. Several varieties of supernormal AV conduction have been identified in clinical electrocardiograms, and their electrophysiologic mechanisms may well differ from one patient to the next.

In this chapter, three varieties will be briefly discussed. In the first, in a second degree AV block showing the Wenckebach phenomenon, one conducted beat is associated with a shorter P–R interval after the P–R intervals of preceding beats show a progressive increase. The second variety of supernormal AV conduction is diagnosed when P waves occurring later in the electrical diastole of the ventricles are not conducted because of a high degree of AV block, whereas the P waves occurring immediately after a QRS complex produced by a subsidiary pacemaker (either AV junctional or idioventricular) are conducted successfully to the ventricles. Alternation of short and long P–R intervals in the presence of regular sinus rhythm and 1:1 AV conduction represents the third type of supernormal AV conduction.

When a phenomenon similar to the first variety of supernormal AV conduction was observed in an experiment on an isolated perfused rabbit heart, transmission of the first several atrial impulses to the ventricles was accompanied by changes in the AV nodal action potentials, suggesting a progressive increase in inhomogeneous conduction in this tissue. The following AV nodal action potential showed a much smoother upstroke, suggesting reorganization of the excitation front, and the AV conduction time was shortened. Although the reason for the recovery of homogeneity of intranodal conduction is still unknown, several mechanisms (e.g., slight variations in atrial cycle length, different modes of invasion of the AV node by atrial impulses resulting from alterations in the atrial excitation process, and temporal fluctuations of conductivity within the AV node) may be postulated.

In contrast, the second variety of supernormal AV conduction has been explained by several investigators on the basis of the concept of a "peeling back" of the refractory barrier. These investigators have demonstrated that a premature atrial impulse that ordinarily is blocked within the AV junction can be transmitted successfully to the ventricles when the AV junctional tissue is depolarized by a retrograde impulse that originates in the ventricles just before the supraventricular impulse arrives in this region.

A possible explanation for these findings is that, since the fibers in the region of propagation failure are prematurely depolarized by the retrograde impulse, both their repolarization process and their refractoriness will be terminated earlier, allowing these fibers to recover their excitability before the atrial impulse arrives. Blockage of premature atrial impulses in these instances is predicated on the presence of markedly prolonged refractoriness in the AV junction. It is, however, still questionable whether the same mechanism can be invoked in the presence of a regular sinus rhythm with high grades of AV block.

The concept of inhomogeneous conduction may provide us with an alternative explanation. When high-grade AV block in the orthograde direction is caused by a marked inhomogeneity of intranodal conduction, invasion of this region by a retrograde impulse may cause more homogeneous depression of conductivity in this area; therefore, the next atrial impulse is associated with a better organized wavefront of excitation and a successful impulse transmission.

Still another explanation for this type of supernormal AV conduction invokes the mechanism of so-called "phase 4 block." When certain fibers of the AV conducting system show marked diastolic depolarization, their transmembrane potential will be progressively decreased later in electrical diastole and their conductivity depressed. When the sinus cycle is relatively long, most of the sinus impulses may arrive at these fibers when their membrane potential is sufficiently reduced to cause orthograde conduction block. Contrariwise, a sinus impulse arriving immediately after the completion of the action potential produced by the impulse from a subsidiary pacemaker may depolarize these fibers at the time their membrane potential is most negative (the maximal diastolic potential), generate an action potential with a greater upstroke velocity and amplitude and sustain a lesser degree of decrement. Further studies are clearly needed to elucidate the true mechanisms of this interesting conduction phenomenon.

The following considerations lead us to believe that the third variety, as described earlier in this section, may not satisfy the criteria for supernormal AV conduction. It has been argued that in the presence of regular sinus rhythm with alternation of short and long P–R intervals, the P wave following a beat conducted with a prolonged P–R interval would appear closer to the preceding QRS and have a shorter interval. This suggests the invasion of an atrial impulse into the AV conducting system after a shorter interval and at a time when the conducting fibers are less fully recovered. Since this should be accompanied by a further prolongation of the AV conduction time, the paradoxic shortening of the P–R interval in the following beat has been considered an expression of supernormal AV conduction. It must be pointed out, however, that the shorter R–P interval may not necessarily indicate an early arrival of an impulse in the AV conducting system. If the preceding QRS complex has been produced by an impulse from a subsidiary pacemaker, a shorter R–P interval definitely indicates an earlier arrival of the impulse with reference to the preceding depolarization of the AV junctional fibers. Under a regular sinus mechanism, however, all the atrial impulses will attempt to invade the AV junction with a constant P–P interval; the R–P interval would have no significance in determining the subsequent conduction phenomena. It is known that a slow propagation of excitation is accompanied by a prolonged action potential in fibers in such regions. If the subsequent atrial impulse arrives immediately after the repolarization of these fibers, and if a diastolic depolarization is present, the concept of "phase 4 block" may again be invoked, as in the previous variety, to explain the shorter P–R interval or a paradoxic improvement in AV conduction. Inhomogeneous conduction again may be offered as an alternative mechanism. If, in the presence of functional longitudinal dissociation of the AV junction, one portion of the AV junctional tissue maintains a 1:1 conduction while the other portion shows a 2:1 block, a better organized excitation front with a higher conduction velocity will alternate with a poorly organized and slowly conducting wavefront. The concept of so-called "dual AV nodal pathways" may have the same significance as long as the term does not necessarily imply two anatomically separated pathways. Admittedly, all these mechanisms are still hypothetical, and the phenomena of supernormal AV conduction require more extensive experimental study.

COMBINED DISTURBANCES OF IMPULSE FORMATION AND CONDUCTION

One can readily understand the close association between abnormal impulse formation and disturbances of conduction in the genesis of cardiac arrhythmias by recognizing that a localized conduction disorder with reentry movements will produce a premature systole or an ectopic tachycardia and that premature depolarization of the AV junction by an ectopic impulse can make the AV junction refractory and block a subsequent atrial impulse. Furthermore, abnormal impulse formation in one portion of the myocardium (atria) may accompany a conduction disturbance in another portion (AV conducting system), as is the case in atrial tachycardia with AV block. In this section, however, the term "combined disturbances of impulse formation and conduction" will be used in the narrower sense in that an arrhythmia is generated by the combination of these two mechanisms in a rather localized area of myocardium.

Two major types of arrhythmia included in this category are (1) ectopic rhythms with exit block and (2) parasystole. Atrial fibrillation and ventricular fibrillation also will be discussed in this section, although their classification within this category may be subject to controversy.

Exit block from an ectopic pacemaker is seen most frequently in the presence of either AV junctional rhythm or nonparoxysmal AV junctional tachycardia, but it is also often seen in idioventricular rhythm in cases of third degree AV block, type B. We have previously demonstrated the actual occurrence of exit block from an AV junctional pacemaker with microelectrode techniques in isolated perfused rabbit hearts (Fig. 13–12). The difficulty in the exit of impulses from an automatic focus may be explained by the concept of phase 4 block, as diastolic depolarization in fibers within and around the pacemaker will cause a gradual loss of membrane potential, thus decreasing the rate of rise and amplitude of the action potential. This will cause decremental conduction. Indeed, phase 4 depolarization was observed in several recording sites adjacent to the point of earliest depolarization or the origin of ectopic impulses. In other words, automaticity in the localized area of the myocardium in this type of arrhythmia produces an ectopic rhythm on the one hand and facilitates the development of exit block on the other.

Regarding parasystole, disturbance of impulse transmission is considered to play a role in the form of so-called "protection block" around the site of impulse formation. The electrophysiologic mechanisms of such protection of the parasystolic pacemaker are still subject to controversy. Certain investigators postulate extremely rapid impulse formation in the parasystolic focus so that the region of the pacemaker remains almost always in the state of refractoriness, thereby preventing depolarization by extrinsic stimuli. Although cases of parasystole with such a high-frequency discharge may indeed exist, the rather slow parasystolic rhythms most commonly seen clinically are not easily explained by this mechanism unless a rather high degree of exit block is postulated.

A second explanation proposes that, since the fibers within the parasystolic focus have a higher stimulation threshold than the surrounding tissue, impulses of the basic rhythm fail to excite the pacemaking fibers, whereas the impulses formed within this focus can depolarize the surrounding fibers with a relatively low threshold of stimulation and can make an exit. Since the difference of excitability between fiber groups is causing a conduction disturbance, this mechanism may be considered one type of protection block. Still another possibility is that the tissue around the site of parasystolic impulse formation has an abnormally prolonged refractory period, which prevents the invasion of extrinsic stimuli into the area. Distinguishing this mechanism from protection block

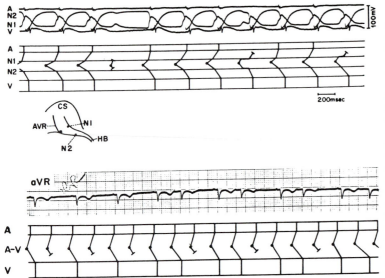

Figure 13–12 An experimental record showing exit block from an AV nodal pacemaker *(top)* and an equivalent clinical electrocardiogram *(bottom)*. Transmembrane potential N1 was recorded from the N region of the AV node, and N2 (with reversed polarity) from the NH region. Site of impulse formation in this AV junctional rhythm (X mark) is shown in the inset. Either conduction delay or block in the exit of impulses from this pacemaker produces notched upstroke of phase 0 or incomplete depolarization in these fibers and dropping out of atrial (A) or ventricular excitation (V). In the bottom record, AV junctional rhythm with exit block in forward direction is diagnosed from regular appearance of positive P waves (this suggests retrograde conduction in lead AVR) and irregular R–R intervals (see the ladder diagram).

due to conduction disturbance again may be rather difficult.

These three theories invoke either refractoriness or lowered excitability in or around the parasystolic pacemaker; however, phase 4 block in surrounding fibers also may explain such a protection mechanism. In this instance, diastolic depolarization in certain fibers of the specialized conducting system produces regular automatic impulse formation and, at the same time, prevents their discharge by extraneous impulses. The electrophysiologic mechanism of parasystole then becomes quite similar to that of ectopic rhythms with exit block. If the site of phase 4 block–induced unidirectional conduction acts mainly to protect this focus from invading sinus impulses, parasystolic rhythm will be produced. Conversely, if the mechanism of unidirectional conduction due to phase 4 block mainly inhibits 1:1 outward spread of automatic impulses, an ectopic rhythm with exit block may ensue. It must be pointed out that parasystole occasionally is associated with exit block, suggesting the development of bidirectional block. We have previously demonstrated that impulse formation in ventricular parasystole in patients with intraventricular conduction disturbances tends to develop in the regions of the bundles, or fascicles, in which conduction is disturbed. Such observations may indirectly suggest the interrelationships between automaticity (diastolic depolarization), intraventricular conduction disorder due to phase 4 block, and the protection block. It may be speculated further that, if a region of unidirectional conduction is indeed playing a major role in protecting a parasystolic pacemaker, transition between simple, coupled premature systoles and parasystolic impulse formation may possibly be observed, as reentry movement also is predicated on the presence of unidirectional block. Reports showing the occurrence of coupled premature systoles, which were considered reentrant in nature, near the site of parasystolic impulse formation appear to support the aforementioned concept.

Regarding the phenomenon of cardiac fibrillation, theories of unifocal impulse formation, multifocal impulse formation, and reentry have been advocated by different investigators. In the first two theories, abnormal impulse formation is considered to play a major role in the genesis of this arrhythmia, whereas the reentry theory invokes mainly disturbances of conduction. Since it is our current feeling that cardiac fibrillation probably is explained either by reentry alone or by the combination of unifocal impulse formation and reentry, discussion of this arrhythmia has been included in this section.

In the theory of multifocal impulse formation, an entire disorganization of the atrial or ventricular excitation process results from the coexistence of numerous foci of impulse formation that cause independent and random depolarization of multiple points. In contrast, the unifocal impulse formation theory postulates a single site of impulse formation at an extremely high frequency through which some fibers cannot respond in a 1:1 fashion. Islands of conduction block will then result in irregular spread of ventricular excitation. In this instance, however, the development of multiple areas of localized conduction block would most likely generate numerous microreentry circuits, and resort to a combination with the reentry theory may become mandatory.

The genesis of fibrillation triggered by a single premature impulse occurring in the so-called "vulnerable period" is explained by the theory of reentry in the following manner. Because of the nonuniformity of the action potential duration as well as the refractory period between fiber groups, a premature stimulus may produce different degrees

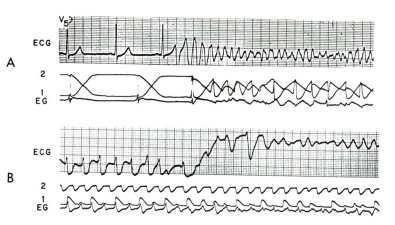

Figure 13–13 Two mechanisms of ventricular fibrillation. *A,* Sudden onset of ventricular fibrillation (V_5) after a ventricular premature complex occurring at the apex of the T wave. Lower strip, experimental record showing premature action potentials (third beat). Note slight delay in the inscription of the inverted action potential followed by marked disorganization of excitation and abnormal action potentials. *B,* Gradual onset of ventricular fibrillation following continued disorganization of excitation process (lower strip). Clinical record shown above.

of response in individual fibers. Thus, the wavefront of excitation will become grossly irregular, leading to multiple areas of microreentry.

Findings that apparently support this concept have been observed experimentally, an example being shown in Figure 13–13*A,* lower record. When ventricular fibrillation was initiated in isolated perfused rabbit hearts with a premature systole, the two adjacent epicardial fibers showed markedly different responses to this premature impulse, with increased asynchrony of depolarization and dissimilar upstroke velocity and amplitude of the action potentials. A rapid transition to ventricular fibrillation is clearly noted in the electrocardiogram. Disorganized spread of ventricular excitation caused by premature stimulation is thus evident, and the development of microreentry circuits may readily be anticipated. Such a rapid development of fibrillatory movement during the vulnerable period (termed *type A* by us) appears to be explained by the reentry theory.

Figure 13–13*B* illustrates another mode of onset of fibrillation observed both clinically and experimentally. In this instance, abnormal spread of ventricular excitation is gradually exaggerated after a more prolonged period of ectopic tachycardia, finally deteriorating into fibrillation. The experimental findings shown in the bottom record revealed that the transmembrane potentials recorded in one of the two adjacent ventricular muscle fibers develop an alternation of action potential amplitude, and asynchrony of depolarization in these two fibers not only becomes greater but also fluctuates from beat to beat. These findings will suggest the development of localized

conduction block and marked variations of the excitation process from one beat to the next. Again, formation of numerous microreentry circuits will be easily envisioned. Hence, also in this concept of onset of fibrillation (termed *type B*), the role of conduction disturbance cannot be disregarded.

Experimental observations, as discussed, as well as numerous reports in the literature, suggest that the role of the reentry mechanism is now widely accepted, at least in the maintenance of fibrillation. However, we have often observed in our experimental studies on the antifibrillatory actions of antiarrhythmic agents that a transition from ventricular fibrillation to what appears to be a ventricular tachycardia occurred after the administration of various antiarrhythmic agents. This was either sustained for a prolonged period or eventually returned to a normal sinus rhythm, which may suggest the possible role of unifocal impulse formation in the initiation of fibrillation. Demonstration of the localized area of high frequency discharge at the beginning of experimental atrial fibrillation produced by premature electrical stimulation, as reported by Sano and Scher, is of great interest in this regard. Furthermore, since the various mechanisms of abnormal impulse formation dependent on slow inward currents are activated when the cell membrane is partially depolarized, and since this latter condition facilitates marked conduction disturbances through the production of so-called "slow responses," increased attention will be directed to the significance of slow channels in the genesis of cardiac fibrillation. A more detailed discussion of the mechanisms of cardiac fibrillation has been published elsewhere.

REFERENCES

Antoni, H., and Oberdisse, E.: Elektrophysiologische Untersuchungen über die Barium-induzierte Schrittmacher Aktivität in der Arbeitsmuskulatur des Säugetierherzens. Arch. Exp. Pathol. Pharmakol. 247:329, 1964.

Arita, M., Nagamoto, Y., and Saikawa, T.: Automaticity and time-dependent conduction disturbance produced in canine ventricular myocardium. New aspects for initiation of ventricular arrhythmias. Jap. Circ. J. 40:1401, 1976.

Aronson, R. S., and Cranefield, P. F.: The effect of resting potential on the electrical activity of canine cardiac Purkinje fibers exposed to Na-free solution or to ouabain. Pfluegers Arch. 347:101, 1974.

Beeler, G. W., Jr., and Reuter, H.: Membrane calcium current in ventricular myocardial fibers. J. Physiol. 207:191, 1970.

Bellet, S.: Clinical Disorders of the Heart Beat. 3rd ed. Philadelphia, Lea & Febiger, 1971.

Bigger, J. T., Jr.: Electrical properties of cardiac muscle and possible causes of cardiac arrhythmias. *In* Dreifus, L. S., and Likoff, W. (Eds.): Cardiac Arrhythmias. New York, Grune & Stratton, 1973, p. 13.

Bigger, J. T., Jr., Bassett, A. L., and Hoffman, B. F.: Electrophysiological effects of diphenylhydantoin on canine Purkinje fibers. Circ. Res. 22:221, 1968.

Brooks, C. McC., Hoffman, B. F., Suckling, E. E., and Orias, O.: The Excitability of the Heart. New York, Grune & Stratton, 1955.

Brooks, C. McC., and Lu, H. H.: Sinoatrial Pacemaker of the Heart. Springfield, Ill., Charles C Thomas, 1972.

Castellanos, A., Jr., Lemberg, L., Johnson, D., and Berkovits, B. V.: The Wedensky effect in the human heart. Br. Heart J. 28:276, 1966.

Chung, E. K.: Principles of Cardiac Arrhythmias. 3rd ed. Baltimore, Williams and Wilkins, 1982.

Cranefield, P. F.: The Conduction of the Cardiac Impulse. Mount Kisco, New York, Futura Publishing Co., Inc., 1975.

Cranefield, P. F., and Hoffman, B. F.: Conduction of the cardiac impulse. II. Summation and inhibition. Circ. Res. 28:220, 1971.

Cranefield, P. F., Klein, H. O., and Hoffman, B. F.: Conduction of the cardiac impulse. I. Delay, block and one-way block in depressed Purkinje fibers. Circ. Res. 28:199, 1971.

delaFuente, D., Sasyniuk, B., and Moe, G. K.: Conduction through a narrow isthmus in isolated canine atrial tissue. A model of the W-P-W syndrome. Circulation, 44:803, 1971.

Dreifus, L. S., Watanabe, Y., Haiat, R., and Kimbiris, D.: Atrioventricular block. Am. J. Cardiol. 28:371, 1971.

Elizari, M. V., Lazzari, J. O., and Rosenbaum, M. B.: Phase-3 and phase-4 intermittent left anterior hemiblock. Report of 1st case in the literature. Chest 63:673, 1972.

Ferrer, M. I.: The sick sinus syndrome in atrial disease. J.A.M.A. 206:645, 1968.

Ferrer, M. I.: The sick sinus syndrome. Circulation 47:635, 1973.

Ferrier, G. R., and Moe, G. K.: Effect of calcium on acetylstrophanthidin-induced transient depolarizations in canine Purkinje tissue. Circ. Res. 33:508, 1973.

Gettes, L. S., and Surawicz, B.: Effects of low and high concentrations of potassium on the simultaneously recorded Purkinje and ventricular action potentials of the perfused pig moderator band. Circ. Res. 23:717, 1968.

Goto, M.: Physiology of Circulation—Heart and Systemic Circulation. Tokyo, Asakura Book Co., 1971.

Hellerstein, H. K., and Turell, D. J.: The mode of death in coronary artery disease. An electrocardiographic and clinicopathological correlation. *In* Surawicz, B., and Pellegrino, E. D. (Eds.): Sudden Cardiac Death. New York, Grune & Stratton, 1964, p. 17.

Hodgkin, A. L., and Huxley, A. F.: A quantitative description of membrane current and its application to conduction and excitation in nerve. J. Physiol. (London) 117:500, 1952.

Hoffman, B. F.: The pathophysiology of failure of impulse transmission to the ventricles. *In* Surawicz, B., and Pellegrino, E. D. (Eds.): Sudden Cardiac Death. New York, Grune & Stratton, 1964, p. 78.

Hoffman, B. F.: The electrophysiology of heart muscle and the genesis of arrhythmias. *In* Dreifus, L. S., and Likoff, W. (Eds.): Mechanisms and Therapy of Cardiac Arrhythmias. New York, Grune & Stratton, 1966, p. 27.

Hoffman, B. F., and Cranefield, P. F.: Electrophysiology of the Heart. New York, McGraw-Hill Book Co., 1960.

James, T. N.: The connecting pathways between the sinus node and A-V node and between the right and left atrium in the human heart. Am. Heart J. 66:498, 1963.

Katz, B.: Electrical properties of the muscle fiber membrane. Proc. Roy. Soc. 135:506, 1948.

Katz, L. N., and Pick, A.: Clinical Electrocardiography. Part I: The Arrhythmias. Philadelphia, Lea & Febiger, 1956.

Kimura, E.: Paroxysmal tachycardias. Heart 3:1395, 1971.

Konishi, T., and Matsuyama, E.: Effect of changes in inputs to atrioventricular node on AV conduction. Jap. Circ. J. 40:1392, 1976.

Matsuda, K.: Significance of slow inward current in the myocardium. Heart 7:617, 1975.

Matsuda, K.: Function of the node of Tawara. Clin. Res. 50:3514, 1973.

Matsuda, K., Hoshi, T., and Kameyama, S.: Effects of aconitine on the cardiac membrane potential of the dog. Jap. J. Physiol. 9:419, 1959.

Miller, H. C., and Strauss, H. C.: Measurement of sinoatrial conduction time by premature atrial stimulation in the rabbit. Circ. Res. 35:935, 1974.

Moe, G. K., and Abildskov, J. A.: Atrial fibrillation as a self-sustaining arrhythmia independent of focal discharge. Am. Heart J. 58:59, 1959.

Moe, G. K., Childers, R. W., and Merideth, J.: An appraisal of "supernormal" A-V conduction. Circulation 38:5, 1968.

Moore, E. N., and Spear, J. F.: Experimental studies on the facilitation of A-V conduction by ectopic beats in dogs and rabbits. Circ. Res. 29:29, 1971.

Müller, P.: Ca- and K-free solution and pacemaker activity in mammalian myocardium. Helv. Physiol. Acta 23:C38, 1965.

Noble, D.: A modification of the Hodgkin-Huxley equations applicable to Purkinje fiber action and pacemaker potentials. J. Physiol. 160:317, 1962.

Ogawa, S., Watanabe, Y., and Dreifus, L. S.: Double ventricular parasystole. Am. Heart J. 93:767, 1977.

Pamintuan, J. C., Dreifus, L. S., and Watanabe, Y.: Comparative mechanisms of antiarrhythmic agents. Am. J. Cardiol. 26:512, 1970.

Pick, A., Langendorf, R., and Katz, L. N.: The supernormal phase of atrioventricular conduction. I. Fundamental mechanisms. Circulation 26:388, 1962.

Reuter, H.: Divalent cations as charge carriers in excitable membranes. Prog. Biophys. Mol. Biol. 26:1, 1973.

Rosen, K. M., Rahimtoola, S. H., and Gunnar, R. M.: Pseudo A-V block secondary to premature nonprogagated His bundle depolarizations: documentation by His bundle electrocardiography. Circulation 42:367, 1970.

Rougier, O., Vassort, G., Garnier, D., et al.: Existence and role of a slow inward current during the frog atrial action potential. Pfluegers Arch. 308:91, 1969.

Ruiz-Ceretti, E., and Ponce-Zumino, A.: Action potential changes under varied Na^+ and Ca^{2+} indicating the existence of two inward currents in cells of the rabbit atrioventricular node. Circ. Res. 39:326, 1976.

Sano, T., and Hiraoka, M.: Studies on the site and mechanism of sinoatrial block. J. Jpn. Med. Assoc. 63:866, 1974.

Sano, T., Iida, Y., and Yamagishi, S.: Changes in the spread of excitation from the sinus node induced by alterations in extracellular potassium. *In* Sano, T., Mizuhira, V., and Matsuda, K. (Eds.): Electrophysiology and Ultrastructure of the Heart. Tokyo, Bunkodo, 1967, p. 127.

Sano, T., and Scher, A. M.: Multiple recording during electrically induced atrial fibrillation. Circ. Res. 14:117, 1964.

Scherf, D., and Bornemann, C: Parasystole with a rapid ventricular center. Am. Heart J. 62:320, 1961.

Scherf, D., and Cohen, J.: The Atrioventricular Node and Selected Cardiac Arrhythmias. New York, Grune & Stratton, 1964.

Scherf, D., and Schott, A.: Extrasystoles and Allied Arrhythmias. London, William Heinemann, Ltd., 1953.

Schmidt, R. F.: Versuche mit Aconitin zum Problem der spontanen Erregungsbildung im Herzen. Pfluegers Arch. 271:526, 1960.

Schmitt, F. O., and Erlanger, J.: Directional differences in the conduction of the impulse through heart muscle and their possible relation to extrasystolic and fibrillary contractions. Am. J. Physiol. 87:326, 1928.

Singer, D. H., Lazzara, R., and Hoffman, B. F.: Interrelationships between automaticity and conduction in Purkinje fibers. Circ. Res. 21:537, 1967.

Singer, D. H., Parameswaran, R., Drake, F. T., et al.: Ventricular parasystole and reentry: Clinical-electrophysiological correlations. Am. Heart J. 88:79, 1974.

Vassalle, M.: Cardiac pacemaker potentials at different extra- and intracellular K concentrations. Am. J. Physiol. 208:770, 1965.

Vitek, M., and Trautwein, W.: Slow inward current and action potential in cardiac Purkinje fibers. Pfluegers Arch. 323:204, 1971.

Watanabe, Y.: Antagonism and synergism of potassium and anti-arrhythmic agents. *In* Bajusz, E. (Ed.): Electrolytes and Cardiovascular Disease. Basel, S. Karger AG Medical Publishers, 1965, p. 86.

Watanabe, Y.: Effects of electrolytes and antiarrhythmic agents on atrioventricular conduction. *In* Sandøe, E., Flensted-Jensen, E., and Olesen, K. H. (Eds.): Symposium on Cardiac Arrhythmias. Södertälje, Sweden, A B Astra, 1970, p. 535.

Watanabe, Y.: Reassessment of parasystole. Am. Heart J. *81*:451, 1971.

Watanabe, Y.: Cardiac Arrhythmias. Electrophysiologic and Clinical Aspects. Tokyo, Bunkodo, 1973.

Watanabe, Y.: Conduction disturbances in cardiac arrhythmias from the electrophysiological standpoints. Clin. Physiol. *3*:575, 1973.

Watanabe, Y.: Extrasystoles and parasystole: mechanisms involved. Triangle *12*:69, 1973.

Watanabe, Y.: Genesis of cardiac arrhythmias. Intensivmed. Prax. *10*:109, 1973.

Watanabe, Y.: Electrophysiology of cardiac arrhythmias. Clin. Res. *51*:607, 1974.

Watanabe, Y.: Mechanisms of A-V conduction. Heart *6*:604, 1974.

Watanabe, Y.: How to read electrocardiograms: arrhythmias (7): high grade A-V block and unidirectional A-V conduction. Clin. All-round *24*:492, 1975.

Watanabe, Y.: Clinical pharmacology of circulatory diseases, 6. antiarrhythmic drugs. *In* I to Y (Ed.): Handbook of Clinical Cardiology. Vol I: Diagnosis and Treatment in General. Tokyo, Kanehara Publishing Co., 1976, p. 276.

Watanabe, Y.: The role of conduction disturbances in cardiac arrhythmias (editorial). Indian Heart J. *28*:3, 1976.

Watanabe, Y., and Dreifus, L. S.: Inhomogeneous conduction in the A-V node. A model for re-entry. Am. Heart J. *70*:505, 1965.

Watanabe, Y., and Dreifus, L. S.: Mechanisms of ventricular fibrillation. Jpn. Heart J. *7*:110, 1966.

Watanabe, Y., and Dreifus, L. S.: Second degree atrioventricular block. Cardiovas. Res. *1*:150, 1967.

Watanabe, Y., and Dreifus, L. S.: Newer concepts in the genesis of cardiac arrhythmias. Am. Heart J. *76*:114, 1968.

Watanabe, Y., and Dreifus, L. S.: Sites of impulse formation within the atrioventricular junction of the rabbit. Circ. Res. *22*:717, 1968.

Watanabe, Y., and Dreifus, L. S.: Antifibrillatory action of antiarrhythmic agents. Fed. Proc. *30*:554 (abstr.), 1971.

Watanabe, Y., and Dreifus, L. S.: Levels of concealment in second degree and advanced second degree A-V block. Am. Heart J. *84*:330, 1972.

Watanabe, Y., and Dreifus, L. S.: Factors controlling impulse transmission with special reference to A-V conduction. Am. Heart J. *89*:790, 1975.

Watanabe, Y., and Dreifus, L. S.: Cardiac Arrhythmias. Electrophysiologic Basis for Clinical Interpretation. New York, Grune & Stratton, 1977.

Watanabe, Y., Dreifus, L. S., and Likoff, W.: Electrophysiologic antagonism and synergism of potassium and antiarrhythmic agents. Am. J. Cardiol. *12*:702, 1963.

Watanabe, Y., Pamintuan, J. C., and Dreifus, L. S.: Role of intraventricular conduction disturbances in ventricular premature systoles. Am. J. Cardiol. *32*:188, 1973.

Weidmann, S.: Effects of calcium and local anesthetics on electrical properties of Purkinje fibers. J. Physiol. *129*:568, 1955.

Weidmann, S.: The effect of the cardiac membrane potential on the rapid availability of the sodium-carrying system. J. Physiol. *127*:213, 1955.

West, T. C.: Effects of chronotropic influences on subthreshold oscillations in the sino-atrial node. *In* Paes de Carvalho, A., de Mello, W. C., and Hoffman, B. F. (Eds.): The Specialized Tissues of the Heart. Amsterdam, Elsevier Press, Inc., 1962.

Zipes, D. P., and Fischer, J. C.: Effects of agents which inhibit the slow channel on sinus node automaticity and atrioventricular conduction in the dog. Circ. Res. *34*:184, 1974.

14 Renal Disease: Water and Electrolyte Balance

Dana L. Shires, Jr. and Yvonne E. Cummings

INTRODUCTION

The opportunity to review, condense, and present information currently pertaining to the pathophysiologic status of the human kidney is an awesome and exciting undertaking. That only the high points can be brushed upon in the space allotted is a statement that needs no further elaboration. As students of nephrology, we have never been disappointed by the continuing amassment of useful information relating to this truly remarkable organ and the role it plays in the regulation of the internal milieu in both health and disease.

The kidneys represent only 0.4 per cent of total body weight. Despite this relatively insignificant mass, they receive, on an average, 20 per cent of the total cardiac output. They play an intricate if not dominant role in the regulation of total body volume, composition of electrolytes and acid-base balance, mineral metabolism, amino acid metabolism, erythropoiesis, blood pressure control, and no doubt many additional undefined metabolic and endocrine functions yet to be described.

THE RENAL CIRCULATION

In humans, the kidneys together receive 20 per cent of the cardiac output, or roughly 500 ml/min of blood. This circulation gives the kidney the highest per-gram blood flow of any organ. Under usual circumstances, each kidney is supplied by a single artery from the aorta that divides into a dorsal and a ventral branch within the hilus. These vessels in turn divide into several interlobar arteries that ascend into the corticomedullary area. At this point the arcuate arteries are formed, from which arise the majority of the interlobular vessels. As the interlobular vessels pass through the cortex they give off the afferent arterioles. These, in turn, supply blood to the functioning filter of the kidney, the glomerulus (Fig. 14–1).

The afferent arteriole contains smooth muscle as well as myoepithelial cells. These cells occur in the distal portion of the afferent arteriole in continuity with the macula densa. This composite structure has been termed the "juxtaglomerular apparatus." Within the glomerulus, the afferent arteriole gives off five to eight branches that further subdivide into 20 to 40 capillary loops. These capillary loops coalesce to form the efferent arteriole, through which the circulation exits the glomerulus. In the superficial cortex, the efferent arteriole from a given glomerulus may exclusively supply the tubule of the parent glomerulus. In the deeper subcortical glomeruli, the efferent arterioles run toward the superficial or deep regions of the cortex and may surround tubules quite distant from their point of origin. In juxtamedullary nephrons, there are two main types of efferent arterioles: (1) the corticomedullary efferent arteriole, a thin-walled vessel that divides into a capillary network in the area of the corticomedullary junction and the outer medulla, and (2) the medullary efferent arteriole, a larger vessel that contains smooth muscle and divides into multiple vasa recta. The corticomedullary efferent arterioles are present in 25 to 40 per cent of the juxtamedullary nephrons and are the major vascular supply to the outer medulla. As the vessels descend into the medulla, most of these arteriolar vasa recta end in the capillary plexus, leaving only two to four branches that enter the inner medulla. These do not branch until they reach the tip of the papillae; they then empty into the ascending venous vasa recta.

Anatomically, the venous circulation generally parallels the course of the arterial system.

Mass blood flow through the renal tissue is not evenly distributed. A number of methods for evaluation of blood flow distribution have been devised and applied. They include both direct and indirect methods—each having built-in discrepancies to make them less than perfect. This subject has been extensively reviewed in various reports from which several important conclusions can be drawn. Under normal physiologic circumstances, the greater circulation is to the cortical areas of the kidney, representing roughly 85 per cent of the total blood flow to the kidney. No more than 15 per cent of blood flow enters the juxtamedullar nephrons. Most, if not all, of blood flow destined for the medulla traverses the juxtaglomerular nephrons. The osmolar concentration at the papillary tip is inversely related to blood flow to that area. Changes in medullary blood flow are an important determinant in the regulation of water balance. There is evidence that alteration in urinary sodium excretion is due, at least in part, to preferential redistribution of renal cortical blood flow to the juxtamedullary nephrons, which have a greater capacity for sodium reabsorption. Conversely, redistribution of blood flow to the outer cortical nephrons results in natriuresis. There are two types of juxtamedullary nephrons: (1) those with a postglomerular circulation that is distributed only in the outer medulla, and (2) those with the larger vasa recta that enter the inner medulla. Nephrons with the larger vasa recta make up 60 to 75 per cent of the glomeruli in the juxtamedullary cortex. There is a direct relationship between renal oxygen consumption and absolute sodium resorption or total renal blood flow. Over a wide range of sodium resorption, the ratio of sodium transport to oxygen utilization remains constant.

The kidney has a remarkable ability to maintain a constant blood flow, regardless of arterial pressure. This capability is independent of renal innervation and has been termed *autoregulation*. Under usual circumstances, autoregulation can be maintained with alterations of mean perfusion pressure from 60 to 180 mm Hg. Mechanisms intrinsic to the kidney for autoregulation are extremely complex. Despite the fact that the kidneys receive a rich supply of both adrenergic and cholinergic nerve fibers, complete denervation of a kidney fails to alter the autoregulatory mechanisms materially. This leads to one of two conclusions: (1) the kidney maintains an intrinsic neural distribution independent of extrinsic neural supply, or (2) intrinsic humoral factors are primarily responsible for autoregulation. There is no doubt that certain humoral mechanisms play an important role in the distribution of renal blood flow. Angiotensin II, generated by the release of renin from the juxtaglomerular apparatus, is the most potent vasoconstrictor known to humans. Prostaglandins have been shown to be powerful renal vasodilators. It seems appropriate to conclude, at this stage of the art, that an intrinsic balance of these two humoral factors and possibly as yet undetermined additional humoral factors play a paramount role in this autoregulatory mechanism so crucial to renal homeostasis.

THE GLOMERULUS

The glomerulus is the primary filtering unit of the kidney. The highest concentration of glomeruli is in the outer cortex; a lesser concentration appears in the juxtaglomerular area. The outer cortical glomerulus, although more frequent, is somewhat smaller in size than the juxtamedullary glomerulus. The juxtamedullary glomerulus has been shown to have a higher filtration rate per glomerular unit than does the cortical glomerulus. Each glomerulus receives its individual blood supply from an afferent arteriole. That arteriole, shortly after entering Bowman's capsule, divides into several branches. These, in turn, produce 20 to 40 capillaries per glomerulus. These capillaries then coalesce to form the efferent arteriole, which exits from Bowman's capsule in proximity to the afferent arteriole. There are roughly two million

glomeruli in each individual. These glomeruli are permanently formed shortly after birth, and, although they may enlarge as the individual matures, no new glomeruli are formed.

The total filtering surface has been calculated for both kidneys to represent roughly one square meter. The thickness of the basement membrane in humans has been established by electron microscopy as being roughly 3500 Å. The membrane itself can be divided into at least three anatomic divisions: (1) the endothelial component of the capillary wall, (2) a continuous basement membrane, and (3) the epithelial portion of the basement membrane. The structure and function of these component parts have been studied extensively. Each component plays an integral role in establishing permeability of the membrane to the various solute components of the plasma. For this discussion, suffice it to say that the membrane is freely permeable to solutes with a molecular weight equal to or less than that of inulin—inulin having a molecular weight of 5200 and an effective radius of 14 Å. Stated another way, molecules of this size and smaller will occur in concentrations when measured in Bowman's capsule equivalent to their concentration in the plasma. Larger molecules will be progressively restricted in their ability to pass this capillary membrane, depending on size and molecular shape.

The glomerulus is composed of three separate cellular elements: (1) the mesangial cell that constitutes the cellular matrix and supporting structures of the glomerulus, (2) the endothelial cell that forms and contributes to the endothelial lining of the basement membrane, and (3) the epithelial cell that forms the external component of the capillary loop as well as the lining of Bowman's capsule.

Under usual circumstances in a 70-kilogram man, 180 liters of glomerular ultrafiltrate will be formed daily, of which less than 1 per cent is normally excreted in the form of urine. This ultrafiltrate, as noted previously, contains small solute particles in roughly the same concentration as they are measured in plasma. It is almost totally free of larger molecular weight substances. It might be noted that the concentration of albumin with a molecular weight of 68,000 is less than 1 per cent of the concentration of inulin in the ultrafiltrate as measured in Bowman's capsule.

THE TUBULES

The human kidney has at least two populations of nephrons. Those nephrons derived from cortical glomeruli are composed of a proximal convoluted segment, a straight descending segment (pars rectus), a short diluting segment (short loop of Henle), and a thick ascending segment terminating at the macula densa, where it becomes the distal convoluted tubule. For the purpose of

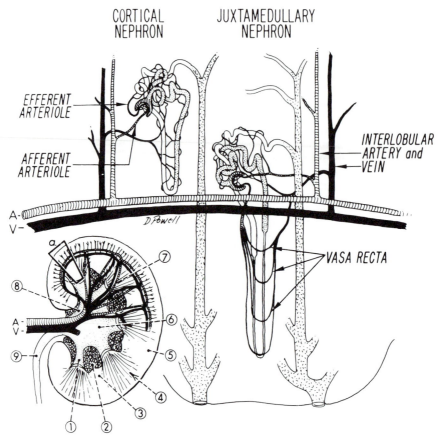

Figure 14–1 The sagittal surface of a bisected kidney is illustrated diagrammatically (lower left). Numbers 1 through 9 indicate the following: (1) minor calix; (2) fat in sinus; (3) renal column of Bertin; (4) medullary ray; (5) cortex; (6) pelvis; (7) interlobar artery; (8) major calix; and (9) ureter. The letter *A* indicates the renal artery; the letter *V* indicates the renal vein. Insert *a* from the upper pole is enlarged to illustrate the relationships between the juxtamedullary and the cortical nephrons and the renal vasculature. (From Brenner, B. M., and Rector, F. C., Jr. [eds.]: The Kidney. 2nd ed. Philadelphia, W. B. Saunders Company, 1981.)

conceptualizing various physiologic events as they relate to tubule function, renal physiologists have assigned functions to specific anatomic areas on the basis of in-vivo and in-vitro studies. It is worthy of mention that nature may not be as anatomically precise as the scientific community would choose; however, for the sake of simplicity, we shall observe the more precise assignments of function and duty.

Nephrons from the juxtamedullary glomeruli have (in addition to the anatomic structures described for nephrons derived from cortical glomeruli) a long descending and ascending medullary thin segment. Some of these segments extend to the very tip of the renal papillae.

The proximal convoluted tubule is lined by thick cuboidal cells with a prominent brush border along the luminal surface. The ultrafiltrate of plasma is delivered in toto to this segment from Bowman's space, where roughly 60 per cent of the transluminal volume is reabsorbed by both active and passive mechanisms. Luminal fluid remains isosmotic to plasma as it transcends this tubule segment.

Within this segment active transport mechanisms have been demonstrated for sodium, potassium, glucose, amino acids, phosphate, and other less prominent cations and anions. The transport of sodium appears to be of major importance in total volume removal, with a lesser role assigned to bicarbonate and potassium. Although a number of investigators have strongly suggested a direct transport mechanism for bicarbonate, the consensus at this writing favors the more classic description of hydrogen ion diffusion from the transluminal cells, formation of carbonic acid, rapid dissociation to CO_2 + H_2O in the presence of abundant carbonic anhydrase, and diffusion of CO_2 intracellularly, where it again becomes available for formation of the bicarbonate ion (Fig. 14–2).

Water passively follows the active transport of solute. The cells of the proximal tubules are aligned with their luminal membranes joined by

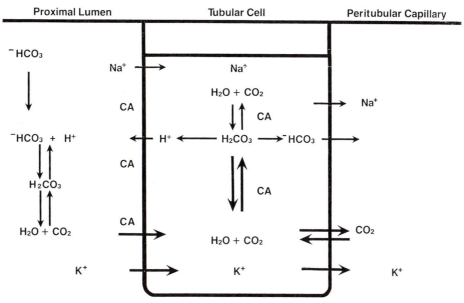

Figure 14–2 Luminal bicarbonate (HCO_3^-), combines with hydrogen (H^+) ion to form carbonic acid (H_2CO_3). In the presence of abundant carbonic anhydrase (CA), H_2CO_3 rapidly dissociates to carbon dioxide (CO_2) and water (H_2O). CO_2 diffuses back into the cells of the proximal tubule, where it is available for conversion to H^+ and HCO_3^-. The result is the generation of HCO_3^- and the excretion of H^+.

so-called "tight junctions" (Fig. 14–3). Between these tight junctions and the contraluminal membrane is an intercellular compartment, a site at which active transport of sodium ion is thought to occur. As sodium enters this paracellular channel, it increases the tonicity of the fluid, and water then moves toward the osmotic gradient thus cre-

ated. These low-resistance paracellular channels may play a major role in passive transfer of water and solute in the proximal tubule.

Each of the nephrons of the juxtamedullary glomeruli has a long descending and ascending thin segment (Fig. 14–4) that extends for a variable distance into the inner medulla. It is this

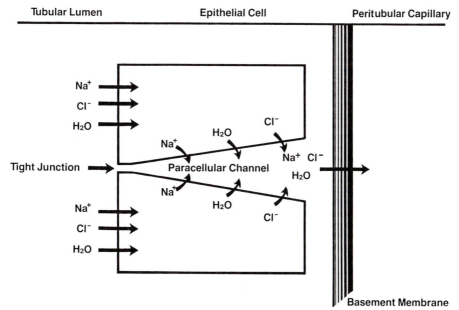

Figure 14–3 The cells of the proximal tubule with the "tight junctions" and the paracellular channel, a site at which active transport of sodium ion (Na^+) is thought to occur, creating an osmotic gradient for water (H_2O) and solute removal.

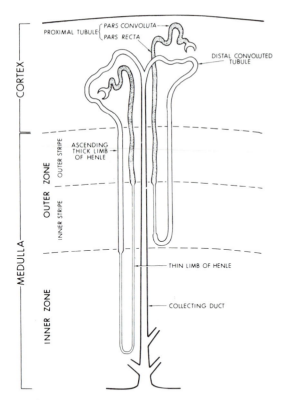

Figure 14–4 Diagram of the structural organization of the mammalian kidney demonstrating the relationships between the various segments of the nephron and the zones of the kidney, especially the medulla. (From Brenner, B. M., and Rector, F. C., Jr. [Eds.]: The Kidney. 2nd ed. Philadelphia, W. B. Saunders Company, 1981.)

highly specialized segment of tubule that in conjunction with its closely associated vasa recta and collecting ducts provides the concentrating mechanism so critical to the mammalian kidney. Many models have been proposed to explain the complexities of this countercurrent system. Most have in common two major factors: (1) selective segmental permeability or impermeability to solute and water, and (2) an energy-dependent active transport mechanism (Fig. 14–5).

A simplified explanation of this countercurrent mechanism follows. Tubule fluid enters the descending thin segment of the loop of Henle from the pars rectus of the juxtamedullary nephron. At the point of entry it is isotonic to plasma. The descending thin segment is freely permeable to water and, to a lesser extent, solute. As the intraluminal fluid proceeds toward the inner medulla it is exposed to increasingly higher osmolalities and, because of the permeability factors noted, becomes progressively more hypertonic.

The ascending limb is highly impermeable to water; however, the active transport of chloride ion allows for the production of an increasingly dilute luminal fluid to a point at which fluid is hypotonic to plasma as it enters the distal convoluted tubule. It is estimated that 25 per cent of the filtered load of sodium is absorbed by this chloride transport mechanism in the ascending thick segment and represents the primary source of energy expenditure for both concentration and dilution of urine.

The anatomic segment of the nephron extending from the macula densa to the point of junction with other tubules to form the collecting duct is

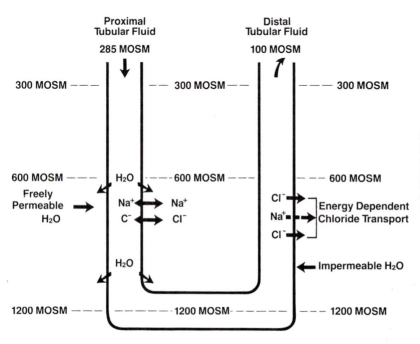

Figure 14–5 The descending limb is freely permeable to water (H$_2$O) and less so to solute. The ascending limb is impermeable to H$_2$O, coupled with an energy-dependent mechanism for the active transport of chloride.

called the *distal convoluted tubule*. The urine at its point of delivery to this tubule segment is hypotonic to plasma. Depending on the state of hydration, urine may be maintained in this hypotonic state or returned toward isotonicity—antidiuretic hormone (ADH) directly affects tubule permeability to water in the distal portions of this nephron segment. In addition to having a role in concentration and dilution, the distal nephron is a major factor in the regulation of potassium and hydrogen excretion by the kidney. Renal handling of potassium and hydrogen will be discussed in greater detail in a later section of this chapter.

The collecting ducts are formed by the coalescence of several distal convoluted tubules and terminate in the ducts of Bellini. The epithelial cells lining this duct are selectively impermeable to the flux of water in the absence of ADH, resulting in the excretion of a highly dilute urine. In the presence of ADH, membrane permeability is greatly enhanced, allowing water to diffuse down a concentration gradient into the hypertonic interstitium of the medulla, resulting in a concentrated urine. ADH has been shown to enhance selectively the diffusion of urea in segments of the collecting duct, further enhancing the establishment and maintenance of medullary hypertonicity. The collecting duct is capable of maintaining hydrogen ion gradients and plays an important role in the active transport of sodium from the tubule fluid. Although the absolute amount of sodium is small when compared with total filtered sodium, the collecting duct may serve as the ultimate "fine-tuning" for sodium excretion.

SUMMARY

Roughly 25,000 mEq of sodium ion are filtered by the normal glomerular mass in 24 hours. Approximately 65 per cent of the filtered sodium ion is absorbed in the proximal tubule by a process of active transfer. Twenty-five per cent is absorbed in the loop of Henle secondary to active transport of chloride ion in the ascending thick segment. Less than 10 per cent is absorbed by an active process in the distal convoluted tubule, approximately 1 per cent is absorbed in the collecting duct, and less than 1 per cent is finally excreted in the urine.

The renal handling of water is entirely passive—movement of water throughout the kidney is dependent on solute concentration. Bulk water movement is dependent on the active transport of sodium ion. The kidney is unique as far as we know in that the ascending loop of Henle and the collecting duct have the capability of remaining impermeable to water despite continued solute transport. It is this property that allows the kidney to form a dilute urine and at the same time to establish osmotic gradients necessary for final urinary concentration.

Potassium is filtered at the glomerulus, with 85 to 90 per cent active reabsorption occurring in the proximal tubule. Some additional absorption occurs in the ascending limb of Henle's loop secondary to chloride transport. Intraluminal fluid reaching the distal tubule is almost potassium-free. In this tubule segment, there is a bidirectional flux of potassium ion. The intracellular potassium ion of tubule cells is high and enters tubule fluid probably by passive flux from the higher concentration in the cell to the lower concentration in the tubule fluid. Final concentration may be determined by the rate at which potassium ion is actively pumped against the gradient back into the cell.

Potassium transport in the distal segment is under partial control of aldosterone. Although there is a loose relationship between potassium ion concentration, sodium, and hydrogen ion, there is not a tightly coupled exchange mechanism as was previously thought to exist.

The kidneys are responsible for the removal of roughly 75 mEq of hydrogen ion per 24 hours under usual conditions of intermediary metabolism. Metabolic derangements associated with various pathologic states may produce a significant increase in hydrogen ion excretion. At least three physiologic mechanisms exist within the kidney to meet this need. There may be more.

Bicarbonate, because of its small molecular size, is freely filterable at the glomerulus and reaches the proximal convoluted tubule in concentration equivalent to that found in plasma (24 to 26 mM per liter). Transcending the early portion of this tubule segment, it is rapidly removed from the tubule fluid as it combines with hydrogen ion entering the lumen from the paratubular cells: $H^+ + HCO_3^- \rightarrow H_2CO_3 \rightarrow H_2O + CO_2$. The CO_2 and H_2O are free to diffuse across the peritubular membrane (Fig. 14–2). By this process, one hydrogen ion molecule has been effectively eliminated and a bicarbonate radical returned to the general circulation to sustain the intact bicarbonate buffering system. As the luminal fluid proceeds down the tubule, there is a slight rise in hydrogen ion concentration as bulk bicarbonate is removed and is no longer available for combination with hydrogen ion. There is little reason to believe that the loop of Henle plays a major role in renal acidification mechanisms.

Tubule fluid reaching the distal segment of the nephron under normal circumstances contains little or no bicarbonate. In certain pathologic or drug-induced states, bicarbonate may be delivered to this segment, and under these circumstances regeneration of bicarbonate takes place in the distal nephron. Under more usual physiologic conditions, hydrogen ion is secreted into tubule fluid against a concentration gradient, allowing the hydrogen ion concentration to rise selectively. Tubule cells here are relatively impermeable to the back diffusion of hydrogen ion, a property also inherent in the cells of the collecting duct.

Ammonia production plays a major role in the

kidney's ability to excrete an excess hydrogen ion load. The capacity to produce ammonia by the selective degradation of the amino acid glutamine is a property inherent in all tubule cells. Ammonia thus formed is free to diffuse into the luminal fluid, where it binds with accessible hydrogen ion and forms the ammonium radical, NH_4^+. The peritubular cell membranes are much less permeable to this radical. In essence it is now trapped in the tubular lumen, has buffered a hydrogen ion, and is excreted in the final urine. Under conditions of excessive hydrogen ion load, this accounts for the major route of hydrogen ion removal.

CLINICAL EVALUATION OF RENAL FUNCTION

The problem facing the physician in diagnosing renal disease is the relatively long asymptomatic period found in almost all types of kidney disorders. When the patient finally seeks attention, it is frequently too late to alter the course of his basic disease process. The importance of finding early disease cannot be overstressed. Only through a complete history and physical examination and the proper use of laboratory procedures does a physician have a chance to offer his patient help before it is too late.

The *urinalysis* is the most helpful and frequently the most overlooked renal function study in clinical medicine. It is often relegated to the least skilled member of the laboratory staff, who does it without interest or skill. In addition, the importance of collection and rapid evaluation after collection is overlooked. The best specimens are collected by the "clean-catch" method and examined promptly. Allowing urine to sit for any amount of time leads to destruction of the formed elements through changes in pH and osmotic pressures. We strongly recommend that in any patient suspected of having renal disease the physician examine each urine specimen under the microscope.

The finding of *protein* in the urine—by any method and in any amount—is reason for further evaluation. Proteinuria is the hallmark of renal disease. The lack of protein in the urine suggests that renal disease is not present; however, even this is not conclusive. A number of disease processes may present with minimal or no proteinuria. Examples are obstruction, hypercalcemia, hypokalemia, chronic pyelonephritis, arteriosclerosis and nephrosclerosis, polycystic disease, congenital diseases of the tubule, analgesic-abuse nephritis, neoplasms, stones, and congenital malformations. The amount of protein found in 24 hours is of prime importance, both diagnostically and prognostically. Persistent proteinuria inevitably indicates renal disease. Even amounts only minimally in excess of normal may be of significance. Under normal circumstances, very little albumin is filtered at the glomerulus. Various investigators

have estimated the rate of albumin filtration at 12 mg per kg per 24-hour period and a normal excretion rate at 2 mg per kg per 24-hour period. The 10-mg per kg per 24 hours represents proximal tubule transport of albumin by an energy-dependent process of pinocytosis. This means that a 70-kg man would be expected to excrete no more than 140 mg of albumin in any 24-hour period. The kidney normally secretes, probably by tubule cells, a globulin (Tamm-Horsfall protein) that occurs naturally in the urine in very minute quantities. The amount of protein excreted in any 24-hour period is useful in making a clinical assessment of the area of the kidney involved in the disease process. Patients with primary tubule disease usually will excrete less than 3 gm per day. Patients with disease processes related to glomerular basement membrane damage may be expected to excrete protein in excess of 3 gm per day and can reach values of 30 to 40 gm per day.

Normally, a small amount of *glucose* appears in the urine in the range of 100 to 200 mg per 24 hours. The appearance of glucose in excess of this amount is an indication that the tubule mechanism for glucose transport has been exceeded. This may indicate that plasma glucose is high or that tubule defects exist that have lowered the renal threshold for glucose. Renal glycosuria is frequently found in association with other proximal tubule transport defects, such as aminoaciduria, uric acid, and phosphate wasting.

The *pH* of the urine is routinely tested in the standard urinalysis. The kidney is capable of excreting urine over a wide range of pHs from 4.5 to 8.5. Humans normally excrete the hydrogen ion produced from the metabolism of carbohydrate, lipids, and sulfa-containing amino acids in two forms. Thirty to 50 mEq of hydrogen ion per 24 hours are excreted in combination with ammonia. Ten to 30 mEq per 24 hours of hydrogen ion are excreted as so-called "titratable acidity." Hydrogen ion in this form is, for the most part, buffered by either phosphate or creatinine. The finding of a pH of 5.5 or below in a urinalysis signifies that tubule mechanisms of acidification are intact. The finding of a value above this in a routine urinalysis does not imply that these mechanisms are defective. This can only be evaluated by stressing the patient with a hydrogen ion load. Failure to acidify may suggest such diseases as renal tubule acidosis, early pyelonephritis, primary aldosterone-secreting tumor, and hypokalemia. The failure of the kidney to excrete hydrogen ion in renal disease results in its retention and leads to chronic metabolic acidosis, which is always seen with severe azotemia. In certain types of renal disease systemic acidosis may develop even though the glomerular filtration rate is well preserved. Renal tubule acidosis and analgesic-abuse nephritis are two examples of disease processes in which a relatively alkaline urine may be excreted in the face of metabolic acidosis.

Specific gravity is an indirect measurement of

urine osmolality and thus of the kidney's ability to concentrate or dilute urine. Because specific gravity depends on the density and number of particles of solute rather than their absolute concentration, at times it may be misleading. Large amounts of protein or glucose in the urine may give the false impression of an ability to concentrate when that ability no longer exists. A direct measurement of urine osmolality is much more specific in establishing concentration or dilution abilities. This is done on as little as 2 ml of urine by freezing-point determination: Osmolalities may range from as low as 40 to as high as 1400 mOsm per kg of water. The finding of a fixed urine osmolality indicates a significant loss of functional renal mass. Tests of concentrating ability are frequently used to determine early damage to the kidney, especially in pyelonephritis and other forms of interstitial nephritis. Ability to form a highly concentrated urine indicates a relatively intact medulla, ascending and descending loop of Henle, collecting duct, and posterior pituitary. In the oliguric patient a specific gravity of 1.020 or an osmolality of 600 or above is considered indication of prerenal etiology for oliguria.

The *microscopic examination* of the urinary sediment is the most important part of the study to be performed by the physician. This should be done only on a fresh specimen of urine. First, an unspun specimen should be searched for bacteria and cells. If bacteria are present, the assumption can be made that their numbers in the urine exceed 100,000 per ml. The urine should then be spun for five minutes at 2000 rpm. Staining is used in some laboratories for cell differentiation; however, in general it is not necessary. The quantitative evaluation of cells and types and number of casts produced by the kidney can be done with a 12- or 24-hour Addis count. In the 12-hour Addis count, one normally expects to see 2000 hyaline casts, 130,000 to 300,000 red cells, and 650,000 to 1,000,000 white cells. In the normal urinalysis, a small number of cells can often be seen: 2 to 3 red cells, 4 to 5 white cells per high-powered field on a spun specimen, and an occasional hyaline cast are accepted as normal. The finding of red blood cells in the urine is indicative only of blood loss. The origin of these red cells cannot be localized to bladder, prostate, urethra, ureter, or kidneys. The finding of red blood cell casts indicates primary renal parenchymal involvement. Red cell casts do not persist in alkaline or hypotonic urine, and, therefore, repeated examinations may be necessary to rule out the presence of casts when one is searching for a primary glomerular lesion. Red cell casts are strongly suggestive of primary glomerular involvement, whether it be glomerulonephritis, angiitis, lupus, or periarteritis. They may also be found in malignant hypertension, in acute tubular necrosis, and following trauma to the kidney. White blood cells and white blood cell casts may be found in increased numbers in any type of renal parenchymal lesion. White cells may be excreted at any point along the urinary tract, and their origin cannot be determined specifically by examination of the urine. The occurrence of large numbers of white cell casts is a strong indication that the renal parenchyma itself is involved in the disease process.

Routine biochemical evaluation of most patients entering the hospital includes a blood urea nitrogen (BUN) as an indicator of renal dysfunction. Unfortunately, as a screening test the BUN lacks sensitivity, as significant rises occur only after substantial loss of renal function. Changes in BUN are also dependent on the state of protein catabolism and may be found artificially low or high on that basis, independent of normal renal function.

A more informative clinical study is a direct or indirect measurement of *glomerular filtration rate*. In order to determine glomerular filtration rate, a substance must have the following characteristics:

1. It should neither be absorbed nor secreted by the renal tubule.
2. It must not be protein bound.
3. It must be easily measured in the serum and urine and be nontoxic.
4. It must have a molecular weight compatible with unimpeded filtration at the glomerulus.

The reference standard for measuring glomerular filtration rate in humans is inulin. Unfortunately, the performance of a clearance evaluation using inulin is cumbersome and necessitates a constant intravenous infusion and catheterization of the bladder. Urea, which is the end product of protein metabolism, does not come close to fulfilling any of the prerequisites of a substance for measuring glomerular filtration rate. Urea is not only filtered—it is also absorbed in significant quantities along the tubule and the collecting duct. Its clearance depends to a large extent on the rate of urine formation. As urine flow decreases, larger amounts of urea are resorbed, leading to significant decreases in clearance rate in the face of a normal glomerular filtration. At high urine flow rates, the clearance of urea is roughly 70 per cent of the clearance of inulin.

A more reliable marker of clinical renal function is creatinine. Creatinine is a normal end product of muscle metabolism. Its plasma concentration and 24-hour urinary excretion are relatively constant. They are not influenced by diet, metabolic rate, exercise, or urine flow. It is these several advantages over urea that have made it acceptable in routine measurement of glomerular filtration rate. The usual formula for calculating the glomerular filtration rate is: GFR is equal to the urinary concentration (U) of creatinine times the volume (V) divided by the plasma concentration (P) of creatinine: GFR = U V/P. In humans, unfortunately, not only is creatinine filtered but also small quantities are secreted by the renal tubule. Fortuitously, the Jaffe chemical determination of plasma creatinine measures not only true creatinine but also a group of substances known as creatinine chromogens. These substances are not secreted and do not appear in the urine. This results in a falsely high plasma creatinine value that is balanced by the increase in creatinine excretion secondary to tubule secretion. As renal function fails, the serum creatinine rises, but the chromogens remain relatively unchanged. The result is that creatinine clearance in patients with renal disease reflects a certain amount of secretion, producing an artificially high creatinine clearance in patients with far advanced renal failure. Serial determinations and observations are therefore superior to any single observation, and the use of multiple determinations allows for a check on accuracy and the rate of progression of the disease. The following substances may interfere with the Jaffe reaction for creatinine: acetone, acetoacetic acid, ascorbic acid, barbiturates, BSP, and PSP. The normal creatinine clearance values are as follows: men, creatinine clearance of 120 ± 25 ml/min.; women, creatinine clearance of 96 ± 13 ml/min. When corrected for body surface area, the values are: men, 103 ± 15 ml/min/1.7 M²; women, 97 ± 9 ml/min/1.73 M².

The creatinine clearance is by far the most sensitive regular clinical test of renal function available today. It is necessary to re-emphasize the importance of obtaining serial values rather than trusting a single determination. The use of serum creatinine values as estimates of renal function is not as accurate as a clearance value, but it is a much more sensitive reflection of early changes of renal function than is the BUN. Normal values of creatinine vary depending on the method and specimen used. When plasma and the Jaffe method are used, the upper limits of normal creatinine values are as follows: men, 0.8 to 1.2 mg/100 ml; women, 0.6 to 1.1 mg/100 ml. A rough estimate of renal function ability can be made using the following schedule: serum creatinine of 1 mg = 100 per cent normal function; serum creatinine of 2 mg = 50 per cent or less of normal renal function; serum creatinine of 4 mg = 25 per cent or less of normal renal function.

The BUN/creatinine ratio is a commonly derived function in many automated clinical laboratories and, under certain circumstances, can be used to draw additional clinical data about the status of renal function. This comparison takes advantage of the two different patterns of excretion of these compounds. Normal individuals are expected to maintain a BUN/creatinine ratio of approximately 10. The following is a list of reasons for values of this ratio over 10:

1. Excessive ingestion of protein in a patient with depressed renal function.
2. Blood in the small intestine.
3. Excessive protein catabolism. This may be due to a variety of factors, such as burns, fever, steroids, wasting, and trauma.

4. Marked glomerulotubular imbalance—a finding most often related to underperfusion of the kidney. The glomerular filtration is relatively maintained, but absorption of urea becomes more complete. Dehydration and congestive heart failure are common examples of this phenomenon.

In certain circumstances, the BUN/creatinine ratio may be less than 10 (e.g., in a patient with very low protein intake in renal disease). Low protein diets are frequently used in the treatment of renal failure, and the BUN in these patients no longer reflects the reduced functional capacity of the kidney. In these incidences, BUNs falling within the normal range may occur in patients with creatinine clearances of less than 20. Other examples can relate to excessive vomiting, diarrhea, or hepatic insufficiency.

The laboratory functions and studies that we have discussed are those commonly available to any physician from a routine reference laboratory. It is beyond the scope of this discussion to evaluate the application of more sophisticated radiologic, immunologic, and isotopic studies in evaluation of renal function. It is pertinent to know that they exist and that their application is often indicated to delineate further the extent of renal embarrassment. The importance of serial testing should always be kept in mind. The use of multiple tests on individual patients will give a better evaluation than any single determination. The rate of change in functional testing is more important than the information gained from a single battery of tests.

DISORDERS OF SODIUM METABOLISM

Sodium is the major extracellular cation. The normal plasma sodium is 142 mEq per liter. The intracellular sodium is less than 10 mEq per liter of cell water (normal muscle cell). The total body sodium of a normal adult male averages 60 mEq per kg of body weight. A 70-kg man contains some 4200 mEq of sodium. Bone contains between 40 and 45 per cent of the total body stores of sodium. Accordingly, about 50 per cent of total sodium is extracellular, 40 per cent is associated with bone, and 10 per cent is intracellular. Exchangeable sodium amounts to 42 mEq per kg of body weight. This fraction includes all extracellular and intracellular sodium and slightly less than half of the bone sodium. If sodium is lost in sweat, urine, or diarrheal fluid, that present in the exchangeable reservoir, including the exchangeable sodium of the cancellous bone, is available to mitigate the decrease in concentration that would otherwise occur when body water is restored. When sodium is retained, it is distributed into the subject's exchangeable reservoir.

The average American diet contains sodium far in excess of usual body requirements calculated at roughly 50 mEq per day. The normal gastrointestinal tract has an almost unlimited capacity for sodium absorption. There is little net transport of sodium in the stomach. The bulk of ingested sodium absorption occurs in the small bowel (both jejunum and ileum), with final conservation occurring in the colon, leaving a residual stool sodium for excretion of between 5 and 10 mEq per 24 hours. It must be recalled that sodium is also a major ionic constituent of gastrointestinal secretions, and the net absorption of sodium by the bowel may, under normal conditions, exceed 1500 mEq per 24 hours. Sodium transport, at least in the colon, is facilitated by the presence of aldosterone.

Under normal physiologic circumstances, the kidney is the major route for excretion of excess body sodium. Under conditions of stress, such as continued vomiting or prolonged diarrhea, the gastrointestinal tract can make a major contribution to the depletion of total body sodium. Cutaneous losses of sodium vary widely with the individual's activity and conditioning and with environmental factors. Sweat sodium varies directly with the rate of sweat formation. An individual in a resting state may have less than 30 mEq of sodium per liter in his sweat. As the ambient temperature rises, or as his endogenous production of heat increases, his rate of sweating increases, as does the concentration of sodium in the sweat. At high rates of sweating (as much as 700 ml/hr under maximal stimulation), sodium losses increase dramatically, sometimes in excess of 100 mEq per liter of sweat. It is apparent that prolonged exposure to conditions associated with sweating at a maximal rate can lead rapidly to severe body depletion of both salt and water. It is important to note that sweat is always hypotonic to plasma, and thus profuse sweating without access to water replacement can lead to a clinical state of hypernatremia. Sodium levels of 165 to 170 mEq per liter have been reported in otherwise healthy athletes undergoing vigorous exercise and denied free access to fluid replacement.

The normal functioning kidney is the ultimate regulatory organ for total body sodium. A 70-kg man will form roughly 180 liters of plasma ultrafiltrate per day at the glomerulus. This means that in excess of 25,000 mEq of sodium are presented to the renal tubule every 24 hours, where more than 99 per cent is selectively reabsorbed. Under conditions of maximum stress and salt loading, individual cases have been reported in which 65 per cent of the filtered load of sodium can be excreted by the appropriately functioning kidney. We have previously discussed the more intricate details of tubule handling of sodium earlier in this chapter.

HYPERNATREMIA

Hypernatremia can be divided into two major classifications: (1) that associated with dehydra-

tion, and (2) that related to the inability to conserve water. Dehydration occurs when excessive body water is lost in comparison to total body sodium. This state of affairs is most commonly associated with disease processes that either limit the access of the individual to water or result in excessive losses of water, usually through the gastrointestinal tract. Increased insensible water losses may also lead to a state of hypernatremia and dehydration. Common causes of this pathologic state are associated with hyperventilation or fever. Inappropriate water loss is usually divided into central and nephrogenic *diabetes insipidus*.

Central diabetes insipidus is always associated with the absence of or less than normal release of antidiuretic hormone (ADH) secondary to appropriate stimuli. Central diabetes insipidus is associated with some form of central nervous system disease, although the idiopathic variety has been recognized with no demonstrable central nervous system pathology. Nephrogenic diabetes insipidus is either an acquired or a hereditary disorder. The hereditary disorder is characterized by insensitivity of the collecting duct to antidiuretic hormone. The disorder usually presents in childhood with recurrent dehydration, a dilute urine, and failure to thrive. In this disorder, ADH has no effect on renal concentration. There is no other demonstrable renal lesion. Proximal tubule anatomic anomalies have been described, but their significance is uncertain. Inheritance is sex-linked dominant, and most cases occur in males; heterologus females may have some limitation of concentrating ability.

A more common form of nephrogenic diabetes insipidus is the acquired variety. This may be related to metabolic anomalies, certain disease processes, or the administration of a variety of drugs. Examples of nephrogenic diabetes insipidus in which the distal nephron and collecting duct have become insensitive to the action of antidiuretic hormone include hypokalemia, hypercalcemia, sickle cell disease, amyloidosis, Sjögren's syndrome, Fanconi's syndrome, post–urinary tract obstruction, acute tubule necrosis, and radiation nephritis. The administration of methoxyflurane, lithium, colchicine, vincristine, and demeclocycline may also produce symptoms. In the syndrome secondary to drug administration, the process is usually a reversible one, and the sensitivity to the actions of ADH returns with the removal of the drug.

HYPONATREMIA

Hyponatremia is one of the more common fluid and electrolyte anomalies seen in the practice of clinical medicine (Table 14–1). The etiologies of hyponatremia can be considered in terms of total body sodium: low, normal, or elevated. The causes of hyponatremia associated with a low total body sodium include renal sodium loss and extrarenal

TABLE 14–1 HYPONATREMIA

1. Dilutional
2. Depletion
3. Factitious
   a. Hyperglycemia
   b. Hyperlipemia
   c. Hyperproteinemia
4. Diuretic-induced
   a. Dilutional
   b. Depletion
   c. Hypokalemia
5. Hypothyroidism
6. Adrenal insufficiency
7. Inappropriate secretion of antidiuretic hormone
   a. Malignant tumors
   b. Central nervous system disease
   c. Pulmonary disease
   d. Drugs

sodium loss. Conditions common to the former include salt-wasting nephropathies, adrenal insufficiency, and disorders related to the use of diuretics. The most common origin of extrarenal sodium loss is the gastrointestinal tract. Common to both groups is solute and water loss, with replacement of only the water losses. Volume losses lead to a decrease in effective circulating volume and stimulation of thirst. Thus, patients with such disorders also have an element of dilution contributing to their hyponatremia. The urine sodium is helpful in the diagnosis of hyponatremia. In hyponatremia due to extrarenal losses, the kidney will sense the decrease in effective circulating volume and will attempt to maintain perfusion by maximal sodium conservation. Therefore, the urine sodium will be low (<10 mEq/L). In hyponatremia due to renal losses, however, the urine sodium will be elevated (>20 mEq/L). Because sodium loss occurs through the kidney, urine sodium will be high, even in the presence of decreased effective circulating volume.

The syndrome of inappropriate ADH secretion is associated with a normal total body sodium and occurs secondary to a variety of clinical diseases. These include various malignant tumors, central nervous system disorders, and pulmonary disease. The pathophysiology that develops is thought to relate to the activation of compensatory mechanisms to maintain volume. The continued and inappropriate elaboration of antidiuretic hormone results in expansion of total body fluid volume. Proximal tubule transport of sodium is depressed, and significant sodium losses result. A number of drugs have also been implicated in the production of this syndrome. The drug may (1) act at the central nervous system level to stimulate excessive elaboration of vasopressin, or (2) facilitate the hormone's action at the distal nephron and collecting duct. Examples of drugs that have been implicated in the production of inappropriate ADH secretion syndrome are barbiturates, morphine, nicotine, chlorpropamide, cyclophosphamide, vincristine, clofibrate, and norepinephrine.

Conditions associated with an elevated total body sodium and hyponatremia include congestive heart failure, liver disease (particularly cirrhosis), and nephrotic syndrome. The underlying pathophysiologic mechanism in all these conditions is decreased effective circulating volume that results from (1) decreased cardiac output in congestive heart failure, (2) portal hypertension and vascular volume loss into the abdominal space in liver disease, and (3) decreased plasma oncotic pressure (hypoalbuminemia) in nephrotic syndrome. Affected patients present with volume expansion as the kidney attempts to maintain effective circulating volume by reabsorption of sodium and water. However, the sodium reabsorbed continues to leave the vascular space as long as the aforementioned mechanisms are not corrected. The urine sodium in these conditions is low (<10 mEq/L).

Factitious hyponatremia may be seen as the direct result of at least three common alterations of internal metabolism. In patients with severe hyperglycemia, the osmotic gradients produced in the interstitial space and plasma volume by excess glucose result in an influx of water in an attempt to maintain osmotic neutrality, and the serum sodium is artificially depressed. Total body sodium is normal, and correction of hyperglycemia results in the correction of hyponatremia.

Factitious hyponatremia may also occur in individuals with hyperlipidemia. In these patients, the distribution of sodium within the water component of the vascular space is entirely normal. That component has been significantly reduced by the high circulating concentration of lipids. A syndrome similar to this has been described with hyperproteinemia exemplified by multiple myeloma and other disproteinemic syndromes. Again, in these conditions, total body sodium is normal.

Hyponatremia may develop in cases of severe hypothyroidism and has long been recognized as a potential component of adrenal insufficiency.

DISORDERS OF POTASSIUM METABOLISM

Potassium is the major intracellular cation. An average man has a total body potassium of 40 mEq per kilogram; a woman has slightly less. Ninety-eight per cent of the potassium pool is concentrated within the cells. Direct measurements of potassium within muscle intracellular water record values of 160 mEq per liter. Normal concentrations of extracellular potassium are recorded between 3.5 and 5.5 mEq per liter of plasma. These transmembrane gradients for potassium are maintained within narrow limits by active transport of sodium from the cell and active transport of potassium into the cell.

The human diet is high in potassium and greatly exceeds daily body requirements. The kidney is the primary organ of excretion, with gastrointestinal losses accounting for less than 10 mEq per day. With prolonged nausea or diarrhea or both, gastrointestinal losses of potassium may be enhanced to the point of producing a clinical state of hypokalemia.

A number of mechanisms contribute to the regulation of total body potassium and its distribution within the body. The status of hydrogen ion concentration has a major impact on distribution and excretion of potassium. With hydrogen ion in excess, there is an increased flux of potassium from the cells as hydrogen ion enters. A direct result is a rise in serum potassium. At the same time, intracellular potassium is lowered, becoming less readily available for secretion by the distal tubule segment or the collecting duct or both, impairing renal mechanisms for potassium excretion.

Bicarbonate has an action on transmembrane potassium transport independent of hydrogen ion concentration. When pH is maintained by elevating the CO_2 and bicarbonate is increased, there is a significant shift of potassium intracellularly. This was suspected by clinicians for many years, but confirmed only later in experimental animals.

The mineralocorticoid aldosterone plays a major role in the internal regulation of potassium. In all probability, aldosterone promotes the intracellular flux of potassium of all cells. This may assume particular significance in the renal handling of potassium. In the presence of aldosterone, cells of the distal nephron and collecting duct are able to concentrate potassium, allowing for its increased flux into the tubular fluid and ultimate excretion. The ability of the distal nephron and collecting duct to secrete potassium depends on the rate of flow of tubule fluid. When the flow rate is diminished, the secretion of potassium also diminishes. In states of potassium depletion the distal nephron and collecting duct have the ability to further the conservation of potassium by selectively removing it from the tubule fluid. In states of chronic potassium overload and perhaps uremia, the ability of these segments to secrete potassium is enhanced. The action of aldosterone on sodium transport mechanisms in these tubule segments is thought to be independent of this effect on potassium.

Insulin has been shown to promote cellular uptake of potassium independently of its action on glucose. Epinephrine infusion is followed by an initial rise in plasma potassium, followed shortly thereafter by a prolonged period of hypokalemia. This action is explained by an initial release of potassium from cells followed by an increase in potassium uptake by the liver.

It is beyond the limited scope of this discussion to review all known clinical disorders with which hypokalemia may be associated (Table 14–2). Rather, we shall concentrate on broad categories based on the mechanisms of potassium regulation.

Hypokalemia. Maintaining a normal potassium balance requires (1) *adequate intake,* (2) *appropriate internal distribution* between intracellular and extracellular fluid compartments, and (3) appropriate control and function of *mechanisms of excretion.* A state of clinical hypokalemia can result from alteration in any of these integrated functions. Hypokalemia may result following upper gastrointestinal disease with associated vomiting or nasogastric suction. Depending on the level of secretion, GI contents may contain potassium concentrations in excess of 20 mEq per liter. Over a prolonged period, losses of this nature can result in serious depletion. With loss of accompanying hydrogen ion, the situation may be complicated by metabolic alkalosis with further depression of serum potassium.

Disease processes associated with alterations of internal mechanisms of control are exemplified by primary hyperaldosteronism, in which hypokalemia results from a combination of inappropriate distribution, excessive excretion, and metabolic alkalosis.

Disease processes associated with alteration in the mechanisms of potassium excretion may result in hypokalemia. A classic example is renal tubule acidosis, type I, in which failure of appropriate hydrogen ion excretion results in excessive losses of potassium. A more complete list of known causes of hypokalemia appears in Table 14–2.

The clinical manifestations associated with hypokalemia relate to the skeletal muscle, smooth muscle, kidneys, and the cardiac conducting system. Reduction in plasma potassium concentration leads to an increase in resting membrane potential by altering the ratio of the concentration of intracellular potassium to extracellular potassium. Membrane excitability is reduced, and muscle weakness, or even paralysis, is the result. Signs and symptoms of muscle weakness do not com-

---

TABLE 14–2 CLINICAL STATES ASSOCIATED WITH HYPOKALEMIA

1. Inappropriate intake
2. Disorders of internal distribution
   a. Metabolic alkalosis
   b. Hyperinsulinism
   c. Periodic paralysis
3. Inappropriate excretion
   a. Renal tubule acidosis
   b. Mineralocorticoid excess
   c. Licorice abuse
   d. Salt-losing nephropathies
   e. Bartter's syndrome
   f. Interstitial nephritis
   g. Diuretic therapy
4. Inappropriate gastrointestinal losses
   a. Vomiting
   b. Nasogastric suction
   c. Diarrhea
   d. Laxative abuse
   e. Villous adenoma

monly occur until plasma potassium values drop below 2.5 mEq per liter; however, many factors such as plasma calcium, hydrogen ion concentration, and the state of intracellular potassium stores may modify response. The distribution of muscular weakness is characteristic, with early involvement of the lower extremities, followed by muscles of the trunk, upper extremities, and, ultimately, the muscles of respiration. In severe cases, rhabdomyolysis and myoglobinuria may occur. Smooth muscle involvement can lead to paralytic ileus.

In the human kidney, potassium deficiency after a period of time leads to a characteristic vacuolar lesion in the tubule cells of the proximal nephron, which rarely may occur in the distal nephron as well. A common clinical manifestation is impairment in the ability to excrete a concentrated urine. This inability to concentrate is secondary to a decreased sensitivity to antidiuretic hormone. The degree of polyuria is less than that described with diabetes insipidus of a central origin.

Metabolic alkalosis is a commonly associated phenomenon in states of hypokalemia. With reduction in intracellular potassium, the hydrogen ion concentration rises. Hydrogen ion is then more available for secretion, thus sustaining the continuing metabolic alkalosis. Hypokalemia reduces the ability of the kidney to excrete or conserve a sodium or water load appropriately. In the face of a high sodium diet, this can lead to fluid retention and edema.

The electrocardiogram reflects the electrical events of the heart. The P wave represents atrial depolarization, the QRS complex ventricular depolarization, and the ST segment, T, and U waves ventricular repolarization. Hypokalemia produces characteristic changes in the electrocardiogram that are primarily due to delayed ventricular repolarization. The result is ST segment depression, decreased amplitude or inversion of the T wave, and increased height of the U wave with prolongation of the Q–U interval. With more severe hypokalemia, increased amplitude of the P wave, prolongation of the P–R interval, and widening of the QRS complex may occur. There may be a variety of associated cardiac arrhythmias, including premature atrial or ventricular beats, sinus bradycardia, paroxysmal atrial tachycardia, Wenckebach block, atrioventricular dissociation, nodal tachycardia, and ventricular fibrillation. The frequency and severity of arrhythmias are increased in the presence of digitalis preparations.

Hyperkalemia. In clinical medicine, hyperkalemia can be divided into only two categories. The first is inappropriate internal distribution between the intracellular and extracellular fluid compartments. A classic example is untreated diabetic ketoacidosis, in which total body potassium is often reduced despite significant elevations in serum potassium.

The second category includes the pathologic states associated with the inability of the kidney to excrete potassium appropriately. Whether as the result of reduction in functioning renal mass or the absence of aldosterone, the end result is the same—inadequate excretion of potassium with all the resultant hazards. A list of common causes of hyperkalemia is presented in Table 14–3.

Clinical signs and symptoms of hyperkalemia relate to the skeletal muscles and conducting system of the myocardium. Muscle weakness is the most common finding. It characteristically begins in the lower extremities. This muscle weakness or paralysis is a result of a reduction in resting membrane potential as the ratio of intracellular potassium to extracellular potassium shifts toward unity. The cell membrane is unable to repolarize after a single depolarization stimulus. Elevations in serum potassium lead to a number of characteristic changes in the electrocardiogram, which may be progressive to the point of ventricular standstill or fibrillation as potassium continues to rise. Although observations of changing electrocardiographic signs are helpful, it is critical to note that there is no clear-cut correlation with serum potassium. Any electrocardiographic changes of hyperkalemia are considered signs of serious intoxication and indicate a need for prompt institution of corrective measures. The earliest changes in the cardiogram are peaking of T waves with shortening of the Q–T segment, reflecting rapid repolarization. More advanced changes include widening of the QRS complex, prolongation of the P–R interval, diminished amplitude, and widening of P waves with eventual disappearance. The QRS complex will finally widen out to blend with the T wave in the so-called "sine-wave."

DISORDERS OF HYDROGEN ION CONCENTRATION

Disorders of acid-base balance are, by today's standards, entirely too commonplace in the practice of clinical medicine. No doubt they have always been present; however, with the advent of

TABLE 14–3 CLINICAL STATES ASSOCIATED WITH HYPERKALEMIA

1. Disorders of internal distribution
   a. Acidosis
   b. Insulin deficiency
   c. Tissue catabolism
   d. Periodic paralysis—hyperkalemic
   e. Succinylcholine
2. Disorders of urinary excretion
   a. Renal failure
   b. Adrenal insufficiency
   c. Administration of potassium-sparing diuretics
      1. Triamterene
      2. Spironolactone
   d. Volume depletion

TABLE 14–4 COMPARISON OF HYDROGEN ION [H+] WITH pH

pH	[H+] nanomoles/L
7.8	16
7.7	20
7.6	26
7.5	32
7.4	40
7.3	50
7.2	63
7.1	80
7.0	100
6.9	125
6.8	160

arterial blood gases and pH as common laboratory determinants, they are more readily recognized, requiring an appropriate understanding and response on the part of the physician. Understanding is critical if response is to be appropriate.

We physicians have been saddled and befuddled with the physical-chemical term "pH" since our thought processes first turned toward an understanding of internal metabolism, and, like so many anachronisms of medicine, the term would best be discarded. However, we are afraid that for the foreseeable future we will unfortunately continue to rely on this word, although we may eventually cease to use it if we learn to think in terms of hydrogen ion concentration [H+]. [H+] is a reciprocal function of pH; therefore, as [H+] rises, pH drops, and vice versa. We can think of [H+] in exactly the same fashion that we consider Na^+, K^+, CO_2^-, HCO_3^-, and Cl^-, recognizing that [H+] is found in the plasma in concentrations at roughly one millionth the concentration of the other commonly measured cations and anions. [H+] can be expressed as either nanomoles or nanoequivalents 10^{-6} millimoles. A value of 40 nanomoles of [H+] per liter equals a pH value of 7.40. The entire range of [H+] compatible with life extends only from a low of 16 nanomoles per liter to a high of 160 nanomoles per liter (Table 14–4).

With this simple understanding, we have taken a giant step forward. When a patient is acidotic [H+] is high; when a patient is alkalotic [H+] is low. These findings are absolutes and never change. We now have only to establish the cause and we are well on our way to appropriate correction.

The concentration of hydrogen ion in the body is interrelated with the concentrations of the major extracellular cation (sodium) and the major intracellular cation (potassium). The absolute status of hydrogen ion concentration is controlled by only three known mechanisms. These mechanisms are as follows: (1) Buffering, which takes place both intracellularly and extracellularly. In simple terms, a buffer is any molecule that can readily give up or receive a hydrogen ion in response to minor changes in concentration. (2) The ability of

the lung to remove CO_2, raising or reducing the alveolar partial pressure of CO_2 and, thus, plasma CO_2. (3) The ability of the kidney to increase or decrease plasma bicarbonate by hydrogen ion secretion in response to changes in [H+]. A brief discussion of each of these mechanisms is in order.

Extracellular Buffers. In the extracellular fluid, bicarbonate is the most important buffer owing to its relatively high concentration and the ability to vary the P_{CO_2} through changes in alveolar ventilation. An appropriate formulation of this reaction is as follows: $CO_2 + H_2O \rightleftarrows H_2CO_3 \rightleftarrows H^+ + HCO_3^-$. All gases dissolve in water to a greater or lesser extent, and the degree to which this occurs is proportional to the partial pressure of the gas in the solution. In the human, the partial pressure of CO_2 in arterial blood is in equilibrium with that in the alveolar space and normally approximates 40 mm Hg. At 37° C, the amount of CO_2 dissolved in the plasma is as follows: dissolved $CO_2 = 0.03\ P_{CO_2} = 0.03 \times 40 - 1.2$ mM/L, where 0.03 is the solubility constant for CO_2. The equilibrium for the reaction for the formation of bicarbonate—dissolved $CO_2 + H_2O = H_2CO_3$—under normal physiologic circumstances favors the reaction to the left. Approximately 500 molecules of CO_2 are in solution for each molecule of H_2CO_3. The degree to which H_2CO_3 dissolves into $H^+ + HCO_3^-$ can be appreciated from the law of mass action for this reaction:

$$K\alpha = \frac{[H^+]\,(HCO_3^-)}{(H_2CO_3)}$$

$$K\alpha = 2 \times 10^{-4} \text{ and the normal } [H^+] - 40 \times 10^{-9} \text{ mol/L}$$

$$\text{thus, } 2 \times 10^{-4} = \frac{40 \times 10^{-9}\,(HCO_3^-)}{(H_2CO_3)}$$

$$\frac{(HCO_3^-)}{(H_2CO_3)} = 5 \times 10^3$$

Thus, there are approximately 5000 molecules of bicarbonate for each molecule of H_2CO_3. From the preceding equation it is obvious that, for all practical purposes, H_2CO_3 does not exist in a physiologic state within the body; therefore, we can focus our thinking on the partial pressure of CO_2 and the concentration of bicarbonate. There are other quantitatively less important buffers in the extracellular space (two of which are plasma proteins and inorganic phosphate); however, their importance is not so critical as the bicarbonate buffering system because of the ability of the lung to vary the concentration of dissolved CO_2 in the plasma.

Intracellular Buffers. The intracellular buffers of importance are proteins, organic and inorganic phosphates, and, within the red cell, hemoglobin.

The buffering of hydrogen ion in the cells has an important effect on plasma K^+ concentration. To maintain electroneutrality, the movement of hydrogen ion into the cells is associated with the movement of sodium and potassium out of the cells. The result may be a potentially serious increase in the plasma potassium concentration from the normal plasma concentration of 4 mEq/L to 7 or 8 mEq/L. If, conversely, the extracellular hydrogen concentration is reduced, hydrogen ions are released from the intracellular buffers and enter the extracellular fluid space. In this setting, sodium and potassium enter the cells, resulting in a fall in the concentration of potassium in the plasma. Similar changes may occur in the concentration of plasma sodium; however, since the normal plasma sodium concentration is 140 mEq/L, small variations in the plasma sodium of several milliequivalents are not of physiologic importance.

Bone Buffers. Bone carbonate represents a large store of buffer which contributes to the buffering of hydrogen ion. For example, after an acid load, bone carbonate is released into the extracellular space. This is accompanied by the uptake of extracellular phosphate or by the release of calcium and sodium from the bone. It is difficult to measure the exact contribution of bone bicarbonate. It has been suggested, however, that as much as 40 per cent of the buffering of an acute acid load takes place in this fashion.

Ventilatory Responses to Changes in Hydrogen Ion Concentration. The main physiologic stimulus to respiration is a change in hydrogen ion concentration in arterial blood. This response is mediated by chemoreceptors sensitive to hydrogen ion concentration located in the medulla of the brain and chemoreceptors in the carotid bodies and in the aortic arch. As hydrogen ion concentration rises, respiration is stimulated, and there is a concomitant drop in arterial CO_2, shifting the reaction in which hydrogen ion is released—dissolved $CO_2 + H_2O \leftrightarrows H^+ + HCO_3^-$—to the left, effectively reducing the hydrogen ion concentration within the arterial circulation. This response occurs within a matter of minutes following a rise in the effective concentration of hydrogen ion in the arterial circulation.

Renal Response to a Change in Hydrogen Ion Concentration. We have previously discussed the handling of hydrogen ion by the kidney. It is important to recognize that the kidney's response to a sudden shift in hydrogen ion concentration within the arterial circulation occurs over a prolonged period of time and is not complete until probably 3 to 5 days after the initial change in hydrogen ion concentration occurred. The kidney responds in a number of interrelated fashions—by the conservation of bicarbonate, by the rise in absolute excretion of hydrogen ion as measured by titratable acidity, and by the production and excretion of increased concentrations of ammonia.

CLINICAL DISORDERS OF HYDROGEN ION CONCENTRATION

There are four clearly defined metabolic states associated with anomalies of hydrogen ion concentration: metabolic acidosis, metabolic alkalosis, respiratory acidosis, and respiratory alkalosis. It is important to remember that the hydrogen ion concentration as determined in the laboratory may be the end result of altered physiologic mechanisms in more than one system of control, and we therefore often see a state of mixed metabolic acidosis-alkalosis or one of a variety of other combinations.

Metabolic Acidosis. A state of metabolic acidosis exists when the ingestion of hydrogen ion or endogenous production of hydrogen ion exceeds the body's capabilities for elimination. This presumes that the respiratory mechanisms for alveolar ventilation are intact. Under these circumstances, we would expect to see an absolute rise in the concentration of hydrogen ion in the general circulation where excess hydrogen ion would combine with the readily available bicarbonate in the reaction $H^+ + HCO_3^-$. Following the law of mass action, this would lead to an increased formation of CO_2 and H_2O. At the same time, the chemoreceptor centers described previously would stimulate respiration and the increased removal of CO_2 by the alveolar mechanism. By this mechanism, P_{CO_2} is reduced, and the hydrogen ion concentration returned toward the normal concentration of 40 nM/L. It is important to note that the respiratory compensation for metabolic acidosis is never complete and that plasma concentration of hydrogen ion will remain elevated. The respiratory response is prompt, occurring within minutes of the initial rise in hydrogen ion concentration. As the intracellular concentration of hydrogen ion rises, the kidney is stimulated to reabsorb more bicarbonate and excrete more hydrogen ion, thus returning the hydrogen ion concentration of the body toward normal. The major causes of metabolic acidosis are listed in Table 14–5.

ANION GAP. The calculation of anion gap is a simple clinical tool and can be derived from the readily available blood electrolytes as determined in any clinical laboratory. The causes of metabolic acidosis can be divided into those that elevate the anion gap and those that do not. Determining the anion gap is then very helpful in the beginning differential diagnosis of a patient with metabolic acidosis. The anion gap is simply determined by adding the chloride and bicarbonate and subtracting the total from the serum sodium. The anion gap normally should measure 10 to 14 mEq per liter. As hydrogen ion accumulates in the body, there is rapid extracellular buffering by HCO_3^-. If the acid is HCl, then that effect is the mEq-for-mEq replacement of extracellular bicarbonate by chloride. Since the sum of chloride and bicarbonate

TABLE 14–5 CAUSES OF METABOLIC ACIDOSIS

I. Inability to excrete the dietary hydrogen load
  A. Diminished ammonia production
    1. Renal failure
  B. Diminished hydrogen ion secretion
    1. Distal renal tubule acidosis
    2. Hypoaldosteronism
II. Increased hydrogen ion load or bicarbonate loss
  A. Ketoacidosis
  B. Lactic acidosis
  C. Ingestions
    1. Salicylates
    2. Ethylene glycol
    3. Methanol
    4. Paraldehyde
    5. Ammonium chloride
    6. Hyperalimentation fluids
  D. Gastrointestinal bicarbonate loss
    1. Diarrhea or fistula
    2. Cholestyramine
    3. Ureterosigmoidostomy
  E. Renal bicarbonate loss
    1. Renal failure
    2. Proximal renal tubule acidosis

concentrations remains constant, the anion gap is unchanged. Because of the increase in the plasma chloride concentration, this is referred to as a "hyperchloremic acidosis." Gastrointestinal or renal loss of sodium bicarbonate produces the same result, the exchange of bicarbonate for chloride, since the kidney retains sodium chloride in an effort to preserve the volume of the extracellular fluid. Conversely, if hydrogen ion accumulates with any ion other than chloride, extracellular bicarbonate is replaced by an unmeasured anion. As a result, there is a decrease in the sum of chloride and bicarbonate concentration and an increase in the anion gap. In disorders of this form, identification of the specific disease process can be obtained by measuring the serum concentration of BUN, lactate, glucose, and pyruvate and by checking for the presence of ketones or exogenous intoxicants (see Table 14–6).

Metabolic Alkalosis. Metabolic alkalosis is characterized by a disorder of hydrogen ion in which there is an absolute decrease in hydrogen ion concentration, an increase in plasma bicarbonate concentration, and a compensatory rise in Pco_2 produced by depressed alveolar ventilation. A state of metabolic alkalosis is produced by either the excessive loss of hydrogen ion or the excessive retention of bicarbonate. It should be pointed out that the retention of bicarbonate will ultimately result in the excessive loss of hydrogen ion and that alkalosis can only exist when total hydrogen ion concentration is depressed, whatever the mechanism of that depression may be. Metabolic alkalosis is most commonly associated with gastrointestinal losses of hydrogen ion. This is usually accomplished by prolonged nasogastric suction.

For every hydrogen ion that is secreted by the gastric mucosa, there is generated a bicarbonate ion that is returned to the extracellular space. If we return to the formula $CO_2 + H_2O \leftrightarrows H_2CO_3 \leftrightarrows H^+ + HCO_3^-$, it is apparent that we are overloading the right-hand side of this reaction and driving the reaction to the left, with an overall reduction of circulating hydrogen ion.

Excessive renal retention of bicarbonate may be stimulated by mineralocorticoid excess, volume contraction, or hypokalemia. Again, for every hydrogen ion loss, we are generating bicarbonate at the renal tubule and effectively decreasing circulating concentration of hydrogen ion. Additional unusual causes of metabolic alkalosis are the chronic ingestion of bicarbonate and the milk-alkali syndrome.

In considering metabolic alkalosis, it usually is not difficult to establish the initial cause; however, recognizing the sustaining events that surround metabolic alkalosis may be more difficult. Two conditions play a major role in sustaining metabolic alkalosis once it has been established: volume depletion and potassium depletion. A state of chronic volume contraction will consistently stimulate the tubule cells of the proximal nephron to reabsorb bicarbonate, despite existing alkalosis. The state of volume deficiency overrides the need for bicarbonate excretion and correction of alkalosis. This results in the facilitation of salt and water conservation despite the persisting state of alkalosis.

With potassium deficiency, we see a similar process. As hydrogen ion moves into cells to replace potassium ions that have been lost, there is

TABLE 14–6 ANION GAP IN METABOLIC ACIDOSIS

Normal Anion Gap
1. Gastrointestinal loss of bicarbonate
  a. Diarrhea and fistulae
  b. Cholestyramine
  c. Ureterosigmoidostomy
2. Renal bicarbonate loss
  a. Proximal RTA
  b. Renal insufficiency
3. Ingestions
  a. Ammonium chloride
  b. Hyperalimentation fluids
4. Renal dysfunction
  a. Pyelonephritis and obstructive uropathy
  b. Hypoaldosteronism
  c. Distal RTA

High Anion Gap
1. Ketoacidosis
2. Lactic acidosis
3. Renal insufficiency
4. Ingestions
  a. Salicylate
  b. Ethylene glycol
  c. Methanol
  d. Paraldehyde

a facilitation of bicarbonate resorption in the proximal tubule produced by the presence of the additional hydrogen ion within these tubule cells. Persistent bicarbonate resorption occurs despite a continuing state of alkalosis. The point to be gained by all this is that if metabolic alkalosis is to be effectively corrected, any existing volume depletion or potassium depletion must be recognized and corrected.

Respiratory Acidosis. Respiratory acidosis is a metabolic state of increased hydrogen ion concentration secondary to CO_2 retention. It may be either acute or chronic. In acute respiratory acidosis, a minimum amount of buffering can occur from the shifts of intracellular bicarbonate, and there will be a small but significant rise in plasma bicarbonate levels, rarely exceeding 3 or 4 mEq. This is extremely helpful in determining whether the respiratory acidosis is of sudden onset or has been a long-standing process. With long-standing respiratory acidosis, renal compensation begins to play a major role with increased resorption of bicarbonate, and the bicarbonate levels may become significantly elevated.

Respiratory Alkalosis. A reduction in alveolar P_{CO_2} secondary to hyperventilation leads to respiratory alkalosis as plasma P_{CO_2} falls concomitantly. Hyperventilation can result from primary central nervous system pathology, primary lung disease, anxiety, various intoxications, or overvigorous artificial ventilation. This metabolic state is characteristically acute in nature and of a readily recognizable etiology. Therapy revolves around treatment of the underlying pathology. Hydrogen ion concentrations are lowered with reduction of P_{CO_2} as follows: $\downarrow P_{CO_2} \leftrightarrows HCO_3^- + H^+$. The kidney responds by decreasing the reabsorption of bicarbonate.

DIURETICS

Diuretics as a group are one of the most widely used categories of drugs in modern medicine. By the very nature of their function, diuretics must alter the physiologic functions of the kidney, and any discussion of basic pathophysiology mechanisms of acid-base balance and fluid and electrolyte disturbances must include at least a brief look at this broad category of drugs. The diuretics can be divided into seven general categories. Although diuretics in each class do not necessarily have a similar formula, their clinical activity can be grouped conceptually into one of these categories, and this provides a reasonable way to remember their clinical application. The seven categories are (1) xanthine compounds, (2) carbonic anhydrase inhibitors, (3) osmotic diuretics, (4) organomercurials, (5) thiazides, (6) spironolactone–triamterene, and (7) ethacrynic acid–furosemide.

Xanthine Compounds. Xanthine compounds in themselves are very weak diuretic agents that have been available to clinicians for many years. They are rarely, if ever, used alone but may have a significant potentiating effect when used in association with the more potent diuretic agents in common clinical use. Their action appears to be threefold. There is an inotropic effect on the myocardium that increases cardiac output and secondarily increases renal plasma flow. There is a suggested mechanism directly affecting renal hemodynamics with increased filtration fraction, and a third possible role in inhibition of active sodium transport in the proximal tubule.

Carbonic Anhydrase Inhibitors. Approximately 90 per cent of the filtered load of bicarbonate is reabsorbed in the proximal tubule. Bicarbonate is absorbed as a direct result of hydrogen ion secretion in the following formulation: $HCO_3^- + H^+ \rightarrow H_2CO_3 \rightarrow CO_2 + H_2O$. The CO_2 diffuses into the paratubular cell, where it is used to reconstitute bicarbonate. These reactions are greatly facilitated by the presence of the enzyme carbonic anhydrase, which is abundantly present in the proximal tubule cells and in high concentration in the brush border of the paraluminal surface of the proximal nephron. Inhibitors of carbonic anhydrase exert a diuretic effect by reducing the efficient reabsorption of bicarbonate and thus sodium. The diuresis induced is characterized by high content of bicarbonate in the urine and the tendency, after prolonged administration, to the development of metabolic acidosis. Diuresis is self-limited in that a new bicarbonate steady state will shortly be re-established and no further diuretic action will occur.

Mannitol. The mechanisms of mannitol diuresis include (1) osmotic retention of water in the proximal tubule, which (2) decreases sodium concentration in the lumen, thus creating a sodium gradient between the lumen and blood sufficiently large to reduce proximal sodium transport, (3) increased renal blood flow and reduced medullary hypertonicity, (4) reduced movement of sodium and water from Henle's loop into the medullary interstitial spaces, and (5) reduced medullary hypertonicity due to osmotic retention of water in medullary tissues. Mannitol enhances excretion of calcium, phosphorus, magnesium, potassium, uric acid, and urea. These effects are brought about by producing osmotic dilution of these substances in the lumen, creating a gradient unfavorable for their transport and favorable for secretion.

Organomercurials. The organomercurials were for many years the most potent diuretics available and the mainstay of diuretic therapy. Because they must be given intramuscularly or intravenously for effective clinical application, the advent of the potent oral loop diuretics, exemplified by ethacrynic acid and furosemide, has significantly reduced their clinical application. Experimental data based primarily on the findings of micropuncture constitute a persuasive argument that this class of drugs acts by the inhibition of active transport of chloride and that the natriuresis is secondary to the chloruresis. The mode of action of the mercurials at the cellular level has not yet been defined. Available evidence strongly suggests that this diuretic has its main site of action on the ascending thick segment of the loop of Henle.

Thiazide Diuretics. The thiazides are the most prescribed group of diuretics in clinical medicine. Micropuncture data suggest that their site of action is in the thick segment of the ascending loop of Henle at some point distal to the site of action of mercurials, ethacrynic acid, and furosemide. They apparently have no effect on proximal tubule transport of sodium and no distal action in terms of sodium or water resorption. Independent of their diuretic effect is their effect on glomerular filtration rate, which in animal experimentation has been shown to produce a reduction in effective glomerular filtration rate by as much as 25 per cent. They exert a primary effect on free water clearance (i.e., the ability of the kidney to form a dilute urine) but do not interfere with the ability of the kidney to achieve maximal water resorption from the collecting duct.

Spironolactone–Triamterene. Spironolactone and triamterene have different sites of action at the cellular level but can be considered together in terms of their clinical action as diuretic agents. Spironolactone acts by blocking the effect of aldosterone in the distal tubule and possibly the collecting duct, whereas the action of triamterene is independent of the presence of aldosterone, although its site of action is similar to that of spironolactone. The major action is to block the distal tubule transport of sodium. At the same time, there is interference with the secretion of potassium at the distal tubule nephron. These diuretics are relatively ineffective when used alone, but become clinically significant when used in conjunction with one or more of the other available diuretic agents or when a potassium-sparing effect is desired.

Ethacrynic Acid–Furosemide. The loop diuretics, exemplified by ethacrynic acid and furosemide, constitute the most recent group of diuretic agents introduced into clinical practice and the most potent currently available. Their site of action is thought to be in the medullary and cortical segments of the ascending loop of Henle. Like the mercurial diuretics, evidence suggests that their major pharmacologic effect inhibits the active transport of chloride in this tubule segment, producing a chloruresis and a natriuresis. Because the site of action is both medullary and cortical in the ascending loop, they interfere with both free water clearance and the ability of the kidney to concentrate maximally. They have not been demonstrated to have a clinical effect on glomerular filtration rate when volume is maintained. In large doses—usually doses in excess of those applied in clinical practice—a proximal tubule effect has been demonstrated in some animal species. This proximal tubule effect appears to be a direct inhibition of active sodium transport, but it plays little or no role in production of diuresis in current clinical practice.

COMPLICATIONS OF DIURETIC THERAPY

The most important complication of diuretic therapy is excessive and unwarranted depletion of extracellular volume. This may lead to hypotension and various complications of organ hypoperfusion, including syncope, confusion, transient ischemic attacks, oliguria, azotemia, and angina. In the cirrhotic patient, hepatorenal syndrome and hepatic coma may be induced by excessive volume reduction. In some cases, particularly in the patient with advanced cirrhosis, elimination of ascites and edema cannot be achieved without an unacceptable reduction of effective plasma volume.

None of the available diuretics is known to enhance potassium secretion directly. The potassium losses and the resulting hypokalemia seen as the direct result of diuretic therapy are secondary to increased delivery of volume to the distal nephron. Increased volume enhances the secretion of potassium at these sites, with excessive potassium losses occurring in the final urine. There may exist slight differences in potassium-losing effect among the various thiazide diuretics, but none are of practical importance. It is suggested that, in addition to potassium loss, a redistribution of potassium from the extracellular to the intracellular space may result from thiazide administration. Whether potassium supplement is a necessity with thiazide or other diuretic therapy has been brought into serious dispute by recent studies that tend to show that total body potassium depletion is minimal and the administration of exogenous potassium salts does little to correct this deficiency.

The risk of hyperkalemia must always be considered in patients with compromised renal function placed on spironolactone or triamterene. These drugs interfere with the secretion of potassium into the distal tubule segments, where the bulk of potassium excretion must occur.

Hyperuricemia has been shown to be associated with the administration of thiazide diuretics, furosemide, ethacrynic acid, and acetazolamide. The effect of mercurials is much less clear. Thiazide diuretics and ethacrynic acid become uricosuric when given in larger doses or after intravenous administration.

Instantaneous sudden deafness may occur with rapid intravenous administration of furosemide or ethacrynic acid. In rare cases, deafness has been reported after the oral administration of these drugs as well. This effect usually lasts for no more than a few hours and seems related to the action of the diuretics on the electrolyte composition of the endolymph. It has been shown that ethacrynic acid can cause a complete reversal of the sodium/potassium ratio in the endolymph 10 minutes after administration.

The occurrence of transient and sometimes fatal arrhythmias has been reported after rapid administration of large doses of furosemide. This is probably due to alterations of sodium/potassium ratios within the heart itself. A number of other complications have been described, including idiosyncratic or hypersensitive reactions, but these are not directly related to the biochemical effects of the diuretic agents themselves.

ADDITIONAL CLINICAL APPLICATION OF DIURETIC AGENTS

Hypertension. Thiazides, chlorthalidone, ethacrynic acid, and furosemide have been used in the management of hypertension. Although it has been definitely established that one effect of diuretic therapy resulting in lower blood pressure is produced by contraction of extracellular volume, additional mechanisms have been suggested. At equipotent diuretic doses, thiazides seem to be somewhat better antihypertensive agents than are the other diuretics available. Their postulated action on arteriolar smooth muscle has not been definitely established.

Acute Pulmonary Edema. Rapid reduction of extracellular volume by furosemide or ethacrynic acid is a frequently used therapy in the emergency treatment of acute pulmonary edema. The major effect is the reduction of preload and afterload on the myocardium in addition to the clearing of the pulmonary transudate.

Acute Renal Failure. Mannitol, furosemide, and ethacrynic acid have been used to induce diuresis during the early phases of acute tubule necrosis in hopes of reversing the underlying process. The effectiveness of this procedure remains in doubt, and there is clinical evidence to suggest that, although volume may be increased acutely by this approach, the long-term effect on the underlying disease process is not a clinically significant one.

Diabetes Insipidus. Diuretics reduce the volume and increase the osmolality of the urine in diabetes insipidus, whether the diabetes insipidus is central or nephrogenic in origin. The urine becomes less hypotonic, but never hypertonic. The effect is not due to any ADH-type activity. One explanation given is enhanced proximal tubule resorption secondary to volume depletion. This results in a reduction in the volume delivered to the distal tubule and the collecting duct. The diuretics most frequently used for this purpose are thiazides, although other diuretics are effective as well. The therapeutic benefit is potentiated by salt restriction and neutralized by high salt intake.

Syndrome of Inappropriate Antidiuretic Hormone Secretion. Under conditions of hyponatremia and inappropriately low free water clearance, furosemide and ethacrynic acid can enhance free water clearance. This is particularly true in the presence of a high glomerular filtration rate. This property has been used to induce diuresis of a dilute urine, which together with the administration of salt corrects the hyponatremia in the syndrome of inappropriate secretion of antidiuretic hormone.

Renal Tubule Acidosis. Hypovolemia produces metabolic alkalosis by enhancing proximal tubule transport of bicarbonate. Diuretic-induced volume contraction can help improve the acidosis of renal tubule acidosis. The action is particularly effective with the administration of thiazide diuretics.

Hypercalcemia. Diuresis induced by furosemide or ethacrynic acid produces calcium loss and a correction of hypercalcemia. It is important to note that thiazides are contraindicated in hypercalcemia and, under certain circumstances, can produce a hypercalcemic state. A possible explanation for the difference lies in the fact that most of the nonproximal calcium resorption takes place in the medullary segment and very little in the cortical segment of the ascending limb of the Henle's loop.

CONGENITAL ABNORMALITIES OF THE KIDNEY

CONGENITAL MALFORMATIONS

Normal Embryology. During embryologic development of the human, three distinct excretory organs are formed. The first is the *pronephros,* the remnants of which rarely persist. The second is the *mesonephros,* parts of which persist in the adult male as epididymis and vas deferens and as vestigial appendages in the female. The third is the *metanephros,* which forms the adult kidney and derives from two sources: (1) the ureteric bud, a diverticulum from the mesonephric duct, which forms the ureter, pelvis of the kidney, and collecting ducts; and (2) mesoderm from the nephrogenic cord, which invests the distal end of the ureteric bud and forms the convoluted tubules and loops of Henle. The glomeruli develop within the mesodermal tissue and obtain arterial supply.

The kidneys are first formed at the fourth lumbar segment and ascend cephalad to the level of T12 or L1, their final position. During ascent, they are squeezed together as they arise from the pelvis and rotate a quarter turn so that the pelves are medial and the convex borders are lateral. Arterial supply for the developing kidneys arises from vessels supplying the segments through which they ascend.

Congenital abnormalities of the adult kidney can be ascribed to errors or abnormalities of development at specific stages.

Bilateral agenesis, which is of course incompatible with life, is rare. The true incidence is difficult to ascertain. It apparently affects males more frequently than females. In true agenesis one would expect to find no ureter. However, in a large reported series, ureters were absent in only about one half the patients. This suggests either that some cases of agenesis were actually extreme hypoplasia or that there was specific failure of the metanephric part of the holonephros. Agenesis of both kidneys is associated with oligohydramnios; fetal malformations of ears, eyes, and legs; and pulmonary hypoplasia.

Unilateral agenesis is not extremely rare and is compatible with normal development. Associated malformations apparently are not common. There may be absence of the fallopian tube or nondescent of the testis on the same side. The single kidney is hypertrophic and prone to infection. Recognition of a single kidney in cases of infection, stones, or tumor is of course, important.

Supernumerary kidneys occur rarely. These by definition should have their own blood supply and own ureter. The supernumerary kidney is usually smaller than normal.

Hypoplastic kidneys are small kidneys with smaller than normal cells and a reduced number of nephrons. The arteries and ureters are likewise hypoplastic. Bilateral hypoplasia usually is incompatible with life. The hypoplastic kidney is prone to infection. The *Ask-Upmark kidney* is one in which there is hypoplasia of a single renal lobule and its calyx.

Fetal lobulation of the adult kidney is a retention of the surface marking of individual lobules. It is of no significance.

The *dysplastic kidney* represents a disturbed differentiation of nephrogenic tissue and consists of nonfunctional cystic structures and may contain cartilage. It may be associated with other organ defects but, if unilateral, has the same significance as unilateral agenesis. A unilateral dysplastic kidney is the most common palpable abdominal mass in the newborn, with a greater incidence than that of Wilms' tumor.

Ectopic kidneys may be located from pelvis to thorax. They may be retained in the pelvis by persistence of vascular attachments or allowed to migrate to the thorax through diaphragmatic defects. They are prone to infection, may cause compression of adjacent structures, and may be mistaken for a tumor.

Fused kidneys occur in two forms: the horseshoe kidney and the cake kidney. The *horseshoe* kidney is the more common, with an incidence of 1:300 to 1:800. The two kidneys are fused at the lower poles in 90 per cent of cases. While horseshoe kidney is not incompatible with a normal life span, it may be associated with symptoms of abdominal pain and vasomotor disturbances. These fused kidneys are susceptible to trauma, infection, and ureteral obstruction and are associated with other urogenital tract abnormalities and defects of the gastrointestinal and cardiovascular systems. *Cake, lump,* or *shield* kidney is quite rare. Symptoms and complications are similar to those associated with horseshoe kidney. It may be palpable and mistaken for a neoplasm.

Malrotation of the kidney may occur to any degree, that is, pelvis of kidney facing anteriorly, laterally, or dorsally. It is of no clinical significance other than its appearance on an IVP.

Otherwise normal kidneys may be supplied with more than the usual one renal artery. They may enter from above or below to supply the upper or lower pole of the kidney. They may cause complications if they pass ventral to the ureter and cause obstruction. There are a large number of anomalies of the ureters. There may be two separate ureters supplying two separate pelves of the same kidney and emptying into the bladder at separate locations. The ureter may divide anywhere along its length from bladder to hilus. There may be an anomaly involving stenosis of a valve or megaloureter. These are of concern because they predispose to infections and can then require urologic evaluation.

Several congenital abnormalities of the kidney have been reported to be hereditary (e.g., hydronephrosis and megaloureter). Available data do not give conclusive evidence of the mechanism of inheritance. Renal tumors have been observed to appear in families.

HEREDITARY RENAL DISEASES

Hereditary renal diseases may be divided into two major classifications: cystic and noncystic. The most common cystic disease affecting the kidney is the so-called "classic polycystic kidney disease of the adult." It is first recognized in adult life, usually in the fourth or fifth decade. In the typical patient, cystic changes are grossly apparent throughout the renal parenchyma, with a wide variation in size. Microscopically, cystic ectasia of all tubule elements abounds. In most instances, adult polycystic disease is inherited as an autosomal dominant trait, but the disorder may also occur without clear-cut evidence of genetic transmission. Polycystic kidney disease is one of the more important causes of recurrent painful hematuria unassociated with nephrolithiasis. Polycystic disease of the liver, a cystic ectasia of the bile duct radicals, frequently attends this syndrome and can result in hepatomegaly as striking as the renomegaly. The common symptom of abdominal fullness in these patients is often a consequence of enlargement of both liver and kidneys. Only rarely does the liver involvement lead to portal hypertension. Progressive azotemia and uremia are characteristic of patients with polycystic disease. Hypertension is a usual and often fatal complication in these patients, and intracranial aneurysm is frequently found in association. The characteristic intravenous pyelogram reveals an overall increase in size of both kidneys. The width of the renal parenchyma is characteristically increased, the pelvocaliceal system is frequently elongated, and the caliceal stalks can be so narrowed by impinging cysts that the pelvocaliceal pattern appears to be stretched out. The prognosis is one of progressive uremia and death unless intervention by dialysis or transplantation occurs.

Infantile polycystic disease refers to a variety of hepatorenal polycystic disorders that occur in infancy and early childhood and are genetically transmitted as autosomal recessive traits. Throughout both kidneys there is a uniform distribution of fusiform cysts. The glomeruli, intratubular tissue, calices, pelves, ureters, and lower urinary tract are normal. In the liver there is a bizarre infolding proliferation and dilatation of well-differentiated portal bile ducts and ductules associated with a variable degree of periportal fibrosis. Various investigators have attempted to subcategorize infantile polycystic disease on the basis of onset and pathology. Unfortunately, regardless of categorization, prognosis appears to be uniformly poor.

Medullary Cystic Disease

Medullary cystic disease is another form of microcystic involvement of the renal medulla and usually manifests itself by the insidious onset of uremia leading to death, frequently in the second or third decade of life. This disease should not be confused with medullary sponge kidney, another form of microcystic disease of the renal medulla, which is compatible with a normal life span and, in most cases, asymptomatic. Medullary cystic disease is predominantly one of youth: The average age at death has been reported to be 27 years, with no predilection for sex. The disease seems to have an autosomal recessive inheritance pattern. Cysts appear to be derived from distal tubules or collecting ducts. They range in size from 100 μ to 1 cm or more in diameter and are restricted to the corticomedullary junction. The cortex is usually thin and poorly demarcated, with the majority of the glomeruli partially or completely hyalinized. The interstitial tissue shows diffuse fibrosis and round cell infiltration. Blood pressure is characteristically normal at the beginning of the disease, but may become moderately elevated later in the clinical course as uremia develops. The urinary sediment may be normal, and daily excretion of protein rarely exceeds 150 mg per 24 hours. The prognosis is poor, with uniform progression to renal insufficiency as the rule.

Medullary Sponge Kidney

Medullary sponge kidney designates a rather benign renal disorder oftentimes diagnosed by intravenous pyelogram. It is quite unlike classic polycystic kidney disease. The intravenous pyelogram is characterized by multiple discrete urographic opacifications clustered around the caliceal cups of the pelvocaliceal system. In most cases, there appears to be no evidence of genetic transmission. Nephrocalcinosis, indistinguishable from that seen with renal tubule acidosis, can occur in these patients. An increased incidence of hypercalciuria has been described. The most common symptoms of patients with medullary sponge kidney relate to urinary tract infection, hematuria, and renal colic, which have been ascribed to their increased propensity for infection and stone formation. In contrast to patients with classic polycystic kidney disease, these patients have no associated hypertension or liver disease.

Hereditary Chronic Nephritis

A second major classification of hereditary renal disorders can be grouped under *hereditary chronic nephritis*. A hereditary form of renal disease often clinically indistinguishable from chronic glomerulonephritis or pyelonephritis has been recognized for many years; however, it was not until 1927 that its association with nerve deafness was first noted by Alport. Males are more severely affected than females, and affected males appear to have a deficiency of affected sons. Affected females often have an excess of both affected sons and daughters. The hereditary complexities of this syndrome have not been firmly established. The syndrome is best regarded, at this point, as being inherited in an autosomal dominant manner. Many females with hereditary nephritis remain asymptomatic for most, if not all, of their lives, but some females and most males develop the progressive symptoms of chronic glomerulonephritis or pyelonephritis. The earliest manifestations of the disease are albuminuria and hematuria. In affected males, death generally occurs in the second or third decade of life, either from renal failure or from the vascular and cardiac complications of hypertension. Death of females usually occurs much later. The basic renal lesion has been variously described as chronic glomerulonephritis, chronic pyelonephritis, interstitial nephritis, or a combination of all these. The principal glomerular abnormalities include cellular proliferation and swelling, capsular adhesions, and thickened basement membranes with periglomerular fibrosis. The characteristic abnormality of the tubules is atrophy, alternating with discrete areas of tubule dilatation, hypertrophy, and regeneration. The prominence of lipid-laden "foam cells" is a characteristic feature of hereditary nephritis. The recognition of foam cells is not limited to this form of renal disease, and to date what role, if any, these cells may play in the pathogenesis of this syndrome has not been defined. The incidence and severity of deafness in this disease appears to be greater in males than in females, and audiometry may be necessary to detect a hearing loss in the latter. The hearing loss is bilateral and usually symmetric. Loss of high-frequency perception is the earliest lesion, and this may progress to profound deafness. Although various eye anomalies including myopia and macular lesions have been described in association with hereditary nephritis, the most characteristic lesions are associated with lens defects. There is no specific treatment and management other than that associated with the care of any patient suffering from advancing renal failure.

A third category of hereditary kidney diseases relates to *primary tubular disorders*. The discussion may be divided into disorders of proximal tubule and disorders of distal tubule. The proximal tubule is concerned with resorption of amino acids, glucose, phosphate, uric acid, and other substances filtered at the glomerulus. Proximal tubule syndromes are characterized by various combinations of glycosuria, aminoaciduria, increased clearance of phosphate, and high uric acid clearance. Distal tubule syndromes more classically relate to abnormalities in the final adjustment of urinary pH, salt, and water balance.

Hereditary Proximal Tubule Defects

Cystinuria. In cystinuria there is a defect in a single amino acid transport system in the proximal tubule resulting in excessive excretion of cystine, lysine, arginine, and ornithine. Until recently these amino acids were thought to be reabsorbed by the same transport system. There is now good evidence that lysine, arginine, and ornithine are reabsorbed by the same transport system, but the abnormal excretion of cystine conforms more closely to a pattern of tubule secretion than to defective reabsorption, the theory being that lysine and cystine interact by sharing an efflux mechanism and that cysteine is the intracellular form of cystine. Thus, a defect in lysine transport inhibits efflux of cysteine into capillaries, causing a buildup of cysteine in cells and inhibiting luminal uptake of cystine. All other renal functions are normal early in life. Cystine is one of the least soluble of the amino acids. Between pH 5 and 7 it is soluble to the extent of only 300 to 400 mg/L. Cystinuric patients excrete on the average of 0.73 gm of cystine per day. The problem occurs when urine is saturated with cystine and calculi form. The other amino acids excreted are freely soluble.

Calculi predispose to obstruction and infection. They may begin to form early and cause symptoms even in infancy. Symptoms of nephrolithiasis most commonly occur between the ages of 20 and 25 years. Cystinuria accounts for a large proportion of stones in infancy. In adults it may account for as much as 1 per cent of renal calculi. The stones are radiopaque but less dense than calcium stones. They can contain calcium in their matrix or may be pure cystine. Symptoms are those ascribed to any type of calculi. Diagnosis is made by stone analysis, and the finding of increased amounts of cystine, lysine, arginine, and ornithine in the urine. Cystine may be excreted in large amounts in other disorders that produce broad tubule damage and generalized aminoaciduria. Cystinuria must also be distinguished from cystinosis. Cystinosis is a defect in protein metabolism resulting in the deposition of cystine in many organs including the kidney. Cystinosis of the kidney results in proximal tubule damage with generalized aminoaciduria. Cystinosis is one of the known causes of Fanconi's syndrome in children.

Cystinuric families can be divided into two distinct groups. In the first group there are two classes of individuals: (1) affected and (2) nonaffected. The hereditary pattern in this group is typical mendelian recessive. The second group, less common than the first, has three types of individuals: (1) severe cystinuric, (2) mild cystinurics who have increased excretion of cystine and lysine but normal amounts of arginine and ornithine, and (3) the unaffected individuals. The disease can be passed from generation to generation in this group, and the hereditary pattern is termed "incomplete recessive."

Hartnup's disease is a rare congenital defect of recessive inheritance. The clinical manifestations are a pellagra-like rash with variable attacks of cerebellar ataxia and other neurologic abnormalities. The biochemical abnormality is a specific aminoaciduria involving glutamine, asparagine, histidine, serine, threonine, phenylalanine, tyrosine, and tryptophan. The four amino acids found in the urine in cystinuria (i.e., cystine, arginine, ornithine, and lysine) are not found in greater than normal amounts. There is a specific defect in renal tubule absorption of the aforementioned amino acids. There is also a defect in jejunal absorption of tryptophan, which results in increased gastrointestinal formation of indoles by bacteria and increased absorption and urinary excretion of these substances.

The pellagra-like rash results from tryptophan deficiency secondary to defective jejunal absorption and increased urinary excretion. The attacks of cerebellar ataxia are due to intoxication of the central nervous system, probably secondary to action of bacteria on intestinal amino acids. The disease is not serious unless the patient develops central nervous system involvement. It shows a tendency to remit with increasing age, especially after adolescence. During attacks, treatment is directed toward reducing bacterial degradation of amino acids by measures similar to those used in hepatic coma: reduction in dietary protein intake and an attempt to sterilize the intestinal tract with neomycin.

Fanconi's syndrome is characterized by multiple proximal tubule defects. Typically, these defects involve the tubule's handling of phosphate, glucose, and amino acids. There is usually proteinuria with a high concentration of globulins, reflecting tubule cell damage rather than increased glomerular permeability to albumin. On occasion, tubule damage is more widespread and associated with difficulties in water absorption, bicarbonate absorption, and absorption of potassium. Children with Fanconi's syndrome develop rickets, fail to thrive, and suffer dehydration. In adults, osteomalacia and weakness associated with acidosis may occur. Symptoms are a result of bone anomalies, acidosis, and potassium depletion. The glycosuria and aminoaciduria produce no symptoms. There appear to be several forms of Fanconi syndrome. An idiopathic congenital type of uncertain inheritance occurs in childhood, with the child developing progressive renal failure terminating in death.

Lowe's syndrome is a rare hereditary renal disorder with diffuse and variable abnormalities. These are similar to those seen in Fanconi's syndrome, with diffuse renal aminoaciduria, proteinuria of the tubule type, systemic acidosis, increased phosphate clearance, and defects in concentration and acidification of the urine. With Lowe's syndrome, there is also mental retardation and severe congenital anomalies of eyes. Tubule atrophy is a pathologic finding frequently associated with thickening of the basement membrane of the tubules. Transmission is sex-linked. The full syndrome occurs only in males.

Hypophosphatemia associated with rickets resistant to vitamin D is characterized by rickets in children and osteomalacia in adults. It is unresponsive to physiologic doses of vitamin D. There is a failure of reabsorption of phosphate in the proximal tubules and, therefore, high phosphate clearance. Kidney function is otherwise normal. Intestinal absorption of calcium and phosphate may be concomitantly affected. It is transmitted by the unusual mode of a sex-linked dominant. Heterozygous females are affected much less severely than homozygous males. Homozygous females are unknown.

Renal glycosuria is a benign congenital condition that requires no treatment. It does not cause polyuria, polydipsia, or ketoacidosis. The main problem is to differentiate it from diabetes mellitus, avoiding inappropriate treatment. It occurs in two forms. The most common is due to an unusual heterogenicity of proximal tubule function regarding glucose resorption. The transport maximum for glucose is normal, but the titration curve exhibits an abnormally marked splay so that glucose is spilled at low serum levels. This appears to be transmitted as a mendelian recessive and is due to a single defect in transport. In the second type, there is a reduction in transport maximum for glucose throughout the kidney. Most cases of the latter type are associated with other generalized proximal tubule defects.

Distal Tubular Syndromes

Nephrogenic diabetes insipidus is a hereditary disorder characterized by an insensitivity of distal tubule and collecting duct epithelium to antidiuretic hormone. This disorder presents in childhood with recurrent dehydration, hypernatremia, a dilute urine, and failure to thrive. Mental and physical retardation and death may occur. With early therapy a normal life span may be possible. Vasopressin has no effect on renal concentration in these individuals. There appears to be no other renal defect. Proximal tubule anatomic anomalies have been described, but their significance is not clear. Inheritance is sex-linked; most cases occur in males. Heterozygous females may have some limitation in concentrating ability.

Renal Tubule Acidosis. The renal acidification process contributes to acid-base balance by regulating the concentration of plasma bicarbonate. In normal humans, this process operates to maintain plasma bicarbonate at physiologic concentrations. Bicarbonate that is filtered by the glomerulus is reabsorbed, and hydrogen ion is excreted in an amount equal to the bicarbonate thus generated. The bulk of bicarbonate resorption occurs in the proximal tubule, and the final regulation of hydrogen ion concentration in the urine occurs in the distal tubule and collecting duct. Metabolic acidosis can occur with defects at either level.

Proximal renal tubule acidosis results from an incomplete reabsorption of bicarbonate in the proximal tubule. The distal tubule cannot absorb the excess bicarbonate, and bicarbonate is lost until the patient becomes acidotic. Distal renal tubule acidosis is the result of an inability to establish or maintain a hydrogen ion gradient at the distal tubule and collecting duct epithelium. Complications of acidosis such as bone disease, nephrocalcinosis, and renal calculi are more common in distal tubule acidosis. In distal renal tubule acidosis the kidney is unable to form an acid urine with a pH below 6. In proximal renal tubule acidosis, an acid urine of pH 5 or less may be formed once severe acidosis has developed and the filtered load of bicarbonate is reduced. Both forms of renal tubule acidosis occur as a primary disorder. Familial distal renal tubule acidosis occurs as an autosomal dominant with variable penetrance with greater expressivity in females. Familial proximal renal tubule acidosis occurs more commonly in males. Secondary causes of proximal renal tubule acidosis are cystinosis, Wilson's disease, Lowe's syndrome, multiple myeloma, heavy metal poisonings, and galactosemia. Secondary causes of distal renal tubule acidosis include vitamin D excess or deficiency, analgesic-abuse nephritis, and pyelonephritis.

PATHOPHYSIOLOGY OF GLOMERULAR DAMAGE

It is now generally accepted that immunologic mechanisms normally concerned with host protection play a major role in the pathogenesis of most, if not all, forms of glomerulonephritis. This appreciation of the role played by the immunologic system is due in large part to studies conducted in experimental animal models. The resemblance of these diseases in the models to those in humans is particularly striking.

Two general mechanisms have been implicated in the genesis of these diseases. The first involves antibodies with a specificity for antigenic components of the glomerular basement membrane (GBM). The second is dependent on the formation of immune complexes, that is, circulating antibody-antigen complexes, in which the antigen is not necessarily of glomerular origin. The focusing of antibodies or immune complexes within glomeruli is not of itself pathogenic. Tissue damage results from the inflammatory response that these components trigger via the activation of the complement system. This in turn may trigger the coagulation system, resulting in additional glomerular damage. Glomeruli destruction, then, is the end result of a vicious cycle of a number of interacting components. The development and severity of glomerulonephritis depend on these various factors and the delicate balance between them. Consideration of only one of these components, for example that of the antibody involved, indicates that the immunoglobulin class, kinetics of appearance, amount, specificity, and avidity may all influence the development and/or severity of the disease.

Moreover, it is now appreciated that antigens foreign to the glomerulus can, if deposited there from the circulation, attract circulating specific antibody to form complexes by a process of in-situ combination. In general these "planted" antigens form immune complexes localized at the subepithelial site. It now seems likely that the predominant mechanism in the formation of subepithelial deposits is in-situ combination of antigen and specific antibody, both in experimental models and in humans. A fourth immunologic mechanism has been implicated more recently in the triggering of the disease process. Antibody may be involved in the activation of the complement cascade by the alternate pathway of the properdin system. Although the triggering event may be different, the end result is the same.

A fifth mechanism, that of cellular-mediated immunity, may also be involved in these disease processes. Although patients with glomerulonephritis possess lymphocytes that are specifically sensitized to glomerular or cross-reactive antigens, their possible role in the pathogenesis is not yet clear. It seems quite likely, however, that all these aforementioned mechanisms may contribute at some point to the disease process. The following outline is not intended to be an all-inclusive summary of the role of immunologic reactions in renal disease. Rather, it is but one of many possible ways to organize our thoughts concerning the triggering events, the role immunologic mechanisms may play, and the points in these sequences that we may logically attack with methods for therapy or possible prevention.

Several types of bacterial infections in humans have been treated by passive immunization with xenogeneic serum, such as horse antitetanus toxin. This particular form of therapy has been largely discontinued. However, use of xenogeneic serum or globulin therapy such as horse antilymphocyte serum is expected to increase. Recipients of such treatment often develop the serum sickness syndrome characterized by fever, enlarged lymph nodes and spleen, erythematous and urticarial rashes, painful joints, and renal involvement. The acute form (or "one-shot") may result in a renal lesion at 10 to 14 days, which usually heals spontaneously. In contrast, a chronic form of the disease may result from continued antigen exposure, in which a severe and progressive glomerular lesion with resultant structural damage is evident. Investigations of the serum sickness syndrome have been the springboard for our understanding of the pathologic immunogenic mechanisms involved in renal disease. These mechanisms have been more carefully delineated in the experimental models discussed subsequently. Their human disease correlates have been well documented.

EXPERIMENTAL MODELS

Heterologous Anti-GBM. This model, first provided by Masugi, involves the injection of heterologous antibody of anti–host kidney specificity into recipient animals (such as rabbit anti–rat kidney serum injected into rats). These immunoglobulins combine with the glomerular basement membrane or with other vascular tissues that are antigenically similar to GBM, such as in the lung. There they trigger a sequence of pathologic events by the activation and fixation of complement, the infiltration of polymorphonuclear (PMN) leukocytes, and destruction of basement membrane. A second round of immunologic insult results when the host makes antibody to the foreign immunoglobulins that are bound to its own basement membrane. This antibody-antigen complex may again trigger an inflammatory response, leading to additional membrane destruction.

Autologous Anti-GBM. In this model, the experimental animal is immunized with homologous or heterologous GBM. Its immunologic response results in a clinical picture very similar to that of the Masugi type of nephritis, except in this case the triggering antibody is of host origin (i.e., an autoimmune phenomenon). That such antibody is pathogenic is demonstrated by the fact that transfer to normal animals of such antibody isolated from the serum of immunized animals (or eluted from their affected kidneys) may result in severe glomerular damage.

Immune Complex. The classic model has involved the single injection of a rather large dose of radiolabeled bovine serum albumin as antigen into the rabbit. Analysis of the immunologic events that followed has been a significant contribution in our understanding of the pathogenesis of glomerulonephritis. The antigen is seen to disappear from the circulation in three phases: equilibration, metabolic decay, and immune elimination. During the last phase, antibody forms complexes with the antigen. These may be deposited in tissues including heart, joints, and kidneys. Renal involvement occurs during the time interval when immune complexes are in slight antigen excess. The presence of such complexes within the glomeruli has been documented. When free noncomplexed antibody make its appearance in the circulation, the complexes disappear along with the manifestations of renal disease. Coincident with the complex formation and renal disease there is a decrease in the serum complement level.

A different course of events is noted if the antigen is given in smaller repeated doses over a prolonged period. This form of chronic stimulation produces a severe and progressive glomerular lesion causing structural damage. In several studies, rabbits undergoing such experimentation fell into three groups according to their antibody response. The first group did not produce antibody and did not have any renal lesions despite the presence of foreign antigen in the circulation and tissues for prolonged periods of time. A second group of animals synthesized very large amounts of antibody that efficiently cleared the reinjected antigen from the circulation. Some of the animals in this second group developed an acute glomerulonephritis within the first 2 weeks, which usually resolved quickly with no further lesions observed. The third group produced an intermediate amount of antibody such that the repeatedly introduced antigen was cleared in a delayed fashion. Most of these animals developed chronic glomerular lesions. Thus it is apparent that soluble immune complexes must be present in the circulation for some period of time to cause glomerular injury. In addition, only complexes of the appropriate size of lattice formation (those in slight to moderate antigen excess) are potentially pathogenic. The fact that not all rabbits developed glomerular lesions indicates that the character of the animal's antibody response also influences the development of such lesions. Quantitative relationships between antigen and antibody appear crucial in determining the eventual response we may expect to see.

Spontaneous Glomerulonephritis in Animals. A particularly interesting animal model that has been useful in unraveling the mechanisms inherent in the development of glomerulonephritis is the New Zealand mouse. F1 hybrids of the black and white strains (NZB/W F1) spontaneously develop a disease process that closely resembles systemic lupus erythematosus (SLE) in humans. Females are more susceptible, beginning to die at 6 months of age. Mortality increases with advancing age, and 98 per cent are dead at 1 year. This fatal autoimmune glomerulonephritis is characterized by the presence of immune complexes within renal tissues. Approximately 50 per cent of the antibody eluted from these immune complexes reacts specifically with host deoxyribonucleic acid (DNA). Another 15 to 20 per cent react with "C" type oncogenic virus endogenous to these animals. Experimentally induced infection—with lymphocytic choriomeningitis (LCM) virus, for example—markedly enhances or accelerates the immune response to DNA and the resultant nephritis. In contrast, rendering these animals tolerant to DNA prevents the disease. Although of the immune complex type (DNA–anti-DNA), this model provides an example of spontaneous development of this disease triggered by endogenous materials.

Heymann Nephritis. It has been shown that when rats are given injections of isologous kidney, a nephritogenic antigen named "renal tubular epithelial (RTE) antigen" can be found in the renal tubular brush border. Crude preparations injected into a host rat induced antibody production and the appearance of chronic membranous glomerulopathy. Renal tubular epithelial antigen was demonstrated in the glomerular deposits. The antigen was detected in a particular fraction of tubule preparation known as "FX1A."

Initially it was assumed that the nephritis so produced resulted from the formation of FX1A–anti-FX1A immune complexes in the circulation and their subsequent deposition within the kidney. However, it has been shown that injection of anti-FX1A antibody could also produce nephritis (passive Heymann nephritis). This observation prompted the search for an alternative explanation to the classic concept of glomerular injury caused by the deposition of circulating immune complexes. More recently, it has been shown that the glomerular basement membrane contains antigens that cross-react with anti-FX1A, and that formation of immune complexes within the glomerular wall follows within seconds of injection of the anti-FX1A antibody. In crucial experiments that involved in vivo perfusion of the isolated kidney with anti-FX1A antibodies and FX1A–anti-FX1A complexes, it was demonstrated that the anti-FX1A fixed to the glomerulus, whereas the FX1A–

anti-FX1A complexes did not. These data support the concept of in-situ antigen-antibody combination as another mechanism of immunologically based renal injury.

MECHANISMS OF IMMUNE INJURY

As we have indicated, the trigger to the sequence of events that terminates in irreversible kidney damage—that of antibody or immune complex deposition within glomeruli—is not pathogenic of or in itself. The destruction is the result of the inflammatory response that follows, which in turn triggers the clotting, fibrinolytic, and kinin-generating systems.

Antibody Specificity. Antibody with GBM specificity produced either endogenously or exogenously reacts directly with these structures. A smooth continuous ribbon-like deposition of antibody along the basement membrane can be visualized by immunofluorescent techniques. The kidney, and occasionally the lung, are specific target tissues for antibodies of anti-GBM specificity. In contrast, the discontinuous granular immunoglobulin deposits of immune complex disease consist of antibodies of varied and widely ranging specificities together with their respective antigens. The complexes visualized in SLE consist of DNA and antibodies to nuclear factors. These tissues are innocent bystanders when immune complexes containing antibody and antigen of nonglomerular origin are deposited within them. Both forms of antibody-antigen interaction are capable of triggering the complement cascade.

Quantity and Quality. The formation of pathogenic immune complexes is dependent on the immune response of the individual to a given antigenic challenge. Those individuals producing minimal or no antibody will have either none or very small nonpathogenic immune complexes formed. Those individuals responding vigorously with large amounts of antibody will form very large complexes in antibody excess that are rapidly cleared by the reticuloendothelial system. Individuals intermediate in their response (i.e., those barely keeping up with the job of clearing antigen) will form immune complexes in slight to moderate antigen excess. Such complexes are of sufficient size to be deposited within glomeruli, are most efficient at triggering the complement cascade, and are thus potentially pathogenic. Recent studies in the NZB/W F1 model suggest that antibody affinity may be of critical importance. The time of onset, time course, and severity of the murine lupus syndrome are associated with the presence of increasing levels of low-avidity anti-DNA antibody. Likewise, avidity of anti-DNA antibody in the serum of SLE patients with renal disease is lower than that in the SLE patient without renal involvement. Low-affinity antibody is less efficient at antigen-clearing and allows for the production

and persistence in the circulation of potentially pathogenic immune complexes. In this sense, the development of immune complex nephritis can be considered a consequence of a relative immunodeficiency, that of making poor quality (low-affinity) antibody.

Immunoglobulin Class. IgM and IgG are capable of triggering the classic pathway of the complement system. IgA, in contrast, employs the alternative (properdin) pathway, in addition to the other properdin-triggering materials such as aggregated immunoglobulins and endotoxins. Involvement of IgE antibody is suggested by some investigators. They propose that antigen induces the release of platelet-activating factors and histamine from basophils sensitized with specific IgE antibody. The clumping of platelets releases vasoactive amines that along with histamine increase vascular permeability, allowing for the entry and deposition of immune complexes along the glomerular basement membrane.

Complex Size. Very large complexes (relative antibody excess) are inefficient at triggering complement. Although they may remain in the circulation for extended periods, they apparently do not have a propensity for accumulation within the glomeruli. Intermediate complexes (slight to moderate antigen excess with molecular weights $>10^6$) are soluble and very efficient at fixing complement, and show a propensity for accumulation within tissues.

THE INFLAMMATORY AND COAGULATION RESPONSE

The Complement (C′) System. Several lines of evidence implicate the complement system in the pathogenesis of nephritis. These include depression of total serum complement levels during immune complex deposition; identification of complement components (usually C′3) within glomeruli in a pattern similar to antibody deposition, either ribbon-like or "lumpy-bumpy" and prevention of arteritis and glomerulitis by depleting or inhibiting complement components (e.g., by the use of cobra venom factor). Activation of the complement system by the classic or alternative pathway results in the liberation of anaphylatoxins, which increase vascular permeability and facilitate deposition of immune complexes. Chemotactic factors attract leukocytes that release their enzymes, causing degradation of the basement membrane and exposing collagen structures. In addition, stimulation of platelet aggregation and the amplification loop of the complement system ensue. The complement system in turn triggers and/or is triggered by the coagulation system.

Clotting and Coagulation Systems. Prevention of glomerulonephritis by depletion or inhibition of components of the coagulation system supports a role for this system in the pathogenesis of nephritis. Hageman factor is activated by the exposed collagen of damaged basement membrane, which in turn leads to the coagulation mechanism. Plasminogen is converted to plasmin, which in turn activates C′1 and C′3. Hageman factor converts prekallikrein to kallikrein, which is chemotactic for leukocytes, and also activates the complement system. The cleavage of kininogen to bradykinin, a vasoactive amine, results in reinforcement of this cycle. A protease released by the leukocyte is also capable of activating C′3. Activated C′3 in turn promotes platelet clumping and fibrin deposition, and so the cycle continues.

CLINICAL EXAMPLES OF COMMONLY OCCURRING GLOMERULAR LESIONS IN HUMANS

We have briefly examined the immune mechanisms recognized as contributing factors in the development of certain glomerular lesions. The basic research is related to experiments performed primarily in animals. There are comparable examples well recognized in humans, and a brief consideration of some of those examples is in order. It is beyond the scope of this text to examine the broad spectrum of recognized glomerular syndromes in their entirety, and we must therefore limit our discussion to classically described examples of disease.

Acute proliferative glomerulonephritis has long been recognized as a syndrome closely associated with streptococcal infections. That this syndrome may be temporally related to infections with many other organisms is well recognized, and documentation exists for bacterial, viral, and fungal infections as antecedent events leading to the development of acute glomerulonephritis. There are, in addition, many cases for which no antecedent infectious agents can be recognized, and these, for lack of better definition, have been lumped into an idiopathic variety. For this discussion, we will reserve our remarks to the well-recognized poststreptococcal glomerulonephritis.

This disease entity occurs with the highest frequency in children, although it may occur at any age. There is a latent period between the recognition of streptococcal infection and the onset of the renal lesion. The classic clinical presentation includes hematuria, proteinuria, a rapidly rising BUN and creatinine, diminution in urinary output, fluid retention, and elevation in blood pressure. The presence of any or all of these clinical findings is highly variable, and in all probability many cases are never clinically recognized. These clinical findings are associated with well-documented pathologic changes within the glomerular tufts. The glomeruli are bloodless, hypercellular, and enlarged, and they fill Bowman's space; there

is marked proliferation of mesangial and endothelial cells and a variable degree of infiltration, with polymorphonuclear leukocytes in the capillary lumina and the mesangial space. All glomeruli are affected, and involvement is relatively uniform. Capillary walls are thin and delicate, except for occasional irregularities that, by light microscopy, can be recognized as discrete deposits on the epithelial surface of the basement membrane. Changes in the parietal epithelial cells are inconspicuous, although a few segmental epithelial crescents may be seen. Necrosis of the tufts and hilus thrombi are unusual. Interstitial edema, focal tubule degeneration, and scattered collections of mononuclear cells may be seen. Blood vessels are usually normal.

By electron microscopy, the most consistent finding is the presence of discrete electron-dense nodular deposits on the epithelial surface of the basement membrane. The overlying epithelial cell cytoplasm is condensed adjacent to the hump, and the deposits are most often located at the site of the epithelial cell slit pore. Leukocytes may be seen impinging upon basement membrane denuded of endothelial cell cytoplasm. Epithelial cell foot processes show coalescence with obliteration of the slit pore complex. Mesangial cells are notably increased in number. Examination by immunofluorescent staining may reveal irregular deposits of IgG, IgM, and, less commonly, IgA. Components of the complement system are found in frequent association with the immunoprotein deposits. Deposits of fibrin may be found distributed in a segmental fashion within the mesangium or in association with epithelial crescent formation.

These clinical, morphologic, and serologic features suggest that classic acute poststreptococcal glomerulonephritis is an immune complex disease. Repeated attempts have been made to localize soluble streptococcal products in association with the immune complex deposits, but results have been negative, inconclusive, or difficult to repeat.

The immediate prognosis for poststeptococcal glomerulonephritis is favorable. With modern management, less than 1 per cent of pediatric patients can be expected to die in the acute stages of the illness. Long-term prognosis, however, remains controversial. Available evidence suggests that in the majority of pediatric patients the prognosis is excellent. The complete disappearance of urinary abnormalities may be delayed for several years; serial biopsies may display focal glomerular abnormalities and persistent deposits within the mesangium of immune globulins or complement or both. The situation in adults is quite different. Collective evidence available suggests that the older the patient is at the onset of disease, the less likely he is to enjoy a total and complete recovery.

The treatment of acute poststreptococcal glomerulonephritis is entirely symptomatic until all clinical signs of disease have abated. Most patients can be expected to undergo a diuresis within 1 to 3 weeks of the onset of illness. Prolonged oliguria and persistent massive proteinuria are indications for serious concern, and under these conditions, a renal biopsy should be performed to assess prognosis and confirmation of the original diagnosis. The administration of cytotoxic agents such as cyclophosphamide and azathioprine has not been demonstrated to alter the course of acute poststreptococcal glomerulonephritis, and to date there is no evidence to recommend the use of steroid preparations.

Rapidly Progressive Glomerulonephritis. This disorder is relatively uncommon and, in one recently reported series, accounted for less than 2 per cent of cases presenting with glomerulonephritis. The patients are usually young to middle-aged males, with a male-to-female predominance of roughly 2:1. The onset of the disease may be abrupt and resemble acute poststreptococcal glomerulonephritis, except severe oliguria occurs much more commonly. A history of streptococcal infection does not exist; more commonly, a history of a recent upper respiratory tract infection or flu-like syndrome will be elicited. In most cases, there is an insidious onset of disease with presenting complaints referable to the development of uremia or fluid retention. The absence of pulmonary hemorrhage distinguishes this syndrome from that of Goodpasture's disease. Examination of the urine classically reveals red blood cells and red blood cell casts in association with a varying degree of proteinuria. Circulating antiglomerular basement membrane antibody may be demonstrated early in the course of the disease. Fibrin degradation products are frequently elevated in plasma and urine; serum levels of complement are usually normal, although $C'3$ may be depressed in some cases. Examination of renal tissue by light microscopy reveals extensive extracapillary proliferation of the parietal epithelial cells that line Bowman's capsules into *epithelial crescents*. In usual cases, more than 50 per cent of glomeruli will evidence crescent formation. The glomerular tufts may be compressed by this proliferation of epithelial cells. Extensive necrosis of glomerular tufts can be seen in association with leukocyte infiltration and collapse of capillary loops. Over a period of days or weeks, progressive sclerosis and fibrosis of glomeruli occur.

Immunofluorescent studies are highly variable, and at least three patterns have been described. A linear IgG deposit, diffuse granular IgG, or, less commonly, IgM accompanied by complements, specifically $C'3$, settles in both the peripheral capillary loops and the mesangial interstitium. Fibrin-related deposits are also found, frequently in the crescents and in Bowman's space and less commonly in the lumina of involved tubules. Electron microscopy may reveal subendothelial deposits of electron-dense material indicative of immune complex disease. Biopsies may fail to reveal any deposits, with the principal pathologic alteration that of increasing mesangial matrix, collapse of denuded capillary walls, and fibrin thrombi. The crescents, by electron microscopy, demonstrate proliferation of parietal epithelial cells.

The diffuse IgG pattern in rapidly progressive glomerulonephritis with or without pulmonary hemorrhage is indicative of an antiglomerular basement membrane pathogenesis. The presence of diffuse granular deposits of IgG is more indicative of an immune complex pathogenesis. The third pattern consisting of scanty or irregular deposits of IgG with extensive fibrin deposition is relatively uncommon. It seems possible that each of the described patterns is compatible with a common pathologic basis, that is, immune complexes leading to initial damage, subsequent exposure of basement membrane antigen, an endogenous immune response to the antigen thus exposed, and a cascading of the complement system in association with fibrin deposits leading to the various described pathologic entities, depending on the time at which tissue is taken for examination.

The outlook for recovery in untreated rapidly progressive glomerulonephritis is extremely poor. Recently, several authors have reported favorably on a combination therapy of cytotoxic agents, steroids, and repeated plasmapheresis.

Membranous Glomerulonephritis. Membranous glomerulonephritis may result from a number of known causes; the majority of cases, however, will fall under the catch-all term of "idiopathic membranous glomerulonephritis" (Table 14–7). This disease process can occur at any age. The majority of patients are over the age of 40 at the time of diagnosis. The onset is insidious, without antecedent upper respiratory tract infection or history of streptococcal or other known infection. An interesting feature is that HLA studies have shown membranous nephropathy strongly associated with HLA DR3. Hypertension and azotemia occur late in the course of the disease. Proteinuria is commonly nonselective. Microscopic hematuria is common; complement levels in the

TABLE 14–7 CLINICAL CONDITIONS COMMONLY ASSOCIATED WITH MEMBRANOUS GLOMERULONEPHRITIS

1. Idiopathic
2. Systemic lupus erythematosus
3. Heavy metals
4. Syphilis (congenital and secondary)
5. Malaria
6. Chronic active hepatitis
7. Sarcoidosis
8. Sjögren's syndrome
9. Sickle cell disease
10. Neoplasia
11. Renal vein thrombosis
12. Diabetes mellitus

plasma are usually normal. Patients classically present with asymptomatic proteinuria or frank nephrotic syndrome. The rate at which the disease progresses to renal failure is highly unpredictable. Examination of tissue by light microscopy reveals the characteristic feature of diffuse and uniform thickening of the capillary walls without significant proliferation of endothelial, mesangial, or epithelial cells. With progression, capillary walls become increasingly thickened; even with advanced progression of the capillary lesion, tubule alterations are minimal. Crescents, if present at all, are focal and are considered a late manifestation of the disease. Electron microscopy reveals small, discrete subepithelial deposits of electron-dense material producing some distortion of the foot processes. As the disease progresses, the electron-dense deposits enlarge, and projections of basement membrane–like material develop, demonstrating the characteristic positive spikes seen by silver staining in light microscopy. This gives an irregular contour to the epithelial side of the basement membrane. With time, the deposits become larger and more heterogeneous in size and distribution, and they may vary in their degree of electron density. Foot processes demonstrate progressive distortion and disruption. By immunofluorescence, IgG is nearly always present in a granular distribution corresponding to the capillary loops sparing the mesangium. In advanced cases, IgG deposits may be weak and irregular or even negative, corresponding to the decreased electron-density seen by electron microscopy. IgM and IgA deposits are scanty; complement is usually found in a pattern similar to that of IgG. The glomerular lesion of the aforementioned autologous immune-complex nephritis in rats (Heymann nephritis) is analogous to that of membranous glomerulopathy in humans. Although there is evidence that, in humans, membranous glomerulopathy can be produced from circulating anti-FX1A antibody (passive Heymann nephritis), the extent to which in-situ complex formation contributes to all membranous nephropathy is unknown. However, in-situ complex formation could explain why circulating immune complexes are not found in the majority of patients with membranous nephropathy. It may also explain the failure of membranous nephropathy to transmit to grafted kidneys. The natural history and course of this disease form a highly irregular progression, punctuated by clinical remissions, which may be spontaneous. Data from one multicenter controlled trial suggest that high-dose alternate-day steroids for 2 to 3 months may be of benefit in preventing progression of renal failure.

Minimal change disease, also known as "lipoid nephrosis" and "no-change by light microscopy," has no clear-cut or documented association with an alteration in immune mechanisms. However, considerable circumstantial evidence implicates immunologic mechanisms in the pathogenesis of minimal change nephropathy. It has been suggested that minimal change disease might represent a defect in the function of thymus-derived lymphocytes (T cells). In particular, the response of this disease to both corticosteroids and cytotoxic agents has been used to support the hypothesis that minimal change nephropathy is caused by a disorder of T-cell function. It is commonly seen in younger age groups, occurring less and less frequently with advancing age. Usually there is a sudden onset of edema associated with massive proteinuria. Males predominate by a ratio of 1.5:1 in most series. Hypoalbuminemia and hyperlipemia are commonly demonstrated in association with the onset of edema. Hypertension is uncommon, and azotemia occurs rarely, unless hypovolemia is severe. Microscopic hematuria may be seen in a minority of cases, C′3 and C′4 levels are usually normal, and C′1q levels may occasionally be decreased. The proteinuria is most often selective in nature, particularly in children. In adults, however, poorly selective proteinuria may be seen in a substantial number of cases. Examination by light microscopy reveals a paucity of pathologic findings. Electron microscopy detects abnormalities of epithelial cells of the glomerular capillaries that are typical but not specific. Juxtaposition of the foot processes of epithelial cells and the obliteration of the slit pore membrane are noted in all glomeruli and glomerular capillaries. There is an associated vacuolation of cell cytoplasm. The glomerular basement membrane is normal in thickness. Examination by immunofluorescence fails to reveal significant deposits of IgG, IgM, or complement. The pathogenesis of this clinical entity remains to be delineated. Spontaneous remissions apparently occur frequently, and a high percentage of cases respond dramatically following the initiation of steroid therapy. In patients who fail to respond to steroids or who relapse following their withdrawal, the administration of cyclophosphamide may be therapeutic. Although the mechanism of action of steroids and cytotoxic agents in minimal change disease is not completely understood, there is evidence that cyclophosphamide produces long-term impairment of suppressor cell function in patients in remission. It has also been postulated that this phenomenon protects against subsequent relapse of minimal change disease.

Nephrotic Syndrome. Nephrotic syndrome is a flexible term that is difficult to define with any degree of accuracy. It has been defined in the past as the association of edema, proteinuria, hypoalbuminemia, and hyperlipemia with renal disease. The presence of all these findings is considered necessary for its diagnosis, but, if these criteria are too rigidly enforced, several forms of the disease may be overlooked. It is true that most patients will exhibit all these manifestations at one time or another during the course of their illness, but it is also true that all manifestations may not be present at the same time, especially at an early stage. A better definition for the nephrotic syndrome is the one offered by Kark, in which he defines it as the metabolic, nutritional, and clinical consequences of massive proteinuria. Its presence does not imply a single disease entity. It can be observed in various forms of primary renal disease, as well as in association with certain generalized systemic diseases.

The nephrotic syndrome may be found at any age, occurring more commonly in children and young adults, but it is still observed frequently in the middle and older age groups. Edema is usually the first clinical manifestation noted and frequently brings the patient to the attention of the physician. It may appear gradually in the course of weeks, or it may be of rapid and sudden onset. The edema is usually pitting in nature and is influenced by gravity. As a consequence, it varies with position, noticed in the face in the morning and in lower extremities in the evening. It may be minimal or extensive, involving the various serous cavities producing hydrocele, ascites, and pleural effusion. Visceral edema can occur in the more advanced cases of anasarca. Cases of acute edema of the larynx have been reported. Retinal sheen and skin pallor are manifestations of local edema. The presence of edema is not necessary for the definition of nephrotic syndrome, and in early stages a moderate proteinuria may be the only clinical manifestation. Weakness, anorexia, and headaches are common complaints. Changes in the fingernails are observed consisting of paired horizontal white lines on the nail bed and pinking of the normally white semilune. These changes are secondary to hypoproteinemia.

The most important change in the urine is proteinuria. Its intensity varies greatly; values range from 2.5 gm to as high as 70 gm per 24 hours. It is usually found in excess of 3.5 gm per 24 hours. Proteinuria is related to an increased permeability of the glomerular basement membrane to plasma proteins. Albumin constitutes the bulk of protein present. Protein losses may be highly *selective*, composed primarily of albumin, or relatively *nonselective*, with the presence of alpha-1 globulin, alpha-2 globulin, and lipoproteins, depending on the basic underlying pathology. The degree of selectivity may have a prognostic value, those with the nonselective type having the worst prognosis. Examination of the urinary sediment will reveal the presence of casts, birefractile bodies, and often minimal concentrations of red and white blood cells. The lowering of the plasma protein level, particularly of albumin, is another characteristic feature of the nephrotic syndrome. Increased lipemia and hypercholesterolemia are consistently present in association with minimal change disease. Hypercholesterolemia may be absent in other forms of the syndrome. The evolution of the nephrotic syndrome will depend on the nature of the underlying renal disease. It may present a wide spectrum of clinical disease,

from the benign course associated with minimal change commonly seen in children to the picture of progressive renal failure and uremia observed in older adults. Infection is a common complication, and before the advent of antibiotics it was the major cause of death. It has been proposed that the propensity for infection is associated with the demonstrated low levels of circulating IgG commonly associated with relapse.

The major pathophysiologic event in the nephrotic syndrome is the increase of the permeability of the glomerular basement membrane to protein. The mechanism of this increased permeability is not well understood, but it appears that the increased filtration of plasma proteins is due to a diffuse change in the basement membrane at the micromolecular level.

TUBULOINTERSTITIAL DISEASES (INTERSTITIAL NEPHRITIS)

Pathologists have long recognized a disease syndrome characterized by renal failure in association with bilaterally small kidneys and a normal caliceal system by gross examination. Microscopic examination reveals relative glomerular sparing, periglomerular fibrosis, a remarkable amount of interstitial fibrosis with or without round cell infiltration, and marked flattening of tubule epithelial cells with dilatation of tubule lumina that are filled with a pink proteinaceous material on staining with hematoxylin and eosin. Distribution of these changes is not uniform, and they occur in varying degrees of severity. It has been common practice to lump all disease patterns that approximated these findings into a single disease process believed to be caused by infection. Although infection apparently may lead to this clinicopathologic state, many other etiologies are now recognized and most probably account for the majority of cases described (Table 14–8).

The onset and progression of interstitial nephritis may be acute and fulminating, with accompanying oliguria and rapidly progressive renal failure. A more common presentation is that of slowly progressive and often unrecognized renal

TABLE 14–8 COMMON CAUSES OF TUBULOINTERSTITIAL DISEASE

1. Antibiotics (e.g., methicillin)
2. Analgesics (phenacetin, acetaminophen, aspirin)
3. Diuretics (furosemide, hydrochlorothiazide)
4. Heavy metals (gold, lead)
5. Metabolic disorders (hypercalcemia, hypocalcemia, hyperuricemia)
6. Hyperproteinemia (multiple myeloma)
7. Anesthetics (methoxyflurane)
8. Infections

failure with clear-cut clinical symptomatology developing only after the renal damage has become far advanced. Many of the recognized and, to some extent, previously discussed physiologic functions of the kidneys predispose them to injuries of the type described in tubulointerstitial diseases. In all probability, as yet undefined functions may make additional contributions to the initiation and progression of disease. Specific factors related to the kidney include the following:

1. The kidneys receive a remarkably high blood flow calculated at 20 per cent of cardiac output. This fluid flow perfuses tissue representing only 0.4 per cent of total body weight. Ninety per cent of that blood flow is directed to the renal cortex. Despite small differences in arteriovenous oxygen, renal oxygen consumption is high. This makes renal tissue susceptible to any factor that interferes with oxygen availability, transport, or utilization.

2. Cells of the renal tubule epithelium have the ability selectively to uncouple protein binding. Many potential cellular toxins are effectively inactivated while circulating bound to plasma proteins. Unbound by the uncoupling mechanism of the kidney, they may become toxic to the cells in which the uncoupling has taken place. At the same time, concentration and acidification of urine is taking place, adding a further burden of susceptibility.

3. Compounds that may be relatively nontoxic at a pH of 6.8 to 7.4 may become highly toxic when hydrogen ion concentration increases and pH values fall to the range of 4.5 to 6.5.

4. Phagocytosis by white blood cells is impeded by rising osmolality and ceases altogether when values exceed 600 milliosmoles.

5. Ammonia production is a usual and important function of normal kidney tissue and rises rapidly in the face of an increased hydrogen ion load. High concentrations of ammonia interfere with complement activation and may interfere with the usual immunologic response to potential injury.

6. The vascular bed of the kidney is extensive per gram of tissue and may in itself predispose to injury beyond that seen in other organs.

The clinical presentation is remarkably variable. In the acute fulminating form, the patient experiences oliguria associated with a rapid rise in BUN and serum creatinine. He may have a concomitant cutaneous rash and peripheral eosinophilia in association with eosinophils in the urine. Protein, WBCs, RBCs and a variety of urinary casts are present in the urine but are in no way diagnostic.

Chronic forms are insidious in onset and, under most circumstances, are associated with no history of an acute episode. As opposed to the usual finding of normal-size or enlarged kidney by x-ray in acute form, kidneys are classically small and scarred. The caliceal system is normal unless papillary necrosis or obstruction is present or has occurred in the past. In many cases anemia may be out of proportion to the degree of uremia. Proteinuria is present, but rarely exceeds 2 gm per 24 hours. White blood cells and, to a lesser extent, red blood cells may be present in the urine.

Although it is beyond the scope of this discussion to consider in detail all the known causes of tubulointerstitial disease, several of the more common categories can be reviewed.

Disorders Due to Hypersensitivity. Agents included in this grouping are methicillin, ampicillin, penicillin, sulfonamides, diuretics, anticonvulsants, and antituberculin drugs. The lesion is not dose-related and often follows the second exposure to the drug. Antibodies to specific agents (e.g., methicillin) have been demonstrated. With appropriate recognition of the inciting agent and its prompt removal, recovery is the rule, although cases have been reported with chronic renal failure as the end result.

Toxic Factors. Agents falling into this category have a direct toxic effect on tissues either alone or in combination. Examples include phenacetin, acetaminophen, and acetylsalicylic acid (disease caused by ingestion of large amounts of aspirin is often referred to as analgesic-abuse nephritis). The usual course is one of injury occurring with prolonged exposure. An individual susceptibility apparently exists, and injury does not occur in every individual so exposed. A wide variety of antibiotics has been implicated. Diuretics have been implicated on occasion.

The nonsteroidal antiflammatory drugs (NSAID), which inhibit prostaglandin synthesis, have gained widespread acceptance in clinical medicine. This class of drugs has been used for treatment of a wide variety of illnesses. However, numerous reports are appearing in the literature documenting the renal complications of these drugs. These complications include sodium retention, impairment of free water clearance, antagonism of diuretics, nephrotic syndrome, and acute and chronic renal failure. The mechanisms by which NSAID cause alterations in renal function are not completely understood, but, in many instances, the effects on renal function may be a direct extension of their pharmacologic effect. NSAID have been shown to decrease renal blood flow and redistribute the flow away from the superficial cortical glomeruli to the juxtamedullary glomeruli. The juxtamedullary glomeruli have an increased capacity for sodium reabsorption. These changes in renal blood flow may alter the kidney's susceptibility to injury.

Metabolic Factors. Hypercalcemia can lead, either abruptly or gradually, to renal failure. Crystallization may occur in the interstitial area with or without intraluminal crystallization. Calcium ion in high concentrations may have a direct toxic effect on tubule cells without any demonstrable crystal formation and produce a concomitant drop in renal blood flow, leading to a rapid fall in glomerular filtration rate. An associated nephrogenic diabetes insipidus syndrome may occur.

Other examples of metabolic factors that may lead to interstitial nephritis include hypokalemia and hyperuricemia. Renal changes usually occur only after prolonged states of potassium deficiency and appear to be largely reversible. Cases of persistent changes have been reported but are difficult to document.

Pyelonephritis. The role of urinary tract infection in the pathogenesis of acute or chronic renal disease has undergone major reassessment. Data currently available suggest that primary infection of the kidney in the absence of other renal pathology is an unusual cause of extensive renal parenchymal damage in the adult.

The bacteria commonly responsible for infections in the urinary system are *Escherichia coli, Proteus, Klebsiella, Enterobacter,* and *Pseudomonas.* Various species of enterococci have been implicated. All these agents are usual and common constituents of bowel flora. The majority of uncomplicated infections are caused by *E. coli.* If the patient has undergone prior antibiotic therapy or instrumentation or has an associated urinary tract anomaly, the prevalence of infection with organisms other then *E. coli* rises sharply.

Infection may occur in any segment of the urinary tract without necessary involvement of other segments. The mere presence of bacteria in the urine cannot directly implicate the area primarily involved.

Spread of infection to involve the renal parenchyma may occur in one of three ways: (1) direct invasion by ascending the urethra, bladder, and ureter, (2) lymphatic invasion, and (3) hematogenous spread. Evidence suggests that lymphatic spread is a rare event. The most common route of infection occurs by direct ascent. Hematogenous infection is much less common, and when it does occur it is related to specific organisms such as *Mycobacterium, Staphylococcus,* and *Pseudomonas.*

The usual site of infection is the medulla, with direct extension into the cortex in a segmental fashion. The susceptibility of the medulla to small numbers of organisms of relatively low virulence can be explained by a number of factors unique to this renal segment. Among these are (1) high ammonia level, (2) hypertonicity, (3) relatively low blood flow, and (4) depressed leukocyte migration.

Renal parenchymal infection without associated pathology is self-limited and can be expected to resolve spontaneously in a period of 6 weeks to 6 months with or without therapy. Underlying pathology such as stones, reflux, obstruction, and scarring can contribute to sustained and widespread infection, resulting in significant and permanent loss of parenchyma.

In our discussion of tubulointerstitial diseases, we have touched on only a small number of known causes of this type of renal damage. No doubt a wide variety of as yet unidentified compounds exists with the potential for producing nephrotoxicity in addition to those already identified. This is particularly disturbing in a society in which new chemical agents in a variety of forms and exposure reach the environment each day. Only after long exposure, as in the case of analgesic-abuse nephritis, will many of these agents be documented as potential toxins to renal tissue. It behooves us all as physicians to keep this point in mind when searching for a potential cause of renal failure and, more importantly, in doing our part to see that exposure is limited to an absolute necessity in an area over which we have control—that is, exposure to prescription drugs.

REFERENCES

REVIEW OF NORMAL RENAL PHYSIOLOGY

Boyer, C. C.: The vascular pattern of the renal glomerulus as revealed by plastic reconstruction from serial sections. Anat. Rec. *125*:435, 1956.

Brenner, B. M., and Galla, J. H.: Influence of postglomerular hematocrit and protein concentration on rat nephron fluid transfer. Am. J. Physiol. *220*:148, 1971.

Brenner, B. M., Troy, J. L., and Daugharty, T. M.: The dynamics of glomerular ultrafiltration in the rat. J. Clin. Invest. *50*:1776, 1971.

Edwards, J. G.: Efferent arterioles of glomeruli in the juxtamedullary zone of human kidney. Anat. Rec. *123*:521, 1956.

Elias, H., Hosman, A., Barth, I. B., and Solmon, A.: Blood flow in the renal glomerulus. J. Urol. *83*:790, 1960.

Forster, R. P., and Maes, J. P.: Effect of experimental neurogenic hypertention on renal blood flow and glomerular filtration rates in intact denervated kidneys of unanesthetized rabbits with adrenal glands demedullated. Am. J. Physiol. *150*:534, 1947.

Hardaker, W. T., Jr., and Wechsler, A. S.: Redistribution of renal intracortical blood flow during dopamine infusion in dogs. Circ. Res. *33*:437, 1973.

Hardwicke, J., Hulme, B., Jones, J. H., and Ricketts, C. R.: Measurement of glomerular permeability to polydisperse radioactively labeled macromolecules in normal rabbits. Clin. Sci. *34*:505, 1968.

Hollenberg, N. K., Solomon, H. S., Adams, D. F., et al.: Renal vascular responses to angiotensin and norepinephrine in normal man. Circ. Res. *31*:750, 1972.

Horster, M., and Thurau, K.: Micropuncture studies on filtration rates of single superficial and juxtamedullary glomeruli in rat. Arch. Ges. Physiol. *301*:162, 1968.

Jamison, R. L.: Intrarenal heterogeneity. The case for two functionally dissimilar populations of nephrons in the mammalian kidney. Am. J. Med. *54*:281, 1973.

Johnson, H. H., Herzog, J. P., and Lauler, D. P.: Effect of prostaglandin E_1 on renal hemodynamics, sodium and water excretion. Am. J. Physiol. *213*:936, 1967.

Kaihara, S., Rutherford, R. B., Schwenker, E. P., and Wagner, H. N.: Distribution of cardiac output in experimental hemorrhagic shock in dogs. J. Appl. Physiol. *27*:218, 1969.

Kirschenbaum, M. A., and Stein, J. H.: The effect of inhibition of prostaglandin synthesis on urinary sodium excretion in conscious dogs. J. Clin. Invest. *57*:517, 1976.

Maddox, D. A., Bennett, C. M., Deen, W. M., et al.: Determinants of glomerular filtration in experimental glomerulonephritis in the rat. J. Clin. Invest. 55:305, 1975.

Maddox, D. A., Deen, W. M., and Brenner, B. M.: Dynamics of glomerular ultrafiltration. VI. Studies in the primate. Kidney Int. 5:271, 1974.

Malnic, G., and Steinmetz, P. R.: Transport processes in urinary acidification. Kidney Int. 9:172, 1976.

Maren, T. H.: Chemistry of the renal absorption of bicarbonate. Canad. J. Physiol. Pharmacol. 52:1041, 1974.

Maude, D. L.: The role of bicarbonate in proximal tubular sodium chloride transport. Kidney Int. 5:253, 1974.

Mitchell, G. D. G.: The nerve supply of the kidneys. Acta Anat. (Basel) 10:1, 1950.

Neutze, J. M., Wyler, F., and Rudolph, A. M.: Use of radioactive microspheres to assess distribution of cardiac output of micropheres. Am. J. Physiol 215:496, 1968.

Smith, J. P.: Anatomical features of the human renal glomerular efferent vessel. J. Anat. 90:290, 1956.

Swain, J. A., Heynkricky, G. R., Boettcher, D. H., and Vatner, S. F.: Prostaglandin control of renal circulation in unanesthetized dog and baboon. Am. J. Physiol. 229:826, 1975.

Stein, J. H., Congbalay, R. C., Karsh, D. L., et al.: Effect of bradykinin on proximal tubular sodium resorption in the dog: evidence for functional nephron heterogeneity. J. Clin. Invest. 51:1709, 1972.

Trueta, J., Barclay, A. E., Daniel, P. M., et al.: Studies of the Renal Circulation. Oxford, Blackwell Scientific Publications, 1948.

Windhager, E., and Giebisch, G.: Proximal sodium in fluid transport. Kidney Int. 9:121, 1976.

Zins, G. R.: Renal prostaglandins. Am. J. Med. 58:14, 1975.

CLINICAL EVALUATION OF RENAL FUNCTION

Anderson, R. J., Linas, S. T., Berns, A. D., et al.: Nonoliguric acute renal failure. N. Engl. J. Med. 269:1134, 1977.

Doolan, P. D., Alpen, E. L., and Theil, G. B.: A clinical appraisal of the plasma concentration and endogenous clearance of creatinine. Am. J. Med. 32:65, 1962.

Healy, J. K.: Clinical assessment of glomerular filtration rate by different forms of creatinine clearance and a modified urinary phenolsulphonphthalein excretion test. Am. J. Med. 44:348, 1968.

Jelliffe, R. W.: Creatinine clearance: bedside estimate. Ann. Int. Med. 79:604, 1973.

Jones, L. W., and Weil, M. H.: Water creatinine and sodium excretion following circulatory shock with renal failure. Am. J. Med. 51:314, 1971.

Spinel, C. H.: The Fe Na test used in the differential diagnosis of acute renal failure. J.A.M.A. 236:579, 1976.

Wesson, L. G.: Physiology of the Human Kidney. New York, Grune & Stratton, 1969.

DISORDERS OF SODIUM METABOLISM

Albrink, M. J., Hald, P. M., Mann, E. B., and Peters, J. P.: The displacement of serum water by the lipids of hyperlipemic serum: a new method for the rapid determination of serum water. J. Clin. Invest. 31:1483, 1955.

Arieff, A., and Guisado, R.: Effects on the central nervous system of hypernatremia and hyponatremic states. Kidney Int. 10:104, 1976.

Bartter, F. C., and Schwartz, W. B.: The syndrome of inappropriate secretion of antidiuretic hormone. Am. J. Med. 42:790, 1967.

Brenner, B. M., Falchuk, K. H., Keimowitz, R. I., and Berliner, R. W.: The relationship between peritubular capillary protein concentration and fluid resorption by the renal proximal tubule. J. Clin. Invest. 48:1519, 1969.

Carter, N. W., Rector, F. C., and Seldin, D. W.: Hyponatremia in cerebral disease resulting from the inappropriate secretion of antidiuretic hormone. N. Engl. J. Med. 264:67, 1961.

DeRivera, J. L.: Inappropriate secretion of antidiuretic hormone from fluphenazine. Ann. Int. Med. 82:811, 1975.

DiScala, V. A., and Kinney, M. J.: Effects of myxedema on the renal diluting and concentrating mechanisms. Am. J. Med. 50:325, 1971.

Earley, L. E., and Friedler, R. M.: The effects of the combined renal vasodilatation and pressor agents on renal hemody-

namics and the tubular resorption of sodium. J. Clin. Invest. 45:542, 1966.

Klahr, S., and Slatopolsky, E.: Renal regulation of sodium excretion. Arch. Int. Med. 131:780, 1973.

Moses, A. M., and Miller, M.: Drug induced dilutional hyponatremia. N. Engl. J. Med. 291:1234, 1974.

Pitts, R. F.: Physiology of the Kidney and Body Fluids. Chicago, Yearbook Medical Publishers, 1974.

DISORDERS OF POTASSIUM METABOLISM

Beck, N., and Webster, S. K.: Impaired urinary concentrating ability and cyclic AMP in potassium depleted rat kidney. Am. J. Physiol. 231:1204, 1976.

Brautbar, N., Levi, J., Rosler, A., et al.: Familial hyperkalemia a probable defect in potassium secretion. Clin. Res., Feb., 1976, p. 125A.

Davidson, S., and Surawicz, B.: Incidence of superventricular and ventricular ectopic beats and rhythms of atrioventricular conduction disturbances in patients with hypopotassemia. Circulation 34(suppl 3):85, 1966.

Flear, C. T. G., Cook, W. T., and Quentin, A.: Serum potassium levels as an index of body content. Lancet 1:458, 1957.

Fordtran, J. S., and Dietschy, J. M.: Water and electrolyte movement in the intestine. Gastroenterology 50:263, 1966.

Gennari, F. J., and Cohen, J. J.: Role of the kidney in potassium homeostasis: lesson from acid-base disturbances. Kidney Int. 8:1, 1975.

Giebisch, G.: Some reflections of the mechanism of renal tubular potassium transport. Yale J. Biol. Med. 48:315, 1975.

Goldfarb, S., Cox, M., Singer, I., and Goldberg, M.: Acute hyperkalemia induced by hyperglycemia: hormonal mechanisms. Ann. Int. Med. 84:426, 1976.

Khuri, R. M., Wiederholt, M., Strieder, N., and Giebisch, G.: Effects of flow rate and potassium intake on distal tubular potassium transfer. Am. J. Physiol. 228:1249, 1975.

Knochel, J. P., Dotin, L. N., and Hamburger, R. J.: The pathophysiology of intense physical conditioning in a hot climate. Mechanisms of potassium depletion. J. Clin. Invest. 1:242, 1972.

Schwartz, W. B., and Relman, A. S.: Metabolic and renal studies in chronic potassium depletion resulting from overuse of laxatives. J. Clin. Invest. 32:258, 1953.

Schwartz, W. B., and Relman, A. S.: Effects of electrolyte disorders on renal structure and function. N. Engl. J. Med. 276:383, 1967.

Simmons, D. H., and Avedon, M.: Acid-base alterations in plasma potassium concentration. Am. J. Physiol. 197:319, 1959.

Tanne, R. L., Wedell, E., and Moore, R.: Renal adaptation to a high potassium intake. The role of hydrogen ion. J. Clin. Invest. 52:2089, 1973.

Wright, F.: Sites and mechanisms of potassium transport along the renal tubule. Kidney Int. 11:415, 1977.

ACID-BASE DISTURBANCES

Brackett, N. C., Cohen, J. J., and Schwartz, W. B.: Carbon dioxide titration curve of normal man. Effect of increasing degrees of acute hypercapnia on acid-base equilibrium. N. Engl. J. Med. 272:6, 1965.

Kurtzman, N. A., White, M. G., and Rogers, P. W.: Pathophysiology of metabolic alkalosis. Arch. Int. Med. 131:702, 1973.

Lemmon, E. J., and Lemann, J., Jr.: Defense of hydrogen ion concentration in chronic metabolic acidosis. Ann. Int. Med. 65:265, 1966.

Morris, R. C., Jr.: Renal tubular acidosis: mechanisms, classification and implications. N. Engl. J. Med. 281:1405, 1969.

Morris, R. C., Jr., Sebastian, A., and McSherry, E.: Renal acidosis. Kidney Int. 1:322, 1972.

Oliva, P. B.: Lactic acidosis, Am. J. Med. 48:209, 1970.

Rector, F. C., Jr., Blommer, H. A., and Seldin, D. W.: Effect of potassium deficiency on the resorption of bicarbonate in the proximal tubule of the rat kidney. J. Clin. Invest. 43:1976, 1964.

Rector, F. C., Jr., Carter, N. W., and Seldin, D. W.: The mechanism of bicarbonate resorption of proximal distal tubules of the kidney. J. Clin. Invest. 44:278, 1965.

Schwartz, W. B., Orning, K. J., and Porter, R.: The internal distribution of hydrogen ion with varying degrees of metabolic acidosis. J. Clin. Invest. 36:373, 1957.

Seldin, D. W., and Rector, F. C., Jr.: Symposium on acid-base homeostasis. The generation and maintenance of metabolic alkalosis. Kidney Int. *1*:306, 1972.

ACTION OF DIURETIC DRUGS

Burg, M.: The mechanism of action of diuretics in renal tubules. *In* Wessen, L., and Fanelli, G. (Eds.): Recent Advances in Renal Physiology and Pharmacology. Baltimore, University Park Press, 1974.

Burg, M., and Green, N.: Effect of ethacrynic acid on the thick ascending limb of Henle's loop. Kidney Int. *4*:301, 1973.

Burg, B. M.: Tubular chloride transport and the mode of action of some diuretics. Kidney Int. *9*:189, 1976.

Cannon, P. J., Heinemann, H. O., Albert, M. S., et al.: "Contraction" alkalosis after diuresis of edematous patients with ethacrynic acid. Ann. Int. Med. *62*:979, 1965.

Clapp, J. R., and Robinson, R. R.: Distal sites of action of diuretic drugs in the dog nephron. Am. J. Physiol. *215*:228, 1968.

Kessler, R. H., Lozano, R., and Pitts, R.: Studies on structure-diuretic activity relationship of organic compounds of mercury. J. Clin. Invest. *36*:656, 1957.

Kunau, R. T., Jr., Weller, D. R., and Webb, H. L.: Clarification of the site of action of chlorothiazide in the rat nephron. J. Clin. Invest. *56*:401, 1975.

Maren, T. H.: Carbonic anhydrase: chemistry, physiology and inhibition. Physiol. Rev. *47*:595, 1967.

Muth, R. G.: Diuretic properties of furosemide in renal disease. Ann. Int. Med. *69*:249, 1968.

Seeley, J. F., and Dirks, J. H.: Micropuncture studies of hypertonic mannitol diuresis in the proximal and distal tubule of the dog kidney. J. Clin. Invest. *48*:2330, 1969.

Suki, W., Rector, F. C., Jr., and Seldin, D. W.: The site of action of furosemide and other sulphonamide diuretics in the dog. J. Clin. Invest. *44*:1458, 1965.

CONGENITAL ANOMALIES OF THE KIDNEY

Alport, A. C.: Hereditary familial congenital hemorrhagic nephritis. Br. Med. J. *1*:504, 1927.

Bigelow, N. H.: The association of polycystic kidneys with intracranial aneurysms and other dilated disorders. Am. J. Med. Sci. *225*:485, 1953.

Bricker, N. S., and Patten, J. F.: Cystic disease of the kidneys. A study of dynamics and chemical composition of cyst fluid. Am. J. Med. *18*:207, 1955.

Bricker, N. S., and Patten, J. F.: Renal function studies in polycystic disease of the kidneys with observation on the effect of surgical decompression. N. Engl. J. Med. *256*:212, 1957.

Dalgaard, O. Z.: Bilateral polycystic disease of the kidneys: follow-up of 284 patients and their families. Acta Scand. *328*:1, 1957.

Hayman, J. M., Jr.: Congenital malformations of the kidney. *In* Strauss, M. B., and Welt, L. G. (Eds.): Diseases of the Kidney. 2nd ed. Boston, Little, Brown & Co., 1971.

Morris, R. C., Jr., McInnes, R. R., Epstein, C. J., et al.: Genetic and metabolic injury of the kidney. *In* Brenner, B. M., and Rector, F. C., Jr. (Eds.): The Kidney. Volume II. Philadelphia, W. B. Saunders Co., 1976.

Morris, R. C., Yamauchi, H., and Palubinskas, A. J.: Medullary sponge kidney. Am. J. Med. *38*:883, 1965.

Osath, A., Nondh, V., and Patter, E. L.: Pathogenesis of polycystic kidneys. Arch. Pathol. *77*:466, 1964.

Perkoff, G. G.: The hereditary renal diseases. N. Engl. J. Med. *277*:79, 1967.

Purriel, P., Drets, M., Pascal, E. E., et al.: Familial hereditary nephropathy (Alport's Syndrome). Am. J. Med. *49*:753, 1970.

Segal, S.: Disorders of renal amino acid transport. N. Engl. J. Med. *294*:1044, 1976.

Stella, F. J., Massry, S. G., and Kleeman, C. R.: Medullary sponge kidney associated with parathyroid adenoma. Nephron *10*:332, 1973.

PATHOPHYSIOLOGY OF GLOMERULAR DAMAGE

Baldwin, D. S., and Gluck, M. C.: The long term course of poststreptococcal glomerulonephritis. Ann. Int. Med. *80*:342, 1974.

Baldwin, D. S., and Schact, R. G.: Late sequelae of poststreptococcal glomerulonephritis. Ann. Rev. Med. *27*:49, 1976.

Cameron, J. S.: Pathogenesis and treatment of membranous nephropathy. Kidney Int. *15*:88, 1979.

Cameron, J. S., and Clark, W. F.: A role for insoluble antibody-antigen complexes in glomerulonephritis? Clin. Nephrol. *18*:55, 1982.

Cattran, D. C., and Chodirker, W. B.: Experimental membranous glomerulonephritis. The relationship between circulating free antibody and immune complexes to subsequent pathology. Nephron *31*:260, 1982.

Cochrane, C. G.: Immunologic tissue injury mediated by neutrophilic leukocytes. Adv. Immunol. *9*:97, 1968.

di Belgiojoso, G. B., Tarantino, A., Bazzi, C., et al.: Immunofluorescence patterns in chronic membranoproliferative glomerulonephritis. Clin. Nephrol. *6*:303, 1976.

Dickson, F. J., Feldman, J. D., and Vasquez, J. J.: Experimental glomerulonephritis. The pathogenesis of a laboratory model resembling the spectrum of human glomerulonephritis. J. Exp. Med. *113*:899, 1961.

Douglas, M. F. S., Rabideau, D. P., Schwartz, M. M., and Lewis, E. J.: Evidence of autologous immune-complex nephritis. N. Engl. J. Med. *305*:1326, 1981.

Hinglais, N., Garcia-Torras, R., Kleinknecht, D.: Long term prognosis in acute glomerulonephritis. Am. J. Med. *52*:56, 1974.

Kark, R. M., Pirani, C. L., Pollak, V. E., et al.: The nephrotic syndrome in adults: A common disorder with many causes. Ann. Intern. Med. *49*:751, 1958.

Kluthe, R., Vogt, A., and Batsford, S. R. (Eds.): Glomerulonephritis: International Conference on Pathogenesis, Pathology and Treatment. New York, John Wiley & Sons, 1977.

Lambert, P. H., Perin, L. H., Mahieu, P., et al.: Activation of complement in human nephritis. Adv. Nephrol. *4*:79, 1974.

Lange, K. and Treser, G.: Acute poststreptococcal glomerulonephritis. Clin. Nephrol. *1*:55, 1973.

Lockwood, C. M., Rees, A. J., and Pearson, T. A.: Immunosuppression and plasma-exchange in the treatment of Goodpasture's syndrome. Lancet *1*:711, 1976.

MacIntosh, R. M., Tinglot, B., Kaufman, D., et al.: Immunohistology in renal disease: diagnostic, prognostic, therapeutic and etiology value and limitations. Q. J. Med. *40*:385, 1971.

McCluskey, R. T., and Classen, J.: Immunologically mediated glomerular tubular and interstitial renal disease. N. Engl. J. Med. *288*:564, 1973.

Merrill, J. P.: Glomerulonephritis. N. Engl. J. Med. *290*:257, 1974.

Peters, D. K., and Williams, D. G.: Complement and mesangial capillary glomerulonephritis: role of complement deficiency in pathogenesis of nephritis. Nephron *9*:189, 1974.

Taube, D., Brown, Z., and Williams, D. G.: Long term impairment of suppressor-cell function by cyclophosphamide in minimal-change nephropathy and its association with therapeutic response. Lancet *1*:235, 1981.

Wilson, C. B., and Dickson, F. J.: Immunopathology and glomerulonephritis. Ann. Rev. Med. *25*:83, 1974.

Wilson, C. B., and Dixon, F. J.: Antiglomerular basement membrane antibody induced glomerulonephritis. Kidney Int. *3*:74, 1973.

TUBULOINTERSTITIAL DISEASES (INTERSTITIAL NEPHRITIS)

Andres, G. A., and McClusky, R. T.: Tubular and interstitial disease due to immunological mechanisms. Kidney Int. *7*:271, 1975.

Drago, J. R., Rohner, T. J., Sanford, E. J., et al.: Acute interstitial nephritis. J. Urol. *115*:105, 1976.

Fuller, T. J., Barcenas, C. G., and White, M. G.: Diuretic induced interstitial nephritis. J.A.M.A. *235*:1998, 1976.

Lavelle, K. J., Aronoff, G. A., and Luft, F. C.: The effect of nonsteroidal anti-inflammatory agents on renal function. J. Ind. State Med. Assn. *75*:334, 1982.

Suki, W. N., and Eknoyan, G.: Tubulo-Interstitial diseases. *In* Brenner, B. M., and Rector, F. C., Jr. (Eds.): The Kidney. Philadelphia, W. B. Saunders Co., 1976, pp. 1113–1137.

Torres, V. E.: Present and future of the nonsteroidal anti-inflammatory drugs in nephrology. Mayo Clin. Proc. *57*:389, 1982.

Pulmonary Ventilation and Blood Gas Exchange*

W. Keith C. Morgan and Douglas Seaton

The primary purpose of the lungs is to maintain the oxygen and carbon dioxide content of the arterial blood within a relatively narrow range. This range must be maintained even though both oxygen need and carbon dioxide production are constantly changing with the degree of activity and metabolic rate of the subject. The lungs achieve this homeostasis by allowing venous blood to come into contact with the alveolar gases; such contact occurs over an enormous surface area, the alveolocapillary bed. Three basic mechanisms are involved in gas exchange: (1) *ventilation,* or, as it is often known, the "bellows" function of the lungs; (2) *diffusion,* or the transfer of gas from the alveolus to the capillary; and (3) *perfusion,* or pulmonary blood flow.

VENTILATION

The ventilatory capacity of the lungs depends first on their size (lung volumes), second on the resistance to flow present in the airways, and third on the elastic properties or compliance of the lungs and the chest wall. Movement of air into and out of the lungs can be compared with the action of a pair of bellows and is dependent on the pressure difference between the mouth and the alveoli at various phases of breathing. At times of no flow, alveolar and mouth pressures are equal. During *inspiration,* the thorax enlarges, the diaphragm descends, and, as a result, the chest cage increases in volume as do the lungs. In contrast, *expiration* is largely passive and depends on the elastic recoil of the chest wall and lungs. The pressure that acts on the lungs and causes them to expand during inspiration is that which exists in the pleural cavity. Intrapleural pressure is negative as compared with the atmospheric pressure, and during normal breathing it ranges between -5 and -9 cm of water. Much larger pressure changes occur during forced expiratory and inspiratory maneuvers; for example, at total lung capacity, the intrapleural pressure is -35 to -40 cm of water, whereas at residual volume the pressure may become slightly positive, especially at the lung bases. A detailed description of the mechanical

events involved in inspiration is beyond the scope of this chapter but can be found in *The Respiratory Muscles* by Campbell et al.

At this stage, it is necessary to point out that there is a gradient in pleural pressure from the top to the bottom of the lung. This gradient is largely gravity-dependent and is thought to be related to the weight of the lung. Pleural pressure increases from the apex to the base; there is a gradient of approximately 7 to 8 cm of water from top to bottom of the lung. This gradient has profound effects on regional ventilation and perfusion and will be discussed in more detail later in this chapter.

STATIC LUNG VOLUMES

Certain lung volumes can be measured with a spirometer; however, others require more complicated apparatus. The volume of each breath exhaled during quiet respiration is known as the *tidal volume (V_T)*. The total volume of air that the lungs and bronchial tree contain after maximal inspiration is known as the *total lung capacity (TLC)*. If the subject then exhales as much air as he can, the volume of air remaining in the lungs after the expiration is known as the *residual volume (RV);* that which has been expelled is known as the *vital capacity (VC)*. It must be stressed that during the measurement of VC, the patient is permitted to take as long as he likes to complete the maneuver. If after maximal inspiration, he exhales as rapidly and as forcibly as possible, then the measurement obtained is known as the forced vital capacity (FVC). In normal persons, the FVC and the VC are not significantly different; however, in certain types of airways obstruction (e.g., emphysema), the FVC may be considerably less than the vital capacity as a result of collapse of the smaller airways during forced expiration—a phenomenon known as air trapping. The volume of air remaining in the lung at the end of a normal expiration is known as the functional residual capacity (FRC), whereas the volume that can be exhaled from FRC is known as the *expiratory reserve volume (ERV)*. Similarly, the volume of air that can be taken in from FRC is known as the *inspiratory capacity (IC);* needless to say, the sum of the ERV and IC equals the VC (Fig. 15–1). The VC, ERV, and IC can be measured with a spirometer; TLC and its derivatives, FRC

*Much of this chapter was previously published in *Occupational Lung Disease* by W. K. C. Morgan and A. Seaton, Philadelphia, W. B. Saunders Company, 1975.

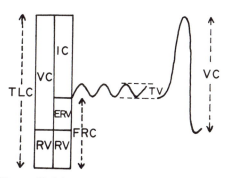

Figure 15–1 Lung volumes and spirometric tracing of a slow vital capacity maneuver in a normal subject.

and RV, require other means, namely, closed circuit helium equilibration, the nitrogen washout, a radiographic method, or plethysmography.

The helium equilibration method requires that the subject rebreathe a known volume of helium in a closed circuit until equilibration is reached. The carbon dioxide produced during the rebreathing is absorbed. If the volume of the helium reservoir is known, and if the initial and final concentrations of helium in the system are known, it is therefore possible to calculate the FRC. The nitrogen washout depends on giving the subject 100 per cent oxygen and collecting all the expired air in a large spirometer. When the nitrogen has been completely washed out from the lungs and collected along with the expired air in a Tissot spirometer, the volume of the expirate and the nitrogen concentration are measured. Since the concentration of nitrogen in the lungs at the start of the maneuver is known, it is possible to calculate the volume of nitrogen present in the lungs and hence the FRC.

The plethysmographic method is probably the best and most accurate way of determining lung volumes, since it measures all the gas in the thoracic cage. In contrast, the helium equilibration and nitrogen washout methods do not include regions of poorly ventilated lung that contain trapped gas (e.g., bullae are not included), and thus falsely low estimates are obtained. A body plethysmograph consists of an airtight box in which the subject sits. As the subject breathes in and out, the pressure inside the box changes and is recorded by sensitive transducers. If the change in lung volume with each breath is also known, then by simple application of Boyle's law it is possible to calculate the intrathoracic gas volume.

Total lung capacity can also be accurately determined from the chest film. Barnhard and his colleagues have described a method that utilizes anteroposterior and lateral films. The method depends on treating the lungs as a series of elliptical cylindroids and calculating the area of each. Allowance is made for heart size, pulmonary blood volume, the spine, and the domes of the diaphragm. The method has been simplified by Reger

and his coworkers. It is accurate and has application to epidemiologic surveys. If the VC is determined by spirometry, it then becomes possible to measure the RV and hence the RV/TLC.

In a healthy young adult, the residual volume (RV) is around 20 per cent of the TLC. As the subject grows older, the RV slowly increases so that by age 60 it may constitute up to 40 per cent of the TLC. The increase in RV is related to the fact that with increasing age the lung loses some of its elasticity. The decreased elastic recoil of the older person is opposed by an unchanged but relatively greater intrapleural pressure that maintains the lungs at a higher level of inflation than that present when the subject was younger. The increased lung volumes and associated increased radiographic translucency that occur with age used to be known as "senile emphysema"; however, since there is neither airways obstruction nor disruption of the alveolocapillary surface, that term is a misnomer.

In obstructive airways disease and emphysema, the RV/TLC is increased, and in many instances the RV may be well over 50 per cent of the TLC (Fig. 15–2). An increased RV/TLC is an almost invariable finding in air flow obstruction, but lesser increases in the ratio are sometimes seen in diffuse fibrosis such as fibrosing alveolitis and asbestosis. Such increases often are more apparent than real and frequently are related either to inadequacies in the predicted values for RV and TLC or, sometimes, to an appreciable decrease in TLC, with the RV being less affected. In most subjects with emphysema, the TLC is increased above the predicted figure owing to a decrease in the elastic recoil of the lungs; however, the increase in TLC is not as dramatic as is the increase in RV. In the diffuse fibroses, all the lung volumes tend to be smaller than the predicted figure, and this is particularly true of the VC and TLC (Fig. 15–3). In contrast, and for the aforementioned reasons, changes in RV are sometimes less spectacular in pulmonary fibrosis. Thus in an individual subject small increases in the RV/TLC are not necessarily diagnostic of any particular type of physiologic impairment. In many subjects,

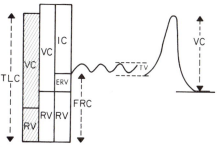

Figure 15–2 Lung volumes and spirometric tracing of a slow vital capacity maneuver in a subject with airways obstruction. The hatched area represents predicted values.

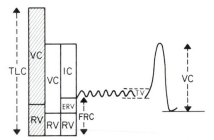

Figure 15–3 Lung volumes and spirometric tracing of a slow vital capcity in a subject with diffuse fibrosis. The hatched area represents predicted values.

there is a mixed effect, the subject having some degree of airways obstruction and subsequently contracting another disease that produces stiff and smaller lungs. In epidemiologic studies a knowledge of the RV/TLC in large groups of persons is much more useful than it is in the individual. Thus, the demonstration of an increased RV/TLC in a particular group of subjects as compared with an analogous control group indicates a higher prevalence of airways obstruction or emphysema.

DYNAMIC LUNG VOLUMES

Ventilatory capacity also depends to a large extent on the resistance to airflow in the bronchial tree. If a normal subject is asked to breathe in as far as possible and then to breathe out as rapidly and as forcibly as possible, he should be able to exhale 80 per cent of his FVC in one second ($FEV_{1.0}$) and 95 per cent in 3 seconds. Although this is true in the young subject, there is a fall in the $FEV_{1.0}$/FVC ratio with age. By the time the subject is 55 years or older, the ratio will often be approximately 65 to 70 per cent. Expiratory flows are most rapid early in the forced expiratory volume maneuver, but as the subject begins to approach RV there is a marked slowing. This is most evident once the subject gets below his FRC. When RV is reached, flow ceases entirely (Fig. 15–4). Subjects with airways obstruction—that is to say, those who have an increased resistance to flow of air into and out of their lungs, e.g., asthmatics, chronic bronchitics, and those with emphysema—

all show a flatter curve with decreased flow rates. In some instances, there is also a loss of VC. In asthma, but not in the other two conditions, the use of bronchodilators such as salbutamol and epinephrine by nebulization will appreciably lessen the obstruction so that the forced expiratory volume curve becomes steeper and more closely resembles that of a normal person. As indices of obstruction, both the 1-second and 3-second timed vital capacity tests (percentage of FVC exhaled in 1 and 3 seconds, respectively) are frequently used. Some workers, on the other hand, prefer to measure the actual volume of air exhaled in the first 0.75 second ($FEV_{0.75}$). A less popular but still commonly used measurement is the maximal expiratory flow rate (MEFR), this being the rate of flow between 200 and 1200 ml on a forced expiratory volume tracing. Another index that has its advocates is the FEF_{25-75} (MMF) or the maximal expiratory flow over the middle of a forced expiratory spirogram. The latter measurement is more sensitive but it is also more variable, and if the forced expiratory volume maneuver is not recorded for an adequate period, spurious results are frequently obtained. All these indices have their proponents, but there are valid reasons for preferring the $FEV_{1.0}$ and the FEF_{25-75}.

An additional method by which the ventilatory capacity can be assessed is the maximal breathing capacity (MBC). Preferably called *maximal voluntary ventilation* (MVV), this capacity is the maximal volume of air breathed over 1 minute. As the test is very tiring to subjects with airways obstruction, the volume is usually measured over a period of 15 to 20 seconds and the result multiplied by the necessary factor. This test is effort-dependent and has little advantage over the single breath tests. The simple expedient of multiplying the FEV_1 by 39 yields an excellent approximation to the measured MVV.

The normal respiratory rate (f) of a young adult is approximately 12 per minute. With increasing age, there is a rise to 14 or 16. Since the tidal volume is normally about 500 ml the minute ventilation is 12×500 ml = 6 L ($V_T \times$ f). Not all of every breath reaches the alveoli; some air remains in the nose, nasopharynx, and bronchi and therefore does not come into contact with the alveolocapillary surface. The non–gas-exchanging

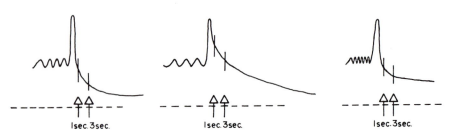

Figure 15–4 Forced expiratory volume maneuvers in a normal subject *(left)* and in subjects with obstructive *(center)* and restrictive *(right)* impairment.

part of the respiratory system is known as the anatomic dead space (V_{D_A}) and is normally about 150 ml. In a normal subject, the volume of gas reaching the alveoli with each breath is 500 − 150 ml = 350 ml ($V_T − V_{D_A}$). Alveolar ventilation per minute therefore equals 350 ml × 12 = 4.2 L. The anatomic dead space must be distinguished from the physiologic dead space (V_{D_P}), which consists of the anatomic dead space plus the fraction of each breath wasted, either to ventilate under-perfused alveolar units or to overventilate alveolar units relative to perfusion. In a normal subject, the anatomic and physiologic dead spaces are approximately the same, but with mismatching of ventilation and perfusion, the V_{D_P} increases. Lung volumes are generally expressed at the subject's body temperature saturated with water vapor and at 760 mm Hg (BTPS). When expressed at BTPS, the various indices represent the actual volume in the lungs.

AIRFLOW RESISTANCE

During quiet breathing, most of the respiratory effort goes toward overcoming the compliance of the lungs and chest wall. By comparison, the work necessary to overcome airflow resistance is small, but when breathing becomes deeper and more rapid, the work expended overcoming airways resistance increases rapidly. When the airways are narrowed or obstructed by mucus, there is a huge increase in airways resistance and the work of breathing, especially at lower lung volumes, at which the lumina of the airways normally are narrower.

Gas flow in the airways is governed by the same factors that regulate the flow of fluid in tubes or, if it comes to that, the flow of the electricity in a conductor. Ohm's law (C = E/R, where C is the current or flow, E the voltage or pressure gradient, and R the resistance) applies equally well to the flow of gas in the airways. Airflow may be either turbulent or laminar. When flow is turbulent, the pressure gradient necessary to produce a certain flow rate is appreciably higher. With laminar flow, the pressure gradient necessary to produce a certain flow is directly proportional to the viscosity of the gas. In contrast, for turbulent flow, the viscosity of the gas becomes less important and the density more important. Under normal circumstances flow in the larger airways tends to be turbulent, with eddy currents being set up at the bifurcation of the airways. In contrast, flow in the smaller airways (viz, from the twelfth generation and distally) is mainly laminar. Thus, flow in the central airways is mainly density-dependent, whereas in the smaller airways it is related more to the viscosity of the gases present. Poiseuille's law (P = K_1V, where P is driving pressure, V is flow, and K_1 is a constant that depends on the viscosity of the gas) applies only to laminar flow

in a straight line in a tube whose cross-sectional diameter does not change. Clearly this situation does not apply in lungs, where the cross-sectional diameter is constantly changing, where the airways are repeatedly dividing, and where, owing to disease, the diameter of the airways may be either narrowed and distorted or occasionally dilated. Nonetheless, despite all these variables, it is useful to apply to clinical situations the concept of airways resistance and the basic physical laws.

Airways resistance depends not only on the number of patent airways but also on the total cross-sectional area of the airways. The intrathoracic resistance of the airways may be partitioned into central and peripheral components. The central component includes the resistance from the trachea to roughly the eleventh generation of bronchi. The peripheral component is made up of the resistance from the twelfth generation to the alveoli. Central resistance in normal subjects constitutes 85 to 90 per cent of the total airways resistance (R_A). Thus, the peripheral resistance accounts for only 10 to 15 per cent of the total resistance and, moreover, at high lung volumes is negligible (Fig. 15–5). It is therefore possible for a subject to have diffuse disease of the small airways and yet have a normal airways resistance and normal spirometry. When the resistance in the peripheral airways is increased, the lungs become less distensible, although total resistance may still be within normal limits. The peripheral airways usually are not uniformly and diffusely affected; rather, the pathologic processes producing small airways disease tend to lead to patchy or regional involvement.

Airways resistance is normally expressed at FRC. This is related to the fact that the cross-sectional diameter of the airways varies greatly with lung volume. Thus, at TLC the airways are widely patent, and with expiration there is a fairly minor change in a cross-sectional diameter until

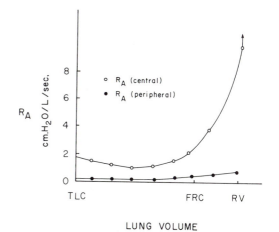

Figure 15–5 Relationship of central and peripheral airways resistance to lung volumes.

FRC is approached, at which time the airways start to narrow rapidly. For this reason, R_A remains relatively unchanged until FRC, at which time it starts to rise geometrically. It is also important to remember that in airways obstruction both the R_A and the FRC are likely to increase, although not always to the same extent.

Airways resistance can be measured directly in several ways. These include the body plethysmograph, the simultaneous recording of alveolar pressure and flow using an esophageal balloon, the interrupter technique, and also the oscillator method. A description of these various techniques is beyond the scope of the present chapter; however, suffice it to say that the plethysmographic method is to be preferred because it is most accurate in the clinical situation. There is little doubt that measurement of R_A in many instances adds little and is not as useful as is spirometry in most clinical situations. However, determination of R_A can be most useful in challenge tests and in the assessment of various bronchodilator drugs. Under the latter circumstances, objective measurements of resistance may be preferable to spirometry.

The normal airways resistance is around 1.5 cm H_2O/L/sec. In comparison, the nasal airflow resistance is two to three times as high. In emphysema, the airways are irreversibly obstructed, and R_A may be increased four- to sixfold, under which circumstances most of the increased resistance is located in the respiratory bronchioles and smaller airways. In asthma, even greater increases in R_A occur, but here the obstructions usually are located in both small and large airways.

COMPLIANCE OF THE LUNGS

Ventilation also depends on the compliance of the lungs. This is a measurement of the distensibility of the lungs and is expressed as the change in lung volume that occurs when the pressure gradient between the pleura and the alveoli is changed by 1 cm of water. It may be measured during breathholding (static compliance) or during regular breathing (dynamic compliance). If the increase in volume were directly proportional to the pressure change through the range of inflation and deflation, then a single value for static compliance would describe the elastic properties of the lungs. In reality this is not the case. The lungs become less compliant at high lung volumes; only in the tidal volume range is the relationship approximately linear. Lung compliance also depends on lung size, and the larger the lungs the more compliant they are. Thus an infant's lung is less compliant than is an adult's; likewise, there is disparity in the compliance of the lungs of large and small men. The reason for this can be clearly seen if one considers the hypothetical case of a man whose vital capacity is 5 L and whose static compliance is 0.2 L/cm H_2O. Under such circum-

stances, increasing his negative intrapleural pressure by 1 cm H_2O increases the volume of his lungs by 200 ml. Were he then to have one lung removed, this would reduce his vital capacity to 2.5 L, and a pressure change of 1 cm would then increase his lung volume by only 100 ml. In short, his compliance would be halved although the elastic properties of his lung would be unchanged. This is an oversimplification of the problem, since following pneumonectomy some compensatory overdistention of the remaining lung occurs. The latter phenomenon, nonetheless, is responsible for only a marginal increase in the volume of the remaining lung.

To get around the problem of lung size, a measurement known as specific compliance has been introduced. This relates compliance to lung volume and is obtained by dividing the static compliance by the FRC. If the lungs become stiff and fibrotic, as frequently occurs in asbestosis, sarcoidosis, berylliosis, and certain other diffuse fibroses, the compliance is markedly reduced, and values of 0.04 L/cm H_2O and less may be found. In subjects who have a marked reduction of compliance, the vital capacity usually is concomitantly decreased. In conditions in which the lung has lost elasticity, a small change of pressure may produce a large increase in lung volumes (Fig. 15–6). Under such circumstances, the lungs are said to be more compliant than normal. This is the usual state of affairs in emphysema and certain other conditions. Measurement of compliance usually is carried out by relating intrapleural pressure changes as reflected by changes in esophageal pressure to volume change in the lungs. Esophageal pressure is recorded by placing a cylindrical balloon attached to a fine plastic tube in the lower third of the esophagus. The measurement of compliance is objective, but care must be taken to see that the balloon is situated correctly.

Dynamic compliance may be defined as the ratio of tidal volume to the difference between pressure at end-inspiration and end-expiration at

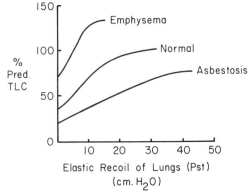

Figure 15–6 Pressure volume curves in a normal subject and in subjects with emphysema and diffuse fibrosis (e.g., asbestosis).

points of no flow during breathing. In normal subjects, measurement of dynamic compliance gives similar values to the static compliance; however, when airways resistance is increased an appreciable difference is often present. This is best explained by considering a state of affairs in which there is partial obstruction of a lobe or lung. In the unobstructed region, flow is maximal and there is an appropriate increase in flow volume for this area. In contrast, the flow of gases into the region with increased airways resistance takes place more slowly, thereby causing smaller increase in volume per head of pressure.

SURFACTANT

The compliance of the lungs also depends on the presence of surfactant. The latter is a substance that lines the alveoli and respiratory bronchioles and tends to prevent their collapse. Radford first demonstrated that animal lungs that had been filled with saline distended more easily than they did with air. This phenomenon suggests that saline either removed or rendered ineffective a substance that regulates the surface tension of the gas-tissue interface. Pattle subsequently showed that pulmonary edema fluid has a much lower surface tension than does plasma, an observation that suggests there is a substance lining the alveoli and influencing surface tension. Subsequently, Clements and his colleagues demonstrated that the surface retractive forces are appreciable during lung expansion; however, during deflation of the lungs and as the surface area contracts these forces decrease.

In normal subjects, there is a difference between the inspiratory and expiratory limbs of a pressure volume curve, a phenomenon usually referred to as *hysteresis*. By way of contrast, the saline-filled lung fails to show hysteresis, which suggests that the difference in the inspiratory and expiratory limbs in the normal subject is a consequence of a substance that regulates surface tension at the air-liquid interface. This substance has been shown to be surfactant, a complex of diapalmitoyl-lecithin with protein. It can be extracted from minced lungs or by washing out the lungs with saline. It appears to be secreted by the alveolar cells and has been shown to be present in decreased amounts in hyaline membrane disease, in conditions in which the blood flow to the lungs is decreased, and in sundry other conditions including the prolonged inhalation of 100 per cent oxygen.

IMPAIRMENT OF THE SMALL AIRWAYS FUNCTION

The detection of changes in air flow resistance and function in the small airways is a challenge

to the ingenuity of the physiologist, and several techniques have been devised that can be used to this end. Moreover, in many subjects such changes have been shown to be reversible and it has therefore been suggested that if the abnormalities are detected early before there are accompanying spirometric abnormalities, and if further exposure to the responsible agent is avoided, irreversible disease may be avoided. Whether such tests will prove useful in prognosticating whether a particular subject is going to develop irreversible airways obstruction remains undecided. Three approaches are at present popular:

1. Flow Volume Loop. The standard method of recording a forced expiratory volume maneuver plots volume against time. In contrast, the flow volume loop, as the name suggests, plots flow against volume. There are several types of flow volume curves and each needs a definition. The maximal expiratory flow volume curve (MEFV) is a plot of maximal expiratory flow (Vmax) against volume during a forced expiratory maneuver. The term flow volume loop refers to a loop obtained when a maximal forced expiration is followed immediately by forced maximal inspiration, both being presented on the same tracing.

The typical flow loops are shown in Figure 15–7. Peak flow is largely effort-dependent and is mainly a reflection of the state of the large airways. Flow at 50 per cent of vital capacity (FEF_{50}) reflects both large and small airways function, with the former probably predominating. The latter part of the curve is felt to represent flow in the smaller airways. Also shown in Figure 15–7 is the curve of a subject with airways obstruction.

Figure 15–8 shows a series of curves with different efforts. Although the peak flow varies, it can be seen that eventually the latter part of the curve blends with that of the MEFV; in short, there is a final common pathway. These phenomena stimulated Hyatt to construct isovolume pressure flow curves (IVPF), in which he measured transpulmonary pressure. These showed that as driving pressure increased, flow concomitantly in-

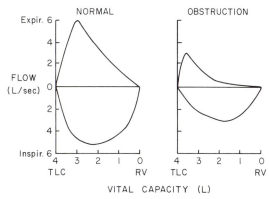

Figure 15–7 Flow volume loops of a normal subject and of a subject with airways obstruction.

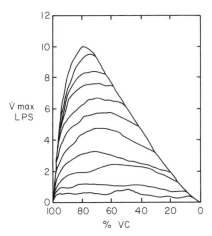

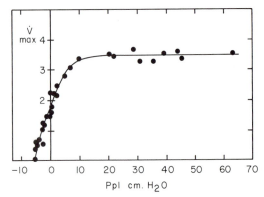

Figure 15–9 Isovolume pressure flow showing limitation of flow at pressure of 15 cm/H_2O.

Figure 15–8 Series of flow volume curves showing graded respiratory efforts and different inspiratory volumes.

creased until a maximal value was attained, after which further increases in pressure produced no further increase in flow (Fig. 15–9). Although flow usually is expressed as a percentage of vital capacity, it is preferable to relate it to total lung capacity (TLC) for the following reasons. When the MEFV is being used to evaluate bronchodilator drugs or to assess changes in air flow resistance over a relatively short period, for example, during challenge tests or when subjects may have been exposed to cotton dust or agents likely to produce an acute change in the airways, in some instances not only the flow rates decline but also lung volumes and VC may likewise show a decrease. Thus it is possible for a "before and after" challenge FEF_{50} when expressed as a percentage of VC to remain relatively unchanged; however, were the FEF_{50} related to TLC, a marked difference would become apparent.

In large airways, because flow is partly turbulent, the pressure necessary to produce a particular flow rate increases with gas density. In contrast, flow in the peripheral airways is for the most part laminar and therefore independent of gas density. If one measures airways resistance (R_A) when the subject is breathing a 4:1 helium and oxygen mixture (HeO_2) it is found that the R_A is substantially decreased. If a subject with peripheral airways obstruction alone breathes a helium-oxygen mixture, there is little change in R_A, since flow in small airways is mainly laminar. Since the effective pressure necessary to produce maximal flow is independent of the gas mixture breathed, and since the difference in flow between breathing air and helium-oxygen mixture is determined by how much the peripheral airways contribute to the total resistance, the higher the resistance to flow in the peripheral airways, the less will be the helium responses (Fig. 15–10).

At a particular lung volume, the flows of HeO_2 and air coincide. This is known as the point of identical flow (PIF). It is usually expressed as a percentage of vital capacity. In normal subjects it ranges from 0 to 6 per cent and is rarely elevated above 10 per cent. In small airways obstruction, it may be elevated to approximately 30 per cent (Fig. 15–10).

The flow volume curve is also useful in detecting obstructing lesions of the right and left

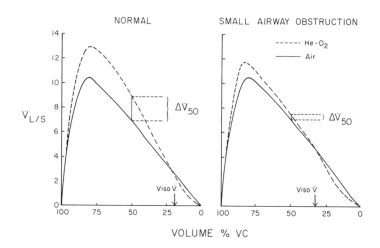

Figure 15–10 Helium-oxygen and air flow volume curves in a normal subject and in a subject with small airways obstruction. Note that the point of identical flow ($V_{iso}\dot{V}$) is farther from RV in the subject with small airways obstruction.

main bronchi, the trachea, and larynx. Figures 15–11, 15–12, and 15–13 show typical examples of the major airways obstruction. Figure 15–11 is a tracing from a subject with a variable extrathoracic obstruction, namely bilateral vocal cord paralysis. It is apparent that inspiratory flows are more affected than are expiratory flows. A variable intrathoracic obstruction (e.g., a tracheal cylindroma) is represented in the tracing shown in Figure 15–12. Expiratory flows are more affected because the trachea is compressed during exhalation. Figure 15–13 shows a fixed extrathoracic obstructive lesion in which inspiration and expiration are both affected (e.g., stenosis of the larynx following surgery or injury).

2. Closing Volume. It has been shown that small airways start to close somewhere between functional residual capacity (FRC) and residual volume (RV). Closure depends on the pressure difference acting on the wall of the airway and on the elastic properties of the small airways. If the lumina of peripheral airways are narrowed by mucus or some pathologic process or if the concentration of surfactant is reduced, the surface forces acting on the airways become greater and a tendency to collapse occurs.

Fowler originally observed that when a person exhaled to residual volume and then took a breath of oxygen and achieved total lung capacity (TLC), then during a subsequent slow expiratory maneuver, a tracing of the percentage of nitrogen exhaled showed four distinct phases (Fig. 15–14). In phase 1 there is an absence of nitrogen owing to the fact that the dead space contains pure oxygen. Phase 2 begins as the subject starts to exhale a mixture of gas from the dead space and alveoli; it is characterized by a sharp increase in the concentration of expired nitrogen. Phase 2 is followed by an alveolar plateau known as phase 3. In phase 4, there is an abrupt increase in the concentration of nitrogen. The junction of phases 3 and 4 is thought

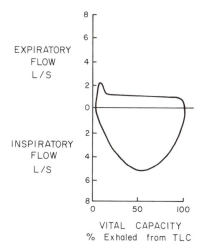

Figure 15–12 Flow volume curve showing variable intrathoracic obstruction.

to be the volume at which the basal airways close, and the volume between the junction of phases 3 and 4 and RV is known as *closing volume (CV)*. CV plus RV is known as *closing capacity (CC)*. The upward inflection at the end of phase 3 is best explained by the effects of gravity on the distribution of inspired gas. In a normal subject, there is a gradient of transpulmonary pressure from the top to the bottom of the lung. When a sitting or standing subject takes a breath from RV, the first portion of the breath is distributed to the apices, whereas the latter portions are distributed to the lower lobes. During a subsequent exhalation, the air that is exhaled first comes from both the upper and lower zones, but toward the end of the breath small airways in the lower zones close and the upper zones make a relatively greater contribution. This principle has been aptly named "first in–last out."

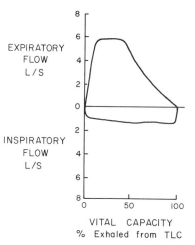

Figure 15–11 Flow volume curve showing variable extrathoracic obstruction.

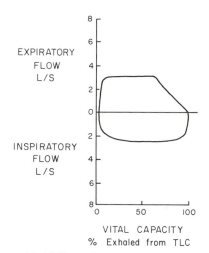

Figure 15–13 Flow volume curve showing fixed extrathoracic obstruction.

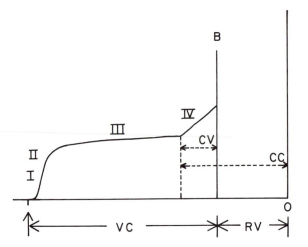

Figure 15–14 Single breath oxygen test showing the four phases.

FULL INSPIRATION

Measurement of closing volume can be carried out in several ways. The most simple is the resident nitrogen method, in which the subject takes a breath of 100 per cent oxygen. The nitrogen remaining in the airways forms a bolus of tracer gas. Other methods involve labeling the inspired air with a foreign gas such as argon, xenon, or helium. Differences in measurement of closing volume in the same subject have been noted according to the method used. A normal closing volume implies that the distribution of inspired gases is mainly dependent on gravity and that the lungs empty relatively homogeneously. When filling and emptying become discordant, the principle of "first in–last out" is broken, and a closing volume may not be apparent on the tracing. Phase 3 represents gas coming from alveoli, and as such the alveoli must contain different concentrations of nitrogen in order to account for the slope. The steepness of the slope is therefore an indication of abnormal distribution, since the concentration of nitrogen in each alveolus after a breath of oxygen depends on how much oxygen enters each alveolus.

Measurement of CV is influenced by the rate at which the inspired breath is taken, by expiratory flow, and by prolonged breath-holding, which leads to absorption of a greater percentage of oxygen. Expiratory flow should be regulated to between 0.4 and 0.5 L/sec. CV, CV/VC%, and CC/TLC% all have higher coefficients of variation than do the FEV_1 and FVC. In this regard, CV and CV/VC% are the most variable, namely, 20 to 25 per cent. Moreover, whereas intelligent subjects have no difficulty in carrying out the CV maneuver, its applicability in field studies is severely limited by the inability of a substantial proportion of the less well-educated population to carry out the respiratory maneuvers in a satisfactory fashion. Abnormalities of CV, in the presence of normal spirometry, have been reported in obese individuals,

cigarette smokers, asthmatics in remission, coal miners, and patients with skeletal deformities such as kyphosis. As such, an elevated CV is thought to indicate early disease; nonetheless, the prognostic significance of CV remains a topic of controversy.

3. Frequency Dependence of Dynamic Compliance. The history of the development of this technique begins with the mechanical time constant theory elaborated by Otis and coworkers and used to explain the relationship between mechanical factors and the intrapulmonary distribution of inspired gas. Theory suggests that differences in time constants (resistance × compliance) between parallel lung units would be associated with a decrease in dynamic compliance as breathing frequency increased. This would mean that a progressively smaller portion of the lung would be ventilated as breathing frequency increased.

Macklem and Mead reported that the time constants of the distal lung units (airways smaller than about 2 mm) were in the order of 0.01 sec. They concluded that a fourfold difference in these time constants would cause dynamic compliance to fall with any increase in respiratory frequency because there would be less time for air to enter and leave the affected regions. Thus, an increased resistance to flow in the smaller airways should lead to a fall in dynamic compliance at faster rates of breathing. This raised the possibility that the frequency dependence of dynamic compliance could be used as a test of obstruction in peripheral airways.

For widespread time constant discrepancies to occur, the obstruction must be unevenly distributed; that is, some airways must remain patent while others are narrowed. Other criteria must be met before it can be assumed that frequency-dependent dynamic compliance is a consequence of peripheral airway narrowing rather than of lesions in large airways or other parts of the lung. If the static pressure/volume (compliance) curve of the lung is normal, then it is not likely that frequency-dependent dynamic compliance is due to abnormal elastic properties of the lung. It has been assumed that regional differences in elastic properties sufficient to cause a detectable fall in dynamic compliance at rapid respiratory rates should result in an abnormal static compliance curve. Thus, if a patient has normal pulmonary resistance, spirometry, and static pressure/volume curve, any fall in dynamic complicance with increased frequency of respiration (frequency-dependent compliance) is assumed to be due to peripheral airways obstruction. The time constants and ventilation of peripheral gas-exchanging units of the lung will be affected by the following:

1. Regional obstruction due to bronchiolar narrowing or obstruction by mucus.

2. Regional increases in elastic recoil produced by the interstitial fibroses; for example, in asbestosis and berylliosis.

3. Regional loss of elastic recoil with airways collapse; for example, in centrilobular emphysema and the focal emphysema of coalworkers' pneumoconiosis (CWP).

All three of these pathologic processes may lead to unequal time constants in the lung and hence to an uneven distribution of ventilation that is more pronounced at faster rates of ventilation. All should produce a fall in dynamic compliance at higher respiratory rates.

The detection of frequency-dependent dynamic compliance involves measuring dynamic compliance at various rates of respiration (e.g., 20, 40, 60, and 80 breaths/minute). The dynamic changes in volume are obtained using a pneumotachograph; the intrapleural pressure changes are measured with an esophageal balloon.

WORK OF BREATHING

A certain amount of energy is expended with each breath we take. Part of the energy expenditure is related to moving air into and out of the lungs, and part to moving the thoracic cage and diaphragm. Normal values for the work of breathing are 0.5 kg./m²/min. at rest and up to 250 kg./m²/min. with a maximal voluntary ventilation maneuver. In asthma and emphysema, the main increase in the work of breathing is related to overcoming the increased airflow resistance; in pulmonary fibrosis the additional work is necessary to overcome the stiffness of the lungs. The respiratory muscles under normal circumstances use about 2 to 4 per cent of the energy requirements at rest, but in disease they may use 30 to 40 per cent.

REGIONAL DISTRIBUTION OF VENTILATION AND PERFUSION

VENTILATION

Quantitative studies of the regional distribution of gas over large zones of excised lung using radioactive xenon have shown relatively even distribution of inspired gas per unit lung volume. The situation in life, with the lungs suspended within the chest wall, is very different in that the intrapleural pressure is no longer uniform as in the isolated preparation. Instead, in the erect posture there is a vertical gradient of intrapleural pressure, with a progressive reduction in pressure from the base to the apex of the lung. As the static transpleural pressure (i.e., pressure difference between pleural surface and atmosphere, during breath-holding with the glottis open) is more negative at the apex, the upper zone alveoli tend to be more expanded than those in the lower zones. An analogy is a loosely coiled spring that, when suspended by its uppermost coil, becomes progressively more expanded by its own weight from bottom to top (Fig. 15–15). The pleural pressure

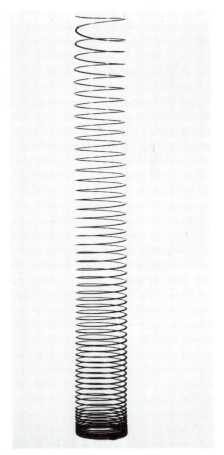

Figure 15–15 A spring suspended by the uppermost coil showing the relative separation of the coils at the top and bottom.

gradient in the chest always occurs in the direction of gravitational pull; thus, in a supine subject the differences in alveolar expansion occur dorsoventrally. Because of these regional differences in alveolar expansion, the static lung compliance of the more stretched upper zones is less than that of the lower zones in the erect posture, and therefore during tidal breathing at low flow rates basal ventilation tends to exceed that of the apices. As inspiratory flow rate increases, regional airways resistance is thought to become more influential than compliance in determining regional ventilation, which is then more evenly distributed. It is of note that in elderly normal subjects, particularly in the supine posture, regional ventilation may be altered by small airways closure occurring in dependent lung zones during tidal breathing and that this may result in a reduction in arterial oxygen tension.

PERFUSION

Studies using a variety of different radioactive tracer techniques have also demonstrated that pulmonary perfusion is not uniformly distributed and that there is a vertical gradient of increasing pulmonary perfusion per unit lung volume from apex to base in the erect posture, apart from some reduction over the most dependent 6 to 10 cm of lung. West and Hughes have explained these regional differences in terms of the interaction of pulmonary arterial, venous, alveolar, and interstitial pressures in the lungs (Fig. 15–16). In zone 1 of the upright lung there is no pulmonary arterial perfusion because pericapillary lung pressure, which under static conditions can be thought of as "alveolar" pressure, exceeds pulmonary arterial pressure at this level, and alveolar vessels therefore collapse. The junction of zones 1 and 2, at which pulmonary arterial perfusion commences, is represented by the height of a column of blood in an open manometer tube connected to the pulmonary artery. Below this level, pulmonary arterial pressure exceeds atmospheric pressure and can therefore open the vessels, perfusion increasing down this zone as the hydrostatic pressure of the column of pulmonary arterial blood rises. The amount of perfusion at any level in this zone is determined by the difference between the pulmonary arterial and alveolar pressures, which still exceeds pulmonary venous pressure. In zone 3, pulmonary venous pressure now also exceeds alveolar pressure. Here there is a continued slower increase in perfusion that is probably due to distention of intra-alveolar vessels as a result of a continued increase in the hydrostatic pressure in both pulmonary artery and pulmonary vein, whereas alveolar pressure remains atmospheric. Zone 4 was added to this scheme when it was observed that there was some fall-off of basal blood flow, particularly at lung volumes below functional residual capacity. This is attributed to a lung volume–related change in the resistance of extra-alveolar pulmonary vessels, whose caliber is related to changes in surrounding interstitial pressure rather than alveolar pressure.

REGIONAL VARIATION IN THE MATCHING OF VENTILATION AND PERFUSION

Although in the normal lung both alveolar ventilation ($\dot{V}_A$) and perfusion ($\dot{Q}$) vary regionally in the same direction, according to vertical gravity-dependent gradients, the rate of increase of perfusion from apex to base is steeper than that for ventilation. Consequently, the regional matching of $\dot{V}_A$ to $\dot{Q}$, which may be conveniently expressed as $\dot{V}_A/\dot{Q}$ ratios, is not uniform, but decreases down the length of the lung. The total $\dot{V}_A/\dot{Q}$ ratio for a normal upright lung with cardiac output of approximately 6 L per minute and alveolar ventilation of 5 L per minute lies between 0.8 and 0.9; however, regional $\dot{V}_A/\dot{Q}$ ratios vary considerably, ranging from about 3.3 at the apex to 0.6 at the lung base. The predilection of postprimary pulmonary tuberculosis for the lung apices has been attributed to the high apical $\dot{V}_A/\dot{Q}$ ratio, which results in an alveolar oxygen tension and hence tissue tension over 40 mm Hg higher than that at the lung base. This idea is supported by observations of a higher incidence of this disease in patients with pulmonary stenosis whose apical perfusion is further reduced. Conversely, tuberculosis usually affects the lung *bases* in bats, since they hang upside down. Regional alterations in the normal pattern of $\dot{V}_A/\dot{Q}$ matching are important as they determine the overall efficiency of the lung in its principal function as a gas-ex-

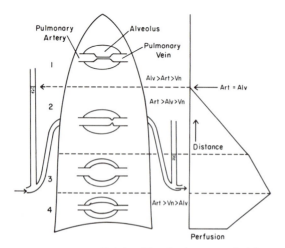

Figure 15–16 Relationship of pulmonary arterial, venous, alveolar, and interstitial pressures in the various zones of the lung. (Based on West, J. B.: J. Appl. Physiol. *17*:893, 1962.)

changer. Exercise and the assumption of the supine position even out the regional differences. In disease, most abnormalities of gas exchange result from mismatching of ventilation and perfusion, and these inequalities may be expressed in terms of wasted blood flow or ventilation.

Wasted Perfusion. If an alveolus is totally unventilated but remains perfused ($\dot{V}_A/\dot{Q} = 0$), the distal end of the capillary supplying it will still contain blood of venous composition, and perfusion will have been useless and is often referred to as a "true shunt." Suppose that the supply of fresh air to the alveolus is not completely interrupted but merely reduced disproportionately to its blood supply. It may be felt intuitively that some of the perfusion is still surplus to the requirements of that alveolus. We can imagine that the reduced amount of inspired gas will be totally accommodated by some fraction of the same volume of perfusing blood, and the rest will remain venous. In both these situations "venous" blood will mix with arterialized blood, reducing its oxygen content and increasing its carbon dioxide content. This process, which is called "shunting," or "venous admixture," may, if sufficient alveoli are involved, produce measurable changes in the gas tensions of arterial blood. It should be noted that both oxygen and carbon dioxide transfer are impaired in shunting; however, usually the respiratory center responds to hypercarbia by increasing ventilation, which lowers the P_{CO_2} of ventilated alveoli. Since the carbon dioxide dissociation curve is nearly linear (Fig. 15–17), this will be accompanied by an approximately equal fall in CO_2 content for a given fall in P_{CO_2} over the physiologic range and, as a result, in shunts a normal arterial P_{CO_2} can usually be maintained. In the absence of a hyperventilatory response, carbon dioxide retention would occur. Arterial oxygen content is less easily maintained because increasing the P_{O_2} of relatively well-ventilated alveoli on the flat part of the nonlinear oxyhemoglobin dissociation curve (Fig. 15–18) will produce only minimal improvement in the oxygen saturation of the blood perfus-

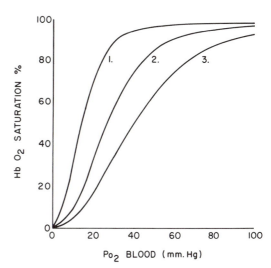

Figure 15–18 Oxygen dissociation curves showing right and left shifts. (See text for explanation.)

ing these units, which cannot therefore compensate for unventilated units. The arterial blood gas abnormality most commonly found in significant shunts is a lowered arterial P_{O_2} in the presence of a normal or low arterial P_{CO_2}.

The direct passage of blood from the arterial to the venous side of the pulmonary circulation without any contact with ventilated alveoli is called "true shunting," and it is physiologically indistinguishable from the small amount of anatomic shunting that occurs in normal individuals through the bronchial circulation and thebesian veins of the heart. Any remaining shunt is due to alveoli with low $\dot{V}_A/\dot{Q}$ ratios and is really a shunt-like effect or physiologic shunt. Total shunt in a resting normal individual does not usually exceed 5 per cent of the cardiac output, of which true shunt accounts for about 2 per cent.

Wasted Ventilation. Now consider the opposite situation of a normally ventilated alveolus receiving no perfusion ($\dot{V}_A/\dot{Q}$ = infinity). This alveolus will act as an extra space in which air is moved to and fro without participating in gas exchange and is therefore dead space or wasted ventilation. In terms of function, this dead space produces the same effect as an enlargement of the anatomic dead space, which comprises the whole of the nonalveolated respiratory tract from the mouth and nose to the respiratory bronchioles. If the perfusion of the alveolus is not completely interrupted but only reduced disproportionately to its ventilation, a fraction of that ventilation will be sufficient to meet the gas-exchanging potential of the reduced blood flow, and the remaining ventilation is therefore useless. This process will also contribute to alveolar dead space. Alveolar dead space is therefore the volume of inspired gas entering alveoli but not taking part in gas exchange due to local $\dot{V}_A/\dot{Q}$ imbalance. It is more conceptual and less tangible than anatomic dead space, which,

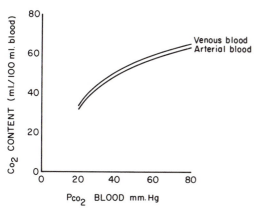

Figure 15–17 Carbon dioxide dissociation curve.

as it is a volume contained within a physical structure, is easier to picture. Alveolar and anatomic dead space together are conventionally referred to as physiologic dead space. The measured physiologic dead space in health is usually not more than 30 per cent of the tidal volume.

If anatomic dead space is increased artificially, for example, by mouth breathing through a length of tube, and if the rate and depth of breathing are unaltered, less fresh air will reach the alveoli with each inspiration. It follows that alveolar P_{O_2} will fall and alveolar P_{CO_2} rise, with consequent hypoxemia and hypercapnia. Suppose now that alveolar dead space is increased by relative underperfusion of a group of normally ventilated alveoli, and that the rate and depth of breathing and overall pulmonary perfusion remain unaltered. Although the oxygen tension of the reduced volume of blood perfusing these alveoli will be increased, it will be insufficient to compensate for a greater reduction of oxygen tension in blood coming from other normally ventilated alveoli, which become overperfused as they receive additional blood that normally would have been directed to the first group of alveoli. The result will be a reduction in arterial oxygen tension. Even though overall alveolar ventilation may remain normal, wasted regional ventilation will also reduce carbon dioxide exchange, tending to produce a raised arterial carbon dioxide tension. In disease this tendency is often corrected by compensatory hyperventilation, although hypoxemia often persists.

ALVEOLOARTERIAL OXYGEN GRADIENT [(A—a)Do₂]

Were the matching of ventilation and perfusion perfect, with the assumption that gas diffusion occurred across the alveolocapillary membrane to equilibrium, arterial and alveolar oxygen tensions would be equal. When mismatching occurs, an alveoloarterial oxygen tension difference (A—a)D_{O_2} will develop. The measurement of arterial oxygen tension is easy, but that of average alveolar oxygen tension presents problems. Although end-expiratory samples of alveolar gas may not be contaminated by dead space air in normal subjects, in pulmonary disease some lung units may take much longer to empty than others, so that end-expiratory P_{O_2} measured at the mouth changes continually, and spot sampling introduces error. Consequently, for clinical purposes "ideal" alveolar P_{O_2} is estimated indirectly. This is the alveolar P_{O_2} that would be found in a given subject if, for the same overall rate of consumption of oxygen and production of carbon dioxide, ventilation and perfusion were to become perfectly matched throughout the lung. The calculation requires the analysis of an expired air and arterial blood sample. A simplified version of the ideal alveolar gas equation is

$$\text{ideal } PA_{O_2} = PI_{O_2} - \frac{Pa_{CO_2}}{R}$$

where PI_{O_2} is the inspired oxygen tension, Pa_{CO_2} is the arterial carbon dioxide tension, and R is the respiratory quotient (rate of production of carbon dioxide divided by the rate of uptake of oxygen, which usually is 0.8). The ideal (A—a)D_{O_2} underestimates true (A—a)D_{O_2} because it fails to account for alveoli with a raised P_{O_2} due to high $\dot{V}_A/\dot{Q}$ ratios. It is used as a nonspecific indicator of impaired gas exchange due to diffusion or distribution abnormalities. It remains normal (4 to 15 mm Hg) in patients with overall alveolar hypoventilation and is increased by hyperventilation, whether voluntary or induced by anxiety (Table 15–1).

ESTIMATION OF SHUNT

Physiologic shunt (anatomic plus alveolar shunt) may be estimated using the following equation:

$$\frac{\dot{Q}s}{\dot{Q}} = \frac{Ci_{O_2} - Ca_{O_2}}{Ci_{O_2} - C\bar{v}_{O_2}}$$

where $\dot{Q}s/\dot{Q}$ is the proportion of total pulmonary flow taking part in the shunt, Ca_{O_2} and $C\bar{v}_{O_2}$ are the arterial and mixed venous oxygen contents, and Ci_{O_2} is the ideal arterial oxygen content (that which would result from an arterial P_{O_2} equal to the ideal alveolar P_{O_2}) which can be obtained from a knowledge of the ideal alveolar P_{O_2}, by use of the oxyhemoglobin dissociation curve. True shunt (anatomic shunt plus shunt through totally ventilated alveoli) may be separated from shuntlike effects (alveoli with low $\dot{V}_A/\dot{Q}$ ratios) by the administration of 100 per cent oxygen for 20 minutes. This washes out all alveolar nitrogen and fully oxygenates even poorly ventilated alveoli (alveolar P_{O_2} approximately 670 mm Hg), thereby abolishing shuntlike effects. The only possible cause for persisting hypoxemia in this situation is a true shunt, where venous blood unexposed to ventilated

TABLE 15–1 CHANGES IN ARTERIAL BLOOD GASES AND (A–a)O₂ GRADIENT IN VARIOUS PHYSIOLOGIC IMPAIRMENTS

	P_{O_2}	P_{CO_2}	(A–a)D_{O_2}
Regional $\dot{V}_A/\dot{Q}$ mismatching	↓	↑ or N or ↓	↑
"Pure" diffusion block	↓	N or ↓	↑
Overall alveolar hypoventilation	↓	↑	N
Overall alveolar hyperventilation	N or ↑	↓	↑

alveoli continues to dilute oxygenated blood. It should be noted that the arterial P_{O_2} will rise to some extent in true shunts owing to the increased alveolar P_{O_2}, and only in large shunts (greater than 25 per cent of the cardiac output) will the blood remain desaturated. A widened $(A—a)D_{O_2}$ will persist in true shunts but not in shuntlike effects.

ESTIMATION OF PHYSIOLOGIC DEAD SPACE AND EFFECTIVE ALVEOLAR VENTILATION

Physiologic dead space (anatomic dead space plus alveolar dead space) may be estimated using Bohr's equation in terms of alveolar and mixed expired P_{CO_2}:

$$V_{DP} = V_T \frac{(PA_{CO_2} - P\bar{E}_{CO_2})}{PA_{CO_2}}$$

The difficulties inherent in measuring average alveolar P_{CO_2} are avoided by equating it to arterial P_{CO_2} (equals ideal alveolar P_{CO_2}). The proportion of the tidal volume (V_T) made up by the physiologic dead space V_{DP} may now be shown by the following equation:

$$\frac{V_{DP}}{V_T} = \frac{Pa_{CO_2} - P\bar{E}_{CO_2}}{Pa_{CO_2}}$$

Alveolar ventilation has already been defined in terms of anatomic dead space and minute ventilation. If the physiologic dead space is known, it is possible to estimate the effective alveolar ventilation, this being the proportion of total ventilation being used effectively in carbon dioxide exchange according to the following equation:

$$\underset{ml/min}{V_A (eff)} = \underset{breaths/min}{f} \times \underset{ml}{(V_T - V_{DA})}$$

In clinical practice, however, arterial P_{CO_2} alone is generally taken as a reliable and readily available indicator of the level of effective alveolar ventilation. Hypoventilation, by reducing the delivery of fresh air to gas-exchanging areas, inevitably reduces arterial P_{O_2} and increases arterial P_{CO_2}. The resultant hypoxemia may be eliminated by the administration of a high concentration of oxygen, but the raised arterial P_{CO_2} cannot be corrected unless the level of alveolar ventilation is increased. Conversely, conditions that result in effective alveolar hypoventilation are associated with a lowered arterial P_{CO_2}. This may be seen in hysterical overbreathing and occasionally following the hyperventilatory response to hypoxemia found in diffusion impairment or ventilation-perfusion mismatching in which sufficient normal lung tissue remains to eliminate carbon dioxide.

THE TRANSPORT OF GASES BY THE BLOOD

In a mixture of different gases, the pressure exerted by each of the constituents—commonly referred to as the partial pressure (P)—is the product of its fractional concentration by volume and the total pressure of the mixture. For inspired air containing 20.93 per cent oxygen, 0.03 per cent carbon dioxide, and 79 per cent nitrogen and other inert gases, whose total pressure is 760 mm Hg (barometric pressure at sea level) and whose water vapor pressure is 10 mm Hg, the P_{O_2} will be as follows:

$$\frac{20.93}{100} \times (760 - 10) = 157 \text{ mm Hg}$$

Water vapor pressure is subtracted because volumes of gases are conventionally estimated dry. Similarly the atmospheric P_{CO_2} will be 0.2 mm Hg and the P_{N_2} 592 mm Hg. If a mixture of gases is brought into contact with a fluid, then the constituent gases will continue to diffuse into it until their partial pressures in solution are equal to those of the gas phase. At this point equilibration is said to have occurred. The partial pressure of a gas in fluid is often referred to as its *tension*.

The content of a gas in a fluid is derived from the product of the gas's solubility coefficient (α) and its partial pressure and is expressed in ml of gas measured at standard temperature and pressure dry (STPD) per 100 ml of liquid or in volumes per cent. The solubility coefficient of oxygen is 0.003 ml/100 ml/mg Hg, and its average partial pressure in the alveoli is approximately 100 mm Hg. This is less than that of atmospheric air because of mixing with oxygen-depleted and carbon dioxide–rich gas already present in the lung and since it also becomes saturated with water vapor during its passage to the gas-exchanging surfaces, the saturated water vapor pressure at 37° C being 47 mm Hg. The average content of dissolved oxygen in pulmonary capillary plasma at equilibrium with alveolar air will therefore be $0.003 \times 100 = 0.3$ ml/100 ml.

A normal resting subject's oxygen requirement is around 300 ml/min, and were all dissolved oxygen in the plasma removed by the tissues on each complete circuit, the minimum cardiac output necessary to support life would be 60 L/min, a level impossible to sustain. This difficulty is overcome by the reversible binding of most oxygen to hemoglobin, of which whole blood contains approximately 15 gm/100 ml. Hemoglobin is a tetramer formed by a globulin molecule bound to four heme molecules, each of which may react with a single oxygen molecule. This complex structure is capable of binding 1.34 ml of oxygen/gm, and the hemoglobin capacity is therefore $1.34 \times 15 = 20.1$ ml/100 ml. Percentage saturation is the oxygen content, which may be measured by Van Slyke's method, and expressed as a percentage of the blood oxygen-carrying capacity.

OXYHEMOGLOBIN DISSOCIATION CURVE

The content of a gas dissolved in fluid, expressed in volumes per cent, is related to its partial pressure in a linear fashion (Henry's law). This contrasts markedly with the S-shaped relationship of blood oxygen tension to saturation that results from the presence of hemoglobin (Fig. 15–18). The curve owes its distinctive shape to the so-called *heme-heme reaction,* in which the oxygenation of each heme molecule in the tetramer in turn affects the oxygen affinity of the other subunits, so that the molecule as a whole has four successive equilibrium constants. Notice that the upper part of the curve is relatively flat, so that a drop in oxygen tension from 100 to 60 mm Hg is associated with a relatively small fall in oxygen saturation. As a result, persons who live at an altitude of 10,000 feet, at which the alveolar Po_2 is about 60 mm Hg, still maintain an oxygen saturation of about 90 per cent, which is clearly to their advantage. Conversely, a rise in the Po_2 of arterial blood in this range produces only a minimal increase in oxygen saturation. Consequently, hyperventilation of normal lung tissue may be unable to compensate for hypoxemia resulting from areas of impaired gas exchange elsewhere. The lower, steeper part of the curve is also physiologically important, as a small fall in the Po_2 of blood is associated with a relatively large change in its oxygen content. Thus, the transfer of oxygen from blood to metabolically active tissues is facilitated.

FACTORS AFFECTING THE OXYHEMOGLOBIN DISSOCIATION CURVE

The relation of the Po_2 of blood to hemoglobin saturation may be altered by a number of factors that are capable of causing a "shift" of the oxyhemoglobin dissociation curve to either the right or the left, so that the flat part of the curve corresponding to high hemoglobin saturations is either expanded or contracted (Fig. 15–18). The most important of these factors are pH, Pco_2, 2,3-diphosphoglycerate level (2,3 DPG), and temperature. These shifts may be defined in terms of the Po_2 of blood at which hemoglobin is half saturated (P_{50}). If the oxyhemoglobin dissociation curve shifts to the right, the P_{50} rises, and with a shift to the left, it falls. Although it might at first seem that a raised P_{50} would be disadvantageous, since a smaller amount of oxygen is being transported for a given Po_2, careful examination of the diagram shows that as a result of the shape of curve 3, a raised P_{50} implies that for a given reduction in arterial Po_2 in the physiologic range, a greater amount of oxygen becomes available to the tissues.

If on passing through the systemic capillaries the Po_2 of arterial blood falls from 90 to 40 mm Hg (arteriovenous O_2 difference), then according to curve 2 the oxygen saturation would fall by only 20 per cent, whereas if curve 3 is applied, the fall would be 40 per cent.

When hemoglobin is oxygenated, hydrogen ions are released from the molecule. If the pH of the red cell, which is linearly related to that of the plasma, is reduced by the addition of hydrogen ions, then by the principle of mass action, this process tends to reverse, hemoglobin reverting to its deoxygenated state with the release of oxygen. In practice metabolically active tissues constitute a more acid environment for the blood perfusing them as a result of the local production of CO_2 and lactic acid, and this low pH therefore assists the transfer of more oxygen to the tissues for the same arteriovenous fall in Po_2. In other words, a fall in pH results in an increase in P_{50}, or shift of the oxyhemoglobin dissociation curve to the right. This is known as the *Bohr effect.* It might be thought that the reduced oxygen affinity of venous blood that is more acid would be detrimental to the uptake of oxygen in the lungs; however, at a higher Po_2, the dissociation curves come closer together and oxygen uptake is little affected. P_{50} may be altered by a change of either pH or Pco_2, for the shift to the right will still occur if pH is kept constant and Pco_2 increased, showing the latter has an effect independent of pH.

The organic phosphate 2,3 DPG is an intermediate in erythrocyte carbohydrate metabolism and constitutes most of the phosphate in red cells. If the concentration of 2,3 DPG is increased, it competes with oxygen for binding sites on deoxygenated hemoglobin, thereby reducing its oxygen affinity, shifting the oxyhemoglobin dissociation curve to the right. The level of 2,3 DPG is regulated by erythrocyte enzyme systems that are pH-dependent, so that acidity or alkalinity tends to suppress or stimulate its production, respectively. We have seen that a fall in plasma pH causes an immediate shift of the curve to the right, thereby reducing the affinity of hemoglobin for oxygen. If this fall in pH persists for several hours, 2,3 DPG production is reduced, exerting a counterbalancing effect on the pH-mediated right shift. Consequently, when long-standing acidosis is quickly corrected with bicarbonate, a persisting low 2,3 DPG level may have a deleterious "overshoot effect" by increasing the oxygen affinity of hemoglobin and reducing its supply to the tissues. Deoxygenated hemoglobin, which is a weaker acid and therefore relatively alkaline, stimulates 2,3 DPG production, reducing the affinity of hemoglobin for oxygen and causing the shift to the right that is associated with long-standing hypoxemic conditions such as cyanotic heart disease and chronic bronchitis. Similarly, the rise in plasma alkalinity that occurs at high altitudes causes a shift to the left with increased hemoglobin-oxygen affinity and also stimulates 2,3 DPG production, which has a counteraction. Other situations in which 2,3 DPG may be depleted with a reduction in blood oxygen-transferring efficiency include the storage of transfusable blood, hypophosphatemia, certain congenital hemoglobinopathies, and the raised blood levels of carboxyhemoglobin associated with cigarette smoking.

A rise in the temperature of blood reduces the oxygen affinity of hemoglobin and facilitates its removal by metabolizing tissues, the temperature of which is slightly higher than that of the lungs.

CARBON DIOXIDE TRANSPORT

The partial pressure gradient between metabolizing tissues and the capillaries perfusing them results in the diffusion of carbon dioxide into the blood, in which it is carried in three forms: (1) in solution in plasma, (2) combined with hemoglobin, and (3) as bicarbonate (Fig. 15–19). Plasma alone is an inefficient carrier of carbon dioxide, and only 5 per cent of total carbon dioxide is carried in this way. Although the volume of dissolved carbon dioxide is linearly related to the P_{CO_2} of blood, the slope of this relationship is not steep enough to enable the elimination of sufficient carbon dioxide by the lungs to keep pace with its production by the tissues. A small proportion of dissolved carbon dioxide in the plasma reacts with water to form carbonic acid, which then ionizes according to the equation:

$$CO_2 + H_2O \rightleftarrows H_2CO_3 \rightleftarrows H^+ + HCO_3^- \text{ (equation 1)}$$

Carbon dioxide also diffuses into red blood cells, and here the aforementioned reaction proceeds

rapidly as a result of the action of the enzyme carbonic anhydrase. This results in a concentration gradient of bicarbonate between the erythrocyte and the plasma, so that bicarbonate diffuses out of the cell in exchange for chloride, which passes in to maintain electrical neutrality, a process known as the *chloride shift*. The hydrogen ions are largely buffered by hemoglobin, although venous blood is rendered slightly more acid than arterial blood. Ninety per cent of total blood carbon dioxide is carried as bicarbonate in this way. The remaining 5 per cent combines reversibly with NH_2 on deoxygenated hemoglobin to form hemoglobin carbamate:

$$HbNH_2 + CO_2 \rightleftarrows HbNHCOOH \rightleftarrows HbNHCOO^- + H^+$$

When venous blood in the lungs comes into contact with alveolar gas, carbon dioxide in the plasma diffuses into the air spaces, causing the equations illustrated in Figure 15–19 to proceed in the opposite direction. It is clear that the red blood cell is essential not only to oxygen transport but also to carbon dioxide transport.

ACID-BASE BALANCE

The acidity or alkalinity of blood is expressed as pH, which is the negative logarithm of the hydrogen ion concentration [H+]. If an acid is added to water (pH 7), it dissociates and the hydrogen ion concentration increases, producing a fall in pH:

$$HCl \rightleftarrows H^+ + Cl^-$$

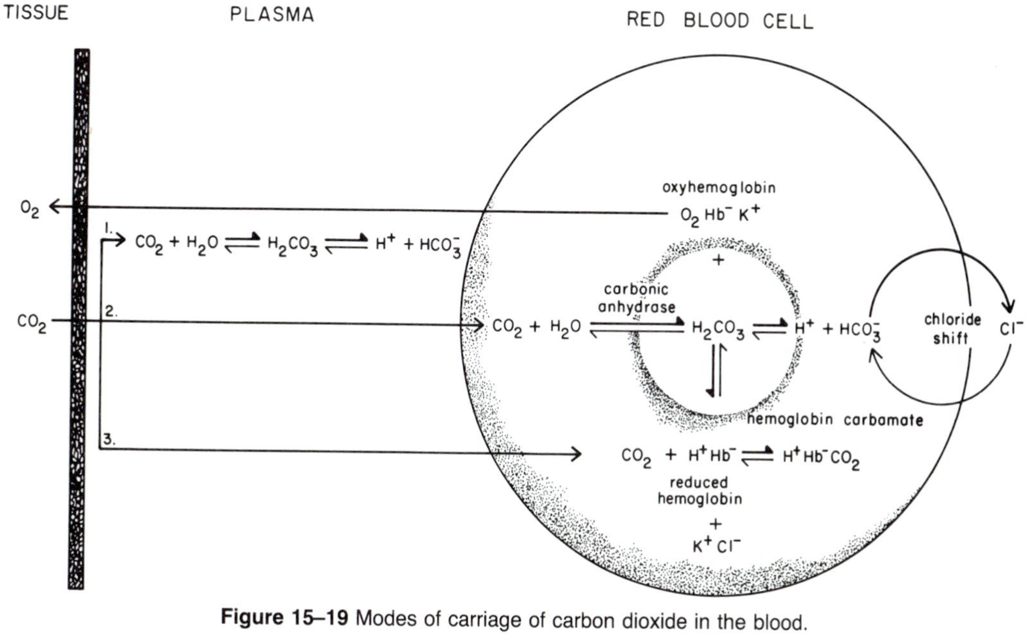

Figure 15–19 Modes of carriage of carbon dioxide in the blood.

The addition of a base has the opposite effect, reducing hydrogen ion concentration and therefore increasing pH:

$$NaOH + H^+ \rightleftharpoons Na^+ + H_2O$$

There is a constant tendency for the body to increase its acidity by the production of both gaseous and nongaseous acid metabolites. This tendency is controlled by the excretion of hydrogen ions indirectly by the lungs and by the kidneys, and it involves a number of chemical buffering systems. These mechanisms are normally able to maintain the pH in a narrow range between 7.36 and 7.44; a departure above or below these limits is referred to as *alkalosis* or *acidosis,* respectively.

A *buffer solution* is one whose pH is relatively unchanged following the addition of an acid or alkali. In general, buffers are effective only over a certain range of pH. An example of such a buffer system is a solution containing a weak acid (by which is meant one that does not completely dissociate in solution) and a salt of that acid. A buffer system replaces the stronger, more dissociable acid with one that is weaker and less dissociable, therefore reducing the hydrogen ion concentration. In humans, there are a number of buffers, the most important of which is the carbonic acid/bicarbonate system, which buffers nongaseous acidic metabolites such as lactic and pyruvic acids. Thus, sodium bicarbonate reacts with lactic acid to produce carbonic acid and sodium lactate:

$$NaHCO_3 + HLac \rightleftharpoons NaLac + H_2CO_3$$

Since carbonic acid is a weaker acid, it is less dissociated than lactic acid, and fewer hydrogen ions are released into solution. The buffer system has therefore "mopped up" a number of hydrogen ions that otherwise would have been released were lactic acid alone dissociated in solution.

In addition to nongaseous tissue metabolites, it can be seen from equation 1 that the continual production of carbon dioxide also has an extremely important influence on pH in that each molecule of carbon dioxide produced releases one hydrogen ion. We have seen (Fig. 15–19) how this is buffered by reduced hemoglobin and its neutral salt:

$$H_2CO_3 + KHb \rightleftharpoons HHb + KHCO_3 \xrightarrow{\text{chloride shift}} Cl^-$$

Reduced hemoglobin is an even weaker, less dissociable acid than carbonic acid, and it necessarily reduces hydrogen ion concentration, thereby preventing acidemia. Although the role of hemoglobin in buffering tissue carbon dioxide is important, the overall level of carbon dioxide retained in the body depends on the rate at which it can be eliminated from the blood; this in turn is dependent on the level of alveolar ventilation. If alveolar ventilation is reduced disproportionately to the

rate of carbon dioxide production, equation 1 moves to the right, with a consequent fall in pH.

The ability of these buffer systems to maintain pH within a given range is related to the readiness or otherwise with which the weak acid dissociates. This may be expressed mathematically:

$$K' = \frac{[H^+] \times [A^-]}{[HA]} \qquad \text{(equation 2)}$$

where K' is the dissociation constant of HA, which is a weak acid, the brackets denoting concentration. The higher the value of the dissociation constant, the more readily the acid dissociates. Just as hydrogen ion concentration is for convenience expressed as the logarithm of its reciprocal, $-\log_{10}[H^+]$ or pH, so the dissociation constant is conventionally written as $-\log_{10}K'$ or pK'. Equation 2 may therefore be rewritten as follows:

$$-\log K' = -\log[H^+] - \log\frac{[A^-]}{[HA]}$$

$$pK' = pH - \log\frac{[A^-]}{[HA]}$$

By adding the last term to both sides of this equation we obtain the following:

$$pH = pK' + \log\frac{[A^-]}{[HA]} \qquad \text{(equation 3)}$$

The relationship of the pH of blood to its carbon dioxide content and tension may be derived by substituting carbonic acid from equation 1 as the weak acid in equation 3:

$$pH = pK' + \log\frac{[HCO_3^-]}{[H_2CO_3]} \qquad \text{(equation 4)}$$

This is the Henderson-Hasselbalch equation. The dissociation constant of carbonic acid at 37° C is 6.10, and measurement of the remaining two factors will allow the pH to be calculated. In practice, the concentration of carbonic acid in plasma is about 700 times lower than that of dissolved CO_2, as the reaction in equation 1 is driven to the left by HCO_3^- ions derived from sodium and potassium salts.

$$NaHCO_3 \rightleftharpoons Na^+ + HCO_3^- \qquad \text{(equation 5)}$$

Dissolved CO_2 also bears a constant relationship to carbonic acid concentration; it can therefore be substituted for it in equation 4:

$$pH = pK' + \log\frac{[HCO_3^-]}{[CO_2]} \qquad \text{(equation 6)}$$

The quantity of CO_2 in solution is the product of its solubility coefficient ($\alpha = 0.03$) and partial pressure, and the latter can be measured directly with a CO_2 electrode. Carbonic acid contributes insignificantly to the plasma concentration of HCO_3^- ions, which are largely accounted for by the reaction shown in equation 5. The plasma bicarbonate of arterial blood may be derived by subtracting dissolved from total carbon dioxide content and is normally 24 mEq/L. With substitution of these values in equation 6 we find the following:

$$pH = 6.10 + \log \frac{24}{40 \times 0.03}$$

$$= 7.4$$

The practical importance of the Henderson-Hasselbalch equation is that in order for pH to remain constant, any change in bicarbonate (the numerator) has to be matched by a proportional change in CO_2 (the denominator). If this ratio, which is normally 20:1, is altered, a change in pH is inevitable. Disturbances of pH primarily due to alteration in CO_2 are referred to as *respiratory;* those primarily due to alteration in HCO_3^- are called *metabolic*. Any primary change in one component of the HCO_3^-/CO_2 ratio leads to a similar change in the other component in an attempt to maintain normal pH. If for some reason the lungs are unable to remove CO_2 as fast as it is produced, arterial P_{CO_2} will rise and pH will fall. In order to correct this respiratory acidosis, the kidneys act by conserving HCO_3^- and excreting H^+ ions, leading to a compensatory rise in HCO_3^-. In disturbances of acid-base balance the compensatory change in HCO_3^- or CO_2 is less than the primary change and is also usually insufficient to return the pH to the normal range. The following analyses of arterial blood samples will illustrate this.

Example One: P_{CO_2} = 60 mm Hg,
plasma bicarbonate = 26 mEq/L

Here the rise in P_{CO_2} is greater than that of bicarbonate and is therefore likely to reflect respiratory acidosis rather than a metabolic alkalosis. The pH of 7.29 confirms this. Normally, a rise in P_{CO_2} leads to an increase in output of the medullary respiratory center, resulting in increased ventilation, that "blows off" CO_2. A failure of this homeostatic mechanism to compensate can commonly occur with widespread airways obstruction, producing ventilation-perfusion mismatching as seen in chronic bronchitis, or with failure of the bellows function due to muscle weakness, as in myasthenia gravis or depression of the respiratory center by drugs.

Example Two: P_{CO_2} = 50 mm Hg,
plasma bicarbonate = 40 mEq/L

Here the greatest rise has occurred in bicarbonate with a smaller compensatory rise in P_{CO_2}

and is therefore likely to result from a metabolic alkalosis rather than a respiratory acidosis. This is confirmed by the pH of 7.53. This situation might follow the excessive ingestion of alkali or after repeated vomiting, and it may also occur in hypokalemia in which depleted intracellular potassium is replaced by hydrogen ions, resulting in extracellular alkalosis.

Example Three: P_{CO_2} = 30 mm Hg,
plasma bicarbonate = 12 mEq/L

Here the major fall is in bicarbonate with a smaller compensatory fall in P_{CO_2}. This is therefore likely to be a nonrespiratory or metabolic acidosis rather than a respiratory alkalosis. This is confirmed by the pH of 7.24. This situation is commonly seen in renal failure and in diabetic ketoacidosis, in which the excretion of hydrogen ions fails to keep pace with the production of nongaseous acid metabolites.

Example Four: P_{CO_2} = 25 mm Hg,
plasma bicarbonate = 20 mEq/L

Here the major change is in P_{CO_2}, with only a small fall in bicarbonate. The fact that this is a respiratory alkalosis is confirmed by the pH of 7.53. This picture may be seen in hysterical hyperventilation or with overbreathing due to other causes such as salicylate poisoning or diffusion defects.

GAS TRANSFER

DIFFUSING CAPACITY

The rate of diffusion of a gas in a gaseous medium is inversely proportional to the square root of its density (Graham's law). Thus, in such a medium CO_2 diffuses less easily than does oxygen; however, diffusion in the lungs involves a gaseous phase and a liquid phase. For this reason, the solubility of the gas in the liquid is an important factor and is governed in this instance by Henry's law. This law states that the volume of the gas that dissolves in a given volume of a liquid is directly proportional to the partial pressure of that gas. Since CO_2 is 24 times more soluble than oxygen, it has a greater rate of diffusion.

Factors Influencing the Diffusing Capacity of the Lungs (Table 15–2)

The Pressure Gradient Between the Alveoli and the Capillary Blood. Under normal circumstances blood remains in the pulmonary capillaries for 0.75 second. Even this short time is more than enough to allow equilibrium to take place, the

TABLE 15–2 PHYSIOLOGIC FACTORS AND DISEASE PROCESSES AFFECTING THE DIFFUSING CAPACITY

	$D_{L_{CO}}$	Principal Determinants
Loss of lung tissue		
e.g., emphysema, lung resection	↓	D_M ⎫
Diffuse infiltrations		⎬
e.g., asbestosis, sarcoid, scleroderma	↓	D_M/V_C ⎭
Altered pulmonary blood volume		
e.g., mitral stenosis	↑ or ↓	V_C/D_M
left to right cardiac shunt	↑	⎫
exercise	↑	⎬ V_C
supine posture	↑	⎭
Valsalva maneuver	↓	
Altered Hb binding capacity		
e.g., anemia	↓	⎫
polycythemia	↑	⎬ θ
reduced Pa_{O_2}	↑	⎭
increased Pa_{O_2}	↓	

latter being reached in 0.3 second in a normal subject breathing ambient air at sea level. Under these conditions, the alveolar P_{O_2} is around 100 mm Hg. With moderate impairment of diffusion, equilibration takes longer to occur; even so, it is still achieved in less than 0.75 second. Only when alveolocapillary block is severe does hypoxemia result. During exercise, however, the time the blood remains in the capillaries is shortened; so although the subject may not be hypoxemic at rest, he may become so with exercise. The pressure difference responsible for the diffusion of oxygen is not, as might be expected, the initial alveoloarterial gradient (100 − 40 = 60 mm) nor the end capillary gradient (100 − 99.9 = 0.01 mm) but is an integrated mean value that depends on a variety of complex factors including the time oxygen takes to traverse the membrane and combine with hemoglobin.

The Length of the Pathway of Diffusion. Before an oxygen molecule can combine with hemoglobin it must traverse the following:

1. Surfactant lining of alveoli
2. Alveolar membrane
3. Capillary endothelium
4. Plasma in the capillary
5. RBC membrane
6. Intracellular RBC fluid

The distance across the membrane is usually about 0.2 μ. In certain disease states, this distance may be increased by edema fluid, fibrous tissue, or the presence of additional alveolar cells.

The Surface Area Available for Diffusion. The area available for diffusion depends on the number of functioning alveoli rather than the total number of alveoli present in the lungs. In humans, it is approximately 70 square meters. Thus, loss of

diffusing surface occurs in emphysema, following resection, and in a fibrothorax with compression of the adjacent lung. Owing to the fact that in exercise many nonfunctioning alveoli open up, the diffusing capacity increases with exercise.

The Number and Character of the Red Blood Cells Available to Accept Diffused Oxygen. Anemia reduces the diffusing capacity because there are fewer red blood cells to take up the diffused gas. In addition, were the red cells affected in some anatomic or physiologic way that impaired the acceptance of diffused oxygen, the diffusing capacity would likewise be reduced. The latter is mainly a theoretic concept.

Measurement of Diffusing Capacity

To measure the capacity, it is necessary that the gas used be more soluble in blood than in the alveolocapillary membrane and in the tissue fluid. Both oxygen and carbon monoxide fulfill this criterion because they combine with hemoglobin. Other gases such as N_2O are equally soluble in tissues and blood and therefore can be used to measure pulmonary capillary blood flow. They are not, however, suitable for the measurement of the diffusing capacity.

The equation for measurement of the diffusing capacity for oxygen is expressed thus:

$$D_{O_2} = \frac{\text{ml } O_2 \text{ taken up by capillaries/min}}{\text{alveolar } P_{O_2} - \text{pulmonary capillary } P_{O_2}}$$

$$= \text{ml } O_2/\text{min/mm Hg}$$

Measurement of D_{O_2} necessitates a knowledge of the mixed venous blood since this datum is essential to calculation of the alveolocapillary gradient. In addition, since the capillary P_{O_2} rises as the blood traverses the capillary, the gradient and hence the rate of diffusion fall. Calculation of D_{O_2} requires that a knowledge of the Pa_{O_2} is available at every moment as the blood traverses the capillary. Although these data can be derived mathematically, the calculations are tedious and many assumptions are made. Thus, for the most part, persons seldom measure the diffusing capacity of the lungs for oxygen. In this regard, CO is far more convenient and is used almost exclusively now. The advantages of the use of CO are that the P_{CO} in the mixed venous blood is zero except in the case of heavy smokers and hence need not be measured. In addition, CO has 210 times the affinity for hemoglobin, and, consequently, only very low concentrations of inhaled CO (0.3%) are necessary to measure the $D_{L_{CO}}$.

There are a number of methods for obtaining $D_{L_{CO}}$, of which the most commonly used is the single breath technique. This requires the subject to make a vital capacity inspiration of a mixture containing 0.3 per cent carbon monoxide, 10 per cent helium, and 21 per cent oxygen and to breath-hold at total lung capacity for 10 seconds so that some of the carbon monoxide diffuses into the blood. A forced expiratory volume maneuver is then made, and once dead space gas has been displaced, an "alveolar" sample is taken and is analyzed for the final carbon monoxide concentration (FE_{CO}). The carbon monoxide concentration that was present in the alveolar gas before transfer had taken place is estimated from the dilution of inspired helium (He) according to the following equation:

$$FIN_{CO} = \frac{\overline{FE}_{He} \times FI_{CO}}{FI_{He}}$$

(initial CO concentration in alveolar gas)

where

$\overline{FE}_{He}$ = He concentration in expired alveolar sample
FI_{He} = Inspired He concentration
FI_{CO} = Inspired CO concentration

The change in carbon monoxide concentration during breath-holding is now known, and thus DL_{CO} can be calculated according to Krogh's equation:

DL_{CO} (ml/min/mm Hg) =

$$\frac{\text{Alveolar Volume (L)} \times 60}{\text{Time (sec)} \times (\text{BaPr} - 47)} \times \log_N \frac{FIN_{CO}}{\overline{FE}_{CO}}$$

Alveolar volume in this equation may be shown as the sum of the inspired volume and the residual volume (measured separately), or the "effective" alveolar volume (V_{Aeff}) may be calculated from the dilution of helium contained in the mixture according to the equation:

$$V_{Aeff} = \frac{FI_{He}}{\overline{FE}_{He}} \times (VI - V_{DA}) \times 1.05$$

where

VI = inspired volume
V_{DA} = anatomic dead space
1.05 = correction for CO_2 absorbed before analysis of expired gas

The effective alveolar volume tends to give a lower value for DL_{CO} in obstructive lung disease than does the former method.

DL_{CO} may also be measured by a steady state technique in which the subject rebreathes a mixture containing a small concentration of carbon monoxide in air, during which the rate of removal of the gas is measured. This method has the advantage that it may be used during exercise; however, errors may occur in the estimation of alveolar P_{CO}, particularly at rest when the tidal volume is small and dead space gas may not be entirely flushed out when sampling is made.

DL is analogous to an electrical conductance, and its reciprocal is therefore comparable to a resistance. Resistances arranged in series may be added to give the overall resistance, and so in the lungs the following equation applies:

$$\frac{1}{DL} = \frac{1}{\text{D alveolar walls}} + \frac{1}{\text{D capillary walls}}$$
$$+ \frac{1}{\text{D plasma}} + \frac{1}{\text{D red cells}}$$

Although it is not possible to estimate each of these smaller values separately, they may be incorporated into two measurable terms to give the following:

$$\frac{1}{D_L} = \frac{1}{D_M} + \frac{1}{\Theta V_c}$$

where D_M is the diffusing capacity of the alveolo-capillary membrane and ΘV_c is the diffusing capacity of the blood (V_c being the volume of alveolocapillary blood to which the gas is exposed in the lungs, and Θ being the rate of reaction of the gas with hemoglobin in ml/min). DL_{CO} falls following oxygen breathing because the value of Θ, which can be determined in vitro, depends on the degree of saturation of hemoglobin, which in turn determines the number of binding sites available for carbon monoxide. If two measurements of DL_{CO} are made after breathing first room air and then oxygen, and Θ is known for each level, simultaneous equations may be solved for the two unknowns D_M and V_c. The membrane component (D_M) falls in diseases in which the surface area available for diffusion is reduced (e.g., emphysema or following lung resection). It is also reduced in conditions causing abnormal thickening of the alveolocapillary membrane, such as fibrosing alveolitis and sarcoidosis. The alveolocapillary blood volume (V_c) is labile because the pulmonary circulation has a large reserve capacity, and it may not fall until pulmonary disease is advanced. It tends to increase in normal subjects when they exercise or lie flat. It is also increased in patients with left-to-right cardiac shunts. In mitral stenosis DL_{CO} may be initially raised due to an elevation of V_c (Table 15–2). This may later fall due to "pruning" of the lungs' vasculature as a result of pulmonary hypertension. The picture may be further complicated by pulmonary edema, which leads to a reduction of D_M. Θ is lowered in anemia and raised in polycythemia, and DL_{CO} may be corrected for hemoglobin concentration by the following equation:

$$DL_C = DL_O (14.6a + Hb) \div (1 + a)Hb$$

where DL_C and DL_O are corrected and observed DL_{CO}, respectively; Hb is the hemoglobin concentration; and a is the D_M/V_c ratio, which is assumed to be 0.7.

In bronchial asthma the DL_{CO} is normal, which is a useful point in distinguishing this condition from irreversible airflow obstruction due to emphysema. The measurements of D_M, V_c, and Θ are laborious, and, for clinical purposes, the simpler measurement of DL_{CO} usually suffices. It should be clear that this is influenced by a variety of factors other than thickening of the alveolocapillary membrane as was once thought, and it is therefore sometimes called the *gas transfer factor* (T_LCO).

Carbon Dioxide

Because of its solubility, carbon dioxide diffuses from the pulmonary capillaries to the alveoli about 20 times more rapidly than does oxygen. For this reason, diffuse pulmonary fibrotic or granulomatous diseases, such as asbestosis or sarcoidosis which are associated with impaired diffusion of oxygen, do not affect the diffusion of carbon dioxide sufficiently to cause a rise in arterial P_{CO_2}. By the time this stage is reached, the arterial P_{O_2} is too low to support life. A raised arterial P_{CO_2} usually indicates alveolar hypoventilation.

Control of Respiration

The regulation of ventilation, by which the arterial P_{O_2} and P_{CO_2} are maintained within a fairly narrow range, is complex and incompletely understood. The involuntary rhythmic nature of breathing depends primarily on the integrity of collections of interrelated, reciprocally acting inspiratory and expiratory neuronal pathways contained in the reticular formation of the medulla oblongata. These are known as the *medullary respiratory centers,* although they have no distinct anatomic boundaries. Their output to the respiratory neurones in the spinal cord is modified by cortical and pontine activity, by the aortic and carotid body chemoreceptors, and by vagus-mediated signals from the lungs and chest wall. They are extremely sensitive to the arterial P_{CO_2} level, and a 5 per cent increase causes the minute ventilation to double. Carbon dioxide will cross the blood-brain barrier more readily than will bicarbonate, and the subsequent dissociation of carbonic acid releases hydrogen ions into the cerebrospinal fluid (CSF), which is less able to buffer them than is blood. The medulla possesses receptors on its ventral surface that, when bathed with acid CSF, respond by increasing first tidal volume and later respiratory rate. If the acidity of the CSF is prolonged, as may occur in respiratory acidosis due to chronic obstructive airways disease, a compensatory change occurs in which CSF bicarbonate is increased, raising the pH again. As a result, a patient with an elevated arterial P_{CO_2} due to chronic bronchitis may have a diminished hyperventilatory response to carbon dioxide and depends instead on hypoxic drive. Uncontrolled oxygen therapy in such a patient may produce apnea by raising arterial P_{O_2} above the normal level,

thereby leading to secondary hypoventilation and a further rise in P_{CO_2}, which raises the intracranial pressure and acts as a respiratory depressant. Depression of the respiratory center also occurs physiologically during sleep and may be deepened by hypnotic drugs or anesthetics.

The carotid body and aortic arch chemoreceptors are stimulated mainly by hypoxia and to a lesser extent by hypercarbia. The carotid bodies are also sensitive to a fall in pH. These peripheral chemoreceptors are highly active metabolically, and it has been suggested that they are stimulated by the local accumulation of products of anaerobic metabolism occurring either as a consequence of a reduction in arterial P_{O_2} or from diminished perfusion in the presence of normoxemia, as may occur in hemorrhagic shock. Their afferent signals are carried to the medulla by the glossopharyngeal and vagus nerves. The peripheral chemoreceptor response to hypoxia is not as sensitive as the medullary carbon dioxide response, and the alveolar P_{O_2} is usually reduced to about 50 mm Hg before the chemoreceptors take over. Variation in the intensity of hypoxic drive among normal individuals has been reported, and it is possible that this might explain the differing clinical presentations of chronic obstructive airways disease, in which the "blue bloater" with a poor hypoxic response may be found at one end of the scale, and the "pink puffer" with a normal response at the other.

A number of vagally mediated afferent stimuli pass to the respiratory centers from the lungs and chest wall. The Hering-Breuer reflex is initiated by receptors in the bronchial and bronchiolar walls and in the diaphragm. Inhibitory signals are generated when these are stretched on inspiration. These do not affect central respiratory drive, but they modify tidal volume and breathing rate during exercise and hypoxic or hypercarbic stimulation. Their role during quiet breathing is minimal. In addition to the brain stem and the cortex, the diaphragm and the intercostal and abdominal muscles, which drive the "respiratory pump," are subject to reflex influences at the spinal level. Like other voluntary muscles, they contain length-sensitive spindle fibers that when stretched produce signals that are transmitted to the spinal cord by γ-afferent fibers. Here these synapse with α-motor neurons supplying the corresponding muscle fibers. It is thought that the γ-afferent system may have a coordinative function, providing proprioceptive information about the respiratory muscles, so that motor output may be modified accordingly.

In *metabolic acidosis,* as occurs in renal failure or diabetic ketosis, nongaseous acid metabolites that do not cross the blood-brain barrier may stimulate respiration by acting on the peripheral carotid body chemoreceptors, leading to Kussmaul breathing. Cheyne-Stokes breathing is characterized by a cyclical waxing and waning of tidal volume and respiratory frequency and is commonly seen in severe cardiac failure associated with hypotension and following cerebrovascular accidents. This instability of the ventilatory control system may result from a variety of causes, such as prolonged circulation time resulting in delayed feedback signals to the respiratory centers, or from increased sensitivity of the CO_2 control system as a consequence of damage to higher centers, or, paradoxically, from depression of CO_2 responsiveness due to brain-stem disease, enabling the less stable O_2 control system to take over.

PARTICLE DEPOSITION AND CLEARANCE

Tyndall first made the observation that inspired air contains numerous bacteria and other particles, whereas expired air is sterile, provided one does not sample the air that has come from the dead space. Both inorganic and organic particles are inhaled with each breath. Included among the latter are bacteria, fungi, and viruses. The vast majority of larger particles (5 to 10 μ) and a varying proportion of smaller particles (1 to 5 μ) are deposited in the nose. Of those particles that pass through the nose, a small but significant number are deposited in the trachea and bronchi, with the majority of such particles being in the range of 5 to 10 μ. Those that are not deposited in the nose or in the trachea and bronchi reach the

gas-exchanging portions of the lung and are likely to be deposited there. A few of the smaller particles are breathed out again.

Deposition depends on three physical processes: (1) sedimentation, (2) inertial impaction, and (3) diffusion, or Brownian movement. Sedimentation is the main cause of deposition of particles of 3 μ or over in size; however, some particles of between 0.5 and 3 μ also settle as a result of this process. In contrast, most small particles between 0.1 and 1.5 μ come into contact with the alveolar walls through Brownian movement. A smaller proportion of the larger particles is deposited through inertial impaction. This process comes into play when a particle is being carried along by an air current and when at a bifurcation of an airway the momentum of the particle is such that it will continue along its original path so that it comes in contact with the wall of the airway and hence is deposited.

Over 99 per cent of deposited particles are removed by the lung-clearing mechanisms. Those that are deposited in the dead space are cleared by the mucociliary escalator; those that are deposited in the parenchyma are taken up by the alveolar macrophages, and either they are transported to the terminal bronchiole and hence to the mucociliary escalator or they migrate into the interstitium of the lung and hence into the lymphatics to be carried to the regional nodes.

REFERENCES

Bake, B., Wood, L., Murphy, B. et al.: The effect of inspiratory flow rate on the regional distribution of inspired gas. J. Appl. Physiol. 37:8, 1974.

Barnhard, H. J., Pierce, J. A., Joyce, J. W., and Bates, J. H.: Roentgenographic determination of total lung capacity. Am. J. Med. 28:51, 1966.

Campbell, E. J. M., et al: The Respiratory Muscles. Philadelphia, W. B. Saunders Co., 1970.

Clements, J. A.: Surface phenomena in relation to pulmonary function. Physiologist 5:11, 1962.

Comroe, J. H.: The Lung. 2nd ed. Chicago, Year Book Medical Publishers, 1962.

Evans, J. W., Wagner, P. D., and West, J. B.: Conditions for reduction of pulmonary gas transfer by ventilation—perfusion inequality. J. Appl. Physiol. 36:533, 1974.

Fahri, L. E., and Rahn, H.: A theoretical analysis of the alveolar oxygen difference with special reference to the distribution effect. J. Appl. Physiol. 7:699, 1955.

Filley, G. F., MacIntosh, D. J., and Wright, G.: Carbon monoxide uptake and pulmonary diffusing capacity in normal subjects at rest and during exercise. J. Clin. Invest. 33:530, 1954.

"First In-Last Out." Editorial. Br. Med. J. 3:119, 1973.

Fowler, W. S.: Lung function studies, III. Uneven pulmonary ventilation in normal subjects and in subjects with pulmonary disease. J. Appl. Physiol. 2:283, 1949.

Glazier, J. B., Hughes, J. M. B., Maloney, J. E., and West, J. B.: Vertical gradient of alveolar size in lungs of dogs frozen intact. J. Appl. Physiol. 23:694, 1967.

Hughes, J. M. B., Glazier, J. B., Maloney, J. E., and West, J. B.: Effect of lung volume on the distribution of pulmonary blood flow in man. Resp. Physiol. 4:58, 1968.

Hyatt, R. E., Schilder, D. P., and Fry, D. L.: Relationship between maximum expiratory flow to degree of lung inflation. J. Appl. Physiol. 13:331, 1960.

Lenfant, C., Wayes, P., Aucutt, C., and Couz, J.: Effect of chronic hypoxic hypoxia on the O_2-Hb dissociation curve and respiratory gas transport in man. Resp. Physiol. 7:7, 1969.

Macklem, P. T., and Mead, J.: Resistance of central and peripheral airways measured by retrograde catheter. J. Appl. Physiol. 22:395, 1967.

Milie-Emili, J., Henderson, J. E. M., Dolovich, M. B., et al.: Regional distribution of inspired gas in the lung. J. Appl. Physiol. 21:749, 1966.

Ogilvie, C. M., Forster, R. E., Blakemore, W. S., and Morton, J. W.: A standardized breath holding technique for the clinical measurement of the diffusing capacity of the lungs for carbon monoxide. J. Clin. Invest. 36:1, 1957.

Otis, A. B., McKerrow, C. B., Bartlett, R. A., et al.: Mechanical factors in the distribution of pulmonary ventilation. J. Appl. Physiol. 26:732, 1969.

Pattle, R. E.: Lining layer of the lung. Br. Med. Bull. 19:41, 1963.

Perutz, M. F.: Stereochemistry of cooperative effects of haemoglobin. Nature 228:726, 1970.

Radford, E. P.: Recent Studies of the Mechanical Properties of Mammalian Lungs. In Remington, J. W. (Ed.): Tissue Elasticity, Washington, D.C., American Physiological Society, 1957.

Reger, R. B., Young, A., and Morgan, W. K. C.: An accurate and rapid radiographic method of determining total lung capacity. Thorax 27:163, 1972.

Riley, R. L., and Cournand, A.: "Ideal" alveolar air and the analysis of ventilation—perfusion relationships in the lungs. J. Appl. Physiol. 1:825, 1949.

Roughton, F. J. W., and Forster, R. E.: Relative importance of diffusion and chemical reaction rates in determining rate of exchange of gases in the human lung, with special reference to true diffusing capacity of pulmonary membrane and volume of blood in the lung capillaries. J. Appl. Physiol. 11:277, 1957.

West, J. B.: Regional differences in gas exchange in the lung of erect man. J. Appl. Physiol. 17:893, 1962.

16   Pulmonary Defense Mechanisms

David Center and Robin McFadden

STRUCTURE-FUNCTION RELATIONSHIPS

THE NASOPHARYNX

The major function of the nose is to modify the temperature and humidity of inspired air; it has a large reserve capacity to perform this function and is remarkably refractile to physical and environmental injury. The ciliated nasal mucosa has an extensive and complex vascular supply that is under autonomic control. This network can take inspired air at temperatures of 20 to 55° C and adjust it to within 10° C of body temperature as well as add enough water to effect 100 per cent humidification. This critical function is performed at the expense of a doubling of total respiratory resistance. In fact, the pressure drop across the narrow anterior portion of the nose can cause enough turbulence to make even quiet breathing audible.

Should nasal resistance be increased, as is often seen with mucosal congestion accompanying allergic rhinitis or the common cold, the demands of ventilation may require the subject to switch to oropharyngeal breathing. This results in suboptimal warming and humidification, and some people demonstrate bronchial hyperreactivity to inspired air, as in cold-induced asthma. A similar mechanism is thought to underlie exercise-induced asthma; although exercise results in a reflex decrease in nasal resistance in normal individuals, with increased ventilatory demand the airways are exposed to cool and relatively dry air from the mouth. This accentuates heat loss across the tracheobronchial epithelium and results in "reflex" bronchospasm.

Another major function of the nose is the filtering of particulate matter from inspired air. This function is served by the vibrissae at the anterior nares and the mucus blanket covering the turbinates and septum. The inspired air stream undergoes changes in direction and velocity, maximizing the chances for particle deposition. Respirable particles of 5 to 10 μm in diameter are effectively filtered by the nose, and a significant number of smaller particles are also deposited here. Infectious droplet nuclei of 2 to 4 μm in diameter or inorganic particulates of a similar size can often traverse the nose and deposit in the bronchial tree. Obviously, bypassing the nasal filter, as with mouth breathing or cigarette smoking, can expose the lower airways to dry air con-taining various sizes of respirable particulates. The nasal mucosa can also remove some or all of inspired gases, such as sulfur dioxide, during passage through the nose.

The adenoids are accumulations of lymphoid tissue with a rich vasculature located in the posterior nasopharynx. They lie in both the nasal airstream and the nasal mucociliary stream. The tonsils are of similar structure; they likely continuously sample all materials that are swallowed while the adenoids monitor inhaled particulates and antigens. It is thought that both structures play an important role in the development of immune mechanisms in childhood. Tonsils contain a full range of immunocompetent cells; they are capable of a local immune response, and they may also serve as a reservoir for antigen-reactive precursor cells to populate the lamina propria of the upper respiratory tract with cells that form IgA antibodies.

TRACHEA AND BRONCHI

The trachea branches into the right and left bronchi, and this pattern of dichotomous division is repeated to the level of the respiratory bronchioles. Here the branching becomes much more extensive and gives rise to alveolar ducts, alveolar sacs, and alveoli. Although the size of airways decreases with each division, total cross-sectional area increases.

Structurally, the trachea and bronchi contain more or less the same elements, although there are quantitative variations. Each is divided into four layers if viewed in cross-section: the epithelial, lamina propria, muscular, and adventitial layers.

The epithelial layer consists of ciliated columnar cells interspersed with goblet cells in a ratio of about 5:1. This pattern persists throughout the trachea and bronchi until bronchioles are reached that are 0.4 mm in diameter. Here the goblet cells disappear, and the ciliated cells become cuboidal and interspersed with nonciliated bronchiolar secretory (Clara) cells. Finally, in smaller bronchioles, the ciliated cells disappear altogether.

Epithelial cells continuously shed into the lumen and are replaced by the basal and intermediate cells; the piling up of these latter cells under the orderly ciliated cell layer gives the epithelium a pseudostratified appearance. After bronchial denudation in humans, regeneration of the epithelial layer begins within 2 to 3 days and is complete in about 2 weeks. Epithelial regeneration is a complex repair process that depends on the integrity of the underlying basement membrane, the number and location of surviving alveolar type II cells, and a number of other factors. Sensory fibers of the trigeminal, glossopharyngeal, and vagal nerves are present at various levels of the respiratory mucosa of the pharynx, larynx, trachea, and bronchi. Stimulation of these fibers by irritating substances results in cough.

The lamina propria lies between the basement membrane, upon which the epithelial cells rest, and the muscular layer. It is composed largely of connective tissue elements, arterioles, venules, and capillaries of the bronchial vasculature. There are also fibers of the vagi and sympathetics distributed to the blood vessels. The lymphatic vascular system is found in this layer and is one of the most extensive in the body.

The muscular layer, composed entirely of smooth muscle, extends from the trachea to the alveoli. The helical turns in criss crossing muscle fibers are almost circular in the larger bronchi, but the turns become steeper peripherally. This more or less circular arrangement of the muscle fibers provides efficiency in constriction as well as strength against high intraluminal pressures. Innervation of the musculature occurs via the vagi and sympathetics, which, by their activity, may produce constriction and relaxation, respectively. Beneath the smooth muscle layer are the longitudinal elastic fibers, which passively resist the expansion of inspiration and by elasticity alone bring the airways back to their resting length on expiration.

The submucosal glands, which extend throughout the three outer layers, produce a mucoprotein secretion of varying viscosity (see further on). Cartilage, which at first is regularly disposed and almost surrounds the trachea and large bronchi, eventually becomes fragmented into irregular plaques and in bronchioles disappears altogether. Where cartilaginous support is absent, the encircling muscle fibers can produce maximal constriction.

Mucociliary Clearance

As first described, the respiratory tract from the proximal trachea to the terminal bronchioles is covered with ciliated epithelium. Each columnar epithelial cell has about 200 surface projections, or cilia, that are approximately 6 μ long and 0.2 μ in diameter. Each cilium on cross-section microscopy can be shown to contain a characteristic 9 + 2 microtubular arrangement, a pattern repeated in the cilia and flagella of many animal species. Two central single fibrils are surrounded by nine outer doublet fibrils (Fig. 16–1). Inner and outer dynein arms are associated with these microtubule doublets. Nexin and radial-spoke linkages provide circumferential and radial links between microtubules.

Cilia beat in a uniplanar fashion, carrying the overlying mucus layer in a cephalad direction. Adjacent cilia beat in a coordinated manner to provide for least interference. Ciliary efficiency is critically dependent on the rheologic properties of the mucus blanket (see further on).

Certain inhalants impair ciliary function by either denuding respiratory epithelium or produc-

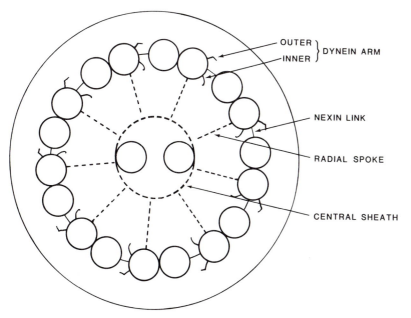

Figure 16–1 Schematic cross-section of a normal cilium.

ing ciliostasis. Cigarette smoking is the most common cause of these and various other defects, such as increased mucus production. Cigarette smokers frequently rely on cough to clear their airways as an effective compensation for impaired mucociliary clearance. Atmospheric pollutants such as sulfur dioxide and nitrogen dioxide are ciliotoxic beyond certain concentrations.

More frequently, a group of acquired and congenital disorders of ciliary motility have been described that are associated with recognizable alterations in ciliary ultrastructure. The first recognized of these dysmotile cilia syndromes was a defect in the dynein arms of outer doublet microtubules; various subcategories of dynein-arm deficiency have been described, and radial-spoke defects and microtubular transportation have also been identified. These defects are associated with ciliary stasis or impaired or discoordinated ciliary beating. Patients with these disorders commonly have sinusitis and serous otitis, reflecting impaired mucociliary clearance of the sinuses and middle ear, as well as chronic bronchitis; superimposed infections may lead to severe bronchiectasis. Kartagener syndrome is a historic eponym describing the combination of bronchiectasis, sinusitis, and situs inversus that has now been explained as a result of immotile cilia. The situs inversus is postulated to result from impaired function of the cilia that help propel the organs in their rotation through the coelom during embryonic development. Male patients also are infertile as a result of immotile spermatozoa, again due to ultrastructural defects in the sperm tail. Nosologic difficulties have arisen because patients with more typical acquired respiratory diseases, such as chronic bronchitis, have been found to have ciliary dysmotility with ultrastructural defects; some of these disorders can apparently be acquired after prolonged bronchial injury or infection. Nonspecific ciliary defects, such as absent or supernumerary tubules or ciliary fusion, are common in patients with recurrent respiratory infection.

The tracheobronchial mucus blanket is produced by the submucosal glands and goblet cells; the latter appear to secrete their mucus droplets upon direct irritation, whereas the submucosal glands release their seromucus content upon parasympathetic stimulation. The mucus blanket is composed of two layers, an inner periciliary layer (sol) and a more viscous mucus layer (gel) on top. The periciliary layer is difficult to demonstrate conclusively in vivo, and its cell of origin is unknown. The mucus layer is normally discontinuous, 5 to 10 μm deep, and interacts with the tips of the epithelial cilia, propelling it in a cephalad direction. The daily volume of respiratory mucus in normal individuals has been estimated to be 10 to 100 ml; mucus is 95 per cent water but contains electrolytes, amino acids, and several macromolecules, including lipids, immunoglobulins, enzymes, and acid or neutral glycoproteins. Disulfide cross-

linking and hydrogen bonding between glycoprotein molecules and water is a major determinant of the viscoelastic, or rheologic, properties of mucus.

The efficiency of mucociliary clearance depends on the thickness and rheologic properties of the mucus layer. Increased mucus production, as seen in patients with chronic bronchial injury, will slow overall mucociliary clearance, but because the reserve capacity of the mucociliary escalator is large, the amounts of excess mucus noted in disease states should not prevent clearance from occurring. Probably more important is the elasticity and viscosity of the mucus blanket; secretions that are excessively viscous and inelastic are cleared much less effectively.

Patients with chronic bronchitis show columnar epithelial atrophy and squamous metaplasia, leading to a reduction in the amount of ciliated epithelium, and the cilia that are present may be short and abnormal according to ultrastructural study. In addition, goblet cell metaplasia and submucosal gland hyperplasia and hypertrophy lead to an increased volume of mucus, often of high viscosity. Both these factors tend to decrease effective mucociliary clearance. However, the altered ventilatory distribution in patients with obstructed airways dictates that particulate deposition will be more central, where mucociliary clearance is more effective. In addition, the chronic cough seen in chronic bronchitis (see further on) may compensate for ciliary dysfunction and adverse mucus rheology. Hence, overall clearance in chronic bronchitis may be decreased, normal, or increased. It is likely, however, that disruption of orderly mucociliary clearance plays a role in the retention of pathogens in the lower airways, contributing to the common occurrence of infectious bronchitis and pneumonia. It has also been hypothesized that local areas of impaired mucociliary clearance, commonly occurring at sites of large airway bifurcation, may promote interaction of inhaled carcinogens with damaged epithelium and result in the recognized propensity for bronchogenic carcinoma to occur in these locations.

Cystic fibrosis is a systemic exocrinopathy, and its historic synonym, *mucoviscidosis,* alludes to the increased tenacity of exocrine secretions. Nasal and tracheobronchial secretions in children with cystic fibrosis have been shown to contain increased amounts of acid mucoglycoproteins, but significant alterations in rheologic properties have been difficult to demonstrate. The relative contribution of abnormal mucus in the pathogenesis of the respiratory complications of cystic fibrosis has not yet been determined.

Normally, the "cleansing" secretions of the lung are handled almost entirely by ciliary action, with some assistance from the expulsive forces of quiet respiration. However, when bronchial or tracheal secretions become excessive, acceleration of the expiratory air flow by clearing of the throat may be necessary to clear the nonciliated vocal cords. If this is ineffective, a more forceful mechanism, the cough, is used. The cough reflex is initiated by stimulation of afferent nerve endings of the vagi and glossopharyngeal nerves in the laryngeal, tracheal, and bronchial mucosa. The act itself can be divided into three parts. First, there is a deep inspiration, followed immediately by closure of the glottis. Second, with the glottis still closed, positive pressure develops in the thorax by contraction of muscles of the chest and the abdominal wall. Third, the glottis is suddenly opened and the air under pressure is rapidly expelled. If the offending substance is eliminated or if it is moved up to an insensitive area, coughing ceases. There may, however, be continuous paroxysms of coughing that move the offensive material little by little until it is eliminated or until the cough reflex is suppressed by medication.

Lymphatic Clearance

The lymphatic system of the lung is one of the most extensive in the body; the gut and respiratory system are constantly sampling environmental organisms and immunogens, and their lymphatic systems have adapted to accommodate such a load. The lymphatic vessels course in the lamina propria throughout the tracheobronchial tree to the level of the alveolar ducts. There are no lymphatics in the septa adjacent to alveoli. The lymphatics form a plexus about the arteries, veins, and airways, and they drain into larger collecting channels that contain one-way valves. Lymph flow in the peribronchovascular lymphatics is centripetal and moves into the tracheobronchial and hilar lymph nodes. Peripheral connections are made with the lymphatic plexus in the pleura. The pleural lymphatics also drain into lymph nodes at the hilum, coursing over the lung surface in a subpleural location. One of the peculiarities of the pulmonary lymphatic system is that nearly all the lymph from both lungs drains into the right lymphatic duct. Only lymph from the left upper lobe drains into the thoracic duct. There are, however, frequent connections between the two sides, so that this separation is not entirely complete. These patterns are of importance in the understanding of metastatic spread of infection and malignant disease. As in other parts of the body, lymph flow in the lungs depends on the movement of tissues. In the central portions of the lung, movement is restricted by large vascular and bronchial structures, with resultant sluggish lymph flow. As a consequence, in certain disease states accompanied by pulmonary edema, the edema, as revealed radiographically, may be more marked centrally and in a "butterfly" arrangement.

Well-developed lymph nodes, with afferent and efferent channels, a limiting capsule, mature follicles, and germinal centers, are found only in the region of the trachea and major bronchi. These nodes drain the pulmonary and subpleural lymphatics; they are identical with lymph nodes elsewhere in the body except for the accumulation of previously inhaled particulates (e.g., carbon particles) and the significant population of IgA- and IgE-producing cells, reflecting their mucosal proximity. Lymphoid nodules are unencapsulated aggregates scattered in the walls of large and medium-sized bronchi, particularly at branching points. Lymphoid nodules are separated from the airspace by a single layer of flattened, nonciliated epithelium that is intimately associated with lymphocytes, the so-called lymphoepithelium. More distal airways contain less well-circumscribed lymphoid aggregates, again associated with specialized overlying epithelium (lymphoepithelial organs), down to the level of the respiratory bronchioles. Aggregates also occur throughout the lobular and subpleural interstitial tissue. Nodules and aggregates have a rich vascular supply and are often associated with the origin of blind lymphatic channels. This supports the concept that such accumulations integrate the immunologic function of the lung by sampling the inhaled air, circulating blood, and providing a site for local production or egress of immunocompetent cells. They are also thought to serve as filters and pathways for the removal of alveolar fluids and particulates (pulmonary sump). This bronchus-associated lymphoid tissue (BALT) is morphologically similar to the Peyer's patches and gut-associated lymphoid tissue (GALT); because they contain a high proportion of incompletely differentiated cells, both areas are thought to function as reservoirs for immunocytes.

In a rare condition termed the "yellow nail syndrome," dystrophic and discolored nails are associated with lymphedema of the face and extremities and bilateral pleural effusions. Some patients present lacking one feature of this classic triad. Although difficult to prove, the underlying pathogenesis is thought to involve congenital hypoplasia of the lymphatics draining the arms, legs, and visceral pleura. Individuals often are asymptomatic until adulthood; commonly a respiratory infection or dermatologic disease will overload the capacity of the hypoplastic lymphatics and result in protein-rich exudates in tissues and the pleural space. Chronic sinopulmonary infections are also commonly seen with this syndrome; some people will have coexisting immunologic defects.

ALVEOLAR STRUCTURE

The majority of the alveolar epithelial lining is composed of the squamous type I cell, adapted for transfer of respiratory gases across their protoplasm. The type I cells have the distinction of being the most susceptible to inhalant injury and as fully differentiated cells are unable to regenerate. The surfactant-secreting cuboidal type II cells are responsible for replicating and repopulating the alveolar surface following injury, and they eventually transform into gas-exchanging type I cells. This repair process forms the basis of the cuboidalization of the alveolar epithelium described during repair and seen after some injuries.

Alveolar Clearance

The respiratory bronchiole divides twice, giving rise to three orders of respiratory bronchioles. The third order then divides into two alveolar ducts, which in turn divide five to eight times and terminate as alveolar sacs. There are occasional small projecting spaces, the alveoli, on the walls of the first-order respiratory bronchioles. With continued branching, the frequency of these alveoli increases markedly until, at the level of the alveolar sacs, the walls are beset solidly with alveoli. The walls of the alveoli are lined by a continuous epithelium consisting of two cell types—flattened, membranous type I cells and larger, cuboidal type II cells—both of which lie on a relatively permeable basement membrane. The alveolar walls also contain interstitial tissue and an extensive network of capillaries; through these layers gaseous diffusion occurs between air and blood.

Minute openings called *alveolar pores of Kohn* exist between adjacent alveoli, and considerably larger epithelium-lined communications exist between bronchioles and alveolar sacs. These two types of communications are important because they permit the direct passage of air from alveolus to alveolus and bronchioles to alveolar sac. This situation is referred to as *collateral ventilation,* a way in which alveoli may continue to be ventilated in the presence of obstruction to their normal ventilatory pathways.

Maintenance of alveolar ventilation requires counteracting the tendency of alveolar spaces to collapse. Negative intrathoracic pressure and the tethering effect of supporting connective tissue cannot, by themselves, prevent airspace closure (atelectasis). The relationship between pressure (P) within a sphere, tension (T) in its wall, and the radius (r) of the sphere is expressed in Laplace's equation: $P = \frac{2T}{r}$. A sphere such as an alveolus, with airway connections to the atmosphere, would tend to collapse as the radius diminishes on expiration were it not for the presence of a phospholipid layer called *surfactant.* This material, produced by alveolar epithelial type II cells, reduces surface tension as the radius of the alveolus decreases, preventing atelectasis. The major constituent of surfactant, dipalmitoyl phosphatidylcholine (DPPC) is largely responsible for the alveolar stability, as it has low surface tension and low surface compressibility. Immaturity of this alveolar stabilizing system is the cause of the respiratory distress syndrome seen in premature infants. One can diagnose the condition prenatally by measuring the phosphatidylethanolamine: phosphatidylcholine ratio in amniotic fluid. Maturity of type II cells and their production of surfactant are augmented by administration of corticosteroids, potential therapy for some infants.

Respirable particles less than 10 μm in diameter can be found after inhalation rather uniformly deposited over the alveolar walls. Disposal of such foreign material at this level of the respiratory tree primarily depends on phagocytosis by alveolar macrophages. These are the most common cells in the alveolar lumen and are derived from less differentiated stem cells in the pulmonary interstitium and from peripheral blood monocytes. If the ingested material is microbial, it may be destroyed within the macrophage. If, as in the case of various dusts, it is resistant to digestion, the phagocyte either migrates or is swept proximally and is cleared on the mucociliary escalator. Particulates in the interstitial space are ingested by local macrophages and cleared through the lymphatic system.

Inhalants such as cigarette smoke, ozone, and nitrogen dioxide have been demonstrated to have direct toxic effects on pulmonary alveolar macrophages; in-vitro studies demonstrate impaired phagocytosis and reduced bactericidal capacity. These effects are thought to predispose an individual to more frequent respiratory infections. Alveolar macrophages obtained from patients with pulmonary alveolar proteinosis (see further on) are filled with large quantities of the lipoproteinaceous alveolar exudate characteristic of this disease. This is presumed to lead to macrophage dysfunction and the increased incidence of unusual infections, such as nocardiosis, seen in these patients.

The introduction of bronchoalveolar lavage in various studies has allowed several insights into the characteristics of the inflammatory cells present in the alveolar spaces. In normal, nonsmoking individuals the alveolar macrophage is the major effector cell present, representing more than 90 per cent of the obtained cells. Very few neutrophils exist in normal alveolar lavage, but the proportion of these cells increases in patients who smoke, along with an increase in total numbers of cells obtained. Less than 10 per cent of the cells are lymphocytes, and of these about 75 per cent are T cells, 10 per cent are B cells, and about 15 per cent are null cells. Of the T-cell population, approximately 50 per cent belong to the helper/inducer cell subpopulation, and about 25 per cent are suppressor/cytotoxic cells. These values are similar to the normal values for lymphocyte subpopulations in peripheral blood. The macrophages and lymphocytes obtained are not thought to represent "activated" cells; the majority of resident B cells are not producing immunoglobulin.

MUCOSAL IMMUNITY

Respiratory secretions are known to contain all classes of immunoglobulins. Secretory IgA is the predominant species in upper respiratory tract fluids; bronchoalveolar lavage has shown that the lower respiratory tract contains mainly IgG, as in serum, although IgA, IgE, and IgM are also present. There is some evidence suggesting that local immunocompetent cells are responsible for the bulk of this immunoglobulin production. In addition, there is enhanced exudation or transudation of serum immunoglobulins into the tracheobronchial tree in the presence of allergic or inflammatory lung disease. Although difficult to document, there is every reason to believe that IgG and IgM function in respiratory secretions the same as they do systematically (i.e., agglutinating particulates, opsonizing bacteria, activating complement, and neutralizing viruses and bacterial exotoxins).

Secretory IgA is the predominant immunoglobulin in most mammalian external secretions; it accounts for more than 80 per cent of the immunoglobulin content of human saliva. Plasma cells resident in the lamina propria and lymphoid nodules secrete IgA as a dimer, consisting of the two IgA molecules joined by a polypeptide J chain. Ninety per cent of IgA in mucus exists as a dimer, and only 10 per cent exists in the monomeric form common in serum. The immunoglobulin molecules enter epithelial cells and covalently bind to a glycoprotein moiety termed secretory component, and the secretory IgA is secreted onto the mucosal surface. Secretory component apparently confers additional resistance to degradation by proteolytic enzymes. A proportion of locally synthesized IgM is also released as dimers or pentamers with a J chain subsequently complexed with secretory component at the epithelial surface.

IgA differs from IgG and IgM in that it is relatively inefficient in Fc-dependent opsonization of bacteria for effective phagocytosis; IgA may play a contributory role in enhancement of phagocytosis by alveolar macrophages by other membrane recognition units. Secreted dimers are very efficient in complement-independent agglutination and neutralization of a wide range of respiratory viruses. IgA may also inhibit microbial growth and neutralize exotoxins. A related important function of secretory IgA is its "blocking" function; the absorption of soluble, potentially immunogenic macromolecules through mucosal surfaces is impeded when IgA combines to form nonabsorbable complexes. Such a function partially prevents the diversified antigenic challenges derived from mucosal surfaces and may reduce the chance of a subject developing hypersensitivity to inhaled or ingested allergens. In an analogous manner, salivary secretory IgA has been shown to inhibit bacterial adherence to respiratory epithelial cells.

Selective IgA deficiency occurs with a frequency of between 1 per 500 and 1 per 800 indi-

viduals. These patients may be entirely healthy, but a proportion suffer from chronic sinopulmonary infections. In addition, these people appear to have an increased incidence of atopic and autoimmune disorders, of intestinal diseases such as gluten-sensitive enteropathy and giardiasis, and of mucosal malignancy. Inherited IgA deficiency likely results from a selective maturation arrest of IgA-producing B-lymphocytes. A more generalized B-cell maturation defect is the most common underlying cause of common variable (adult-onset) hypogammaglobulinemia. Some cases have been associated with excess T-suppressor cells, deficient T-helper cells, or serum inhibitory factors. These patients respond poorly, if at all, to antigenic impaired host defense. Patients with this disorder suffer from recurrent sinopulmonary infections with encapsulated pyogenic organisms (Streptococcus pneumoniae, Hemophilus influenzae) and have an increased incidence of infection with protozoan organisms (Pneumocystis carinii, Giardia lamblia). Bronchiectasis is a common complication. These individuals also suffer from various gastrointestinal disorders and have an increased incidence of autoimmune diseases and malignancy.

In addition to the aforementioned humoral immune mechanisms, cell-mediated immunity is an important component of lung defense. This type of immune response is most important in the host's response to intracellular facultative bacteria, such as Listeria monocytogenes and Mycobacterium tuberculosis. T-lymphocyte deficiency, as seen in children with congenital immunodeficiency syndromes (severe combined immunodeficiency, DiGeorge syndrome) results in severe life-threatening infections by organisms that are usually of low virulence (e.g., Candida). Infections with more pathogenic organisms pursue a more aggressive and lethal course (e.g., disseminated mycobacteriosis). More recently, an acquired immunodeficiency syndrome has been described that appears to represent a selective depletion of a subset of T-lymphocytes, those serving a helper or inducer function. The precise etiology of the cellular immunodeficiency is unknown. Initially described in male homosexuals and drug abusers, the lymphocyte deficiency is thought to underlie the common and particularly aggressive infections these patients experience; cytomegalovirus and herpesvirus infections, candidiasis, Pneumocystis carinii pneumonia, and disseminated mycobacteriosis. Patients with these diseases also have a profoundly increased incidence of an unusual soft-tissue neoplasm, Kaposi's sarcoma.

PULMONARY INFECTIONS

Under normal circumstances, pulmonary clearance mechanisms maintain the alveoli essentially free of particulate matter such as dust and bacteria. This situation is in striking contrast to that seen in the upper respiratory tract, where there is a wide variety of viruses and bacteria that, if permitted to seed the alveoli, could produce serious disease. However, like all defense mechanisms, those of the lung are not perfect, and infectious disease of the lung is a major cause of morbidity and mortality.

Since particles are removed from the air from the moment the air enters the nares until the time it reaches the alveoli, one would expect that the major affected regions would be the trachea and bronchi. Experimentally, this theory is supported by numerous radiologic studies in which opaque dusts insufflated into lungs did not appear to enter the alveoli, although bronchi were rendered opaque. Clinically, the theory is supported by the fact that the majority of respiratory tract infections actually are limited to the trachea and bronchi. Ordinarily, the lining of the trachea and bronchi is constantly being swept upward for elimination of foreign material deposited on it. When the foreign material is irritating and produces inflammation of the larger airways, the cough mechanism moves the sheet more rapidly. Yet this constant cleansing action is not impregnable. During sleep, for example, septic material from the nose and pharynx, particularly if it is abundant, is commonly aspirated into the lungs. Other factors that must be taken into consideration when there is a breakdown of protective mechanisms are the virulence of the organisms inhaled, the dosage of the infectious material, and variation in the patient's native resistance to pathogenic organisms. Once an organism invades and produces an inflammatory reaction, secondary defenses involving humoral and cellular immunity, still assisted by the expulsive mechanisms, are manifested.

ACUTE TRACHEOBRONCHITIS

Acute tracheobronchitis is most often the result of viral infection. It is a common occurrence in normal individuals, in whom the respiratory complaints may be minimized in the presence of considerable extrapulmonary flulike symptoms. Infectious tracheobronchitis takes on greater significance in patients with underlying lung disease, especially those with chronic bronchitis. Here the additional insult may result in significant morbidity and mortality, as evidenced by the great influenza pandemics. There is some suggestive evidence that childhood tracheobronchitis, especially pertussis and respiratory syncytial virus infections, predispose an individual to chronic bronchitis in adulthood.

Cigarette smoke and other inhaled pollutants may also lead to an irritative tracheobronchitis in susceptible individuals. A number of people will manifest bronchospasm during episodes of tracheobronchitis, and short-term bronchodilator therapy may be beneficial. A degree of bronchial hyperreactivity to various stimuli may persist for weeks to months after an otherwise routine tracheobronchitis.

ASPIRATION PNEUMONIA

Aspiration pneumonia refers to the various pulmonary sequelae of the entry of endogenous secretions and exogenous substances into the lower respiratory tract. Most normal people aspirate small amounts of oral secretions daily, particularly while asleep.

Although not invariably true, more significant aspiration generally occurs when the patient's state of consciousness is further depressed, commonly in association with administration of an anesthetic agent, debilitation, stroke, brain tumor, ingestion of drugs, and alcoholic intoxication. Each of these conditions may either depress or eliminate the normal protective mechanism of reflex glottic closure associated with vomiting and swallowing. When large solids are aspirated, bronchi may be occluded, with consequent distal pulmonary collapse or infection.

Aspiration usually occurs into dependent lung segments—the basal segments of the lower lobes when the patient is upright and the posterior segment of the upper lobe and superior segment of the lower lobe when supine. The most virulent form of aspiration pneumonia results from the aspiration of acidic gastric fluid. When the pH of the aspirate is below 2.5 and the volume is sufficiently large, the mortality rate is high, over 70 per cent in some reports. After aspiration, acid is rapidly dispersed throughout the lungs and damage begins. Areas of atelectasis are seen early; surfactant activity is destroyed, diluted, or altered by acid. Pathologic examination reveals epithelial degeneration in the bronchi and alveoli with pulmonary edema and hemorrhage. A marked polymorphonuclear leukocyte infiltration results in alveolar consolidation with hyaline membrane formation. Within 72 hours, repair has begun, with regeneration of bronchial epithelium and fibroblast proliferation. The lungs of survivors show parenchymal scarring with pleural retraction and areas of bronchiolitis obliterans and atypical bronchial regeneration.

Reflex airway closure usually occurs soon after aspiration of gastric contents, regardless of whether the substance is acidic or bland; bronchospasm may be prominent. A decrease in compliance and reduction in lung volumes is seen in the exudative phase of acid injury. Pulmonary artery pressure rises rapidly and then begins to drop with the fall in cardiac output and systemic blood pressure as a result of diminished intravascular volume. Pulmonary vascular resistance remains high, reflecting anatomic destruction and hypoxic vasoconstriction. Acid aspiration is one cause of, and may merge with, the adult respiratory distress syndrome (ARDS).

In the presence of an anatomic or functional defect of the upper respiratory and gastrointestinal tracts, chronic aspiration may result. This may result in an indolent, often bilateral pneumonitis; foci of granulomatous inflammation with incorporated lipids or vegetable fragments may be seen. Some individuals may chronically aspirate animal, vegetable, or mineral oils into the lungs, the latter usually taken as a laxative. Oil entering the alveoli becomes emulsified, is engulfed by macrophages, and induces an inflammatory and fibrogenic reaction. This lipid pneumonia often produces a single basilar infiltrate.

For a discussion of other pneumonias, see Chapter 21.

LUNG ABSCESS

Aspiration of infectious material from the upper air passages is the most common cause of lung abscess. Cuffed endotracheal tubes have greatly decreased the incidence of aspiration during surgery, but the extubated postoperative patient is still at risk. Secretions along with organisms from the mouth are inhaled into the lungs at a time when the cough reflex is depressed by general anesthetics and sedatives. There is a simultaneous increase in the viscosity of the bronchial secretions as a consequence of premedication, anesthesia, and dehydration, rendering ciliary action less effective. With the inactivation of these mechanisms for clearing the foreign material, the groundwork is laid for bacterial multiplication and abscess formation.

Several studies have shown that the anaerobic commensal organisms in the mouth are responsible for the majority of necrotizing infections following aspiration. Similar infections may also be seen in alcoholic stupor, dementia, and other neurologic and muscular diseases impairing orderly deglutition. Abscesses resulting from aspiration are most commonly found in the right lung, owing to the shorter and straighter mainstem bronchus found there, and in the posterior segment of the upper lobe and superior segment and the lower lobe, since most aspirations occur in the supine position.

Various forms of intrinsic bronchopulmonary disease may predispose an individual to infection from small inocula of aspirated material. For example, intrabronchial tumors may disrupt the processes that normally remove foreign material from the lower respiratory tract. Necrotizing vasculitis of Wegener's granulomatosis and polyarteritis nodosa may also result in abscess. Occasionally, abscesses arise from hematogenous spread of organisms in septicemias and in septic pulmonary infarcts, as from right-sided endocarditis. Even aseptic infarcts, by devitalizing pulmonary parenchyma, may predispose the lung to abscess for-

mation by permitting multiplication of small numbers of bacteria that would ordinarily be cleared. Occasionally, necrotizing pneumonia can be the result of infections with overwhelming numbers of gram-negative bacilli or staphylococci without anaerobes. Infrequently, pulmonary abscess may result from transdiaphragmatic spread of infectious material. Amebic hepatic abscess is generally considered in this situation if the abscess is in the base of the right lung, but this same route may be taken by any subdiaphragmatic abscess. Progress of the infection is usually slow enough to allow symphysis of the pleura, so that the lung is invaded without empyema occurring first.

In most cases of simple abscess the intrinsic defense mechanisms, when aided by antibacterial agents, will be adequate. The abscess wall subsequently collapses, and scar formation occurs. The chronic abscess with a thick fibrous wall that will not collapse even on adequate bronchial drainage is seen less frequently than in the past, even in tuberculosis, because of earlier diagnosis and effective antibiotic agents.

MYCOBACTERIAL INFECTIONS

Tuberculosis

In primary pulmonary tuberculosis, the bacilli are inhaled and arrive at the alveoli in the same manner as other small particulate matter. Because ventilation is greater in the lower two thirds of the lungs, most bacilli and consequent primary lesions occur in this area, where, depending on the number and virulence of organisms and the native resistance of the host, there may be little reaction or the formation of a relatively acute inflammatory exudate. The latter develops into a patch of bronchopneumonia with bacillary proliferation and inflammatory changes that are not unique to tuberculosis. However, whatever the initial reaction, multiplication of tubercle bacilli results in a zone of tuberculous granulation tissue consisting of blood vessels, lymphocytes, epithelioid, Langhan's cells, and connective tissue. Bacilli become scarce in the areas of caseous central necrosis. As adequate acquired resistance develops, the lesions become quiescent, with the formation of a hyalinized connective tissue capsule from the zone of granulation and a consequent reduction in the size of the lesion. The caseous material may be resorbed, inspissated, calcified, or subsequently liquefied. Bacilli in such a primary lesion may be completely eliminated or they may remain quiescent but virulent for years.

As the pulmonary lesion develops, bacilli appear in the hilar lymph nodes, and some individuals become mycobacteremic. The progressive inflammatory changes are similar in all anatomic locations. The pulmonary parenchymal tubercle and hilar nodal involvement together form the primary complex; if both become calcified, a Ghon complex is formed.

Following primary infection, tubercle bacilli are phagocytosed by alveolar and parenchymal macrophages but continue to multiply. Within 3 weeks, T-cell sensitization occurs, as demonstrated by the inflammatory indurative response to intradermal injection of tuberculoprotein (purified protein derivative, PPD). Pleural effusions, reflecting reaction to either intact bacilli or tuberculoprotein, can be seen at this stage. It is important to realize that up until now, the patient may be entirely asymptomatic or may manifest significant constitutional complaints like fever, malaise, and weight loss. A proportion of patients with primary infection do not manifest a skin test response; they are termed *anergic*. This is more likely to be seen in the elderly, in the malnourished, in patients receiving corticosteroids or other immunosuppressive drugs, and in individuals with Hodgkin's disease, other cancers, or recent viral infections or vaccinations.

It is believed that, in the evolution of the primary lesion, bacilli reach the blood stream either directly from the parenchyma or indirectly via the hilar lymph nodes and thoracic duct into the subclavian vein. Generally, the seeding is slight, the lesion is minute, and the end result is encapsulation, calcification, or complete absorption. Infrequently, persistent viable bacilli in these extrapulmonary sites later may give rise to progressive disease in the organ in which they are situated. Tissues with a high oxygen tension constitute a preferential site for the bacilli to proliferate, hence the prime frequency of apical pulmonary infections with a lesser tendency to metastatic lesions of the kidney, brain, and epiphyses of bones before maturation. Infrequently, hematogenous dissemination is massive; constitutional and extrapulmonary symptoms predominate. This co-called "miliary tuberculosis" occurs predominantly in the elderly and immunosuppressed and is associated with a high mortality rate.

The tendency of tubercle bacilli to localize in the posterior portions of the upper lobes is well recognized, but the mechanism of this localization has not been clearly defined. It is most likely because in the upright human the upper lung zones have a higher partial pressure of oxygen. Postprimary adult tuberculosis occurs as a result of reactivation in these foci, despite the defense mechanisms of specific immunity walling off the necrotic lesions.

The functional alterations in advanced pulmonary tuberculosis are secondary to parenchymal infiltration, loss of lung parenchyma, fibrosis, and pleural disease. Although the loss of lung substance in itself is infrequently serious owing to the large pulmonary reserve, it may be critical when combined with extensive fibrosis of the lung parenchyma and pleura, resulting in loss of compliance, subsequent defects in gas mixing, and compensatory emphysema. Pulmonary function tests reveal these pathologic changes as a decrease in vital capacity, an increase in dead space, and a decrease in arterial oxygen saturation on exercise. Although cor pulmonale is less common in tuberculosis than in chronic bronchitis and emphysema, it does occur in long-standing cases as a consequence of extensive vascular destruction from inflammation and fibrosis and increased shunting of blood from the bronchial arteries into the pulmonary veins.

There has been a slow decline in the prevalence of tuberculous infection and the resultant morbidity and mortality during this century in developed countries. This is largely attributable to improved sanitation and general living conditions, with some added benefit from the use of various chemotherapeutic agents since 1950. In the United States today, tuberculous infection during childhood is rare, with the majority of primary infections occurring in midadulthood. This is in contrast to the picture in underdeveloped countries, where childhood infection is common and all too frequently lethal and an adult with a negative tuberculin skin test is unusual. There is still a considerable reservoir of tuberculous infection in North America, however. There is a higher frequency of tuberculosis among recent immigrants, especially those from the Far East and the Caribbean, ghetto dwellers, Amerindians, and alcoholics. A factor contributing to persistent infection in these groups and their contacts is a greater prevalence of strains of *M. tuberculosis* that are resistant to conventional chemotherapy.

Various mycobacteria other than *M. tuberculosis* have been reported to cause disease in humans (formerly called *atypical mycobacteria*). Such organisms are very common in nature, inhabiting soil and water. Acid-fast bacilli may occasionally be seen in the gastric aspirates of healthy individuals. The majority of species are nonpathogenic. Inhalation is the most common form of human exposure; no convincing evidence of human to human spread exists, and there is no animal vector. Pulmonary disease is the most common manifestation, which is indistinguishable from disease caused by *M. tuberculosis*. As a group, these organisms are less susceptible to standard antituberculosis chemotherapy.

Mycobacteria are thought to possess inherently low pathogenicity. They are most frequently found colonizing damaged lung with bronchiectasis. It can be very difficult to differentiate simple commensalism from tissue invasion without pathologic material. Frequency of exposure to these bacilli is very much related to place of residence; for instance, many people in the southeastern United States can be shown to have cutaneous hypersensitivity to members of the *M. avium-intercellularis* group. This can cause confusion when interpreting the results of standard tuberculin skin tests in exposed individuals; considerable antigenic similarities exist between the organisms and this can cause weakly positive or indeterminate tuberculin skin test responses in patients unexposed to *M. tuberculosis*.

The reason that some people develop clinical disease due to these ubiquitous organisms is unknown, but it is thought to relate to relative impairment of bacterial clearance and other host defenses. *M. kansasi* infection usually leads to pulmonary disease that very much resembles classic tuberculosis. The *M. avium-intercellularis* group produces particularly indolent and destructive lung disease, notoriously resistant to drug therapy. *M. scrofulaceum* can cause isolated cervical lymphadenitis in children, likely via introduction through the upper airways or gingiva. Other mycobacteria may be responsible for localized skin infections. Occasionally, any of these organisms may cause a systemic mycobacteriosis if the host defenses are severely impaired by other diseases or immunosuppresive therapy.

OBSTRUCTIVE LUNG DISEASE

ASTHMA

Asthma is discussed in Chapters 4, 5, and 18.

CHRONIC BRONCHITIS AND EMPHYSEMA

Chronic obstructive pulmonary disease (COPD) is a commonly used term in pulmonary medicine; it suffers from imprecision but is clinically useful in that it implies that, most often, chronic bronchitis and emphysema occur together. The two can exist separately, and, in fact, neither need be accompanied by "significant measurable" airflow obstruction on physiologic testing. Complicating matters clinically is the fact that patients with "COPD" may have a degree of easily reversible airflow obstruction (or asthma) or areas of distorted and destroyed bronchial architecture (bronchiectasis).

Chronic bronchitis is defined as the presence of a productive cough for most days of at least 3 months during consecutive years. Pathologically, airways show mucus gland hyperplasia with some mucus plugging, and the ciliated epithelium undergoes squamous metaplasia. These changes result in defective mucociliary clearance, leaving patients susceptible to infectious bronchitis and pneumonia.

Emphysema is defined as dilatation of airspaces associated with alveolar wall destruction. Pathologically, several types have been described. Centrilobar emphysema begins in the first-order respiratory bronchioles and is patchy in distribution. There is scarring, irregularity, and local

dilatation of the airways and of adjacent alveoli, resulting in formation of central microbullae. This is the form most commonly associated with chronic bronchitis. Panlobular emphysema describes destruction and dilatation of all of the terminal respiratory airways. Patients with severe α_1-antitrypsin (α_1-PI) deficiency have a particularly severe and diffuse panlobular emphysema (see further on). *Paraseptal emphysema* refers to blebs or bullae along intralobular septa, and *subpleural emphysema* describes airspace dilatation just beneath the pleural surface. Although subpleural blebs may be important in the etiology of spontaneous pneumothorax, these latter two forms seldom interfere with overall lung function. Commonly, there are localized areas of airspace dilatation in the region of fibrotic scars (paracicatricial emphysema) that, if small, may represent little physiologic impairment.

Cigarette smoking serves as a common pathogenetic factor for both chronic bronchitis and emphysema. No other single factor has been demonstrated to have as strong an association with the presence of chronic productive cough, airflow obstruction on physiologic testing, and emphysema on autopsy studies. Smoking accounts for most of the observed increase in mortality from COPD in men and in women. Frequent respiratory infections in childhood predispose an individual to chronic bronchitis, and the incidence is higher in urban areas than in rural settings. The latter finding is considered suggestive evidence for the importance of some types of air pollution. Airway hyperreactivity and damage can certainly be seen with inhaled pollutants such as sulfur dioxide and ozone; deleterious effects of gas-burning stoves have also been postulated.

In certain occupational groups (e.g., coal, asbestos, gold and metal miners; cement manufacturers; and cotton and foundry workers), a nonspecific chronic bronchitis is common. Such industrial bronchitis is likely a response to prolonged deposition of respirable particulates in conducting airways, leading to mucus gland and goblet cell hypertrophy and excess mucus secretion. Although there may be evidence of large airways obstruction, industrial bronchitis does not appear to predispose one to emphysema.

Whatever the etiology of the initial injury, the ensuing process of lung inflammation and repair is presumed to follow a relatively standard progression. Cigarette smoke and other pollutants likely cause epithelial cell injury by the production of toxic oxidating metabolites, overwhelming the tissue and cellular antioxidants that normally control such generation. Early in the resultant inflammatory response, granulocytes are seen in the airways, along with increased numbers of alveolar macrophages. These cells presumably release elastase and other proteases that cause tissue destruction.

Various theories regarding the pathogenesis of emphysema consider the "checks and balances" that are in place to prevent excessive destruction as a result of the initial bronchial injury (Fig. 16–2). Alpha$_1$-antitrypsin (a$_1$-PI) is a major serum glycoprotein that inhibits several proteases. It is postulated that it is a major defense against the proteases and elastases released from inflammatory leukocytes. As already mentioned, a small subgroup of people have been identified to have a serum deficiency of this antiprotease, apparently due to impaired release from hepatocytes. These patients develop severe panlobular emphysema at an early age with little exposure to bronchial irritants; the process is accelerated in cigarette smokers.

Patients with very low circulating levels of a$_1$-PI (<15 per cent of normal, corresponding to phenotype PiZZ) have been shown to have undetectable a$_1$-PI in bronchoalveolar lavage fluid, and this may allow any elastolytic load unchecked. Patients with less complete deficiencies of a$_1$-PI (<40 per cent of normal circulating level, e.g., phenotypes PiMZ and PiSZ) usually have some demonstrable pulmonary dysfunction (particularly the smokers). In contrast, patients with normal PiMM phenotype or other heterozygotes generally have greater than 40 per cent of the normal circulating a$_1$-PI level; because these patients cannot be demonstrated to have lung destruction, such concentrations are considered sufficient to neutralize routine loads of proteases released from neutrophils.

In contrast to those relatively few patients who have inherited antiprotease deficiency, the vast majority of people with emphysema have normal a$_1$-PI levels in the blood and bronchoalveolar fluid. Accelerated neutrophil influx is one way that such patients could be exposed to excess elastase. There is also evidence, however, that a$_1$-PI can be functionally inactivated in the lung by exposure to oxidant injury. Activated alveolar macrophages have been shown to produce oxidative products (superoxide radical, O$_2$, hydrogen peroxide, H$_2$O$_2$, and oxygen free radicals) that can directly oxidize and inactivate various enzymes and antiproteases. In addition, H$_2$O$_2$ can serve as a cofactor, along with a halide ion, for the myeloperoxidase of monocytes or neutrophils, which can form other very powerful oxidizing agents. It has been shown that the elastase-inhibitory activity of a$_1$-PI can be blocked by the oxidation of its active methionyl residues. The presence of oxidants in the lung could thus favor a$_1$-PI inactivation. In addition to the production of these oxidizing agents by phagocytic cells, various strong oxidants can be identified in cigarette smoke, potentially resulting in direct a$_1$-PI inactivation (Fig. 16–2).

Cigarette smoke has been shown to block the three-dimensional covalent cross-linking of elastin catalyzed by the enzyme *lysyl oxidase;* interference with this vital structural step could prevent orderly elastin repair and contribute to the development of emphysema. Several enzymes administered intratracheally to experimental animals can produce a picture of emphysema; a common denominator appears to be the ability of these enzymes to degrade elastin.

Airflow Pathophysiology

In normals, the negative intrapleural pressure generated with inspiration results in airway widening, making breathing relatively effortless. Even though COPD patients have hyperexpanded

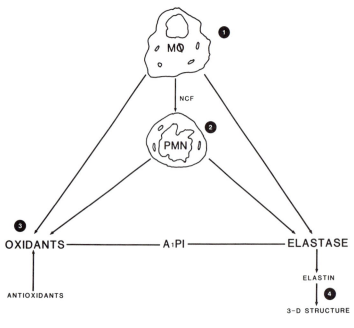

Figure 16–2 Schematic representation of potential protease-antiprotease interactions in the alveolar walls. (1) Activated macrophages secrete (3) oxidants and elastase and NCF, which attracts (2) neutrophilic polymorphonuclear leukocytes to the lung, which secretes similar degradative factors. Ultimately, excess elastolytic activity unchecked by antiprotease alters (4) the elastin matrix of the lung, causing emphysema.

lungs that deflect the main inspiratory muscle, the diaphragm, downwards into a mechanically disadvantageous position, there is still usually little airflow obstruction on inspiration. With expiration, however, flow deteriorates dramatically. In chronic bronchitis, peripheral airways in which there are excessive mucus accumulation, mucosal inflammation, and edema and smooth-muscle thickening lack substantial cartilaginous support. The increase in intrapleural pressure seen with expiration causes the lumen of these airways to close prematurely. In emphysema, the destruction of the alveolar framework that has occurred causes a reduction of the elastic recoil pressure of airway walls, resulting in collapse of normal airways in expiration. Thus, reduction in expiratory flow rates is the hallmark physiologic feature of both forms of COPD. Increasing expiratory effort by increasing intrathoracic pressure (contraction of the expiratory intercostal and abdominal muscles) makes the airway narrowing worse; there is a maximum flow rate that can be achieved, and expiration is characteristically slow and prolonged (low forced vital capacity and forced expiratory volume in 1 second). In contrast, total lung capacity and especially residual volume may be greatly increased, representing air-trapping in distal airways.

In emphysema, the same air-space destruction that results in loss of lung connective tissue causes measurable impairment of oxygen diffusion across the respiratory membrane, primarily by coexistent pulmonary microvascular destruction. In chronic bronchitis, alveolar hypoxia is a potent stimulus to the pulmonary vascular hypertension that is seen with this condition. Right-sided heart failure secondary to the pulmonary hypertension resulting from progressive lung dysfunction (cor pulmonale) is a terminal feature in patients with all types of COPD. In addition to being hypoxemic, end-stage individuals usually reveal hypercarbia, reflecting relative alveolar hypoventilation.

BRONCHIECTASIS

Bronchiectasis is defined as permanent dilatation of the bronchi associated with bronchial wall destruction. Bronchiectasis most commonly occurs in the varicose form, in which dilatation is irregular and there are areas of focal constriction. Cylindrical bronchiectasis describes uniform bronchial dilatation. Saccular or cystic bronchiectasis is a severe form in which the dilatations are large and central with an impressive reduction in distal bronchial branching.

Pathologically, mucus gland hypertrophy and squamous metaplasia, as in chronic bronchitis, are universal. In addition, destruction of the elastic and muscular layers in the bronchial wall is prominent, and the epithelium may be ulcerated. Acute and chronic inflammatory cell infiltrates are present in the bronchial walls. Occasionally, amyloid deposition in the bronchi (and even systemically) speaks for the chronicity of the inflammation.

The most important etiologic factor in the development of bronchiectasis is bronchial infection. Childhood viral pneumonias and staphylococcal pneumonia are notorious. The primacy of infection as a cause of bronchiectasis is demonstrated by the rather striking decline in incidence since the advent of antibiotics. Once a portion of the bronchial tree is rendered ectatic, there is a predisposition to recurrence of infection. Mucociliary clearance is ineffectual, and peripheral parenchymal destruction and dilatation of the airways prevent effective cough. Recurrent infectious bronchitis and bronchopneumonia are the clinical hallmarks of bronchiectasis.

Other etiologies include the postobstructive bronchiectasis and atelectasis seen with bronchial tumors or foreign bodies. Upper lobe fibrosis due to inactive tuberculosis is a form of cicatricial bronchiectasis. A subgroup of asthmatics develop recurrent parenchymal infiltrates, central saccular bronchiectasis, and evidence of immune hypersensitivity to *Aspergillus* species or other fungi, so-called "allergic bronchopulmonary aspergillosis" (ABPA).

A number of genetic and acquired systemic defects are commonly associated with bronchiectasis. In cystic fibrosis there is an increase in the viscosity of pulmonary secretions and recurrent bacterial pneumonias (especially *Pseudomonas* species) leading to particularly severe bronchiectasis. Bronchiectasis has also been associated with cases of immunoglobulin deficiency, and the "dysmotile cilia syndrome."

Physiologically, these patients usually manifest some decrease in expiratory flow rates. Loss of effective ventilating lung regions results in a reduction in lung volumes. Hypoxemia can be impressive, reflecting not only loss of parenchyma but also significant shunting of blood through unventilated lung units. Therefore, cyanosis and clubbing can be seen. With each successive infection, some pulmonary function is lost, and patients with late cases show hypercarbia, acidemia, and cor pulmonale, characteristic findings in severe obstructed airways disease.

DISEASES OF THE PULMONARY CIRCULATION

HYDROSTATIC PULMONARY EDEMA

The pulmonary vascular endothelium is a semipermeable membrane; fluid and small solutes continuously leak across into the lung interstitium. Fluid movement across capillaries is determined by the same forces as are operative elsewhere in the body, as outlined by Starling (see Chapter 6). The pulmonary vasculature is a low-pressure system, thus reducing capillary hydrostatic pressure, and the effect of surfactant on reducing alveolar surface tension is also thought to reverse what would be an important force drawing fluid out of capillaries. Interstitial hydrostatic pressure is difficult to measure in the lung as elsewhere, but it may be that pulmonary interstitial pressure is normally more negative, reflecting the negative intrapleural pressure throughout quiet respiration. This would lead to an increase in capillary fluid efflux.

The lymphatic system is normally capable of handling any fluid in the interstitial space and has a capacity several times what is needed in most circumstances. When one of the components of the Starling equation is altered sufficiently, the lymphatics may be overloaded, leading to a buildup in interstitial fluid, which by itself has no physiologic or clinical importance. With continued imbalance, however, there is a backup of fluid into the perivascular connective tissue and into the airspaces themselves. The presence of alveolar edema has very definite deleterious effects on pulmonary mechanics and gas exchange. An area of the lung can be particularly susceptible to edema if its lymphatics have been damaged by previous infection or other injury.

The most common cause of pulmonary edema is postcapillary hypertension due to elevated left heart pressures (e.g., ischemic heart disease with left ventricular dysfunction). Left-sided valvular heart disease is also an important cause, with mitral stenosis being the classic example. Changes in capillary hydrostatic pressures are also thought to underlie both neurogenic and high-altitude pulmonary edema; the former usually occurs in the postictal state or following head trauma, whereas the latter characteristically occurs when people actively ascend to altitudes greater than 2750 meters.

Pathologically, lungs are heavy and moist, and transudative pleural effusions are often present. Cut sections of lung show increased fluid in the peribronchovascular and interlobular interstitial spaces; the alveoli may contain proteinaceous fluid with red cells. Total lung capacity and vital capacity are usually reduced in cardiogenic pulmonary edema, reflecting the decrease in lung compliance. There may be mild to moderate airflow obstruction. Since elevated hydrostatic pressures dictate that fluid will settle most in the dependent lung (lower lobes if the patient is upright, posteriorly if supine, and unilaterally if on one side), there is a shunting of pulmonary blood flow to the nondependent portions in an attempt to minimize ventilation/perfusion inequality. Such mismatch is responsible for the hypoxemia observed; in most patients, this is accompanied by dyspnea and subsequent alveolar hyperventilation with hypocarbia.

PERMEABILITY PULMONARY EDEMA (PPE)

The variables in the Starling equation can be predicted and, to some extent, manipulated only when the diffusion constant for the pulmonary capillary endothelium does not change. Since the mid 1960s, a form of acute respiratory failure characterized by pulmonary edema in the presence of normal left ventricular filling pressures has been increasingly recognized. There are many known causes of this adult respiratory distress syndrome (ARDS). The disease was initially described in trauma victims (soldiers in Vietnam, motor vehicle casualities) and in patients with shock, either hemorrhagic or septic. Other causes include drug reactions or overdose, aspiration of gastric contents, near-drowning, smoke inhalation, massive blood transfusions, pancreatitis, uremia, and viral pneumonias. In all cases, an injury to the alveolocapillary membrane is the underlying pathologic defect, leading to increased capillary permeability and pulmonary edema.

In most cases of PPE, the actual agent responsible for the injury to the alveolocapillary barrier is not known. Systemic complement activation is a common accompaniment of many of the diseases that underlie ARDS; complement fragments such as C5a have been shown to promote neutrophil aggregation and adherence. These aggregates accumulate in the lungs of experimental animals, and the neutrophils can then release superoxide radicals and other reactive oxidant by-products that may injure endothelial cells. The neutrophils also release various neutral and acid proteases that disrupt the underlying structural proteins. The increase in capillary permeability seen in experimental models of endotoxemia and pancreatitis is not seen in granulocytopenic animals. There has also been a proposed pathogenic role for the platelet fibrin thrombi that are frequently seen in the lungs of patients with ARDS, since both the particulate and soluble products of intravascular coagulation and fibrinolysis can cause microvascular injury resembling ARDS in laboratory animals. These systems likely have interdependent roles in the genesis of the acute lung injury. There is evidence of deficient or defective surfactant in ARDS patients, which promotes atelectasis; this is likely not a primary pathogenic defect but simply a result of lung injury.

A related but somewhat separate issue is the reparative process occurring after injury, seen as a severe interstitial and intra-alveolar fibrosis centered around the alveolar ducts. With more effective management of the initial acute alveolitis, this pulmonary fibrosis appears to be the major determinant of survival in ARDS patients. The fibrosis resembles that seen in idiopathic pulmonary fibrosis (see further on), but the factors that tie this proliferative response to the initial acute alveolitis are unknown. It is likely that some intermediate regulator cells (perhaps alveolar macrophages or lymphocytes) play some role by stimulating fibroblast proliferation and collagen synthesis. It has also been conclusively demonstrated that therapy with high partial pressures of oxygen, sometimes unavoidable in ARDS, can potentiate or augment the fibrotic response. This may occur by direct oxygen toxicity to a select subpopulation of cells, such as the regenerating type II epithelial cells, causing structural disarray and disruption of the normal cell-to-cell interactions inherent in the reparative process.

In spite of the many etiologies, the pathologic changes are relatively consistent. Initially, there is patchy edema and alveolar hemorrhage with consolidation that progresses to a more homogenous picture with significant atelectasis. The lungs become dark red and airless, with a consistency resembling that of liver. The early leukocytic and proteinaceous alveolar exudate often leads to "hyaline membrane formation," and lung repair results in epithelial cell hyperplasia with cuboidalization of the alveolar type II pneumocytes. After a few days, mononuclear cell infiltration and collagen formation herald the onset of interstitial and perialveolar fibrosis. Early changes in precapillary pulmonary arteries include reduced number and volume of small arteries, some showing muscularization. Larger muscular arteries show medial hypertrophy.

Atelectasis and consequent consolidation cause irregularly distributed increases in lung compliance resulting in maldistribution of ventilation. In severe cases, pulmonary hypertension develops in response to local and systemic hypoxemia and intravascular clotting. Subsequent venoarterial shunting and deadspace ventilation result in a widening of the alveolar-arterial oxygen tension gradient and hypoxemia refractory to oxygen therapy. In time, carbon dioxide retention and respiratory acidosis ensue; with profound reductions in blood oxygen tension, tissue hypoxia and lactic acidosis develop.

PULMONARY HYPERTENSION

Sustained elevation of pulmonary artery pressures can lead to hypertrophy of the muscular arteries in the lung, followed by intimal thickening and proliferation. If the cause of the pulmonary hypertension can be corrected, these changes are reversible; if not, permanent luminal narrowing occurs, with fibrinoid necrosis and dysplastic changes. Pulmonary hypertension is most often secondary to primary diseases of the heart and lungs.

Congenital heart diseases characterized by large left-to-right shunts (atrial and ventricular septal defects, patent ductus, etc.) lead to markedly increased flow through the pulmonary circulation. Elevated pulmonary artery pressures are produced by an increase in vasomotor tone, which, after a period of time, gives way to more permanent morphologic changes in the vasculature. In terminal stages of uncorrected disease, pulmonary arterial pressures exceed those in the systemic circulation, causing a reversal of flow through the abnormal connection that leads to progressive hypoxemia and cyanosis (Eisenmenger syndrome). A degree of passive pulmonary hypertension often accompanies acquired heart diseases that elevate left-sided filling pressures (e.g., ischemic left ventricular failure). In severe mitral stenosis, passive pulmonary vascular congestion can be followed by active pulmonary arterial vasoconstriction. In some cases, permanent morphologic changes occur, with the site of the increased resistance to blood flow actually shifting from the mitral valve to the pulmonary arteries.

The most commonly encountered form of pulmonary hypertension is that secondary to chronic structural or functional derangement in the respiratory system, so-called *cor pulmonale* (pulmonary hypertension with right ventricular hypertrophy). Most often, this is associated with diseases producing chronic alveolar hypoxia, which is a potent stimulus to pulmonary vasoconstriction. Chronic bronchitis, bronchiectasis, and cystic fibrosis are diseases in which structural derangements and ventilation/perfusion inequalities lead to alveolar hypoventilation and chronic alveolar hypoxia. Cor pulmonale is a common late manifestation of all these obstructive lung diseases.

There is also a group of respiratory disorders in which, in the absence of significant parenchymal lung disease, ventilation is still inadequate (global alveolar hypoventilation). Such dysfunction may be intermittent; patients with the sleep apnea syndrome have periodic upper airway obstruction while asleep and pulmonary vasoconstriction, which, with time, yields to fixed pulmonary hypertension. Fixed upper airway obstruction, central alveolar hypoventilation, and neuromuscular diseases that impair the function of the respiratory bellows can all lead to pulmonary hypertension as a result of alveolar hypoxia.

Other respiratory disorders lead to pulmonary hypertension by reducing the size of the vascular bed available to blood flow. Diffuse parenchymal infiltrative diseases, such as pulmonary fibrosis, sarcoidosis, and the pneumoconioses, may destroy or severely compromise the pulmonary arterial system. Extensive focal fibrosis, as in tuberculosis, or surgical resection of large quantities of lung tissue may have the same effect. Diseases of the pulmonary vasculature may result in severe pulmonary hypertension without affecting airway function. Widespread vascular obstruction as seen in chronic thromboembolism and schistosomiasis can obliterate enough pulmonary vasculature to result in elevated pulmonary artery pressures.

Lastly, in some cases of pulmonary hypertension, no associated cardiac or lung disease can be identified. This is most commonly seen in young females and is termed *primary pulmonary hypertension*. Pathologically, medial hypertrophy of the pulmonary arteries is often accompanied by fibrinoid necrosis, and arteritis is occasionally present. Organizing thrombi may be seen in involved areas.

Pulmonary-function testing in pulmonary hypertension is directed at defining underlying airway or interstitial disease, even though the pulmonary hypertension itself may have little measurable impact. With exercise, patients with all forms of pulmonary hypertension tend to increase the deadspace to tidal-volume ratio, accompanied by worsening hypoxemia and widening of the arterial–to–end-tidal carbon dioxide difference. This may reflect portions that are ventilated but not adequately perfused owing to vascular bed restriction or an inability to raise cardiac output appropriately. Cardiac catheterization is generally necessary for documentation of pulmonary hypertension and for measurement of pulmonary capillary wedge pressure, right-sided pressures, cardiac output, and left-to-right shunts to determine underlying etiology. In primary pulmonary hypertension, pulmonary function tests will be normal, and cardiac catheterization will fail to reveal a cardiac cause.

PULMONARY EMBOLISM

The pulmonary vascular tree is an efficient filter that can remove emboli of neoplastic cells, bacteria, blood clots, fat globules, injected particulates, and the debris of amniotic fluid. By far the most common form of pulmonary embolism is that due to a bland blood clot, usually arising in the deep venous system of the legs or pelvis. Depending on the size and frequency of such thromboemboli, there may be insignificant or profound effects on pulmonary physiology. The majority of thromboemboli resolve spontaneously, over days to weeks, largely as a result of the fibrinolytic activity of the circulating blood or the pulmonary arterial wall. The thrombus may also organize and recanalize. Occasionally, the thrombi will not resolve, and with repeated episodes will lead to chronic obliterative pulmonary hypertension, as mentioned previously.

Pulmonary infarction, the death of lung tissue due to vascular obstruction, is not an invariable accompaniment of embolism, probably occurring in less than 10 per cent of all cases of thromboembolism. The collateral bronchial circulation is, in many cases, adequate to maintain viability of the area involved. In the presence of conditions such as diminished ventilation, pulmonary infection, and congestive heart failure, all of which

tend to produce vascular stasis, an embolus is much more likely to result in infarction. Embolic obstruction leads to hyperemia and edema, which, if some of the aforementioned conditions are present, will progress in about 24 hours to infarction with alveolar wall necrosis and hemorrhage into the alveoli and associated bronchi. Within 2 weeks, fibroblastic proliferation is in progress, and the end result is a contracted scar that may or may not be visible on radiographs.

The severity of response to embolism is a function of the previous cardiovascular status and the subsequent degree of blood pressure elevation in the pulmonary arterial tree. In general terms, the obstruction of a small pulmonary artery may be silent, whereas occlusion of the main trunk of the pulmonary artery may be followed by cessation of cardiac output and death. Between these extremes is a spectrum of pathophysiologic responses.

If the vascular bed obstructed is of intermediate size, the systemic blood pressure may fall in association with a concomitant rise in the pulmonary artery pressure, the right ventricular end-diastolic pressure, and the systemic venous pressure. The mechanism or mechanisms producing the pulmonary hypertension continue to be a source of considerable controversy. Although some experimental studies indicate that the extent of embolism, or the reduction in cross-sectional area of the pulmonary vascular bed, is the most important factor, there is also evidence for neural reflex or humoral mechanisms for the pulmonary hypertension seen following embolism, but these are not well understood.

With embolism, there is a sudden onset of dypsnea that is due in part to hypoxia and reflexes from stimulation of receptors in the pulmonary artery. The degree of symptomatology may be far in excess of what might be expected based on the cross-sectional area occluded. Tachycardia occurs as a response to the fall in systemic blood pressure, hypoxemia, and perhaps apprehension. Cyanosis is occasionally seen following massive embolism, perhaps the result of shunting of blood through arteriovenous anastomoses bypassing areas of ventilated lung. With smaller emboli, such deadspace ventilation is minimized by reflex constriction of the bronchial smooth muscle in the area of embolism, thus reducing ventilation to that area. There is also a reduction of surfactant synthesis in oligemic lung, which leads to alveolar instability, atelectasis, and a further reduction in ventilation. Pulmonary embolism per se is generally not accompanied by fever and leukocytosis; however, both may occur as a consequence of an underlying infection or pulmonary infarction. When cough occurs, it is probably in response to the inflammation of the bronchial mucosa within the area of infarction. With involvement of the pleural surface by infarction there is frequently pleuritic pain, but there may also be substernal discomfort of myocardial ischemia. This may be attributable to the mechanical block of pulmonary arteries reducing, in turn, the cardiac output and coronary blood flow. Distention of the right cardiac chambers may also impede coronary flow by interfering with coronary venous return. Since other types of pulmonary hypertension have been noted to produce similar pain, it is also possible that some of the pain may result directly from distention of the pulmonary arteries.

INTERSTITIAL LUNG DISEASES

The interstitial lung diseases are a heterogeneous group of disorders that affect primarily the alveolar wall structures; over 100 different interstitial lung diseases have been described. The most common are those associated with inhalation of inorganic or organic dusts, idiopathic pulmonary fibrosis, sarcoidosis, and connective tissue diseases. Independent of the type or specific etiology, the initiation of most of these diseases occurs through an "alveolitis" (i.e., the infiltration of the alveolar wall by inflammatory cells). Bronchoalveolar lavage in patients with interstitial lung disease is characterized by an increased total number of cells. In addition, there is often a change in cell distribution such that one or more effector cell types are emphasized, and frequently these effector cells show evidence of "activation." These activated inflammatory cells possess the potential to augment parenchymal toxicity, alter the numbers of resident and inflammatory cells, activate immunocompetent cells, and participate in the derangements of connective tissue metabolism underlying the fibrotic process.

PNEUMOCONIOSIS

If large airborne particles are inhaled, they impinge on the walls of the tortuous airways and are either swept out in the mucus sheet by ciliary action or expelled by the cough mechanism. However, if the particles are small, less than 10 μm in diameter, some will reach the alveoli. These particles are engulfed by phagocytes and transported toward the respiratory bronchioles. Even in normal lungs this is a relatively inefficient process, and silting up of these dust cells occurs in the respiratory bronchioles. Thus, not all of the material reaches the continuous layer of ciliated epithelium that could expel the dust from the lung. Macrophages containing inorganic particulates enter the interstitial tissues, where the dust particles may remain in situ or from which they enter the lymphatics. Much of the dust is arrested in foci of lymphatic collections at the division of the airways or vessels, and the remainder is carried to the tracheobronchial and hilar lymph nodes. There is not clear-cut evidence that phagocytes have any destructive action on most inorganic particles. Apparently, they act merely as vehicles to free the alveoli from foreign matter.

Although the precise mechanism of fibrosis is not clear, the early fibrotic lesion is localized in the small bronchioles. This can lead to impairment of airflow at these sites, distortion and disruption of alveoli, and the development of focal emphysema. Thus, early in the pulmonary fibrotic response to inorganic material, small airways obstructive disease can be seen (independent of cigarette smoking). This also appears in several animal models of pneumoconiosis (asbestosis). As most pneumoconioses advance, lung volumes decrease from interstitial scarring, and compensatory paracicatricial emphysema may occur in other areas. If the process is extensive, there is not only disturbance of the ventilatory function but also disruption of the pulmonary capillary bed. Fibrosis occurring around the lymphatics impedes lymph flow, so that the irritating dust and phagocytes escape into the alveolar tissue about the blood vessels. In this position, further fibrosis, with the added element of decreased capillary bed, contributes to the development of pulmonary arterial hypertension. Thus, a patient with this condition will have a diminished total lung capacity, decreased forced vital capacity (with a normal forced expiratory volume in 1 second to forced vital capacity ratio; FEV_1/FVC), diminished diffusing capacity, and evidence of pulmonary hypertension.

Although many inorganic particulates are inert, others have been demonstrated to have significant effects at the cellular level, and they demonstrate striking pulmonary pathology. Extensive aerosol exposure to free crystalline silica (as occurs with mining, foundry working, and sandblasting) has long been known to produce fibrotic lung disease (silicosis). The development of lung disease is dose-related. Silica particles have been demonstrated to have direct cytotoxic effects on alveolar and tissue macrophages, leading to the release of destructive enzymes and oxidants. Ingestion of particles may also result in the release of soluble mediators (monokines) that may activate lymphocytes and stimulate the proliferation of, as well as collagen production by, fibroblasts. Pathologically, birefringent crystals appear in the center of the characteristic silicotic nodules, surrounded by whorled, hyalinized collagen. With extensive disease, areas of fibrosis may coalesce, forming conglomerate masses of dense scar tissue. Some central cavitation may occur, and it is generally thought that silicotics are associated with an increased incidence of pulmonary tuberculosis.

Carbon dust encountered during the mining and processing of coal has also been demonstrated to produce a chronic fibrotic pulmonary process (pneumoconiosis of coal workers, or "black lung disease"). Carbon-laden macrophages in the respiratory bronchioles cause focal emphysema, and accumulating connective tissue produces pulmonary fibrosis. Conglomeration of these collagenous foci in a subset of patients leads to the most severe form of this disease, progressive massive fibrosis.

The most widely publicized pneumoconiosis is that due to asbestos. This particularly indestructible silicate is used in the manufacture of insulation material, brake and pipe linings, cement, and some fabrics. Contamination of the surrounding atmosphere with asbestos fibers may occur, so that persons removed from the mining and manufacturing of asbestos may be susceptible to disease. Inhalation of fibers results in alveolar deposition, predominantly in the lower lobes. Asbestos fibers have been shown to have direct cytotoxic effects on alveolar macrophages and to have suppressive effects on the cell-mediated immune response. Soluble mediators again likely mediate fibroblast proliferation and collagen production. The level and length of exposure to aerosolized asbestos are related to subsequent development of progressive peribronchiolar pulmonary fibrosis (asbestosis), usually 15 to 20 years after the first exposure. The asbestos particles are only slowly degraded, and the pathophysiologic process perpetuates; interstitial pulmonary fibrosis continues long after exposure has ended.

Asbestos is notorious for causing other distinct pathologic processes. Benign pleural disease, in the form of nondescript effusion or pleural thickening or plaque formation, is relatively common 5 to 15 years after what may be comparatively small asbestos exposures. More sinister is the malignant tumor of the pleura, mesothelioma. Almost all patients with this aggressive, uniformly fatal tumor have a history of asbestos exposure, again sometimes slight. In addition, recent studies suggest an increased risk of bronchogenic carcinoma among asbestos-exposed patients; often this is related to a potentiating effect of the known carcinogenicity of smoking cigarettes.

HYPERSENSITIVITY PNEUMONITIS

The inhalation of various organic dusts can result in both acute and chronic changes in pulmonary function. Farmer's lung was the first of these diseases to be well described. The storage of wet hay in warm places allows the growth of microorganisms such as *Micropolyspora faeni* and the thermophilic actinomycetes, which may be inhaled. Bird-breeder's lung occurs in individuals handling pigeons or domestic fowl, and it is thought to result from inhalation of avian serum proteins found in excreta. Bagassosis is seen in workers in the sugar-cane industry; contaminating mold spores are thought to be responsible. Thermophilic actinomycetes can also contaminate humidifiers used in heating or air-conditioning systems and can cause hypersensitivity pneumonitis in exposed individuals (humidifier lung). There are several other etiologies described, most

with colorful names describing the appropriate occupational exposure.

Some patients manifest subacute episodes of dyspnea 4 to 6 hours after an unusually heavy exposure to organic dust antigen. Another pattern of response is an acute asthmatic reaction immediately following exposure that clears spontaneously, only to be followed 6 hours later by an episode of dyspnea, fever, and systemic symptoms. The last presentation is observed in patients who have had prolonged low-grade or repeated exposures. The pattern, then, is that of an insidious restrictive lung disease indistinguishable from other forms of interstitial pneumonitis, except by careful occupational and environmental investigation.

The immunopathogenesis of hypersensitivity pneumonitis is quite complex. The presence of precipitating antibodies to the antigen in question in the serum and bronchoalveolar fluid of many patients suggests a possible role for immune complexes (type III reaction) in this disease. However, the presence of these antibodies in the serum of the majority of exposed but asymptomatic workers argues for an important role for individual host susceptibility factors. The pathology of the lung disease strongly suggests a major role for type IV, or delayed, hypersensitivity. Initially, there is a widespread alveolar infiltration of mononuclear cells, followed by interstitial accumulations of histiocytes and plasma cells and subsequent fibrosis. Granuloma formation is characteristic in the fibrotic lung. Bronchoalveolar lavage of patients with hypersensitivity pneumonitis reveals a preponderance of small lymphocytes, with an increased T-suppressor to T-helper ratio in some individuals.

The alterations in pulmonary function depend on when in the course of the disease the patient is tested. Occasionally, the process may mimic asthma, with severe reductions in expiratory flow rates and evidence of air-trapping. More often, a restrictive defect is seen early in the disease process. Patients with the insidious form usually manifest a decrement in all lung volumes, a reduced diffusing capacity, and hypoxemia.

IDIOPATHIC PULMONARY FIBROSIS (IPF)

The histologic appearance of IPF demonstrates widespread but inhomogeneous involvement. It is thought that early stages involve interstitial edema with some hemorrhage and neutrophil infiltration. Over time, mononuclear cells (lymphocytes and macrophages) predominate. Organization of the alveolar exudate and destruction of the alveolar epithelium result in attenuated and irregularly thickened alveolar septa. There is not only an increase of the connective tissue elements (collagen, elastin, and glycosaminoglycans) but also, as revealed by electron microscopy, a disordered arrangement of collagen fibers. Bronchiolar inflammation may occur, and varying degrees of vascular bed obliteration may be seen. Smooth-muscle hyperplasia is common. In end-stage fibrotic lung disease, large airspaces (0.5 to 1.0 cm diameter) lined by hyperplastic epithelium are surrounded by dense connective tissue (honeycomb lung). Any clues to the underlying etiology are usually lost at this stage.

A subset of patients with IPF are described who have a paucity of interstitial fibrosis when first seen but who manifest an impressive alveolar cellular exudate. The alveoli are packed with polyclonal cells, some showing mitotic figures; the majority appear to be alveolar macrophages. This "desquamative interstitial pneumonia" (DIP) is thought to represent a more treatable form of alveolitis. This is in contrast to "usual interstitial pneumonia" (UIP), in which there is less intra-alveolar and alveolar wall cellularity, the majority of which is mononuclear. This form is not particularly responsive to corticosteroid therapy.

Another distinguishable form of IPF is characterized by recurrent peripheral infiltrates on chest radiographs, fever, and eosinophilic alveolar and interstitial infiltrates. This eosinophilic pneumonia is seen in individuals in the sixth and seventh decades of life, frequently in association with asthma. It can be exquisitely sensitive to corticosteroid therapy. Other rarer forms of IPF have been described with a lymphocytic inflammatory component (LIP) that in some cases is associated with connective tissue disorders; in others, it may be an early form of lymphoma.

In the early stages of interstitial lung disease, minimal hypoxemia at rest and a widened arterial-alveolar oxygen gradient are usually seen. The diffusing capacity for carbon monoxide is usually low, but Pa_{O_2} often increases with exercise, demonstrating the importance of ventilation/perfusion mismatch at rest. With disease progression, there is a reduction in all lung volumes and in lung compliance. Flow rates are usually normal. Resting hypoxemia and stimulation of interstitial stretch receptors combine to produce tachypnea and alveolar hyperventilation with hypocapnia. In time, the work of breathing is strikingly increased, and further oxygen desaturation with exercise occurs. In end-stage disease, hypercapnia and pulmonary hypertension are manifest.

SARCOIDOSIS

Sarcoidosis is a disease of unknown etiology characterized by the presence of noncaseating epithelioid cell granulomas involving multiple organs. At least 90 per cent of all patients have lung involvement, and, for most, the pulmonary manifestations have the most serious consequences. The characteristic morphologic feature of pulmonary sarcoidosis is the presence of noncaseating granulomas; these are sharply circumscribed and are present in the alveolar septa and often in the walls of bronchi and pulmonary arteries and veins as well. The center of the granuloma consists of nodules of lightly packed epithelioid cells; these are cells derived from the mononuclear-phagocyte system. Multinucleated giant cells, primarily of Langhan's type, and discrete macrophages are also found in the central region; the latter morphologically resemble secretory cells more than phagocytic cells. These macrophages and epithelioid cells may be responsible for secreting the large amounts of lysozyme and angiotensin-converting enzyme (ACE) found in the blood and bronchoalveolar lavage (BAL) of some sarcoid patients. Surrounding the central follicle is a perimeter of lymphocytes, macrophages, monocytes, and fibroblasts. Those lymphocytes present appear large and "activated." Any necrosis in the center of these granulomas is minimal and never caseous.

There is increasing evidence that the typical granulomatous pulmonary reaction is preceded by a more diffuse interstitial alveolitis. Early in their development, granulomas are composed of a loose collection of inflammatory and immune effector cells and few epithelioid cells; with maturation, the relative numbers of epithelioid cells increase. Sampling of the alveolar space by BAL has served to define the cellular interactions during the inflammatory response. The relative proportion of activated T-lymphocytes in lavage samples is increased in patients with sarcoidosis. Further subdivision demonstrates that there is an excess of T-helper cells in lavage samples, with few T-suppressor cells. The lymphocyte profile contrasts with that seen in the peripheral blood of such patients; most are relatively lymphopenic, with a decreased proportion of T cells. This systemic lymphopenia is thought to be important in the skin-test anergy seen in these patients. The lymphocyte distribution in the hilar and mediastinal lymph nodes more closely resembles that seen in the lung. This serves to magnify the role of the pulmonary inflammatory response in the pathogenesis of sarcoidosis. Lavaged T cells from sarcoid lungs, but not peripheral blood lymphocytes, have been shown to release spontaneously significant quantities of monocyte chemotactic factor (MCF), which may underlie the observed accumulation of monocytes in the inflammatory interstitial foci. The proportion of T cells obtained on lavage has also been shown to correlate with excess immunoglobulin-secreting cells in lavage samples. It has been suggested that the polyclonal hyperimmunoglobulinemia seen in these patients is a result of lung T-helper cells augmenting locally produced immunoglobulin.

The fate of the underlying lung interstitium with sarcoid granuloma can progress along two pathways: It can remain normal, or it can undergo progressive fibrosis. In about 20 per cent of patients with sarcoidosis, there is progression to interstitial fibrosis with distortion and replacement of the pulmonary architecture. Eventually, the end-stage fibrotic lung disease is indistinguishable from other causes of fibrosing alveolitis.

Patients with radiographically evident parenchymal lung disease may have some reduction in lung volumes; the vital capacity is often proportionately lower than the residual volume. The diffusing capacity for carbon monoxide at rest may be normal or low; exercise often reduces the DLCO further and may also widen the alveolar-arterial oxygen gradient. In addition to demonstrating these standard findings, a proportion of these patients will show a significant obstructive component thought to represent granulomatous inflammation of the small airways, on pulmonary-function testing.

ALVEOLAR DISEASES

PULMONARY ALVEOLAR PROTEINOSIS

This chronic disease of the lungs, characterized by the accumulation of eosinophilic material in the alveoli, was described first by Rosen and coworkers in 1958. It occurs most commonly in males between the ages of 20 and 50 years. Efforts to isolate infectious agents or to identify an inhalant or aspirant common to all cases have also been unsuccessful. Alveolar material of similar composition has been found in acute silicoproteinosis, which occurs in sandblasters exposed to high concentrations of silicon dioxide. The material has a chemical composition similar to that of pulmonary surfactant but has decreased surface-active properties. At present, the disease is believed to result from decreased clearance of surfactant rather than from overproduction of the agent.

In the early stages of pulmonary alveolar proteinosis, septal cells in the walls of alveoli increase in both size and number. Increasing further, they may line the alveoli, project into the lumina, slough, disintegrate, and give rise to PAS-positive granular and floccular material with numerous small acicular spaces. Continuation of this sequence leads to the filling of the alveoli and distal airspaces, including respiratory bronchioles. In these areas of consolidation there is a striking absence of cellular infiltration into the interalveolar septa, and there is no evidence of vascular congestion. The ultimate histologic fate is not clearly defined, although it is known from clinical studies that regression may occur. Biopsy studies of areas believed to have been involved previously have shown slight interstitial fibrosis of questionable significance and some residual granularity of the alveolar lining cells.

In this disease, although the distal parenchyma is not normal and air-containing, there is no primary involvement of the airways. Hence, spirographic studies show little evidence of obstruction to air flow. There is, however, filling of alveoli by "proteinaceous" material and replacement of functioning lung volume by consolidation. As a consequence of this, there is a restrictive pattern of ventilation with a decrease in vital capacity. The patient may complain of dyspnea, which frequently is not as severe as one might expect, considering the level of hypoxemia or extent of radiographic findings.

The increase in size and number of alveolar septal cells and the early partial coating of alveoli with eosinophilic material interfere with the diffusion of oxygen across the alveolocapillary membrane. This does not permit full saturation of hemoglobin passing such alveoli and results in various degrees of arterial unsaturation and its clinical manifestation, cyanosis. Further arterial oxygen unsaturation is caused by venous blood passing through the intact vasculature of consolidated alveoli, which contain no air at all. Thus, the pathophysiology of pulmonary alveolar proteinosis is a consequence of a ventilation/perfusion imbalance. There is no evidence of impaired carbon dioxide excretion. If clinical improvement occurs, the oxygenation of blood may return to normal.

From clinical studies thus far published, it appears that patients with pulmonary alveolar proteinosis are unusually susceptible to superimposed infections, especially from *Nocardia, Aspergillus,* and *Cryptococcus* organisms; steroid treatment favors infection and is of little efficacy. In the presence of pulmonary insufficiency, such infections, even though minor in extent, may lead to death. Bronchopulmonary lavage has been of value in reducing the level of hypoxemia in some patients. Those who have died without recognized infection showed progressive respiratory failure in the forms of dyspnea and cyanosis.

PLEURAL DISORDERS

The pleura is a double layer of thin, mesothelial serous membrane; the visceral pleura coats the surface of the lung, and the parietal pleura lines the inside of the chest wall. Lying beneath the mesothelial monolayer is a connective tissue layer, composed of elastic and collagenous fibers, blood vessels, and lymphatics. The parietal pleura is also supplied with sensory nerve endings. The pleural space is normally only a potential space; approximately 30 ml of serous fluid serves as a lubricating layer, facilitating ventilatory movements of the lungs against the adjacent hemithorax.

PLEURITIS AND PLEURAL EFFUSIONS

The pleural membranes are permeable to gas and liquid. Under normal circumstances, the small amount of pleural fluid present filters out of the arterial end of the parietal pleural capillaries, and the majority is reabsorbed at the venous end of visceral pleural capillaries. If there is an excessive amount of pleural fluid or if such fluid has a high protein concentration, the visceral pleural lymphatics play an increasingly critical part in maintaining a clear pleural space.

The balance between fluid formation and absorption is governed by the same Starling forces that determine transport across other capillary beds. In the presence of inflammation, the filtration coefficient of the pleural membrane, a measure of its permeability, increases. This change may be due to damage of the vascular endothelium or the action of various soluble mediators of inflammation. Commonly, a coexistent increase in blood flow elevates capillary hydrostatic pressure, and this combines with the elevated temperature to augment fluid and protein filtration. An increased amount of protein in the pleural space elevates colloid osmotic pressure, thus retarding fluid absorption; it has been shown that a pleural fluid protein concentration of about 4 gm/100 ml overloads the absorptive capacity of the visceral pleural capillaries and requires active lymphatic drainage for clearance. Bacterial or viral pneumonia with contiguous pleuritis is the most common cause of such a high-protein pleural effusion (exudate). Other causes include pulmonary infarction, the inflammatory pleuritis seen in patients with uremia or collagen vascular diseases, and actual pleural-space infection, empyema.

An elevation of capillary hydrostatic pressure is the mechanism of the pleural effusions commonly accompanying the systemic venous hypertension seen in congestive heart failure. Such effusions are normally of low protein content (transudates) and are most often right-sided or bilateral. A decrease in the colloid osmotic pressure of blood, as seen in patients with hypoproteinemia (e.g., cirrhosis, nephrotic syndrome, congestive heart failure) may also contribute to effusion formation. With plasma albumin levels below 1.5 gm/dl, diffuse edema formation (anasarca) may be accompanied by ascites and bilateral pleural effusions of low protein content. Thus, patients with ascites may have coexistent pleural effusions. Lymphatic vessels lie beneath the serosal membrane on both sides of the diaphragm and have extensive communications. In addition, small defects have been demonstrated in the dome of the diaphragm in many individuals, and they can serve as pathways for fluid transport. Patients with ascites due to liver failure or Meigs syndrome (ascites and pleural effusion associated with benign ovarian solid tumors) and patients with hydronephrosis accumulate pleural fluid by a combination of these two mechanisms.

Since lymphatic drainage is one of the two ways that pleural fluid can leave the thorax and the only way that protein can leave, disruption of the lymphatic system can result in pleural effusion. When mediastinal lymph nodes are infiltrated by tumor or fibrous tissue, lymph flow decreases and lymphatic pressure increases. Obstruction or disruption of the thoracic duct will have a similar effect. Hypoplasia of the lymphatics, as in the yellow nail syndrome, also results in pleural effusions.

Neoplasms in the thorax cause pleural effusions by a variety of mechanisms. Central tumors or mediastinal invasion may impair lymphatic drainage. Pleural seeding in metastatic deposits is a common cause of exudative pleural effusion; there may be increased permeability of the capillaries supplying the tumor explant or actual fluid and protein production by the tumor itself. Obstructive pneumonitis and peripheral blood and lymphatic vessel invasion are other potential pathogenic contributors.

EMPYEMA

When pleural fluid becomes infected, its volume and consistency and the coexisting inflammatory changes may prevent adequate resorption. In empyema, the pleural surfaces represent abscess walls that are thickened, inflamed, and granular. Infectious agents most often gain entry into the pleural space via spread from the underlying lung. Less commonly, direct spread from other contiguous primary sites of infection occurs; mediastinitis, vertebral osteomyelitis, and hepatic and subdiaphragmatic abscess can lead to empyema. The next most common mechanism of seeding is direct passage through the chest wall, as with penetrating trauma or after surgical intervention, including simple thoracentesis. Lymphohematogenous seeding of pleural fluid as a cause of empyema is uncommon, except perhaps in primary tuberculosis.

The frequency with which bacteria gain access to the pleural space is unknown. Some aberration of the host-parasite relationship is necessary for empyema to develop, such as a large or particularly virulent inoculum or impaired pleural drainage or host defense. Positive pleural-fluid bacterial cultures are seen in patients who do not progress to develop empyema; the fluid is turbid but usually easily drained by thoracentesis. The thick, grossly purulent, often foul-smelling fluid of empyema patients is usually easily recognized; it has also been suggested that a low pleural-fluid pH (< 7.10) and a low pleural-fluid glucose level may serve to distinguish infected exudates requiring tube thoracostomy. Once the organism becomes established, the previously glistening pleura becomes a dull, thickened, granulating surface. Further progression of the inflammatory process results in fibrous bands criss-crossing the empyema space and loculation of the exudate so that complete removal by thoracentesis is not possible. The wall of the empyema becomes organized into fibrous tissue, which may effectively limit the infection or necessitate external drainage.

Even if the empyema is small, a decrease in the excursions of the diaphragm and ribs secondary to pain may reduce the vital capacity and maximal breathing capacity. If the empyema is large, the lung is compressed and the mediastinum is shifted toward the opposite lung, decreasing its volume also. The total pulmonary volume is reduced, vital capacity is decreased and pulmonary blood flow is diminished. Reduced oxygenation of the blood is generally evident. Although the loss of volume may not be great, the development of a nonelastic fibrous peel over the pleura will reduce ventilatory function by mechanically limiting changes in volume. With maturation of the fibrous tissue, contraction occurs, which may reduce the lung volume severely by pulling the mediastinum toward the affected side and elevating and fixing the diaphragm. When this develops in early life, there may be a deforming scoliosis. With the decrease in volume on the side of disease, there is an absolute increase in volume in the normal hemithorax that results in compensatory emphysema.

EPIDEMIC PLEURODYNIA

Epidemic pleurodynia, or Bornholm disease, is an acute febrile illness due to infection with coxsackievirus B. In experimental animals, the typical lesion in striated muscle resembles Zenker's hyaline degeneration. In humans, the histologic changes are unknown because the illness is self-limited and followed by complete recovery. There may be severe pain and tenderness of muscles in the trunk and extremities, suggesting that the basic lesion is perhaps a myositis that also involves the diaphragm. Pleuritis, pleural effusion, exanthems, orchitis, diarrhea, hepatitis, meningitis, and pulmonary infiltrations have been noted. There are no significant alterations in pulmonary function. Recovery is characterized by a rise in specific neutralizing antibodies.

PNEUMOTHORAX

Pneumothorax is defined as the presence of air in the pleural space. Normally, throughout respiration, the pressure in the pleural space is subatmospheric. Any breach in the visceral pleura allows leakage of air from the adjacent alveoli into the pleural cavity. Trauma is a common cause of pneumothorax. Penetrating chest injury and fractured ribs may tear the pleura, as may a thoracentesis needle. Pneumothorax is the most common complication of blind transbronchial biopsy, which is performed with small forceps advanced through the inner channel of a fiberoptic bronchoscope. Air may also enter the pleural space from the mediastinum as a result of tracheal or esophageal rupture or spontaneous pneumomediastinum.

When pneumothorax occurs in the absence of trauma, the process is termed *spontaneous pneumothorax*. In older individuals, such an airleak is usually a complication of severe underlying lung disease and is termed *complicated spontaneous pneumothorax*. In contrast, pneumothorax in young people is most commonly due to the rupture of the localized apical bullae unaccompanied by other lung disease, so-called *simple spontaneous pneumothorax*. This latter condition is most common in tall men, is more common on the right side, and is frequently of a recurrent nature. Both the genesis of the bulla and the precipitating cause of the rupture are unknown. Although the majority of episodes occur at rest, rapid changes in ambient pressures do precipitate pneumothoraces, as during rapid ascent to high altitude or during decompression after diving.

Complicated spontaneous pneumothorax is most often due to widespread bullous emphysema; a coexistent bronchopleural fistula often makes reexpansion notoriously difficult. Other underlying causes of pneumothorax include severe asthma, rupture of a pneumatocele in staphylococcal pneumonia, rupture of subpleural cavities in necrotizing lung disease, and eosinophilic granuloma. Rupture of a lung abscess into the pleural space results in pyopneumothorax.

If the rent in the pleura is small, the size of the pneumothorax will be self-limiting, with the defect tending to close as the lung collapses. If the defect is large, complete lung collapse may occur. A proportion of individuals go on to develop "tension pneumothorax"; positive expiratory airways pressure forces air into the pleural space, but its escape is prevented by a flap-valve phenomenon. There is a theoretic limitation to the amount of positive pleural pressure that can be generated by this mechanism, but because only 15 to 20 cm H_2O pleural pressure can lead to pulmonary vascular hypotension, reduction in functional residual capacity of the contralateral lung, and significant ventilation/perfusion mismatch, these patients develop severe dyspnea and respiratory failure. The mediastinum shifts, compressing the contralateral lung and death will ensue if the hemithorax is not decompressed.

To a large extent, the physiologic consequences of pneumothorax depend on the extent of underlying lung disease. Young healthy individuals may have very little dyspnea after traumatic or simple spontaneous pneumothorax, since lung collapse leads to a reduction in both ventilation and perfusion and the contralateral lung is normally functioning adequately. In the presence of severe lung disease, however, even small pneumothoraces may compound the gas exchange problems and lead to severe hypoxemia and respiratory failure.

REFERENCES

Black, L. F.: The pleural space and pleural fluid. Mayo Clin. Proc. *47*:493, 1972.

Bowden, D. H.: Alveolar response to injury. Thorax *36*:801, 1981.

Crystal, R. G., Roberts, W. C., Hunninghake, G. W., et al.: Pulmonary sarcoidosis: A disease characterized and perpetuated by activated lung T-lymphocytes. Ann. Intern. Med. *94*:73, 1981.

Daniele, R. P., Dauber, J. H., and Rossman, M. D.: Immunologic abnormalities in sarcoidosis. Ann. Intern. Med. *92*:406, 1980.

de Shazo, R. D.: Current concepts about the pathogenesis of silicosis and asbestosis. J. Allergy Clin. Immunol. *70*:41, 1982.

Divertie, M. B.: The adult respiratory distress syndrome. Mayo Clin. Proc. *57*:371, 1982.

Farrell, P. M., and Avery, M. E.: Hyaline membrane disease. Am. Rev. Respir. Dis. *109*:287, 1974.

Gaensler, E. A., Carrington, C. B., Couter, R. G., et al.: Radiographic, physiologic, pathologic correlations in interstitial pneumonias. Prog. Respir. Dis. *8*:223, 1975.

Gustman, P., Yerger, L., and Wanner, A.: Immediate cardiovascular effects of tension pneumothorax. Am. Rev. Respir. Dis. *127*:171, 1983.

Holland, W. W.: Beginnings of bronchitis. Thorax *37*:401, 1982.

Karlinsky, J. B., and Goldstein, R. H.: Fibrotic lung disease: A perspective. J. Lab. Clin. Med. *96*:939, 1980.

Keogh, B. A., and Crystal, R. G.: Alveolitis: The key to the interstitial lung diseases. Thorax *37*:1, 1982.

Killen, D. A., and Gobbel, W. G.: Spontaneous Pneumothorax. Boston, Little, Brown & Co., 1968.

King, R. J.: Pulmonary surfactant. J. Appl. Physiol. *53*:1, 1982.

Morgan, W. K. C.: Industrial bronchitis. Br. J. Industr. Med. *135*:285, 1978.

Rinaldo, J. E., and Rogers, R. M.: Adult respiratory-distress syndrome: changing concepts of lung injury and repair. N. Engl. J. Med. *306*:900, 1982.

Rosen, S. H., Castleman, B., and Liebow, A. A.: Pulmonary alveolus proteinosis. N. Engl. J. Med. *258*:1123, 1958.

Snider, G. L.: Clinical Pulmonary Medicine. Boston, Little, Brown & Co., 1981.

RHEUMATOLOGY, ALLERGY, INFECTIOUS DISEASE, AND HEMATOLOGY

Rheumatic Diseases **17**

Giles G. Bole, Jr.

The rheumatic diseases are grouped together because they produce symptoms in and impairment of function of the musculoskeletal system as well as other body systems. The musculoskeletal system can be visualized as a highly integrated apparatus consisting of (1) the bones, which provide the skeletal supports of the body, (2) the joints between the osseous structures, which permit mobility while maintaining the capacity for stability, and (3) the neuromuscular apparatus for moving or stabilizing the supporting structures as needed. This chapter will be concerned primarily with the articulations and with the disturbances in function of the musculoskeletal system produced by diseases of the joints and closely related structures. It will also deal with other closely related diseases of connective tissue.

The joints and the tendinous structures, which transmit the motivating forces to permit smooth and efficient motion, represent specialized forms of connective tissue. Basic information regarding the structure and function of connective tissues, immune reactions, and the inflammatory response is needed for an understanding of normal function of these structures and the alteration produced by disease.

STRUCTURE AND FUNCTION OF CONNECTIVE TISSUES

It is no longer possible to regard connective tissue as an inert stuffing material, supporting and binding together the parenchymatous, neural, and vascular structures of multicellular organisms. As a result of numerous investigations, there has emerged a concept emphasizing the complex and dynamic state of these tissues, their importance in maintaining the physiologic integrity of the musculoskeletal system, and the significance of pathologic alterations in diseases of the connective tissues. The several types of connective tissues that differentiate from the mesenchyme include loose (areolar) connective tissue, dense fibroelastic connective tissue, reticular, adipose and elastic connective tissue, as well as bone, cartilage, and synovium.

Connective tissue can be regarded as composed of *cellular* and *intercellular* elements, with the intercellular components consisting of an *amorphous ground substance* interlaced with extracellular *fibrillar* materials. The proportion of these three constituents varies greatly with ana-

tomic location and functional requirements: tendons and fascia are largely fibrillar, Wharton's jelly of the umbilical cord is predominantly ground substance, and cartilage and synovium are relatively rich in cells.

Connective tissue has the obvious important function of mechanical support and protection. In addition, it is essential to the smooth transmission of mechanical energy derived from muscle contraction to move the organism or its parts, facilitated by lubrication from ground substance components located in the gliding planes of joints, bursae, and tendon sheaths. Since connective tissue is everywhere interposed between capillaries and cellular structure, it has an important transport function, influencing the passage of essential nutrients to the cells and the return of metabolic wastes to the circulation. Particularly noteworthy is the remarkable potential of connective tissue in the process of anatomic repair. Following tissue injury, cellular components usually neutralize or destroy noxious agents, remove debris, and produce a framework of fibers and ground substance that bridges the anatomic defect and frequently restores functional capacity.

CONNECTIVE TISSUE CELLS

The cellular elements of connective tissue control the formation, maintenance, and breakdown of the extracellular components. Primordial mesenchymal cells may differentiate to become macrophages, mast cells, plasma cells, lymphocytes, and fibroblasts. Fibroblasts are capable of mitotic division and are not dependent on a "stem cell" for their perpetuation. Tissue macrophages, widely distributed throughout the connective tissue, arise from hematogenous precursors and serve a scavenger role, ingesting foreign substances and removing debris. These cells form an important element in the immune system and also constitute the mononuclear phagocytic system, which includes the Kupffer cells of the liver, alveolar macrophages of the lung, and splenic and bone marrow mononuclear phagocytes. Tissue mast cells, also diffusely distributed, may be present in significant numbers in certain tissues. They represent 3 per cent of the cells in the superficial aspect of the synovial membrane. Their role in the physiology of connective tissue is not clear; they contain heparin, histamine, and 5-hydroxytryptamine. Plasma cells, lymphocytes, and eosinophils, derived from the bloodstream, are sparsely and irregularly distributed throughout connective tissue.

Fibroblasts are responsible for the formation and maintenance of fibrous and fibroelastic connective tissues. Specialized variants of fibroblasts—the chondrocytes, osteocytes, and synoviocytes—are responsible for the formation of cartilage, bone, and the synovial fluid, respectively. The fibroblast appears as a stellate or spindle-shaped cell with a large pale nucleus and faintly staining cytoplasm under conventional light microscopy. Ultrastructural studies demonstrate that these cells are equipped for complex biosynthetic activities. By tissue culture it has been convincingly demonstrated that the fibroblast synthesizes the glycosaminoglycans (acid mucopolysaccharides) of the ground substance. In addition, the fibroblast produces collagen and elastic fibers, which are first detectable in aggregated form outside, but close to, the cell periphery.

FIBRILLAR COMPONENTS

Three types of intercellular fibers can be distinguished by staining techniques and light microscopy. The most abundant is collagen, composing one third of total body protein. With conventional histologic techniques this appears as wavy bundles of fibers, with the smallest units appearing to be nonbranching fibers with a uniform diameter of 0.3 to 0.5 μ. Under the electron microscope, these fibers appear to be made up of submicroscopic fibrils with a characteristic periodic banding measuring 68 nm.

The formation of collagen and its molecular characteristics have been intensively investigated. The fundamental unit is referred to as *tropocollagen,* which is rod-shaped (1.5 × 300 nm) and consists of three α (alpha) chains in triple helical configuration. Five different α chains with distinctive amino acid sequences are recognized: α 1 (I), α 2, α 1 (II), α 1 (III), α 1 (IV). Each chain has a molecular weight of 95,000 to 100,000 daltons and contains high concentrations of the unique amino acids hydroxyproline and hydroxylysine, as well as glycine, alanine, lysine, and proline. At least five distinct collagen molecules have now been identified as unique gene products: type I in molecular form $[\alpha1(I)]_2\alpha2$; type II $[\alpha1(II)]_3$; type III $[\alpha1(III)]_3$; type IV $[\alpha1(IV)]_3$; and type V in molecular form A and B. These collagens demonstrate differences in carbohydrate content number of cross-links, and the degree of hydroxylation of prolyl and lysyl residues. Tissue distribution of the five major types of collagen can be related to these structural differences and the functional requirements within each tissue. Type I collagen contains fibrils of high tensile strength and occurs in tissues that contain sparse amounts of ground substance materials. It is the most common type of collagen and is found in large amounts in bone,

skin, and tendons. In cartilage the collagen is type II, contains a high concentration of carbohydrate, does not form prominent fibrils, and is complexed with large amounts of proteoglycan. Chondroblasts are the only cells known to synthesize this form of collagen. Type III collagen is found in fetal tissues, skin, arteries, and uterus; occurs in association with type I collagen, and contains the amino acid cysteine and a high content of hydroxyproline. Basement membranes contain type IV collagen, which is rich in carbohydrates, including mannose and hexosamines. In addition, this form of collagen contains 3-hydroxyproline and large amounts of cysteine, plus hydroxylysine. Type V collagen is found in basement membranes and around smooth muscle cells, chondrocytes, and other tissues in pericellular location.

The biosynthesis of collagen molecules follows the general process established for proteins that are to be secreted from the cell. Collagen messenger RNA (mRNA) is transcribed from structural genes specific for each α chain. The precursor of α chains is a larger molecule (pro α chain, 150,000 daltons) that contains noncollagenous sequences at the N- and C-terminals of the molecule. These parts of the molecule are cleaved after secretion and are thought to maintain solubility, to facilitate orientation of troprocollagen, and to inhibit cross-link formation. Within the endoplasmic reticulum each pro α chain is synthesized, then three chains form triple helix protropocollagen, lysyl and prolyl residues are hydroxylated, glycosylation occurs, and the molecule is secreted from the cell. This process is schematically outlined in Figure 17–1.

After secretion of protropocollagen, proteolysis of the noncollagen N-terminus peptides occurs first (procollagen peptidase), followed by cleavage of the C-terminus peptides, leaving helical tropocollagen. The latter polymerizes into fibrils in a highly specific fashion in types I and II collagen, with each tropocollagen molecule overlapping its neighbor by 68 nm or a multiple of this length. Cross-linking occurs through action of lysyl oxidase on lysine to form an aldehyde (allysine) that interacts with a hydroxylysine residue on an adjacent chain. These steps can be inhibited by copper deficiency, β-aminoproprionitrile, or penicillamine. Other cross-linking reactions also occur, and their number determines the tensile strength of the collagen fibrils in different connective tissues.

Collagen in triple helical configuration resists degradation by most proteases. Specific collagenases degrade types I, II, and III collagens. They are synthesized in latent form by macrophages, polymorphonuclear leukocytes, and fibroblasts and are activated by proteinases. These collagenases are less active against denatured collagen, inhibited by serum alpha globulins (except granulocyte-derived collagenase), and cleave tropocollagen between glycine-isoleucine three fourths of the distance from the N-terminus of the molecule. Both

Figure 17–1 Diagrammatic representation of collagen biosynthesis and extracellular formation of collagen fibrils. The major steps in the process are outlined:

1. *Transcription* of structural genes produces messenger ribonucleic acid (mRNA) specific for each α chain type.

2. *Translation:* The mRNA molecules are transported to ribosomes lining the rough endoplasmic reticulum. Pro–α chain synthesis includes N-terminal ☐ and C-terminal ■ noncollagen peptides.

3. *Hydroxylation:* The middle collagen pro α chains are enzymatically hydroxylated at certain prolyl and lysyl residues.

4. *Triple helix formation:* Three pro α chains are aligned and form protocollagen.

5. *Glycosylation* involves addition of galactose (Gal) and the disaccharide glucosylgalactose (Glu-Gal).

6. *Secretion:* The completed molecule is transported to the Golgi apparatus (not shown) and secreted from the cell.

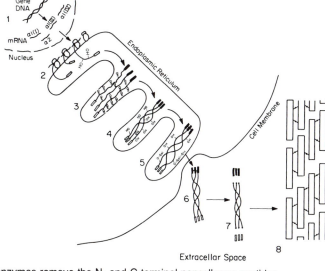

7. *Propeptide cleavage:* Extracellular protolytic enzymes remove the N- and C-terminal noncollagen peptides.

8. *Collagen fibril* polymerization and cross-link formation. Interchain cross links (—·—) are initiated by the enzyme lysyl oxidase. The degree of cross-linking depends on the collagen type.

fragments of the molecule are then susceptible to denaturation at 37°C, and in nonhelical form they can be degraded by a broad spectrum of extracellular proteases active at neutral pH or in phagolysosomes at acid pH. Type IV basement membrane collagen is also susceptible to degradation by polymorphonuclear leukocyte elastase, and type V collagens are degraded by specific proteinases that have been isolated from macrophages. These mechanisms are visualized as responsible for collagen turnover and tissue destruction within an inflammatory focus.

The second type of intercellular fiber, reticulin, defined by its intense black appearance after reaction with silver methionine stain under light microscopy, has no certain counterpart identifiable by electron microscopy. These fibers are found around blood and lymph vessels, nerves, and muscle fibers; in basement membranes; and in the lymphoid organs. The exact composition of reticulin has not been determined, but it appears to consist of collagen, noncollagen proteins, lipid, and proteoglycans. The fibers are labile to collagenases but resist proteolytic digestion by trypsin.

Elastic fibers, the third type of intercellular fibers, quite clearly differ from collagen. They have less tensile strength than collagen fibers but have a much greater tendency to return to their previous fiber length after removal of a distorting force. The elastic fiber viewed by electron microscopy consists of a fibrillar and an amorphous component. Most of the classic efforts to characterize elastic fibers have utilized bovine ligamentum nuchae, although large blood vessels, lung, and most tissues also contain this fibrillar protein. The extreme insolubility of elastic fibers has made their biochemical characterization difficult. The

two components of the elastic fiber differ in chemical composition. The microfibrils are rich in polar and sulfur-containing amino acids, but no hydroxyproline or cross-links are present. In the amorphous component the amino acid composition conforms to that of "elastin." It contains nonpolar amino acids and no cysteine or methionine, but cross-links and hydroxyproline have been detected. The precursor to elastin is tropoelastin, which is synthesized by fibroblasts and smooth muscle cells. A high content of lysine in tropoelastin is critical to the development of the three major cross-links in elastin (desmosine, isodesmosine, lysinonorleucine). The enzyme lysyl oxidase is responsible for aldehyde formation (as in collagen), which leads to the development of cross-links between tropoelastin chains. In copper deficiency or osteolathyrism the cross-linking is impaired and elastic fiber tensile strength reduced. Cross-linked elastin invests the microfibrils to form mature elastic fibers. The microfibrils contain cystine disulfide bonds, and as just noted differ in chemical composition from elastin. They are glycoproteins that contain hexose and hexosamines that are labile to a fairly broad spectrum of proteases. Turnover of elastin and presumably elastic fibers occurs slowly (as studied in aortic tissue). The enzyme elastase is involved in the degradation process; it is susceptible to inhibition by naturally occurring substances in phagocytic cells.

GROUND SUBSTANCE

The cellular and fibrillar components of connective tissue are embedded in an amorphous sol-gel continuum known as *ground substance*. In routine histologic preparations much of the ground substance is leached out, leaving empty spaces between cells and fibers. By special fixation and appropriate histochemical procedures a dramatic staining of ground substance is produced. Although these methods are not specific for glycosaminoglycans, they identify the acidic nature of the extracellular materials. Information concerning its chemical composition has increased considerably in recent years, but much remains to be learned about variations with anatomic location and alterations with aging and in disease states. It is clear that this optically structureless sol-gel is an aqueous solution of electrolytes, proteins, highly polymerized carbohydrate-containing substances known as *glycosaminoglycans* that (except perhaps for hyaluronic acid) are covalently linked to protein and called *proteoglycans,* combinations of amino acids and carbohydrate substances known as *glycoproteins,* and lipoproteins.

By extraction procedures, the proteins of ground substance have been characterized as quite distinct in amino acid content from the fibrillar proteins and as very similar to certain of the plasma proteins in electrophoretic properties. The glycoprotein content of connective tissue is somewhat higher than in plasma, and there is evidence that at least some of these glycoproteins are synthesized by connective tissue cells.

The best characterized constituents of ground substance are the proteoglycans, which contain protein covalently linked to glycosaminoglycans (GAG). The structure of the protein portion is partially defined, and the ester linkage to GAG is through the amino acid serine, or threonine. The GAG chains are arranged perpendicular to the protein "core" and are visualized as bristles on a test tube brush. In most instances, 30 to 100 GAG chains are attached to the protein molecule. Within the GAG chain a repeating disaccharide unit consists of specific monosaccharides: glucosamine or galactosamine (with acetyl and sulfate substituents) plus glucuronic or iduronic acid. In keratan sulfate the simple sugar galactose replaces the uronic acid. In the hyaluronic acid polymer the presence of protein is disputed; however, the number of disaccharide units may approximate 2500. Currently, seven different GAG have been recognized: hyaluronic acid, chondroitin-4-sulfate, chondroitin-6-sulfate, dermatan sulfate, heparin, heparan sulfate, and keratan sulfate. The proteoglycans are named for the GAG contained in the molecule; their structure is outlined in Table 17–1.

The initiation of biosynthesis of the protein core of proteoglycans is believed to follow the mechanisms responsible for development of a protein destined for secretion. Attachment of individual sugars is initiated at the serine, or threonine, residue of the core protein through the action of specific transferases that utilize nucleotide sugars as precursor molecules. Before development of the

TABLE 17–1 COMPOSITION OF GLYCOSAMINOGLYCANS AND THE CARBOHYDRATE PORTION OF CERTAIN PROTEOGLYCANS

Glycosaminoglycan	Hexosamine	Hexuronic Acid	Hexose	Disaccharide Units
Hyaluronic acid	N-acetyl-D-glucosamine	D-glucuronic	—	500–2500
Chondroitin-4-sulfate	N-acetyl-D galactosamine 4- or 6-sulfate	D-glucuronic	—	60
Dermatan sulfate	N-acetyl-D galactosamine 4-sulfate	L-iduronic + D-glucuronic 5–15%	—	40–60
Heparin*	N-sulfamido-glucosamine 6-sulfate	D-glucuronic + L-iduronic trace	—	10–20
Heparan sulfate*	N-sulfamido-glucosamine or N-acetylglucosamine 6-sulfate	D-glucuronic	—	10–20
Keratan sulfate	N-acetyl-D-glucosamine	—	D-galactose	10–20

*The degree of sulfation of heparin and heparan sulfate varies in the disaccharide units. For heparin SO_3^- radical can occur at the 2-position of the uronic acid and/or 2- and 6-position of the hexosamine. For heparan sulfate SO_3^- radical can occur at the 2- and/or 6-position of the hexosamine.

repeating disaccharide portion of the GAG chain a "linkage region" of monosaccharides is attached to the protein core through action of individual enzymes. All the enzymes responsible for growth of the carbohydrate chains, including the addition of sulfate groups, are found in the endoplasmic reticulum and the Golgi apparatus. It has been shown that fibroblasts, synoviocytes, chondrocytes, and endothelial cells synthesized certain of the GAG or proteoglycans. Heparin is synthesized by mast cells. Degradation of GAG has been shown to occur in several of the heritable diseases of connective tissue (mucopolysaccharidoses) through action of specific lysosomal enzymes. In these situations, GAG are degraded in phagolysosomes. Phagocytic cells such as macrophages are probably responsible for the intracellular breakdown of GAG or proteoglycans or both.

Tissue culture and isotope studies indicate that connective tissue cells from many sources synthesize glycosaminoglycans locally from simple precursors, including glucose. Cultures of human synovial tissue synthesize hyaluronic acid from the components of a chemically defined medium. Turnover rates determined with isotopes indicate that in connective tissue GAG or proteoglycans or both are continuously in active flux, in contrast to the relatively static collagen. The half-life of hyaluronic acid is 2 to 4 days, and that of chondroitin sulfate(s) is 7 to 10 days.

The anatomic distribution of GAG and proteoglycans has considerable functional significance. Synovial fluid and vitreous humor contain only hyaluronic acid. Cartilage ground substance contains chondroitin-4 and 6-sulfate and keratan sulfate. The major glycosaminoglycan in adult bone is chondroitin-4-sulfate. Mixtures of the chondroitin sulfates and hyaluronic acid occur in diverse tissues such as umbilical cord, skin, tendon, heart valve, and aorta. Heparan sulfate, a family of compounds with variable acetyl and sulfate ratios, has been isolated from aorta, lung, liver, and amyloid tissue. Certain of these substances are excreted in large amounts in the urine by some patients with a hereditary disease of connective tissue. Heparin can be isolated from lung and aorta as well as liver. Keratan sulfate I or II has been identified in cornea, nucleus pulposus, aging cartilage, and growing bone. Chondroitin has been found only in the cornea.

FORMATION OF CONNECTIVE TISSUE

An orderly sequence of connective tissue formation has been demonstrated in the healing wound and in a variety of experimental granulomas. The connective tissue defect is promptly flooded with plasma proteins and leukocytes from the circulatory system. Early in the reparative phase there is an impressive increase in the number of cells. This active proliferation of connective

tissue cells is accompanied by a striking change in the tinctorial properties of the ground substance, characterized by prominent metachromatic staining that indicates high local concentrations of acidic substances, including glycosaminoglycans. Soon fine intercellular collagen fibers can be detected. As the repair continues, the fibers become more numerous and individually larger, the cellular elements decrease in size and number, and the metachromatic hue of the ground substance subsides. Chemical analyses along the time course of this process show the hexosamine content (from glycoproteins and glycosaminoglycans) to peak in the first few days and then fall steadily, whereas hydroxyproline (an index of collagen content) rises steadily.

Protein depletion prior to wounding is known to retard healing and decrease wound tensile strength. The granulation tissue in healing wounds of protein-depleted animals contains decreased amounts of hexosamine and hydroxyproline, suggesting that fibroblastic synthesis of both ground substance and collagen has been retarded. Ascorbic acid deficiency in guinea pigs and in humans results in the failure to form collagen fibers, probably owing to the inability to hydroxylate proline to hydroxyproline. Correction of the vitamin C deficiency is followed within hours by the appearance of collagen fibers.

The effect of adrenal glucocorticoids on connective tissue has been extensively studied. An excess of hydrocortisone (in many studies doses exceed maximum pharmacologic doses in humans) will interfere with wound healing and the formation of granulation tissue. Cell culture studies show that near-physiologic concentrations of hydrocortisone induce multiple effects on fibroblasts, including accelerated mitosis, suppression of collagen deposition, and depression of the specific rate of hyaluronate synthesis.

Recently, several peptide or other mediators have been identified that link the activities of the major cell types found in both acute and chronic inflammation with the function of specialized connective tissue cells (synoviocytes, chondrocytes, bone cells, etc.). These substances act as mediators that bridge the gap between the exudative and reparative phase of inflammation. In pathologic states of inflammation they can play a critical role in perpetuating the inflammatory response along with immune mediators that amplify the inflammatory reaction.

STRUCTURE AND FUNCTION OF JOINTS

Simple gliding joints (diarthroses) consist of two bone ends covered by articular hyaline cartilage and held together by a sleeve of white fibrous connective tissue—the joint capsule (Fig. 17–2). The inner layers of this capsule consist of spe-

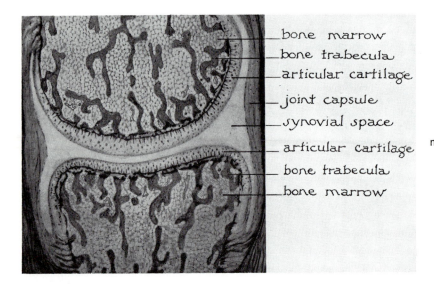

- bone marrow
- bone trabecula
- articular cartilage
- joint capsule
- synovial space
- articular cartilage
- bone trabecula
- bone marrow

Figure 17–2 Sketch of a normal diarthrodial joint.

cialized connective tissue cells—the synovium or synovialis. Within the joint space is a small amount of synovial fluid. In the human embryo, the future joint can be identified by the fifth to seventh week as a remnant of mesenchyme interposed between two chondrogenous zones. Later, the center of this zone appears to liquefy, owing to elaboration of soluble ground substance, and the mesenchyme appears to retract peripherally and to produce large numbers of closely packed fibrils. This is the future joint cavity, and its lining is the embryonic equivalent of the synovium.

JOINT CAPSULE

The joint capsule consists largely of fibrous collagenous tissue with few elastic fibers. It is reinforced in areas by ligaments. It blends with periosteum of the bone shaft above and below the joint and with tendinous and ligamentous periarticular structures. Stability and normal movement of the joints require that the relationships of the articulating bones maintain a normal alignment. This is accomplished to some extent by the anatomic configuration of the articulating surfaces ("congruity"), by the slight negative pressure in the joint cavity (-2 to -12 cm water), and by the molecular cohesive properties of the synovial fluid. But the most important stabilization is provided by the strong fibrous outer part of the joint capsule and its reinforcing ligaments. When the joint capsule is weakened, joint stability and function are threatened or destroyed. The collagenous layers determine the mechanical properties of the joint capsule. It has very little elasticity, but its resistance to a stretching force is 30 times that of a sheet of pure rubber of equal thickness. Like tendinous connective tissue it has a high resistance to tear. The pliability of the synovium helps it to withstand the stresses of joint motion.

The blood vessels that supply the joint usually arise in common with those supplying adjacent bone and form a prominent arterial circle around the joint. Those that supply the joint ultimately pass into a rich capillary network that is prominent in the cellular and areolar areas of the synovium.

Articular nerves carry fibers from several spinal nerves and may supply more than one joint. They contain sensory fibers and autonomic fibers. The branches are widely distributed to joint capsule, ligaments, and synovium. The larger sensory fibers form proprioceptive endings in the capsule and ligaments that are very sensitive to position and motion. They play an important role in reflex control of posture, locomotion, and kinesthetic sensation. The smaller sensory fibers form pain endings in the capsule and ligaments and along the blood vessels. Twisting and stretching are the most effective pain stimuli to the joint capsule. Joint pain is perceived as diffuse and poorly localized; when severe, it may be felt distally over most of the extremity. Like visceral pain, it may be referred to another anatomic location. Joint pain not uncommonly leads to reflex contraction of adjacent muscles, which may take the form of a protective spasm.

ARTICULAR CARTILAGE

Cartilage is tough, resilient connective tissue consisting of cells embedded in a firm extracellular matrix that is made up of a spongelike network of type II collagen fibers into which proteoglycans are tightly packed. The proteoglycans exist in large aggregates of molecular weight of a million or more, which consist of a highly polymerized chain of hyaluronate and tissue glycoproteins that stabilize the interaction of 30 to 40 proteoglycan molecules with the hyaluronate chain (Fig. 17–3).

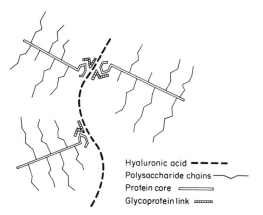

Hyaluronic acid ▬ ▬ ▬
Polysaccharide chains ◠◠◠
Protein core ▭▭▭
Glycoprotein link ▭▭▭

Figure 17–3 Diagrammatic representation of a proteoglycan aggregate.

Since the collagen fibers have nearly the same refractive index as the matrix, they are not visualized by conventional light microscopy. With polarized light the fibers are seen to be arranged so as to provide optimal resilience (Fig. 17–4). They extend as a looping curve resembling a croquet wicket with the ends anchored in the deeper calcium-rich zone of cartilage adjacent to the underlying bone. In relation to the cartilage surface this provides a surface zone of closely packed fibers parallel to the surface, an intermediate zone where the fibers are tangential, and a deeper zone where the direction is perpendicular to the surface. The proteoglycan aggregates can bind large amounts of water but are constrained by the collagen mesh from binding excess amounts of it. This arrangement restricts access of molecules larger than 70,000 daltons, such as proteolytic enzymes. This capacity of the cartilage mass to change in shape and "weep water" under pressure provides a cushioning effect protecting the subchondral bone and is the major method of buffering the blows and jolts received by the skeleton. The surface arrangement of the fibers assists the cartilage in providing a smooth gliding surface for the opposing bone ends. Under frequent intermittent pressures cartilage continues to be elastic, but with continuous compression its expansile power is decreased and the time for recovery becomes longer. Elasticity is also reduced as water content decreases.

Articular cartilage has no blood supply. It receives most of its nourishment from the synovial fluid, probably augmented by the pumping action of intermittent compression and decompression. Some nutrition may be derived from diffusion from vessels in the underlying subchondral bone or subsynovial vessels located at the junction of the capsule and cartilage at the periphery of the joint.

Articular cartilage contains relatively few cells; therefore, the rate of respiration is relatively low. However, the rate of metabolism per cartilage cell is in the range exhibited by other connective tissues. New cartilage is formed interstitially by chondrocytes, which are most numerous in the deeper layers of the cartilage. The cells of adult articular cartilage have restricted mitotic ability. Consequently, the capacity of this tissue to repair itself or to regenerate after injury is distinctly limited. Nevertheless, there is evidence that in normal use some replacement of articular cartilage may occur and that opposition of articular surfaces is necessary for maintenance of cartilage integrity. Reaction to injury depends on the depth of the damage of the cartilage. Superficial cuts show little or no reaction. Peripheral lesions reaching the joint capsule or central lesions extending to the subchondral bone are promptly filled with fibrous tissue. Sclerosis of the subchondral bone is a response to altered biomechanical forces and is augmented by microfractures that stiffen the tissue. This reduction in elasticity adversely affects the function of the overlying cartilage.

THE SYNOVIUM

Synovial tissue, a vascular connective tissue basically similar to connective tissue elsewhere in the body, lines the inner surface of the joint capsule but does not cover the articular cartilage. It consists of cells, fibers, and ground substance. The cells near the surface have long cytoplasmic processes that overlap and intertwine. They may be one to several layers thick, forming a relatively smooth surface from which villi, folds, and fat pads may project into the joint cavity. Tissue deep to the surface may be fibrous, fatty, or areolar. The surface cells do not form a complete lining, so that

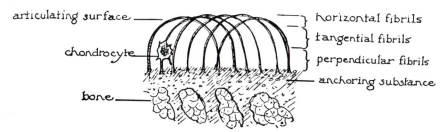

Figure 17–4 Sketch showing arrangement of collagen fibrils in articular cartilage as seen with polarized light. Note the three zones of fibrils aligned in horizontal, tangential, and radial positions.

intercellular material may be directly adjacent to the synovial space. Thus, the joint cavity is not a body cavity like the pleura, pericardium, and peritoneum. It is a specialized connective tissue space.

The synovium is richly supplied with blood vessels, lymph vessels, and some nerve fibers. The capillary network and lymphatic network are adjacent to the joint cavity, and diffusion takes place readily between these vessels and the joint cavity. Most substances in the bloodstream enter the joint cavity easily, and many substances injected into the joint cavity readily enter the blood. The size and configuration of large molecules appear to influence the ease with which they may pass. Colloidal solutions, fine suspensions, and proteins, when injected into the joint cavity, enter into the subsynovial tissue and are removed chiefly by the lymphatics. Large particles are removed with difficulty and leave the joint by way of the lymphatics after phagocytosis. Motion of the joint definitely facilitates removal of materials injected into the joint cavity by both vascular and lymphatic routes.

Since the synovium is quite cellular and has an excellent blood supply, it is not surprising that it has a very good capacity for regeneration. After surgical removal, it will be formed again either from remnants of synovial tissue or from the joint capsule.

SYNOVIAL FLUID

The fluid within the joint cavity is highly viscous and sticky, resembling egg white in consistency. It is slightly alkaline and ranges from colorless to pale yellow. It contains relatively few cells (Table 17–2), predominantly mononuclear cells derived from the synovium. Normal fluid is 95 per cent water and has a specific gravity around 1.010. In normal joints the amount of synovial fluid present is small; one can expect to aspirate only about 1 ml of fluid from a normal knee.

The relative viscosity of normal joint fluid ranges from 50 to 200 or more times that of water. This viscosity is due to the hyaluronic acid content, which averages 3.5 mg per gram of fluid. The viscosity increases exponentially with increases in concentration of hyaluronic acid and is also clearly related to the degree of polymerization of this polysaccharide. The viscosity of hyaluronic acid is due to the complex, highly asymmetric long-chain structure of the high molecular weight polymer. This structure confers the property of binding large amounts of water to form a viscous sol. Thus, the joint fluid is provided with high viscosity with negligible osmotic properties. A protein solution with comparable viscosity would produce an osmotic pressure far beyond the physiologic range.

In joint fluid, the hyaluronic acid is conjugated with but easily separated from a protein component; the protein content is less than 2 per cent of the total complex. This protein-polysaccharide forms a clotted precipitate when treated with dilute acids, forming *mucin*. The characteristics of the mucin clot formed on addition of dilute acetic acid provide a crude index of the degree of polymerization of the hyaluronic acid. In normal joint fluids, a tight adherent clot is formed. Such good mucin clot formation is also seen in fluids from traumatized joints, in degenerative joint disease, and in most types of acute inflammatory arthritis. In more chronic types of inflammatory joint disease this "mucin clot test" produces a flocculent, loosely adherent precipitate or even a powdery precipitate (Table 17–2).

The electrolyte content of joint fluid is comparable to that of the blood plasma. The amount of nonprotein nitrogenous substances and uric acid is lower than in plasma. The glucose content varies with the level in the plasma, with changes in joint fluid sugar lagging behind fluctuations in blood sugar. The total protein content is lower than plasma, ranging from 1 to 2 grams per 100 ml. In normal joint fluids, the protein is largely albumin, with albumin:globulin ratios as high as 20:1. This is attributed to the smaller size of the albumin molecule.

Thus, synovial fluid, aside from its hyaluronic acid content, can be considered as a dialysate of plasma. Just as the joint cavity can be considered a specialized connective tissue space structurally and functionally, the synovial fluid can be visualized as a specialized type of ground substance, composed of a dialysate of plasma to which the synovial cells have added a characteristic polysaccharide.

JOINTS AS FUNCTIONAL UNITS

The structure of joints appears to be well adapted to serve the primary purposes of bearing weight and providing motion. Stability with motion is afforded by the fibrous joint capsule, ligaments and tendons, and muscle tone. The elasticity of articular cartilage permits adaptation to changing pressures and buffers impacts to which the skeleton is subjected. Viscous synovial fluid forms a strong fluid interface with the cartilage surface, so that motion can occur with negligible friction. At reduced load a trypsin-sensitive protein in synovial fluid acts as a boundary lubricant between the cartilage surfaces. The hyaluronic acid molecule does not make a major contribution to cartilage lubrication. At high loads the "weeping action" of cartilage also helps protect the surfaces and attenuates the force of impact. During impact loading the muscle and bone, rather than the cartilage, absorb most of the biomechanical force that is applied to the joint.

Joint lubrication is so extremely efficient that the coefficient of friction is less than that of ice sliding on ice. It is usually considered to be an example of fluid film, or "floating," lubrication.

Since the articular surfaces do not fit perfectly throughout the whole range of motion, this incongruity permits the development of wedge-shaped spaces filled with synovial fluid. The intra-articular pressure increases during motion, and it is greatest where the articular cartilages are closest together. Since this pressure is great enough to keep the articular surfaces apart, the intervening film of synovial fluid, rather than the bearing surfaces, takes up the effects of friction. In many joints, intra-articular fibrous and fibrocartilaginous structures such as menisci and disks, as well as fat pads and synovial folds, aid in distributing the synovial fluid. In the joints, this classic concept of hydrodynamic lubrication must be modified to take into consideration the fact that synovial fluid is absorbed by articular cartilage and oozes from the cartilaginous surfaces under pressure. This, along with the trypsin-sensitive protein, provides an element of boundary lubrication where the moving surfaces are separated by a layer of lubricant that is adherent to or incorporated into the surface and need be only a few molecules thick.

Like all moving mechanical systems, the human joint wears with time. Some wear and tear is inevitable with normal activity. The most evident result is wearing away of the articular cartilage to some degree. Articular cartilage is subjected to wear and tear unequaled by any other tissue except the skin. Since articular cartilage has no blood supply and since adult cartilage cells have largely lost the power of mitosis, the potential for regeneration of cartilage is limited.

In contrast, the highly vascular and cell-rich synovium has great capacity for regeneration. But alterations in the synovium can result in modifications in exchange equilibria between plasma and synovial fluid and changes in the characteristics of the protein-polysaccharide of synovial fluid. Since the articular cartilage is dependent primarily on the synovial fluid for its nutrients, sooner or later the cartilage can be expected to reflect the results of functional aberrations of the synovialis.

FUNDAMENTAL PATHOLOGIC CHANGES OF JOINT DISEASE

Virtually all forms of joint disease can be understood in terms of two pathologic processes—degeneration and inflammation. Degenerative changes are dependent primarily on the limited capacity of articular cartilage to repair itself. Inflammation may be predominantly exudative or predominantly proliferative or a combination of the two. It is not surprising that both degenerative and inflammatory changes can often be seen in the same joint. Cartilage that has been damaged as a result of inflammation is rendered more vulnerable to subsequent degenerative changes. In

TABLE 17–2 CHARACTERISTICS OF SYNOVIAL FLUID IN NORMAL JOINTS AND IN COMMON FORMS OF ARTHRITIS

		Appearance	Viscosity	Mucin Clot	Cell Count (per mm³)	Crystals	Bacteria (on stain or culture)
Group I Noninflammatory	Normal	Straw-colored, clear	High	Good	±200 WBC 20% PMN	0	0
	Traumatic arthritis	Yellow to bloody, often turbid	High	Good	±2000 WBC 30% PMN Many RBC	0	0
	Osteoarthritis	Yellow, clear	High	Good	±1000 WBC 15–25% PMN	0	0
Group II Inflammatory	Rheumatoid arthritis	Yellow to greenish, cloudy	Low	Fair to poor	15,000 to 40,000 WBC 60–90% PMN	Occasionally cholesterol	0
	Rheumatic fever	Yellow, slightly cloudy	Low	Good	10,000 to 12,000 WBC ±50% PMN	0	0
	Systemic lupus erythematosus	Straw-colored, slightly cloudy	High	Good	±5000 WBC 10–15% PMN	0	0
	Gout	Yellow to milky, cloudy	Low	Fair to poor	10,000 to 30,000 WBC 60–80% PMN	Urate +	0
	Pseudogout	Yellow, clear to slightly cloudy	Low	Fair to poor	1000 to 10,000 WBC 25–50% PMN	Calcium pyrophosphate +	0
Group III Septic	Tuberculous arthritis	Yellow, cloudy	Low	Poor	±25,000 WBC 50–60% PMN	0	+
	Septic arthritis	Grayish or bloody, turbid to purulent	Low	Poor	80,000 to 200,000 WBC 75–90% PMN	0	+

older persons, degenerative changes that have developed over the years do not render the joint immune to superimposed inflammation.

DEGENERATIVE JOINT CHANGES

Much of the knowledge of the sequence of degenerative changes has been obtained from studies of the normal aging process in the joints. Abnormality of articular structure can be seen first in the second decade and increases with advancing age. The first changes appear in the articular cartilage and show a predilection for those areas that are subjected to weight-bearing or shearing pressures. These are seen as localized areas of softening of the cartilage associated with a fine velvety disruption of the surface. In these areas, dehiscence of the cartilage occurs along the planes of the collagen fibers. The most superficial dehiscences are oriented parallel to the surface and, when confined to the tangential layers at the surface, produce "flaking." As the dehiscences proceed to the deeper layers they arch downward in a more vertical direction, producing "fibrillation" of the cartilage. An early change in the ground substance in these areas of cartilage is indicated by decrease in proteoglycan content in perichondrocyte regions and more conspicuous fibrillar elements—the "unmasking" of the collagen fibrils. Chemical studies show an increase in tissue water and a decrease in the proteoglycan content and size of aggregates relative to the collagen in such areas.

With abrasion of the fibrillated cartilage, clefts and fissures develop, followed by erosion and progressive denudation of the underlying bony cortex. Associated with the progressive wearing away of the cartilage is new bone formation in two separate locations relative to the joint surface: (1) exophytic growth at the margins of the articular cartilage, and (2) formation in the marrow and cortex of the subchondral bone immediately underlying the articular cartilage. The latter has been proposed as a primary event that leads to microfractures in the subchondral bone and disruption of the integrity of overlying cartilage. The marginal osteophytes develop at the periphery of the articular cartilage, where the joint capsule blends with the periosteum covering the shaft of the bone. They may extend into the joint cavity and tend to develop within capsular and ligamentous attachments to the joint margins, generally growing in a direction governed by the lines of mechanical forces exerted on the area. Such marginal bony lipping may be seen in the knee joint as early as the fourth decade of life. The osteophyte consists largely of bone that merges imperceptibly with the cortical and cancellous structure of subchondral bone. Proliferation of bone in the subchondral area results in increased density of the bony structure underlying cartilage. It is most marked in areas that have been denuded of their covering of cartilage. Here the exposed bone becomes dense and hardened and takes on a highly eburnated appearance.

The synovial tissue itself is largely unaffected in degenerative joint disease. This conventional view has recently been modified to take into account the release of low molecular weight peptides called *catabolins* from synovial and other connective tissue cells. The catabolins have been shown in vitro to stimulate living cartilage cells to degrade their extracellular matrix. These mediators may play a role in both osteoarthritis and in cartilage degeneration associated with inflammatory forms of joint disease.

Because of the development of marginal osteophytes and sclerosis of subchondral bone, degenerative joint disease is called *osteoarthritis* or *osteoarthrosis*. Predisposing factors may be grouped as (1) those that influence the integrity of the articular cartilage and (2) those that accentuate or accelerate normal wear and tear. One hypothesis suggests that abnormal stress or tissue injury or both stimulate increased formation and release of hydrolytic enzymes from chondrocytes. This leads to degradation of matrix with concomitant proliferation of chondrocytes and synthesis of proteoglycan and collagen. When reparative processes fail to keep pace with cartilage breakdown, the manifestations of osteoarthritis appear (Fig. 17–5).

Genetic influences may be important determinants of the resistance of cartilage to wear and tear. Stecher demonstrated a hereditary pattern in the occurrence of *Heberden's nodes,* osteophytes that form at the base of the distal phalanges of the fingers and that are more common in women than in men. *Acromegaly,* in which there is excessive proliferation of cartilage, is associated with osteoarthritis with an unusual degree of bony overgrowth. In ochronosis that complicates alkaptonuria, an abnormal pigment discolors articular cartilage and intervertebral discs, with gross alterations of their physical properties; this is often associated with unusually severe osteoarthritis. A disease of growing children characterized by defective growth and maturation of the epiphyses results, despite the age of the patient, in joint changes indistinguishable from osteoarthritis. This disorder, known as *Kaschin-Beck disease,* is seen in Manchuria and eastern Siberia and is clearly the result of improper nutrition. In *hemophilia,* repeated hemorrhage into the joint leads to deposition of hemosiderin in the articular cartilage and eventually results in severe osteoarthritis. These rare forms of degenerative joint disease suggest that extreme endocrine, metabolic, and dietary influences may alter the integrity of articular cartilage and predispose to the development of osteoarthritis. Whether more subtle influences of the same nature are operative in the more common types of degenerative joint disease remains undetermined.

It is much easier to document the role of

predisposing factors that accentuate or accelerate the wear and tear on the joints. *Secondary osteoarthritis* can result from excessive or abnormal stresses and strains related to postural or orthopedic abnormalities. A variety of structural abnormalities of the hip joint in childhood such as congenital dysplasia, Legg-Calvé-Perthes disease, slipped femoral epiphysis, and congenital coxa vara lead to premature osteoarthritic degeneration. It may be a late result of trauma to the joint structures or of chronic irritation produced by derangement of internal joint structures—for example, a torn semilunar cartilage in the knee. It may appear in joints previously damaged by other types of inflammatory arthritis.

The clinical features of osteoarthritis are read-

ily explained by the underlying pathologic changes in the joint. It affects chiefly older individuals and characteristically involves weight-bearing joints. It is a localized disease of the joints and is not accompanied by systemic symptoms. The most common complaint is an aching pain that occurs on use, is rarely intense, and is diminished by rest. Stiffness after sitting is noted, particularly with the first few motions involving use of the part. Such stiffness is dissipated rapidly and rarely persists more than a few minutes. Objectively, the joints may appear normal, but bony enlargements may be felt around the joint margins. Occasionally these are tender. Crepitus, creaking, or grating on motion can usually be detected. Increase in synovial fluid is uncommon; when it does occur—

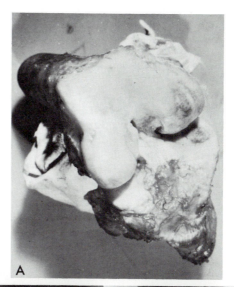

Figure 17–5 *A,* Osteoarthritic erosions of the medial and lateral femoral condyles and tibial plateau of the knee. *B,* Roentgenograms of the knee joint of a patient at ages 45, 52, and 61 years demonstrating progressive changes due to osteoarthritis. Over this 16-year interval, there has been loss of joint space owing to cartilage degeneration, development of marginal osteophytes, and irregularity and eburnation of subchondral bone.

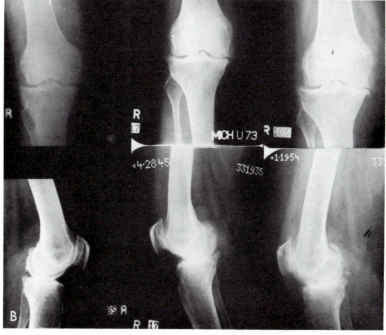

usually in the knees—it subsides within a few days after elimination of weight bearing. The range of motion is usually only slightly impaired except in osteoarthritis of the hip. The radiographic features of osteoarthritis are decrease in thickness of articular cartilage (erroneously termed *loss of joint space*), formation of intra-articular and marginal osteophytes (*lipping*), and increased density of the subchondral bone. In advanced disease, there may be crumbling and remodeling of the subchondral bone.

Neurologic disorders that result in loss of proprioceptive and pain sensation may be complicated by *neuropathic joint disease* which has many features of osteoarthritis. Deprived of its protective reflexes the joint is subject to severe and cumulative injury. There is relaxation of supporting structures with chronic instability of the joint. The degenerative changes progress rapidly, and cartilage damage is extensive. With relative absence of pain, continued use results in extensive damage to cartilage and subchondral bone. These structures fragment, leaving loose bodies of cartilage and bone free in the joint cavity. These loose bodies and the extensive erosion of bone stimulate the synovium, with a resulting proliferative synovitis and persistent joint effusion. Subluxations and dislocations are common, as are intra-articular and juxta-articular fractures. The degenerative changes are accompanied by exuberant overgrowth of bone. The characteristic clinical features are the relative absence of pain and remarkable hypermotility of the affected joint. Radiographic features are the combination of extensive destructive and hypertrophic changes.

Classically, neuropathic joints occur as a complication of tabes dorsalis (*Charcot's joints*). Syringomyelia and spinal cord degeneration accompanying diabetes and pernicious anemia may also be the basis. Usually one joint only is affected—most often the hip, knee, ankle, midtarsal joints, and the lumbar and the lower spine. In syringomyelia, joints in the upper extremity may be involved.

EFFECTS OF TRAUMA

The simplest type of joint abnormality is that which results from injury. The trauma may be slight and cause only a strain on the fibrous capsule or ligaments. The response of edema and congestion produces swelling around the joint, with pain and stiffness from stimulation of the nerve endings, which are abundant in the periarticular tissues. Since the tissues affected have a good blood supply, healing is usually rapid and complete. With more severe trauma, the synovium may be injured, followed by traumatic synovitis and effusion within the joint cavity. In the absence of repeated trauma, such sterile inflammation persists for a relatively short time, and recovery is

usually complete. More severe trauma can damage the cartilage and, at times, the underlying bone and may provoke changes in the dynamics of the joint that, after a period of time, result in post-traumatic degenerative changes. If the injury is to the cartilage located centrally in the joint, little regeneration takes place and the irregularity of the joint surface places a strain on the periarticular structures at the joint margins, stimulating proliferation of bone. If the injury is at the articular margin of the cartilage, abnormal bone formation may develop rapidly. The late changes resulting from severe joint trauma are those of osteoarthritis, with rapidity of development determined by severity and location of the damage to joint structures.

JOINT INFLAMMATION—SYNOVITIS

The vascular phase of inflammation can be visualized as a progressive impairment of the microcirculation of a tissue, initiated by a variety of agents and mediated by mechanisms that are incompletely characterized. The classic manifestations of heat, redness, swelling, pain, and impaired function correlate with alterations in the microcirculation, predominantly increased local blood flow, and increased vascular permeability ("leaks"). Since the vascular and lymphatic supply to the joint is predominantly in and just beneath the synovium, it is this tissue that is initially and principally involved in joint inflammation.

In acute synovitis, exudative inflammation predominates. The joint is swollen, warm, tender to touch, and painful to move. Redness and heat over the joint vary with the type and severity of inflammation. The joint capsule is distended by an outpouring of synovial fluid with an increased content of inflammatory cells, nearly always polymorphonuclear neutrophils. Microscopically, the venules and capillaries of the synovium are dilated; the synovium and subsynovial tissues are edematous and infiltrated to a varying degree with inflammatory cells. Some types of arthritis such as the synovitis of serum sickness and acute rheumatic fever, which are self-limited and subside without residual joint damage, can be regarded as examples of purely exudative inflammation of the synovium.

However, in the more chronic forms of arthritis, the proliferative phase of inflammation develops and may dominate the pathologic and clinical features of the disease. Rheumatoid arthritis is the prototype of such combined exudative and proliferative inflammation, with extensive formation of granulation tissue accounting for the joint destruction and disability (Fig. 17–6). The synovium is swollen and deep red in color, and there is hypertrophy of the villous processes. There is reduplication of the synovial lining cells and proliferation of fibroblasts. The inflammatory cells are chiefly lymphocytes (T cells predominating), plasma cells, and macrophages, and they may appear in a follicle-like arrangement. Many of the cells found in the tissue lesions are designated as *immunocompetent*. The fibroblastic and angioblastic proliferation forms granulation tissue that replaces the synovium and invades the joint capsule and periarticular structures. Particularly significant is the invasion of the interior of the joint by a reddish, roughened, tongue-like protrusion of granulation tissue, growing over the articular cartilage from the joint margins (pannus formation).

By lysis of cartilage ground substance and fibers, interference with nutrition of the cartilage, and actual invasion, this inflammatory tissue

slowly destroys the articular cartilage. It may join with similar granulation tissue arising from subchondral marrow. The capsular inflammation and proliferative granulation tissue tend to persist and to progress slowly, with remissions and exacerbations leading to cumulative damage to cartilage and subchondral bone. This damage, consequences of the original inflammation, accounts for the deformities and crippling that characterize the later stages of rheumatoid arthritis. In these later stages, the evidences of exudative inflammation usually lessen and may appear to subside completely. The granulation tissue becomes primary fibrous and is converted to a dense scar. This tough fibrous scar limits or prevents joint motion (fibrous

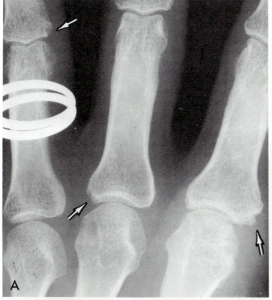

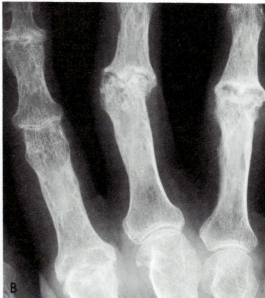

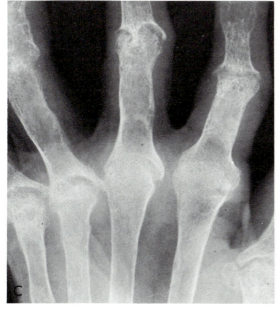

Figure 17–6 Progressive changes in the proximal interphangeal (PIP) and metacarpophalangeal (MCP) joints of patients with rheumatoid arthritis. In *A,* early marginal inflammatory erosions are identified by the arrows. In *B* and *C,* progressive destructive changes due to rheumatoid pannus are shown. In addition, secondary osteoarthritic alterations and bony ankylosis of PIP and MCP joints have developed as sequelae of the rheumatoid process.

ankylosis). On occasions, this scar becomes calcified and is converted to osseous tissue (bony ankylosis).

ALTERATIONS IN JOINT FLUID PRODUCED BY DISEASE

It is to be expected that changes in the permeability of the synovial tissues and vessels will be reflected by changes in the joint fluid. The increased permeability accompanying inflammation permits more ready passage into the joint cavity of water, electrolytes, and easily diffusible colloids. The passage of protein molecules is enhanced, and the increase in total protein content of the joint fluid is proportional to the intensity of the inflammation. Increased permeability also accounts for the presence of fibrinogen, immune globulins, leukocytes, and proteins with enzymatic activity in the joint fluid during inflammation. The glucose content tends to decrease as the leukocyte content increases, and it is characteristically low or absent in septic joints. This is attributed to the increased glycolytic activity of the leukocytes and synovial cells.

The viscosity of joint fluid is reduced in inflammatory disease, particularly in rheumatoid arthritis. This is explained in part by a decrease in concentration of hyaluronate; however, since the volume of joint fluid is increased severalfold, the total amount of hyaluronate is considerably greater than that in the normal joint. Some of the decrease in viscosity is also due to the presence of less highly polymerized molecules of hyaluronate. These changes are usually considered to reflect alterations in metabolic activity of synovial cells during inflammation, a concept supported by the observation that rheumatoid synovial cells in culture produce larger amounts of less highly polymerized hyaluronate as compared with synovial cell cultures from noninflamed joints. The possibility of degradation in vivo by enzymes released from leukocytes and synovial lining cells into the synovial fluid cannot be ruled out.

The characteristic changes in the synovial fluid in the more common forms of arthritis are listed in Table 17–2. As an aid in differential diagnosis, examination of the synovial fluid by simple methods is of greatest help in differentiating noninflammatory from inflammatory synovial effusions, in the detection of septic arthritis, and in the demonstrations of characteristic crystals in gout and calcium pyrophosphate dihydrate deposition disease (pseudogout). Effusions in traumatic and degenerative joint disease are relatively clear, do not clot, and characteristically show only a modest increase in number of white blood cells but may contain increased numbers of red blood cells. Viscosity is well maintained and the mucin clot is firm, ropy, and nonfriable. Inflammatory fluids are more turbid, may clot on standing owing to the

presence of fibrinogen, and usually contain more than 5000 leukocytes per mm^3, sometimes ranging as high as 60,000 to 80,000 in chronic inflammation. The leukocytes are predominantly polymorphonuclear neutrophils. Varying degrees of deterioration in viscosity and characteristics of the mucin clot reflect alterations in the hyaluronate. In septic joints, the fluid is turbid to frankly purulent, the leukocyte count is 80,000 to 200,000 per mm^3 (almost all of which are polymorphonuclear leukocytes), and the responsible microorganism may be demonstrated by direct staining or by culture.

PATHOGENESIS OF JOINT INFLAMMATION

Extensive investigation has defined many of the physiologic, immunologic, and biochemical mechanisms by which inflammation is produced. Since the joint in an extremity is a well-demarcated tissue space that can be sampled easily and repeatedly by needle aspiration or biopsy, studies of joint inflammation have contributed significantly to concepts relating inflammatory mechanisms to human disease. Present knowledge permits what must be regarded as an evolving concept of the mechanisms and mediators of the changes in the microcirculation, which is the "final common pathway" of inflammatory damage. Factors that have been considered mediators of the microcirculatory effects can be conveniently grouped under headings of *small molecular mediators, plasma factors, leukocyte factors, immune mechanisms,* and *tissue necrosis,* with full appreciation of the interplay between such factors and others yet to be identified.

The biologic activities of immune complexes, lymphokines, immunocompetent cells, phagocytic cells, complement components, and lysosomal enzymes, have been shown to be of importance in the pathogenesis of rheumatic disease (see Chapter 5).

Plasma factors implicated in inflammatory reactions include Hagemen factor, the kininogen system, and the fibrinogen and plasminogen systems. Each of the systems involves specific substrates, enzyme activators, cofactors, and inhibitors.

Small molecular mediators include histamine, the kinin peptides, serotonin, cyclic nucleotides, leukotrienes, and prostaglandins. Several of these chemicals, produced by body cells, have profound effects on the microcirculation in extremely small concentrations. In model systems, injections of histamines, bradykinin, and serotonin produce only an immediate and transient effect on the microcirculation. Whether such substances serve only to initiate the inflammatory response or whether continued production of them may sustain the inflammation is not clear. Kinin peptides in synovial fluids from inflamed knees have been demonstrated by bioassay. High concentrations of prostaglandins have been identified in inflammatory tissues, including rheumatoid synovium. They are synthesized from arachidonic acid, with the first enzyme in the sequence, cyclooxygenase, being susceptible to specific inhibition by most of the nonsteroidal antiinflammatory drugs. Another important pathway of arachidonic acid metabolism involves the enzyme lipoxygenase; this enzyme catalyzes production of the leukotrienes. These compounds are potent chemotactic factors and include slow reactive substance, a mediator of allergic reactions.

Among leukocyte factors, the concept of *lysosomes* has attracted much attention in recent years. This concept, originated by DeDuve, visualizes many types of cells to contain small subcellular aggregates (granules) of hydrolytic enzymes active against a variety of substrates. These enzymes are active only when leaks develop in the wall of the lysosomal structure that contains them. Once released, the enzymes all have optimal activity at an acid pH. The key to the lysosome is its lipoprotein membrane, which can be either stabilized or weakened by a number of exogenous factors. The lysosomal membrane can be disrupted by mechanical means, by chemical means, and by enzymes. It may be stabilized by compounds such as corticosteroids, cholesterol, and chloroquine.

It is convenient to measure the activity of one or more of these enzymes as an index of lysosomal disruption; acid phosphatase and beta glucuronidase are most often measured. It is of interest that lysosomal hydrolyases have been demonstrated in the cytoplasm of proliferating fibroblasts. Several lysosomal hydrolyases have been found in the synovial fluid from inflamed joints, with levels paralleling the number of polymorphonuclear leukocytes.

Although lysosomes are found in many types of cells, the polymorphonuclear leukocytes are particularly rich in them, and they constitute the familiar neutrophilic granules seen with Wright's stain. Three mechanisms of disruption of the lysosomes of these cells have been described:

1. During phagocytosis of particulate matter, the cell membrane invaginates to surround the ingested particle, forming an autophagic vacuole; the lipid wall of the lysosome fuses with the vacuole and discharges the hydrolytic enzymes into the vacuole as well as to the extracellular environment. Leukocytes exuding in response to particulate matter such as bacteria and crystals die in a few hours.

2. Certain bacterial exotoxins, such as streptolysin O and S, can rupture lysosomes within the cytoplasm of the leukocyte, resulting in rapid death of the cell. This phenomenon has led some workers to refer to lysosomes as "suicide bags."

3. A staphylococcal exotoxin, "leukocidin," causes the granules to swell into vesicles, some of which fuse with the cell membrane and rupture to the outside. The end product in each case is a degranulated leukocyte showing the nuclear and cytoplasmic changes of cell death, and nearly every exudate rich in polymorphonuclear leukocytes has shown elevation of the activity of those enzymes that serve as an index of lysosomal disruption.

The interrelations among various factors and their relative importance in producing the microcirculatory alterations and tissue changes characteristic of inflammation are not completely understood at the present time. Nevertheless, it is possible to examine these mechanisms as they apply to the various types of inflammatory joint disease. Much of the remainder of this chapter represents an attempt to do this.

SPECIFIC INFECTIOUS ARTHRITIS

Almost every type of microorganism can infect joint tissues and cause inflammation. Rarely, the entry to the joint is directly by laceration or by extension of infection from contiguous bone. Usually, the infection is carried by the bloodstream, with initial localization of the microorganism in the synovial and subsynovial tissues. The inflammatory reaction in the joint has the same characteristics as that provoked by the particular microorganism in other body tissues.

Bacteria most commonly responsible for purulent inflammation of the joint are staphylococcus, streptococcus, gonococcus and several other gram-negative species. Infection by these organisms in their more usual habitat may be evident but at times must be searched for carefully. The large joints, such as the hip, knee, and wrist, are most commonly affected, although any articulation, either spinal or peripheral, can be involved. The process usually involves only one or a few joints, although with gonococcal infection there may be an early migratory phase with pain in several joints before the bacteria settle down to provoke a true septic arthritis. The inflammation is dominated by the purulent exudate, and the "leukocyte factors" are undoubtedly principally responsible for the intensity of the inflammatory reaction. These factors also account for the rapid destruction of articular cartilage that accompanies the presence of pus in the joint cavity. Proteolytic and other hydrolytic enzyme activity can be demonstrated in leukocyte autolysates and purulent synovial fluids. Fluids containing 110,000 or more leukocytes per mm^3 are capable of digesting small pieces of cartilage, whereas synovial fluids with leukocyte counts of 6000 to 20,000 are not. If septic arthritis is not recognized promptly and treated with appropriate antibiotics, extensive joint destruction may occur. Also, the natural repair of joint tissue that has harbored prolonged purulent inflammation results in granulation tissue with ensuing scar formation, and fibrous ankylosis may result.

Tuberculous infection usually involves only one joint, provoking a slowly progressive low-grade synovitis dominated by the granuloma formation and proliferative inflammation characteristic of the response to the tubercle bacillus. Doughy swelling of the joint with slight to imperceptible increase in local heat may be present, owing to the thickened synovium rather than increase in synovial fluid. The tuberculous synovitis forms a pannus of granulation tissue that tends to spread over and destroy the cartilage and also infiltrates under the cartilage, resorbing the bony articular cortex and the lower layers of the cartilage. In some cases this results in detachment of the articular cartilage. Since the synovial fluid in tuberculous arthritis is not rich in proteolytic and other hydrolytic enzymes, such loosened cartilage may persist for months but is eventually destroyed. Early destruction of periarticular bone is one of the radiographic features of tuberculous arthritis. An exception is the knee joint, where tuberculous synovitis of low grade may persist for months or years with little discomfort and little bone destruction. However, in almost all cases the joint tuberculosis should be regarded as involving synovium, cartilage, and bone. The tuberculous process may extend into periarticular tissues, producing a "cold abscess" about the joint, or it may travel between muscle and fascial planes and drain to the exterior or through sinus tracts.

Mycotic infections of the joints, which develop in the disseminated granulomatous phase of coccidioidomycosis, histoplasmosis, blastomycosis, cryptococcosis, and actinomycosis, provoke an inflammatory reaction that has many of the clinical, radiographic, and pathologic features of tuberculous arthritis.

CRYSTAL-INDUCED SYNOVITIS

ACUTE GOUTY ARTHRITIS

The rediscovery in 1960 of the vital role of urate crystals in the acute gouty attack stimulated extensive studies of mechanisms involved in acute joint inflammation. Crystals of monosodium urate monohydrate were demonstrated to be a constant finding in synovial fluid of patients with gout. The presence of such crystals within leukocytes is characteristic of acute gouty inflammation. The crystals are seen in wet preparations as short rod shapes with rounded ends or as needle-like entities. Under polarized light, they show a strong negative birefringence, which is definitive. Injection of urate crystals (0.5 to 8μ in length) into the joints or subcutaneously into experimental animals or human subjects (both normal and gouty) produces an acute inflammatory response, whereas amorphous urates produce only a mild response,

and urates in solution produce no response. Other crystalline substances of similar configuration produce a similar inflammatory reaction, indicating that the phenomenon is dependent on the physical rather than the chemical nature of the crystal.

It has been convincingly demonstrated that this inflammatory response requires leukocytes. Dogs rendered profoundly leukopenic by prior administration of vinblastin or by the use of specific antileukocyte serum displayed suppression of the inflammatory response to intra-articular injection of urate crystals. The ability to respond was restored when the injected joint was perfused by blood from a normal animal. Following intra-articular injection of microcrystalline urate, the joint pressure increases and the pH of the synovial fluid falls, owing to a rise in the concentration of lactic acid that results from increased metabolic activity of the leukocytes. The crystals are phagocytized and either destroyed or released if the leukocyte ruptures and may be reingested by others. After entry into a phagosome, the plasma-derived protein (immunoglobulin) coating of the crystal may be digested away by lysosomal enzymes, leading to crystal perforation of the lysosomal membrane with escape of hydrolytic enzymes into the cell sap, which is responsible for death of the cell and extracellular escape of hydrolytic enzymes.

Such observations support the concept of the pathogenesis of acute gouty arthritis as originally proposed by Seegmiller and associates. This is illustrated in Figure 17–7. The initial event is precipitation or release of urate crystals locally. The presence of even a few crystals in supersaturated body fluids promotes further crystallization. The crystals provoke a polymorphonuclear leukocyte response. These leukocytes phagocytose the urate crystals; simultaneous phagocytosis occurs, leukocyte metabolic activity increases, and lactic acid production increases, producing a lowering of local pH. Because urate solubility decreases at a more acid pH, this change tends to promote further precipitation of urate crystals, and a self-perpetuating cycle is produced. Colchicine, the drug that for centuries has been the classic and highly specific treatment for the acute gouty attack, appears to interrupt this cycle by a direct effect upon the leukocyte, with inhibition of its metabolic and biologic activity. One specific action has been shown to be related to inhibition of organization of microtubules within the cell. These subcellular constituents are essential to the structure and mobility of cells.

This system has also permitted study of possible mediators of the inflammatory response. Considerable evidence has accumulated to support the role of kinin polypeptides in this response. It has been demonstrated that urate crystals are capable of activating Hageman factor (factor XII). In addition to its role in initiating coagulation, Hageman factor has the ability to activate kallikrein, the enzyme regulating the formation of bradykinin from kininogen. It has been established that Hageman factor is present in the synovial fluid in acute gout (and in other inflammatory joint diseases), decreasing in concentration as the inflammation subsides. There is evidence that Hageman factor (and urate crystals without the intervention of Hageman factor) can activate C1-esterase; this in turn promotes activation of complement components that produce increased vascular permeability, phagocytosis, and chemotaxis. The leukocytes may also significantly contribute to the production of kinins. It has also been demonstrated that phagocytosis of crystals leads to rapid release of a chemotactic protein from the leukocyte. Alternatively, or in addition, they contribute to the inflammatory process by release of lysosomal enzymes. It has also been demonstrated that immunoglobulin coating of extracellular urate crystals may alter their phlogistic properties.

Gout is fundamentally a disorder of purine metabolism, usually genetically determined but sometimes acquired, characterized by persistent elevation of urate in the plasma.

A detailed description of the mechanisms responsible for hyperuricemia will not be attempted; however, a brief review of major advances in our understanding of human purine metabolism will be undertaken. The reader is referred to various reviews for more detailed discussion. It is now evident that hyperuricemia occurs as a result of excessive production of uric acid, reduced renal excretion, or a combination of these two events.

Identification of specific enzyme defects leading to both uric acid over- and underproduction have helped to clarify the regulatory mechanism that operates in the purine pathway. Although these enzymatic defects account for only a small fraction (1 to 3 per cent) of gouty overproducers (10 to 15 per cent) within the total population of patients with primary gout, their recognition is important. Key reactions relevant to this discussion are outlined in Figure 17–8. The synthesis of purine nucleotides (adenylic, guanylic, inosinic acid) occurs directly from purine bases (adenine, guanine, hypoxanthine) or de novo from precursors that lead to the formation of inosinic acid (IMP). The latter is a common intermediate for the other purine nucleotides used in the formation of nucleic acids and critical nucleotide intermediates. Degradation of purine nucleotides leads to the formation of xanthine and, finally, uric acid. The enzyme *amidophosphoribosyltransferase* is the rate limiting step in de novo purine synthesis, which is itself regulated by the intracellular concentration of PRPP (Fig. 17–8). When PRPP levels in the cell are increased, the rate of uric acid synthesis is increased, and vice versa.

Clinical disorders leading to overproduction of uric acid and gout include the Lesch-Nyhan syndrome, which is due to complete deficiency of hypoxanthine-guanine phosphoribosyltransferase (HGPRT). This X-linked disorder afflicts children and is further characterized by self-mutilation, spasticity, choreoathetosis, and mental retardation. Partial deficiency of HGPRT leads to onset

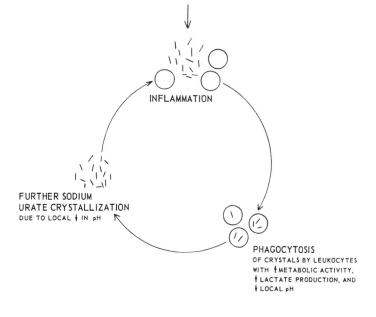

Figure 17–7 Concept of pathogenesis of acute gouty arthritis as a self-propagating inflammatory reaction. (From Seegmiller, J. E., and Howell, R. R.: Arthritis Rheum. 5:616, 1962.)

PRECIPITATION
OF SODIUM URATE CRYSTALS
FROM HYPERURICEMIC BODY FLUIDS

INFLAMMATION

FURTHER SODIUM
URATE CRYSTALLIZATION
DUE TO LOCAL ↓ IN pH

PHAGOCYTOSIS
OF CRYSTALS BY LEUKOCYTES
WITH ↑METABOLIC ACTIVITY,
↑LACTATE PRODUCTION, AND
↓LOCAL pH

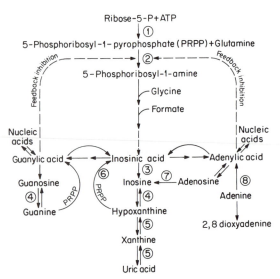

Figure 17–8 The purine pathway in humans. The following enzymes are identified: (1) PRPP synthetase; (2) amidophosphoribosyltransferase; (3) 5'-nucleotidase; (4) purine nucleoside phosphorylase; (5) xanthine oxidase; (6) hypoxanthine-guanine phosphoribosyltransferase; (7) adenosine deaminase; (8) adenine phosphoribosyltransferase.

of acute gout and renal stone formation in patients 15 to 25 years of age who are neurologically normal. Another enzyme abnormality leading to gout has been shown to be due to overactivity of PRPP synthetase in a small number of patients. Deficiency of this enzyme has been associated with hypouricemia, orotic acidemia, and mental retardation. The first two manifestations can be traced to the deficiency of intracellular levels of PRPP. Xanthine oxidase deficiency leads to increased urinary excretion of oxypurines and reduced plasma levels and urinary excretion of uric acid. Patients with a homozygous deficiency of adenine phosphoribosyltransferase were found to have renal calculi composed of the compound 2,8-dioxyadenine. Adenosine deaminase deficiency has been identified in patients with severe combined immunodeficiency (severe T-cell and mild B-cell dysfunction). Other patients with immune deficiency disease have defects in the enzyme purine nucleoside phosphorylase. These abnormalities unrelated to aberrations in uric acid metabolism have linked purine metabolism with regulation of the immune system. Elucidation of other genetic defects relevant to gouty arthritis and their relation to the larger population of patients with primary gout are to be anticipated. The renal mechanisms of handling uric acid also require further investigation.

Clinically, gout is manifested by recurrent attacks of a characteristic type of acute arthritis, by depositions of sodium urate monohydrate in and around joints of the extremities and by renal disease that may include deposits of urate crystals in the kidney and formation of urate calculi. The clinical manifestations are ultimately dependent on the fact that, even in normal humans, uric acid is present in concentrations near the limit of its solubility in body fluids.

Acute attacks of gout are characterized by abrupt onset and extremely severe inflammation that may easily be mistaken for a septic joint. Although the victim of this disease may be totally incapacitated, the synovitis subsides in several days to a week or two, with complete resolution of the inflammation and restoration of normal joint function. The aforementioned concepts provide an explanation for many features of the acute episodes, including the abruptness of onset, the severity of the synovitis, and the intermittent pattern of attacks. However, the events leading to the initial crystallization of sodium urate from the supersaturated fluid are incompletely defined. Furthermore, these concepts do not clarify how and why the untreated attack resolves spontaneously.

CHRONIC GOUTY ARTHRITIS

In gout, urates tend to deposit in cartilage, epiphyseal bone, periarticular structures, and the kidneys. Such deposits may form visible tophi and may be responsible for permanent joint damage or chronicity of symptoms. Such urate deposition is dependent on the height of the serum uric acid concentration, the severity of the renal involvement, and the duration of the disease. Tophi are seen most often in patients who have had gout for 6 to 10 years or more. Lowering of the serum urate concentration with appropriate medication can prevent urate deposition and can actually lead to disappearance of tophi that have previously developed.

Deposition of urates produces a local necrosis and (unless the tissue is avascular) an ensuing foreign-body reaction with proliferation of granulation tissue. In the joint, synovial proliferation with pannus formation may develop, producing chronic synovitis with capsular fibrous thickening. Deposits of urate on the surface of the articular cartilage are often present with associated cartilaginous degeneration and accelerated appearance of degenerative joint changes. Destruction of subchondral bone with depositions of urate in the marrow results in the punched-out lesions of bone commonly seen in radiographs of gouty patients. These marrow tophi often communicate with the urate crust on the articular surface through erosions and defects in the articular cartilage.

CALCIUM PYROPHOSPHATE DIHYDRATE DEPOSITION DISEASE (PSEUDOGOUT)

When, stimulated by the findings in gout, microscopic examination of wet preparations of synovial fluid by compensated polarized light was applied to examination of many synovial fluids, nonurate crystals were discovered in the joint fluids of patients whose clinical diseases had many features of gout. The crystals appeared as rodlike or rhomboid forms with sharp corners, and under polarized light they demonstrated weakly positive birefringence. By x-ray diffraction these crystals were identified as *calcium pyrophosphate dihydrate (CPPD)*. Fluids removed from acutely inflamed joints with pseudogout invariably showed CPPD crystals within polymorphonuclear leukocytes, indicating that they had been phagocytosed. Crystals with morphologic features identical with the natural crystals were synthesized. Injection of synthetic or natural crystals into human and canine joints was followed by acute inflammation associated with phagocytosis of the crystals by polymorphonuclear and mononuclear leukocytes. The inflammation was related in severity to the dose of crystals injected and was completely reversible. Although the details of mediation of the inflammation in this condition have not been studied as completely as in gout, it is clear that this condition is another example of crystal-induced synovitis.

As this disease was recognized, its association with miliary calcium deposits in fibrocartilaginous structures, articular cartilage, ligaments, and joint capsule visible on radiographs (chondrocalcinosis) soon became apparent. Now it is established that these punctate and linear densities are seen most frequently in the menisci of the knee; other fibrocartilaginous structures calcified in this fashion are the articular discs of the distal radioulnar articulation, the symphysis pubis, the glenoid and acetabular labra, and the annulus fibrosus of the intervertebral discs. Calcification in the hyaline articular cartilage appears as a midzonal radiopaque line paralleling the contour of the underlying bone. Calcification may also be seen in the articular capsules of the larger joints. The deposits visualized radiographically have been studied at necropsy and have been convincingly demonstrated to be calcium pyrophosphate dihydrate crystals.

The clinical pattern of the arthritis ranges from intermittent acute attacks with complete remission between attacks, to clusters of almost continuous acute episodes in a number of joints, to a chronic progressive arthritis with superimposed acute episodes. Synovial biopsy shows inflammatory and reparative changes consistent with the clinical appearance of the joint. Some patients show only a chronic progressive arthritis without acute episodes; in such patients the crystals often cannot be demonstrated in the synovial fluid. Some patients with chondrocalcinosis are completely asymptomatic, and many patients will show calcific deposits in the tissues of joints that have never been the site of acute or chronic inflammation.

The mechanism for deposition of the calcium pyrophosphate crystals in cartilage and periarticular structures is unknown. Undoubtedly, local tissue changes must be favorable for the physical-chemical formation of the crystals. Aside from the occasional patient with hyperparathyroidism, serum values for calcium and phosphorus are normal. Diseases associated with calcium pyrophosphate crystal deposition disease include hemochromatosis, hyperparathyroidism, degenerative and destructive joint disease, and possibly hypophosphatasia and neuropathic joints. The relationship between hydroxyapatite crystals and the onset of acute inflammation in tendons, bursae, or joints is discussed in the next section.

CALCAREOUS TENDINITIS (WITH SUBACROMIAL BURSITIS)

Inflammatory involvement of tendons and contiguous bursae associated with deposition of calcium in and about the tendon is presumably another example of crystal-induced inflammation. This commonly occurs around the shoulder, with calcium deposition in one or more of the tendons in the rotator cuff, notably the supraspinatus tendon. Such deposits, visualized radiographically, are the most frequent abnormality encountered in acutely and subacutely painful shoulder. However, similar calcifications are found in many asymptomatic patients. The deposition of calcium is believed to be associated with degenerative changes in the tendon, perhaps related to wear and tear. As long as the calcium is confined to the relatively avascular fibrous tendon, it excites little or no reaction. But with encroachment into more vascular areas, a severe acute inflammatory reaction with hyperemia and edema is aroused. In the shoulder, the floor of the subacromial bursa forms part of the sheath for the supraspinatus tendon. Fluid collects within the tendon sheath and bursa and produces pressure, pain, and muscle spasm.

The calcium deposits in calcareous tendinitis have been found to resemble hydroxyapatite, although the characteristics of the local inflammatory response have only been partially defined. Most recently, apatite crystals have been found by electron microscopic study in synovial effusion cells in acute undiagnosed arthritis and exacerbation of synovitis in patients with osteoarthritis. This suggests that apatite found as the principal normal mineral of bone can under certain circumstances induce an acute inflammatory reaction. The inflammation in calcareous tendinitis is self-limited, and subsidence may be accelerated by removal of the calcium by needle aspiration or by the injection of anti-inflammatory agents. Often, as a result of the hyperemia of the inflammation, the calcium densities seen radiographically may appear to be resorbed.

IMMUNOLOGICALLY MEDIATED INFLAMMATION

As immunologic observations have been correlated with clinical experience, a workable system of general classification of the immunologic reactions producing tissue injury has emerged. As proposed by Gell and Coombs, the system is based on four general types of reactions. Those of principal interest in rheumatic diseases are types II, III, and IV, or a combination thereof. Humoral antibody responses are mediated by B-lymphocytes, and cellular immune responses by subsets of T-lymphocytes and their influence on mononuclear phagocytes (macrophages). Type II reactions (complement-dependent cytotoxic reactions) are dependent on the interaction of antibody with cell-bound antigen, with consequent activation of the complement system to produce cell damage or lysis. Type III reactions (immune-complex reactions) are mediated by the deposition of soluble antigen-antibody complex at a reaction site. Following complex formation, complement fixation occurs, with sequential activation of the complement system accounting for the biologic alterations of the reaction. Among the diverse biologic consequences of the interaction of antigen, antibody, and the complement system are activation of the kallikrein-kinin system, the attraction of polymorphonuclear leukocytes, and increase in capillary permeability. The kinin peptides induce vasodilatation, pain, and increased vascular permeability. The infiltrating leukocytes have been shown to ingest complexes, then to degranulate and release their lysosomal enzymes, which in turn act as even more powerful chemotactic agents and mediators of the inflammatory response.

Type IV reactions (delayed or cellular reactions) depend on the interaction of specifically sensitized subsets of lymphocytes (T cells) with the antigen. Developmentally, these small lymphocytes with the capacity for immunologic memory are thymus-dependent. A brief and undoubtedly oversimplified summary of the mechanism of this type of delayed reaction is as follows. Contact of these small lymphocytes with antigen leads to blast transformation and biosynthetic events producing a "sensitized lymphocyte." Cell-free extracts of disrupted leukocytes from individuals displaying delayed hypersensitivity are capable of transferring this capacity to sensitize the small lymphocyte (transfer factor). Upon recurrent contact with the antigen, these sensitized lymphocytes can recruit other mononuclear cells to the reaction site by the elaboration of effector substances called *lymphokines*. The lymphokines can be subdivided into groups according to their biologic activity. They include cytotoxic factors, chemotactic substances, inhibitory factors, and a group of substances that activate or alter the function of macrophages. Cytolysis of antigen-bearing cells may

then result from adherence of sensitized cells and elaboration of lytic substances. Under the microscope, the delayed or cellular reaction may show variable accumulation of fluid and polymorphonuclear leukocytes for the first 24 hours but thereafter is dominated by mononuclear cells, predominantly macrophages and monocytes with occasional small lymphocytes. The macrophages may coalesce to form giant cells. In severe reactions, necrosis in the central portion of the lesion may develop (see also Chapter 5).

SERUM SICKNESS

The basic mechanism of serum sickness is a type III antigen-antibody interaction. In studies with suitably tagged foreign protein, the concentration of circulating antigen shows a gradual decrease for 10 to 14 days. This corresponds to the latent period between introduction of the foreign protein and the appearance of symptoms, a period of development of the immune response. Circulating antibody is not easily detected at this time because of the formation of soluble complexes with the circulating antigen. This is indicated by a sudden drop in the level of circulating antigen, and onset of the inflammatory lesions corresponds to the appearance of circulating soluble immune complexes. The disease continues until complexes are entirely removed from the circulation. Antibodies to the foreign protein are easily demonstrated in the patient's serum during convalescence and for long periods of time thereafter. Readministration of the foreign antigen leads to prompt formation of antibodies and immune complexes and recurrence of the clinical disorder.

In experimental animals, localization of immune complexes containing antigen, antibody, and complement has been demonstrated in the endothelium of vessels of several organs. In synovial tissue this immune complex deposition leads to inflammatory infiltration, edema, and tissue necrosis.

Clinically, serum sickness is characterized by fever, arthralgia, skin eruptions, and edema. Objective evidence of synovitis may be present. It is a self-limited disease, the manifestations usually subsiding in 1 to 3 weeks. With the advent of antimicrobial therapy the use of serum for the treatment of bacterial infection has declined markedly. At the present time the most common cause of serum sickness is an administered drug, most often an antibiotic.

RHEUMATIC FEVER

Rheumatic fever is an uncommon but by no means rare sequela to an upper respiratory tract infection caused by group A hemolytic streptococci. Although most, if not all, serologic M types of group A streptococcal infections of the pharynx can lead to rheumatic fever, only 3 per cent or less of all patients who do not receive adequate antimicrobial treatment for streptococcal infection will develop subsequent rheumatic fever. There is a latent period of 2 to 4 weeks between the streptococcal infection and the appearance of signs and symptoms. Multiple focal aseptic inflammatory lesions are the basis of the acute manifestations. These include migratory arthritis, carditis, chorea, skin lesions, and subcutaneous nodules. The acute disease is of limited duration, but the carditis can lead to permanent valvular damage.

The arthritis in rheumatic fever is characterized by an inflammation that develops and subsides in the joints first affected, only to occur in other joints that were initially spared ("migratory polyarthritis"). The inflammation can be mild, with only vague discomfort in the region, but is often severe, with acutely inflamed joints that are very painful to touch or on attempted motion. The fluid in such joints is turbid and contains inflammatory leukocytes (Table 17–2) but is sterile on bacteriologic culture.

An immunologic mechanism in the production of at least the acute inflammatory lesions in rheumatic fever is strongly suggested in the production of the synovitis by the intriguing parallelism between the latent period of serum sickness and rheumatic fever and by the fact that the inflammation in both conditions is self-limited, subsiding completely and without residual joint damage. Antibodies to numerous components of streptococcus appear in the circulation of patients during pharyngeal infection by this organism, regardless of whether these individuals subsequently develop rheumatic fever. Therefore, an increase in the titer of antistreptococcal antibodies is evidence of a recent streptococcal infection and is not diagnostic of rheumatic fever. Most of but not all those who develop rheumatic fever have a higher antibody response that may persist longer than in those who do not develop this complication after streptococcal pharyngitis.

The mechanism for production of the carditis and the late valvular lesions has been proposed. Autologous antibodies that react with mammalian muscle including myocardial elements occur in the sera of patients with rheumatic fever in concentrations greater than those in the sera of patients who do not develop this complication. This autologous antibody cross-reacts with a streptococcal antigen. The source of the antigenic stimulus for this antibody and the role that it plays in the pathogenesis of the disease remain to be determined.

RHEUMATOID ARTHRITIS

Much evidence has accumulated implicating immunologic mechanisms in the pathogenesis of rheumatoid arthritis. This dates from the identification at the end of the 1950s of autologous immune globulins ("rheumatoid factors") in the serum of most patients with rheumatoid arthritis. This immune globulin has the characteristics of an antibody to normal human gamma globulin. The presence of complexes of this antigen and antibody in the leukocytes of rheumatoid synovial fluid has also been demonstrated. In addition, impressive evidence for activation of the complement system by way of both the classic and alternate pathways in rheumatoid synovial fluid has emerged. These findings correlate with the presence of immune complexes in the synovial fluid.

It has long been recognized that the sera of some patients with rheumatoid arthritis could cause the agglutination of a number of different particles. It has also been found that the particle involved is nonspecific and that the essential reaction is between the gamma globulin coating the particle and a factor in rheumatoid serum. The factor responsible for these reactions is gamma globulin with a sedimentation constant in the ultracentrifuge of a macroglobulin (19S). It is frequently found in serum in a complex with 7S gamma globulin. Thus, classic rheumatoid factor has been defined as IgM with antibody binding sites directed toward determinants of IgG. Also, globulins of the IgG and IgA classes have been found to have anti-IgG activity, and polymorphism among the rheumatoid factors is well established. Rheumatoid factors react most avidly with IgG that has been partly denatured or aggregated, presumably owing to exposure of additional binding sites by the alteration in molecular configuration. Immunofluorescent studies indicate that rheumatoid factor is produced by lymphoid tissues in the "large pale cells" in the germinal centers of lymph nodes and in plasma cells surrounding the germinal centers. The same distribution of staining is seen in the lymphoid nodules within the synovial membrane of rheumatoid joints.

Immunofluorescence studies have also demonstrated certain components of complement in tissue sections of rheumatoid synovium along with deposits of immunoglobulins. Although the serum level of complement in patients with rheumatoid arthritis is in the normal range, the complement activity of the synovial fluid usually is definitely lower in rheumatoid fluids as compared with that of other joint effusions. This lowered complement activity is most consistently found in the fluids from seropositive patients. Methods for quantitative studies of the sequential activation of this system have become available as a result of identification of the 12 serum proteins constituting the complement system (nine "components" and three "inhibitors," or "inactivators"). Several investigators have applied such methods to measure the activities of components of the complement sequence involved in both the classic and alternate (properdin) pathways in synovial fluids from pa-

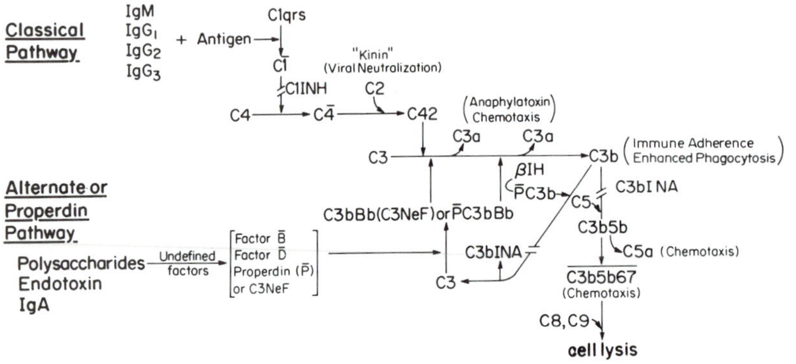

Figure 17–9 Pathways of complement activation and some of the biologic factors generated during the process of activation.

tients with seropositive or seronegative rheumatoid arthritis or osteoarthritis. In these studies, certain of the fluids from seropositive patients have demonstrated marked reduction in activity of the first component (C1). Although depressed activities of C1 have not been uniformly found, there has been ample evidence of activation of this component in the striking reduction in the second (C2) and fourth (C4) components. It has also been found that these two components are the natural substrates for activated C1 (C$\overline{1}$). In addition, reduction of the third component (C3), indicating generation of C3 convertase by the action of C1 on C4 and C2, has been demonstrated. Additional products of complement activation—namely, C3a, which increases vascular permeability, and chemotactic fragments C5a and the trimolecular complex C567—have been found in rheumatoid synovial fluid. Taken together, these alterations in complement component activities are consistent with the intrasynovial activation of the complement system in rheumatoid synovial fluids by an immune complex or its equivalent. At the present time, the specific antigen(s) in the complex is obscure. Although such evidence for complement activation has been most impressive in fluids from seropositive patients, borderline reductions in activities of the C2 and C4 components suggest that activation of C1 also occurs in fluids from seronegative patients. The reaction sequences and some of the biologic activities of complement by-products generated by activation of the complement system are outlined in Figure 17–9.

These observations have led to the concept that immune complexes activate the complement system within the joint, with diverse biologic consequences that lead to the inflammatory response. The role of rheumatoid factor of the 7S class (7S-anti-IgG) may be particularly important in activating the complement system. Complexes of IgG-7S-anti-IgG are demonstrable in rheumatoid synovial fluid, and the extent of complement depletion can be correlated with the quantities of these complexes contained in the fluid. There is evidence that the presence of 19S (IgM) rheumatoid factor may greatly augment the activating effects of

these complexes. This would account for the fact that the most profound alterations in the complement system are observed in synovial fluids from seropositive patients.

It is clear that several steps need further elucidation before a completely satisfactory immunologic explanation of rheumatoid arthritis can be established. The nature of the original antigenic stimulus is unknown. The question remains whether it is an exogenous foreign antigen or an autoantigen. If the rheumatoid factors are antibodies, presumably IgG should be the antigen. Several observations suggest that some alteration in the molecular configuration of IgG is required to provide such antigenic properties. There is ultrastructural evidence that mononuclear cells within the rheumatoid synovium are undergoing blast cell transformation. There is also evidence that the synovium is heavily infiltrated with T-lymphocytes that generate immune mediators (lymphokines). Several of the latter act upon polymorphonuclear and mononuclear phagocytic cells. These cells release lysosomal enzymes (collagenases, elastase, cathepsins, other glycosidases, proteases) that can mediate damage to articular cartilage, soft tissues, and bone. These responses encompass almost every immune reaction found in the several forms of chronic immunologic disease.

One of the most important findings related to rheumatoid arthritis is that the genes of the major histocompatibility complex (HLA system of humans), specifically at the HLA-D region, show strong correlation with this disease. This association is with immune response genes (Ir genes), which exercise control over the entire immune system. It has been shown that HLA-D4 and -DR4, identified by mixed lymphocyte culture reaction, occurs more commonly in white and black patients with rheumatoid arthritis than in control groups. It is presumed that through further study a locus with even higher association will be found. It is assumed that the frequent association of ankylosing spondylitis and Reiter's disease (not discussed in this chapter) with the HLA-B27 antigen (>90 per cent) is a similar marker for a yet unidentified Ir gene abnormality. Further details regarding the HLA system and disease can be found in other recent publications on this topic.

In contrast to some of the other immunologically mediated forms of arthritis, rheumatoid synovitis is characterized by fluctuating but continuing inflammatory activity with predominance of the proliferative and granulomatous reaction. The basis for this chronicity is not easily explained. There may well be continuing release of biologically active substances by the aforementioned mechanisms, but the process may also be perpetuated by other means. Several differences in the biologic activity of fibroblasts from patients with rheumatoid synovium as compared to that in normals have been reported. These "abnormalities" are reproducible on successive subculture. The prospect that exogenous substances derived from infectious agents or endogenous materials such as proteoglycans or collagen function as an antigenic stimulus in this disease remains a distinct possibility.

Rheumatoid arthritis, however, is not just a localized disease of the joints. It is a systemic disease, and constitutional manifestations such as ease of fatigue, weight loss, weakness, and at times fever and anemia are common. The outstanding characteristic is a chronic proliferative synovitis in multiple joints with a predilection for smaller joints such as the proximal interphalangeal, the metacarpophalangeal, and the metatarsophalangeal and a tendency for symmetric distribution of the joint involvement once the disease has become established. Yet inflammatory lesions are seen throughout the connective tissues of the body. Both the constitutional symptoms and the inflammatory activity are subject to fluctuations in severity, with a strong tendency to remission and exacerbation without apparent reason.

Prominent among the extra-articular manifestations is the rheumatoid nodule. These nodules occur in 20 to 25 per cent of patients at some time during the course of their disease. They arise as a microvascular lesion and are found most frequently in patients positive for rheumatoid factors. These are granulomas with a characteristic microscopic appearance (Fig. 17–10). They are most common over bony prominences and often are attached to the articular capsule or to bursae, but they may be attached to the periosteum, lie loose in the subcutaneous tissue, or involve the deeper layers of the skin. They may persist for months or years. Such nodules are occasionally seen in pleura and pulmonary tissue and actually have been found in virtually every connective tissue structure throughout the body. Other systemic manifestations include pericarditis, pleuritis with or without effusion, rheumatoid pneumoconiosis, scleritis, uveitis, peripheral neuropathy, and vasculitis. Vasculitis may be found in about 10 per cent of patients with rheumatoid arthritis, and an arteritis, at times difficult to distinguish from polyarteritis nodosa, is occasionally encountered in severe cases. The occurrence of these extra-articular lesions can be correlated in many instances with the presence of serum antinuclear antibodies and with deposition of immunoglobulins and complement in vessel walls in affected tissues. It may also be significant that more than 95 per cent of patients with nodules are seropositive for rheumatoid factor and that patients with the severe complications of rheumatoid arthritis usually have uncommonly high titers for rheumatoid factors in their circulating blood.

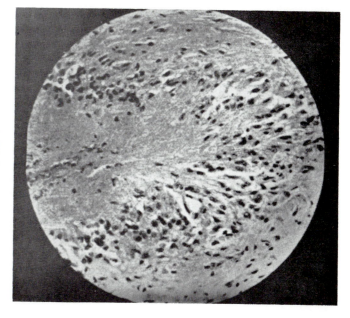

Figure 17–10 An extra-articular inflammatory lesion in rheumatoid arthritis: a subcutaneous rheumatoid nodule. Note the central zone of fibrinoid necrosis, the middle palisading zone of epithelioid cells, and the outer fibrous zone.

SYSTEMIC LUPUS ERYTHEMATOSUS

Systemic lupus erythematosus (SLE) is a chronic autoimmune disease affecting connective tissue, cells, and many organ systems, either individually or in various combinations. The clinical course may be fulminating or indolent but usually is characterized by periods of remission and exacerbation. Typically, patients with this disease manifest a host of immune phenomena, with circulating antibodies to their own cells, cell constituents, and proteins. Among these, particular significance is usually attributed to antibodies to nuclear materials. One of these antinuclear antibodies (deoxyribonucleoprotein, anti-DNP) is responsible for the LE cell phenomenon—an in-vitro "happening" dependent on the traumatization of some leukocytes with release of nuclear material, then the binding of the antibodies to nuclear material, and the subsequent phagocytosis of this complex by white blood cells, usually polymorphonuclear neutrophils. In the sera of patients with SLE there are multiple antinuclear antibodies with specificities to various nuclear constituents. These include double stranded DNA (ds DNA); single stranded DNA (ss DNA); histones; and nonhistone acidic nuclear proteins (Sm, RNP, others). Antibodies to ds DNA are felt to be almost specific for SLE; however, antibodies to ss DNA and denatured DNA may react with incompletely purified test antigen. Detection of antibodies to Sm antigen have been found to be highly diagnostic of SLE. Identification of antinuclear antibodies using cell or tissue section substrates and indirect immunofluorescent techniques is positive in 95 to 100 per cent of patients with SLE.

Clinically, SLE has a bewildering array of acute and chronic manifestations. Nearly all patients have constitutional symptoms, ranging from malaise and weight loss to high fever and prostration in fulminating cases. Ninety per cent will have joint and muscle pain, and of these about 70 per cent will have objective evidence of synovitis. Most characteristic is episodic inflammatory arthritis, especially of joints around the hands and feet, which develops rapidly and persists for only a few days. Although more persistent synovitis can occur, major joint swelling, capsular thickening, development of deformities, and ankylosis are uncommon. A variety of skin and mucous membrane lesions occur, especially in skin areas exposed to the sun. The identification of multiple immunoglobulin deposits in the basement membrane of biopsies of normal and involved skin ("Band test") by direct immunofluorescence is a useful diagnostic procedure. The classic erythematous "butterfly rash" on both cheeks and over the bridge of the nose is seen in less than half the patients. Involvement of serosal surfaces with pleuritis, pericarditis, or, less often, peritonitis may dominate the clinical picture. There may be pulmonary infiltrates. The myocardium and endocardium can be involved as well as the pericardium. Depression of one or more of the formed elements in the blood with anemia, neutropenia, or thrombocytopenia is common. The Coombs' antiglobulin test is frequently positive. Involvement of the central nervous system may be reflected in organic neurologic disturbances or psychiatric syndromes, and peripheral neuropathy is not uncommon. Elevations of spinal fluid gamma globulin levels occur during CNS involvement; however, detection of depressed C4 complement content is unreliable as an index of cerebritis owing to technical problems. Renal involvement occurs in about half the patients with SLE, presenting as either nephritis or the nephrotic syndrome. SLE is frequently the explanation for false-positive serologic reactions for syphilis. Rarely do all these manifestations occur at the same time in any one patient, but they may present at the same time in various combinations. When it is possible to follow patients with SLE over long periods of time, the sequential development of these varied manifestations is impressive. Such acute episodes, dominated at one time by one manifestation and later by another, are often separated by months or years of apparent good health.

The pathologic changes of SLE, even in organs and tissues known to be clinically involved, are often minor when examined by usual histologic techniques. Vasculitis and perivascular injury produced by immunologic mechanisms are the most common findings in inflammatory sites such as pleura, pericardium, synovium, skin lesions, and in Libman-Sacks nonbacterial verrucous endocarditis. Vasculitis can involve venules, capillaries and arterioles, and occasionally arteries. By immunofluorescent methods, fibrin and serum proteins, including immunoglobulins, complement, and DNA, have been detected in the tissue lesions. Deposits of immune complexes have been eluted from glomeruli taken from patients with SLE. The only in-vivo analogue of the LE cell is the "hematoxylin body," a rounded hematoxylin-stained mass, roughly the size of nuclei, occasionally seen in areas of inflammation.

Renal involvement in SLE is of special interest. From a practical point of view, progressive impairment of renal function terminating in uremia is still a cause of death in this disease. The renal involvement also provides the best insight into immunologic mechanisms that are important in the pathogenesis of SLE. The renal lesions may vary from mild to severe. The mildest form consists of deposits of immunoglobulins (chiefly IgG) and complement (especially C3) in the mesangium and along the glomerular basement membrane, without any other apparent abnormality. The most common renal lesion is focal glomerulitis with fibrinoid change, focal thickening of basement membrane, and slight increase in cellularity. These changes have been found in patients in the absence of clinical evidence of nephritis. In SLE glomerulonephritis, these lesions are more generalized and severe, with a mixture of proliferative and membranous changes and hypercellularity leading to crescent formation. Some kidneys show only a diffuse membranous glomerulonephritis with considerable thickening of the glomerular basement but little hypercellularity.

It is in SLE nephritis that the most definite changes in the immune mechanisms have been noted. The LE cell phenomenon and the titer of antibody to nucleoprotein do not correlate closely with clinical activity of the disease or with the presence or absence of renal involvement. However, the titers of antibodies to DNA are characteristically higher during periods of clinical activity, especially nephritis, than during remissions. Minute amounts of DNA have been demonstrated in serum at the same time that anti-DNA antibodies are present. Markedly decreased levels of circulating complement are seen primarily in active lupus glomerulitis. This can be measured as whole complement (CH50) or complement components (C3 and C4). Less impressive decreases in complement levels occur at some time during the course of SLE in 95 per cent of patients. These low levels are evidence of in-vivo activation of the complement system and fixation of complement components by circulating immune complexes.

The demonstration of these immunologic phenomena has led to the concept that these antibodies with determinants directed against the patient's own cells, cell constituents, and proteins are "autoantibodies," and that SLE, rheumatoid arthritis, and related disease are "autoimmune" diseases. The nature of the antigenic stimulus in SLE remains a mystery. A viral etiology for SLE has long been suspected. This possibility has received added impetus by the study of animal models of SLE (NZB/NZW mouse) in which type C virus is present and by detection, under the electron microscope, of cytoplasmic microtubules in the glomerular endothelium of patients with this disease. Although not specific or pathognomonic for SLE, such virus-like particles are demonstrable very frequently in the kidneys and other tissues of patients with the disease, and their recognition has some diagnostic value. However, these particles may represent ultrastructural manifestations of endothelial cell injury due either to secondary imposition of a viral infection in a more vulnerable host or tissue or to some other deleterious mechanism. The pathogenic significance of virus infection in the initiation of SLE may be clarified by further studies of excellent animal models (mouse, dog) that simulate human SLE.

OTHER RHEUMATIC DISEASES

Diseases grouped together with rheumatoid arthritis, rheumatic fever, and SLE under the heading of *the rheumatic or connective tissue diseases (collagen diseases)* are progressive systemic sclerosis, polymyositis, and polyarteritis nodosa. An additional disorder referred to as *mixed connective tissue disease* has been described. These diseases of unknown etiology are grouped together because of common or overlapping clinical and histopathologic features. An estimate of prevalence of these diseases per 1.0 million population per year compared with that of rheumatoid arthritis (500) and SLE (30) is 12 cases of progressive systemic sclerosis, 10 cases of polymyositis, and an undetermined number of cases of polyarteritis nodosa. The common histologic feature is widespread inflammatory damage to connective tissues and blood vessels, often associated with deposition of immune material. Clinical findings that justify a common grouping include the occurrence of major features of more than one entity in the same patient; sequential transitions between one entity and another in the same patient; suggestions of familial aggregation of more than one disease; and serologic abnormalities that predominate in one entity but that have an appreciable incidence in others. For example, approximately 15 per cent of patients with rheumatoid arthritis have positive tests for antinuclear antibodies, whereas 15 to 20 per cent of patients with SLE have positive serologic reactions for rheumatoid factor.

Progressive systemic sclerosis (scleroderma) was first recognized as a disease of the skin characterized by dermal fibrosis and fixation of the skin to underlying structures. Later, involvement of visceral organs (notably gastrointestinal tract, lungs, kidney, and heart) were recognized as part of the same process. The pathologic lesions are essentially those of mild to moderate vascular inflammation followed by excessive laying down of collagen in both appropriate and inappropriate sites, with ensuing fibrosis. There is limited evidence of a qualitative abnormality in this excessive collagen. In-vitro cultures of scleroderma fibroblasts show augmented synthesis of collagen that is sensitive to serum supplementation. About 70 per cent of patients with progressive systemic sclerosis have circulating antinuclear antibodies, usually of the type directed against various components of the nuclear material rather than against nucleoprotein. Also in contrast to patients with SLE, individuals in whom immunochemical analysis of vascular lesions in systemic sclerosis has been undertaken have not demonstrated deposition of immunoglobulins or complement. However, evidence that endothelial cell injury and damage to the microvasculature is important in the pathogenesis of this disease is now well established. Nailfold capillary abnormalities occur with high frequency in this disorder and have diagnostic specificity as well. Rheumatoid factor is present in 20 to 40 per cent of patients with systemic sclerosis. A cell-mediated immune abnormality has been ascribed to a subclass of T cells in some patients. Perhaps a cell-mediated immune reaction involving endothelial cell injury may prove to be involved in the pathogenesis of this disease.

Polymyositis (also termed *dermatomyositis* if there is an associated dermatitis) is a less common disease in which weakness of skeletal muscle is the outstanding clinical feature. Although inflammatory degenerative and regenerative changes are seen in the muscle, inflammation and pain are rarely prominent among the clinical manifestations. Dysphagia results from involvement of muscle in the pharynx and upper third of the esophagus; visceral involvement also includes cardiopulmonary complications in some patients. Occasionally, patients show features of both polymyositis and systemic sclerosis. Overlapping with features of rheumatoid arthritis and SLE also occurs at times. The muscle biopsy may show edema and inflammatory cells, particularly around blood vessels in the connective tissue between muscle fibers, with degeneration of muscle fibers and phagocytosis of remnants of muscle necrosis. Other features include evidence of efforts at muscle regeneration, non-necrotizing perivasculitis, and interstitial fibrosis.

Evidence of muscle involvement can be documented by electromyographic abnormalities and by characteristic biochemical changes. Release of several enzymes normally found in muscle is reflected by elevated serum levels of creatinine phosphokinase, aldolases, transaminases, and lactic dehydrogenases. There is usually creatinuria. Measurement of serum myoglobin levels provides an additional approach to evaluation of disease activity. An immunologic mechanism has been suggested by the association of malignant disease in 15 to 20 per cent of adults with dermatomyositis, but attempts to demonstrate antibodies to the patient's own tumor have rarely been successful. In-vitro studies indicate that lymphocytes from polymyositis patients are cytotoxic for skeletal muscle cells, suggesting that a cell-mediated abnormality is present in this disease. In addition, high antibody titers to *Toxoplasma gondii* are found in the serum of many patients, but the pathogenic significance of this abnormality remains unclear.

Mixed Connective Tissue Disease (MCTD) is defined as a disorder characterized by overlapping features of systemic lupus erythematosus, progressive systemic sclerosis, and polymyositis. Serologically, patients with this disorder have a high titer of antibody to ribonucleoprotein (RNP), a ribonuclease-sensitive antigenic component of extractable nuclear antigen (ENA). ENA, isolated chemically from calf thymus, has been reported to be a loose molecular complex with several antigenic sites. Two major antigenic components are RNP and a ribonuclease-resistant non-nucleoprotein fraction termed *Sm*. Besides Sm, other minor antigenic components have been found in the ribonuclease-insensitive ENA fraction. The antibody to RNP, although found in high titer in MCTD, has been found in patients with SLE, in individuals with progressive systemic sclerosis, and in some series in patients with polymyositis and in those with "undifferentiated connective tissue disease." A multicenter study of MCTD demonstrated that the most common clinical features of this disorder include Raynaud's phenomenon, polyarthralgia and arthritis, swollen hands, esophageal hypomobility, abnormal pulmonary diffusion capacity, inflammatory myositis, speckled nuclear fluorescent antinuclear antibodies, and high titers of RNP antibodies. It is now clear that not all patients with overlapping features of the several major forms of connective tissue disease can be accounted for as individuals with MCTD.

POLYARTERITIS (POLYARTERITIS NODOSA, NECROTIZING VASCULITIS)

The term *polyarteritis* is applied to a disorder characterized pathologically by inflammation and fibrinoid necrosis of medium-sized or small arteries. The widespread distribution of these arterial lesions produces a diversity of clinical manifestations that depend on the particular organ system that has suffered impairment of its arterial supply. Common presentations include renal disease, hypertension, abdominal symptoms that may simulate conditions requiring emergency surgery, coronary artery disease, cerebrovascular disease, peripheral neuritis, and fever of unknown origin with weight loss. A majority of patients complain of migratory muscle and joint aching, but true synovitis is uncommon.

The pathologic lesions typically involve one or more segments of small or medium-sized arteries with necrosis, fibrinoid change, and infiltration with polymorphonuclear neutrophils and varying numbers of eosinophils. The media is involved with extension to the intima and adventitia. Weakening of the arterial wall may lead to dissection or aneurysmal dilatation with rupture and hemorrhage. As the areas of fibrinoid necrosis are replaced by cellular granulation tissue, proliferation of the intima may lead to thrombosis with arterial occlusion and infarction. As the involved segment is finally replaced by scar tissue, the periarterial fibrosis may be sufficient in rare instances to produce gross nodules and partial vascular occlusion. Characteristically, both fresh and healing inflammatory lesions are found together in an individual case.

No clear line of demarcation can be drawn between the pathologic lesions of polyarteritis and other types of systemic necrotizing vasculitis, including those that may be associated with any of the other connective tissue diseases. Necrotizing vascular lesions resembling those of human polyarteritis can be produced in rabbits by repeated injections of foreign protein. Indeed, it was from such studies that the current understanding of the mechanism of serum sickness and the concept of the type III immunologic reaction developed. Evidence that some patients with polyarteritis have chronic hepatitis B (HBs) antigenemia has led to the demonstration that vascular lesions result from deposition of immune complexes containing HBs antigen. The circulating immune complexes form in the presence of excess viral antigen. The clinical findings in these individuals compared with those in patients who were HBs-negative were quite comparable. The extent to which this important finding can be correlated with all cases of "classic form" polyarteritis remains undetermined. In recent series HBs positive cases have accounted for as few as 10 per cent to as many as 54 per cent of patients with polyarteritis. Some of the HBs-positive patients were found to have chronic active hepatitis. Response to treatment did not differ among HBs-positive and HBs-negative cases. There is a very low incidence of positive tests for either rheumatoid factor or antinuclear antibodies in patients with polyarteritis. Some pathologists distinguish the angiitis (hypersensitivity vasculitis) related to hypersensitivity to serum and drugs from classic polyarteritis on the basis of inflammatory and necrotic changes in arterioles and venules (which are characteristically spared in classic polyarteritis); the development of changes first in the intima and then by extension involving the entire vessel wall; the relatively uniform character of the lesions at any particular evolutionary stage; and the frequent involvement of pulmonary vessels. Other syndromes associated with necrosis and inflammation of arteries include Wegener's granulomatosis, giant cell arteritis, aortic arch arteritis, and infective vasculitis. The reader is referred to other sources for a detailed description of these entities.

NONARTICULAR RHEUMATISM

In addition to the diseases that affect the joints themselves, disorders of the muscles that move the joints, neurologic diseases, and circulatory disturbances can cause discomfort and dysfunction of the musculoskeletal system. Pain and interference with joint function can also be produced by disorders in periarticular connective tissue structures such as tendons, tendon sheaths, bursae, and fascia; these are termed *nonarticular rheumatism.*

Inflammation of tendon sheaths (tenosynovitis) and bursae can result from specific infections,

with or without accompanying joint involvement. Sterile inflammation of these structures occurs in rheumatoid arthritis, gout, and systemic lupus erythematosus; it may also develop as a local disturbance without other disease. Bursitis around the shoulder has been discussed with calcareous tendinitis. Inflammation of tendons and bursae located around the elbows, knees, ischial tuberosities, hips, and Achilles' tendons can cause similar pain and interference with function of the adjacent joint, although seldom as troublesome as that produced by bursitis around the shoulder. Tenosynovitis may interfere with free motion of the enclosed tendon, impairing motion of the joint moved by the tendon. The sheaths of the flexor tendons of the fingers are common sites of such inflammation, with fibrous tissue reaction leading to adhesive tenosynovitis, so that if the finger is flexed, it cannot be extended without assistance ("trigger finger"). In some cases, inflammation of the flexor tendon sheaths and palmar fascia may result in adhesions so strong that the fingers become fixed in a partially flexed position. A fibroblastic reaction in the palmar fascia may cause adhesions with contractures resulting in flexion deformities of the fourth and fifth fingers (Dupuytren's contracture).

Primary fibrositis is the term applied to a symptom complex characterized by generalized or localized muscle stiffness and discomfort, particularly after rest, made worse by cold and usually alleviated by heat, massage, and exercise. It is also called *muscular rheumatism.* It may occur in acute attacks, accounting for the "stiff neck" or low back pain of "lumbago," which nearly everyone experiences at some time in life. It may also occur in more chronic forms, involving many structures at one time, or it may migrate from one part to another. Although the name *fibrositis* implies an inflammation of fibrous tissue, biopsies have failed to show histologic abnormalities in either connective tissue or muscle. The symptom complex is presumed to be an expression of a localized abnormality in the muscle or connective tissue. Sleep disturbances have been demonstrated in some patients with fibrositis syndrome; however, the exact significance of this finding remains uncertain.

Like any other system in the body, the musculoskeletal system may serve as the means of somatic expression of psychiatric disorders. Such expression is more common in psychoneurosis than in psychosis, although complaints referred to the musculoskeletal system are not uncommon in depression. Such manifestations are sometimes termed *psychogenic rheumatism.*

REFERENCES

STRUCTURE AND FUNCTION OF CONNECTIVE TISSUE
Brandt, K. D.: Glycosaminoglycans. *In* Kelley, W. N., Harris, E. D., Ruddy, S., and Sledge, C. B. (Eds.): Textbook of Rheumatology. Philadelphia, W. B. Saunders Co., 1981.
Castor, C. W.: Regulation of connective tissue metabolism. *In*

McCarty, D. J. (Ed.): Arthritis and Allied Conditions. Philadelphia, Lea and Febiger, 1979.
Copenhaver, W. M., Kelly, D. E., and Wood, R. L. (Eds.): Bailey's Textbook of Histology. 17th ed. Baltimore, Williams & Wilkins Co., 1978.

Eyre, D. R.: Collagen: molecular diversity in the body's protein scaffold. Science 207:1315, 1980.

Gallop, P. M., Blumenfeld, O. O., and Seifter, S.: Structure and metabolism of connective tissue proteins. Annu. Rev. Biochem. 41:617, 1972.

Harris, E. D.: Collagenases. In Cohen, A. S. (Ed.); Rheumatology and Immunology. New York, Grune and Stratton, 1979.

Hascall, V. C.: Interaction of cartilage proteoglycans with hyaluronic acid. J. Supramol. Struct. 7:101, 1977.

Kang, A. H.: Connective tissue: collagen and elastin. In Kelley, W. N., Harris, E. D., Ruddy, S., and Sledge, C. B. (Eds.): Textbook of Rheumatology. Philadelphia, W. B. Saunders Co., 1981.

Muir, H.: Proteoglycans: state of the art. Semin. Arthritis Rheum. 11(Suppl):7, 1981.

Pras, M., and Glynn, L. E.: Isolation of a noncollagenous reticulin component and its primary characterization. Br. J. Exp. Pathol. 54:449, 1973.

Ross, R.: The elastic fiber: a review. J. Histochem. Cytochem. 21:199, 1973.

Wahl, L. M., Wahl, S. M., Mergenhagen, S. E., and Martin, G. R.: Collagenase production by lymphokine-activated macrophages. Science 187:261, 1975.

STRUCTURE AND FUNCTION OF JOINTS

Barland, P.: Synovial membrane. In Cohen, A. S. (Ed.): Rheumatology and Immunology. New York, Grune and Stratton, 1979.

Engin, A. E., and Korde, M. S.: Biomechanics of normal and abnormal knee joint. J. Biomechanics 7:325, 1974.

Harris, E. D.: Biology of the joint. In Kelley, W. N., Harris, E. D., Ruddy, S., and Sledge, C. B. (Eds.): Textbook of Rheumatology. Philadelphia, W. B. Saunders Co., 1981.

Mankin, H. J., and Radin, E.: Structure and function of joints. In McCarty, D. J. (Ed.): Arthritis and Allied Conditions. Philadelphia, Lea and Febiger, 1979.

Radin, E. L.: Mechanical aspects of osteoarthrosis. Bull. Rheum. Dis. 26:862, 1975–76.

Simon, S. R.: Biomechanics of joints. In Kelley, W. N., Harris, E. D., Ruddy, S., and Sledge, C. B. (Eds.): Textbook of Rheumatology. Philadelphia, W. B. Saunders Co., 1981.

Woodburne, R. T. (Ed.): Essentials of Human Anatomy. 7th ed. New York, Oxford University Press, 1983.

FUNDAMENTAL PATHOLOGIC CHANGES OF JOINT DISEASE

Barrett, A. J., and Saklatvala, J.: Proteinases in joint disease. In Kelley, W. N., Harris, E. D., Ruddy, S., and Sledge, C. B. (Eds.): Textbook of Rheumatology. Philadelphia, W. B. Saunders Co., 1981.

Bennett, G. A., Waine, H., and Bauer, W.: Changes in the Knee Joint at Various Ages, with Particular Reference to the Development of Degenerative Joint Disease. New York, Commonwealth Fund, 1942.

Dingle, J. T.: Recent studies on the control of joint damage: the contribution of the Strangeways Research Laboratory. (Heberden Oration, 1978.) Ann. Rheum. Dis. 38:201, 1979.

Howell, D. S., and Talbott, J. H.: Osteoarthritis Symposium. Semin. Arthritis Rheum. 11(Suppl):1, 1981.

Lichtenstein, L.: Diseases of Bone and Joints. St. Louis, C. V. Mosby Co., 1975.

McCarty, D. J.: Synovial fluid. In McCarty, D. J. (Ed.): Arthritis and Allied Conditions. Philadelphia, Lea and Febiger, 1979.

Muir, H.: Molecular approach to the understanding of osteoarthrosis. (Heberden Oration, 1976.) Ann. Rheum. Dis. 36:199, 1977.

Pinals, R. S.: Traumatic arthritis and allied conditions. In McCarty, D. J. (Ed.): Arthritis and Allied Conditions. Philadelphia, Lea and Febiger, 1979.

Ropes, M. W., and Bauer, W.: Synovial Fluid Changes in Joint Disease. Cambridge, Harvard University Press, 1953.

Ziff, M.: Symposium on rheumatoid arthritis. Arthritis Rheum. 20:S31, 1977.

PATHOGENESIS OF JOINT INFLAMMATION

DeDuve, C.: The lysosome. Sci. Am. 208:64, 1963.

Harris, E. D., Vater, C. A., Mainardi, C. L., and Werb, Z.: Cellular control of collagen breakdown in rheumatoid arthritis. Agents Actions 8:36, 1978.

Ilardi, C. F., and Sokoloff, L.: The pathology of osteoarthritis: ten strategic questions for pharmacologic management. Semin. Arthritis Rheum. 11(Suppl.):3, 1981.

Kuehl, F. A., and Egan, R. W.: Prostaglandins, arachidonic acid, and inflammation. Science 210:978, 1980.

Ruddy, S.: Plasma protein effectors of inflammation: complement. In Kelley W. N., Harris, E. D., Ruddy, S., and Sledge, C. B. (Eds.): Textbook of Rheumatology. Philadelphia, W. B. Saunders Co., 1981.

Stossel, T. P.: Phagocytosis. N. Engl. J. Med. 290:717, 1974.

Ward, P. A.: Part V. Acute and chronic inflammation. The inflammatory mediators. Ann. N.Y. Acad. Sci. 221:290, 1974.

Weissmann, G.: Lysosomes and rheumatoid joint inflammation. Arthritis Rheum. 20:S193, 1977.

Wiggins, R. C., and Cochrane, C. G.: Immune complex–mediated biologic effects. N. Engl. J. Med. 304:518, 1981.

Zimmerman, T. S., Fierer, J., and Rothberger, H.: Blood coagulation and the inflammatory response. Semin. Hematol. 14:391, 1977.

SPECIFIC INFECTIOUS ARTHRITIS

Berney, S., Goldstein, M., and Bishko, F.: Clinical and diagnostic features of tuberculous arthritis. Am. J. Med. 53:36, 1972.

Goldenberg, D. L., and Cohen, A. S.: Acute infectious arthritis. Am. J. Med. 60:369, 1976.

Handsfield, H. H., Wiesner, P. J., and Holmes, K. K.: Treatment of the gonococcal arthritis-dermatitis syndrome. Ann. Intern. Med. 84:661, 1976.

Karten, I.: Septic arthritis complicating rheumatoid arthritis. Ann. Intern. Med. 70:1147, 1969.

Rosenthal, J., Bole, G. G., and Robinson, W. D.: Acute nongonococcal infectious arthritis. Arthritis Rheum. 23:889, 1980.

Sharp, J. T., Lidsky, M. D., Duffy, J., and Duncan, M. W.: Infectious arthritis. Arch. Intern. Med. 139:1125, 1979.

Ward, J. R.: Infectious arthritis. Med. Clin. North Am. 61:313, 1977.

CRYSTAL-INDUCED SYNOVITIS

Fessel, W. J.: Renal outcomes of gout and hyperuricemia. Am. J. Med. 67:74, 1979.

Howell, D. S.: Deposition of calcium pyrophosphate and hydroxyapatite. In Kelley, W. N., Harris, E. D., Ruddy, S., and Sledge, C. B. (Eds.): Textbook of Rheumatology. Philadelphia, W. B. Saunders Co., 1981.

Kelley, W. N.: Gout and related disorders of purine metabolism. In Kelley, W. N., Harris, E. D., Ruddy, S., and Sledge, C. B. (Eds.): Textbook of Rheumatology. Philadelphia, W. B. Saunders Co., 1981.

Klinenberg, A. R. (Ed.): Proceedings of the second conference on gout and purine metabolism. Arthritis Rheum. 18(Suppl.):659, 1975.

McCarty, D. J. (Ed.): Proceedings of the conference on pseudogout and pyrophosphate metabolism. Arthritis Rheum. 19(Suppl.):275, 1976.

McCarty, D. J.: Calcium pyrophosphate dihydrate crystal deposition disease: nomenclature and diagnostic criteria. Ann. Intern. Med. 87:240, 1977.

McCarty, D. J., Jr., and Hollander, J. L.: Identification of urate crystals in gouty synovial fluid. Ann. Intern. Med. 54:452, 1961.

Rodnan, G. P.: Treatment of the gout and other forms of crystal-induced arthritis. Bull. Rheum. Dis. 32:443, 1982.

Schumacher, H. R., Somlyo, A. P., Tse, R. L., and Mauer, K.: Arthritis associated with apatite crystals. Ann. Intern. Med 87:411, 1977.

Seegmiller, J. E., and Howell, R. R.: The old and new concepts of acute gouty arthritis. Arthritis Rheum. 5:616, 1962.

Thompson, G. R., Ting, Y. M., Riggs, G. A., Fenn, M. E., and Denning, R. M.: Calcific tendinitis and soft tissue calcification resembling gout. J.A.M.A. 203:464, 1968.

IMMUNOLOGICALLY MEDIATED INFLAMMATION

Barnett, E. V., Knutson, D. W., Abrass, C. K., et al.: Circulating immune complexes: their immunochemistry, detection, and importance. Ann. Intern. Med. 91:430, 1979.

Cochran, C. G.: Mediating systems in inflammatory disease. J. Invest. Dermatol. 70:40, 1978.

Cohen, S., Pick, E., and Oppenheim, J.: Biology of the Lymphokines. New York, Academic Press, 1979.

Coltan, H. R., Alper, C. A., and Rosen, F. S.: Genetics and biosynthesis of complement proteins. N. Engl. J. Med. *304*:653, 1981.

Dubois, E. L. (Ed.): Lupus Erythematosus. A Review of The Current Status of Discoid and Systemic Lupus Erythematosus and Their Variants. 2nd ed. Los Angeles, University of Southern California Press, 1976.

Evans, R. L., Beard, J. M., Lazarus, H., et al.: Detection, isolation, and functional characterization of two human T-cell subclasses being unique differentiation antigens. J. Exp. Med. *145*:221, 1977.

Fearon, D. T., and Austen, K. F.: The alternative pathway of complement—a system for host resistance to microbial infection. N. Engl. J. Med. *303*:259, 1980.

Ferrell, P. B., Aitcheson, C. T., Pearson, G. R., and Tan, E. M.: Seroepidemiological study of relationships between Epstein-Barr virus and rheumatoid arthritis. J. Clin. Invest. *67*:681, 1981.

Gell, P. G. H., and Coombs, R. R. A. (Eds.): Clinical Aspects of Immunology. 2nd ed. Philadelphia, F. A. Davis Co., 1969.

Glynn, L. E., and Schlumberger, H. D. (Eds.): Experimental Models of Chronic Inflammatory Diseases. Berlin, Springer-Verlag, 1977.

Guttmann, R. D. (Ed.): Immunology. Kalamazoo, Upjohn, 1981.

Hargreaves, M. M.: The L.E. cell phenomenon. Adv. Intern. Med. *6*:133, 1954.

Hurd, E. R.: Extra-articular manifestations of rheumatoid arthritis. Semin. Arthritis Rheum. *8*:151, 1979.

Karsh, J., Klippel, J. H., Balow, J. E., and Decker, J. L.: Mortality in lupus nephritis. Arthritis Rheum. *22*:764, 1979.

Kunkel, H. G.: The immunologic approach to SLE. Arthritis Rheum. *20*:S139, 1977.

McDevitt, H. O.: Regulation of the immune response by the major histocompatibility system. N. Engl. J. Med. *303*:1514, 1980.

Mellors, R. C., Heimer, R., Corcos, J., and Korngold, L.: Cellular origin of rheumatoid factor. J. Exp. Med. *110*:875, 1959.

Miescher, P. A., and Müller-Eberhard, H. J. (Eds.): Textbook of Immunopathology. 2nd ed. (Vols. I and II). New York, Grune & Stratton, 1976.

Morimoto, C., Reinherz, E. L., Schlossman, S. F., et al.: Alterations in immunoregulatory T cell subsets in active systemic lupus erythematosus. J. Clin. Invest. *66*:1171, 1980.

Movat, H. Z. (Ed.): Inflammation, Immunity and Hypersensitivity. Hagerstown, Harper and Row, 1979.

Pollack, V. E., and Pirani, C. L.: Renal histologic findings in SLE. Mayo Clin. Proc. *46*:630, 1969.

Snyderman, R., and McCarty, G. A.: Role of macrophages in the rheumatic diseases. Clin. Rheum. Dis. *4*:499, 1978.

Stastny, P.: HLA-D typing in rheumatoid arthritis. Arthritis Rheum. *20*:S45, 1977.

Stollerman, G. H.: Rheumatic Fever and Streptococcal Infection. New York, Grune & Stratton, 1975.

Tisher, C. C., Kelso, H. B., Robinson, R. R., et al.: Intraendothelial inclusions in kidneys of patients with systemic lupus erythematosus. Ann. Intern. Med. *75*:537, 1971.

Williams, R. C.: Rheumatoid Arthritis as a Systemic Disease (Major Problems in Internal Medicine, Volume IV). Philadelphia, W. B. Saunders Co., 1974.

Winchester, R. J. (Ed.): Conference on new directions for research in systemic lupus erythematosus. Arthritis Rheum. *21*:S1, 1978.

Yoshiki, T., Mellors, R. C., and Strand, M.: The viral envelope glycoprotein of murine leukemia virus and the pathogenesis of immune complex glomerulonephritis of New Zealand mice. J. Exp. Med. *140*:1011, 1974.

OTHER RHEUMATIC DISEASES

Adams, R. D. (Ed.): Diseases of Muscle. 3rd ed. New York, Harper & Row, 1975.

Callen, J. P., Hyla, J. F., Bole, G. G., and Kay, D. R.: The relationship of dermatomyositis and polymyositis to internal malignancy. Arch. Dermatol. *116*:295, 1980.

Christian, C. L., and Sergent, J. S.: Vasculitis syndromes: clinical and experimental models. Am. J. Med. *61*:385, 1976.

Farber, S. J., and Bole, G. G.: Antibodies to components of extractable nuclear antigen. Arch. Intern. Med. *136*:425, 1976.

Fauci, A. S., Haynes, B. F., and Katz, P.: The spectrum of vasculitis: clinical, pathologic, and therapeutic considerations. Ann. Intern. Med. *89*:660, 1978.

Gocke, D. J., Hsu, K., Morgan, G., and Christian, C. L.: Association between polyarteritis and Australia antigen. Lancet *1*:1149, 1970.

Kenik, J. G., Maricq, H. R., and Bole, G. G.: Blind evaluation of the diagnostic specificity of nailfold capillary microscopy in the connective tissue diseases. Arthritis Rheum. *24*:885, 1981.

LeRoy, E. C.: Scleroderma (systemic sclerosis). *In* Kelley, W. N., Harris, E. D., Ruddy, S., and Sledge, C. B. (Eds.): Textbook of Rheumatology. Philadelphia, W. B. Saunders Co., 1981.

LeRoy, E. C., Maricq, H. R., and Kahaleh, M. B.: Undifferentiated connective tissue syndromes. Arthritis Rheum. *23*:341, 1980.

Rodnan, G. P.: When is scleroderma not scleroderma? Bull. Rheum. Dis. *31*:7, 1981.

Sharp, G. C.: Mixed connective tissue disease, current concepts. Arthritis Rheum. *20*:S181, 1977.

NONARTICULAR RHEUMATISM

Berges, P. U.: Myofascial pain syndromes. Postgrad. Med. *53*:161, 1973.

Canoso, J. J., and Yood, R. A.: Reaction of superficial bursae in response to specific disease stimuli. Arthritis Rheum. *22*:1361, 1979.

Smythe, H. A.: Fibrositis as a disorder of pain modulation. Clin. Rheum. Dis. *5*:823, 1979.

Weiss, E.: Psychogenic rheumatism. Med. Clin. North Am. *39*:601, 1955.

18 Allergy and Asthma

Charles E. Reed

PATHOPHYSIOLOGY OF ALLERGY

Allergy is the converse of immunity. Immunity evolved in animals as protection from a myriad of toxins and infections by viral, bacterial, fungal, protozoan, and metazoan parasites. These mechanisms that so effectively dispose of foreign invaders do so at the cost of inflammation that often injures surrounding tissues of the host. At times, innocuous foreign antigens call forth these same immune defenses, with tissue injury being the only result. The antigen by itself is harmless. This inflammatory process is called *allergy*. Thus, an allergy occurs when lesions are generated as a result of an antigen's initiation of the cellular and humoral reactions of immunity. In many individual cases of allergic diseases, no antigen can be identified despite diligent investigation. In such cases, it seems likely that the chain of biochemical reactions involved in immunity is activated at a step distal to antigen-antibody reactions. The complexity of immunity with countless cellular and humoral interactions that include multiple feedback amplification and inhibition loops provide ample opportunity for biochemical initiation of allergic inflammation without the need for an antigen. Identification of these biochemical events has only just begun, but several drugs cause "allergic" reactions by their pharmacologic effects rather than by acting as haptenes binding to antibodies. Aspirin-provoked attacks of asthma and anaphylaxis following radiographic contrast injections are examples.

Early in this century, before the mechanisms of immunity were so well known, several authors suggested that allergy might be responsible for a variety of conditions of obscure cause. Research has confirmed some of these suggestions and explained their mechanisms. Unfortunately, however, the concept of allergy is not yet completely understood. Although there are yet many facts to be discovered, the broad outline of allergic diseases is quite distinct. Because allergy is an inflammatory process, it does not cause headaches, fatigue, behavorial disorders, or other noninflammatory conditions.

ALLERGIC MECHANISMS

Immunity is discussed thoroughly in Chapters 4 and 5. Here it is sufficient to mention that there are four broad categories of effector systems of immunity (Table 18–1). Three of these systems have similar organizations. Recognition protein (antibodies or antibody-like receptor proteins on lymphocytes) activate intermediary molecules through a cascade of enzymes (lymphokines, complement, and mast cell mediators) that attract and activate effector cells adapted to dispose of the invading organism. Two of the effector cell types, macrophages and neutrophils, ingest and kill organisms in phagolysomes. The third, eosinophils, kill multicellular parasites by exocytosis of their granules that contain toxic proteins. Many of the intermediary molecules themselves contribute to inflammation, acting as vasodilators, increasing capillary permeability, and lysing cells. The fourth immune system, mucosal immunity, does not seem to have an inflammatory component.

Cell-mediated immunity is phylogenetically the most ancient effector system. It has evolved from simple killing of foreign cells by unicellular organisms to the complex multicellular network that operates in mammals. It seems especially effective against intracellular parasites, particularly viruses, that express antigens on cell surfaces. It can also operate against extracellular infections, such as parasites and fungi, and can even be evoked by soluble antigens, such as tuberculin. Ordinarily, the infective agent or the virus-infected cell is killed by cytotoxic lymphocytes or by macrophage lysosomal enzymes either inside the macrophage after phagocytosis or outside after the lysosomal enzymes have been secreted. At times, when the antigen persists and macrophage stimulation continues, the macrophages assume the appearance of epithelioid cells and ultimately become giant cells. Thus, granulomas are unique examples of cell-mediated immunity.

Humoral immunity appeared in early vertebrates and has also evolved in complexity from sharks to mammals. In its simplest form, antibody binds a bacterial antigen and initiates the classic complement cascade. The activated complement enzymes lyse the cell. Other pathogens, e.g., bacteria, are coated with antibody and complement, ingested by neutrophils, and killed by peroxidases. Cells coated with antibody may also be killed by macrophages or certain lymphocytes by a process known as *antibody-dependent cellular cytotoxicity*. Some organisms have polysaccharides or other macromolecules that activate complement, not through antibody, but through the alternate pathway.

Anything truly complex resists simple classifications. Allergy is no exception. Sometimes antibodies develop to the host's own cell surface receptor proteins and may bind to the receptors without injuring the cell, but either stimulates or inhibits the receptor. Long-acting thyroid-stimulating substance (LATS), found in hyperthyroidism, is an example of an antibody stimulating a hormone receptor. Antibody to the acetylcholine receptor blocks its stimulation by the neurotransmitter and is responsible for the muscle weakness seen with myasthenia gravis. Whether or not this process should be called *allergy* is a question of definition of terms rather than understanding of pathophysiology.

Anaphylactic immunity, like the other forms of immunity, has been studied most thoroughly in mammals. It exists in some birds but seems to have evolved later than the other forms. Immunoglobulin E is the major antibody involved, although in guinea pigs a class of IgG functions in a similar way. Whether in some situations IgG antibodies, especially IgG$_4$, cause anaphylactic reactions in humans is still controversial. Transient production of IgE antibody commonly follows the first contact with antigens, but it is usually promptly terminated by immunoglobulin E class-specific suppressor cells. In some situations, such as after pertussis immunization or during infection with nematodes, IgE antibody production is enhanced and prolonged. Patients with IgE-mediated diseases, such as allergic rhinitis and asthma, continue to make IgE for many years. The explanation is unknown, but the prolonged IgE production during nematode infections in animals is a fruitful model for study. The mechanisms of anaphylaxis are discussed more thoroughly in Chapter 4.

Amplification and inflammation are not part of mucosal immunity. A more or less separate compartment of the lymphoid system located primarily in the gut is responsible for the development of mucosal immunity and IgA antibody production. After primary contact with the antigen in the gut, lymphocytes migrate to other organs such as lung and breast, where mucosal immunity is important. There is some evidence that cell-mediated immunity may be relatively specifically expressed on mucosal surfaces after mucosal immunization.

For purposes of classification and introduction of concepts, I have described these systems as if they were independent, but in reality they are quite intertwined. In numerous ways, components of one system recruit or inhibit components of another. For instance, chemotactic factors among the lymphokines released from sensitized lymphocytes attract eosinophils. IgE bound to macrophages may participate in killing metazoan parasites. Products of the complement cascade, particularly C5a, stimulate mast cell mediator release.

Immunity to any specific infection usually involves several of the immune effector systems simultaneously, although for some specific infections one particular factor seems to be especially important. For example, immunization with killed measles virus elicited primarily an antibody response without cellular immunity. Some of the children immunized with the killed virus had more severe than average illness, with pneumonia when they subsequently became infected. This attempt at immunization backfired. On the other hand, immunization with live attenuated virus evokes both cellular and humoral immunity and protects fully against disease. Thus, cellular immunity seems essential in measles. Tetanus immunization regularly evokes both cellular and humoral immunity. Only the humoral immunity is needed for protection. The cellular immunity, however, involves an antigen that can be conveniently included in a battery of skin tests for evaluating the integrity of the cellular immune system. Very rarely, anaphylactic immunity dominates the response to immunizing injections of toxoid. Interestingly, an IgE antibody response occurs much more frequently to diphtheria toxoid than to tetanus toxoid.

Anaphylactic immunity characterizes metazoan infestations, but humoral and cell-mediated immunity also play an important part in immunity to schistosomiasis and other parasitic diseases.

ALLERGIC DISEASES

Similarly, allergic diseases often involve more than one category of immunity. For example, the proteinuria of experimental immune complex ne-

TABLE 18–1 IMMUNE EFFECTOR SYSTEMS

Type of Immunity	Antigen Recognition	Amplification and Intercellular Signal	Effector Cells	Typically Protective Against
Cell mediated	Lymphocyte membrane antigen-specific binding patterns	Lymphokines	"Killer" lymphocytes, macrophages	Intracellular parasites
Humoral	Immunoglobulin antibodies, IgM and IgG	Complement	Neutrophils	Extracellular bacteria and toxins
Anaphylactic	Immunoglobulin E bound to mast cell surface receptors	Mast cell mediators and arachidonic acid metabolites	Eosinophils	Metazoan parasites
Mucosal	Immunoglobulin A, gut-associated lymphoid tissue			Mucosal pathogens, absorption of intact proteins

phritis in rabbits requires both IgE and IgG antibody, as do the urticaria and kidney disease seen with serum sickness in humans.

In other situations, absence of normal redundancy in immune response may increase the severity of an allergic reaction. For example, beekeepers who are stung many times develop high titers of both IgG and IgE antibody. Apparently, the IgG antibody is protective because they have no allergic reaction to the stings. Occasional members of their families, however, develop only the IgE antibody and suffer with anaphylaxis after stings.

Isolated IgA deficiency usually causes no illness, but subjects with IgA deficiency have an increased risk for various autoimmune diseases and may develop IgE antibody to heterologous IgA contained in gamma globulin or other blood products. Severe anaphylaxis has been reported.

Many diseases are known or suspected of being allergic in the two senses already defined: immunologic inflammation initiated (1) by otherwise innocuous antigens, or (2) in the absence of an antigen by a biochemical reaction (Table 18–2). In some diseases (e.g., bee sting anaphylaxis and contact dermatitis to poison ivy), the antigen is known and the immunologic mechanisms are quite well understood. In others (e.g., asthma), the allergic features are known but contribute only partially to the overall pathogenesis of the disease. In still others (e.g., rheumatoid arthritis), allergic mechanisms are reasonably suspected from the cellular architecture of the lesions or the deposition of immunoglobulins and complement, but the responsible antigens, if they exist, have not been identified.

For a more complete discussion of these disorders, the reader is referred to textbooks of clinical immunology and allergy.

DRUG ALLERGY

Drugs are frequent causes of allergic reactions operating through one or more of the basic immune mechanisms. Some, like insulin, act as complete protein antigens. Others, like penicillin, are haptenes forming complete antigens after reacting with a body protein. Penicillin is an example of a drug that can elicit several different types of allergy: anaphylaxis, humoral (hemolytic anemia) or cell mediated (contact dermatitis). The details of immunologic reactions in allergy to most drugs are incompletely understood except in the case of penicillin.

Some drugs, notably aspirin and radiographic contrast agents, initiate allergic diseases by acting not as haptenes combining with antibody but as drugs inhibiting enzymes that are important in the sequence of biochemical events in the allergic reaction. Patients who react to aspirin react also to indomethacin and the other nonsteroidal anti-inflammatory agents. A few patients also react to tartrazine, a common yellow dye for foods and drugs. Some drugs (e.g., alpha-methyldopamine) induce antibodies that react with autoantigens, in this case Rh antigens on erythrocytes. Common drug reactions are classified in Table 18–3. Reports of the varieties of allergic reactions that have been observed in isolated cases create the impression that any drug can cause virtually any kind of reaction. However, many of these reports do not establish a strong cause and effect relationship. In reality, allergic reactions to specific drugs seem quite consistent.

PATHOPHYSIOLOGY OF ASTHMA

From the physiologic viewpoint, asthma is, as defined by a joint committee of the American Thoracic Society and American College of Chest Physicians, "a disease characterized by an increased responsiveness of the trachea and bronchi to various stimuli and manifested by widespread narrowing of the airways that changes in severity either spontaneously or as a result of therapy." For the physiologic diagnosis of asthma, two measurements of the airway obstruction are needed, one before and one after treatment with a bronchodilator or glucocorticoids. In mild cases in which the initial values are normal, spirometry before and after a bronchoconstrictive stimulus (e.g., methacholine or isocapneic hyperventilation) will demonstrate increased responsiveness.

From the pathologic viewpoint, asthma is characterized by an inflammation of the bronchial wall with infiltration by mononuclear cells and eosinophils. Often there is vacuolization of the epithelium that progresses to desquamation of the ciliated epithelium. Hypersecretion of mucus occurs, and with loss of function of the mucocilliary escalator the lumen becomes occluded with plugs of inflammatory exudate and desquamated epithelium in a matrix of viscous mucus. In addition to these reversible inflammatory changes, there is collagen deposition in a band beneath the basement membrane, hypertrophy of bronchial smooth muscle, and hyperplasia of bronchial mucous glands.

From the immunologic viewpoint, asthma is an example of immunoglobulin E–mediated anaphylactic allergic reaction to airborne antigens, although in many patients no allergen can be identified, and patients whose attacks are often provoked by an antigen also have attacks provoked by nonallergic stimuli (e.g., exercise or airborne irritants).

PATHOGENESIS

The cause of asthma is unknown. It is not even clear whether asthma is a single disease with

TABLE 18–2 SELECTED ALLERGIC DISEASES AND THEIR IMMUNE MECHANISMS

Disease	Mechanisms
Skin	
Contact eczematoid dermatitis	Cell-mediated
Contact urticaria	Anaphylactic
Atopic dermatitis	Uncertain. Anaphylactic? Cell-mediated? Both?
Acute urticaria and angioedema	Anaphylactic
Subacute urticaria and angioedema (3 days to 3 wks)	Anaphylactic or humoral, usually to microbial antigens
Chronic urticaria and angioedema (longer than 3 wks)	Unknown. Biochemical activation of anaphylactic pathways?
Cutaneous vasculitis	Anaphylactic and humoral
Lung	
Hay fever	Anaphylactic
Nasal polyps and hyerplastic sinusitis	No antigens identified. Biochemical initiation of anaphylactic pathways?
Asthma	Anaphylactic. Biochemical activation of anaphylactic pathways?
Hypersensitivity pneumonitis (allergic alveolitis)	Cell-mediated? Humoral?
Allergic bronchopulmonary aspergillosis	Anaphylactic? Humoral? Cell-mediated?
Pulmonary infiltrate, with eosinophilia	Unknown
Pulmonary fibrosis in SLE rheumatoid arthritis	Unknown
Cardiovascular system	
Rheumatic fever	Unknown. Humoral? Cell-mediated?
Necrotizing vasculitis:	Humoral
cranial (giant cell) arteritis	Unknown. Cell-mediated?
Eosinophilic granulomatous arteritis (Churg-Strauss syndrome)	Unknown. Anaphylactic and cell-mediated?
Polyarteritis nodosa	Unknown
Granulomatous arteritis	Unknown. Cellular?
Kidney	
Glomerulonephritis	Humoral
Goodpasture syndrome	Humoral
Interstitial nephritis	Unknown. Humoral? Cell-mediated? Both?
Gastrointestinal system	
Pernicious anemia	Humoral. And cell-mediated?
Eosinophilic gastritis	Anaphylactic
Eosinophilic gastroenteritis	Unknown. Anaphylactic?
Crohn disease	Unknown
Chronic ulcerative colitis	Unknown
Chronic active hepatitis	Unknown. Humoral?
Joints	
Rheumatoid arthritis	Humoral? Cell-mediated?
Systemic lupus erythematosis	Humoral? Cell-mediated?
Blood cells	
Autoimmune hemolytic anemia	Humoral
Hemolytic disease of the newborn	Humoral
Neutropenia	Humoral
Thrombocytopenia	Humoral
Nervous system	
Mononeuritis	Humoral. And anaphylactic?
Postvaccinial encephalitis	Cell-mediated
Multiple sclerosis	Cell-mediated?
Myasthenia gravis	Humoral
Endocrine glands	
Thyroiditis	Humoral. And cell-mediated?
Adrenalitis	Humoral. And cell-mediated?
Juvenile diabetes	Humoral. And cell-mediated?

TABLE 18–3 SOME COMMON ALLERGIC DRUG REACTIONS

Reaction	Drug	Mechanisms
Skin		
Contact dermatitis	Ethylenediamine	Cell-mediated
	Neomycin	"
Erythroderma	Gold salts	Cell-mediated?
	Phenytoin	"
	Phenobarbital	"
	Allopurinol	"
Urticaria and	Penicillin	Anaphylactic
angioedemas	Sulfa	"
	Nonsteroidal antiinflammatory agents	Enzyme inhibition?
Morbilliform	Ampicillin	Unknown
		"
Photosensitivity	Phenothiazines	"
	Griseofulvin	"
	Thiazides	"
Fixed eruption	Phenophthalein	Unknown
Lung		
Asthma	Aspirin and other antiinflammatory agents	Enzyme inhibition
Pneumonitis or pleural effusion	Nitrofurantoin	Cell-mediated?
	Busulfan and other antineoplastic drugs	Unknown
	Cromolyn	"
Cardiovascular system		
Vasculitis	Sulfa	Unknown
	Penicillin	Humoral
Liver		
Cholangitis,	Phenothiazines	Unnown
hepatocellular injury	Gold salts	Unknown
	Isoniazid	
Kidney		
Interstitial nephritis	Penicillin, especially methicillin	Unknown

Table continued on opposite page

a single cause or a symptom complex with many separate causes. There is clearly a familial risk associated with asthma. The symptom complex of allergic rhinitis, allergic asthma, and eczematous dermatitis has been called "atopy." However, the genetic basis for atopy is unknown. Genetic control over several processes probably accounts for the familial clustering. These processes include the level of serum IgE, immune response genes, and variability of the irritability of the airways.

For the present, it is best to consider asthma a disease of three components: (1) *stimuli* that provoke episodes, (2) the *response* of airways to these stimuli, and (3) *pathways* that link the stimuli to the response (Table 18–4).

Stimuli

The first three stimuli listed in Table 18–4 act in all patients; the last three affect only some individuals. However, in any particular patient the same stimulus regularly evokes the same response. A stimulus cannot be identified for every episode of asthma, and in a few patients chronic asthma persists in the absence of identifiable stimuli.

Response

Although airway obstruction is widespread it is patchy, involving some parts of the bronchial tree more than others.

During severe episodes, central as well as peripheral airways are obstructed. As the episode responds to treatment, the central airways clear first. It is likely that patients vary in the degree of central and peripheral obstruction. Typically, central obstruction causes cough and tickle; peripheral obstruction causes chest tightness. Patchy peripheral obstruction may persist even in asymptomatic periods, when up to half the alveoli lie behind completely occluded airways. This nonun-

TABLE 18–3 SOME COMMON ALLERGIC DRUG REACTIONS (*Continued*)

Reaction	Drug	Mechanisms
Blood		
Hemolytic anemia	Penicillin	Humoral
	Quinidine	"
	Alpha-methyldopamine	"
	Levodopa	"
Aplastic anemia	Phenylbutazone	Unknown
	Phenytoin	"
	Gold salts	"
	Chloramphenicol	"
	Penicillamine	
Thrombocytopenia	Gold salts	Humoral
	Phenytoin	
	Levodopa	"
	Methyldopa	"
	Quinidine	"
	Thiazides	"
	Acetaminophen	"
Granulocytopenia	Aminopyrine	Unknown
	Phenothiazines	"
	Phenylbutazone	"
	Penicillin	"
		"
Anaphylaxis	Chymopapain	Anaphylactic
		"
		"
		"
	Penicillin	
	ACTH	
	Insulin	
	Blood products	IgA deficiency
	Radiographic contrast agents	Complement activation
	Sulfites	Unknown
	Opiates	Direct mast cell histamine release
	Local anesthetics	Unknown

iform obstruction explains the hypoxemia that occurs during acute attack. Although compensatory local vasoconstriction partially adjusts blood flow to match ventilation, compensation is incomplete, and the alveoli behind occluded airways still receive a small fraction of the normal blood flow. Mixture of this poorly oxygenated blood with blood from other areas that are actually hyperventilated accounts for the hypoxemia with respiratory alkalosis that characterizes mild attacks. Only when the asthma is so severe that total alveolar ventilation is impaired does carbon dioxide retention occur. Respiratory acidosis is therefore much more dangerous in asthma than in other chronic obstructive lung diseases. It is often an indication for intubation and assisted ventilation. The characteristic high-pitched musical wheeze of asthma is another manifestation of the uneven ventilation. The musical sound arises from individual airways that are almost but not completely occluded. As air moves through the airway, it vibrates like an oboe, opening and closing with the frequency of the pitch of the sound. Most wheezes arise in the peripheral airways. Partial narrowing of central airways is indicated by increased bronchovesicular

breathing, best heard at the mouth. This sound results from increased turbulence due to increased velocity of airflow through the narrowed airway.

The airway obstruction also varies in tempo. Some attacks, such as those resulting from exercise or brief exposure to certain antigens (e.g., a friend's cat) start promptly and subside promptly. At times, there is a second wave of obstruction 4 to 12 hours after exposure to an antigen, especially if the exposure is heavy and the patient is highly sensitive. Quite rarely only the late response occurs. Still a third tempo can occur after an antigen exposure. Asthma may recur nightly for several nights. This kind of response has been studied most thoroughly in various occupational allergies. Because the close temporal connection between exposure and symptoms may be obscured, this response sometimes makes the diagnosis of occupational asthma difficult.

During the attack, the pathologic change may be either simple bronchospasm or inflammation of the bronchial wall with plugging of the lumen. Most often, it is a combination of both. Acute brief attacks are chiefly due to bronchospasm and respond to theophylline or adrenergic bronchodila-

TABLE 18–4 ASTHMA AS A DISEASE OF STIMULUS-RESPONSE

Stimuli
1. Exercise, cold air, hyperventilation
2. Viral respiratory infections
3. Airborne irritants (dusts and fumes)
4. Emotionally charged situations
5. Airborne allergens
6. Chemicals such as aspirin, sulfite, diisocyanates

Response variables
1. Location
2. Tempo
3. Pathology

Pathways linking stimulus to response
1. Neurohumoral control of airway smooth muscle
2. Anaphylactic allergy (immediate and late)

tors. Other attacks, such as those associated with viral respiratory infection, begin insidiously, persist for days or weeks, and respond poorly to bronchodilators. This airway obstruction is principally due to inflammation and mucus plugs. It responds slowly to treatment with glucocorticoids.

Linkage Pathways

There has been great progress in understanding the two major pathways that link stimulus to response. The first involves neurohumoral regulation of the smooth muscle of the airways, which is predominantly controlled by the vagus. Different fibers of the vagal bronchoconstrictive reflex arise in the rapidly adapting irritant receptors located between mucosal epithelial cells. These receptors are most numerous in the central airways, and are particularly concentrated at bifurcations. Similar afferent receptors are present in the esophagus and perhaps in the nasal and paranasal sinus mucosa. The efferent limb of this reflex arc arises in the brain stem, passes down the vagal trunk, and synapses in autonomic ganglia located in the bronchial wall. Postganglionic cholinergic fibers innervate the smooth muscle. Most of the postganglionic myoneural junctions are on the adventitial side of the muscle layer; the impulse spreads through the muscle from there. Normally, there is some vagal tone in the airways, but during acute attacks of asthma, vagal bronchoconstriction greatly increases. Cholinergic fibers also innervate bronchial glands and stimulate secretion. In dogs and some other animals, postganglionic adrenergic fibers arising in the cervical ganglia innervate bronchial muscle and produce adrenergic bronchodilation. In humans, however, postganglionic adrenergic synapses cannot be

found in bronchial muscle. Physiologic adrenergic bronchodilation is due to circulating catecholamine, not sympathetic innervation. There is, however, a nonadrenergic inhibitory nervous innervation of the airways similar to that in the gut. The neurons arise in the cholinergic bronchial ganglia. The neurotransmitter has not yet been identified with certainty but is probably a peptide. It is not known whether abnormal function of these neurons contributes to asthma.

Increased activity of vagal reflex bronchoconstriction is characteristic of asthma and accounts for the hyperreactivity of the airways. But the reason for the increased reactivity is not known. Irritant receptors respond to tactile stimuli (dusts), chemical stimuli (sulfur dioxide, ozone), and to mediators of anaphylaxis (e.g., histamine). Asthmatics react at concentrations 10- to 100-fold less than normal subjects do, and the magnitude of their response is greater. The evidence is still conflicting, concerning whether or not two common stimuli that cause acute bronchoconstriction, exercise and antigen inhalations, do so through reflexes. Histamine and other bronchoconstrictive mediators probably act directly on bronchial muscle as well as indirectly by stimulating irritant receptors. Exercise and isocapneic hyperventilation cause bronchoconstriction through cooling of the central airways by evaporation of water, but the subsequent steps have not yet been identified. Not only do asthmatics react to stimulation of the irritant receptors but they also react excessively to cholinergic agonists (e.g., methacholine) that act directly on bronchial smooth muscle.

The other major pathway is anaphylactic allergy. A specific receptor protein located in the membrane of mast cells and basophils binds the Fc portion of IgE molecules. When IgE is crosslinked by an antigen molecule with two or more combining sites, enzymes in the cell membrane are activated, calcium flows into the cell, the mast cell granule fuses with the cell membrane, and the granule contents are extruded from the cell. Phospholipases in other cells as well as in the mast cell are activated, producing arachidonic acid and various products of arachidonic acid metabolism.

The acute bronchoconstriction that follows antigen exposure presumably results from the activity of bronchoconstrictive mediators. Histamine comes from the mast cells, and leukotrienes are produced by arachidonic acid metabolism, chiefly in other nearby cells. The second wave of airway obstruction, occurring 4 to 12 hours following antigen challenge, is less well understood. Histamine and leukotrienes have only a brief effect, as they are rapidly metabolized and readily reversed by bronchodilators. Since the late phase of obstruction responds poorly to bronchodilators but does respond to glucocorticoids, it seems likely that the late phase is the result of airway inflammation. Possibly, there are continued syntheses and release of mast cell products, but this is an open question. Bronchial biopsy has not been obtained, so direct information about histology is lacking. However, IgE is both necessary and sufficient for a similar late reaction at skin test sites. Biopsy of these test sites shows eosinophil and lymphocyte infiltration. This observation suggests that the late phase of anaphylactic allergy in the lung may also be responsible for the similar inflammatory changes in the airways seen in severe asthma.

Eosinophils are prominent in the lesions of asthma and presumably contribute importantly to the epithelial damage. The major basic protein of the eosinophil granule, which is lethal to schistosomules and *Trichinella* larvae, also damages ciliated respiratory epithelium in vitro. The levels required to produce this damage are found in the sputum of patients admitted to the hospital for treatment of severe asthma. At autopsy, the mucus plugs and the bronchial walls contain not only eosinophils but also free eosinophil granules and free major basic protein lying outside the granules. Major basic protein is especially concentrated along the basement membrane at sites of epithelial desquamation. It is not yet known what accounts for this eosinophil accumulation and degranulation in patients who have normal amounts of IgE and who have no demonstrable allergies to environmental allergens. Presumably, some other stimulus is operating to initiate a process similar to the late phase of the IgE-mediated reaction. The mast cell mediators responsible for the late phase have not yet been identified. Possibly there are several. Potential candidates include eosinophil chemotactic tetrapeptide, platelet-activating factor, neutrophil chemotactic factor, and several products of the lipoxygenase pathway of metabolism of arachidonic acid.

These neural and immunologic pathways interact. For a time after a late bronchial response to an antigen, presumably while the inflammation persists, the airways show increased reactivity to methacholine. Similar increased reactivity follows respiratory infection and exposure to irritant gasses. In addition, these two systems share with each other and indeed with all reactive cells the processes of cellular response to an extracellular signal by intracellular second messengers. The biochemistry of the stimulus-response coupling of mast cells, lymphocytes, neutrophils, autonomic neurons, and smooth muscle is remarkably similar. In mast cells, for example, the first event following cross-linking of IgE molecules is activation of enzymes that methylate phosphatidylethanolamine on the inner surface of the cell membrane to phosphatidylcholine, translocating it to the outer surface. The phosphatidylcholine is the precursor of arachidonic acid. Shortly afterwards, there is a burst of activity of adenylate cyclase followed by a slow flux of calcium into the cell and release of histamine.

Because intracellular calcium ion and cyclic AMP serve such central roles as second messengers in all responses to cholinergic and adrenergic agonists, prostaglandins, leukotrienes, and other substances, and because they modulate critical cell functions such as secretion, contraction, and neurotransmission, reactions involving calcium ion and cyclic AMP deserve continued attention. Fruits of investigations of these membrane reactions in asthma are likely to include not only better understanding of the disease but also new approaches to treatment.

REFERENCES

GENERAL

Lockey, R. F. (Ed.): Clinical Immunology and Allergy for Students and Practicing Physicians. New York, Medical Examination Publishing Co. Inc., 1978.
Middleton, E., Reed, C. E., and Ellis, E.: Allergy Principles and Practices. 2nd. ed. St. Louis, C. V. Mosby, 1983.
Samter, M. (Ed.): Immunologic Diseases. 3rd. ed. Boston, Little Brown & Co., 1978.
Stiles, D. P., Stobo, J. D., Fudenberg, H. H., and Wells, J. V.: Basic and Clinical Immunology. 3rd. ed. Los Altos, Lange Medical Publications, 1982.

BASIC MECHANISMS

David, J. R., and David, R. R.: Cellular hypersensitivity and immunity: inhibition of macrophage migration and lymphocyte mediators. Prog. Allergy 16:300, 1972.
Plaut, M., Lichtenstein, L. M.: Cellular and chemical basis of the allergic inflammatory response. In Middleton, E., Reed, C. E., and Ellis, E. (Eds.): Allergy Principles and Practices. 2nd ed. St. Louis, C. V. Mosby Co., 1983.
Tomasi, T. B., Larson, L., Challcombe, S., and McNabb, P.: Mucosal immunity. The origin and migration patterns of cells in the secretory system. J. Allergy Clin. Immunol. 65:12, 1980.

ALLERGIC DISEASES

Mathews, K. P.: Chronic urticaria revisited. J. Allergy Clin. Immunol. 61:347, 1978.
Parker, C. W.: Drug allergy. N. Engl. J. Med. 292:732, 1975.
Patterson, R., et al.: Serum immunoglobulin levels in pulmonary allergic aspergillosis and certain other lung diseases, with special reference to immunoglobulin E. Am. J. Med. 54:16, 1973.
Roberts, R. C., and Moore, V. L.: Immunopathogenesis of hypersensitivity pneumonitis. Am. Rev. Resp. Dis. 116:1075, 1977.
Sullivan, T. J.: Antigen specific desensitization of patients allergic to penicillin. J. Allergy Clin. Immunol. 69:500, 1982.
ACCP–ATS Joint Committee on Pulmonary Nomenclature: Pulmonary terms and symbols. Chest 67:385, 1975.

ASTHMA

Austen, K. F., and Lichtenstein, L. M. (Eds.): Asthma: Physiology, Immunopharmacology and Treatment. New York, Academic Press, 1973.

Austen, K. F., and Lichtenstein, L. M. (Eds.): Asthma II: Physiology, Immunopharmacology and Treatment. New York, Academic Press, 1977.

Austen, K. F., Lichtenstein, L. M., and Kay, A. B. (Eds.): Asthma III: Physiology, Immunopharmacology and Treatment. New York, Academic Press, 1983.

Butterworth, A. E., Wassom, D. L., Gleich, G. J., et al.: Damage to schistosomules of *Schistosoma mansoni* induced directly by eosinophil major basic protein. J. Immunol. *122*:221, 1979.

Frigas, E., Loegering, D. A., and Gleich, G. J.: Cytotoxic effects of the guinea pig eosinophil major basic protein on tracheal epithelium. Lab. Invest. *42*:35, 1980.

Frigas, E., Loegering, D. A., Solley, G. O., et al.: Elevated levels of the eosinophil granule major basic protein in the sputum of patients with bronchial asthma. Mayo Clin. Proc. *56*:345, 1981.

Hirata, F., and Axelrod, J.: Phospholipid methylation and biological signal transmission. Science *209*:1082, 1980.

Ishizaka, T., Conrad, D. H., Schulman, E. S., et al.: Biochemical analysis of initial triggering events of IgE mediated histamine release from human lung mast cells. J. Immunol. *130*:2357, 1983.

Nadel, J. A.: The parasympathetic system and its role in asthma. Adv. Asthma Allerg. Pul. Dis. *4*:15, 1977.

Parker, C. W.: Prostaglandins and slow-reacting substance. J. Allergy Clin. Immunol. *63*:1, 1979.

Piper, P. J.: SRS-A and Leukotrienes. Oxford, John Wiley, 1981.

Rasmussen, H.: Calcium and cAMP as Synarchic Messengers. New York, John Wiley & Sons Inc., 1981.

Richardson, J. B., and Ferguson, C. C.: Neuromuscular structure and function in the airways. Fed. Proc. *38*:202, 1979.

Spector, S. L., Wangaard, C. H., and Farr, R. S.: Aspirin and concomitant idiosyncrasies in adult asthmatic patients. J. Allergy Clin. Immunol. *64*:500, 1979.

Szentivanyi, A.: The beta adrenergic theory of the atopic abnormality in bronchial asthma. J. Allergy *42*:203, 1968.

Pathogenic Properties of Invading Microorganisms

19

Louis Weinstein and Morton N. Swartz

INTRODUCTION

Although the terms "health" and "disease" are mutually exclusive, "health" and "infection" are not. For example, within a few days of birth an infant is "infected" with a variety of bacteria and remains so infected throughout his lifetime. Thus, bacterial (and viral) colonization of body surfaces and the intestinal tract is the early and inevitable consequence of the ubiquitous distribution of microorganisms in human surroundings. A delicate but peaceful balance is ordinarily maintained between the host and his normal flora through the operation of a variety of natural antibacterial defenses. These serve to limit the flora to areas in which it may be tolerated safely, such as the surfaces of the upper respiratory tract, the skin, and the intestinal tract. However, there are two ways in which microorganisms may gain access to tissues not normally colonized: (1) The intrinsic pathogenicity of the organism may be such that it is capable of breaching the natural protective physical or biochemical barriers. *Streptococcus pyogenes* (group A streptococcus) is an example of a bacterial species with such potential. (2) Natural defenses may be sufficiently compromised (trauma, immunosuppression, phagocytic malfunction, etc.) to allow commensal organisms to enter tissues not normally infected and to produce disease. This situation has become increasingly familiar during the past several decades as advances in the treatment of a variety of diseases have been won at the price of decreasing the host's natural resistance to invasive infection by elements of his own flora. Such infections have been designated "opportunistic." In this setting, ordinarily bland organisms such as *Staphylococcus epidermidis, Serratia,* and *Acinetobacter* may produce life-threatening invasive infection.

Whatever the mechanism of microbial invasion, once invasion has taken place the clinical manifestations of the infection are the result of the interaction of several major factors: (1) the intrinsic virulence of the microorganisms, (2) the nature of the host response to infection, and (3) specific anatomic features at the site of infection. The role of these factors in the pathophysiology of the infectious process and thus in the development of characteristic signs and symptoms will be the theme of this and the succeeding chapters in this section. An attempt will be made not to be encyclopedic but rather to examine some of the impor-

tant examples of the aforementioned interactions. Since the presentation of most infections is that of involvement of a specific organ, and since this is necessarily the focus of the clinician's initial attention, considerable emphasis will be given to the particular pathophysiologic features of infection at specific sites, such as the heart, central nervous system, skeletal system, and so on.

BASIC MECHANISMS OF PATHOGENICITY

Bacteria produce disease by either (1) the elaboration of toxins or (2) the invasion of tissues. The pathogenicity of certain bacterial species appears to reside exclusively in their ability to elaborate a potent toxin (e.g., *Clostridium tetani,* the causative organism in tetanus), whereas that of other species appears to be due to bacterial multiplication and invasiveness alone (e.g., *Streptococcus pneumoniae*). However, the combination of invasive and toxigenic potential accounts for the pathogenicity of many other species (e.g., *Streptococcus pyogenes*).

TOXIN PRODUCTION

There are two major types of bacterial toxins: *exotoxins* and *endotoxins*. The former are produced within the interior of the cell and appear in filtrates of growing cultures and in infected tissues. Some exotoxins diffuse readily through the bacterial cell wall and appear in greatest concentration in culture filtrates toward the end of the logarithmic phase of growth (e.g., alpha toxin of *Clostridium perfringens*). Others, sometimes designated "protoplasmic toxins," do not diffuse through the cell wall as easily and do not appear in appreciable amounts in culture fluid until the cells have autolyzed (e.g., tetanus and botulinum toxins). Those toxins that have been purified thus far appear to be proteins. In contrast, endotoxins are lipopolysaccharides of the cell wall of many gram-negative bacteria and are released into culture media only on autolysis or disruption of the organisms. In the case of several of the potent bacterial exotoxins, rather specific mechanisms of action have been elucidated at both the gross physiologic and subcellular levels. Although endotoxins have been studied extensively and although a variety of consequences of their administration have been demonstrated, their exact role in human disease is less specific and remains unclear.

EXOTOXINS

The number of bacterial exotoxins that have been reasonably well characterized is now rather extensive. Most of these, but not all, are produced by gram-positive bacteria, and they are listed in Table 19–1. No attempt is made here to provide a complete catalogue. In several instances, a given organism produces a variety of toxic products, but only an illustrative example of clear clinical import is listed. Thus, *Clostridium perfringens* produces, in addition to the α toxin (lecithinase), κ toxin (collagenase) and λ toxin (protease), and so on. A variety of exotoxins similar to those produced by *C. perfringens* are produced by other clostridial species. More recent additions to the list of toxigenic bacteria include enterotoxigenic strains of *Escherichia coli* and certain enterotoxigenic strains of *Shigella*. In the case of certain exotoxins, the altered physiology they produce is now understandable at a subcellular or molecular level (diphtheria toxin, α toxin of *Clostridium perfringens*,

Vibrio cholerae enterotoxin); in other instances, the biochemical lesion is not as clearly understood, but the cellular localization of the toxin and the ensuing functional alterations have been reasonably well characterized (botulinum and tetanus toxins). On the basis of their mechanisms of action, certain of the exotoxins can be characterized as *general cytotoxins, neurotoxins,* or *enterotoxins.*

GENERAL CYTOTOXINS

Diphtheria Toxin. The variety of clinical manifestations that may develop in the course of diphtheria are directly due to the production of toxin at the site of the pharyngeal (or, rarely, cutaneous) infection. The hallmark of the disease, the gray faucial membrane, is due to the local effect of the potent necrotizing exotoxin and the inflammatory response of the body. This membrane may progress downward and involve the larynx and trachea, causing airway obstruction. Absorption of exotoxin into the general circulation may lead to abnormalities in many distant organ systems.

Cardiac involvement (in the second week or later) occurs in about two thirds of patients with diphtheria, as judged by electrocardiographic ob-

TABLE 19–1 SOME TOXIGENIC BACTERIA AND THEIR EXOTOXINS

Bacterial Species	Disease	Toxin	Mechanism of Action
Corynebacterium diphtheriae	Diphtheria	Diphtheria toxin	Neurotoxic; generally cytotoxic
Clostridium tetani	Tetanus	Tetanus toxin	Neurotoxic (spastic)
Clostridium botulinum	Botulism	Botulinum toxin (5 immunologic types)	Neurotoxic (paralytic)
Clostridium difficile	Pseudomembranous colitis ("antibiotic-associated" diarrhea)	*C. difficile* enterotoxin	Cytotoxic
Clostridium perfringens	Gas gangrene; bacteremia	Alpha toxin	Lecithinase (necrotizing, leukotoxic, hemolytic)
Streptococcus pyogenes (group A streptococcus)	Pyogenic infections; scarlet fever	Streptolysin O and DPNase	Leukotoxic (?)
		Erythrogenic toxin	Vascular dilatation and injury
Staphylococcus aureus	Pyogenic infections; food poisoning; "toxic shock syndrome"	Alpha toxin	Necrotizing
		Leukocidin	Leukotoxic (?)
		Enterotoxin	Enterotoxic (vomiting; diarrhea)
		"Exfoliatin"	Exfoliation
		Pyrogenic exotoxin type C	
Bacillus anthracis	Anthrax	Lethal toxin	Lethal; edema production
Pasteurella pestis	Plague	Plague toxin	Necrotizing (?); vascular injury causing shock
Vibrio cholerae	Cholera	Cholera enterotoxin	Intestinal loss of water and electrolytes
Escherichia coli (enterotoxigenic strains)	Gastroenteritis	*E. coli* enterotoxin	Intestinal loss of water and electrolytes
Shigella	Gastroenteritis	*Shigella* enterotoxin	Intestinal loss of water and electrolytes
Pseudomonas aeruginosa	Pyogenic infections	Exotoxin A	Lethal; necrotizing

servations. Frank myocarditis is seen in 10 to 25 per cent of patients. Conduction abnormalities are prominent features: bundle branch block (commonly), complete heart block, sinus tachycardia, atrial fibrillation, increased ventricular irritability or ventricular tachycardia, and fibrillation. Congestive heart failure and cardiogenic shock may occur owing to the toxic myocarditis and are ominous developments. Diffuse involvement of the myocardium with granular and hyalin myofiber degeneration, mononuclear cell infiltration, and scarring has been found on pathologic examination of the heart in fatal cases. These findings are consistent with the expected effects of a potent cytotoxin (see further on).

Nervous system complications occur in about 10 per cent of patients with diphtheria. Postdiphtheritic paralysis affects cranial and peripheral nerves. In severe cases, paralysis of the soft palate may appear early (first 1 to 2 weeks) and is probably due to the direct action of the toxin on the pharyngeal motor nerve endings. More commonly, neuritis involving cranial nerves III, VI, VII, IX, and XI or peripheral nerves occurs in the second to sixth week. Motor loss is the predominant feature. A late (2 to 3 months) form of peripheral neuritis, initially characterized by symmetrically distributed sensory loss and identical with the Guillain-Barré syndrome, also may occur. Very rarely, diphtheria is associated with encephalitis.

Hepatitis and nephritis are occasionally seen in diphtheria and are probably due to effects of the toxin. Necrosis, fatty infiltration, and cellular degeneration are demonstrable histologically in the liver, kidney, and adrenal glands.

Diphtheria toxin is highly toxic for many species (human, guinea pig, rabbit); but a few (rat, mouse) are notably resistant. As little as 50 to 100 nanograms per kg is lethal in a sensitive species. Diphtheria toxin is a single polypeptide chain of 62,000 daltons, which on cleavage of a single peptide bond and a disulfide linkage is split into two fragments. Fragment A (21,000 daltons) is the toxic moiety; fragment B (40,000 daltons) is nontoxic by itself but is required for recognition of specific surface receptors in susceptible cell membranes. The cell surface receptor responsible for internalization of the toxin (or its toxic moiety) appears to have the oligosaccharide-binding properties of a lectin. In the absence of the B portion of the molecule (or of fragment B), fragment A is not toxic because it cannot cross the plasma membrane and gain entry into the cell. A number of other toxins (cholera, *Escherichia coli* enterotoxin) consist, similarly, of an A and a B polypeptide chain where the latter interacts with membrane receptors and the former is the "toxic" fragment.

Clinical evidence suggests that a variety of types of body cells are injured by diphtheria toxin. The work of Pappenheimer and his colleagues on the molecular basis of the action of diphtheria

toxin is in keeping with these observations. The toxin interferes with mammalian cell protein synthesis, a process common to all cells of the body. Diphtheria toxin at a concentration of approximately 1 μg per ml completely suppresses protein synthesis when added to HeLa cells or to cell cultures derived from animal species that are sensitive in vivo to the toxin. In cell-free systems from mammalian sources, the toxin (or fragment A) promptly inhibits the incorporation of amino acids into protein in the presence of the cofactor nicotinamide adenine dinucleotide (NAD). Transfer of amino acids from aminoacyl-tRNA to the growing polypeptide chains on the polyribosomes is blocked. This inhibition of polypeptide chain elongation is the result of the specific inactivation of the eukaryotic translocating enzyme (elongation factor-2 [EF-2], also known as transferase II), a soluble protein required for the guanosine triphosphate (GTP)–dependent translocation of peptidyl transfer RNA from the aminoacyl ("A") site to the peptidyl ("P") site on the ribosome (Figs. 19–1 and 19–2). An inactive adenine diphosphate ribosyl (ADPR) derivative of EF-2 is formed in a reaction catalyzed by diphtheria toxin:

$$NAD^+ + EF\text{-}2 \underset{(active)}{\xrightarrow{\text{Diphtheria toxin}}} ADP\text{-ribosyl } EF\text{-}2 + (inactive)$$

$$nicotinamide + H^+$$

The effect of toxin can also be demonstrated in cell-free extracts prepared from a diphtheria toxin–susceptible species such as the guinea pig. Relatively small amounts of toxin (less than 25 M.L.D.) administered parenterally render inactive the "soluble enzyme fraction" (EF-2), prepared from heart and skeletal muscle, that is an essential component of the in-vitro protein synthesizing system. Polyribosomes prepared from intoxicated guinea pigs function normally in in-vitro protein synthesis, provided that the "soluble enzyme fraction" is obtained from animals that have not been treated with toxin.

The toxin is extremely potent. Only a few molecules located in the cell membrane of an HeLa cell in the presence of the internal NAD concentration are capable of converting the entire cell content of free EF-2 to its inactive ADP-ribosyl derivative. In vivo, certain tissues, such as the heart and skeletal muscle, are particularly sensitive to small amounts of toxin. The inhibition of protein synthesis in subcellular components is consistent with the clinical and pathologic findings. Since the turnover rate of protein in muscle is slow, the toxin may inhibit synthesis at a functionally critical site (the S-A node or conduction system) or of specific enzymes involved in maintaining normal cardiac function. In vitro, the direct addition of diphtheria toxin to brain and liver tissue extracts of the susceptible guinea pig

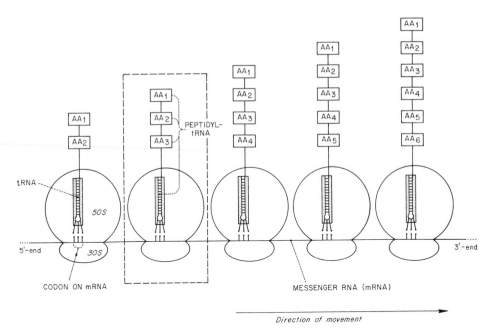

Direction of movement

Figure 19–1 Polypeptide synthesis on polyribosome. Schematic representation showing polypeptide chain elongation during movement of the ribosomes (made up of 30S and 50S subunits) along the messenger RNA (mRNA) molecule. Five ribosomes are shown bound to the mRNA. Initiation of protein synthesis begins at the 5′ end of the mRNA, and polypeptide chain elongation proceeds on each ribosome as it moves toward the 3′ end of the mRNA. The ribosomes shown on the right of the diagram (toward the 3′ end of the mRNA) bear the longer polypeptide chains. The tRNA molecule is shown in a specific site (darkened area) on each ribosome, positioned in relation to the codon on the mRNA by its complementary codon (anticodon). The tRNA serves as an "adapter" to which an amino acid is attached, so that the latter can be adapted to the triplet-based (nucleotide) genetic code. When an incoming amino acid is added to the initiating aminoacyl-tRNA, the latter is converted to a peptidyl-tRNA. The initial amino acid is designated as AA₁. Subsequent amino acids added to the nascent polypeptide chains are designated AA₂, AA₃, and so on. Because each of the five ribosomes above are traveling down the same mRNA molecule, the same five polypeptide chains will ultimately be made. The detailed steps involved in the addition of a single amino acid to form the peptidyl-tRNA shown in the boxed area in the figure are illustrated in Figure 19–2. The molecular site of action of diphtheria toxin is located there.

inhibits polypeptide synthesis. However, the protein-synthesizing ability of the in-vitro system prepared from brain tissues of intoxicated guinea pigs is not significantly impaired. This is in contrast to the aforementioned results with heart and skeletal muscle. The reason for this apparent difference is obscure. A possible explanation may lie in the number of surface receptors for the toxin on brain cells. It would be informative to study the protein-synthesizing system in peripheral nerves, since the major impact of diphtheria toxin is registered there rather than in the brain. Nonetheless, the available body of evidence is sufficient to suggest strongly that diphtheria toxin acts in the susceptible animal in a manner analogous to its action in cell cultures and in cell-free systems, namely, by inactivation of EF-2. The biochemical basis for the resistance to diphtheria toxin of certain species, such as the rat and mouse, is unclear. The defect does not appear to be due to an absence or deficiency of surface membrane receptors for the toxin. It is likely that the toxin insensitivity of these species stems from a deficiency in the transport process.

Clostridium Perfringens Toxins. *Clostridium perfringens* is an obligate anaerobe normally inhabiting the lower gastrointestinal tract of humans. Wound contamination with this organism is very common; however, significant infection is rare. Clostridial infections are not due to uniquely pathogenic strains but rather to local circumstances such as low oxidation-reduction potential, ischemia, and necrosis that are favorable for multiplication. The critical pathogenic step that transforms the relatively mild gas-forming infection (anaerobic cellulitis) into the devastating, rapidly advancing anaerobic myositis ("gas gangrene") capable of involving healthy muscle is as yet unknown. Several of the exotoxins produced by the organisms, such as κ toxin and λ toxin, may contribute to the rapid advance of the highly lethal infection through their collagenolytic and proteolytic activities respectively. However, it is important to recognize that the mere fact of production of these toxins is not sufficient evidence to establish their role in the pathogenesis of the infection. The alpha toxin, or lecithinase (phospholipase-C), of *C. perfringens* has been implicated

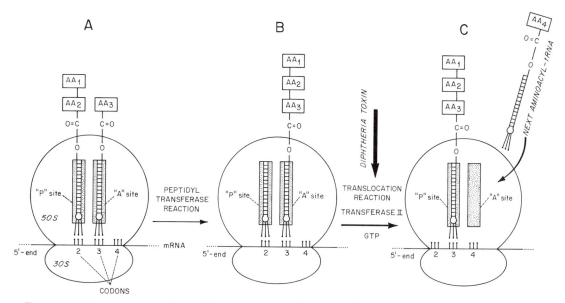

Figure 19–2 Schematic view of the individual steps involved in polypeptide chain elongation on an individual ribosome.

A, A ribosome (made up of its 50S and 30S subunits) is shown bound to a segment of mRNA. Two sites (aminoacyl, or "A"; peptidyl, or "P") are shown on the ribosome. The incoming aminoacyl-tRNA (bearing AA_3) is bound to the "A" site, positioned in accordance with the complementary nucleotide sequence it bears to the next codon (codon 3) of the mRNA. The "P" site is occupied by a peptidyl-tRNA (in this case bearing the two amino acids. AA_1 and AA_2).

B, The addition of AA_3 to the growing polypeptide chain involves peptide bond formation between the amino group of AA_3 and the esterified carboxyl group of AA_2 of the peptidyl-tRNA. This reaction is catalyzed by the enzyme peptidyl transferase, a part of the 50S subunit of the ribosome. As a result of this reaction, AA_1 and AA_2 are displaced from their tRNA in the "P" site to the tRNA in the "A" site, forming a new, elongated peptidyl-tRNA. The tRNA portion of the peptidyl-tRNA formerly in the "P" site (tRNA-AA_2-AA_1) remains (without its amino acid charge) bound to the "P" site.

C, The next step in polypeptide chain elongation is the translocation reaction, a complex step involving a specific protein (elongation factor-2 in mammalian cell systems, also designated "transferase II") and the ribonucleoside triphosphate GTP. This reaction involves the physical movement of peptidyl-tRNA (tRNA-AA_3-AA_2-AA_1) from the "A" site to the "P" site, with resulting displacement of the empty (uncharged) tRNA from the latter site. As a result of this movement, the "A" site is now open and available to receive a new incoming aminoacyl-tRNA coded for by codon 4. The cycle can then be repeated. Diphtheria toxin acts to inhibit the transferase II–requiring translocation reaction by causing the adenosine diphosphate ribosylation of the protein (see text).

in both the local tissue necrosis and toxemic features of gas gangrene. However, it should be noted that some strains of *C. perfringens* isolated from severe gas gangrene have been poor producers of alpha toxin. Furthermore, specific antitoxin to the lecithinase will not protect against the development of gas gangrene, not stop its spread, and not alleviate the toxemia and shock that are features of this disease. The interaction of alpha toxin or other extracellular enzymes with injured muscle is thought by some to be the source of the as yet unidentified toxic factor in gas gangrene. Although the direct role of alpha toxin has been somewhat de-emphasized in the foregoing discussion, it should be appreciated that it is nonetheless an extremely potent and lethal product. Intravenous administration in experimental animals produces fever, hypotension, intravascular hemolysis, jaundice, hemoglobinuria, renal shutdown, and death. The clinical counterpart with the identical constellation of findings develops in the course of high-grade *C. perfringens* bacteremia. This does not occur ordinarily in gas gangrene but is a fairly

common complication of clostridial infection of the uterus following a septic abortion. The lethal effects of the lecithinase are due to splitting of lecithin (Fig. 19–3), which is present in the membranes of a variety of cells in the body. These cells include erythrocytes, which are hemolyzed by this enzyme; leukocytes are probably similarly injured, accounting for the paucity of these cells in the exudate of gas gangrene. Various studies indicate that purified phospholipase-C does not have primary hemolytic activity; rather, it acts in concert with the theta toxin (an hemolysin) of *C. perfringens*. The initial action of the theta toxin on erythrocyte membranes exposes buried phospholipid groups to subsequent phospholipase-C action; the latter in turn renders the red blood cell more susceptible to hemolysis.

Pseudomonas Aeruginosa Exotoxin A. This protein exotoxin can be demonstrated in the blood of experimental animals moribund with systemic infection due to *P. aeruginosa*. Injection of purified toxin intraperitoneally in mice produces leukopenia, hepatic necrosis, renal tubular necrosis and

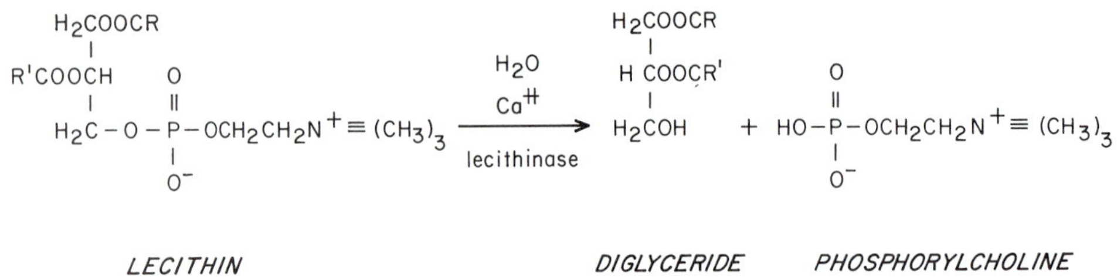

$$
\begin{array}{c}
\text{H}_2\text{COOCR} \\
| \\
\text{R'COOCH} \quad\quad \text{O} \\
| \quad\quad || \\
\text{H}_2\text{C}-\text{O}-\text{P}-\text{OCH}_2\text{CH}_2\text{N}^+\equiv(\text{CH}_3)_3 \\
| \\
\text{O}^-
\end{array}
\xrightarrow[\text{lecithinase}]{\substack{\text{H}_2\text{O} \\ \text{Ca}^{++}}}
\begin{array}{c}
\text{H}_2\text{COOCR} \\
| \\
\text{H COOCR'} \\
| \\
\text{H}_2\text{COH}
\end{array}
+
\begin{array}{c}
\text{O} \\
|| \\
\text{HO}-\text{P}-\text{OCH}_2\text{CH}_2\text{N}^+\equiv(\text{CH}_3)_3 \\
| \\
\text{O}^-
\end{array}
$$

LECITHIN   *DIGLYCERIDE   PHOSPHORYLCHOLINE*

Figure 19–3 Action of *Clostridium perfringens* lecithinase (α toxin) on lecithin. Cleavage of the bond between the phosphoric acid and glycerol moieties yields a diglyceride and phosphorylcholine. R and R' represent fatty acids esterified with glycerol.

death. This toxin is more than 20,000 times as toxic (on a weight basis) as *Pseudomonas* endotoxin. Although a role of the toxin in the clinical manifestations of localized (pneumonia, pyelonephritis, etc.) and systemic (bacteremia) *Pseudomonas* infection in humans is as yet unclear, a potential involvement is suggested by (1) the lethality of exotoxin A for multiple species of animals, (2) the protection of animals against subsequent challenge with toxigenic strains of *Pseudomonas,* and (3) the decreased virulence of *P. aeruginosa* infections due to mutants lacking toxin A. This toxin appears to act at a molecular level like diphtheria toxin: It interferes with protein synthesis by effecting ADP-ribosylation of eukaryotic elongation factor-2 (EF-2). However, clinically these two toxins appear to have different cellular specificities. Whether these variations stem from differences in cell membrane receptors remains to be elucidated.

Tetanus Toxin. Tetanus is an intoxication with the exotoxin of *Clostridium tetani* and is characterized by intense, severe muscle spasms. The toxin, known as *tetanospasmin,* is one of the most potent bacterial toxins known. Spores of the etiologic agent, *C. tetani,* are introduced by contamination of a wound. The wound may be an extensive laceration, gun shot or puncture wound, or a very trivial lesion into which spores of the organism have been introduced. The mere presence of *C. tetani* in a wound does not mean that tetanus will develop. Transformation of the spores into toxin-producing vegetative forms requires a lower oxidation-reduction potential than is present in normal tissues. Necrotic tissue produced by the trauma or by invasion by pyogenic bacteria simultaneously present and the introduction of foreign material can lower the oxidation-reduction potential sufficiently to allow this to occur. There is little or no capacity of the organism to invade tissues, and often the wound hardly appears to be infected. All the clinical manifestations of the disease are due to the physiologic changes produced by the toxin in the nervous system—spinal cord, brain stem, and sympathetic nervous system. Toxin introduced into muscle spreads centrally along motor nerves and up the spinal cord. Toxin may also be spread via the bloodstream, and this route may be the more important one in generalized tetanus. Despite the violent and widely distributed symptoms of the disease, no lesions are detectable in the nervous system (or other tissues), even with the electron microscope.

The major clinical manifestation of tetanus is muscular rigidity. This may be mild in "local tetanus," in which rigidity affects only one limb or one group of muscles (the site of injury) and usually occurs in patients with a limited degree of immunity. More often, the initiating injury is followed within a matter of days by local muscular spasm about the wound and then trismus. Stiffness of the facial muscles may produce a bizarre sneering expression *(risus sardonicus).* Stiffness of the back, neck, and abdomen may become marked enough to produce pain as a prominent symptom. Dysphagia and hydrophobia are due to spasm of the pharyngeal and glottal muscles. With the progression of generalized tetanus, opisthotonos and violent spasmodic contractions of the neck, trunk, and limb muscles occur. Despite the severity of such manifestations, the sensorium is still clear. Sudden stimuli (noise, bright light, an injection) may precipitate a generalized tonic convulsion, with accompanying spasm of the larynx and respiratory muscles, resulting in respiratory arrest. Thus, afferent stimuli appear to produce an exaggerated effect. This suggests that the toxin produces its characteristic effects by disturbing the normal regulation of the reflex arc. Reciprocal innervation is abolished, and, as a result, both the stimulated muscle groups and the opposing groups contract simultaneously. This produces the characteristic muscular spasm. The particular features of this spasm are determined in each area by the relative bulk (strength) of the opposing muscle groups. Thus, since the masseters are stronger than the opposing mylohyoid and digastricus muscles, trismus results. The masseters generally show greater sensitivity to tetanus toxin than the muscles of the extremities. It has been suggested that this is because the masseters are normally maintained in a state of partial contraction when an individual is awake. In the lower extremities, the strength of the extensor groups exceeds that of the flexors, and the predominant posture in tetanus is that of extension at the hips and knees.

The neurophysiology of the action of tetanus toxin now seems reasonably clear, particularly as a result of the studies of Sir John Eccles. The main impact of the toxin is on the spinal cord. Grossly, the effects of the toxin are very similar to those of strychnine. The toxin does not act on reflex arcs that include only sensory and motor neurons (two-neuron or monosynaptic reflexes). It profoundly affects the more complex reflexes (polysynaptic reflexes that involve interneurons), blocking the normal postsynaptic inhibition of spinal motorneurons that results from afferent impulses. This action of the toxin in selectively blocking inhibitory synapses in the central nervous system results in multiplication of excitatory impulses that run in unchecked fashion and are not coordinated by inhibitory mechanisms. This produces the muscular spasms (tetanic seizures) characteristic of tetanus.

In the normal resting state, muscle tone is maintained by the constant mild tension of opposing muscle groups. Thus, motion at the elbow is controlled by two sets of muscles—the extensor (triceps) and the flexor (biceps). When the biceps contracts slightly, the triceps is stretched, activating stretch-sensitive receptors. These, in turn, send afferent impulses to the spinal cord, where they stimulate the motor neurons and cause contraction of the triceps opposing the stretch. The stretch reflex thus plays an important role in maintaining postural tone. However, for proper functioning of the elbow joint, for example, it is essential that the biceps not be opposed too vigorously by the triceps. Otherwise, the forearm would be locked into spasm by the action of the opposing muscles, and voluntary movement would be impossible. Therefore, the afferent impulse that causes the activation of the biceps must facilitate relaxation of the triceps. This inhibition is effected in the spinal cord by branching of the axon carrying the afferent impulse. One branch excites the biceps and the other excites the internuncial neuron ("inhibitory cell") to release an inhibitory transmitter (Fig. 19–4). This inhibitory transmitter in turn acts on the anterior horn cells innervating the triceps, thus opposing the action of the excitatory transmitter released there from the stretch-sensitive afferent nerve. The net result is that triceps motor neurons are not excited and the triceps does not contract; the biceps is then able to flex the forearm unhindered. Tetanus toxin acts in the spinal cord to disrupt this balanced reciprocity by suppressing the normal inhibition through the internuncial connections. The toxin appears either to reduce the amount of inhibitory transmitter (glycine) available for release or to block its release. As a result, in the absence of inhibition the normal stretch reflex of the triceps is unopposed, and when the biceps contracts, the antagonist muscle, the triceps, does likewise, locking the forearm in spasm.

An unusual form of tetanus results from ac-

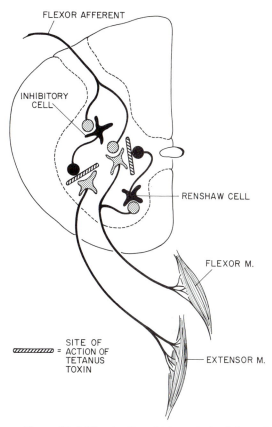

Figure 19–4 Site of action of tetanus toxin. Schematically shown are neural connections involved in controlling the action of opposing flexor and extensor muscle groups such as the biceps and triceps. Contraction of the biceps normally stretches the triceps, activating receptors that pass to the spinal cord (this afferent is not shown on the illustration) and stimulating the motor innervation of the triceps. Another afferent to the biceps is shown that synapses with an inhibitory cell ("interneuron"). The latter releases an inhibitory transmitter, preventing the stretch-induced excitation of the triceps. Also shown is a second inhibitory pathway, involving an axon collateral from the flexor motor neuron extending to a Renshaw cell. This cell, in turn, synapses with the flexor motor neuron, producing postsynaptic inhibition, controlling the stimulation of flexor contraction. Tetanus toxin appears to act by blocking both the above inhibitory pathways in the spinal cord.

tion of the toxin primarily on the motor innervation (in the brain stem) of the facial, glossal, pharyngeal, jaw, and ocular muscles. Whether the toxin reaches these areas by the neural or hematogenous route is not clear. This form of tetanus is known as "cephalic tetanus." It occurs when the spores of C. tetani are introduced into wounds involving the eye, during tonsilloadenoidectomy, during the course of chronic otitis media, or following trauma to the head or neck. In this form of tetanus, the affected muscles appear to be paralyzed, especially those involving facial and ocular movements. The apparent facial palsy in reality is a pseudoparalysis. Hypertonia involves all the muscles supplied by the facial motor neurons, and voluntary movements are prevented. Although "cephalic tetanus" may be the only clinical presentation, it is important to emphasize the fact that generalized disease may develop subsequently.

Overactivity of the sympathetic nervous system has been observed in patients with severe tetanus, suggesting that tetanus toxin may also directly affect this portion of the nervous system. Among the manifestations that may develop, in any combination, are labile hypertension, tachycardia, peripheral vasoconstriction, irregularities of cardiac rhythm, profuse sweating, increased respiratory rate, increase in the urinary excretion of catecholamines, and, in some instances, during the late stage of the disease, hypotension. These manifestations do not appear to be related to hypoxia secondary to involvement of the innervation of the muscles of respiration or to pulmonary infection. Such evidences of sympathetic overactivity are not generally observed in other paralyzed patients treated in identical fashions to support respiration and maintain adequate oxygenation.

"Localized tetanus" is an unusual clinical form of tetanus in which intermittent twitching and spasm of muscles occur in a circumscribed area of the body, with or without a known wound or injury in that area. Stiffness of the muscles in the involved area, usually a limb, may be the initial symptom. The manifestations may persist over several weeks or months restricted to the initial area of involvement, or the process may progress to generalized tetanus within a few days. Although it was originally believed that this form of tetanus was due to the local action of the toxin on muscle near the site of injury, it is now thought that the manifestations of this form of tetanus are also due to suppression of spinal inhibitory mechanisms. Toxin reaching the spinal cord either by passage along regional nerves or by hematogenous spread (as seems more likely) produces an increased central excitatory state. This, however, is so slight in localized tetanus as to be inapparent if it were not for the increased afferent inflow from the periphery provided by the local skin and muscular lesion at the site of trauma.

The pathophysiology of the action of tetanus toxin at the molecular level is unknown. However, Van Heyningen has demonstrated that the site of toxin binding in nervous tissue is the synaptic membrane of the nerve endings. The chemical substance binding the toxin is a ganglioside, a compound containing fatty acid, sphingosine, sialic acid, and several sugars. The role of toxin binding in clinical tetanus is not clear; there is no detectable change in the ganglioside molecule where the toxin is bound. Binding may not be an essential feature of the action of toxin but may simply be a means of channeling this toxin to the central nervous system. Like diphtheria toxin, tetanus

toxin can be dissociated by proteolytic cleavage and thiol-reducing agents into two polypeptide chains (α and β). The ganglioside-binding site of the intact toxin molecule resides in its β chain. A 50,000 dalton fragment of proteolytic cleavage of the β chain of tetanus toxin forms pores in phospholipid vesicle membranes in vitro. A similar action has been ascribed to a similar fragment of diphtheria toxin. The formation of these pores may be integral to the transport of such toxin fragments across lipid membranes into the cytosol.

Botulinum Toxin. Botulism is an intoxication with the exotoxin of *Clostridium botulinum* and is characterized by profound weakness of both skeletal and smooth muscle. The disease results from the ingestion of food (canned meats and vegetables, packaged fish, sausages) in which the organism has grown under anaerobic conditions and elaborated its potent exotoxin. There is absolutely no invasive potential to the organism itself, and all the clinical manifestations are due solely to the toxin. The toxin is heat labile; cooking at boiling temperature for a few minutes destroys it. Clinical symptoms usually develop 18 to 36 hours after ingestion of contaminated food. The cranial nerves are involved earliest, resulting in paresis of accommodation, diplopia due to weakness of the external ocular muscles, dysphagia, difficulty in talking, and weakness of the jaw muscles. Subsequently, the muscles of the trunk and limbs become weak. The deep tendon reflexes remain normal; sensory abnormalities are absent. A curious neurophysiologic response, a facilitated muscle-action potential after repetitive nerve stimulation, is typical of botulism.

Like tetanus toxin, botulinum toxin is extremely potent yet produces no apparent structural damage. There is no evidence of involvement of the central nervous system. In contrast to the diffuse muscular overactivity of tetanus, the characteristic feature of botulism is a flaccid weakness; this is not due to any loss of contractile power of the muscles themselves, since they respond normally to direct electrical stimulation.

After absorption from the gastrointestinal tract, toxin reaches susceptible neurons via the circulation and there becomes bound to presynaptic terminals. The molecular nature of the toxin receptor in the presynaptic membrane is not certain but is suggested by the finding that certain gangliosides bind botulinum toxin. Burgen, Dickens, and Zatman have reported that the toxin acts at the neuromuscular junctions, preventing release of acetylcholine, the excitatory transmitter. They noted that the quantity of acetylcholine liberated by stimulation of phrenic nerve-diaphragm preparations of rats was very much smaller in the presence of botulinum toxin than in control preparations. Thus, excitatory impulses are blocked between the efferent nerve endings and the muscle; this leads to flaccid weakness. Electron microscopic studies indicate that the toxin blocks exocytosis of acetylcholine-containing vesicles at presynaptic release sites.

ENTEROTOXINS

Cholera Enterotoxin. Cholera, an infection due to *Vibrio cholerae,* is characterized by dramatic and devastating diarrhea, resulting in enormous fluid and electrolyte losses. It occurs endemically and epidemically in Asia but recently has spread to Africa and southern Europe. The disease is usually transmitted by contaminated water but occasionally by fruits or vegetables contaminated with human feces. Its onset is sudden, and the course is, as a rule, fulminant. Chills and fever are not prominent features; the body temperature may, in fact, be depressed. Abdominal pain and vomiting may accompany the initial diarrhea. Later, however, the striking feature of the disease is the prodigious fluid loss from the intestine. This may exceed one liter of fluid per hour. The "rice water" stool is watery, odorless, and mucoid. The various clinical manifestations that develop later are secondary to the severe degree of dehydration and the loss of electrolytes. These manifestations include hypotension and shock, metabolic acidosis, muscle cramps, stupor and coma, hypokalemic flaccid paralysis, acute tubular necrosis, and, occasionally, myocardial infarction.

The primary pathophysiologic disturbance in cholera is severe loss of fluid and electrolytes from the small intestine. These changes occur in the absence of any invasion of the intestinal mucosa by the organisms or a significant inflammatory response. The initial outpouring of large volumes of fluid into the lumen of the intestine occurs at a time when there is no disruption of the intestinal mucosa. Denudation of the mucosa is a late phenomenon and is secondary to severe hypovolemia in the end stages of cholera. The only histologic changes noted consistently in early human cases and in the experimental animal (rabbit) are mild hyperemia of the mucosal capillaries and edema of the tunica propria of the small intestine.

The fluid lost from the intestine is isotonic and has a low protein content similar to that found in the intestinal fluid of normal persons. The bicarbonate concentration of this fluid is about twice and the potassium concentration about four times that of normal plasma. All the clinical manifestations of the disease can be corrected by prompt intravenous administration of appropriate fluid and electrolytes.

Several studies of the effects of cholera enterotoxin indicate that it produces increased fluid and electrolyte movement across the small intestine from plasma to the gut lumen. This could be due either to increased filtration of electrolytes from intestinal capillaries across the mucosal cells or to active secretion of one or more electrolytes by the epithelial lining cells. Present evidence suggests that the former is not the case. For example, decreasing the mesenteric blood flow in the dog by as much as 70 per cent does not reduce the rate of fluid production by intestinal loops treated with cholera enterotoxin. Even more telling evidence against the filtration hypothesis is provided by the examination of the intestinal clearance of mannitol and sodium in patients with acute cholera. Gordon has demonstrated that the clearance of intravenously administered ^{14}C mannitol is only 25 per cent of the clearance of sodium, indicating less resistance to the flow of sodium than of mannitol.

Considerable insight into electrolyte movement across the normal and cholera enterotoxin–treated intestine has been provided by study of the isolated rabbit ileal mucosa. Normally, the net secretory flux of HCO_3^- balances the net absorptive flux of Cl^-. There is also a net absorptive flux of Na^+, and this can be increased by the addition of glucose to the solution on the luminal side of the isolated ileum. (This experimental observation has a very important therapeutic implication. Indeed, orally administered glucose-containing solutions can reduce considerably the electrolyte loss of patients with the disease.) The addition of cholera enterotoxin to the mucosal side of such an in-vitro preparation produces distinct changes after a latent period of about an hour. These consist of (1) complete disappearance of the net absorptive flux of Na^+, and (2) reversal of the direction of chloride transport, the net absorptive flux being replaced by a net secretory flux. The HCO_3^- net secretory flux remains unchanged. *Thus, the effect of enterotoxin on solute transport consists of stimulation of chloride secretion and inhibition of sodium absorption.* The toxin-induced secretion of anion would then cause isosmotic accumulation of water. Fluid pouring into the intestine in the cholera patient or in the rabbit ileal loop is indeed isotonic. Large losses of HCO_3^- occur when the reabsorptive capacity of the colon for diarrheal fluid is exceeded. The same mechanism may be responsible for substantial losses of potassium.

Cyclic AMP (3',5'-AMP), when applied to the isolated rabbit ileal mucosa preparation, produces changes in ion flux similar to those produced by cholera enterotoxin. This suggests that the cholera enterotoxin-induced fluid and electrolyte loss may be mediated by cyclic 3',5'-AMP. There is a large body of evidence in support of this concept: (1) Adenylate cyclase, the enzyme involved in the synthesis of 3',5'-AMP from ATP, is demonstrable in the mucosa at all levels of the small intestine but is present in highest concentration in the duodenum. Outpouring of fluid and solute in response to cholera enterotoxin occurs at all levels of the small bowel; the highest rate of secretion is in the duodenum. (2) Theophylline, an inhibitor of the phosphodiesterase that normally breaks down 3',5'-AMP to 5'-AMP, produces effects similar to those of cholera enterotoxin: Infusion of theophylline into the superior mesenteric artery of dogs produces fluid and solute secretion into the small intestine comparable to that produced by cholera enterotoxin, and theophylline produces alterations of ion flux similar to those produced by cholera enterotoxin on the isolated rabbit ileal mucosa. (3) Cholera enterotoxin increases the adenylate cyclase activity of membranes prepared from rabbit small intestine. (4) 3',5'-AMP levels in intestinal mucosa are increased several-fold after preincubation with the toxin either in vitro (membrane preparations) or in vivo (intact mucosal cell in the experimental animal).

The detailed molecular events in the action of cholera toxin are currently in the process of being defined in many laboratories. Cholera toxin, molecular weight 84,000, consists of two subunits (or protomers): A and B. The entire toxin molecule is necessary for intoxication of intact cells through activation of adenylate cyclase. The first step in the activation process appears to be the binding of the B protomer of the toxin to cell surface receptors containing the monosialoganglioside G_{M1}. The A protomer then appears to penetrate the cell membrane at least as far as the inner surface, where it activates the adenylate cyclase. The lag between exposure of intact cells to toxin and the first rise in adenylate cyclase activity probably represents the time needed for the A protomer to cross the membrane and reach its site of action. In disrupted cell preparations the initial B protomer binding step is unnecessary, and the A protomer alone can activate adenylate cyclase. Cholera toxin and its A protomer catalyze the hydrolysis of nicotinamide adenine dinucleotide (NAD) to ADP-ribose and nicotinamide. It can also catalyze the ADP-ribosylation of the amino acid L-arginine. It has, therefore, been proposed that activation of adenylate cyclase by cholera toxin involves ADP-ribosylation of an arginine or similar amino acid residue in some acceptor protein (even adenylate cyclase itself). This would be analogous to the mechanism of action of diphtheria toxin (or its active fragment A) that catalyzes the ADP-ribosylation of a protein, elongation factor-2.

Several other acute infectious diarrheal diseases of humans may be produced by a mechanism identical with that operative in cholera. These are disorders in which bacterial invasion of the bowel wall does not take place but in which exotoxins may have a major pathogenic role. These include the gastroenteritides due to enterotoxin-producing strains of *Escherichia coli, Shigella,* and *Clostridium perfringens*. Extracellular products of these organisms have been shown experimentally to stimulate small intestinal fluid secretion. *E. coli* enterotoxin has been shown to cause diarrhea by increasing adenylate cyclase levels in intestinal mucosa. A peptide released from enterotoxic *E. coli* appears very similar to the A protomer of cholera toxin and, like the latter, is able to activate adenylate cyclase in vitro.

ENDOTOXINS

Bacterial endotoxins are integral parts of the bacterial cell wall and are released only upon disruption of the bacterial cell. Endotoxins differ in a variety of ways from bacterial exotoxins: (1) Endotoxins are particulate macromolecules. Although originally isolated as phospholipid-polysaccharide-protein complexes, their biological activity resides in an extractable lipopolysaccharide fraction. Their toxicity appears to reside predominantly in the phospholipid component; the major antigenic determinants are in the polysaccharide fraction. However, bacterial exotoxins are proteins, usually of relatively small size (M.W. 50,000 to 100,000, occasionally as large as 1,000,000). (2) True endotoxins are found predominantly, if not exclusively, in gram-negative bacteria. In contrast, exotoxins are produced by many types of bacteria, most frequently by gram-positive bacilli. (3) Endotoxins are less potent by at least several orders of magnitude than most exotoxins. (4) Endotoxins from a variety of bacterial species elicit the same responses after parenteral administration, even though the intrinsic pathogenicity of the organism from which they were derived shows considerable differences. (5) Endotoxins are relatively heat-stable, unlike bacterial protein exotoxins (with the exception of the enterotoxin of *Staphylococcus aureus*). (6) Bacterial endotoxins are much more varied in their activity and less specific in their cytotoxic actions. Thus, no effects of endotoxin can compare with the exquisite selective neurotropism of the toxins of C. *tetani* and C. *botulinum*.

Endotoxins have been identified in *E. coli, Salmonella, Shigella, Vibrio cholerae, Brucella, Neisseria gonorrhoeae,* N. *meningitidis,* and other gram-negative organisms. When injected intravenously in experimental animals, they produce a variety of biologic effects. These include fever, diarrhea, hypotension, shock, transient leukopenia followed by leukocytosis, hyperglycemia, abortion, capillary hemorrhages, diffuse intravascular coagulation, altered resistance to bacterial infections, and the Shwartzman phenomenon. Despite this large number of physiologic derangements produced by endotoxins, their role in the clinical features of illnesses due to gram-negative bacteria remains speculative. Tolerance, or refractoriness to the pyrogenic and other biologic effects of endotoxin, develops on repeated injection. The state appears to be independent of the development of demonstrable circulating antibody, since it subsides after 1 to 2 weeks following a course of repeated injections, whereas active immunity persists much longer. Tolerance results from an increased clearance of injected endotoxin by cells of the reticuloendothelial system (RES); it can be prevented by prior injection of particulate material (Thorotrast, India ink) that is readily taken up by the RES, resulting in "blockade" of its ability to clear subsequently injected endotoxin. It has been suggested that circulating endotoxin plays an important role in sustained gram-negative infection and that the development of tolerance is an important aspect of recovery from the illness. Tolerance to endotoxin is not a feature of human infections produced by gram-negative bacteria (brucellosis, typhoid, tularemia). There is, in fact, an enhanced reactivity to its effects. Indeed, in experimental typhoid fever an enhanced pyrogenic response to injected endotoxin can be elicited from late in the incubation period through the early phase of convalescence. As the convalescent phase progresses, tolerance to the pyrogenic effects of endotoxin develops. Tolerance to endotoxin, induced in humans by daily injections, disappears during the active stage of typhoid fever and reappears when chemotherapy has produced a favorable response.

Biologic Effects

1. *Fever* is produced by the intravenous injection of endotoxin in most laboratory animals and humans. The febrile response occurs in humans after a lag period that may be as long as 90 minutes. Clearer understanding of the febrile response to endotoxin has come from the animal studies of Atkins and Wood. Immediately following the injection of endotoxin, blood was found to contain a weak pyrogen that had all the properties of the originally injected material. This then disappeared from the blood, which became non-pyrogenic; 90 to 120 minutes after the endotoxin injection a second pyrogen appeared in the circulation. The properties of this substance differed in many ways from those of endotoxin and appeared to be identical with those of endogenous (leukocytic) pyrogen (EP, or IL-1) (see Chapter 20). The marked neutropenia produced by the injection of endotoxin has been presumed to be evidence of direct damage to leukocytes by this macromolecule. Release of EP is the most likely cause of the later fever. The non-identity of EP and endotoxin has been demonstrated in several ways. Endogenous pyrogen is active in animals previously rendered tolerant to the pyrogenic effects of bacterial endotoxin. Unlike endotoxin, endogenous pyrogen produces a single febrile peak after a very brief lag period when injected into animals.

2. *Granulocytopenia* appears promptly after intravenous injection of endotoxin, persists for 3 to 6 hours, and is followed by a marked leukocytosis. The short period of granulocytopenia is associated with impairment of leukocytic migration into areas of active inflammation. Granulocytopenia develops as neutrophils shift from the circulating pool to the marginal one, as a result of increased adherence of leukocytes to the vascular endothelium, particularly in the lung.

3. *Hypotension and shock* are produced in animals by the injection of large doses of endotoxin. Species difference among animals with regard to the pattern of vascular response to this substance has been a source of confusion in attempts to understand the pathophysiology of endotoxic shock and to relate the circulatory changes in bacteremia due to gram-negative organisms in humans to "endotoxic shock." For example, in the dog the early systemic hypotension that develops after injection of endotoxin stems from a decreased cardiac output. This follows a marked decrease in venous return that is due primarily to pooling in the portal system secondary to constriction of hepatic veins produced by release of histamine. Recovery from the initial hypotension occurs within a few minutes. A second fall in blood pressure occurs in 1 to 2 hours; this is more gradual, and spontaneous recovery is not usual. There is gradual slowing of blood flow in the microcirculation and vasospasm of arterioles and venules. Decreased perfusion of many organs ensues, with the greatest effects occurring in the renal and splanchnic circulation. Catecholamines are released and produce an increase in total peripheral arterial resistance. When endotoxic shock has gone on for several hours in the dog, the process becomes irreversible. This stage is featured by arteriolar and capillary dilatation, venular contraction, stasis, and morphologic evidences of damage to capillaries and veins (hemorrhage and edema, especially of the intestine). In contrast to the response to endotoxin in the dog, the circulatory changes in humans are less clear and well-defined. The cause of the circulatory changes occurring in patients with sepsis due to gram-negative bacteria is uncertain. Many of the features may be attributed to the bacteremia itself or to endotoxemia alone.

4. *Coagulation* may be profoundly altered following injection of endotoxin into experimental animals. The changes in hemostasis are biphasic. After a lag period, there is a hypercoagulable state (associated with an increased amount of circulatory fibrinogen), followed in a matter of hours by a prolonged hypocoagulable period. The latter is characterized by depletion of plasma fibrinogen, thrombocytopenia, and other changes associated with intravascular clotting. In-vitro studies of human and animal plasma suggest that endotoxin initiates intravascular clotting by activating Factor XII (Hageman factor), which appears to be capable of activating plasma prekallikrein to the active protease kallikrein. This in turn releases bradykinin (an extremely powerful vasodepressor) from its inactive plasma precursor kininogen. Bradykinin, with its ability to increase vascular permeability and its vasodepressor effects, may be responsible for many of the circulatory effects of septic shock. Thus, it is likely that the same site of endotoxin action (activation of Factor XII) may initiate both the coagulation and hemodynamic

alterations associated in some instances with shock.

5. The *Shwartzman phenomenon* is a peculiar toxic reaction observed in rabbits following two injections of endotoxin. Two types of this phenomenon have been described. The *local Shwartzman reaction* consists of gross hemorrhage and necrosis in the skin. It occurs after an initial *cutaneous* injection of endotoxin (or endotoxin-containing bacteria), which is then followed in some hours by an *intravenous* injection of endotoxin. The initial ("preparatory") and second ("eliciting") injections may utilize endotoxin from different bacterial species. Non-bacterial materials such as washed antigen-antibody precipitates may be employed for the "eliciting" reaction. Polymorphonuclear leukocyte "cuffing" develops about the small veins at the skin site following the "preparatory" injection. Peripheral vasoconstriction, particularly at the prepared skin site, is produced by the intravenous injection. Leukocyte-platelet thrombi develop and occlude capillaries and small veins, resulting in necrosis of vessel walls and secondary hemorrhage.

The *generalized Shwartzman reaction* develops when both the "preparatory" and the "eliciting" injections of endotoxin are given intravenously approximately 24 hours apart. The typical histologic lesion that develops is characterized by deposition of fibrinoid material within capillaries. This occurs most dramatically in the kidney and produces bilateral renal cortical necrosis. The histologic findings appear to be the result of disseminated intravascular coagulation. Polymorphonuclear leukocytes are essential to the development of the Shwartzman phenomenon; the prior induction of leukopenia will prevent both the localized and generalized forms of the reaction.

The striking incidence of purpuric skin lesions in meningococcemia, in comparison with the incidence in bacteremias due to gram-negative bacilli, appears to be related to the properties of meningococcal endotoxin (lipopolysaccharide). Whereas the lipopolysaccharides (LPS) from the meningococcus and from enteric gram-negative bacilli (*Escherichia coli, Salmonella typhimurium*) are of comparable potency for the general Shwartzman reaction and for mouse lethality, the meningococcal LPS is five to ten times more potent in inducing the localized (dermal) Shwartzman reaction. Histologic examination of purpuric skin lesions of patients with acute meningococcemia reveal large numbers of meningococci in endothelial cells and neutrophils, endothelial necrosis, and thromboses. Immunoglobulins and complement are present in the vascular walls, suggesting possible immunologic factors in the genesis of the skin lesions. Although it is tempting to ascribe the characteristic hemorrhagic necrotic skin lesions of meningococcemia to the Shwartzman reaction, convincing proof that this reaction occurs during disease in humans is still lacking.

INVASION OF TISSUES

Local Effects

Most infectious agents produce demonstrable damage to host cells in the area immediately surrounding their site of invasion. In many instances, this is due primarily to multiplication of the infecting agent (usually bacteria or fungi) or to its growth (parasites). Among the invasive bacteria, *Streptococcus pneumoniae* (pneumococcus) is an example of an agent whose pathogenicity appears to be solely related to its capacity to multiply rapidly and successfully in the susceptible host. No toxins capable of producing local or distant effects have been demonstrated in infections produced by this organism. The essential ingredient in its pathogenicity is the antiphagocytic activity of its capsular polysaccharide. Thus, smooth encapsulated strains are capable of resisting surface phagocytosis, the first line of host defense, prior to the appearance of specific antibody. Pneumococci invading the lung are thus capable of extensive multiplication and of eliciting marked edema and an acute inflammatory response in the alveoli. The extensive lobar involvement that occurs is responsible for the characteristic dyspnea and tachypnea due to both arterial oxygen undersaturation (secondary to continued perfusion of the poorly ventilated area of lung) and splinting of the chest (secondary to spread of the bacterial inflammation to the pleural surface with its attendant pain). Rarely, the unrestrained growth of pneumococci may be so extensive that frank tissue destruction and abscess formation occur. This is almost invariably due, when present, to type 3 pneumococci, strains that, because they produce unusually abundant capsular material, are almost totally insulated from surface phagocytosis.

Localized pyogenic foci (abscesses) due to a large variety of bacteria may develop almost anywhere in the body and increase in size sufficiently to produce obstructive or pressure phenomena. However, when they occur in the central nervous system their effects may be most dramatic because of their anatomic location and the lack of elasticity of the surrounding structures. Thus, an abscess in the cerebrum or cerebellum can produce marked neurologic deficit by two mechanisms: (1) neuronal destruction by the invading microorganisms, and (2) swelling of surrounding brain tissue due to edema and the inflammatory response. The abscess may be satisfactorily walled off by a thick capsule, and there may be little or no fever or other manifestations of infection. The clinical picture may then mimic that of an enlarging cerebral mass lesion such as a brain tumor. Manifestations of increased intracranial pressure such as headache, papilledema, and sixth and third cranial nerve palsies may dominate the clinical picture. If untreated, the lesion may go on to cause herniation of the temporal lobe and midbrain compression, or it may rupture into the ventricular system and cause fulminating meningitis. A temporal lobe lesion that may present in a similar way may occasionally be seen in viral infection of the central nervous system, especially encephalitis due to *Herpes hominis*.

The dramatic mass effects of infection are particularly prominent in certain parasitic infestations. Heavy loads of adult *Ascaris* may produce abdominal pain and even intestinal obstruction. Migration of these worms into the biliary tree may produce obstruction and ascending cholangitis. Cysticercosis represents the invasion of various tissues by the larval form of the pork tapeworm, *Cysticercus cellulosae*. The brain is most commonly involved. The parasitic cyst surrounded by a thick capsule can mimic a neoplasm and cause seizures, personality changes, long tract signs, or increased intracranial pressure. The larvae of *Toxocara canis* may migrate in humans to a variety of organs such as liver, lung, and eye. In the ocular form, a space-occupying granulomatous mass resembling a retinoblastoma may develop and distort the retina.

Effects of Widespread Dissemination of Infection

Bacteremia may result when initial host defenses are insufficient to contain the invading microorganism locally. Thus, *Staphylococcus aureus* bacteremia following an initial skin or other focus of infection may produce abscess formation in distant organs such as kidney, bone, and brain. The symptoms and signs of the infection that develops in this situation are related to dysfunction of the particular organ involved. A transient bacteremia may become high grade and continuous when staphylococcal infection is superimposed on a previously damaged (or entirely normal) heart valve to produce acute bacterial endocarditis (see Chapter 21). Rarely, the density of staphylococci in the blood may be sufficiently high as to be visible in Gram-stained smears of a "buffy-coat" preparation of venous blood. The nature of the factors that contribute to staphylococcal pathogenicity is unclear. Clinical isolates do not appear to contain an antiphagocytic capsule component.

Another organism that, in the setting of nosocomial infection, is notoriously capable of producing abscesses in multiple organs following bacteremia is *Pseudomonas aeruginosa*. It is an aggressive secondary invader in open wounds, in decubiti, at the sites of foreign bodies (e.g., indwelling venous catheters), and particularly in extensive third-degree thermal burns. It is an opportunist par excellence in patients suffering from complicated, debilitating illness, in premature or malnourished infants, in individuals whose normal bacterial flora has been altered by prior

antibiotic therapy, and in persons with neoplastic disease (especially leukemia) whose antibacterial defenses are compromised by deficiencies of circulating or cellular immunity (or both) or by defective circulating granulocytes. Invasion of the bloodstream by *P. aeruginosa,* unlike that due to *S. aureus,* is frequently followed by the development of widespread bacterial vasculitis. Growth of the organism in the walls of small and medium-sized arteries leads to thrombosis and septic infarction in many organs. Nodular, necrotic septic lesions occur, particularly in lung, kidney, heart, and brain. Unusual but characteristic bullous, hemorrhagic, and necrotic lesions of a similar pathogenesis may develop in the skin. Involvement of the lung results in pneumonia characterized by multiple nodular areas of consolidation that may rapidly undergo abscess formation. Dyspnea, pleuritic pain, and hemoptysis are prominent clinical manifestations. Involvement of the heart may lead to endocarditis, myocardial infarction secondary to coronary artery occlusion by the arteritis, or pericarditis, as a result of spread of infection to the pericardial sac by the bacteremic route or by contiguity from a septic myocardial infarct. The cellular or extracellular factors involved in the invasive propensity of *P. aeruginosa* in the compromised host have not been characterized. The very recent isolation and characterization of *P. aeruginosa* exotoxin A (see earlier section on General Cytotoxins) as a lethal toxin may provide valuable insights into the pathogenicity of this highly invasive organism. The role of exotoxin A in the production of the striking bacterial arteritis that occurs in *P. aeruginosa* is not known at present. In view of the extensive bacterial proliferation in and about blood vessels in such infections, direct bacterial invasiveness must be an important, if not the only, determinant of pathogenicity.

Widespread dissemination of infection leading to involvement of multiple organs is not restricted exclusively to bacterial disease. Although viral infections often demonstrate rather remarkable tropism for specific organs (poliomyelitis for anterior horn cells, infectious hepatitis for the hepatocytes, influenza for respiratory epithelial cells), certain viruses may, under special circumstances, proliferate in many organs and produce tissue damage. Thus, *Herpes hominis* infection in the neonate may eventuate in viremia that is followed by invasion of multiple sites. Destruction of cells of the skin, brain, liver, lung, and adrenal glands may occur as a result and contribute to the usually lethal outcome. Overt, clinically evident pneumonia, encephalitis, and hepatitis may dominate the picture.

Widespread involvement of organs may also occur in protozoan disease such as malaria. In infection due to *Plasmodium vivax*, up to 2 per cent of erythrocytes may be parasitized; in disease produced by *P. malariae*, such involvement usually does not exceed 1 per cent. *P. falciparum* has the greatest invasive propensity of the three major species of malarial parasites and may parasitize as many as 10 per cent of the red blood cells of a patient. The consequences of such marked multiplication may be extensive and produce a variety of organ dysfunctions secondary to circulatory changes. Hemolysis produced by red cell rupture at the time of schizogony leads to the rapid development of severe anemia. Evidence suggests that the hemolysis in malaria is related to the loss of erythrocyte membrane function. This appears to be the consequence of the usurpation by the parasite of the metabolic machinery of the red cell needed for the maintenance of the membrane. Further, hemolysis may be related to splenic removal of parasitic inclusions from the erythrocytes ("pitting") as they pass between the walls of splenic sinusoids. The red cells that survive this procedure re-enter the circulation as spherocytes. Some of these spherocytes are damaged in the process and subsequently exhibit a shortened survival in the circulation. Capillary distention and blockage by parasitized red cells result in anoxia that may produce irreversible damage in brain, liver, and kidneys. Pulmonary edema may develop as a consequence of cerebral, pulmonary, and cardiovascular injury in patients with acute falciparum malaria.

COMBINATION OF TOXIN PRODUCTION AND INVASIVENESS AS BASIS OF PATHOGENICITY

The clinical manifestations of certain infections are due exclusively to the effects of potent exotoxins in the absence of bacterial invasion (tetanus, botulism). The primary features of other infectious processes, on the basis of current evidence, appear to be related almost exclusively to the local or disseminated proliferation of the invading microorganism itself. A third class of infectious diseases is one in which clinical manifestations appear to be related both to the activity of exotoxin and to the multiplication of and invasion by bacteria. Three different diseases produced by three distinct bacterial species serve as examples of this type of infection.

Scarlet fever is a syndrome characterized by a localized infection, usually of the pharynx but occurring anywhere in the body, accompanied by a toxic rash. The eruption is produced by an erythrogenic toxin elaborated by the organisms at their site of multiplication and absorbed into the bloodstream. This toxin is produced by the majority of strains of group A and by occasional strains of groups C and G streptococci. Its production is related to the presence of a temperate bacteriophage in the streptococcus, a phenomenon very similar to that involving diphtheria toxin elaboration by lysogenic strains of *Corynebacterium diphtheriae*.

The signs and symptoms of scarlet fever consist of two groups: (1) The *local manifestations of infection* in the pharynx are the result of the inflammatory reaction and response of the lymphoid tissues to bacterial invasion. These account for the redness of the pharyngeal mucosa, the development of soft, yellow exudate that fills the crypts of the tonsils and may overflow onto the pharynx and over the uvula, and the edema and enlargement of lymphoid tissues, including those of the posterior pharynx. In an occasional patient with streptococcal tonsillitis, bacteremia may develop as a complication. Although an abundance of extracellular products are produced by group A streptococci and although it is tempting to assign them a role in the invasiveness of the organism (e.g., streptolysin O and DPNase are leukotoxic; hyaluronidase may assist in breaking down tissue barriers; streptokinase is fibrinolytic and might account for lack of localization of many streptococcal infections), there is no clear evidence to establish such a role. (2) *The manifestations of scarlet fever due to the erythrogenic toxin* are a characteristic skin eruption and various peripheral signs. This agent acts primarily on the capillary bed to produce dilatation, congestion, and increased fragility.

The typical scarlatiniform eruption, a punctate rash superimposed on an erythematous base, the bleeding lines (Pastia's lines), the suggestive early "strawberry" and later "raspberry" tongue, the increased excretion of red blood cells in the urine, and the swelling of the hands and feet that may be present at the onset of the disease are all due to activity of erythrogenic toxin in the vascular bed. The generalized abdominal pain, nausea, and vomiting that may be early features have a similar pathogenesis. The diffuse erythema of the skin is related to the dilatation of the capillaries; the punctate erythematous lesions are manifestations of the same effect on the tufts of blood vessels in the dermal papillae, causing them to be raised and somewhat darker than the surrounding skin. Histologic study reveals dilatation of small blood vessels that are surrounded by an accumulation of neutrophilic exudate. When injected into the skin of normal nonimmune subjects, purified erythrogenic toxin produces a localized area of erythema (Dick test). The action of the toxin on the capillary tuft in the papillae may be sufficiently intense to cause increased fragility and the appearance of petechiae. The effect of the toxin on the integrity of the capillary vasculature is readily shown by the occurrence of "bleeding lines" and hematuria. Because of increased fragility, vessels in skin folds (e.g., inguinal, axillary, and antebrachial areas), which are subjected to considerable movement and minor trauma, rupture and produce linear extravasations of blood (Pastia's lines). The renal glomerular capillaries are also injured by the toxin and leak small numbers of red cells in the urine early in the disease and for as long as a week.

The changes in the tongue characteristic of

scarlet fever are also due to the effects of the erythrogenic toxin on the capillary bed of this organ. The "strawberry" tongue, present at the onset of the disease, is not pathognomonic of scarlet fever. It represents the early effect of toxin on the capillaries in the lingual papillae, which become enlarged and reddened and protrude through the white coat on the surface of the tongue, giving the appearance of an unripe strawberry. The "raspberry" tongue appears after 3 to 4 days and is much more characteristic of the disease. It is the result of continued activity of the toxin on the blood vessels, which are now diffusely dilated, accounting for the deep red color of the tongue after the coat has been shed. Because of the greater number of capillaries in the lingual papillae, these become large and deeper in color than the surrounding tissue, standing out as strikingly elevated structures.

Within a week or so, desquamation of the skin and tongue begins. This represents shedding of superficial dermal and lingual layers of these organs that have borne the brunt of the activity of the erythrogenic toxin and have eventually been destroyed. This leads to separation of large patches of skin from the hands and feet, "brawny" desquamation on the trunk, and loss of lingual papillae (to such an extent that the surface of the tongue becomes quite smooth).

The diffuse abdominal pain, nausea, and vomiting that often characterize severe scarlet fever are probably the result of the effects of erythrogenic toxin on the capillary vasculature of the intestinal tract as well as on the lymphoid tissues in the intestinal wall and mesenteric nodes. The fact that lymph nodes may be affected by erythrogenic toxin in the absence of bacteremia is strongly suggested by the presence of generalized lymphadenopathy in most cases and splenomegaly in about 10 per cent of patients.

Jaundice, accompanied by evidence of dysfunction of the liver, may be a feature of severe scarlet fever and is probably due to a toxic hepatitis produced by the erythrogenic toxin.

When scarlet fever is severe, it is not uncommon for patients to complain of arthralgia and to exhibit a considerable degree of swelling of the hands and feet. Since these findings appear during the first 1 or 2 days of the disease, it is clear that they are not manifestations of rheumatic fever but are manifestations of the activity of erythrogenic toxin on blood vessels, resulting in the development of edema. An unusual feature of the early stage of scarlet fever is the presence of meningeal irritation, with stiff neck and back and positive Kernig and Brudzinski signs. Examination of the cerebrospinal fluid discloses a pleocytosis (up to 1000 cells per mm^3, practically all of which are lymphocytes), a moderate increase in the concentration of protein, and a normal content of sugar. This is the "serous meningitis" of scarlet fever and has been considered to be due to the effect of the erythrogenic toxin or other extracellular products of Streptococcus pyogenes.

Toxic epidermal necrolysis ("scalded-skin" syndrome) is a dramatic and serious skin disease, usually occurring in infancy. It is characterized by tenderness of the skin and striking erythema, followed by desquamation in sheets over most of the body. Because of the extensive exfoliation, temperature regulation and fluid balance are particular problems in the newborn. The characteristic histologic changes are the formation of a cleavage plane high in the epidermis, in the granular cell layer, and separation of the epidermal layer by edematous fluid producing typical bullae. This disorder has been associated with the presence on the epidermis or at other sites of infection of large numbers of S. aureus of phage group II. Such strains produce an extracellular toxic protein ("exfoliatin") capable of causing exfoliation in neonatal mice following subcutaneous or intraperitoneal administration; this is presumed to be the agent responsible for the scalded-skin syndrome in infants. This toxin is separate and distinct from the alpha and delta toxins of the organism. It has been proposed that the rare case of scarlatiniform eruption associated with some infections due to S. aureus is a forme fruste of the scalded-skin syndrome in which systemic spread of the toxin has occurred without the full picture of exfoliation, due to less toxin production or to undefined host factors.

Anthrax is a disease in which bacterial multiplication and dissemination and toxin production in vivo proceed pari passu. Evidence has suggested a predominant role for a toxin in the pathophysiologic changes that occur in the lethal form of the disease. Anthrax is an infection, primarily of animals, caused by Bacillus anthracis. It is occasionally transmitted to humans by exposure to animal products (wool, bone, etc.). The commonest manifestation of the disease in humans is a necrotic skin or mucous membrane ulcer ("malignant pustule") surrounded by a wide zone of gelatinous edema. Dissemination of infection from the original focus may occur via the bloodstream and may lead to the development of a hemorrhagic mediastinitis or hemorrhagic meningitis. Following inhalation of anthrax spores, a fulminant form of the disease may occur, characterized by a hemorrhagic mediastinitis and meningitis. When dissemination of the infection occurs, blood cultures are usually positive. The bacteremia is often high grade, and it may be possible to identify the bacilli on stained smears of centrifuged sediment of blood. No quantitative data are available on the number of organisms per milliliter of human blood. However, in the experimental animal, 10^8 to 10^9 organisms per ml of blood may be found terminally. Although it was originally thought that death was due to widespread capillary blockage produced by the large number of bacilli in the circulation, this hypothesis is no longer accepted.

A toxin has been demonstrated in the edematous fluid of the anthrax lesion and in the plasma of animals dying of anthrax. This substance appears to be made up of a complex of three serologically distinct components: an *edema-producing factor,* a *protective antigen,* and a *lethal factor.* The level of the toxin in the blood roughly parallels the degree of bacteremia. The most recent experimental evidence strongly suggests that the exotoxin contributes significantly to the patho-physiology of the infection. Purified anthrax toxin complex is lethal for several animal species. Its main effect is to increase vascular permeability; this may account for the gelatinous edema about the local lesion and the terminal pulmonary edema in fatal disease in experimental animals. The molecular mechanism of action of the toxic moiety is unknown. It is now generally believed that death from anthrax is due to the effects of this toxin.

REFERENCES

GENERAL CYTOTOXINS

Bartlett, J. G.: Antibiotic-associated diarrhea. *In* Remington, J. S., and Swartz, M. N. (Eds.): Current Clinical Topics in Infectious Disease. New York, McGraw-Hill Book Co., 1980.

Bornstein, D. L., Weinberg, A. N., Swartz, M. N., and Kunz, L. J.: Anaerobic Infections: review of current experience. Medicine 43:207, 1964.

Bowman, C. G., and Bonventre, P. F.: Studies on the mode of action of diphtheria toxin III. Effect on subcellular components of protein synthesis from the tissues of intoxicated guinea pigs and rats. J. Exp. Med. 131:659, 1970.

Chang, T., and Neville, D. M., Jr.: Demonstration of diphtheria toxin receptors on surface membranes from both toxin-sensitive and toxin-resistant species. J. Biol. Chem. 253:6866, 1978.

Collier, R. J.: Effect of diphtheria toxin on protein synthesis: Inactivation of one of the transfer factors. J. Mol. Biol. 25:83, 1967.

Collier, R. J., and Pappenheimer, A. M.: Studies on the mode of action of diphtheria toxin II. Effect of toxin on amino acid incorporation in cell-free systems. J. Exp. Med. 120:1019, 1964.

Cross, A. S., Sadoff, J. C., Iglewski, B. H., and Sokol, P. A.: Evidence for the role of toxin A in the pathogenesis of infection with *Pseudomonas aeruginosa* in humans. J. Infect. Dis. 142:538, 1980.

Davis, B. D., et al.: Anaerobic spore-forming bacilli. *In* Microbiology. 3rd ed. New York, Hoeber Medical Division of Harper and Row, 1980.

Draper, R., Chin, D., and Simon, M. I.: Diphtheria toxin has the properties of a lectin. Proc. Natl. Acad. Sci. (USA) 75:261, 1978.

Gill, D. M., Pappenheimer, A. M., Brown, R., and Kurnick, J. T.: Studies on the mode of action of diphtheria toxin. J. Exp. Med. 129:1, 1969.

Honjo, T., Nishizuka, Y., Kato, I., and Hayaishi, O.: Adenosine diphosphate ribosylation of aminoacyl transferase II and inhibition of protein synthesis by diphtheria toxin. J. Biol. Chem. 246:4251, 1971.

Iglewski, B. H., and Kabat, D.: NAD-dependent inhibition of protein synthesis by *Pseudomonas aeruginosa* toxin. Proc. Natl. Acad. Sci. 72:2284, 1975.

Lehninger, A. L.: Ribosomes and protein synthesis. *In* Biochemistry—The Molecular Basis of Cell Structure and Function. New York, Worth Publishers, Inc., 1970.

Liu, P. V.: Extracellular toxins of *Pseudomonas aeruginosa.* J. Infect. Dis. 120(S):594, 1974.

MacLennan, J. D.: The histotoxic clostridial infections of man. Bact. Rev. 26:177, 1962.

Pappenheimer, A. M., and Brown, R.: Studies on the mode of action of diphtheria toxin VI. Site of the action of toxin in living cells. J. Exp. Med. 127:1073, 1968.

Pappenheimer, A. M., Jr.: Diphtheria toxin. Ann. Rev. Biochem. 46:69, 1977.

Young, L. S.: The role of exotoxins in the pathogenesis of *Pseudomonas aeruginosa* infections. J. Infect. Dis. 142:626, 1980.

NEUROTOXINS

Boquet, P., and Duflot, E.: Tetanus toxin fragment forms channels in lipid vesicles at low pH. Proc. Natl. Acad. Sci. (USA) 79:7614, 1982.

Burgen, A. S. V., Dickens, F., and Zatman, L. J.: The action of botulinum toxin on the neuromuscular junction. J. Physiol. 109:10, 1948.

Eccles, J. C.: The Physiology of Synapses. Berlin, Springer-Verlag Publishers, 1964.

Koenig, M. G., Spickard, A., Cardella, M. A., and Rogers, D. E.: Clinical and laboratory observations of type E botulism in man. Medicine 43:517, 1964.

Prys-Roberts, C., Kerr, J. H., Corbett, J. L., et al.: Treatment of sympathetic overactivity in tetanus. Lancet 1:542, 1969.

Simpson, L. L.: The action of botulinal toxin. Rev. Infect. Dis. 1:656, 1979.

Struppler, A., Struppler, E., and Adams, R. D.: Local tetanus in man. Arch. Neurol. 8:162, 1963.

Wright, G. P.: The Neurotoxins of *Clostridium botulinum* and *Clostridium tetani.* Pharmacol. Rev. 7:413, 1955.

Young, R. R., and Delwaide, P. J.: Drug therapy: spasticity. N. Engl. J. Med. 304:28, 1981.

Zacks, S. I., and Sheff, M. F.: Tetanism: pathobiological aspects of the action of tetanal toxin in the nervous system and skeletal muscle. Neurosci. Res. 3:209, 1970.

ENTEROTOXINS

Field, M.: Intestinal secretion: effect of cyclic AMP and its role in cholera. N. Engl. J. Med. 284:1137, 1971.

Gill, D. M.: Involvement of nicotinamide adenine dinucleotide in the action of cholera toxin *in vitro.* Proc. Natl. Acad. Sci. 72:2064, 1975.

Gill, D. M., Evans, D. J., Jr., and Evans, D. G.: Mechanism of activation of adenylate cyclase *in vitro* by polymyxin-released, heat-labile enterotoxin of *Escherichia coli.* J. Infect. Dis. 133 (S):S103, 1976.

Gordon, R. S.: Moderator-Combined Clinical Staff Conference at the National Institutes of Health. Ann. Intern. Med. 64:1328, 1966.

Keusch, G. T., Grady, G. F., Mata, L. J., and McIver, J.: The pathogenesis of *Shigella* diarrhea. I. Enterotoxin production by *Shigella dysenteriae.* J. Clin. Invest. 51:1212, 1972.

Kimberg, D. V., Field, M., Johnson, J., et al.: Stimulation of intestinal mucosal adenyl cyclase by cholera enterotoxin and prostaglandins. J. Clin. Invest. 50:1218, 1971.

Moss, J., and Vaughan, M.: Mechanism of action of choleragen. J. Biol. Chem. 252:2455, 1977.

Moss, J., Manganiello, V. C., and Vaughan, M.: Hydrolysis of nicotinamide adenine dinucleotide by choleragen and its A protomer: possible role in the activation of adenylate cyclase. Proc. Natl. Acad. Sci. 73:4424, 1976.

Pierce, N. F., Greenough, W. B., III, and Carpenter, C. C. J.: *Vibrio cholerae* enterotoxin and its mode of action. Bact. Rev. 35:1, 1971.

ENDOTOXINS

Cluff, L. F.: Effects of endotoxins on susceptibility to infections. J. Infect. Dis. *122*:205, 1970.

Davis, C. E., and Arnold, K.: Role of meningococcal endotoxin in meningococcal purpura. J. Exp. Med. *140*:159, 1974.

Elin, R. J., and Wolff, S. M.: Biology of endotoxin. Ann. Rev. Med. *27*:127, 1976.

Greisman, S. E., Hornick, R. B., Carozza, F. A., and Woodward, T. E.: The role of endotoxin during typhoid fever and tularemia in man. I. Acquisition of tolerance to endotoxin. II. Altered cardiovascular responses to catecholamines. III. Hyper-reactivity to endotoxin during infection. J. Clin. Invest. *42*:1064, 1963, and *43*:986, 1774, 1964.

Landy, M., and Braun, W. (Eds.): Bacterial Endotoxins. Institute of Microbiology. New Brunswick, Rutgers University Press, 1964.

Munford, R. S., Hall, C. L., Lipton, J. M., and Dietschy, J. M.: Biological activity, lipoprotein-binding behavior, and in vivo disposition of extracted and native forms of *Salmonella typhimurium* lipopolysaccharides. J. Clin. Invest. *70*:877, 1982.

Nowatny, A. (Ed.): Symposium on Molecular Biology of Gram-Negative Bacterial Lipopolysaccharides. Ann. N. Y. Acad. Sci. *133*:277, 1966.

Sotto, M. N., Langer, B., Hoshino-Shimizu, S., and deBrito, T.: Pathogenesis of cutaneous lesions in acute meningococcemia in humans: light, immunofluorescent, and electron microscopic studies of skin biopsy specimens. J. Infect. Dis. *133*:506, 1976.

Thomas, L.: The physiologic disturbances produced by endotoxins. Ann. Rev. Physiol. *16*:467, 1954.

Zweifach, B. W., and Janoff, A.: Bacterial endotoxemia. Ann. Rev. Med. *16*:201, 1965.

INVASIVE INFECTIONS

Brooks, M. H., Malloy, J. P., Bartelloni, P. J., et al.: Pathophysiology of acute falciparum malaria. I. Correlation of clinical and biochemical abnormalities. Am. J. Med. *43*:735, 1967.

Conrad, M. E.: Pathophysiology of malaria. Ann. Intern. Med. *70*:134, 1969.

Lincoln, R. E., and Fish, D. C.: Anthrax toxin. *In* Montie, T. C., Kadis, S., and Ajl, S. J. (Eds.): Microbial Toxins. Vol. III. New York, Academic Press, 1970.

Melish, M. E., Glasgow, L. A., and Turner, M. D.: The staphylococcal scalded-skin syndrome: isolation and partial purification of the new exfoliative toxin. J. Infect. Dis. *125*:129, 1972.

Melish, M. E., Glasgow, L. A., Turner, M. D., and Lillibridge, C. B.: The staphylococcal epidermolytic toxin: its isolation, characterization, and site of action. Ann. N. Y. Acad. Sci. *236*:317, 1974.

Neva, F. A., Sheagren, J. N., Shulman, N. R., and Canfield, C. J.: Malaria: host defense mechanisms and complications. Combined Clinical Staff Conference of the National Institutes of Health. Ann. Intern. Med. *73*:295, 1970.

Nungester, W. J.: Proceedings of the Conference on Progress in the Understanding of Anthrax. Fed. Proc. *26*:1491, 1967.

Rabin, E. R., Graver, C. D., Vogel, E. H., et al.: Fatal *Pseudomonas* infection in burned patients: a clinical, bacteriologic, and anatomic study. N. Engl. J. Med. *265*:1225, 1961.

Rogers, D. E.: The current problem of staphylococcal infections. Ann. Intern. Med. *45*:748, 1956.

Symposium on Toxic Shock Syndrome. N. I. H. Conference. Ann. Intern. Med. *96*:835, 1982.

Wood, W. B., Jr.: Studies on the cellular immunology of acute bacterial infections. The Harvey Lectures, *Series XLVII*:72 1951–52.

20 Host Responses to Infection

Louis Weinstein and Morton N. Swartz

INTRODUCTION

The host response to an invading microorganism may be varied in nature, in extent, and in pathophysiologic consequences.

1. *In some circumstances the response may be minimal.* The majority of individuals exposed to *Mycobacterium tuberculosis* do not develop symptomatic pulmonary involvement or manifestations of disseminated infection. The host response is sufficient to contain the infectious process without progression to overt clinical disease. The only evidence that infection has taken place is the development of delayed hypersensitivity to antigens of *M. tuberculosis* as indicated by positive skin tests. A similar situation prevails in certain areas of the western United States in which a fungus, *Coccidioides immitis,* is present in the soil; the majority of the population in such areas are infected with the organism (positive skin reactions) but do not develop an identifiable illness.

2. *In other circumstances, the response of the host may be significant, but the major impact of the infection is the result of the organism's invasive properties or toxigenicity or both.* Examples of such infections (anthrax, cholera, streptococcal and staphylococcal sepsis) have been discussed in Chapter 19.

3. *In another group of infectious processes, the host response may be so exaggerated and troublesome, or so specific in nature, that it alone induces pathophysiologic consequences of considerable magnitude.* These responses may then account for various disorders that dominate the clinical picture. The invasive or toxin-producing phase of the infection may never develop, or if it does, it is concluded by the time symptoms become manifest. The signs and symptoms due to the host response become paramount or, in effect, constitute the entire clinical illness itself. It is this third category of infection that is the focus of discussion in this chapter. A variety of general responses may be elicited by most infections. Some, such as fever, are so common as to be considered a hallmark of this kind of disease. Others, such as disseminated intravascular clotting, are relatively uncommon but are recognized more and more frequently as the laboratory criteria for their diagnosis have been clarified.

GENERAL HOST RESPONSES

Fever

Fever is an almost universal response of warm-blooded animals to infection. The normal oral body temperature is 98.6° F (37° C). However, this represents a mean value derived from studies of large numbers of normal people, and the "normal" for occasional individuals may deviate from this value by as much as 0.5° to 1.0° F. During the course of the day, body temperature varies over a range of 0.5° to 2.0° F, the low point occurring in the early morning hours during sleep and the peak being reached late in the afternoon. In addition to disease, a variety of physiologic and environmental factors may transiently elevate the temperature by temporarily overwhelming the mechanism available for heat loss. For example, in very warm weather body temperature may rise 0.5° to 1.0° F. Similarly, after vigorous exercise or a hot shower even greater increases may occur. Commencing at the time of ovulation and persisting during the second half of the menstrual cycle, a more prolonged physiologic rise in morning temperature (0.50° to 0.75° F) occurs and continues until the onset of menstruation. Basal and maximal "normal" daily temperatures decrease with increasing age. Such elevations are minor and, in most instances, only transitory. The term "fever" is commonly reserved for more sustained elevations of greater magnitude occurring in the course of disease.

The role of fever as a potential defense mechanism is obscure. There is as yet no clear evidence that a rise in body temperature confers a selective advantage to the host over the invading microorganism. However, this may be the case in a few infections. The optimal temperature for the retention of the infectivity of *Treponema pallidum* in vitro is 34° to 35° C. Higher temperatures are progressively more unfavorable for the spirochete. It is not unreasonable to suggest that this sensitivity to temperature is involved in the predilection of this organism for the skin. In addition, the occasional favorable response of certain forms of syphilis subjected to fever therapy in the preantibiotic era may be accounted for on this basis. It is very difficult to design an experiment with ordinary laboratory animals to determine whether the febrile response of the host augments resistance to infection because the measures required to suppress fever are themselves capable of producing complicating side-effects. However, an interesting study of the role of fever in survival from bacterial infection has been carried out in lizards, reptiles whose body temperature can be kept constant over a wide range by simply controlling the ambient temperature. In lizards inoculated with the pathogenic bacteria *Aeromonas hydrophila,* an elevation of body temperature from 34° to 40° C increased survival from 0 to about 70 per cent, suggesting enhanced host defenses at the elevated temperature. (The in-vitro bacterial growth rate was stable between these two temperatures.) Similarly, when goldfish are infected with the same bacteria they will, if provided the opportunity, elevate their body temperature by 1° or 2° by swimming into an adjoining warmer container. The higher body temperature thus produced is associated with greater survival from the infection. Limited data from studies with mammals (rabbits infected with bacteria, dogs and rats infected with viruses) also suggest that moderate, but not extreme, fever is associated with decreased mortality from certain experimental infections. The elevations of body temperature commonly observed with infection have been noted to enhance, in vitro and in vivo, specific components of normal host defenses such as leukocyte mobility, leukocyte bactericidal activity, interferon action, and T-cell proliferation and antibody production induced by interleukin-1 (formerly designated "lymphocyte-activating factor"). If the febrile response to infection *is* beneficial, then the common use of antipyretic agents in the treatment of mild infectious fevers might be ill advised.

Although fever is usually associated with infection, this is by no means an exclusive relationship. Thus, it may be a manifestation of neoplastic disease (e.g., lymphoma), noninfectious inflammatory disorders (e.g., vasculitis, rheumatoid arthritis, ulcerative colitis, regional enteritis), or excess catabolism in certain metabolic states (e.g., pheochromocytoma, thyrotoxicosis). However, severe infection may exist without eliciting hyperpyrexia. Hypothermia (accompanying hypotension) may be present in the course of overwhelming infections. The presence of certain metabolic abnormalities (myxedema, uremia) may completely quench the usual febrile response to infection.

Normal Thermoregulation. Normal body temperature is the result of a delicately maintained balance between heat production and heat loss. In the resting state, the major sites of heat production, under normal circumstances, are the liver and skeletal muscles; during exercise or in disease-associated febrile states, the latter is the major site. Loss of heat takes place at the surface of the body (skin and lungs) through radiation, convection, and vaporization. The primary mechanisms

by which control of temperature is maintained involve the nervous system. Generation of heat is produced through the somatic motor efferents (shivering); conservation or loss of heat is achieved through the control, by the autonomic nervous system, of cutaneous blood supply (loss of heat), and sudomotor activity (sweating). The central guidance for these efferent connections is the thermoregulatory center in the anterior hypothalamus. It responds to stimuli from two sources: (1) the superficial thermoreceptors of the skin that respond to changes in surface temperature, and (2) the deep thermoreceptors located in or near the hypothalamus that respond to slight changes in the temperature of the blood perfusing this part of the central nervous system. The thermoregulatory center in the hypothalamus operates as a thermostat, with a "set point" at about 98.6° F, and responds to superficial and deep stimuli from external heat load (e.g., high environmental temperature) by initiating loss of heat via sweating and vasodilatation.

Injury to the anterior hypothalamus by tumor growth or tissue destruction results in erratic regulation of body temperature. Individuals with such lesions are subject to unexplained fevers or to dangerously low body temperatures when exposed to a cold environment.

The specific setting of the hypothalamic thermostat varies somewhat from person to person (96° to 99.6°F), with lower "set points" being more frequent in older individuals.

Thermoregulation in Febrile Disease States. An endogenous febrile reaction consists of four phases that are fairly sharply defined and that follow in regular sequence: (1) prodrome, (2) chill, (3) flush, and (4) defervescence. During the prodrome, there are only nonspecific complaints such as fleeting aches and pains, mild headache, nausea, and malaise; the circulation through the skin is normal. The initial discernible event in the chill phase is cutaneous vasoconstriction—the patient complains of being cold and often covers up with more bedclothes. He becomes increasingly pale, and the extremities appear somewhat cyanotic. The skin is cool and dry, except perhaps for a little perspiration of the forehead or upper lip. This phase lasts approximately 1½ hours. These changes suggest that during the early phases of a febrile illness, the hypothalamic thermostat responds as though its "set point" has been raised to a new higher maintenance level. If the decrease in surface temperature due to reduced blood flow is of sufficient magnitude, the superficial cutaneous thermoreceptors are triggered. Feedback from the latter to the hypothalamus reflexly produces increased muscular activity in the form of shivering or, when this is maximal, a shaking chill. Production of heat is markedly increased by this muscular activity. During the chill phase the low skin temperature makes the patient feel cold even though the rectal temperature is rising. In fact, since the most severe chills are associated with the most marked rises in rectal temperatures, patients feel coldest when they are storing the most heat. The patient continues to feel cold; a disproportion between internal and cutaneous temperatures may be responsible in part for the sensation of cold. The clinical and physiologic manifestations of chills may be precipitated or aggravated by exposure to cold when the subject is in the chill phase of a febrile reaction.

The effectiveness of shivering as a means of increasing heat production for the maintenance of the body heat balance can be gauged in a quantitative way. Thus, in an experiment in a calorimeter at 23° C reported by Hardy, production of heat prior to a chill was 63 kcal over an hour, and heat loss was 87 kcal. In the next half hour, during a chill, the rate of heat production was 164 kcal per hour and heat loss was 116 kcal per hour. Shivering is a more efficient means of increasing body temperature than exercise because loss of heat can be minimized by reducing the body surface area (site of convection loss) by curling up and by maintaining some degree of insulation by simultaneous vasoconstriction.

As the temperature of the skin rises with prolonged shivering, a sensation of warmth develops, and the shivering ceases. Cutaneous vasodilatation proceeds rapidly, and the flush phase begins. The increased flow of blood in the skin causes an increase in the rate of heat loss, balancing the abnormally high level of heat production. As a result, body temperature remains poised at the newly established higher level. When the skin temperature reaches about 34° C, sweating occurs and marks the defervescent phase of the febrile response. Stimulation of the sweat glands is produced by efferent impulses from the hypothalamus, stimulated itself both by afferent impulses from the skin and by the elevated temperature of the blood flowing through the brain.

As already suggested, deviations of body temperature from the "set point" initiate mechanisms that tend to restore body temperature to the programmed level. Fever appears to represent, in essence, a rise in the "set point." In keeping with this is the observation of Cooper and coworkers that in humans, when body temperature is elevated but stable, the skin vasomotor responses to a heat load are normal. In a normal subject infused with endogenous pyrogen (see further on), prepared by preincubation of the subject's blood with bacterial endotoxin, an abrupt rise in temperature ensues and reaches its peak in about an hour. This is associated with marked cutaneous vasoconstriction, myalgias, and chills. Following this, there is a stable period (several hours) during which the peak temperature level is maintained. An additional heat load (generated by immersion of an arm in warm water) during the phase of rising temperature causes no cutaneous vasodilatation measured in the other hand. In contrast, immersion during the stable phase at the peak temperature produces a transient rise in oral temperature with increased elimination of heat on the other hand. The elevation of temperature required to induce vasodilatation is very small (0.10° to 0.15° C) in contrast to the increase (1.70° C) induced by the administration of pyrogen. Further evidence bearing on the hypothalamic "set point" is provided by the observations of MacPherson on the effects of intermittent exercise on rectal temperature in humans, including a subject who developed a mild infection with fever while participating in the study. The aforementioned subject, during repeated periods of calibrated exercise in a warm environment, showed fixed elevations of rectal temperature (0.4° to 0.5° C) essentially identical with those of afebrile individuals. However, his baseline temperature, attained before each of the repeated bouts of exercise, was about 1.0° C higher (38° C) than that of similar subjects without fever. These observations are compatible with the view that fever represents an alteration in the level at which the thermostat is set, and that, at this new setting, thermostatic control is as well regulated as at the former lower setting.

A variety of pathophysiologic changes involving the cardiorespiratory system accompany the febrile state. Changes in respiration may be prominent. In the chill phase, respiratory rate and minute volume increase, and the tidal volume decreases. There may be a small decrease in arterial Po_2 owing to rapid shallow breathing, but respiratory alkalosis is the more common finding. The increased respiratory activity during fever serves to eliminate some of the heat. The stimulus for this is thought to be the increased temperature of the blood supplying the respiratory center; accumulation of carbon dioxide in the respiratory center as a result of decreased cerebral blood flow during the chill phase may also play a role.

Cardiac output differs in the various phases of the febrile state. With severe chills a considerable decrease in cardiac output may occur, resulting in hypotension. During the flush phase, the cardiac output is increased in excess of the rise in oxygen consumption. During defervescence, cardiac output and oxygen consumption return toward normal. During the febrile period, the pulse rate in humans roughly parallels the temperature; a rise of nine beats per minute occurs for each Fahrenheit degree increase in rectal temperature. However, the pulse rate is a poor indicator of changes in cardiac output during fever, since it often increases disproportionately and may rise when the cardiac output falls.

Mediators of Fever. The well-known clinical association of fever with inflammatory processes led to an early examination of purulent exudates for materials capable of evoking a febrile response in experimental animals. The results of such studies were obscured by the probable presence, in the soluble fractions of the exudates, of endotoxin, a pyrogenic lipopolysaccharide from the cell envelopes of contaminating gram-negative bacilli. In 1948, Beeson, employing procedures to exclude endotoxins, was able to extract from granulocytes a fever-producing material that he termed *endogenous pyrogen* (EP). Since then, this substance has been the subject of considerable interest and study by many investigators. Most of the current knowledge concerning EP has been derived from investigations of experimental fever in animal models. When rabbits are given injections of endotoxin (typhoid vaccine) intravenously, fever develops and lasts for 5 to 8 hours. Serum obtained at intervals during the febrile period elicits a febrile response when injected into normal animals. Except for the serum obtained early in the experiment, the development of fever in the recipient animals is not due to carry-over of endotoxin, since elevation of temperature is produced in endotoxin-refractory (tolerant) animals as well. Thus, the febrile response is induced by another pyrogenic material that appears to have properties indistinguishable from those of the pyrogen obtained from sterile exudates containing predominantly granulocytes.

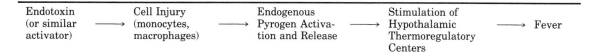

Studies by Bennett and Beeson and by Wood initially provided evidence that the leukocytes (the granulocytes, they and others believed) in sterile rabbit peritoneal exudates were the principal source of EP. The EP could be released from such exudates on incubation in vitro in isotonic saline. Human EP can be produced in vitro following incubation of buffy-coat cells with endotoxin. Injection of the supernatant into human subjects produces fever within 20 minutes. In contrast, fever does not occur for more than 45 minutes after the injection of endotoxin alone or of the supernatant from incubations with leukocyte-deficient plasma with endotoxin. Human EP is, like rabbit EP, a rapidly acting pyrogen that is heat labile.

EP derived from both rabbit and human leukocytes has been purified and appears to be made up of several proteins—one with a molecular weight of 15,000 is the predominant species; a second with a molecular weight of 40,000 may represent an oligomer or some form of posttranscriptional modification. Two nanograms/kg or less of EP can produce fever in rabbits. Little if any active EP is present preformed in peripheral blood leukocytes; disruption of such cells does not release EP. Such cells are activated to produce EP in vitro by exposure to endotoxin or a phagocytic stimulus. Activation of EP production requires protein synthesis; addition of inhibitors of protein synthesis that do not prevent phagocytosis (puromycin, cycloheximide) at the time of exposure to endotoxin or a phagocytic stimulus prevents the subsequent production of EP. Synthesis of new messenger RNA appears to be necessary as well for EP synthesis, since actinomycin D, an inhibitor of DNA transcription, similarly prevents the production of EP in vitro.

Sources of Endogenous Pyrogen. A prominent role of granulocytes in the production of EP was originally suggested by the association of an initial leukopenia (mainly granulocytic) with the experimental fever induced by endotoxin. (Margination of polymorphonuclear leukocytes along blood vessel walls occurs at the same time.) Although early studies with peritoneal exudates of rabbits had also indicated an essential role for the granulocyte in the production of EP, other cell sources of this substance were suggested by the occurrence of fever in granulocytopenic patients and in nitrogen mustard–treated rabbits who lack significant numbers of circulating granulocytes. The role of other cell types in the generation of EP was further suggested by the observation that peripheral blood leukocytes from patients with severe agranulocytosis or monocytic leukemia, when stimulated in vitro, produced large quantities of EP, accounting for fever occurring in patients lacking circulating granulocytes. Early investigations reporting EP production from either rabbit neutrophilic exudates or human blood neutrophils involved granulocyte preparations containing 1 to 5 per cent contamination with monocytes. Rabbit granulocytes separated quantitatively from mononuclear cells by Ficoll-Hypaque gradients have been shown by Hanson and coworkers to produce little or no EP but to exhibit normal chemotaxis and generate normal amounts of superoxide and bactericidal activity on phagocytic (staphylococci) stimulation. The rabbit macrophage produces 100 times or more the amount of EP produced by a rabbit granulocyte; similarly, the human peripheral blood monocyte produces 20 to 40 times more EP than the human circulating granulocyte. Thus, it appears that only bone marrow–derived mononuclear phagocytes produce EP. Kupffer cells in the liver and other fixed phagocytic cells are probably also sources of EP. Alveolar macrophages obtained from the lungs of rabbits sensitized to tuberculin by intravenous injection of BCG release abundant EP when incubated with tuberculin in vitro. This observation may provide an explanation for the occurrence of fever in patients with pulmonary tuberculosis.

Inducers of Production of Endogenous Pyrogen. Intravenous injection of bacterial endotoxins, various bacteria, or viruses in normal or specifically sensitized rabbits has been followed by fever and the appearance of demonstrable EP in the circulation. Release of EP from suspensions of rabbit granulocytes occurs when they have been incubated in vitro with bacteria, viruses, tuberculin, or antigen-antibody complexes. Successful phagocytosis appears to be an important feature of the bacteria-induced EP release.

Many agents that produce fever in humans have been shown to stimulate the production of EP by human leukocytes in vitro. In addition to the aforementioned bacteria, endotoxin, viruses, and so forth, these agents include chemically diverse biologically active materials such as the synthetic adjuvant *N*-acetyl-muramyl-L-alanine-D-isoglutamine (MDP) (the basic unit of the peptidoglycan polymer found in most bacterial cell walls), etiocholanolone (a product of human steroid metabolism), and bleomycin. Phagocytosis is required in order for bacteria (alive or dead) to be active as inducers in vitro. For endotoxin, MDP, etiocholanolone, or bleomycin to stimulate EP production, exposure to leukocytes for varying periods of time is necessary: as little as 45 minutes for endotoxin; as long as 6 to 8 hours for etiocholanolone.

Relation of Endogenous Pyrogen to Immunostimulatory Mediators. Lymphocyte activating factor, now known as interleukin-1 (IL-1), is a monokine, a protein produced by macrophages that amplifies the mitogenic response of T-lymphocytes to certain lectins (e.g., concanavalin A) and antigens. Thus, IL-1 serves as a modulator of lymphocyte activation and may be essential to immune responses. IL-1 made by rabbit alveolar macrophages and EP made by rabbit peritoneal exudate cells appear to be identical as judged by a substantial body of biochemical, functional, and immunologic evidence obtained on study of purified material. Evidence from studies of human peripheral blood monocytes also indicates that EP is probably identical with IL-1.

It appears likely that a functional interrelation occurs between the two biologic properties (pyrogenicity and T-cell mitogenicity) of IL-1. Duff and Durum have shown that the T-cell proliferative response to IL-1 is considerably increased at 39° compared with 37°C. Thus, the pyrogenic activity (EP) of IL-1 acts on the central nervous system to produce fever, which is then capable of enhancing the clonal expansion of T-lymphocytes produced by IL-1. Depending on the T-cell subsets principally affected, the interactions of the two biologic functions of IL-1 might be expected to alter immunoregulation considerably. For example, the temperature elevation just cited has been shown to augment the primary in vitro humoral immune response, mainly by the increased generation of T-helper cells (rather than by augmented B-cell activation or reduction of suppressor T-cell function).

If the febrile response to infection plays as important a role in vivo as in vitro in modulating the immune response, then more evidence will be at hand indicating a role for fever as an important part of the host defense. The widespread use of antipyretic agents in the symptomatic treatment of infectious fevers may be unwise when considered in this light.

Other Effects of Endogenous Pyrogen in the Acute Inflammatory Response. EP appears to have a central role in the host's coordinated response to an invading microorganism, a response considered to produce a less favorable environment for the multiplication of the pathogen. This response has been recognized for some time, although its relation to EP has only recently been suggested, and has been designated "acute phase reaction." It is characterized by a complex of changes including (1) polymorphonuclear leukocytosis, (2) increases in plasma levels of fibrinogen (responsible for the elevated sedimentation rate that occurs with infections or inflammatory processes), C-reactive protein, haptoglobin, ceruloplasmin, and alpha-1-acid glycoprotein, (3) increases in plasma levels of lactoferrin, and (4) decreases in plasma iron and zinc levels and increases in plasma copper levels. A macrophage product known as leukocyte endogenous mediator (LEM) is capable of inducing all of the aforementioned changes. Various studies suggest that EP and LEM either are the same protein or at least share multiple biochemical and functional characteristics. The increased levels of C-reactive protein, fibrinogen, and other circulating proteins that occur in animals following injection of EP are due to increases in the rate of hepatic synthesis of these proteins. EP increases the release of lactoferrin, an avid iron-binding protein, from secondary granules of polymorphonuclear leukocytes and thus probably accounts for the increased circulating levels of lactoferrin observed in some infections. The fall in plasma iron concentration plus the associated increased circulating levels of iron-binding lactoferrin is of potential benefit to the host, since many microorganisms require iron for growth. In addition, the ability of bacteria to obtain this needed iron from the environment depends on their production of bacterial iron-binding proteins (siderophores), which is reduced at the temperatures associated with febrile states. Thus, on several scores, in the febrile patient the invading bacterial pathogen may be lacking in iron. The possible survival value of fever-induced hypoferremia has been shown in lizards. The mortality rate in bacteria-infected lizards that became hypoferremic was low, but when they were injected with iron the mortality increased.

Site of Action of Endogenous Pyrogen. The

introduction of endotoxin or any of many other activators of EP in a susceptible animal or human appears to set off the following sequence of events in which EP is the final common pathway (see formula given previously). The central site of action of EP has been demonstrated in rabbits. When this substance is infused slowly into the carotid artery to perfuse the brain directly, a more rapid and greater febrile response is generated than when it is given intravenously. In contrast, the degree of fever produced by endotoxin is the same when given by either route. These observations are consistent with the concept that EP acts directly on the hypothalamus and that endotoxin activates circulating leukocytes to release EP. Direct perfusion of the anterior hypothalamus of rabbits with extremely small amounts of EP via microcannulas causes an immediate rise in body temperature.

Possible Role of Chemical Mediators in the Central Nervous System Response to Endogenous Pyrogen. The mechanism by which EP causes thermosensitive neurones in the preoptic hypothalamus to fire is unknown. EP is a 15,000-dalton protein, and there is no evidence that it can cross the blood-brain barrier. It is possible that its pyrogenic effects are produced by intermediary substances such as neurotransmitters. The most likely candidates would be prostaglandins, monoamines, cyclic nucleotides, and Na^+ or Ca^{++} ions. Although prostaglandins are the leading contenders for this role, the evidence is as yet inconclusive. Prostaglandins, particularly PGE_1, do produce fever promptly (more promptly than similar injections of EP) when injected into the brain of animals, but only in the preoptic anterior hypothalamus. This suggests that increases in hypothalamic prostaglandin E levels might be a consequence of the effects of EP on the thermoregulatory center. Also, prostaglandin E levels in the cerebrospinal fluid do increase during fever produced by peripheral infusions of EP. Furthermore, purified human EP does increase the in-vitro synthesis of prostaglandin E from brain tissues. The well-known antipyretic effects of prostaglandin synthetase inhibitors such as salicylates and indomethacin would also be consistent with a role for prostaglandins as hypothalamic mediators of fever. However, inconsistent with this putative role for prostaglandins is evidence that although intravenous injection of EP or endotoxin results in a rise in cerebrospinal fluid levels of prostaglandin E, intravenous injection of sodium salicylate or indomethacin prevents the rise in prostaglandins but does not block the fever. Also, in animals with anterior hypothalamic lesions in whom local application of prostaglandin E or EP does not produce fever, instillation of EP, but not prostaglandin E, into the lateral ventricles results in a febrile response.

In primates, serotonin is the major thermo-genic monoamine, and norepinephrine is the predominant thermolytic monoamine; both are present in high concentrations in the preoptic hypothalamus. Their possible role in mediation of fever is suggested by (1) increases in concentrations of monoamines in the hypothalamus produced by EP, and (2) significant modification of experimental EP-induced fever following pretreatment with monoamine-depleting agents.

Evidence implicating cyclic AMP as a mediator in the hypothalamus in the production of fever is of several types. First, cyclic AMP produces fever if injected into the third ventricle or anterior hypothalamus of experimental animals. Secondly, cerebrospinal fluid levels of cyclic AMP double during EP-induced fevers. Thirdly, theophylline, an inhibitor of phosphodiesterase that breaks down cyclic AMP, enhances endotoxin- and prostaglandin E–induced fevers.

It has been postulated that many of the mediators mentioned act in a sequential fashion in the pathogenesis of fever: (1) EP reaches the hypothalamus via the circulation; (2) there, it induces synthesis of a prostaglandin; (3) the prostaglandin, in turn, stimulates local synthesis of norepinephrine; and (4) cyclic AMP directly stimulates temperature-sensitive neurons that alter the body's heat conservation and production.

Mechanism of Fever Production During Overt Infections. Crucial to the definition of the role of EP in fever production is the demonstration of its presence in some common infectious processes. In experimental pneumococcal peritonitis produced in rabbits, the substance is present in the peritoneal cavity in the early stages of infection; it is detectable in thoracic-duct lymph and in blood later in the course of the fever. When the infection is controlled by therapy with penicillin, fever subsides and EP can no longer be demonstrated.

The possible role of continuing endotoxemia from *Salmonella typhosa* in typhoid fever has been studied by Greisman and coworkers in human volunteers. Endotoxin tolerance, induced immediately before or during experimental typhoid fever, did not inhibit the febrile course or toxemia characteristic of the disease. This appeared to eliminate continuing circulation of endotoxin as responsible for the sustained fever in this infection. Thus, it seems likely that in this disease persistence of fever is due to the production of EP by phagocytes in areas of inflammation.

Headache

Headache is a common symptom of systemic infection and is usually associated with fever. We are concerned here only with elevations of temperature unrelated to specific infections of the central nervous system such as meningitis or brain abscess. The febrile headache is usually throbbing in character at the onset of the febrile reaction and then becomes a deep dull ache of varying severity. It is usually generalized but may be predominantly in the frontotemporal, occipital, or suboccipital areas. It is aggravated by bodily movement. Several mechanisms may be active in the pathogenesis of headache occurring in the course of fever related to infection. First, there may be microscopic evidence of central nervous system inflammation without obvious meningeal signs. Thus, an occasional patient with mumps and a more severe than usual headache will have a small (but abnormal) number of lymphocytes in the cerebrospinal fluid. In most other infections in which febrile headaches occur, however, there is no evidence of active infection of the central nervous system or its linings. Such headaches may be a particularly prominent feature of influenza, typhoid fever, typhus and other rickettsial diseases, mycoplasma pneumonia, and infectious mononucleosis. It usually parallels the fever but may precede or outlast it.

The pain-sensitive structures in the central nervous system are the dural sinuses and their principal branches, the arteries in the dura and the areas immediately surrounding them, and the large intracranial arteries. It seems reasonable to suggest that disturbance of one or more of these structures during infection is responsible for febrile headaches.

Present evidence strongly suggests that pyrexial headaches result from stretching of sensitive structures about the intracranial arteries due to dilatation of these vessels. Sutherland and Wolff have reported that after intravenous administration of typhoid vaccine an increased amplitude of pulsations of the cerebrospinal fluid preceded the onset of headache, the severity of which closely paralleled the magnitude of the oscillations that occurred synchronously with the pulse. In addition, a direct relation was noted between the intensity of the headache and the amplitude of pulsations in the temporal artery. Direct visualization of pial vessels through skull windows in experimental animals has shown that intravenous administration of typhoid vaccine is followed by cerebral vasodilatation. The immediate factor or factors directly responsible for the cerebral vasodilatation are unknown at present. It is of interest that the headache following injection of histamine is similar in character and that dilatation of intracranial arteries is the basis of the pain.

It appears reasonable to consider the following sequence of events in the development of the headache produced by infections in which direct invasion of the central nervous system is not a feature: Phagocytosis of the infecting agent → Activation of mononuclear pyrogen (EP) → Action of EP on the thermoregulatory center, generating a febrile response → Cerebral vasodilatation mediated in some way directly by EP or through alterations secondary to the EP-induced fever.

Hypotension and Shock

Shock associated with bacteremia is the major cause of mortality in infections otherwise amenable to antibiotic therapy. Although gram-negative bacteria are the most frequent offending organisms, the syndrome may develop in the course of disease produced by viruses, fungi, and rickettsiae. Shock in bacteremia is not due simply to endotoxin; studies with the Limulus amebocyte gelation assay for circulating endotoxin have revealed no correlation between positive assays and the number of circulating gram-negative bacilli or the occurrence of shock or death. The pathophysiology of the changes observed in bacteremia and septic shock in humans are still incompletely understood. It was formerly believed that the fundamental problem was a low pressure state due to loss or paralysis of vasomotor tone. Thus, treatment in the past was directed at restoration of circulating blood volume and correction of defective vasomotor tone by administration of vasopressor agents. The more recent concept of the mechanism of septic shock is that it is due to redistribution of blood within the vascular bed in a manner precluding maintenance of an adequate circulating blood volume. Tissue ischemia and anoxia are a consequence of this pooling and lead to decreased renal function, myocardial failure, lactic acidemia, and ultimately to cell death.

Commonly, when hypotension develops during the course of bacteremia due to gram-negative bacilli, the patient is febrile and the extremities are warm. During this early pyrogenic phase of acute circulatory failure, cardiac output, stroke volume, and pulse pressure are increased, and arterial vasodilatation predominates. This is the syndrome that has been labeled "warm shock." Adrenergic effects are not prominent at this stage. There is an increased circulatory demand that cannot be met. As a result, hypoxia, oliguria, and alterations in the sensorium begin to occur. With progression of shock, cardiac output is decreased secondary to a reduction in effective blood volume due to what appears to be pooling of blood in the venous capacitance bed. At this stage (so-called "cold shock") the more typical clinical changes of shock (pallor; cold, clammy extremities; peripheral cyanosis) are observed, and adrenergic response dominates the picture. This stage of shock is characterized by reduced cardiac output, increased peripheral arterial resistance, decreased central venous pressure, and decreased tissue perfusion and oxygenation. Decline in renal perfusion results in reduction of urine output. As tissue hypoxia increases, serum lactic acid levels rise, and blood pH and bicarbonate fall. If the shock is of severe degree and persists for a protracted period, the picture of "shock lung" develops. "Shock lung" is one form of a distinctive clinical picture of acute respiratory failure (developing in previously normal lungs) that has been recognized since the late 1960s in adults and has been designated "adult respiratory distress syndrome" (ARDS). The process is often initiated by hemorrhagic or septic shock but may be a consequence of a variety of diverse processes such as acute pancreatitis, aspiration of gastric contents, or drug overdosage. The common thread here is the ability to damage the pulmonary microcirculation and to cause leakage of fluid eventuating in pulmonary edema. Pulmonary edema is magnified by increases in hydrostatic pressure in the lung microvasculature, often occurring as a consequence of the administration of large quantities of fluid required to maintain adequate blood pressure and urine flow. Another factor in ARDS is atelectasis, probably secondary to damage to type II lining cells and their capacity to form surfactant. The lungs become stiff, and ventilation is driven reflexly by juxtacapillary reflexes (J reflex) and by arterial hypoxemia. Increasing venous admixture is caused by the combination of pulmonary edema, atelectasis, and ventilation-perfusion abnormalities. The accompanying elevation of pulmonary vascular resistance increases the work load on the right ventricle and raises the right ventricular end-diastolic volume. Patients in whom prolonged septic shock has been reversed may nevertheless die from acute respiratory insufficiency as a result of this type of pulmonary difficulty. Persistence of shock leads to intense vasoconstriction of both the arterial and venous sides of the microcirculation. Eventually, the precapillary arterial vasoconstriction diminishes without a concomitant decrease on the venous side. A consequence of this is a high degree of congestion in the pulmonary capillary bed. Hypoxia and lactic acidosis intensify.

Other Circulatory Changes

The elevation of body temperature accompanying infection is usually associated with a proportional increase in heart rate. Relative bradycardia is seen during infections due to gram-negative bacilli (e.g., typhoid fever, tularemia). Endotoxin has been suggested as the element inducing this peculiar response. The definition of the actual microbial component inducing the response seems more complex than this, however, since relative bradycardia is also observed in viral diseases (dengue, yellow fever), mycoplasma infections (primary atypical pneumonia), and during illness due to *Chlamydia* (psittacosis). Bradycardia (accompanied by hypertension) may be present in infections of the central nervous system (meningitis, subdural empyema, brain abscess, and encephalitis) as a consequence of increased intracranial pressure.

Reversible Alterations of Sensorium—Confusion, Delirium, Stupor, and Coma

Alterations of sensorium occur in many infectious diseases in the absence either of cerebral invasion by the attacking microorganism or of histologic evidence of inflammatory brain disease. Stupor and coma are usually more evident and more severe in systemic infections in which high fever and hypotension are prominent features. However, such changes may occur in the absence of hypotension or extreme hyperthermia. They are usually reversible and disappear when the infection is brought under control. The usual sequence involves a progressive change from a state of drowsiness and confusion to stupor and finally coma. The pathophysiologic alterations producing these changes are not well understood.

In the presence of severe hypotension (systolic level below 70 to 75 mm Hg), the cerebral metabolic rate is reduced as a result of decreased blood flow to the brain. This may account for the stupor or coma often seen in septic shock. Extremes of hyperthermia (106° F or higher) or hypothermia (below 97° F) may develop during bacteremia or septic shock and are thought to induce coma by altering neuronal metabolism nonspecifically. Hyperthermia due to any cause may initiate a convulsion (febrile seizure) in infants and young children, presumably through temporary alterations in cerebral cortical function. Alterations in sensorium that occur in some bacterial infections are thought to be due to "toxins" elaborated by the organisms. However, such toxins have not been isolated, and their role remains hypothetical. Cerebral metabolic rate is reduced while blood flow remains normal in the course of coma associated with some systemic infections.

A severe and extreme example of alteration of cerebral function during the course of infection is *acute toxic encephalopathy*. This syndrome occurs during or following bacterial or viral disease. It is characterized by fever, confusion, stupor, and coma. Generalized convulsive seizures are prominent and, unlike simple febrile convulsions, are recurrent. Focal disease of the cerebrum or brain stem is absent. Although bacterial "toxins" have been proposed as the cause of the cerebral changes, no clear-cut substantiating evidence is available. There does not appear to be a close correlation between the severity of the initiating infection and the degree of neurologic dysfunction. Contributing factors initiating the process may be fever, hypoxia, and cerebral edema secondary to water intoxication.

Skin Reactions in Disseminated Infection

Skin eruptions of differing morphology are frequently associated with systemic bacterial or viral infections. The cutaneous changes may be produced in several different ways:

1. Bacteremic or viremic spread to the skin, with local proliferation of the organism (subcutaneous abscesses in *Staphylococcus aureus* bacteremia, cutaneous vesicles in disseminated Herpes simplex infection of infants).

2. Development of a cutaneous vasculitis. The etiologic agent (bacteria or virus) may or may not be found in the vessel wall or surrounding dermis.

3. The damaging effect of antigen-antibody complexes on the skin or, possibly, the development of delayed hypersensitivity to the infecting agent.

Staphylococcal infections are an example of bacteremic skin lesions due to direct invasion of skin. Frank, fluctuant subcutaneous abscesses, nodular subcutaneous lesions, pustules, and purulent purpura (a small area of hemorrhage with a white purulent center) may be present. *S. aureus* can be demonstrated without any difficulty in any of these lesions. Vasculitis involving small blood vessels of the skin may occur in the absence of demonstrable localization of bacteria. The macular, papular, nodular, and petechial lesions of chronic meningococcemia are examples of this phenomenon. The painful, nodular pretibial lesions of erythema nodosum exhibit a prominent element of vasculitis, but the instigating organism in certain cases is located at a distance from the subcutaneous lesions (e.g., streptococcal pharyngitis). Vasculitis of the skin may also be associated with direct invasion of the vessel wall by bacteria. A characteristic example of this is the widespread involvement of blood vessels that occurs in the course of *Pseudomonas* bacteremia. Bullous, hemorrhagic, and necrotic skin lesions develop as a result of intramural bacterial proliferation, which leads to occlusion of vessels by fibrin thrombi.

Immunologic factors may play a role in the production of the skin lesions in certain systemic infections, particularly in the case of some viral exanthems. Measles is a good example of this. The pathogenesis of the rash in this disease is not clearly established. It could be the result either of direct viral invasion of the epidermal and vascular endothelial cells or of damage induced locally by a virus-antibody complex. There is some evidence in support of the latter concept. The time of appearance of the rash coincides with the appearance of circulating antibody. Another intriguing bit of evidence is the absence of rash in some children, usually those with leukemia, who develop chronic measles with giant cell pneumonia but do not produce specific antibody. The use of inactivated measles virus vaccine has suggested an altered cutaneous reactivity in the host. Individuals pre-viously immunized with this agent develop an atypical measles syndrome characterized by unusual skin lesions (petechiae, purpura, urticaria, or vesicles superimposed on a maculopapular rash) following exposure several years later to the natural disease. Local reactions, consisting of erythema and vesicle formation, have developed at the site of live measles vaccine injection in patients who had previously received inactivated measles vaccine. Little is known of the exact basis of these reactions. It is of interest in this regard, however, that a high incidence of delayed hypersensitivity to antigens in inactivated measles vaccine has been demonstrated in recipients of the killed vaccine.

Hematologic Changes

A variety of alterations of blood elements occur during the course of human infectious diseases. They are common; the magnitude of the changes is usually minor and contributes little to the overall symptomatology or clinical findings. On occasion, however, they may be so profound as to dominate the clinical picture completely or to influence significantly the host response to the infection.

Changes in Circulating Neutrophils. Most infections due to pyogenic bacteria are accompanied by a polymorphonuclear leukocytosis. A relation between this response and the inflammatory reaction at the site of the infectious process has been inferred from the known phagocytic function of these cells and their presence in abundance in the early stages of inflammation. The best insights into the dynamics of the neutrophil response to infection have evolved from studies of neutrophil kinetics employing radioactive isotopic techniques.

Polymorphonuclear leukocytes are produced continuously in the bone marrow through the differentiation of precursor myeloid cells. Upon maturation, the granulocytes enter the marrow storage pool, one of several "pools" in the body. From the *marrow pool* they are discharged into the circulation, where they enter either the *circulating granulocyte pool* (CGP) or the *marginal granulocyte pool* (MGP). The former is made up of actively circulating cells, whereas the latter consists of granulocytes that are sequestered, or "marginated," in various capillary beds. Prompt increases in numbers of circulating granulocytes that result from exercise or injection of catecholamines involve movement of the marginated leukocytes into the circulating pool. The size of the CGP depends on three concurrent processes: (1) rate of release from marrow, (2) proportion of granulocytes held in MGP, and (3) rate of loss of granulocytes into tissues.

It has been difficult to study leukokinetics in acute infections of humans because patients are not seen until disease is well established and treatment initiated. However, acute infections have been studied in experimental animals (pneumococcal pneumonia in the dog) and have provided valuable insights into the kinetics of the response. The sequence of events that takes place is as follows: (1) Infection produces an increased demand for migration of granulocytes from the CGP. (2) Egress from the blood is via diapedesis from the MGP; an increase in the size of this pool is required for this. However, migration from the MGP to the tissues is a one-way street; there is no evidence that the granulocytes re-enter the circulation from infected areas. (3) The marrow responds to the foregoing with acceleration of the rate of release of cells from the marrow storage pool. This might involve a feedback loop mediated by a serum factor. Also contributing to the marrow response is a subsequent wave of differentiation down the myeloid pathway to the granulocyte level. (4) Enlargement of the CGP occurs only after the acceleration of release from the marrow storage pool has exceeded the enhanced rate of movement from the blood into the tissues. Within 4 hours of inoculation of pneumococci, an accelerated rate of release of neutrophils from bone marrow to blood, as indicated by an increase in the ratio of band forms to segmented forms, can be observed. This can sometimes be detected before there is an increase in the numbers of circulating neutrophils in venous blood. This lag period before the rise in neutrophil count appears to be the result of restoration of the MGP before the CGP.

An occasional patient with severe pneumococcal pneumonia will develop severe neutropenia. When this same response occurs in the experimental animal, it is associated with an acceleration of marrow neutrophil release and a marked increase in the ratio of band to segmented forms. Neutropenia in this situation stems from inability of the marrow to replenish the accelerated cell loss to the sites of tissue inflammation. Data from kinetic studies with labeled cells as well as examination of marrow (loss of mature neutrophils) suggest exhaustion of the marrow granulocyte pool. There is no evidence that infection blocks release of neutrophils from the marrow. The well-known poor prognosis of such severe pneumococcal (and other bacterial) infections is more readily understandable if the mechanism of the neutropenia is depletion of the marrow granulocyte reserve.

In certain bacterial infections, particularly typhoid fever, leukopenia is a common finding. The basis for this phenomenon is not known. However, it is of interest that a similar blood picture features the initial response in rabbits and humans to the injection of gram-negative bacilli or of bacterial endotoxin. This occurs at the time of the chill and is followed by leukocytosis in ½ to 4 hours. The initial leukopenia is due to enlargement of the MGP before that of the CGP. The subsequent leukocytosis is secondary to release of cells from both the MGP and the marrow storage pool.

Anemia of Infection. Anemia is a common feature of chronic infections but may occasionally complicate acute ones. In the latter case, the anemia is usually hemolytic. High-grade bacteremia with *Clostridium perfringens* may produce massive intravascular destruction of erythrocytes, with shock and anuria. The production by this organism of a lecithinase (α toxin) and hemolysins (e.g., θ toxin) which act on the membranes of red cells and cause their lysis is the basis for the hemolytic anemia of clostridial bacteremia (see Chapter 19). Primary atypical pneumonia due to *Mycoplasma pneumoniae* is, on rare occasions, complicated by severe hemolysis related to the development of autoantibodies, the cold agglutinins. These are IgM antibodies, most often directed against the I antigen on red blood cells. There is some evidence that certain infectious agents like *M. pneumoniae* may interact with the red blood cell, thus altering the I antigen and making it immunogenic. In patients with congenital deficiency of the erythrocyte enzyme glucose-6-phosphate dehydrogenase (G6PD), episodes of hemolysis may be precipitated by a variety of infections. Bacterial infections (pneumonia) and viral infections (infectious hepatitis) have been associated with hemolytic episodes. Accumulation of metabolites capable of oxidizing glutathione, and thus decreasing the concentration of the reduced form of this compound, has been suggested as the basis for the hemolysis. However, direct exposure of G6PD-deficient erythrocytes to influenza virus produces increased hemolysis; this suggests a direct effect on the red cell rather than an indirect one due to toxic metabolites produced in the host.

The anemia associated with chronic infections is usually normocytic and normochromic but may be normocytic and hypochromic. The infectious process is usually of many weeks' duration, since the life span of the normal erythrocyte is 120 days. Anemia is common in cases of subacute bacterial endocarditis, tuberculosis, brucellosis, and chronic pulmonary infections such as lung abscess and empyema. A decrease in serum iron, serum iron-binding capacity, and saturation of transferrin with iron are the biochemical changes characteristic of this type of anemia. Ferrokinetic and erythrokinetic studies have revealed the following:

1. A rapid rate of clearance of injected iron from the plasma.

2. Normal or only moderately increased erythropoiesis.

3. Mildly shortened erythrocyte survival. The latter finding suggests a *hemolytic process,* yet the usual evidences of increased blood destruction (increased serum bilirubin and urobilinogen excretion) are not present.

4. Increased iron stores in bone marrow and reticuloendothelial system (RES). The reason for this avidity of the RES for iron is unclear. The serum transferrin levels are low, and its turnover rate is increased, findings thought to be due to increased catabolism and decreased synthesis of transferrin.

The pathophysiologic basis for the anemia of infection is not clear. The defect may be in erythropoietin production (the bone marrow has more than enough potential for the replacement of the red cells lost as a result of the shortened red cell survival), RES function, transferrin metabolism, or a combination of these factors. The manner in which bacterial products or the inflammatory response affects any or all of these targets remains a mystery.

Coagulation Defects. Isolated thrombocytopenia may develop during the course of some acute gram-positive and gram-negative bacterial infections. It may also appear immediately before, during, or after some systemic viral diseases such as measles. During bacteremia and viremia, platelets tend to adhere to each other and the vascular endothelium; this probably accounts for their depletion. This adherence may be due to the action of bacterial toxins or other products on the platelet. For example, staphylococcal alpha toxin causes agglutination and lysis of rabbit platelets in vitro. The extent of thrombocytopenia may be sufficient to cause bleeding, usually in the form of petechiae and purpura. Bone marrow depression secondary to the infection may also contribute to the thrombocytopenia to a lesser degree.

A more profound coagulation defect, *disseminated intravascular coagulation* (DIC), may occur as a complication of infections with a variety of agents: gram-positive organisms (group A and group B streptococci, *Pneumococcus*, *Staphylococcus aureus*, *Clostridium perfringens*); gram-negative bacteria (*Meningococcus*, *Escherichia coli*, *Proteus*, *Pseudomonas*, etc.); viruses (varicella, variola, rubella, rubeola, hemorrhagic fevers, etc.); rickettsiae (*Rickettsia rickettsii* of Rocky Mountain spotted fever); protozoa (malaria, *Leishmania donovani* of kala-azar). DIC is a distinct clinical entity in which the clinical manifestations are fever, petechial or purpuric eruption, hypotension, and a widespread hemorrhagic diathesis. Renal failure is usually evident secondary to hypotension or, occasionally, to renal cortical necrosis. Histologically, there is evidence of fibrin deposition in blood vessels of various organs, particularly in the capillaries and venules of the skin. The basic pathophysiology of DIC involves a host response to an underlying illness (many processes other than infection may also trigger this response) that sets off a generalized activation of the normal clotting mechanism. As a result of systemic infection, endothelial damage and inflammation of blood vessel walls occur. The subsequent depletion of fibrinogen

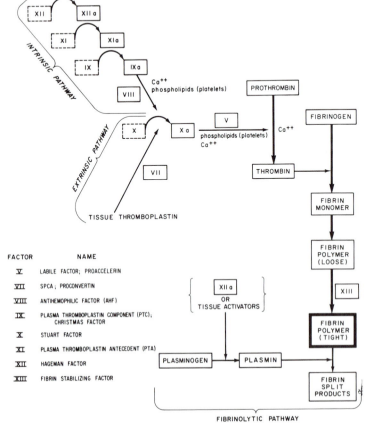

FACTOR	NAME
V	LABILE FACTOR; PROACCELERIN
VII	SPCA ; PROCONVERTIN
VIII	ANTIHEMOPHILIC FACTOR (AHF)
IX	PLASMA THROMBOPLASTIN COMPONENT (PTC); CHRISTMAS FACTOR
X	STUART FACTOR
XI	PLASMA THROMBOPLASTIN ANTECEDENT (PTA)
XII	HAGEMAN FACTOR
XIII	FIBRIN STABILIZING FACTOR

Figure 20–1 Coagulation cascade and fibrinolytic pathway. Clotting factors in [- - - -] represent inert precursor forms of the factors. Clotting factors with subscript "a" in [ ] represent activated forms of the factors. *Intrinsic pathway* for prothrombin conversion to thrombin is initiated by conversion of Hageman factor to its activated form. Cascade follows, in which various clotting factors are sequentially converted from their precursor form to their active form. Activated Factor X with Factor V, platelet phospholipids, and Ca^{++} forms a *prothrombin converting principle,* which liberates thrombin from its precursor, prothrombin. Once thrombin forms, it converts fibrinogen to the fibrin monomer, which after several steps becomes a tight fibrin polymer (clot). *Extrinsic pathway* is initiated by tissue thromboplastins (present in many tissues, particularly blood vessel walls, lung, and brain) that interact with Factor VII, calcium ions, Factor X, and Factor V to form the prothrombin converting principle. This then converts prothrombin to thrombin.

The *fibrinolytic pathway* is initiated by the conversion of the inactive proteolytic enzyme plasminogen, present in all body fluids, to its active form, plasmin. This conversion is activated either by Factor XIIa or by activators present in tissues and vascular endothelium. Plasmin then cleaves fibrin, releasing fibrin split products.

and other clotting components and the ensuing clinical bleeding diathesis are the results of two fundamental processes: (1) activation, by endothelial damage, of the coagulation sequence, leading to the generation of thrombin; and (2) activation of the natural defense of the body (fibrinolytic system) against widespread clotting initiated by uncontrolled thrombin production.

The current state of knowledge suggests that the following sequence of events is involved in the coagulation aspect of DIC. The initiating event is a vascular injury such as occurs in meningococcemia, Rocky Mountain spotted fever, and so on. This can activate the clotting mechanism in three ways:

1. *Activation of the Intrinsic Clotting System.* Loss of integrity of the vascular endothelium exposes the circulating blood to collagen, which converts Factor XII (Hageman factor) from an inert precursor to its enzymatically active form, which then initiates the intrinsic clotting cascade (Fig. 20–1) by converting Factor XI, plasma thromboplastin antecedent (PTA), from the precursor to the active form. Activated Factor XI then activates Factor IX (Christmas factor, or plasma thromboplastin component [PTC]). Activated Factor IX forms a complex with Factor VIII (antihemophilic factor) and with platelet phospholipids (platelet Factor III). This complex then activates Factor X (Stuart factor). Activated Factor X, in the presence of platelet phospholipids and Factor V (proaccelerin), forms a complex that converts prothrombin (Factor II) into thrombin. Thrombin then transforms soluble fibrinogen (Factor I) to the still soluble fibrin monomer. The latter then polymerizes and is converted to the stable insoluble fibrin polymer by the action of the Factor XIII (fibrin-stabilizing factor). Factor XIII exists as an inert precursor and must be activated by thrombin before it can act on the fibrin polymer. In addition to converting fibrinogen to fibrin and to activating Factor XIII, thrombin enhances the activities of both the activated Factor IX–Factor VIII–phospholipid complex and the activated Factor X–Factor V–phospholipid complex, thus accelerating its own formation.

2. *Activation of the Extrinsic Clotting System.* Vascular injury secondary to infection releases tissue thromboplastin (probably from the walls of blood vessels) which interacts with calcium and Factor VII (serum prothrombin conversion accelerator) to form a complex capable of activating Factor X. At this point, the extrinsic clotting system joins the intrinsic system, and the steps leading to the formation of fibrin are identical.

3. *Activation of the Plasma Kallikrein System.* Shock may occur during the course of infections with a wide variety of organisms. However, shock per se, regardless of its cause, can induce intravascular coagulation. Endothelial damage due to infection or due to endotoxin is capable of activat-

ing Factor XII (Fig. 20–2). Activated Factor XII or its derivatives are able to activate plasma prekallikrein to the active enzyme kallikrein. This results in elaboration of bradykinin, a highly potent vasodepressor, from its precursor plasma kininogen. Thus, the same trigger point, Factor XII activation, appears capable of initiating both activation of the coagulation pathway directly and bacteremic shock via the kallikrein-kinin system. Once developed, shock itself may elicit further intravascular coagulation. In keeping with this interrelation is the clinical observation that DIC commonly occurs in patients with bacteremia and hypotension but does not develop when infection is unaccompanied by hypotension. However, it is still not clear whether the intravascular coagulation appears first and causes shock and hypoxia, or vice versa.

Once thrombin has been generated into the circulation during the coagulation process, several mechanisms come into play to limit its unimpeded action. One is its rapid removal by adsorption to the newly formed fibrin gel and another is its slow inactivation by a serum factor, antithrombin III. The most important mechanism for interfering with the action of thrombin involves plasmin (fibrinolysin), which destroys fibrinogen, the substrate for thrombin. Plasmin is a potent but relatively nonspecific proteolytic enzyme that degrades many proteins, including fibrinogen. Activation of the plasmin system involves cleavage of an inert circulating protein, plasminogen, by activated Factor XII. This results in the conversion of plasminogen to the active enzyme plasmin, which then acts on fibrinogen to degrade it into a series of large and small fragments. It also digests fibrin; this results in the production of polypeptides (fibrin split products). A potent anticoagulant activity is produced when fibrinogen is cleaved by plasmin. The anticoagulants are two large fragments of fibrinogen that act as (1) competitive inhibitors of fibrinogen for thrombin, and (2) blockers of the formation of a tight fibrin gel by interposing between fibrin polymers as they are forming.

The inappropriate and extensive clotting process proceeds at an accelerated rate in DIC. Fibrin deposition extends throughout the vascular tree, causing local tissue necrosis and more extensive organ damage. Soon, hemorrhage becomes a major clinical feature as blood coagulation factors are depleted (V, VIII, prothrombin, fibrinogen), and fibrin can no longer be formed. Aggravating the coagulation picture is the activation of the fibrinolytic system. Five major events are involved to produce the net result—incoagulable blood: (1) depletion, during coagulation, of blood clotting components, (2) depletion of fibrinogen by the intravascular clotting, (3) plasmin-mediated digestion of fibrinogen and possibly Factors V and VIII, (4) suppression of thrombin action by the split

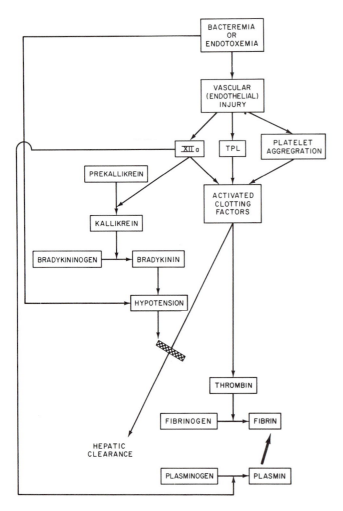

Figure 20–2 Pathogenesis of disseminated intravascular coagulation (DIC). The chain of events initiated by bacteremia is shown schematically. Vascular injury has a central role. It causes activation of Factor XII, release of tissue thromboplastins (TPL), and aggregation of platelets. All three then initiate activation of clotting factors, XIIa by the intrinsic pathway, and TPL and platelet aggregation by the extrinsic pathway. Thrombin generation and fibrinogen conversion to fibrin occur intravascularly.

Activation of Factor XII contributes to intravascular coagulation by another mechanism as well. Factor XIIa (activated factor XII) interacts with the kallikrein-kinin system, converting prekallikrein (kallikreinogen) to its active form, kallikrein. Plasma kallikrein, in turn, acts on its major substrate, bradykininogen, releasing the nonapeptide bradykinin, a powerful vasodilator. Hypotension and shock develop as a result of the activity of bradykinin. The effects of these circulatory changes are to decrease the hepatic clearance rate of activated clotting factors and to induce additional intravascular clotting. Hypotension induced directly as a result of bacteremia by mechanisms other than the kinin pathway similarly decreases hepatic processing of clotting factors and enhances intravascular coagulation.

Activation of Factor XII has a third major effect, one related to its role in the activation of plasminogen to plasmin. Plasmin furthers the incoagulability of blood in DIC by attacking fibrinogen and fibrin to produce split products that inhibit thrombin and fibrin polymerization.

products of fibrinogen and fibrin, and (5) inhibition of fibrin polymerization by the split products of fibrinogen and fibrin.

Treatment of DIC is aimed at control of the underlying infection with the appropriate antibiotic and management of any accompanying shock. The potent anticoagulant heparin has been used in the treatment of DIC accompanying septicemia when there have been evidences of bleeding, but it appears to have been effective in only a minority of patients.

SPECIAL HOST RESPONSES

Eosinophilia and Eosinopenia

Eosinophils are present in all species above the most primitive vertebrates, and their appearance in evolution roughly parallels that of complex lymphocyte-mediated immune systems. Although eosinophils do not seem important in defense against most invading microorganisms, they do appear to confer some protection against certain helminthic parasites. In addition, eosinophils serve to modulate tissue reactions in which mast cells or basophils degranulate and release potent mediators of inflammation (histamine, slow-reacting substance of anaphylaxis). Previously it was thought that phagocytosis of immune complexes was a unique function of the eosinophil, but it is now clear that such complexes are readily phagocytosed by polymorphonuclear neutrophils and mononuclear cells as well. The fact that eosinophils are not commonly present in tissues in immune-complex diseases (glomerulonephritis, lupus nephritis) further indicates that the eosinophil does not have a special role in the removal of such complexes. Infection can profoundly affect the number of circulating eosinophils: A striking eosinophilia develops in the course of infection with certain metazoan helminths, and a marked diminution occurs during acute bacterial infections.

The circulating eosinophil is believed to be an end-cell. Its maturation takes place in the bone marrow, where it enters a reserve pool several orders of magnitude larger than the total of circulating eosinophils. Upon release from the marrow, it circulates for only a few hours in the blood before migrating into tissue sites, where it dies or is extruded from a mucosal surface.

Much of current knowledge of the eosinophilic response has developed from the studies of Beeson and his coworkers on parasitic infection of the rat with the nematode *Trichinella spiralis*. Following intravenous injection larvae are trapped (and die) in the lungs, where they elicit a granulomatous response. Eosinophilia develops in about 3 days and appears to be the result of interaction between intact parasites and host cells, since it does not occur if homogenized larvae (fragments small enough to pass through the pulmonary vessels) are infused intravenously.

Production of eosinophils by the bone marrow consists of an inductive and a proliferative stage analogous to the phases of antibody production to a specific antigen. A role for the lymphocyte in the inductive phase is suggested by the fact that depletion of the pool of recirculating lymphocytes (antilymphocyte serum, cortisone) a few hours before (but not 24 hours after) the intravenous injection of *T. spiralis* blocks the development of eosinophilia. More direct evidence of a role for the lymphocyte in inducing an eosinophilic response is provided by lymphocyte transfer studies: Injection of thoracic duct lymphocytes from animals in the early (intestinal) phase of the natural form of trichinosis into recipients causes an eosinophilia 3 or 4 days later. Also, a role for the lymphocyte can be shown in the test model employing intravenous injection of *T. spiralis* larvae. Whole-body irradiation blocks development of the eosinophilic response, which can be restored by infusion of bone marrow cells and lymphocytes from normal syngeneic donors. An enhanced response occurs in irradiated animals reconstituted with normal bone marrow and lymphocytes from animals with trichinosis, suggesting a cooperative interaction between lymphocytes (exhibiting "memory" from prior contact with *T. spiralis*) and eosinophil precursors in the marrow. Analogous to the secondary antibody response, a second intravenous challenge with *T. spiralis* larvae produces an enhanced eosinophil response as an indication also of immunologic memory. The stimulation of eosinopoiesis by lymphocytes appears to be mediated by a diffusible product: Thoracic-duct lymphocytes from rats with naturally acquired trichinosis evoke eosinophilia in syngeneic recipients when placed into the peritoneal cavity with a millipore diffusion chamber.

The T-lymphocytes (thymus-processed) appear to be the ones involved in inducing the eosinophilic response. Thymectomized mice fail to develop an eosinophilic reaction to trichinosis but do respond to acute bacterial infections with an increase in neutrophils. Reconstitution of these animals with graft of thymus tissue permits a normal eosinophil response to trichinosis. The use of antisera to effect selective removal of B- or T-lymphocytes further supports the role of the T-cell.

Following the induction phase, the proliferative phase of the eosinophilic response occurs, characterized by a 16- to 64-fold increase in formation of eosinophils. This phase cannot be blocked by antilymphocyte serum, but it is inhibited by immunosuppressive drugs, such as methotrexate and cyclophosphamide, administered 24 hours after the antigen. A role for "eosinophilopoietin," a small polypeptide described by Mahmoud and coworkers, in the proliferative phase has been suggested. This material is found in the serum of mice rendered eosinopenic by repeated administration of rabbit anti-mouse eosinophil serum. Injection of serum from such eosinopenic mice into normal mice produces an increased production of marrow eosinophils. It is not yet known whether "eosinophilopoietin" is a product of T-lymphocytes.

Eosinopenia is a characteristic feature of the host response to acute bacterial infections. A similar response occurs in experimental animals with pneumococcal, *Escherichia coli,* and coxsackievirus infections and with sterile inflammation due to turpentine. This suggests that the effect is not due to a specific pathogen or toxin but rather to an acute inflammation, but this can be reversed by elimination of the inflammatory (infectious) stimulus. Such inflammation can markedly suppress the eosinophilia of trichinosis. Eosinopenia is part of the normal response to stress. Since administration of glucocorticosteroids causes eosinopenia, it had been assumed that the eosinopenia of acute infection is a nonspecific aspect of the hormonal response to the stress of acute infection. However, recent studies indicate that the eosinopenia of acute infection is independent of the adrenal response to nonspecific stress: The eosinopenic response to acute inflammation occurs prior to the rise in serum corticosterone level and occurs normally in adrenalectomized animals. The marked decrease in circulating eosinophils during acute inflammation is due to both a rapid accumulation of eosinophils at the periphery of the inflammatory lesion and a suppression of the discharge of eosinophils from bone marrow. Prolongation of the inflammation causes suppression of eosinopoiesis as well. A protein (molecular weight of greater than 30,000 daltons) capable of producing an eosinopenic response when injected into mice with trichinosis has been found in inflammatory exudates. The response it induces is so rapid as to suggest a direct effect on eosinophils (e.g., by inducing intravascular margination).

The best evidence for the possible role of the eosinophil in defense against multicellular parasitic invaders comes from studies of schistosomiasis and trichinosis. Resistance to reinfection with *Schistosoma mansoni* develops in mice and rats after primary infection, and it can be passively transferred with serum (but not cells). This immune response is directed mainly at the migration of young worms (schistosomules) following cercarial penetration of the skin. Such penetration elicits a prompt eosinophilic inflammatory response in the immune animal. Within 12 hours, degenerating schistosomules can be observed in the dermis surrounded by masses of eosinophils. Pretreatment of immune mice with nonspecific antieosinophil serum (but not antilymphocyte, antimacrophage, or antineutrophil serum) abrogates the immunity, and the numbers of schistosomules and adult worms increase to the levels found in nonimmune animals. Sera from partially immune mice, passively transferred to uninfected mice, confer marked resistance to infection as measured by decreased recovery of schistosomules. Antieosinophil serum administered to the recipient blocks this passively transferred immunity. Thus, it appears that antibody-dependent, cell-mediated immunity to schistosomiasis occurs in vivo and involves the eosinophil. A similar role for the eosinophil in defense against *T. spiralis* is suggested by the markedly increased number of viable encysted larvae found in muscles of animals depleted of eosinophils by treatment with antieosinophil serum.

Lymphocytosis

An absolute lymphocytosis of great magnitude and consisting of mature lymphocytes is characteristic of two infectious diseases: pertussis and infectious lymphocytosis (an unusual viral disease of children). The parenteral injection of killed virulent *Bordetella pertussis* organisms produces a marked lymphocytosis in a variety of vertebrate species. Lymphocytosis-promoting factor (LPF), a polypeptide of molecular weight approximately 70,000 released into the supernatant of cultures of *B. pertussis*, evokes a lymphocytosis on intravenous injection. Morse and his coworkers have elucidated the mechanism of this lymphocytosis by demonstrating that the peripheral lymphocytosis is accompanied by depletion of small lymphocytes in thymus, spleen, and lymph nodes. The lymphocyte content of thoracic duct lymph is markedly reduced, indicating that the cells enter the circulation from lymphoid organs by a more direct route. Once in the circulation, lymphocytes no longer migrate back to lymph nodes and other areas across postcapillary venules. It appears that migration is impaired owing to changes on the lymphocyte surface, possibly produced by adsorption of LPF onto the cell membrane. Lymphocytosis featured primarily by atypical lymphocytes ("viral cells") develops in other diseases such as infectious mononucleosis and infectious hepatitis. The Epstein-Barr virus, the etiology of infectious mononucleosis, infects only B-lymphocytes. The atypical lymphocytes that are so prominent in this disease are T-cells, suggesting that these uninfected cells play an important role in the immune response to this viral agent.

Alterations Due to the Immune Response of the Host

One of the major defenses of the host against bacterial and viral disease is the mounting of an antibody response. This may be of great importance in the complement-dependent bactericidal reaction against gram-negative bacilli and in the phagocytosis and intracellular killing, by polymorphonuclear leukocytes, of various species of bacteria and viruses. The presence of specific circulating antibody also provides protection against reinfection on re-exposure to the same microorganism. The role of type-specific antibody to the pneumococcal capsular polysaccharide in the response of the host to pneumococcal infection (pneumonia) was manifest, during the preantibiotic era, in the dramatic clinical improvement that occurred coincident with the appearance of circulating antibody. The development of an immune response against an invading organism is, however, not invariably a salutary event. Occasionally, this may result in injury to the host and the appearance of overt clinical disease. Several examples will be cited here to illustrate this phenomenon, but no attempt will be made to be encyclopedic.

Immune Complex Disease. Circulating antigen-antibody complexes contribute to the pathophysiology and pathology of at least several human diseases such as acute poststreptococcal glomerulonephritis and viral hepatitis.

Poststreptococcal glomerulonephritis appears to be primarily an immunologic disorder in which antigen-antibody complexes are produced and subsequently trapped in or adjacent to the glomerular capillary walls. Evidence for this is the following: (1) The appearance of the disease after a latent period following streptococcal infection. (2) The high titers of antibodies to streptococcal products present in the sera of patients. (3) The involvement of only certain type-specific strains of group A streptococci in outbreaks of acute glomerulonephritis. (4) The reduction of complement levels in the sera of patients. (5) The presence of granular and lumpy deposits of complement and bound gamma globulin in the glomerular capillary walls and near the renal basement membrane. These deposits are similar to those observed on electron microscopy and by immunofluorescence in experimentally induced immune complex glomerulonephritis. (6) Demonstration of streptococcal antigen (cell wall rather than cell membrane in origin) in the glomeruli. However, the presence of streptococcal antigen in the nodular, gamma globulin and complement-containing deposits in the kidney must be proved by elution techniques. (7) Development of a possible laboratory model in the rat of experimental poststreptococcal glomerulonephritis. This involves intraperitoneal implantation of millipore chambers containing group A streptococci. Proteinuria develops a short time after the appearance of type-specific antibodies in the serum and simultaneous with the demonstration of bound gamma globulin, complement, and streptococcal M protein in the region of the glomerular basement membrane.

The circulating soluble immune complexes appear capable of mediating immunologic injury following deposition on the glomerular basement membrane through activation of complement and stimulation of an inflammatory response consisting of polymorphonuclear leukocytes. This glomerular inflammation accounts for many of the clinical manifestations of acute glomerulonephritis such as hematuria, proteinuria, edema, hypertension, and azotemia.

Immunopathologic mechanisms appear to be involved also in the development of glomerulonephritis following pneumococcal infection. Glomerular bound C3, pneumococcal polysaccharide, and properdin are observed as well as subepithelial and intramembranous electron-dense deposits, suggesting that activation of the alternate complement pathway by the pneumococcal capsular antigen has occurred.

Circulating immune complexes appear to be involved in the pathogenesis of the glomerulonephritis that occurs in other infections such as bacterial endocarditis, quartan malaria, infected ventriculoatrial shunt pathways, and possibly secondary syphilis. With the exception of secondary syphilis, the feature common to these disorders is a chronic relapsing course. Instances of diffuse glomerulonephritis as a complication of bacterial endocarditis due to a variety of organisms have been reported. These include *Streptococcus viridans*, *Staphylococcus aureus*, *S. epidermidis*, and group G streptococci.

Antibody-Induced Agglutination and Hemolysis of Erythrocytes. Cold agglutinins develop in 50 per cent or more of individuals with primary atypical pneumonia due to *Mycoplasma pneumoniae*. They may also appear in high titer in patients with the protozoan disease trypanosomiasis. Although the incidence of these antibodies in mycoplasma pneumonia is high, acute hemolytic anemia develops only rarely, most often toward the end of the second week of illness and is featured by fever, prostration, and hypotension. The latter or, less commonly, hemoglobinemia and hemoglobinuria may lead to renal failure.

Amyloid Disease. A variety of chronic infectious diseases may be complicated by the development of amyloidosis. These include tuberculosis, leprosy, chronic osteomyelitis, and chronic bronchiectasis. The clinical manifestations and pathophysiologic consequences depend on the major sites of deposition of the amyloid. The kidneys, spleen, liver, and adrenal glands are most commonly affected, but the nervous system, gastrointestinal tract, blood vessels, and heart may be damaged as well. Deposition in the kidney is usually manifest by proteinuria and the nephrotic syndrome and

may lead to progressive renal insufficiency. Nervous system amyloidosis is characterized by a peripheral combined sensory-motor polyneuropathy involving the distal extremities initially. Involvement of the heart usually occurs in the older age group, and its clinical correlates include myocardial failure, conduction disturbances, coronary artery insufficiency, and restrictive cardiomyopathy presenting a clinical picture of chronic constrictive pericarditis.

Several studies have established that, in some instances, amyloidosis consists of the deposition in various organs of specific fragments of immunoglobulins. The insolubility of partially purified amyloid fibrils had raised some question as to the relation of amyloid to the immunoglobulins and presented problems in its further purification. However, it has been possible to solubilize these fibrils and to analyze their composition. Such amyloid fibrils are made up of the amino-terminal variable portion of the kappa or lambda light chain of immunoglobulin molecules as determined by amino acid sequencing studies. Further support for the immunoglobulin origin of amyloid fibrils is derived from the in-vitro conversion, by proteolytic digestion, of a soluble light chain (Bence Jones protein), with production of insoluble fibrils having the staining properties of amyloid and a partial amino acid sequence derived from the amino-terminal variable region of the Bence Jones protein.

The mechanism of formation and the specific localizations in tissues of amyloid are not clearly understood. It has been reported that Bence Jones proteins from patients with amyloidosis have a greater tendency to bind to kidney, liver, and heart muscle than those from individuals with myeloma uncomplicated by amyloidosis. The possible route for generation of the amyloid fibril is unclear. It has been suggested that antigen-antibody complexes may be processed by macrophages and the immunoglobulin degraded in such a manner as to produce fibrils that are then deposited in the macrophage-rich organs such as liver and spleen. It has also been postulated that free whole immunoglobulins (as in chronic infections) or free light chains (as in myeloma) circulating in increased concentrations may be the immediate source of the fibrils in the vascular system.

Another protein, unrelated to known immunoglobulins and designated "amyloid A (AA) protein," is present in the amyloid of patients with secondary amyloidosis, that form of the disease associated with chronic infectious diseases such as osteomyelitis, leprosy, and tuberculosis. In human serum, there is normally a protein (SAA) antigenically related to the AA protein of secondary amyloid. Circulating SAA is increased in infection and inflammation and appears to act like an acute phase reactant. Thus, it is possible that the prolonged production of endogenous pyrogen in association with chronic infection can cause continuation of the acute phase response (including increases in SAA) and ultimately lead to secondary amyloidosis.

Unusual Responses of the Host to Viral Disease

Hypersensitivity Induced by Viral Agents— Postinfectious Encephalomyelitides. Demyelinating encephalitis occasionally follows some viral infections, particularly measles, vaccinia, rubella, and varicella. The disorder occurs most commonly on the fourth or fifth day after the rash but may develop earlier or later. The histologic pattern is that of a lymphoplasmacytic infiltration of the adventitia of cerebral blood vessels with microglial proliferation in the perivascular spaces. Distinctive perivenous demyelinization is a prominent feature. The infecting virus has not been isolated from the brain or spinal cord of patients with this disease. However, it is important to note that in a few cases of measles encephalitis, cytoplasmic and nuclear inclusion bodies as well as small multinuclear giant cells have been found, suggesting direct viral invasion of brain tissue.

Similar histologic lesions are observed in the brain and spinal cord of laboratory animals in which experimental allergic encephalomyelitis has been produced by a single injection of brain or spinal cord tissue suspended in Freund's adjuvant. The immunologic basis of this disease is suggested by several features: (1) It occurs nine days or more following the injection; there is a shorter latent period when animals that have recovered are reinjected, as would be expected in a secondary response. (2) The inciting ingredient is specific, namely, myelin-containing tissues. (3) The pathologic changes are distinctive and are limited, for the most part, to the white matter. (4) Brain-reactive antibodies are demonstrable in serum, and lymphoid cells cause cytopathic effects on myelinated brain tissue and glial cells in tissue culture. Although antibodies are present in serum, the lesions appear to be due to the cellular type of immunity as judged by (a) a delayed type skin response to intradermal injection of myelinated tissue in affected animals and (b) transfer of the disease from affected animals by lymphocytes but not by serum. The neurologic signs are extremely varied, reflecting the patchy distribution of the lesions; they may include pyramidal tract involvement, akinetic mutism, cortical blindness, cerebellar ataxia, choreiform movements, and so on.

It is tempting to relate the experimental disease to the naturally occurring encephalomyelitis that develops following viral infections. Release of, and hypersensitivity to, myelin basic protein may constitute the common denominator.

Chronic Viral Infections of the Central Nervous System. There are four known chronic viral infections ("slow virus" diseases) of humans: subacute sclerosing panencephalitis (SSPE), kuru, Creutzfeldt-Jakob disease, and progressive multifocal leukoencephalopathy. Common to all these are an incubation period of many months to years and a clinical course of prolonged motor and mental deterioration. The unusual features may be related primarily either to unique properties of the virus or to an unusual host response to a typical viral agent. The agents of kuru and Creutzfeldt-Jakob disease have been transmitted to chimpanzees but have not been cultivated in tissue culture, and they thus are not yet well characterized. However, the agent of SSPE has been identified as the measles virus in tissue culture. (A syndrome of progressive rubella panencephalitis with insidious deterioration of mental and motor function in the second decade of life also has been described.) This disease is uncommon (1 case per million population in the United States), with the onset in childhood. Clinically, it is characterized by progressive motor and mental dysfunction with myoclonic movements. Extremely high levels of measles antibody are present in the spinal fluid and blood. SSPE (measles) viruses have been isolated from lymph nodes as well as from the brains of patients with the disease, suggesting that the infection may be a disseminated one. These viruses have biologic properties that are more characteristic of the laboratory-adapted vaccine strains of measles than of isolates of the wild virus. It has been suggested that these features may be the result of defective viral replication in nondividing neurons. Another, perhaps more appealing, suggestion is that the disease represents an unusual host response to the virus, one characterized by a specific defect in cellular immunity to the agent of measles.

Metabolic Alterations in Infection

A variety of metabolic changes accompany systemic infection. Some may be the direct result of the activity of the infecting agent, some may represent the consequences of epiphenomena such as fever and infection-induced glucocorticoid and aldosterone excess, and others may be related to specific organ dysfunction due to localization of the infectious process (e.g., hepatitis or pyelonephritis). The sorting out of the contributions to the overall picture by each of these elements has not thus far been achieved.

Changes in electrolyte metabolism have been described in a variety of infectious diseases due to extracellular and intracellular agents. Increased urinary losses of sodium and chloride occur in the immediately prefebrile and early symptomatic periods. This may be due to increased renal perfusion and sodium delivery to renal tubules secondary to increased cardiac output early in the febrile phase. Poor dietary intake, vomiting, diarrhea, and sweating may contribute to electrolyte loss. In sum, these factors probably account for the hyponatremia and hypochloridemia observed at the height of symptoms. The initial heightened urinary sodium and chloride loss is followed by renal retention of sodium coincident with increasing compensatory aldosterone secretion.

In chronic infections involving the lung (slowly resolving pneumonias, pulmonary tuberculosis) and central nervous system infections (tuberculous meningitis), water retention and hyponatremia may develop secondary to inappropriate antidiuretic hormone activity (ADH). The role of hyponatremia in the symptoms of acute infections is not established, but it may contribute to the asthenia and malaise that commonly occur.

The most obvious metabolic consequences of acute infection are catabolic. A negative nitrogen balance occurs regularly during infections but does not begin until after the onset of symptoms. It is usually paralleled by potassium losses. The role of these catabolic changes in the not infrequent occurrence of the troublesome and prolonged postinfectious asthenia is still speculative.

Alterations in whole blood amino acid concentrations have been observed during the course of a variety of experimentally induced infections in humans. An increase in the total amino acid concentration occurs during the incubation period of typhoid fever. This is followed by a decrease in amino acid concentrations, accompanying the development of overt clinical illness. It is not clear whether these alterations are the direct effect of the infectious agent on host amino acid metabolism or the consequence of a nonspecific host response to stress mediated by adrenocorticosteroids. No clinical manifestations have been directly attributable to these biochemical changes.

Diffuse myalgias are common symptoms in patients with a variety of infections. Occasionally, as with meningococcal disease, they are conspicuous manifestations. Rarely, muscle involvement in the course of systemic infection is extreme, resulting in the picture of rhabdomyolysis. Accelerated catabolism of skeletal-muscle protein is a feature of severe infection and undoubtedly accounts in a large measure for the marked weakness observed during the interval following such illnesses. The catabolic response of skeletal muscle has been ascribed to endogenously produced mediators. Clowes and coworkers have observed in the plasma of patients with sepsis a peptide (approximately 4300 daltons and possibly a degradation product of endogenous pyrogen) that stimulates protein degradation in rat or human muscle specimens. Baracos and colleagues have noted that EP (IL-1) produces a rapid increase in muscle proteolysis but does so without affecting the simultaneous rate of muscle protein synthesis. This accelerated proteolysis is mediated through the increased synthesis of prostaglandin E_2 in muscle. Both the enhanced synthesis of prostaglandin E_2 and the accelerated protein breakdown can be blocked by incubation of the muscle with the prostaglandin synthetase inhibitor indomethacin. The accelerated skeletal muscle proteolysis associated with infection may be part of an integrated "protective" host response (acute phase response) directed by IL-1. IL-1 stimulates hepatic protein synthesis (including acute phase plasma proteins) while it accelerates muscle proteolysis. IL-1 seems capable of acting through prostaglandin E both centrally (in generating fever) and peripherally (in stimulating proteolysis) as the key element in the host response to a variety of infecting agents.

Marked elevations in the concentrations of total serum lipids have occurred in patients with severe infections, particularly bacteremia, due to gram-negative bacilli. The lipid pattern consists of a predominant increase in free fatty acids accompanied by lesser increases in triglycerides and phospholipids. In contrast, similar changes in serum lipids have not been observed in severe infections caused by gram-positive cocci. In experimental animals, injection of endotoxin has produced hyperlipidemia, and this component of gram-negative bacilli may be responsible for the changes in lipids during bacterial infections.

REFERENCES

FEVER

Altschule, M. D., and Freedberg, A. S.; Circulation and respiration in fever. Medicine 24:403, 1945.

Atkins, E.: Pathogenesis of fever. Physiol. Rev. 40:580, 1960.

Atkins, E., and Bodel, P.: Fever. N. Engl. J. Med. 286:27, 1972.

Bennett, I. L., Jr., and Beeson, P. B.: The properties and biological effects of bacterial pyrogens. Medicine 29:365, 1950.

Cooper, K. E.: Temperature regulation and the hypothalamus. Br. Med. Bull. 22:238, 1966.

Cooper, K. E., Cranston, W. I., and Snell, E. S.: Temperature regulation during fever in man. Clin. Sci. 27:345, 1964.

Dinarello, C. A., and Wolff, S. M.: Molecular basis of fever in humans. Am. J. Med. 72:799, 1982.

Duff, G. W., and Durum, S. K.: Fever and immunoregulation: hyperthermia, interleukins 1 and 2, and T-cell proliferation. Yale J. Biol. Med. 55:437, 1982.

Greisman, S. E., Hornick, R. B., Carozza, F. A., and Woodward, T. E.: The role of endotoxin during typhoid fever and tularemia in man. I. Acquisition of tolerance to endotoxin. II. Altered cardiovascular responses to catecholamines. III. Hyperreactivity to endotoxin during infection. J. Clin. Invest. 42:1064, 1963; 43:986, 1774, 1964.

Hanson, D. F., Murphy, P. A., and Windle, B. E.: Failure of rabbit neutrophiles to secrete endogenous pyrogen when stimulated with staphylococci. J. Exp. Med. 151:1360, 1980.

Hardy, J. D.: Physiology of temperature regulation. Physiol. Rev. 41:521, 1961.

Hornick, R. B., Greisman, S. E., Woodward, T. E., et al.: Typhoid fever: pathogenesis and immunologic control. N. Engl. J. Med. 283:686, 739, 1970.

Kluger, M. J., Ringler, D. H., and Anver, M. R.: Fever and survival. Science 188:166, 1975.

MacPherson, R. K.: The effect of fever on temperature regulation in man. Clin. Sci. 18:281, 1959.

Murphy, P. A., Simon, P. L., and Willoughby, W. F.: Endogenous pyrogens made by rabbit peritoneal exudate cells are identical with lymphocyte-activating factors made by rabbit alveolar macrophages. J. Immunol. *124*:2498, 1980.

Wood, W. B., Jr.: Studies on the cause of fever. N. Engl. J. Med. *258*:1023, 1958.

Wood, W. B., Jr.: The pathogenesis of fever. *In* Mudd, S. (Ed.): Infectious Agents and Host Reactions. Philadelphia, W. B. Saunders Co., 1970.

HEADACHE ASSOCIATED WITH FEVER

Scott, R. B., and Warin, R. P.: Observations on the headache accompanying fever. Clin. Sci. *6*:51, 1948.

Sutherland, A. M., and Wolff, H. G.: Experimental studies on headache: further analysis of the mechanism of headache in migraine, hypertension, and fever therapy. Arch. Neurol. Psychiat. *44*:929, 1940.

Wolff, H. G.: Headache and Other Head Pain. New York, Oxford University Press, 1963.

SEPTIC SHOCK

Blain, C. M., Anderson, T. O., Pietras, R. J., and Gunnar, R. M.: Immediate hemodynamic effects of gram-negative vs. gram-positive bacteremia in man. Arch. Intern. Med. *126*:260, 1970.

Christy, J. H.: Pathophysiology of Gram-negative shock. Am. Heart J. *81*:694, 1971.

Fishman, A. P.: Adult respiratory distress syndrome. *In* Fishman, A. P. (Ed.): Pulmonary Diseases and Disorders. New York, McGraw-Hill Book Co., 1980.

Gilbert, R. P.: Mechanisms of the hemodynamic effects of endotoxin. Physiol. Rev. *40*:245, 1960.

Mills, L. C., and Moyer, J. H. (Eds.): Shock and Hypotension: Pathogenesis and Treatment (The 12th Hahnemann Symposium). New York, Grune and Stratton, 1965.

Nishijima, H., Weil, M. H., Shubin, H., and Cavanilles, J.: Hemodynamic and metabolic studies on shock associated with gram-negative bacteremia. Medicine *52*:287, 1973.

ALTERATIONS OF SENSORIUM

Lyon, G., Dodge, P. R., and Adams, R. D.: The acute encephalopathies of obscure origin in infants and children. Brain *84*:680, 1961.

HEMATOLOGIC CHANGES

Bass, D. A.: Behavior of eosinophil leukocytes in acute inflammation. II. Eosinophil dynamics during acute inflammation. J. Clin. Invest. *56*:870, 1975.

Bass, D. A.: Reproduction of the eosinopenia of acute infection by passive transfer of a material obtained from inflammatory exudate. Infect. Immunol. *15*:410, 1977.

Basten, A., Boyer, M. H., and Beeson, P. B.: Mechanism of eosinophilia. II. Role of the lymphocyte. J. Exp. Med. *131*:1288, 1970.

Basten, A., Boyer, M. H., and Beeson, P. B.: Mechanism of eosinophilia. I. Factors affecting the eosinophil response of rats to *Trichinella spiralis*. J. Exp. Med. *131*:1271, 1970.

Beeson, P. B., and Bass, D. A.: The Eosinophil. Vol XIV: Major Problems in Internal Medicine. Philadelphia, W. B. Saunders Co., 1977.

Cartwright, G. E., and Wintrobe, M. M.: The anemia of infection XVII. A review. *In* Dock, W., and Snapper, I. (Eds.): Advances in Internal Medicine. Vol. V. Chicago, Year Book Medical Publishers, Inc., 1952, p. 165.

Coleman, R. W., Girey, G. J. D., Zacest, R., and Talamo, R. C.: The human plasma kallikrein-kinin system. Progr. Hematol. *VII*:255, 1971.

Corrigan, J. J., Ray, W. L., and May, N.: Changes in the blood coagulation system associated with septicemia. N. Engl. J. Med. *279*:851, 1968.

Deykin, D.: Thrombogenesis. N. Engl. J. Med. *276*:622, 1967.

Marsh, J. C., Boggs, D. R., Cartwright, G. E., and Wintrobe, M. M.: Neutrophile kinetics in acute infection. J. Clin. Invest. *46*:1943, 1967.

Mahmoud, A. A. F., Warren, K. S., and Peters, P. A.: A role for the eosinophil in acquired resistance to *Schistosoma mansoni* infection as determined by anti-eosinophil serum. J. Exp. Med. *142*:805, 1975.

Mahmoud, A. A. F., Stone, M. K., and Kellermeyer, R. W.: Eosinophilopoietin: a circulating low-molecular-weight peptide-like substance which stimulates production of eosinophils in mice. J. Clin. Invest. *60*:675, 1977.

Minna, J. D., Robboy, S. J., and Coleman, R. W.: Disseminated Intravascular Coagulation in Man. Springfield, Ill., Charles C Thomas Co., 1974.

Morse, S. I., and Riester, S. K.: Studies on the leukocytosis and lymphocytosis induced by *Bordetella pertussis*. II. The effect of pertussis vaccine on the thoracic duct lymph and lymphocytes of mice. J. Exp. Med. *125*:619, 1967.

Rodriguez-Erdmann, F.: Bleeding due to increased intravascular blood coagulation. N. Engl. J. Med. *273*:1370, 1965.

Taub, R. N., Rosett, W., Adler, A., and Morse, S. I.: Distribution of labeled lymph node cells in mice during the lymphocytosis induced by *Bordetella pertussis*. J. Exp. Med. *136*:1581, 1972.

Wilhelm, D. L.: Kinins in human disease. Ann. Rev. Med. *22*:63, 1971.

MISCELLANEOUS

Baracos, V., Rodemann, P., Dinarello, C. A., and Goldberg, A. L.: Stimulation of muscle protein degradation and prostaglandin E_2 release by leukocytic pyrogen (interleukin-1). N. Engl. J. Med. *308*:553, 1983.

Beisel, W. R., Sawyer, W. D., Ryll, E. D., and Crozier, D.: Metabolic effects of intracellular infections in man. Ann. Int. Med. *67*:744, 1967.

Clowes, G. H. A., Jr., George, B. C., Villee, C. A., Jr., and Saravis, C. A.: Muscle proteolysis induced by a circulating peptide in patients with sepsis or trauma. N. Engl. J. Med. *308*:545, 1982.

Feigin, R. D., Klainer, A. S., Beisel, W. R., and Hornick, R. B.: Blood amino acids in experimentally induced typhoid fever. N. Engl. J. Med. *278*:293, 1968.

Gallin, J. I., Kaye, D., and O'Leary, W. M.: Serum lipids in infection. N. Engl. J. Med. *281*:1081, 1969.

Glenner, G. G.: Amyloid deposits and amyloidosis. The B-fibrilloses. N. Engl. J. Med. *302*:1283, and 1333, 1980.

Glenner, G. G., Ein, D., and Terry, W. D.: The immunoglobulin origin of amyloid. Am. J. Med. *52*:141, 1972.

Gutman, R. A., Striker, G. E., Gilliland, B. C., and Cutler, R. E.: The immune complex glomerulonephritis of bacterial endocarditis. Medicine *51*:1, 1972.

Lennette, E. H., Magoffin, R. L., and Freeman, J. M.: Immunologic evidence of measles virus as an etiologic agent in subacute sclerosing panencephalitis. Neurology *18*:21, 1968.

Miller, H. G., Stanton, J. B., and Gibbons, J. L.: Parainfectious encephalomyelitis and related syndromes. Q. J. Med. *25*:427, 1956.

Payne, F. E., Baublis, J. V., and Itabashi, H. H.: Isolation of measles virus from cell cultures of brain from a patient with subacute sclerosing panencephalitis. N. Engl. J. Med. *28*:585, 1969.

Swartz, M. N., and Weinberg, A. N.: Infections due to gram-positive bacteria. Gram-negative coccal and bacillary infections. *In* Fitzgerald, T. B. (Ed.): Dermatology in General Medicine. New York, McGraw-Hill Book Co., 1971.

Zabriskie, J. B.: The role of streptococci in human glomerulonephritis. J. Exp. Med. *134*:180, 1971.

Pathophysiologic Changes Due to Localization of Infections in Specific Organs

21

Louis Weinstein and Morton N. Swartz

The major impact of a number of human infections is directly related to the specific anatomic site of disease, and the pathophysiologic abnormalities that develop are due primarily to dysfunction of the single or principal organ involved. In some instances, a wide variety of organisms are capable of localizing at the same site, where they produce roughly similar pathophysiologic changes (e.g., infective endocarditis due to any of a number of bacterial and mycotic species). In others, a specific discrete site may be involved by only a very limited group of infectious agents (e.g., involvement of the motor neurons of the spinal cord in disease due to poliomyelitis or coxsackieviruses).

The pathophysiology of many of the common infectious diseases represents, in effect, the changes due to dysfunction of a particular organ. These are little different from those that might be induced in the same area by noninfectious processes. Thus, the abnormalities that develop in viral hepatitis have much in common with those that appear in acute alcoholic hepatitis. This is also true for chronic pyelonephritis and chronic renal disease due to other causes such as hypertension and chronic glomerulonephritis. The cardiovascular alterations associated with myocarditis are much the same whether it is due to viral infection or alcoholic cardiomyopathy. Likewise, the dramatic circulatory consequences of cardiac tamponade are similar whether this is the result of viral or tuberculous pericarditis on the one hand or pericardial invasion by a neoplastic process on the other. The pathophysiology of these and many other infectious diseases is considered in sections devoted to organ-system physiology elsewhere in this book. The focus in this chapter is on selected organ involvement in which the pathophysiologic changes, although reflecting primarily organ dysfunction, are quite uniquely produced by infectious agents. Emphasis is placed on a limited number of illustrative examples rather than on a comprehensive listing of infectious diseases appropriate to this category.

The characteristic pathophysiologic changes to be considered may be centered about one organ primarily (e.g., osteomyelitis), or the ramifications may be broad, involving many other organs in a specific fashion (e.g., infective endocarditis, syphilis with its multiple stages).

INFECTIONS WITH PATHOPHYSIOLOGIC CONSEQUENCES IN MULTIPLE ORGAN SYSTEMS

Infective Endocarditis

Although this infection involves primarily the heart valves or mural endocardium, the peripheral changes secondary to bland (or septic) emboli, associated vasculitis, or antigen-antibody complexes may be so striking as to become pre-eminent. Thus, neurologic dysfunction, skin and joint changes, or renal failure may dominate the picture and draw attention to organs other than the heart.

Pathogenesis of Endocarditis. The pathophysiologic processes involved in the development of subacute bacterial endocarditis are strikingly different from those operative in the development of the acute form of the disease. Four mechanisms are responsible for the initiation of the subacute infection: (1) a previously damaged cardiac valve, or a hemodynamic situation in which a "jet effect" is produced by blood flowing from an area of high pressure to one of relatively low pressure; (2) a sterile platelet-fibrin thrombus; (3) bacteremia (often transient); and (4) a high titer of agglutinating antibody for the infecting organism.

By the introduction of a bacterial aerosol into an air stream moving through an agar Venturi tube, Rodbard has shown clearly how high pressure drives an infected fluid into a low-pressure sink and produces a characteristic pattern of colony distribution, concentrating in the low-pressure region just distal to the orifice (Fig. 21–1). This model helps account for the distribution of lesions observed in endocarditis complicating various cardiac valvular and septal defects (Fig. 21–2). In mitral insufficiency, a "jet effect" is produced when blood is driven from a high-pressure site (left ventricle) into a low-pressure area (left atrium); vegetations of endocarditis are typically located on the atrial (low-pressure) side of the valve and on

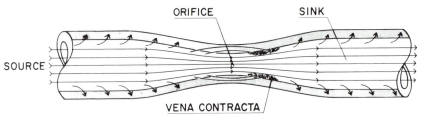

Figure 21–1 Venturi model of high-pressure source driving a bacterial aerosol into a low-pressure sink. Typical location of bacterial colonies is noted at the vena contracta. (From Rodbard, S.: Blood velocity and endocarditis. Circulation 27:18, 1963. Reproduced with permission of the publisher.)

the adjacent atrial endocardium, where the impacting regurgitant stream produces a fibrous area, MacCallum's patch. In aortic insufficiency, the aorta is a high-pressure area, and the left ventricle is a low-pressure zone; vegetations of endocarditis characteristically are located on the

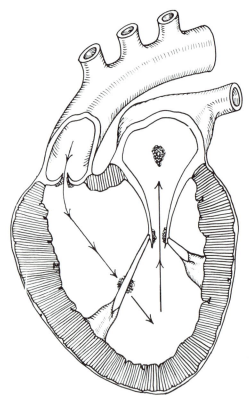

Figure 21–2 High-velocity streams in mitral and aortic insufficiency and locations of endocarditic lesions. Arrows at the left indicate regurgitant flow from aortic high-pressure area into left ventricle. Endocarditic lesions appear at the ventricular surface of the aortic valve. The "jet" stream through the incompetent aortic valve may produce secondary lesions on the chordae tendineae of the anterior leaflet of the mitral valve. In the presence of mitral insufficiency, the regurgitant "jet" stream (arrow at right) will enter the sink of the left atrium during ventricular systole, and bacterial vegetations will tend to develop on the atrial surface of the mitral valve and on the site of impact on the atrial endocardium. (Adapted from Rodbard, S.: Blood velocity and endocarditis. Circulation 27:18, 1963. Reproduced with permission of the publisher.)

ventricular (low-pressure) surface of the aortic cusps. In addition, in the presence of active infection on the aortic valve, a regurgitant "jet" of blood can inoculate bacteria onto the adjacent anterior leaflet of the mitral valve, where a secondary infection can result in mitral insufficiency and further compromise left ventricular function. In a small ventricular septal defect with a left-to-right shunt, a Venturi effect can result in the development of vegetations around the orifice on the right ventricular side or on the right ventricular wall opposite the defect at the site of jet impact.

As blood flows over a valve leaflet that has been distorted by acquired heart disease, such as acute rheumatic fever, or malformed because of a congenital defect, a "whipping" effect is produced, inducing platelet deposition. Platelet aggregation occurs, initiating coagulation factor activation and local fibrin formation. A platelet-fibrin thrombus is thus deposited at the site of the deformity on the valvular surface. The valvular defect responsible for this phenomenon is occasionally of insufficient magnitude to cause enough turbulence of flow to produce a murmur. Although transient bacteremias probably occur very frequently in humans, they are usually without clinical significance, even in the individual with abnormal cardiac valves on which sterile platelet-fibrin thrombi may be situated. In most instances, the failure of implantation of organisms on such a valve is related to the small number of bacteria in the circulation at any given time. A factor that possibly plays an important role in the development of valvular infection is the level of circulating antibody, especially agglutinins. These may result in conglutination of a sufficiently large number of bacterial cells to allow their successful multiplication and the establishment of infection within the platelet-fibrin thrombus. This phenomenon may be of particular importance in the pathogenesis of subacute endocarditis because of the relatively low invasive capacity and the small number of organisms of the bacterial species usually present during an episode of transient bacteremia.

The pathophysiologic changes involved in the development of acute bacterial endocarditis are, in most respects, quite different. In at least 50 to 60 per cent of cases of acute endocarditis, previously normal valves are the site of infection. It appears, therefore, that the presence of a sterile platelet-fibrin thrombus is unnecessary in the pathogenesis of this form of the disease. Because the organisms responsible for this type of infection (*Staphylococcus aureus,* pneumococci, meningococci, gonococci, *Streptococcus pyogenes,* and *Haemophilus influenzae*) are highly invasive, only small numbers are required to establish infection. Thus, the only requirement for the establishment of acute endocarditis is bacteremia due to an invasive organism. It should be pointed out, however, that in the instances in which underlying valvular damage, either acquired or congenital, is present, sterile platelet-fibrin thrombi may develop and facilitate the initiation of this type of infection. The exact mechanism by which "pathogenic" bacteria invade normal valve leaflets is unknown in some instances. It is now clear, however, that some organisms, for example *Staphylococcus aureus,* have the capacity to adhere to the surface of normal valvular leaflets. In a great many cases of subacute bacterial endocarditis, the bacteremia responsible for the infection originates not from an infectious process but from trauma to an area in which the causative organisms normally reside as components of the indigenous flora (e.g., the teeth, urinary tract, and intestine). This is in sharp contrast to some cases of acute infective endocarditis, in which the inducing bacteremia has its origin in an active infection at a site remote from the heart.

Support for the concept that nonbacterial thrombotic endocarditis is the initial lesion that is converted to subacute bacterial endocarditis comes from studies of an experimental model of this disease by Durack and Beeson. In this model, nonbacterial thrombotic endocarditis is produced by insertion of a polyethylene catheter into the right side of the heart of a rabbit. Subsequent intravenous injection of *S. viridans* results in adherence of the bacteria to the vegetation, where they multiply rapidly and serve as a source of continuing bacteremia. Microcolonies appear beneath and within a superficial layer of material that appears to be fibrin.

Selective bacterial adherence to valvular endothelium has been suggested as an important characteristic of bacteria capable of causing endocarditis in humans. On incubation in vitro with excised valve leaflets, strains of enterococci, viridans streptococci, and *S. aureus* adhere more readily than *Escherichia coli* and *Klebsiella*. These gram-positive organisms are the commonest causes of endocarditis, whereas *E. coli* and *Klebsiella* are rarely implicated, despite their frequency as causes of bacteremia. Although these findings are suggestive, adherence is not the sole determinant of bacterial pathogenicity in endocarditis, as is indicated by the fact that *Pseudomonas aeruginosa,* a rare cause of endocarditis, exhibits marked adherence.

Pathophysiology of the Clinical Features of Endocarditis. Four mechanisms are responsible

for the clinical features of infective endocarditis: (1) the infectious process on the involved valve; (2) the occurrence of emboli; (3) metastatic infection; and (4) the deposition of immune complexes and clinical manifestations of immunologic injury, including vasculitis. All these are not found in every patient. There are also striking qualitative and quantitative differences in their roles in the acute and subacute forms of the disease.

THE INFECTIOUS PROCESS ON THE INVOLVED HEART VALVE. The striking differences in the clinical course of subacute and acute endocarditis can be related almost entirely to the pathoanatomic and pathophysiologic changes induced at the primary site of infection, the heart valve. Microscopic study of the lesions in subacute bacterial endocarditis reveals evidence of both slowly progressive activity and early or complete healing. Neutrophils, lymphocytes, plasma cells, and Anitschkow cells compose the cellular infiltrate. The impression is one of simultaneous slow destruction and healing, with the latter not quite "catching up" with the former. In contrast to this are the anatomic changes characteristic of acute endocarditis. Grossly, the vegetations on the involved valve surface are often larger, softer, and more friable than the smaller, harder thrombi observed in the subacute infection. In the more fulminant forms or when the lesion has been present for some time, a variety of destructive changes may occur in proximity to the valvular vegetation (Table 21–1). Tears, aneurysms, and/or perforation of one or several cusps of the aortic valve may take place during the course of active infective endocarditis. Eversion or extreme distortion of the aortic valve cusps may occur in some instances after bacteriologic cure has been achieved. Free aortic regurgitation is produced, and marked acute left ventricular failure ensues.

A mycotic aneurysm of the sinus of Valsalva may develop in the course of acute or subacute bacterial endocarditis involving the aortic valve. The aneurysm occasionally enlarges by burrowing through the commissure into the wall of the ventricle and there forms an abscess, destroying myocardial fibers. The aneurysmal sac may even dissect into the septum and rupture into the right atrium. This occurrence is characterized by the sudden development of a roaring continuous thrill and murmur over the upper left sternal border along with peripheral signs of aortic and tricuspid regurgitation, the sudden onset of congestive failure, and the absence of radiologic findings of marked pulmonary edema. Infection of the aortic valve may also burrow into the root of the aorta (erosion of aortic annulus; aortic ring abscess), and the inflammation may extend posteriorly to the pericardial wedge between the aorta and pulmonary artery, producing fibrinous or hemorrhagic pericarditis. A ring abscess may secondarily involve the mitral-aortic intervalvular fibrosa (the junctional zone between the aortic and mitral valves) and form an expanding false aneurysm,

TABLE 21–1 INTRACARDIAC COMPLICATIONS OF INFECTIVE ENDOCARDITIS

Aortic Valve
1. Eversion or distortion of a cusp
2. Fenestration, rupture, or avulsion of a cusp
3. Erosion of aortic annulus; aortic ring abscess
   a. Rupture into pericardium → tamponade
4. Mycotic aneurysm of sinus of Valsalva or of the mitral-aortic intervalvular fibrosa
5. Dissection of a valve ring abscess or of a mycotic aneurysm into the upper (membranous) interventricular septum
   a. Perforation of the septum producing a shunt between left ventricle and right atrium
   b. Perforation of the septum producing a shunt between left ventricle and right ventricle
6. Occlusion of the valve orifice by vegetations (fungal endocarditis; prosthetic valve endocarditis)

Mitral Valve
1. Distortion of leaflet
2. Mycotic aneurysm of mitral valve
3. Rupture of chordae tendineae
4. Papillary muscle dysfunction
5. Dissecting infection involving mitral annulus
6. Occlusion of valve orifice by vegetation (fungal endocarditis; prosthetic valve endocarditis)

Tricuspid Valve
1. An uncommon site of endocarditis; distortion, etc., of leaflets producing valvular insufficiency

Pulmonic Valve
1. A rare site of endocarditis; distortion, etc., of leaflets producing valvular insufficiency

Myocardium
1. Abscess (wall or septum)
2. Diffuse myocarditis
3. False aneurysm
4. Rupture of abscess → cardiac tamponade

Pericardium
1. Pericarditis
   a. Fibrinous or hemorrhagic pericarditis secondary to aortic annulus erosion or to burrowing of aortic root abscess into the epicardium

Septal Abscess
1. Dissection of infection from aortic ring abscess or from infection involving mitral annulus
2. Bacteremic or embolic infection of septum

Coronary Arteries
1. Embolus → myocardial infarction
2. Mycotic aneurysm

ultimately rupturing with hemorrhage into the pericardial cavity and causing death from cardiac tamponade.

Similarly destructive changes may involve the mitral valve and produce rupture of the chordae tendineae or of a head of a papillary muscle. Catastrophic mitral regurgitation with a loud pansystolic murmur then develops, accompanied by sudden dyspnea and attacks of acute pulmonary edema. Infection involving the mitral valve may burrow into the mitral annulus and even become superimposed on degenerative calcification of the mitral annulus.

Myocardial abscesses may develop not only by extension from valvular vegetations but also as a result of seeding of the coronary circulation with organisms from the vegetations on the aortic valve or as a consequence of septic embolization. Hectic fevers with or without positive blood cultures

(while the patient is receiving antibiotic therapy) and rapidly progressive left-sided heart failure are prominent features. Myocardial abscesses in a strategic location in the septum may cause striking changes in conduction. Infection that involves this area may have (1) spread down the septum from the aortic valve to the A-V bundle, causing disruption of A-V conduction; (2) spread from the mitral valve through the annulus to the region of the A-V bundle or node; or (3) reached the septum by embolization through the coronary circulation. The proximity of the aortic valve (right and noncoronary cusps) to the conduction system and of the mitral annulus to the atrioventricular node and the common bundle of His accounts for the development of conduction defects when infection has extended beyond the valve annulus (Fig. 21–3). Prolongation of the PR interval, a new left bundle branch block, or a new right bundle branch

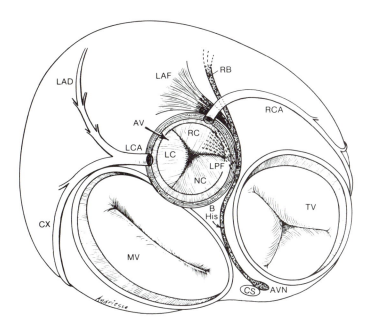

Figure 21–3 Anatomic relationships between cardiac valves and conduction system as viewed from above (superiorly). MV indicates mitral valve; TV, tricuspid valve; AV, aortic valve; LC, left coronary cusp; RC, right coronary cusp; NC, noncoronary cusp; LCA, left coronary artery; LAD, left anterior descending artery; CX, circumflex artery; RCA, right coronary artery; CS, coronary sinus; AVN, atrioventricular node; B His, common bundle of His; LPF, left posterior fascicle of left bundle branch; LAF, left anterior fascicle of left bundle branch; RB, right bundle branch. (Adapted from Hutter, A. M., and Moellering, R. C.: Assessment of the patient with suspected endocarditis. J.A.M.A. *235*:1603, 1976. Reproduced with permission of the publisher.)

block with left anterior hemiblock could indicate extension of infection from the mitral valve into the interventricular septum. Extension of infection from the aortic annulus into the atrioventricular node or proximal bundle of His might be indicated by the onset of nonparoxysmal junctional tachycardia, second degree A-V (Wenckebach) block, or complete heart block with a narrow QRS on the electrocardiogram. Rupture of the interventricular septum secondary to a septal abscess occurs very rarely and is characterized by the abrupt appearance of a pansystolic murmur and thrill as well as by rapidly developing cardiac failure.

The constitutional reaction to the valvular infection is manifested by elevated temperature, rigors, and generalized malaise; it is, in general, less intense in subacute than in acute endocarditis. Although the level of fever may be the same in either type of disease, it is lower, as a rule, in the chronic form and may never exceed 100° to 101° F; in about 5 per cent of cases, particularly in patients with azotemia, it may be absent entirely. In contrast, the temperature is very often high in the acute disease and commonly reaches 103° to 104° F or more. Although rigors may occur at the beginning or during the course of untreated subacute bacterial endocarditis, they are more frequently present in acute endocarditis. Anemia is usually present in both types of disease and may develop quite rapidly in the absence of overt intravascular hemolysis; it is usually the anemia of infection (see Chapter 20).

A changing murmur has been considered a common and characteristic feature of subacute endocarditis. However, broad experience has made it clear that this is rarely the case when *Streptococcus viridans,* the usual cause of this disease, is involved. In contrast, murmurs often undergo

rapid and striking changes in intensity and quality in patients with acute valvular infections. This is due to several factors: (1) decrease or increase in size of the relatively soft valvular thrombi, (2) tears or fenestration of valve leaflets, (3) rupture of chordae tendineae or papillary muscles, (4) perforation of the ventricular septum, or (5) development of an aneurysm in an aortic cusp or in the sinus of Valsalva. Of great importance is the fact that murmurs may be absent in patients with subacute bacterial endocarditis, even when the disease has been present for some weeks. Also, about one third of patients with *acute* valvular infections involving the left side of the heart or patients with right-sided endocarditis (commonly acute) may have no detectable murmurs early in the course of the disease.

Valvular infection due to enterococcus occupies a clinical position between that produced by *Staphylococcus aureus* (acute) and *Streptococcus viridans* (subacute). Distant septic complications may develop but are most uncommon in endocarditis due to *S. viridans.*

Although the white blood count may be elevated (10,000 to 20,000 per mm³), it is commonly not increased in patients with subacute bacterial endocarditis. Indeed, the presence of a leukocytosis usually suggests the occurrence of embolic complications or an infecting organism other than *S. viridans* (e.g., enterococcus). Leukocytosis is common in the acute type of disease; however, the number of white cells in the peripheral blood may be normal or even strikingly decreased.

The interval between the onset of infection and the establishment of the diagnosis, as well as the duration of disease in untreated patients with endocarditis, is directly related to the character of the valvular lesion. The progression of the infectious process in the acute form is so rapid that severe constitutional manifestations force the patient to seek early medical attention. If the infection is undetected and therefore untreated, death may occur in 1 or 2 weeks as the result of marked destruction of the involved valve, multiple metastatic infections, or embolization to a vital area. The course of subacute endocarditis is strikingly different. In this, the symptoms of infection are often very insidious in onset, mainly low-grade fever and slowly developing anemia. The patient's only complaints may be loss of appetite, increasing fatigue, weight loss, or night sweats. The interval between the onset of symptoms and definitive diagnosis in 100 cases of subacute bacterial endocarditis was about 3.5 months. Life expectancy after development of this disease is usually rather long, even in the absence of antimicrobial therapy, unless rupture of a mycotic aneurysm or lethal embolization occurs. The chronicity of the disease reflects the slow progress of the pathologic process on the infected valve. Survival for 3 to 6 months is common. It may be even longer (over 1 year) when *Staphylococcus epidermidis* is the responsible organism.

EMBOLIC PHENOMENA. Embolic episodes are common in both acute and subacute bacterial endocarditis. Although they occur most often when infection is still present, they may supervene at any time in the course of the disease, even well into convalescence when the active process has been eliminated. Almost any organ may be the site for embolic deposition. However, the kidneys, heart, brain, spleen, and eyes are more frequently involved than other organs. The areas of resulting infarction may be solitary and large or multiple and quite small; the clinical manifestations that develop as well as the risk of death depend on the organ involved and the extent of damage. Cerebral embolism is the most common of the neurologic complications of bacterial endocarditis and occurs in 15 to 20 per cent of patients with this disease; it is particularly common in patients with mitral valve involvement and in those with infection due to pyogenic organisms such as *Staphylococcus aureus* and enteric gram-negative bacilli. Although emboli in both acute and subacute endocarditis usually contain organisms early in the course of infection, there is a striking difference in the changes that develop at the sites of deposition. The areas of infarction that occur in the subacute disease are, as a rule, sterile. Thus, in a subacute endocarditis one observes the paradox of an infected embolus producing a bland infarct. In contrast, infarcts that develop in the course of acute valvular infections, especially those caused by *S. aureus*, rapidly suppurate. Emboli that occur in patients with fungal endocarditis or atrial myxoma tend to be large. Occlusion of major vessels should, therefore, suggest the presence of these diseases rather than the commoner bacterial infections of valves.

Myocardial infarction secondary to coronary embolization may occur in the course of bacterial endocarditis. Pericarditis may result from extension of the area of infarction to the pericardial surface. Although this is the basis of the pericardial involvement in some patients with endocarditis it is not the only cause for pericardial inflammation in this setting. Other causes include myocardial abscess, erosion of a mycotic aneurysm of the sinus of Valsalva, extension of aortic valve infection into the pericardial wedge between the root of the aorta and the pulmonary artery, uremia, bacteremic spread of infection to the pericardium, and reactivation of acute rheumatic fever.

METASTATIC INFECTIONS. One of the most striking differences between subacute and acute bacterial endocarditis is the high frequency with which metastatic infection occurs in the latter. Infarcts in subacute infection usually do not become infected. This may be attributed to several factors: (1) the invasive capacity of the organisms involved is relatively low, (2) the number of organisms present in the embolus is insufficient to establish metastatic infection, and (3) a high titer of specific antibody results in killing of the few bacteria that are deposited at the local site. Thus, while infarction of the kidneys, heart, and brain occurs in patients with subacute bacterial endocarditis, abscesses in these organs, meningitis, pyelonephritis, or suppurative myocarditis develop only very rarely. However, a sterile meningitis, with the biochemical and cellular characteristics of "aseptic" meningitis, is not an uncommon occurrence in the subacute form of the disease. Mycotic aneurysms of the aorta and its branches that may develop in the course of subacute valvular infection are usually not due to suppuration in and about the vessel walls. In most instances, the vascular necrosis, mural weakening, and aneurysmal dilatation result from sterile occlusion of the vasa vasorum; histologic study of such lesions rarely reveals evidence of active inflammation. Mycotic aneurysms may occur intracranially, particularly in the distribution of the middle cerebral artery. Leakage or rupture of such aneurysms may produce neurologic dysfunction secondary to intracerebral or subarachnoid bleeding. Cerebral mycotic aneurysms now tend to occur more frequently in the course of acute than subacute endocarditis; when they occur in the latter it is late in the course of the disease. Healing of mycotic aneurysms, as shown on sequential angiography, can occur during the course of effective antimicrobial therapy. Mycotic aneurysms may also develop in a coronary artery, in the mesenteric arterial tree, or in arteries of the extremities. Because the organisms contained in emboli in acute infective endocarditis are usually highly invasive, they are able to multiply successfully and establish infection in the infarcted areas. Thus, when valvular disease is due to *Staphylococcus aureus*, multiple abscesses are often detectable, particularly in the kidney and myocardium.

Brain abscesses, often small and multiple,

may complicate acute endocarditis, particularly when *S. aureus* is the cause. Purulent meningitis may occur also owing to seeding during bacteremia. It is important to recognize that the symptoms of headache, nuchal rigidity, and a mild cerebrospinal fluid pleocytosis during endocarditis do not necessarily represent pyogenic meningitis; they may result from cerebral emboli. Such emboli may involve relatively silent areas of the cortex and produce few if any localizing neurologic findings.

IMMUNOLOGIC ASPECTS AND HYPERSENSITIVITY PHENOMENA. Agglutinating, complement-fixing, and opsonizing antibodies specific for the infecting bacteria in subacute bacterial endocarditis are regularly present. There is an increased level in the serum of both IgG and IgM. Over 50 per cent of patients develop some type of antiglobulin factor. The latex fixation test for rheumatoid factor is positive in about 50 per cent of cases when the disease has been present for 6 weeks or longer. Large amounts of cryoglobulins and macroglobulins may be present. About one third of patients with endocarditis have high levels (about 100 µg per ml) of circulating immune complexes; high levels are much more frequent in patients with extravalvular manifestations of endocarditis (arthralgias, sterile arthritis, splenomegaly, Roth spots in the retina, glomerulonephritis) than in those without such signs. This suggests, but does not prove, that immune complexes may be important in the pathogenesis of all these features of endocarditis. It has been suggested that the articular symptoms, a prominent feature in some patients with subacute endocarditis, are related to the presence of the rheumatoid factor. Arthralgia or florid arthritis may occur early or late in the course of subacute endocarditis. The synovial fluid is usually sterile. Changes in serum globulins are much less marked and less frequently present in the acute endocarditis because death occurs early if the disease is untreated.

Renal lesions often develop in the course of bacterial endocarditis, particularly the subacute variety. These are of several types: (1) diffuse membranous glomerulonephritis, both acute and subacute, in which immune complexes consisting of antigen, antibody, and complement are deposited as "lumpy-bumpy" aggregates on the glomerular basement membrane (see Chapter 20); (2) renal infarcts, both large and small; and (3) so-called "focal embolic glomerulonephritis," an entity presumed in the past to be the result of multiple small emboli but now also considered to be due to an immune complex mechanism. The renal lesions appear to play an important role in death from prolonged and untreated endocarditis. Disease that has persisted for protracted periods may no longer require the active participation of viable bacteria. A "bacteria-free stage" of chronic bacterial endocarditis has been described, the predominant features of which are those of chronic renal failure.

The classic peripheral signs of subacute bacterial endocarditis, originally considered to be of embolic origin, have been thought more recently to represent lesions of allergic vasculitis involving small arteries. Among such signs are *Osler's nodes* (painful and tender bluish-red lesions in the pulp spaces over the terminal phalanges of the fingers or toes); *Janeway's lesions* (nontender, irregular, erythematous or hemorrhagic lesions situated most often in the skin over the thenar and hypothenar eminences of the hands or on the soles of the feet); *Roth's spots* (boat-shaped exudates with a surrounding zone of hemorrhage in the retina); *subungual* or *"splinter"* hemorrhages in the nail beds; and *petechial skin lesions*. Histologic and bacteriologic studies of Osler's nodes have been performed in only a few patients with endocarditis. Pathogenic organisms have been isolated from aspirates of Osler's nodes in four patients (*Staphylococcus aureus* in three patients and *Candida albicans* in one); histologic examination of the skin lesion from one of these patients with *S. aureus* endocarditis revealed a microabscess in the dermis and microemboli in adjacent arterioles. These four patients had acute bacterial endocarditis due to virulent organisms. Thus, in acute bacterial endocarditis Osler's nodes may be due to septic microemboli. In contrast, in subacute bacterial endocarditis due to viridans streptococci and other microorganisms of limited pathogenicity, convincing proof of an embolic origin for Osler's nodes is lacking. It is thought that Osler's nodes are painful because of the location of the lesion in the densely-packed, extensively innervated tissues of the digital pulp space.

Salmonella Infections (Salmonellosis)

Infections caused by different species of *Salmonella* have in common a number of clinical features such as fever, chills, and diarrhea. However, careful consideration of the pathophysiologic processes involved in the syndromes of "acute gastroenteritis," "enteric fever," and isolated "bacteremia" produced by this group of organisms clearly indicates striking differences that sharply distinguish one disease pattern from another. In fact, these are distinct disorders in most respects, the only common denominator being invasion by *Salmonella,* some species of which are more commonly responsible for certain clinical pictures.

Salmonella Gastroenteritis. A very large number of species of *Salmonella* are capable of producing acute gastroenteritis. This form of infection is usually limited to the intestine. Unlike cholera, this enteritis appears to be related to bacterial invasion of the intestinal mucosa and not to elaboration of a specific enterotoxin. The presence of polymorphonuclear leukocytes in the feces is consistent with an inflammatory reaction in the bowel. Only salmonella strains capable of penetrating the intestinal mucosa induce the appearance of inflammatory cells or of enhanced fluid electrolyte loss; noninvasive strains that merely proliferate in the bowel lumen do not produce these changes. Not all invasive strains induce fluid secretion. Evidence suggests that some strains of *Salmonella* that cause fluid secretion may induce intestinal prostaglandin secretion, which in turn stimulates adenylate cyclase, resulting in fluid and electrolyte loss. Bloodstream invasion is very uncommon except in young infants and elderly individuals. Metastatic infections of the hepatobiliary and other organ systems is also very infrequent. Several abnormal states appear to be of importance in increasing susceptibility to this type of intestinal infection. Among these are *subtotal gastrectomy* (probably related to a decrease in gastric acid production that permits viable organisms to pass through the stomach), *neoplastic diseases, hemoglobinopathies,* the *administration of antimicrobial agents* (related to suppression of competing components of the normal intestinal flora), and the *use of corticosteroids* (possibly due to alteration in immune mechanisms).

Enteric Fever. The enteric fevers include typhoid *(Salmonella typhi)* and the paratyphoid *(S. paratyphi, S. schottmülleri,* and *S. hirschfeldii)* fevers. A similar clinical picture may be produced occasionally by others of the more than 1500 *Salmonella* species. The pathogenesis and pathophysiologic phenomena involved in this group of infections are quite distinct and different from those that characterize *Salmonella* gastroenteritis. The enteric fevers are not primary diseases of the intestinal mucosa but rather affect principally the lymphoid tissues in certain areas of the small intestine. The clinical manifestations of dysfunction of the intestine that occur are secondary to this anatomic localization of the infection. The following sequence takes place after ingestion of an inoculum of one of the *Salmonella* species causing enteric fever. Organisms in contaminated water or food pass through the stomach into the small intestines, where they enter the smaller lymphatic channels and are deposited in the lymphoid tissues within the bowel wall. The organisms multiply in the lymph follicles and are often found intracellularly within plasma cells. This intracellular location may be responsible for persistence of infection in the presence of circulating antibodies. A marked macrophage response is induced locally, and a varying degree of necrosis of the nodes occurs. At the end of about 2 weeks, the average length of the incubation period for the enteric fevers, the organisms invade the bloodstream from the lymphatics. At this point, clinical manifestations of disease (fever, chills, and other constitutional reactions to infection) appear. The bacteremic phase may, in fact, be made up of two periods, as suggested by studies of experimental typhoid fever in the mouse. The initial bacteremia is a transitory one, rapidly brought to an end by the removal of the bacilli by the reticuloendothe-

lial system, particularly in the liver and spleen. This is followed by a period of very active bacterial proliferation in the reticuloendothelial cells of these organs. A secondary and more intense bacteremia then ensues, resulting in widespread dissemination of the bacteria. The bacteremia usually persists for several days but may last as long as 10 days; during this time salmonellae ordinarily cannot be recovered from the feces. However, after this they are demonstrable in fecal cultures. During the bacteremic phase, salmonellae reinvade the intestine via the gallbladder and bile ducts. Ulcerations occur in Peyer's patches in the ileum, and salmonellae appear in the feces. Because of the location of the collections of lymphoid tissue in the intestinal wall, the ulcerations are not linear but encircle the bowel. The fact that intestinal involvement is secondary to disease in the lymphoid structures is supported by the absence of diarrhea in over half the patients with enteric fevers. The two commonest complications of this type of *Salmonella* infection, intestinal hemorrhage and perforation, are directly related to the active inflammatory and destructive process in the submucosal aggregations of lymphoid cells. Despite the prominent bacteremia, it is uncommon for metastatic infections of various organs to occur in the course of typhoid and paratyphoid fever.

Salmonella Bacteremia. A number of unrelated factors play important roles in the pathogenesis of *Salmonella* bacteremia. Although not known for some, the pathophysiology of others has been partly defined. *Advancing age* appears to predispose to this type of disease. Individuals with *hepatic cirrhosis* are also more prone to develop this syndrome. This may be related to their greater susceptibility to bacteremia in general because of the decreased effectiveness of the liver in removing members of the intestinal microflora from the portal circulation. *Various types of neoplastic disease* predispose to this type of salmonellosis; although not proved, it is likely that this is related to the immunosuppressive effects of certain malignant diseases. The *administration of antimicrobial agents and corticosteroids* may play a role in the pathogenesis of *Salmonella* bacteremia; the former by eradicating competing elements of the normal flora, and the latter by decreasing immunocompetence. A group of disorders characterized by *chronic or acute episodes of hemolysis*—malaria, sickle cell anemia (or other hemoglobinopathies), louse-borne relapsing fever *(Borrelia recurrentis),* and Oroya fever *(Bartonella bacilliformis)*—are associated with a markedly increased risk of intestinal infection and bacteremia due to *Salmonella.* The loading of macrophages with large quantities of hemoglobin breakdown products may make it possible for these cells, the major defense against salmonellae, to ingest and kill the organisms. It has also been suggested that hyperferremia, consequent on acute hemolysis, is responsible for the increased susceptibility to invasion by salmonellae. There is some evidence, from animal studies, that hypoferremia may be associated with some increase in resistance to certain infections, whereas excessive levels of iron in the serum may be associated with a decrease in resistance. The association of *Salmonella* osteomyelitis with hemoglobinopathies is well recognized. The microscopic areas of bone infarction that commonly occur in sickle cell anemia appear to serve as a nidus for the engraftment and multiplication of salmonellae that have previously entered the circulation. An increased susceptibility to invasion by salmonellae occurs in patients with schistosomiasis. Chronic *Salmonella* urinary tract infection can complicate *Schistosoma hematobium* infection in this area. Salmonellae are able to penetrate and multiply within schistosomes *(S. mansoni),* protected from the effects of antibody and antimicrobial agents. From this sanctuary they may be the source for persisting or recurrent bacteremias.

One of the most interesting pathophysiologic phenomena that may play a very important role in the pathogenesis of continuing *Salmonella* bacteremia is an *arteriosclerotic aneurysm of the aorta* or one of its major branches. The aneurysmal sac or the clot may become infected during a transient *Salmonella* bacteremia. This then becomes the site of a bacterial endarteritis, which thereafter is a source for a continuous intense bacteremia. However, in some patients with this syndrome, neither clot nor infection of the aneurysmal wall can be demonstrated. An aortic aneurysm in a rare patient with *Salmonella* infection of a vertebral body may become infected as the result of direct spread of infection to its outer wall from the adjacent area of osteomyelitis. The pathophysiologic changes in *Salmonella* bacteremia consist of three groups of phenomena: (1) those due to the presence of viable gram-negative bacilli in the circulation; (2) those related to circulating endotoxin (myalgias, fever, and even disseminated intravascular coagulation in an occasional patient); and (3) the tendency for metastatic infections to develop. The lungs, meninges, synovial membranes, bones, and endocardium (valvular) are most often involved.

Syphilis

Syphilis may involve any part of the body, particularly in its late stages, and may produce profound functional changes in many organs. The pathophysiologic phenomena in this disease are the result of inflammatory and vascular changes in organs where *Treponema pallidum,* the etiologic agent, has been deposited during the early phase of invasion of the bloodstream. The changes are conveniently considered under three major groupings: *early, late, and congenital* syphilis. The relative impact of the disease on various organ systems depends on the stage of the process; the latter is determined to a large measure by the effective-

ness of the immunologic response to the invading spirochete. Certain organs such as the heart and aorta, the central nervous system, and the eye are prominently involved; important functional derangements occur as a result. The natural history of untreated early syphilis, as observed at the turn of this century, suggested that in about two thirds of individuals the disease became latent and produced no major manifestations. However, it was found, 50 to 60 years later, that 10 per cent of these patients had syphilitic cardiovascular disease and another 6.5 per cent had neurosyphilis.

Early Syphilis. The usual portal of entry for *T. pallidum* is skin or mucous membrane. Symptomatic early syphilis comprises two stages. The initial lesion of *primary syphilis* is a papule that evolves into a painless, eroded or crusted lesion (chancre), usually located on the genitals but occasionally at extragenital sites. The chancre develops 2 to 6 weeks after inoculation of the organism. Painless regional lymphadenopathy appears shortly thereafter. Pathologically, the primary lesion shows a dermal infiltrate (lymphocytes and plasma cells), a proliferation of capillaries, and endarteritis. *T. pallidum* is present in the lesion and in the regional nodes. The chancre, even if untreated, slowly heals over the next 2 to 6 weeks. During the evolution of the primary lesion and extension of infection to regional lymph nodes, the treponemes enter the circulation and are widely disseminated. Metastatic foci develop, particularly in the skin, the mucous membranes, and the nervous system.

Secondary syphilis occurs 5 to 6 weeks after the appearance of the chancre and is a manifestation of treponemal multiplication in metastatic foci. The principal features are a generalized measles-like rash (often accompanied by erosive superficial lesions in the oral, genital, or anal mucous membranes) and generalized lymph node enlargement. The *secondary eruption,* even if untreated, disappears within several weeks, and the treponemes in other foci appear to die out, presumably as a result of the immunologic response of the host. Occasionally, sufficient numbers of the organisms survive to initiate another round of treponemia. This is responsible for one or more recurrent episodes of secondary syphilis (mucocutaneous relapse). Meningitis due to invasion by treponemes is not uncommon in secondary syphilis. In addition to the usual findings common to many types of aseptic meningitis, delirium and seizures occasionally occur. Damage to the third, sixth, seventh, and eighth cranial nerves may develop as a result of reactive fibrosis of the leptomeninges about the base of the brain. Acute hydrocephalus with papilledema may rarely complicate the process. The cerebrospinal fluid shows a pleocytosis of up to 500 cells, predominantly lymphocytes. The duration of the meningitis is usually less than a month. Other areas that may be involved in secondary syphilis are the *eye* (visual loss due to iritis or optic perineuritis secondary to meningitis); *kidney* (interstitial nephritis; nephrotic syndrome due to membranous glomerulonephritis, with proteinuria and edema); *liver* (hepatitis mimicking viral hepatitis in its manifestations); and *bones* (pain and tenderness of long bones due to periostitis).

Late Syphilis. In about one third of patients with untreated early syphilis, sufficient immunity does not develop to render the disease asymptomatic (latent) for the remainder of the patient's life. Instead, chronic destructive inflammatory and vascular changes slowly progress over many years and produce late manifestations. These occur principally in the skin and mucous membranes, bones, joints, central nervous system, and heart and great vessels.

The characteristic lesion in late syphilis is the gumma, a granulomatous lesion in which there is coagulation necrosis due to obstructive inflammation of small arteries; treponemes are usually absent.

SKIN AND MUCOUS MEMBRANES. The changes of late syphilis in the skin consist of gross, nodular, ulcerating lesions. Gummas also may occur in the oral mucosa and cause perforation of the palate and destruction of the nasal septum.

SKELETAL SYSTEM. Gummatous periosteal involvement of bones produces pain and swelling, particularly of the tibia and clavicle. Destructive involvement of weight-bearing joints ("Charcot's joints") is not due to invasion of the synovia by treponemes but rather to the effects of constant trauma on joints lacking pain sensation because of the neurologic changes of syphilis (tabes dorsalis).

CENTRAL NERVOUS SYSTEM. There are five definable patterns of late syphilis of the central nervous system:

1. *Meningovascular syphilis.* This develops a few years after the primary lesion and lacks the usual features of acute bacterial meningitis. The fundamental lesion is an arteritis. The clinical features result from arterial thromboses and fibrosis. A variety of neurologic syndromes may develop, depending on the site of vascular occlusion. These may be located in the cerebral cortex and produce hemiplegia, aphasia, homonymous hemianopia, or seizures. Occlusions of the anterior spinal artery may lead to paraplegia. Other vascular lesions may produce sensory loss and impairment of bowel and bladder function. A mild lymphocytic pleocytosis (up to 100 cells) of the cerebrospinal fluid is common.

2. *Tabes dorsalis.* This occurs 10 to 30 years after the initial infection. Atrophy of the dorsal roots and demyelinization of the sensory fibers that ascend in the posterior columns of the spinal cord are the characteristic pathologic changes. These are produced by the inflammatory arteritis in the meninges and not by direct invasion of the cord substance by treponemes. As a result of posterior column involvement, position sense is grossly impaired. Patients have difficulty walking, particularly in the dark. Sharp stabbing pain over the extremities or trunk occurs episodically and is due to the changes in the dorsal roots. Involvement of the sacral nerve roots causes impotence, incontinence, and constipation. Atrophy of the optic nerve and changes in function of the pupil (poor responsiveness to light but normal reaction to accommodation—Argyll Robertson pupil) is common.

3. *Primary optic atrophy.* This may occur in the absence of tabes dorsalis. Damage to the optic fibers results from continuous leptomeningitis. This is confirmed by the observation that the outer portions of the optic nerve are first affected, causing impairment of peripheral vision. Subsequent decrease in central visual acuity develops, owing to involvement of the deeper placed fibers in the optic nerve.

4. *General paresis.* This is a very serious form of central nervous system syphilis, involving primarily the cerebral cortex, meninges, and cerebral arteries. Large numbers of *T. pallidum* are found in the cortex, and diffuse neuronal destruction with reactive gliosis is prominent. Atrophy of the frontal and temporal lobes and dilatation of the ventricles are marked. As a result of these extensive pathologic changes in the cerebral cortex, evidence of a wide range of mental and neurologic dysfunction is present. Delusions, hallucinations, hypomania, and paranoia may be prominent. As in tabes dorsalis, patients with paresis may have the Argyll Robertson pupil (irregular miotic pupil responsive to accommodation but not to light). Seizures and strokes secondary to the syphilitic endarteritis are not uncommon. Once developed, general paresis progresses rapidly, with profound mental deterioration followed by physical incapacitation. If untreated, the disease is uniformly fatal.

5. *Gummas of the central nervous system (intracranial or intraspinal).* These are rare and present with manifestations consistent with an expanding lesion, such as a tumor.

Very rarely, *T. pallidum* appears to persist (as evidenced by dark-field microscopy and immunofluorescent antibody techniques) in cerebrospinal fluid or aqueous humor of the eye (or even lymph nodes) following heretofore considered adequate penicillin treatment of latent or late syphilis. Progression of central nervous system syphilis in an occasional patient after conventional penicillin therapy may be related to persistence of the spirochete in areas where antibiotic penetrance is poor. Higher penicillin dosage to provide maximal treponemicidal concentrations in the cerebrospinal fluid is now recommended for such patients.

CARDIOVASCULAR SYSTEM. Cardiovascular syphilis takes the form of either an aortitis of the ascending aorta, producing the clinical features of aortic insufficiency with left ventricular strain, or an aneurysm of the ascending aorta. Involvement of the coronary ostia in the aortitis may lead to coronary insufficiency. Syphilitic aortic aneurysms cause hoarseness (impingement on the recurrent laryngeal nerve); cough and dyspnea (pressure on the trachea and bronchi); dysphagia (compression of the esophagus); and pain (erosion of ribs, sternum, or vertebrae).

Congenital Syphilis. As a result of treponemia occurring after the fourth month of pregnancy, the fetus becomes extensively infected. The placenta is enlarged, and there is extensive proliferation of fibrous connective tissue. Similar fibrotic lesions with mononuclear cell infiltrations are present in many viscera. The most characteristic findings are in the lungs ("pneumonia alba"), which show a marked increase in fibrous tissue and poorly developed alveoli filled with macrophages. Periostitis and osteochondritis are also common.

Late congenital syphilis is a prenatally acquired infection that has been less acute and the clinical manifestations are not evident until the child is over 2 years of age. Osseous changes (saddle nose, saber-shaped tibia from periostitis), synovitis of the knees, dental deformities (upper central incisors), and eighth nerve deafness are usually present. The most common manifestation is interstitial keratitis, an inflammatory process of the cornea complicated by neovascularization, which may progress to blindness. Central nervous system involvement may occur, as in the acquired disease, and result in meningitis, meningovascular disease, juvenile paresis, and, rarely, tabes dorsalis.

INFECTIONS WITH PATHOPHYSIOLOGIC CONSEQUENCES IN A SINGLE ORGAN OR ORGAN SYSTEM

Lobar Pneumonia

The pneumococcus is the commonest cause of lobar pneumonia, but other organisms such as *Klebsiella pneumoniae* may produce a similar lesion. The onset of pneumococcal infection of the lung is usually preceded by a viral upper respiratory tract infection of several days' duration. Aspiration of the infected mucus from the nasopharynx into the distal ramifications of the bronchial tree, usually in the lower lobes, sets up the initial focus of pulmonary infection. The occurrence of such an aspirational event is enhanced by alcoholic intoxication, anesthesia, or depressant drugs, all of which are known to diminish the epiglottal reflex.

Following establishment of infection in the alveoli, a characteristic sequence takes place in the evolution of pneumococcal pneumonia. First, bacterial invasion by the encapsulated diplococci evokes an outpouring of edematous fluid. This thin fluid serves as a vehicle for carrying the organisms into terminal bronchioles and through the alveolar pores of Kohn into adjoining alveoli. Inspiratory movements aid the rapid spread of infection toward the lung periphery. Polymorphonuclear leukocytes quickly enter the infected area and soon reach sufficient numbers to fill the alveoli completely and produce frank consolidation. At this stage, phagocytosis by leukocytes begins to take place even though type-specific opsonizing capsular antibodies have not yet appeared. Such early phagocytosis ("surface phagocytosis") follows the trapping by the leukocytes of pneumococci against alveolar walls or against the surface of other leukocytes. Unspecific heat-labile opsonins (capable of acting on bacteria in general) contribute to the effectiveness of this early phagocytic process and the subsequent destruction of the organisms. After the untreated patient has been ill for some days, monospecific anticapsular antibody appears. By neutralizing the antiphagocytic properties of the capsular polysaccharide, this antibody considerably enhances phagocytosis and intracellular killing. Once most of the organisms have been ingested, macrophages derived from the monocytes of the blood and the lining cells of the alveoli enter the lesion to clear away the bacterial and leukocytic debris.

Although the aforementioned events occur sequentially in a given area of involvement, all are going on simultaneously when the entire spreading lobar process is considered. Three areas of activity are discernible. The peripheral portion of the lesion, the edema zone, is composed of alveoli filled with bacteria and serous fluid containing few, if any, cells. Inside this is a second zone characterized by the presence of leukocytes and red blood cells that have entered through injured alveolar walls. These two peripheral areas, exhibiting edema and hemorrhage together, present the gross appearance of "red hepatization." The third or central zone is one in which the alveoli are crowded with polymorphonuclear leukocytes and in which the appearance of macrophages may herald early resolution. This dense consolidation, when viewed in the gross, is the area of "gray hepatization."

The spreading pneumonic process may rapidly involve a whole lobe, extending as far as the pleural surface. Aspiration of infected edematous fluid into the bronchial tree may spread the infection to several lobes. The infection may not be contained by the pleural boundaries but may enter the pleural space and produce empyema.

Clinical Manifestations of Pneumonia. A variety of clinical manifestations develop in association with the progression of the histologic changes in the lung. The pathophysiologic basis of the signs and symptoms that characterize this kind of pneumonia is understood to a varying degree.

COUGH. This is usually an important feature

of the disease. The cough reflex is stimulated by irritation of the lower respiratory tract and by the accumulation of purulent exudate in the bronchial tree. Pink, bloody, or "rusty" sputum is produced by the majority of patients and is the result of the bleeding into alveoli that characterizes the early inflammatory process.

CHILL AND FEVER. The first major symptom of lobar pneumonia is frequently a single shaking chill that is temporally related to the stage of bacterial invasion of the lung. Phagocytosis stimulates the production and release of EP and thus may be the responsible mechanism. Bacteremia is present in approximately one third of cases of pneumococcal lobar pneumonia and is usually detectable when patients enter the hospital some time after the chill has occurred.

PLEURITIC PAIN. Severe chest pain occurs in the majority of patients with pneumococcal pneumonia. It often occurs at the onset of the disease and is the result of inflammation of the pleural surface following peripheral extension of the pneumonia. The pain is usually referred directly to the overlying chest wall. However, when the diaphragmatic pleura is involved, it is referred to the shoulder. The discomfort is strikingly accentuated by inspiratory movement; this leads to splinting of the affected side of the chest and rapid, shallow, and grunting respiration.

CYANOSIS. Cyanosis of the lips and nail beds is commonly present, in the absence of shock, in pneumococcal lobar pneumonia. This indicates a significant degree of arterial hypoxemia. Several mechanisms may be involved in the pathogenesis of this phenomenon:

1. *Shunting of blood through consolidated lung tissue.* The extensive exudate that completely fills the alveoli in much of the involved lobe decreases or abolishes effective gas exchange in this area. However, blood flow to the consolidated, poorly aerated lobe continues. Thus, venous blood perfusing the area is not exposed to high oxygen tensions and is, in effect, physiologically shunted into the pulmonary veins, and then to the systemic circulation.

2. *Postpulmonary shunting.* This results from admixture of unsaturated blood that occurs distal to the pulmonary capillaries from such venous channels as thebesian vessels, bronchial veins, and anastomoses between portal vein collaterals and the pulmonary circulation (portopulmonary shunt).

3. *Ventilation-perfusion disturbances in unconsolidated areas of the lung.* Most of the hypoxia in patients with lobar pneumonia is accounted for by a right-to-left shunt. When the disease is moderately severe, essentially all of the shunt is pulmonary. When it is severe, both pulmonary and postpulmonary shunting is markedly accentuated. The increase in the postpulmonary shunt in severe pneumonia has been attributed to an increase in bronchial circulation. However, a more likely explanation is that the heightened tissue metabolism in the area of infection causes an increase in the observed total shunt (without affecting the pulmonary shunt) by decreasing the oxygen content of pulmonary venous blood. Later in the course of pneumonia (after 4 days), the magnitude of the shunt declines. After 4 days of illness, ventilation-perfusion disturbances begin to contribute relatively more to the observed hypoxia in some instances. This may be due to altered lung mechanics known to be present in acute pneumonia (decrease in lung compliance out of proportion to the amount of lung tissue involved as observed in roentgenograms of the chest). The reason for this increased rigidity of apparently normal parts of the lung may be the reduction of surface activity that has been noted in grossly normal areas from lungs containing lobar consolidations. The causes of hypoxemia in lobar pneumonia clearly appear to depend to some extent on both the severity and the duration of the pulmonary infection.

CIRCULATORY CHANGES. Cardiovascular function may be taxed heavily by the stress of pneumonia. The impact on the heart may be so severe that death results. The adequacy of the circulation and tissue perfusion can be appraised by measurement of the arteriovenous (A-V) oxygen difference. A normal (not exceeding 5.5 vol per cent) or narrowed A-V difference is an indication of a physiologically adequate circulation. In the presence of fever, the cardiac output is normally increased in parallel or in excess of the increase in oxygen consumption. The net effect is that the A-V O_2 difference remains normal or is narrowed. In two thirds of patients with pneumonia, tissue perfusion is adequate as judged by evidence of an appropriate circulatory response—an increased cardiac output associated with increased oxygen consumption and an A-V O_2 difference not in excess of 5.5 vol per cent. In the other one third of patients, there is an inadequate hemodynamic response, consisting of a relatively low cardiac output that results in a widened A-V O_2 difference. This occurs in patients who have no apparent evidence of pre-existing heart disease and whose venous pressure is normal. These individuals also have an abnormally high total peripheral resistance and an increased hematocrit. The hypodynamic state in this group appears to be due principally to depressed myocardial function that returns to normal during convalescence. Relative hypovolemia due to decreased fluid intake, fluid losses secondary to fever, and shifts out of the vascular compartment may also contribute to the lowered cardiac output. The underlying nature of the myocardial dysfunction is unknown. T-wave changes have been reported in the EKG during pneumonia; infiltration of the myocardium with inflammatory cells has been noted in some fatal cases. Whether these represent direct effects of a bacterial product or of hypoxia is not known.

ILEUS. Adynamic ileus and gastric dilatation

may be prominent features in pneumococcal pneumonia. They may be of sufficient magnitude to add to the patient's discomfort and interfere with respiration. The cause of the ileus is not established, but it may result from the low O_2 saturation of the blood supplying the bowel.

HERPES LABIALIS. Pneumococcal pneumonia is frequently accompanied by an attack of herpes labialis. By means not yet understood, this pulmonary infection (as well as a variety of other events) can stimulate herpes simplex virus release from trigeminal ganglia in which it resides quiescently. After passage of the virus down the nerve fibers to the skin, infection of epidermal cells occurs, with development of characteristic vesicles on the lips.

Complications of Pneumococcal Pneumonia. A variety of complications may occur and produce pathophysiologic consequences depending on their location.

PULMONARY AND PLEURAL INVOLVEMENT. Lung abscess is a rare complication of pneumococcal pneumonia and is almost always due to infection with type III strains. These organisms possess an abundant "slime layer" of antiphagocytic capsular polysaccharide. This interferes with initial surface phagocytosis, as a result of which the density of bacteria in the pneumonic focus may reach an extremely high level and produce local necrosis of the lung. Pleural involvement may lead to the development of an effusion or a frank empyema. Fever and evidence of infection will persist if the latter is not properly drained. Compression of the lung may become chronic owing to fibrosis and produce restrictive changes in pulmonary function.

CARDIAC INVOLVEMENT. Purulent pericarditis and acute bacterial endocarditis are the serious cardiac complications of pneumococcal pneumonia and are due to direct bacterial invasion. Pericarditis may produce cardiac tamponade, with limitation of venous return and cardiac output as the physiologic consequences of this constrictive process.

MENINGITIS. This complication is the result of bacteremic spread of infection.

ARTHRITIS. This is a suppurative process due to growth of pneumococci in the synovia and extension into the joint space.

PERITONITIS. Although pneumococcal peritonitis may occur in the course of pulmonary infection due to this organism, it is rare. Patients with either postnecrotic hepatic cirrhosis or the nephrotic syndrome are particularly susceptible to the development of peritoneal involvement. The clinical picture is that of a septic process complicated by adynamic ileus.

FULMINANT PNEUMOCOCCAL BACTEREMIA. Splenectomized patients, particularly children whose spleens have been removed because of thalassemia or other hemolytic anemia, are particularly susceptible to severe pneumococcal infections with intense bacteremia complicated by shock and disseminated intravascular coagulation.

Interstitial Pneumonia

Interstitial pneumonia is a diffuse inflammatory process of the lung in which the pathologic changes are located mainly in the alveolar walls and, to a varying degree, within the alveoli. There is involvement of the alveolar ducts and bronchioles to a lesser extent. Histologically, there is an extensive interstitial inflammatory infiltration, usually consisting of mononuclear cells, in the walls of alveoli and in the connective tissue septa about the small pulmonary vessels. This process usually accompanies or immediately follows an initial intra-alveolar inflammatory reaction. It may be manifest clinically as an acute process and resolve completely or occasionally lead to severe interstitial fibrosis and run a subacute or chronic course.

A wide range of infectious agents may be involved in the pathogenesis of interstitial pneumonia: (1) viruses, such as influenza, varicella, adenovirus, and herpes hominis; (2) *Mycoplasma pneumoniae* (the cause of the common type of "atypical pneumonia"); (3) *Chlamydia* (psittacosis or ornithosis); (4) *Rickettsia,* principally *Coxiella burnetii* (Q fever); (5) bacteria, primarily *Haemophilus influenzae;* (6) fungi such as *Histoplasma capsulatum;* and (7) protozoa *(Pneumocystis carinii)*. However, a somewhat similar clinical and pathophysiologic picture can also be produced by a variety of noninfectious processes. These include (1) *infiltrative disorders* (sarcoidosis, histiocytosis); (2) *pneumoconioses;* (3) *collagen vascular diseases;* (4) *radiation pneumonitis;* (5) *drug sensitivity* (busulfan, methotrexate); and (6) *unusual pathologic process of unknown etiology* ("desquamative interstitial pneumonia," "lymphocytic interstitial pneumonia").

Nonproductive cough, fever, and slight shortness of breath are the principal symptoms in mild cases of interstitial pneumonia. Breathing is rapid and shallow, even at rest, in more severe cases. Radiographic changes are usually minimal and consist of fine mottling and a reticular pattern. The oxygen saturation of arterial blood may be markedly reduced, and cyanosis, incompletely relieved by oxygen administration, may be present. The P_{CO_2} of arterial blood is normal or decreased (owing to hyperventilation). The low arterial oxygen tension (P_{O_2}) was originally interpreted to be the result of impairment of diffusion of oxygen through a thickened alveolar membrane ("alveolar-capillary block" syndrome). However, physiologic studies have indicated that it is unlikely that this can account for the observed arterial oxygen unsaturation. A more likely explanation stems from the finding that there are irregularly distributed areas of lung with altered mechanical properties in this disease. Alveoli in such areas of reduced compliance have somewhat decreased ventilation but are still normally perfused. Thus, abnormalities of ventilation-perfusion and ventilation-diffusion ratios result in inadequate oxygenation of blood leaving certain areas of the lung (venous admixture).

Physiologic studies of patients with acute interstitial pneumonias have been very limited. Varicella pneumonia, a disease seen almost exclusively in adults, has been examined more extensively than others. Dyspnea, nonproductive cough, and cyanosis are common features due to pulmonary involvement in patients with extensive and severe chickenpox. Death may occur from respiratory failure. Radiographic examination discloses prominent bronchovascular markings and diffuse nodular densities. There is no evidence of obstructive ventilatory difficulty. Increased venous admixture has been found during the acute phase of illness. There may be chronic impairment of gas transfer after resolution of the pneumonia. Scattered, small nodular pulmonary calcifications may develop some time after recovery.

Bacterial Meningitis

The syndrome of uncomplicated bacterial meningitis represents a combination of the *nonspecific manifestations of infection* (fever, malaise, headache), the *signs of meningeal irritation* (stiff neck and back, positive Kernig's and Brudzinski's signs), and *abnormalities of the spinal fluid* (variable numbers and types of cells, and changes in content of sugar and protein). These alterations are induced by pathophysiologic processes that are, for the most part, reasonably well understood.

Manifestations of Infection. As with infections of most types, fever is an almost universal accompaniment of meningitis; chills are often, but not invariably, present. Generalized malaise, often with pain in the muscles and joints, is common. Myalgia appears to be a more prominent feature during the prodromal stages of meningococcal meningitis than during other bacterial meningitides. This may be a manifestation of the accompanying meningococcemia or of endotoxemia.

Manifestations of Meningeal Irritation and Intracranial Infection. The signs of meningeal irritation are produced by the inflammatory reaction about the pain-sensitive spinal roots and nerves. As attempts are made to flex the neck or back or to extend the lower legs on the flexed thighs, traction occurs on the spinal roots and nerves; this produces pain and results in involuntary spasm of the muscles innervated by these nerves. The inability to flex or extend respective muscle groups is responsible for the stiffness of the neck and back and the positive Kernig's and Brudzinski's signs.

Headache, often extremely severe and "pounding" in character, is the most common symptom of meningitis. Although an increase in intracranial pressure is relatively frequent, the pain in the head is usually not due to this, but appears to be related to distortion of the meningeal vessels, which are usually encased in the inflammatory exudate.

A common occurrence in the course of the bacterial meningitides is the development of *cerebral edema.* This may be of a degree severe enough to produce changes in the state of consciousness, confusion, or even localizing neurologic signs. It may develop early during meningitis and may be accentuated by excessive administration of parenteral fluids in the course of treatment. The primary danger is herniation of the temporal lobe or cerebellum with compression of the midbrain at the tentorium, producing respiratory arrest. Removal of cerebrospinal fluid in the presence of heightened intracranial pressure may precipitate herniation. Marked brain swelling is usually reflected clinically by coma, by signs of third nerve dysfunction (irregularity of the size or fixation of the pupils), or by respiratory arrest. Papilledema may occur in various types of meningitis. However, the majority of patients with meningitis and increased CSF pressure do not have papilledema. Elevated CSF pressure in the early stages of bacterial meningitis is, in most instances, due to brain swelling and not to obstructive hydrocephalus or intraspinal block. It is important to remember, however, that meningeal infection may be the consequence of intraventricular leakage of a cerebral abscess or may be accompanied or complicated by subdural empyema. Both cerebral abscess and subdural empyema are space-occupying lesions that can produce increased intracranial pressure and papilledema. Since their treatment is different from that of meningitis, early diagnosis is essential.

Seizures frequently complicate bacterial meningitis. The incidence is higher in infants. However, convulsions are known to be frequent in young children with fever due to a variety of causes. The seizures associated with meningeal infection may be focal or generalized. A common type of focal episode consists of rhythmic jerkings of the eyes conjugately to one side. Seizures may occur during the peak of the meningitis or may appear for the first time during the second or third week of the disease, when evidence of active meningeal infection has all but disappeared. Delayed thrombosis of cortical veins is responsible for late seizure activity; it can also account for seizure activity that develops earlier in the disease. Brain swelling may be responsible for seizures during the course of meningitis. Seizures during treatment of meningitis may be a manfestation of penicillin neurotoxicity if this antibiotic is being administered in high dosage to a patient with reduced renal function.

Focal cerebral signs, aside from seizures and alterations of consciousness, occur in meningitis infrequently. Focal cerebral signs that appear early are commonly due to cortical necrosis or occlusive vasculitis (usually venous). Among these are hemiparesis, quadriparesis, visual field defects, disorders of conjugate gaze, and dysphasia. Temporary hemiparesis (persisting up to several hours or longer) can occur as a postictal phenomenon, and its significance can be considerably different from that of a true dense hemiplegia. Prominent and persisting focal cerebral signs always raise the spectre of an associated pyogenic process such as brain abscess, subdural empyema, or possible cerebral embolism from bacterial endocarditis.

Cranial nerve dysfunction is not uncommon in bacterial meningitis. Impaired ocular movement (paresis of third or sixth cranial nerve) is the most frequently encountered evidence of such dysfunction. Facial weakness (seventh nerve) and deafness (eighth nerve) are the other principal signs of cranial nerve involvement. In general, dysfunction of the cranial nerves is transient and disappears shortly after recovery from the meningitis. It is generally assumed, but not yet proved, the damage to these nerves results from their entrapment by the meningeal exudate. Deafness and labyrinthine deficits tend to persist, in contrast to the transient character of the disturbance of other cranial nerve functions. This suggests the possibility that damage to the inner ear is the result of the activity of bacteria or their products. Deafness is not correlated with the presence of otitis media. In fact, deafness is observed more frequently after meningococcal than after other types of meningitis; yet otitis media is much less common in meningococcal meningitis than in meningitis due to *Streptococcus pneumoniae* or *Haemophilus influenzae.*

Sterile subdural effusions occur in about 10 per cent of patients under the age of 2 years with bacterial meningitis. They are only rarely reported in children older than this. Repeated vomiting, persistence or recurrence of fever, increasing irritability, seizures, fullness of the fontanelle, or increasing cranial circumference have been attributed to subdural effusion when they occur later in the course of meningitis. Transillumination has proved a useful means of making the diagnosis, but CT scanning is now also available. In many infants with meningitis, such sterile subdural effusions disappear without the need for subdural tap. Indeed, they may be found (on routine transillumination of infants with meningitis) in the absence of any clinical manifestations attributable to the process. Rarely, subdural effusions are invaded by bacteria as a result of penetration of the arachnoid by the infectious process. The resulting subdural empyema is characterized by high fever, considerable toxicity, and a variety of cortical signs (seizures, hemiplegias, visual field defects). The latter signs are due to (1) inflammation and thrombosis of the cortical veins that run through the subdural space, and (2) pressure phenomena secondary to the often large accumulation of pus over one or both cerebral hemispheres.

Abnormalities of Cerebrospinal Fluid. An increase in the number of cells is demonstrable, with very rare exceptions, in patients with bacterial meningitis. Almost without exception, the predominant cell in the early stages of the disease is the neutrophil. In rare instances, mobilization of inflammatory cells into the spinal fluid may not occur, and culture of the spinal fluid may yield organisms that are too few in number to be detectable in stained preparations. Although not frequent, this phenomenon appears to be most common in the early stage of meningococcal infection. This may be due to the fact that insufficient time had elapsed for the developing inflammatory exudate in the meninges to extend into the spinal fluid. Rarely, the cerebrospinal fluid may be strikingly turbid in the absence of cells; the turbidity then is due entirely to large numbers of organisms. The pneumococcus is the usual etiologic agent in these circumstances. In such cases, studies of bone marrow and peripheral blood have revealed no abnormalities; in fact, a leukocytosis with a shift to the left is commonly present. Patients with leukemia may develop meningitis with similar findings; in this instance, the lack of cerebrospinal fluid pleocytosis is attributable to the marked reduction in circulating neutrophils.

The increased content of protein in the spinal fluid in cases of meningitis is the result of leakage of serum proteins, the release from the meninges of the products of inflammation, and the breakdown of leukocytes introduced during the infectious process. The pathophysiologic basis of very high levels of protein (up to 1 gm or more per dl) in fluid removed from the lumbar sac is intraspinal block, usually complicating more chronic forms of meningitis such as that due to *Mycobacterium tuberculosis;* excessive concentrations in ventricular fluid are suggestive of block in the internal circulation of spinal fluid, most commonly due to obstruction of the sylvian aqueduct.

Reduction of the concentration of glucose in the spinal fluid is usually, but not always, observed in the active, untreated phase of bacterial meningitis. Although levels may be normal in the very early stage of the disease, these decrease, as a rule, as the infection progresses. It must be stressed that the content of glucose in the cerebrospinal fluid in healthy individuals is directly related, except in uncommon instances, to the concentration of glucose in the blood. High blood sugar levels in a patient with diabetes may be accompanied by a normal or elevated concentration in the spinal fluid. In contrast, quite low levels of glucose in the spinal fluid of young infants do not necessarily indicate infection but may reflect hypoglycemia due to vomiting or poor food intake.

Although extensive bacterial multiplication may play some role in the fall in cerebrospinal fluid glucose concentration in certain types of experimentally produced meningitis (pneumococcal) in animals, it is clear that the metabolic demands of the bacteria or of the leukocytes alone do not account for the lowered levels of glucose. The limited surface phagocytosis that occurs in early bacterial meningitis may contribute in a small measure to lowering CSF glucose through augmented glucose utilization, a characteristic of the phagocytic event. However, interference with the transport of glucose from blood to cerebrospinal fluid appears to be the major factor contributing to the lowering of the concentration of glucose in the spinal fluid. Under physiologic conditions, the transfer of glucose from blood to spinal fluid is mediated by two processes: simple diffusion and carrier-facilitated diffusion. The facilitated diffusion of glucose from blood to the cerebrospinal fluid and outward diffusion of glucose from spinal fluid to blood are impaired in bacterial meningitis. This may be secondary to alterations in the blood-CSF barrier due either to increased metabolism of the cells involved or to structural changes produced by the inflammatory process. In addition, there may be greater utilization of glucose by the brain in the course of meningeal infection.

An increase in the concentration of cerebrospinal fluid hydrogen ion has been reported in some patients with bacterial meningitis or subarachnoid hemorrhage. The decrease in pH is associated with a rise in the level of lactic acid in the CSF. It has been suggested that some of the changes in respiration and sensorium that occur in the course of bacterial infection of the meninges may result from this. The decreased pH of CSF may stimulate medullary chemoreceptors and induce hyperventilation, an event that occurs occasionally in severe meningitis. The respiratory alkalosis produced by hyperventilation may then reduce cerebral perfusion, and, in this way, exacerbate the CSF acidosis.

The aforementioned pathophysiologic processes are common to practically all the bacterial meningitides. However, each etiologic type of meningeal infection has individual physiologic and anatomic features that may account for some of their special clinical characteristics.

Meningococcal Meningitis. Meningococcal infection may have its sole impact as a meningeal disease. However, there may also be widespread effects on other organ systems. Infection of the upper respiratory tract is the most common form of meningococcal disease in humans but produces few, if any, symptoms. In a small percentage of these patients, there is a sequential development of clinical manifestations: bacteremia, meningitis, and/or other metastatic localizations. The presence of circulating antibodies specific for the various serologic groups of meningococci affords protection against bloodstream invasion.

The occurrence of meningococcal bacteremia (meningococcemia) precedes the development of meningococcal meningitis. The pathophysiologic consequences of meningococcemia vary.

MILD MENINGOCOCCEMIA. The onset is usually acute, with fever, chilliness, myalgias, arthralgias, nausea, and vomiting. Macular skin lesions, particularly on the extremities, are replaced by petechiae and, at times, purpuric lesions. The petechiae that are so common in this disease often contain a necrotic center surrounded by a small zone of hemorrhage. Meningococci may sometimes be demonstrated in Gram stains or culture of material obtained by needle from the pale center of such lesions. The pathophysiologic basis of the lesions in the skin may be a bacterial vasculitis, an endotoxin-induced Shwartzman-like reaction, or thrombocytopenia secondary to the bacteremia. Meningitis quickly follows the bacteremia in some cases; in others, meningeal infection never develops. Some patients develop meningitis without even exhibiting any manifestations in the skin, despite the presence of organisms in the circulation.

ACUTE FULMINATING MENINGOCOCCEMIA (WATERHOUSE-FRIDERICHSEN SYNDROME). The striking feature of this process is the abruptness of its onset and the rapidity with which it inexorably progresses. Shock, extensive purpura, and rapid death (within 24 hours of the intrusion of meningococci into the bloodstream) are attributable to the overwhelming bacteremia and the effects of endotoxin. Circulatory collapse, coma, and disseminated intravascular coagulation (see Chapter 20) may occur within a few hours of onset of the disease. The coagulopathy is responsible for widespread but patchy gangrene of the skin, digits, ears, and nose that may lead to spontaneous amputation of the involved areas. Gastrointestinal bleeding may occur secondary to mucosal lesions of the bowel. Bilateral hemorrhages of the adrenal glands are often present in fatal cases. Levels of corticosteroids in the circulation are usually normal or elevated in fulminant meningococcemia. Thus, acute adrenal insufficiency is probably not the major pathophysiologic basis of the shock occurring in this form of disease.

METASTATIC INFECTIONS SECONDARY TO MENINGOCOCCEMIA. The meninges are the commonest sites of metastatic infection in the course of meningococcemia. However, the organisms may be deposited at many other sites. This usually occurs early in the disease and most often coincides with the meningitis. Metastatic infections of joints, endocardium, myocardium, pericardium, eyes, testes, and lungs have been recorded.

CHRONIC MENINGOCOCCEMIA. This is a rare syndrome characterized by recurrent episodes of fever, chills, arthralgias (or arthritis), and an erythematous papular rash. These tend to occur at intervals of 48 to 72 hours and last for 1 to 2 days. Blood cultures usually yield meningococci early in the febrile stage. The source of the organisms cannot be defined in every case; in some instances, however, they may be recovered from the upper respiratory tract. Recurrent attacks may go on for weeks to months if treatment is not instituted; meningitis or endocarditis may develop in patients who are not treated.

The clinical characteristics of the meningitis due to *Neisseria meningitidis* are, in general, similar to those present in other types of pyogenic meningeal infections. However, several features are more often associated with disease caused by the meningococcus than with that in which the pneumococcus or *Haemophilus influenzae* is involved. Among these are severe agitation, delirium, and maniacal behavior in the early stages of the meningitis; acute brain swelling also appears to be more common and, indeed, may be the pathophysiologic basis of the cerebral signs.

An interesting group of late complications may appear in a small percentage of patients in the course of meningococcal bacteremia or meningitis. Among these are marked arthralgia or frank arthritis, pericarditis (usually with effusion), and myocarditis (primarily electrocardiographic abnormalities). These usually develop during convalescence and are not prevented or abolished by effective antimicrobial therapy. The synovial or pericardial fluids contain a moderate number of polymorphonuclear leukocytes but are sterile. This process is distinct from the septic arthritis or pericarditis that accompanies or complicates the acute phase of meningococcemia or meningitis. It has been suggested that these manifestations represent immunologic reactions, involving complexes of meningococcal polysaccharide antigens and antibody deposited in various tissues. In several patients who developed sterile arthritis during recovery from meningococcal meningitis, circulating immune complexes have been demonstrated in sera and synovial fluid. Deposits of meningococcal antigen, immunoglobulin, and complement (C3) have been detected in leukocytes in synovial fluid and in skin lesions. Host responses to the antigen-antibody complexes are thought to produce the ensuing sterile inflammation in the involved areas.

Haemophilus influenzae Meningitis. The age distribution of *H. influenzae* meningitis is striking, with the vast majority of cases occurring in patients between the ages of 6 months and 3 years. The presence of bactericidal antibody appears to be a crucial determinant in this predilection of the disease for the young. Antibody to type B *H. influenzae*, the strain principally responsible for human infection, is transferred across the placenta to the fetus and persists at effective levels in the infant until somewhere between the ages of 3 and 6 months. Thereafter, children are without this protective antibody until they are 3 years of age, when they begin to acquire it as a result of contact or of relatively minor infections. By the time most individuals are 12 to 15 years old, they are immune to invasion by the type B organism. This accounts for the relative infrequency of this type of meningitis in otherwise normal adults.

The pathophysiology of meningitis due to *H. influenzae* is, for the most part, similar to that produced by the meningococcus. Bacteremia originating from the respiratory tract occurs frequently in this type of infection but is not necessary for initiation of meningeal infection. Suppurative arthritis is a rare complication. Petechial rashes may develop rarely in patients in whom the organisms have invaded the bloodstream.

Seizures and sterile subdural effusions occur more commonly with meningitis due to *H. influenzae* than with that caused by the meningococcus. This does not stem from a difference in the invasive properties of the organisms but rather from the age distribution of the two types of meningitis. *H. influenzae* meningitis commonly occurs in infants or young children, whereas the peak age incidence of meningococcal meningitis is in older children and young adults. The prominence of seizures in *H. influenzae* meningitis may reflect merely the frequency of "febrile convulsion" in young infants prone to develop this disease. The higher incidence of subdural effusions with *H. influenzae* meningitis may similarly reflect the age distribution of this type of meningitis and the availability of easy methods of detecting the presence of subdural fluid (transillumination or subdural tap) in children less than 2 years of age.

Pneumococcal Meningitis. Many, but not all, instances of pneumococcal meningitis are secondary to bacteremia. This is particularly so when the source of the organisms is pneumonia. In about 25 per cent of patients, the primary infection involves the middle ear or paranasal sinuses from which it extends to the lining of the central nervous system along venous channels that drain these areas, or the disease reaches the meninges by direct invasion of bone (e.g., the mastoid).

Most instances of recurrent bacterial meningitis are caused by the pneumococcus; as many as 20 episodes have occurred in the same patient. The anatomic basis for this disease is the presence of a cranial lesion that permits communication between the external environment and the meninges. Organisms then can pass directly from the upper respiratory tract, most commonly the nose and its accessory structures, to the central nervous system. The predisposing conditions are usually tears in the dura, fractures of the cribriform plate, nasal meningoceles, and osteomyelitis of the floor of the anterior fossa of the skull.

Meningitis due to the pneumococcus tends to be a more severe disease with a significantly higher mortality than that due to the meningococcus or *H. influenzae*. The exudate tends to be thicker, particularly over the convexity of the brain, in pneumococcal meningitis. Cerebral venous and arterial occlusions leading to hemiplegia or other syndromes appear to be more common in this type of meningeal infection than in the other two types, probably reflecting the effect of the markedly purulent exudate that is often present.

Tuberculous Meningitis. Bacteremia is probably not the immediate predisposing event in tuberculous meningitis. The most likely focus from which *Mycobacterium tuberculosis* reaches the meninges is a pre-existing small tuberculoma within the cerebral substance or abutting on the meninges. These lesions usually develop during the course of a transient postprimary tubercle bacillemia. The tuberculoma is quickly walled off by host defenses and then remains quiescent for many years or for the lifetime of the patient; however, in a rare instance, breakdown of the lesion occurs later and leads to spread of organisms to the meninges. Meningitis may develop occasionally as a complication of disseminated (miliary) tuberculosis, particularly in children. Even under these circumstances it is probable that the meningeal infection is not the result of direct implantation of organisms but is secondary to the development of microscopic tuberculomas within the central nervous system. In support of this is the observation that injection of tubercle bacilli into the carotid arteries of dogs produces tuberculomas of the brain and meninges but not tuberculous meningitis. Overt pulmonary tuberculosis is not a prerequisite for the development of meningitis; infection of the lung is not apparent in about one third of instances of central nervous system disease. Two pathophysiologic features of tuberculous meningitis account for several characteristic aspects of this form of meningitis. These are the basilar location of the inflammatory exudate and the common involvement of blood vessels, particularly in the form of an occlusive arteritis. These are responsible for the frequent development of cranial nerve dysfunction, especially bilateral paralysis of the sixth nerve, and the sudden appearance of signs of vascular thrombosis, including hemiplegia and other manifestations of localized brain or spinal cord damage. Ventricular block or spinal block may occur secondary to the chronic inflammatory process and may lead to obstructive hydrocephalus.

The abnormalities in the spinal fluid in tuberculous meningitis differ from those found in meningitis due to pyogenic bacteria. The cellular response consists predominantly of lymphocytes, whereas in untreated pyogenic meningitis over 80 per cent of the cells are polymorphonuclear leukocytes. While the cell count in meningitis caused by other bacteria is usually between 1000 and 10,000 per mm³, it rarely exceeds 500 per mm³ in tuberculous meningitis. The other changes in the spinal fluid in this disease are qualitatively the same as those in the other bacterial meningitides; they are, however, quantitatively different. In contrast to other infections of the meninges, the sugar content of spinal fluid falls much more slowly and the quantity of protein usually increases to appreciably higher levels. Although it was formerly thought that a reduced concentration of chloride in the cerebrospinal fluid was characteristic and even diagnostic of tuberculous meningitis, this is now known not to be the case. Decreased levels of chloride may occur in other types of meningeal infection and are directly related to hypochloremia, a not uncommon phenomenon in this disease due to the loss of chloride from the profuse sweating and vomiting that frequently occur in the early stages of infection. The syndrome of inappropriate antidiuretic hormone secretion, though not common, occurs more frequently in tuberculous than in other types of meningitis, perhaps related to its longer course and the accompanying chronic pulmonary tuberculosis. It may contribute significantly to the low levels of chloride in the serum and spinal fluid.

Serous tuberculous meningitis is an unusual clinical entity that occasionally develops in children with tuberculosis. The clinical features associated with this syndrome are similar to those characteristic of the early stage of infection of the meninges by the tubercle bacillus—fever, apathy, irritability, headache, vomiting, and stiff neck. Cranial nerve abnormalities do not occur. Serous meningitis differs from caseous tuberculous infection in several ways:

1. It may resolve spontaneously in several weeks or less, whereas true tuberculous meningitis is almost invariably fatal without antimicrobial therapy.

2. Tubercle bacilli are not found in the cerebrospinal fluid.

3. Chemical alterations are generally not observed in the CSF: The glucose concentration is normal and the protein level is, at most, only slightly increased.

4. The number of cells, usually predominantly lymphocytes, is sometimes normal but is frequently increased to as high as 300 per mm³.

Serous meningitis is thought to be an inflammatory response of the meninges to the presence of localized adjacent (parameningeal) caseous foci, the result of hematogenous infection. These foci induce a "sympathetic" response in the meninges that is similar to that which occurs in pyogenic intracranial infections (brain abscess, subdural empyema), without creating a diffuse meningitis due to seeding with tubercle bacilli. Another interesting, but unproved, hypothesis for the mechanism of serous meningitis is based on the concept of a tuberculin reaction restricted to the meninges. The setting for this process is thought to be an individual with an "inactive" pulmonary lesion and a quiescent tuberculoma of the meninges. Release of tuberculoprotein into the circulation when the pulmonary process becomes active may initiate a response of delayed hypersensitivity (tuberculin reaction) in the meningeal focus. This results in development of fever, signs of meningeal irritation, and CSF pleocytosis.

Since the introduction of effective antituberculous drugs, calcification of intracranial tuberculous lesions (located in the basal meninges and in the brain itself) has been observed more frequently. In occasional patients the late onset (several years after recovery from tuberculous meningitis) of dysfunction of the hypothalamic-pituitary axis (diabetes insipidus, hypopituitarism, precocious puberty) has become evident, apparently related to chronic scarring or necrosis secondary to the meningeal inflammation.

Poliomyelitis

Poliomyelitis virus, acquired by a nonimmune person from a patient with active disease or from a healthy carrier, enters the body by the oral route. It multiplies in the oropharynx for a short period, then disappears from this site. At the same time that the virus becomes established in the upper respiratory tract, it also is implanted in the intestine. There it continues to replicate throughout the incubation period and active stage of the disease and for some time during and after convalescence. From the intestine, the infectious agent invades the regional lymphatic channels; from there, it reaches the bloodstream. The virus enters the central nervous system at many points by direct passage from capillaries to the motor neurons.

A number of physiologic processes play important roles in determining susceptibility and response to infection by poliomyelitis virus. The mechanism by which these processes operate is obscure in most instances. Listed subsequently are a few of these physiologic factors:

1. Age is an important determinant of severity of the disease. Young children with spinal involvement usually have paralysis of one extremity, most commonly a leg. In contrast, a quadriplegia is the most frequent consequence of involvement of the spinal cord in adults. Paralysis of the bladder is about 10 times more common in older individuals than in youngsters.

2. Pregnancy increases the risk of developing poliomyelitis. Women who come in contact with the virus at about the time of ovulation are more prone to infection than if they are exposed at other times in the menstrual cycle.

3. Muscles that have been subjected to trauma or intense exercise may be particularly vulnerable. Muscles that are sites of injection of vaccines, particularly those containing *Bordetella pertussis,* are prone to becoming paralyzed, if immunization is carried out during a period of endemicity of poliomyelitis.

4. Patients who have undergone tonsilloadenoidectomy are much more susceptible to the development of the bulbar form of the disease than those not subjected to this procedure, regardless of when the operation was performed.

The clinical pictures that characterize poliomyelitis are primarily the direct result of pathophysiologic phenomena involving areas of the nervous system invaded and injured by the virus. The sore throat, often present as a prodromal manifestation of the disease, is due to the growth of and accompanying local inflammatory reaction initiated by the virus. The gastrointestinal manifestations (nausea, vomiting, diarrhea) are related to multiplication of the agent in this area and to its effect on the function of the plexuses of Meissner and Auerbach. The anterior horn cells of the spinal cord are the site of predilection for viral invasion, but this occurs in a scattered ("skip") fashion, with variation in the degree and distribution of neuronal involvement. This is manifested by varying degrees of asymmetric paresis or paralysis of extremities and of weakness of the muscles of respiration. The neurologic findings are characteristic of a lower motor neuron lesion: flaccid weakness, loss of reflexes, and fasciculation of muscles. Sensory modalities are unimpaired. Alterations in blood pressure, irregularity of cardiac rhythm, variation in skin and muscle temperature, and a variety of skin rashes may be related to invasion of autonomic ganglia by the virus.

When neurons in the medulla are involved, two pathophysiologic consequences are observed. Striking irregularity in the rate and depth of breathing (Biot respiration) is the result of involvement of the respiratory center. As the disease progresses, there are longer periods of apnea until breathing ceases completely. Hiccupping, probably related to irritation of the respiratory center, is often present in the early phase of involvement of this area. Hypoxia, without visible cyanosis, is common and may produce transient elevations of blood pressure. Viral injury to the neurons in the vasomotor center in the medulla is manifested by hypertension initially, followed by fluctuations in the level of blood pressure, and finally by severe hypotension together with the clinical manifestations of shock. Myocarditis is not uncommon in poliomyelitis; it is probably due to direct invasion by the virus. Electrocardiographic abnormalities, mainly T and ST and P–R alterations, are present in from 10 to 20 per cent of cases. Irregularities in cardiac rhythm, including sinus tachycardia or bradycardia, atrial fibrillation, premature ventricular contractions, and ventricular fibrillation, may supervene. Hyperpyrexia, with temperatures of 106° or higher, often develops in the late stages of the type of disease in which the medulla is involved.

The brain may be affected, to a varying degree, by poliomyelitis. Encephalitic manifestations occur as isolated syndromes or together with bulbar or spinal disease. The diffuse form of encephalitis is featured by confusion, agitation, anxiety, or somnolence. Quivering and jerking of the facial muscles and extremities, flushing of the face, tremor of the hands, and restless movements occur.

In focal polioencephalitis, there may be clinical evidence of dysfunction, or the lesions may be silent and demonstrable only at necropsy. Visual-verbal agnosia, myoclonic jerks, grand mal seizures that occasionally persist long after recovery, spastic hemiparesis, ataxia of one arm or leg, and hydrocephalus have been described.

Dysfunction of the peripheral vascular tree may accompany severe poliomyelitis in some cases. This is probably related to invasion of the sympathetic ganglia by the virus. A variety of skin eruptions including miliaria, morbilliform rashes and scarlatiniform eruptions may develop in the severely paralyzed patient; these are usually transient but tend to recur. Abnormalities of sweating are quite common. Autonomic disturbances may be reflected in coldness, pallor, and even cyanosis of the paralyzed limbs. These have been attributed to persisting spasm of the peripheral blood vessels. However, it has been suggested that, although peripheral vasoconstriction is probably a very common phenomenon in chronically paralyzed muscles, angiospasm may not be a feature of the early phase of poliomyelitis. The exact mechanism involved in this phase is not clear.

There is considerable evidence that artificial respiration effected in a tank respirator under negative pressure is physiologically the same as that produced by application of positive pressure to the upper airway. Positive airway and negative intratank pressures produce identical changes in intrapulmonary, intrapleural, intracardiac, and systemic arterial and venous pressures. These result in (1) impairment of the circulation and decrease in cardiac output, (2) increase in cerebral venous and spinal fluid pressures, (3) rise in central venous pressure, (4) loss of blood volume, and (5) increased filling of the venous bed and arteriolar constriction. In the individual who has normal hemodynamics at the time of institution of artificial respiration, compensatory mechanisms tend to counteract these deleterious circulatory effects. Positive pressure applied to the airway results in transmission of a large fraction of the increase to the pleural space, great veins, and right atrium. The elevated pressure in the right atrium produces a momentary decrease in the venous gradient. Although venous return and cardiac output are momentarily decreased, they return to normal rapidly because there is a rise in peripheral venous pressure that reconstitutes the venous gradient and reestablishes venous return. The reconstitution of the venous gradient depends on the existing vascular tone, the capacity for reflex vasoconstriction, and the presence of a normal circulating blood volume. The increase in peripheral venous pressure required to establish the venous gradient causes a rise in capillary filtration pressure; this results in a reduction of the circulating blood volume. When the sympathetic pathways are affected in severe poliomyelitis, reestablishment of the venous gradient after the application of positive pressure to the airway

is greatly hindered. Because of this, venous return, cardiac output, and blood pressure fall in direct proportion to the degree of pressure applied. When intense generalized vasoconstriction is present in poliomyelitis because of diffuse involvement of the autonomic nervous system, positive pressure breathing produces a decline in arterial pressure because the mechanisms responsible for re-establishing the venous gradient are already maximally active. Although this discussion has been limited to the pathophysiologic changes in the circulation that develop when respiratory assistance is required during poliomyelitis, it must be pointed out that similar phenomena are present in other situations that require the use of artificial respiration.

Life-threatening pulmonary edema develops in some individuals with poliomyelitis, especially those who are severely ill because of medullary involvement or because of difficulty in respiration as a result of paralysis of the diaphragm and intercostal muscles. Although the exact mechanisms involved in the pathogenesis of this phenomenon are unknown, several factors that may contribute to its development have been suggested. Among these are hypoxia, oxygen toxicity (overuse of 100 per cent oxygen), constriction of the pulmonary vessels, pulmonary infection, circulatory changes produced by artificial respiration, and myocardial dysfunction.

An interesting and clinically important pathophysiologic phenomenon that develops in practically all patients severely paralyzed by poliomyelitis is mobilization of calcium from the bones. This is responsible for the nephrolithiasis that commonly complicates the prolonged course of illness in these cases. The presence of stones is often the factor responsible for infection of the urinary tract that leads, if untreated, to chronic pyelonephritis and subsequent renal failure. The stones that are formed may be so large as to produce sufficient obstruction to require nephrostomy.

Some of the clinical features of poliomyelitis may have as their basis direct viral involvement of extraneural tissues. Thus, some of the cardiovascular abnormalities are unquestionably related to invasion of the myocardium resulting in interstitial lymphocytic infiltration in most instances or in severe necrosis in others. Generalized lymphadenopathy, a common feature of the disease, is probably due to multiplication of the virus in lymph nodes.

Herpes Zoster

Herpes zoster and varicella are produced by the same virus, and the initial event in the natural history of the herpetic syndrome is an episode of chickenpox at any age, but usually in childhood. It has been proposed that recovery from varicella is sometimes accompanied by passage of the virus from the lesions in the skin and mucous membranes into the sensory nerve endings of these tissues. From here, it is thought, the agent is transported up the sensory fibers to the sensory ganglia, where it may become established in the nuclei of the ganglion cells and remain quiescent for varying periods, often for many years. During this latent period, small quantities of virus might possibly enter the circulation from the ganglia but would be quickly and effectively neutralized by specific antibody. Such periodic intrusions of the virus into the circulation, when they occurred, would be expected to stimulate production of neutralizing antibody.

It appears most likely that activation of the latent varicella-zoster agent is responsible for clinical herpes zoster. In most instances, provoking factors are not readily apparent. However, a variety of disorders that lead to generalized immunosuppression (or drugs such as corticosteroids and cytotoxic agents that produce the same effect) seem to predispose to the development of clinical herpes zoster, presumably by activating the latent virus. Among such diseases are the lymphomas, leukemia (usually lymphatic), and multiple myeloma.

It has been postulated (but not proved) that when antibody levels are reduced, the virus, which has remained latent in the nucleus of sensory ganglia, emerges and travels antidromically down the sensory nerve. In its passage from the ganglia along the sensory nerve it may produce a severe neuritis; this is thought to account for the severe pain commonly present in the pre-eruptive stage (before skin lesions are apparent) of herpes zoster. The virus may travel over only a portion of the length of the nerve and may not reach the skin; the only manifestation in this situation is severe root pain without dermal lesions, so-called *herpes zoster sine eruptione,* or *zoster sine herpete.* If, as is the case in most patients, the virus reaches the dermal sensory nerve endings, the typical vesicular eruption develops; the lesions are always in the most precise anatomic relation to the neurons of the sensory ganglia that have been involved or destroyed. Virus is shed from the vesicles and may lead to the development of characteristic varicella if acquired by nonimmune individuals.

Although the spinal ganglia are most frequently involved, others may be the site for presumed long-term residence of the virus. Activation of the virus may produce a variety of syndromes characterized by neurologic dysfunction related to the area affected. The fifth cranial nerve is the apparent pathway for transport of the virus from its ganglion (gasserian). When virus in this location is activated, any one of the three main branches of the fifth nerve may be involved; pain and skin lesions are distributed along the course of the mandibular, maxillary, or ophthalmic divisions. Involvement of the latter *(herpes zoster ophthalmicus)* produces lesions of the cornea; the earliest sign is loss of the corneal reflex. Enlargement of the ipsilateral preauricular lymph nodes and conjunctivitis (Parinaud's syndrome) are com-

mon. When the nasociliary branch of the ophthalmic division is affected, the skin lesions usually appear at the end of the nose; other manifestations of this syndrome include conjunctivitis, keratitis, retinopathy, and retrobulbar neuritis, which may lead to blindness. The necrotizing retinopathy is presumed to be the result of migration of virus along the ophthalmic branch of the fifth cranial nerve, along the nasociliary branch, and ultimately to the long ciliary nerve extending to the retina. Typical intranuclear inclusions have been identified in the involved sensory retina. The geniculate ganglion may be involved (Ramsay Hunt syndrome). In this situation, the skin lesions are present on the pinna, tympanic membrane, or external ear canal. The accompanying neurologic abnormalities are facial palsy alone or together with diminished hearing and tinnitus. If the chorda tympani is involved, there is loss of the sensation of taste over the anterior two thirds of the tongue.

In rare instances, paralysis of the muscles of the arms, legs, abdomen, and diaphragm has been described. This suggests involvement by the virus of anterior horn cells, but proof is lacking as yet. An unusual syndrome of ophthalmic herpes zoster followed in a few weeks by an acute contralateral hemiparesis or aphasia has occurred in rare patients. An unusual segmental granulomatous arteritis (possibly due to varicella-zoster virus) confined to the central nervous system is believed to be responsible for the contralateral neurologic findings. Bladder hypertonia results from mild inflammation in dorsal root ganglia; urinary retention may develop with more extensive involvement of parasympathetic fibers innervating the bladder (second, third, and fourth sacral segments) as well as meninges and possibly anterior-horn cells. Vesicles and hemorrhagic cystitis may be observed on the bladder mucosal surface. Transient ileus may rarely occur in herpes zoster. On occasion, the lesions of herpes zoster may be diffusely distributed in the skin in a centripetal fashion similar to that of initial episodes of varicella. "Cropping," that is, the continuing appearance of new lesions of varying structure in the same area of skin, as is the case in varicella, does not occur in the disseminated form of herpes zoster. These lesions are practically always painless. This is probably so because the virus has reached the skin as a result of viremia rather than spread from local sensory ganglia.

Osteomyelitis

Osteomyelitis may take the form of either an acute or a chronic infection. However, there is no abrupt shift from acute to chronic disease but rather a gradual blending of one into the other. On the basis of the pathogenesis of the lesion, cases of osteomyelitis fall into one or another of three categories: (1) *hematogenous osteomyelitis;*

(2) *osteomyelitis secondary to a contiguous focus of infection* (including postoperative wound infections, osteomyelitis in which bacteria have been introduced following a puncture wound, and bone involvement from an adjoining soft tissue focus of infection); and (3) *osteomyelitis associated with peripheral vascular disease.*

Hematogenous Osteomyelitis. Acute hematogenous osteomyelitis most frequently involves rapidly growing bone, as evidenced by the fact that over 85 per cent of cases occur in children. There is often a history of antecedent trauma to the area subsequently involved in the septic process. The disease characteristically affects the metaphysis of long bones. The anatomic features of the microvasculature adjacent to the metaphyseal side of the growth plate provide the most satisfactory explanation for the localization of blood-borne bacteria and initiation of infection. The capillary ramifications of the nutrient arteries supplying bone loop sharply just below the epiphyseal growth plates and then enter large sinusoidal veins, where the flow of blood is sluggish (Fig. 21–4). These sinusoidal vessels connect with the venous channels of the medullary cavity. In experimental animals (and probably also in humans) the inability of the metaphysis to handle infection is related to several factors:

1. The afferent loop of the metaphyseal capillary lacks phagocytic lining cells, and the phagocytic cells present in the efferent loop (a sinusoidal structure) are functionally inactive.

2. Flow in the descending loops of the metaphyseal capillaries is slower and more turbulent because the descending loops are often multiple and have a diameter two to seven times as great as that of the ascending loops.

3. The capillary loops adjacent to the epiphyseal growth plates are nonanastomosing branches of the nutrient artery, and obstruction (by bacterial growth or microthrombi) would be expected to result in small areas of avascular necrosis, a mechanism conducive to progressive infection.

Once infection has started, the local decrease in pH, the edema, and the accumulation of leukocytes (and possibly their collagenase) all contribute to tissue necrosis and breakdown of bone trabeculae. The infection extends to the neighboring bone through the haversian and Volkmann canals, occludes vascular channels, and causes the death of more osteocytes in the process. Larger segments of bone, deprived of blood supply by this process of vascular compromise, may become separated and form sequestra. These act as foreign bodies, converting the infection into a chronic one and rendering eradication by antibiotic therapy impossible until the devitalized bone is removed. Osteoblastic apposition can take place on smaller pieces of already dead bone, further compounding the problem by burying the infection behind a rampart within which bacteria can multiply uninhibited by circulating bactericidal factors and phagocytic cells. The suppurative process may also produce a septic thrombophlebitis of the diaphys-

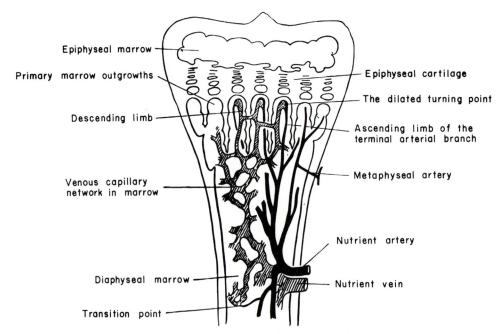

Figure 21–4 Schematic representation of the blood supply of a long bone in the region of the metaphyseal growth plate (epiphyseal cartilage). (From Waldvogel, F. A., Medoff, G., and Swartz, M. N.: Osteomyelitis: A Review of Clinical Features, Therapeutic Considerations and Unusual Aspects, 1971. Courtesy of Charles C Thomas, Publisher, Springfield, Illinois.)

eal vessels, impairing venous return and increasing the high pressure created within bone. Upon reaching the outer part of the cortex the infection causes an inversion of the slow periosteal blood flow and enters the subperiosteal space. This then may progress to formation of subperiosteal abscess that is associated with considerable local pain, tenderness, and swelling because of accumulation of pus under pressure. The local presence of heat, pain, and erythema may be so prominent that a subcutaneous abscess is erroneously suspected. Incision and drainage may be carried out in the mistaken belief that the process is a soft-tissue infection, when, in fact, the process merely represents extension from a focus of acute osteomyelitis. Subperiosteal infection may induce exuberant circumferential growth of the periosteum (involucrum). Progressive chronic destruction of the cortex is followed by spontaneous pathologic fracture in some instances.

MANIFESTATIONS IN DIFFERENT AGE GROUPS. The clinical course of hematogenous osteomyelitis may vary somewhat, depending on the age of the patient. These differences are related to certain anatomic features and their changes during growth. In the infant below the age of 1 year, infection begins in the metaphyseal sinusoidal veins. However, at this age some patent capillaries still perforate the epiphyseal growth plate, and infection can spread rapidly via this route to the epiphysis. This results in septic arthritis, thrombosis of nutrient vessels, and possible destruction of the epiphyseal growth anlage. Such destruction may result in loss of hip joint function and eventual shortening of the involved leg. *Between the age of 1 year and puberty,* the initial metaphyseal infection is contained by the epiphyseal growth plate and spreads laterally through the paths of least resistance. It commonly perforates the cortex, lifting off the periosteum (which is loosely adherent) and produces a subperiosteal collection of pus. The epiphysis in this age group is protected from the spread of infection by the epiphyseal plate, and normal growth is usually not impaired. *In the adult,* because resorption of the growth cartilage has occurred, anastomoses between metaphyseal and epiphyseal blood vessels are reestablished and make spread of the infection to the subarticular space a distinct possibility. Subperiosteal abscess formation and extensive periosteal proliferation are unusual in this age group, since the periosteum is firmly attached to the underlying bone.

About one third of patients with acute hematogenous osteomyelitis have demonstrable bacteremia and exhibit a toxic, febrile course. *Staphylococcus aureus* is the most common etiologic agent, but other pyogenic gram-positive cocci (pneumococcus, group A streptococcus) are occasionally implicated. *Salmonella* infections are a relatively common complication of sickle cell anemia. If *Salmonella* bacteremia occurs in patients with this disease, it is almost always associated with subsequent localization in bone. It has been suggested that the small "bone infarcts" that occur in sickle cell anemia secondary to occlusion of small blood vessels by the deformed red cells are favorable sites for the initiation of infection.

FEATURES DUE TO SPECIFIC SITES OF INVOLVEMENT. Vertebral body involvement in hematogenous osteomyelitis has been seen with increasing frequency, usually in adults, and often complicating pelvic surgery and urinary tract infections. Infection of the vertebral body spreads readily to adjacent ligaments and adjoining vertebral bodies by anastomosing venous channels. Thus, this type of osteomyelitis frequently involves two adjacent vertebral bodies and the intervening intervertebral disk. Special problems may arise with this type of osteomyelitis because of proximity to the spinal cord. Infection may extend through the thin vertebral periosteum, and pus may accumulate between the periosteum and the dura mater (spinal epidural abscess). Further extension of infection through the dura, either directly or through venous channels, into the subarachnoid space may lead to acute bacterial meningitis. The initial site of bone infection may, not infrequently, fail to produce prominent manifestations. In this situation, the illness is heralded by the sudden onset of the complicating spinal epidural abscess (compressing the spinal cord) or bacterial meningitis. Compression of the cord with concomitant paraplegia may result from the epidural extension of the infectious process itself, from secondary vascular impairment with infarction of the cord, or from compression fractures of the involved vertebrae.

The particular anatomic features of the hip and shoulder joints account for the common occurrence of septic arthritis secondary to osteomyelitis of the femur and humerus in children. Although the epiphyseal plate serves as an effective barrier to the direct extension of infection from the metaphysis to epiphysis (and thence to the joint space) in this age group, an alternative route is available. The synovial capsules in these joints reach beyond the epiphyseal growth plate; thus, infection can rupture through the cortex and spread directly from the metaphyseal focus into the joint.

Osteomyelitis Secondary to a Contiguous Focus of Infection. This type of disease is at present most common after surgical procedures such as open reduction of fractures, craniotomy, and reconstruction of joints severely affected by degenerative arthritis. However, it may follow burns, infection of the ears or paranasal sinuses, animal bites, and infection of soft tissue produced by trauma. Because the route of infection is different than in hematogenous osteomyelitis, metaphyseal localization of the process is much less frequent. In contrast to hematogenous osteomyelitis, which is predominantly a disease of the young, most patients with this form of bone disease are over 50 years old. These infections tend to be chronic, recurrent, and difficult, if not impossible, to eradicate until all foreign bodies (plates, screws, and other orthopedic appliances) have been removed. The most frequent clinical manifestations are local pain and drainage from a sinus tract. *Staphylococcus aureus* is the organism most commonly involved. However, less invasive bacteria can produce this syndrome when infection of an orthopedic prosthesis takes place. The usual manifestations of acute infection are often absent in this setting. There may be only minimal local erythema and only low-grade fever. Pain and limitation of motion secondary to spasm of muscle due to inflammation in and around bone may be important features.

Osteomyelitis Associated With Vascular Insufficiency. The pathogenesis of the process in this situation involves extension of infection to bone secondary to ischemic ulceration of the skin. The toes or the small bones of the feet are almost invariably involved. This is a problem almost always in patients with long-standing diabetes mellitus, occasionally in individuals with severe atherosclerosis, and rarely in persons with vasculitis secondary to a connective tissue disorder. Local symptoms (pain, swelling, erythema) dominate the clinical picture. There are few systemic manifestations of infection.

REFERENCES

INFECTIVE ENDOCARDITIS

Alpert, J. S., Krous, H. F., Dalen, J. E., et al.: Pathogenesis of Osler's nodes. Ann. Intern. Med. 85:471, 1976.

Angrist, A. A.: Pathogenesis of bacterial endocarditis. J.A.M.A. 183:249, 1963.

Arnett, E. N., and Roberts, W. C.: Valve ring abscess in active infective endocarditis. Circulation 54:140, 1976.

Bayer, A. S., Theofilopoulos, A. N., Eisenberg, R., et al.: Circulating immune complexes in infective endocarditis. N. Engl. J. Med. 295:1500, 1976.

Durack, D. T., and Beeson, P. B.: Experimental bacterial endocarditis. I. Colonization of a sterile vegetation. Br. J. Exp. Path. 53:44, 1972.

Garvey, G. T., and Neu, H. C.: Infective endocarditis—an evolving disease: a review of endocarditis at the Columbia Presbyterian Medical Center. Medicine 57:105, 1978.

Gould, K., Ramirez-Ronda, C. H., Holmes, R. K., and Sanford, J. P.: Adherence of bacteria to heart valves in vitro. J. Clin. Invest. 56:1364, 1975.

Hutter, A. M., and Moellering, R. C.: Assessment of the patient with suspected endocarditis. J.A.M.A. 235:1603, 1976.

Karchmer, A. W., and Stinson, E. B.: The role of surgery in infective endocarditis. In Remington, J. S., and Swartz, M. N. (Eds.): Current Clinical Topics in Infectious Disease. 1. New York, McGraw-Hill Book Co., 1980.

Kaye, D. (Ed.): Infective Endocarditis. Baltimore, University Park Press, 1976.

Lerner, P. I., and Weinstein, L.: Infective endocarditis in the antibiotic era. N. Engl. J. Med. 276:199, 323, 388, 1966.

Phair, J. P., and Clarke, J.: Immunology of infective endocarditis. Prog. Cardiovasc. Dis. 22:137, 1979.

Pruitt, A. A., Rubin, R. H., Karchmer, A. W., and Duncan, G. W.: Neurologic complications of bacterial endocarditis. Medicine 57:453, 1978.

Rodbard, S.: Blood velocity and endocarditis. Circulation 27:18, 1963.

Weinstein, L., and Schlesinger, J. J.: Pathoanatomic, pathophysiologic and clinical correlations in endocarditis. N. Engl. J. Med. 291:832 and 1122, 1974.

Ziment, I.: Nervous system complications in bacterial endocarditis. Am. J. Med. 47:593, 1969.

SALMONELLA INFECTIONS

Bennett, I. L., Jr., and Hook, E. W.: Infectious diseases (some aspects of salmonellosis). Ann. Rev. Med. 10:1, 1959.

Black, P. H., Kunz, L. J., and Swartz, M. N.: Salmonellosis—a review of some unusual aspects. N. Engl. J. Med. 262:811, 864, 921, 1960.

Giannella, R. A.: Importance of the intestinal inflammatory reaction on Salmonella-mediated intestinal secretion. Infect. Immun. 23:140, 1979.

Giannella, R. A., Gots, R. E., Charney, A. N., et al.: Pathogenesis of salmonella-mediated intestinal fluid secretion: activation of adenylate cyclase and inhibition by indomethacin. Gastroenterology, 69:1238, 1975.

Gill, F., Kaye, D., and Hook, W.: The influence of erythrophagocytosis on the interaction of macrophages and salmonella in vitro. J. Exp. Med. 124:173, 1966.

Greisman, S., Hornick, R. B., Carozza, F. A., Jr., and Woodward, T. E.: The role of endotoxin during typhoid fever and tularemia in man. I. Acquisition of tolerance to endotoxin. J. Clin. Invest. 42:1064, 1963.

Hook, E. W.: Salmonellosis: certain factors influencing the interaction of salmonella and the host. Bull. N. Y. Acad. Med. 37:499, 1961.

Hornick, R. B., Greisman, S. E., Woodward, T. E., et al.: Typhoid fever: pathogenesis and immunologic control. N. Engl. J. Med. 283:686, 739, 1970.

Kaye, D., and Hook, E. W.: The influence of hemolysis on susceptibility to salmonella infections: Additional observations. J. Immunol. 91:518, 1963.

Rubin, R. H., and Weinstein, L.: Salmonellosis—Microbiologic, Pathologic, and Clinical Features. New York, Stratton Intercontinental Medical Book Corporation, 1977.

SYPHILIS

Clark, E. G., and Danbolt, N.: The Oslo study of the natural history of untreated syphilis. J. Chronic Dis. 2:311, 1955.

Merritt, H. H., Adams, R. D., and Solomon, H.: Neurosyphilis. New York, Oxford University Press, 1946.

Sparling, P. F.: Diagnosis and treatment of syphilis. N. Engl. J. Med. 284:642, 1971.

Turner, T. B.: Syphilis and the treponematoses. In Mudd, S. (Ed.): Infectious Agents and Host Reactions. Philadelphia, W. B. Saunders Co., 1970.

Yobs, A., Clark, J. W., Jr., Mothershed, S. E., et al.: Further observations on the persistence of Treponema pallidum after treatment in rabbits and humans. Br. J. Vener. Dis. 44:116, 1968.

PNEUMONIA

Benson, H., Akbarian, M., Adler, L. A., and Abelmann, W. H.: Hemodynamic effects of pneumonia. I. Normal and hypodynamic responses. J. Clin. Invest. 49:791, 1970.

Bocles, J. S., Ehrenkranz, N. J., and Marks, A.: Abnormalities of respiratory function in varicella pneumonia. Ann. Intern. Med. 60:183, 1964.

Davidson, F. F., Glazier, J. B., and Murray, J. F.: The components of the alveolar-arterial oxygen tension difference in normal subjects and in patients with pneumonia and obstructive lung disease. Am. J. Med. 52:754, 1972.

Herzog, H., Staub, H., and Richterich, R.: Gas-analytical studies in severe pneumonia. Observations during the 1957 influenza epidemic. Lancet 1:593, 1959.

Marshall, R., and Christie, R. V.: The visco-elastic properties of the lungs in acute pneumonia. Clin. Sci. 13:403, 1954.

Mellemgaard, K.: The mechanism of hypoxemia in lobar pneumonia. Scand. J. Resp. Dis. 48:109, 1967.

Triebwasser, J. H., Harris, R. E., Bryant, R. E., and Rhoades, E. R.: Varicella pneumonia in adults. Report of seven cases and review of the literature. Medicine 46:409, 1967.

Wood, W. B., Jr.: Studies on the cellular immunology of acute bacterial infections. The Harvey Lectures, *Series XLVII*:72, 1951-52.

INFECTIONS OF THE CENTRAL NERVOUS SYSTEM

Bodian, D.: Histopathologic basis of clinical findings in poliomyelitis. Am. J. Med. 6:563, 1949.

Controni, G., Rodriguez, W. J., Hicks, J. M., et al.: Cerebrospinal fluid lactic acid levels in meningitis. J. Pediatr. 91:379, 1977.

Denny-Brown, D., Adams, R. D., and Fitzgerald, P. J.: Pathologic features of *Herpes zoster*. Arch. Neurol. Psychiat. 51:216, 1944.

Dodge, P. R., and Swartz, M. N.: Bacterial meningitis. II. Special neurological problems, post meningitic complications and clinicopathological correlations. N. Engl. J. Med. 272:954, 1003, 1965.

Feigin, R. D., and Dodge, P. R.: Bacterial meningitis: newer concepts of pathophysiology and neurologic sequelae. Pediatr. Clin. North Am. 23:541, 1976.

Fishman, R. A.: Carrier transport of glucose between blood and cerebrospinal fluid. Am. J. Physiol. 206:836, 1964.

Greenwood, B. M., Whittle, H. C., and Brynceson, A. D. M.: Allergic complications of meningococcal disease. II. Immunological investigations. Br. Med. J. 2:737, 1973.

Harter, D. H., and Petersdorf, R. G.: A consideration of the pathogenesis of bacterial meningitis: Review of experimental and clinical studies. Yale J. Biol. Med. 32:280, 1960.

Hope-Simpson, R. E.: The nature of *Herpes zoster*. A long-term study and a new hypothesis. Proc. Roy. Soc. Med. 58:9, 1965.

Horstmann, D. M., McCollum, R. W., and Mascola, A. D.: Viremia in human poliomyelitis. J. Exp. Med. 99:355, 1954.

Horwitz, S. J., Boxerbaum, B., and O'Bell, J.: Cerebral herniation in bacterial meningitis in childhood. Ann. Neurol. 7:524, 1980.

Lincoln, E. M., and Sewell, E. M.: Tuberculosis of the meninges and central nervous system. *In* Tuberculosis in Children. New York, McGraw-Hill Book Co., 1963.

Miller, L. H., and Brunnel, P. A.: Zoster, reinfection or activation of latent virus? Observations on the antibody response. Am. J. Med. 49:480, 1970.

Petersdorf, R., and Harter, D.: The fall in cerebrospinal fluid sugar in meningitis. Arch. Neurol. 4:21, 1961.

Scheld, W. M., Dacey, R. E., Winn, H. R., et al.: Cerebrospinal fluid outflow resistance in rabbits with experimental meningitis. Alterations with penicillin and prednisolone. J. Clin. Invest. 66:243, 1980.

Swartz, M. N., and Dodge, P. R.: Bacterial meningitis—a review of selected aspects. I. General clinical features, special problems, and unusual meningeal reactions mimicking bacterial meningitis. N. Engl. J. Med. 272:725, 779, 843, 898, 1965.

Weinstein, L.: Cardiovascular disturbances in poliomyelitis. Circulation 15:735, 1957.

Weinstein, L.: Influence of age and sex on susceptibility and clinical manifestations in poliomyelitis. N. Engl. J. Med. 257:47, 1957.

Weller, T. H., Witton, H. M., and Bell, E. J.: The etiologic agents of varicella and *Herpes zoster*. Isolation, propagation, and cultural characteristics *in vitro*. J. Exp. Med. 108:843, 1958.

OSTEOMYELITIS

Collins, D. H.: *In* Dodge, O. G. (Ed.): Pathology of Bone. London, Butterworth, 1966.

Diggs, L. W.: Bone and joint lesions in sickle cell disease. Clin. Orthop. 52:119, 1967.

Trueta, J.: The three types of acute hematogenous osteomyelitis: a clinical and vascular study. J. Bone Joint Surg. 41B:671, 1959.

Waldvogel, F. A., Medoff, G., and Swartz, M. N.: Osteomyelitis—clinical features, therapeutic considerations, and unusual aspects. N. Engl. J. Med. 282:198, 260, 316, 1970.

Waldvogel, F. A., and Vasey, H.: Osteomyelitis: the past decade. N. Engl. J. Med. 303:360, 1980.

Leukocytes and Hematopoietic Stem Cells

22

John C. Marsh and Dane R. Boggs

INTRODUCTION

NORMAL VALUES FOR BLOOD LEUKOCYTES

The leukocytes (white cells) of the blood comprise a heterogeneous population of nucleated cells that differ from one another with respect to morphology and function. They share the common property of being less dense than red cells and, along with platelets, constitute the so-called "buffy coat" when blood is centrifuged in a suitable tube such as the hematocrit. The number of blood leukocytes in adults normally is maintained between 4500 and 10,000 cells/mm³ or 4.5 to 10.0 × 10⁹/liter. The values are remarkably similar in the same individual over long periods of time. Black subjects have a somewhat lower range because they have fewer neutrophils. In the newborn and during the first few days of life, there may be moderate leukocytosis, with a range of 9 to 30 cells/mm³ at birth and 5 to 20 cells/mm³ by 2 weeks, owing to increased numbers of neutrophils and nucleated red blood cells, the latter not normally being found in adult blood.

Classically, blood leukocytes have been counted under a microscope in a counting chamber. For reasons of both speed and accuracy, the majority of investigators now employ automated electronic cell counters, using either an impedance or darkfield technique.

Although the total leukocyte count is useful to know, it represents incomplete information unless the individual types of white cells that constitute the total population are known. In a "differential" evaluation of a stained dried blood smear, the nucleated cells are counted and classified into the various types. The distribution of each type is then calculated as a percentage. The absolute number of each leukocyte type circulating in the blood should then be determined from the differential and total counts. Consideration should be given to five major cell types as to whether the absolute number is increased or decreased (Table 22–1). One can readily appreciate that deviations from normal within a given population may not always be reflected in any change in the total blood leukocyte count. One most commonly derives differential counts from visual examination of the blood smear using a Romanovsky stain (e.g., Wright or May-Grünwald-Giemsa), but again in

the interest of speed, automated units are often used. These are based on pattern recognition or staining properties of the various normal cell types. Some of the automated differential counting systems are extremely accurate with respect to enumerating normal leukocytes indicating the presence of abnormal cells. However, no currently available systems can identify abnormal cells as to type, although pattern recognition systems will identify these as "unclassified" and locate them automatically so that the operator can then look at them.

All of the normal blood leukocytes except lymphocytes are derived exclusively from the bone marrow. Lymphocytes are formed in other areas of the body as well, including the spleen, thymus, and lymph nodes. Although a common function of leukocytes is defense against "foreignness," the various populations function differently and separately, and thus separate consideration is important. The cells most frequently seen in the blood are neutrophilic granulocytes, both relatively old ("segs") and young ("bands", "stabs"), followed by lymphocytes, monocytes, eosinophilic granulocytes, and basophilic granulocytes. Sometimes the latter two types are not seen if only a few cells

TABLE 22–1 CONCENTRATION OF LEUKOCYTES IN VENOUS BLOOD SAMPLES*

	Cells/mm³	
	Mean	*Normal Range*
Neutrophils: White subjects	3700	2000–7000
Black subjects	3400	1300–7000
Lymphocytes	2500	1500–4000
Monocytes	400	400–1000
Eosinophils	150	0*–700
Basophils	30	0*–150

*Total leukocyte count (Coulter Counter) times the percentage of each cell type as determined in a 200-cell differential count of Wright-stained blood smear equals concentration of each cell type (291 normal subjects). A true zero value for eosinophils and basophils is not normal. A few can always be found if the blood is truly normal. However, the technique used for counting may yield a zero value, and this will occur more frequently when only 100 cells are enumerated in the differential examination. Many laboratories are converting to automated differential counting systems and results obtained with these may differ somewhat from those obtained by manual methods. (Adapted from Orfanakis et al.: Am. J. Clin. Pathol., 53:647, 1970.)

(i.e., 100 or less) are counted, but it is abnormal for none to be present in the blood, and evaluation of a larger sample will usually disclose them. The accuracy of counts of some automated machines is based primarily on the ease with which they classify large numbers of leukocytes. Plasma cells, megakaryocytes (the precursors of platelets), nucleated red cells, and immature forms of the normal blood leukocytes are but rarely found in normal blood.

In contrast to the other formed elements in the blood (red cells and platelets), leukocytes function almost entirely in the tissues and body cavities, with the blood functioning primarily as a transport medium. Leukocyte function can be classified very broadly into ingestion of foreign particles, or phagocytosis, and development of an immune response, which in turn can be subdivided into cellular and humoral immunity. The chief phagocytic cells are neutrophils, monocytes, and eosinophils; the so-called "immunocytes" are lymphocytes and their derivatives, plasma cells. The two systems interrelate closely; for example, antigens are "processed" by monocytes and their derivatives, macrophages, for presentation to the lymphoid system for antibody production, and ingestion of some particles by neutrophils is markedly enhanced when those particles are coated with an opsonin-type antibody, made by lymphocytes or plasma cells or both.

MORPHOLOGY OF BLOOD LEUKOCYTES

The following descriptions and figures refer to the normal blood leukocytes as they are seen with light microscopy of a suitably stained blood film. Electron microscopy, phase microscopy, and special stains are useful in certain situations but are not usually required for normal recognition. The pattern of nuclear chromatin, the shape of the nucleus, and the appearance and relative quantity of cytoplasm are all helpful. Granulocytes are those cells that have specific granules, which may be light pink or ground-glass in appearance (neutrophils), bright orange-red (eosinophils), or dark blue (basophils). Monocytes are also "granulocytes" in the sense that they contain large numbers of lysosomes, usually smaller than those of the neutrophil, but they are not conventionally classified with the aforementioned cells.

Mature neutrophils (polymorphonuclears, PMNs, "segs") have at least two nuclear segments, separated by a fine, threadlike filament. The median number of segments is three, but up to five may occasionally be seen. More segments suggest disorders of nucleic acid biosynthesis, such as vitamin B_{12} or folate deficiency. The nucleus usually is dark purple with coarse, condensed chromatin. The cytoplasm is faint pink with small primary and secondary granules, which are, in fact, lysosomes. The cells are of uniform size.

Band neutrophils are virtually identical in appearance with PMNs except for a nonfilamented, or sausage-shaped, nucleus. Bands are somewhat less mature than those of PMNs. The absolute number of bands is normally a small fraction (2 to 30 per cent) of the number of segmented neutrophils, and an increase in the band/PMN ratio may be an indication of an increased rate of input of neutrophils from the marrow into the blood (e.g., as a response to infection or hemorrhage).

Lymphocytes vary considerably in size, but many of them are the smallest of white cells, being only slightly larger (10 μm or less in diameter) than red cells. Typically, they are round or oval with round or oval nuclei as well. The nucleus may be slightly indented or even cleft. Cytoplasm of the small cells is very sparse, but in the larger lymphocytes it may be abundant with occasional pink granules. The cytoplasm may be various shades of blue. Nuclear chromatin is heavily clumped, and there are occasional nucleoli. Although lymphocytes may be classified as "T" (thymus-derived) or "B" (bone marrow–derived) by special techniques, these types are not discernible with routine blood smears. Plasma cells, important lymphocyte derivatives that make and secrete antibody, are not normally found in the blood.

Monocytes are somewhat larger (16 to 20 μm) cells with a highly variable appearance. They are often confused with large lymphocytes and immature neutrophil precursors. The cell is usually round but may have a wavy cytoplasm, at times with small pseudopodia. The nucleus is large and may be round, oval, kidney-shaped, or even segmented. The nuclear chromatin is delicate, often appearing reticular (lacy), and nucleoli are rare. The cytoplasm is typically bluish-gray or blue and often contains vacuoles. Granules usually appear very small and are fewer than those of granulocytes. This is a phagocytic bone marrow–derived cell, and it is the precursor of the tissue macrophage and, probably, of the osteoclast.

Eosinophils have nuclei similar to those of neutrophils and may have band or segmented forms; more than three segments are rare. The characteristic granules are large and are a striking red or reddish-orange, owing to a high content of basic protein.

Basophils have nuclei similar to those of the other granulocytes but seldom more than two lobes. The granules are large and bluish-black or purple, tend to fill the cytoplasm, and often overlie the nucleus. Similar cells in tissues, mast cells, differ from basophils in terms of enzyme content, ultrastructure of the granules, and method of discharge of granule content but also are derived from a precursor originating in the bone marrow.

BONE MARROW

Except in fetal life, all blood cells except lymphocytes are formed exclusively in the bone marrow. In infants, the hematopoietically active red marrow extends into all the extremities, but normal adult hematopoiesis is confined to the axial skeleton and only the most proximal portions of the limbs. The inactive, or yellow, marrow constitutes a reserve of potential blood formation that may be called into activity under conditions requiring more production, such as chronic hemolytic anemia or damage to the active marrow, such as that produced by irradiation. More than 60 per cent of normal hematopoiesis is in the pelvis and vertebrae, with 10 per cent in the skull and another 10 per cent in the ribs and sternum. The active marrow is moderately rich in fat, whereas inactive marrow is primarily fat. The marrow vasculature is unique, consisting of a rich system of postcapillary venous sinusoids that empty into a central vein. Newly formed blood cells, which are formed outside the sinusoids in islands of active blood cell formation, pass through an endothelial membrane to enter the sluggish flow of blood in the sinuses. This endothelial layer seems to be the only continuous lining of the sinusoids. Basement membranes and adventitial cells are only intermittently present. Newly formed blood cells passing into the sinusoids pass through the endothelial cell, where it is not lined by basement membrane and adventitial cells, via temporary pores called *fenestrations* (Fig. 22–1 and 22–2). What controls the development of fenestrations is not yet known. Adventitial cells often contain fat and are capable of phagocytosis and forming reticulin. They are classified as reticulum cells (mac-

rophages) on marrow aspirates and account for less than 1 per cent of the nucleated cells.

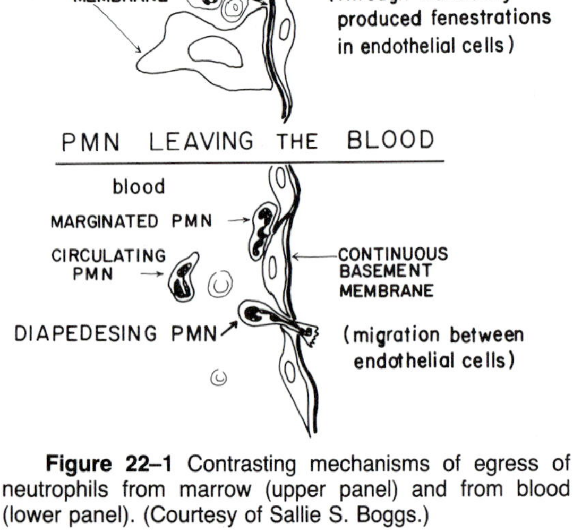

Bone marrow is often aspirated for diagnostic purposes. In addition, a biopsy producing a small core of marrow is often done as well, which gives a useful estimate of marrow cellularity and aids in detection of infiltration by various processes, such as lymphoma, carcinoma, and granuloma. An estimate of fat spaces to active hematopoietic cells can be made; the normal ratio of fat to marrow is between 1:1 and 2:1. The aspirate is evaluated from a Romanovsky-stained smear, and usually at least 500 nucleated cells are counted from which a marrow differential is derived (Table 22–2). From this, a determination of the myeloid: erythroid ratio can be made. This may range normally from 1 to 3.5:1, which is the ratio of all the granulocytes and their precursors to nucleated red cells of all degrees of maturity. Both biopsy and aspirate are useful in detecting and quantitating abnormal cells or increased amounts of apparently normal cells.

The cells normally present in the marrow include red cell precursors, of which there are four major types; granulocyte precursors, including two nonspecific and four specific for neutrophils, eosinophils, and basophils; mast cells; monocytes; lymphocytes; plasma cells; reticulum cells; and immature and mature megakaryocytes, large cells that are platelet precursors. Thus, there are 24 normal categories of bone marrow cells (Table 22–2). The total number of nucleated cells in the bone marrow has been estimated to be 14 to 18 × 10^9 cells/kg body weight. Thus, the active marrow constitutes a diffusely distributed organ, approximately the same size as the liver. Red cell production has been estimated to be 8 to 12 times normal in some congenital, hemolytic anemias; platelet production has been reported to be increased 8-fold in idiopathic thrombocytopenic purpura; and neutrophil production has been shown to be increased 4-fold in chronic infection and as much as 10-fold in Felty syndrome. Increased demands can be met by cellular hyperplasia with a decrease in the marrow:fat ratio of existing marrow parenchyma in normally active bones and also by distal extension of "red" marrow into the bones of the extremities. Shortening of cellular generation and maturation time may also occur.

It is unclear what regulates the rate of flow of newly formed blood cells from the hematopoietic parenchyma into the sinusoids and thence into the blood stream. The more mature cells of each line, reticulocyte or nonreticulated, non-nucleated red cell; segmented or band granulocyte; and platelet, are all relatively deformable and thus better able to squeeze through the fenestrations of the endothelial cells than their precursors are. Under conditions that require more cells, more and presumably larger fenestrations can be formed. That marrow release is, at least in part, mediated by a humoral signal has been shown in animals and

Figure 22–1 Contrasting mechanisms of egress of neutrophils from marrow (upper panel) and from blood (lower panel). (Courtesy of Sallie S. Boggs.)

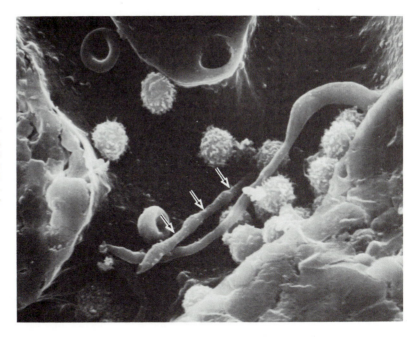

Figure 22–2 Electron micrograph of a marrow sinus with snakelike protrusions of a portion of a megakaryocyte. These processes emerge through pores created in endothelial cells (Fig. 22–1), and platelets break off at the constrictions indicated by arrows. (Courtesy of P. De Bruyn.)

humans rendered acutely or chronically neutropenic. The plasma from such individuals has been shown to contain a "neutrophil-releasing factor" by reinfusion studies. How this works is not known. Changes in the position of adventitial cells of the sinusoids to allow a larger surface for the potential development of fenestrations have been reported in acute hemorrhage, which results in an increased input of red cells, neutrophils, and platelets into the sinusoids.

The accelerated release of red cells from the marrow is often accompanied by the accelerated release of granulocytes and platelets, whereas release of granulocytes or platelets can occur as independent events. This suggests that a more specific mechanism is involved in release of the

TABLE 22–2 DIFFERENTIAL COUNTS OF BONE MARROW ASPIRATES FROM 12 HEALTHY MEN*

	Mean (Per Cent)	Observed Range (Per Cent)	95 Per Cent Confidence (Per Cent)
Neutrophilic series (total)	*53.6*	*49.2–65.0*	*33.6–73.6*
Myeloblast	0.9	0.2–1.5	0.1–1.7
Promyelocyte	3.3	2.1–4.1	1.9–4.7
Myelocyte	12.7	8.2–15.7	8.5–16.9
Metamyelocyte	15.9	9.6–24.6	7.1–24.7
Band	12.4	9.5–15.3	9.4–15.4
Segmented	7.4	6.0–12.0	3.8–11.0
Eosinophilic series (total)	*3.1*	*1.2–5.3*	*1.1–5.2*
Myelocyte	0.8	0.2–1.3	0.2–1.4
Metamyelocyte	1.2	0.4–2.2	0.2–2.2
Band	0.9	0.2–2.4	0–2.7
Segmented	0.5	0–1.3	0–1.1
Basophilic and mast cells	*< 0.1*	*0–0.2*	
Erythrocytic series (total)	*25.6*	*18.4–33.8*	*15.0–36.2*
Pronormoblasts	0.6	0.2–1.3	0.1–1.1
Basophilic	1.4	0.5–2.4	0.4–2.4
Polychromatophilic	21.6	17.9–29.2	13.1–30.1
Orthochromatic	2.0	0.4–4.6	0.3–3.7
Lymphocytes	*16.2*	*11.1–23.2*	*8.6–23.8*
Plasma cells	*1.3*	*0.4–3.9*	*0–3.5*
Monocytes	*0.3*	*0–0.8*	*0–0.6*
Megakaryocytes	*< 0.1*	*0–0.4*	
Reticulum cells	*0.3*	*0–0.9*	*0–0.8*
M:E ratio	*2.3*	*1.5–3.3*	*1.1–3.5*

(From Clinical Hematology. 8th ed. Philadelphia, Lea and Febiger, 1982.)

latter cells. The release of red cells may be determined by mechanical factors such as flow, but erythropoietin, the hormone that controls red cell production, also can induce accelerated red cell release from marrow. Diseases of bone marrow such as myelofibrosis and invasion by cancer cells may result in release of immature cells into the blood, presumably owing to disruption of the normal mechanical barriers. Similar changes in the blood (i.e., the presence of nucleated red blood cells, early granulocyte forms, and young platelets) may result from extramedullary hematopoiesis.

Extramedullary Hematopoiesis

Extramedullary hematopoiesis occurs normally in fetal life. Blood formation begins in the yolk sac, then develops in the liver at 6 weeks' gestation, occurs in the spleen at 12 weeks, and begins in the marrow by 20 weeks. By the time of birth, nearly all blood formation is in the marrow. Production of lymphocytes in lymphoid tissues begins at about 20 weeks. When postnatal extramedullary hematopoiesis does occur, it is most commonly in spleen and liver; but lymph nodes and, rarely, other tissues such as cartilage, adrenal glands, and kidney may contain small islands of hematopoietic tissue. It occurs in some, but not all, diseases characterized by increased production of blood cells such as hemolytic disease of the newborn, pernicious anemia, thalassemia, and sickle cell disease but is not routinely present in any of these diseases. Extramedullary hematopoiesis is present in virtually all patients with idiopathic myelofibrosis and in most with the myeloid leukemias. In infantile osteopetrosis, characterized by failure of normal bone resorption by osteoclasts resulting in near obliteration of the marrow cavity, extramedullary hematopoiesis persists throughout life. What causes the development of extramedullary blood formation in some conditions and not others is not known, but it clearly does not develop simply in response to a demand for increased blood production, perhaps because the ability of the normal bone marrow to increase production is very great or because a change in the poorly defined microenvironment of the extramedullary tissue is required for hematopoiesis to be permitted. Idiopathic myelofibrosis and the myeloid leukemias are clonal diseases involving an abnormal stem cell, so one of its abnormalities may be the ability to grow in nonmyeloid tissue.

HEMATOPOIETIC STEM CELLS (HSC)

Stem cells are defined as cells that are capable of self-renewal. Differentiation (i.e., maturation into more functional cells with specific tasks) is also a necessary characteristic of a normal HSC. Under normal conditions, the population of stem cells remains constant in number. For every cell that differentiates and leaves the compartment of stem cells, another must take its place through mitosis of a second cell. An alternate mechanism could be the differentiation of one of the two progeny resulting from the cell division of each stem cell (Fig. 22–3).

All hematopoietic cells ultimately are derived from a single class of HSC, the totipotent HSC (THSC). Following maturation from this compartment, there is a concatenation of HSC, with each successive compartment having a more restricted potential for direction of differentiation (Fig. 22–3). Stem cells are not recognizable as such because they are present in very low numbers among more differentiated progeny; some superficially resemble medium-sized lymphocytes but, in fact, have no other "lymphoid" characteristics.

The first quantitative assay for an HSC was that of Till and McCulloch, who demonstrated the formation of nodules in the spleens of lethally irradiated mice injected with bone marrow from syngeneic mice. These nodules contained granulocytes, nucleated red cells, and megakaryocytes, sometimes mixed together but more often separate. The number of nodules formed was proportional to the number of marrow cells injected, and later studies in which chromosome markers were used demonstrated the clonal nature of the nodules, or colonies. Thus, each colony was derived from one cell, which was capable of producing all myeloid cells. At least certain colonies, when injected into secondary recipients, contained cells that could repopulate the entire hematopoietic system. Thus, most such colonies are formed by either pluripotent myeloid stem cells (PMSC) or THSC (Fig. 22–3). This cell has become known as the CFU_s (colony-forming unit, spleen) and fulfills the requirement for a pluripotent stem cell, since it has also been shown to be capable of self-replication. It is present in normal bone marrow in concentrations of only about one in 10,000. The CFU_s is also present in blood and in fetal liver. Such experiments obviously cannot be done in humans, but the presence of multipotent stem cells for the erythroid, granulocytic, and megakaryocytic lineages is suggested (1) by the presence of a characteristic chromosomal abnormality (the Philadelphia, or Ph^1 chromosome) in those cells but not in nonhematologic cells in chronic myeloid leukemia, (2) by the growth of clonal "mixed" colonies from normal marrow in vitro, and (3) most particularly from glucose-6-phosphate dehydrogenase (G6PD) isozymes (see further on).

A few years after the demonstration of the CFU_s in rodents, several workers demonstrated, first in mice and then in humans, the ability of bone marrow (and blood) to form colonies composed of granulocytes and macrophages or of eosinophils in a semisolid medium (e.g., agar or methylcellulose). Again, the number of colonies was proportional to the number of cells plated, and they were

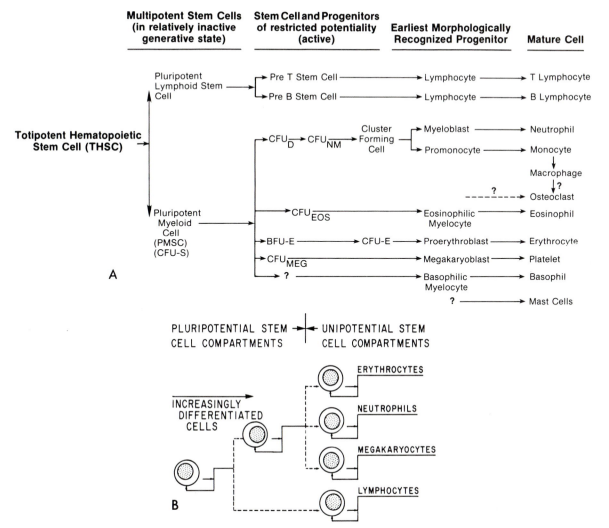

Figure 22–3 The hematopoietic stem cell compartments. *A,* Seemingly complex but probably oversimplified diagram. *B,* Markedly oversimplified diagram. The illustrated concept of a series of concatenated compartments of increasingly restricted potentiality is fairly well established, as are the compartments shown in the figure: BFU, burst-forming unit; CFU, colony-forming unit; D, diffusion chamber; E, erythroid; EOS, eosinophil; MEG, megakaryocte; NM, neutrophil-monocyte; S, stem cell.

derived from one cell (i.e., were clonal). This clearly demonstrated a common origin for granulocytes and monocytes (the blood precursor of the macrophage). The precursor cell has been referred to as the *colony-forming unit in culture, or CFU$_C$.* It has been shown to be quite distinct from the CFU$_S$ by various fractionation studies. These in-vitro studies require a specific growth factor or factors. This glycoprotein, derived from various sources including fetal tissue, the monocyte itself, activated T-lymphocytes, and certain endothelial cells, has been called the *colony-stimulating factor (CSF)* or *colony-stimulating activity (CSA).* It may be a physiologic leukopoietin (i.e., a factor or factors required for normal granulocyte-macrophage production in vivo).

A possible intermediate stem cell between the CFU$_S$ and CFU$_C$ is a cell that gives rise to granulocytes and monocytes when suspended in a diffusion chamber in the peritoneal cavity of a mouse, the CFU$_D$.

Colony-forming cells for red cells, megakaryocytes, eosinophils, and basophils and for T- and B-lymphocytes have also been demonstrated in semisolid media under appropriate conditions (e.g., addition of a specific red-cell growth factor, the glycoprotein erythropoietin, to produce red cell colonies). At least two types of erythroid colony-forming cells have been described: (1) cells that form large colonies, or "bursts" (BFU$_E$), and (2) cells that form small colonies, or "clusters" (CFU$_E$). The BFU$_E$ is thought to be a precursor of CFU$_E$, which in turn gives rise to the earliest recognizable erythroid cell in the marrow, the pronormoblast.

Although the aforementioned stem cells and growth factors seem to be specific for myeloid cells (i.e., red cells, granulocytes-monocytes, platelets, and eosinophils), there is compelling evidence for a totipotent stem cell that is capable of differentiation into lymphoid precursors as well as myeloid (CFU_s) precursors. These data have been obtained from studies of G6PD isozyme distribution in clonal hematopoietic neoplastic diseases in humans and from transplantation of HSC with induced chromosomal abnormalities in mice. Evidence is also available to suggest that there are cells committed to T-, B-, and non–T-, non–B-lymphocyte formation as well (Fig. 22–3). The more differentiated and committed HSC tend to be more active mitotically, as shown by susceptibility to such inhibitors of DNA synthesis as tritiated thymidine, hydroxyurea, and cytosine arabinoside, than are the more primitive ones, such as the totipotent cell and pluripotent myeloid stem cell (CFU_s). Stem cells for every type of bone marrow–derived cell have not yet been found, and the interrelationships noted in Figure 22–3 are tentative, undoubtedly to be refined by future studies; nevertheless, the concept is quite useful in understanding normal physiology of hematopoiesis and diseases that may be considered stem cell disorders.

Assay methods for the definition of HSCs are listed in Table 22–3. The various HSC compartments will normally be constant in size, indicating the balance between self-replication and differentiation to mature nonreplicating cells. Cell death may also occur in the compartment and is a major factor for kinetic consideration of lymphocyte precursors in the thymus; however, for HSC compartments cell death and differentiation are equivalent kinetic events. When there is a parent compartment, there is an input from the parent compartment as well. The rates of each of these processes will determine the size of the compartment. It should be emphasized that these "compartments" are conceptual and probably diffuse entities rather than anatomic "boxes."

The mature myeloid cells, granulocytes, red cells, and platelets are end cells, incapable of division. Monocytes and macrophages, however, are capable of cell division and perhaps of self-replication, as are lymphocytes.

Thus, under normal conditions, the mature blood cells are maintained by the relatively rapidly proliferating stem cell compartments such as CFU_c and BFU_E and by doubling divisions in subsequent compartments. If these compartments are damaged (e.g., by chemotherapy for cancer or other drugs or through irradiation) or if there is an increased demand for mature cells, more primitive compartments, such as CFU_s, in which most cells are normally not in cell cycle, will be triggered into proliferation until the appropriate needs are met, if that is possible. The signals are poorly defined but probably are both humoral, allowing distant cells to exert an influence, and cellular, relying on cell to cell contact, the absence of which could either trigger or depress proliferation. It is probable that marked reduction of a specific compartment is followed first by HSC self-replication in order to refill that compartment partially, after which differentiation is allowed to proceed. Humoral factors have been defined and partially characterized for the committed compartments involved in producing red cells, granulocytes, macrophages, eosinophils, and platelets but not as yet for multipotent or totipotent stem cells.

The "soil" for hematopoiesis has been studied, the hematopoietic microenvironment (HM). There are certain mutant mice in which either defective HSC or defective HM has been demonstrated. The concept of favorable "hematopoietic inductive microenvironment" (HIM) existing in the marrow has been proposed. This suggests that there are favorable "niches" in which local conditions allow production of specific types of blood cells, with these conditions normally being absent elsewhere.

THE SPLEEN

The spleen is an important phagocytic and immunologic organ. Although neither its removal in the event of trauma or disease nor its congenital absence generally produces any significant clinical problem, there are characteristic changes in the blood that occur as a result of its absence. Most

TABLE 22–3 METHODS OF ASSAY FOR DEFINITION OF HEMATOPOIETIC STEM CELLS

Type of Stem Cell	Assay System
Totipotent	Murine chimerism; lethally irradiated or congenitally anemic recipients of cells
Pluripotent myeloid	Murine chimerism; spleen colonies in irradiated recipients, in-vitro "mixed" colonies*
Cell producing granulocytes and monocytes in diffusion chambers*	Cells† in cell tight diffusion chamber are implanted in an irradiated rodent
Stem cells* limited in their potentiality to B- or T-lymphocytes, neutrophils and monocyte-macrophages, eosinophils, basophils, erythrocytes, megakaryocytes	Cells† added to semisolid media in presence of appropriate stimulus, and each stem cell proliferates and its differentiated progeny form colonies. The number of colonies formed is a measure of the number of stem cells added

*Indicates that human stem cells can be analyzed; mouse is the index mammal in which all techniques were devised.

†Nucleated cells from marrow (all techniques) or from blood (most techniques).

commonly and persistently, there are Howell-Jolly bodies, which are round, purple-staining bits of residual nuclear DNA of red cells, normally removed or "pitted" in the spleen as a result of the sluggish flow through an organ filled with many phagocytic macrophages. The absence of Howell-Jolly bodies provides one with sufficient cause to doubt the absence of the spleen or to suspect the growth of a functioning auxiliary one. Other changes include the presence of nucleated red cells in the blood, reticulocytosis, macrocytosis, and siderocytosis. Leukocytosis occurs transiently, initially due primarily to neutrophilia, but the leukocytosis found several months after splenectomy often is due to lymphocytosis and monocytosis. Thrombocytosis commonly develops in asplenic subjects and may persist for years.

Increased susceptibility to infection in adults following splenectomy is disputed but is a real hazard in very young children (younger than 2 years) during the first 2 years following surgery and if the underlying disease carries a high risk of infection. The most frequent infecting organism is the *Pneumococcus,* which requires opsonization for effective phagocytosis. The loss of the antibody-producing function of the spleen and the loss of large numbers of phagocytic cells in that organ (composing part of the reticuloendothelial system, or monocyte-macrophage phagocyte system) presumably are the major factors explaining this increased susceptibility to bacterial infection.

The structure of the spleen (Fig. 22–4) is such that a portion of the blood travels through it very slowly, with maximum exposure to its numerous phagocytic cells (macrophages). Arteries branch so that after they leave the connective tissue bands, or trabeculae, they pass through the white pulp, composed largely of lymphoid follicles consisting primarily of lymphocytes and a few macrophages and plasma cells. Some vessels bypass the white pulp to enter the adjacent red pulp directly, made up of splenic sinuses and splenic cords. These arteries actually terminate without capillary connection (unique to the spleen), and blood percolates through a loose network of cells by entering the open, proximal end of sinuses or of the "cords" (Fig. 22–4). The sinuses enter the venous system and are lined by endothelium. The cords are lined by specialized macrophages, or reticulum cells, and the endothelium separating them from the sinuses contains permanent fenestrations, smaller in diameter than red blood cells. Red cells that enter cords (<10 per cent passing through the spleen) rather than sinuses must pass through these fenestrations in order to reenter the general circulation. The circulation of platelets through the spleen is quite slow; normally about one third of extramedullary platelets are found in the spleen. The spleen is extremely rich in lymphocytes and monocytes, many of which can enter the general circulation from the spleen. The kinetics of neutrophil movement through the spleen and sequestration by this organ are poorly defined.

An important activity of the white pulp, where there is evidence for lymphocyte recirculation, is antibody formation in response to particulate antigen, initially processed by the phagocytic cells present primarily in the red pulp. Differentiation

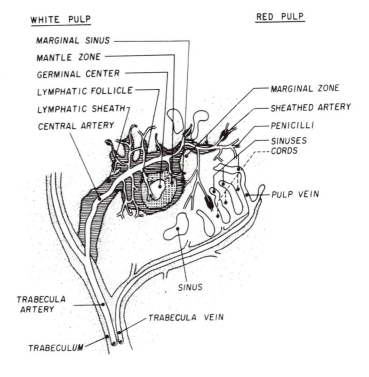

WHITE PULP   RED PULP

MARGINAL SINUS
MANTLE ZONE
GERMINAL CENTER
LYMPHATIC FOLLICLE
LYMPHATIC SHEATH
CENTRAL ARTERY

MARGINAL ZONE
SHEATHED ARTERY
PENICILLI
SINUSES
CORDS

PULP VEIN

SINUS

TRABECULA ARTERY

TRABECULA VEIN

TRABECULUM

Figure 22–4 Diagram of the splenic structure and circulation. The components of the white pulp are listed on the left; those of the red pulp are shown on the right. (From Wintrobe, M. M., et al.: Clinical Hematology. 8th ed. Philadelphia, Lea and Febiger, 1971.)

of the lymphocytes in the spleen into plasma cells, the direct sources of antibody, has been observed. Although the spleen is not necessary for antibody production, its importance is indicated by the fact that the antibody response in its absence is less rapid and not as marked; that is, the defect is a quantitative one. This is particularly important for circulating antigens. This function probably explains, at least in part, such observations as the deficient antibody response to pneumococcal vaccine of Hodgkin's disease patients, previously splenectomized as part of the initial staging of their disease, and of a similar deficient response in patients who have sickle cell anemia with "functional asplenia."

One potential function of the spleen is hematopoiesis. However, even though splenic hematopoiesis is normally found in the mouse (particularly erythropoiesis, but also some granulocyte and platelet production), this function has not been proved in humans. Lymphocytes and perhaps macrophages are produced in the spleen on a regular basis, although part of the evidence for this is indirect, based on animal rather than human studies. It is thought that the basis for this proliferation of cells is a stimulation by increases in the filtered load of particulate matter and subsequent phagocytosis that the spleen is called on to perform.

The spleen is able to trap and phagocytose mildly damaged red cells, presumably owing to its unique circulation, which allows prolonged contact with phagocytic cells in the splenic cords. This process is referred to as *culling* and probably represents a normal disposal mechanism for senescent cells of all types. Normally, disposal of old cells certainly occurs elsewhere as well, such as in marrow and perhaps in liver or other sites, but the spleen is especially skilled at it. "Pitting" of red cells refers to the removal of various particles such as siderotic granules, Howell-Jolly bodies, and Heinz bodies (particles of degenerated hemoglobin) from the red cell without destruction of the whole cell. In the past, the spleen was thought to exert some inhibitory control over marrow production of cells, but no direct evidence for this exists.

PHAGOCYTES

NEUTROPHILS

One half to two thirds of the cells in the normal bone marrow are neutrophils and neutrophil precursors (Table 22–2). The two most immature morphologically recognizable ones, the *myeloblast* and the *promyelocyte,* are shared with the far less frequent eosinophil and basophil series and probably with the monocyte as well. These cells together with *myelocytes,* which represent the first stage at which the neutrophil, eosinophil, and basophil lines can be distinguished by ordinary microscopy, constitute the mitotic pool of granulocyte precursors (Fig. 22–5). About 30 per cent of neutrophil precursors are, therefore, capable of cellular division. The remainder, the neutrophilic *metamyelocytes, band cells,* and *segmented cells* (in order of maturation), are not able to divide. They make up the neutrophil maturation and storage pools. The immediate precursor of the myeloblast is probably the CFU_C, defined earlier. This is a functional entity and has been characterized morphologically by complex cell isolation and concentration studies but cannot be "routinely" identified.

The myeloblast, normally found only in the marrow and accounting for 0.5 to 2.0 per cent of nucleated cells, is a round or oval cell 10 to 20 μm in diameter, with a prominent round or oval nucleus and little cytoplasm. The cytoplasm is blue, with no granules. The nuclear chromatin is fine and evenly dispersed, with no clumping around the thin nuclear membrane, an observation that can be helpful in distinguishing it from the lymphoblast in acute leukemia. There are usually two to five pale blue nucleoli. Although Auer rods (thin, red, oval or spindle-shaped cytoplasmic structures) may be seen in acute myeloid leukemia (AML), they are not present in normal myeloblasts. It is quite difficult at times to distinguish the myeloblast from the earliest recognizable red cell precursor, the pronormoblast, although the latter has a more deeply colored blue cytoplasm and chromatin structure differs subtly.

The promyelocyte, about three times as numerous as the myeloblast, is somewhat larger and has azurophilic, or primary, granules in the prominent cytoplasm, which appear dark pink to purple. The nucleus is very similar to that of the myeloblast except that the nuclear chromatin is somewhat more clumped. Nucleoli are still prominent. The azurophilic granules are characteristic and differ for neutrophils, eosinophils, and basophils by electron microscopy but not by light microscopy. These granules contain peroxidase, an important antimicrobial enzyme that stains characteristically and acts as a marker for the granulocyte series and monocytic series. The granules also contain numerous other enzymes, such as acid phosphatase, esterases, lysozyme and β-glucuronidase, but not alkaline phosphatase. The granules are membrane-bound lysosomes and persist during the maturation of the cell to segmented neutrophils, being sequentially diluted with each succeeding mitotic division, since all are synthesized at the promyelocyte stage. (The monocyte—and the macrophage—are capable of continued lyposomal synthesis and changing lysosomal enzyme content, even after leaving the bone marrow.)

The neutrophilic myelocyte, about four times as common in the marrow as its predecessor, is slightly smaller and has a more clumped nuclear chromatin, and nucleoli usually are not evident by light microscopy. The nucleus is round or very slightly indented. Light pink or "neutral" (specific, secondary) granules are assembled at this stage,

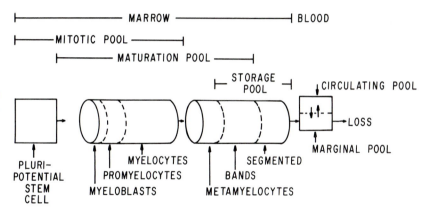

Figure 22–5 An overall model of neutrophil production, storage, and circulation.

which give the series its name. These differ from primary granules not only in color but in chemical composition. They are about two to three times as numerous as primary granules. They do not contain peroxidase or acid phosphatase but do contain lysozyme and various other basic proteins. They contain or at least are associated with alkaline phosphatase, which also is present in nongranular portions of the cytoplasm. Staining mature neutrophils for alkaline phosphatase and scoring the amount of staining is of some value in the differential diagnosis of conditions associated with neutrophilia (see further on).

The metamyelocyte, the next step in the series, has a clearly indented nucleus, but one that has not yet reached the halfway point of indentation. It is no longer capable of mitosis, and granule formation, seen at the earlier two stages, has ceased. Chromatin is coarse and clumped, and nucleoli are absent. These cells are capable of active movement and are occasionally seen in the blood. They are the most frequent neutrophil precursor in normal marrow.

Band forms and segmented neutrophils have been described earlier; their ratios to one another in the blood and marrow are reversed. The prominent, dark-staining primary granules are difficult to discern in mature, segmented neutrophils, but electron microscopy demonstrates that they are still present. The number of lobes in a mature neutrophil does not serve as an indicator of its age.

"Drumsticks" corresponding to one of the X chromosomes are present in a few of the PMN of normal females. These are not found in normal men, but they may be seen in men with Klinefelter syndrome or other conditions in which there is more than one X chromosome. They are absent in females with the XO (instead of XX) chromosome constitution (ovarian dysgenesis, or Turner syndrome).

Neutrophil Kinetics

Following derivation from multipotent and committed stem cells, neutrophil life may be di-

vided into bone marrow, blood, and tissue phases (Fig. 22–5). The bone marrow phase is divided into mitotic and postmitotic maturation and storage phases, each of which lasts about 6 to 8 days. Thus, the maximum effect of most cytotoxic agents used in cancer chemotherapy, which primarily affect dividing cells, is seen at 10 to 14 days after administration and is manifested by a decreased number of blood neutrophils (neutropenia). About five cell divisions occur during the mitotic phase.

Cells pass through these marrow compartments in an orderly fashion, with cells being released from the latter part of the storage pool as bands and segs on demand. When rate of release increases acutely, there is an increase in the proportion of young cells in the blood, the so-called "shift to the left." There are about 15 to 20 times as many bands and segs in the marrow as in the blood.

Distribution studies of radioactively labeled blood neutrophils have demonstrated the existence of two blood pools of approximately equal size. The circulating granulocyte pool (CGP) is in equilibrium with the marginated granulocyte pool (MGP), which is composed of granulocytes marginated along the walls of capillaries and postcapillary venules, especially those in the lungs, spleen, and liver. One determines the CGP by multiplying the absolute granulocyte count by the blood volume. The total blood granulocyte pool (TBGP) can be determined by isotope dilution studies of labeled blood granulocytes, and the MGP is determined by the difference; thus, TBGP = CGP + MGP. The two blood pools are in rapid equilibrium and have the same band:seg ratio. Cells may be demarginated from the MGP into the CGP by an event such as voluntary muscular exercise, convulsions, or secretion of epinephrine, resulting in neutrophilia, but there will be no change in the size of the TBGP or band:seg ratio. Neutropenia can follow an increase in margination at the expense of the CGP. This may occur in the early phase after endotoxin injection or its release from bacteria or in any type of beginning inflammation. Such a "shift" accounts for the neutropenia associated with malaria and probably that seen with typhoid fever.

Neutrophils normally pass through the blood within 10 hours; isotopic studies have shown that the disappearance is random, not age-related, and that there is a half-life of 6.5 to 7 hours. Once neutrophils enter the tissues by passing between endothelial cells (Fig. 22–1), they do not return to the blood. Their life span in the tissues is not known with certainty, but most are quickly destroyed there or migrate into various body cavities, or potential cavities, as virtually no extravascular neutrophils are seen in any normal tissue. Others may be recognized in the bronchial secretions, urine, saliva, and feces, but the relative quantitative importance of these different routes of loss is not known.

Blood neutrophils are replaced from the marrow, then, about 2½ times per day, in marked contrast both to red cells, which are replaced about every 120 days, and to platelets, which are replaced about every 10 days. The granulocyte turnover rate (GTR) ranges normally from 60 to 400 cells × 10^7/kg/day. Since the concentration of blood neutrophils is normally constant, the rate of input from the marrow is equal to the rate of departure to the tissues. When an acceleration in the rate of neutrophil release by the bone marrow occurs, it is usually manifest by an increase in the band:seg ratio, since bands are relatively more numerous in the marrow storage pool.

Physiologic variations in blood neutrophil concentration include higher levels with activity or with virtually any "stressful" situation, and such neutrophilia is thought to be mediated by increased secretion of epinephrine or cortisol or both. Administration of adrenal glucocorticosteroid increases the CGP by decreasing the rate of egress into the tissues, increasing the rate of release of cells from the marrow, and slightly shifting the balance of cells from MGP to CGP. Pregnancy is also associated with a slight neutrophilia.

Control mechanisms of neutrophil production and release are incompletely understood. They probably consist of a mixture of humoral and cellular interactions. Processes affected by controlling factors may include the proliferation rate of the usually slowly dividing multipotent stem cell (CFU_s), the degree of commitment of this cell to the immediate granulocyte precursor (CFU_C), the rate of proliferation of CFU_C, the proliferation rate of recognizable neutrophil precursors, the maturation time of the postmitotic cells, and the rate of release from the bone marrow. Negative and positive feedback loops may be involved; thus, a decreased number of neutrophils in the blood must somehow stimulate an increased rate of release from the storage pool as well as an increase in the rate of production within the marrow. However, we would emphasize that the control by number of neutrophils in the blood must be by some secondary, indirect regulating system, since there are many reasons for believing that their blood number per se cannot be the primary control

point. This also is true for blood platelets; that is, their number in circulating blood is decreased when an increased percentage is circulating very slowly through the spleen, but this provides no apparent stimulus to increased platelet production.

The primary candidate for a humoral factor that may be important for stimulation of in-vivo granulocytopoiesis is the glycoprotein, CSF. Actually, multiple CSFs have been described, even from the same species. At least four, of differing molecular weights, have been found in humans. They are required in vitro for granulocyte-macrophage colony development, and, as noted previously, they are derived from a variety of cells. CSF can be found in human urine and serum. There is good but not conclusive evidence for a key physiologic role for these substances as granulopoietic regulators. Inhibiting substances of possible physiologic significance also have been described.

There are, then, three major processes that determine blood neutrophil concentration: (1) the rate at which cells leave the blood for the tissues, (2) the rate at which they are released by the marrow into the blood, and (3) the ratio of circulating to marginated cells. Thus, apparent neutrophilia or neutropenia may represent only a redistribution of cells between the MGP and CGP, the later pool being the only one counted directly. The accelerated marrow release produced by endotoxin, corticosteroids such as prednisone, or the androgenic steroid etiocholanolone makes it possible to gauge the adequacy (but not the actual size) of the marrow storage pool of neutrophils. Injection of one of these substances produces an increment of several thousand blood neutrophils per mm^3 within a few hours in a person with normal marrow function. This information may be useful when cancer chemotherapy or radiation therapy is contemplated.

Neutrophil Function

The major function of neutrophils, known for many years, is to seek and destroy foreign materials and microorganisms, classically bacteria, that may be noxious to the parent organism. Neutrophils are motile, increasingly so as they mature (Fig. 22–6). Foreign substances are taken into the cell by the process of *endocytosis*, in which portions of the cell membrane invaginate around them and move them into the cell as vacuoles or vesicles. Endocytosis of liquid droplets is called *pinocytosis* and that of solid particles is *phagocytosis*. Once foreign substances enter the cell, the structure thus formed (phagosome) may be fused with the primary or secondary granules, forming a digestive vacuole that leads in most instances to breakdown of the ingested material. Once this process is complete, the undigestable material may then be extruded from the cell either by exocytosis of

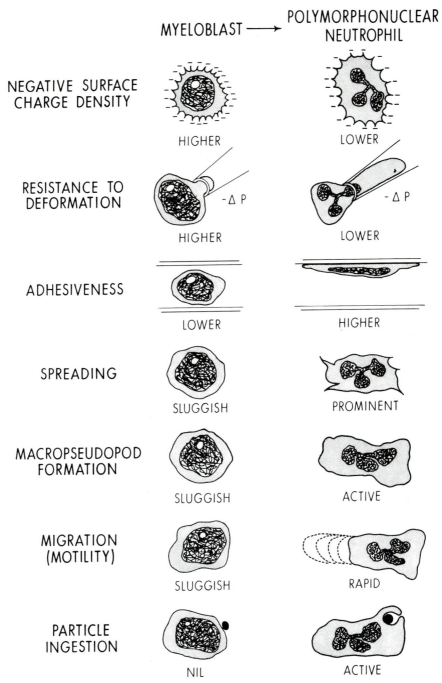

MYELOBLAST ⟶ POLYMORPHONUCLEAR NEUTROPHIL

NEGATIVE SURFACE CHARGE DENSITY — HIGHER / LOWER

RESISTANCE TO DEFORMATION — HIGHER / LOWER

ADHESIVENESS — LOWER / HIGHER

SPREADING — SLUGGISH / PROMINENT

MACROPSEUDOPOD FORMATION — SLUGGISH / ACTIVE

MIGRATION (MOTILITY) — SLUGGISH / RAPID

PARTICLE INGESTION — NIL / ACTIVE

Figure 22–6 Changes in functional properties of neutrophils during maturation in the bone marrow. (Courtesy of Marshall A. Lichtman.)

the phagosome or by refusion of the phagosome membrane with the cytoplasmic membrane and expulsion of its contents.

In considering neutrophil function, one should remember that most studies have been carried out in vitro and are sometimes of uncertain physiologic significance. Typically, a drug may be added to isolated PMNs whose function, such as migration,

phagocytosis, or intracellular killing, is then measured. In-vivo studies, however, consist of administration of the substance to be studied to intact animals or patients, removal of their cells, and assessment of their function by comparison with normal cells.

Although neutrophils entrap some microorganisms more efficiently with the aid of specific antibody, the presence of antibody is not necessarily required in the phagocytic process. Phagocytosis can occur anaerobically and is not sensitive to inhibitors of glycolysis.

Neutrophil function can be broadly subdivided into the migration cascade, or sequence, and the killing cascade (Fig. 22–7). The former includes the processes of margination, adherence and aggregation, diapedesis through the vessel wall, and migration, directed through a chemotactic stimulus. The killing cascade includes recognition, attachment, phagocytosis, granule fusion, degranulation, and the respiratory burst associated with intracellular killing, digestion, and exocytosis.

The Migration Cascade. Margination is increased by histamine, iron oxide, and dextran. It is part of the early phase of a variety of inflammatory processes. In the process of adherence, the PMN attaches to the vascular endothelium and spreads out on its surface. When multiple cells attach to one another, the process is referred to as *aggregation.* Adherence requires normal intracellular microtubule and microfilament function. Colchicine inhibits the adherence process, presumably through its effect on microtubules. Complement and Mg^{++} are required for adherence.

The next step, diapedesis through the vessel wall, occurs when the cell moves through the junction between endothelial cells and breaks the basement membrane (Fig. 22–1). This is to be contrasted with release from the marrow, which

occurs in temporary pores *within* the endothelial cells lining the sinuses (Fig. 22–1).

Once into the tissues, PMNs migrate toward their objective in response to a concentration gradient of a mediator, called a *chemotactic stimulus,* for which the cell has a receptor. Chemotaxis in vitro is commonly studied with a chamber in which the cells to be studied are separated from the chemotactic stimulus by a filter that can then be examined for the extent of PMN migration through it. The in vivo counterpart is the "skin window" in which coverslips or chambers are placed over a skin abrasion, with or without a chemotactic stimulus, and examined quantitatively over a period of time for the rate of appearance of PMNs or monocytes or both. If a patient is afflicted with numerous bacterial infections, his cells can be evaluated for response to known chemotaxins by one of these methods. The skin window gives information regarding the function of the entire migration cascade. There are many chemotaxins, both natural and synthetic, and the latter have been studied extensively in vitro. Chemotaxins stimulate neutrophil adherence and aggregation as well as directed motion. Among the natural chemotaxins are culture filtrates of microorganisms, certain cleavage components of complement (C5a), casein, and some low molecular weight peptides purified from bacteria, notably those with *N*-formyl attachments. Other chemotaxins include activated Hageman factor from the coagulation

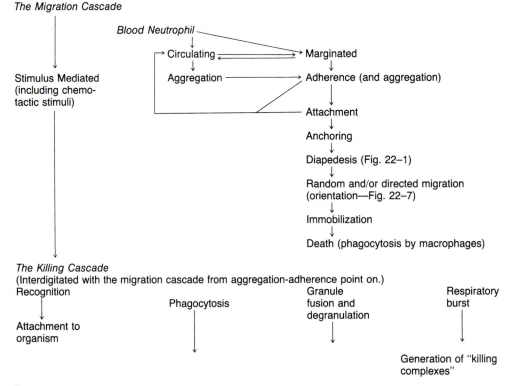

The Migration Cascade

Blood Neutrophil

Stimulus Mediated (including chemotactic stimuli)

Circulating ⇄ Marginated

Aggregation → Adherence (and aggregation)

Attachment

Anchoring

Diapedesis (Fig. 22–1)

Random and/or directed migration (orientation—Fig. 22–7)

Immobilization

Death (phagocytosis by macrophages)

The Killing Cascade
(Interdigitated with the migration cascade from aggregation-adherence point on.)

Recognition

Attachment to organism

Phagocytosis

Granule fusion and degranulation

Respiratory burst

Generation of "killing complexes"

Fig. 22–7 A diagram of the interlocking steps of neutrophil migration into exudates and bacterial killing.

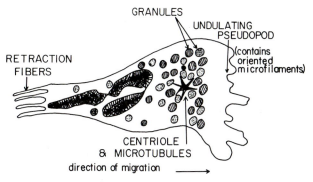

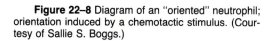
Figure 22–8 Diagram of an "oriented" neutrophil; orientation induced by a chemotactic stimulus. (Courtesy of Sallie S. Boggs.)

cascade, cyclic nucleotides, and certain prostaglandins. Endotoxin, antigen-antibody complexes, and lysosomes from various cells may generate chemotactic activity following interaction with plasma or serum.

The identification of many receptors on the surface of cells has led to the suggestion that these in turn, when occupied, somehow signal the cell motion machinery. In the presence of an effective chemotaxin, the cell's movements, normally random, become unidirectional in the direction of the concentration gradient, and the cell is said to be "oriented" (Fig. 22–8). A series of metabolic events occurs after chemotaxin binding, including hyperpolarization of the cell membrane, an increased flux of Ca^{++}, changes in the membrane synthetic rate of phospholipids, an increase in cyclic nucleotides, and generation of prostaglandins through the activation of phospholipase. Actin-myosin contractile proteins are involved in the movement of the cell, as are the aforementioned microtubules and microfilaments.

Among the in-vivo inhibitors of chemotaxis are hydrocortisone and colchicine. In-vitro inhibitors include methyl prednisolone, chloroquine, quinine, and phenylbutazone. Aspirin has no such effect. Other inhibitors are tetracycline, rifampin, chloramphenicol, amphotericin B, chlorpromazine, ethanol, heparin, and caffeine.

During the migration process, some events that normally are considered part of the "killing cascade" can occur, such as degranulation. The release of some enzymes in this fashion from the cell may actually enhance the cell's movement through tissues containing a substrate for the released enzyme (e.g., collagen).

The Killing Cascade. The process of particle recognition by and attachment to the cell must precede ingestion. Attachment is facilitated by immunoglobulins, whose F_C fragment can attach to cell receptors and whose F_{ab} fragment can attach to a particle, such as a bacterium. Complement, a heat-labile material, may serve a similar linking role to some organisms, and C3b receptors are also found on PMNs. *Opsonin* is the general term for materials that can attach to particles, making them attractive to phagocytes, and includes specific antibody, complement, other heat-labile substances, and lysozyme. Divalent ions such as Mg^{++} and Ca^{++} also play a role in attachment.

Phagocytosis is the engulfment of a particle and its sequestration in an intracellular vacuole. One can quantitate it by measuring the rate of uptake of particles over a period of time or the number of particles ingested per cell at a specific time. The percentage of cells that contain ingested particles can also be measured. The process begins with portions of membrane (pseudopods) surrounding the particle and fusing. This movement of the membrane is probably initiated and carried out by the actin-myosin microfilaments. The process is associated with a burst of anaerobic glycolysis that involves an increase in lactate production and an increase in membrane lipid synthesis, presumably to replace that portion of cytoplasmic membrane that is pinched off to surround the ingested particle. Phagocytosis is inhibited by increased concentrations of galactose and glucose, thus providing a possible explanation for the increased susceptibility to infection seen in galactosemia as well as in the much more frequent, uncontrolled diabetes mellitus. Cyclic AMP (cAMP) inhibits and cyclic GMP enhances phagocytosis, and the inhibitory effects of histamine, certain prostaglandins and some β-adrenergic agents, are thought to be mediated by cAMP.

During particle ingestion, the various granules (lysosomes) begin to fuse with each other and with the phagosome. The specific (secondary) granules apparently precede the primary granules in this process, but the net result is exposure of the ingested particle to the many enzymes contained within both types of granules. This degranulation can also occur into the extracellular environment as the phagosome is forming or even preceding phagocytosis during the migration cascade. Intracellular degranulation is inhibited in vivo and in vitro by colchicine (used to reduce the inflammation of acute gout), the anticancer drug vinblastine, histamine, and β-adrenergic agents. In vitro, cholinergic agents enhance degranulation, and extracellular degranulation is inhibited by corticosteroids and chloroquine.

The granule enzymes are probably not the major killers of ingested particles but are important in facilitating the digestive process once killing has occurred. Ingestion and degranulation may occur in the absence of killing, as in chronic granulomatous disease (see further on).

Intracellular killing by neutrophils may be considered in two broad categories: oxygen-dependent and oxygen-independent. The "respiratory burst," mediated by a membrane oxidase, results in increased hexose monophosphate shunt (HMP) activity, an increase in oxygen consumption, the production of superoxide from oxygen, and the production of hydrogen peroxide (H_2O_2) from superoxide by a dismutase enzyme. When H_2O_2, a halide ion, and myeloperoxidase from primary granules combine, they form a potent antimicrobial killing system. Some patients with myeloperoxidase deficiency have an increased incidence of infection, although most do not; compensatory killing mechanisms that are not dependent on peroxidase have been invoked to explain the relative benignancy of the disorder. These include H_2O_2 itself and possibly some of the other intermediates in peroxide generation, such as superoxide and free, or singlet, oxygen.

The peroxidase-halide-H_2O_2 complex has been reported to inhibit the chemotactic effect of activated complement product, thus preventing the cell from moving off again while killing microbes. The peroxidase killing system is inhibited by various sulfonamides and antithyroid agents in vitro; the clinical significance of this is unclear.

Oxygen-independent mechanisms of antimicrobial killing include various components of granules, for example, lysozyme, various cationic proteins, lactoferrin, arginase, glucosidase, and an acid environment that develops in the phagosome. These are all probably important to varying degrees against different organisms. Most patients exhibiting the various functional defects of neutrophils with respect to killing show susceptibility to certain microorganisms but not to others. When an organism has been killed by a PMN, typically it is digested, and any indigestible debris is discarded outside the cell. The latter two processes actually are less important for neutrophils than for macrophages, as neutrophils are rather short-lived, dying not long after killing microorganisms. Many dying or dead neutrophils are phagocytosed by macrophages.

Patients who have unexpected, serious infections and particularly those who have recurrent bacterial or fungal infections, even minor ones, require evaluation of both the immune system or systems (see further on) and the phagocyte system or systems. The integrity of the phagocyte system, in a patient in whom the obvious problem is not neutropenia or monocytopenia or both, is best accomplished by testing the migration cascade with a "skin window" and assessing the killing cascade by adding bacteria to blood neutrophils (and monocytes) and studying bacteriocidal rates by the cells. If at all possible, a bacterium (or fungus) grown from an actual infection in that patient should be studied. If one or both are defective, detailed studies are required that may involve referral of the patient to an investigator who is particularly interested in such problems.

Among the important *secretory products* of neutrophils is a B_{12}-binding protein, transcobalamin III (TC III). This and other B_{12}-binding proteins may be elevated in the serum of patients with acute and chronic myeloid leukemia and correlate well with the TBGP. They are often decreased in patients with neutropenia.

Diseases and Drugs That Routinely Affect Neutrophil Function or Number or Both

Only a few drugs and diseases that affect neutrophils will be discussed. Lithium carbonate has well-defined stimulatory effects on neutrophil production, possibly by stimulating CSF, and has some effect in protecting against the neutropenia produced by various antineoplastic agents. Ethanol has multiple inhibitory effects on neutrophil function, including decreases in cellular adherence, chemotaxis in vitro, and phagocytosis. Diabetes, when significant hyperglycemia is present, has been associated with decreased PMN adherence, chemotaxis, phagocytosis, and intracellular killing. Renal disease with uremia has been reported to cause impaired chemotaxis, but phagocytosis and intracellular killing are normal.

Diseases of Neutrophil Function. There are numerous types of congenital and acquired diseases that are associated with defective neutrophil function (Table 22–4). We will discuss only a few representative examples.

CHRONIC GRANULOMATOUS DISEASE (CGD). This is a lethal, X-linked recessive, fairly uncommon disease affecting the intracellular neutrophil killing process. Affected boys usually die in childhood of recurrent bacterial infections that are often caused by organisms that are of low-grade virulence in normal persons. Skin is involved most frequently, but liver and lung infections are also common, with the progressive chronic infection and granuloma formation that give the disease its name. PMN migration and phagocytosis are normal, and degranulation is probably normal, with normal enzyme contents in the granules. The respiratory burst fails to occur with phagocytosis, with consequent faulty generation of H_2O_2 and related metabolites; this is due to a defect in cytoplasmic oxidase or its activation. The result is faulty killing of certain bacteria, primarily those that are catalase-positive, and of certain fungi and viruses. Catalase-negative bacteria can supply peroxide to the phagosome, thus bypassing the preceding steps of the respiratory burst and contributing to their own death. If the bacteria also generate catalase, their peroxide is inactivated. There are also defects in macrophage and eosino-

TABLE 22–4 EXAMPLES OF DEFECTS INVOLVING NEUTROPHIL FUNCTION

Defects in the Migration Cascade
  Congenital complement deficiency
  Generation of chemotactic factors
    Is inhibited in uremia, and congenital absence of chemotactic lymphokines has been described.
  Acquired production of chemotactic inhibitors
    In cancer, renal dialysis, chronic infections, and so forth, as well as idiopathic (? usually an IgG).
  Congenital absence of a membrane glycoprotein
    Defective attachment, absent migration, associated with marked neutrophilia and increased neutrophil
    production, but with severe, recurrent infection.
  The Job syndrome
    Defective chemotactic response with "boils" (also increased IgE, eosinophila, eczema).
    Levamisole seems to restore chemotaxis to normal, but does not improve recurrent boils.
  "Lazy leukocyte" syndrome
    The neutrophil defect (undefined) that leads to neutropenia (reduced release from marrow) also is associated
    with reduced adhesion and migration.

Defects in the Killing Cascade
  Chronic granulomatous disease
  Glucose-6-phosphate dehydrogenase deficiency
    If severe, there is inefficient NADPH generation with a killing defect and infectious problems.
  Myeloperoxidase deficiency
    Minimal problems, mostly with *Candida* infections. Alternate means of generating oxydizing radicals are
    generally sufficient for killing.
  Deficiency of H_2O_2 detoxifying enzymes
    Detectable changes in duration of killing-associated events, but not associated with increased frequency of
    infection (glutathione reductase, catalase, dismutase).

Defects with Significant Influence on Both Cascades
  Congenital absence of specific granules
    Adherence and aggregation were supranormal, and chemotaxis, killing, and respiratory burst were decreased in
    a patient with severe infection.
  Congenital absence of actin polymerization
    Cells can adhere, but adherence is not stimulated by chemotaxins, and migration and phagocytosis are
    inhibited.
  Defects in microtubule assembly
    Congenital increase in assembly with increased infection, defective orientation, chemotaxis, and phagocytosis.
    Decreased assembly is seen with the Chediak-Higashi syndrome.
    Various drugs (such as vincristine, vinblastine, colchicine) poison microtubules.
  Diabetes and other causes of hyperosmolality
    Virtually all neutrophil responses are sluggish but return to normal when severe hyperglycemia is corrected.
  Alcohol intoxication
    Virtually all neutrophil responses are sluggish but are corrected quickly when the cell "sobers up," secondary to
    the patient doing the same.

phil function. The simplest way to demonstrate the defect is to observe the failure of affected PMNs to reduce the dye *nitroblue tetrazolium (NBT)*, which normal neutrophils reduce from colorless to bluish-black. Therapeutic measures include vigorous treatment of infection with antibiotics, but bone marrow transplantation has been curative when a compatible donor was available.

MYELOPEROXIDASE DEFICIENCY. This is a relatively common, usually benign disease that is inherited as an autosomal recessive or acquired with clonal myeloid neoplasms. Neutrophils and monocytes are both affected. Clearly, there are efficient alternate microbial killing pathways that do not require peroxidase, since myeloperoxidase deficiency is so much less serious than CGD. The major organisms infecting patients with myeloperoxidase deficiency are *Candida* species.

Other, very rare defects in intracellular killing include the severe form of glucose-6-phosphate dehydrogenase (G6PD) deficiency, with impaired generation of NADPH (which is required for peroxide generation) and abnormalities in glutathione peroxidase and glutathione synthetase (which are involved in the intracellular metabolism of peroxide).

There are a number of conditions associated with defects in PMN migration with or without associated defects in killing. Some newborns, especially prematures, have transient defects in chemotaxis and bacterial killing, sometimes associated with clinical infections. Congenital deficiency of some of the components of the complicated sequence of proteins known collectively as *complement* can result in pyogenic infections due to effects on PMN. C3 deficiency can impair phagocytosis, and it also interferes with the generation of C5a, an important component of the chemotactic stimulus.

Congenital defects limited to the migration

sequence are rare but include (1) a defect in a membrane glycoprotein with defective PMN attachment to endothelium; (2) the Job syndrome, which is known to be associated with recurrent pyogenic skin infections and defective chemotaxis, but whose basic defect is still uncertain; and (3) the "lazy leukocyte" syndrome, associated with neutropenia that is due to a decreased rate of release of PMNs from the marrow in conjunction with impaired cell adherence and migration.

Morphologic Abnormalities of Neutrophils. The Chediak-Higashi (C-H) syndrome is a rare autosomal recessive disease characterized by skin and eye albinism, a bleeding tendency with abnormal platelet function associated with defective storage of serotonin, and an increased susceptibility to infection, due to defective granulocytes that are abnormal both in appearance and in function. The PMN granules are larger and fewer than normal and are thought to arise from abnormal fusion and malformation of both primary and secondary (specific) granules. A defective assembly of microtubules in the PMN is also present, and both these abnormalities have been implicated as possible causes of the increased infection, defects in cell migration and killing having been demonstrated. Transient improvement has been seen in PMN function after induction of an increase in cellular cGMP or exposure to ascorbic acid, normal platelets, or serotonin. Abnormal granules may also be found in other leukocytes, such as eosinophils and monocytes, and in other cells, such as melanocytes and osteoclasts.

The Pelger-Huët anomaly is inherited as an autosomal dominant trait or, occasionally, is acquired with neoplasms of myeloid tissue. The heterozygous form is a benign condition characterized by decreased segmentation of nuclei and increased coarseness of nuclear chromatin. The nuclei are round, oval, or bilobed, resembling spectacles or dumbbells. The cytoplasm is normal, and the cells function normally. Affected persons have little or no evidence of increased susceptibility to infection. Three or more lobes in the nuclei of the PMN are distinctly rare, accounting for less than 5 per cent of the population, compared with more than 50 per cent for normal blood PMN. Apparently identical "pseudo-Pelger" cells may be seen as an acquired abnormality in certain types of myeloid leukemia, idiopathic myelofibrosis, or the "preleukemia syndromes." Homozygous inheritance of the Pelger-Huët gene results in all "mature" neutrophils having a round, oval, or indented (but not segmented) nucleus. Although the homozygous form is lethal in utero in rabbits, it causes little difficulty in humans.

Other rare familial abnormalities of leukocyte morphology include the May-Hegglin anomaly, hereditary hypersegmentation of the nuclei, giant neutrophils, cytoplasmic vacuolization, and Alder's anomaly. None of these morphologic changes is associated with an evident increase in frequency or severity of infection.

Neutrophilia. An increase in the concentration of PMN in the blood can result from a variety of causes. It is well to recall that this may occur through (1) an increased rate of input of cells from the marrow; (2) a decrease in the outflow from the blood to the tissues; (3) a decrease in the marginal granulocyte pool (MGP), with an increase in the circulating granulocyte pool (CGP) but no change in the overall blood granulocyte pool; or (4) any combination of these three factors. The MGP to CGP shift is merely a redistribution and may occur, as noted previously, in response to either endogenous or exogenous epinephrine or muscular exercise. No significant change in band:seg ratio occurs. This redistribution has been referred to as *pseudo- (shift) neutrophilia.* Also, as noted previously, the neutrophilia following administration of corticosteroids and presumably an *acute* increase in their endogenous production is a result of accelerated bone marrow release, a decrease in the rate of egress of PMN out of the blood into the tissues, and a slight MGP:CGP shift.

The most common cause of sustained neutrophilia is infection. In controlled studies in animals, the first change is increased margination of cells and increased egress in response to the inflammatory stimulus, with a transient "pseudoneutropenia." A rapid increase in the rate of marrow input quickly follows, with a consequent increase in the blood concentration when marrow input exceeds the rate of output of cells from the blood into the tissues. If the infection is very severe, depletion of the marrow storage pool may occur, and "exhaustion neutropenia" may develop. This is especially true if the marrow storage pool is already abnormally small, as may occur in patients receiving cancer chemotherapy, in those with infiltrative disease of the marrow such as tumor, or in those with folic acid or vitamin B_{12} deficiency. Neutropenia developing in the face of a severe pyogenic bacterial infection is an ominous prognostic sign. During such strong inflammatory stimuli, the half-life of neutrophils in the blood has been shown to be considerably shortened.

Neutrophilia is expected with acute infections with bacteria such as *Pneumococcus, Streptococcus,* and *Staphylococcus;* with certain fungi; and with viruses such as zoster-varicella. However, many viral and parasitic infections and some bacterial infections, such as typhoid fever, are characterized by normal or even reduced neutrophil counts, an observation that may be of some diagnostic help. Clearly, neutrophilia is not diagnostic of infection or of any particular type of infection.

In the presence of chronic infection or other stimuli of long duration (e.g., with some cancers), neutrophilia may persist for a long period (throughout life in many patients with sickle cell anemia), with increased production and increased rates of input and output from the blood. A new steady state of neutrophil kinetics is thus reached.

Acute bleeding and acute destruction of red

cells (hemolysis) are often associated with neutrophilia, as is tissue damage due to burns, myocardial infarction, intestinal obstruction, and surgery. Other causes of inflammation giving rise to neutrophilia include gouty arthritis, scarlet fever, acute glomerulitis, and rheumatic fever. Uremia, diabetic acidosis, toxemia of pregnancy, jaundice due to alcohol-induced cirrhosis of the liver, poisoning by snake or insect venoms or by lead or other heavy metals, and ingestion of some drugs and chemicals can also cause neutrophilia. Convulsions and labor may cause neutrophilia, largely through demargination.

Patients with untreated chronic myeloid leukemia (CML) always have leukocytosis with neutrophilia, except for the rare patient whose leukocytes "cycle." The degree of myeloid immaturity is proportional to the height of the total white blood cell count, and more than 100,000/mm³ neutrophils and neutrophil precursors are commonly present at diagnosis. Neutrophilia, mimicking the blood picture seen in CML, often is observed in patients with idiopathic myelofibrosis (IMF), but less than 100,000/mm³ usually are present. In polycythemia vera (PV), characterized typically by an increase in all the formed elements of the blood, the leukocytosis is less and there is relatively little or no "shift to the left." Hodgkin's disease, other lymphomas, and some carcinomas may have associated neutrophilia. This may be due either to complicating infection, necrosis, and tissue damage with inflammation or to a factor produced by the tumor. The latter is well documented in animals but less so in humans.

The common denominator in most causes of neutrophilia is inflammation. The neutrophilia is the response of a normal marrow to such a stimulus. Neutrophilia of CML, PV, or IMF is due to abnormalities of the neutrophil series itself (i.e., inappropriate proliferation in the absence of the usual stimuli, such as inflammation due to tissue damage or infection).

When the total blood leukocyte concentration exceeds 50,000/mm³, the term *leukemoid reaction* is often used. This term also is often applied to lesser degrees of leukocytosis in which there are abnormal immature cells in the blood. This merely is an extreme instance of the neutrophilia that may be seen with any of the aforementioned causes, which superficially may resemble leukemia because of the magnitude of the leukocytosis. Most cases of leukemia are readily distinguishable from leukemoid reactions. The overall clinical pattern usually is quite different. Chromosomal changes usually are absent in leukemoid reactions, and the leukocyte alkaline phosphatase is high in most leukemoid reactions and low in CML. The proof of a leukemoid reaction is its disappearance when the offending condition is corrected. In Table 22–5, certain useful measures in the differential diagnosis of CML and diseases and reactions mimicking CML are listed.

TABLE 22–5 CERTAIN COMPARATIVE FEATURES OF "LEUKEMOID REACTIONS,"* CHRONIC MYELOID LEUKEMIA, POLYCYTHEMIA VERA,† AND IDIOPATHIC MYELOFIBROSIS

	Leukemoid Reactions	Chronic Myeloid Leukemia	Polycythemia Vera	Idiopathic Myelofibrosis
Physical findings				
Enlarged spleen	Rare‡	Expected	Expected	Expected
Enlarged liver	Rare‡	Common	Rare	Common
Sternal tenderness	Rare	Common	Rare	Rare
"Routine" laboratory				
Neutrophils	(↑ by definition)*	↑↑↑↑	↑–N	↑–N–↓
Red cells	↓–N	↓–(N)§	↑↑	↓–(↑)
Platelets	N–↑–↓	↑–N	↑–N	↑–N–↓
Basophils	N	↑–(N)	↑–(N)	↑–(N)
Eosinophils	↓–N	↑–(N)	↑–N	↑–N
Monocytes	N–↑–↓	↑–(N)	N–↑	↑–N
Lymphocytes	↓–N	↑–N	N	N–↓
Uric acid	N	↑–N	↑–N	↑–N
Chromosomal abnormality	None	Ph¹ (90%)	Various (50%)	Various (50%)
Leukocyte alkaline phosphatase	↑–(N)	↓ (90%)	↑–(N)	↑–(N)–(↓)
Growth of CFUc (granulocyte colonies)	Normal	Normal–↑	Normal	Normal
CFUc in blood	N–↑	↑	N	↑↑–(N)

*Those reactions mimicking myeloid leukemia, not applicable to those mimicking lymphoid leukemias.
†Excludes patients who have developed secondary myelofibrosis and those entering a blastic phase of the disease.
‡Rare, unless the finding is a part of the underlying disease producing the leukemoid reaction (e.g., with visceral tuberculosis, hepatosplenomegaly would be common).
§Indicates an uncommon finding.

Neutropenia (Table 22–6). A decrease in the normal concentration of blood neutrophils may be caused by decreased production, by increased demand for neutrophils in the presence of an inadequate increase in production by either a normal or subnormally functioning marrow, or by a shift from the CGP into the MGP (Fig. 22–9). Increased demand may be due to increased destruction of PMN by antibodies or severe infections; decreased production may be observed in many conditions. An absolute blood PMN count of less than approximately 500 cells/mm³ renders the patient quite susceptible to severe infection, and the risk increases with increasing severity of neutropenia. Patients who develop fever in the face of neutropenia must be assumed to have infection. This often is due to gram-negative bacteria and can be rapidly fatal. Patients who have this complication should be treated promptly with broad-spectrum antibiotics in the hospital following appropriate procurement of cultures. Granulocyte transfusions, although logistically difficult to procure and lasting a very short time in the blood, may prove

of some benefit in certain instances in which a return of the patient's own PMN can be anticipated within a few days.

Neutropenia may be congenital or acquired. There are several congenital varieties that are characterized by inadequate production. There are a variety of forms of dominantly inherited neutropenia, almost all of which are relatively benign with little or no evidence of an increased frequency of infection. All have been associated with decreased production. However, stem cells (CFU$_C$) have been increased in the form that is very common in Yemenite Jews but low-normal or decreased in most other families that have been studied. In most forms, neutrophils often exceed 500/mm³, and other blood leukocytes are present in normal concentration. However, the members of one family have been reported to have virtually no neutrophils, but in these individuals there is a striking monocytosis, and they have little difficulty with infection.

One of the most severe forms of neutropenia is infantile agranulocytosis (Kostmann syndrome),

TABLE 22–6 EXAMPLES OF TYPES OF NEUTROPENIA*

Kinetic Defect and Its Cause:

Decreased production
  Congenital*
    Dominantly inherited—reduced feed-in from stem cells.
    Recessively inherited (Kostmann syndrome)—increased feed-in from stem cells but either cell death or "maturation arrest" beyond the promyelocytic stage.
    Cyclic—cyclic variation in feed-in from stem cells, so that blood neutrophils "cycle" from normal to ± zero levels every 21 days and other myeloid hematopoietic cells also cycle.
  Drug-induced
    Cytotoxic therapy or accidental exposure—all dividing cells or even resting stem cells may be damaged or killed or both.
    Idiosyncratic—an occasional patient develops neutropenia (often severe) that is due to loss of neutrophil precursors at doses that have no effect in most patients.
  Associated with other diseases
    Acute leukemias—? leukemic stem cell is recognized by the normal control mechanisms as if it were a normal cell, and stem cell output declines?
    Vitamin B$_{12}$ and folate deficiency—number of neutrophil precursors in the marrow is actually increased, but they die in the marrow (ineffective hematopoiesis).

Increased destruction or loss of neutrophils from blood
  Immune-mediated
    Idiopathic—antineutrophil antibody, usually IgG, coats the neutrophil so that it is phagocytosed by macrophages.
    Neonatal (transient)—mother sensitized against fetus neutrophils by previous pregnancy or by receipt of blood products, and her resultant antibody crosses placenta.
  Drug-induced
    Hapten type—drug as antigen induces antibody that cross-reacts with neutrophils. Accidental passenger"—antibody is to drug but drug binds to neutrophil so antibody also affects neutrophil.
    Associated with other diseases
      Felty syndrome (rheumatoid arthritis with neutropenia and splenomegaly) antibody develops that may also react with marrow precursors as well as with blood neutrophils, so production is highly variable.
  Severe pyogenic infection

Pseudoneutropenia—shift from circulating to marginal pool without change in total number of blood neutrophils.

Reduced release from marrow (production and size of the storage pool are normal or increased)
  Congenital diseases in which the mature neutrophil seems functionally abnormal, termed "myelokathexis" and "lazy leukocyte syndrome" (the latter has also been reported as an acquired disease).

---

*This is a very incomplete list; for example, there are at least three varieties of dominantly inherited neutropenia of variable severity, but all have been associated with decreased production.

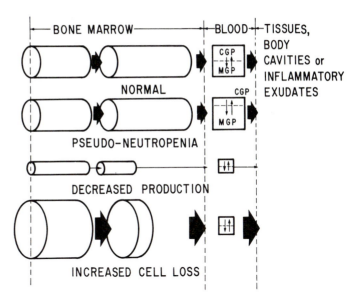

Figure 22–9 The three basic kinetic mechanisms of neutropenia.

which is inherited as an autosomal recessive. Death due to infection usually occurs in infancy. The absolute PMN concentration approaches or reaches zero, and the marrow shows few neutrophil precursors beyond the myelocyte stage. There are at least three forms; certain patients have been able to respond to infection with significant production of neutrophils, whereas others have not. There is one infant with the blood and marrow neutrophil picture of Kostmann syndrome but with extreme eosinophilia and an in-vitro growth pattern different from that of other patients. At least one patient with the Kostmann syndrome has been cured by allogeneic marrow transplantation. Some rare forms of granulocytopenias have coexisted with immunodeficiency (severe combined immunodeficiency), a doubly dangerous combination.

A fairly severe, nonfamilial form of chronic neutropenia of childhood is associated with repeated infections, but survival is possible, and recovery can eventually occur. Mature neutrophils are absent from the marrow, but metamyelocytes and a few bands are found. Increased destruction rather than decreased production may be the pathologic mechanism.

Cyclic neutropenia with a remarkable periodicity of the formed elements of the blood may be acquired or congenital. An autosomal dominant pattern has been observed in some families, whereas in others it appears to be recessively inherited. Episodes of severe neutropenia occur on the average of every 21 days, with 3 to 4 days of fever, malaise, and infection, which is sometimes fatal. Neutrophils, monocytes, eosinophils, reticulocytes, platelets and perhaps lymphocytes all have a periodicity, suggesting an intermittent failure of pluripotent stem cell production. The timing of the peak and nadir of the cycle varies from cell to cell. A phenotypically similar disorder in grey collies can be cured by appropriate bone marrow transplantation, and the disease has been trans-

mitted by marrow transplantation in both humans and dogs. Thus, it seems clear that at least certain of the inherited syndromes of cyclic hematopoiesis are due to abnormally functioning HSC. Cyclic hematopoiesis also has been induced in normal dogs by administration of chronic low doses of the cancer chemotherapeutic agent cyclophosphamide, presumably resulting in a reduction of the stem cell pool to a critical level at which cycling is the response. The acquired condition in humans has been reported to improve following the administration of adrenal corticosteroids. Androgens, endotoxin, and lithium have been effective in dogs, but, to date, the congenital form or forms in humans have been unresponsive to any medication. The recurrent infections should be treated with antibiotics, but there are always periods of good health, when the PMN count is normal and many episodes of neutropenia are not associated with infection.

CANCER CHEMOTHERAPY. The pharmacologic treatment of cancer is perhaps the most common cause of neutropenia encountered clinically. Various drugs cause damage to rapidly proliferating cells in the neutrophil series but are capable of killing stem cells as well, such as CFU_C and CFU_S. Busulfan and the nitrosoureas, such as BCNU and CCNU, have a profound and somewhat selective effect on pluripotent stem cells, as evidenced by the fact that their time to maximum neutrophil nadir is late (35 to 42 days) and by the observation that patients experience a slow recovery, whereas the typical nadir for most agents is about 12 to 14 days. Cytotoxic effects on red cells and platelets are also observed, but these are not as devastating as the effects on neutrophils because red cells and platelets have longer life spans and can be easily replenished via transfusions.

The potential for a specific drug to produce neutropenia is a function of the dose, the route of administration, the schedule, the metabolic integrity of the host, and the proliferative state of the bone marrow. The potential for inducing neutropenia varies widely among different drugs and from patient to patient. Patients with a limited bone marrow reserve due to stem cell depletion by prior therapy or the tumor itself are often more sensitive to a given dose and may require a long recovery period. The regaining of a normal neutrophil count may not always mean that the marrow has returned to normal; if adequate recovery time has not elapsed, the marrow precursors may still be actively proliferating at a greater than normal rate, and the reserve may not be replenished. Such a marrow may be more sensitive to a dose of drug that was easily tolerated previously. Although complete recovery of the marrow occurs with most drugs, some agents (e.g., the nitrosoureas and the alkylating agent busulfan) can produce irreversible changes over a period of time, probably as a result of destruction of multipotent stem cells.

What clues can be used to help the physician decide whether a specific dose of chemotherapy can be given safely? The integrity of the bone marrow may be presumed to be compromised if neutropenia develops earlier than 1 week after the administration of a myelotoxic agent in a previous course. The normal marrow granulocyte storage pool should be able to maintain a normal circulating neutrophil level for that time, even if the production of mitotically active cells is completely halted. The total leukocyte count may be misleading if considered alone, since the differential count may reveal a preponderance of mononuclear cells. Tests of marrow granulocyte reserve with predni-

sone, etiocholanolone, or endotoxin may be used, and an increased band:seg ratio (more than 0.3) may indicate that the marrow storage pool is inadequate and that relatively young cells are being released into the circulation to maintain a normal blood granulocyte pool. The relatively simple procedure of obtaining and examining marrow biopsy and aspirate specimens can be quite useful. The biopsy will indicate overall cellularity, and the adequacy of the granulocyte reserve can be judged from the presence or absence of a normal percentage of bands and segs in the aspirate. The latter correlates quite well with the use of the endotoxin test for adequacy of the reserve.

Although evaluation of the concentration of mature blood cells is the most commonly used method of monitoring hematopoietic toxicity of chemotherapeutic agents, it is an "after the fact" measure. By the time the blood cells decline, severe damage has developed in the marrow (Fig. 22–10).

Factors that determine the potential for bone marrow toxicity of a specific cancer chemotherapeutic agent include its biochemical mechanism of action; the concentration required for cell killing; its pharmacokinetics as determined by the volume of distribution, metabolism, and excretion; and the target stem cells in the bone marrow that are sensitive to its action. Most agents in common clinical use are more toxic to rapidly cycling stem cells, such as those found in a recovering bone marrow, than resting ones, although the nitrosoureas and busulfan (and irradiation) are more effective against resting cells. It is now theoretically possible to evaluate the potential for myelotoxicity

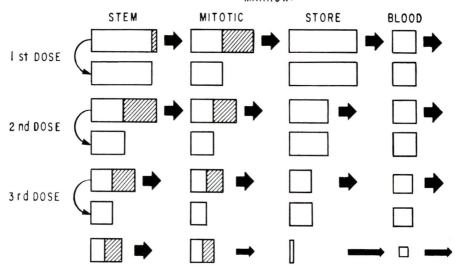

Figure 22–10 The effect of repetitive doses of a cycle-active agent (i.e., one affecting only those cells that are in an active generative cycle) upon the neutrophilic system. Note that the last event is a decrease in blood neutrophils that develops only after the overall system has sustained severe damage.

of new agents that are candidates for cancer chemotherapy by measuring their effect on bone marrow granulocyte-macrophage colony-forming cells and other colony-forming cells in various species, including humans. The results predicted from such studies have correlated to some degree with clinical effects. Dose-response curves are of two main shapes: (1) Drugs may kill with first-order kinetics and produce an exponential curve when the survival is plotted as a function of dose (Fig. 22–11), or (2) the curve will plateau after only about 50 per cent of the population has been killed (Fig. 22–12). The latter curve is typical of cycle-specific (phase-specific) agents, which kill only those cells that are in active cell cycle when they are exposed to the drug. The linear, exponential curve is representative of those drugs that are cycle-nonspecific.

IDIOSYNCRATIC REACTIONS TO DRUGS AND CHEMICALS. The examples of drug effects from cancer chemotherapy are predictable and are a function of dose. Another important type of neu

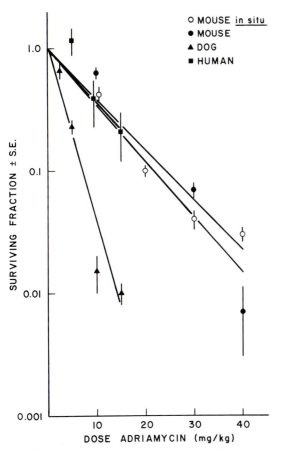

Figure 22–11 Dose-response curves of leukocyte-committed bone-marrow colony-forming cells from various species after exposure to doxorubicin (Adriamycin) in the agar diffusion chamber system. (From Marsh, J. C.: Cancer Res. *39*:360, 1979.)

tropenia is due to the idiosyncratic effect of drugs on neutrophil production. This too may be accompanied by evidence of damage to other formed blood elements or it may be isolated. Perhaps the best known of drugs that have such effects is the tranquilizer chlorpromazine. At least several weeks are required after administration for neutropenia to develop, which complication is seen in only a small proportion of patients treated. The drug interferes with the synthesis of RNA and DNA by marrow cells in vitro, and it has been suggested that sensitive subjects are unable to overcome this effect. Two types of neutropenia are seen. In one, severe neutropenia develops rapidly, and if one examines the marrow before or just after administration of the drug is discontinued, no neutrophil precursors are seen; recovery of production begins almost immediately after administration ceases. The second, perhaps more common type is one in which a modest degree (500 to 1500 neutrophils/mm³) of quite stable neutropenia develops and does not worsen unless the drug dosage is increased; marrow examination suggests it is due to decreased production. Many other drugs can cause neutropenia by decreasing production. Among them are antimicrobials, such as chloramphenicol, oxacillin, INH, the sulfonamides, and cephalothin; the anticoagulant phenindione; the anticonvulsant phenytoin; and the anti-inflammatory agents phenylbutazone and aspirin.

Some drugs, such as aminopyrine, produce a rapid onset of neutropenia in which there is sudden disappearance of neutrophils from the blood almost immediately following drug administration, suggesting an immune mechanism. It has been proposed that the drug combines with neutrophils and thus makes them antigenic, with production of antibody to the combination, or alternatively, that the drug combines with a protein to become an antigen to which antibodies are formed. With the latter mechanism, the immune complex may be attached to the neutrophil and the cell then destroyed. In either case, sudden onset of neutropenia shortly following drug ingestion would represent the continuing presence of the preformed antibody, identifying the drug as antigen. Sulfonamides and antithyroid drugs, such as propylthiouracil and methimazole, can act to produce abrupt neutropenia through a similar immunologic mechanism as well as by an effect on production as already described.

NEUTROPENIA SECONDARY TO DISEASE. Neutropenia due to decreased production may be seen in various diseases of the bone marrow, such as infiltration by certain types of carcinoma (breast, prostate, small-cell lung); granulomatous disorders such as tuberculosis, Paget's and Gaucher's disease; and certain intrinsic marrow neoplasms, such as the leukemias, lymphomas, and multiple myeloma.

In certain instances, effective production appears to be decreased owing to intramedullary

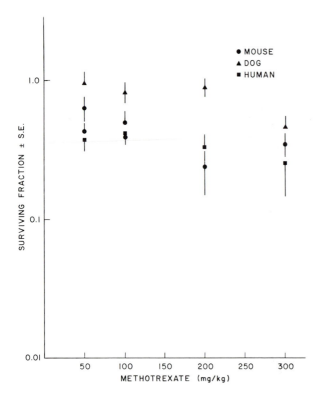

Figure 22-12 Dose-survival curves of bone marrow agar diffusion chamber precursor cells from different species 18 hours after administration of methotrexate. (Marsh, J. C.: Cancer Treat. Rep. *66*:499, 1982.)

destruction of abnormal neutrophils, analogous to "ineffective erythropoiesis." The seeming presence of granulocyte hyperplasia in marrow in association with neutropenia in B_{12} and folate deficiency and in IMF probably represents such "ineffective granulocytopoiesis."

Neutropenia in infection has been discussed. Some patients with severe malnutrition may have neutropenia, but the mechanism is unknown.

Neutropenia also may develop in association with a large spleen, and in some the question of neutrophil destruction or sequestration by the spleen can be raised ("hypersplenism"). However, with systemic lupus erythematosus and rheumatoid arthritis with splenomegaly (Felty syndrome), an immune mechanism may be the culprit. With malignant lymphoma as well as neutropenia and splenomegaly, there also may be a production defect that is due to the lymphoma per se or that is secondary to therapy with radiation or drugs. However, neutropenia (as well as anemia and thrombocytopenia) often is associated with congestive splenomegaly secondary to portal hypertension. Neutropenia usually is corrected by splenectomy for this condition, suggesting that "pure" hypersplenism may involve increased sequestration and/or destruction of neutrophils by the spleen.

Sequestration of neutrophils in the lungs with consequent neutropenia has been described in association with the early stages of hemodialysis and harvesting of cells by filtration for granulocyte transfusion. The mechanism in both cases is due to activation of complement ($C5a_{des arg}$) by a component of the dialysis coil or filtration material that is capable of causing neutrophil aggregation and adhesion. Recovery usually occurs rapidly by marrow PMN release and by subsequent demargination of some of the cells.

Several immunologic mechanisms have been described that result in neutropenia. One of these produces severe but transient neutropenia in newborn infants as a result of isoimmunization of the mother to fetal incompatible neutrophils. The antibodies formed by the mother are then able to cross the placenta and destroy mature cells in the fetal blood and marrow. The mechanism is similar to that invoked to explain the more frequent erythroblastosis fetalis involving maternal isoimmunization by fetal red cells. Some cases of chronic neutropenia have been associated with a factor or factors capable of agglutinating neutrophils in vitro. Plasma factors that can facilitate the ingestion of human neutrophils by various types of macrophages have also been described, suggesting that there is an autoimmune type of neutropenia, with inappropriate, accelerated destruction of neutrophils by the macrophage system that is initiated or enhanced or both by immunoglobulins to one's own PMNs. This is usually an IgG antibody.

Some apparent neutropenias are due to an increased fraction of cells in the MGP, seen without any change in the TBGP. This has not been proved as a cause of otherwise unexplained, chronic neutropenia but, as noted previously, occurs transiently in a number of situations. With chronic neutropenia, as the severity of neutropenia increases, the CGP:MGP ratio decreases. Thus, a degree of "shift" appears to be a physiologic mechanism accompanying most, if indeed not all, forms of neutropenia.

MONOCYTES AND MACROPHAGES

Monocytes are phagocytic cells, originating in the marrow, passing through the blood, and, for the most part, taking up residence in the tissues for relatively long periods of time. In the tissues, they mature into cells known as *macrophages*. In this form, they may be seemingly fixed in one place or may move about to different areas ("wandering macrophages"). All tissue macrophages ultimately are derived from blood monocytes, but at least some macrophages are capable of replicating independently in the tissues, thus expanding or maintaining their number without input from new monocytes. The relative importance of input to the macrophage system from blood monocytes versus macrophage self-replication in maintaining homeostasis of the compartment is poorly delineated. However, when an acute inflammation is initiated, virtually all macrophages in the resultant inflammatory exudate are derived from chemotactically mediated blood monocytes.

Phylogenetically, the macrophage, or at least a macrophage-like cell ("amoebocyte"), is the "oldest" of blood cells; species that remain unchanged after millions of years (e.g., the limulus, or horseshoe crab) have macrophage-like cells as their only blood cells.

The close relationship between the monocyte and neutrophil is demonstrated by the following findings: (1) they are both capable of phagocytosis; (2) in-vitro colonies may contain both types of cells; (3) early precursors of both in the marrow are very similar morphologically, usually requiring electron microscopy to distinguish them; and (4) many acute leukemias are characterized by the presence of cells resembling both cell types.

Monoblasts and promonocytes have been described in the marrow, but their distinction from myeloblasts and promyelocytes is difficult if not impossible with Romanovsky-stained smears. Some subtle differences between promonocytes and promyelocytes exist: The former have fewer primary granules, a more indented nucleus, and bundles of filaments in the cytoplasm. The mature monocyte has been described earlier; various degradative enzymes including peroxidase and lysozyme are present. It is larger and tends to have more cytoplasm and cytoplasmic organelles than other leukocytes.

Macrophages are larger still (20 to 80 μm), with very abundant cytoplasm, often filled with granules and vacuoles. There tends to be a differ-ent appearance, depending on the location. Thus, alveolar and peritoneal macrophages may differ considerably in appearance as well as in enzyme content. Macrophages transform into large epithelioid and giant cells in response to some types of inflammation (classically tuberculosis), and giant cells are multinucleated, primarily as the result of fusion of several macrophages. Other types of specialized macrophages include fat storage cells and Kupffer cells in the liver. The multinucleated osteoclast, the surface cell of bone that is responsible for surface bone resorption, may also be derived from the monocyte-macrophage system. The entire system of macrophages lining vascular spaces has been referred to as the reticuloendothelial system, and the term histiocyte has been used synonymously with macrophage.

Monocyte Kinetics

Labeling studies with tritiated thymidine (^{3}H-TdR) and DF^{32}P have been critical in working out the kinetics of monocytes. A marrow mitotic pool of precursors consists of monoblasts and promonocytes. The data suggest that there are two generations of promonocytes, the development of each taking about a day, with subsequent production of monocytes that pass directly to the blood. There is no significant marrow storage pool for monocytes, as exists for neutrophils. In the blood, a marginal pool of monocytes has been described similar to that of neutrophils, although it seems to be 3 to 4 times the size of the circulating pool. Monocytes leave the blood at a similar rate to that of neutrophils, and in a random fashion, with a half-life of about 8 hours. With an inflammation, monocytes migrate from blood more slowly than neutrophils but remain in the inflammatory area for longer periods. The turnover rate of monocytes in the blood is increased in severe infection; steroids produce a marked reduction of blood monocytes, and the rate of their migration into tissues in response to inflammation is also reduced, with the latter effect being similar to the steroid effect on neutrophils.

In contrast to neutrophils, which seem to live only a brief time in the tissues after leaving the blood, macrophages live quite a long time. They account for a much larger total number of cells than is present in the blood. One study suggests a steady-state life span of alveolar macrophages of 80 days. In another, a life span of 100 days was found for Kupffer cells. Macrophages may reenter the blood, since they are seen in some types of infection (e.g., the "histiocytes" of bacterial endocarditis). However, it is possible that the monocyte-macrophage transformation may occur in the blood, not in the tissues, under these conditions. Factors that stimulate the in-vitro growth of macrophage colonies have been purified from a variety of sources and may be distinct from the CSF required for neutrophil or neutrophil-macrophage colony formation.

Monocyte and Macrophage Function

Extremely diverse functions have been elucidated for the macrophage system. They include the phagocytosis and killing of microorganisms; the phagocytosis of effete cells, cellular debris, and particles; the synthesis and secretion of a number of biologically active substances; antitumor activities; and a major role in the initiation and regulation of the immune system through direct and indirect interaction with lymphocytes. Many of these functions are interrelated and are not clearly separable. Monocytes, therefore, although less numerous in the blood than neutrophils, their close relatives, are a more versatile population of cells. Macrophages, the tissue form of monocytes, are capable of cell division and transformation to "activated macrophages," epithelioid, and giant cells, and they can also synthesize new quantities of enzymes and adapt metabolically to their environment. Pulmonary alveolar macrophages, for example, rely more on aerobic glycolysis than their peritoneal counterparts. Another difference between monocyte and macrophage is the loss of peroxidase from the lysosomes in the latter.

Monocytes and macrophages are capable of chemotaxis. Of the numerous chemotaxins, some are excellent attractants for both neutrophils and monocytes-macrophages, whereas others primarily attract one or another type of cell. Factors primarily chemotactic for monocytes include a product of interaction of sensitized lymphocytes and antigen and the immune stimulant levamisole.

Monocyte-macrophages have been shown to have several binding sites for immunoglobulins (IgG) as well as the C3 component of complement. These are thought to be important in allowing the cell to recognize and ingest foreign particles. Monocytes are more effective in ingesting fungi, sensitized red blood cells, and inert particles than PMNs, but they are less effective than PMNs in dealing with certain types of bacteria. Monocytes can form rosettes with sensitized red cells in suspension, but neutrophils cannot. The phagocytic process seems to depend largely on oxidative phosphorylation in the monocyte and the alveolar macrophage, but it apparently derives more energy from anaerobic glycolysis in the PMN and the peritoneal macrophage.

Intracellular killing of some bacteria in monocytes is enhanced by serum factors for which these cells have receptors, namely the F_c fragments of certain IgG immunoglobulins and C3. In a manner similar to PMN, phagosomes are formed with fusion of intracellular lysosomes (granules) to carry out the killing process. Unlike PMNs, monocytes and macrophages can resynthesize new granules and the enzymes contained within them. One of the important factors accounting for macrophage efficacy in killing of PMN-resistant organisms such as mycobacteria, protozoa, helminths, viruses, and fungi is *activation,* in which the cell becomes larger and synthesizes new granules. The metabolism of glucose by the hexose-monophosphate shunt is increased. The activation process is produced by certain soluble products of T-lymphocytes called *lymphokines* and also by interferon. It can be demonstrated that unactivated macrophages can be colonized by certain bacteria that will survive in them; these colonized cells can be activated to kill the indwelling bacteria by incubation with activated T cells (exposed to the same or different bacteria) or by incubation with soluble products from the same T cells.

Macrophages in inflammatory exudates ingest the debris produced by earlier PMN ingestion and killing of the inciting microorganisms. They also can ingest immune complexes, denatured protein, and activated, presumably useless clotting factors. As cells lining vascular channels, they perform this function efficiently as the components of the "reticuloendothelial system." Aged red cells, platelets, and various leukocytes are also removed in this way, with conservation and reutilization of iron from the red cells. When these formed elements of the blood are inappropriately coated with antibody, as in autoimmune hemolytic anemia or idiopathic thrombocytopenic purpura (ITP), the macrophage system is the immediate cause of the premature destruction. The macrophage system may become less active following extensive trauma or various viral infections. It may be made temporarily more active (as one can demonstrate by measuring the rate of clearance of aggregated albumin) by infections such as typhoid fever or pneumococcal pneumonia.

A large number of active substances are synthesized and secreted by monocytes and macrophages. Among them are CSF, required for neutrophil-monocyte colony development in vitro, and, quite possibly, a physiologic regulator in vivo. Under certain circumstances, they synthesize and release erythropoietin, the hormone primarily responsible for control of RBC production. They also make interferon, an important antiviral agent and endogenous pyrogen, which is probably *not* made by neutrophils as previously thought. Endogenous pyrogen is released following phagocytosis or in response to macrophage exposure to bacterial endotoxin. It causes fever and changes in iron kinetics, notably a fall in plasma iron levels by interfering with the release of iron into the plasma by macrophages. It may be identical with interleukin 1 (IL-1), which stimulates T-lymphocytes to secrete another factor (IL-2), which stimulates the proliferation of more T-lymphocytes. Lysozyme, transcobalamin II (a transport protein for vitamin B_{12}), prostaglandins, and certain components of complement are all synthesized by these busy cells.

Macrophages have been shown to kill cancer cells in vitro and may be an important defense mechanism against tumor development. Activated macrophages can kill tumor cells directly or through the mediation of cytotoxic antibodies to which the macrophages bind by F_c receptors. Attempts to increase macrophage cytotoxicity in cancer therapy by the use of nonspecific immunotherapy (e.g., with Calmette-Guerin bacillus, or BCG, an attenuated mycobacterium) have met with equivocal success. Many tumors, when examined histologically, are found to be infiltrated by macrophages, and the degree of infiltration has been related to prognosis of certain cancers but not of others. Circulating monocytes are often increased above normal in a variety of cancers. Phagocytosis of inert particles by monocytes from cancer patients is generally normal, as is bactericidal capacity. However, there are a number of reports of depressed chemotaxis of monocytes in cancer patients, and a plasma factor inhibitory for chemotaxis has been described in some of them. This material may be produced directly by the tumor or by the host in response to it, since the degree of inhibition has been decreased by surgical removal of the tumor.

The immune response (to be discussed in more detail in the section on lymphocytes) is a complex, incompletely understood, coordinated effort that occurs principally between macrophages and lymphocytes. The latter may be considered broadly as T-, or thymus-derived, lymphocytes, responsible largely for cellular immune responses, and B- (avian *bursa*–equivalent, or *bone* marrow–derived) lymphocytes, which subserve the humoral immune response characterized by immunoglobulin synthesis and secretion. One of the key roles of macrophages is to "process" various antigens for presentation to reactive T- and B-lymphocytes. Macrophages accomplish this processing by breaking down the antigens and chemically changing them. The immunization process is rendered considerably more efficient in this way. Another form of macrophage-lymphocyte communication involves the secretion by macrophages of IL-1, which results indirectly in the proliferation of specific T-lymphocytes. Prostaglandins released by macrophages have been implicated in the inhibition of certain functions of activated lymphocytes, thus constituting a physiologic "brake" on their activity. Overactivity of this process may be one explanation for the impaired cellular immune response seen in Hodgkin's disease, other cancers, and some chronic infections.

Macrophages are influenced in turn by products of T-lymphocytes (lymphokines) as the latter respond to antigens. Among the many lymphokines are chemotactic factor; migration inhibiting factor (MIF), which helps direct the phagocytic cell; and macrophage activating factor, which makes the macrophage a more efficient killer of intracellular organisms.

The normal range for blood monocytes is from 200 to 950/mm³. An increased number (monocytosis) may be found in various malignancies, such as Hodgkin's disease, non-Hodgkin's lymphoma, myeloma, chronic myelocytic leukemia (CML), carcinomas (e.g., those of the lung, breast, stomach, and ovary), and melanoma. Absolute monocytosis may characterize lipid-storage diseases, such as Gaucher's disease; collagen vascular disease, such as lupus erythematosus, rheumatoid arthritis, and polyarteritis nodosa; sarcoidosis; inflammatory bowel disease; and the early recovery from neutropenia. It also occurs in certain infections such as typhus, malaria, Rocky mountain spotted fever, syphilis, tuberculosis, brucellosis, and subacute bacterial endocarditis, especially that due to *Streptococcus viridans*.

Diseases of Monocytes and Macrophages

Since the monocyte and neutrophil are so closely related, one might expect that they would share some enzyme defects. The monocyte is affected by the oxidase deficiency seen in the PMN of chronic granulomatous disease. They also share some clonal neoplasms, such as acute leukemia. The terminology applied to certain tumors is inaccurate with respect to cell origin. Most of the tumors that have been called "histiocytic lymphoma" or "reticulum cell sarcoma" are, in fact, tumors of the lymphoid system rather than of the monocyte-macrophage system.

Several peculiar diseases of unknown cause, characterized by diffuse or focal collections of macrophages, often with an admixture of eosinophils, were grouped together as one entity, "histiocytosis X," because of their similar histologies. This term is not very useful because of great variations in clinical course, treatment implications, and prognosis, and thus the original three names—*eosinophilic granuloma of bone, Hand-Schüller-Christian disease,* and *Letterer-Siwe disease*—are still widely used. Unifying features include the tendency to occur in children and the presence of large, foamy histiocytes in various organs. The etiology of each disease is unknown, although current opinion favors an unknown infection, and indeed some response to antibiotics has been seen. Eosinophilic granuloma of bone usually involves only bone, although sometimes other tissues such as the lungs may become involved. Of these three diseases, eosinophilic granuloma is the only one that often affects adults, and cure is often effected by curettage of the tissue or low doses of radiation. Hand-Schüller-Christian disease is typically characterized by multiple bone lesions, exophthalmos, and diabetes insipidus due to pituitary dysfunction. There are defects in membranous bones, liver and spleen enlargement, enlarged lymph nodes, skin and mucous membrane lesions, and, often anemia. The prognosis is fair and related to the extent of disease when first diagnosed. Sometimes, bone lesions alone are the presenting problem. Adrenal corticosteroids, a variety of anticancer drugs, and radiotherapy for local bone lesions are all effective to varying degrees. Letterer-Siwe disease occurs primarily in infants or very young children. It is associated with erosive bone lesions, lymphadenopathy, organomegaly, anemia, variable thrombocytopenia, and prominent skin lesions. Compared with eosinophilic granuloma and Hand-Schüller-Christian disease, this disorder is uncommon. Although it is usually fatal, patients sometimes respond to vinca alkaloids or alkylating agents.

Several other conditions constituting the *lysosomal storage diseases* involve an overloading of mononuclear phagocytes with lipid or lipid-containing cellular products. Most of these disorders are familial and due to inherited enzyme deficiencies that prevent the normal catabolism of classes of lipids called *sphingolipids,* which are important components of neural tissue (gangliosides) and of cell membranes (globosides). Blood group antigens are sphingolipids. Among these disorders are Gaucher disease, Niemann-Pick disease, Fabry disease, and the syndrome of "sea-blue histiocytes." A related disorder, Tay-Sachs disease, has such devastating neurologic effects, culminating in death during infancy, that a macrophage component warrants little attention.

Gaucher disease is a chronic familial disorder associated with organomegaly, brown pigmentation of the skin, pingueculae, varying degrees of anemia, thrombocytopenia and leukopenia due to hypersplenism, and bone lesions. Inheritance is autosomal recessive. Severity varies according to the degree of β-glucocerebrosidase deficiency, which results in the accumulation of glucose-ceramide within macrophages. The cells have a characteristic appearance. They are large and pale blue with numerous cytoplasmic whorls or fibrillae. They contain acid phosphatase, and indeed the serum level of this enzyme is increased. The spleen, liver, lymph nodes, and bone marrow are packed with these "Gaucher" cells. Patients with the adult onset form of the disease can live fairly normally; the infantile form is lethal, and the cases in which onset occurs during childhood are quite severe. Splenectomy can ameliorate the blood abnormalities. Bone marrow transplantation has been tried with some initial reports of success. Gaucher-like cells have also been seen as part of several other hematologic diseases such as CML and hemolytic anemia in the absence of any enzyme defect. This suggests that overloading of macrophages can occur if there is an accelerated turnover of cellular lipid. However, these can be distinguished from the cells of Gaucher disease by specialized study (e.g., transmission electron microscopy).

Niemann-Pick disease is also inherited as an autosomal recessive trait. It is due to a deficiency of sphingomyelinase, with consequent overloading of macrophages by sphingomyelin, a phosphorylcholine derivative of an acyl sphingosine, or ceramide. The storage cells are large but foamy, contain small cytoplasmic droplets, and lack the lamellar structure of Gaucher cells. The cells may be seen in the blood as well as in the marrow, nodes, liver, spleen, and central nervous system. There are several different clinical forms, most running a fulminant course with severe neurologic deterioration. Some patients have lived to early adulthood. There is no effective treatment.

Fabry's disease is an X-linked disorder shown to be due to a deficiency of the enzyme α-galactosidase, which leads to a block in the degradation of ceramide trihexose, a component of the normal membrane lipid globoside. This material accumulates in many cells, including macrophages, giving rise to foamy cells in the marrow and urine. Significant accumulation occurs in other cells, such as vascular endothelium, renal epithelium, and heart muscle. Very characteristic skin lesions around the scrotum, thighs, and umbilicus in males may be mistaken for purpura. However, unlike petechiae, they are raised and palpable and their purple color does not fade with time. Proteinuria and renal failure commonly develop, with death occurring in young adulthood.

"Sea-blue histiocytes" have been seen as part of an apparently familial recessive disorder and in sporadic cases of other illnesses such as CML and ITP. The primary disorder seems to arise in association with the accumulation of excess cerebroside and sugars within macrophages, but a specific enzyme defect has not been demonstrated. There is splenomegaly, thrombocytopenia secondary to the enlarged spleen, and consequent purpura. The cells are found in the marrow, liver, and spleen. Their color, a very deep blue, is due to the large number of pigmented granules found in these cells. The disorder usually is not lethal, but some patients have died of complications such as severe hemorrhage.

EOSINOPHILS

Maturation of eosinophils is similar to that of PMNs, with corresponding cells termed *myelocytes, metamyelocytes, bands,* and *segmented cells* after they begin to synthesize the characteristic large, bright red to orange granules that give them their name. Like neutrophils, eosinophils are made only in the marrow, and there is a marrow storage pool of mature cells. Both types of cells respond to chemotactic stimuli, although these vary in attractive strength for the two types of cells. Eosinophils are capable of margination, migration, phagocytosis, and intracellular killing. They are as motile as PMNs and tend to appear most prominently at sites of foreign protein deposition, to participate in allergic reactions, and to be especially suited to interaction with parasites.

Eosinophils differ from PMNs in several prominent ways. For example, eosinophils are able to recirculate from the blood into the marrow and from the tissues into the blood. The blood clearance time has tended, therefore, to be longer, although the disappearance is random, similar to that of PMNs. Eosinophils are formed in specific colonies in vitro when stimulated by their own CSA, formed by activated T-lymphocytes, a role that may be of physiologic significance. Their primary granules have a crystalline structure quite distinct from those of PMNs when examined by electron microscopy, and the enzyme content is also different, with a different kind of peroxidase, various cationic, basic proteins (which cause the attraction for eosin), but no lysozyme or alkaline phosphatase. Eosinophils generally have only two lobes, whereas many PMNs typically have more.

One of the most notable characteristics of eosinophils is their disappearance from the blood following the acute administration of adrenal corticosteroids or during stress, such as acute infection. The mechanism is not clear, but it does not appear to be cell lysis or inhibition of release of cells by the marrow. Some type of sequestration or return to bone marrow has been postulated. The eosinopenia is not chronic, with near-normal levels being regained after several days in the face of continued steroid administration.

Eosinophil Function

It has been known for many years that eosinophils are attracted to antigen-antibody complexes and may then phagocytize them. Histamine is one of the chemotactic substances for eosinophils as well, and the interaction of histamine with eosinophils suggests that basophils produce histamine, which attracts and is then destroyed by eosinophils. Immune complexes react with the complement system to produce chemotactic substances for both eosinophils and PMNs. Specific receptors on each cell type undoubtedly play critical roles in determining which substances attract which cells. Eosinophils are less potent than PMNs in killing bacteria and in ingesting them. They have a well-established role in certain parasitic infestations, particularly when larvae are invading tissues. In general, they are more effective against flatworms than roundworms. They are active as *useful* defensive cells, primarily when the host has been previously immunized and is making immunoglobulin, such as IgG or IgE, which coats the parasite. In the presence of immune globulin or activated complement, the eosinophil attaches to the parasite, its granules fuse, and their contents are extruded into the area between the cell and the attached worm, which is usually too large for

ingestion by the eosinophil. The products of the killing cascade and the various cationic proteins can degrade the parasitic wall and may eventually kill the larvae. Tissue damage can, however, result from the granulomas around parasites, formed by macrophages and eosinophils. Whether the role of the eosinophil is helpful or harmful depends on prior immunization in experimentally induced schistosomiasis. If animals are previously immunized, the eosinophil plays a helpful role in killing larvae before extensive tissue invasion is accomplished. If they are not immunized, eosinophils are attracted only after antibodies appear and tissue invasion is already established; at this point, the eosinophil's attack contributes to more extensive granuloma formation, with most damage occurring in tissues such as the liver.

Charcot-Leyden crystals are eight-sided, elongated, pointed structures 20 to 40 μm long that are often found in acute asthmatic sputum. They are thought to be formed from material in eosinophil granules. The eosinophil has no known secretory function but is capable of inactivating excretory and potentially dangerous products of mast cells (see further on).

Eosinophilia

An increase in the absolute number of eosinophils in the blood, more than 700 cells/mm³, is found in a variety of conditions. It must be distinguished from relative eosinophilia (an "increase" in percentage), which is insignificant. Parasitic infestations, usually with tissue invasion, are a classic cause. Among them are schistosomiasis, trichinosis, malaria, toxoplasmosis, ascariasis, and hookworm disease. However, others such as trypanosomiasis, amebiasis, and pinworm infestation, usually are not associated with eosinophilia.

Loeffler's syndrome and the pulmonary infiltration with eosinophilia (PIE) syndrome are both combinations of lung involvement with eosinophilia, differing only in the duration of illness, and both are often associated with infections, either parasitic or bacterial. Both snydromes are presumably related to hypersensitivity to a foreign substance. Allergic reactions, such as bronchial asthma, hives, hay fever, angioneurotic edema, and reactions to various drugs, are often associated with eosinophilia and certain skin diseases, such as pemphigus, psoriasis, eczema, dermatitis herpetiformis, and scabies. Eosinophilia is sometimes seen as a hereditary, benign condition.

With certain hematologic malignancies, such as CML, IMF, and PV, eosinophilia is very common. Patients with pernicious anemia, sickle cell disease, and various kinds of collagen disease may have eosinophilia. Eosinophilia is not a common characteristic of any type of cancer of nonmyeloid origin, even Hodgkin's disease, in which it is more often written about than seen. However, it can be a manifestation of virtually any type of cancer; if one surveys a general hospital population for the presence of eosinophilia, cancer probably is the most common underlying disease.

"Tropical eosinophilia" is a febrile disease associated with pulmonary infiltration and splenomegaly and is possibly due to filariae. It involves an impressive increase in eosinophils and often responds promptly to filaricides.

Some types of eosinophilia appear to be neoplasms of the myeloid series and are therefore properly termed *eosinophilic leukemia*. Some of these appear to be CML variants, and numerous eosinophils coexist with a great number of neutrophils, with or without a Ph[1] chromosome. Others appear to be more acute, with enlargement of liver, spleen, and nodes; pulmonary infiltrates; and often subendocardial fibroelastosis with mural thrombi, congestive heart failure, and thrombophlebitis. The eosinophils often show various abnormalities such as decreased granulation and vacuolization, but these may also be seen in "secondary" forms of eosinophilia. It is probable that the endocardial fibrosis is secondary to damage produced by eosinophil contents, since it has been observed in other conditions associated with marked eosinophilia.

Eosinopenia

Virtually complete disappearance of eosinophils from the blood is more common than eosinophilia, since it occurs with many kinds of acute infection or inflammation. It is caused by a combination of factors, including migration of eosinophils to the inflamed area, margination, cessation of release from marrow, and perhaps return to it. As already noted, steroid administration causes acute eosinopenia. Eosinopenia is such a "routine" finding during the early phases of pyogenic bacterial infection that this diagnosis should be carefully re-evaluated if eosinophils are found easily on blood smears.

BASOPHILS AND MAST CELLS

Basophils are the least numerous type of blood leukocyte, normally not exceeding 150/mm³. Thus, one will not see any basophils in the majority of 100 cell differential counts of blood smears. They are formed in the marrow in a similar fashion as the other granulocytes. Their morphology has been described. The large, bluish-black granules are formed primarily at the myelocyte stage. Heparin and histamine in the primary granules are thought to cause the characteristic staining. The granules also contain eosinophil chemotactic factor, a slow-reacting substance causing anaphylaxis, and a platelet-activating factor. They are fairly motile.

Mast cells are found in tissues and resemble basophils in their granule appearance and content. However, they are larger, and the electron microscopic appearance of the granules is different, as is the chemical content. The nucleus is round, rather than segmented as in the basophil, and there tend to be more granules in the cell. Mast cells in the tissues are certainly more numerous than basophils in the blood and marrow. In spite of these differences, however, the two possibly share a common stem cell in the marrow, and their functions are very similar.

Blood basophils are capable of phagocytosis but it is not clear that this is their prime function. They release their granular content outside the cell, as do mast cells. Histamine is released in the degranulation process after reaction with certain antigens or with IgE, for which they have receptors. Numerous other substances that cause bronchoconstriction, vasoconstriction, and chemotaxis are released as well by mast cells and basophils (Table 22–7). The release of heparin from these cells, which activates lipoprotein lipase, is thought to play a role in triglyceride metabolism (e.g., clearance of postprandial hyperlipemia). Eosinophils are thought to regulate or modify the various mediators of basophils and mast cells by phagocytosing granules and by releasing enzymes that neutralize or degrade some of these mediators. Sudden, massive release of mast cell (and basophil) granules and their contents is thought to be the principle mediator of such dire and sometimes fatal events as anaphylactic shock. Mast cells and basophils which have released granules are capable of resynthesizing them.

Basophilia and Basopenia

Increased numbers of basophils in the blood are seen in hypothyroidism; reduced numbers often are observed in hyperthyroidism. Increases have also been seen in chickenpox, ulcerative colitis, some types of renal disease, postsplenectomy, and Hodgkin's disease. However, striking increases in blood basophils rarely are seen in any condition except for the clonal myeloid neoplasms (myeloid leukemias, IMF, PV). Corticosteroids reduce the numbers of basophils, as does pregnancy, whereas estrogen and antithyroid drugs cause an increase. Basophilic and mast cell leukemias have been described. In urticaria pigmentosa, a congenital disorder, increased numbers of mast cells are present in the skin. These cause pigmented nodules or macules that produce redness and edema on rubbing. This is due to the release of histamine from the mast cells; some patients develop flushing, itching, hypotension, headache, dizziness, nausea, vomiting, and diarrhea due to the systemic effects of histamine. The disorder usually disappears by adolescence. Systemic mastocytosis is an

TABLE 22–7 CERTAIN MAST-CELL–DEPENDENT MEDIATORS

Mediator:

Released as preformed substance

Histamine	Smooth muscle contraction
	Increase in vascular permeability
	Modulation of chemotaxis, prostaglandins, cyclic nucleotides
Serotonin	Smooth muscle contraction
	Increase in vascular permeability
Eosinophil chemotactic factors (various)	Attract and deactivate eosinophils and neutrophils
Heparin	Anticoagulation
	Neutralizes major basic proteins of eosinophils
Enzymes (chymase, peroxidase, arylsulfatase)	Proteolysis, hydrolysis, cleavage
Chondroitin sulfate	Interacts with platelets

Newly generated on release

Leukotrienes (slow-reacting substances of anaphylaxis)	Smooth-muscle contraction
	Increase in vascular permeability
	Chemotactic
	Modulates histamine, prostaglandins
Platelet activating factor	Promotes platelet aggregation, adhesion

Preformed or generated or both

Prostaglandins and other arachidonic metabolites	Smooth-muscle contraction and relaxation
	Chemotaxis
	Modulation of cyclic nucleotides

acquired disorder of adulthood in which mast cells progressively invade the skin, resulting in papules, nodules, telangiectasia, involvement of mucosal surfaces, and bone lesions. Enlargement of liver, spleen, and nodes; bone marrow infiltration; and pancytopenia in more severe cases due to mast cell proliferation suggest a neoplastic cause. Large amounts of histamine may be seen in serum and urine, and systemic symptoms due to histamine are often present.

MYELOID STEM CELL NEOPLASMS

A number of neoplastic diseases are clonal tumors of hematopoietic stem cells; that is, the

abnormal cell line arises from one abnormal stem cell, which may or may not be capable of differentiation, often distorted. Fairly firm proof of the clonal nature of these (and most) neoplasms comes from the demonstration that gene products of the X chromosome in heterozygous individuals are homogeneous in the neoplastic cells. The best example of this is the enzyme glucose-6-phosphate dehydrogenase (G6PD) in black women whose normal cells carry one or the other of two separable isoenzymes. When such patients develop a tumor, such as acute leukemia, all the neoplastic cells have but one type of enzyme, rather than two (Fig. 22–13). Abnormal chromosome patterns for neoplastic cells have also borne out this hypothesis, classically the Ph[1] chromosome in CML.

The best known neoplasms of myeloid stem cells include acute myeloid leukemia (AML), chronic myeloid leukemia (CML), polycythemia vera (PV), idiopathic myelofibrosis (IMF) with myeloid metaplasia, and paroxysmal nocturnal hemoglobinuria (PNH). These diseases have been referred to as *myeloproliferative disorders,* a broad term that has little meaning with regard to specificity and should therefore *not* be used as a diagnostic term. Recent evidence suggests that Hodgkin's disease may be more a neoplasm of macrophages than lymphocytes and thus also be a "myeloid" neoplasm. We have discussed Hodgkin's disease with the other "lymphomas" according to traditional classification schemes, recognizing that it is primarily a tumor involving lymph nodes. The true "histiocytic" neoplasms (those that arise from the monocyte-macrophage arm of the myeloid system) also are mentioned with the lymphomas, as their clinical manifestations often are more

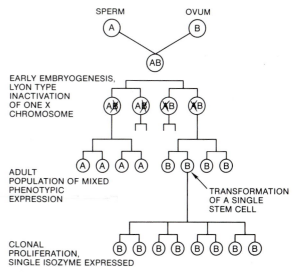

Figure 22–13 Schematic representation of the basis for the use of G6PD analysis in isozymic heterozygotes in the determination of the clonal origin of neoplasms. *A* indicates the isozyme Gd^A and *B* indicates Gd^B.

representative of these diseases than of the afore-mentioned myeloid neoplasms.

All the stem cell neoplasms are characterized by an inappropriate expansion of one or more hematopoietic cell compartments in the absence of an excess of the usual stimuli for proliferation. In some of the disorders, the tumor cells are morphologically identical with their normal counterparts, whereas in others, definite abnormalities are seen.

The tumor cell expansion is not due to abnormally rapid cell growth, but the tumor cells are clearly at a growth advantage relative to the normal stem cells. Normal and tumor stem cells often coexist, and the normal cells often become predominant with induction of a complete remission. The leukemic clone may produce a substance or substances that inhibit the proliferation of normal stem cells. Leukemic stem cells retain some characteristics of the normal cells and may respond to normal stimuli, but they are relatively independent. The fact that PV erythroid colonies in vitro are independent of erythropoietin, which is required for normal erythroid colony growth, is a case in point. However, the stem cell of PV is not completely autonomous with respect to erythropoietin. It is abnormally sensitive to the hormone, responding to levels that will not detectably affect normal erythroid cells. It will respond with increased production to increasing levels of erythropoietin.

The terms *acute* and *chronic* no longer accurately refer to the duration of life in patients with various forms of leukemia but are useful with regard to the speed of onset and type of predominant cell to be expected, the prognosis, and the choice of therapy. "Leukemia" does not mean leukocytosis in all situations, although it is required for a diagnosis of chronic leukemia. In many of the acute leukemias, there is a low or normal number of white cells in the blood, although abnormal ones usually are present. When there are no abnormal cells in the blood ("aleukemic leukemia"), they are disclosed by bone marrow examination. Transitions may occur. The most charac-

teristic is the change of CML into a clinical entity resembling acute leukemia ("blast crisis"); another is the evolution of PV into an IMF-like picture. Both of these, as well as PNH, occasionally terminate in AML.

The myeloid stem cell neoplasms are somewhat more common in males than in females. CML is a disease largely of early adulthood and middle age; PV and IMF occur most frequently in the elderly; and AML can occur at any age, although it is less common in children than in adults and becomes more common with increasing age.

ACUTE MYELOID LEUKEMIA

Many features of acute myeloid leukemia (AML) are shared by other hematologic neoplasms; thus we have discussed this disease in some depth as an "index" type of disease.

This disorder and its morphologic variants are rapidly fatal when untreated, and, even with modern therapy, median survival is only about 1 year, depending largely on whether a complete remission can be achieved. AML *must* be distinguished from acute lymphoblastic leukemia (ALL), as the treatment for each is quite different. Although at least seven different morphologic variants can be recognized (Table 22–8), they are similar in mode of onset, course, and response to treatment.

The French-American-British (FAB) classification of AML is a morphologic one, identifying six AML variants (Table 22–8). In many instances, various mixtures of the cell types listed in Table 22–8 are encountered, and if one wishes to classify such cases of AML with regard to morphologic variant, this usually is done on the basis of the most common of the leukemic cells in blood or marrow or both. Many investigators have adopted the term "acute nonlymphocytic leukemia" as a substitute for AML. Our opinion of this term apparently is shared by H. E. M. Kay, author of the following "Poem to the Editor":*

---

*New England Journal of Medicine, February 25, 1982.

TABLE 22–8 MORPHOLOGIC SUBCLASSIFICATION OF ACUTE MYELOID LEUKEMIA AND CORRESPONDING FRENCH-AMERICAN-BRITISH (FAB) CLASSIFICATION

Cell Type	FAB Designation	Relative Frequency (674 Patients)* (Per Cent)
Myeloblastic (AMbL)		
("Undifferentiated")	M1	13
("Myeloblastic")	M2	45
Promyelocytic (APL)	M3	7
Myelomonocytic (AMML)	M4	14
Monocytic (AMoL)	M5	18
Erythroleukemic (AEL)	M6	3
Megakaryoblastic (AMegL)	None	?

*(From combined series in Clinical Hematology. 8th ed., Philadelphia, Lea & Febiger, 1982, p. 1537).

HEY NONNY NO

I'm feeling a trifle non-normal,
I wonder just what it could be;
Not, I hope, non-A or non-B,
Or, supposing there is one, non-C.

I trust that it's not a leukemia,
Especially a non-LL,
(Better a non-T or non-B)
Of course not non-HD as well.

To disprove that it's not neoplastic,
Nor yet not non-infective too,
Analysis not non-stochastic,
Can tell what's not false nor untrue;

I'll negate all the non-information,
Which, as non-inessentials, I must.
It's not that I'm not non-agnostic,
But this nonsense has got me nonplussed.

A major defect is the failure of the leukemic stem cell to differentiate normally, and this indeed may account for its unrestrained proliferation through lack of feedback inhibition by mature cells. Normally formed elements of the blood are not produced in adequate numbers, and the consequences are lethal. At diagnosis, there is usually anemia (>90 per cent), contributing to fatigue; thrombocytopenia (80 to 90 per cent), causing hemorrhage; and neutropenia (80 to 90 per cent), with a risk of severe infection. Furthermore, there is evidence that the mature cells are not derived from residual normal stem cells but are part of the leukemic clone (this is *not* the case in ALL). That is, a few of the immature AML cells do mature, producing PMNs, red cells, and platelets that are part of the clone and further supporting the concept that the disease operates phenotypically at the level of a pluripotent myeloid stem cell. However, these neutrophils and platelets often are functionally abnormal, further adding to problems of bleeding and infection associated with their decreased numbers. The major components of supportive care are identification and treatment of these problems. Therapy is continued until the leukemic clone can be eradicated or, at least, suppressed and normal cells can grow again.

Prominent clinical features include fatigue, shortness of breath, pallor, weight loss, bone or joint pain, organomegaly due to leukemic cell infiltration, purpura, and fever, either because of or independent of, infection. Sternal and other bone tenderness is common and is thought to be due to leukemic cell hyperplasia within the marrow. Bleeding, particularly but not exclusively in APL (M3), may be due to intravascular coagulation triggered by a clotting factor in the leukemic granules. Gum infiltration is particularly common in the monocytic leukemia variants (M4, M5). Meningeal infiltration can occur but is not as common as in ALL.

The white cell count is highly variable, but immature cells ("blasts") are nearly always pres-ent in the blood and always present in increased numbers in the bone marrow. The marrow is usually highly cellular. However, hypocellular, fibrotic, or even necrotic marrow may be present, and in these circumstances it may occasionally be difficult for one to make an unequivocal diagnosis of AML. Auer bodies are abnormal forms of azurophilic granules and may be seen in the cytoplasm of blasts and more mature cells. The morphologic diagnosis of AML can be made with certainty when these entities are seen, as their presence has been limited to patients with AML, to individuals in blast crisis of CML, and perhaps to the fetus. Auer bodies are seen in a high frequency of cells in only about 10 per cent of patients with AML, but a prolonged, careful search of slides will disclose them in as many as 40 per cent.

Hyperuricemia is seen in about half the patients at diagnosis. This disorder is due to increased production of uric acid resulting from increased nucleic acid turnover due to cell breakdown and ineffective hematopoiesis. With vigorous chemotherapy, virtually all patients will develop hyperuricemia, often to levels that will lead to acute renal insufficiency unless proper, prophylactic measures are instituted. Elevated serum lysozyme is seen in the monocytic variants, and hypokalemia may result from the renal tubular damage produced by increased lysozyme excretion.

Etiology

The cause of AML is not known. Because of viral etiologies for some animal tumors and leukemias, the search for viruses has been intensive but not conclusive. Some AML cells contain the enzyme reverse transcriptase, which can utilize RNA as a template for DNA synthesis, a characteristic "footprint" of certain viruses.

AML has followed exposure to irradiation, as a result of atomic bombing or of therapy for arthritis or other malignancies. Chemical agents such as benzene can be implicated in a few patients. A fairly common sequel to successful therapy for malignant disease such as myeloma, Hodgkin's disease and other lymphomas, and cancer of the ovary and breast has been AML. A common denominator is the use of chemotherapeutic drugs, particularly alkylating agents, often in combination with irradiation. These secondary leukemias may have a long "preleukemia" phase and as a group are less responsive to therapy than AML that arises de novo. AML is a common terminal phase of CML and occurs in a few patients with PV and IMF, but in these diseases the contribution of therapy to the AML genesis is debatable.

Biology

Gross cytogenic abnormalities are present in about 50 per cent of patients (karyotype abnormalities), but newer techniques indicate a still higher frequency of more subtle chromosomal changes. The defects are seen only in malignant cells and disappear during remission. Their incidence relative to the normal karyotype in marrow cells has prognostic value with respect to the frequency of remission induction and duration. Patients in whom virtually all metaphases examined from bone marrow are aneuploid (an abnormal number of chromosomes) or pseudodiploid (a normal number of chromosomes—46—but with loss of one or more balanced by reduplication of others) have a poorer prognosis than those in whom no such defects are noted. Those in whom abnormalities are present in some, but not all, cells examined have an intermediate prognosis. The patterns vary considerably among patients but are nonrandom. A gain of chromosome 8 and a loss of chromosome 7 are fairly common. A translocation between chromosomes 8 and 21 has been found only in M1 and M2 AML, more frequently in children, and is associated with a large number of Auer bodies. This translocation is an exception to the generality that karyotype changes mean a bad prognosis. A translocation between chromosomes 15 and 17 has been seen only in APL (M3).

In-vitro growth of neutrophil-macrophage colonies (CFU_{NM}, discussed previously) is abnormal in AML and shows one of three patterns: (1) no growth at all (least common); (2) cluster formation (groups of eight to 50 cells, most common); and (3) colony formation (more than 50 cells, intermediate frequency). The colonies, unlike normal CFU_{NM}, are composed of immature cells. Colony growth returns to normal in remission.

Survival

Median survival in AML is a matter of 2 to 3 months in the untreated or nonresponsive patient. An increment in survival is seen in direct proportion to the incidence of complete remission, which is now achievable in as many as 80 per cent of patients under 60 years of age, with median survival in that group in the range of 1½ years. Unfortunately, the induction of complete remission usually does not mean cure, since relapse occurs in the vast majority of patients. Clinical factors that have been associated with a low remission rate include older age (death during induction), low platelet count, and an extremely high blast count at diagnosis. Patients with a rapidly rising blast count in the blood are at high risk to die of intracerebral hemorrhage that is secondary to lodging of rapidly growing blasts within the cerebral circulation. These form macroscopic tumors that rapidly erode the vessels in which they initially lodge and grow (a form of "leukostasis").

Therapy

The key to treatment of AML is the rapid production of marrow hypoplasia by killing leukemic cells so that normal stem cells may have an opportunity to repopulate the marrow. Unfortunately, selective killing of leukemic rather than normal cells does not occur with current therapy, in contrast to the situation in ALL, in which such agents as vincristine and prednisone are relatively selective in killing lymphoblasts.

Equally important are certain ancillary measures that should be instituted concurrently or before initiation of induction therapy. If leukocytosis in excess of $100 \times 10^3/mm^3$ is present, one must assume that this represents a rapidly rising count and that leukostasis with intracerebral tumor formation is underway or imminent (as discussed previously). This must be considered a medical emergency, and intensive antileukemic chemotherapy should be begun immediately. Emergency irradiation to the entire brain is recommended by some. Whether leukapheresis should also be initiated is less clear; the primary problem appears to be the potential growth rate of the blasts in the blood that lodge in vessels rather than the actual number of blasts in the blood. Patients who are severely thrombocytopenic ($<20 \times 10^3/mm^3$) should immediately receive platelet transfusions, irrespective of the number of blasts in the blood.

Allopurinol is used to reduce the hyperuricemia that is often already present and that may be exacerbated by killing a large number of leukemic cells. This drug inhibits xanthine oxidase, the enzyme that produces uric acid from the breakdown of the purines of RNA and DNA as cell lysis occurs. Hypoxanthine and xanthine (which are more soluble) are formed instead, thereby causing less risk of the obstructive uropathy that can follow excretion of large amounts of uric acid in the urine. Secondary gout, a less common problem, is also prevented.

A variety of chemotherapeutic agents useful in AML have evolved over several decades, but the pyrimidine analogue cytosine arabinoside (ara-C) and anthracyclines such as daunorubicin and doxorubicin are the keystones of treatment. Other active agents are the thiopurines, 6-mercaptopurine (6-MP) and 6-thioguanine (6-TG); 5-azacytidine; and the acridine dye derivative, amsacrine (m-AMSA). Single-agent therapy has not produced durable remissions or high response rates, but certain drugs have shown promise when used in combination therapy. Newer ways of using established agents have also improved results. Ara-C is considerably more active when given either continuously over 5 to 7 days or twice daily than when given as a single daily dose. This is presumably due to more leukemic cells entering into the DNA synthesis (S phase) of the cell cycle, during which they are most sensitive to ara-C. The best known and most widely used current regimen is a combination of ara-C, daunorubicin, and 6-TG. Complete-remission rates of 70 to 80 per cent have been reported in some series involving patients less than 60 years of age. However, the problem of how to maintain such a remission has not been solved. Current evidence suggests that very intensive maintenance therapy for at least the first year or so that the patient is in complete remission will significantly prolong this remission as compared with either no maintenance or less toxic maintenance regimens.

Killing leukemic cells is essential to successful therapy, but the administration of agents used for this purpose acutely worsens an already bad situation with respect to inadequate numbers of normally functioning red cells, neutrophils, and platelets. Red cell transfusions are needed by virtually every AML patient. Transfusions have been associated with the transmission of infectious hepatitis, cytomegalovirus, and toxoplasmosis. Platelet transfusions are also widely used to prevent hemorrhage. The risk of life-threatening bleeding rises acutely at platelet counts below 20,000/mm³, and this level is used as an indication for prophylactic treatment. With repeated transfusions of random donor platelets, immunization may occur with almost immediate destruction of the platelets by the host. Matching of donors within the HLA system (see Chapter 3) can be useful in dealing with refractoriness to random donor transfusions but must not be used if marrow transplantation is a possibility, since the recipient may become sensitized to minor (non-HLA) histocompatibility antigens.

Infection continues to be the leading cause of death in AML. The risk of severe infection begins to rise abruptly as the absolute neutrophil count falls below 500 cells/mm³. The type of infection is largely a function of the external environment and of the nature of the patient's endogenous flora. Infections acquired outside the hospital by patients who have not recently received antibiotics usually are from staphylococci, pneumococci, or normal gram-negative inhabitants of the gut such as *Escherichia coli* and *Klebsiella*. Patients who have recently received antibiotics and particularly those who are in the hospital are more likely to be invaded by organisms that are less common causes of overall infection in the general population, such as *Pseudomonas, Serratia, Aspergillus* and *Candida*. Immunosuppression further enhances susceptibility to infection in patients in complete remission who are on an intensive maintenance regimen or in the post–marrow-transplant period. In these circumstances, there is also a risk of infection with agents such as *Pneumocystis* and cytomegalovirus.

The complexity of the management of fever and infection in the patient who is severely neutropenic or immunosuppressed or both, and the controversies surrounding such management, are beyond the scope of this text. However, the following are general principles that are applicable to patients with AML as well as to those with other diseases. With the onset of fever in a severely neutropenic (<500 × 10³/mm³) patient, broad-spectrum antibiotics should be begun immediately. If the fever disappears or declines during the first 2 to 3 days and subsequently disappears, the antibiotic regimen should be continued until fever recurs or until blood neutrophils increase. If fever persists for 2 to 3 days and the patient appears toxic, consideration should be given to initiating systemic antifungal therapy and to giving transfusions of neutrophils. If fever persists, but the patient does *not* appear toxic, consideration should be given to stopping antibiotic therapy after 3 to 4 days and obtaining further blood cultures. Obviously, blood cultures, a urine culture, and cultures of any area of suspected inflammation should be obtained before initiation of antibiotic therapy, and the aforementioned plans should be altered if positive cultures are obtained. Neutrophil transfusion is of benefit under well-controlled, experimental conditions, but its "routine" usefulness is less clear. Large numbers of neutrophils are needed, and the cells from about 10 to 20 units of blood are required to provide any increment in neutrophils in an adult recipient.

Disseminated intravascular coagulation (DIC) can be a problem in any type of acute leukemia but most commonly is seen in APL (M3 type of myeloid leukemia). It is thought to be due to triggering of the coagulation process by the release of thromboplastic substances by leukemic cells, particularly from the large, abnormal granules of APL. It has been treated, and perhaps prevented, during remission induction through the careful administration of heparin, although such usage is somewhat controversial. Heparin is an activator of the antithrombin III system, which inhibits multiple steps of the coagulation pathway that have been inappropriately activated. Such activation causes the DIC syndrome of bleeding, hypotension, renal failure, and clots in various blood vessels.

With proper, vigorous therapy, failure to achieve remission occasionally is due to resistance of leukemic cells to chemotherapy. More commonly, death occurs during induction, usually from infection. Occasionally, the leukemic cells regrow at a more rapid rate than normal cells following the aplastic period, resulting in failure to induce remission.

Bone marrow transplantation has been attended by increasingly better results in AML since the early 1970s. Sufficient cytotoxic chemotherapy (and often irradiation as well) must be given to eradicate the leukemia, and much better results are obtained when patients are transplanted while in remission rather than in relapse. Most commonly, the transplant is allogeneic (i.e., from a different, non-twin person, usually an HLA-matched sibling). Vigorous supportive care is required, and patients older than 40 years do not do well for a variety of reasons. The commonest cause of death in marrow transplant recipients is graft-versus-host disease (GVHD), which is due to immunologically competent cells from the donor attacking somewhat dissimilar recipient tissues. Despite these problems, allogeneic marrow transplantation appears to be at least as effective in patients for whom suitable donors are available as modern chemotherapy in prolonging life and, at present, appears to be associated with a higher number of cures.

With syngeneic transplants (identical twins) there is no GVHD and no rejection. The principal problem has been recurrent leukemia, due either to insufficient killing of the original tumor cells or to the same factors giving rise to leukemia in the donor cell that caused the original disease. It has been known for many years that the incidence of leukemia in identical twins of affected patients is high and that the recurrent disease may be due to development of the disease in the transplanted cells. Leukemia in the transplanted cells has been proved in at least five allogeneic transplants.

"Immunotherapy" involving treated leukemia cells used as antigen or the nonspecific immunostimulant BCG has been attended by some suggestively positive results, particularly with regard to survival and frequency of induction of a second remission. However, immunotherapy is, as yet, of no proven benefit in this or in any other human cancer.

Factors Determining Success of Treatment

Older patients (over 60 to 65 years) do less well than younger patients, particularly with respect to surviving the initial attempts at remission induction. The primary problem in elderly patients is death from infection, often combined with hemorrhage due to severe thrombocytopenia. Other adverse clinical factors include hyperleukocytosis, sternal tenderness, 100 per cent karyotype abnormalities, a high serum lactic dehydrogenase (LDH), and leukemia that develops after treatment for another malignancy.

In-vitro tests of leukemia-cell sensitivity to various chemotherapeutic agents are still in the data-collection stage and have not yet become part of the standard armamentarium for treatment.

PRELEUKEMIA

The term *preleukemia* has been used broadly to describe diseases in which there is a higher than normal incidence of acute leukemia (e.g., PV, IMF, and Down's syndrome) but also to refer to a hematologic abnormality for which no specific diagnosis is possible and which in retrospect has evolved into leukemia, usually AML. One cannot be certain that a particular patient has preleukemia until after the leukemia has developed, but certain findings are suspicious enough that the diagnosis can be considered probable. This syndrome is sometimes referred to as *myelodysplasia*. Anemia is almost universal, with a varying frequency of thrombocytopenia and leukopenia. The presence of a hypercellular or normocellular marrow increases the likelihood that leukemia will develop. Chromosomal abnormalities are common, as are "ringed sideroblasts"; these are red cell precursors with abnormal quantities and location of iron, which is deposited in mitochondria, forming a partial or full "ring" around the nucleus. This is a consequence of abnormal heme synthesis, and the finding characterizes a somewhat diverse group of disorders, collectively referred to as *sideroblastic anemias,* some of which terminate in acute leukemia. Growth in vitro is often abnormal in preleukemia and is similar to that seen in AML. About 75 per cent of patients destined to develop leukemia with the preleukemia syndrome do so within 2 years. The typical patient is an older man. No specific number of blasts in the marrow can be used to distinguish AML from preleukemia, but a progressive increase in blasts or major complications due to cytopenia or both generally help one make a diagnosis.

Although the criteria for preleukemia are inexact, it seems clear that the disease represents an early, relatively stable phase of a stem cell disorder characterized by abnormal growth and differentiation and that it probably represents one end of a spectrum of the somewhat diverse group of diseases known as AML. All descendants of the myeloid stem cell line are involved, and chromosome abnormalities and growth disorders in vitro as well as in vivo support the relationship. Whether such patients, when they can be identified with relative certainty, should receive chemotherapy suitable for AML or simply supportive treatment aimed at alleviation of symptoms as long as possible is still unknown. The typically older age of patients makes aggressive therapy, with its associated risks, less desirable.

ALL very rarely has a preleukemic phase. When it does, this phase usually is quite different from the aforementioned one: The patient develops what appears to be typical, idiopathic aplastic anemia that then remits spontaneously, followed shortly by the development of ALL.

CHRONIC MYELOID LEUKEMIA (CML)

The hallmark of this disease is neutrophilic leukocytosis; typically, total white counts are approximately several hundred thousand per mm³, but they may range from 20,000 to over 1 million.

The entire series of neutrophil precursors is found in the blood, with the more mature ones being most numerous. The degree of myeloid immaturity, the severity of associated anemia, and the extent of splenic enlargement are directly related to the magnitude of the total white blood cell count. There are varying degrees of excessive numbers of eosinophils, basophils, monocytes, lymphocytes, and platelets in the blood. Thus, this is a disorder not only of the myeloid stem cell but also, probably, of the totipotent hematopoietic stem cell. The characteristic Ph¹ chromosome, found in 90 per cent of patients, is present in the precursors of red cells and granulocytes and in megakaryocytes. It was not initially found in lymphocytes, but later studies have indicated its presence in some lymphocyte populations. All myeloid components and at least some portion of the lymphoid populations are part of the leukemic clone in patients studied by G6PD isozyme analysis (Fig. 22–13). The lymphoblastic characteristics of some instances of the terminal acute phase support the totipotent concept as well.

Some patients with CML have a history of exposure to excessive irradiation, but most do not. The Ph¹ chromosome, loss of a portion of the long arms of chromosome 22, is a reciprocal translocation, usually with chromosome 9. Exactly what changes characteristic of the disease this produces is not known, but it does not correlate well with such abnormalities as low leukocyte alkaline phosphatase (LAP). Observations in Japanese survivors of the atomic bombings who subsequently developed CML have shown that the Ph¹ chromosome becomes established long before clinical onset of the disease and that it may coexist with normal marrow elements initially. The leukemic cells clearly have a growth advantage over normal cells. However, the Ph¹ chromosome is not necessarily in all of the leukemic cells of a given patient. Cells that are without the Ph¹ but that are part of the leukemic clone, as defined by G6PD analysis, may coexist with cells with Ph¹.

A general rule for chromosomal abnormalities can be formulated that is applicable to the acute leukemia as well as to CML (Fig. 22–14). If a cell in a patient with leukemia has a noninherited chromosomal abnormality, that cell can be assumed to belong to the leukemic clone. However, the converse is not true; the chromosomal abnormality is not necessarily present in all cells in the clone. This concept makes it very unlikely that the grossly visible chromosomal change is necessary for clonal growth. This presumption has been proved correct in murine AKR leukemia. Trisomy of chromosome 15 is a very common finding in the spontaneously arising AKR clone, but cells lacking the abnormality will transmit the disease. Trisomy 15 may be acquired or lost by clones in the mouse or in tissue culture, without changing the phenotypic characteristics of leukemia induced by transplantation of the cells into nonleukemic AKR.

○ Clone

◑ Chromosomally abnormal cells

◉ Morphologically identifiable cells

Figure 22–14 Schematic representation of the relationship of chromosomal abnormalities to the clone of tumor cells. It is based on the hypothesis that all cells in the clone need not share the chromosomal abnormality (see text).

However, these data, general rules, and hypotheses in no sense exclude the possibility (probability?) that an abnormal change in DNA content or DNA arrangement in the chromosome is the primary oncogenic event. Indeed, the hypothesis that gene substitution, loss, or rearrangement in such a manner that existing "oncogenes" are expressed in a cell resulting in its "cancerous" growth has strong experimental support.

Symptoms at diagnosis commonly are those of fatigue, weight loss, abdominal fullness or pain due to splenomegaly, and, rarely, easy bruising or bleeding. Splenomegaly is seen in 95 per cent of patients, hepatomegaly in 50 per cent, sternal tenderness in 75 per cent, and slightly enlarged nodes in a few. The bone tenderness probably reflects increased cellularity of the marrow, and the organomegaly suggests leukemic cell infiltration. Anemia is observed in 85 per cent of patients, thrombocytosis in about 60 per cent, and thrombocytopenia in 15 per cent. Fever and sweats may be seen in association with an increased metabolic rate. A high incidence of peptic ulcer has been attributed to elevated levels of histamine released by the increased numbers of basophils.

There is a tendency in most patients for the markedly increased leukocyte count to increase with time, with proportionately more myelocytes and younger cells entering the blood. The usual release mechanism that keeps immature cells in the marrow is somewhat disordered, perhaps because of the hyperplasia of marrow cells and consequent increased pressure. However, there continue to be more immature cells relative to mature ones in the marrow than in the blood, indicating that the mechanism is not entirely deranged. Occasionally, untreated patients will exhibit extreme rises and falls of the leukocyte count occurring in fairly regular cycles. However, such cycles are often of 2 to 3 months duration, as compared with approximately 21 days in the congenital or acquired forms of cyclic hematopoiesis (see earlier discussion).

Cytoplasmic maturation is somewhat faster than nuclear maturation, as shown by the greater than normal numbers of granules in promyelocytes and the acquisition by younger cells of some ability to perform phagocytosis. The enzyme LAP is decreased in mature neutrophils in approximately 95 per cent of patients, and abnormalities of other enzymes may occur. The Pelger-Huet anomaly of nuclear shape (mentioned earlier) may also be seen. The number of CFU_{NM} in the blood is markedly increased, although maturation is essentially normal in the colonies produced. Marrow CFU_{NM} are normal to moderately increased, with a higher than normal proportion in the S phase of the cell cycle. Mature neutrophils in CML have been reported to produce less colony-inhibitory activity, measurable in vitro, than normal neutrophils. Also, the CML target for this material is reported to be less sensitive to the inhibitory effects of this substance than normal target cells. Thus, a double defect in the normal regulation of neutrophil growth may be present.

Hyperuricemia is present for the same reason as in AML, and gout may occur. Urate nephropathy is less common than in AML, but allopurinol probably should be used routinely during periods of treatment. Serum B_{12} is elevated, reflecting the large amounts of B_{12}-binding proteins released by the enlarged pool of granulocytes and monocytes. Granulocyte kinetic studies have shown a blood half clearance time (t ½) that is three to ten times normal probably because of the delayed clearance of immature cells and some degree of recirculation to the spleen and bone marrow.

Therapy and Survival

Patients in the chronic phase of their disease are relatively easily controlled with oral alkylating agents (e.g. busulfan or the DNA synthesis inhibitor hydroxyurea) or even with splenic irradiation. These measures will reduce the elevated white count, improve the anemia, and shrink the spleen so that the patient looks and feels normal and becomes hematologically normal. The chromosomal abnormality remains, in contrast to what happens during complete remission in AML, and the therapy merely suppresses the disease, without any clear benefit with regard to survival. The median survival has been about 3 years, determined almost entirely by the time that the dreaded acute transformation, or "blast crisis," develops. Some patients present for the first time in this phase, but in general there is a chronic phase first. There is a 25 per cent chance each year that a patient will enter the acute phase, for which there is no particularly effective therapy. Since onset of blast crisis appears to be a random event, some patients remain in the chronic phase for 5 or even 10 years and, very rarely, even longer. The rapidity of the rise in the white count after the first course of therapy has been discontinued has been inversely correlated with survival, suggesting a more aggressive disease. Patients with the Ph^1-negative form of the disease have a worse prognosis and develop the acute stage earlier than Ph^1-positive patients (Fig. 22–15).

Since the early 1950s, administration of busulfan (Myleran) in a daily oral dose of 4 mg/day has been the most common therapy. This drug kills resting stem cells as well as rapidly dividing cells of the bone marrow; it is still more effective than other drugs in its class. Virtually any chemotherapeutic agent that will kill normal cells will also kill CML cells, unless the CML cell has developed resistance to that agent or class of agents. Unlike AML and ALL cells, chronic phase CML cells rarely develop drug resistance. With busulfan therapy, the white count usually starts to fall within 2 or 3 weeks, and its rate of fall is usually exponential. A recommended method is to stop treatment when the white count reaches 10,000/mm³; if the drug is continued beyond this point, there is a substantial risk of marrow aplasia, with subsequent infection or hemorrhage or both. Often the patient can then merely be observed until there is a rise in the white count to the point at which symptoms reappear, usually in the range of 50,000/mm³. Multiple courses can be given this way, often only once or twice a year. If the count begins to rise rapidly after the drug is stopped, small daily doses may be given continuously to maintain the leukocyte count at normal levels. Intermittent therapy is better when the disease can be controlled satisfactorily, since it is more convenient for physician and patient and because the risk of drug side effects such as marrow aplasia, pulmonary dysfunction due to fibrosis, and a syndrome resembling adrenal insufficiency is less. Splenic irradiation can produce remissions, probably by killing stem cells residing in or passing through the spleen at the time of radiation exposure. Remissions can also be achieved by extracorporeal irradiation of the blood or by administration of radioactive phosphorus, which localizes to some degree in the marrow. Splenic irradiation has been shown to be less effective than busulfan in terms of survival. Leukapheresis, the removal of large numbers of leukocytes by continuous-flow centrifugation, is temporarily effective in lowering the white count, but it does not affect the large proliferating cell mass and actually worsens the anemia. It is, therefore, not a satisfactory long-term solution and is rarely needed to control the high white cell count, since leukocytosis per se rarely presents any evident problem in CML.

Attempts to eradicate the malignant clone by aggressive chemotherapy in CML, although of great experimental interest, have not been successful enough to warrant use as standard therapy, nor has splenectomy.

Acute Phase ("Blast Crisis") of CML

The acute phase of CML typically fails to respond to busulfan or indeed to most other agents.

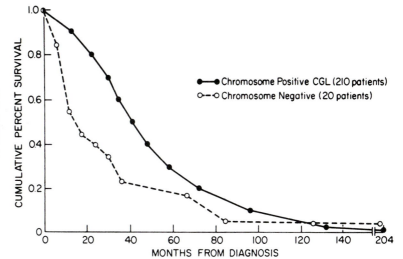

Figure 22–15 Actuarial survival among 230 patients with chronic granulocytic leukemia according to the presence of the Philadelphia chromosome. All cases were followed at NCI. (From Canellos, G. P., et al.: Am. J. Clin. Pathol. *65*:467, 1976.

The event occurs randomly and cannot be predicted with any accuracy, although chromosomal changes and alterations of the pattern of in-vitro growth of CFU_{NM} may precede it by some months. Numerous myeloblasts and promyelocytes develop in the marrow, and neutropenia, anemia, and thrombocytopenia become severe. Splenomegaly, increased lymph node size, fatigue, pain in various locations, and fever are prominent findings. Interestingly, the LAP often becomes normal or even increased; marrow fibrosis is not unusual. Most patients (80 per cent) develop new abnormalities in addition to the Ph[1] in their chromosome pattern. This may precede the clinical transformation by years but most commonly does so by 2 to 4 months when sought frequently. Certain specific types of chromosomal abnormalities in addition to the Ph[1] do not indicate impending blast crisis, but most do. The most common changes involve chromosomes 8 and 17, or duplication of the Ph[1] (chromosome 22). Multiple clones may be present.

Some acute transformations (approximately 20 to 30 per cent) are lymphoid instead of myeloid, as shown morphologically and more specifically, by the demonstration of lymphoid antigens on the cell surface and the presence in the blasts of the lymphoid enzyme terminal deoxynucleotidyl transferase (TdT). Patients with lymphoid blast crisis may respond to prednisone and vincristine, drugs that generally are helpful only in ALL. When the blast crisis is myeloid, attempts to use the standard treatments for AML are often fruitless, for although marrow hypoplasia can often be achieved, subsequent normalization of the marrow or return to the chronic phase occurs in a minority of patients. If a "remission" is induced in a patient with blast crisis, this usually is not a complete remission as defined for most other hematopoietic neoplasms; rather, the patient usually reenters a chronic phase picture of CML. Unfortunately, such remissions are short, rarely lasting more than 1 year. In some instances, the picture is of a mixed myeloid-lymphoid blast crisis or one that alternates between the two over time.

There have attempts to store *autologous bone marrow* during the chronic phase of CML for use as a transplant during blast crisis. This has been successful in reinstituting the chronic phase but generally only for brief periods of time. The success in the chronic phase of syngeneic marrow transplants in apparently curing the disease has led to the use of *allogeneic transplants*. They have not been successful in the acute phase but are beginning to show promise during the chronic phase. Since there is a 30 per cent or greater risk of mortality from the transplant procedure, it is clear that this must be balanced against the risks (about 25 per cent annually) of developing blast crisis. What is needed is a reliable way to predict with certainty those patients who are about to transform into the acute phase as candidates for transplantation. This presupposes the availability of an HLA-matched donor.

LEUKEMIC RETICULOENDOTHELIOSIS ("HAIRY CELL LEUKEMIA," HCL) AND HISTIOCYTIC MEDULLARY RETICULOSIS (HMR)

These two chronic "leukemias" are considered together because they are often quite similar in their clinical manifestations. HCL is quite possibly a disease of a pluripotent hematopoietic stem cell, whereas HMR is somewhat more differentiated, with the malignant cell resembling mature macrophages and monocytes in some respects.

HCL has been variably defined by immunologic studies to be a neoplasm of B-lymphocytes (most often), T-lymphocytes, or monocyte-macrophages. Perhaps most significantly, the neoplastic cells from the same patient when studied over time have appeared to change from one type to another or even to be hybrids, suggesting a pluripotent nature. Abnormalities in red cells and platelets reinforce this theory.

HCL patients are most often men in their mid fifties. Splenomegaly is almost universal, and modest lymphadenopathy is seen in one fourth to one third of patients. There are thrombocytopenia and anemia in 85 per cent, leukopenia in 50 per cent, and leukocytosis in 15 to 20 per cent. The typical cell, found in the bone marrow and spleen and, less often, in the blood (65 to 85 per cent) resembles a lymphocyte and is of variable size. There are characteristic projections of the cytoplasm, seen best in phase microscopy or with electron microscopy, although in Romanovsky stains some irregularity of the cell makes the diagnosis debatable. A diagnostic feature is the presence of a tartrate-resistant acid phosphatase in the leukemic cells. Bone marrow aspiration is often difficult but biopsy is helpful, nearly always showing increased reticulum fibers with variable fibrosis in addition to the typical cells. Fever is common and is usually due to infection associated with neutropenia, but in a significant proportion no infection is identified. Death is usually from infection or hemorrhage. Although not curative, significant improvement results from splenectomy in those patients for whom some evidence of splenic pooling or destruction of the normal blood cells exists. Other methods of treatment, including chemotherapy and corticosteroids, have been of variable benefit. The disease may be acute and fulminant but more often is chronic, with median survival in the range of 4 to 5 years.

HMR is clinically very similar to HCL. The major difference is the presence of significant erythrophagocytosis by histiocytes in HMR, easily seen with marrow examination and contributing substantially to the anemia. Phagocytosis of platelets and PMN by the malignant histiocyte may also take place. The malignant cells are normally not seen in the blood but are found in enlarged lymph nodes and bone marrow. Patients tend to be somewhat younger than those with HCL, and the disease is more fulminant, with median survival of between 6 months and 1 year. Splenectomy has been helpful in a few patients, as has chemotherapy. Certain children with ALL have developed a disease resembling HMR. Some of them were in remission when this developed. That this is the same disease as seen de novo seems unlikely, as spontaneous resolution of the HMR picture in the child with ALL has been reported.

POLYCYTHEMIA VERA

Polycythemia vera (PV) is a relatively benign neoplasm arising from a multipotent HSC, proba-

bly the THSC (Fig. 22–1). It is characterized by excessive production of red cells and is usually accompanied by overproduction of granulocytes, monocytes, and platelets as well. G6PD studies (Fig. 22–13) support the inclusion of all myeloid cells in the neoplastic clone, and a few reports of an ALL-like termination of PV suggest that the THSC rather than the PMSC may be the HSC site of origin. Nonrandom chromosomal defects are present in as many as 50 per cent of patients before any treatment is given but almost invariably are present in a minority of metaphases examined in an individual patient. Unlike the situation in CML or preleukemia, these defects have no evident prognostic significance (i.e., they have no predictive implication for the development of acute leukemia).

Relative autonomy of cellular growth has been observed in in-vitro culture studies of the bone marrow. Red cell and mixed (erythroid, granulocyte, macrophage) colonies normally require the addition of erythropoietin (EP) to the culture for erythroid maturation to develop. Erythroid colonies from marrow (and blood) of patients with PV will grow in the absence of added, exogenous EP, but a larger number is seen after EP addition. However, if an antibody to EP is added to PV cultures, growth ceases. The EP mechanism appears to be intact in vivo in that phlebotomy in PV patients resulting in anemia produces an appropriate increase in EP levels in serum and urine. These observations suggest that the abnormal HSC system leading to PV is not truly autonomous with respect to EP regulation but that the cells are exquisitely responsive to the hormone.

There is a marked increase in marrow cellularity involving all elements except lymphocytes. Labeled glycine turnover and plasma iron turnover rates indicate the greater erythropoiesis, and $DF^{32}P$ studies of granulocytes show an increased TBGP with a normal or longer half-life and an increased GTR. The blood volume is expanded, owing entirely to the increased red cell mass, and the blood viscosity is also markedly greater. Hyperuricemia is due to the increased cellular turnover, and secondary gout is common. The serum vitamin B_{12} and B_{12}-binding protein are increased owing to the greater number of neutrophils or monocytes or both. Blood histamine levels are elevated secondary to the basophilia, which is thought to play a role in the marked itching so often present, as well as an increased incidence of peptic ulcer.

The most common symptoms are headache, weakness, itching, and dizziness, seen in about half the patients. Sweating, visual disturbances, weight loss, dyspnea, joint pains, and epigastric pain are seen in one fourth to one third of patients. Gum bleeding, purpura, and abdominal fullness due to an enlarged spleen are seen in some affected individuals. Intense redness of the skin, particularly of the head, is characteristic. Hepatomegaly is seen in half the patients, and splenomegaly occurs in 75 to 90 per cent. The increased blood volume is thought to be a major factor contributing to organomegaly, but extramedullary hematopoiesis may also contribute. The oxygen saturation usually is normal and helps one rule out secondary polycythemia, which is generally confined to red cell overproduction ("erythrocytosis"). However, PV itself may lead to a modest decrease in pulmonary function (viscosity ?, thrombi?) so that a decrease in arterial O_2 may be the result of PV as well as the primary cause of secondary polycythemia.

Other noteworthy laboratory studies include a normal or increased LAP and absence of the Ph[1] chromosome, findings that differ from those observed in CML. The leukocyte count usually is lower than in CML, and the hemoglobin level is considerably higher, but some overlapping (and confusion) may occur (Table 22–5).

The course of PV is chronic, with median survival ranging from 10 to 15 years in treated patients but only 2 to 3 years in untreated patients. Therapy is tailored to the patient's symptoms as well as to the severity of laboratory findings. The major complications include thrombosis secondary to the increased blood viscosity and decreased flow and, probably, thrombocytosis as well as hemorrhagic episodes, associated with functional abnormalities of platelets and perhaps with chronic DIC. Late complications include progressive myelofibrosis and myeloid metaplasia, notably in the spleen (about 25 per cent), and acute leukemia, which may be seen in untreated individuals or in patients whose treatment consists only of phlebotomy but which is more frequent in patients treated with alkylating agents, most notably clorambucil, or with the marrow-seeking isotope ^{32}P.

Therapy

There is little doubt that treatment both improves symptoms and enhances survival, but the disease is not curable at the present time. Marrow transplantation presumably would cure PV. However, the hazard of this procedure, the chronicity of PV, and the age of the population with PV presently excludes marrow transplantation unless the patient has an unaffected identical twin. Lowering of the increased red cell mass has been a mainstay of treatment for many years. This may be done acutely and sometimes exclusively by removal of several units of blood, which results in remissions of several months. This does not affect the increased rate of blood cell production and often is inadequate treatment in that thrombocytosis may be accentuated. Iron deficiency (see Chapter 23), with absent marrow iron stores and microcytic, hypochromic red cells, may be present at diagnosis, particularly in women with PV, and

develops in almost all patients who are treated with multiple phlebotomies. Even patients who had normal iron stores before PV developed may exhaust these stores simply by expanding the red cell mass. Whether iron deficiency should be treated in a patient with PV or should be allowed to persist and thus impede expansion of red cell volume is a point of contention. There are data that suggest that iron deficiency without significant anemia produces symptoms of fatigue and decreased exercise tolerance; iron content of certain enzymes in various tissues may diminish with declining total iron in the body prior to any decrease in the amount of iron utilized for hemoglobin production.

Systemic irradiation with radioactive inorganic phosphorus (^{32}P) is a very effective form of therapy. Given intravenously, the chemical localizes to a large extent in bone, with a physical half-life of 14 days. Doses of 3 to 5 millicuries gradually decrease the elevated volume of packed red cells within 1 to 2 months. Phlebotomy is often used initially and followed by ^{32}P. Examination every 3 months and retreatment as needed have been recommended. Chemotherapeutic agents, such as melphalan, busulfan, cyclophosphamide, and chlorambucil, have all been used. In a randomized trial in which phlebotomy alone was compared with phlebotomy in combination with ^{32}P or phlebotomy plus chlorambucil, after a median of 6½ years, the incidence of acute leukemia was 1, 6, and 11 per cent, respectively. Clearly, chlorambucil cannot be recommended over ^{32}P, and it remains to be seen whether any of the other alkylating agents is safer. In this study, the frequency of thrombosis appeared to be slightly higher and the duration of survival seemed somewhat shorter in those treated with phlebotomy plus ^{32}P as compared with those treated with phlebotomy alone.

Surgery for any condition in PV has been associated with very high mortality rates in the patients who have uncontrollably elevated blood volumes and should be avoided unless absolutely necessary.

Allopurinol has been quite effective in controlling hyperuricemia that is seen either in the untreated state or as a result of cytotoxic treatment. Itching has been controllable in some patients with antihistamines such as cyproheptadine, but better control is achieved by treatment of the increased cellular proliferation.

IDIOPATHIC MYELOFIBROSIS (IMF) WITH MYELOID METAPLASIA

This disorder, also known as *agnogenic myeloid metaplasia* and various other descriptive names, is also a neoplasm involving pluripotent HSC, as judged by G6PD analysis (Fig. 22–13). Whether it arises from the totipotent or pluripotent myeloid stem cell is unclear, but occasional lymphoblastic termination suggests it may be of totipotent origin. Chromosomal changes in IMF are very similar to those previously described for PV (i.e., they are nonrandom, occur in one half or less of patients, are present in a minority of cells in a given patient and have no prognostic significance).

Increased fibrosis in marrow is a hallmark of the disease. However, the marrow fibroblast is *not* part of the neoplastic clone. The fibroblast is not derived from the HSC system and is not part of the neoplastic, HSC-derived clone, as judged by either G6PD or chromosomal analysis. It has been suggested that marrow fibroblast and osteoblast proliferation is triggered by an unknown stimulus resulting from multiplication of the marrow stem cells, perhaps associated with the highly ineffective hematopoiesis of red cells, leukocytes, and platelets that is observed in the disease. The release by such cells (particularly from platelets or megakaryocytes or both) of a stimulus that induces fibrosis is supported by in-vitro studies.

Colony studies have shown an increased number of both erythroid colony-forming cells and CFU_{NM} in the blood, although this can be seen in PV as well, particularly when it is complicated by secondary fibrosis. Other studies have shown an increased number of colony-forming cells for all three cell lines in blood and marrow.

IMF is seen in older patients and has no predilection for either sex. Patients complain of symptoms related to anemia and massive splenomegaly. Hyperuricemia and gout may be seen, and bleeding due to thrombocytopenia or platelet function defects or thrombosis, usually associated with thrombocytosis, may occur. Hepatomegaly is seen in about half the patients, whereas splenomegaly is nearly universal. Sternal tenderness is uncommon. The characteristic changes in the blood are marked poikilocytosis (abnormal shape including "teardrops") of the red cells and immaturity of all cell lines (i.e., nucleated red cells, increased reticulocytes and immature neutrophils, basophilia and eosinophilia, and abnormally large platelets, with megakaryocyte fragments). The differential count reveals all degrees of myeloid immaturity including myeloblasts. This is one of the very few conditions in which myeloblasts in the blood do not necessarily indicate AML, although AML can evolve from IMF. All these findings are ascribed to insufficient and ineffective hematopoiesis by the marrow, which becomes more fibrotic with time, and a large degree of extramedullary blood formation, without the usual marrow release mechanisms. Anemia is nearly universal and becomes more severe with time. Red cell production as measured by iron incorporation studies is reduced, with more of the iron taken up by liver and spleen than by marrow. Some shortening of red cell survival is also seen, with splenic sequestration and destruction demonstrable in some. Sometimes the plasma volume is increased as well, thereby reducing the apparent volume of packed red cells, even though this does not influence the actual red cell mass. Thus, anemia represents "ineffective erythropoiesis" (see Chapter 23) as perhaps the primary factor, with decreased red cell survival, increased splenic pooling, and increased plasma volume. The white cell count may be of almost any value: low in 25 per cent of patients, normal in another 25 per cent, and increased in the remaining 50 per cent. The LAP tends to be high in most patients but may be normal or low. The platelet count is often increased initially but may decrease to hazardous levels over time. The spleen also has a tendency to increase in size with time.

The bone marrow may be hypercellular at first, but with time often becomes increasingly fibrotic or may be fibrotic at presentation. Aspirations are often difficult and nondiagnostic, and biopsies are frequently required to clarify the issue. Many patients have osteosclerosis due to increased bone formation that is significant enough to be visible on bone radiographs. Survival is quite variable (median of 4 to 5 years) and tends to be shorter with greater degrees of marrow fibrosis, organomegaly, thrombocytopenia, and anemia.

There is no specific therapy of proven benefit; treatment is directed at symptoms and certain complications. Anemia may be treated with transfusions; splenectomy, although associated with a high risk, is valuable if there is significant pain or general discomfort from the enlarged organ (rare) or if the degree of sequestration of red cells or platelets or both in the spleen is thought to outweigh its production component. These can be measured by various isotopic studies. The liver may increase greatly in size after splenectomy, reflecting increased hematopoiesis in that organ as "compensation" for the missing spleen. Cytotoxic agents such as busulfan and ^{32}P may help reduce the spleen size and lower elevated platelet counts or neutrophil counts, but they seldom correct the anemia, and are therefore seldom indicated. Androgen therapy may help relieve the anemia in a small number of patients. Allopurinol is indicated for hyperuricemia.

Termination of PV in IMF is a common problem, and AML may develop in IMF in as many as 5 per cent of patients. Fibrosis of the marrow is seen in many other diseases (including CML, AML, ALL, the lymphomas, various cancers, tuberculosis, and osteomyelitis) and following benzene exposure. Sometimes a blood picture of myeloid and erythroid immaturity is seen as well, but the mechanisms are obscure. The combination of a large spleen, fibrosis of the marrow, typical blood smear, evidence for extramedullary hematopoiesis, and the absence of one of the associated causes (tumor, infection) confirm the diagnosis of IMF.

APLASTIC ANEMIA

Aplastic anemia can be regarded as hematopoietic stem cell failure resulting in varying degrees of pancytopenia, a hypocellular marrow, and a major risk of death from infection or bleeding. No abnormal cells are apparent, and there is no organomegaly, lymph node enlargement, or sternal tenderness. It tends to be chronic and in many patients is of unknown cause. In others, it results from chemical or drug exposure. The myelosuppression from cancer chemotherapeutic drugs produces aplastic anemia, but this is transient and quickly reversible in almost all instances, and this situation is not usually described as aplastic anemia.

The basic defect is a failure of production of blood cells. That most, if not all, of the problem resides in the stem cell itself is strongly suggested (1) by the fact that colony formation of red cells, granulocytes, and macrophages in vitro is decreased, and (2) by the ability of bone marrow transplantation between identical twins to be curative in most instances. Attempts to implicate components of the marrow stroma as a cause of aplastic anemia are less convincing.

There are conflicting data about the importance of immunologic suppression of hematopoiesis as a cause of aplastic anemia. Lymphocytes from patients with aplastic anemia have been reported to inhibit erythroid colony formation by normal marrow when cocultured. Some patients have benefited when treated with immunosuppressive agents such as cyclophosphamide or with antithymocyte globulin. Blood lymphocytes from a large group of patients with aplastic anemia have exhibited reactivity against their own lymphocytes in vitro about 30 per cent of the time, which is ten times higher than for normal controls. These data can be interpreted to indicate an immunologic mechanism for the autoreactivity, with the disappearance of a suppressor cell as the primary event, which leads to reactivity against the stem cell as well. An alternate explanation would explain the autoreactivity as a *result* of aplastic anemia, with the loss of a monocyte-like suppressor as part of the disease. Other experiments have shown the failure of in-vitro red cell colony development in 20 per cent of peripheral blood cells in aplastic anemia until T-lymphocytes (possibly suppressor cells) were removed. Thus, it is possible that deranged immunologic mechanisms play a role in some, but probably not all, cases of aplastic anemia.

About half the patients with aplastic anemia have experienced exposure to some type of chemical agent. Drugs such as chloramphenicol, phenylbutazone, gold compounds, quinacrine, methylphenylhydantoin, trimethadione, and the industrial solvent benzene have all been associated with a significant number of cases of aplastic anemia; many other drugs have been implicated several times. The effect of any specific drug in a particular patient is unpredictable, and the evidence for its role in aplastic anemia is circumstantial at best. No test for predicting individual sensitivity is available. The risk with chloramphenicol, the agent most frequently implicated as a cause of aplastic anemia, is in the range of one in 8000 to 20,000 persons exposed to the drug. There is no dose relation; most patients are women. Reversible depression of erythropoiesis occurs in half the patients given large doses of the drug, and, less commonly, there is inhibition of granulopoiesis and thrombopoiesis. However, these dose-related toxic effects bear no apparent relationship to the development of aplastic anemia after drug exposure, and much smaller doses often produce aplastic anemia that results in death. The only available defense against this type of drug reaction is the careful judgment of the physician who initially prescribes the drug. All too often, this agent and other potentially lethal drugs are used for trivial and inappropriate reasons.

In addition to the administration of various drugs, certain viral infections, such as hepatitis, may precede development of aplastic anemia. About half of all patients with the disease have no history of infection or significant drug ingestion.

Clinical features are those that might be expected from anemia, thrombocytopenia, or neutropenia. Most white cells that are present are lymphocytes. The marrow is hypocellular or acellular on biopsy and aspiration, usually with a preponderance of lymphocytes.

The prognosis and course are related to the severity at initial examination. With conservative measures, about half the patients will die within 1½ years, but the 5-year survival is about 30 per cent. The disease is judged to be severe if two of the three following criteria are present: (1) the reticulocyte count is less than 1 per cent, (2) the platelet count is less than 20,000/mm³, or (3) the neutrophil count is less than 500/mm³.

Symptomatic treatment includes red cell transfusions and prompt treatment of infection with antibiotics. Platelet transfusions should be reserved as treatment for severe bleeding, since their prophylactic use will lead to rapid development of platelet isoantibodies in the recipient. Sensitization is usually avoided if HLA-matched platelets are given, but this in turn can sensitize the patient to other histocompatibility antigens, and HLA-matched cells should never be given to any potential candidate for marrow transplantation.

Marrow transplantation can be curative, and if an identical twin is available as a donor, virtually all cases should be so treated. Allogeneic transplants are restricted to patients with severe disease (i.e., those presenting with two of the three aforementioned criteria), since there is a significant risk associated with the transplant. An HLA-identical donor ordinarily is used. The recipient's immune system is suppressed (virtually destroyed) with large doses of cyclophosphamide before the graft is attempted. Marrow is harvested from the donor by multiple punctures obtaining at least 5 × 10⁸ nucleated cells/kg of recipient. Evidence of engraftment occurs within 2 to 3 weeks, and vigorous support is needed up to that time. Sterile environments help prevent infection. Rejection of the graft is more common in aplastic anemia than in acute leukemia, presumably because immune destruction is more complete with the more vigorous preparatory regimen designed to eradicate the leukemia. Rejection is more frequent in the patient who has been transfused with any blood product more than a few days before transplantation preparation is begun than in nontransfused patients. GVHD has been prevented in the past with methotrexate; a newer agent, cyclosporin, holds much promise and is being evaluated. Seventy to 80 per cent of patients appear to have good long-term, disease-free survival if they receive transplants before any transfusions have been given, with the figure falling to about 50 per cent if they have been previously transfused. As in AML, transplantation has generally not been productive in patients over 40 years of age.

Other methods of treatment include adrenocorticosteroids (rarely effective) and androgens, which may be of some benefit in patients who do not have severe disease at the outset. Antithymocyte globulin has also been beneficial in a small but encouraging number of patients.

LYMPHOCYTES

PHYSIOLOGY

Lymphocytes constitute the second largest population of blood leukocytes. They are also found in large numbers throughout the body in lymphoid tissue, notably lymph nodes, spleen, bone marrow, thymus (a special organ for lymphopoiesis, more active in fetal than in adult life), and in focal areas in the gastrointestinal epithelium known as *Peyer's patches*. Their rather inconspicuous appearance in Wright-stained blood smears, described earlier, belies their active role as the central cell population in the immune system. Most lymphocytes are small, with very little cytoplasm, and are in an intermitotic phase of long duration. A small number of these cells are larger and actively engaged in nucleic acid and protein synthesis. Various stimuli (mitogens) can trigger this process, called *transformation,* both in vivo and in vitro.

Generally, diseases of the lymphoid system may be considered to result from *inadequate* immune responses (immunodeficiency diseases), *inappropriate* immune responses (autoimmune diseases), or neoplasms (lymphatic leukemias, lymphomas, plasma cell dyscrasias).

Although lymphocytes cannot be distinguished in simple blood smears, there are three main categories of these cells in the blood: B cells, T cells, and null cells. They have their own functions that can interrelate closely with each other and to other leukocytes, especially macrophages. Lymphocytes share a common stem cell with the myeloid system but then branch into separate cellular compartments, with B cells and T cells probably being supplied from separate and distinct stem cell compartments (Fig. 22–1). In all probability, "mature" lymphocytes can self-replicate, serving as their own stem cell.

B-Lymphocytes, Plasma Cells, and Immunoglobulins (Ig)

B-lymphocytes account for about 5 to 20 per cent of the blood lymphocytes. They are *bone* marrow–derived, although in birds they arise in an organ called the *bursa* of Fabricius. They are identified by the presence of immunoglobulin (Ig) on their surface, detectable with fluorescent antibody. With appropriate antigenic stimulation and with help from T cells, processing of antigen by macrophages, or direct contact with certain types of antigen for which the surface immunoglobulin (sIg) may be a receptor, they transform into plasma cells, which are committed antibody (Ig) factories. B-lymphocytes, plasma cells, and their products make up the humoral component of the immune response that is most effective against the pyogenic, encapsulated bacteria whose phagocytosis is more efficiently carried out in the presence of antibody. These include streptococci, pneumococci, meningococci, staphylococci, and *Haemophilus influenzae*. Antiviral antibodies are also of great importance, and vaccinations against various infectious diseases depend largely on an intact humoral response. Antibodies also play a possible role in tumor immunity in conjunction with cellular components of the immune response and acute rejection of transplanted organs, and in some circumstances they can block rejection or antitumor effects ("blocking antibodies").

The stages of development of B cells are still incompletely known, but one well-defined cell is the "pre-B cell". These are found in large numbers during fetal life in the liver and bone marrow. B cells develop somewhat later. Pre-B cells are much less common in adulthood. They can be identified with some certainty by the presence of *cytoplasmic* immunoglobulin (cIg), most of which is IgM, but they do not yet have the surface Ig characteristic of B cells. The immunoglobulin in the cytoplasm may be incomplete, composed only of the heavy chain portion, which is identifiable with the techniques used. Even at this early stage, the cell is thought to be committed to react to a single antigen. Pre-B cells are large, but with maturation they become smaller, lose cIg, and acquire sIg.

This can occur in the marrow or in other lymphoid tissues. The sIg is still IgM, but other immunoglobulins can develop on the surface to replace it in some cells: IgG, IgD, IgE, IgA. Other membrane receptors develop on the surface, including complement receptors, receptors for T cell–activating factors, and antigens that give it histocompatibility specificity. Each B cell is still able to react with only one antigen; that is, it is monoclonal in orgin.

B-lymphocytes react in vitro to pokeweed mitogen (PWM), which both stimulates their proliferation and causes them to synthesize immunoglobulins. They react to a lesser extent with T-cell stimuli such as concanavalin A (Con-A) and phytohemagglutinin (PHA).

B-lymphocytes, like T cells, may be either short-lived or long-lived, with considerable recirculation in and out of the blood. Lymphocyte populations reenter the blood via the lymphatic vessels, which drain lymph nodes. The largest of these is the thoracic duct. In the lymphoid tissue, there is a tendency for separation of B and T cells. B cells are found primarily in the follicular and medullary region of nodes, the primary follicles and red pulp of the spleen, and the follicular areas of lymphoid tissue in the gastrointestinal tract.

B-cell response to most antigens is mediated by soluble signals from T cells. One group, the so-called "helper T cells," transmit a signal to the B cells after interacting with antigen or antigen that has been processed first by macrophages. This signal is required for many antigens to trigger B-cell proliferation and ultimate Ig synthesis. An-

other group of T cells, suppressor cells, act as a brake on the antibody synthetic process by B cells, which may have either been triggered by T cells or acted independently, depending on the antigen. This mechanism prevents too much Ig from being produced and, it is thought, prevents inappropriate response to the individual's own antigens. With such a complex interacting system, the opportunities for derangement are many.

The receptors on B cells that recognize antigen are surface immunoglobulins that are specific for that antigen, fitting it as a lock fits a key. Once stimulated, either directly by some antigens or indirectly by T cell–mediated stimuli, the B cells enlarge, proliferate, and form plasma cells, as well as a series of small B-lymphocytes that act as stem cells for future challenges by the same antigen. These account for the relative speed with which a repeat antigenic challenge can produce a secondary humoral response: The memory is already coded in a B cell population that is ready to move into action (Fig. 22–16).

Serum antibodies, or immunoglobulins (Ig), may be evaluated in several ways. The most common methods are serum electrophoresis (SEP), immunoelectrophoresis, and quantitative immunoglobulin analysis. The first technique involves subjecting the serum proteins to an electric charge and measuring the area under the resulting curves. Normally, albumin travels most rapidly, followed by four globulin peaks labeled *alpha*$_1$, *alpha*$_2$, *beta*, and *gamma*, respectively. Most immunoglobulins are in the gamma region, but some

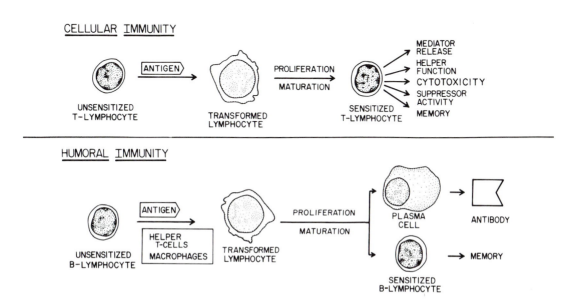

Figure 22–16 Responses of mature lymphocytes to antigens. In both the T- and B-cell systems, stimulated cells undergo a dedifferentiation process that produces immature-appearing lymphoblasts. (Courtesy of A. Winkelstein.)

migrate more rapidly in the beta or alpha$_2$ regions. SEP can identify a decrease in Ig as hypogammaglobulinemia; an increase may be diffuse owing to an increase in the number of proteins ("polyclonal gammopathy") or it may result from production of a single protein in a very large amount, giving rise to a large peak ("monoclonal gammopathy"). SEP is quantitatively more accurate than immunoelectrophoresis. Immunoelectrophoresis allows recognition of the approximate amounts of the different types of immunoglobulin, which SEP does not; that is, it allows one to determine whether the specific amounts of IgG, IgA, or other immunoglobulins are increased or decreased. Changes in the concentration of a monoclonal protein over a period of time are most accurately and easily assessed with serum electrophoresis.

Immunoglobulins are composed of four polypeptide chains, two identical small or light (L) chains and two heavy (H) chains, and all are held together by disulfide bonds. The heavy chains are specific for each of the five known classes of immunoglobulin and are variable in structure: gamma (IgG), alpha (IgA), mu (IgM), delta (IgD), and epsilon (IgE). This order corresponds to the normal serum concentration. All light chains of the Ig are of either the kappa or lambda type.

The antigenic specificity of each immunoglobulin is determined by the N terminal of both the light and heavy chains; these areas make up the variable region of the Ig, whereas the other ends of the chains are a constant region. When the immunoglobulins are digested with the proteolytic enzyme papain, two identical fractions composed of the light chains and the attached piece of the heavy chains result, called the F_{ab} *(antigen-binding) fragments;* the piece that is left is the F_c *(crystallizable) fragment,* which determines binding to such substances as complement. The F_c fragment therefore contains the carboxy terminal of the heavy chains, the attached carbohydrate that is present in all Ig, and the class determinant.

All the Ig monomers, IgG, IgD, and IgE, are Y-shaped. IgA may be a dimer when secreted at various mucosal surfaces; IgM consists of five monomers held together by other polypeptides.

The serum half-lives are variable, with IgG having the longest, and IgD and IgE the shortest, corresponding to and in part determining their relative serum concentrations. IgM, which has a very high molecular weight, is almost entirely intravascular, whereas the other immunoglobulins exist both in and out of the vascular space. All the immunoglobulins are too large to be filtered by the normal kidney, but light chains are not, and the latter are made in excess in some plasma cell dyscrasias, "Bence Jones protein." The excess light chains occur as a result of production by plasma cells of light and heavy chains on different polyribosomes; and in the dyscrasias (e.g., multiple myeloma) light chains may be made in excess and secreted or, indeed, may be the only product of the malignant clone. In normal plasma cells, there is balanced production of light and heavy chains, which are combined before they are secreted by the cell.

There are four subclasses of IgG, designated numerically according to their highest concentration, and their distinction results from differences in amino acid sequences of the F_c fragments. The subclasses perform different tasks, such as binding to complement, F_c receptors of macrophages, PMNs, and rheumatoid factor (an antibody to IgG). Antibodies to various antigens are represented within the different subclasses. IgG is the only immunoglobulin that passes the placenta and provides antibody protection to the newborn child until his own system matures sufficiently. IgG is the major component of the secondary response to antigen.

IgA has its major role in various secretions, such as tears and saliva, and in bronchial, pharyngeal, gastrointestinal, seminal vesicle, and cervical secretions. It is secreted as a dimer, with some linking pieces and a secretory piece made by the epithelial cells in the vicinity of the plasma cells in which the IgA is made. Another IgA system releases monomeric protein into the blood, spinal fluid, synovial fluid, and mesothelial fluids. This is a system for internal secretions in contrast to the one for external secretions. Both have antimicrobial activity, and the external secretion system may block various antigens and microorganisms that otherwise would be absorbed.

IgM, or macroglobulin, is unique in its large size and intravascular state. It is usually the first immunoglobulin synthesized in the initial humoral response to particulate antigen (primary response), but it typically is succeeded by higher concentrations of IgG that last longer. There may be a regulatory interaction between these two types of immunoglobulins. Macroglobulins form the major component of molecules such as heterophils, seen in infectious mononucleosis; Wassermann antibodies, which act against syphilis; and cold agglutinins. Monomers of IgM are predominant on the B-cell surface during its development and may occur as an antinuclear factor in lupus erythematosus and various immunodeficiency disorders and neoplasms, such as Waldenström macroglobulinemia.

The function of IgD, present in small quantities, is obscure. It is a prominent immunoglobulin on the surface of some B cells.

IgE, or reagin antibody, is a critical participant in allergic reactions. Its F_c fragment binds to basophils and mast cells, and when two such molecules are bound by an antigen ("bridged"), the cell degranulates, releasing histamine and other substances, which cause bronchospasm, the wheal-flare reaction of the skin, vasodilation, and hypotension.

Plasma cells are antibody-synthesizing descendants of B cells and have a characteristic appearance. Their cytoplasm is abundant and deep blue, owing to the large content of ribosomal RNA. There is a well-defined perinuclear clear zone, and the nucleus is usually eccentric. The nuclear chromatin is often arranged in a configuration resembling the spokes of a wheel if examined in histologic sections. Intermediate forms between lymphocytes and plasma cells with respect to morphologic appearance may be seen, especially in the lymphoid neoplasms. Normal, mature plasma cells are formed by the proliferation and mitosis of B-lymphocytes and are incapable of further mitosis. They must be replaced by further B-lymphocyte differentiation, a process thought to require the continued presence of antigen.

Antibody is synthesized in locations in which antigen would be expected to come into contact with lymphoid tissue: in the spleen and marrow after intravenous injection of antigen, in regional nodes draining a subcutaneous or intradermal area, and in subepithelial lymphoid tissue when an antigen enters the respiratory or gastrointestinal tract.

T Cells

T-lymphocytes, programmed by the *t*hymus gland, account for some 60 to 80 per cent of blood lymphocytes. They probably have a stem cell in common with B-lymphocytes, but their pathways diverge early in development (Fig. 22–1). Cooperation between these two major classes is a major part of the immune response, the cellular component of which is effected by T cells. T cells are identified by their ability to form rosettes with sheep red blood cells in vitro and indeed can be distinguished from other blood mononuclear cells in this way or by monoclonal antibodies specific for various stages and classes of T cells. Like B-lymphocytes, T cells may be long-lived or short-lived and recirculate freely. T cells tend to inhabit those areas of lymphoid tissue that B cells do not: the interfollicular areas of gastrointestinal- and respiratory-tract lymphoid tissue, the periarteriolar region of the spleen, and the paracortical areas of lymph nodes.

The functions of T cells are quite diverse (Fig. 22–16). They are active in defending against intracellular pathogens, such as *Mycobacterium tuberculosis, Salmonella,* and numerous fungi, viruses, and protozoa. *Candida albicans, Pneumocystis carinii,* and cytomegalic inclusion virus are only a few of the pathogens found in patients with defects in T-cell function. T cells are responsible for the rejection of tissue transplants involving organs such as kidneys, hearts, livers, and bone marrow. A major problem following allogeneic marrow transplantation, graft-versus-host disease (GVHD), is mediated by donor T-lymphocytes that recognize recipient tissue as foreign. T cells have an uncertain role in the body's defense against

cancer. Whether cytotoxic defense mechanisms, mediated by T cells, are in some way defective in the genesis of malignant tumors is not clear.

Transformation of T cells in vitro is induced by mitogens such as phytohemagglutinin (PHA) and concanavalin A (Con-A). T-cell receptors probably are similar to B-cell receptors, being composed of some type of Ig. The mitogens are thought to react with particular subpopulations of T cells (e.g., Con-A) acting primarily on suppressor cells. T-lymphocytes can be stimulated in vitro by similar cells from other individuals, with the degree of the response being proportional to the degree of tissue incompatability, particularly for HLA-D antigen. This mixed leukocyte culture (MLC) reaction is used to test the utility of prospective donors for bone marrow transplantation. The less strong the reaction between two otherwise HLA-matched siblings, the more effective and less prone to GVHD a transplant is likely to be.

As mentioned earlier, T cells help modulate the response of B cells in the response to antigenic stimuli (Fig. 22–16) and the production of antibodies. Helper T cells encourage this process, and suppressor T cells inhibit it.

Lymphokines, chemical mediators that influence other cells, are elaborated by T cells. Among these are substances influencing macrophages, such as a chemotactic factor, a migration inhibition factor, and an activating factor, all of which increase the ability of the macrophage to kill intracellular organisms. Monocytes produce a substance called *interleukin I,* which transforms T cells. *Interleukin II* is produced by T cells and supports the growth of other T cells. It is also known as *T-cell growth factor.*

Technology involving monoclonal antibody production has served to identify certain classes, or subsets, of T cells and to trace the development of T cells in the thymus and elsewhere. These antibodies are produced by "hybridomas," fused cells of mouse myeloma cells and mouse spleen cells sensitized to the specific antigen to be tested. They are grown in culture and produce large amounts of antibody to that specific antigen. Such "monoclonals" will detect specific antigens that are found on the surface of T cells of various capacities and maturation. For example, T3 antibodies react with T cells as a whole; T4 antibodies react with helper T cells; and T8 antibodies react with suppressor cells. The normal ratio of T4 (helper) to T8 (suppressor) reactive blood lymphocytes is 2:1, and various immunopathologic conditions are associated with an alteration in this ratio.

T-cell precursors may be found in the yolk sac and liver in the embryo and in the bone marrow in adults. They migrate to the thymus, where they develop under the influence of the thymic hormone thymopoietin, made by the thymic epithelial cells. The earliest thymic cells contain the T9 and T10 antigens, and about 10 per cent of thymocytes bear one or both of these antigens (Fig. 22–17). T9 is lost during the maturation process, but T6, T4, and T8 are gained. Cells with these four markers account for about 70 to 80 per cent of thymic lymphocytes. These cells are located in the cortical region of the thymus. At this stage, they are not immunologically reactive. During the final stage of the maturation process within the thymus, the T6 antigen is lost; T3, characteristic of mature T cells is gained, and either T4 or T8 is lost. These mature thymocytes, then, contain T10, T3, and either T4 or T8. They are located at this stage in the medullary region of the thymus. When they enter the blood, the T10 antigen is lost. Most T-cells precursors appear to die within the thymus or shortly after leaving it.

Various T-cell malignancies bear antigens that help identify them as derivatives of a specific cellular stage of the T-cell maturation pathway.

In addition to assisting in the modulation of B-cell function by stimulating production of antibodies through helper and suppressor cells, T cells are active in various autoimmune states and in the cellular reactions that constitute contact sensitivity (e.g., in the skin rash of poison ivy).

One often assesses T-cell function by testing for various delayed hypersensitivity skin reactions, which measure the capacity of the immune system to respond to antigens to which the individual has been exposed previously. When such an antigen is injected into the skin, a reaction develops, characterized by redness and induration, with a peak at 48 hours. The cellular infiltrate is composed largely of macrophages and T-lymphocytes. Purified protein derivative of tuberculin, used in the diagnosis of tuberculosis, is the best

known of these antigens. Other commonly used antigens that are likely to reside within an individual's immunologic "memory" include mumps, *Candida,* and streptokinase-streptodornase. An antigen that is not likely to have been encountered naturally, but that may be used to test the system by a sequential series of patch tests, is dinitrochlorobenzene (DNCB). Failure to respond to antigens that would be expected to evoke a response is called *anergy.*

Certain enzymes have been identified in T-cell populations. Thymocytes, but not blood lymphocytes, contain the enzyme terminal deoxynucleotidyl transferase (TdT), which can serve as a marker for the lymphoid nature of malignancies. It can help identify patients likely to respond to certain types of chemotherapy, as in blast crisis of CML. Another T-cell enzyme is purine nucleoside phosphorylase; lack of this enzyme results in failure of certain T-cell functions. Adenosine deaminase is important in purine synthesis, and its absence is described in some patients with a combined immunodeficiency, affecting both T and B cells.

Null Cells

Those 10 to 30 per cent of blood lymphocytes that bear neither T- nor B-cell markers are referred to as *null cells.* They include precursors of the more differentiated T and B cells, natural killer cells, and cells that are able to carry out cell killing with the aid of antibodies (antibody-dependent cellular cytotoxicity, ADCC).

Natural Killer (NK) Cells. These thymus-inde-

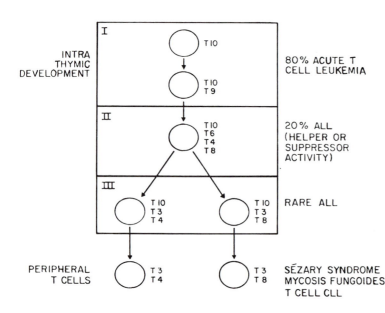

Figure 22–17 Maturation of T cells through the thymus. As can be seen, there is progressive acquisition and loss of antigens in association with cellular development. Different types of T-cell neoplasms can be equated with arrest at various stages of maturation. (Courtesy of A. Winkelstein.)

pendent cells can attack tumor cells or virus-infected cells and destroy them without prior education by antigenic exposure. They cross-react with a monocyte monoclonal antibody, and some of them contain receptors for sheep red cells. Morphologically, they appear to be large lymphocytes.

Killer (K) cells are also capable of killing cells without prior sensitization but require antibody to do so. They contain F_c and complement receptors but no sIg. The antibody serves to bind the K cells to the target cell. The role of null cells in antitumor reactions or autoimmune phenomena has not yet been fully determined.

LYMPHOCYTOSIS

An increase in the blood lymphocyte concentration to more than 4000 cells/mm³ is defined as *lymphocytosis* (Table 22–1). It is to be distinguished from the relative lymphocytosis seen in many conditions associated with neutropenia. This condition is seen in the recovery phase of bacterial infections and during the acute phase of a few viral infections. Infectious mononucleosis, and lymphoid neoplasms, including acute and chronic lymphocytic leukemia and non-Hodgkin's lymphoma.

Pertussis, or whooping cough, is capable of causing a very impressive lymphocytosis, particularly within the first 2 to 3 weeks of infection. Counts of 10,000 to 50,000 cells/mm³ may be found. The morphology is that of normal small lymphocytes. A lesser degree of lymphocytosis may be seen in chronic infections with brucellosis, tuberculosis, and syphilis.

Viral infections causing lymphocytosis include infectious hepatitis and cytomegalovirus. Toxoplasmosis, a protozoal infection, may be associated with lymphocytosis. These, as well as infectious mononucleosis (discussed subsequently) are characterized by many atypical as well as normal lymphocytes in the blood. The infecting agent of mononucleosis, the Epstein-Barr virus (EBV), infects B cells; however, the atypical cells in the blood are transformed T cells. Acute infectious lymphocytosis, usually seen in children, is almost certainly of viral origin, but an agent has not yet been identified. Small lymphocytes that appear normal are in the blood at levels of 10,000 to 100,000/mm³ for several weeks; there are often no symptoms or only vague ones. There is no splenomegaly or lymphadenopathy.

The lymphoid malignancies, to be discussed later, can generally be distinguished morphologically from benign lymphocytosis by the appearance of the abnormal cells. In chronic lymphocytic leukemia, cells often appear quite normal; however, this picture is seldom, if ever, seen in children or young adults, in whom benign infectious disease is much more common.

INFECTIOUS MONONUCLEOSIS

Infectious mononucleosis is a generally benign disorder that is usually seen in young adults. It is characterized by fever, sore throat, lymphadenopathy, splenomegaly, lymphocytosis with atypical cells, and the development of antibodies against the causative EBV and certain heterologous red cells. These heterophil antibodies, known for many years to accompany infectious mononucleosis transiently, have been found to be accompanied by a rise in EBV antibodies that endure longer and that confer permanent immunity. Most cases of infectious mononucleosis probably are expressed as subclinical infections or are so mild in clinical expression that they are not detected.

EBV is a herpesvirus, first isolated in lymphoblasts from patients with Burkitt lymphoma. Infectious mononucleosis appears to be spread most commonly by intimate oral contact, with infections being acquired mainly from carriers rather than acutely ill individuals. The virus is thought to infect B cells, although very few infected cells are seen in the blood. Large numbers of noninfected B cells are increased in the blood in the early stages of the disease, and a polyclonal rise in immunoglobulins is seen. Certain types of T cells are thought to recognize the EBV-containing B cells and to proliferate rapidly. These are thought to be primarily suppressor T cells and are responsible for the many atypical lymphocytes seen in the blood as well as the lymphadenopathy, splenomegaly, and infiltration of various other organs, including the liver, which is often enlarged and functionally abnormal. These cells are capable of suppressing the proliferation of B cells producing the various immunoglobulins as well as preventing their response to in vitro stimulants such as pokeweed mitogen.

The lymphocytosis usually peaks at the second or third week of the illness. Atypical cells account for 20 per cent or more of the lymphocytes. In infectious mononucleosis, the bone marrow usually does not show an increased number of abnormal cells, and there is usually no anemia or thrombocytopenia. This picture contrasts with that seen in acute leukemia, with which infectious mononucleosis is sometimes confused.

Anti-EBV antibodies are produced in a sequence similar to that found for many other infections: IgM antibodies that are transient, followed by IgG antibodies of longer duration. The "heterophil" antibodies, which have been of great diagnostic value in infectious mononucleosis, include agglutinins against sheep and horse red cells and lytic antibodies for beef red cells. These IgM antibodies are not identical. The specific pattern of the heterophil antibody, reacting with sheep red cells after absorption by guinea-pig kidney and beef red cells, helps distinguish the serum of infectious mononucleosis from that of serum sickness, which also may contain anti–sheep cell agglutinins. It has been suggested that the antigen that stimulates the heterophil antibodies in infectious mononucleosis is a new antigen on lymphocytes transformed by the EBV.

Formalized horse red cells are somewhat more specific for heterophil antibodies in infectious mononucleosis than are sheep red cells and are the basis for a widely used slide test for this disease ("Monospot").

Both the heterophil and the Monospot test can be used to make a fairly firm diagnosis of infectious mononucleosis, but false-negatives are fairly common, particularly in early stages of disease and in children. Thus, tests for EBV may be more definitive in certain circumstances.

Other antibodies may sometimes be seen, including antinuclear antibodies, cryoglobulins, rheumatoid factor, and several red-cell antibodies, including anti-i cold agglutinins and cold hemolysins. The latter two antibodies sometimes may cause hemolytic anemia, but anemia is usually absent, even with demonstrable anti–red cell antibodies. The cause of the production of all these antibodies is unknown, but a disorder of normal T-cell function causing an imbalance of helper and suppressor cells can be postulated. A generalized elevation of immunoglobulins, especially IgM, is common in infectious mononucleosis. Complications requiring steroid therapy include pharyngitis severe enough to threaten airway obstruction, severe hepatitis, severe generalized malaise and fever, and severe autoimmune hemolytic anemia or thrombocytopenia. The autoimmune thrombocytopenia seen in a few cases of infectious mononucleosis is managed like any form of "ITP" (see Chapter 24), including prompt splenectomy if a steroid response is not seen and if the thrombocytopenia is of life-threatening severity ($< 10,000$ to $20,000/mm^3$).

Infection with cytomegalovirus can cause a clinical picture that is very similar to infectious mononucleosis but that is not associated with heterophil antibodies. Sore throat and severe fatigue are usually not present, and the infection is often associated with massive blood transfusion (e.g., after open heart surgery). Anti-CMV antibodies instead of anti-EBV antibodies are found. The blood smear is similar to that of infectious mononucleosis.

HYPERGLOBULINEMIA

The concentration of immunoglobulins may be increased in the serum either as a diffuse increase in many antibodies (polyclonal) or as a large amount of one antibody (monoclonal). Monoclonal disorders, or gammopathies, may be benign or malignant.

A polyclonal gammopathy manifests as a broad, rounded or irregular peak on serum electrophoresis. This may be seen in many conditions, such as infectious mononucleosis, Hodgkin's disease, tuberculosis, brucellosis, and cirrhosis of the liver. Polyclonal gammopathies involve numerous kinds of antibodies and thus will contain various heavy chains and a fairly equal distribution of kappa and lambda light chains.

Monoclonal antibodies are composed of one type of heavy chain and one type of light chain, either kappa or lambda. Although the peak typically is seen on serum electrophoresis, its type must be identified by immunoelectrophoresis. The "M" (myeloma", "macroglobulin") antibodies may be complete molecules formed of heavy and light chains in the same molecule, complete molecules in association with excess light chains, heavy chains only, or light chains only. Light chains are not usually seen as peaks on serum electrophoresis, since their small size allows prompt glomerular filtration. They are detected as Bence Jones proteins in urine by heating and disappearance with further heating or identified as light chains in urine concentrates subjected to the aforementioned tests for serum proteins.

LYMPHOPENIA

Reduction of the blood lymphocyte concentration below $1500/mm^3$ may occur in a variety of conditions. Radiation therapy, systemic chemotherapy, administration of adrenal steroids, and various acute infections are among the most common causes. It is quite common in various types of cancer and in some of them is a bad prognostic sign, associated with advanced disease and failure of the T-cell system. Many patients with advanced cancer are anergic and have no response to DNCB. Lymphopenia is particularly common in Hodgkin's disease, but here it does not indicate a poor prognosis.

Patients with various immunologic deficiency syndromes, either congenital or acquired, may have either lymphopenia or abnormalities in the relative number of B, suppressor, or helper T cells.

PRIMARY IMMUNE DEFICIENCY DISEASES

Diseases characterized by various deficiencies of lymphocyte function may be either congenital or acquired; they may be primary, in which case there is no other disease process, or secondary to another disorder, most commonly a neoplasm of the lymphoid system. Any type may be characterized by a failure of humoral immunity (B cells), cellular immunity (T cells), or both.

An increasing number of congenital immune deficiencies have been described since the early 1950s, beginning with Bruton's description of congenital agammaglobulinemia, the prototype of absent B-cell function.

The deficiencies may be partial or complete. Mechanisms for their production include insufficient stem cells; failure of stem cell differentiation and maturation along specific pathways; specific lymphocyte enzyme defects, such as those involving adenosine deaminase (ADA) or purine nucleoside phosphorylase (PNP); and failure of cellular interaction. Various metabolic abnormalities and autoimmune diseases have been observed in patients with pre-existing primary immune deficiencies, most commonly B-cell disorders. Imbalance of T-cell function is presumably to blame. An increased incidence of malignant disease is also found in affected individuals with immune deficiencies; most often these are lymphomas or leukemias (75 per cent), and gastric cancer is the most commonly associated type of carcinoma. Whether the excessive cancers are due to a breakdown in surveillance function by T cells or result from the same cause as the immune deficiency is unknown.

The agammaglobulinemia of Bruton is an X-linked disorder of males, appearing as an infantile susceptibility to infection, usually from pyogenic bacteria. Although infections with fungi and most viruses are handled well, infectious hepatitis (viral) infection is not. Lymphopenia is generally not present; response to skin tests and other tests of T-cell function are normal, but there are no B cells in the blood or nodes; and antibody synthesis is lacking, with extremely low levels of serum Ig. Lymph-node follicles are poorly developed, and plasma cells are absent. Immunoglobulin replacement therapy can be given, allowing survival to adulthood. IgA is not effectively replaced in this way, since its injection does not replete the gastrointestinal and respiratory surfaces where it normally functions.

Severe combined immune deficiency (SCID) results in poor function of both T and B cells, perhaps owing to a lack of or an abnormality in lymphocyte stem cells. Several forms exist, distinguishable by their mode of inheritance, association with enzyme (ADA) deficiency, appearance of the thymus, and response to therapy. ADA deficiency results in the accumulation of deoxyadenosine, which may inhibit DNA synthesis in T cells. All SCID patients are susceptible to infection, and many die in infancy, of almost all kinds of infection, both those due to organisms normally of low virulence and those that are more aggressive. Lymphopenia is present, and T cells are reduced. B cells may be present in one type of SCID, but synthesis of Ig is poor in all types, regardless of the presence or absence of B cells. Skin tests show anergy, PHA response in vitro is low, and Ig in the serum is very low after the loss of the maternal contribution at 3 months of age. The thymus contains epithelial but no lymphoid elements, and there is virtually no peripheral lymphoid tissue. SCID is fatal at 6 to 12 months. Bone marrow transplantation from an HLA-compatible donor can be life-saving, achieving immunologic reconstitution. In the ADA-deficient patients without marrow donors, it has been possible to supply the enzyme by red cell transfusions from normal donors, since these cells are a rich source of enzyme. Repeated transfusions are necessary.

A transient delay in infant Ig synthesis at 3 to 5 months of age, when it normally occurs, can result in a syndrome similar to X-linked agammaglobulinemia. Recovery can occur at about 1 year of age with judicious use of antibiotics and gamma-globulin administration.

Common variable hypogammaglobulinemia, or dysgammaglobulinemia, is a heterogeneous group of disorders in which the common denominator is low levels of immunoglobulin; the variation relates to which immunoglobins are low and to what extent. In some patients, the defect is acquired, whereas in others it is congenital. Some immunoglobulins may be present, but new antibodies may not be formed effectively. Abnormalities include absent B-lymphocytes, B-lymphocytes present but unable to transform into antibody-synthesizing plasma cells, a lack of helper T cells, and an excess of suppressor T cells. Cyclic neutropenia is seen in some patients with these disorders. The incidence of pernicious anemia is also very high, and other autoimmune disorders are seen with increased frequency.

Selective deficiency of IgA may be totally benign or may cause an increased susceptibility to sinus and respiratory tract infections, celiac disease, and a large number of autoimmune diseases. It may be sporadic or inherited. It is fairly common, occurring in one per 600 or 700 people. IgA in the serum and secretions is low. IgM may help take up the slack at mucosal surfaces and protect from infection. B cells are present in the blood in normal numbers, as are total lymphocytes. IgA-coated B lymphocytes are found, but plasma cells do not produce IgA, suggesting a selective block in differentiation. In some patients, it has been possible to show increased suppressor T-cell activity specific for IgA production. Gamma-globulin administration is not helpful.

Selective IgM deficiency is somewhat less common but produces more problems with infections than IgA deficiency does. B cells with IgM surface markers are present but seem to be unable to secrete the immunoglobulin. T-cell function is normal.

DiGeorge syndrome of thymic hypoplasia results from failure of the development of the third and fourth pharyngeal pouches during fetal life, with resultant hypoplasia not only of the thymus but also of the parathyroid glands. Neonatal tetany due to hypocalcemia from parathyroid hormone deficiency may be the first clue to the diagnosis. The immunologic defect, diminished to markedly absent T cells, results in severe infections and death, usually within the first year. The organisms responsible are those normally controlled by the cellular immune system: *Candida, Pneumocystis carinii, Listeria, Mycobacterium tuberculosis,* and viruses such as cytomegalovirus and vaccinia. Failure of growth is seen. Interestingly, there is no increased incidence of autoimmune disease or cancer. Total lymphocyte counts are normal, but T cells are greatly decreased, and B cells are elevated. T-cell regions of nodes are poorly developed. Skin tests show no responsiveness, and PHA reactivity in vitro is diminished. Immunoglobulins are normal, and antibody production can proceed normally. T-cell precursors are apparently present, since thymic extract treatment can produce normal T cells. Transplantation of fetal thymic tissue is often successful and a humoral factor responsible for the recovery is probable, as the thymic tissue can be enclosed in a millipore chamber without loss of effectiveness.

A deficiency of purine nucleoside phosphorylase, inherited as an autosomal recessive trait, has been shown to cause T-cell deficiencies, presumably because of the accumulation of deoxyguanosine, resulting in an inhibition of T-cell DNA synthesis. T-cell function is deranged, as with thymic hypoplasia, but the onset of infection with the same kinds of organisms occurs somewhat later, in early childhood rather than infancy. Lymphopenia is present with absent or markedly reduced T cells but normal B cells and immunoglobulins. Suppressor cells are more severely affected than helper cells, and, possibly as a result, autoimmune disease is fairly common. Thymic replacement has not been effective, but some patients may respond to enzyme replacement by red cell transfusion, as in ADA deficiency.

The Wiskott-Aldrich syndrome combines thrombocytopenia, severe eczema, and an immune defect. Lymphopenia develops during the course of the disease; the proportion of B cells is variable, but T-cell levels are low. IgM is reduced, but other Igs are normal. Tests of T-cell function are abnormal, such as DNCB, other skin tests, rejection of skin grafts, and response to allogeneic cells in vitro. Paradoxically, the PHA response is normal. Neutrophil function is normal, but macrophage chemotaxis is defective. Patients are at risk for bacterial sepsis from organisms normally causing an IgM response as well as from the intracellular organisms already mentioned under thymic hypoplasia. Patients can die during early life as a result of infections, bleeding from the platelet defect, or a malignancy, commonly lymphoma. Irradiation of blood products to be transfused is necessary because of the T-cell defect, which allows proliferation of donor lymphocytes with consequent GVHD. Marrow and thymus transplantation does not seem to be effective, although thymic extracts have been said to be helpful in some cases. The defect is clearly located in many types of hematopoietic cells.

Ataxia telangiectasia is associated with an immune deficiency that involves both B and T cells and with a very high incidence of malignancy of all kinds. Autoimmune disease is common in this autosomal recessive condition. Severe cerebellar degeneration and conjunctival and skin telangiectasia give the syndrome its name. The immune defect is characterized by low levels of IgA and IgE, with normal to increased numbers of IgA-bearing B cells (i.e., a failure of Ig secretion). Other variable defects are low T cells (with a decreased helper:suppressor ratio), decreased, delayed hypersensitivity, low IgG levels, and poor antibody response. Sinus and lung infections are common, and the outlook for survival beyond adolescence is poor. No treatment has been shown to be effective.

OTHER ACQUIRED IMMUNE DEFICIENCY DISEASES

A variety of malignant neoplasms of the lymphoid system (e.g., leukemia and lymphoma) produce immune deficiencies, and these will be discussed subsequently. Other, nonlymphoid malignancies, when advanced, are often associated with lymphopenia and decreased T-cell function.

Patients with intestinal lymphangiectasia may have obstruction of intestinal lymph drainage or a lymphatic fistula into the bowel, the result being loss of both serum proteins and lymphocytes into the stool. Loss of albumin produces edema and ascites, and a rather mild combined immunodeficiency syndrome develops. There is lymphopenia, low serum Ig of all types, and skin test anergy, but serious infections are rare. The basic defect can sometimes be repaired by surgery or improved by a low-fat diet.

Sarcoidosis, a granulomatous disease of unknown etiology, is often accompanied by a defect in T-cell function, with skin anergy the most prominent feature. This is not too severe, and infections usually are not a major problem. The degree of anergy fluctuates, and anergy may disappear when the disease enters a remission. Serum IgG is usually normal or even increased.

The acquired immune deficiency syndrome (AIDS) is a remarkable, recently described disease found in homosexuals, hemophiliacs, intravenous drug abusers, and Haitian immigrants. The defect is one of cellular immunity, with lymphopenia and a decreased helper:suppressor ratio. Anergy is often present. B cells and Ig are normal to increased, as is neutrophil function. Natural killer cells are variably decreased. The deficiency is associated with a variety of serious, often lethal infections, including those caused by *Pneumocystis carinii, Aspergillus, Candida, Cryptococcus, Toxoplasma,* herpes simplex, and cytomegalovirus. Chronic progressive multifocal leukoencephalopathy, a devastating brain disease, possibly of viral origin, has also been seen. A somewhat uncommon neoplasm, Kaposi sarcoma, has been seen in very large numbers of patients, especially homosexuals, provoking much speculation about its cause and that of cancer in general. Over 4,000 cases of AIDS were observed between 1981 and 1984, with death resulting in more than half the patients. Among hemophiliacs, lyophilized factor VIII concentrates have been implicated as a possible cause. Most investigators hypothesize that AIDS is due to a virus, probably a T-cell leukemia virus. Other proposed causes of AIDS include cytomegalovirus, exposure to foreign antigens (spermatozoa in the case of homosexuals), and nitrites inhaled during drug abuse.

Benign monoclonal gammopathies, which may be seen in a wide variety of conditions, occur most commonly in elderly people. They are associated with a "spike" on electrophoresis but with no other evidence of a malignant plasma cell neoplasm. The concentration of protein does not increase but tends to be constant and is usually lower than that seen in myeloma (less than 3 gm/dl), and the concentration of the nonmonoclonal immunoglobulins is normal or increased. Anergy to skin tests and defective in-vitro responses to T-cell mitogens support the notion that this is an age-related deficiency of suppressor T-cell function, allowing a single clone of B cells to proliferate inappropriately in an autonomous fashion. Only a few patients demonstrating such findings progress to develop malignant plasma cell neoplasms, but it is possible that more of them would eventually develop malignancy if their advanced age did not cause them to die of other illnesses. The bone marrow contains 10 per cent or less of plasma cells that are usually normal morphologically, and some have completely normal marrows. Free light chains are seldom present, so renal dysfunction is rare. Bone destruction, hypercalcemia, and anemia, which are common features of myeloma, are not seen. Associated diseases may be present that are *not* benign, such as carcinomas. It is important to recognize this condition so that affected patients are not treated with aggressive therapy appropriate for myeloma or macroglobulinemia. The cause of the clonal plasma cell proliferation, by definition a neoplasm, is presumably some type of antigenic challenge developing from a chronic infection or a tumor, with failure of clonal development to cease, but not continuing to proliferate beyond a certain number of cells. Transient M proteins have appeared with various infections, tumors, hypersensitivity reactions, and autoimmune diseases.

PRIMARY MALIGNANT NEOPLASMS OF LYMPHOID CELLS

Hyperglobulinemia caused by proliferation of a malignant clone of plasma cells occurs in multiple myeloma (plasma cells), macroglobulinemia (of Waldenström), and heavy chain disease (cells often resembling lymphocytes), the so-called "plasma cell dyscrasias." Monoclonal gammopathies also occur in some lymphomas and in CLL as well.

A large amount of immunoglobulin in the plasma may cause a marked increase in its resistance to flow, or viscosity, producing the so-called "hyperviscosity syndrome." This is more common in monoclonal IgM diseases because of the high molecular weight associated with such disorders, but it can also be seen in IgA disease due to polymer formation and in IgG myeloma with a very high protein concentration. Viscosity is measured as a ratio of flow of the fluid in relation to water; patients with a viscosity of more than 5 (normal plasma being 1.5 to 1.7) are quite likely to be symptomatic. The syndrome includes headache, dizziness, sleepiness, stupor or coma due to sluggish intracerebral flow, and, sometimes, thrombosis. Visual disturbances are common, with characteristic changes seen in the retinal veins (i.e., alternate bulging and constriction, often with retinal hemorrhages and exudates). Deafness and peripheral neuropathies are also seen. Cardiac failure may develop owing to an increased plasma volume. Excessive bleeding is due to interaction of the immunoglobulin component with various clotting factors. The acute treatment of the hyperviscosity syndrome consists of plasmapheresis: removal of large amounts of plasma and substitution of normal plasma. Since IgM is contained largely within the intravascular space, this technique is fairly efficient. Removal of several liters of plasma weekly can reduce the viscosity to tolerable levels. Treatment of the underlying plasma cell dyscrasia with chemotherapy is required to bring the syndrome under long-term control, but this may require weeks or even months to become effective.

MULTIPLE MYELOMA

Multiple myeloma is a fatal disease characterized by the inappropriate, continuous proliferation of a clone of plasma cells. The cells often are morphologically abnormal and found primarily in the bone marrow, although soft-tissue masses attached to, or distant from, bones are sometimes seen (plasmacytomas). In more than 95 per cent of cases, there is a monoclonal protein, which may be complete, composed of a light chain only, or the combination of light chains and complete protein. The amount of protein measured in the serum or urine or both is related to the total number of plasma cells, and various clinical measurements have been used to quantitate the approximate number of malignant cells in the body and to estimate the prognosis of the patient. Lytic lesions of bone probably are not produced by mechanical destruction from local collections of plasma cells but by their production of osteoclast-activating factor, a substance that stimulates osteoclasts to resorb abnormal amounts of bone. Hypercalcemia is thus seen as a consequence. Diffuse osteoporosis rather than discrete lesions is often seen. Bone lesions are widespread but seen primarily in the areas of normal red marrow distribution. Anemia is very common, and granulocytopenia and thrombocytopenia may be seen. Myeloma cells have been reported to produce a substance that causes macrophages to suppress B-cell function inappropriately, perhaps an exaggeration of a normal regulatory mechanism. In any event, the concentration of the nonmyeloma immunoglobulin is generally decreased, with consequent susceptibility to infection. Both primary and secondary humoral antibody response to antigens is depressed (or absent) and is the primary cause of susceptibility to infection. Complicating this is mild granulocytopenia due to the disease and often accentuated by treatment. Abnormal opsonization has been observed, and myeloma patients are afflicted with such encapsulated organisms as pneumococci as well as the ubiquitous gram-negative bacteria.

Renal disease in myeloma is common and is a determining factor in length of survival. Bence-Jones proteinuria (light-chain excretion) is the major cause; proximal tubular cells are damaged by this protein, and casts form within the entire nephron, composed of all kinds of protein, producing ultimate destruction. Uric acid and calcium are often excreted in excess and add to the renal insult.

Vertebral disease can lead to compression of nerve roots and of the spinal cord, with pain, loss of sensation, paralysis, and loss of bladder and bowel function. Disease of the vertebrae can complicate any of the hematologic neoplasms but is most common in myeloma; approximately 20 per cent of patients may be threatened by compression symptoms, which constitute a "medical emergency." Cord compression requires immediate radiotherapy or surgical decompression or both. Myeloma is quite sensitive to radiation and some types of chemotherapy, and the judicious use of these modalities has been responsible for an impressive prolongation of life in this disease. The tumor is ultimately fatal, as chemotherapeutic resistance eventually develops. A small number of patients eventually develop AML, probably attributable in part to therapy. The increased incidence of AML may also be due to the increased survival with myeloma coupled with an increased AML risk secondary to myeloma itself.

Amyloidosis may complicate plasma cell dyscrasias and is an adverse prognostic factor when present. It refers to the deposition of an insoluble protein substance having a specific configuration in many tissues and interfering with their function. Some amyloid is derived from certain light chains or fragments of immunoglobulins, creating fibrils, which are thought to be formed and secreted by macrophages that process the light chains formed by neoplastic plasma cells. A macrophage protease may be responsible. When this variety of amyloid is deposited, it affects renal, cardiac, and gastrointestinal function adversely. Macroglossia (large tongue) may be diagnostic; cardiac failure refractory to the usual measures may occur. Peripheral neuropathy, especially the carpal tunnel syndrome with compression of the median nerve, may be present and should be distinguished from spinal cord or nerve root compression by vertebral or paravertebral tumor. Patients with myeloma who develop amyloid almost always demonstrate excess light-chain production, but only some of these individuals develop amyloid. There may be something structurally unique about their light chain and/or a combined processing and secreting ability of their macrophages. The only satisfactory approach is treatment of the associated myeloma.

Myeloma is best treated with systemic chemotherapeutic agents. Local radiation is used to palliate local disease, such as pain or spinal cord compression. Administration of short, periodic "bursts" of combination therapy consisting of the alkylating agent melphalan and prednisone has become the standard treatment, although various other agents are active. Survival is determined by the number of cells present at outset (indirectly assessed by the concentration of M protein or amount of light-chain excretion or both), the degree of anemia, hypercalcemia, renal function, and extent of bone lesions. Survival is also very dependent on the response to therapy. Median survivals range from 2 to 4 years, with considerable variation. The presence of compromised renal function is perhaps the most important determinant of survival. The class of monoclonal immunoglobulin is also important in the following order of worsening prognosis: IgM, kappa light chain only, IgG, IgA, lambda light chain only, and IgD. Those with *no* abnormal protein, the nonsecretors, probably have the worst prognosis and usually have very rapidly advancing disease, demonstrating marked destruction of bone.

Macroglobulinemia of Waldenström

This is a plasma cell dyscrasia characterized by the monoclonal production of IgM, with large quantities in the serum, often leading to the hyperviscosity syndrome. The malignant cells, often referred to as *plasmacytoid lymphocytes*, are transitional between lymphocytes and plasma cells. They frequently contain abundant amounts of carbohydrate, as shown by a positive PAS reaction. Carbohydrate accounts for a large proportion of IgM. That the neoplastic cells are transitional in the B-cell series is shown by their content of immunoglobulin both on the cell surface and in the cytoplasm. The clinical findings are those of a malignant lymphoma, with enlarged lymph nodes, liver, and spleen and either a diffuse or nodular pattern of lymphoid infiltrate in the bone marrow.

Fatigue and other manifestations of hyperviscosity (e.g., blurred vision) are common, but bone lesions, hypercalcemia, and renal failure are not. Although Bence-Jones proteinuria can occur in a small proportion of patients, this does not usually cause renal failure. Amyloidosis is also unusual. A bleeding tendency has been attributed both to abnormal platelet function caused by the interaction of platelets with IgM and to interaction of the abnormal protein with coagulation factors.

Anemia is common; leukopenia and thrombocytopenia are less frequent. Rouleaux formation of red cells causes a greatly increased sedimentation rate, and this too is due to macroglobulin. In some patients, the IgM is also a cryoglobulin that precipitates at low temperatures, causing cold sensitivity and Raynaud's phenomenon.

The diagnosis is made by identification of the monoclonal protein in the serum, accomplished with electrophoresis and immunoelectrophoresis coupled with evaluation of the overall clinical picture. Therapy of this disease, found largely in the elderly, is directed at amelioration of the hyperviscosity syndrome with plasmapheresis and reduction of the size of the malignant clone with chemotherapy. About half the patients will demonstrate a good response to alkylating agents such as chlorambucil, cyclophosphamide, and melphalan. Most patients survive for 3 to 4 years, but some individuals show no symptoms and have stable protein levels; they may be left untreated, sometimes for years.

Heavy Chain Disease

This is a plasma cell dyscrasia in which the monoclonal cells (lymphocytes or plasma cells) produce incomplete heavy chains without connected light chains. The three types that have been described correspond to immunoglobulins IgA, IgG, and IgM, in order of frequency. As with macroglobulinemia, the clinical picture resembles that of malignant lymphoma more than that of myeloma. The heavy chains are usually incomplete and often exist as dimers or polymers. Light chains may also be synthesized but are not joined to the heavy chains.

Alpha–heavy chain disease involves the usual site of IgA secretory production, the gastrointestinal tract. Patients are usually young adults, in the second and third decades, and have abdominal pain, diarrhea, and malabsorption. Most cases occur in the Middle East and Mediterranean basin. Weight loss and bowel obstruction are common. Peripheral adenopathy and hepatosplenomegaly are unusual, as is marrow involvement. The disease is largely confined to the intestine and regional lymph nodes, and it consists of varying degrees of infiltration by lymphocytes and plasma cells. There is some indirect evidence that the disease may be a reaction to an unidentified mi-

croorganism or parasite, and antibiotic treatment of early stages has been reported to result in improvement. T-cell functional defects and low levels of normal immunoglobulins have been described. Combination chemotherapy, similar to that used in other lymphomas, has been used in more advanced cases with some improvement. Some patients in the Mediterranean area with a clinically similar gastrointestinal lymphoma do *not* have heavy chain formation; in general, the histology is more malignant, a so-called "immunoblastic sarcoma." It has been suggested that this and IgA-type heavy chain disease are part of a spectrum in which a gastrointestinal pathogen initially incites lymphoid proliferation of benign-appearing cells that can make heavy chains but that then become increasingly immature, more invasive, autonomous, and devoid of their capacity for immunoglobulin fragment synthesis.

IgG-type heavy chain disease has no such racial predilection and occurs in all age groups. Lymphadenopathy, hepatosplenomegaly, and a peculiar swelling of the uvula are common. Some patients have an autoimmune disease such as rheumatoid arthritis, hemolytic anemia, lupus, thyroiditis, myasthenia gravis, or Sjögren's syndrome. The bone marrow is usually infiltrated by lymphocytes, plasma cells, or large blasts, and cytopenias are generally seen. The heavy chains often are present with other abnormalities, and normal immunoglobulins are depressed. The prognosis and response to treatment are quite variable but are generally unfavorable.

ACUTE LYMPHOBLASTIC LEUKEMIA (ALL)

Acute lymphoblastic, or lymphocytic, leukemia is the most common leukemia of childhood, with the incidence peaking at about age 3 years. It can occur at all ages but tends to become less common with age, accounting for 80 to 90 per cent of acute leukemias in patients under age 20 years and representing only a small fraction of the acute leukemias in patients over age 40 years. There is no particular relationship to chemical exposure or irradiation. Classification can be made morphologically, but of perhaps more significance with respect to prognosis is an immunologic classification. The morphologic classification in the "French-American-British" (FAB) system is as follows: L1 is composed of blast cells that are homogeneous in appearance and relatively small, no larger than twice the diameter of normal lymphocytes. L2 cells are large and very heterogeneous, with nucleoli that tend to be larger and more prominent and cytoplasm that is more abundant than in L1. L3 cells, the least common type, are large and homogeneous and often demonstrate cytoplasmic vacuolation. Many L3 cells have surface immunoglobulin, are in the B lineage, and resemble the cells of the Burkitt lymphoma.

Researchers have extensively studied membrane surface markers using sheep red cell rosetting (E +), sIg, complement receptors (CR), the F_c portion of Ig, and sheep red cell rosette formation after treatment with complement and anti–sheep red cell antiserum (EAC rosettes). Specific antibodies to T cells and their subtypes, B cells, and "common" ALL (CALLA) are also widely used. The most frequent type of ALL (70 to 85 per cent of cases) was originally called the "null cell variety," as none of the first five aforementioned markers was present, although many of these react with the CALLA antibody (Table 22–9). These are thought to be pre-B cells, but they do not yet have immunoglobulin expression and are thus more immature than the pre-B cell identified by its cytoplasmic Ig (cIg) (see previous discussion).

Twelve to 30 per cent of patients have T-cell markers on their cells; 2 to 4 per cent have differentiated B markers (sIg); and a very few have both T and B markers. In general, the prognosis is best for the less differentiated cells (i.e., the "null but CALLA +" type).

Distinguishing ALL from AML is not always easy (Table 22–10) but is essential to selecting the appropriate therapy. Age helps determine the probability of one or the other type in the general population but is of *no* help in the individual. Morphologic appearance of the cells usually is characteristic, and special stains for peroxidase, Sudan black, and PAS (periodic acid–Schiff's) reagent are occasionally helpful. Lymphoblasts tend to show more clumping of chromatin and nuclear clefting; myeloblasts demonstrate very fine chromatin and may have Auer bodies or some granule formation. In AML many immature cells resemble monocytes, and morphologic abnormalities of erythroid and megakaryocytic systems are common (as discussed earlier), whereas such cellular appearances are not part of the process of ALL. Hypodiploidy is more common in ALL, and the pattern of CFU_c and CFU_e in-vitro colony formation is usually normal in ALL and abnormal in AML. Patients with ALL are more likely to have prominent lymph node enlargement and mediastinal masses. The degree of hepatosplenomegaly, the blood leukocyte count, the severity of anemia or thrombocytopenia, and the extent of marrow infiltration are not very helpful distinguishing features.

The symptoms and signs of ALL are similar to those of AML, being due primarily to anemia, neutropenia, and thrombocytopenia. In fact, the similarities are so great that the common clinical and laboratory features of AML, reviewed on page 615 will not be reconsidered for ALL. However, certain special features of ALL will be mentioned.

Very high white counts and mediastinal masses suggest T-ALL. Anergy, suggesting deranged T-cell function, is common. However, unlike other lymphoid neoplasms, ALL is rarely associated with hypogammaglobulinemia, and

monoclonal Ig spikes on serum electrophoresis are infrequent in this disease.

Drugs that are particularly useful in ALL remission induction, but not very effective in AML, are vincristine, prednisone and L-asparaginase. The anthracyclines doxorubicin and daunorubicin are used in both diseases. In ALL, combination chemotherapy with these agents has produced complete remissions in 90 to 95 per cent of children. Achievement of a significant number of cures depends on maintenance of remissions with continued chemotherapy for several years. This is accomplished with such drugs as 6-mercaptopurine and methotrexate administered in various ways, with invisible disease treated for an arbitrary (approximately 2.5 years) but necessary period of time. As with AML, supportive care with platelet transfusions, prompt antibiotic treatment of infections, and granulocyte transfusions when necessary during the induction phase are critical.

The development of neurologic symptoms and demonstration of leukemic cells in the meninges during times of remission suggest that the central nervous system (CNS) can be a "sanctuary" for ALL cells, presumably because of the failure of penetration of the drugs into these tissues when given intravenously or orally. Therapy designed to prevent this problem consists of cerebral irradiation and instillation of chemotherapy, usually methotrexate, into the subarachnoid space by lumbar puncture or intraventricular reservoir. The

TABLE 22–9 TYPE AND APPROXIMATE FREQUENCY OF SUBDIVISIONS OF ALL BASED ON SURFACE MARKERS*

	Approximate Percentage of Patients in Subset	Approximate Percentage of Total Patients
B-cell lineage (Ia +)		75
sIg	95	
CALLA +	80	
CALLA −	20	
ClgM +	20	
sIg +	5	
T-cell lineage (Ia −)		20
E +, T-Ab +	90	
E −, T-Ab +	10	
TH2 +	20	
TH2 −	80	
Indeterminate (no identifiable markers)		2
T- and B-cell markers		2

Abbreviations: Ia, antibody directed against cells of B-cell lineage; sIg, surface immunoglobulin; CALLA, common acute lymphoblastic leukemia antigen; ClgM, cytoplasmic IgM; E, rosetting with sheep red blood cells; T-Ab, antibody specific for cells of T-cell lineage; TH2, antibody against T-cell subset.

TABLE 22–10 STEPS IN A COMPLETE EVALUATION OF PATIENTS WITH ALL TO DISTINGUISH ACUTE LYMPHOBLASTIC FROM ACUTE MYELOID LEUKEMIA

Steps	Results
I. "Routine" morphology or special stains to aid in forming an opinion as to cell type	
A. Auer rods	Pathognomonic for AML
B. Azurophilic, eosinophilic, or basophilic granules that are peroxidase positive	Pathognomonic for AML if present in ≥ 10% of cells
C. Nuclear chromatin pattern	
1. Fine, stippled, or lacy	Favors AML
2. Irregularly clumped	Favors ALL
D. Nuclear configuration	
1. Folded	Favors AML
2. Clefted	Favors ALL
E. Megakaryocyte and platelet abnormalities	Favors AML
F. Megaloblastic erythroblasts	Favors AML
G. Other	
1. Mature neutrophils, low LAP	Favors AML
2. Mature neutrophils, pseudo-Pelger-Hüet	Favors AML
3. Peroxidase-negative azurophilic granules	Favors ALL
4. Special stains	
Sudan black B +, Napthal-ASD—Chloracetate +	Favors AML
PAS + in a "block" pattern	Favors ALL
II. Leukemic cell surface markers	
A. E rosette +, anti-T-Ab +	Indicates T-ALL
B. Ab against common form ALL (CALLA)	Indicates ALL, usually pre-B variety
C. Detection of surface immunologloblulin	Favors B-ALL, also seen in AML
D. Detection of Ia-like Ag	Either ALL or AML
E. Detection of antigen prepared against AML cells	Indicates AML
F. Detection of B1 antigen with monoclonal Ab_2	Indicates ALL
III. Positivity for terminal transferase	Strongly favors ALL
IV. Cell growth in semisolid media	
A. Marrow	
1. CFU-C—normal colonies	Favors ALL
—abnormal growth	Favors AML
2. BFU-E and CFU-E—normal colonies	Favors ALL
—no growth	Favors AML
B. Blood	
1. CFU-C—increased concentration of normal colonies	Favors ALL
—abnormal growth	Favors AML
2. BFU-E—increased concentration	Favors ALL
—no growth	Favors AML
V. Cytogenetics—hypodiploid cells	Favors AML
VI. If in doubt (should be only 1–2% at this point) treatment with prednisone and vincristine. Response:	Favors AML

testes have also been a sanctuary for microscopic foci of leukemic cells in a small number of patients.

Prognosis, independent of patient age, depends primarily on duration of the first remission. Duration of first complete remission is dependent to a large degree on age and immunologic type. The prognosis for ALL is best in patients between 3 and 5 years of age. As age increases (or decreases) prognosis worsens. Over half of young children are cured with current therapy, but adults seldom are cured, although complete remissions are the rule. CALLA-positive disease is slightly more common in children, whereas B-cell ALL and null-cell ALL are slightly more common in adults.

However, these differences cannot account for the marked differences in duration of remission or rate of cure. T-ALL is associated with a predominance of males, higher white cell counts, mediastinal masses, organomegaly, and a shorter duration of complete remission than T-negative ALL. Females, whites, and patients with low WBC counts at diagnosis have better survivals, apparently independent of immunologic type and age. Patients with CNS disease at the outset do poorly, as do patients who are anergic.

In a population of young children who have ALL, one can anticipate cure rates in the group of as high as 80 per cent (1) if the patients demonstrate no more than modest leukocyte elevation, modest node and organ enlargement, and cells that are CALLA-positive but negative for T and B markers; and (2) if the patients receive induction therapy consisting of 4 weeks of prednisone and vincristine (>90 per cent complete remission rate), perhaps with added asparaginase, CNS prophylaxis with intrathecal methotrexate, and usually cranial irradiation as well as maintenance therapy for 2½ years with daily 6-MP and bolus, oral methotrexate once or twice a week.

Since relapse after initial remission induction is seldom associated with subsequent cure, this is a subgroup of patients, for whom bone marrow transplantation is a suitable option. The second remission, when the number of leukemic cells is once again low, is the optimal time for transplantation. Patients in whom there is little anticipation of cure with the aforementioned regimen (e.g., any patient with T-cell ALL or adults with any form of ALL) are candidates for transplantation during first remission.

CHRONIC LYMPHOCYTIC LEUKEMIA (CLL)

CLL is characterized by blood lymphocytosis, usually with B cells that are morphologically normal. It is a disease of individuals in late middle age and of the elderly, with male predominance (approximately 2:1). Survival may be quite long,

with the median ranging from 5 to 8 years in different series (Fig. 22–18), and for long periods of time no therapy may be required. However, it is not curable. The usual cause of death is infection, due to the immunologic abnormality that results in hypogammaglobulinemia and failure to produce antibody; the risk is enhanced in some by therapy-induced neutropenia or adrenal corticosteroids or both. A significant number of patients, about one third, die of other causes related to age but with no evident direct relation to CLL. Acute transformation rarely occurs.

B-cell markers (sIg, usually IgM) are present. Serum Ig levels may be normal or reduced at diagnosis, but severe hypogammaglobulinemia, particularly for IgM and IgA, eventually develops in most patients. Response to mitogens in vitro is impaired and delayed. There is poor antibody synthesis, even if normal serum Ig levels are present. IgM response to an antigenic challenge is slow, and the usual changeover to IgG is delayed. Some patients have decreased ratios of helper:suppressor T cells, but most patients have normal T-cell function as measured by delayed hypersensitivity tests. Function of natural killer cells and antibody-dependent cytotoxicity are impaired.

Increased incidences of "autoimmune" disease and cancer have been reported in CLL. This may be due to inappropriate production of antibodies directed against native antigens by the malignant B cells or a failure of T-cell suppressor function. Hemolytic anemia, immune thrombocytopenia, or

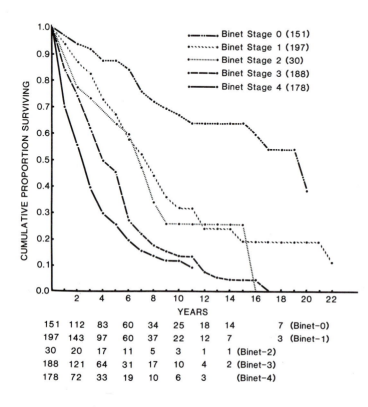

Figure 22–18 Survival of 745 patients with chronic lymphocytic leukemia. Each stage represents increasingly severe disease as judged by physical findings and laboratory studies. (From Skinnider, L. F., et al.: Cancer *50*:2951, 1982.)

immune neutropenia may result. The Coombs'-positive hemolytic anemia, which develops in approximately 20 per cent of patients, and the immune thrombocytopenia (approximately 5 per cent) are managed with steroids and splenectomy in the same manner as when these syndromes develop de novo (see Chapters 23 and 24). Occasionally, patients develop "selective red cell aplasia" (see Chapter 23), but this is *not* associated with an immunoglobulin directed against erythroid precursors, as is the case with most such acquired aplasia.

Large numbers of lymphocytes accumulate and seem to be blocked in their differentiation into plasma cells. More than 80 per cent of patients have lymphadenopathy, which may be massive. Normal node architecture is destroyed. Splenomegaly is present in 75 per cent of patients, hepatomegaly in half, and sternal tenderness in one third. There may be few if any symptoms in 40 per cent. Fatigue, node enlargement, and infection are the most common presenting symptoms.

By our definition, all CLL patients have lymphocytosis; one third have counts higher than 100,000/mm^3. About one half are anemic at diagnosis, and 40 per cent have thrombocytopenia. The lymphocytes are usually typical, normal-appearing small cells, but small numbers of larger cells with fine nuclear chromatin may be seen. Bone marrow examination shows moderate to marked infiltration by mature lymphocytes in virtually all patients. A poor prognosis has been reported for those patients with marrow infiltration out of proportion to the degree of blood lymphocytosis.

When the cells have T surface markers (<10 per cent of patients), there are some clinical differences from B-cell disease, but it is not clear that there is any difference in survival. Patients tend to have a greater blood lymphocytosis and more impressive organ enlargement, and skin infiltration is more common with T- than with B-CLL.

Some patients have striking bone marrow infiltration with small lymphocytes in the absence of blood lymphocytosis. Their prognosis is significantly worse than that of CLL patients, and their disease is usually classified as diffuse, well-differentiated non-Hodgkin's lymphoma primarily involving bone marrow, rather than CLL. Such patients often present with pancytopenia.

Several staging systems have been proposed that involve various combinations of adenopathy, organomegaly, anemia, and thrombocytopenia (Fig. 22–18). It is clear that patients with lymphocytosis alone at diagnosis have the best prognosis, with a median survival of greater than 10 years. The presence of a few regions of lymphadenopathy does little to change this figure, but when many node areas are involved the median survival decreases significantly. The presence of organomegaly at the outset further decreases survival, and with severe anemia and particularly with significant degrees of thrombocytopenia, the median survival may be less than 2 years.

It is not clear that therapy prolongs survival, and the current policy of most (but not all) physicians is to give no treatment if the patient is asymptomatic or only modestly symptomatic. Anemia and thrombocytopenia are most effectively treated with steroids. Splenectomy can sometimes be helpful, particularly if autoimmune cell destruction is present. During the response to steroids, the blood lymphocyte count may increase temporarily while nodes, spleen, and liver are shrinking and anemia and thrombocytopenia are improving. Steroids can increase the susceptibility to infections, so they should not be given without a clear indication, usually severe anemia or thrombocytopenia or both. Steroids should be used in a *short* intensive course preceding or concurrent with alkylating agents.

Alkylating agents have been the mainstay of treatment for CLL since the 1950s. They are useful in reducing enlarged lymph node masses and organs, but they may sometimes exacerbate other hematologic abnormalities. Chlorambucil and cyclophosphamide are the most widely used, and the former is probably the safest of these agents; combining these with prednisone or with vincristine and prednisone has also been tried, but it is not clear that these programs, or indeed any therapy, have prolonged survival. Complete remissions are uncommon; hematologic toxicity is not.

Leukapheresis can be used to reduce the number of circulating blood lymphocytes and may be employed in patients who cannot tolerate cytotoxic chemotherapy, but the results are transient. Monoclonal antibodies directed against cell surface antigens can also temporarily reduce the degree of lymphoid infiltration, but they are not yet of any long-term value. Perhaps more specific antibodies will be more useful. Total body irradiation can produce remissions but often is quite toxic. The routine replacement of deficient immunoglobulins with gamma globulin is of no proven benefit in CLL, but it is sometimes used in desperation in the patient with recurrent infections due to hypogammaglobulinemia; a controlled trial of immunoglobulin therapy in myeloma failed to disclose any evidence of an effect of such therapy on frequency of infection.

THE LYMPHOMAS

HODGKIN'S DISEASE

Hodgkin's disease, described by Thomas Hodgkin in the mid-nineteenth century, has been considered to be a malignant lymphoma for many years because it clearly is a disease of lymph nodes, causing their enlargement and often progressing from one nodal area to contiguous ones. It can involve non–lymph node areas as well, commonly the spleen, bone marrow, and liver. The characteristic cell is the Reed-Sternberg cell, which is a large, binuclear or multinuclear cell with vesicular nuclei and prominent nucleoli. It has been likened to an owl's eyes. The malignant nature of the cells is shown by indefinite growth in tissue culture, production of tumors in immunosuppressed mice, and aneuploidy.

Evidence is accumulating that the Reed-Sternberg cell is a derivative of the monocyte-macrophage line rather than a malignant lymphocyte. The type and distribution of immunoglobulin and complement on the cell surface resemble those of macrophages rather than lymphocytes. The cells are capable of phagocytosis. With electron microscopy, the cytoplasm resembles that of macrophages and monocytes more than that of lymphocytes. The nucleus does, however, resemble that of lymphocytes, and typical macrophage enzymes are not present. Thus, the issue is not closed. The other strong possibility is that the Reed-Sternberg cell is a malignant T-lymphocyte. There are some characteristic immunologic abnormalities that certainly implicate the T-cell system. Thus, there may be skin test anergy, failure to reject grafts, and failure of Hodgkin's lymphocytes both to cause GVHD and to react to various mitogens in culture or to allogeneic lymphocytes. Lymphopenia is frequent, except in the most early stages, with reduction of both T and B cells. Abnormalities are found in the ratio of suppressor:helper cells, which is increased in the blood and nodes but decreased in the spleen. The abnormal T-cell function and distribution have been attributed to the secretory activity of suppressor monocytes, perhaps the Reed-Sternberg cells themselves, but the basic cause is unknown. For the most part, B-cell function (as measured by circulating immunoglobulin and antibody synthesis) is normal, as is macrophage and neutrophil function, although there have been scattered reports of minor abnormalities.

Patients with Hodgkin's disease are susceptible to a variety of infections (e.g., herpes zoster, tuberculosis, *Cryptococcus*, and other fungi and viruses), which is expected because of the T-cell defect. These patients also have a large number of infections with bacteria, but these have usually followed therapy.

Hodgkin's disease can be seen at all ages but is most common in young adults. There are four major types of disease, classified according to histologic features. They all contain the Reed-Sternberg cell and varying amounts of lymphocytes, histiocytes, eosinophils, plasma cells, neutrophils, and fibrous tissue. The lymphocyte-predominant and lymphocyte-depletion types represent the two ends of the spectrum and account for 15 to 35 per cent of cases, with the mixed-cellularity type intermediate and making up about 40 per cent. Histologic progression from the lymphocyte-predominant variety to the mixed-cellularity and lymphocyte-depletion types over time is fairly common. The nodular sclerosis variety is rather unique and may be a "separate" type of disease. It does not often change to other types and is distinctive in that large amounts of collagen tissue separate the lymphoid tissue into islands. The Reed-Sternberg cells of nodular sclerosis have a unique histologic appearance and a peculiar "lacunar" placement, being separated from neighboring cells by apparently empty spaces, due to shrinkage from fixation or possibly cellular lipid. This type of Hodgkin's disease is most often found in young adults, especially in females. It commonly involves the neck or mediastinal nodes or both and accounts for 30 to 70 per cent of cases in various series.

Since Hodgkin's disease can usually be cured with a choice of therapy appropriate to disease location and extent, careful clinical staging is of paramount importance. Varying combinations of chemotherapy alone, radiotherapy alone, or combined modality therapy are used, depending on the clinical and often the pathologic stage.

The clinical staging classification most widely used is the "Ann Arbor" system (Table 22–11). Stages I and II represent Hodgkin's disease that is localized to one side of the diaphragm, and they are treated with radiation therapy to encompass the nodes involved and contiguous node-bearing areas. Stage IV is best treated with chemotherapy and often with radiation in low doses to areas originally involved with disease; stage III is increasingly being treated with chemotherapy as well. The results in IIIB disease treated with chemotherapy are better than those of IIIA disease treated with radiotherapy, at least in some series. Since the best treatment depends on an accurate assessment of where the disease is located, aggressive staging should be done, including lymphangiography to define para-aortic and inguinal node involvement, bone marrow aspiration and biopsy, and perhaps a gallium scan, which can often detect areas of disease not previously detectable. In many instances, if the results will determine the choice of therapy, a staging laparotomy in which the spleen is removed, suspicious nodes are sampled, and the liver is biopsied.

An enlarged but painless node in the neck is the most common initial presentation. Fever, sweats, weight loss, itching, and immediate alcohol-induced pain at the site of involvement may also be seen. Some of these complaints represent the so-called "B" symptoms used in the staging classification (Table 22–11). The enlarged node may be the only one, or it may be found that the patient has generalized adenopathy or disease in several areas. In most, but not all, patients the pattern of spread is most compatible with the disease beginning in one node region, usually the neck or supraclavicular areas, and then spreading to contiguous areas. Lung involvement is most commonly from adjacent mediastinal or hilar

TABLE 22–11 CLINICAL STAGES OF HODGKIN'S DISEASE

Stage	Criteria
I	Involvement of a single node-bearing area (I) or a single extralymphatic site (IE)
II	Involvement of two or more node-bearing areas on the same side of the diaphragm (II) or localized involvement of a single extralymphatic site in addition to two or more node-bearing areas on the same side of the diaphragm (IIE)
III	Involvement of node-bearing areas on both sides of the diaphragm (III). The spleen is considered a lymph node. In addition, there may be localized involvement at a single extralymphatic site (IIIE)
IV	Diffuse, disseminated involvement of one or more extralymphatic organs or tissues by multiple lesions with or without lymph node disease

In addition to Roman numeral stages, a letter designation is assigned to all patients: A = no fever, night sweats, or weight loss; B = either fever (greater than 100°F), significant loss of weight (at least 10%), or night sweats, or any combination of the three within 6 months of diagnosis and of at least 1 month's duration.

nodes or both, and liver involvement is seen almost entirely in conjunction with splenic involvement.

Anemia is seen in about one half the patients and is due to a combination of inadequate red cell production and a slightly increased rate of destruction. Occasionally, an autoimmune hemolytic anemia (positive Coombs' test) is present. Leukocytosis due to neutrophilia is present in 30 to 50 per cent of patients, and lymphopenia is seen in 45 to 65 per cent, except in stage I disease, in which it is rare. Monocytosis and eosinophilia are less common but are seen in 5 to 10 per cent of patients. The platelet count is usually normal or increased but may be low, with evidence of bone marrow involvement. The bone marrow is involved in less than 10 per cent of patients at diagnosis, and myelofibrosis even without evident Reed-Sternberg cells is considered adequate evidence of marrow involvement in an untreated patient with proven Hodgkin's disease. In contrast, granulomas in liver, marrow, or spleen that lack Reed-Sternberg cells do *not* represent Hodgkin's disease of that organ. Elevations of the serum copper, the erythrocyte sedimentation rate, and alpha$_2$-globulins are often seen.

A relationship between histologic type and clinical stage exists. Thus, 90 per cent of patients with lymphocyte-predominant disease are likely to be in stage I or II; and approximately 70 per cent with nodular sclerosis, less than 50 per cent with mixed cellularity, and almost all with lymphocyte depletion are in stage IV.

Prognosis is very much a function of clinical stage. In addition, the histologic type, sex, and age are important. Within a given clinical stage, the most dismal prognoses are associated with mixed-cellularity and lymphocyte-depletion types, with males compared with females, with patients over the age of 40 years, and with those demonstrating systemic "B" symptoms. Approximate overall 5-year disease-free survivals for the four clinical stages from 1971 to 1975 were 90, 73, 65, and 52 per cent, respectively. Relapse after 5 years, indeed after 3 years, is uncommon. Thus, Hodgkin's disease must be approached as a potentially curable disease.

Much of the progress in Hodgkin's disease has been due to the utilization of modern, megavoltage radiotherapeutic equipment; the adherence to the principle of treating areas adjacent to those involved; and the development of four-drug combination regimens. Such chemotherapy combinations are clearly better than single drugs or even two or, probably, three drugs, and they are associated with a much higher frequency of complete remission and long-term control. The best known combinations are MOPP (nitrogen *m*ustard, vincristine [*O*ncovin], *p*rednisone, and *p*rocarbazine), and ABVD (doxorubin [*A*driamycin], *b*leomycin, *v*inblastine and *D*TIC [Dacarbazine]). These are associated with comparable complete remission rates and relapse-free rates. Using them alternately is one strategy currently under investigation. One of the unfortunate outcomes of "cured" Hodgkin's disease is the occasional development of acute leukemia in those patients given alkylating agents, often in conjunction with radiotherapy.

NON-HODGKIN'S LYMPHOMA

This name obviously reflects the frustration experienced by many investigators engaged in a continuing attempt to arrive at a classification of a group of diverse diseases that is meaningful both to the clinically oriented hematologist-oncologist and to the hematopathologist. In most cases, these heterogeneous neoplasms are composed of lymphocytes in various stages of proliferation and differentiation. We have passed through eras of several confusing histologic and immunologic classifications, and the end is not in sight. A very old scheme described "lymphosarcoma," "reticulum cell sarcoma," and "giant follicle lymphoma." A more recent one, described in 1956 by Rappaport, was based strictly on morphology and is still widely used (Table 22–12). It is based on the nodular or diffuse histologic appearance of the tumor and the type of cell. A "nodular" pattern, slightly reminiscent of normal nodal architecture, is associated with better prognosis than a "diffuse" pattern. Large cells (some erroneously called "his-

TABLE 22–12 A WORKING FORMULATION OF NON-HODGKIN'S LYMPHOMA FOR CLINICAL USAGE: RECOMMENDATION OF AN EXPERT INTERNATIONAL PANEL; COMPARISONS WITH THE RAPPAPORT SCHEME

Working Formulation	Rappaport Terminology
LOW GRADE	
A. Malignant lymphocytic small lymphocytic consistent with chronic lymphocytic leukemia plasmacytoid	Diffuse, well-differentiated, lymphocytic
B. Malignant lymphoma, follicular Predominantly small cleaved cell diffuse areas sclerosis	Nodular, poorly differentiated, lymphocytic
C. Malignant lymphoma, follicular Mixed, small cleaved and large cell diffuse areas sclerosis	Nodular, mixed lymphocytic histiocytic
INTERMEDIATE GRADE	
D. Malignant lymphoma, follicular Predominantly large cell diffuse areas sclerosis	Nodular histiocytic
E. Malignant lymphoma, diffuse Small cleaved cell	Diffuse pooly differentiated lymphocytic
F. Malignant lymphoma, diffuse Mixed, small and large cell sclerosis epitheloid cell component	Diffuse mixed lymphocytic-histiocytic
G. Malignant lymphoma, diffuse Large cell cleaved cell non-cleaved cell sclerosis	Diffuse histiocytic
HIGH GRADE	
H. Malignant lymphoma Large cell, immunoblastic plasmacytoid clear cell polymorphous epitheloid cell component	Diffuse histiocytic
I. Malignant lymphoma Lymphoblastic convoluted cell non-convoluted cell	Diffuse lymphoblastic
J. Malignant lymphoma Small non-cleaved cell Burkitt's follicular areas	Diffuse undifferentiated

Modified from Rosenberg, S. A. et al.: Cancer 49:2112, 1982.

tiocytes," but really lymphoblasts) are associated with a worse prognosis than small cells resembling normal lymphocytes. Lukes and Collins devised a system based on immunologic principles as inferred from lymph node morphology, with classifications based on probable T- or B-cell derivation. Thus, there are "immunoblastic sarcomas" of the B- or T-cell type and B lymphomas of the follicular center cell type (FCC) that may be either large or small, cleaved or noncleaved. A more recent attempt to reconcile all of these classifications has resulted in an international working formulation (Table 22–12) that, it is hoped, will provide a common language, at least for pathologists. However, the overall clinical utility of such a complex classification of a relatively rare disease (or diseases) is necessarily of limited value. If one couples clinical staging and A and B symptoms with this, *hundreds* of varieties exist, so that correlation with survival, response to therapy, and so forth for individual types is mathematically impossible without a central registry involving populations of hundreds of millions of persons.

Increasingly, lymph node tissue from patients with non-Hodgkin's lymphoma is being subjected to immunologic study, and it is possible to categorize a malignant population with specific markers other than morphology alone, which is highly subjective, thus contributing to substantial error and lack of agreement among pathologists. Several series have shown that 65 to 70 per cent of non-Hodgkin's lymphomas are of the B-cell type, 6 to 10 per cent are of the T-cell variety, 15 to 25 per cent are of the "null" type, and 2 to 5 per cent are undefined. In one series, patients with the B type had a mean survival of 58 months, whereas those with the null and T types had a mean survival of only 14 months. Typing the immunoglobulin also seemed to have significance: Those patients in the B category who had both IgM and IgD on cell surfaces did much better than those with IgM only, IgM plus either IgA or IgG, or only IgA or IgG. Combining this type of study with a simplified morphologic classification may help resolve the puzzle of why patients with the same type of pathology may differ widely in their disease course and may assist in the selection of those for whom aggressive therapy is justified. It is noteworthy that all nodular lymphomas and well-differentiated diffuse lymphomas, as well as the Burkitt type, are B-cell neoplasms. The identification of various other markers on lymphoma cells, such as differentiation antigens, may also help.

There is no consistent pattern of immunologic defects in non-Hodgkin's lymphoma. Some patients, particularly those with diffuse histiocytic lymphoma, may be lymphopenic. Lymphocytosis with abnormal cells can occur in the late stages of some of the lymphomas ("lymphosarcoma cell leukemia"). Hypogammaglobulinemia can be found in a small number of patients, especially late in the disease, as is the case with CLL. The Burkitt lymphoma, a B-cell neoplasm, is often associated with hypogammaglobulinemia. Antibody responses are often depressed, and anergy may be present, particularly with advanced disease. Other measures of T-cell function may also be depressed.

In contrast to Hodgkin's disease, non-Hodgkin's lymphoma is often widespread at diagnosis (90 per cent of cases) and does not seem to spread by contiguity. Well-differentiated lymphocytes are capable of recirculation in the blood, a fact that may account for early, widespread dissemination of this cellular type. The more poorly differentiated cell types have a tendency to be localized at first but eventually to spread via lymphatics and the blood in a fashion similar to that seen with epithelial neoplasms.

Most patients with non-Hodgkin's lymphoma present with lymphadenopathy. Systemic symptoms are somewhat less common than in Hodgkin's disease, and patients are generally older. Mesenteric nodes and nonlymphoid tissue are more commonly involved in non-Hodgkin's lymphoma than in Hodgkin's disease. The spleen is less often involved but bone lesions are more common in non-Hodgkin's lymphoma.

The blood is normal in about half the patients, more frequently in those 60 per cent of patients without bone marrow involvement. Anemia may be seen in this group, but neutropenia and thrombocytopenia are minimal in those without obvious marrow infiltration. Lymphopenia is present in about half of each group. Some of the normal-appearing lymphocytes are actually monoclonal when tested and are thus presumably part of the tumor-cell population. Bone marrow involvement is relatively uncommon (15 per cent of cases) in diffuse histiocytic lymphoma but common in the poorly differentiated and well-differentiated lymphocytic lymphomas.

Serum copper and lactate dehydrogenase are often elevated; uric acid levels are less frequently increased. Serum proteins are usually normal at the outset, but albumin may decrease with time. When a monoclonal protein spike is found in the serum, it is usually IgM. Neurologic involvement with meningeal infiltration or spinal cord compression can occur. The former is especially seen in patients with diffuse histiocytic lymphoma with bone marrow involvement. Cranial nerve lesions

or cerebral symptoms such as headache, nausea, or vomiting predominate, and treatment consisting of cranial irradiation and intrathecal chemotherapy must be directed at the CNS, as in ALL.

Infection, the major cause of death, is due to a combination of factors. These include deficient antibody synthesis, seen with advancing disease; neutropenia due to marrow infiltration and, commonly, to chemotherapy and radiotherapy; adrenal corticosteroid therapy; and organ damage due to tumor infiltration, especially in the lung and bowel. Bacterial infection is most frequent, but fungal infections also occur often.

Survival for patients with this heterogeneous group of diseases is a function of histologic type, immunologic type (as noted earlier), clinical stage, and the presence of systemic symptoms. Adults do better than children, and females fare better than males. Individuals with the nodular histologic subtype do better than patients with diffuse disease. The achievement of a complete remission provides superior survival to a partial remission; these patients in turn do better than those who have no response to therapy.

Treatment is generally systemic, involving some type of chemotherapy. For the small number of patients with truly localized disease (stage I), radiotherapy is appropriate. Laparotomy is seldom indicated in non-Hodgkin's lymphoma, since treatment is unlikely to be influenced by the results. Patients with a poor prognosis are likely to benefit from combination chemotherapy including such drugs as cyclophosphamide, doxorubicin, vincristine, prednisone, and bleomycin. Patients with favorable histology, such as the nodular type, may do just as well with less aggressive combinations (cyclophosphamide, vincristune, prednisone) or a single alkylating agent or even no therapy until symptoms develop.

About 40 per cent of those with diffuse histiocytic lymphoma treated with aggressive combination chemotherapy involving four or more drugs appear to have a long-term survival and probably are cured. Patients with certain of the more indolent lymphomas have a median survival of as long as 7 to 8 years, but they rarely, if ever, are cured.

REFERENCES

GENERAL

Boggs, D. R., and Winkelstein, A.: White Cell Manual. 4th ed. Philadelphia, F. A. Davis, 1983.
DeBruyn, P. P. H.: Structural substrates of bone marrow function. Semin. Hematol. 18:179, 1981.
DeVita, V. T., Jr., Hellman, S., and Rosenberg, S. A.: Cancer. Principles and Practice of Oncology. Philadelphia, J. B. Lippincott, 1982.
Fialkow, P. J.: Cell lineages in hematopoietic neoplasia studied with glucose-6-phosphate dehydrogenase cell markers. J. Cell Physiol. Suppl. 1:37, 1982.
Fischer, D. S., and Marsh, J. C.: Cancer Therapy, Boston, G. K. Hall, 1982.

Gallo, R. C., et al.: Review: Retroviruses as etiologic agents of some animal and human leukemias and lymphomas and as tools for elucidating the molecular mechanism of leukemogenesis. Blood 60:545, 1982.
Wintrobe, M. M., Lee, G. R., et al.: Clinical Hematology. 8th ed. Philadelphia, Lea & Febiger, 1981.

PHAGOCYTES

Bass, D. A.: Behavior of eosinophils in acute inflammation. J. Clin. Invest. 56:870, 1975.
Butterworth, A. E., and David, J. R.: Current concepts: eosinophil function. N. Engl. J. Med. 304:154, 1981.
Cline, M. J., Lehrer, R. I., Territo, M. C., and Golde, D. W.:

Monocytes and macrophages: functions and diseases. Ann. Intern. Med. *88*:78, 1978.

Fauci, A. S., Harley, J. B., Roberts, W. C., et al.: The idiopathic hypereosinophilic syndrome: Clinical, pathophysiologic and therapeutic considerations. Ann. Intern. Med. *97*:78, 1982.

Gabig, T. G., and Babior, B. M.: The killing of pathogens by phagocytes. Annu. Rev. Med. *32*:187, 1981.

Gallin, J. I., Wright, D. G., Malech, H. I., et al.: Disorders of phagocyte chemotaxis. Ann. Intern. Med. *92*:520, 1980.

Harlan, J. M., Killen, P. D., Harker, L. A., et al.: Neutrophil-mediated endothelial injury in vitro—mechanisms of cell detachment. J. Clin. Invest. *68*:1394, 1981.

Lowe, D., Jorizzo, J., and Hutt, M. S. R.: Tumour-associated eosinophilia: a review. J. Clin. Pathol. *34*:1343, 1981.

Marsh, J. C.: Chemical toxicity of the granulocyte. Environ. Health Perspect. *39*:71, 1981.

Marx, J. L.: The leukotrienes in allergy and inflammation. Science *215*:1380, 1982.

McLaren, D. J.: The role of eosinophils in tropical disease. Semin. Hematol. *19*:100, 1982.

Shiffmann, E.: Leukocyte chemotaxis. Ann. Rev. Physiol. *44*:553, 1982.

Tauber, A. L.: Current views of neutrophil dysfunction. An integrated clinical perspective. Am. J. Med. *70*:1237, 1981.

Wasserman, S. I.: The mast cell and the inflammatory response. *In* Pepys, J., and Edwards, A. M. (Eds.): The Mast Cell. Baltimore, University Park Press, 1979, pp. 9–20.

MYELOID STEM CELLS

Bertazzoni, U., et al.: Prognostic significance of terminal transferase and adenosine deaminase in acute and chronic myeloid leukemia. Blood *60*:685, 1982.

Beutler, E., McMillan, R., and Spruce, W.: Brief review: the role of bone marrow transplantation in the treatment of acute leukemia in remission. Blood *59*:1115, 1982.

Bevan, D., Rose, M., and Greaves, M.: Leukemia of platelet precursors: diverse features in four cases. Br. J. Haematol. *51*:147, 1982.

Brincker, H.: Population based age- and sex-specific incidence rates in the four main types of leukaemia. Scand. J. Haematol. *29*:241, 1982.

Buckner, C. D., Clift, R. A., and Thomas, E. D.: Bone marrow transplantation. Leuk. Res. *6*:381, 1982.

Cervantes, F., and Rozman, C.: A multivariate analysis of prognostic factors in chronic myeloid leukemia. Blood *60*:1298, 1982.

Dick, F. R., Armitage, J. O., and Burns, C. P.: Diagnostic concurrence in the subclassification of adult acute leukemia using French-American-British criteria. Cancer *49*:916, 1982.

Gaetani, G. F., Ferraris, A. M., Galiano, et al.: Primary thrombocythemia: clonal origin of platelets, erythrocytes and granulocytes in A Gd^B/Gd^{mediterranean} subject. Blood *59*:76, 1982.

Gomez, G. A., Sokal, J. E., and Walsh, D.: Prognostic features at diagnosis of chronic myelocytic leukemia. Cancer *47*:2470, 1981.

Goto, T., Nishikori, M., Arlin, Z., et al.: Growth characteristics of leukemia and leukemic and normal hematopoietic cells in Ph^{1+} chronic myelogenous leukemia and effects of intensive treatment. Blood *59*:793, 1982.

Jacobson, R. J., Salo, A., and Fialkow, P. J.: Agnogenic myeloid metaplasia: a clonal proliferation of hematopoietic stem cells with secondary myelofibrosis. Blood *51*:189, 1978.

Keating, M. J., McCredie, K. B., Bodey, G. P., et al.: Improved prospects for long-term survival in adults with acute myelogenous leukemia. J.A.M.A. *248*:2481, 1982.

Najean, Y., DeDanvic, M., and Pecking, A.: Present results of the cooperative studies on aplastic and refractory anemias. Acta Haematol. *61*:325, 1979.

Partanen, S., Ruvtu, T., and Vuopio, P.: Circulating haematopoietic progenitors in myelofibrosis. Scand. J. Haematol. *29*:325, 1982.

Rowley, J. D.: General report on the second international workshop on chromosomes in leukemia. Int. J. Cancer *26*:531, 1980.

Rowley, J. D., Alimena, G., Garson, O. M., et al.: A collaborative study of the relationship of the morphological type of acute non-lymphocytic leukemia with patient age and karyotype. Blood *59*:1013, 1982.

Sullivan, R., Quesenberry, P. J., Parkman, R., et al.: Aplastic anemia: lack of inhibitory effect of bone marrow lymphocytes on in vitro granulopoiesis. Blood *56*:625, 1980.

Thomas, E. D., Clift, R. A., and Buckner, C. D.: Marrow transplantation for patients with acute nonlymphoblastic leukemia who achieve a first remission. Cancer Treat. Rep. *66*:1463, 1982.

Van Der Reijden, H. J., Van Rhenen, D. J., Lansdorp, P. M., et al.: A comparison of surface marker analysis and FAB classification in acute myeloid leukemia. Blood *61*:443, 1983.

Weber, R. F. A., Geraedts, J. P. M., et al.: The preleukemia syndrome. I. Clinical and hematological findings. Acta Med. Scand. *207*:391, 1980.

LYMPHOCYTES

Cho, Y., and DeBruyn, P. H.: Transcellular migration of lymphocytes through the walls of the smooth-surface squamous endothelial venules in the lymph node: evidence for the direct entry of lymphocytes into the blood circulation of the lymph node. J. Ultrastruct. Res. *74*:259, 1981.

Herberman, R. B., and Ortaldo, J. R.: Natural killer cells: their ·role in defenses against disease. Science *214*:24, 1981.

Hooper, W. C., Buss, D. H., and Parker, C. L.: Leukemic reticuloendotheliosis (hairy cell leukemia): a review of the evidence concerning the immunology and origin of the cell. Leuk. Res. *4*:489, 1980.

Jansen, J., Schuit, H. R. E., Meijer, C. J. L. M., et al.: Cell markers in hairy cell leukemia studies in cells from 51 patients. Blood *59*:52, 1982.

Kay, N. E., Ackerman, S. K., and Douglas, S. D.: Anatomy of the immune system. Semin. Hematol. *16*:251, 1979.

Reinherz, E. L., and Schlossman, S. F.: Regulation of immune response—inducer and suppressor T-lymphocyte subsets in human beings. N. Engl. J. Med. *303*:370, 1980.

Rosenthal, A. S.: Regulation of the immune response—role of the macrophage. N. Engl. J. Med. *303*:1153, 1980.

Ruscetti, F. W., and Gallo, R. C.: Human T-lymphocyte growth factor: regulation of growth and function of T lymphocytes. Blood *57*:379, 1981.

Unanue, E. R.: Cooperation between mononuclear phagocytes and lymphocytes in immunity. N. Engl. J. Med. *303*:997, 1980.

Waldman, R. H., and Ganguly, R.: Role of immune mechanisms, on secretory surfaces in prevention of infection. *In* Allen, J. C. (Ed.): Infection and the Compromised Host. Baltimore, Williams & Wilkins, 1976, p. 29.

Waldmann, T. A., Blaese, R. M., Broder, S., et al.: Disorders of suppressor immunoregulatory cells in the pathogenesis of immunodeficiency and autoimmunity. Ann. Int. Med. *88*:226, 1978.

Winkelstein, A.: The anatomy and physiology of lymphocytes. *In* Lichtman, M. A. (Ed.): The Science and Practice of Clinical Medicine. Vol. 6. Hematology and Oncology. New York, Grune & Stratton, 1980, p. 165.

Zacharski, L. R., and Linman, J. W.: Lymphopenia: its causes and significance. Mayo Clin. Proc. *46*:168, 1971.

LYMPHOID NEOPLASMS

Bennett, J. M., Catovsky, D., Daniel, M. T., et al.: (The French-American-British (FAB) Co-Operative Group): The morphological classification of acute lymphoblastic leukaemia: concordance among observers and clinical correlations. Br. J. Haematol. *47*:553, 1981.

Berard, C. W., Greene, M. H., Jaffe, E. S., et al.: A multidisciplinary approach to non-Hodgkin's lymphomas. Ann. Intern. Med. *94*:218, 1981.

Berger, C. L., Morrison, S., Chu, A., et al.: Diagnosis of cutaneous T-cell lymphoma by use of monoclonal antibodies reactive with tumor-associated antigens. J. Clin. Invest. *70*:1205, 1982.

Bowman, W. P., Melvin, S., and Mauer, A. M.: Cell markers of lymphomas and leukemias. Adv. Intern. Med. *25*:391, 1980.

Brittinger, G.: Histopathology and clinical problems in non-Hodgkin lymphomas. Blut *43*:139, 1981.

Broder, S., Muul, L., Marshall, S., et al.: Neoplasms of immunoregulatory T cells in clinical investigation. J. Invest. Dermatol. *74*:267, 1980.

Camitta, B. M., Pinkel, D., et al.: Failure of early intensive chemotherapy to improve prognosis in childhood acute lymphocytic leukemia. Med. Pediatr. Oncol. *8*:383, 1980.

Colby, T. V., Hoppe, R. T., and Warnke, R. A.: Hodgkin's disease: a clinicopathologic study of 659 cases. Cancer *49*:1848, 1982.

Durie, B. G. M., Persky, B., Soehnlen, B. J., et al.: Amyloid production in human myeloma stem-cell culture, with morphologic evidence of amyloid secretion by associated macrophages. N. Engl. J. Med. *307*:1689, 1982.

Greaves, M. F.: "Target" cells, cellular phenotypes, and lineage fidelity in human leukemia. J. Cell. Physiol. Suppl 1:113, 1982.

Hoppe, R. T., Coleman, C. N., Cox, R. S., et al.: The management of stage 1-11 Hodgkin's disease with irradiation alone or combined modality therapy: The Stanford experience. Blood *59*:455, 1982.

Hubbard, S. M., Chabner, B. A., DeVita, V. T. et al.: Histologic progression in non-Hodgkin's lymphoma. Blood *59*:258, 1982.

Levine, P. H., Kamaraju, L. S., Connelly, R. R., et al.: The American Burkitt's lymphoma registry: eight years' experience. Cancer *49*:1016, 1982.

Lutzner, M., Edelson, R., Schein, P., et al.: Cutaneous T-cell lymphomas: the Sezary syndrome, mycosis fungoides, and related disorders. Ann. Intern. Med. *83*:534, 1975.

Mauer, A. M.: Review: Therapy of acute lymphoblastic leukemia in childhoood. Blood *56*:1, 1980.

McNutt, N. S., Heilbron, D. C., and Crain, W. R.: Mycosis fungoides: diagnostic criteria based on quantitative electron microscopy. Lab. Invest. *44*:466, 1981.

Portlock, C. S.: Deferral of initial therapy for advanced indolent lymphomas. Cancer Treat. Rep. *66*:417, 1982.

Rosenberg, S. A.: The non-Hodgkin's lymphoma pathologic classification project. National Cancer Institute Sponsored Study of Classification of non-Hodgkin's lymphomas: summary and description of a working formulation for clinical usage. Cancer *49*:2112, 1982.

Rozman, C., Montserrat, E., Feliu, E., et al.: Prognosis of chronic lymphocytic leukemia: a multivariant survival analysis of 150 cases. Blood *59*:1001, 1982.

Rudders, R. A.: Surface markers in non-Hodgkin's lymphoma. Hosp. Pract. *18*:161, 1982.

Skinnider, L. F., Tan, L., Schmidt, J., and Armitage, G.: Chronic lymphocytic leukemia: a review of 745 cases and assessment of clinical staging. Cancer *50*:2951, 1982.

Solanki, D. L., McCurdy, P. R., et al.: Chronic lymphocytic leukemia: a monoclonal disease. Am. J. Hematol. *13*:159, 1982.

Wiernik, P. H.: Book review. Hairy cell leukaemia, by Cawley J.C., Burns G. F., Hayhoe F. G. J. Leuk. Res. *5*:437, 1981.

23

The Erythrocyte

Carlos E. Moya, Sheila Shah,
and Thomas M. Sodeman

Primary disorders of the erythrocyte result in profound effects on human physiology. The classification of red cell diseases is based on disorders of red cell mass that may be mediated by normal or disturbed regulatory mechanisms. Increased red cell mass, or polycythemia, may be compensatory or idiopathic with altered erythropoietic regulation. Decreased red cell mass, or anemia, may be secondary to impaired production, blood loss, increased red cell destruction, or a combination of several mechanisms. The following discussion reviews the pathophysiology of these processes, and, where relevant, correlates the clinical manifestations with their pathogenesis and the pathophysiologic bases.

GENERAL ANEMIA

The definition of anemia is usually based on measures of the loss of red cell mass. The ultimate definition, however, appears to relate to a state in which oxygenation of tissue is not maintained. Such a definition then encompasses not only the loss of red cell mass but all related changes in the physiology of the system. Routine laboratory measures of red cells, hemoglobin and packed volume, may not reflect the true physiologic state. The clinical effects of the gradual loss of red cell mass, whether from hemorrhage or anemia, will be reflected in the loss of tissue oxygenation. The oxygen gradient must be maintained from central circulation to the peripheral capillary bed. In the anemic state the need to meet oxygen demands requires a greater extraction from the red cell. The arteriovenous oxygen difference increases, and the capillary oxygen tension falls. The pressure head of oxygen is therefore decreased, and the diffusion of oxygen at the terminal end is reduced. The body defense mechanisms adjust for this problem by shunting blood to increase flow and return for reoxygenation. This is partially accomplished by vasoconstriction, which in chronic anemia is directed at the skin circulation and the kidney. Increases in both pulmonary and cardiac function occur. In severe chronic anemia with hemoglobin levels below 7 g/dl, the cardiac output is increased. The rate of blood flow is increased, the circulation time shortened, and the peripheral resistance lowered. When the anemia is severe, dyspnea may occur with an increase in respiratory rate and depth. Palpitations and a bounding pulse

are frequently found. Cardiac murmurs, usually systolic, are encountered. The oxygen affinity of red cells is also altered. This change appears to be related to an increase in 2,3-diphosphoglycerate (2,3-DPG). Hemoglobin's ability to discharge oxygen is increased in the presence of 2,3-DPG. The bonding site for 2,3-DPG is in a central cavity formed by the N-termini of the beta chains. The level of 2,3-DPG is almost equimolar with hemoglobin. Its oxygen affinity binds it to hemoglobin in the deoxygenated state, reducing the affinity of hemoglobin for oxygen by forming a bridge between the subunits stabilizing the T configuration. As the 2,3-DPG level falls (for example, in the storage of blood), oxygen is less easily given up from hemoglobin (oxygen-tissue exchange is discussed in detail in Chapter 15). Why 2,3-DPG levels increase as a response to anemia is unclear. Proposed reasons are a shift to an alkaline intracellular pH with the greater deoxygenation of blood and increased production as more 2,3-DPG is bound to deoxygenated hemoglobin. The role of 2,3-DPG in compensating for anemia appears critical and can be equivalent to an increase in cardiac output or in hemoglobin. The response of the marrow to anemia—to return the red cell mass to the optimum level—can bring the physiologic processes back into balance. The ideal hematocrit involves the influences of the appropriate number of red cells for oxygen-tissue exchange and the influence of increasing viscosity of blood as the hematocrit increases. The increasing viscosity, associated with decreased blood flow, hampers oxygen exchange. The optimum point between viscosity, hematocrit, and oxygen exchange will vary for each person.

HEMOGLOBIN FUNCTION

Hemoglobin has four sites for oxygen binding. These sites lie in a crevice associated with the globin chain and controlled by two histidine molecules. One gram of hemoglobin can bind a maximum of 1.39 ml of oxygen. A plot of the partial pressure of oxygen against the percentage of hemoglobin gives a sigmoid curve. The oxygen affinity of hemoglobin is expressed as the oxygen tension at which half of the hemoglobin is saturated, P_{50}. For the normal red cell this is 26 mm Hg. High P_{50} levels reflect a low affinity for oxygen. In arterial blood, hemoglobin is almost fully saturated. Approximately 25 per cent of the oxygen is removed by tissues, the hemoglobin returning to the lung 75 per cent saturated. The binding at each of the four sites in the hemoglobin molecule influences the others. As each unit is bonded to oxygen, the strength of the next bonding is increased. The steep slope of the sigmoid curve reflects the small change in partial pressure required as oxygen is released from hemoglobin. In essence, the saturation of hemoglobin changes more rapidly with changes in partial pressure than it would if each binding site operated independently. In addition pH, carbon dioxide, and temperature all are biologically important in oxygen binding. Both acidity and increasing concentration of carbon dioxide enhance the release of oxygen and increase the P_{50}. The effect of pH on oxygen affinity is known as the Bohr effect. The lowering of pH results in stabilization of the T configuration and a lower oxygen affinity. Such a fall in pH is encountered as blood passes through the peripheral circulation in metabolically active tissues. The reverse occurs in the lung, where the pH rise improves the uptake of oxygen. High levels of oxygen force hemoglobin to unload carbon dioxide. Binding of oxygen to hemoglobin results in changes in the quaternary structure. The hemoglobin tetramer in deoxygenated hemoglobin is stabilized by intersubunit salt bonds as well as hydrogen bonds. This configuration is commonly referred to as the T, or taut, configuration. It has a low oxygen affinity. Iron must be brought into the plane of the porphyrin to form a strong bond with oxygen. The $alpha_2$-$beta_2$ dimer rotates relative to the $alpha_1$-$beta_1$ dimer. This rotation narrows the cavity for 2,3-DPG, preventing its binding. Prior to the quaternary changes, tertiary structural changes in the subunits take place. Upon oxygenation of one subunit of hemoglobin, they are transmitted to the other subunits. The eight salt links between the four subunits of deoxygenated hemoglobin must be broken for iron to move up in the plane for maximum oxygen binding. The molecule is said to form an R configuration, or relaxed mode. With binding of the first oxygen molecule, more salt links must be broken to permit entry of oxygen. With acquisition of each subsequent oxygen molecule, fewer salt links must be broken. Less energy is required with each oxygen molecule, accounting for the sigmoid dissociation curve. The binding of one oxygen molecule then makes the likelihood of binding a second greater. A right shift in the oxygen dissociation curve occurs in most types of anemia.

Certain inherited abnormal hemoglobins are associated with increased affinity for oxygen. This results in a relative anoxia with stimulation of erythropoietin. The red cell mass is increased and problems of viscosity may be encountered. More than 40 different high-affinity hemoglobins have been reported. The substitutions in the molecule occur near the C-terminal of the globin chain and

disrupt the configurational change in hemoglobin associated with oxygen release. Low-affinity hemoglobins have also been reported. These defects are in a similar region of the molecule. The patients present with chronic cyanosis; the red cell mass, however, is usually normal.

Besides changes in tissue oxygenation and blood volume, anemias are accompanied by a variety of signs and symptoms. Marrow adjustment to the anemia may be sufficient for the patient to avoid experiencing any symptoms; when the hemoglobin level falls below 8 g/dl, however, symptoms usually begin to appear. Cardiopulmonary adjustments have already been referred to earlier. Pallor of skin and mucous membranes, headaches, vertigo, and muscle weakness are common in severe anemia. A hemolytic process may be accompanied by jaundice, splenomegaly, cholelithiasis, and leg ulcers.

ACUTE BLOOD LOSS

The initial threat of acute blood loss is decreased blood volume. This occurs with the loss of more than 30 per cent of blood volume. For the 70 kg normal man, this is equal to 1500 ml of blood. Sudden loss of this amount of blood leads to circulatory collapse manifested by a fall in cardiac output and signs of shock. Tachycardia and postural hypotension, early signs of acute blood loss, appear with a loss of 1000 ml, or approximately 20 per cent of blood volume. These signs are usually present only with exertion. The sudden loss of less than 1000 ml of blood for an average man will not cause symptoms. Loss of more than 50 per cent of blood volume is accompanied by severe shock and, without intervention, may result in death. Ability to withstand severe hemorrhage is obviously dependent on the state of health of the patient prior to the bleed. The cardiovascular response can be seriously hampered by cardiac or vascular insufficiency. The body responds to the blood loss by mobilization of extravascular albumin. Because of the combined loss of both red cell mass and plasma, the relative hematocrit may give a false impression of the extent of the loss. As the body gradually replaces fluid over 2 to 3 days following hemorrhage, the hematocrit will fall to reflect the true loss of red cell mass. In gradual blood loss, this adjustment is continuous and the hematocrit provides a reasonable picture of the red cell mass. With the loss of red cell mass in acute hemorrhage, the need to maintain tissue oxygenation is controlled by adjustments in cardiovascular dynamics that send blood to the oxygen-sensitive tissues. This is reflected in the signs of shock and cold clammy skin. Erythropoietin levels rapidly increase following the bleeding episode. While the effect of erythropoietin is to stimulate the marrow, there is no immediate pool of mature red cells to replenish those lost. The response then is gradual over several days as red cells mature in the marrow and are released into the circulation. The stimulated premature delivery of reticulocytes can be seen in a peripheral smear. Erythroid hyperplasia is evident in the marrow in 2 days, peaking at 8 to 10 days. The intensity of the marrow response usually reflects the degree of anemia, assuming iron availability is not a limiting factor. Under normal conditions the marrow will respond by a two- or threefold increase. In cases of slow gradual bleeding, iron can become a major limiting factor in the ability of the marrow to maintain its response. Under these circumstances the marrow will be unable to maintain the increased production and may fall behind the loss of red cell mass. With iron therapy, marrow response can be maintained and exceed the normal response by a twofold increase.

RED CELL MEMBRANE

The ability to free the red cell membrane from other cellular elements has provided an ideal tool for study of membrane architecture. The red cell membrane consists of lipids and proteins arranged to provide a highly selective, permeable barrier essential to the regulation of intracellular constituents. Like that of other cells, the red cell membrane controls the flow of information between the cell and its environment. This is accomplished through molecular pumps and gates as well as specific receptors on the membrane surface. The membrane is in essence its own microcosm. It is composed of approximately 50 per cent protein, 40 per cent lipid, and 10 per cent carbohydrate.

BASIC MEMBRANE MODEL

The basic model of the red cell membrane has primarily been developed through biochemical analysis and a varied electron micrographic approach. The red cell membrane is approximately 800 nm thick. The outer layer consists of a lipid bilayer in which the phosphoric acid moieties form the outer and inner molecular surfaces. In the need to conserve energy by the hydrocarbon or fatty acid hydrophobic chains, these hydrophilic components are forced outward. The bilayer clustering of the lipid components minimizes the number of exposed hydrophobic units in a water environment. The hydrophobic interactions are favored by their clustering and are critical for the formation of the lipid bilayer. Phospholipids and nonesterified cholesterol are key constituents, forming 95 per cent of the total lipids, which include small amounts of glycolipids and free fatty acids. The molecular arrangement has the decided advantage of tending to be self-sealing with very little permeability for ions and polar groups. The high protein content of the red cell will exert osmotic effects

that result in water influx and ultimately red cell lysis. This is prevented by active transport systems that regulate ion distribution.

MEMBRANE LIPIDS

Biochemical analysis of the red cell membrane demonstrates a variety of lipids (Table 23–1). While triacyglycerol and diol derivatives have been identified, they do not appear to play the major role that phosphoglycerides, sphingolipids, and nonesterified cholesterol play. The phosphoglycerides have glycerol molecules to which a phosphoric acid is esterified at the alpha carbon, forming the polar head, and two long-chain fatty acids forming the hydrophobic tails. Attached to the phosphodiester bridge are common alcohol moieties choline, ethanolamine, serine, and inositol in descending percentages.

Lysophosphatides represent a group of phospholipids with one fatty acid group. These have both lipophilic and hydrophilic characteristics that make them ideal at fluid interfaces. Red cell membranes contain only small amounts of lysophosphatides. Mechanisms are available to control their level in the membrane, without which membrane distortion occurs, echinocyte and spherocyte forms develop, and hemolysis may result. Sphingomyelin contains sphingosine instead of glycerol. This amino alcohol is linked to two fatty acids. The primary hydroxyl group of sphingosine is esterified to phosphoryl choline. Some sphingomyelin molecules have sugar moieties attached rather than choline, forming glycolipids. These amphipathic lipids with their polar heads at the aqueous interface form a very stable structure held together by noncovalent interactions. Water is essentially excluded from the inner hydrophobic units. These lipid molecules appear to be in a fluid state. A single lipid may diffuse rapidly in the plane of the membrane, unless fixed for specific purposes. Movement from one side of the membrane to the other, however, is a very slow process. This creates an asymmetric distribution of lipids between the inner and outer layers. The hydrophobic nature of the tails tends to prevent the flip-flop of the polar head. Phosphoglycerides, phosphatidylcholine and sphingomyelin tend to be lo-

TABLE 23–1 RED CELL MEMBRANE LIPID CONTENT

Lipid	Per Cent
Cholesterol	25
Glycolipids	15
Phospholipids	60
Phosphatidylcholine	30
Phosphatidylserine	14
Phosphatidylethanolamine	28
Sphingomyelin	25

cated in the outer leaflet, while phosphatidyl-ethanolamine, inositol, and serine tend to be on the inner leaflet, creating an excess positive charge on the inner surface. The asymmetry may play a role in the relationship between lipids and the inner protein network. Cholesterol appears evenly distributed between the inner and outer lipid layers and is important in providing a degree of rigidity to the membrane. Cooper has discussed the effect of cholesterol in the red blood cell membrane on the cell shape in disease. Increasing cholesterol in the membrane produces a less fluid layer. In severe liver disease with an associated increase in cholesterol, acanthocytes result. The mature red cell cannot de novo synthesize lipids, but turnover and reuse mechanisms exist. Some equilibrium exists between plasma lipids and the membrane components, so plasma levels can influence the cell membrane as in the case of phosphatidylcholine. Red cell cholesterol appears to be in equilibrium with plasma unesterified cholesterol.

MEMBRANE PROTEIN

Membrane proteins have been analyzed by sodium dodecylsulfate digestion and polyacrylamide-gel electrophoresis. They have been grouped into peripheral and integral types. The peripheral proteins are loosely bound by hydrogen and electrostatic bonds. The integral proteins, thought to be globular, require strong agents to be released and are bound with the hydrocarbon units (Fig. 23–1). The integral proteins include bands 3, 7, and all PAS bands (Table 23–2). They lie in the lipid bilayer. The peripheral proteins, bands 1, 2, 4.1, 4.2, 5, and 6, appear to be weakly bound to the surface of the integral proteins, where they form a latticework on the inner surface of the lipid layer. Spectrin, bands 1 and 2, along with bands 4.1, 4.2, and 5, probably stabilizes and to a certain extent shapes the red cell membrane. Spectrin accounts for about 35 per cent of membrane protein. In the absence of the protein network, the red cell is spherical. Pathophysiologic abnormalities in this network account for some of the hereditary hemolytic anemias to be discussed later. Integral proteins, about 40 per cent of total membrane protein, are seen as globular masses in the inner membrane on freeze-etch electron microscopic studies. Usually lipoproteins, they interact extensively with the hydrocarbon chains of the membrane lipids. A major integral protein, glycophorin A, is a transmembrane protein relatively free of lipids and associated with enzymatic activity. This protein, PAS 1, contains carbohydrate units that extend outside the membrane and has a hydrophobic region in the membrane and a terminal carboxyl portion projecting into the cell. Its function is unknown. Band 3 provides an anion channel essential for CO_2 transport and permeability to HCO^{3-} and Cl^-. There are 10 molecules of band 3 for each complex of spectrin 1 and 2, and about 200 lipid molecules for each unit of band 3.

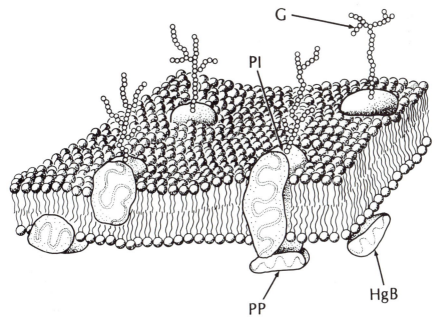

Figure 23–1 Diagrammatic representation of red cell membrane architecture. The membrane lipid bilayers with polar heads project to the surface. Imbedded in the membrane are integral proteins (PI) to which carbohydrates (G) are attached along the external surface. Peripheral proteins (PP) form a latticework on the inner surface. Hemoglobin (HgB) may attach to the inner surface.

TABLE 23–2 RED CELL MEMBRANE PROTEINS

Band	Name	Molecular Weight	Type
1	Spectrin	240,000	Peripheral
2	Spectrin	235,000	Peripheral
2.1	Ankyrin	195,000	Peripheral
3	Anion channel	88,000	Integral
4.1,4.2	Protein kinase	78,000, 72,000	Peripheral
5	Actin	43,000	Peripheral
6	Glyceraldehyde-3-	35,000	Peripheral
7	phosphate dehydrogenase	29,000	Integral
PAS 1	Glycophorin	55,000	Integral
PAS 2	———	55,000	Integral
PAS 3	———	———	Integral
PAS 4	———	———	Integral

Protein enzyme systems exist to control sodium-potassium movement across the membrane and to regulate calcium. The ATPase system for sodium-potassium has about 200 to 400 sites per cell. The system pumps sodium out of the cell while pumping potassium into the cell and is activated by either ion. This pump is a transmembrane protein composed of two subunits. The channel is not available to divalent cations or anions. Movement of sodium out and potassium in is associated with a configuration change in the protein carrier molecule. Sodium reacts with the channel, causing phosphorylation of ATPase by ATP, while potassium causes dephosphorylation. Three sodium and two potassium ions are transported per ATP hydrolyzed. The process is tightly coupled so that sodium and potassium must be present to hydrolyze the ATP. The hydrolysis site is on the inner side of the membrane. Numerous enzymes are also attached to or are part of the red cell membrane. Band 6, glyceraldehyde-3-phosphate dehydrogenase, is the most common membrane enzyme and is also present in the cytoplasm of the red cell.

Glycoproteins are mostly found on the exterior surface of the membrane and are important in maintaining the asymmetry of the membrane. The sugar residues are attached to the side chains of proteins. They clearly play a vital role in cell recognition and account for the negative charge on the exterior of the cell. The carbohydrate chains that extend from glycophorin A, accounting for PAS bands 1 and 2, form the A, B, and H substance of blood group antigens. Acetylcholinesterase is another glycoprotein located on the surface of the red cell. It is an externally oriented enzyme. Its activity is decreased in paroxysmal nocturnal hemoglobinuria and autoimmune hemolytic anemia. The protein element thus provides structure, recognition, transport, and enzymatic activity. The filamentous helical protein spectrin appears to be bound with hemoglobin.

RED CELL SHAPE

After extrusion of the nucleus the polychromatophilic normoblast II matures as a reticulocyte in the marrow for 24 hours and is released into the circulation. Electron microscopy demonstrates that no endoplasmic reticulum remains, though mitochondria, ribosomes, and Golgi vesicles are found. This cell, slightly larger (10 μm) than the mature red cell, synthesizes its remaining hemoglobin and over the next 24 to 48 hours gets rid of unnecessary organelles by autophagy. The mature red cell with a life span of 100 to 120 days is biconcave, 7.5 to 8.3 μm in diameter, 2.5 μm at its maximum thickness, and has a surface area of 160 μm. At least a 5 to 10 per cent variation is expected among the red cell population. The basic shape depends on a variety of influences, including the surrounding milieu, surface tension, membrane elasticity, age, and metabolic status. In an energy-deprived system, the red cell will assume a spherical shape. The normal disc shape provides an excellent ratio of surface to volume, facilitating gas transfer. The ability to deform depends on the flexibility of the membrane, the geometry of the cell, and the internal viscosity. Fragmentation will occur if the cell surface is stretched by more than 5 per cent. Cellular dehydration due to water or ion loss can raise the usual low viscosity of hemoglobin and alter the deformability of the red cell. Studies of the biconcave shape suggest that shape dependency is partially based on ATP-calcium interaction. ATP provides a protective effect by preventing calcium-induced changes in the contractile protein elements of the membrane and prevents a sol-gel effect on proteins and hemoglobin. Calcium appears to be membrane-based in the red cell. A gradient is maintained between the outside and inside by a calcium-ATP pump different from the sodium-potassium pump. The inside of the red cell contains little, if any, calcium. The calcium pump is ATP-dependent and is located on the inner surface of the membrane. The pump plays no role in maintaining the inner membrane calcium level but rather controls cytoplasmic levels. Increased red cell cytoplasmic calcium is deleterious to the cell, reacting with membrane proteins to increase the rigidity of the cell wall. Excess calcium also causes potassium to leak, resulting in increased viscosity. ATP competes with membrane protein for calcium. Declining levels of ATP are accompanied by increased calcium membrane binding and loss of elasticity. Responding to the stresses of flow, red cells may assume a variety of shapes, at times catching along the endothelial surface to stretch out like teardrops. A red cell is capable of squeezing through holes one twentieth its size. With aging the red cell undergoes fragmentation and a slow loss of membrane, becoming spherocytic in shape. The loss of flexibility and the exhaustion of metabolic processes, including ATP, which contributes to the rigidity through its influence on calcium, are recognized by the reticuloendothelial system, and the cell is removed from circulation. This picture is far from clear, as studies have demonstrated that little lipid is lost in the last half of the red cell's life. While the spleen is a major site of removal of old red cells, splenectomy does not affect the life span of cells.

ECHINOCYTE—DISCOCYTE—STOMATOCYTE

The transformation to a series of classic shapes recognized in peripheral blood smears and associated with specific abnormalities has been studied intensely. In Table 23–3 the standard nomenclature for these red cell shapes is presented. The biconcave red cell, the discocyte, is converted through a series of stages to an echinocyte or stomatocyte. The volume of the cell is not altered in this process, and the conversion is reversible in the early stages. In the final stages, the red cell transforms to a spherocyte. In the in vivo state echinocytes have been associated with

TABLE 23–3 NOMENCLATURE OF RED CELL SHAPES

Specific Name	Synonyms
Acanthocyte	Spur cell
Codocyte	Target, hat
Dacryocyte	Teardrop, poikilocyte
Discocyte	Biconcave
Drepanocyte	Sickle
Echinocyte	Burr, crenated
Elliptocyte	Ovalocyte
Leptocyte	Thin cell
Schizocyte	Helmet, fragmented
Spherocyte	Sphere
Stomatocyte	Cup, mouth

uremia, peptic ulcers, neonatal liver disease, pyruvate-kinase deficiency, and carcinoma. Lysolecithins are known to induce echinocytes in vitro. Echinocyte production in aged plasma has been postulated to be based on decreases in cell ATP, increases in calcium, and the membrane content of lysophosphatides. The tonicity of the surrounding environment plays little role.

The stomatocyte forms from a discocyte through a series of transformation steps and in its end stage forms a spherocyte. It can be induced by a number of chemical agents, low pH, and a decrease in ATP. Stomatocytes are also associated with Rh null cells, immune anemias, hydrocytosis, and a hereditary autosomal dominant stomatocytosis. In the last named, movement of sodium into the red cell is increased in relation to potassium movement out. With sodium, water is drawn into the cell. The membrane defect responsible for the increase in sodium permeability is unclear. Osmotic fragility is increased, and glucose consumption rapid. At times a reverse pump change occurs, resulting in increased viscosity that may contribute to hemolysis. The anemia is probably based on splenic trapping of abnormal cells. Splenectomy, however, will not cure the anemia.

ABNORMAL RED CELL SHAPES

Poikilocyte indicates a variable-shaped red cell. Many of these shapes have their pathophysiologic origin in biochemical abnormalities of the membrane or metabolic process within the cell. Acanthocytes are red cells with 3 to 12 spicules of uneven length versus the 10 to 30 of echinocytes. The mechanism of formation is unknown. The cell volume, life span, contents, and osmotic fragility appear normal. Acanthocytes are associated with abetalipoproteinemia, liver disease, particularly alcoholic cirrhosis, and disorders of lipid metabolism. Studies of red cells from patients with abetalipoproteinemia have not defined a clear-cut lipid membrane disorder associated with the plasma abnormalities. Cholesterol and phospholipid contents of red cells are normal or vary only slightly. The sphingomyelin level, however, is increased in respect to lecithin and may account for the increased rigidity. Normal red cells transfused into a patient become abnormal, and this change is not reversible. The red cells from patients with severe liver disease demonstrate an increase in membrane cholesterol and a shortening of the life span, possibly due to increased rigidity. Phospholipids are normal quantitatively; however, relative changes in the amount of specific lipid types are found. No abnormality of glycolysis or permeability has been demonstrated. Osmotic fragility is normal, and autohemolysis is increased and not corrected by glucose or ATP. As opposed to acanthocytes, the spur cells associated with liver disease have an increase in lecithin and a decrease in sphingomyelin. Similar changes are seen in target cells. The increased exposure of the red cell to the increased free cholesterol in the plasma results in an imbalance in membrane lipid. Transfused red cells will acquire the same defect. During passage through the spleen, the spur cells lose membrane and are slowly removed, giving rise to the anemia.

Dacryocytes are pear-shaped or teardrop-shaped red cells that occur in fibrotic states of the marrow, hemolytic anemia in thalassemia, and as a result of certain drugs. Their origin is thought to be in the pitting function involved in removing red cell inclusions. The cells are stretched beyond their ability to reconform. Even following hemolysis, they do not return to their biconcave shape.

Codocytes, bell-shaped red cells when seen in peripheral smears, appear as targets. The form develops from excess membrane or a decrease in hemoglobin that results in a relative membrane increase. The life span of the cell varies with the pathologic condition responsible. Codocytes are associated with thalassemia, hemoglobinopathies, and iron deficiency anemia. They also appear with lipid abnormalities associated with obstructive liver disease and cirrhosis. There is an increase in membrane cholesterol. Lecithin levels are also increased, so the microviscosity of the membrane is not greatly altered as in acanthocytes. Sphingomyelin is decreased. Leptocytes and microcytes also are seen in circumstances in which membrane is increased.

Macrocytes, red cells greater than 100 μm^3, result from premature release of red cells, usually in periods of erythropoietic stress. Because of the stress element they are to be expected in hemolytic anemias and hyperthyroidism. They are also seen in circumstances in which accelerated hemoglobin synthesis occurs, as in megaloblastic anemia. Microcytes represent red cells less than 80 μm^3 and are found in iron deficiency anemia related to a decrease in hemoglobin. They occur in metabolic disorders such as pyruvate-kinase deficiency in which ATP is decreased and fluid balance is upset in the red cell.

Schizocytes, fragmented red cells, result from membrane damage. The usual mechanism involves trapping of red cells in the circulation by fibrin. As the red cell is forced past the obstruction, it fractures. The membrane, if not irreparably damaged, self-seals. If damage is severe, a spheroschizocyte develops and is rapidly removed by the spleen or liver. Osmotic fragility is increased, and the cells are microcytic because of membrane loss. They are associated with microangiopathic anemia, thrombotic thrombocytopenic purpura, disseminated intravascular coagulation, mechanical problems of vascular disease, valve prostheses, and march hemoglobinuria.

SPHEROCYTOSIS

Spherocytes are red cells with increased central thickness. They are usually not truly spherical until just prior to lysis. Membrane depletion, accelerated aging from pathologic processes, immune hemolytic anemia, heredity, and hydrocytosis are the major causes of spherocytes. In hereditary spherocytosis the cause of their formation is unknown. Not all the red cells in the peripheral circulation will be spherocytic. The total lipid content of the membrane appears to be decreased, though the relative ratios between lipid types are normal. An abnormality of lipid and protein may be responsible but is not yet explained. While a specific quantitative protein abnormality has yet to be defined, there appears to be a functional metabolic problem. As discussed earlier, the membrane proteins are intimately involved in maintaining permeability of the membrane and the osmotic regulation of the cell. Anions and water pass freely, while permeability to cations and glucose is controlled. This requires an energy-dependent system in which ATP and calcium play vital roles. The energy is derived from glucose. Without glucose the red cell will slowly swell as sodium influx increases and ATP level drops. It appears that in the red cell in hereditary spherocytosis there is an acceleration of metabolic processes, possibly to compensate for increased permeability of the membrane. Glucose is used at a high rate in the glycolytic pathway. Sodium leaking into the cell because of increased permeablity must be pumped out. The increased need for ATP may be the stimulus for the glycolytic pathway. The deformability of the membrane is associated with membrane protein. The ATP-calcium link discussed earlier, if altered, can result in calcium accumulation, which upon binding to membrane protein, decreases elasticity. In hereditary spherocytosis the elasticity is lessened even at normal ATP levels. Other membrane protein abnormalities have been suggested. The specific nature of the protein defect remains elusive; it is thought to be the cause of the membrane defect. The shortened life span of the red cell is directly related to splenic removal. In the spleen the spherocyte, less able to deform because of the altered ratio of surface area to volume and the decreased elasticity, appears to take longer to traverse the splenic circulation. The spleen has two circulation paths, one in which cells pass through rapidly, accounting for 75 per cent of the flow, and a second path that is slow. The reduced pH and glucose during the stasis compounds the metabolic problems of the cell, so repeated exposure in the spleen results in a subpopulation of true spheroidal cells with less cell membrane and greater osmotic fragility. This population of true spheroidal cells is not found in patients after removal of the spleen. Normal cells transfused into a patient with hereditary spherocytosis have a normal life span, showing that the defect is not acquired but intrinsic to the cell. As an autosomal dominant non–sex-linked transmitted disease, it affects both sexes equally. Variations in the degree of penetrance and expression are found. The disease is expressed as a hemolytic anemia with jaundice and increased bone marrow erythropoiesis. The anemia depends on the degree of bone marrow compensation. The spherocytic nature of the red cells can be demonstrated by the osmotic fragility test in which cells exposed to a hypotonic medium are more quickly hemolyzed owing to their already spherical shape than are normal cells. Depending on the number of cells already in a full spheroidal shape, a bimodal population may be found. Splenectomy provides a permanent cure of the anemia.

ELLIPTOCYTOSIS

Elliptocytes are oval cells that vary in form from slightly spherical to rodlike. The mechanism of formation is unclear. The cells assume a more elliptical shape as they age. As in spherocytes, there appears to be a membrane defect that leads to increased metabolic activity and use of ATP. Glycolytic processes and hemoglobin are normal. It has been noted that, at bends in the cells, there is a greater concentration of cholesterol. No other lipid abnormality has been found. The disease is transmitted equally to both sexes as an autosomal dominant trait. In some families, it appears to be linked to the Rh blood group. Up to 15 per cent of the cells in a normal patient may be elliptocytes, while in elliptocytosis 25 per cent or more will be abnormal. The anemia is mild.

BIOCHEMISTRY OF THE RED CELL

The dominant component of the red cell cytoplasm is hemoglobin. Biochemically, the basic role of the cell is to maintain the function of hemoglobin and the integrity of the cell membrane. The mature red cell has lost its nucleus and most of its organelles. It is not able to produce proteins or lipids de novo, although systems to reuse lipids are available. The mature cell lacks a tricarboxylic acid cycle, a major source of energy in a cell. The ability to synthesize DNA is lost early in development in the polychromatophilic normoblast stage. RNA synthesis is detectable until the orthochromatic stage because of the ability of the mechanism to restore RNA. With this, protein synthesis carries on into the reticulocyte stage. The basic synthesis of protein is no different than in other cells reviewed earlier in the core section of the book. Upon maturation, the cell enters the

circulation without the ability to produce more protein or enzymes for its life.

PURINE METABOLISM

The production of ATP is critical to the red cell, as seen in the discussions of the red cell membrane. Red cells incubated in systems that reduce ATP lose their control of the membrane systems and with that their osmotic regulation. The cells accumulate sodium and lose potassium. The major source of ATP in the mature red cell is the glycolytic pathway (anaerobic glycolysis) discussed in the first chapter of this book. The hexose monophosphate shunt (HMP), an oxidative pathway, is also active; but the electron transport systems are absent, as no mitochondria remain in the mature red cell. While certain enzymatic steps are intact for purine synthesis in the red cell, key steps in the pathway are lacking. The production of adenosine nucleotides is limited to salvage pathways. The adenine nucleotide salvage pathway requires phosphoribosyl pyrophosphate (PRPP) derived from the HMP shunt; in the presence of adenine and phosphoribosyl transferase, PRPP reacts to give rise to AMP. A second pathway involves conversion of adenosine to AMP by the action of adenosine kinase. The purine adenine may be derived from plasma or liver. Adenosine can pass the red cell membrane by both active and passive mechanisms to feed the salvage pathway. Extensive studies in the preservation of blood for transfusion have demonstrated that ATP levels fall during storage while the levels of ADP and AMP increase. Irreversible changes will occur in time. As ATP levels decrease, glucose conversion to lactate, and therefore ATP production, becomes further impaired. The salvage pathways to produce nucleotides sustain ATP by providing adenine in storage solutions. Blood stored with adenine can sustain itself for at least 35 days. The decrease in ATP during storage is associated with a loss of membrane lipid, an increase in membrane rigidity, and transformation of red cells to spherocytes. As ATP levels fall, ATP-calcium balance is altered, with increasing binding of membrane protein spectin by calcium and a loss of deformability. Adenine can sustain red cells in storage for at least 4 to 8 weeks. The production of ATP by the glycolytic pathway is essential to the integrity of the red cell. Hereditary abnormalities of purine in the red cell have been reported. A dominantly transmitted hyperactive form of adenosine deaminase has been described in which adenosine is irreversibly converted to inosine. Patients with this disorder have lowered levels of ATP as the adenosine is diverted from conversion by adenosine kinase to ATP by the hyperactive adenosine deaminase. Adenosine deaminase deficiency has also been reported with the reverse effect of increased adenine nucleotide levels. It is inherited as an autosomal recessive trait and results in the clinical picture of combined immunodeficiency disease. The enzyme deficiency is found in red cells and lymphocytes.

PYRIMIDINE METABOLISM

The synthesis of pyrimidine nucleotides, nicotinamide adenine dinucleotide (NAD^+) and nicotinamide adenine dinucleotide phosphate ($NADP^+$) is essential for the glycolytic process. As with purines, pyrimidine nucleotides are not synthesized de novo in the red cell, but a salvage mechanism involving pyrimidine phosphoribosyl transferase is available by conversion of pyrimidine to the nucleotide. Orota, uracil, and thymine, but not cytosine, can be used as substrates. Pyrimidine nucleoside kinase also provides a salvage mechanism by diverting nucleosides from degradation to pyrimidine nucleotide. Both hereditary and acquired deficiencies of pyrimidine nucleotidase have been reported. A hemolytic anemia occurs in the homozygous deficiency of pyrimidine-5'-nucleotidase (PN) deficiency that is accentuated by lead exposure. Beutler (1979) proposed that this is one of the most common hereditary red cell enzyme deficiencies. The anemia is chronic and ongoing, with a distinctive feature of basophilic stippling of red cells. Pyridine nucleotides that would normally be dephosphorylated by PN and diffused from the red cell build up during maturation. The impaired cellular processing of RNA by the reticulocyte results in basophilic stippling. Patients usually develop enlarged spleens. In the acquired form, exposure to lead inactivates pyrimidine-5'-nucleotidase, resulting in the same basophilic stippling seen in the hereditary form. The basophilic stippling appears to be altered ribosomes. Hemolysis and the shortened red cell life span may be due to suppression of ATP and related functions. The accumulation of pyrimidine nucleotides accompanies reduction in the ATP pool. Abnormalities in pyrimidine nucleotide occur in association with other enzyme defects. In glucose-6-phosphate dehydrogenase deficiency, concentrations of $NADP^+$ are increased with the reduction of the HMP shunt and the decreased capacity to reduce $NADP^+$ to NADPH.

GLYCOLYTIC PATHWAY

Besides maintenance of the membrane and membrane systems, energy is essential to keep iron in the divalent form and enzymes and hemoglobin reduced. The glycolytic, or Embden-Meyerhof, pathway was discussed in the first chapter, and the details will not be reviewed again. In essence glucose, which enters the red cell by a carrier system, is converted to lactate anaerobically with a net yield of two moles of ATP. Certain critical points need to be discussed in relation to the red cell. The red cell does not require insulin actually to enter the cell. There are approximately 30,000 glucose binding sites on the red cell associated with protein band 3. Between the conversion of 1-3 diphosphoglyceride and 3-P-glycerate is a branch that bypasses production of one ATP with conversion to 2,3-diphosphoglycerate (2,3-DPG). Glucose passing through the 2,3-DPG pathway has no net increase in ATP. The limiting enzyme step is very pH-dependent, so with an acid pH hydrogen ions inhibit the enzyme and 2,3-DPG levels fall. As will be discussed later, 2,3-DPG plays a critical role in oxygen transfer in the red cell. The reduction of NAD^+ to NADH in the glyceraldehyde-3-phosphate conversion assists in reducing methemoglobin to hemoglobin. The end products, pyruvate and lactate, diffuse out of the red cell. A major rate-limiting factor in glucose utilization is the hexokinase step. Hexokinase is susceptible to product inhibition by glucose-6-phosphate (G6P). Such inhibition within the red cell may occur when the pH falls below 7.0 as G6P accumulates secondary to inhibition of phosphofructokinase. Hexokinase is also the most age-dependent enzyme in the pathway. Approximately 95 per cent of glucose is metabolized via the anaerobic pathway. This pathway yields 75 per cent of the available red cell energy. In addition, both fructose and mannose can be converted to enter the glycolytic pathway and provide energy.

HEXOSE MONOPHOSPHATE SHUNT

The hexose monophosphate shunt, also discussed in detail in the first chapter, provides an alternate pathway for glucose metabolism. Under in vitro circumstances 10 per cent of G6P passes through the HMP shunt. No high-energy phosphate bonds are produced; however, reducing energy in the form of NADPH is produced. HMP is critical for reduction of glutathione to protect hemoglobin against methemoglobin formation and oxidative denaturation. It also prevents oxidation of critical sulfhydryl groups on membrane proteins. The relative activity of the HMP shunt is governed by the availability of $NADP^+$, the level of which is controlled in part by the oxidation-reduction state of glutathione. Reduced glutathione (GSH) plays a vital role in reduction of the hydrogen peroxide that may accumulate in the red cell. Hydrogen peroxide is converted to water by the action of glutathione peroxidase. Glutathione also reduces sulfhydryl groups on proteins, enzymes, and hemoglobin that have become oxidized. The oxidized form of glutathione (GSSH) can be reduced to GSH by glutathione reductase with NADPH serving as an electron donor. It can also leave the cell by active transport. Normally, the HMP shunt is relatively inactive but may be stimulated in stress situations or by an oxidizing drug or agent. Glutathione has a short half-life, a turnover rate of 4 days. Its synthesis requires glutamic acid, cysteine, glycine, ATP, and the enzyme glutathione synthetase. NADPH and GSH may serve as electron donors in the presence of methylene blue for the reduction of methemoglobin. Glutathione appears essential for stabilization of red cell proteins, promptly reversing oxidative changes that may occur by offering a preferential substrate. NADPH is also essential in preventing oxidative injury to detoxifying oxidant compounds. In the absence of a functional HMP shunt, there is disruption in the intracellular reducing mechanisms and a failure to maintain GSH levels. Hydrogen peroxides and other oxidants that build up form insoluble complexes with hemoglobin (Heinz bodies), result in excessive amounts of oxidized ferric-porphyrine complexes (methemoglobin), and oxidize the sulfhydryl groups on proteins important for cell wall integrity. While the red cell has high levels of catalase that would be expected to detoxify H_2O_2, catalase appears ineffective at the low levels of H_2O_2 generated in the red cell. At low levels of H_2O_2, detoxification occurs through the glutathione-mediated pathway.

RED CELL AGING

The death of red cells ultimately appears to be based on a number of events. The reduction in protein, lipids, and other compounds in the aging red cell provides one basis for death. As already discussed, the red cell has little or no capability for forming many vital substances in the absence of a nucleus and cellular organelles. The resulting alterations in membrane and biochemical energy pathways limit the life of the cell. Many enzymes in the glycolytic and HMP pathways are known to decline with age. The resulting decreases in ATP, NADH, and NADPH change the ability of red cell pumps to work and reduce the energy needed to maintain hemoglobin and membrane proteins. The lipid contents of the membrane decrease with red cell age. Membrane changes with clumping of intracellular material along the inner membrane surface have been demonstrated by electron microscopy. Approximately 80 per cent of normal red cell destruction is extravascular in the reticuloendothelial system. Heme is separated from the globin molecule and degraded to bilirubin. Intravascular hemolysis accounts for 20 per cent of normal red cell loss. The free hemoglobin is quickly bound to haptoglobin to be processed by the liver, saving iron. The nonbound hemoglobin disassociates into dimers, which are filtered by the kidney with some reabsorption in the proximal tubule.

ENZYME DISORDERS OF RED CELLS

The hereditary enzyme defects that are associated with hemolytic anemia first came to light with the definition of a deficiency of glucose-6-phosphate dehydrogenase (G6PD). Approximately 15 enzymatic defects have been defined in red cells. They have in common the absence of detectable abnormal hemoglobin, a negative antiglobulin test, only rare spherocytes, normal osmotic fragility, and only partial benefit from splenectomy. They represent the congenital nonspherocytic hemolytic anemias. The degree of hemolysis is quite variable and exhibits no relationship to the severity of enzyme deficiency.

The deficiencies in red cell enzymes due to inborn errors have been categorized as deficiencies in enzymes of the HMP shunt, deficiencies of nonglycolytic enzymes, and deficiencies of enzymes in the glycolytic pathway. These deficiencies may result in alterations in the maintenance of the red cell membrane or the hemoglobin-oxygen relationship, or in a failure of detoxification. Since deficiencies in any one of the three areas may have repercussions on the others, multiple molecular and functional abnormalities can be expected. Any resultant change to the larger molecules, such as proteins or lipids, can result in early destruction of the red cell. In Table 23–4 are listed the deficiencies that have been reported in all three categories as well as their frequency, genetic basis, and degree of anemia, and the availability of screening tests. Deficiencies in the glycolytic pathway result in moderate to severe anemia, while those in the HMP shunt often require oxidants before there is expression of any defect. Drug-induced hemolysis is found in deficiencies of the enzymes in the HMP shunt. While there have been reports of drug-induced hemolysis in enzymatic deficiencies of the glycolytic pathway, most have been accompanied by concomitant defects in the HMP shunt.

GLUCOSE-6-PHOSPHATE DEHYDROGENASE

The most common of the disorders involves the first step in the HMP shunt, i.e., a deficiency of G6PD. This is estimated to involve 100 million people. G6PD has been purified and crystallized from mammalian tissue. The enzyme bound with $NADP^+$ consists of two subunits, but up to six subunits have been reported. With removal of $NADP^+$, G6PD disassociates into monomeric inactive units of 40,000 to 50,000 daltons. G6PD is strongly, but not absolutely, specific for G6P. Numerous variants of G6PD have been described on the basis of electrophorectic mobility, Michaelis

TABLE 23–4 HEREDITARY ENZYME DEFICIENCIES

	Frequency	Genetic Basis	Anemia	WBC	Screening Tests	Autohemolysis Type
Hexose-monophosphate shunt						
Glucose-6-phosphate dehydrogenase (G6PD)	Common	X-linked	None–severe	Normal	Yes	I
6-Phosphogluconate dehydrogenase (6-PED)	Rare	AR*	None	Normal	Yes	I
Nonglycolytic enzymes						
Glutathione reductase (GSSG-R)	?	AD†	?		Yes	II
Glutathione peroxidase (GSH Px)	Rare	AR*	Mild–moderate		Yes	
Glutathione synthetase	Rare	AR*	Mild		Yes	
ATPase	?	AD†	Moderate		No	
Adenylate kinase (AK)	?	AR*	Moderate		No	
Ribosephosphate pyrophosphokinase (RPK)	?	AR*	Moderate		No	II
Embden-Meyerhof pathway						
Hexokinase (HK)	Rare	AR*	Mild–severe	Normal	No	I
Glucosephosphate isomerase (GPI)	Rare	AR*	Moderate–severe	Low	Yes	I
Phosphofructokinase (PFK)	Rare	X-linked	Mild	Normal		
Triosephosphate isomerase (TPI)	Rare	AR*	Severe	Low	Yes	
2,3-Diphosphoglyceromutase (2,3-DPGM)	Rare	AR*	Severe–moderate		No	I
Phosphoglycerate kinase (PGK)	Rare	X-linked	Severe–moderate		No	I
Pyruvate kinase (PK)	Common	AR*	Mild–severe	Normal	Yes	II
Lactate dehydrogenase (LDH)		AR*	None		No	

*AR, autosomal recessive.
†AD, autosomal dominant.

constant determination, ability to utilize alternate substrates, heat stability, optimum pH, susceptibility to inhibition by sulfhydral reagents, and chromatographic mobility. At least 78 variants of G6PD have been well characterized. Two major types of G6PD, A⁺ and B⁺, have been fingerprinted, with the A⁺ differing from the B⁺ by a change of asparagine to aspartic acid. Electrophoresis demonstrates three G6PD types in normal people. In Caucasians it presents as a single B band. Thirty to forty-five per cent of normal Negroes have a faster A band. Ten to twenty per cent of normal Negro females are heterozygous for A and B types. The Mediterranean variant has a mobility similar to normal B, but its activity is 0 to 7 per cent of that of normal B. The Canton variant is faster than normal A, with activity of 4 to 24 per cent of that of normal B. The A⁻ variant closely resembles normal A⁻ type except for its decreased level in red cells. In fact, immature red cells have levels approaching normal; however, there is a rapid deterioration resulting in a low average red cell level. Even in the normal red cell G6PD activity decreases with age.

A deficiency of G6PD may result from formation of a less active molecule, as in the Oklahoma variant; decreased production, as in the Mediterranean variant; or production of a less stable molecule, as in the A⁻ or Chicago I variants. G6PD

deficiency is most often clinically expressed among males and shows an intermediate degree of expression in females. The deficiency is sex-linked with the gene locus on the X chromosome. Its expression in males is therefore understandable, as is the absence of father to son transmission. The expression of G6PD activity in heterozygous females suggests that only one X chromosome is functional or that there is a preferential activation. Depending on which chromosome is inactive, a heterozygous female may show normal activity, or intermediate or homozygote levels in red cells. The dominance of a cell line is crucial in the expression of G6PD levels, as cell lines with an active deficient X chromosome or active nondeficient heterozygous partner will result in varying levels of G6PD in the red cell in the female. In fact, two cell populations can be demonstrated and in each population only one gene is active. The degree of dominance on one cell line will set the level of G6PD in the heterozygous female. At times, it may be difficult to demonstrate the heterozygosity for the mother. In the United States, the most common deficiency is the A⁻ type in Negro subjects. The incidence of G6PD deficiency in Caucasian Sephardic Jews is 2 to 36 per cent, in Ashkenazi Jews 0 per cent, in Turkish Jews 60 per cent, in Italians 0.35 per cent, in Greeks 3 per cent in Arabs 3 to 13 per cent, in North American

Negro males 12 to 15 per cent, in female Negro homozygotes 1 to 3 per cent, in female Negro heterozygotes 16 to 20 per cent, in African Negroes 0 to 28 per cent, and in Chinese 2 to 5 per cent. The clinical course of the A⁻ patient usually suggests some inciting agent or stress, that within 2 or 3 days precipitates an acute hemolytic process associated with falling hematocrit, hemoglobin, and red cell count, an increase in reticulocytes, darkening urine, and in more severe cases clinical jaundice. Heinz bodies may be found in red cells in the early phase. The attack is self-limiting, lasting approximately 1 to 2 weeks, followed by a recovery phase despite continued exposure to the inciting agent. Hemolysis continues as long as the agent is present but is limited to cells that age and have falling G6PD levels. In most cases erythropoiesis maintains a normal hematocrit, and hemolysis is clinically inapparent. An increase in the agent can cause a second hemolytic crisis. Not all agents produce the same degree of hemolysis in each variant. For example, fava beans will not cause hemolysis in the A⁻ type but will in the more severe Mediterranean type. Congenital nonspherocytic hemolytic disease has been associated with the Chicago, Oklahoma, Ohio, Milwaukee, and Mediterranean variants in which G6PD depression is 0.5 to 14 per cent of normal.

Depression of G6PD leads to a deficiency of red cell NADPH and GSH. In milder variants the G6PD level in the cell drops with aging, and the older cells (63 to 73 days) are unable to withstand the stress. In some variants even young red cells are sufficiently deficient to be hemolyzed. In milder variants, the hemolysis is self-limiting as the older cells are destroyed. The young cells have sufficient G6PD activity to withstand the insult. The half-life of G6PD B is 62 days. Reticulocytes then will have twice the level of old cells. Abnormal variants have a shorter half-life, 13 days for G6PD A⁻. In fact, elevated levels of G6PD have been reported in hemolytic periods because of the selection of young cells. If G6PD-deficient cells are exposed to one of the agents listed in Table 23–5, the HMP shunt is stimulated. At the same time the available GSH is oxidized in response to the presence of the agent and its effect on hemoglobin and proteins in the membrane. The degree of activity of the shunt, however, in G6PD-deficient cells is less than normal and sufficient reduced NADP⁺ to maintain GSH is not available (Fig. 23–2). A major role of NADPH is to reduce the disulfide form of glutathione to the sulfhydryl form. GSH maintains the cysteine residues of hemoglobin and other red cell proteins in the reduced state. Oxidation of sulfhydryl groups in the membrane can result in alteration in ATPase and the sodium-potassium pump. Within 36 hours of administration of the agent the GSH level begins to fall and continues to fall over 5 to 7 days to approximately 20 per cent of normal. It will return to pre-agent levels in 14 to 18 days. Additional functions associated

TABLE 23–5 AGENTS ASSOCIATED WITH HEMOLYSIS

Antimalarials	Sulfones
Primaquine	Sulfoxone
Pamaquine	Thiazolsulfone
Pentaquine	Diaminodiphenyl
Quinacrine	sulphone
Quinocide	
Plasmoquine	
Quinine	Nitrofurans
Chloroquine	Nitrofurantoin
	Furaltadone
	Furazolidone
Antipyretics	Nitrofurazone
Acetanilid	
Acetophenetidin	
Aminopyrine	Miscellaneous
Antipyrine	Phenylhydrazine
Acetylsalicylic acid	Acetylphenylhydrazine
	Probenecid
	Dimercaprol
	Methylene blue
Sulfonamides	Naphthalene
Sulfanilamide	Vitamin K
Sulfacetamide	Aminosalicylic acid
Sulfapyridine	Trinitrotoluene
Salicylazosulfapyridine	Quinidine
Sulfisoxazole	Chloramphenicol
Sulfamethoxypyridazine	Fava beans
N₂ acetylsulfanilamide	Neosalvarsan

with GSH or NADPH, such as methemoglobin reduction, are decreased. ATP level also decreases, possibly through indirect effects on glyceraldehyde-3-phosphate and hexokinase by the decrease in reduced glutathione.

Most of the hemolytic drugs are oxidation-reduction substances that catalyze the oxidative denaturation of hemoglobin with oxygen and stimulate the HMP shunt. There are more than 40 known drugs capable of causing hemolysis. Oxidation of the sulfhydryl groups of the membrane protein interferes with membrane function, leading to early removal by the spleen and in more severe cases also by the liver. Drugs that are more lipotropic tend to damage the membrane proteins more than the hemoglobin. G6PD-deficient cells may also be deficient in NADPH-diaphorase and pyrophosphatase. The degree of susceptibility to hemolysis is not predictable from the G6PD level. In some cases the damaging agent is a metabolite of the drug; for example, primaquine is thought to cause hemolysis by its metabolite 8-amino-5,6-quinolinediol. Administration of such an agent results in increased red cell H_2O_2, either by oxidation of hemoglobin or autooxidation. Reduced glutathione mediated through glutathione peroxidase detoxifies the H_2O_2. The level of utilization of GSH is markedly increased, and the HMP shunt is stimulated both directly and indirectly. In G6PD-deficient cells the regeneration of GSH is hampered. Just prior to hemolysis, GSH levels drop and GSSH increases. The oxidized glutathione diffuses out of the cell, resulting in a fall in total glutathione in the cell.

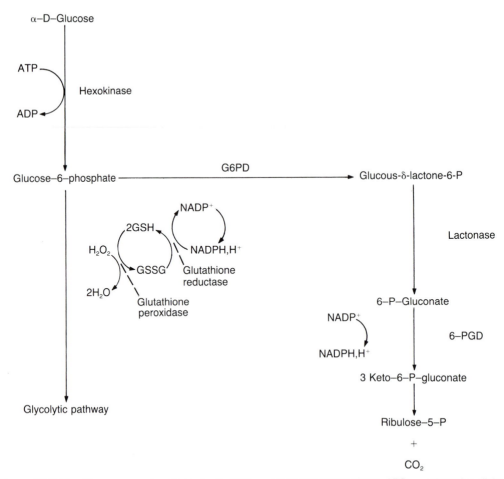

Figure 23–2 The Hexose-monophosphate shunt. ATP = adenosine triphosphate, ADP = adenosine diphosphate, G6PD = glucose-6-phosphate dehydrogenase, GSH = glutathione, GSSG = glutathione reductase; NADP = nicotinamide adenine dinucleotide phosphate; 6PGD = 6-phosphogluconate dehydrogenase.

In drug-induced hemolysis with oxidative injury to hemoglobin, methemoglobin may be produced. The intermediate role of methemoglobin and Heinz body formation is unclear and may be of no significance. The methemoglobin level is not universally elevated in patients with G6PD deficiency; in vitro induced methemoglobin does not lead to an increase in Heinz bodies or hemolysis, and stabilization of methemoglobin does not prevent hemolysis. If Heinz bodies do form, they can be responsible for some hemolysis as a result of splenic pitting and membrane alteration by binding of the denatured hemoglobin to the membrane. As a result of the binding, permeability is changed, intracellular sodium increases, and ATP decreases. In addition to decreased GSH and NADPH, possible secondary inhibition of other enzymes has been demonstrated, and decreased levels of NADP+, NAD+, ATP, and other intermediate enzymes occur. Oxidation of free sulfhydral radicals on the membrane may be responsible in part for some of the hemolysis due to increased membrane rigidity. Under stress, such as infections, a build-up of oxidative substances, for example, ascorbic acid, can precipitate hemolysis. In some cases the enzyme defect is severe enough to give rise to lifelong anemia.

Deficiencies of glucose-6-phosphate dehydrogenase, phosphogluconic dehydrogenase, glutathione reductase, glutathione synthetase, and glutathione peroxidase, all of which are associated with drug-induced hemolysis, appear to have their hemolytic effect mediated through glutathione.

PYRUVATE KINASE DEFICIENCY

The second most common inherited hemolytic anemia is pyruvate kinase deficiency. Pyruvate kinase (PK) catalyzes the conversion of phosphoenolpyruvate to pyruvate with the production of ATP. It is one of the rate-limiting steps in the glycolytic pathway. A deficiency in this terminal stage obviously results in a build-up of glycolytic intermediates and a decrease in ATP. An accumulation of 2,3-DPG leads to low oxygen affinity and easy release of oxygen in tissue. This partially compensates for the anemia. Of critical importance is the decrease in metabolism of glucose and therefore of ATP production. Like G6PD deficiency, PK deficiency demonstrates varying degrees of inactivity based either on lower levels of enzyme, reduced enzymatic activity, or reduced affinity for the substrate. There are three distinct PK isoenzymes in tissues. Its structure appears to be tetrameric, like lactate dehydrogenase. The red cell form is a heterotetramer of L type. In the severe forms of PK deficiency, hemolysis is probably the result of marked reduction of ATP and the inability of the cell to maintain membrane and cytoplasmic functions. The red cell life-span is shortened. Deficiency in ATP may be more strongly manifested in the more metabolically active reticulocyte, particularly in the static blood flow in which pH rises and glucose availability is decreased. Reticulocytes with severe PK deficiency particularly appear to be sequestered in the spleen and destroyed. Osmotic fragility is usually normal in red cells of patients with PK deficiency. The autohemolysis test demonstrates a type II pattern, poorly corrected by glucose or adenosine. Other cell lines in the body may also be affected but, in the presence of a nucleus and RNA, can better withstand the deficiency. PK deficiency is inherited as an autosomal recessive trait, both sexes being equally affected. Expression occurs in the homozygote; the heterozygote is usually asymptomatic. Polymorphism is expressed, some symptomatic heterozygotes having two different PK mutants. In severe forms, hemolysis and hyperbilirubinemia are seen in the neonate. In milder forms, hemolysis occurs in periods of stress. There is no distinguishing feature of the anemia. An aplastic crisis may be precipitated. Splenomegaly is the rule. Unlike G6PD deficiency, PK deficiency is not associated with denaturation of hemoglobin or membrane by oxidation. The HMP shunt is functional. Acquired forms of PK deficiency have been reported in a variety of other hematologic disorders such as refractory anemia and acute leukemia. Among the proposed pathophysiologic mechanisms are the presence of an inhibitor, loss of an activator, or alteration in protein synthesis.

MISCELLANEOUS HEREDITARY ENZYME DEFECTS

The remaining enzyme defects listed in Table 23-4 are uncommon. Their basic pathophysiologic action is similar to either that of G6PD by disruption of the HMP shunt, or of NADP+ resulting in easy oxidative injury, or of PK deficiencies causing reduction of anaerobic glycolysis or nucleotide metabolism or both. The general expression of one of these deficiencies is similar to G6PD or PK deficiency, although some are more generalized owing to involvement of other cell types, as in triose phosphate isomerase deficiency in which there is neuromuscular dysfunction. Glucose phosphate isomerase deficiency appears to be the third most common red cell enzyme defect and is transmitted as an autosomal recessive trait, expressed in the homozygote or double heterozygote. The deficiency is usually apparent in infancy with a pattern of anemia similar to PK deficiency. Stress is the usual inciting agent. The life-span of red cells is decreased. The defect in the enzyme appears to be predominantly one of increased instability. All tissues are affected. Glycolytic intermediates accumulate in the red cell and other tissues. Hexokinase deficiency, like PK deficiency, presents with different mutations. Glycolytic intermediates are decreased and ATP levels low. The enzymatic defect may be either quantitative or qualitative. Its inheritance is autosomal recessive. Triose phosphate isomerase deficiency results in only half of the glucose molecule being used in the glycolytic pathway. This limits the production of ATP and NADH. The HMP shunt is stimulated. A deficiency in 2,3-diphosphoglycerate results from a defect in diphosphoglycerate mutase. The effect on oxygen affinity reduces release to tissues. Defects in glutathione and its metabolism also give rise to hemolytic anemia. As in G6PD deficiency, oxidative drugs set off the hemolytic process. The anemia has a pathophysiologic basis similar to that in G6PD deficiency. Patients with acatalasia usually do not have associated hemolytic anemia. Under stress of oxidative drugs, however, the cells may not have sufficient reducing energy from NADPH to meet the needs. Under these circumstances the HMP shunt is stimulated, but the oxidative drug stresses the capacity of glutathione peroxidase with no backup system available. Not all enzyme deficiencies cause hemolytic anemia, as for example, defects of lactate dehydrogenase, adenosine triphosphatase, 6-phosphogluconate, and catalase.

RED CELL DEVELOPMENT

The development of red cells in the marrow takes place in the stroma, outside the blood-filled sinusoids. The sinusoidal bed is formed by capillaries and venules as they are distributed radially to a central vein. The red cell forming elements lie outside the sinuses in a reticular stroma. The wall of the sinuses is composed of three layers, an inner lining cell, a basement membrane, and an adventitial layer. Fat accumulates in the adventitial cells and less often in the endothelial cells. The sinusoidal layer varies in thickness and has discontinuous areas. In the areas composed only of endothelial cells, openings allow newly formed blood cells to enter the circulation. Erythroblasts lie just outside the sinusoids in clusters. These islands contain centrally located macrophages with erythroid elements arranged around the sides. Between the projections of the macrophages, the proerythroblasts, or pronormoblasts, develop through a series of stages, finally releasing themselves into the marrow sinuses as reticulocytes. The macrophages appear to provide nutrients to the developing red cell. Entry of the marrow elements into the circulation is by migration and diapedesis. The stimulus for entering the circulation is unclear, although erythropoietin is known to increase the release of reticulocytes. Red cells arise from a yet to be identified stem cell in the bone marrow. Once committed, the cell line progresses through a series of microscopically definable stages.

From its earliest microscopically recognizable stage, the pronormoblast, the cell constricts in size, the nucleus becomes pyknotic, and the cytoplasm takes on a pinkish stain as RNA is replaced by hemoglobin. The stages are recognized as basophilic normoblast, polychromatophilic normoblast, orthochromatic normoblast, and reticulocyte. In the first three stages the cell is capable of division and protein synthesis. The capacity to divide results in more late-stage than early-stage red cells in the marrow. The developmental stages from a single pronormoblast to orthochromatic normoblast take 3 days, when the nucleus is extruded. Three to four divisions take place during this process, yielding 8 to 16 orthochromatic normoblasts per pronormoblast. The cell decreases in size with each division. When extruded, the nucleus carries a small amount of cytoplasm with it. Once released, the nucleus is quickly phagocytized. Two additional days are spent in the reticulocyte phase. During this last phase, the reticulocytes are sticky and frequently bound together in clumps. This stickiness is felt to be due to transferrin on the surface. The extrasinusoidal area of marrow development is free of mature red cells. A pool of reticulocytes exists in the extrasinusoidal space, however, ready for release. The final phase of development for many of these cells appears to take place in the spleen. Ten to fifteen per cent of the cells die during maturation, representing ineffective erythropoiesis.

ERYTHROPOIESIS

In the fetus, red cell production begins in the yolk sac, shifting after 6 weeks to the liver and spleen. About the fifth month, early bone marrow activity occurs, the marrow ultimately becoming the dominant site by birth. Adult hemoglobin is detectable by the eleventh week, becoming the predominant hemoglobin in the last 6 weeks. The hepatic site can be reactivated after birth if hematopoiesis requirements exceed the limited space provided in a child's marrow cavities. Red cell production is mediated by a glycoprotein hormone, erythropoietin. Control begins in the fetus under the influence of tissue oxygenation. Erythropoietin does not cross the placental barrier, being produced by the fetus in a number of sites but primarily the liver. At birth, production is taken over by the kidney, with 5 to 10 per cent of the production remaining in the liver. Control of erythropoietin production is related to the oxygen tension in the kidney, although the exact cell of origin is not known. The juxtaglomerular apparatus has been implicated. In patients with progressive renal damage, there is decreased ability to respond to anemia. The association between tension and erythropoietin production is supported by the fact that patients who have hemoglobin abnormalities with a high affinity for oxygen have high levels of erythropoietin. Reduction in blood flow to about 40 per cent is required before erythropoietin is stimulated. The end organ effect of this hormone is to increase the number of stem cells and the proliferation of early stages of normoblasts, shortening the transit time. Activity is thought to be directed against committed cells rather than pluripotential cells. Erythropoietin appears to act on receptor sites on the cell, resulting in new synthesis of RNA. This is followed by production of DNA and cell division. Red cell generation is also shortened, suggesting action on more mature cells as well. The levels of erythropoietin appear to fluctuate in the plasma, and yet marrow production is steady, the number produced being balanced with the number of red cells destroyed. An erythropoietin releasing factor produced in the central nervous system has been postulated but not substantiated. Other workers have proposed that the kidney produces an erythropoietin activating enzyme that acts on a substrate produced elsewhere, for example, in the liver. Also postulated is the theory that a pro-hormone is produced in the kidney and is activated in plasma. Lastly, it has been proposed that the kidney produces both the hormone and an inhibitor, the latter inactivated by plasma. The final answer as to how erythropoietin is produced is yet to come. Following stimulation, erythropoietin levels increase in 12 hours with a peak level at 72 hours. In the face of hemolysis, red cell production appears to increase to a greater degree than that produced by acute bleeding. The possibility of a second stimulus exists. Negative feedback also appears to occur in polycythemia, possibly caused by an inhibitor. In many patients with anemia or hypoxemic polycythemia, the level of erythropoietin activity is increased. Some of the highest levels are found in cases of aplastic anemia. Erythropoietin is also increased in pregnancy. On the other hand, in anemia of chronic renal disease, infection, and cancer, erythropoietin levels are not usually raised.

Examination of marrow by aspiration and differential counting demonstrates a ratio of myeloid to erythroid cells of 3:1 to 5:1. The marrow can be stimulated to increase production to at least six times normal. The effectiveness of erythropoiesis can be easily measured by the degree of reticulocytosis. Other more complicated methods include measurement of bilirubin turnover and ferrokinetics. At times, despite marrow hyperplasia, the reticulocyte count is not increased, suggesting ineffective erythropoiesis, such as is seen in sideroblastic anemia and thalassemia. The intramedullary red cell pool has been determined to be 13×10^9 per kilogram body weight. The red cell volume is approximately 29 ml/kg in adult males and 25 ml/kg for females. Erythroid hyperplasia in the marrow is an indication of the need for erythropoiesis. In mild cases of anemia, the marrow red cell production can compensate for destruction. If destruction reduces red cell survival to less than one sixth normal, the red cell balance will fall behind unless other factors come into play. In hemolytic anemia, red cell survival is decreased. The marrow may compensate to bring the equilibrium back into balance, but if unable to do so because of severe shortening of life span, decompensated anemia, the inability of the marrow to respond, or dyserythropoietic anemia, a progressive anemia, develops.

RED CELL SURVIVAL

The life span of red cells can be measured by either random labeling with ^{51}Cr, immunologic markers, or cohort labeling by radioactive glycine or ^{59}Fe. In the cohort procedure, the label is incorporated by red cell precursors measuring the total life span of the red cell. This requires considerable time and a large dose of radioactivity. The Ashby technique utilizes a nonradioactive system of immunologic cell markers with a normal life span of 110 to 135 days. The random labeling method is most commonly used. Radioactive chromium penetrates the red cell membrane to bind to hemoglobin. The high-energy gamma rays permit ease in sample preparation and direct measurement in the patient. Its main disadvantage is the slow elution from the red cell that must be accounted for by a correction factor. This elution rate is 1 per cent per day and leads to a nonlinear curve. The technique provides a rapid measure of red cell survival but is not sensitive enough to pick up low-level destruction. The average life span of the red cell in man is accepted as 120 days. Daily destruction is 0.06 to 0.4 per cent per day. A plot of per cent survival against time can give a clue to the reason for shortening of the red cell life. A corrected linear relationship is seen under normal circumstances of aging red cells. In a hemolytic process the normal aging process has superimposed upon it a random destruction of red cells. This mixed pattern gives rise to an exponential effect. The normal half-life by ^{51}Cr is 28 to 38 days.

Below 26 days abnormal destruction is present. Red cell survival can be tested by using the patient's own cells, transfused normal cells in the patient, or the patient's cells in someone else. The first method does not distinguish between intrinsic and extrinsic factors. The second method indicates an extrinsic factor, and the third method, an intrinsic factor as shown in survival curves by the ^{51}Cr technique. Mixed patterns are to be expected where both extrinsic and intrinsic defects exist. Such situations can provide data that are most difficult to interpret.

DISORDERS OF RED CELL MASS

PATHOPHYSIOLOGY

Disorders of red cell mass can be defined as hematologic alterations in which too many or too few red cells are present in the circulation; they are classified as polycythemias and anemias.

Normal values for erythrocytes are defined within relative broad ranges and have significant physiologic variations related to age, sex, hydration, physical activity, posture, high altitude, and diurnal fluctuations.

Functionally, polycythemia refers to an increase in concentration of erythrocytes in the peripheral blood above 5.7 million/mm^3 in women and 6.4 million/mm^3 in men and elevations of hematocrit above 54 per cent. Consequently, the clinical manifestations are due to hypervolemia and hyperviscosity rather than changes in oxygen delivery. In contrast, the anemias are characterized as a reduction in red cell mass, with decreased erythrocyte and hemoglobin concentration in peripheral blood, and clinical manifestations dependent on the oxygen carrying capacity of the decreased erythrocytes.

Both polycythemias and anemias can be classified as relative or absolute on the basis of whether the size of the red cell mass is due to changes in plasma volume or to real changes in the red cell volume. From the clinical point of view, relative polycythemias and anemias play important roles but should not be considered as primary hematologic disorders.

Traditionally, absolute polycythemias were subdivided into primary (polycythemia vera) and secondary (erythrocytosis). The absolute anemias were classified into two large groups: those due to decreased red cell production and those due to decreased red cell survival.

DISORDERS OF INCREASED RED CELL VOLUME

Increases in red cell volume, more correctly erythrocytoses, have been classified under the broad clinical term *polycythemias,* which have been further classified as absolute and relative. *Polycythemia* is a descriptive term employed to indicate an increase in the concentration of the packed erythrocyte volume (hematocrit) and hemoglobin concentration in the peripheral blood. It should be emphasized that these measurements are an expression of a ratio between erythrocytes and plasma, and do not represent their absolute concentration in the intravascular space.

Under physiologic conditions, it has been demonstrated by radioisotopic labeling techniques that the red cell mass is maintained at approximately 30 ml/kg of body weight. Hume and Goldberg observed that determinations of venous hematocrit alone can be very misleading in the evaluation of actual red cell mass. Therefore, it is essential that if an increase is observed, these findings be documented by in vivo direct measurement of red cell volume by radioisotopic labeling technique. If by this method the red cell volume exceeds 30 ml/kg of body weight, the existence of an absolute erythrocytosis is confirmed. Cases in which the hematocrit is elevated but the red cell volume is normal fall into the category of spurious erythrocytosis due to decreased plasma volume.

Once the presence of a true polycythemia is established, the differential diagnosis between primary and secondary can be established by measurement of arterial oxygen saturation and serum and urine levels of erythropoietin. In polycythemia vera, oxygen saturation is essentially normal and erythropoietin levels are usually low to absent. In secondary polycythemias, oxygen saturation is decreased and erythropoietin levels are elevated owing to an appropriate response to tissue hypoxia.

One major complication of an increased circulating red cell mass is the rise in whole blood viscosity, an event responsible for the sluggish blood flow and the cause of many of the pathophysiologic manifestations of the disease. This increase in blood viscosity leads to an increase in blood volume with subsequent increase in cardiac workload, vasodilatation, and increased oxygen supply to the tissues, therefore facilitating adjustments between red cell mass and oxygen transport.

Regulation of red cell mass is exerted at the level of production and is governed by the hormone erythropoietin. Erythropoietin is a glycoprotein with a molecular weight between 30,000 and 60,000 daltons. The hormone not only stimulates erythropoiesis but also is responsible for its regulation. When animals or humans are subjected to cellular hypoxia, an immediate blood increase of erythropoietin is found, reaching maximum serum levels between 12 and 18 hours after the exposure and decreasing thereafter.

The elegant studies by Jacobson and coworkers in 1957 demonstrated that most of the erythropoietin is produced in the kidneys, since nephrectomized animals, after exposure to low ambient Po_2, produce very little or no erythropoietin. The site and biochemical details of its renal production have not been clarified. It has, however, been postulated that renal hypoxia stimulates production of the hormone. Cardiac and vascular adjustments are relatively insensitive to moderate decreases in hemoglobin oxygen binding capacity and to changes in oxygen affinity of red cells. Pronounced changes in red cell mass are compensated for by blood flow changes, but erythropoietin production could be partially reduced by the acute stimulation. It is evident that this erythropoietin response during moderate anoxia and its reduction during severe hypoxia is due to changes in red cell oxygen affinity. Parer has demonstrated the importance of red cell oxygen affinity for the production of erythropoietin in patients whose blood hemoglobins have abnormally high oxygen affinity. In general, these patients develop polycythemia. In contrast, it has been also demonstrated by Stamatoyannopolous' studies of hemoglobin Seattle that the presence of significant amounts of hemoglobin with abnormally low oxygen affinity results in low hemoglobin concentration without increases of erythropoietin production or signs of anemia.

When humans are exposed to high altitude, the chemoreceptor mechanisms are activated by the low ambient Po_2. The individual hyperventilates, causing a gradual decrease of Pco_2 that immediately leads to an increase in oxygen affinity of the red cells. This, combined with low arterial oxygen content, hinders oxygen supply to erythropoietin production sites and subsequently stimulates erythropoietin production.

A decrease in oxygen saturation of the red cells and an increase in pH stimulates red cell metabolism. During short-term exposure to high altitude there is a significant reduction of inorganic blood phosphate, which results in reduced synthesis of 1,3-DPG and, therefore, of 2,3-DPG. These metabolic changes promote red cell synthesis of 2,3-DPG, and its slow accumulation inside the red cells is followed by a reversal of carbon dioxide–induced increase in oxygen affinity of hemoglobin. In the following days after high altitude exposure, bicarbonate excretion in the urine is increased as pH returns to normal. The oxygen affinity is reduced compared with pre-exposure levels. As erythropoietin increases, these metabolic changes take place, and when oxygen affinity is normalized, erythropoietin levels begin to fall.

Absolute Polycythemias

Polycythemia Vera. Polycythemia vera comprises several closely related hematologic syndromes, grouped under the name of myeloproliferative disorders, that are characterized by an abnormal proliferation of the hematopoietic pluripotential cell precursor elements and stroma. Each cell line may be differently involved and may display a gamut of abnormalities of growth or arrested maturation, depending on the myelodysplastic syndrome. This concept was developed by Dameshek in 1951, and each syndrome is identified according to the predominant line of proliferation. When the disorder presents itself as an increased bone marrow erythrocyte production with elevated circulating levels of mature erythrocytes, despite other clinical and laboratory manifestations of other myeloproliferative disorders, the syndrome is called polycythemia vera.

The disease was described by Vaquez in 1892 and further redefined by Türk. Many hypotheses as to its origin have been postulated, but these investigations have been more fruitful in aiding differential diagnosis rather than determining the cause of the disease. Much attention has focused on the search for abnormalities of the normal mechanisms that regulate erythropoiesis through the erythropoietin–erythroid controlled stem cell axis. Erythropoiesis in polycythemia vera is autonomous and appears to be independent of erythropoietin stimulation. Levels of erythropoietin in serum and urine are found to be below the detectable ranges, and normal production is suppressed by the elevated hematocrit. Ward and Robinson described a factor from plasma of patients with polycythemia vera that was capable of stimulating red cell precursors in laboratory animals. The presence of such a factor, however, is still unproved.

Recent studies suggest the existence of clonal or biclonal populations of erythroid precursors in patients with polycythemia vera. One clone is autonomous and proliferates in the absence of erythropoietin, while the other behaves in a normal fashion and requires the presence of erythropoietin for proliferation and differentiation. Continuous erythroid activity of the autonomous clone could explain the steady increase of red cell mass, while the second clone could be responsible for increased erythropoietin and red cell production in anoxic or anemic patients with polycythemia vera.

Extensive chromosomal abnormalities have been reported in approximately 25 per cent of cases. They are varied in type and include aneuploid deletions, and the presence of an extra C group chromosome. Unfortunately, these extensive chromosomal abnormalities have been reported in patients under myelosuppressive therapy and are probably the end result of treatment with phosphorus 32 (^{32}P). Normal and abnormal chromosomal studies have been also reported in patients with polycythemia vera prior to myelosuppressive therapy.

The use of radioactive iron has proved invaluable in elucidating the complex mechanisms of iron metabolism and erythropoiesis in health and disease. Ferrokinetic studies in patients with polycythemia vera have demonstrated that erythropoiesis is effective and the released red blood cells have a normal life span. In order to maintain the peripheral red cell mass, the erythroid marrow is also increased. As a consequence there is an accelerated iron turnover with depletion of tissue iron stores. This trend is further complicated by the bleeding tendencies of these patients and the therapeutic use of phlebotomies.

Polycythemia vera is a rare disease, and its incidence rate ranges from 0.6 to 1.6 per 100,000 population according to Silverstein and Lanier. There is a male predominence of approximately 1.5:1. With advancing age, there is an annual increase in specific incidence, the median age of onset being 50 to 60 years. The disease appears to have a preponderance in patients of Jewish ancestry, and blacks have a significantly smaller incidence.

The onset is insidious, and the disorder may be accidentally discovered when laboratory studies demonstrate an elevated red cell count, hemoglobin content, and hematocrit. At other times clinical complications such as thrombosis or severe hemorrhage may be the initial presentation.

As stated before, the disease is basically a myeloproliferative disorder characterized by abnormal proliferation of the erythroid, the myeloid, or the megakaryocytic elements. Each of these proliferations is responsible for certain signs, symptoms, and complications.

As a consequence of the increased red cell mass, the plasma volume is increased and hypervolemia and hyperviscosity appear, compromising cardiovascular integrity. Cardiac output decreases, peripheral vascular resistance increases, and the interaction of these factors produces hypertension. Symptoms and signs of vascular involvement constitute 30 to 45 per cent of presenting complaints. Plethora, redness or cyanosis of digits, vertigo, dizziness, and headaches are noted first. Injection of conjunctival and retinal vessels, peripheral cyanosis, and transient coronary or cerebral ischemia may develop into major complications such as retinal vein thrombosis and blindness, hemiplegia, and gangrene. Venous thrombosis of abdominal vessels or splenic infarctions may present as acute surgical abdominal disease.

The marrow biopsy is hypercellular with very little fat and with an increase of cells of the granulocytic, eosinophilic, erythroid, and megakaryocytic lines. Iron is generally absent to markedly decreased. Squash preparations demonstrate a large number of cells of all types with usually normal percentile values. Reactivation of dormant tissue produces an expansion of the functioning hematopoietic organ with a centrifugal and axial bone marrow increase.

Splenic enlargement is an important distinguishing feature between myeloproliferative polycythemia and secondary erythrocytosis, and has been attributed to extramedullary hematopoiesis and vascular congestion.

Liver enlargement occurs less frequently and tends to develop late in the course of the disease. Liver function is usually not compromised.

In its early stages, the circulating erythrocytes are generally normochromic, normocytic; however, as the disease progresses hypochromia and microcytosis may develop because of iron depletion. Abnormal red blood cells such as teardrop, elliptocytic, and nucleated red blood cells appear as the panmyelosis progresses to the myelofibrotic stage.

The megakaryocytic hyperplasia is usually followed by an increase in the effective rate of platelet production with an absolute increase of total platelet mass. Survival studies have given conflicting results. Functional abnormalities have been detected by in vitro aggregation studies and are characterized by impairment of normal aggregating agents. Small groups of patients have demonstrated excessive ability of platelets to aggregate. The role of these abnormalities in the origin of bleeding and thrombosis is still not well understood.

Qualitative and quantitative changes in the granulocyte population are present in polycythemia vera. Granulocyte production is increased, as is the absolute circulating granulocyte count, rarely exceeding 30,000/mm^3. The differential count reflects a "left shift" with increased number of bands and occasional metamyelocytes and myelocytes. An increase in leukocyte alkaline phosphatase activity is seen in approximately 80 per cent of cases, and the abnormality appears to be strictly quantitative owing to an increase in the bulk of enzyme contained in the specific granules. Leukocyte metabolic activity is also increased with elevated phagocytic index, increased oxygen consumption, and greater total reduction of nitroblue tetrazolium. Increased granulocyte turnover often manifests itself as an increase in the concentration of vitamin B_{12} and B_{12} binders in serum as well as an increase in urinary muramidase. An absolute increase in basophils is also present.

Histidine decarboxylase, an enzyme involved in the production of histamine from histidine, is increased in leukocyte lysates and correlates with the number of basophils present. This may explain the common complaint of untreated patients of itching that may appear spontaneously after baths or showers.

Few problems are specifically attributable to the increase of granulocytes in the disease process. Granulocyte involvement is, however, responsible for the most serious terminal complication of the disease: the progression into acute myeloblastic leukemia. The transition is a late complication that can occur at any time. Whether acute leukemia arises from the actions of myelosuppressive therapy or is due to the presence of abnormal myeloid line precursors is still not well understood, but good evidence has accumulated regarding the leukemogenic influence of radiation and alkylating agents.

Acute myelogenous leukemia develops in approximately 15 per cent of patients. Once it develops it is well known to be associated with short survival, very low remission rate, and poor response to antileukemic therapy.

After several years and owing to massive splenomegaly, a decrease in hematocrit and platelet count may occur because of waning proliferative activity in the bone marrow and pooling, sequestration, and destruction by the spleen. Splenic infarctions are observed, and anemia may become a major symptom. An increased nucleoprotein turnover, resulting from the myelodysplastic process, results in an elevated uric acid serum level in more than 50 per cent of patients. Secondary gout, tophi, renal stones, and severe kidney damage develop in 50 per cent of these patients.

Secondary Polycythemia (Erythrocytosis)

Secondary polycythemia, also known under the more descriptive term of *erythrocytosis*, is an absolute elevation above normal in the number of erythrocytes in the circulating blood, caused by intensified stimulation of erythrocyte production. As stated before, erythropoietin is responsible for the intensified stimulus as a compensatory mechanism to minimize tissue hypoxia. In such cases the hormone release is appropriate, as seen in high altitude acclimatization, chronic pulmonary disease, congenital or acquired cardiovascular diseases, and defective oxygen transport of abnormal hemoglobins.

When increased erythropoietin production is not related to generalized tissue hypoxia, the hormone release is inappropriate, as seen in certain tumors and structural or functional abnormalities of the kidney. Therefore secondary polycythemias have been divided into those related to compensatory type, appropriate; and those due to pathologic type, inappropriate.

Appropriate Secondary Polycythemias

ERYTHROCYTOSIS DUE TO LOW ATMOSPHERIC PRESSURE (HIGH ALTITUDE). Secondary polycythemias due to low atmospheric pressure are considered an appropriate physiologic adaptation of the human body to anoxia and are perhaps the most common cause of secondary polycythemias.

Human beings and most domesticated animals under normal physiologic conditions can easily adapt to atmospheric pressure as low as to two thirds of normal. Studies on high altitude polycythemia have been carried out in the small mining town of Morococha at 15,000 feet above sea level in the Peruvian Andes. Settlements above 15,000 feet are few; the highest perhaps being Aucanquilcha at 17,500 feet in the Chilean Andes, which physiologically borders on the upper limit of human long-term endurance of high altitude. At such altitude the pressure of the atmospheric oxygen is not greater than the mean capillary oxygen pressure at sea level, compromising the downhill gradient for oxygen from the air to the cells. Attempts by Sir Edmund Hillary to acclimate at 18,750 feet to an atmospheric pressure of slightly less than half normal failed after several months (Bishop 1962). Continuous physical deterioration and cases of severe thrombotic complications were observed in the mountain climbers.

The inhabitants of Morococha live active vigorous lives, and their health and longevity appear to be similar to their fellow countrymen at sea level. At these altitudes, the tissue oxygen demands are similar to those at lower altitudes. The ventilatory stress, however, leads to an expansion of the pulmonary parenchyma and an increase in vital capacity that is responsible for an increase in the alveolocapillary diffusing surface and a decrease in the alveoloarterial gradient from 9 mm to 1.5 mm, almost eliminating the alveolocapillary gradient. In the beginning, in order to minimize the arteriocapillary gradient, there is an increase in cardiac output. When acclimatization begins, a high mean capillary oxygen pressure is accomplished by a mild shift to the right of the oxygen dissociation curve, resulting in moderate impairment of hemoglobin oxygen binding and increased hemoglobin oxygen release. This physiologic adaptation appears to be beneficial in short-term acclimatization, but its benefits in long-term acclimatization have been questioned, since studies in llamas and vicuñas, animals indigenous to these areas, demonstrate oxygen dissociation curves situated far to the left. This suggests that loading of oxygen in the lungs by a hemoglobin with high oxygen affinity is more important than hemoglobin oxygen release. The mechanisms by which the tissues of these animals receive oxygen from such a high oxygen affinity hemoglobin are still not well understood, but polycythemia is not characteristic of such animals.

In less adapted mammals, high altitude hypoxia induces the release of erythropoietin, which in turn stimulates erythropoiesis and red cell production. This compensatory mechanism induces polycythemia, which eventually enhances oxygen carrying capacity and expansion of the total blood volume with dilatation of vessels and an increase in tissue perfusion.

The clinical manifestations of high altitude polycythemia are characteristically ruddy cyanosis and physiologic emphysema. The vascular dilatation is characterized by capillary and venous engorgement of the conjunctiva, oral mucosa, and skin; a feature that may be responsible for the capacity of the Sherpas to walk barefoot or sleep on ice or snow.

The blood picture demonstrates a normo-chromic normocytic erythrocytosis with essentially normal white blood cell and platelet counts. The absolute reticulocyte count as well as iron turnover and iron absorption is increased. Serum and urine erythropoietin levels are increased, and the spleen is within normal limits in contradistinction to polycythemia vera.

Chronic mountain sickness, or Monge's disease, is a syndrome characterized by a slow decompensation of the balancing mechanism of high altitude dwellers leading to alveolar hypoventilation and anoxia. This in turn results in cardiovascular decompensation due to a markedly increased red cell mass and serum viscosity. It manifests clinically with marked cyanosis, physical and emotional deterioration, hepatomegaly, and edema. Therapeutic phlebotomies produce temporary improvement, but complete relief cannot be achieved until after return to sea level.

Acute mountain sickness is characterized by anoxic symptoms such as headaches, mental dullness, nausea, and vomiting associated, especially while sleeping, with Cheyne-Stokes respiration. Abnormal accumulation of fluids may lead to pulmonary or cerebral edema or both.

ERYTHROCYTOSIS OF CHRONIC HYPOXEMIA. Erythrocytosis of chronic hypoxemia can be seen in chronic pulmonary disease that seriously impairs the normal saturation of arterial blood with oxygen or those diseases that alter the alveolar ventilation perfusion relationship. Erythrocytosis leads to an increased blood viscosity that, associated with an increased pulmonary vascular resistance, elevates the right ventricular pressure. This further aggravates the cor pulmonale, retention of water, and an increase in plasma volume that may be responsible for the hidden increase of red cell mass. In some cases, for unknown reasons, erythrocytosis is never present.

Abnormal ventilatory conditions due to alveolar hypoventilation lead to arterial oxygen unsaturation, hypercapnia, somnolence, cyanosis, and increased red cell mass. These changes may be due to decreased atmospheric pressure, as previously described, or to the pickwickian syndrome in very obese individuals. The syndrome has been also described in nonobese individuals.

ERYTHROCYTOSIS OF HEART DISEASE. Congenital heart disease occurs in approximately 8 per 1000 live births, and the defect is well tolerated in utero. After birth, however, the abnormalities become apparent, and the severity of the disease depends on the spectrum of the malformation and the duration of disease.

Congenital heart disease with shunting of blood from right to left is characteristically associated with cyanosis and elevated red cell mass, with counts exceeding 10 million/mm^3 and packed red cell volumes as high as 86 per cent. The most common congenital cardiac diseases associated with right-to-left shunt and polycythemia are tetralogy of Fallot, pulmonary atresia, tricuspid atresia, transposition of great vessels, and persistent truncus arteriosus. There are other less common abnormalities. In severely symptomatic patients phlebotomies with fresh frozen plasma replacement result in temporary reduction of blood viscosity. Peripheral and cerebral thromboses are seen as complications of increased blood viscosity due to extreme polycythemia; they may be precipitated by dehydration. Other coagulation disorders have been also described.

An increase in red cell mass is rare in acquired heart disease, although some studies have demonstrated a mild increase. Chronic decompensation leads to fluid retention and increased plasma volume, which leads to spurious low determinations of red cell count and packed red cell volume.

ERYTHROCYTOSIS DUE TO DEFECTIVE OXYGEN TRANSPORT. This type of polycythemia is observed in patients with congenital or acquired hemoglobin abnormalities. The congenital type is subclassified according to those hemoglobins causing cyanosis and those with altered oxygen affinity.

In the group causing cyanosis there are five hemoglobins that have been designated as hemoglobin M's. Owing to amino acid substitutions near the heme group, oxidation of the ferric form occurs with production of methemoglobin and cyanosis. The disease is dominantly transmitted, and hemoglobin M disease can be distinguished from other forms of methemoglobinemia by hemoglobin electrophoresis or hemoglobin spectral analysis.

More than 20 abnormal hemoglobins have been described as having an increase in oxygen affinity, demonstrated by a shift to the left of the oxygen dissociation curve, and decreased oxygen release to the tissues, leading to tissue hypoxia. This in turn causes release of erythropoietin and erythrocytosis.

Erythrocytosis due to acquired defective oxygen transport of hemoglobin is generally caused by exposure to certain drugs and toxins that can cause clinically significant methemoglobinemia. Such agents include nitrites and nitrates, aniline dyes, phenacetin and acetanilid, sulfonamides, and a few other drugs currently in use. The degree of methemoglobinemia depends on dose and individual susceptibility, since heterozygotes for the disease are more likely to develop it than normal individuals. In general, erythrocytosis is mild without significant increase in blood viscosity.

Sulfhemoglobin is a derivative of unknown composition found in erythrocytes under normal circumstances as an inert oxygen carrier that cannot be converted to normal hemoglobin. As with methemoglobin, there are certain oxidizing drugs that are the most common causative agents, and the degree of anoxia and erythrocytosis is generally mild.

Carbon monoxide combines with hemoglobin and forms carboxyhemoglobin, a hemoglobin that is incapable of carrying oxygen and interferes with normal oxygen release. In heavy smokers carboxyhemoglobin may produce enough anoxia to stimulate erythropoietin and mild erythrocytosis.

Elements such as cobalt can cause cellular anoxia and secondary erythrocytosis.

Inappropriate Secondary Polycythemia. Erythrocytosis has been reported in association with multiple benign and malignant renal and extrarenal tumors as well as in cases of parenchymal renal disease and is not associated with leukocytosis or thrombocytosis.

Narrowing of the renal arterial system impairs blood supply to the kidney, producing tissue anoxia and stimulating erythropoietin. Only in rare cases of vascular disease, however, does increased erythropoietin stimulation lead to erythrocytosis.

The most common causes of inappropriate secondary erythrocytosis due to benign and malignant space-occupying lesions have been reported in association with renal cell adenocarcinoma (hypernephroma), cerebellar hemangioblastoma, pheochromocytoma, hepatocellular carcinoma, virilizing tumors of the ovary and adrenal cortex, and uterine fibromas.

Numerous studies have demonstrated that erythrocytosis associated with tumors is due to a real increase in red cell mass with production of erythropoietin or erythropoietin-like substance, erythroid hyperplasia of the bone marrow, increased clearance of radioactive iron, and a normal red cell life span. The mechanisms for erythropoietin production are still not well understood. Fluid material and extracts of renal cysts, renal cell adenocarcinomas, and cerebellar hemangioblastomas have, however, demonstrated that the cells can produce erythropoietin and erythropoietin-like substances that can be inactivated by erythropoietin antibodies and that appear to be biologically and immunologically identical to renal erythropoietin.

Other benign and malignant tumors of renal cell origin as well as hydronephrosis appear to stimulate erythropoietin production through pressure-induced hypoxia of the adjacent normal renal parenchyma. The same hypothesis has been postulated for some cerebellar hemangioblastomas, since the respiratory center is located in the proximity of the tumor.

The largest series of cases of erythrocytosis associated with hepatocellular carcinomas was reported in 1958 by McFadzean and associates, who demonstrated an increased red cell mass in about 10 per cent of the patients. Despite numerous studies, the cause of erythrocytosis is still unknown.

Erythrocytosis associated with large uterine fibromas has been sporadically documented, but erythropoietin or erythropoietin-like substances have not been demonstrated. It has been suggested that the large tumor mass may interfere with the kidney blood supply or pulmonary ventilation, resulting in anoxia and erythropoietin production.

Erythrocytosis associated with endocrine disorders appears to be of a different nature. In general, because erythrocytosis is moderate and the tumors involved are virilizing in nature, the effect of androgens has been invoked to explain its origin. The erythropoietic activity of androgens has been well documented both in female patients with carcinoma of the breast treated with pharmacologic doses of androgens and in patients with Cushing's syndrome.

In summary, it should be emphasized that in polycythemia vera, erythropoietin levels are normal or decreased and leukocyte alkaline phosphatase and serum vitamin B_{12} levels are elevated. On the other hand, in secondary polycythemia with hypoxia, erythropoietin levels are elevated, leukocyte alkaline phosphatase and serum vitamin B_{12} are normal, and arterial Po_2 is low.

DISORDERS OF DECREASED RED CELL MASS

Structure of Normal Hemoglobin

Understanding the structure of hemoglobin is one of the milestones of molecular biology. Hemoglobin structure and function are so closely interrelated that, in most cases, clinical abnormalities of function can be directly attributed to lesions at a molecular level.

Hemoglobin is a conjugated protein formed by globin, the protein portion, and heme, a complex of iron and protoporphyrin. It is a tetramer of approximately $50 \times 55 \times 64$ Å, with a molecular weight of 64,000 daltons. It is composed of two pairs of nonidentical polypeptide chains and four molecules of heme. The heme group, ferroprotoporphyrin IX, is linked covalently at a specific site to each globin polypeptide chain. When heme iron is in the reduced (ferrous) state, it can bind reversibly with oxygen, whereas in the oxidized (ferric) state it is incapable of oxygenation. Each globin polypeptide chain is composed of specific amino acids; the exact sequence and composition of these amino acids is referred to as the *primary structure. Secondary structure* refers to the organization of amino acids into helices stabilized by hydrogen bonds between the CO and NH groups of adjacent coils. The manner in which the polypeptide chains are folded to form a three-dimensional, spherical unit is termed the *tertiary structure,* and the term *quaternary structure* refers to the fit, contact points of, and way in which the four polypeptide chains join to form a single molecule.

Normal Human Hemoglobins. The heme group is identical in all human hemoglobin phenotypes. The protein part of the molecule, globin, comprises two nonidentical polypeptide chains (α, β, γ, or δ chains). Of normal adult hemoglobin, 97 per cent is hemoglobin A_1, which is composed of

two alpha and two beta chains (structure referred to as $\alpha_2\beta_2$). Approximately 2.5 per cent of adult hemoglobin is Hb A_2, composed of two alpha and two delta chains ($\alpha_2\delta_2$), and 1 per cent is Hb F ($\alpha_2\gamma_2$). A newborn infant, on the other hand, generally possesses about 80 per cent Hb F, 20 per cent Hb A_1, and 0.5 per cent Hb A_2. The level of Hb F falls steadily following birth, approaching the adult level at about 6 months of age. The main component during human fetal development after the first trimester is Hb F. In the very early stages of gestation, primitive erythroblasts in the yolk sac produce embryonic hemoglobins, Gower 1 ($\zeta_2\epsilon_2$) and Gower 2 ($\alpha_2\epsilon_2$). During fetal development there is an orderly switch from ϵ to γ chain production, followed by β and δ chain production after birth; α chain synthesis occurs throughout development.

Genetic Control of Globin Chain Production. Synthesis of each of the known normal polypeptide chains is controlled by distinct, separate genetic loci. There are two pairs of identical α genes located on chromosome 16, whereas there appears to be only one pair each of genes coding for β and δ chains, located on chromosome 11. The heterogeneous F (γ) chains are controlled by at least two different pairs of γ genes, both located on chromosome 11. One, G_γ, provides coding for an F chain with glycine at position 136, whereas another, A_γ, produces F chain with alanine at position 136. The α chain consists of 141 amino acids, whereas the β, γ, and δ chains consist of 146 amino acids each. At birth the ratio of G_γ chains to A_γ chains is about 3:1, whereas the hemoglobin F of the normal adult contains G_γ and A_γ chains in the ratio of 2:3.

Human Hemoglobin Variants. There are several different molecular and genetic mechanisms that give rise to the various abnormal hemoglobin syndromes, as depicted in Table 23–6. More than 300 structurally different human hemoglobin variants have been discovered. Many of these are secondary to a single amino acid substitution in one of the globin polypeptide chains. Generally, this is due to substitution of a single nucleotide base in the deoxyribonucleic acid or messenger ribonucleic acid codon. Many of these were discovered fortuitously during population surveys, and their clinical manifestations, if any, are not known.

Functional abnormalities in association with abnormal hemoglobins can be classified as shown in Table 23–7. Sickle hemoglobin (Hb S, $\alpha_2\beta_2$ 6 Glu $\to$ Val) is the most frequently encountered variant and in the homozygous state gives rise to the most severe clinical manifestations.

Sickle Cell Disease

Hemoglobin S is a classic example of genetic mutation that is the result of the substitution of a

TABLE 23–6 HUMAN HEMOGLOBIN ABNORMALITIES

Molecular Basis	Hemoglobin Example
I. Structurally abnormal polypeptide chains, single amino acid substitution	β chain–S,C,D,E (177 variants)
	α chain (92 variants)
	γ chain (16 variants)
	δ chain (10 variants)
Double amino acid substitution	C-Harlem, J-Singapore
Deletion of 1 to 5 amino acids	Gun Hill
Elongation of polypeptide chains	α chain–Constant Spring
	β chain–Cranston
	Hb H (β_4)
Tetramers (all 4 chains identical)	Hb Bart's (γ_4)
II. Absence or decreased production of one or more Hb polypeptide chains	β–Beta thalassemia syndromes
	α–Alpha thalassemia syndromes
Decreased synthesis with structurally abnormal hemoglobin	Hb Lepore syndromes
III. Continuation of fetal hemoglobin synthesis	Hereditary persistence of Hb F
IV. Combinations of two or more of the foregoing	

single amino acid in one of the globin polypeptide chains. Hb S differs from Hb A_1 only in the substitution of valine for glutamic acid in the sixth position from the N-terminal end of the beta chain. The sickle gene is a common mutant, being fairly prevalent in Central Africa, the Mediterranean region, and parts of India. The average incidence among American blacks is approximately 8 per cent, whereas the average frequency of the sickling trait in a belt extending from west to east across the middle third of Africa approaches 20 per cent.

The substitution of valine in the sixth position for glutamic acid occurs on the surface of the hemoglobin molecule, thereby changing its charge and its electrophoretic mobility. Hemoglobin S is freely soluble when fully oxygenated; however, when oxygen is removed from Hb S, polymerization of the abnormal hemoglobin occurs, forming

TABLE 23–7 FUNCTIONAL EFFECTS OF ABNORMAL HEMOGLOBINS

I. Hemolysis due to decreased hemoglobin solubility
    Hemoglobin S disease (homozygous)
    Hemoglobin C disease (homozygous)

II. Unstable hemoglobins with hemolysis due to reduced solubility
    Congenital Heinz body hemolytic anemia, Hb Köln

III. Methemoglobinemia, familial cyanosis
    The M hemoglobins

IV. Hemoglobins with increased oxygen affinity
    Erythrocytosis as in Hb Chesapeake

V. Hemoglobins with decreased oxygen affinity
    Cyanosis as in Hb Kansas

VI. None or unknown as in Hb G

tactoids (fluid crystals) that are rigid and deform the cell into the curved sickle shape that gave the cell its name. Electron micrographs of sickled red cells show long, thin bundles of Hb S fibers that run parallel to the long axis of the cell.

Hemoglobin monomers are stable in solution when Hb S concentration, pH, ionic strength, and temperature are strictly maintained within certain narrow limits. Changes beyond these limits result in precipitous appearance of Hb S gel, which is the basic change that leads to the viscosity changes, distortion of cell morphology, sludging, and organ infarction that result in the classic clinical manifestations of sickle cell disease.

Various studies have demonstrated a delay time in the deformation of cells containing deoxygenated hemoglobin S. Cells maintain normal shape in the oxygenated arterial circulation; when they enter the capillary circulation, however, the oxygen saturation decreases rapidly together with the hemoglobin solubility. If the delay time in the cell deformation is less than the time spent in the capillary circulation, the cell will sickle in and occlude the capillary. If the transit time in the capillary is shorter than the delay time, however, occlusion will not occur. This is thought to reflect the situation in the myocardium, where occlusion does not occur in spite of the high degree of oxygen extraction. Low pH, high ionic strength, and high hemoglobin concentration shorten the delay time and lengthen the capillary transit time, resulting in capillary occlusion. The hypertonic renal medulla and the acidotic, high-hematocrit environment in the spleen make these organs highly susceptible to sickling and vaso-occlusive episodes.

The cells that undergo reversible polymerization and shape change are called reversibly sickled cells. When oxygenated, these cells resume normal shape and viscosity and contain no hemoglobin polymers. Upon deoxygenation, they develop electron-dense areas consistent with early hemoglobin polymerization and show increased viscosity. A few seconds later, long polymers are visible with protuberances in the biconcave disc shape. By 30 seconds, most cells assume a "holly-leaf" shape. Upon reoxygenation, there is a rapid decrease in the hemoglobin polymers, with resumption of normal shape in the majority of the cells. The cells that do not change shape in spite of a change in polymerization are known as irreversibly sickled cells. These are slender, elongated, crescent-shaped sickle cells that are visible on an oxygenated peripheral blood smear. These rigid cells have a shortened life span and are responsible in part for the increased viscosity of oxygenated whole blood. The number of such irreversibly sickled cells correlates well with the hemolytic rate and spleen size in patients. The rigid cells are more vulnerable to trauma and are readily trapped by the reticuloendothelial system, particularly the spleen, resulting in hemolysis. As a result of the hemolysis and shortened red cell survival, severe continued bone marrow hyperplasia occurs, giving rise to the expansion of the marrow space, thinning of bone cortex, and radial striations seen on skull x-ray.

Clinical Manifestations of Sickle Cell Disease. Sickle cell disease, homozygous Hb S, is characterized by chronic hemolytic anemia and intermittent "crises" of variable severity and frequency. There are episodes of pain, acute vaso-occlusive episodes resulting in infarctions, and aplastic marrow crises. There is increased susceptibility to certain bacterial infections. The clinical manifestations, however, are quite variable. Some patients remain relatively asymptomatic, whereas many others become severely disabled or succumb in infancy or early childhood. The majority of patients have long asymptomatic periods punctuated by occasional acute crises.

The infant born with homozygous sickle cell disease has no symptoms in the first few months of life owing to the high concentration and protective effect of Hb F ($\alpha_2\gamma_2$, non β chain). At birth, Hb F constitutes 80 to 85 per cent of the hemoglobin and subsequently drops off at the rate of 3 to 4 per cent each week. By about 4 to 5 months of age, the infant's red cells contain predominantly Hb S and are capable of being sickled. The most common presenting problems between 6 months and 2 years of age are infection, dactylitis, severe anemia, colic, and irritability. The painful "hand-foot syndrome" is commonly the first clinical manifestation, resulting from ischemic necrosis of the small tubular bones of the hands and feet. There is soft-tissue swelling, heat and tenderness over the metacarpals and proximal phalanges, with fever and frequently leukocytosis. After a week or two, x-ray changes of subperiosteal new bone formation, irregular areas of radiolucency, cortical thinning, or complete bone destruction may be seen.

Vaso-Occlusive Crises. These are acute, painful episodes resulting from local intravascular sickling, stasis, and vaso-occlusion leading to tissue necrosis and infarction. These occur most commonly in the bones, lungs, liver, mesenteric vessels, spleen, brain, and penis. Painful bone crises are the most common acute vaso-occlusive events and give rise to severe pain, with frequent joint effusions. Episodes of "acute chest syndrome" with chest pain due to infection or infarction may occur. Severe acute abdominal pain frequently occurs, particularly in children. One of the leading causes of death in children with sickle cell anemia is the acute splenic sequestration crisis in which there is sudden, rapid, and massive enlargement of the spleen with trapping of large volumes of red cells and resulting in profound hypovolemia and shock.

Aplastic Crisis. In response to the decreased red cell survival of 15 to 60 days (normal 120 days), bone marrow production of red cells is increased six- to eightfold. Periods of temporary cessation of red cell production are referred to as aplastic crises. This generally occurs with viral or bacterial infections and is followed by spontaneous recovery.

Infections. Bacterial infection is a major cause of morbidity and death, particularly in infants and young children. The reasons for the increase in incidence and severity of infection are only partly understood. There is certainly a state of defective host immunity. In sickle cell anemia, the spleen is ineffective in its phagocytic function as well as in antibody synthesis. The unique susceptibility of children with sickle cell disease to bacterial infections (e.g., pneumococcal infection) is similar to that seen in young children who have undergone splenectomy. The younger child who has not yet developed type-specific antibodies is particularly dependent on the splenic function of clearing bacteria from the circulation, which is severely impaired in sickle cell disease. There is also a deficiency of heat-labile opsonizing activity related to an abnormality of the properdin pathway in at least some sickle cell anemia patients.

Chronic Organ Damage. Cardiovascular manifestations in sickle cell anemia are generally related to chronic anemia with compensatory increased cardiac output, pulmonary arterial occlusions leading to cor pulmonale, and myocardial damage resulting from small infarcts as well as from iron deposition. Kidneys are particularly vulnerable because of the hypertonic environment. Hyposthenuria is the principal manifestation, but hematuria, nephrotic syndrome, and uremia may ocur. Cholelithiasis wih bilirubin stones is very frequent, and there may be repeated episodes of hepatic infarction leading to hepatic fibrosis. Leg ulcers are frequent in adolescence and adulthood, occuring most often over the medial surface of the lower tibia. Sensorineural hearing loss may occur following sickling in the cochlear vasculature with obstruction of hair cells. Skeletal changes due to marked expansion of the marrow cavity are common. Repeated infarction with aseptic necrosis and prominently increased susceptibility to osteomyelitis, particularly with salmonella species, cause additional abnormalities. Repeated infarcts of the spleen lead to fibrosis and "autosplenectomy."

Sickle Cell Trait (Heterozygous A₁S). Sickle cell trait is a benign condition not associated with any significant increase in morbidity or mortality rates. The only consistent abnormality found in sickle cell trait is the inability to concentrate urine. There is no anemia, abnormal morphology, or decreased red cell survival. Most patients show about 60 per cent Hb A, and 40 per cent Hb S.

As the red cells contain less than 50 per cent Hb S, only severe deoxygenation can cause sickling. This may occur in the renal medulla, with painless hematuria. For similar reasons, flying at high altitudes in an unpressurized airplane, extreme physical exercise, and complex cardiopulmonary procedures with great risk of deoxygenation should be avoided.

RELATIONSHIP TO MALARIA. Young children with sickle cell trait infected with *Plasmodium falciparum* appear to have an advantage over similarly infected normal children. It is possible that the infected red cell is preferentially sickled and destroyed in the reticuloendothelial system so that the infection is of shorter duration, with a smaller incidence of cerebral malaria and death.

HB C Disease. Hemoblogin C, like sickle hemoglobin, is inherited as an autosomal gene, and is found in about 17 to 28 per cent of West African blacks and 2 to 3 per cent of American blacks. Glutamic acid in the sixth position of the chain is replaced by lysine in Hb C. Homozygous Hb C disease is characterized by a moderate chronic hemolytic anemia (8 to 12 gm/dl) and splenomegaly. There are many target cells on the blood smear, and some contain intracellular crystals. Cholelithiasis secondary to hemolysis may occur.

Hb C trait (heterozygous) is not associated with anemia. The blood smear may show increased numbers of target cells.

HB S-C Disease. Due to the frequency of sickle hemoglobin gene and hemoglobin C gene in the same geographic areas, a doubly abnormal heterozygous state can occur in which the red cells contain a mixture of Hb S and C with no hemoglobin A₁. Many patients remain relatively asymptomatic; however, some experience severe symptoms with crises similar to Hb S disease. Splenomegaly is present along with hemolytic anemia.

Thalassemias

Thalassemias constitute a heterogeneous group of hereditary disorders of the rate of synthesis of hemoglobins in persons of Mediterranean, African, and Asian ancestry. As described earlier, the predominant adult hemoglobin is composed of two polypeptide chains, α and β globins forming HbA₁ ($\alpha_2\beta_2$) in association with heme. In the α thalassemia there is a decrease or complete lack of α globin chain synthesis, whereas in β thalassemias there is decrease or absence of synthesis of β chains. Alpha thalassemias occur predominantly in China, Malaysia, Indochina, and Africa, whereas β thalassemias occur in persons of Mediterranean, African, and Asian ancestry. Deficient α or β chain synthesis leads to a decrease in total red cell hemoglobin concentration (hypochromia) and microcytosis. Some cells are destroyed within bone marrow (ineffective erythropoiesis), whereas the other cells contain a relative excess of one of the globin chains owing to unbalanced chain synthesis. The excess unpaired chains form intracellular aggregates or inclusions that reduce cell deformibility, may act as an oxidant stress causing irreversible membrane damage, or may mediate reticuloendothelial destruction of the cell and lead to decreased survival of red cells and hemolytic anemia.

There is considerable variation in the severity of disease, depending on the nature of the genetic defect and whether the individual is homozygous or heterozygous for the mutation. Patients heterozygous for thalassemia generally show only a mild to moderate hypochromic microcytic anemia; homozygotes demonstrate severe anemia secondary to hemolysis as well as ineffective erythropoiesis. Physical properties of the excess chains play an important role in determining the severity. Beta chains form rather stable tetramers called Hb H (β_4), which become insoluble only when the red cell ages; therefore there is only mild hemolysis in α thalassemia. Alpha chains, on the other hand, are insoluble, precipitating intracellularly immediately. The precipitates interfere with erythroid maturation, giving rise to severe intramedullary hemolysis, ineffective erythropoiesis, and hemolytic anemia.

Beta Thalassemia

HOMOZYGOUS β THALASSEMIA (THALASSEMIA MAJOR). There may be a marked decrease (β^+) or absence (β^0) of beta chain production with excess of α chains in the two types of homozygous β thalassemia. As just discussed, the α chain aggregates precipitate readily, giving rise to ineffective erythropoiesis and severe hemolytic anemia. There appear to be diverse molecular lesions responsible for various types of β thalassemia. In the β^+ type, there is a slower rate of β chain synthesis with deficiency in β globin mRNA, whereas in the β^0 type there may be a total absence of β globin mRNA or there may be a total block in translation.

CLINICAL FEATURES. Affected infants present between 6 months and 2 years of age with failure to thrive, progressive anemia, and splenomegaly. Stunted growth, bossing of the skull, and prominent frontal and maxillary bones impart a mongoloid appearance. There is a marked widening of the diploë with the trabeculae arranged in vertical rows, giving rise to a "hair on end" or "sunray" appearance on skull x-ray. Severe expansion of the marrow cavities causes marked cortical thinning with frequent fractures. There are also masses of extramedullary hematopoietic tissue, causing spinal compression or simulating neoplasms. Severe anemia with hepatosplenomegaly, jaundice, cholelithiasis, and susceptibility to infections occurs. Severe growth retardation demands routine blood transfusions to maintain hemoglobin at 8 g/dl or higher. Unfortunately, nearly all patients develop iron overload and demonstrate all its complications. As iron accumulates, hemosiderin granules are formed and stored in the tissues. Thalassemia patients with significant iron overload have a "free" non–transferrin-bound iron pool, which causes toxic damage such as lipid peroxidation and lysosomal and mitochondrial poisoning. Most patients indeed die of cardiac complications of iron overload. Hemosiderin deposits occur in myocardial fibers, hepatocytes, pancreas, kidney, thyroid, adrenal glands, and the reticuloendothelial system. Patients who have not received transfusions may have hemoglobin levels of 3 g/dl or lower. Reticulocyte count is elevated, with nucleated red blood cells in peripheral blood. Methyl violet stain demonstrates stippling or red cell inclusions. Fetal hemoglobin content is usually elevated, sometimes up to 90 per cent.

THALASSEMIA INTERMEDIA. Some patients with homozygous β thalassemia show milder manifestations of the disease and are able to maintain higher hemoglobin concentrations (6 to 10 g/dl). These patients have thalassemia intermedia, which is a clinical term. There is some variation in the severity of hemolysis, and many patients do show retardation, skeletal abnormalities, and tumor-like masses of extramedullary hematopoiesis. Iron overload may develop over a long period of time owing to increased iron turnover producing greater gastrointestinal iron absorption.

THALASSEMIA TRAIT. The heterozygous state for β thalassemia is associated with mild anemia (9 to 11 g/dl) that is hypochromic and microcytic. Hb A_2 level is increased to 3.5 to 7 per cent, with mild elevation of Hb F level in some patients. Stress of pregnancy or severe infection may give rise to more severe anemia with megaloblastosis secondary to folic acid deficiency.

Alpha Thalassemia Syndromes. Several genetic inheritance patterns exist because of the duplication of the α gene. The most severe results from deletion of all or a large part of the α chain genes. There is complete absence of α chain synthesis, resulting in death of the fetus in utero from severe anemia, referred to as hydrops fetalis. The fetal blood contains only Hb Bart's ($α_4$) and some Hb H ($β_4$). The next syndrome in which three of the alpha globin genes are affected produces Hb H disease. This results from a mixed heterozygote

$α^0/α^+$ or $α^0$/Hb Constant Spring, in which the α chain is elongated with 31 extra residues attached to the C-terminal end. Hemoglobin Constant Spring contains an α chain with 142 rather than 141 amino acids, with glutamine at position 142. Hb H disease patients show moderate to severe anemia with moderate erythroid hyperplasia. Precipitated β globin inclusions can be best seen in red cells after splenectomy. Red cells containing Hb H are sensitive to oxidative stress, which results in hemolysis. These patients show 5 to 30 per cent Hb H and 1 to 2 per cent Hb Constant Spring, the remainder being Hb A_1.

Alpha thalassemia trait, in which two alpha globin chains are affected, is referred to as α thal ($α^0$ thal), and patients demonstrate mild anemia with hypochromic, microcytic cells. At birth, 5 to 10 per cent Hb Bart's ($α_4$) may be present. A silent carrier state, $α^+$ thalassemia, (α thal₂), is characterized by no anemia, normal red cells, and the presence of 1 to 2 per cent Hb Bart's at birth. Both these α thalassemia traits may be associated with 1 to 2 per cent Hb Constant Spring.

HEMOGLOBIN LEPORE. Hemoglobin Lepore is composed of α and hybrid non-α chains that are the product of δβ fusion genes formed by unequal crossing-over between the δ and β globin loci during meiosis (non-α genes lie in a linked cluster in the order $G_γ$-$A_γ$-δ-β). Depending on the exact site of the cross-over, there may be different structural configurations. The δβ fusion chains are inefficiently synthesized and give rise to clinical manifestations of δβ thalassemia. Hemoglobin Lepore shows the same electrophoretic mobility as Hb S.

The abnormal crossing-over that gives rise to Lepore hemoglobins may also give rise to a chromosome that contains normal δ and β globin gene in addition to a fusion δβ gene, the products of which combine with α chains to produce anti-Lepore hemoglobins. These are not associated with clinical manifestations of thalassemia.

Hereditary Persistence of Fetal Hemoglobin (HPFH)

A heterogeneous group of inherited conditions is associated with continuation of Hb F production into adult life. Most patients with HPFH do not manifest significant anemia, hemolysis, or ineffective erythropoiesis. HPFH is currently classified according to the distribution of Hb F in red cells into pancellular and heterocellular syndromes.

Pancellular HPFH. Hb F is present in all the red cells in both homo- and heterozygotes. Individuals homozygous for this form of HPFH have 100 per cent Hb F, and their red cells show mild microcytosis and hypochromia. There may be deletion of β and δ globin chains. Homozygous δβ thalassemia patients will also have only Hb F, but they manifest a more severe anemia than do homozygous patients with HPFH because they synthe-size much more α globin with excess α chains that lead to hemolysis and ineffective erythropoiesis. HPFH is found predominantly in blacks and in Greeks; the homozygous form, however, has been described only in blacks. Heterozygotes for HPFH have 25 per cent to 30 per cent Hb F distributed in normal-appearing red blood cells, whereas heterozygotes for δβ thalassemia show hypo-chromic microcytic cells with variable distribution of Hb F.

Heterocellular HPFH. By definition, this group of inherited conditions is associated with increased amount of Hb F in some of the red blood cells. A few red blood cells in normal adults contain small amounts of Hb F and are referred to as F cells. Their number is increased in heterocellular HPFH syndromes, and the increase is genetically trans-mitted. Swiss, British, and other forms have been described. The homozygous state described only in the British type of HPFH has about 20 per cent Hb F present in 50 to 60 per cent of red cells. Heterozygotes have 6 to 12 per cent Hb F distrib-uted in 20 to 30 per cent of red blood cells.

The Unstable Hemoglobins

Unstable hemoglobinopathy has an autosomal dominant pattern of inheritance, thereby produc-ing manifestations in the heterozygous individual. The homozygous state for this disorder would gen-erally be incompatible with life. About 70 struc-turally different unstable hemoglobin variants have been described. Some of these show only mild instability in vitro, whereas others give rise to significant hemolysis. Many are amino acid sub-stitutions in the vicinity of the heme pocket, pro-ducing perturbations in the hydrophobic interior of the molecule, and preventing normal heme-globin linkage. Precipitated hemoglobin attaches to the red cell membrane (Heinz bodies) and short-ens its survival. The cells become inflexible. Heinz bodies are removed by the spleen. The oxygen affinity is usually abnormal. When the oxygen affinity is increased (e.g., Hb Köln, Hb Gun Hill), patients have relatively high hemoglobin concen-trations with a high reticulocyte count. Those with low oxygen affinity (e.g., Hb Hammersmith) have rather low hemoglobin concentrations and low reticulocyte counts. Heinz bodies are not seen in peripheral blood unless the spleen has been re-moved.

Hemoglobinopathies Producing Cyanosis. Cyanosis is caused by an excess of deoxyhemoglo-bin or methemoglobin in blood. Methemoglobine-mia is discussed elsewhere. A more uncommon cause of methemoglobinemia is the presence of Hb M, which is inherited in the autosomal dominant pattern. Many forms of Hb M show substitution of tyrosine for histidine in the proximal and distal sites of the α and β chains. Dusky color at birth is seen in infants with α chain variants, whereas in the β chain variants, cyanosis is apparent at 6 to 9 months of age. Another group of abnormal hemo-globins cause cyanosis secondary to decreased ox-ygen affinity. This causes a right shift in the oxygen dissociation curve so that less erythropoi-etin is produced, resulting in lower hemoglobin content. Some of these hemoglobins are also mildly unstable, giving rise to hemolysis.

Hemoglobinopathies Producing Erythrocy-tosis. A heterogeneous group of structurally ab-normal hemoglobins cause increased oxygen affin-ity, a shift to the left of the oxygen dissociation curve, and compensatory erythrocytosis. Some of the hemoglobin variants have substitutions at the C-terminal end of the subunit; others show substi-tutions at the $\alpha_1\beta_2$ interface.

IRON METABOLISM

Approximately 70 per cent of the iron in the human body is in the hemoglobin, the oxygen-carrying protein of the red blood cells, and iron metabolism is largely related to the synthesis and breakdown of this protein. The oxygen binding protein of muscle, myoglobin, accounts for another 5 per cent, and enzymes containing iron account for smaller amounts. The remaining body iron is called "storage iron" and is available for the syn-thesis of the iron-containing proteins. The amount of storage iron is variable and under physiologic conditions represents a balance between iron in-take and losses.

Iron losses and absorption are relatively con-stant, approximately 1 mg/dl. Women during child-bearing years have very low to no iron stores because of menstruation and childbirth, while men have between 1 and 2 g of storage iron. These stores are made up of a soluble component, ferritin, and hemosiderin, a degraded form of ferritin, but most is in the ferritin form. When iron load in-creases, the hemosiderin also increases.

Ferritin is roughly a spherical protein shell containing an iron core with a molecular weight of approximately 450,000 daltons. It is considered to play two major roles in iron metabolism: it prevents accumulation of high levels of free iron in cells, and functions as an iron reserve for hemoglobin when needed. The amount of iron stored in the body is reflected by and correlates very well with serum ferritin levels. In health, serum ferritin concentration is relatively stable, with levels ranging from 15 to 300 μg/L, but these ranges depend on age and sex. As far as is known, low ferritin serum levels reflect decreased to ab-sent reticuloendothelial iron stores. Patients with ferritin serum levels of less than 10 to 15 μg/L have a history of continued loss of iron and eventu-ally develop iron deficiency anemia, the most common form of anemia throughout the world.

High serum levels of ferritin have been observed in patients with liver disease, especially those with acute hepatic cell necrosis, in patients with malignant solid tumors and leukemia, and in patients with acute and chronic inflammatory diseases as well as patients with idiopathic or secondary iron overload.

Iron is a vital element in human metabolism, is present in all cells of the body, and plays its most important role in erythropoiesis. It is secured from the environment as an insoluble hydroxide, and almost all organisms have developed specific iron binding molecules for its transport and storage. The management of iron is remarkably efficient, re-utilizing the iron released from the breakdown of hemoglobin and other iron-containing proteins while maintaining its levels within very narrow limits.

Daily iron losses from hemoglobin and from desquamated epithelial cells from skin and intestinal mucosa account for 1 to 2 mg, but such losses are carefully balanced by iron absorption through the gastrointestinal tract. The entire gastrointestinal tract is capable of absorbing iron; however, maximal activity is seen in the duodenum and upper jejunum. The amount of iron available for absorption depends on the amount released by the digestive process and in general is less than half of the total iron present in food. Most of the iron released is in the form of ionizable inorganic iron. Since only iron in the ferrous form can be absorbed, ferric ions undergo increasing polymerization as the pH rises toward neutrality and are reduced to the ferrous form. An acid pH provided by gastric hydrochloric acid regulates the rate of absorption, prevents precipitation of iron phosphates, and aids in the reduction of food iron from ferric to ferrous. As iron is absorbed by the intestinal cells it is immediately oxidized and temporarily stored as ferritin.

The molecular mechanisms of iron absorption are still not well understood. Marx divided iron absorption into phases of mucosal uptake and mucosal transfer. It appears that initial mucosal uptake is predominantly a passive process in which large amounts of iron are taken up by the intestinal mucosal cell vesicles but later released through the lumen if the concentration gradient driving uptake is removed (Eastham et al.). The intestinal mucosal cells have been shown to contain ferritin and transferrin-like proteins, the latter displaying an iron-binding behavior similar to that of the serum protein, while the amounts of ferritin in the cells are directly proportional to body iron stores.

The mechanisms for intestinal iron absorption respond rapidly to changes in the body iron pool. Lack of iron, increased turnover, or ineffective erythropoietic activity results in increased iron absorption. Iron overload promptly reduces iron absorption. The regulatory mechanisms for iron absorption are still not well known.

Experimentally, the intestinal cell may respond to humoral factors by regulating the number of iron-binding sites in the brush border of the cells or by controlling the cell's iron transporting molecules. In addition to cellular mechanisms, there are a variety of luminal factors that may increase or decrease intestinal iron absorption. Ascorbic acid and other reducing substances, sugars, and some iron chelators stimulate iron absorption, while naturally occurring phytates and tannic acid can decrease it.

Vertebrates developed a complex molecule called transferrin to manage the internal transport of iron that is responsible for carrying iron between sites of absorption, storage, and utilization. This single chain polypeptide protein has a molecular weight of approximately 80,000 daltons and contains two specific iron binding sites that have been designated as A and B by some investigators. These iron binding sites differ in their affinity to bind iron and their accessibility to the chemical forms of iron present. These two sites may function in different ways as iron acceptors from absorption and storage sites. Under physiologic conditions, transferrin is only 30 per cent saturated, retains iron more tightly than other iron-binding molecules, and is perhaps the only source of iron to immature erythroid elements for synthesis of hemoglobin. Unlike other glycoproteins, transferrin is neither altered by hepatic clearance nor destroyed during interaction with iron-requiring cells and undergoes many iron-transporting cycles during its 8-day lifetime.

Frieden and Aisen have demonstrated that the distribution of iron between the two binding sites is not random and that the weaker binding site located in the N-terminal segment of the polypeptide is the one that is perferentially occupied. If iron turnover is increased, however, the stronger site in the C-terminal polypeptide exhibits greater occupancy.

Iron receptors are required for transferrin to donate iron to the receptor cell. Such receptors have been identified in red cell precursors, hepatocytes, and many other benign and malignant human cells.

In disorders characterized by iron overload, transferrin binding capacity is exceeded, and nonspecific protein complexes of iron appear in the serum. Some studies indicate that such nonspecific protein-binding complexes may be taken up and deposited by the liver cells and perhaps play an important role in hepatic cirrhosis due to iron overload.

The hepatocyte plays a role in iron metabolism and storage. The exchange of iron between transferrin and the hepatocyte is mediated through specific plasma membrane surface receptors similar to the reticulocyte receptors for transferrin, and the uptake may be controlled in part by the number of available receptors. The net uptake of iron by the liver may depend on total serum iron concentration, transferrin saturation, or both. The Kupffer cell contains little ferritin, and its chief function is to recycle iron from senescent erythrocytes or from hemoglobin. Other than utilization and storage of iron, the liver plays an important role in the synthesis of transferrin, which is increased in response to iron depletion and inhibited by a surplus of the metal.

IRON METABOLISM IN THE ERYTHROCYTE

It is now believed that the transferrin iron complex enters the cell obligatorily; however, the site for final utilization for heme synthesis and the transport of iron to the mitochondrion is still uncertain. Non-heme cytosolic iron-binding intermediates that include ferritin have been proposed. The iron in mitochondria is in the heme and non-heme sulfur iron protein forms; no free iron is stored. Under such circumstances, cytosol-iron appears to be the source for the ferrochelatase reaction, the final step of heme biosynthesis. Iron must be in a ferrous form and must be transported through both mitochondrial membranes in order to reach ferrochelatase, which is located in the inner mitochondrial membrane (Romslo). The mechanism by which ferric iron is reduced for this process is still not understood. The iron is thought to be transported across mitochondrial membranes in association with phospholipids and via an electrogenic carrier. Ferrochelatase binds the ferrous iron, and the complex combines with protoporphyrin to form heme, which binds with the globin to form hemoglobin.

DISORDERS OF IRON METABOLISM

IRON DEFICIENCY

Iron deficiency is present when the content of body iron is decreased. As stated before, under normal conditions, iron is distributed throughout the body among numerous functional compounds. These functional compounds and their metabolism are carefully regulated through a sophisticated mechanism of iron recycling and intestinal absorption to balance iron losses and body iron storage. While body iron storage varies from population to population because of dietary differences, it is usually adequate in normal individuals, and a negative balance results in a state of iron deficiency. If the negative iron balance persists, various clinical degrees of severity develop that merge imperceptibly into each other. In the earlier stages, the negative balance is designated as iron deficiency without anemia, while the more advanced has been called iron deficiency anemia.

Factors Affecting Prevalence of Iron Deficiency

The factors affecting prevalence of iron deficiency in the general population can be classified as physiologic, pathologic, and nutritional (Table 23–8).

Physiologic factors are those related to the body's normal requirement for iron from childhood to adulthood. During the first year of life, the iron needs for adequate erythropoiesis are approximately 180 mg per day in a full-term infant, while premature infants usually require about 240 mg. This demand for iron is increased during the rapid growth from infancy to adolescence, and the great demand plays a very important role in the prevalence of iron deficiency in this population. When adulthood is reached, the requirement is greater in women than in men. In the adult man, 1 mg per day is needed if iron stores are adequate. In women, during the reproductive years, the need for iron is greater because iron is lost from bleeding during menstruation, and many normal women need more than 1 mg per day. When menopause is reached, the daily iron requirements fall, since the menstrual bleeding ceases and in general the female body frame is smaller. In pregnancy, larger amounts of iron are required to supply the expansion of the maternal red cell mass, the needs of the placenta, and fetal erythropoiesis. The needs during the first trimester are essentially the average normal daily requirements. During

TABLE 23–8 FACTORS IN IRON DEFICIENCY

Physiologic factors
  Infancy
  Adolescence
  Menstruation
  Pregnancy
  Delivery
  Lactation

Pathologic factors
  Chronic blood losses
    Gastrointestinal
    Genitourinary
    Pulmonary
    Phlebotomies
    Coagulation disorders
  Iron malabsorption
    Gastric hypochlorhydria
    Intestinal malabsorption

Nutritional Factors
  Decreased iron intake
    Low dietary iron content
  Iron bioavailability
    Dietary heme iron
    Dietary non-heme iron
    Enhancing ligands
    Inhibitory ligands

the second trimester, additional iron is needed and the daily requirements rise to approximately 4 mg per day. During the third trimester, needs are still greater and daily requirements are up to 6 mg per day. During pregnancy, delivery, and lactation, iron deficiency in this population is more prevalent than among any other adult group and approximately 950 mg over and above the normal obligatory losses is required to correct it.

Pathologic factors contributing to iron deficiency are those related to bleeding and poor absorption of dietary iron. The most common causes of pathologic bleeding are those related to diseases of the gastrointestinal, genitourinary, and respiratory tracts. Diseases of the gastrointestinal tract are the most frequent causes of iron deficiency in the adult male and postmenopausal female. In Western countries, benign and malignant neoplasms, ulcers, inflammatory diseases of the bowel, acquired or congenital vascular malformations, and the chronic use of aspirin most commonly cause bleeding. Throughout the world parasitic infestation, especially with hookworm, most frequently cause bleeding and iron deficiency.

Intestinal malabsorption of iron has not been shown to be an important factor in the origin of iron deficiency, except in those patients with hypochlorhydria due to gastric atrophy or gastric resection or those with malabsorption syndromes, especially tropical sprue.

Nutritional factors are very important in the individual requirement for iron. While the amount of iron in the diet is relevant for iron nutrition, its bioavailability is of greater significance. In order to understand this concept one must distinguish between heme iron, which is easily absorbed, and non-heme iron, which is also absorbed, but only under certain conditions.

Iron complexes are dissociated during acid digestion, but heme iron is readily absorbed intact because the iron in the heme is not released from the porphyrin ring until after it has been absorbed by the intestinal mucosal cells. Non-heme iron is dependent on reducing systems and is susceptible to inhibitory ligands that form nonabsorbable complexes with the free iron, such as those found in cereals, certain vegetables, eggs, and tea. Some promoters of non-heme iron absorption such as ascorbic acid, fish, and meat, form small molecular complexes with iron, enhancing its bioavailability. The average Western diet, rich in heme iron, supplies iron needs of up to 3 to 4 mg per day, while cereal diets in less-developed areas of the world supply small amounts of non-heme, more difficult to absorb, iron. This results in great prevalence of iron deficiency in such populations.

Cook and associates, using several populations as a model for studies of iron nutrition, demonstrated that by measuring plasma ferritin concentration, transferrin saturation, red cell protoporphyrin level, and hemoglobin concentrations, an accurate evaluation of iron nutrition can be obtained, and that such populations can be classified as normal, iron depleted, iron deficient erythropoietic, and iron deficiency anemic.

Iron Deficiency Without Anemia

In a state of negative iron balance, iron is gradually mobilized from iron stores to meet metabolic activities and hemoglobin synthesis until iron stores are completely depleted. This state has been called "pre-latent iron deficiency," and its hallmark is increased iron absorption without decrease in hemoglobin or serum iron concentration and the absence of stainable iron in the bone marrow. If iron depletion continues, serum iron concentrations begin to fall, but erythropoiesis is still intact and a "latent" iron deficiency results. When depletion continues, reduction of iron to the bone marrow leads to iron deficiency erythropoiesis, and iron deficiency anemia appears.

Iron deficiency is often associated with nonspecific and specific tissue abnormalities that become clinically obvious, depending on the severity of the state of deficiency. Many tissue abnormalities have been described in experimental animals and iron-deficient patients. Many metabolic processes involve enzymes that either contain iron or require it as a co-factor. Decreased activity appears in such important iron-dependent systems as cytochrome *c*, cytochrome oxidase, catalase, peroxidase, succinic dehydrogenase, tyrosine hydroxylase, phenylalanine hydroxylase, monoamino oxidase, aconitase, proline hydroxylase, and myoglobin. Disturbances in cellular metabolism and function have been described and are associated with defects of tissues characterized by rapidly proliferating cells. The gastrointestinal tract is the most susceptible to such changes, clinically manifest as atrophic mucosal changes that give origin in the mouth to angular stomatitis and glossitis. In the laryngopharynx these mucosal changes have given rise to formation of webs of the postcricoid region clinically manifest as dysphagia and known as the Plummer-Vinson and Patterson-Kelly syndromes. Sideropenic dysphagia syndromes have been found to lead to pharyngeal and esophageal carcinomas. These findings have been confirmed by histologic examination of such webs.

The gastric mucosa has shown extensive atrophic changes that in some cases have been associated with antibodies to parietal cells. Sprue-like histologic changes of the small intestine with widening, blunting, fusion of villi, and chronic inflammatory infiltrate have been also reported.

Oski and Judish and their co-workers reported growth retardation and skeletal muscle abnormalities proportional to the severity of iron deficiency as well as changes in nails (koilonychia) and bones.

Iron Deficiency Anemia

The end stage of a negative iron balance is iron deficiency anemia. It is perhaps the most common manifestation of disease throughout the world and affects persons irrespective of age, sex, or economic status. Several factors affect its prevalence and its clinical manifestations. As the iron deficiency progresses, compensatory mechanisms develop that are responsible for most patients being asymptomatic. As iron deficit increases, clinical manifestations and morphologic features appear. The earliest and most common finding is anemia.

In the beginning, the peripheral red blood cells do not change morphologically, and they are normochromic and normocytic. As these cells are replaced and iron deficiency increases, microcytosis and hypochromia due to a decrease in total hemoglobin concentration appear; the mean corpuscular volume (MCV) falls below the normal levels of 80 μm^3, the mean corpuscular hemoglobin (MCH) drops below 27 pg, and the red cell diameter to thickness ratio rises above 3.2. Fragmented red blood cells, elliptocyte and target cells may also appear. The morphologic changes of the bone marrow are variable. The degree of erythroid hyperplasia does not correlate well with the severity of the anemia, and the normoblasts in the marrow are, in most cases, essentially normal. Only in severe cases do the smaller normoblasts with little hemoglobin demonstrate ragged cytoplasmic rims. Marked decrease to absence of iron stores in the bone marrow is the hallmark of iron deficiency. Siderotic granules, found in some normoblasts, become rare to absent.

Clinical manifestations are pallor, easy fatigability, tachycardia, headaches, ankle edema, and exertional dyspnea. Compensatory mechanisms within the red cell lead to decreased oxygen affinity and an increase in cardiac output in order to provide optimal tissue oxygenation. Several studies have suggested that such symptoms are related to metabolic cell changes and that physical work capacity is markedly impaired. Other studies have given contradictory results. Pica, a peculiar appetite abnormality for clay, dirt, and the like, is an unusual manifestation of iron deficiency and is usually cured by iron therapy.

The symptoms may be related to the manifestations of the primary pathologic factors, to the anemia itself, or to the metabolic cell changes of the impaired iron proteins other than hemoglobin, as previously described.

IRON OVERLOAD

Iron overload occurs when excessive iron enters and is deposited in the body by increased intestinal absorption, parenteral administration of iron complexes, or therapeutic blood transfusions in patients with severe anemias.

Jacobs (1977) demonstrated that resistance of parenchymal cells to damage by iron depends on the ability of the cells to take iron in a nontoxic form. The increase is conducive to an expansion in the cellular iron pool of low molecular weight iron with an increase in ferritin deposition in lysosomes and displacement of most of the cellular components. There is some evidence that iron-loaded lysosomes may play a very important role in cell damage and exaggerated collagen deposition when the lysosomes rupture.

When the enormous ability of the reticuloendothelial cells to store iron is exceeded, transferrin saturation rises and synthesis is inhibited. It has been suggested that under such circumstances, non-protein-bound iron is available for uptake and retention, and that this form of iron is toxic to parenchymal cells. The most frequent, but less severe, form of body iron overload is seen in chronic inflammatory processes and other conditions associated with liver disease, especially cutaneous porphyria, iron-containing alcoholic beverages, and therapeutic use of iron and blood transfusions.

The most clinically prominent disorder of iron metabolism is hemochromatosis.

Primary Hemochromatosis

This disorder of iron metabolism is clinically characterized by skin pigmentation, endocrinopathies, hepatic cirrhosis, cardiomyopathy, and arthropathy due to excessive intestinal absorption of iron leading to an abnormal high deposition in all parenchymal cells of the body.

Cartwright and associates in 1979 and Simon and associates in 1980 demonstrated that hemochromatosis is an inherited disorder and presented evidence that transmission is recessive and that homozygosity is required for full clinical expression of the disease. The mutant gene is closely associated with the HLA, A3, B7, and B14 alloantigens located in the short arm of chromosome 6.

In the past the disease was considered relatively rare, but recent calculations estimate its frequency as greater than 2 per 1000. Beaumont and Edwards estimate the gene frequency at about 50 to 70 per 10,000 with a heterozygote frequency of 10 per 100 of population.

As a result of HLA data, patients with hemochromatosis can be classified as homozygotes and heterozygotes. Homozygotes develop a full-blown clinical disease, while heterozygotes demonstrate the laboratory abnormalities without clinical manifestation of the disease.

The most common symptoms are weakness, arthralgia, and weight loss, and as the disease progresses, cardiac complaints and loss of libido reflect specific organ damage. The physical findings are multisystemic, ranging from hepatomegaly to skin pigmentation and arthropathy. Liver biopsy demonstrates moderate cirrhosis with extensive iron deposits, especially in the periportal areas. Liver function tests may be normal to markedly abnormal, depending on the stage of the disease. Hepatomas occur in approximately 29 per cent of patients with terminal disease.

The most common endocrine disorder reported is diabetes mellitus with pancreatic fibrosis. Iron deposition within islet cells and exocrine tissues is always present in end-stage disease. When glucose tolerance tests are used as the diagnostic criteria in hemochromatosis, the incidence of diabetes mellitus is approximately 80 per cent. In young patients, however, diabetes is not necessarily a feature of the disease.

Hypogonadism is the second most common endocrinopathy, and its etiology is related to inadequate pituitary secretion of gonadotrophic stimulating hormones due to fibrosis and iron deposits in the hypothalamic-pituitary axis and the gonads. Panhypopituitarism with hypothyroidism, hypoadrenalism, and hypogonadism as an end-stage disease have been also reported.

Bronze-colored skin pigmentation is due to increased epidermal melanin and subcutaneous iron deposits. Pigmentation is present in approximately 85 per cent of cases. A progressive polyarthropathy, which does not correlate with iron deposits in the joints, is present in about 50 per cent of patients. Cardiac arrhythmias with congestive heart failure due to extensive myocardial fibrosis and iron loading are also seen in approximately one third of patients.

The average homozygote has accumulated 20 to 40 g of iron by the time end-stage hemochromatosis is diagnosed. The average iron plasma is 250 μg/dl with a transferrin saturation close to 100 per cent. Plasma ferritin concentration is always increased, with levels above 500 ng/ml.

Detection of iron overload would be best achieved by direct measurements of total body iron. No satisfactory technique is as yet available, however. Indirect information is obtained when the patient is given 200 mg of ascorbic acid daily for a week followed by an intramuscular injection of 10 mg/kg of body weight of the chelating agent deferoxamine, and 24-hour urinary iron is measured. Normally, less than 2 mg of iron is excreted, but when the disease is present, urine iron levels are over 5 mg. The most accurate way of estimating iron overload is by direct measurement of iron concentration in biopsies of liver tissue.

Long and coworkers, using computed tomography as a noninvasive method of measuring iron, demonstrated an increased attenuation coefficient of the liver and other organs, which has proved to correlate well with iron concentration in liver tissue obtained by biopsy.

Secondary Hemochromatosis (Hemosiderosis)

In hemosiderosis the iron loading occurs first in the macrophages and later in the parenchymal cells, in contrast to primary hemochromatosis in which iron loading is predominantly a parenchymal cell disorder. Serum iron is widely distributed in ferritin and hemosiderin forms and has been found in all tissues of the body. The internal iron distribution and pattern of organ damage, as well as clinical presentation of the disease, is similar to that of primary hemochromatosis. Cardiac disease, however, is the most frequent cause of death in patients with hemosiderosis, while endocrine deficiencies and other miscellaneous complications are of secondary importance. The plasma ferritin level is elevated early in the course of disease, while increased plasma iron and transferrin saturation occur later.

Disorders of erythropoiesis are also present as a complication of hemochromatosis and are due to improper utilization of iron for hemoglobin synthesis. In such cases, anemia is the result of ineffective erythropoiesis, and iron accumulates in the cytoplasm of the erythroid precursors, giving origin to iron-loading anemias.

Sideroblastic Anemia

Sideroblastic anemia is a comprehensive syndrome that occurs under diverse conditions and is characterized by defective hemoglobin production, the presence of hypochromic microcytic erythrocytes in the peripheral blood, ring sideroblasts in the bone marrow, and a variable iron overload in the mitochondria. The mechanism underlying sideroblastic anemia is thought to be defective heme synthesis, since iron supply to erythroid precursors and globin synthesis appear normal. Vitamin B_6 in the form of pyridoxal phosphate (PLP) is known to be an essential cofactor of δ aminolevulinic acid synthetase for heme synthesis in mitochondria.

The spectrum of sideroblastic anemia has been expanded considerably since its initial description (Table 23–9). It is a rare inherited congenital disorder that most often occurs in young males and, in an acquired form, after the third decade with or without predisposing causes.

The herditary X-linked sideroblastic anemia is overt in males and has a recessive inheritance pattern in female relatives. The erythroid defect appears uniformly as a hypochromic microcytic population of erythrocytes and numerous siderocytes that correlates with the degree of anemia. This contrasts with the acquired sideroblastic anemia in which the ring sideroblast abnormality is found in nondividing erythrocytes.

Cases of undetermined inheritance, mostly seen in females, may represent sporadic cases of homozygotes for an autosomal or X-linked gene with clinical and hematologic features undistinguishable from the X-linked form.

Acquired sideroblastic anemias range from mild to severe and are seen in middle aged to older individuals. Typically, the erythrocytes demonstrate two extreme populations of cells, one microcytic hypochromic and the other, macrocytic. Usually, the latter predominates and the red cell index is macrocytic. Basophilic stippling predominates, and siderocytes are seen less often. In the bone marrow a large percentage of erythroblasts are ring sideroblasts, in contrast with the pattern of the congenital disorder.

As stated in Table 23–9, acquired sideroblastic anemia can be idiopathic or drug-induced. Antituberculous agents, ethanol, chemotherapeutic agents, and chloramphenicol have been associated with the development of sideroblastic anemia. Anemia is promptly and fully reversed, however, after withdrawal of the drug or after administration of vitamin B_6.

Idiopathic sideroblastic anemia and some myeloproliferative disorders share some of their features, clinical presentation, and course (Riedler 1972) and have the potential for leukemic transformation (Linman 1978). In such cases their course resembles that of a chronic granulocytic leukemia, and chromosomal alterations may be seen.

Anemia of Chronic Disorders

Chronic infection, inflammation, and neoplasms are frequently associated with anemia. Although it is a very common disorder, it is usually asymptomatic and overshadowed by the symptoms of the underlying disease.

During the early part of the century, numerous reports associated severe debilitating chronic inflammatory diseases with anemia. During the last two decades it has been recognized that noninfectious inflammatory diseases such as collagen diseases and malignant proliferation are also associated with anemia, hence the designation of anemia of chronic disorders (Table 23–10).

The anemia is usually mild and begins to develop in the first 2 months of the underlying disorder. Although it is characteristically normochromic and normocytic, hypochromia and microcytosis due to decreased mean corpuscular hemoglobin may be seen. The reticulocyte count is usually normal; however, red cell survival is slightly decreased.

TABLE 23–9 CLASSIFICATION OF
SIDEROBLASTIC ANEMIAS

Congenital
  (a) Hereditary, X-linked
  (b) Inheritance undetermined

Acquired
  Idiopathic
    Pyridoxin responsive
    Pyridoxin nonresponsive
    Preleukemic
  Drug-induced
    Antituberculosis drugs
    Ethanol
    Chemotherapeutic agents
    Chloramphenicol

TABLE 23–10 ANEMIAS SECONDARY TO
CHRONIC SYSTEMIC DISORDERS

Anemia of chronic inflammation
  Infection
  Connective tissue disorders
  Malignant proliferation
Anemia of chronic renal disease
Anemia of chronic liver disease
Anemia of endocrine disorders

Serum iron concentration is characteristically low, and the total serum transferrin is also reduced, since the saturation of transferrin is slightly decreased. The bone marrow is generally morphologically normal with sequential erythroid maturation. The most characteristic finding is a reduction of the iron-containing red cell precursors (sideroblast), while bone marrow iron stores are increased. It appears that in anemia of chronic disorders there is no good correlation between iron stores and serum ferritin concentration, which can be normal or elevated. Birgegård and coworkers (1978) found that serum ferritin concentrations closely followed acute-phase reactant proteins such as haptoglobin and that it is possible that serum ferritin elevations are misleading for evaluating serum iron in patients while inflammation is still present.

The anemia is nevertheless characterized by impairment of the compensatory increase in production of red blood cells due to ineffective erythropoiesis and is associated with a slightly shortened red cell life and disturbed iron metabolism. Even though the mechanisms of anemia remain an enigma, studies have demonstrated that perhaps several factors play important roles in the disorder.

Studies by Ward and by Firat and their associates demonstrated that in patients with rheumatoid arthritis and cancer, serum erythropoietin levels were not elevated and that erythropoietic activity was directly rather than inversely related to hemoglobin concentrations, suggesting that the anemia is perhaps due to defective erythropoietin production, and indeed to a decrease in bone marrow sensitivity to erythropoietin stimulation. Whether anemia of chronic disorders is a primary defect of the oxygen sensing device or a failure to produce biologically active erythropoietin is still not well understood, since both anoxia and the administration of exogenous erythropoietin have been shown to correct the anemia in experimental animals (Gutnisky and Van Dyke 1963, Lukens 1973).

It also has been postulated that in chronic inflammatory disease, low serum iron and increased iron stores are due to blockage of iron released from the storage, which limits its supply to the erythroid marrow. The cells apparently can handle the available iron, since the utilization of radioactive iron is normal.

DISORDERS OF HEMOPOIETIC STEM CELL

APLASTIC ANEMIA

Aplastic anemia is defined as a peripheral blood pancytopenia associated with markedly decreased multipotential stem cells in a hypocellular marrow. The fat to marrow ratio is markedly increased, and only small islets of hyperactive marrow are present.

The clinical manifestations of the disorder are directly associated with the pancytopenia. The anemia, like any other anemia, is characterized by pallor, weakness, and easy fatigability. The granulocytopenia increases the possibilities for infection and may cause fever; the thrombocytopenia increases the bleeding time and is associated with severe hemorrhage, hematomas and petechiae.

The anemia, a reflection of the erythroid stem cell deficiency, is generally macrocytic; the reticulocytes are markedly decreased to less than 1 per cent after correction for hematocrit, and plasma erythropoietin and iron levels are elevated. Radioactive iron studies demonstrate reduced plasma iron turnover and prolonged iron clearance due to a markedly reduced bone marrow mass and rate of red cell production. This pattern of iron clearance is characteristic of all anemias due to a decrease in erythropoietic tissues and differentiates them from anemias characterized by ineffective red cell production. In those, intramedullary destruction of erythropoietic precursors causes poor utilization of iron and short iron clearance time resulting from excess of erythropoietic precursors in the bone marrow.

The peripheral blood expression of the granulocytic stem cell deficiency is an absolute granulocytopenia. Patients can be characterized as having mild, moderate, or severe granulocytopenia if the counts range from 2000 to 500 cells/mm³. In cases in which the counts are less than 500/mm³, isolation procedures are recommended to improve immediate prognosis, since the risk of and susceptibility to infections in such patients are very great.

Peripheral thrombocytopenia is the reflection of the megakaryocytic line deficiency with platelet counts lower than 20,000/mm³ and clinical manifestations of mild to severe hemorrhage. Platelet survival in the peripheral blood is essentially normal, indicating that the cytopenia is due to the decreased rate at which platelets enter the circulation rather than to increased turnover.

The diagnosis of aplastic anemia includes a heterogeneous group of conditions with many etiologies and backgrounds that can occur at any of the multiple steps of hematopoiesis. The pluripotential stem cell may be defective in its ability for cell renewal or in its absolute number, may not respond to humoral factors that normally induce differentiation, or the environment may be inadequate to support hematopoiesis. There may be humoral inhibitors of hematopoiesis or cellular inhibitors for specific cell lines, which could explain specific single cell aplasias.

Classification of Aplastic Anemia

From the clinical point of view, aplastic anemias can be classified into two large categories, those expressed clinically as pancytopenias and those with a clinical single cell deficiency. With respect to etiology, aplastic anemias can be further subclassified as acquired, constitutional, and preleukemic (Table 23–11).

Clinical Pancytopenias

Acquired Aplastic Anemias. Medical literature is full of reports concerning the possible causes of acquired aplastic anemias and confirms the fact that the etiology of the disease can only be suspected and is not established. Cases in which no causal agent is suspected or found have been designated as idiopathic. A case is assigned to such a category by exclusion after thorough clinical investigation. Many patients are found to have been exposed to multiple potentially etiologic agents.

Drug-induced Aplastic Anemia. Numerous drugs suspected of causing aplastic anemia have

TABLE 23–11 CLASSIFICATION OF APLASTIC ANEMIAS

Acquired
Idiopathic
Drugs
Idiosyncratic
Dose related
Chemotherapeutic
Chemicals and toxins
Radiation
Infection
Viral
Bacterial
Pregnancy
Thymomas
Constitutional
Fanconi's anemia
Familial aplastic anemia
Amegakaryocytic thrombocytopenia
Dyskeratosis congenita
Shwachman-Diamond syndrome
Preleukemic
Acquired aplastic anemia
Fanconi's anemia
Familial
Single cell deficiencies
Pre-acute lymphocytic leukemia

been listed and published by the American Medical Association (Table 23–12). Drugs that induce aplastic anemia can be grouped into three different categories. The first is related to those chemotherapeutic agents that have myelosuppressive effects that are predictable in relation to dosage.

The second group of drugs includes those that may produce marrow depression during their administration, but after discontinuation of which a full recovery is expected. They rarely cause significant pancytopenia.

Aplastic anemias caused by the third group of drugs can be "idiosyncratic" or due to "hypersensitivity reaction" and may appear several weeks or months after use of the drug. Yunis reported that the same drug may cause dose-related and idiosyncratic aplasias, but the mechanisms may be different, because both reactions have not been seen in the same patients. The drug most frequently associated with aplastic anemia of either type is chloramphenicol. In the dose-related bone marrow depression, one of the first observations is vacuolization of the erythroblast. These changes appear more rapidly in patients treated with large doses of chloramphenicol or in patients with impaired liver and renal function. Rosenthal reported the appearance of idiosyncratic aplastic anemia and suspected genetic predisposition to the reaction in a patient who used chloramphenicol eyedrops and his niece who died of chloramphenicol-related marrow aplasia. Yunis and Bloomberg demonstrated that in patients who have recovered from chloramphenicol-induced idiosyncratic aplastic anemia, DNA synthesis in the marrow was inhibited in vitro by low concentrations of the drug. The same mechanisms have been reported for phenytoin (Dilantin), chlorpromazine, and quinine drug-induced marrow aplasia.

Bone marrow failure and leukemia have been related to certain chemicals and toxins, most of them implicating benzene or nitrobenzene radicals, which are present in many of commercial solvents, coal derivatives, petroleum products, and

TABLE 23–12 COMMON DRUGS ASSOCIATED WITH APLASTIC ANEMIA*

Azathioprine
Carbamazepine
Carbonic anydrase inhibitors
Chloramphenicol
Ethosuximide
Indomethacin
Lymphocyte immune globulin
Penicillamine
Probenecid
Quinacrine
Sulfonamides
Sulfonylurea
Thiazides
Trimethadione

*AMA Drug Evaluations

insecticides. Benzene-induced blood dyscrasias are related to duration and intensity of the exposure. These substances may play an important role in some environmental hazards, many of which involve use of products that contain a petroleum based medium.

Radiation-induced Aplastic Anemia. Radiation-induced aplastic anemia is in the same category as that caused by chemotherapeutic agents. High-energy or prolonged moderate radiation can cause acute or chronic marrow failure and aplastic anemia. All cells can be injured by radiation, but those such as germinal and hematopoietic cells, which have an accelerated turnover of nucleic acid, are more prone to injury. Exposure to high-energy radiation causes acute marrow failure and pancytopenia. If the patient survives the acute radiation injury, the dormant stem cells repopulate the marrow. On the other hand, in patients exposed to prolonged moderate doses, radiation may lead to irreversible damage of the microcirculation and perhaps to the hematopoietic cells as changes in the bone marrow environment prevent repopulation. These changes have been reported in patients with ankylosing spondylitis, in watch-dial painters who accidentally ingested long half-life radioactive paint, and in radiologists exposed to low radiation for many years.

Infection-induced Aplastic Anemia. Numerous cases of infection, whether viral or bacterial, have been linked to aplastic anemia. More than one hundred cases of aplastic anemia associated with viral hepatitis but without other reasons for myelosuppression have been also reported, and the clinical picture of aplastic anemia was found within several months to years after the onset of the disease. Many such patients are also exposed to other drugs and toxins, including chloramphenicol, which makes it unclear whether the aplastic process is due to viral infection or is drug-induced. Williams suggested several possible mechanisms to explain the hepatitis-induced aplasia. Those mechanisms may be related to failure of the liver to detoxify drugs or toxins, direct damage to the marrow, damage to the marrow environment, or an autoimmune response to the virus. Support for the autoimmune concept is found in a case of posthepatitis aplasia in which bone marrow transplants of an identical twin were at first rejected but became successful after the patient was treated with cyclophosphamide.

Pancytopenia has also been seen in patients with bacterial infections, especially tuberculosis, and may happen during or following the infection. The marrow, however, is rarely hypoplastic. Since such patients are often treated with antibiotics and other drugs, the anemia could be related to direct injury to the marrow cells by the drugs or to the compound effects of the infectious agents and the drugs.

Pregnancy and Aplastic Anemia. The precise relationship between pregnancy and aplastic anemia is still unclear. The first report was of aplastic anemia in a pregnant woman, but in many cases reported, the anemia preceded pregnancy and therefore was not the etiologic factor. Cases of aplastic anemia have, however, been reported to begin during pregnancy and remit after delivery. In some of these, the aplastic condition reappeared during a second pregnancy. It has been postulated that the disorder is due to an imbalance between the erythropoietic effects of erythyropoietin and placental lactogen, and the suppressive effects of estrogen on the marrow.

Aplastic anemia associated with thymoma is rare, and most of the cases reported have been associated with pure red cell aplasia. Only a few patients develop marrow hypoplasia and pancytopenia, and most of them are over 50 years of age.

Constitutional Aplastic Anemia. The term *constitutional aplastic anemia* is applied to a group of diseases with an inherent predisposition to cause bone marrow failure, which includes Fanconi's anemia, familial aplastic anemia, amegakaryocytic thrombocytopenia, dyskeratosis congenita, and the Shwachman-Diamond syndrome. The anemia can be congenital, genetic, or familial and can be induced by most of the previously mentioned etiologic agents.

Fanconi's anemia is the best-known aplastic anemia of the group and occurs as an inborn defect associated with congenital physical abnormalities that include skin pigmentation, renal hypoplasia, cardiac defects, absence or hypoplasia of thumbs and radius, microcephaly, and mental retardation. Not all abnormalities need to be present, and the hematologic abnormalities usually do not develop before the age of 5. Random chromosomal abnormalities of the bone marrow cells and lymphocytes have been described. It has also been suggested that such patients have a defect in DNA repair, which may account for the hematologic and physical abnormalities. The bone marrow defect appears to be at the level of the stem cell.

Familial cases in which siblings developed aplastic anemia but without the physical findings of Fanconi's anemia have been reported and may represent an incomplete expression of the disease, which when full blown, has an autosomal recessive inheritance pattern. Numerous cases of atypical familial aplastic anemias have been reported, and it is still not well known whether such cases should be included in this category.

In a small group of patients with neonatal thrombocytopenia who later developed aplastic anemia the disease has been called amegakaryocytic thrombocytopenia. It is not clear whether this is a separate entity or represents variants of Fanconi's anemia.

Other patients with dyskeratosis congenita who demonstrated dermatologic manifestations consisting of hyperpigmentation, dystrophic nails, and leukoplakia, and who developed pancytopenia in the second to third decades, do not appear to have any relationship with Fanconi's anemia.

The Shwachman-Diamond syndrome is characterized by pancreatic insufficiency and neutropenia. Over half the patients have high levels of fetal hemoglobin and less than a third develop pancytopenia.

Acute myelogenous leukemia has followed the diagnosis of aplastic anemia after one to several years in cases of acquired aplastic anemia, Fanconi's anemia, and single cell deficiencies. Whether the first phase of the aplastic process is a preleukemic stage characterized by slow growth of the hematopoietic elements is still not known. It should be considered, however, that many of the drugs and environmental toxins known to induce aplastic anemia are also associated with the development of leukemia.

Pure red cell aplasia, a single cell line deficiency, can also be acquired or congenital. It is a rare disorder characterized by anemia, low reticulocyte count, normal white cells and platelets, and decreased erythropoietic activity in the marrow associated with selective erythroid hypoplasia. Acquired red cell aplasia can be secondary to tumor, severe hemolytic disorders, systemic lupus erythematosus, infections, and renal failure or drug-induced. Approximately 50 per cent of cases are associated with thymomas.

Safdar, Krantz, and Brown demonstrated that some cases of pure red cell aplasia and a history of thymoma were associated with serum inhibitors directed against bone marrow erythroid precursors or erythropoietin.

The congenital form of red cell aplasia is also known as Diamond-Blackfan anemia and demonstrates the same characteristics as the acquired form except that eythropoietin levels are elevated. It therefore is not a disorder of hormone deficiency but perhaps a deficiency of erythroid stem cells.

DISORDERS OF DNA REPLICATION

MEGALOBLASTIC ANEMIAS

The megaloblastic anemias all have in common certain diagnostic abnormalities characterized by impairment of deoxyribonucleic acid (DNA) synthesis, affecting primarily those cells having a relatively rapid turnover such as the hematopoietic precursors in the bone marrow and the epithelial cells of the gastrointestinal mucosa. The epidermis and the germinal epithelium of the testis also involve a continuous and constant loss and production of cells, in order to maintain these tissues in a normal state. Although cell division is sluggish because of the impaired DNA synthesis, cytoplasmic development continues in a normal manner, thus giving origin to an increased ribonucleic acid (RNA) to DNA ratio. Therefore, megaloblastic (*megalo,* large; *blast,* precursor cell) cell changes appear. Megaloblastic anemia is a morphologic entity characterized by asynchronous nuclear/cytoplasmic maturation of all three lines of the hematopoietic elements of the bone marrow and the release of macrocytic red blood cells into the peripheral circulation. In the bone marrow, ineffective erythropoiesis leads to extensive destruction of megaloblastic cells, especially those of the erythroid line precursors, which may reach up to 90 per cent before they are released.

To obviate any confusion, the term *megaloblastic* is used to connote morphologic changes in any of the three lines, while *megaloblast* has come to connote those specific changes that are seen in the erythroid line. The hallmark of the disease is the megaloblastic changes seen in the bone marrow cell precursors of the erythroid line in which the cytoplasmic differentiation outstrips the nuclear maturation. The most immature cell in the series is the promegaloblast, a cell that can be easily recognized by its larger size, its abundant, granule-free, patchy colorless, basophilic cytoplasm and its round to ovoid nucleus with fine delicate, open, lavender colored chromatin surrounded by abundant pink parachromatin and large blue nucleoli, contrasting with the normal characteristics of the pronormoblast. As the cell matures toward the polychromatophilic and the orthochromatic megaloblast, the nuclear chromatin retains its granular but coarser chromatin, the nucleoli disappear, and the cytoplasm is pink to orange and abundant. The complete hemoglobinized orthochromatic megaloblast may contain two or three abnormal nuclei with coarse, dense chromatin masses, and it may be three to four times as large as the regular orthochromatic normoblast.

Megaloblastic granulocyte precursors also demonstrate the nuclear/cytoplasmic asynchronism. The changes, when present, are seen in the late-stage white cell precursors and are characterized by giant metamyelocytes and bands. The metamyelocytes have a large U-shaped, ragged, punched-out, poorly stained nucleus and an immature basophilic cytoplasm that contains fewer granules than the regular metamyelocytes and bands. Abnormally large megaloblastic megakaryocytes are occasionally present and display unattached multilobulated nuclei and poor platelet degranulation.

The peripheral blood picture is one of normochromic macrocytic erythrocytes with mean corpuscular volumes above 100 μm^3 and absolute and relative reticulocyte counts lower than normal. The red cells are variable in size and shape with typical ovalocytes and in severe cases contain intracellular inclusions such as basophilic stippling, Howell-Jolly bodies, and Cabot ring cells. As the anemia progresses, rare multinucleated red blood cells with typical megaloblastic changes appear. The granulocytic line demonstrates large hypersegmented neutrophils that average more than six lobules per cell and are an early sign of the megaloblastic process. The total white blood cell and platelet count may be decreased and

bizarre; irregularly shaped platelets may also be present.

As a consequence of ineffective erythropoiesis, increased destruction of erythroid precursors results in plasma elevations of indirect bilirubin and lactic acid dehydrogenase (LDH) and flipped LDH_1-LDH_2 isoenzymes. Plasma iron and iron turnover are increased, but incorporation of radioactive iron into the red cells is low. Classic examples of megaloblastic anemias are pernicious anemia, which is a reflection of inadequate absorption of vitamin B_{12} due to lack of secretion of gastric intrinsic factor, and folate deficiency megaloblastic anemia. These two are morphologically and biochemically indistinguishable from megaloblastic anemias due to pure deficiency of vitamin B_{12}. The clinical presentation, the cellular morphologic and biochemical similarities, as well as the therapeutic overlaps, suggest a closely related metabolic denominator in the pathogenesis of the disease.

Metabolism of Vitamin B_{12}

Vitamin B_{12} is a complex organometallic compound asymetrically built around cobalt with a corrin nucleus and a nucleotide lying at right angles to the corrin group. The centrally located cobalt is linked to the four pyrrol rings, in a fifth position to the benzimidazole nitrogen, and in a sixth position by one of several different ligands (Fig. 23–3). Cobalamin is the vitamin B_{12} molecule without the anionic ligand. When the sixth position is occupied by cyanide, the resulting compound is called cyanocobalamin. During biosynthesis of coenzyme forms of vitamin B_{12}, the cobalt atom is enzymatically reduced from a trivalent to a monovalent state prior to the attachment of the organic anionic ligands. Cobalamin is exclusively synthesized by bacteria and is present in normal animal liver as 5-desoxyadenosyl cobalamin, while in plasma, methyl-cobalamin is the major form of vitamin B_{12}. The intestinal absorption is mediated by specific receptors on the surface of the microvilli of the terminal ileum and requires cobalamin to be bound to a highly specific glycoprotein, the intrinsic factor (IF). Other cobalamin-binding proteins are known as R-proteins, and the name is related to the "rapid" mobility in electrophoresis. The intrinsic factor is a glycoprotein that consists of two polypeptide chains with a molecular weight of approximately 60,000 daltons and that is produced by the parietal cells of the stomach. Vitamin B_{12}, the "extrinsic factor," binds very avidly to the intrinsic factor, and the complex is very resistant to proteolytic digestion.

The R-proteins carry the bulk of vitamin B_{12} in plasma and are found in food, in saliva and other body fluids, and in the granulocytes. They share a common peptide structure but differ in their carbohydrate content and have been assigned the name *transcobalamin* (TC) (Fernandez-Costa

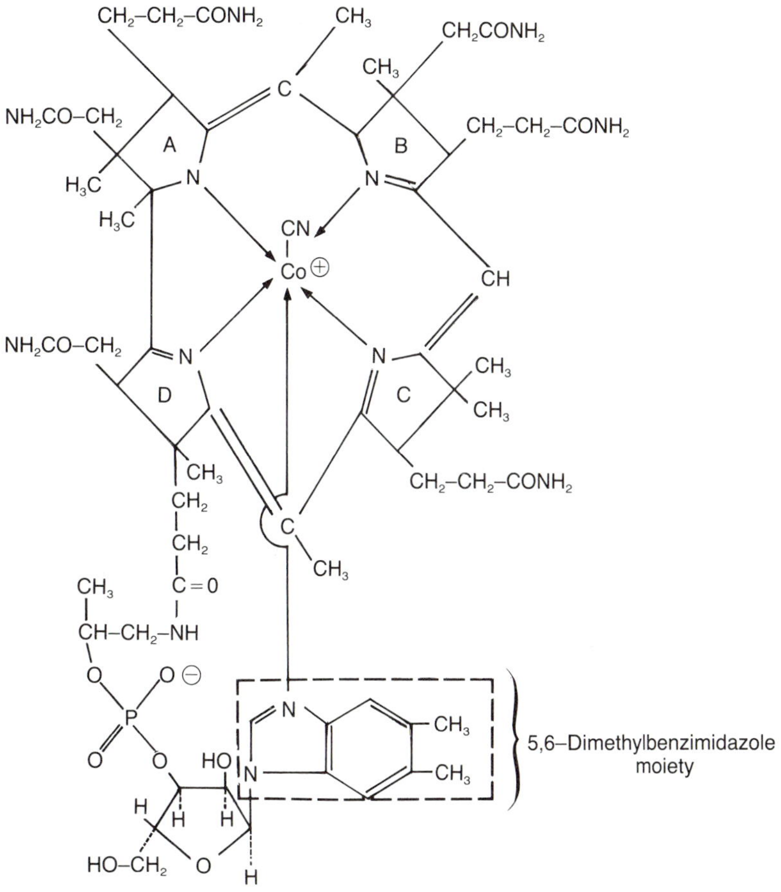

Figure 23–3 Structure of vitamin B_{12} and different ligands. R1 = CH_2CONH_2; R2 = $CH_2CH_2CONH_2$; X = CN, cyanocobalamin; X = OH, hydroxycobalamin; X = CH_3, methylcobalamin; X = 5'-Desoxyadenosylcobalamin.

and Metz). The ileal mucosa receptors have a high affinity for the IF-B_{12} complex, and the binding reaction requires ionized calcium and a pH close to neutral. Very little is known about what happens to the IF-B_{12} complex inside the cell and until it enters the blood, but the process appears to be very complex. After the vitamin is absorbed, it is bound to transcobalamin II (TCII), which is responsible for the transport and delivery of vitamin B_{12} to the liver and other tissues. The process of TCII-B_{12} uptake by the cells is biphasic, the first being the binding to the cell membrane receptors and the second a pinocytotic process for internalization of the complex. Transcobalamin TCI and TCIII are also present in plasma, but their role is still unknown, and their biochemical distinction is still unclear. Two metabolically active forms of the vitamin have been identified by the alkyl group attached to the sixth position of the cobalt atom, and those are adenosylcobalamin and methylcobalamin.

There are in humans two enzymatic reactions in which vitamin B_{12} serves as a coenzyme. The first is the methylation of homocysteine to methionine. Methylcobalamin is utilized as a coenzyme and N^5-methyltetrahydrofolate as the methyl source to be transferred to the cobalamin prosthetic group, which is then transferred to homocysteine to generate methionine. The absence of cobalamin produces a block in this reaction and an accumulation of N^5-methyltetrahydrofolate.

The second enzymatic reaction utilizes adenosylcobalamin for the isomerization of L methylmalonyl-CoA to succinyl-CoA. Succinyl CoA enters the citric acid cycle and is metabolized to CO_2 or provides a pathway for gluconeogenesis via oxaloacetate into pyruvate. This pathway forms a link between lipid and carbohydrate metabolism and has allowed speculation as to its possible role in the biosynthesis of myelin.

In some bacteria vitamin B_{12} is necessary for the reduction of ribonucleotides of DNA synthesis, but there is no evidence that such a function exists in humans.

Metabolism of Folate

Folic acid and folate are generic names for any member of a family of related compounds of which pteroylglutamic acid is the parent form. Chemically, the major portion of the molecule consists of a pteridine moiety linked by a methylene group to paraminobenzoic acid (PABA) that is joined to glutamic acid. Animal cells are unable to synthesize PABA or to attach the pteroid acid; hence folate is required in the diet. Folic acid is found in leafy vegetables and exists as a polyglutamate conjugate with a γ-linked polypeptide chain of serum glutamic acids. It is resistant to hydrolysis by the intestinal proteolytic enzymes, but for efficient intestinal absorption, the polyglutamate form is broken down to monoglutamates by intestinal folyl polyglutamate hydrolase. Only the monoglutamate form is absorbed, further reduced to tetrahydrofolate, and methylated to N^5-methyltetrahydrofolate (Fig. 23–4).

Tetrahydrofolate is the basic reduced folate compound that serves as a carrier in the transfer of single carbon units required for several biosynthetic reactions. In order to do so folate is reduced by the enzyme dehydrofolate reductase. The source of the one carbon unit is generally serine, which reacts with tetrahydrofolate to produce glycine and N^5,N^{10}-methylenetetrahydrofolate. An alternative pathway is formiminoglutamic acid (FIGLU), a catabolite of histidine that releases its formimino group to tetrahydrofolate to produce N^5-formiminotetrahydrofolate and glutamic acid. In folate deficiency, FIGLU accumulates and is excreted in the urine. These products supply an interconvertible pool of tetrahydrofolate derivatives carrying one-carbon units at different levels of oxidation. These donate their carbon units to appropriate acceptors in biosynthetic reactions to form metabolic intermediates for the synthesis of biologic macromolecules. The most important of these transfer reactions include de novo purine synthesis, synthesis of deoxythymidylate monophosphate (dTMP) from N^5,N^{10}-methylenetetrahydrofolate and deoxyuridylate monophosphate (dUMP); and synthesis of methionine from homocysteine by the transfer of a methyl group from N^5-methyltetrahydrofolate. Tetrahydrofolate is produced in all these one-carbon reactions and immediately accepts one carbon unit to reenter the pool—except for the reaction dUMP to dTMP in which dihydrofolate is produced. Dihydrofolate reductase reduces it to tetrahydrofolate to reenter the pool. Folate antagonists block the enzyme, diverting folate from the pool, and thus creating a state of folate deficiency.

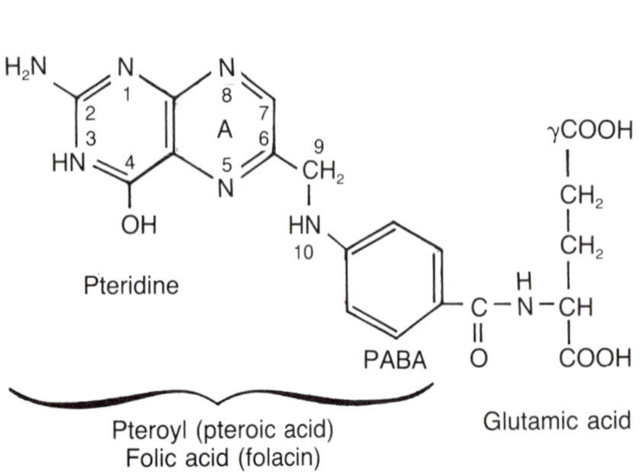

As stated before, methylcobalamin is a vital cofactor in the synthesis of homocysteine to methionine. If this reaction is disturbed, the metabolism of folate is interrupted, and it is at this level of the common biochemical pathway that the impairment of DNA synthesis is thought to be, which leads to an explanation of the characteristic megaloblastic changes seen in the rapidly dividing cells and clinical similarities between vitamin B_{12} deficiency and folate deficiency in man. These close interrelationships between vitamin B_{12} and folate deficiencies have been postulated under the name of the "folate trap" (Katzen and Buchanan 1965, Herber and Zalusky 1961–1962). The trap has two aspects: the inadequate or impaired conversion of N^5-methyltetrahydrofolate to tetrahydrofolate by the vitamin B_{12}–dependent reaction and the defective cellular uptake of N^5-methyltetrahydrofolate in vitamin B_{12} deficiency.

Clinical Features of Megaloblastic Anemias

The clinical manifestations of megaloblastic anemias are related to hematopoiesis and the gastrointestinal tract and are common to all of them. In general the anemia develops slowly and produces very few symptoms to the point that many patients are symptom-free until severe anemia develops. Then the symptoms are the usual ones for anemia: weakness, fatigue, light-headedness, shortness of breath, and palpitations. Characteristically, on physical examination the patient demonstrates severe pallor and mild conjunctival jaundice. The pulse is fast, and murmurs and cardiomegaly may be present when· congestive heart failure develops. The gastrointestinal manifestations are the reflection of rapid cell turnover due to folate or vitamin B_{12} deficiency. The tongue is sore, smooth, atrophic, and beefy red; and the intestinal epithelium is atrophic. The neurologic manifestations of vitamin B_{12} deficiency are related to demyelinization of the nerve followed by axonal degeneration. These changes may not remit completely, and the final stage is irreversible. The spinal cord is the site of involvement, and the posterior and lateral columns typically undergo degeneration. The peripheral nerves and cerebrum also are affected, and the symptoms are numbness and paresthesias in the extremities, poor coordination and sphincter disturbances. Decreased and abnormal reflexes may be present, and impaired mentation may vary from irritability to severe dementia.

Clinical Disorders

The etiologic conditions of megaloblastic anemias are diverse and depend on many factors

Figure 23–4 Structure of folic acid.

(Table 23–13). In temperate zones, pernicious anemia is the most common, while in the tropics, malabsorption due to tropical sprue is a major cause. The usual dietary intake of vitamin B_{12} is very adequate, and only pure vegetarians and diet faddists may have a dietary deficiency. Most cases of megaloblastic anemia are due to vitamin B_{12} malabsorption associated with deficient production and uptake of the specific binding proteins produced in the stomach and the specific cell binding receptors of the distal ileal mucosa. On the other hand, dietary deficiency of folate is common in the poorly fed, "tea and toast" older individuals, breast fed infants, alcoholics, and pregnant women in whom body reserves are already low. If metabolic demands increase, folic acid deficiency may ap-

pear. Combined deficiencies of vitamin B_{12} and folic acid are not uncommon, especially in those patients with malabsorption syndromes. Whichever vitamin is the cause, the megaloblastic changes in the epithelial cells of the intestinal tract lead to pathologic changes similar to those seen in malabsorption syndromes and result in malabsorption of the other.

Megaloblastic anemias may be related to factors other than vitamin deficiency as in drug-induced cases or those rare cases due to congenital protein binding deficiencies, inborn errors of metabolism, or acquired defects of erythroid cell precursors.

The evaluation of patients with megaloblastic anemias requires that one determine whether the deficiency is of vitamin B_{12} or folate. New sensitive radioimmunoassays, able to measure very low levels of these vitamins, are now available. Normal serum levels for vitamin B_{12} range from 200 to 900 pg/ml and for folate from 6 to 20 ng/ml. Values lower than 100 pg/ml for vitamin B_{12} and 4 ng/ml for folate are considered diagnostic. If vitamin B_{12} deficiency is confirmed, the pathogenesis of the disease can be established by the Schilling test. Radioactive vitamin B_{12} is given by mouth and followed in 2 hours by an intramuscular injection of nonradioactive vitamin B_{12}. A carefully timed 24-hour urine collection is required, and the radioactivity for the 24 hours is calculated. If radioactivity is low, the second part of the Schilling test is performed and the patient is given radioactive vitamin B_{12} bound to intrinsic factor. If the absorption is normal, the patient has pernicious anemia. If absorption is low, the cause is intestinal malabsorption.

Vitamin B_{12} Deficiency. Pernicious anemia is the most common cause of vitamin B_{12} deficiency in temperate zones. The disease is more common in individuals of Northern European ancestry and less common in blacks and Orientals and is equally seen in men and women over the age of 60. It can occur under the age of 30 and in children (Cooper). The disease is still not well understood but appears to have an immune basis. Endogenous and exogenous factors such as genetic makeup, associated immune and nonimmune diseases, and diet need to be related to the autoimmune reaction against the gastric parietal cells (Taylor). Serum parietal cell antibodies are present in 90 per cent of patients with pernicious anemia, and circulating intrinsic factor antibodies are present in 60 per cent of those patients. Patients with other immune disorders and relatives of patients with pernicious anemia have a higher incidence of the disease. The gastric lesions in pernicious anemia constitute a chronic gastritis that can be superficial or atrophic, multifocal or diffuse, and that is characterized by a chronic inflammatory mononuclear infiltrate associated with intestinal and antral metaplasia. These changes are more severe at the level of the parietal cells, resulting in achlorhydria. Extensive damage to the gastric mucosa or

TABLE 23–13 CLASSIFICATION OF MEGALOBLASTIC ANEMIA

Vitamin B_{12} deficiency
  Decreased intake
  Malabsorption
    Gastric atrophy (PA)
    Gastrectomy
    Secretion of abnormal IF
    Congenital absence of IF
  Disorders of terminal ileum
    Malabsorption syndromes
    Regional enteritis
    Ileal resection
    Congenital malabsorption of B_{12}
  Competition for vitamin B_{12}
    Fish tapeworm
    Bacteria (blind loop)
  Drugs
    p-Aminosalicylic acid
    Colchicine
    Neomycin

Folic acid deficiency
  Inadequate intake
    Poor diet
    Alcoholism
    Infancy
  Malabsorption
    Malabsorption syndromes
    Associated with anticonvulsants
  Increased requirements
    Pregnancy
    Infancy
    Malignant disease
  Metabolic inhibition
    Purine synthesis
    Pyrimidine synthesis
    Thymidylate synthesis
    Deoxyribonucleotide synthesis
  Errors of metabolism
    Orotic aciduria
    Lesch-Nyhan syndrome
    Transcobalamin II deficiency
    Others
  Acquired
    Erythroleukemia
    Refractory megaloblastic anemia

total gastrectomy is followed, after several years, by megaloblastic anemia due to removal of the source for intrinsic factor.

INTESTINAL ABNORMALITIES. Megaloblastic anemia related to anastomosis diverticula, intestinal strictures, or blind loop syndrome is attributed to massive colonization of the bowel by bacteria that compete with the host for vitamin B_{12}. Therapy with broad-spectrum antibiotics produces a good hematologic response. The same mechanism is attributed to megaloblastic anemia seen in patients harboring the fish tapeworm *Diphyllobothrium latum*. Elimination of the parasite resolves the hematologic problem. Extensive surgical ablation of the ileum or any disorder that compromises the absorptive capacity of the ileal mucosa such as tropical sprue, regional enteritis, Whipple's disease, lymphomas, or tuberculosis causes malabsorption of vitamin B_{12} and megaloblastic anemia. Certain drugs may also interfere with vitamin B_{12} absorption (Stebbins and Bertino 1976).

Folate Deficiency. The most common cause of megaloblastic anemia due to folate deficiency is a folate-poor diet. This is especially characteristic of alcoholics whose regular diet of alcohol and congeners lacks folate and other essential nutrients. These deficiencies are also seen in the poor, the elderly, and the faddist. Prolonged food storage and excessive cooking inactivates folate enzymes and polyglutamates. Under certain circumstances, folate requirements are increased, and if the diet cannot meet those requirements, a megaloblastic anemia appears. The classic example is pregnancy, in which folate is required to supplement the rapidly growing products of conception. The same mechanisms are also seen during infancy and adolescence. Patients with chronic hemolytic anemia and chronic exfoliative dermatitis have greatly increased folate demands due to very active erythropoiesis and epidermal cell regeneration.

INTESTINAL MALABSORPTION OF FOLATE. Malabsorption syndromes are characterized by a reduction in absorption of all nutrients by the affected bowel, but folate malabsorption is especially seen in patients with tropical and nontropical sprue. As with vitamin B_{12} malabsorption, extensive surgical resection of the small bowel, lymphomas, Whipple's disease, regional enteritis, blind loop syndromes, and the like may be associated with folate malabsorption.

Megaloblastic Anemias Associated with Drugs. These are the next most common anemias after vitamin B_{12} and folate deficiencies and can be classified into three different categories (Table 23–14). Those that are direct inhibitors of DNA synthesis and used in the treatment of malignant disease include purine and pyrimidine analogues, alkylating agents, and other drugs that inhibit DNA synthesis through different mechanisms. The folate antagonists, also used in the treatment of certain malignant neoplasms, are powerful inhib-

TABLE 23–14 MOST COMMON DRUG-INDUCED MEGALOBLASTIC ANEMIAS

Drug Interference with DNA Synthesis
Direct inhibitors of DNA synthesis
  Alkylating agents
    Nitrogen mustard
    Cyclophosphamide
    Chlorambucil
    Busulfan
  Purine and pyrimidine analogues
    5-Fluorouracil
    6-Mercaptopurine
    6-Thioguanine
    Adriamycin
    Bleomycin

Drug Interference with Folate Metabolism
Folate antagonist
  Strong dehydrofolate reductase
    Methotrexate
  Weak dehydrofolate reductase
    Pentamidine
    Pyrimethamine
    Triamterene
    Trimethoprim

Drug Interference with Vitamin B_{12} or Folate Metabolism (Uncertain Mechanisms)
B_{12} absorption
  Colchicine
  Ethanol
  Neomycin
  Oral contraceptives
  Para-aminosalicylic acid
Folate, uncertain mechanisms
  Phenobarbital
  Dilantin
  Primidone
  Alcohol
  Oral contraceptives
  Para-aminosalicylic acid
  Cycloserine
  Isoniazid
  Neomycin
  Other

itors of dyhydrofolate reductase, the indispensable enzyme for regeneration of tetrahydrofolate. Methotrexate is the most toxic of these. A number of other drugs that antagonize folate by mechanisms that are poorly understood appear to involve the absorption of folate in a manner similar to that of vitamin B_{12}. Most common of this group are some anticonvulsants, antibiotics, pain relievers, and estrogens. In general, drug-induced megaloblastic anemias are mild. The exception is methotrexate, which in the presence of toxic concentrations produces a florid megaloblastosis, severe painful stomatitis, and extensive necrosis of the gastrointestinal tract.

Idiopathic Megaloblastic Anemias. Rare and most often seen in patients with acquired sideroblastic anemias, the megaloblastic changes are related to the red cell series without alteration of the granulocytic or megakaryocytic series. The anemia fails to respond to vitamin B$_{12}$, folic acid, and pyridoxine and is associated with a greater incidence of leukemia. Megaloblastic anemia is also associated with erythremic myelosis (Di-Guglielmo's syndrome), in which malignant red cell precursors are present, and with several poorly understood hereditary disorders.

CONGENITAL DYSERYTHROPOIETIC ANEMIAS (CDA)

Congenital dyserythropoietic anemias are rather uncommon inherited disorders characterized by refractory anemia with morphologic erythropoietic abnormalities such as multinucleation, karyorrhexis, bizarre nuclei resulting in ineffective erythropoiesis, and secondary hemochromatosis. The degree of anemia is variable, with intense marrow erythroid hyperplasia and normal or only slightly elevated reticulocyte counts. There may be some decrease in red cell survival; however, the major pathogenetic factor is dysplastic erythropoiesis resulting in severe intramedullary erythroid destruction. Three different types have been described.

Type I

This rather rare disorder is an autosomal recessive trait and manifests itself in infancy or later in life with moderate macrocytic anemia, splenomegaly, and mild jaundice. Bone marrow demonstrates extreme erythroid hyperplasia with megaloblastoid features, binucleated cells, or multilobulated nuclei with prominent erythrophagocytosis. Long-term survival has been reported if transfusions are avoided to prevent secondary hemochromatosis.

Type II

The most common type, this was described as hereditary erythroblastic multinuclearity associated with a positive acidified serum test (HEMPAS). There appears to be a higher incidence in northwest Europe, Italy, and North Africa, with autosomal recessive transmission. Normochromic anemia of variable severity and variable jaundice are present with secondary cholelithiasis and hemochromatosis. Bone marrow demonstrates about 10 to 40 per cent of erythroblasts to be binucleated or have multilobulated nuclei. Erythrophagocytosis is present with Gaucher-like histiocytes. The HEMPAS red cells are lysed by some group-compatible sera at pH 6.8; however, unlike paroxysmal nocturnal hemoglobinuria cells, the HEMPAS cells are not lysed by their own acidified serum, and the sucrose hemolysis test is negative. The HEMPAS cells also demonstrate a strong reaction with anti-i, generally characteristic of fetal red cells.

Type III

There appears to be an autosomal dominant inheritance pattern. The patients described so far have been asymptomatic with minimal, if any, anemia. Bone marrow demonstrates multinucleated giant erythroblasts constituting up to 30 per cent of erythroid precursors.

RED CELL DESTRUCTION

The mechanisms of red cell destruction include changes in red cell membrane, a decrease in cell deformability, alteration in intracellular viscosity, and splenic hyperfunction. Throughout this chapter the pathophysiology of these different mechanisms is discussed in relation to specific diseases, for example, hemolytic lysis associated with paroxysmal nocturnal hemoglobinuria. The following discussion is directed to immune-based hemolytic processes. Immune hemolytic anemia (IHA) may result from antibodies directed against the red cell or against elements coating the red cell. IgM antibodies usually cause direct agglutination in vitro because of their large size and multiple binding sites to bridge the red cell gap. These antibodies are capable of causing direct intravascular hemolysis of sensitized cells, usually accompanied by complement activation. IgG antibodies are small molecules that, unable to bridge the gap between binding sites of red cells, instead coat the surface. These antibodies usually cause extravascular hemolysis by sequestration in the spleen. The cornerstone of the diagnosis of IHA is the antiglobulin (Coombs) test used to detect the IgG coating. This test was first applied to blood grouping procedures by Coombs, Mourant, and Race in 1945. For the coated cells to agglutinate, a bridge must be provided. This is done in the antiglobulin test by supplying antihuman globulin, which will react with the IgG on adjacent red cells. A critical level, usually >500 molecules of IgG, is necessary for the antiglobulin test to be positive. In the initial studies the antiserum was developed in rabbits. Now antisera from many animals are available. Antiglobulin reagents are known as broad-spectrum or polyspecific antisera and usually contain anticomplement. Specific antiserum has been produced for each of the classes of immunoglobulins and various complement components. Specific IgG antiserum is particularly useful to define whether a positive antiglobulin reaction with polyspecific antiserum is due to IgG or complement. Subclasses of IgG may also be determined by specific reagents. Weak reactions with polyspecific antiserum are frequently encountered with cells coated with complement alone, often owing to cold agglutinins. Blood bank technology has developed a number of ways to enhance the Coombs reaction by using different temperatures, enzyme-treated cells, and low ionic strength reagents. Two kinds of antiglobulin tests are performed, the direct and the indirect. The direct antiglobulin test determines whether the red cell has been coated in vivo. The red cells are tested directly with antiserum, and a positive reaction indicates that the cells are coated with IgG or complement or both. The indirect test is used to detect antibodies in the serum by causing red cells to react with the patient's serum to sensitize them. Once sensitized, they react with antiserum as in the direct test. The special techniques used for the direct Coombs test can be used to enhance the indirect reaction. The most common uses for the direct antiglobulin test are in hemolytic disease of the newborn, autoimmune hemolytic anemia, incompatible transfusion- and drug-induced reactions.

Antibody reactions demonstrate thermal relationships. Some antibodies react best at body temperature, 37°C, while others react in the cold, 4°C. If the antibody is warm-reacting, i.e., active above 30°C, usually IgG can be demonstrated with or without complement. Complement alone without IgG is less common. In true cold-reacting antibodies, those active below 30°C, the antibody is usually IgM. Incomplete antibodies of IgA and IgM may coat red cells and are usually accompanied by IgG antibodies. Positive antiglobulin tests are seen in IHA associated with a variety of diseases listed in Table 23–15. With cold-reacting antibodies, complement may be the only element found on the cell. During the cold phase, an immunoglobin binds with complement; however, in the process of warming and testing it is removed. Complement is stable and remains attached. The direct antiglobulin reaction is usually weak and is enhanced by albumin. The indirect antiglobulin test has its use in detection of antibody in plasma. Usually this is due to a specific blood group antibody formed in response to prior transfusion or pregnancy. The antibody is specific for an antigen not on the patient's cells. The direct antiglobulin test will be negative. The specificity of antibody,

whether cold or warm, may be demonstrated by using a panel of cells with known antigenic composition. In essence, there are three basic immune hemolytic processes. In the first, the hemolytic process results from an antibody, the isoantibody, formed by one individual attacking the red cells of another, as in hemolytic anemia of the newborn. The second is an autoimmune hemolytic anemia in which the patient makes an antibody directed at his own red cells. The third situation is one in which the antibody produced by the individual is directed against a modified red cell or is not specifically directed against the red cell but involves it as an innocent bystander.

The mechanism of hemolysis, generally extravascular, involves trapping of cells in the spleen with fragmentation and spherocyte formation. The reticuloendothelial system in the liver removes those cells most severely damaged. The Fc portion of the IgG molecule on the red cell is recognized by the Fc receptor on the macrophage membrane, resulting in partial or complete phagocytosis of the red cell. The receptors on the macrophage membranes are felt to be integral proteins. Receptors are also found on neutrophils, lymphocytes, and monocytes. The monocyte contains approximately 20,000 receptors on its surface. How the actual attachment of the immunoglobulin and receptor site stimulates phagocytosis is unclear. Unlike IgG, IgM does not appear to be recognized by the receptor, and complement is required for IgM recognition. In addition, coating of the cell with IgG or complement acts to increase macrophage phagocytosis in the spleen. Cells coated with both IgG and complement are cleared faster than those coated with either alone. IgG_1 and IgG_3 stimulate phagocytosis, as does complement component C3b. Specific receptor sites for IgG_1 and IgG_3 exist on the macrophage membrane. The receptor site is strongly activated by polymers of IgG and only weakly by a single molecule. Clearance of IgG-coated cells can be blocked by circulating free IgG. Complement appears to play a role in augmenting phagocytosis of the coated cells. Phagocytosis is frequently partial, adding to spherocytosis. Upon phagocytosis the red cell is in a phagosome. Lysosomal granules are released into the vacuole with resulting rupture of the red cell. The various elements of the hemoglobin molecule are then metabolized. Intravascular complement lysis of cells in warm autoantibodies is uncommon, usually requiring high levels of sensitizing antibody. While the complement components C3b and C4 may coat the red cell in over half the cases, activation of the terminal phase is uncommon. Direct cytotoxic lysis by macrophages and lymphocytes has also been demonstrated in IHA. These killer cells have receptors for IgG and C3b. Cytotoxicity appears independent of phagocytosis. Cases in which IgG_3 coats the cells are always associated with hemolysis. IgG_1, IgG_2, and IgG_3 are capable of activating complement and there-

TABLE 23–15 DISORDERS ASSOCIATED WITH POSITIVE ANTIGLOBULIN TEST

Drug-induced antibodies
Lymphoma
Leukemia
Collagen disorders
Cancer
Ulcerative colitis
Incompatible transfusion
Infections, viral and bacterial
Sarcoidosis
Storage diseases
Liver disease

fore can cause intravascular hemolysis. Two molecules of IgG are necessary to activate complement, and they must be within 250 to 400 Å of each other. In vivo, many IgG molecules per red cell are required to activate complement. Antigens whose sites are widely separated on the red cell, for example, Rh antigens, are less likely to activate complement.

Under what circumstances will an individual develop antibodies to himself as in the autoimmune form? The first obvious way is for a cell or cell line to be altered so that it appears foreign. The second possibility is based on the concept that during development certain lines of cells become recognized as self while others are inhibited from developing. If one of these lines is later activated, the development of autoantibodies is possible. Such a process could develop in a patient who becomes immunodeficient. Also in an immunodeficient patient, cell lines that normally might develop and be removed could establish a foothold. Lastly, an antigen might react with a compound to form a complex, hapten, to which an antibody could develop.

HEMOLYTIC ANEMIA

Classification

Hemolytic anemias are generally classified as warm antibody–type and cold antibody–type with both idiopathic and secondary forms (Table 23–16). Cold-acting antibodies are frequently referred to as complete because they can cause direct agglutination. They are usually IgM immunoglobulins, frequently naturally occurring, and can cause direct intravascular hemolysis accompanied by complement activation. They react strongly at 0°C and are usually harmless, being active up to 10° to 15°C. Harmless cold autoagglutinins are common in most people. If their thermal amplitude extends up to 30°C or above, symptoms can develop. A commonly encountered cold antibody that can express itself under stress is anti-I. Warm antibodies are usually IgG, react strongly at 37°C, require an albumin medium to agglutinate, and result from immunization. Hemolysis is usually extravascular. As is so often the case in medicine, nothing is that simple, and exceptions to these statements are common; for example, the cold antibody in PNH is IgG, not IgM.

Isoimmune Hemolytic Anemia

The isoimmune antibodies are those directed against the red cell, usually demonstrating a blood group specificity. These are the common antibodies directed against blood group antigens A, B, Rh, M-N-S, Duffy, Kell, Lewis, I-i, and Lutheran. A hemolytic anemia can result from administration

TABLE 23–16 CLASSIFICATION OF ACQUIRED HEMOLYTIC ANEMIA

Autoimmune hemolytic anemia
  Warm antibody
    Idiopathic
    Secondary
  Cold antibody
    Idiopathic
    Secondary
  Isoimmune
    Hemolytic disease of newborn
    Transfusion incompatibility

Paroxysmal cold hemoglobinuria

Drug-induced hemolytic anemia
  Immune complex
  Drug–antibody adsorption
  Membrane alteration
  Autoantibody induction

Traumatic
  Prosthetic valve, vascular grafts
  Hemolytic uremic syndrome
  Thrombotic thrombocytopenic purpura
  Diffuse intravascular coagulation

Infectious agents

Chemical agents

Venomes

Thermal

of an incompatible unit of blood in which either the donor contains antibodies to the recipient red cells or vice-versa. Table 23–17 lists red cell antigens and their frequency of reaction at body temperature. Different antigens stimulate antibodies to varying degrees, so when a recipient receives red cells with a foreign antigen, not all patients will develop clinical antibodies. The importance of an antibody lies in whether or not it can cause hemolysis. On this basis, the A-B-O system is the most important. The Rh system falls next in line. Naturally occurring antibodies in the blood banking system refer to those that develop without prior exposure via blood transfusion or pregnancy. Many feel the stimulus to be bacterial in origin.

TABLE 23–17 RED CELL ANTIGEN LIKELIHOOD REACTION

Antibodies Always Significant	Antibodies Sometimes Significant	Antibodies Rarely Significant
ABO	Le^a	Le^b
Rh	P$_{la}$	York
Duffy	Lu	Xq^a
Kell	MN	Chido
Kidd		

Anti-B, anti-K, and anti-T have all been associated with such origins. With the exception of anti-A and anti-B, most natural red cell antibodies are not of routine significance, since they react in the cold. They represent IgM immunoglobulins. These IgM antibodies will cause rapid removal of incompatible transfused red cells. Most of the hemolysis results from extravascular phagocytosis in the liver stimulated by the size of aggregates and complement coating. The warm antibodies of A-B-O and Rh are usually IgG. The red cell antigens are on the surface of the membrane. In the case of A, B, H antigens they are determined by sugars attached to proteins and lipids in the membrane. The Rh antigens are less well-defined in their biochemical form but appear to be dependent upon lipid in the membrane. The antigenic determinant, the complementary area to the antibody, is usually the terminal sugar residues or terminal amino acid. Different antigenic determinants for the same family may be located on the same molecule. Hemolytic disease of the newborn is a classic isoimmune hemolytic anemia caused by IgG antibodies that can cross the placental barrier. A pregnant woman develops in her circulation antibodies to a foreign antigen acquired from leakage of fetal blood across the placenta, usually at parturition. The greater the bleeding, the more likely clinically significant antibodies will be formed. A single injection of Rh positive cells of 0.5 to 1.0 ml will produce antibodies 50 per cent of the time in an Rh-negative patient. The amount of antigen required to cause immunization is variable. It takes approximately 8 weeks for antibodies to be detected by routine procedures after exposure. A second exposure in a later pregnancy will be associated with a greater response to smaller amounts of blood. Usually, but not always, the initial immunoglobulin response is IgM followed by IgG. If the immune response is strong, usually because of repeated pregnancies, and the antibody crosses the placenta into the fetal circulation, hemolysis can occur. If severe enough, death may result. In the past most hemolytic disease of the newborn was caused by Rh antigens, which have strong immunization properties. The direct antiglobulin test demonstrates the coating of IgG antibodies. In recent years following the introduction of a prophylactic injection of anti-D at the time of birth when most leakage of fetal blood into the mother occurred, the incidence of hemolytic disease of newborn due to Rh has fallen. At this time it appears to have plateaued. Most cases recognized today are due to A-B-O incompatibilities. Unlike Rh hemolytic disease, ABO incompatibility often follows the first pregnancy. The anemia is usually less severe than with Rh disease. The antiglobulin test is positive in most cases of both Rh and ABO disease. The same is true for antibody formation after transfusion or as transfusion reactions in that the most significant is A-B-O followed by Rh, Kell, Duffy, and Kidd. It has been calculated that more antibody is developed by transfusion than by pregnancy, particularly to low-frequency antigens. The risk in pregnancy is based on the single father, while in transfusion, multiple donors are encountered. In addition, in pregnancy antibody formation is based generally on fetal-maternal hemorrhage, which does not always occur. Patients who respond to one antigen are more likely to respond to others. In studies of Rh-D negative patients who are exposed to Rh-D, those who develop anti-D also form more antibodies to other antigens than those who do not form anti-D. Some patients fail to respond even to extensive exposure to an antigen. Poor responders also tend to develop lower titers.

Warm Immune Hemolytic Anemia

In acquired hemolytic anemia due to warm-reacting antibodies the antiglobulin test is frequently positive. It is the most common form of IHA, found in 70 to 80 per cent of cases. The incidence of positive direct antiglobulin tests in the population varies from 1 in 10,000 to 1 in 30,000. Ten per cent will be anemic, and over half demonstrate shortened red cell survival. The strength of the antiglobulin response by routine methods does not correlate well with the extent of hemolysis. With highly sensitive techniques, such correlation is achieved. Most of these have IgG alone (80 per cent) or in combination with complement (50 per cent); complement alone (C3d and C4d) at low levels is not uncommon (10 per cent). While complement may be present on the red cell, the final phase of activation accompanied by hemolysis is not usually activated. The general response to anemia is seen as an increase in reticulocytes, jaundice, and hepatosplenomegaly and decreased haptoglobin. Haptoglobin is an important laboratory monitor of hemolysis. It is an alpha$_2$-glycoprotein that increases as an acute-phase protein. A number of subtypes of haptoglobin have been defined by electrophoresis. The normal values vary with the phenotypic type but can be generalized to 0.4 to 2.0 g/L. Haptoglobin binds plasma oxyhemoglobin on the alpha chain. It will not bind deoxyhemoglobin. Haptoglobin is synthesized and destroyed in the liver, with a half-life of 5 days unbound to hemoglobin. When bound to hemoglobin, the half-life falls to less than 30 minutes. With intravascular hemolysis, the binding and degradation of haptoglobin results in falling levels. The haptoglobin-hemoglobin complex is too large for renal filtration, and it is broken down in the liver; the hemoglobin elements are preserved. Hemoglobin not bound by haptoglobin may be oxidized to methemoglobin and disassociated to heme and globin. Free heme binds to either albumin or a glycoprotein, hemopexin. Hemopexin is produced in the liver and has a half-life of 7 days. Once bound to heme, the complex is removed by the liver, and the half-life falls to 8 hours. The mild forms of IHA may be asymptomatic. The extent of anemia varies. In some patients, bone marrow compensation may maintain the hematocrit. Spherocytes are common in the peripheral smear. Red cell survival is decreased with sequestration in the spleen and liver. The main laboratory feature is the presence of a positive direct antiglobulin test. The patterns in this test, discussed earlier, may reflect IgG coating or complement (C3d or C4), or both. Monospecific antisera can be used to define the other immunoglobulins that may be on the red cell. Using an indirect antiglobulin test, antibodies may also be found in the plasma, as there is an equilibrium between the cell and plasma. In most cases, attempts to identify the antibody on the cell are unsuccessful, and the cause remains idiopathic. This nonspecific reaction may result from an antibody to one or more antigens or some universal antigen. In some studies there is a suggestion of Rh specificity, demonstrated by reaction of the autoantibody with all red cells of common Rh genotype but their failure to react with Rh null cells. In a few cases strong specificity can be demonstrated, also usually to Rh antigens, particularly when IgG alone is found on the cell. This can be critical in transfusion therapy, as identification of the specific antibody permits use of type-specific blood, which results in prolonging red cell survival. Specificity to other antigens have been reported, for example, anti-U, anti-AB, anti-Kell, but these are uncommon. IHA is frequently associated with disturbances of the immune system such as seen in leukemia, lupus erythematosus, rheumatoid disease, infections, and lymphomas. In some of these disorders, antibodies to a variety of cells or cellular elements can also be clearly demonstrated.

The drug alpha-methyldopa can induce a warm IgG autoantibody against red cells, causing IHA. The mechanism is unclear; however, T suppression abnormalities are known to result from the drug. The abnormality of B cells and perhaps the loss of T-cell suppressor function may result in uncontrolled antibody production by the B cells. Others have suggested that the antibody may react with Rh precursor substances or that an alteration in the stem cell results in the loss of recognition of the red cell itself. With the removal of the drug, the process subsides. In 10 to 15 per cent of patients receiving this drug the direct antiglobulin test will be positive; in some patients a positive indirect antiglobulin test is also found. Antibodies to antinuclear material, rheumatoid factor and anti–parietal cells are also encountered. The anemia appears to be dose dependent and takes 3 to 6 months to develop. About 1 per cent of patients develop IHA secondary to splenic sequestration. The antiglobulin test will revert to negative with withdrawal of the drug, but it can remain positive for 2 years afterward.

The course of IHA is unpredictable, with periods of remission and relapses. Treatment may involve steroids, transfusion, immunosuppressive drugs, splenectomy, or plasma exchange. Approximately 20 per cent of patients will go into remission with steroid therapy. Splenectomy can further improve the number of patients who will have remission; relapses are common, however.

Cold Immune Hemolytic Anemia

If serum is mixed with red cells, both from the same patient, agglutination occurs at 0° C. This agglutination is associated with the presence of anti-I and, less frequently, anti-Pr. The red cells of most adults have I antigens and small amounts of i antigens. The cold temperature effect may be related to changes in the configuration of the glycoprotein containing I/i antigens. At birth the reverse, little i dominance, is true; however, during the first 18 months red cells become strongly reactive with anti-I. Cold autoagglutins have been reported to other antigens but are rare. The titer of anti-I normally is low, but under certain circumstances is enhanced in vitro by albumin. The reaction can be reversed by warming the agglutinated cells to 20° C. Cold antibodies have been associated with hemolysis and vascular disturbances with a peak incidence after age 50. Transient forms in which the cold antibody reacts to warming, and idiopathic chronic forms exacerbated on exposure to cold, occur. In cases of IHA, cold antibodies account for 15 to 20 per cent and are usually IgM molecules. These IgM antibodies are usually present in sublytic levels and result in extravascular hemolysis. The most common antibody associated with cold IHA is anti-I, with a small number of cases due to Pr, Pi, or i. At low temperature (0° to 5° C) cold autoagglutinins bind complement to red cells. If the autoagglutinins are strongly complement binding, lysis or sequestration of cells is seen at higher temperatures, 20° to 25° C. At 37° C the antibody is not usually found on the surface of the cell, being eluted off at the warmer temperature; complement C3b and C4d remain, however. The thermal amplitude may vary among patients. Some patients experience problems at room temperature, while others must be exposed to significant chilling. Agglutination or complement binding (or both) can occur in the superficial microcirculation where temperature can reach 20° C. Patients with strong titers of high-amplitude antibodies may have continuous hemolysis, while others develop only episodic hemolysis. In the peripheral circulation, sludging due to agglutination can result in thrombosis. In the chronic form most examples of anti-I and anti-i are IgM, although a warm IgG or IgA autoagglutinin of the same or another specificity may be found. A single molecule of IgM can activate complement. The complement-coated cell is usually cleared by the liver RE system. In man, as few as

20 IgM molecules per cell can result in clearance by the RE system. For direct lysis 25,000 complement complexes are required. IgM-coated cells will not be cleared in the absence of complement. As indicated earlier, the macrophage receptor is not stimulated by IgM in the absence of complement. Not all coated cells will be removed in a single pass through the liver. Some survive and re-enter the circulation, released from the macrophage by a C3 inactivator present in plasma. The cell remains coated but will not be recognized by the hepatic macrophage. Studies of experimental models have shown that splenectomy will increase red cell survival of cells coated with IgG but not IgM. Steroids have been demonstrated to decrease the removal of IgG- and IgG-C3b–coated cells. Secondary cold autoagglutinins are associated with acute infections, particularly by *Mycoplasma pneumoniae*. These are usually transient (1 to 3 weeks), with increasing titers and thermal range of anti-I. The possibility is that *M. pneumoniae* and the I antigen share antigenic properties. Infectious mononucleosis has been associated with anti-i IHA. Chronic forms of cold agglutinins, also i-specific, have been associated with lymphoproliferative disease. A classic pattern of cold-related IHA is paroxysmal cold hemoglobinuria (PCH). In PCH the first phase of complement fixation occurs below 25° C; as the temperature rises in the central circulation the remaining complex is formed and lysis occurs. The antibody involved is an IgG molecule directed against P antigen. Acute forms associated with viral illness and chronic forms associated with congenital syphilis have been reported.

Drug-Induced Hemolytic Anemia

Approximately 12 per cent of IHA is associated with drugs. Most cases are due to alpha methyldopa, whose role in anemia is discussed earlier. Most drug molecules are not sufficiently large to induce an immune response unless complexed with a macromolecule. The drug, a hapten, is usually bound to a protein by weak ionic bonds. There are several ways in which drugs induce anemia (Table 23–18). In the first form, drug antibody adsorption, the basic element is the irreversible combination of drug with plasma protein to form an antigenic unit to stimulate antibody formation. In the case of penicillin the major haptenic determinant is benzylpenicilloyl. Penicillin is nonspecifically adsorbed on the red cell surface. A preformed IgG antibody attacks the drug–red cell complex, causing red cell destruction. Complement may be activated in the process, but usually is not, with hemolysis being extravascular. Cephalosporins are common causes of this type. In approximately 3 per cent of patients receiving large doses of penicillin, a positive direct antiglobulin test is found. Anemia is not always present, occurring in about 5 per cent of the

TABLE 23–18 DRUG-INDUCED POSITIVE ANTIGLOBULIN TEST

Drug antibody adsorption	Immune complex
Penicillin	Quinidine
Cephalothin	Quinine
Streptomycin	p-Aminosalicylic acid
Tetracycline	Phenacetin
	Stibophen
Autoantibody induction	Sulfonamides
α-Methyldopa	Thiazides
Levodopa	Isoniazid
Mefenamic acid	Chlorpromazine
	Aminopyrine
	Altered membrane
	Cephalothin
	Ibuprofen

patients. Hemolysis develops slowly over a week's time. The antibody responsible for the anemia is usually IgG, but may be mixed IgG and IgM. A second mechanism, immune complex, is based on drug-antibody adsorption on the red cell. The drug-antibody complex forms before attachment to the red cell, and the association is a weak one. The complexes are usually IgM. Complement is usually activated in the process. The drug-antibody complex elutes from damaged cells and can then attach to other red cells, causing complement fixation. Quinine, chlorpromazine, aminopyrine (Pyramidon), phenacetin, sulfonamides, and rifampicin are associated with this type of IHA. Leukocytes and platelets may also be affected. Drug dosage does not have to be high. The antiglobulin test is usually positive if anticomplement activity is present in the antisera. Another mechanism is for the drug to alter the red cell membrane, causing a nonimmunologic adsorption of plasma proteins on the red cell surface. The proteins generally include fibrinogen, albumin, and immunoglobulins. Cephalosporins are a common cause of this type.

Nonimmune Hemolytic Anemia

Exposure to large doses of oxidative drugs may cause hemolysis of normal red cells. Accidental irrigation of wounds with water or intravenous administration of water is associated with hemolysis due to the osmotic change. Heavy metals such as lead, copper, and arsenic may also cause hemolysis. Progressive increase in the industrial use of lead has led to significant environmental contamination and human exposure. Other sources of contamination are from canned foods, beverages, water, and paint. As much as 40 per cent lead can be present in dried old paints, of particular concern where young children might ingest flaking old paint. Lead has an affinity for SH groups, causing significant damage to many enzymes and essential cellular structures such as mitochondria. The biologic and clinical effects of lead poisoning are multiple, with predominant central nervous system abnormalities, peripheral neuropathy, abdominal colic, and anemia. The anemia of lead poisoning is attributed to both impaired synthesis and decreased red cell survival. Lead interferes with heme synthesis at several stages, mediated predominantly by inhibition of enzymes such as delta-aminolevulinic acid synthetase, delta-aminolevulinic acid dehydratase, and ferrochelatase. Increased levels of delta-aminolevulinic acid and coproporphyrin are present in the urine. Lead exposure also results in red cell membrane defects, inhibition of ATPase, alteration in alpha and beta globin chain synthesis, and inhibition of pyrimidine 5'-nucleotidase. The latter impairs degradation of RNA, with accumulation of pyrimidine nucleotide characterized by the basophilic stippling seen in the red cells.

Infection-Induced Hemolytic Anemia

Infectious agents may also induce hemolysis. The most common cause of infection-induced anemia in the world is malaria. Malaria is caused by a protozoan parasite transmitted by female mosquitoes. The mosquito injects sporozoites into the blood stream, which in turn infect hepatic cells. The developmental form in the hepatic cell, the exoerythrocytic stage, after a species-specific period of development, ruptures and releases merozoites into the blood stream. These infect red cells and establish a cyclic pattern of development leading to increased numbers and recurrent red cell infection. Four species account for most human infections in man, *Plasmodium falciparum, P. vivax, P. malariae,* and *P. ovale.* The latter three species may persist in the liver phase with recurrent reinfection based on exoerythrocytic development. *P. falciparum,* on the other hand, ruptures and releases all its liver stage organisms at one time, and recurrent infection is based solely on the intraerythrocytic phase. Infection of the red cell by the malaria parasite results in alterations in red cell shape, membrane defects, and increased osmotic fragility. The anemia results from the rupture of infected red cells and pitting of the malaria parasite by the spleen.

Another intraerythrocytic infection is that caused by the protozoan *Babesia microti* or *B. divergens.* Transmitted by a tick, infections have been reported along the eastern coast. The anemia develops for the same pathophysiologic reasons seen in malaria.

Infection of the red cell by *Bartonella bacilliformis* also results in hemolysis. Transmitted by the sandfly, it results in Oroya fever in Peru. Unlike malaria, the organism attaches to the outside of the red cell; however, the anemia develops because of splenic removal, as in malaria. The anemia may be severe and rapid. An underlying chronic granulomatous lesion in lymph nodes is present.

Systemic infection with a variety of viruses and bacteria have been associated with a mild autoimmune anemia, probably resulting from shared antigenic characteristics, adsorption of immune complex onto the red cell surface, or direct toxic effect. Infection by *Clostridium perfringens* results in the release of lecithinase that alters red cell membranes, causing hemolysis. The lecithinase splits phosphorylcholine in the membrane. Snake venom also contains a phospholipase that splits fatty acids from lecithin to form lysolecithin, disrupting the membrane and leading to hemolysis. A role for complement has also been postulated for snake venom. Certain bacteria and viruses produce neuramindase, which can produce polyagglutinability in red cells. Red cells normally have a T antigen hidden on the red cell surface. Removal of n-acetyl neuraminic acid by bacterial neuraminidase exposes the antigen. All human blood contains anti-T, which will result in agglutination. In vivo this process is usually transient, lasting a few weeks. The antiglobulin test is negative, yet red cells agglutinate in serum.

Microangiopathic Hemolytic Anemia

Hemolytic anemia resulting from fragmentation of red cells is associated with physical damage from fibrin meshworks that develop in intravascular coagulation. Damage results from the shearing effect fragmenting the red cells as they pass through the meshwork. If the injury is not too severe, the fragment may reseal, forming a schistocyte. Direct hemolysis as well as splenic removal accounts for the anemia. Mechanical trauma due to defective prosthetic cardiac valves or vascular grafts may also cause hemolysis. The trauma is felt to be caused by the eddy currents that result from the defects. Prolonged chronic anemia due to the mechanical hemolysis can lead to iron deficiency, while the excessive red cell turnover can lead to folic acid deficiency. Hemolytic anemia is also associated with severe burns and is due to the immediate heat injury as well as to the small vessel damage. Damage to small vessels and fibrin activation associated with widespread cancer, malignant hypertension, vasculitis, arteriovenous fistulae, thrombotic thrombocytopenia, and hemolytic uremic syndrome can cause hemolysis. Besides the mechanical injury, it is likely that stasis results in pH changes, anoxia, and substrate deficiency. Direct chemical injury to the red cell membrane may also occur as lysosomes are released into the static area.

METHEMOGLOBINEMIA

Iron resides in the heme molecule in the ferrous state (Fe^{2+}). Upon oxygenation, an electron may be loosely donated from the ferrous ion to oxygen, converting the iron to the oxidated ferric state (Fe^{3+}). The oxygen exists as a superoxide anion. As the oxygen is released, the electron is returned to iron, and the ferrous form is assumed. At times, the oxygen escapes with the electron, leaving hemoglobin with iron in the ferric state, methemoglobin. Both acid and alkaline forms exist. In the acid form the iron has five unpaired electrons with the sixth position taken by water. The iron is in a high-spin state. In the alkaline form, a hydroxyl group is in the sixth position, and iron is in a low-spin state. Methemoglobin is unable to bind oxygen. At levels greater than 1.5 to 2.0 g/dl cyanosis is present. Oxidation of ferrous heme takes place continuously, 1 per cent per day, but is balanced by systems that keep it to a minimum. In the discussion on red cell membrane and biochemistry, systems for handling oxidants, for example, catalase and glutathione, were described. Methods of reducing methemoglobin and the pathophysiologic changes associated with defects are presented here.

Methemoglobinemia results from either congenital abnormalities of metabolic processes associated with methemoglobin reduction, abnormal hemoglobin that resists enzymatic reduction, or toxic oxidation of the ferrous ion in hemoglobin. Clinically, patients demonstrate cyanosis and sometimes a mild polycythemia. Methemoglobin levels of 10 to 20 per cent are tolerated well without oxygen insufficiency; at levels of 30 to 40 per cent symptoms become apparent. At a level of 60 per cent, serious anoxia may occur. Further oxidation of methemoglobin results in the sixth position of iron being attached to the globin molecule, forming hemichromes. The reaction at this point is reversible. With further disruption of the protein structure, irreversible changes result in formation of Heinz bodies.

There are four methods of reducing methemoglobin to hemoglobin. Under normal circumstances these systems provide many times the reducing capability necessary. The four pathways are listed in Table 23–19 in their order of significance. The reduction of methemoglobin, regardless of the substrate, appears to be mediated by pyridine nucleotides. In the glycolytic pathway, NADH can be produced at two points. The major source is in the oxidation of glyceraldehyde-3-phosphate. The reduction of methemoglobin with NADH is mediated by NADH-cytochrome b_5 reductase. This process in the red cell appears to be in competition with conversion of pyruvate to lactate. The latter has 100 times as great an affinity for NADH as methemoglobin. Cytochrome b_5 reductase, a flavoenzyme, functions as an intermediate step, passing the electron to cytochrome b_5. This enzyme is known under many names and accounts for 95 per cent of methemoglobin reduction. In congenital methemoglobinemia, it is this enzyme that is deficient. NADPH-dehydrogenase provides an alternate pathway, accounting for 5 per cent of methemoglobin reduction. In enzyme defects of G6PD in which NADPH is depressed and in cases of congenital absence of the enzyme, methemoglobin reduction capabilities are not lost, supporting the minor role played by NADPH-dehydrogenase. Its importance lies in being an alternate pathway by which to treat NADH-methemoglobin reductase (cytochrome b_5 reductase) deficiency. Methylene blue is reduced by this system to leucomethylene blue, which can function as an electron donor to ferrihemoglobin for conversion to ferrohemoglobin. In the red cell, riboflavine may be the natural activator of this system. Reduced glutathione and ascorbic acid also provide alternate pathways for reduction of methemoglobin. GSH can react via an enzyme to reduce the iron, though the process is slow. GSH also may reduce ascorbic acid to dehydroascorbic acid in the presence of an enzyme. The dehydroascorbic acid may react directly to reduce the iron.

The mode of inheritance for the enzyme deficiency of NADH-cytochrome b_5 reductase is autosomal recessive. Heterozygous patients with the enzymatic inherited form are usually not symptomatic, retaining sufficient reserve reducing capacity even under stress. An exception is seen in the newborn in whom, because of a transient deficiency, the problem is compounded. Newborns exposed to oxidants, nitrite, for example, can develop significant methemoglobinemia. Fetal hemoglobin also is more easily converted to the methemoglobin form than adult hemoglobin. Homozygotes, except those with severe forms, have sufficient reducing power to handle routine activity but not under stress. Cases of both quantitative and qualitative enzyme abnormality have been reported.

In the abnormal hemoglobin form, hemoglobin M, the inheritance is autosomal dominant. Iron is fixed in a partly oxidized state. The heterozygote has a methemoglobin level in the 20 to 30 per cent range. Homozygote states are not compatible with life. Five types of hemoglobin M have been described. The amino acid substitution results in an unstable chain without the ability to maintain the heme iron in the reduced state. In four, there is substitution of tyrosine for histidine, and in the fifth, valine for glutamate.

Toxic forms of methemoglobinemia are associated with normal enzyme levels and can be related to a specific exposure to oxidative chemicals. The most common are nitrites, aniline derivatives, and sulfonamides. Under most toxic conditions methemoglobin will be reduced in 5 to 12 hours; only in severe cases is methylene blue required. The latter will not work in patients with G6PD deficiency.

TABLE 23–19 METHEMOGLOBIN REDUCTION

NADH-cytochrome b_5 reductase	67%
Ascorbic acid	16%
Glutathione	12%
NADH-dehydrogenase	5%

PAROXYSMAL NOCTURNAL HEMOGLOBINURIA

Paroxysmal nocturnal hemoglobinuria (PNH) is characterized by passage of a red to brown urine upon rising from sleep. Not all patients demonstrate this classic pattern; most manifest chronic intravascular hemolysis, sometimes associated with pancytopenia. It is an acquired disorder embodying abnormalities of platelets, granulocytes, and erythrocytes. The hemoglobinuria is variable in occurrence and frequently associated with stress, i.e., infection.

The pathophysiologic state of the red cell is expressed by its increased sensitivity to complement. The complement pathways are reviewed in Chapter 5 and are not repeated here. The intrinsic defect of red cell membrane that leads to the increased sensitivity to complement is unclear. No antibody to red cells has been detected in PNH. Some studies have suggested a membrane protein abnormality; consistent results have not been produced, however. The membrane defect brings about activation of the alternative pathway (properdin system). This system can directly activate complement without an antibody. PNH red cells will fix more complement than normal cells. The system leads to cleavage of C3, which binds and cleaves C5. Reaction with the rest of the classic pathway forms C5b-C9 complex, which is responsible for lysis. This C5b-C9 complex binds to the phospholipids in the membrane. The lytic effect appears to start at the C8 stage and is accelerated by C9. The binding to the lipid membrane is thought to result in a molecular rearrangement, causing holes that reach 100 Å. The C3b component attached to the cell without activation of C5-C9 complex leads to phagocytosis. Acetylcholinesterase on the surface of the cell is depressed in PNH patients. The degree of depression appears to correlate with the severity of the disease. It appears, however, to be a secondary problem as acetylcholinesterase absence in patients without PNH is not associated with complement sensitivity. No lipid membrane deficiency has been consistently found. Pits and folds in the membrane are seen by electron microscopy. The basic glycolytic pathways are normal. These patients demonstrate a pancytopenia suggesting an abnormality in stem cell development. It is possible that an abnormal clone of the pluripotential stem cells develops consequent to injury to the marrow. In some patients the process leads to aplastic anemia. Platelets and granulocytes also show a membrane defect that induces complement sensitivity and alteration of chemotactic response. Both bleeding and thrombotic complications are found as a result of the platelet and granulocytic abnormality and complement activation. Iron deficiency as a result of hemoglobin lost in urine is frequently found. The extent of hemolysis depends on the size of the clone of cells involved. Generally three cell populations can be identified by in vitro tests with different degrees of sensitivity. PNH I cells react normally, and PNH II and PNH III cells demonstrate progressively greater sensitivity. Most patients, about 75 per cent, have a mixed population of PNH I and PNH III cells. The rest have mixtures of PNH I, II, and III cells. With populations of less than 20 per cent PNH III cells, hemolysis is mild. If more than 50 per cent of the cells are PNH III, hemolysis is usually ongoing. The nocturnal hemolysis is believed to occur as a result of pH changes associated with stasis and hypoventilation during sleep. Hemolysis is not, however, always associated with sleep, and in most patients there is a chronic hemolytic anemia in the background. The disease is marked by periods of remission with exacerbations associated with infections or stress. The most serious complications are aplastic anemia and intravascular thrombosis. The mechanical and osmotic fragility are usually normal, haptoglobin is decreased, and hemosiderin is present in the urine. Hemolysis by complement is enhanced in an acid pH and by antibody-mediated hemolysis. The most commonly used test to demonstrate the complement sensitivity is the Ham's, or acid hemolysis, test. In this test complement either from the patient or someone else is allowed to react with the patient's washed red cells at an acid pH (6.8 to 7.0) for an hour at 37 C°. In PNH 10 to 50 per cent of the red cells will lyse. The test is a differential test and will distinguish between lysis that requires serum, that is increased by acidification, that is specific to the patient's red cell, and that is inhibited by heating. The lysis depends on the presence of magnesium but not calcium, unlike immune hemolytic reactions. A second test, the sugar water test, depends on hemolysis in a low ionic strength sucrose solution that promotes complement binding.

MYELOPHTHISIC ANEMIA

This term refers to the anemia and other hematologic abnormalities frequently associated with infiltrative disorders of the bone marrow. There is generally a mild to moderate anemia with thrombocytopenia or thrombocytosis, and leukocytosis with left shift. Red cells are characteristically misshapen, many being teardrop cells (dacryocytes), and nucleated red blood cells may be present. The presence of immature granulocytic cells and nucleated red blood cells is frequently referred to as leukoerythroblastosis. Platelets may be abnormally large. The usual types of infiltrative marrow processes associated with myelophthisic anemia are listed in Table 23–20. Leukemias and lymphomas are by far the most commonly associated conditions.

The extent of marrow replacement has no relation to the degree of anemia or leukoerythroblastosis; however, extensive marrow infiltration and replacement may cause mechanical "crowding-out" of normal hematopoietic cells. The anemia

TABLE 23–20 CONDITIONS ASSOCIATED WITH MYELOPHTHISIC ANEMIA

Tumors
  Leukemias
  Malignant lymphomas
  Multiple myeloma
  Metastatic carcinoma from breast, prostate, lung, etc.
  Neuroblastoma

Myelofibrosis

Infections
  Tuberculosis
  Fungal infection

Sarcoidosis

is multifactorial in origin with ineffective erythropoiesis, inhibitory effects of chronic disease, diminished availability of nutrients such as folic acid and vitamin B_{12}, blood loss from thrombocytopenia or primary disease, and decreased red cell survival due to poikilocytosis. A reactive marrow fibrosis, particularly in association with metastatic carcinoma, may produce myeloid metaplasia with splenomegaly resulting in hypersplenism and further pancytopenia. Alteration of the normal marrow architecture results in disruption of the normal barrier mechanisms and release of immature cells such as nucleated red blood cells, megakaryocytes, myelocytes, promyelocytes, and even some myeloblasts.

THE PORPHYRIAS

The porphyrias are a group of disorders that result from inherited or acquired abnormalities in heme biosynthesis. Porphyrin compounds are widely distributed in nature and form physiologically essential pigments and enzymes when they combine with various metallic ions. Chlorophyll, the plant pigment, for example, is a magnesium porphyrin essential in carbohydrate synthesis. The human pigment hemoglobin contains iron porphyrin. The porphyrin nucleus is also found in myoglobin and essential respiratory enzymes such as cytochromes, peroxidases, and catalases. Erythropoietic cells form 80 per cent of the body's porphyrins, and liver parenchymal cells synthesize the rest. Porphyrins are photosensitizing agents and exhibit a strong absorption in the region of Soret's band at about 400 nm. Most of the porphyrias may be accompanied by cutaneous photosensitivity reactions.

Understanding the hemebiosynthetic pathway and its regulatory mechanisms is essential in the study of porphyrias. Heme synthesis is summarized in Figure 23–5. Primary regulation of heme

synthesis involves a negative feedback mechanism by heme on δ-aminolevulinic acid (ALA) synthetase. Exogenous iron and sex hormones such as testosterone and progesterone increase ALA synthetase activity. Certain drugs can induce or increase ALA synthetase activity; this, in combination with a partial metabolic block at a further stage in heme synthesis, results in porphyrias. The type of porphyria and its manifestations depend on the site of the block and the specific precursor accumulation. Porphyrias may be classified as erythropoietic, hepatic, and erythrohepatic. In the latter type, porphyrins accumulate in both erythroid and hepatic tissues.

Congenital Erythropoietic Porphyria (Gunther's Disease)

This is the only true erythropoietic porphyria and is extremely rare in occurrence. It is an autosomal recessive disorder, and the genetic defect involves uroporphyrinogen cosynthetase. The disease is generally manifested shortly after birth with cutaneous lesions of photodermatitis and hemolysis with porphyrinuria. Uroporphyrinogen I accumulates in red blood cells and is converted to coproporphyrinogen I, which is then stored in other tissues along with coproporphyrin. The urine, bones, and teeth are pink to red to color.

Hepatic Porphyrias

Several types of hepatic porphyrias have been described. The most common of these is porphyria cutanea tarda (PCT).

Porphyria Cutanea Tarda (PCT). The hallmark of this disease is photodermatitis with chronic skin lesions. PCT is frequently associated with alcoholism and liver disease. A deficiency of uroporphyrinogen III decarboxylase has been demonstrated; this may be inherited or acquired. Alcohol and therapeutic hormone administration, such as estrogens, can precipitate PCT in patients with familial predisposition. Toxic exposures, such as hexachlorobenzene and polychlorinated hydrocarbons, precipitate an acquired form of PCT. Photosensitivity with increased susceptibility of skin to minor mechanical damage, hypo- or hyperpigmentation, and hypertrichosis are present. Liver disease occurs frequently, particularly in association with alcoholism. Liver biopsy shows fluorescence with ultraviolet light and bifurcated, needlelike inclusions. Iron storage is increased, frequently resulting in cirrhosis. Urine may be pink to brown with increased uroporphyrin and coproporphyrin.

Acute Intermittent Porphyria (AIP). This hepatic disorder is not associated with increased production of porphyrins or porphyria. There are increased quantities of porphyrin precursors such

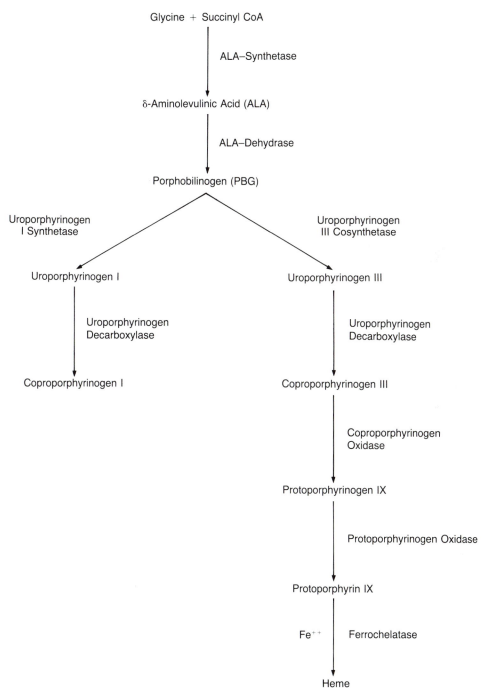

Figure 23–5 Heme biosynthesis.

as ALA amd PBG in urine. There is no photosensitivity or dermatitis; however, neurotoxicity of porphyrin precursors or heme deficiency results in the acute attacks. AIP is inherited as an autosomal dominant trait, and the genetic defect is decreased uroporphyrinogen I synthetase. Many patients have clinically silent (latent) disease. Certain drugs, alcohol, hormones such as estrogens, fasting, and infections can convert the latent disease to active disease. Inciting drugs include barbiturates, meprobamate, sulfonamides, griseofulvin, and imipramine, which are inducers of hepatic ALA synthetase activity. The clinical disease is more common in women after menarche, often cyclically related to menstrual periods, and increased in frequency of acute attacks during pregnancy. The acute attacks show manifestations of autonomic neuropathy such as abdominal colic, constipation, vomiting, hypertension, tachycardia, peripheral motor neuropathy with paresis, and central nervous system manifestations with hypothalamic dysfunction such as abnormal ADH, ACTH and growth hormone secretion, psychoses, delirium and coma. Inability to swallow or breathe may occur and may prove fatal. Porphyrin precursor excretion may be increased in the latent phase; however the most sensitive indicator of latent AIP is decreased uroporphyrinogen I synthetase in erythrocytes or hepatic tissue.

Variegate Porphyria. This hepatic porphyria is inherited as an autosomal dominant trait and is characterized by chronic cutaneous porphyria of variable severity with acute intermittent attacks. Protoporphyrinogen oxidase and ferrochelatase deficiencies have been demonstrated. Patients with acute attacks may appear to have AIP; however, there is increased coproporphyrin and protoporphyrin in feces with increased coproporphyrin, ALA, and PBG in urine.

Erythrohepatic Protoporphyria

This disorder is also thought to be inherited as an autosomal dominant trait with variable penetrance. There is marked reduction in ferrochelatase. Clinical manifestations include cutaneous symptoms such as burning and itching with solar urticaria, resulting in scarring and thickening of skin. There is greater incidence of gallstones containing protoporphyrin. Liver failure occurs in later stages, leading to life-threatening complications. Increased free erythrocyte protoporphyrin and a characteristic clinical history are necessary for diagnosis.

REFERENCES

GENERAL HEMATOLOGY

Babior, B. M., and Stossel, T. P.: Hematology: A Pathophysiological Approach. Chruchill Livingstone, New York, 1984.

Harris, J. W., and Kellermyer, R. W.: The Red Cell. Rev. Ed. 1970. Cambridge, Harvard University Press, 1970.

Henry, J. B.: Clinical Diagnosis and Management by Laboratory Methods. 17th Ed. Philadelphia, W. B. Saunders, 1984.

MacKinney, A. A., Jr.: Pathophysiology of Blood. New York, John Wiley & Sons, 1984.

Miale, J. B.: Laboratory Medicine Hematology. 6th Ed. St. Louis, C. V. Mosby, 1982.

Nathan, D. G., and Oski, F. A.: Hematology of Infancy and Childhood. 2nd Ed. Philadelphia, W. B. Saunders, 1981.

Williams, W. J., Beutler, E., Erslev, A. J., and Lichtman, M. A.: Hematology, 3rd Ed. New York, McGraw Hill, 1983.

Wintrobe, M.: Clinical Hematology. 8th Ed. Philadelphia, Lea & Febiger, 1981.

ANEMIA AND ACUTE BLOOD LOSS

Duke, W., and Abelman, W. H.: The hemodynamic response to chronic anemia. Circulation 39:503, 1969.

Finch, C. A., and Lenfaut, C.: Oxygen transport in man. N. Engl. J. Med. 286:407, 1972.

Hillman, R. S.: Characteristics of marrow production and reticulocyte maturation in normal man in response to anemia. J. Clin. Invest. 48:443, 1969.

Nagel, R. L., and Bookchin, R. M.: Human hemoglobin mutants with abnormal oxygen binding. Semin. Hematol. 11:423, 1974.

Sohmer, P. R., and Dawson, R. B.: The significance of 2,3-DPG in red blood cell transfusion. CRC Crit. Clin. Lab. Sci. 11:107–174, 1979.

Thomas, H. M., Lefrak, S. S., Irwin, R. S., Fritts, H. W., and Caldwell, P. R. B.: The oxyhemoglobin dissociation curve in health and disease. Am. J. Med. 57:331, 1974.

RED CELL MEMBRANE

Bessis, M.: Blood Smears Reinterpreted. Translated by George Brecher. New York, Springer International, 1977.

Bessis, M., Weed, R., and Leblond, P.: Red Cell Shape, Physiology, Pathology, Ultrastructure. New York, Springer Verlag, 1973.

Cohen, C. M., and Branton, D.: The normal and abnormal red cell cytoskeleton: a renewed search for molecular defects. Trends Biochem. Sci. 6:266, 1981.

Cooper, R. A.: Abnormalities of cell membrane fluidity in the pathogenesis of disease. N. Engl. J. Med. 297:371, 1977.

Dacie, J. V.: The Hemolytic Anemias Congenital and Acquired. Part I, The Congenital Anemias. New York, Grune & Stratton, 1960.

Lux, S. E., and Wolfe, L. C.: Inherited disorders of the red cell membrane skeleton. Pediatr. Clin. North Am. 27:463, 1980.

Marchesi, V.: Functional proteins of the human red blood cell membrane. Semin Hematol. 16:3, 1979.

Smith, J. A., Lonergan, E. T., and Sterling, K.: Spur cell anemia: hemolytic anemia with red cells resembling acanthocytes in alcoholic cirrhosis. N. Engl. J. Med. 271:396, 1964.

Weed, R. I.: Hereditary spherocytosis. Arch. Intern. Med. 135:1316, 1975.

Wiley, J. S., Ellory, J. C., Shuman, M. D., Shaller, C. C., and Cooper, R. A.: Characteristics of the membrane defect in hereditary stomatocytosis syndrome. Blood 46:337, 1975.

RED CELL BIOCHEMISTRY

Beutler, E.: Red Cell Metabolism. A Manual of Biochemical Methods. 2nd Ed. New York, Grune & Stratton, 1975.

Beutler, E.: Hemolytic Anemia in Disorders of Red Cell Metabolism. New York, Plenum, 1978.

Beutler, E.: Red cell enzyme defects as nondisease and as diseases. Blood 54:1, 1979.

Jaffe, E. R.: Methemoglobinemia. Clin. Haematol. 10:99–122, 1981.

Paglia, D. E., and Valentine, W. N.: Haemolytic anemia associated with disorders of the purine and pyrimidine salvage pathways. Clin. Haematol. 10:81, 1981.

Valentine, W. N.: Hemolytic anemia and inborn errors of metabolism. Blood 54:549, 1979.

Yoshikawa, H., and Rapoport, S. M.: Cellular and molecular biology of erythrocytes. Baltimore, University Park Press, 1974.

ERYTHROPOIETIN–MARROW DEVELOPMENT

Clinics in Haematology, Vol. 8: No. 2. Cellular Dynamics of Haemopoiesis. Philadelphia, W. B. Saunders, 1979.

DeBruyn, P. P., Michelson, S., Thomas, T. B., et al.: The microcirculation of the bone marrow. Anat. Rec. 168:55, 1970.

Erslev, A. J., Cavo, J., Miller, O., and Silver, R.: Plasma erythropoietin in health and disease. Ann. Clin. Lab. Sci. 10:250, 1980.

Ganzoni, A. M., Oakes, R., and Hellman, R. S.: Red cell aging in vivo. J. Clin. Invest. 50:1373, 1971.

Graber, S. E., and Krantz, S. B.: Erythropoietin and control of red cell production. Annu. Rev. Med. 29:51–66, 1978.

Mohandas, N., and Prenaut, M.: Three-dimensional model of bone marrow. Blood 51:633, 1978.

POLYCYTHEMIAS

Bishop, B. C.: Wintering in the high Himalayas. National Geographic 122:503, 1962.

Dameshek, W.: Some speculations on the myeloproliferative syndromes. Blood 6:372–375, 1951.

Gilbert, H. S.: Definition, clinical features and diagnosis of vera. Clin. Haematol. 4:263–290, 1975.

Hume, R., and Goldberg, A.: Actual and predicted normal red cell and plasma volumes in primary and secondary polycythemia. Clin. Sci. 26:499–508, 1964.

Jacobson, L. O., Goldwasser, E., Fried, W., and Plzak, L.: Studies on erythropoiesis VII. The role of the kidney in the production of erythropoietin. Trans. Assoc. Am. Physicians 70:305–317, 1957.

Lennert, K., Nagai, K., and Schwarze, E. W.: Patho-anatomical features of the bone marrow. Clin. Haematol. 4:331–351, 1975.

Lipsett, M. B.: Hormonal syndromes associated with neoplasia. Adv. Metab. Dis. 3:111–152, 1968.

McFadzean, A. J. S., Todd, D., and Tsang, K. C.: Polycythemia of primary carcinoma of the liver. Blood 13:427, 1958.

Parer, J. T.: Oxygen transport in human subjects with hemoglobin variants having altered oxygen affinity. Resp. Physiol. 9:43–49, 1970.

Peñalosa, D., and Sime, F.: Chronic cor pulmonale due to loss of altitude acclimatization (chronic mountain sickness). Am. J. Med. 50:728, 1971.

Rørth, M., Nygaard, S. F., and Parving, H. H.: Effect of exposure to simulated high altitude on human red cell phosphates and oxygen affinity of hemoglobin. Influence of exercise. Scand. J. Clin. Lab. Invest. 29:329–333, 1972.

Silverstein, M. N., and Lanier, A. P.: Polycythemia vera, 1935–1969: An epidemiologic survey in Rochester, Minnesota. Mayo Clin. Proc. 46:751–753, 1971.

Stamatoyannopoluos, G., Parer, J. T., and Finch, C. A.: Physiologic implications of a hemoglobin with decreased oxygen affinity (hemoglobin Seattle). N. Engl. J. Med. 281:915–919, 1969.

Türk, W.: Beiträge zur Kenntnis des Symptomenbildes Polycythämine mit Milztumor und "Zyanose." Wein Klin. Wochenschr. 17:153–160, 1904.

Valeri, C. R., and Collins, F. B.: Physiologic effects of 2,3-DPG depleted red cells with high affinity for oxygen. J. Appl. Physiol. 31:823–827, 1971.

Vaquez, M. H.: Sur une forme speciale de cyanose s'accompagnant d'hyperglobulie excessive et persistante. C. Soc. Biol. 44:384–388, 1892.

Ward, H. P., and Robinson, W. A.: Presence of a myelostimulatory factor in polycythemia vera (PV) and agnogenic myeloid metaplasia (AMM). Proceedings of the American Society of Clinical Investigation, 64th Annual Meeting, 1972, p. 100a.

SICKLE HEMOGLOBINOPATHY

Barnhart, M. I., Henry, R. L., and Lusher, J. M.: Sickle Cell (Scope Publication). Kalamazoo, Michigan, The Upjohn Co., 1976.

Eaton, W. A., Hofrichter, J., Ross, P. D., et al.: Delay time in gelation: A possible determinant of clinical severity in sickle cell disease. Blood 47:621, 1976.

Finch, C. A.: Pathophysiologic aspects of sickle cell anemia. Am. J. Med. 53:1, 1972.

Messner, M. J., Hahn, J. A., et al.: The kinetics of sickling and unsickling of red cells under physiologic conditions: rheologic and ultrastructural correlations: Symposium on Molecular and Cellular Aspects of Sickle Cell Disease, December, 1975. DHEW (NIH) Pub. 76-1007.

Motulsky, A. G.: Frequency of sickling disorders in U.S. Blacks. N. Engl. J. Med. 288:31, 1973.

THALASSEMIA

Benz, E. J., Jr.: Molecular pathology of the β-thalassemia syndromes. In Nienhuis, A. W., moderator: Thalassemia major: molecular and clinical aspects. Ann. Intern. Med. 91:883–897, 1979.

Modell, C. B.: Total management of thalassemia major. Arch. Dis. Child. 52:489, 1977.

Nienhuis, A. W., and Benz, E. J., Jr.: Regulation of hemoglobin synthesis during the development of the red cell. N. Engl. J. Med. 297:1318–1328, 1371–1381, 1430–1436, 1977.

Ottolenghi, S., Giglioni, B., Comi, P., et al.: Globin gene deletion in HPFH, delta (o) beta (o) thalassemia and Hb Lepore disease. Nature 278:654–657, 1979.

Wood, W. G., Stamatoyannopoulos, G., Lim, G., et al.: F-cells in the adult: normal values and levels in individuals with hereditary and acquired elevation of Hb F. Blood 46:671, 1975.

Wood, W. G., Old, J. M., Roberts, A. V., et al.: Human globin gene expression: Control of beta, delta and delta beta chain production. Cell 15:437, 1978.

IRON METABOLISM

Aisen, P.: Current concepts in iron metabolism. Clin. Haematology, 11:241–257, 1982.

Beaumont, C., Simon, M., Fauchet, R., Hespel, J. P., Brissot, P., Genetet, B., and Bourel, M.: Serum ferritin as a possible marker of the hemochromatosis allele. N. Engl. J. Med. 301:169–174, 1979.

Bentley, D. P.: Anaemia and chronic disease. Clin. Haematol. 11:465–479, 1982.

Birgegård, G., Hallgren, R., Killander, A., Stromberg, A., Venge, P., and Wide, L.: Serum ferritin during infection. A longitudinal study. Scand. Hematol. 21:333–340, 1978.

Bottomley, S. S.: Sideroblastic anaemia. Clin. Haematol. 11:389–409, 1982.

Cartwright, G. E., Edwards, C. Q., Kravitz, K., Skolnick, M., Amos, D. B., Johnson, A., et al: Hereditary hemochromatosis. Phenotypic expression of the disease. N. Engl. J. Med. 301:175–179, 1979.

Charlton, R. W., and Bothwell, T. H.: Definition, prevalence and prevention of iron deficiency. Clin. Haematol. 11:309–325, 1982.

Christensen, B. E.: Red cell kinetics. Clin. Haematol. 4:393–405, 1975.

Cook, J. D., and Finch, C. A.: Assessing iron status of a population. Am. J. Clin. Nutr. 32:2115–2119, 1979.

Cook, J. D., Finch, C. A., and Smith, N.: Evaluation of the iron status of a population. Blood 48:449–455, 1976.

Cook, J. D., Lipschitz, D. A., Miles, L. E. M., and Finch, C. A.: Serum ferritin as a measure of iron stores in normal subjects. Am. J. Clin. Nutr. 27:681–687, 1974.

Eastham, E. J., Bell, J. I., and Douglas, A. P.: Iron-transport characteristics of vesicles of brush-border and baso-lateral plasma membrane from the rat erythrocyte. Biochem. J. 164:289–294, 1977.

Edwards, C. Q., Dadone, M. M., Skolnick, M. H., and Kushner, J. P.: Hereditary haemochromatosis. Clin. Haematol. 11:411–435, 1982.

Edwards, C. Q., Skolnick, M. H., and Kushner, J. P.: Hereditary hemochromatosis. Contributions of genetic analyses. Progr. Hematol. 12:43–71, 1981.

Edwards, C. Q., Cartwright, G. E., Skolnick, M. H., and Amos, D. B.: Homozygosity for hemochromatosis: clinical manifestations. Ann. Intern. Med. 93:519–525, 1980.

Firat, D., and Banzon, J.: Erythropoietic effect of plasma from patients with advanced cancer. Cancer Res. *31*:1355–1359, 1971.

Frieden, E., and Aisen, P.: Forms of iron transferrin. Trends in Biochemical Sciences *49*:XI, 1980.

Gutnisky, A., and Van Dyke, D.: Normal response to erythropoietin or hypoxia in rats made anaemic with turpentine abscess. Proc. Soc. Biol. Med. *112*:75–78, 1963.

Jacobs, A.: Non-haematological effects of iron deficiency. Clin. Haematol. *11*:353–364, 1982.

Jacobs, A.: Low molecular weight intracellular iron transport compounds. Blood *50*:433–439, 1977.

Judisch, J. M., Naiman, J. L., and Oski, F. A.: The fallacy of the fat iron deficient child. Pediatrics *37*:987–990, 1966.

Ley, T. J., Griffith, P., and Nienhuis, A. W.: Transfusion haemosiderosis and chelation therapy. Clin. Haematol. *11*:437–464, 1982.

Linman, J. W., and Bagby, G. C.: The preleukemic syndrome (haematopoietic dysplasia). Cancer *42*:854–864, 1978.

Long, J. A., Doppman, J. L., Nienhuis, A. W., and Mills, S. R.: Computed tomographic analysis of beta-thalassemia syndromes with hemochromatosis: pathologic findings with clinical and laboratory correlations. J. Comput. Assist. Tomog. *4*:159–165, 1980.

Lukens, J. N.: Control of erythropoiesis in rats with adjuvant induced chronic inflammation. Blood *41*:37–44, 1973.

McLaren, G. D., Muir, W. A., and Kellermeyer, R. W.: Iron overload disorder: natural history, pathogenesis, diagnosis, and therapy. Crit. Rev. Clin. Lab. Sci. *19*:205–266, 1983.

Marsh, W. L., and Koenig, H. M.: The laboratory evaluation of microcytic red blood cells. Crit. Rev. Clin. Lab. Sci. *16*:195–254, 1982.

Marx, J. J. M.: Iron absorption and its regulation. A review. Acta Haematol. *64*:479–493, 1979.

Oski, F. A.: The non-hematological manifestations of iron deficiency. Am. J. Dis. Child. *133*:315, 1979.

Oski, F. A., and Horning, A. S.: The effects of therapy on the developmental scores of iron deficient infants. J. Pediatr. *92*:21, 1978.

Riedler, G. F., and Straub, P. W.: Abnormal iron incorporation, survival, protoporphyrin content and fluorescence of one red cell population in preleukemic sideroblastic anemia. Blood *40*:345–352, 1972.

Romslo, I.: Intracellular transport of iron. *In* Jacobs, A., and Worwood, M. (Eds.): Iron in Biochemistry and Medicine II. London, Academic Press, 1980, pp. 325–362.

Rørth, M.: Hypoxia, red cell oxygen affinity and erythropoietin production. Clin. Haematol. *3*:595–607, 1974.

Simon, M., Bourel, M., Fauchet, R., and Genetet, B.: Association of HLA-A3 and HLA-B14 antigens with idiopathic haematochromatosis. Gut *17*:332–334, 1976.

Szur, L., and Lewis, S. M.: Iron kinetics. Clin. Haematol. *4*:407–425, 1975.

Ward, H. P., Kurnick, J. E., and Pisarczyk, M. J.: Serum levels of erythropoietin in anaemias associated with chronic infection, malignancy and primary haematopoietic disease. J. Clin. Inves. *50*:332–335, 1971.

Woodson, R. D.: Red cell adaptation in cardiorespiratory disease. Clin. Haematol. *3*:627–648, 1974.

Worwood, M.: Serum ferritin. Crit. Rev. Clin. Lab. Sci. *10*:171–204, 1979.

Worwood, M.: Ferritin in human tissues and serum. Clin. Haematol. *11*:275–307, 1982.

APLASTIC ANEMIAS

Alter, B. P., Potter, N. U., and Li, F. P.: Classification and aetiology of the aplastic anaemias. Clin. Haematol. *7*:431–465, 1978.

AMA Drug Evaluations, 5th Ed. Chicago, American Medical Association, 1983.

Court-Brown, W. M., and Doll, R.: Leukemia and aplastic anaemia in patients irradiated for ankylosing spondylosis. Special Report Series, Great Britain, Medical Research Council, No. 295, 1957.

Freedman, M. H., and Saunders, E. F.: Deficient erythroid colony growth (CFU-E) in constitutional (congenital) aplastic anemia. Abstracts of the 18th Annual Meeting of the American Society of Hematology, Dallas, Texas, 1975.

Kirshbaum, J. D., Matsuo, T., Sato, K., Ichimaru, M., Tsuchimoto, T., and Ishimaru, T.: A study of aplastic anemia in an autopsy series with special reference to atomic bomb survivors in Hiroshima and Nagasaki. Blood *38*:17–26, 1971.

Krantz, S. B.: Diagnosis and treatment of pure red cell aplasia. Med. Clin. North Am. *60*:945–958, 1976.

Krantz, S. B.: Pure red cell aplasia. N. Engl. J. Med. *291*:345–350, 1974.

Lewis, E. B.: Leukemia, multiple myeloma, and aplastic anemia in American radiologists. Science *142*:1492–1494, 1963.

Rosenthal, R. L., and Blackman, A.: Bone marrow hypoplasia following use of chloramphenicol eye drops. J.A.M.A. *191*:148–149, 1965.

Rosse, W. F.: Paroxysmal nocturnal haemoglobinuria in aplastic anaemia. Clin. Haematol. *7*:541–553, 1978.

Royal Marsden Hospital Bone Marrow Transplantation Team: Failure of syngeneic bone marrow graft without preconditioning in post-hepatitis marrow aplasia. Lancet *2*:742–744, 1977.

Safdar, S. H., Krantz, S. B., and Brown, E. B.: Successful immunosuppressive treatment of erythroid aplasia appearing after thymectomy. Br. J. Haematol. *19*:345–443, 1970.

Williams, D. M., Lynch, R. E., and Cartwright, G. E.: Drug-induced aplastic anemia. Semin. Hematol. *10*:195–223, 1973.

Yunis, A. A.: Chloramphenicol toxicity. *In* Girdwood, R. H. (Ed.): Blood Disorders Due to Drugs and Other Agents. Amsterdam, Excerpta Medica, 1974, pp. 107–126.

Yunis, A. A.: Chloramphenicol-induced bone marrow suppression. Semin. Hematol. *10*:225–234, 1973.

Yunis, A. A.: Drug-induced bone marrow injury. Adv. Intern. Med. *15*:357–376, 1969.

Yunis, A. A., and Bloomberg, G. R.: Chloramphenicol toxicity: clinical features and pathogenesis. Prog. Hematol. *4*:138–159, 1964.

MEGALOBLASTIC ANEMIA

Cooper, B. A.: Megaloblastic anaemia and disorders affecting utilization of vitamin B12 and folate in childhood. Clin. Haematol. *5*:631–659, 1976.

Das, K. C., and Herbert, V.: Vitamin B12-folate interrelations. Clin. Haematol. *5*:697–725, 1976.

Eichner, E. R.: The hematologic disorders of alcoholism. Am. J. Med. *54*:621–630, 1973.

Fernandez-Costa, F., and Metz, J.: Vitamin B12 (transcobalamins) in serum. Crit. Rev. Lab. Sci. *18*:1–30, 1982.

Frater-Schroder, M., Nissen, C., Gmur, J., Kierat, L., and Hitzig, W.: Bone marrow participates in the biosynthesis of human transcobalamin II. Blood, *56*:560, 1980.

Gullberg, R.: Review: classification of human vitamin B12 binding proteins. Scand. J. Gastroenterol. *10*:561, 1975.

Hall, C. A.: Transcobalamins I and II as the natural transport proteins of vitamin B12. J. Clin. Invest. *56*:1125, 1975.

Herbert, V., and Zalusky, R.: Interrelations of vitamin B12 and folic acid metabolism: folic acid clearance studies. J. Clin. Invest. *41*:1263–1276, 1962.

Herbert, V., and Zalusky, R.: Pteroylglutamic (PGA) clearance after intravenous injection: Studies using two microbiologic assay organisms. Clin. Res. *9*:161, 1961.

Hoffbrand, A. V., Ganeshaguru, K., Hooton, J. W. L., and Tripp, E.: Megaloblastic anaemia: initiation of DNA synthesis in excess of DNA chain elongation as the underlying mechanism. Clin. Haematol. *5*:727–745, 1976.

Katzen, H. M., and Buchanan, J. M.: Enzymatic synthesis of the methyl group of methionine. VIII. Repression-depression, purification, and properties of 5-10-methylenetetrahydrofolate reductase from *E. coli*. J. Biol. Chem. *240*:825–835, 1965.

Kolhouse, J. F., and Allen, R. H.: Recognition of two intracellular cobalamin binding proteins and their identification as methylmalonyl-CoA mutase and methionine synthetase. Proc. Nat. Acad. Sci. U.S.A. *74*:921, 1977.

Mollin, D. L., Anderson, B. B., and Burman, J. F.: The serum vitamin B12 level: its assay and significance. Clin. Haematol. *513*:521–546, 1976.

Reynolds, E. H.: Neurological aspects of folate and vitamin B12 metabolism. Clin. Haematol. *5*:661–696, 1976.

Rosenberg, I. H.: Absorption and malabsorption of folates. Clin. Haematol. *5*:3:589–618, 1976.

Scott, J. M., and Weir, D. G.: Folate composition, synthesis and function in natural materials. Clin. Haematol. *5*:547–568, 1976.

Stebbins, R., and Bertino, J. R.: Megaloblastic anaemia produced by drugs. Clin. Haematol. *5*:619–630, 1976.

Stenman, U. H.: Intrinsic factor and the vitamin B12 binding proteins. Clin. Haematol. *5*:473–495, 1976.

Taylor, K. B.: Immune aspects of pernicious anaemia and atrophic gastritis. Clin. Haematol. *5*:497–519, 1976.

IMMUNE HEMOLYTIC ANEMIA

Antman, K. H., Skarin, A. T., Mayer, R. J., Hargrave, H. K., and Canellos, G. P.: Microangiopathic hemolytic anemia and cancer: a review. Medicine *58*:377, 1979.

Beutler, E.: Drug induced hemolytic anemia. Pharmacol. Rev. *21*:73, 1969.

Bentley, S. A.: Red cell survival studies interpreted. Clin. Haematol. *6*:601, 1977.

Bowman, J. M.: Neonatal Management in Modern Management of Rh Problem. 2nd Ed. Queenan, J. T. (Ed.). Hagerstown, MD, Harper & Row, 1977.

Bowman, J. M., Chown, B., Lewis, M., and Pollock, J. M.: Rh-isoimmunization during pregnancy: antenatal prophylaxis. Can. Med. Assoc. J. *18*:623, 1978.

Clin. Haematol. *4*:No. 1: Hemolytic Anemia. Philadelphia, W. B. Saunders, 1975.

Clin. Haematol. *10*:No. 1: Enzymopathies. Philadelphia, W. B. Saunders, 1981.

Clin. Lab. Med. *2*:No. 1: Blood Banking and Hematherapy, Philadelphia, W. B. Saunders, 1982.

Coombs, R. R. A., Mourant, A. E., and Race, R. R.: A new test for the detection of weak and "incomplete" Rh Agglutinins. Br. J. Exp. Pathol. *26*:255, 1945.

Dacie, J. V.: The Haemolytic Anemias. 2nd Ed. New York, Grune & Stratton, 1967.

Frank, M. M., Schreiber, A. D., Atkinson, J. P., and Jaffe, C. J.: Pathophysiology of immune hemolytic anemia. Ann. Int. Med. *87*:210–222, 1977.

Garraty, G., and Petz, L.: Drug-induced immune hemolytic anemia. Am. J. Med. *58*:398–405, 1975.

Jandl, J. H., Jones, A. R., and Castle, W. B.: The destruction of red cells by antibodies in man. I. Observations on the sequestration and lysis of red cells altered by immune mechanisms. J. Clin. Invest. *36*:1428, 1957.

Kirtland, H. H., Mohler, D. N., and Horwitz, D. A.: Methyldopa inhibition of suppressor-lymphocyte function, a proposed cause of autoimmune hemolytic anemia. N. Engl. J. Med. *302*:825–832, 1980.

Mollison, P. L.: Blood Transfusions in Clinical Medicine. 7th Ed. Oxford, Blackwell, 1979.

Petz, L. D., and Garraty, G.: Acquired Immune Hemolytic Anemias. New York, Churchill Livingstone, 1980.

Rubin H.: Autoimmune hemolytic anemias. Am. J. Clin. Pathol. *68*:638, 1977.

METHEMOGLOBIN

Beutler, E.: Hemoglobinopathies producing cyanosis. *In* Williams, W. J. and Beutler, E. (Eds.): Hematology. 3rd Ed. New York, McGraw Hill, 1983, p. 706.

Jaffe, E. R.: Hereditary methemoglobinemias associated with abnormalities in the metabolism of erythrocytes. Am. J. Med., *41*:786, 1966.

PAROXYSMAL NOCTURNAL HEMOGLOBINURIA

Oni, S. B., Osunkoya, B. O., and Luzzatto L.: Paroxysmal nocturnal hemoglobinuria: evidence for monoclonal origin of abnormal red cells. Blood *36*:145, 1970.

Sirchia, G., and Lewis, S. M.: Paroxysmal nocturnal haemoglobinuria. Clin. Haematol. *4*:199, 1975.

MYELOPHTHISIC ANEMIA

Contreras, E., Ellis, L. D., and Lee, R. E.: Value of the bone marrow biopsy in the diagnosis of metastatic carcinoma. Cancer *29*:778, 1972.

THE PORPHYRIAS

Brodie, M. J., and Goldberg, A.: Acute hepatic porphyrias. Clin. Haematol. *9*:253, 1980.

Loftin, E. B.: Porphyrias: Demons in disguise? Diagnostic Medicine, *21*:Oct., 1984.

Moore, M. R.: The biochemistry of the porphyrins. Clin. Haematol. *9*:227, 1980.

Pathophysiology of Hemostasis and Thrombosis

24

Rodger L. Bick

Health-care professionals are frequently faced with the awesome responsibility of diagnosing and treating thrombohemorrhagic disorders. The consequences of these disorders usually consist of acute insults to normal body function, long-term end-organ damage, and, too frequently, death of the patient. Researchers are beginning to appreciate the delicately modulated interplays of the hemostasis system and the abnormal mechanisms by which a variety of apparently unrelated disease processes may precipitate these catastrophic events—thrombosis, thromboembolism, or hemorrhage. Patients may develop hemorrhage or thrombosis or both because of a variety of identifiable abnormalities in the hemostasis system that may involve the vasculature, the platelets, the blood proteins, or any combination of these. Logical and effective therapy of these catastrophic disorders depends on rapid and proper clinical and laboratory identification of the thrombohemorrhagic disease process that is present. Only by developing a firm understanding both of the physiology of hemostasis and thrombosis and of thrombohemorrhagic disorders can the health-care professional appreciate the development and interpretation of sophisticated techniques for assessing hemostasis and begin to formulate logical, sequential, and precise therapeutic modalities. The goals of this chapter are to acquaint the reader with basic concepts of hemostasis, thrombosis, and thrombohemorrhagic disorders. For the sake of brevity and convenience to the reader, only key references have been included in this chapter.

BASIC PHYSIOLOGY OF HEMOSTASIS

MECHANISMS OF HEMOSTASIS

The marked complexities of the hemostasis system have begun to unfold with an explosion of knowledge in basic mechanisms of hemostasis and thrombosis. The hemostasis system can no longer be thought of as simply a "cascade," or a "waterfall," system; this concept is untenable with current concepts of physiology, and, in fact, such a structure is incompatible with mammalian life. However, these historic concepts of "cascade" and "waterfall" have been teleologically useful in developing current understanding of the system. These more archaic concepts of hemostasis have

neglected important contributions of the vasculature, platelets, inhibitory systems, and fibrinolysis. The hemostasis system is actually composed of three *equally important* and *interrelating* hemostasis compartments: (1) the platelets, (2) the blood proteins, and (3) the vasculature. For normal hemostasis to occur, platelets must be normal in number and in function; the blood protein system is of central importance and can no longer be thought of as simply the "coagulation proteins"; the vasculature now assumes major importance in physiology as well as in the pathophysiology of hemorrhage and thrombosis. Figure 24–1 provides a realistic, updated, although complex overview of the hemostasis system. It is suggested that the reader become familiar with this scheme as it encompasses all three hemostasis compartments, their individual functions, and the key interrelationships between the three compartments.

THE VASCULATURE

For many years, the vasculature was the most neglected area of hemostasis, but now the key role of the vascular compartment in hemostasis is recognized. The vascular wall is composed of three morphologic layers: the intima, the media, and the adventitia. The intima consists of (1) a monolayer of *nonthrombogenic* endothelial cells that contact flowing blood, and (2) the internal elastic membrane. The media is composed of smooth muscle cells, the thickness of which depends on the type (arterial, venous) and size of the vessel. The adventitia consists of an external elastic membrane and connective tissue that provides support for the vessel. A common vascular insult is that of endothelial cell "sloughing" with exposure of subendothelial collagen and basement membrane. This occurs via several physiologic and pathologic mechanisms, including shock, acidosis, circulating endotoxin, and circulating antigen/antibody complex. When endothelial sloughing occurs and subendothelial collagen is exposed, platelets are immediately recruited to fill this "endothelial gap" to stop seepage of blood outside the vascular tree. If this is a successful event, a repair process occurs. During repair, muscle cells from the media dedifferentiate, migrate through the internal elastic membrane, and then redifferentiate into endothelial cells, thus forming a new monolayer of endothelial cells to provide again a nonthrombo-

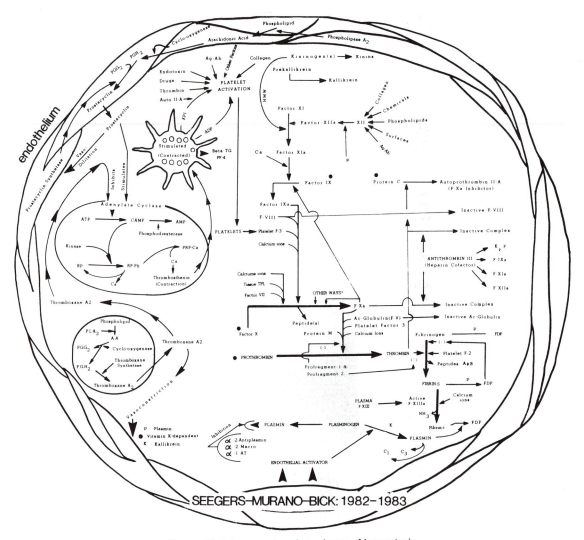

Figure 24–1 A comprehensive scheme of hemostasis.

genic surface. If this is a one-time event, it may occur without serious consequences. However, with progressive uncontrolled deposition of platelets and fibrin, a thrombus and subsequent vascular occlusion may result. If the event occurs constantly over a protracted period of time, the end result may be atherosclerosis. Alternatively, with derangements in the platelet or blood protein system the result will be hemorrhage—blood outside the vascular tree. Functions of the vasculature are listed in Figure 24–2. Three key vascular functions are (1) permeability—an increase may lead to leakage of blood from the vasculature; (2) fragility—an increase may lead to vascular rupture; and (3) vasoconstriction, which may lead to vascular occlusion. Vasoconstriction is under neural, local, and humoral control. Humoral control is primarily mediated by compounds released from platelets, especially biogenic amines. Properties of endothelial cells include contraction when

stimulated by histamine, serotonin, or kinins; release of plasminogen activator activity; and synthesis of high molecular weight factor VIII (von Willebrand factor). Endothelial plasminogen activator activity provides a major mechanism of fibrinolytic system activation.

THE PLATELETS

Like the vasculature, the platelets are now recognized as extremely important and increas-

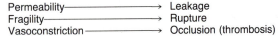

Figure 24–2 Vascular functions. Vasoconstriction is controlled by the following factors: neural (sympathetic system), local (temperature, pH, P_{CO_2}), and humoral (catecholamine, ADP, FDP, kinins).

ingly complex components of the hemostasis system. Platelets are more than simply "buds of cells" derived from megakaryocytes. Platelets display discrete morphology and are similar to most cells except that they lack nuclei. Platelets are composed of a peripheral zone consisting of an outer glycocalyx, a plasma membrane, and an open canalicular system. Inside the peripheral zone is a "sol-gel zone," composed of microtubules, microfilaments, a dense tubular system, and thrombosthenin, the platelet contractile protein. The organelle zone consists of dense bodies, alpha granules, and mitochondria. As platelets become reactive from contact with a foreign surface or exposure to constituents in the immediate environment, they undergo contraction, with resultant pseudopod formation. The process of contraction is mediated by the thrombosthenin; the process of contraction forces organelles and other platelet constituents to the center of the platelet. As this occurs, the contents of the organelles are expelled and extruded through the open canalicular system to the outside of the platelet to become

TABLE 24–1 PLATELET FACTORS

Platelet Factor	Synonym
1	Factor V
2	Thromboplastic substance
3	Phospholipoprotein ("Thromboplastin")
4	Antiheparin factor
5	Fibrinogen clotting factor
6	Antifibrinolytic factor
7	Platelet cothromboplastin

a part of the microenvironment in circulating blood and thus react with adjacent platelet membrane receptors. These compounds are ADP, epinephrine, serotonin, histamine, and kinins, which attach to membrane receptors of adjacent platelets and induce new platelet reactivity. Numerous platelet factors have been described and are depicted in Table 24–1. The most important of these are platelet factor 3 (platelet membrane phospholipoprotein) and platelet factor 4 (antiheparin fac-

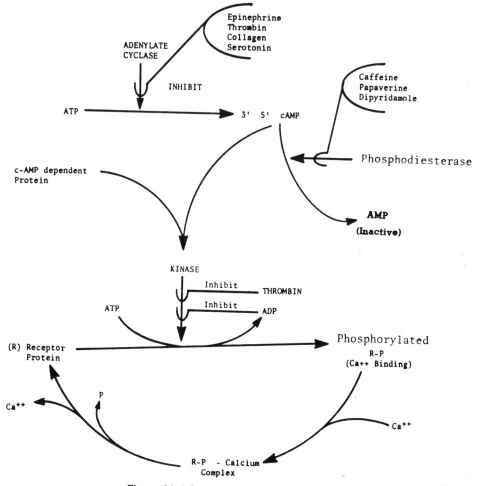

Figure 24–3 Summary of platelet biochemistry.

tor). As platelets become reactive, they first undergo a process of *platelet adhesion,* which refers to platelets adhering to a foreign surface such as subendothelial collagen. As this occurs, there is a release reaction (reverse or primary aggregation), with subsequent release of ADP. As ADP contacts adjacent platelets, the process of *platelet cohesion* (platelets adhering to other platelets) begins. This is associated with a subsequent amplification of ADP release. In addition, serotonin and other biogenic amines are now also released, causing vascular constriction as well as enhanced platelet cohesion. This latter process is also referred to as *irreversible (secondary) aggregation.* At this point, a conformational change in the platelet membrane occurs, with platelet factor 3 (platelet membrane phospholipoprotein) becoming available. Platelet factor 3 then reacts at key points in the coagulation protein system, with resultant coagulation activation, fibrin formation, and the development of a "primary hemostatic plug." Figure 24–3 represents a simplified scheme of the biochemical reactions. As platelet reactivity occurs, platelet factor 4 and beta-thromboglobulin, a low molecular weight form of platelet factor 4, are released. The laboratory measurement of released platelet factor 4 and beta-thromboglobulin provides indices of the degree of platelet reactivity in a variety of thrombohemorrhagic disorders.

The key modulator of platelet biochemistry is cyclic AMP, which is responsible for the generation of an intraplatelet kinase. Intraplatelet kinase functions to phosphorylate a receptor protein in the platelet. Phosphorylated receptor protein binds ionized calcium in the platelet; thus, ionized calcium is not available to thrombosthenin, thrombosthenin thus cannot contract, and the platelet thus cannot adhere or aggregate. Prostaglandin derivatives are key modulators of this platelet biochemical reaction and lead to increased or decreased platelet reactivity. In addition, endothelial cell–platelet interaction is highly dependent on prostaglandin derivatives. Both the endothelial cell membrane and the platelet membrane contain membrane phospholipids that are metabolized by phospholipase A_2 into arachidonic acid, which is subsequently converted into two endoperoxides, PGG_2 and PGH_2. The enzyme responsible for this conversion is cyclo-oxygenase, which is inhibited by aspirin and sulfinpyrizone, two commonly used antiplatelet agents. In the platelet, PGH_2 is converted into thromboxane A_2 by a platelet specific enzyme, thromboxane synthetase. Thromboxane A_2 is a potent vasoconstricting and platelet aggregating agent. Conversely, in the endothelial cell PGH_2 is converted into prostacyclin by an endothelial cell–specific enzyme, prostacyclin synthetase. Prostacyclin is a potent aggregation inhibitor and a potent vasodilator. Thus, the platelet synthesizes thromboxane A_2, whereas the endothelial cell synthesizes prostacyclin, with both compounds being derived from the same parent endoperoxides

(PGG_2 and PGH_2) and demonstrating diametrically opposed actions. In summary, the endothelial cell synthesizes a compound that inhibits platelet aggregation and enhances vasodilatation, whereas the platelet synthesizes a compound that promotes platelet aggregation and vasoconstriction. Platelet and endothelial synthesis of prostaglandins is outlined in Figure 24–4. The mechanisms of action of thromboxane A_2 and prostacyclin have been elucidated. Thromboxane A_2 inhibits adenylate cyclase, whereas prostacyclin stimulates adenylate cyclase, the enzyme responsible for converting ATP to cyclic AMP and thus the modulator of intraplatelet cyclic AMP concentration. By previously outlined mechanisms, the concentration of intraplatelet cyclic AMP will determine the concentration of intraplatelet free ionized calcium that is available to thrombosthenin for the promotion or inhibition of thrombosthenin contraction required in platelet adhesion and aggregation. Figure 24–5 summarizes the role of prostacyclin and thromboxane in modulating platelet adhesiveness and aggregability.

BLOOD PROTEIN FUNCTION

Blood proteins involved in hemostasis include (1) the coagulation proteins (factors) (Table 24–2), (2) the fibrinolytic enzyme proteins, (3) the kinin system, (4) the complement system, and (5) inhibitors to the first four systems. The coagulation protein system is centered on three key reactions, with all other reactions serving to accelerate or inhibit these three key reactions. These three key reactions are: (1) the formation of Factor Xa, (2) the formation of thrombin, and (3) the formation of fibrin.

The Formation of Factor Xa. In considering these reactions, the reader must appreciate that "activated clotting factors" are serine proteases; the active site for enzyme activity is the amino acid serine, and the conversion of a clotting factor precursor to its active form involves the exposure of serine. The formation of factor Xa is a five-component system and requires a substrate, an enzyme, a cofactor, a phospholipid, and calcium. The substrate is Factor X, the enzyme required is Factor IXa, the cofactor is Factor VIII, and the phospholipoprotein is platelet factor 3. These components are held together by calcium and form an enzyme substrate complex that generates a specific product, Factor Xa.

The Formation of Thrombin. Thrombin is formed similarly to Factor Xa and is also composed of a five component system: substrate, enzyme, cofactor, phospholipoprotein, and calcium. In this reaction the substrate is prothrombin (Factor II), the enzyme is Factor Xa (the enzyme generated in the first key reaction), the cofactor is Factor V, and the phospholipoprotein is again platelet factor 3. An enzyme substrate complex is formed and the

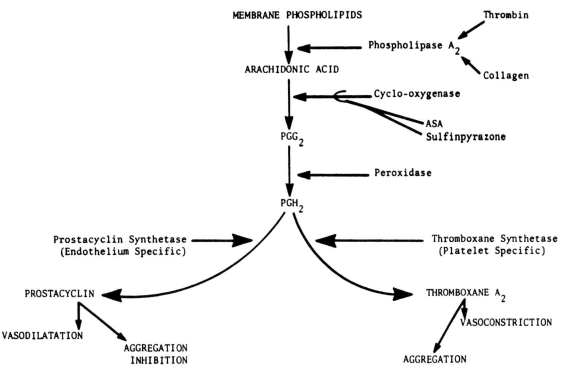

Figure 24–4 Prostaglandin modulation of the platelet-endothelial interaction.

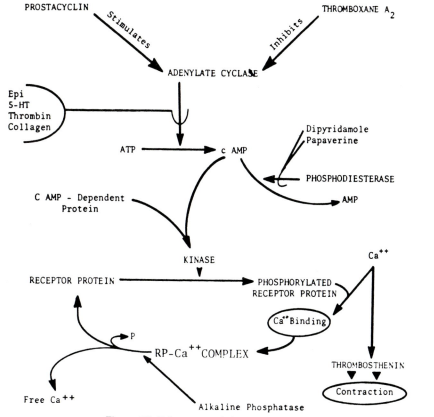

Figure 24–5 Summary of platelet physiology.

TABLE 24–2 COAGULATION FACTORS AND SYNONYMS

Coagulation Factor	Synonym
I	Fibrinogen
II	Prothrombin
III	Tissue procoagulant material
IV	Calcium Ion
V	Accelerator globulin
VI	Not assigned
VII	Serum prothrombin conversion accelerator
VIII	Antihemophilic factor/globulin
IX	Plasma thromboplastin component; Christmas factor
X	Stuart-Prower factor
XI	Plasma thromboplastin antecedent, Rosenthal factor
XII	Hageman factor, contact activation factor
XIII	Fibrin stabilizing factor, Laki-Lorand factor, profibrinoligase
XIV	Protein C
Fletcher Factor	Prekallikrein
Fitzgerald Factor	High molecular weight kininogen, Williams factor, Fleaujac factor, Fujiwara factor

product, thrombin (also a serine protease), is generated. Figure 24–6 depicts these first two key reactions.

The Formation of Fibrin. The enzyme thrombin, generated in the second key reaction, is responsible for the formation of fibrin from its precursor fibrinogen. This reaction is summarized in Figure 24–7. Thrombin is a specific serine protease that cleaves first fibrinopeptide A and then fibrinopeptide B from fibrinogen. The laboratory measurement of fibrinopeptide A by radioimmunoassay provides an indication of the degree of thrombin activity in blood. Fibrinogen minus fibrinopeptides A and B is referred to as *fibrin monomer*. With the removal of the aforementioned peptides, fibrin monomer begins to aggregate end to end and side to side; these aggregates then begin to polymerize and are held together by hydrophobic bonds. This fibrin is referred to as *soluble fibrin,* or *fibrin-s,* and is soluble in urea or monochloracetic acid, the laboratory reagents used to detect the presence of Factor XIII. Concomitant with thrombin-induced removal of fibrinopeptides A and B from fibrinogen, thrombin activates Factor XIII, or fibrin stabilizing factor, rendering Factor XIIIa, or fibrinoligase. Factor XIIIa replaces hydrophobic bonds on polymerized fibrin with solid peptide bonds, resulting in strongly

cross-linked fibrin, known as *insoluble fibrin,* or *fibrin-Is*. This fibrin will not dissolve in urea or monochloracetic acid.

CONTACT ACTIVATION

The contact activation phase of hemostasis leads to initiation of the first key reaction, the generation of Factor Xa. The process starts with Hageman factor, which is then converted to active Hageman factor (Factor XIIa), also a serine protease. This activation may occur by many routes but primarily involves exposure of Factor XII to collagen, phospholipids, or kallikrein. The reaction appears to be accelerated by the presence of Fitzgerald factor (high molecular weight kininogen). Active Hageman factor converts Factor XI into Factor XIa, also a serine protease. This reaction also appears to be accelerated by Fitzgerald factor. Factor XIa then converts Factor IX to Factor IXa, the enzyme responsible for the first key reaction, the conversion of Factor X to Factor Xa. Factor XII activation provides another key pathway for activation of the fibrinolytic system. In addition, activation of the Hageman factor system may eventually generate kinins. The contact activation reactions are depicted in Figure 24–8.

THE FIBRINOLYTIC SYSTEM

Fibrin deposition plays a major role in hemostasis as well as in the inflammatory response and in subsequent wound healing. The hemostasis system is constantly being "driven to the right," with subsequent fibrin formation; this event may occur quite rapidly both physiologically and pathologically. In humans, the price of this protective mechanism is potential accumulation of enhanced fibrin deposits, which may constitute a hazard (i.e., thrombosis and subsequent multiple end-organ damage secondary to impedence of blood flow, ischemia, and infarction). Counterbalancing this potential danger of enhanced fibrin deposition is the fibrinolytic system, which lyses both fibrinogen and fibrin. Plasmin is the enzyme responsible for lysis (degradation) of fibrinogen and fibrin and is derived by activation of its inactive precursor protein plasminogen. Plasminogen is a single polypeptide chain with a molecular weight of approximately 90,000. The precise site or sites of plasminogen synthesis are not clear, but the process may occur in eosinophils. The conversion of plasminogen to plasmin involves the cleavage of peptide bonds, resulting in a molecule with two polypeptide chains: a light chain and a heavy chain. Plasmin, unlike many other serine proteases in the blood coagulation system, is a nonspecific proteolytic serine protease. Plasmin has equal affinity for fibrinogen and fibrin and also hydrolyzes other clotting factors (e.g., active Hageman factor, Fac-

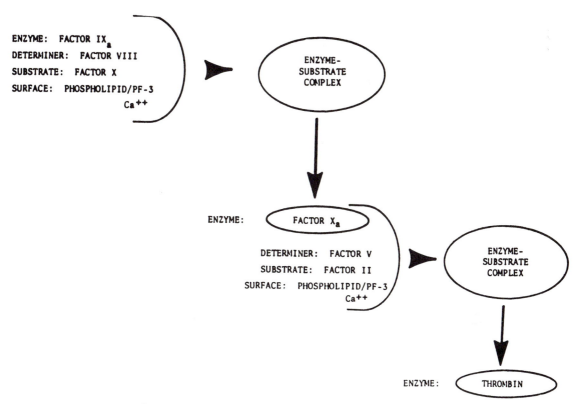

Figure 24–6 Thrombin generation by the first two key reactions.

tor V, Factor VIII, Factor IX, and Factor XI), is capable of activating the complement system, and may indirectly liberate kinins from kininogens. In addition, plasmin is capable of biodegrading ACTH, growth hormone, and insulin. There are many activators of plasminogen, and two key activators appear to be predominant in normal physiology: (1) the Hageman factor (Factor XIIa) pathway of activation, and (2) vascular endothelial plasminogen activator activity. However, there are other activators that are used pharmacologically and that may act physiologically as well. Urokinase, a proteolytic enzyme synthesized by the kidney and found in normal urine, is one such activator. Various tissue activators have also been isolated. Streptokinase, produced by beta-hemolytic streptococci, is a known activator. Urokinase and streptokinase are currently utilized as thera-

peutic thrombolytic agents. Basic physiology and activation of the plasminogen/plasmin system are depicted in Figure 24–9. The Hageman factor activation pathway is indirect, involving the interaction of Factor XIIa or fragments thereof with a plasma factor (plasminogen proactivator). This interaction results in the formation of an active component (activator), which in turn converts plasminogen to plasmin.

Inhibitors of the fibrinolytic system consist of a rapid acting $alpha_2$-antiplasmin and a slower acting $alpha_2$-macroglobulin in presumed descending order of importance. This process of sequential digestion of fibrin(ogen) by plasmin is responsible for formation of the four major clinically recognized fibrinogen/fibrin degradation products (FDPs), the X, Y, D, and E fragments. These fragments are readily measured in the clinical

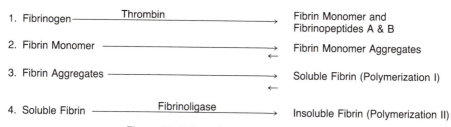

1. Fibrinogen ———— Thrombin ————→ Fibrin Monomer and Fibrinopeptides A & B

2. Fibrin Monomer ————————→ ←— Fibrin Monomer Aggregates

3. Fibrin Aggregates ————————→ ←— Soluble Fibrin (Polymerization I)

4. Soluble Fibrin ———— Fibrinoligase ————→ Insoluble Fibrin (Polymerization II)

Figure 24–7 Steps in the formation of fibrin.

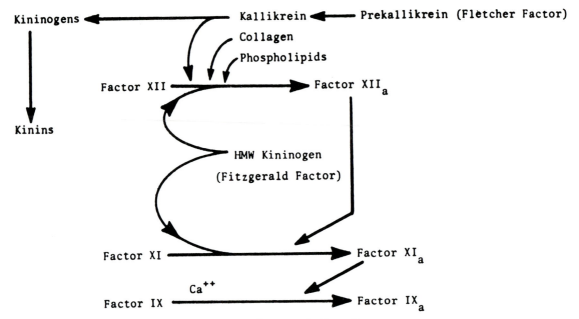

Figure 24–8 Contact activation pathways.

laboratory for assessment of the activation of the fibrinolytic system. During any type of intravascular fibrino(geno)lysis, whether it be a primary or secondary event or therapeutically induced, the titer of these four degradation products becomes significantly increased, as the rate of formation exceeds ability of the reticuloendothelial system to clear them from the circulation. Thus, the FDP

titer can be used as an indirect approximation of the extent of fibrino(geno)lysis. Fibrinogen degradation by plasmin, including the formation of the X, Y, D, and E fragments, is depicted in Figure 24–10. These four degradation products exert significant biologic effects, many of which have major deleterious effects on hemostasis and may enhance hemorrhage. As FDPs are formed from the plas-

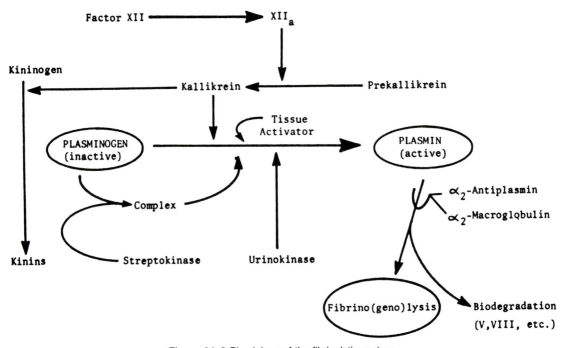

Figure 24–9 Physiology of the fibrinolytic system.

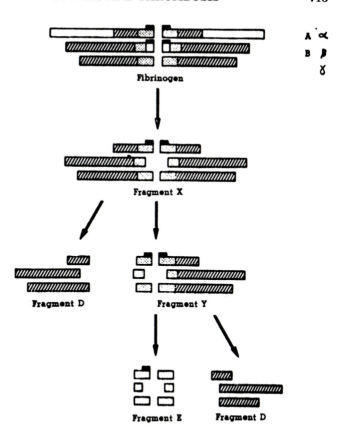

Figure 24–10 Creation of fibrin(ogen) degradation products by plasmin.

min-induced lysis of fibrinogen and fibrin, the biologic consequences are inhibition of the hemostasis system by interference with fibrin monomer polymerization, an antithrombin effect, and interference with platelet function. In addition, FDPs may induce hyperpyrexia.

KININS, COMPLEMENT, AND COAGULATION

The relationship of blood-clotting processes with the immunologic, fibrinolytic, and kinin generating systems has been noted for many years. The first direct evidence associating clotting and other hemostatic mechanisms with immunologic events was derived from the observation that the enzyme plasmin can initiate the primary pathway of complement activation by activating C1s to C1 esterase and can activate the so-called "alternate," or "properdin" pathway by cleavage of C3 to yield anaphylatoxin, which is chemotactic for polymorphonuclear neutrophils and causes release of histamine from mass cells, resulting in increased vascular permeability. C3b generated during alternate pathway activation exhibits many functions. Its presence on the cell membrane permits binding to specific receptors on polymorphonuclear leukocytes, erythrocytes, and platelets in the immune inherence phenomena, leading to release of

lysosomal enzymes that can produce C5a (anaphylatoxin) from C5 and can fragment basement membranes, thereby possibly contributing to Factor XII activation. The involvement of platelets may result in thrombocytopenia and, with their disruption, the release of phospholipids, serotonin, ADP, and so forth, all of which may serve to accelerate the procoagulant clotting process. The activation of complement by plasmin indirectly involves Hageman factor, as Hageman factor is a key activator of the fibrinolytic system that may subsequently activate the complement system.

A third role of Factor XII is the induction of substances responsible for inflammatory states and pain. There exist in human plasma multiple forms of an alpha globulin known as *kininogen*. Two major classes have been identified: low molecular weight (LMW) kininogen and high molecular weight (HMW) kininogen. The latter is also known as *Fitzgerald, Flaujeac,* or *Williams factor.* Its molecular weight is approximately 120,000, and it functions in the activation of Factor XII, as previously discussed. The proteolytic enzyme kallikrein (which exists in plasma as an inactive precursor—prekallikrein or Fletcher factor) has the property of splitting off biologically active polypeptide fragments from high molecular weight kininogen. These fragments are known generically as *kinins*. They can enhance vascular permeability and dilate certain blood vessels (resulting in hy-

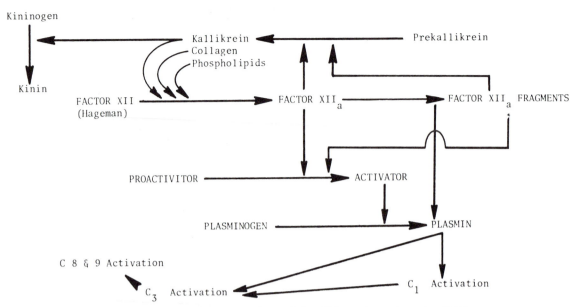

Figure 24–11 Interrelationships of coagulation, kinin, and complement systems.

potension), cause contraction of some smooth muscles, and may bring about the migration of leukocytes in the extravascular space. In addition, kallikrein is also capable of activating Factor XII. Thus, the initiating event in the generation of kinins in human plasma is the activation of Factor XII. Evidence has accumulated indicating that Factor XIIa and/or fragments thereof resulting from plasmin digestion may directly activate prekallikrein to kallikrein, thus causing the conversion of kininogens to kinins. The interrelationships of coagulation, complement, and kinins are depicted in Figure 24–11.

INHIBITORY MECHANISMS

Like most other physiologic processes, the hemostasis system is constantly "driven to the right" (fibrin formation) and thus requires inhibitory mechanisms to limit the extent of the various biochemical reactions previously discussed. Regulation of hemostasis and, in particular, the activated coagulation proteins is effected by a number of negative feedback mechanisms, the involvement of specific inhibitors, and the compartmentalization of function designed to restrict clotting to a localized process. Physiologic inhibition of hemostasis is summarized in Table 24–3.

Antithrombin III. The activity of the various enzymes (serine proteases) involved in hemostasis (thrombin, Factor IXa, Factor Xa, Factor XIa, and Factor XIIa) is controlled primarily by a plasma protein generally known as *antithrombin III (heparin cofactor)*. This inhibitor, synthesized by the liver, inactivates the aforementioned serine proteases (activated clotting factors) by forming an

irreversible complex that effectively blocks the active serine center. Antithrombin III inhibitory activity is optimized in the presence of heparin. The exact mechanism or mechanisms of heparin are not clear; however, it has been proposed that heparin modifies either the enzyme molecule or the antithrombin III molecule in such a way as to facilitate complex formation. Heparin therapy is essentially ineffective in the absence of antithrombin III. It should be noted that other inhibitors, including alpha₁-antitrypsin and alpha₂-macroglobulin, also neutralize the activity of the serine proteases in coagulation; however, their role is much less significant than that of antithrombin III.

Thrombin. The enzyme thrombin, in addition to its ability to convert fibrinogen to fibrin and to activate Factor XIII, also has the potential to enhance temporarily the activity of Factors V and

TABLE 24–3 PHYSIOLOGIC INHIBITORS OF HEMOSTASIS

Antithrombin III: Irreversible complex formation with thrombin, Factors IXa, Xa, XIa, and XII.
Thrombin: Activation, then destruction of Factors V and VIII.
Protein C: Degradation of Factors V and VIII.
FDP: Interference with fibrin monomer polymerization and normal platelet function.
Fibrin(ogen): Absorption and removal of thrombin.
Alpha₂-Macroglobulin: Minor inhibition of activated clotting factors.
Alpha₂-Antitrypsin: Minor inhibition of activated clotting factors.
C1 Esterase inhibitor: Minor inhibition of activated clotting factors.

VIII, followed by immediate destruction of their procoagulant activity. In addition, thrombin hydrolyzes prothrombin to form prothrombin I and prothrombin fragment I, which interfere with the coagulation process.

Activated Protein C. Thrombin converts the newly discovered vitamin K dependent factor (Protein C) to an active protease that appears to degrade Factors V and VIII. In addition, this protein may participate in activation of endogenous fibrinolysis.

Fibrinogen Degradation Products. The products of fibrino(geno)lysis function as inhibitors (as previously discussed) by interfering with conversion of fibrinogen to fibrin, with fibrin monomer polymerization, and with platelet function. Thus, it is evident that the clotting sequence is highly regulated by a series of inhibitory forces, resulting in a highly modulated response limited to the site of vascular injury.

In summary, understanding of hemostasis testing methods and associated pathologies as well as knowledge and development of particular plasma concentrates and specific "hemotherapy" can be derived only from a precise comprehension of basic concepts of hemostasis and thrombosis.

VASCULAR DISORDERS

The vasculature remains one of the most poorly understood components of hemostasis. All three components of hemostasis have been elucidated and their interrelationships discussed earlier in this chapter. This section summarizes vascular disorders that may present as thrombohemorrhagic phenomena. The clinical features of these vascular defects will be characterized with emphasis on the thrombotic or hemorrhagic manifestations or both. Pathophysiology is highlighted where it is known. Acquired vascular defects are now being diagnosed with increasing frequency; nevertheless, when a patient with a known vascular defect is subjected to stress such as trauma or surgery, hemorrhagic or thrombotic complications or both may ensue. The formidable diagnostic and management aspects of a patient with an unrecognized vascular disorder who experiences trauma or undergoes surgery and develops hemorrhagic or thrombotic manifestations are immediately apparent. Some unfortunate cases may end disastrously.

CLINICAL MANIFESTATIONS

The types of hereditary and acquired vascular disorders are highly varied; thus, it is not surprising that clinical manifestations of vascular disorders may also vary greatly. An adequate evaluation of the vasculature requires a thorough examination of the integument. Defects in the integument are usually found in patients with hereditary or acquired vascular disorders; however, the findings may be highly varied, depending on the type of disorder present. Often, the findings are not diagnostic of a vascular disorder but are suggestive. The few exceptions to this are hereditary hemorrhagic telangiectasia, in which one will note the classic nonpulsatile pinpoint; nodular, or spider-like, telangiectasia; giant cavernous hemangiomata; scleroderma; and Behçet's syndrome. Other vascular disorders usually display nondiagnostic features. The most common clinical findings of a vascular defect are petechiae and purpura, which are usually, but not always, dependent on the type of disorder. Platelet function defects and thrombocytopenia, however, usually present as petechiae and purpura throughout the integumentary system and are usually not dependent on the kind of disorder present. Additional common findings in the vascular disorders are a history of gingival bleeding with tooth brushing, a history of epistaxis, a history of easy and spontaneous bruisability, and a history of other mild to moderate mucosal membrane bleeding, often from the gastrointestinal or genitourinary tract.

Although these are the most common and most easily recognized findings, there are other less subtle findings that may also be noted. One must always recall that what is noted in the integument may potentially be occurring in the parenchyma of vital organs as well in patients with generalized vascular disorders. Findings in the integument that again may be assumed to be occurring in the vasculature of vital organ parenchyma as well depend on two factors: (1) the host reaction to a vascular insult or vascular disease or both, and (2) the severity of the vascular insult or damage. The host reaction to a vascular insult or vascular disorder is the product of numerous interrelationships with respect to the coagulation proteins, fibrinolytic enzyme system, complement system, kinin generating system, and cellular response, including migration of leukocytes and response of the immediate normal perivascular cellular elements.

The severity of the insult, in combination with varied host reactions, will determine the degree of vascular permeability, with the usual attendant manifestations of increased vascular permeability or the development of intravascular thrombosis or both. A mild vascular insult usually results in increased vascular permeability with effusion of serum, giving rise to the usual clinical findings of wheals of urticaria, bullae, and some purpura. A moderate insult to the vasculature, in contrast, will usually give rise to effusion of serum as well as blood, and attendant activation of coagulation and resultant microthrombi with petechiae and purpura will be found. A more severe insult will give rise to significantly increased vascular permeability, resulting in endothelial death, surrounding tissue damage and death, local large or small vessel thrombosis, and varying degrees of end-organ ischemia, and it may result in diffuse disseminated intravascular coagulation. Manifestations of a moderate to severe vascular insult will also depend somewhat on the degree of leukocyte migration and release of clot-promoting and clot-lysing enzymes. When many leukocytes migrate into a damaged area, the usual manifestations of painful, erythematous vasculitis will result. Alternatively, few leukocytes are usually found when the vascular insult slowly progresses to occlusive thrombosis with all of its usual associated findings, such as skin necrosis, ulceration, and varying degrees of end-organ damage in vital organs. Table 24–4 summarizes pathogenic mechanisms.

The laboratory diagnosis of a vascular disorder is quite taxing, commonly requiring an autoimmune investigation, connective tissue biopsy, and specific immunofluorescence staining techniques as well as investigation of the kinin system. The most common abnormal laboratory findings in a vascular disorder are an abnormal Rumpel-Leede tourniquet test and, more important, an abnormal template bleeding time. If the template bleeding time is borderline (9 to 12 minutes) following an aspirin tolerance test, the patient is given 600 mg of aspirin, and the test is repeated. A normal individual will usually prolong only by 2 to 3 minutes after ingesting aspirin. Vascular disorders are characterized by an abnormal template bleeding time or an abnormal aspirin tolerance test or both in the face of normal platelet function as defined by aggregation studies. Thus, the finding of one or both of these abnormalities in the face of normal platelet aggregation (in the absence of thrombocytopenia) is strongly suggestive of a vascular disorder. The more specific laboratory findings of the numerous hereditary and acquired vascular defects are outside the scope of this review and can be found in several authoritative reviews.

CLINICAL VASCULAR DISORDERS

Vascular disorders are most conveniently divided into two categories: hereditary and acquired. The acquired types are much more common and a much more frequent cause of hemorrhage.

Hereditary Vascular Disorders. The following are the most common hereditary vascular (or collagen-vascular) disorders that may present as thrombotic, hemorrhagic, or mixed disorders of hemostasis and thrombosis:

The *Ehlers-Danlos Syndrome (ED syndrome)* is a rare connective tissue disorder inherited by autosomal dominance. Interestingly, one of the earliest descriptions of this syndrome may have concerned the violin virtuoso Paganini; this disorder was thought to contribute to his remarkable dexterity and talent. The ED syndrome is characterized by extreme vascular fragility, skin fragility, hypermobile joints, and molluscoid pseudotumors of the knees and elbows. Bleeding may be highly variable; however, easy and spontaneous bruisability are hallmark findings. Patients commonly suffer gingival bleeding with tooth brushing and demonstrate undue bleeding following dental extraction. Also, petechiae, purpura, gastrointestinal bleeding, and hemoptysis are frequent. The bleeding diathesis may be severe enough to suggest hemophilia. In addition, numerous patients demonstrate platelet function defects as well as the characteristic vascular defect. Other characteristics commonly noted in this syndrome are blue sclerae and angioid streaks. In addition, aortic insufficiency and the "floppy" mitral valve syndrome often occur. The common laboratory findings are a prolonged template bleeding time and, in some instances, abnormal platelet aggregation if the patient has an associated platelet function defect (often storage pool in type). The basic pathology of the ED syndrome is poorly understood but appears to represent a decrease in collagen and an increase in elastic tissue. In addition, the collagen from these patients is thought to contain an abnormal amino acid composition.

Marfan's syndrome is well described and is the most common of the hereditary collagen vascular disorders. Marfan's syndrome is inherited as an autosomal dominant trait and is characterized by skeletal defects (long extremities and arachnodactyly), cardiovascular abnormalities (ascending aortic aneurysm or dissection or both), and ocular defects (ectopia lentis). In addition, hyperextensible joints are present. Of all the hereditary collagen vascular disorders, Marfan's syndrome is least likely to be characterized clinically by a hemorrhagic diathesis. However, many patients demonstrate easy and spontaneous bruisability,

TABLE 24–4 PATHOGENESIS OF VASCULAR DISORDERS

A. Host response to vascular disorder
   1. Antigenic response
   2. Activation of coagulation
   3. Activation of fibrinolysis
   4. Activation of kinins
   5. Activation of complement
   6. Activation of other enzymes
   7. Migration of leukocytes
B. Degree of severity of vascular disorder
   1. Mild
     (a) Serum effusion: bullae and erythema
   2. Moderate
     (a) Bullae, erythema, wheals
     (b) Petechiae and purpura
   3. Severe
     (a) Effusion of blood and endothelial cell death
     (b) Petechiae and purpura
     (c) Gross hemorrhage
     (d) Small/large vessel thrombosis

and some may show a poorly characterized platelet function defect (usually storage pool in type) as well.

Osteogenesis imperfecta (brittle bones and blue sclerae) is inherited as an autosomal dominant trait and is characterized by a patchy lack of bone matrix. However, the matrix that does exist undergoes normal calcification. Osteogenesis imperfecta is clinically manifest as deformed, brittle bones that fracture easily. In addition, skin and subcutaneous hemorrhages are characteristic. Death not infrequently occurs at childhood as a result of intracranial hemorrhage caused by an abnormal calvarium coupled with a vascular hemorrhagic diathesis. Easy and spontaneous bruising, hemoptysis, epistaxis, and intracranial bleeding are common. An abnormal template bleeding time is characteristic. In addition, many patients have been described with abnormal platelet function and may demonstrate aggregation patterns suggestive of storage pool defects. The basic pathophysiology of osteogenesis imperfecta appears to be related to an inability of reticulin to mature into collagen. In addition, the collagen present demonstrates an abnormal amino acid composition.

Pseudoxanthoma elasticum (PE syndrome) often does not become manifest until the second or third decade. This very rare disorder is inherited as an autosomal recessive trait. The PE syndrome is commonly characterized by significant hemorrhage, since abnormal elastic fibers affect the entire arterial system. Hemorrhage may occur in any organ, most commonly the skin, eyes, kidneys, and gastrointestinal tract. In addition, patients have a marked tendency to demonstrate easy and spontaneous bruisability and commonly are noted to have petechiae and purpura. In addition, these individuals have a strong predisposition to thrombosis, especially cerebral vascular thrombosis, acute myocardial infarction, and peripheral vascular occlusion with resultant gangrene and loss of extremities. Other clinical characteristics include relaxed, inelastic, and redundant skin in facial, cervical, axillary, orbital, and inguinal areas. Hyperkeratotic plaques develop in these areas, and subcutaneous calcinosis is also commonly found. Death is frequently caused by gastrointestinal hemorrhage. Excessive uterine bleeding and intra-articular bleeding, with formation of characteristic hemarthroses, are also common. The basic vascular pathology of this disorder is poorly understood and thought to be due to metabolic (enzyme) defects in elastic fibers.

Patients with *hemocystinuria,* a rare hereditary collagen vascular defect, bear a superficial resemblance to those with Marfan's syndrome, as these individuals usually have long limbs, kyphoscoliosis, and classic thoracic deformities. In homocystinuria, however, these is joint restriction rather than an increase in mobility. Homocystinuria is inherited as an autosomal recessive trait.

Elevated levels of methionine and homocystine demonstrated in the urine are usually diagnostic. This disorder is most likely due to a specific enzyme deficiency, and successful treatment has occasionally been rendered with a low-methionine and high-cystine diet. Arterial and venous thromboses are common, as is gastrointestinal hemorrhage. However, therapy aimed at controlling vascular thrombosis has been relatively unsuccessful.

Giant cavernous hemangiomas are tumorous masses of dilated thin-walled vessels and sinuses lined by an abnormal endothelium. These masses are usually engorged with venous blood that may be in a semistatic state, thus providing a potential mechanism for hemostasis activation. These giant hemangiomas are commonly found in the skin and subcutaneous tissue. They are usually present at birth but occasionally appear later in life. Also, these hemangiomatous lesions are frequently multiple and widespread, capable of involving any organ or group of organ systems. Recurrent acute thromboses may occur, especially if there is significant involvement of a particular extremity. The development of disseminated intravascular coagulation in many of these patients is the Kasabach-Merritt syndrome. The vast majority of patients with giant cavernous hemangiomata will usually demonstrate chronic disseminated intravascular coagulation, which not uncommonly becomes acute, explosive DIC. Several mechanisms for the development of chronic or acute disseminated intravascular coagulation in patients with giant cavernous hemangiomas have been proposed, including blood stasis with initiation of the contact activation phase of coagulation, as well as abnormal endothelium contacting the blood and perhaps resulting not only in contact phase activation but also in the initiation of a platelet release reaction. These patients may prove extremely difficult to manage once they have developed either chronic or acute disseminated intravascular coagulation, but they often respond to heparin or miniheparin therapy. After coagulation is controlled, radiation therapy or surgery may be considered to remove these giant hemangiomatous masses. However, if surgery is performed before the disseminated intravascular coagulation process has been successfully controlled, the bleeding consequences may prove disastrous.

Hereditary hemorrhagic telangiectasia (HHT, *Osler-Weber-Rendu* disease) is a relatively common disorder and, in fact, is the most common hereditary vascular disorder associated with a hemorrhagic diathesis. HHT is inherited as an autosomal dominant trait, but only 70 per cent of individuals have a positive family history. The homozygous state is thought to be lethal. In addition, there is evidence that the gene responsible for HHT may be linked to blood group O. The hallmark characteristic of this disease is epistaxis, which may be profuse and usually begins in early childhood. If a patient complains of epistaxis, inquiry should always be made as to whether it is always the same side or whether it is bilateral or alternating. The classic telangiectatic lesions of HHT may not appear until later in life, commonly the second or third decade. The classic diagnostic triad of HHT is (1) a hereditary basis, (2) telangiectasia, and (3) bleeding from telangiectatic lesions. Chronic blood loss, commonly from the gastrointestinal tract, is often severe enough to be manifest as a marked iron deficiency anemia of unknown etiology.

The telangiectatic lesions of HHT may be of three types: pinpoint, nodular, and spider-like. Unlike telangiectasia associated with chronic liver disease, those of HHT are nonpulsatile. Telangiectasia and bleeding usually increase with advancing age, although epistaxis often decreases with age. Bleeding with HHT may be occult but a common cause of gastrointestinal hemorrhage, genitourinary hemorrhage, hemoptysis, or heavy menstrual flow. Approximately 20 per cent of patients develop pulmonary arteriovenous fistulae. In addition, there is an inordinately high incidence of Laennec's cirrhosis among these patients. Hamartomas of the liver and spleen may also be associated with HHT. The basic pathophysiology of this disorder is poorly understood. Most studies have shown that elastic fibers are missing from the vascular walls. There are few characteristic laboratory findings in HHT. The template bleeding time may be normal or abnormal, depending on integrity of the vascular wall in the particular area in which the test is performed. The diagnosis is strongly suggested by a history of recurrent epistaxis; occult gastrointestinal bleeding; and nonpulsatile pinpoint, nodular, and/or spider-like telangiectasia, most commonly found in the skin, subungual areas, sublingual areas, or buccal mucosa.

HHT appears to be closely associated with other defects in hemostasis. Abnormal platelet aggregation has been noted in many individuals with HHT. In addition, a poorly defined defect in the fibrinolytic system may be present. Of major importance and not commonly appreciated is that many patients with HHT (approximately 50 per cent) have an associated classic disseminated intravascular coagulation syndrome. This is usually present in chronic form but may periodically become acute. In some individuals, bleeding may be severe enough that spontaneous intra-articular bleeds with resultant hemarthroses may develop. Thus, HHT may be somewhat similar to the syndrome of giant cavernous hemangiomas, and disseminated intravascular coagulation and a "mini–Kasabach-Merritt syndrome" are present in many of these cases, although, as mentioned, they are not usually recognized. When this occurs, treatment should be aimed at acute or chronic disseminated intravascular coagulation.

Therapy of uncomplicated HHT depends on the particular clinical situation and the age of the patient. Localized epistaxis may often be controlled with local supportive measures and vasoconstrictive nasal sprays. However, electrocauterizations may become necessary. Many instances of troublesome bleeding in HHT, such as gingival bleeding with tooth brushing, spontaneous bruising, and gastrointestinal/genitourinary bleeding, can often be controlled with preparations of carbazochrome salicylate (Adrenosem). This agent is usually administered orally in a 5- to 10-mg dose every 3 to 4 hours during waking hours and is not associated with any significant toxicity. High doses of estrogens may be used to scarify telangiectatic lesions and control bleeding. However, this modality should be used as a last resort, especially in younger patients.

Specific therapy for significant bleeding associated with congenital vascular defects other than HHT is generally satisfactory and depends primarily on supportive measures in control of the underlying disease process.

Acquired Vascular Disorders. The acquired vascular disorders that may be complicated by, or give rise to, a thrombotic or hemorrhagic tendency are far more common than the hereditary disorders. It is especially in these acquired disorders that careful attention must be paid to the patient who has a known diagnosis of one of the acquired diseases to be discussed so that the potential of significant hemorrhage and/or thrombosis can be evaluated if trauma or surgery occurs. In addition, one must recall the possibility of these acquired disorders in the differential diagnosis of a patient who presents with vascular type bleeding.

Malignant paraprotein disorders and amyloidosis are associated with numerous thrombotic and hemorrhagic tendencies. The spectrum of these tendencies depends on host response, size and site of the vasculature involved, and response of a particular end-organ. There have been numerous proposed mechanisms for the vascular complications of paraprotein disorders, but only the salient features will be discussed here. Increased circulating levels of IgG and IgM are complement-fixing and thus lead to histamine release, chemotaxis of leukocytes, and platelet aggregation and lysis; these events may then result in increased vascular permeability, effusion of serum or blood or both, and, in some instances, small vein thrombosis.

Hyperviscosity in the malignant paraprotein disorders is a well-known cause of stasis with resultant ischemia and acidosis. This may progress to increased vascular permeability, the consequences of which may be retinal hemorrhage and exudates, epistaxis, and petechiae and purpura of the skin, as well as hemorrhage into other organs. Frank necrotizing vasculitis may occur via unclear mechanisms in the malignant paraprotein disorders. The clinical manifestations, consisting of thrombosis or hemorrhage or both, will depend on the site and severity of the necrotizing vasculitis.

When the malignant paraprotein disorders are associated with cryoglobulinemia (IgG and IgM paraprotein disorders), paraprotein may be found in the walls of small vessels, leading to frank vasculitis with clinical manifestations ranging from effusions, bullae, petechiae, purpura, or frank end-organ damage (especially glomerulonephritis) to ischemia, cellular death, and end-organ damage. In addition, the malignant paraprotein disorders may be associated with a high incidence of thrombosis, often manifest as diffuse recurrent deep vein thrombosis, thromboembolism, pulmonary emboli, and renal vein thrombosis. Mechanisms of thrombosis remain unclear but need not be related to the development of hyperviscosity, except in cases of retinal vein thrombosis. Disseminated intravascular coagulation may be seen in patients with malignant paraprotein disorders. Whether this is due to endothelial damage by paraprotein or by other unexplained mechanisms remains unclear. In addition, the fibrino(geno)lysis that occurs in many individuals with malignant paraprotein disorders is initiated via as yet undefined mechanisms. This may represent fibrinolysis secondary to disseminated intravascular coagulation, due to endothelial damage, or alternatively may be caused by deranged endothelial plasminogen activator activity.

Amyloidosis further complicates the vascular changes of malignant paraprotein disorders, and may further enhance the incidence of hemorrhage or thrombosis or both by vascular disruption. Classically, primary amyloidosis is associated with an unknown etiology or the malignant paraprotein disorders and characteristically involves the skin, tongue, heart, and gastrointestinal tract. Secondary amyloidosis is seen with chronic inflammatory/infectious diseases and characteristically involves the liver, spleen, kidney, and adrenals. However, many "crossovers" and mixtures of the two are also commonly seen, and, in fact, amyloidosis often cannot be precisely defined as primary or secondary. There are numerous proposed mechanisms for vasculitis in patients with primary and secondary amyloidosis, but the precise mechanisms remain unclear. Hemorrhage due to vascular defects is a classic hallmark of primary amyloidosis, especially petechiae, purpura, ecchymoses, and easy and spontaneous bruising, along with spontaneous hemorrhage into lymph nodes, recurrent hematuria, and spontaneous hemorrhage into other vital organs. Several pathophysiologic events have been proposed as causes of generalized vasculitis, including endothelial damage induced by circulating antigen-antibody complex and the deposit of amyloid in the endothelium and in perivascular areas. Endothelial and perivascular amyloid deposits, especially in arterioles, appear to be more commonly noted in secondary forms. This leads to a hemorrhagic as well as a thrombotic tendency. In secondary amyloidosis, amyloid deposits are noted along the endothelium, and intimal deposits are noted to start in the intima and to progress to the media, with amyloid being deposited in parallel with reticulum fibers rather than around the collagen fibers, as is more commonly seen in primary amyloidosis. In addition, in primary amyloidosis the deposits are usually seen along the collagen, with progression from the adventitia to the media of arterioles and veins. The same process appears to occur in veins, thus possibly accounting for the thrombotic tendencies seen in these individuals.

In some patients with systemic amyloidosis, a selective, acquired Factor X deficiency is noted. In two patients similarly afflicted, an acquired combined deficiency of Factors IX and X has been noted. In 1977, Furie and coworkers investigated the mechanisms of Factor X deficiency in such cases by use of ^{131}I-labeled Factor X. They discovered a triphasic plasma clearance pattern such that 85 per cent of the labeled Factor X cleared in less than 30 seconds, about 10 per cent in less than 90 seconds, and the remaining 5 per cent in 10.5 hours. Subsequent surface scanning of the patients 24 hours after the labeled infusion showed high concentrations in hepatic and splenic regions. This observation, coupled with the rapid clearance of the label on initial transit in the circulation, led these investigators to conclude that Factor X is deposited at prior tissue sites of amyloid. At first glance, it may seem that these cases should respond to therapeutic infusions with Factors II, VII, IX, and X concentrates.

The wide variability of hemorrhagic and thrombotic manifestations in patients with paraprotein disorders and amyloidosis will depend on the particular end-organ involved as well as the degree of vessel permeability or occlusion or both.

In summary, patients with malignant paraprotein disorders as well as amyloidosis may develop a diffuse vascular disease that may manifest as hemorrhage or thrombosis or both. A high variability of end-organ damage may be seen. In dealing with these patients, physicians must recognize that such individuals may suffer undue vascular bleeding, as well as bleeding from obvious other causes, when subjected to surgery or trauma. Alternatively, for a patient with a vascular disorder presenting as hemorrhage or thrombosis or both, malignant paraprotein disorders as well as amyloidosis should be considered in the differential diagnosis. When a selective acquired Factor X deficiency in an adult is found, underlying systemic amyloidosis should be strongly suspected.

Autoimmune disorders associated with circulating immune complexes, especially those associated with circulating cryoglobulins, are of paramount importance as disorders associated with a diffuse vasculitis and thus thrombosis or hemorrhage or both.

At least three potential mechanisms by which circulating immune complexes, circulating cryoglobulins, or circulating antibodies may lead to vasculitis have been proposed by Stefanini, Dixon, and Markowitz. First, there may be production of an antibody that is directed specifically against the endothelium. This is probably the least common mechanism. Second, there may be production of a nonspecific antibody or immune complex that attacks and damages endothelium as well as other cellular systems. Third, there may be generation of an antibody or immune complex that attaches to and damages perivascular tissues (including basement membrane) and secondarily causes endothelial damage and thus increased vascular permeability. The vascular response and clinical manifestations will depend on severity, duration, and degree of repetition of the endothelial or periendothelial insult and damage. If the attack is mild, increased vascular permeability, fibrin deposition, and a fibrinolytic response may occur. This will lead to minimal hemorrhage and thrombosis. If, however, the insult is persistent, there will be excessive endothelial damage, depletion of fibrinolytic enzymes and endothelial fibrinolytic activators, increased fibrin and platelet deposition, more pronounced thrombosis or hemorrhage or both, and secondarily, more enhanced and perpetuated endothelial damage. In yet more severe attacks on the endothelium or surrounding tissue by antibody, immune complex, or cryoglobulins, endothelial death, sloughing, and more severe thrombosis, hemorrhage, and end-organ damage may occur. As already mentioned, an antibody directed specifically against the endothelium is a rare mechanism of autoimmune-induced vasculitis and is limited to the allergic purpuras (Henoch-Schönlein, etc.) and polyarteritis nodosum. However, further immunologic investigations may, in the future, define other disorders in this class.

The other two mechanisms of immune complex–induced vasculitis are much more common and are seen in a wide variety of "autoimmune disorders." In many of these diseases, circulating immune complexes (IgG and IgM) attach to the endothelium, fix complement, and induce migration of leukocytes, which may disintegrate and destroy the vessel. For example, all are familiar with the results of antistreptococcal antibody attaching to the glomerular endothelium or basement membrane, thus causing renal vascular damage. An extension of this is, of course, Goodpasture's syndrome, in which case antibody or immune complex is directed against both renal and pulmonary basement membrane with associated endothelial damage and thrombohemorrhagic manifestations.

Many infectious agents are also known to be associated somewhat infrequently with vasculitis and the aforementioned attendant clinical manifestations. These include numerous infections caused by bacteria, viruses, and *mycoplasma*. The mechanisms, where known, include the inducement of specific antiendothelial antibody by the invading microorganism and the development of

TABLE 24–5 INFECTIOUS AGENTS CAUSING VASCULITIS

Viruses (CMV, Epstein-Barr, hepatitis)
Leprosy
Lymphogranuloma venereum
Syphilis
Subacute bacterial endocarditis

circulating immune complexes. These mechanisms have already been described. Table 24–5 lists the most common infectious agents known to be associated with a vasculitis.

In most circulating immune complex diseases, the injury is nonspecific, and not only the endothelium but also many other cellular systems are damaged. Diseases involving vasculitis induced by circulating antibody, immune complex, or cryoglobulin are highly varied and include the collagen vascular disorders, drug reactions, serum sickness, and a large group of seemingly unrelated disorders. Table 24–6 lists the most common autoimmune diseases associated with endothelial damage, vasculitis, and clinical thrombohemorrhagic phenomena.

Thrombohemorrhagic manifestations are associated with *malignant hypertension, eclampsia, Cushing's disease,* and *diabetes.* In patients with malignant hypertension, advancing age, and diabetes mellitus, lipohyaline material is deposited in the subendothelium of arteries and arterioles. In addition, fibrinoid necrosis is an important feature in malignant hypertension. As constant, unrelenting damage occurs, the vessels eventually develop increased vascular permeability with plasma seepage and fibrin deposition. This leads to thrombosis and thromboembolism, a common clinical manifestation of these disorders. The resultant downstream capillary stasis leads to the development of chronic purpura and local hyperpigmentation of the skin. The reader is referred to the authoritative reviews of Farber and Kazmier

TABLE 24–6 CIRCULATING IMMUNE COMPLEXES AND VASCULITIS

A. Collagen vascular disorders and cryoglobulinemia
   1. Systemic lupus erythematosus
   2. Rheumatoid arthritis
   3. Dermatomyositis
   4. Scleroderma
   5. Polyarteritis nodosa
   6. Wegener's granulomatosis
B. Drugs (penicillin)
C. Sjögren syndrome
D. Glomerulonephritis (proliferative)
E. Malignant hypertension
F. Chronic infections
G. Lymphoreticular disorders
H. Allergic vasculitis (Henoch-Schönlein syndrome)
I. Subacute bacterial endocarditis

for more complete descriptions of pathophysiologic events in these disorders.

The features of eclampsia are similar to those findings just cited, with hypertension and localized intravascular coagulation (fibrin deposition) developing in the placental and renal microvasculature. Some women develop classic findings of either chronic or acute disseminated intravascular coagulation with any or all of the attendant clinical manifestations of this secondary syndrome.

The vascular changes in Cushing's disease remain poorly defined, but they include loss of subcutaneous elastic tissues. This leads to poor endothelial support, increased vascular fragility and permeability, and the loss of elastic tissue in the vascular walls. In addition, advanced atherosclerotic changes occur in the larger vessels in these patients. All clinicians should be well aware of the easy and spontaneous bruising seen in most individuals with Cushing's syndrome and the increased incidence of thrombosis and thromboembolic disease in this patient population. Also, all should know that many patients with Cushing's syndrome will suffer profuse bleeding when subjected to surgery or trauma.

Behçet's syndrome is a poorly defined disorder characterized by a typical triad of aphthous stomatitis, gingival ulcerations, and iritis. In addition, many patients develop recurrent deep vein thromboses of unexplained pathophysiologic origin; these usually involve large veins, the saphenous veins, calf veins, and the superior and inferior vena cava. Many of these patients develop a widespread, poorly defined arteritis. Several well-studied patients demonstrated fibrinoid necrosis of the arterial tree. In numerous case studies, impaired fibrinolysis has been reported, and some patients have responded to thrombolytic (fibrinolytic) therapy. However, thus far the pathophysiologic mechanisms for the recurrent deep vein thrombophlebitis, arteritis, and hemorrhage, usually manifest as petechiae and purpura, have remained undefined.

Vascular defects occur in association with *cardiopulmonary bypass (CPB)*. A syndrome of mild to moderate nonthrombocytopenic purpura, accompanied by splenomegaly and atypical lymphocytosis following CPB, has been reported by Behrendt. In this series, purpura was benign, self-limiting, and frequently manifest only after discharge from the hospital. One patient in the series developed classic glomerulonephritis of the type often seen with allergic vasculitis. In addition, one case of fatal purpura fulminans has been reported by Bick following extracorporeal circulation for coronary artery bypass. These two studies suggest that an inflammatory vasculitis may be associated with cardiopulmonary bypass; the mechanisms, however, remain unclear.

Drug-induced vasculitis is a common occurrence in clinical medicine and often forgotten as a cause of petechiae, purpura, skin necrosis, and frank gangrene. There are numerous mechanisms by which drugs may induce vasculitis, and most are similar to the mechanisms operative in circulating immune complex diseases. In many instances, however, the precise mechanisms are poorly understood. There are at least three mechanisms by which drugs may induce a vasculitis. These include the development of a specific anti-vessel antibody, the development of circulating immune complexes (in some instances associated with cryoglobulinemia), and, more rarely, drug-induced independent changes in vascular permeability. Those drugs that are commonly associated with vasculitis are depicted in Table 24–7. A classic and poorly recognized vasculitis due to warfarin anticoagulants has been reviewed and summarized by Nalbandian and coworkers. This peculiar and not uncommon hemorrhagic vasculitis is manifest by hemorrhagic skin infarction and in some instances has been associated with intravascular coagulation. Virtually all warfarin derivatives have been incriminated: 90 per cent of the patients have been women, and gangrene of the breast has occurred in at least 25 per cent of cases. Nalbandian and coworkers have described the histologic features of this syndrome quite well, showing perivascular accumulations of inflammatory cells predominantly involving the venules, with extensive thrombosis of the draining veins, and little or no involvement of arterioles. Typically, the syndrome develops 3 to 10 days after initiation of therapy and bears little relationship to the prothrombin time. The proposed mechanism is thought to be a direct toxic effect on the endothelium by warfarin and its derivatives. Many patients will respond to heparin therapy.

This discussion has summarized the more common disease entities that may be accompanied

TABLE 24–7 DRUGS CAUSING VASCULITIS

Acetylsalicylic acid
Allopurinol
Arsenicals
Chloramphenicol
Chlorothiazide
Chlorpropamide
Digoxin
Estrogens
Furosamide
Gold salts
Indomethacin
Iodine
Isoniazid
Meprobamate
Methyldopa
Piperazine
Quinidine
Quinine
Reserpine
Sulfonamides
Tolbutamide
Warfarin and related compounds

by or may lead to a vascular disorder of hemostasis or thrombosis or both. It is to be emphasized that the vascular component of hemostasis is often overlooked by clinicians caring for individuals with disorders of hemostasis and thrombosis. Abnormalities of the vasculature are equal in importance to those of the coagulation protein system and platelets in leading to a hemorrhagic or thrombotic diathesis.

PLATELET DEFECTS

Platelet defects are most conveniently divided into quantitative and qualitative disorders. Like the vascular defects, the qualitative, or platelet function, defects are best characterized as those that are hereditary or acquired. The classic clinical findings of a platelet defect, be it functional or quantitative, are petechiae and purpura and mild mucosal membrane bleeding, especially manifest as epistaxis and mild to moderate gastrointestinal and genitourinary bleeding. In addition, there is often a history of easy and spontaneous bruising and gingival bleeding with toothbrushing. The petechiae and purpura are usually symmetric and not dependent, as is commonly seen in vascular disorders.

QUALITATIVE PLATELET DEFECTS

Many laboratory modalities are available for assessment of platelet function. Evaluation of a bleeding diathesis associated with platelet defects is initiated by examination of a peripheral smear and quantitative platelet count. Prolongation of the template bleeding time or the aspirin tolerance test is the main form of laboratory screening used in the determination of a platelet function defect; template bleeding time and aspirin tolerance test should not be performed in a thrombocytopenic individual, as little or no information will be obtained, and bleeding may be significant. A platelet function defect should immediately be suspected when there is a prolonged template bleeding time or an abnormal aspirin tolerance test in the face of a normal platelet count. When this combination of laboratory abnormalities is noted, the differential diagnosis is that of a vascular defect versus a platelet function defect, and the next test to be performed should be platelet aggregation. Platelet adhesion in glass bead columns has been utilized in the past; however, this test is of historical interest only and is without clinical relevance. Platelet aggregation to various aggregating agents, as will be discussed, is the definitive test used to confirm the presence or absence of

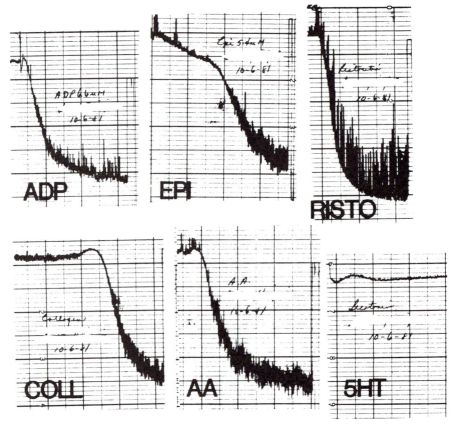

Figure 24–12 Normal aggregation patterns. (EPI = epinephrine; RISTO = ristocetin; COLL = collagen; AA = arachidonic acid; 5HT = serotonin.)

abnormal platelet function. The clot retraction test, also popular in the past, is no longer advocated as a screening test for platelet function, as it is only uniformly abnormal in Glanzmann's thrombasthenia, an extremely rare hereditary condition. Thus, the main laboratory tests for evaluation of platelets and their function are the following: (1) platelet count and evaluation of a peripheral smear, (2) template bleeding time and aspirin tolerance test, and (3) platelet aggregation to various agents. The template bleeding time is best performed with a disposable double-bladed device. Platelet aggregation is performed with a standardized modified photometer. Platelet-rich plasma is placed in a reaction well, and the change in optical density is noted as various platelet aggregating agents are added. As platelets aggregate, the percentage of light-transmission increase is charted on a strip recorder, giving rise to typical aggregation "patterns." The most commonly utilized agents for assessing platelet aggregation are ADP, epinephrine, serotonin, ristocetin, collagen, and arachidonic acid. Normal patterns induced by these aggregating agents are depicted in Figure 24–12. A refinement of platelet aggregometry is platelet lumiaggregation. A lumiaggregometer utilizes two reaction wells, a photometric well and a fluorometric well. As platelet aggregation is induced by the aforementioned reagents, simultaneous ATP release is measured in the opposing well. Typical normal lumiaggregation patterns are depicted in Figure 24–13.

The hereditary platelet function defects may be characterized as abnormalities of (1) platelet adhesion, (2) primary aggregation, and (3) secondary aggregation. A typical abnormality of platelet adhesiveness is that of the Bernard-Soulier syndrome. Abnormalities of primary aggregation are characterized by Glanzmann's thrombasthenia and essential athrombia, and abnormalities of secondary aggregation include the storage pool diseases, the aspirin-like defect, and other rare platelet-release abnormalities. In addition, disorders of platelet function may be associated with severe plasma coagulation factor deficiencies, including afibrinogenemia, severe Factor VIII or Factor IX deficiency.

Hereditary Platelet Function Defects. *Glanzmann's thrombasthenia* and *essential athrombia* are both inherited as autosomal recessive traits and present remarkably similar clinical and laboratory characteristics. Numerous constituents are noted to be abnormal in platelets from these individuals, including glyceraldehyde-3-phosphodehydrogenase, glutathione peroxidase, glutathione reductase, and thrombosthenin. Clinically, patients with these disorders present with spontaneous mucosal and cutaneous hemorrhage as well as petechiae, purpura, and occasional intra-articular bleeds with resultant hemarthroses. As with many hereditary hemorrhagic defects, the bleeding tends to decrease in severity with age. From the laboratory standpoint, these disorders are characterized by a prolonged template bleeding time, an absent ADP-induced primary aggregation wave, and totally absent thrombin-, collagen-, or epinephrine-induced aggregation. In addition, both disorders display decreased platelet factor 3 availability. There is normal subendothelial platelet adhesion. Clot retraction is noted to be abnormal in Glanzmann's thrombasthenia; however, it is normal in essential athrombia. Therapy for both these disorders, as it is in the vast majority of hereditary platelet function defects, is infusion of platelet concentrates until bleeding ceases.

Bernard-Soulier syndrome, a rare but important syndrome, is inherited as an autosomal recessive trait. This syndrome bears a superficial resemblance to von Willebrand's disease and thus is important in the differential diagnosis of von Willebrand's syndrome. Pathophysiologically, this disorder is characterized by an abnormal platelet membrane glycoprotein content and the lack of a platelet membrane ristocetin receptor. In addition, Bernard-Soulier platelets fail to bind plasma coagulation Factors V and XI. Clinically, individuals with this disorder present with easy and spontaneous bruising, profuse epistaxis, and other mucosal membrane bleeding such as hypermenorrhagia. Petechiae and purpura are also commonly noted. The homozygous state is asymptomatic. From the laboratory standpoint, these individuals display borderline to moderate thrombocytopenia in association with giant platelets on a peripheral smear. Platelets from patients with the Bernard-Soulier syndrome fail to aggregate with ristocetin. In addition, these individuals demonstrate a prolonged template bleeding time. Therapy for this disorder is infusion of platelet concentrates until bleeding is controlled.

Storage pool disorders are seen in association with many rare clinical syndromes, such as Wiskott-Aldrich syndrome, Chediak-Higashi syndrome, Hermansky-Pudlak syndrome, and the TAR syndrome. However, most instances of hereditary storage pool disease are unassociated with any such defined clinical syndrome. The inheritance is highly variable. There is an increased ATP/ADP ratio in the dense bodies of platelets from patients suffering from storage pool disease. In addition, there is decreased intraplatelet serotonin and calcium as well as abnormal platelet lipids. There appears to be abnormal release of compounds contained in dense bodies and alpha granules. Clinically, individuals with this disease present with significant mucocutaneous hemorrhage and mucosal membrane bleeding, including hematuria and epistaxis. Petechiae and purpura are found but are uncommon; however, easy and spontaneous bruising is extremely common. Laboratory evaluation reveals absent second-wave aggregation induced by ADP and epinephrine, totally absent collagen-induced aggregation, and normal ristocetin-induced aggregation. The template

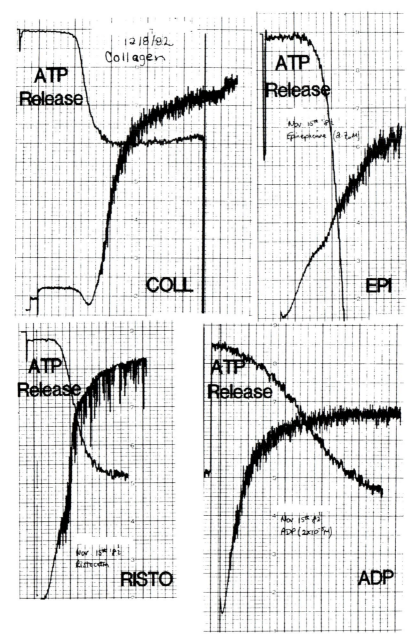

Figure 24–13 Normal lumiaggregation patterns. (COLL = collagen; EPI = epinephrine; RISTO = ristocetin; ATP = adenosine triphosphate; ADP = adenosine diphosphate.)

bleeding time is prolonged. In addition, decreased platelet dense bodies are noted by electron microscopy. When life-threatening hemorrhage occurs, the mainstay of therapy is platelet concentrate infusion. Figure 24–14 reveals typical aggregation patterns from a patient with storage pool disease.

A rare hereditary *aspirin-like defect* has been described. This defect is thought to be inherited as an autosomal dominant trait that becomes clinically evident when a patient ingests aspirin. Pathophysiologically, individuals with this disorder

demonstrate abnormal platelet factor 3 availability and a defect in either the enzyme cyclo-oxygenase or the enzyme thromboxane synthetase. In addition, electron microscopy has revealed an abnormal open canalicular system in the platelets of individuals with the "aspirin-like" defect. Clinically, these individuals present with easy and spontaneous bruising, epistaxis, and other mild mucosal membrane bleeding such as hypermenorrhagia and gastrointestinal bleeding. Laboratory evaluation reveals a prolonged template bleeding time, absent secondary wave to ADP and epinephrine, and absent collagen-induced aggregation. Therapy consists of platelet concentrate–infusion when life-threatening bleeding occurs; occasionally, patients have responded to steroid therapy.

It should be emphasized that the hereditary platelet function defects are extremely rare clinical oddities. However, all should be familiar with their existence and the typical characteristics of each. Hereditary platelet function defects are summarized in Table 24–8.

Acquired Platelet Function Defects. Unlike the hereditary platelet function defects, acquired platelet function defects are extremely common. These disorders should immediately enter into the differential diagnosis of an individual demonstrating easy and spontaneous bruising, mild mucosal membrane bleeding, and a normal platelet count. The acquired platelet function defects are listed in Table 24–9.

Uremia is commonly associated with a significant platelet function defect; most physicians are familiar with the bleeding that may occur in uremic patients as a result of this defect. Mechanisms of platelet dysfunction in uremic patients have been well studied, and it appears that the "toxic" material responsible for altering platelet function is guanidinosuccinic acid.

All the *myeloproliferative disorders* may be associated with a platelet function defect; however, the specific aggregation abnormalities tend not to be characteristic of the particular disease state. The myeloproliferative syndromes that are associated with a platelet function defect include es-

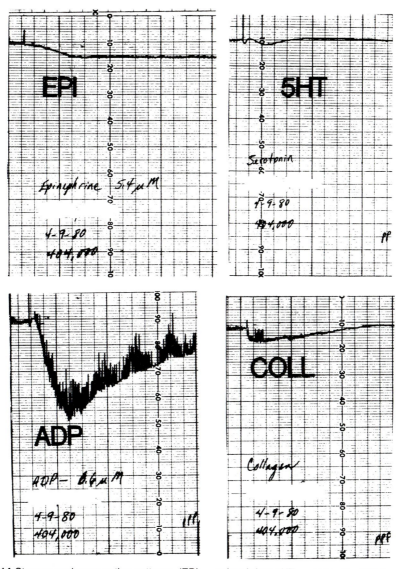

Figure 24–14 Storage pool aggregation patterns. (EPI = epinephrine; 5HT = serotonin; COLL = collagen.)

TABLE 24–8 HEREDITARY PLATELET
FUNCTION DEFECTS

A. Defects of platelet adhesion
  1. Bernard-Soulier syndrome
  2. Impaired adhesion to collagen
    (a) Platelet membrane defect
    (b) Intrinsic collagen defect
B. Defects of primary aggregation
  1. Glanzmann's thrombasthenia
  2. Essential athrombia
C. Defects of secondary aggregation
  1. Storage pool disease
    (a) Unassociated defect (most common)
    (b) TAR syndrome
    (c) Hermansky-Pudlak syndrome
    (d) Chediak-Higashi syndrome
    (e) Wiskott-Aldrich syndrome
  2. Aspirin-like defect
    (a) Cyclo-oxygenase deficiency
    (b) Thromboxane synthetase deficiency
  3. Release reaction defects
    (a) Hereditary collagen disorders
    (b) Glycogen storage disease, type I
    (c) May-Hegglin anomaly
    (d) Hurler's syndrome
    (e) Hunter's syndrome
D. Isolated deficiency of platelet factor 3
E. Severe plasma coagulation factor deficiency
  1. Afibrinogenemia
  2. Hemophilia A
  3. Hemophilia B

TABLE 24–9 ACQUIRED PLATELET
FUNCTION DEFECTS

A. Myeloproliferative syndromes
  1. Essential thrombocythemia
  2. Agnogenic myeloid metaplasia
  3. Paroxysmal nocturnal hemoglobinuria
  4. Polycythemia rubra vera
  5. Chronic myelogenous leukemia
  6. RAEB syndrome
  7. Sideroblastic anemia
B. Uremia
C. Malignant paraprotein disorders
  1. Myeloma
  2. Waldenström's macroglobulinemia
  3. Leukemic reticuloendotheliosis
D. Autoimmune disorders
  1. Systemic lupus erythematosus
  2. Antiplatelet antibodies
E. Presence of FDPs
  1. Disseminated intravascular coagulation
  2. Primary fibrino(geno)lysis
F. Anemia
  1. Severe iron deficiency
  2. Severe folate or B_{12} deficiency
G. Drug-induced
H. Scurvy

sential thrombocythemia, myelofibrosis with agnogenic myeloid metaplasia, polycythemia rubra vera, DiGuglielmo's syndrome, paroxysmal nocturnal hemoglobinuria, sideroachrestic anemias, and the so-called "preleukemic syndromes." Platelet function defects associated with myeloproliferative syndromes may, not uncommonly, give rise to clinically significant diffuse hemorrhage.

The *paraprotein disorders* are commonly associated with platelet function defects. Malignant paraprotein appears to have a high affinity for the platelet surface and readily attaches to the platelet membrane. When this occurs, a clinically significant platelet function defect is commonly noted that can lead to significant hemorrhage, especially if the patient undergoes a surgical procedure or is stressed by trauma. The platelet function defect does not demonstrate characteristic aggregation abnormality patterns, and all combinations of abnormalities have been noted. In addition, the magnitude of the defect does not depend on the particular type of paraprotein present, and a severe defect may occur in Waldenström's macroglobulinemia as well as in plasma cell myeloma, of IgG, IgA, or IgM type.

Fibrinogen/fibrin degradation products (FDP), especially the D and E fragments, appear to have a high affinity for platelet membrane and, when attaching to the platelet membrane, may induce a platelet function defect leading to clinically significant hemorrhage. This occurs regardless of

whether the FDPs are primary or secondary to DIC and thus appears in the primary hyperfibrino(geno)lytic syndromes as well as in disseminated intravascular coagulation syndromes. The disorders giving rise to hyperfibrino(geno)lysis and DIC will be discussed subsequently.

A clinically significant platelet defect may be seen in severe pernicious anemia and in severe iron deficiency anemia; presumably, the megakaryocyte, like the red cell, depends on adequate vitamin B_{12} and iron levels.

TABLE 24–10 COMMON DRUGS CAUSING
PLATELET FUNCTION DEFECTS

Antiflammatory drugs	*Antibiotic drugs*
Aspirin	Ampicillin
Colchicine	Carbenicillin
Ibuprofen	Gentamicin
Indomethacin	Nitrofurantoin
Mefenamic acid	Penicillin G
Phenylbutazone	Ticarcillin
Sulfinpyrazone	
Psychiatric drugs	*Anesthetics*
Phenothiazines	Cocaine
Tricyclic amines	Procaine
	Gaseous anesthetic
Cardiovascular drugs	*Miscellaneous drugs*
Clofibrate	Antihistamines
Dipyridamole	Dextrans
Nicotinic acid	Furosamide
Papaverine	Glycerol guaiacolate
Phenoxybenzamine	(cough syrup)
	Hydroxychloroquine
Propranolol	Nitroprusside
Theophylline	Vinblastine

The list of *drug-induced platelet function defects* has become impressive and immense. The common clinically used drugs that induce such defects are depicted in Table 24–10. This list is by no means complete, and for extensive lists the reader is referred to reviews by Weiss and Deykin. It should be noted that the most common offending drugs leading to a clinically significant platelet function defect and hemorrhage are aspirin, aspirin-containing compounds, sulfinpyrazone, dipyridamole, diphenhydramine, ibuprofen, and papaverine-containing vasodilators. A knowledge of drug-induced platelet function defects is important. First, drugs need to enter into the differential diagnosis of a documented platelet function defect; second, when attempting to evaluate a patient with a platelet function defect a careful drug history needs to be elicted to rule out the ingestion of any drug known to alter results of platelet function testing (aggregation).

QUANTITATIVE PLATELET DEFECTS

Clinical Findings. The clinical findings of thrombocytopenia are similar to those for platelet function defects, consisting of easy and spontaneous bruising, gingival bleeding with toothbrushing, and mild to moderate mucosal membrane bleeding, especially gastrointestinal and genitourinary, found in association with petechiae and purpura. Thrombocytopenia is considered to be present when there are less than 100,000 platelets per cubic millimeter. Thrombocytopenia is probably the most common cause of bleeding encountered by the clinician. The degree of thrombocytopenia correlates very poorly with actual platelet count; some patients may bleed profusely at a platelet count slightly less than 100,000/mm³, and other patients will not demonstrate significant bleeding even at a platelet count of less than 10,000/mm³. The propensity to bleeding most likely depends on two factors: (1) how fast the thrombocytopenia developed, and (2) the percentage of young, more hemostatically active platelets in the patient's platelet population. There are many causes of thrombocytopenia; however, etiologic mechanisms can be divided into three forms: (1) decreased platelet production, (2) increased peripheral platelet utilization, and (3) metabolic/maturation defects.

Platelets are produced by fragmentation from megakaryocytes in the bone marrow; megakaryocytes account for approximately 1 per cent of nucleated cellular elements of normal human marrow. Megakaryocytes are derived from multipotential stem cells capable of maturing into erythroid, myeloid, and megakaryocytic precursors. The mature platelet-producing megakaryocyte is characterized by several nuclear lobes (usually eight, but there may be between four and 16), a granular eosinophilic cytoplasm, and a "demarcation membrane," outside which can be seen numerous

"platelet buds." Approximately 50 per cent of the marrow megakaryocytes are mature. It has been estimated that each megakaryocyte is capable of releasing between 2000 and 8000 platelets under physiologic circumstances. However, this number may increase approximately eightfold in pathologic instances. Platelet production is under control of a hormone, thrombopoietin, which appears to be a glycoprotein. When there is stimulation for increased platelet production, presumably via thrombopoietin, young, large, hemostatically hyperactive platelets are released into the systemic circulation. With the use of various in vitro radioactive labeling techniques, it has been noted that normal platelet life span varies from 9 to 12 days. In addition, similar labeling techniques have demonstrated that approximately two thirds of the total peripheral platelets are located in peripheral blood and approximately one third reside in the spleen. Older (senile) platelets are sequestered and destroyed in the spleen.

Thrombocytopenia. Thrombocytopenia is defined as a decreased number of platelets in the peripheral circulation, and, as discussed previously, this can occur via three independent mechanisms: (1) decreased production, (2) increased peripheral utilization, and (3) maturation/metabolic defects. Characteristic examples of each of these mechanisms will be discussed.

DECREASED PRODUCTION. Decreased production of platelets, or so-called "amegakaryocytic thrombocytopenia," is characterized by decreased numbers of megakaryocytes on bone marrow examination. A decrease of bone marrow megakaryocytes may be selective or may involve any or all combinations of marrow precursor elements. This may be seen in a wide variety of clinical situations, including congenital and acquired states. The congenital thrombocytopenias include Fanconi's syndrome, the TAR syndrome, and suppression of the marrow as a result of intrauterine viral infection, often rubella. In addition, maternal ingestion of thiazide diuretics may cause fetal marrow megakaryocytic hypoplasia. Acquired marrow hypoplasia, involving either megakaryocytes selectively or any combination of marrow precursor elements, may be due to exposure to various physical agents, chemicals, and myelotoxic drugs. In addition, ionizing radiation, chemotherapeutic agents, antimetabolites, and other cytotoxic drugs may be at fault. In addition to agents that usually cause nonselective suppression of the entire marrow, certain drugs appear to suppress megakaryocytes more selectively. These include chlorothiazides and estrogenic hormones, including diethylstilbestrol. This effect may also be seen with heavy ethanol ingestion.

Another common cause of acquired marrow suppression and resultant thrombocytopenia is infiltration of the marrow, such as will occur in disseminated malignancy, acute leukemias, lymphomas, Hodgkin's disease, and disseminated granulomatous disease. Common causes of congen-

TABLE 24–11 THROMBOCYTOPENIA DUE TO DECREASED PLATELET PRODUCTION

Congenital Decreased Production
Alport's syndrome
Bernard-Soulier syndrome
Congenital "thrombopoietin"
    deficiency
Fanconi's syndrome
Gray platelet syndrome
May-Hegglin anomaly
Tar syndrome
Wiskott-Aldrich syndrome
Congenital marrow infiltration
Rubella and other viruses
Maternal drug ingestion
Maternal infections

Acquired Decreased Production
Aplastic anemia
Isolated megakaryocyte aplasia
    (rare)
Marrow infiltrative diseases
Drug-induced marrow suppression
Cyclic thrombocytopenia
Renal failure
Myeloproliferative syndromes
Maturation/metabolic defects
Metastatic malignancy
Leukemia and lymphoma
Myelofibrosis
Tuberculosis
Histiocytosis
Myelosuppressive drugs
Radiation

ital and acquired decreased production of platelets leading to thrombocytopenia are depicted in Table 24–11.

INCREASED PERIPHERAL UTILIZATION. Nonimmunologic peripheral utilization of platelets most commonly arises from splenomegaly and associated hypersplenism. The splenic platelet pool normally contains one third of the total peripheral platelet mass. However, when the spleen becomes enlarged, the splenic pool may or may not increase; if it does, the number of platelets sequestered in the spleen may increase. When thrombocytopenia occurs as a result of splenomegaly, there is commonly an inadequate to minimal thrombopoietin response. Hypersplenism in association with splenomegaly may come about through numerous mechanisms; the most common is that associated with hepatic cirrhosis causing portal hypertension leading to splenomegaly and hypersplenism. However, this may also be seen in Felty's syndrome, lymphomas, Hodgkin's disease, and chronic granulomatous states. Other common causes of nonimmunologic peripheral platelet utilization include disseminated intravascular coagulation and thrombotic thrombocytopenic purpura. DIC will be discussed in detail in subsequent sections. Thrombotic thrombocytopenic purpura is a syndrome characterized by hemolytic anemia associated with microangiopathic peripheral blood smear findings, fluctuating neurologic defects, and severe throm-

bocytopenia. Characteristic pathologic changes include widespread intravascular hyaline deposits. For a thorough discussion of TTP, the reader is referred to recent reviews. Nonimmunologic peripheral utilization may also occur in cardiac surgery, prosthetic heart valve replacement, and other instances of peripheral vascular disease, including arterial and venous graft surgery. Nonimmunologic peripheral utilization of platelets may also come about through systemic infections. However, it should be noted that nonselective bone marrow suppression may also occur in these situations. Enhanced peripheral utilization of platelets most commonly occurs in Rocky Mountain spotted fever, typhus, mumps, malaria, and gram-negative septicemia. Causes of nonimmunologic peripheral utilization of platelets are summarized in Table 24–12.

Immune-induced peripheral utilization of platelets arises via several mechanisms, the most common of which is the induction of platelet antibodies by a variety of causes giving rise to increased splenic sequestration; in most instances, the combination of platelet and antibody (or, where appropriate, platelet, drug, and antibody) is recognized by the spleen as "foreign," thus leading to splenic sequestration and platelet destruction. Isoimmune thrombocytopenia is the result of platelet antibodies arising from active immunization of a patient to platelet antigens. Fetal isoimmune thrombocytopenia occurs after immunization to specific isoantigens. The first-born child is affected in approximately 50 per cent of cases. The affected infant usually develops petechiae and purpura as a result of thrombocytopenia shortly after birth; the thrombocytopenia usually persists for 2 to 3 weeks. Platelet isoantibodies may occur in patients who have received multiple blood transfusions; patients thought to need long-term platelet replacement should be provided with closely matched platelets.

Drug-induced immunologic thrombocytopenia

TABLE 24–12 THROMBOCYTOPENIA DUE TO NONIMMUNOLOGIC PERIPHERAL PLATELET UTILIZATION

Cardiovascular disorders
Cardiopulmonary bypass surgery
Disseminated intravascular coagulation
Drugs
Eclampsia
Hemodialysis
Hemolytic-uremic syndrome
Hypersplenism
Infections
Prosthetic devices
Renal diseases
Thrombotic thrombocytopenic purpura
Bacterial, viral, rickettsial, mycotic,
    and protozoal infections
Acute hemolysis
Kasabach-Merritt syndrome
Mononucleosis
Waring-Blender syndrome

TABLE 24–13 DRUGS THAT INDUCE IMMUNOLOGIC THROMBOCYTOPENIA*

Quinidine	Chlorothiazide
Quinine	Chloroquine
Gold salts	Furosemide
Sulfonamides	Chlorthalidone
Indomethacin	Rifampicin
Sedormid	Valproic acid

*Drugs listed in descending order of probability.

has been reported with numerous drugs. Drug-induced platelet antibodies are most often the result of an idiosyncratic reaction occurring in only a minority of patients given a drug. In most instances, the drug acts as a hapten, and the interaction among drug, antibody, and platelet leads to splenic recognition of this combination as abnormal (foreign), thus resulting in splenic sequestration and platelet destruction. The most common drugs causing immunologic thrombocytopenia include quinidine, quinine, sulfonamides, and gold. Drug-induced immunologic thrombocytopenia is summarized in Table 24–13.

Post-transfusion thrombocytopenia most commonly occurs approximately 1 week after blood transfusion. The antibody is specific for a genetically determined platelet antigen, PL^{A1}, which is present in approximately 98 per cent of the normal population but lacking in the platelets of patients who develop this unique post-transfusion thrombocytopenia with resultant petechiae and purpura. In these individuals, platelet transfusions are generally ineffective. Other disorders not uncommonly associated with immunologic thrombocytopenia due to peripheral utilization by the aforementioned mechanisms include autoimmune hemolytic anemia, chronic lymphocytic leukemia, lymphocytic lymphoma, rheumatoid arthritis, and systemic lupus erythematosus.

Idiopathic thrombocytopenic purpura (ITP) is an immunologic-induced peripheral utilization of platelets made by diagnostic exclusion. In this instance, the thrombocytopenia can be ascribed to no other apparent underlying disease. ITP is a relatively common clinical syndrome and occurs more commonly than all other secondary forms of thrombocytopenia combined. The syndrome of ITP appears to be due to platelet destruction as a result of an immunologic process, presumably caused by an IgG antiplatelet antibody produced by the spleen. In acute idiopathic thrombocytopenia purpura, the disorder is usually self-limited, and spontaneous remissions occur in approximately 90 per cent of patients. However, chronic ITP is characterized by a fluctuating clinical course, and spontaneous remissions are uncommon. Characteristically, the bone marrow demonstrates an increase in megakaryocytes; megakaryocytes reveal an increase in size and a finely granular cytoplasm void of peripheral platelet buds. ITP usually responds to high-dose steroid therapy, with approximately 70 per cent of patients responding. Nonresponders are usually treated by splenectomy followed by

steroid tapering. More recently, patients failing to respond to steroids or splenectomy or both have been treated with vincristine with reasonable success. In general, acute ITP in children does not require steroid therapy or splenectomy, as spontaneous remission, unassociated with life-threatening bleeding, is usual. It should be noted that the incidence of infection, especially pneumococcal pneumonia, is significantly increased in children under 2 years of age who have undergone splenectomy. However, this does not appear to be the case in adults. In general, patients with ITP fail to respond to platelet transfusions, and even massive transfusions of platelets usually produce only a slight or transient increase in the platelet count. However, patients with ITP often do not suffer significant bleeding, even in the face of a markedly reduced platelet count. This is presumably due to the primary platelet population consisting of hemostatically hyperactive young platelets. Table 24–14 summarizes types of immune-induced peripheral utilization of platelets and resultant thrombocytopenia.

Thrombocytopenia may occur via abnormal maturation of megakaryocytes or megakaryocyte precursors in the bone marrow or from abnormal marrow metabolism of nutrients required by the megakaryocytic cell line. Defective platelet synthesis and production are common findings in patients with severe megaloblastic anemia, including pernicious anemia and severe folate deficiency. Thus, although there is an increased marrow megakaryocyte number in many individuals with megaloblastic marrows, there is diminished platelet production due to metabolic/maturation defects, presumably secondary to impaired nucleic acid synthesis. In addition, many of the myeloproliferative syndromes are associated with maturation/metabolic defects leading to ineffective thrombopoiesis and peripheral thrombocytopenia. This is commonly seen in erythroleukemia, paroxysmal nocturnal hemoglobinuria, preleukemia, and the acute granulocytic leukemias. In these instances, the basic change (presumably malignant) appears to affect early megakaryocytic precursors also. In addition, severe iron deficiency anemia may also occasionally be associated with severe abnormalities of platelet production. However, severe iron deficiency anemia may also be associated with marked thrombocytosis in some instances.

Thrombocytosis refers to a nonmalignant increase in the peripheral platelet count, usually due to marrow reactivity. In these instances, the thrombocytosis is best thought of as secondary and usually is transient. In contrast, thrombocythemia

TABLE 24–14 IMMUNE THROMBOCYTOPENIA

A. Idiopathic thrombocytopenic purpura
B. Isoimmune thrombocytopenia
   1. Newborns
   2. Massive transfusions
C. Drug-induced
D. Post-transfusion purpura syndrome

refers to an increase in peripheral platelet count due to a malignant transformation in the bone marrow. Perhaps the most common cause of thrombocytosis occurs in the postsplenectomy syndrome. In this instance, a significant elevation in the platelet count typically reaches a peak 2 weeks postsplenectomy and abates over a 2- to 3-month period. Only rarely is there persistence of thrombocytosis following splenectomy. Thrombocytosis may also be seen after other major surgical procedures, and the elevated platelet count is usually noted between the third and tenth day following surgery, commonly returning to normal in less than 1 month. Acute blood loss may also be associated with reactive thrombocytosis. In addition, reactive thrombocytosis may be noted in rapidly developing iron deficiency anemia; however, chronic iron deficiency anemia is usually associated with thrombocytopenia. It has been noted that unexplained thrombocytosis may be due to occult malignancy, and in one study by Davis more than 30 per cent of patients with unexplained thrombocytosis were found to have an underlying occult malignancy, usually carcinoma. Thus, observation of unexplained thrombocytosis should prompt a search for occult malignancy.

Thrombocytosis is usually not associated with an enhanced propensity to thrombosis, and platelet-suppressive therapy is rarely needed; however, if indicated, it is usually not instituted until the platelet count is greater than 750,000/mm³. In addition, it should be noted that almost all instances of secondary or reactive thrombocytosis are transient and will abate after several months.

Thrombocythemia involves an increased peripheral platelet count secondary to a malignant transformation of the bone marrow and may be seen to accompany any or all of the myeloproliferative syndromes, including polycythemia rubra vera, agnogenic myeloid metaplasia, chronic myelocytic leukemia, and any of the varieties of granulocytic leukemia. In addition, the syndrome of essential thrombocythemia is thought to represent a primary malignant transformation of the megakaryocytic cell line. Unlike a reactive thrombocytosis, thrombocythemia may commonly be associated with thrombosis or hemorrhage. Hemorrhage is far more common than thrombosis in patients with thrombocythemia due to a myeloproliferative syndrome. An elevated platelet count (thrombocythemia) occurs in approximately 50 per cent of patients with polycythemia rubra vera, and, indeed, thrombosis or hemorrhage or both account for approximately 50 per cent of deaths in patients with polycythemia rubra vera. In addition, thrombocythemia may accompany myelofibrosis in approximately 25 per cent of patients. Thirty per cent of patients with chronic myelogenous leukemia will present with thrombocythemia. Essential thrombocythemia is one of the myeloproliferative syndromes and is most commonly seen in the fifth to seventh decade of life.

TABLE 24–15 CAUSES OF THROMBOCYTOSIS AND THROMBOCYTHEMIA

I. Thrombocytosis
  A. Reactive (transient)
    1. Acute blood loss
    2. Adrenal hyperplasia
    3. Drugs
    4. Infection
    5. Oral contraceptives
    6. Osteoporosis
    7. Postpartum state
    8. Recovery from thrombocytopenia
    9. Sarcoidosis
    10. Splenectomy
    11. Surgery
    12. Testosterone
    13. Trauma
  B. Chronic
    1. Collagen vascular disease
    2. Chronic inflammatory bowel disease
    3. Malignancy
    4. Iron deficiency
    5. Splenic infarction/atrophy
II. Thrombocythemia
  A. Essential thrombocythemia
  B. Chronic myelogenous leukemia
  C. Agnogenic myeloid metaplasia
  D. Polycythemia rubra vera

Patients may present with either thrombotic or hemorrhagic symptoms, although hemorrhage is the more common expression. A recent patient seen by this author presented with a massive intra-articular bleed of the knee in association with thrombosis of the sinoatrial artery leading to a sick sinus syndrome and severe cardiac arrhythmias. When bleeding or thrombosis occurs with thrombocythemia, both these complications usually abate when the platelet count is normalized with the use of cytotoxic therapy, usually busulfan or hydroxyurea. Typically, patients with essential thrombocythemia will demonstrate markedly abnormal platelet aggregation patterns. Treatment of patients with active bleeding associated with thrombocythemia requires the liberal use of platelet concentrates. Thrombotic complications may require therapy with antiplatelet agents; however, this must be done prudently owing to the hemorrhage that may ensue. Causes of thrombocytosis and thrombocythemia are summarized in Table 24–15.

HEREDITARY COAGULATION PROTEIN DEFECTS

HEMOPHILIA

The hemophilias are characterized as hereditary coagulation factor defects with clinical bleeding tendency, a prolonged activated partial thromboplastin time, and a normal prothrombin time.

Hemophilia was first recognized in Talmud writings of the second century. It was forbidden to circumcise the sibling male of a male who had bled at circumcision. These ancient Jewish writings not only recognized hemophilia but also recognized its mode of transmission from mother to son, as this law applied only to the same mother; the father could differ. The disease was first noted in the medical literature in 1803 after being recognized by Otto, a Philadelphia physician. The name *hemophilia,* however, was not attached to these disorders until 1828, and it is credited to a German physician named Hopff. In the 1800s, the diagnosis of hemophilia was established by demonstrating a positive family history and abnormal whole-blood clotting time. In 1947, antihemophiliac factor (Factor VIII, AHF, or AHG) was recognized. This began an era of active investigation into the nature of classic hemophilia and led to the development of efficacious therapeutic products. In 1952, a form of hemophilia differing from classic hemophilia was described. The new missing clotting factor was named plasma thromboplastin component (Factor IX, or PTC). In the same year, a similar case was found in England. The surname of the family was *Christmas,* and the disorder became known as *Christmas disease,* or *hemophilia B.* In 1953, a third form of hemophilia was reported by Rosenthal. The thromboplastic factor missing in this disorder was called *plasma thromboplastic antecedent* (Factor XI, or PTA). The disorder is now known as *hemophilia C.*

Hemophilia A (classic hemophilia), inherited as a sex-linked recessive trait (transmitted by the female and manifest in the male), accounts for approximately 85 per cent of all forms of hemophilia. Hemophilia A may occur in females through nondisjunction of the X chromosome or from a marriage between a male hemophiliac and female carrier. Hemophilia B (Christmas disease, or Factor IX deficiency), also inherited as a sex-linked recessive trait, accounts for approximately 10 per cent of cases of hemophilia. Hemophilia C, (PTA deficiency, or Factor XI deficiency) accounts for only 5 per cent of all hemophilias, is inherited as an autosomal dominant trait, and is most commonly seen in Jewish people of Russian descent. All three forms of hemophilia occur in approximately one of every 10,000 male births, although regional variations have been noted.

Hemophilia A (Classic Hemophilia, Factor VIII Deficiency). In order to understand and appreciate the differences between classic hemophilia and von Willebrand disease, familiarity with the Factor VIII molecule is necessary; there are at least three discrete functions that can be attributed to the Factor VIII macromolecular complex. Factor VIII procoagulant activity is measured in the partial thromboplastin time (PTT) assay system or the specific PTT-derived Factor VIII assay. This function is depicted as VIII:C. It is this protein (function) that is abnormal in classic hemophilia. This

small procoagulant portion is attached to a larger portion of the Factor VIII complex; the larger portion is detected immunologically and is commonly referred to as *cross-reacting material,* or *Factor VIII antigen.* This function is depicted as Factor VIII:Ag. Attached to or a portion of the larger immunologic part of the protein is the so-called "von Willebrand factor," which is depicted as Factor VIII:vW, or ristocetin cofactor, Factor VIII:R. It can be found attached to platelet surfaces in the normal patient but not in the von Willebrand patient. In addition, it normally circulates in association with the procoagulant portion. Factor VIII:vW is responsible for vascular integrity and normal platelet function and plays a major role in the platelet-endothelial interaction. Current concepts of the Factor VIII macromolecular complex are illustrated in Figure 24–15. Knowledge of the Factor VIII macromolecule complex allows one to understand the numerous clinical and laboratory differences between classic hemophilia and von Willebrand disease.

Techniques for the immunologic detection of Factor VIII have allowed for the detection of carriers for classic hemophilia. Discriminant analysis and comparison of functional Factor VIII activity versus immunologic activity in a particular female allows for the detection of a carrier state with greater than 80 per cent accuracy. Consistent with the Lyon hypothesis, the female carrier will have 100 per cent of her X chromosomes coding for the synthesis of immunologic Factor VIII. However, only 50 per cent of the X chromosomes will be coding for the synthesis of procoagulant activity. Immunologic assays are also used to define the rare patient with von Willebrand disease who has extremely low Factor VIII procoagulant activity as well. This allows for the differential diagnosis between von Willebrand disease and hemophilia A. In hemophilia A, there will be normal VIII:Ag, and VIII:C will be decreased.

The clinical picture of hemophilia A is characterized by deep tissue bleeding, primarily intra-articular, intramuscular, and intracerebral bleeding. The disease is usually diagnosed in early childhood, when intra-articular bleeding due to crawling can occur. Intra-articular bleeds may later develop into crippling hemarthroses. Some cases are diagnosed at circumcision or tonsillectomy, when profuse bleeding is suddenly noted. In general, classic hemophilia exists in three forms

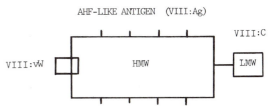

Figure 24–15 AHF macromolecular complex.

(severe, moderate, and mild), and the clinical course correlates quite well with levels of functional Factor VIII.

Severe hemophiliacs have between 0 and 5 per cent of functional Factor VIII (Factor VIII:C). These individuals suffer spontaneous intramuscular, intra-articular, and, sometimes, intracerebral bleeds. Usually, no trauma is required to initiate hemorrhage. Profuse bleeding occurs with minor trauma or surgery. Moderate hemophiliacs have about 5 to 10 per cent functional Factor VIII. Spontaneous intra-articular, intramuscular, and, at times, intracerebral bleeding may occur, but less frequently than in severe patients. Major bleeding occurs with trauma or surgery. Mild hemophiliacs have 10 to 25 per cent functional Factor VIII levels. These individuals rarely have spontaneous bleeding but may bleed profusely when subjected to trauma or surgery.

The diagnosis of hemophilia A is suggested by typical bleeding and a positive family history. However, only 60 per cent have a positive family history. In approximately 40 per cent of patients, the gene appears spontaneously. As noted, the bleeding manifestations are characteristic. The finding of an abnormal activated thromboplastin time and a normal prothrombin time in a patient with a positive bleeding history is highly suggestive of Factor VIII (85 per cent), Factor IX (10 per cent), or Factor XI (5 per cent) deficiency. An abnormal activated partial thromboplastin time in the face of a normal prothrombin time and a negative bleeding history is suggestive of Factor XI, Factor XII, Fletcher factor, or Fitzgerald factor deficiency. These diseases will be covered in detail in subsequent sections. A differential PTT will allow one to differentiate quickly among Factor VIII, IX, and XI deficiency. In this assay system, the abnormal PTT is corrected with reagents that are rich in Factor VIII or Factor IX. The latter reagent consists of aged normal human serum (rich in Factor IX and depleted of Factor VIII). If the Factor VIII–rich reagent corrects the prolonged PTT, the disorder is hemophilia A. If the Factor IX reagent corrects the abnormal PTT, hemophilia B is present. If both reagents partially correct the abnormal PTT, Factor XI deficiency is present. If both reagents totally correct the activated PTT, Hageman (Factor XII) deficiency is present. Differential PTT findings in the hemophilias are summarized in Table 24–16. Once a diagnosis of hemophilia A is established by the differential PTT method, the actual level of Factor VIII should be determined. If the patient is a severe hemophiliac with Factor VIII levels approximately 1 per cent of normal or less, an inhibitor screen should be performed, and, if present, its concentration quantitated by appropriate assay procedures.

In general, mild hemophilic bleeds are best managed by cold compresses and topical thrombin, if needed. Minor bleeds usually do not require

TABLE 24–16 THE DIFFERENTIAL PTT

Defect	PTT	PT	AHF Reagent	PTC Reagent
Hemophilia A	Long	Normal	Total correction	No correction
Hemophilia B	Long	Normal	No correction	Total correction
Hemophilia C	Long	Normal	Partial correction	Partial correction
XII Deficiency	Long	Normal	Total correction	Total correction

infusion of cryoprecipitate or Factor VIII concentrate, although such management is required for significant bleeding. The discovery of cryoprecipitate and its subsequent use in hemophilia were major milestones in management. The disadvantage of cryoprecipitate is the high protein content and variable Factor VIII content. Most centers now utilize commercially available potent Factor VIII concentrates for the management of significant hemorrhage. Concentrates offer the advantage of low volume, low protein content, and a predictable Factor VIII titer. By knowing the initial level of Factor VIII, one can calculate the amount of Factor VIII concentrate needed for infusion. Serious hemophiliac bleeding will cease when the patient's Factor VIII level reaches approximately 30 per cent of normal. As a general rule, the infusion of 25 units of Factor VIII concentrate per kilogram of body weight will increase the Factor VIII level to approximately 50 per cent of normal. The exact amount of Factor VIII needed to raise the patient's level to a predetermined "desired level" can be calculated by a simple formula. The desired level of Factor VIII, minus the initial level, represents the percentage of Factor VIII required. Thus, the desired level minus the initial level multiplied by 0.6 times body weight in kilograms will give the exact number of units required to take the patient to the desired level of Factor VIII activity. This formula is depicted in Table 24–17.

Approximately 10 per cent of hemophilia A patients develop antibodies to Factor VIII. In most instances, these cases are IgG type 4 with a kappa

TABLE 24–17 CALCULATION OF FACTOR VIII OR IX REPLACEMENT

$$U_t = (L_d - L_i) \times 0.6 \times W$$

and

$$C = \frac{R_f}{U_c}$$

U_t = Total units needed
L_d = Level desired
L_i = Initial level
W = Body weight (kg)
C = Milliliters of concentrate needed
U_c = Units/ml in concentrate

light chain. They usually develop spontaneously, and a classic anamnestic response may be seen if individuals with this disorder are treated with Factor VIII concentrates or cryoprecipitate. Immunosuppressive therapy with cyclophosphamide, azathioprine, or prednisone appears to be of minimal efficacy in controlling inhibitors. A newer approach to therapy of severe inhibitor patients is the use of "activated" prothrombin complex concentrates; these contain an "active principle" that bypasses the necessity of Factor VIII and allows for hemostasis. Clinical trials using commercially available "activated" prothrombin complex concentrates in patients with high inhibitor titers have proved successful. Screening tests for the detection of anti-VIII antibodies are now available and quite simple to perform.

Hemophilia B (Christmas Disease, PTC Deficiency, Factor IX Deficiency). The clinical manifestations of Factor IX deficiency are similar to those seen with classic hemophilia. Intra-articular and intramuscular bleeding usually occur in infancy. The disease, like classic hemophilia, can be present in severe, moderate, or mild forms, with mildly affected patients experiencing few if any spontaneous bleeds; however, severe bleeding may occur with trauma or surgery. Like classic hemophilia, Factor IX deficiency should be suspected in the face of a positive bleeding history, an abnormal activated partial thromboplastin time, and a normal prothrombin time. The disease is inherited as a sex-linked recessive trait and is therefore manifest in males. This disorder is much less common than Factor VIII deficiency and accounts for approximately 10 per cent of hemophilia. One diagnoses Factor IX deficiency by utilizing the differential partial thromboplastin time, as described previously. Once a diagnosis of Factor IX deficiency has been made, a specific Factor IX assay should be performed to quantitate the level of circulating Factor IX. Patients with very low levels of Factor IX should be screened for the presence of an inhibitor. The incidence of inhibitors to Factor IX is less frequent than that for inhibitors to Factor VIII.

Much less is known about the pathophysiology of hemophilia B. It is known, however, that variants of hemophilia B exist. Researchers discovered the first variants using ox brain thromboplastin times. Previous work revealed that some patients with Factor IX deficiency had a prolonged ox brain thromboplastin time, whereas others had normal times. Patients with prolonged ox brain thromboplastin times have been designated hemophilia B_m, the "m" being derived from the surname of the first family found with this disorder.

Some cases of Factor IX deficiency resemble classic hemophilia in that Factor IX–like antigen or dysfunctional Factor IX protein is present. Thus, patients with this disorder are positive for cross-reacting material (CRM). The majority of patients with hemophilia B, however, have no

TABLE 24–18 HEMOPHILIA B VARIANTS

Immunologic Status	Ox-Brain Thromboplastin Time	Designation
CRM$^+$	Normal	B$^+$
CRM$^+$	Long	B^+_m
CRM$^-$	Normal	B$^-$
CRM$^-$	Long	B^-_m

detectable Factor IX levels by currently available immunologic techniques. Thus, there are hemophilia B patients who are CRM$^+$ and CRM$^-$. Therefore, at least four genetic variants of hemophilia B exist. These are delineated in Table 24–18. The clinical significance of these variances is not known. Evidence suggests that patients who are CRM$^+$ have a milder form of the disease.

As with hemophilia A, minor bleeding is best managed by supportive therapy, cold compresses, and topical thrombin, when necessary. For life-threatening bleeding, several Factor IX–containing concentrates are commercially available (prothrombin complex concentrates). These preparations are not without hazard of hepatitis, and clinical use should be weighed against this danger. In addition, numerous reports have indicated that these materials can be thrombogenic and may lead to the development of a disseminated intravascular coagulation syndrome. As with hemophilia A, the exact amount of concentrate needed can be calculated according to the formula given in Table 24–17.

Hemophilia C (PTA Deficiency, Rosenthal Disease, Factor XI Deficiency). Hemophilia C is inherited as an autosomal dominant trait and can be expressed in both males and females. In addition, the clinical course can be highly variable, with some patients experiencing no bleeding and other patients suffering profuse bleeding. Interestingly, there is often no correlation between the levels of assayable circulating Factor XI and the bleeding tendency of the patient. Indeed, many patients are noted to change their clinical course, with bleeders becoming nonbleeders and vice versa; this may or may not be correlated with any change in the Factor XI levels. Hemophilia C need not necessarily become manifest in early childhood and commonly becomes evident in adult life.

Little is known about the pathophysiology of hemophilia C. There are no data to indicate whether individuals suffering from this disease have an absolute lack of Factor XI or a circulating, dysfunctional Factor XI. Variants of the disease have not yet been described.

The mainstay of therapy for clinically significant bleeding is the infusion of plasma. A dose of 10 ml/kg usually suffices to control significant bleeding. It has recently been noted that certain lots of commercial prothrombin complex concentrate contain high levels (10 to 30 units per ml) of

Factor XI. This has been used to control life-threatening bleeding in patients who fail to respond to infusions of plasma. Prothrombin complex concentrates are potentially thrombogenic, and a stability check should always be performed on every bottle before this material is infused. The stability check consists of adding 0.1 ml of concentrate to 1 ml of citrated patient's plasma and observing for clot formation for a period of 5 minutes. If no clot forms during that period, it can be assumed that no thrombin is generated. A more predictive assay of thrombogenicity of these concentrates has been advocated by Blatt and coworkers. Prothrombin complex concentrates are less thrombogenic if antithrombin III is added to them.

VON WILLEBRAND SYNDROME

Von Willebrand syndrome is a hemorrhagic disorder inherited as an autosomal dominant trait. Von Willebrand syndrome is a plasma protein defect, with the defect residing in high molecular weight Factor VIII or von Willebrand factor (Factor VIII:vW). A positive family history can be identified in approximately 70 per cent of individuals. Typical bleeding is that of epistaxis, which usually begins in early childhood. In addition, patients present with easy and spontaneous bruising and mild to moderate mucosal membrane bleeding, including hypermenorrhagia as well as gastrointestinal and genitourinary bleeding. Typically, severity of bleeding decreases with age. Thus, the syndrome behaves clinically like a platelet function/vascular defect rather than a strict plasma protein defect, as is seen in the hemophilias. These clinical characteristics are explained by the demonstration of the properties of von Willebrand factor or the high molecular portion of the Factor VIII macromolecular complex. Von Willebrand factor supports ristocetin-induced aggregation of normal human platelets and is necessary for normal platelet function. This is further demonstrated by the fact that von Willebrand factor is essential to normal platelet adhesion to subendothelial collagen. In addition, von Willebrand factor is necessary for normal bleeding times. Thus, in the absence of von Willebrand factor, one notes prolonged template bleeding times, abnormal platelet aggregation to ristocetin, and abnormal platelet adhesion to collagen.

Typical abnormalities and aids in the diagnosis of von Willebrand syndrome are depicted in Table 24–19. The template bleeding time is characteristically prolonged if a modified Ivy or template bleeding time (TBT) is performed. The Duke bleeding time is commonly normal in patients with von Willebrand syndrome. There is a decrease in procoagulant Factor VIII and in Factor VIII–related antigen in von Willebrand syndrome. Abnormal platelet adhesion may be noted by the Bowie technique; however, this technique, al-

TABLE 24–19 CLINICAL AND LABORATORY CHARACTERISTICS OF von WILLEBRAND SYNDROME

Clinical findings
Childhood bleeding
Positive family history
Epistaxis
Easy and spontaneous bruising
Mild mucosal membrane bleeding
Petechiae and purpura
Laboratory findings
Template bleeding time prolonged
Ristocetin aggregation abnormal
PTT moderately prolonged
Factor VIII:C decreased
Factor VIII:Ag decreased
Factor VIII:vW decreased
Sustained rise in Factor VIII:C after plasma infusion

though of historic interest, is no longer recommended in clinical medicine and has no clinical relevance. Typically, normal platelet aggregation to the usual aggregating agents, except ristocetin, will be noted. Ristocetin aggregation is usually abnormal in patients with von Willebrand syndrome. In addition, there is a characteristic and sustained rise in Factor VIII procoagulant activity (Factor VIII:C) after transfusion of the von Willebrand patient with normal plasma, hemophilia A plasma, or cryoprecipitate. In the past, many patients with clinical findings suggestive of von Willebrand syndrome have failed to demonstrate clear-cut and characteristic laboratory findings. Thus, it was postulated that there were several different forms of von Willebrand disease, and at least seven different forms were proposed, depending on the particular laboratory features present. However, evidence suggests that the classic laboratory features associated with von Willebrand syndrome are waxing and waning in the vast majority of patients. In fact, it is now appreciated that in approximately 90 per cent of patients with von Willebrand syndrome, the laboratory features are constantly changing. This suggests that in approximately 10 per cent of patients, variance may exist. However, of more importance is the suggestion that if a patient with suspected von Willebrand syndrome does not display characteristic laboratory features, the laboratory studies should be repeated in several weeks. The mainstay therapy of von Willebrand syndrome is infusion of cryoprecipitate, which is rich in von Willebrand factor. When von Willebrand syndrome is compared with classic hemophilia, it will be noted that both are inherited by different modes; von Willebrand syndrome is under autosomal control, and hemophilia A is under sex-linked control. The template bleeding time is typically normal in the hemophilic patient and prolonged in the von Willebrand patient. In addition, Factor VIII procoagulant activity (Factor VIII:C) is decreased in both disorders but usually much more so in hemophilia A. Factor VIII–related antigen is normal in patients with hemophilia A and typically decreased in the patient with von Willebrand syndrome. In addition, von Willebrand factor (Factor VIII:vW) is decreased in the patient with von Willebrand syndrome and normal in the hemophilia patient. Platelet function studies are typically normal in both disorders, with the exception of ristocetin-induced aggregation, which is normal in the hemophiliac and abnormal in the von Willebrand patient. In addition, clinical features are markedly different in these two disorders. The hemophilia A patient suffers from deep tissue bleeding manifest as intra-articular, intramuscular, and intracranial bleeding; however, the von Willebrand patient suffers platelet function/vascular defect bleeding manifest as petechiae, purpura, epistaxis, and mild to moderate mucosal membrane bleeding in association with easy and spontaneous bruising. It has been suggested that high molecular weight Factor VIII is responsible for induction of the synthesis or release (from hepatocytes?) of low molecular weight Factor VIII, accounting for the sustained rise in Factor VIII procoagulant activity noted when the von Willebrand patient is infused with plasma, cryoprecipitate, or hemophilia A plasma. Von Willebrand factor appears to be synthesized in the endothelial cell.

RARE CONGENITAL COAGULATION PROTEIN DEFECTS

Congenital Fibrinogen (Factor I) Deficiency. Congenital afibrinogenemia is extremely rare, with only 60 cases having been reported. This disorder is inherited as an autosomal recessive trait. It is thought that afibrinogenemia represents the homozygous state and hypofibrinogenemia represents the heterozygote. Afibrinogenemic patients may suffer severe hemophilia-like bleeding, including intra-articular bleeding with crippling hemarthroses. In addition, umbilical stump bleeding at childbirth is characteristic. These patients also suffer cutaneous bruising and have life-threatening bleeding following trauma or surgery. Hypofibrinogenemic patients may suffer only minor bleeding, usually never spontaneous, but may bleed significantly with surgery or trauma. The diagnostic laboratory findings of afibrinogenemia are an infinite thrombin time, reptilase time, prothrombin time, and partial thromboplastin time. These same tests are significantly prolonged, but not infinite, in hypofibrinogenemia.

Dysfibrinogenemia. Congenital dysfibrinogenemia is a disorder characterized by normal fibrinogen levels (immunologically), but the molecule is abnormal. There have been several types of dysfibrinogenemias described. By international agreement, these are named for the location where first discovered. All appear to be inherited by autosomal dominance, and all are characterized by a long or infinite thrombin time, with the exception of fibrinogen Oslow, which demonstrates a short thrombin time, and fibrinogen Oklahoma, which has a normal thrombin time.

More than 50 per cent of patients with congenital dysfibrinogenemias demonstrate no clinical bleeding diathesis. Of the remainder, however, many do demonstrate bleeding similar to that seen with hypofibrinogenemic states. Several of the dysfibrinogenemias are characterized by thrombosis only.

In most of these disorders, the pathophysiology is poorly understood. There are different types of dysfibrinogenemias, and varying characteristics are noted for each. Immunologic methods reveal fibrinogen levels to be normal or increased. Various defects have been described for each particular type of dysfibrinogenemia and have included such findings as abnormal immunoelectrophoretic mobility, abnormal carbohydrate content, and slow release of fibrinopeptide A or B with thrombin. The most completely characterized dysfibrinogenemia is fibrinogen Detroit. In this instance, the amino acid serine is substituted for arginine in position 19 of the A-alpha chain. This unique and laborious discovery represents the second disease state to be defined by a single amino acid substitution (the first, of course, being sickle cell anemia).

Except for fibrinogen Oslow and fibrinogen Oklahoma, all the congenital dysfibrinogenemias have a prolonged or infinite thrombin and reptilase time. In these disorders, a normal amount of immunologic fibrinogen is noted.

Cryoprecipitate or fresh plasma is usually used to treat bleeding episodes in patients with afibrinogenemia, hypofibrinogenemia, or dysfibrinogenemia. To achieve hemostasis, one need only raise and maintain the functional fibrinogen level to 50 to 100 mg/dl. Since the half-life of fibrinogen is about 4 days, infusions need not be frequent. It is of interest to note that bleeding episodes often do not recur when the infused fibrinogen disappears from the patient's plasma. Table 24–20 summarizes congenital fibrinogen disorders.

TABLE 24–20 CONGENITAL FIBRINOGEN DEFECTS

Type	Fibrinogen Protein	Clotting Assays
Afibrinogenemia (Homozygote)	Absent	Infinite
Hypofibrinogenemia (Heterozygote)	Decreased	Prolonged
Dysfibrinogenemia (Homozygote)	Normal	Prolonged–infinite
Dysfibrinogenemia (Heterozygote)	Normal	Normal–prolonged

Congenital Prothrombin (Factor II) Deficiency. This disorder is extremely rare, with only 15 to 16 cases having been reported. Congenital prothrombin deficiency appears to be inherited as an autosomal recessive trait. Clinically, patients with this disorder have numerous hematomas and ecchymoses. In addition, they experience mucosal membrane bleeding and may manifest severe bleeding with surgery or trauma. Intra-articular bleeding and hemarthroses have not been reported. In those instances in which appropriate studies have been performed, a true prothrombin deficiency (CRM⁻) has been found, but at least two cases of dysfunctional Factor II (CRM⁺) have been reported.

Congenital Factor V Deficiency (Parahemophilia). This extremely rare disorder was first found in Oslow in 1947. Subsequently, 30 more cases have been noted. Some have been associated with classic hemophilia and von Willebrand syndrome. Like patients with congenital prothrombin deficiency, many individuals with parahemophilia have mucosal membrane bleeding as well as hematomas and ecchymoses. Intra-articular bleeding and hemarthroses have not been reported. Thus far, evidence suggests this to be a true deficiency (CRM⁻) rather than a dysfunctional Factor V. This deficiency must be treated with fresh plasma when significant bleeding occurs.

Congenital Factors VII and X Deficiencies. These two disorders are extremely rare, with only 60 to 70 cases of congenital Factor VII deficiency having been reported. One in 100,000 patients has Factor X deficiency. Both deficiencies are inherited as autosomal recessive traits, and both manifest a similar clinical bleeding diathesis. Patients suffer intra-articular bleeding and hemarthroses but more commonly demonstrate only mild mucosal bleeding, manifest by epistaxis and genitourinary and gastrointestinal bleeding. Significant bleeding can occur with surgery or trauma. In several instances, no bleeding manifestations whatsoever have been present. In both congenital Factor VII and congenital Factor X deficiency, two variants exist. Some patients with congenital Factor VII deficiency have been reported to have a true deficiency (CRM⁻), whereas others have a dysfunctional Factor VII molecule (CRM⁺). The same situation appears to exist for congenital Factor X deficiency. In both these disorders, the prothrombin time is prolonged. The PTT is normal in Factor VII deficiency and prolonged in Factor X deficiency. The differential diagnosis is based on the Stypven time (prothrombin time performed with Russell's viper venom), which will be normal in congenital Factor VII deficiency and prolonged in Factor X deficiency. Bleeding in both these disorders, if it reaches significant or life-threatening proportions, may be controlled with prothrombin complex concentrates.

Congenital Factor XIII (Fibrin Stabilizing Factor, Laki-Lorand Factor, Transglutaminase) Deficiency. Factor XIII deficiency is extremely rare, with only 50 cases having been reported. This disorder is inherited as an autosomal recessive trait. The clinical hallmark of this disorder is poor wound healing after trauma or surgery, which is found in at least 50 per cent of patients. As in the congenital afibrinogenemias, umbilical cord bleeding at birth is extremely common in Factor XIII deficiency. Other bleeding manifestations are hematomas, ecchymoses, and, more rarely, intra-articular bleeding. Mucosal membrane bleeding has not been described in this disorder. In the vast majority of patients with this disorder, a true deficiency does not exist, but a dysfunctional Factor XIII is present. Thus, the patients are CRM⁺. A few cases have been reported that are truly deficient in Factor XIII (CRM⁻). In congenital Factor XIII deficiency, platelets, as well as plasma, are void of functional Factor XIII. This is in contrast to acquired Factor XIII deficiency, in which plasma is void of functional Factor XIII but Factor XIII is found in platelets.

Factor XIII levels of between 3 and 5 per cent are adequate for normal hemostasis. Since the half-life of Factor XIII is 4 to 6 days, clinically significant hemorrhage due to Factor XIII deficiency can usually be managed with infusion of plasma given at 10 ml/kg every 7 to 10 days. The laboratory diagnosis of Factor XIII deficiency is supported by the finding of fibrin solubility in 1 per cent monochloracetic acid or in 5 M urea.

Contact Activation Defects. Factor XII (Hageman) deficiency was first described by Ratnoff and Colopy in 1955. This disorder is relatively rare; since the original description, fewer than 200 cases have been described. Hageman deficiency is inherited as an autosomal recessive trait and usually is not associated with any bleeding diathesis. However, several patients have had a mild bleeding tendency. Of particular significance, however, is the fact that an inordinately high number of patients with Hageman trait have died as a consequence of thrombosis (usually coronary artery thrombosis or acute pulmonary embolism). This may be related to the known role of Factor XII in activation of the fibrinolytic system.

The pathophysiology of Hageman deficiency is poorly understood; however, in all patients studied thus far there appears to be a true deficiency, as all have been CRM⁻ when subjected to immunochemical studies. Hageman deficiency assumes major importance, since it causes marked prolongation of the activated partial thromboplastin time. The disorder is also characterized by an abnormal whole-blood clotting time and a prolonged clotting time in glass or siliconized tubes. The prothrombin time is normal. Numerous patients with Hageman trait have undergone major surgical procedures and not only have required no preoperative treatment but also have demonstrated no significant bleeding during or after surgery.

Another coagulation factor, Fletcher factor, was described by Hathaway in 1965. This interesting disorder was first observed in a family from eastern Kentucky involved in a fire that necessitated hospitalization of several of the children. During hospitalization, adenoidectomy was contemplated for one child. A preoperative hemostasis screen revealed a markedly prolonged PTT. Four of 14 siblings had markedly prolonged activated partial thromboplastin times. Careful investigation of the family failed to reveal evidence of any hemorrhagic tendency. The family surname is Fletcher, and thus the defect is now known as *Fletcher factor deficiency.* Subsequently, six to eight cases of Fletcher factor deficiency have been found. Investigations into Fletcher factor deficiency have revealed this defect to be characterized by a normal prothrombin time, a long activated partial thromboplastin time, and long plasma recalcification time. Both these latter tests are completely corrected by longer incubation with kaolin, celite, or glass. A screening test for Fletcher factor deficiency is simple, consisting of correction of a markedly prolonged PTT by incubation of the mixture with kaolin for 10 minutes, rather than 2 to 3 minutes.

Decreased Fletcher factor has been found in newborns, patients with severe liver disease, individuals with uremia, and patients with Fitzgerald factor trait, which is discussed subsequently. Fletcher factor is the same as plasma prekallikrein.

It has been noted that a mixture of Factor XII, Factor XI, Fletcher factor, and kaolin fails to activate Factor XI. Because of this, it has been proposed that other "factors" must also be necessary. Fitzgerald factor appears to be one such factor, first reported in 1964. This deficiency was found after observation of a normal prothrombin time and a markedly prolonged activated partial thromboplastin time in an asymptomatic 71-year-old male. Approximately five cases of Fitzgerald factor deficiency have been reported, and preliminary evidence suggests that it is an autosomal recessive trait. This disorder is characterized by a prolonged activated partial thromboplastin time, which is not corrected by longer incubation with kaolin. The defect is, however, corrected with the addition of plasmas that are deficient in Factor XII, Fletcher factor, and Factor XI. Kallikrein ("activated" Fletcher factor) also fails to correct the defect. However, activated XI or XII will correct the disorder. Similar to individuals with Fletcher factor and Factor XII deficiency, these patients have defects in surface-activated fibrinolysis, in kaolin-induced kinin generation, and in vascular permeability. Fitzgerald factor has been shown to be identical with high molecular weight kininogen.

An additional "activation phase" factor was reported in 1974 by Bick. In this instance, a patient with the Hughes-Stoven syndrome (pulmonary arterial aneurysms, deep vein thrombophlebitis, and dural sinus thromboses) was found to have a markedly prolonged kaolin-activated partial thromboplastin time. This individual had a normal bleeding time and normal levels of other known clotting factors, including Fletcher factor. The abnormal kaolin-activated PTT was partially corrected, and the celite-activated PTT was completely corrected by longer incubation times. The addition of normal plasma, aged serum, or barium sulfate–absorbed plasma shortened the activated PTT by 15 to 20 seconds but never corrected it to normal. Circulating anticoagulants could not be found in this patient, suggesting an additional factor in the contact activation phase.

ACQUIRED HEMOSTASIS DEFECTS

DISSEMINATED INTRAVASCULAR COAGULATION (DIC) AND RELATED SYNDROMES

Disseminated intravascular coagulation (DIC, consumption coagulopathy, or defibrination syndrome) is an intermediary mechanism of disease. DIC is usually associated with well-defined clinical entities and may be manifest as a wide clinical spectrum. If the intravascular clotting process is dominant and secondary fibrino(geno)lysis is minimal, DIC may be expressed primarily as diffuse thromboses, as in malignancy; however, if the secondary fibrinolysis that occurs with DIC is dominant and the drive toward procoagulant activity is minimal, the clinical manifestation will be hemorrhage, the most common expression of DIC. Patients usually demonstrate combinations of hemorrhage and thrombosis. Thus, DIC represents a wide spectrum of clinical findings, with patients presenting anywhere in the continuum between diffuse thromboses and hemorrhage. The clinical conditions most commonly associated with DIC are depicted in Table 24–21.

A common trigger for DIC is an obstetric accident, primarily amniotic fluid embolism, retained fetus syndrome, abruptio placentae, and, less commonly, placenta previa. Amniotic fluid has procoagulant (clot-promoting) activity and can initiate the clotting sequence, thus leading to DIC. When a dead fetus remains in utero for longer than 5 weeks, the incidence of DIC approaches 50 per cent. The trigger is thought to be necrotic fetal tissue released into the uterine and, subsequently, into the systemic maternal circulation. Necrotic fetal tissue has procoagulant activity and initiates the clotting sequence. In abruptio placentae, placental tissue or enzymes with procoagulant activity or both may be released into the uterine and then systemic maternal circulation to initiate the clotting sequence.

Another common triggering event for DIC is intravascular hemolysis of any etiology. Two

TABLE 24–21 CONDITIONS ASSOCIATED WITH DISSEMINATED INTRAVASCULAR COAGULATION (DIC)

A. Obstetric vents
 1. Retained fetus syndrome
 2. Amniotic fluid embolism
 3. Placental abruption
 4. Saline-induced abortion
B. Hemolysis
 1. Hemolytic transfusion reaction
 2. Minor hemolysis
 3. Massive transfusions
C. Septicemia
 1. Gram-negative (endotoxin)
 2. Gram-positive (bacterial coat mucopolysaccharide)
D. Viremia
 1. CMV
 2. Varicella
 3. Hepatitis
E. Acute leukemia
 1. Acute promyelocytic
 2. Acute myelomonocytic
F. Disseminated malignancy
 1. Lung
 2. Gall bladder
 3. Gastric
 4. Colon
 5. Ovary
 6. Breast
 7. Prostate
 8. Melanoma
G. Burns, tissue necrosis, crush injuries
H. Shock/acidosis
I. Vascular disorders

mechanisms have been proposed: The release of red cell ADP may initiate a platelet release reaction with generation of platelet factor 3 activity and subsequent activation of the coagulation system, or the release of red cell membrane phospholipoprotein during hemolysis may independently initiate the clotting sequence and perhaps also a platelet release reaction. Sepsis may be associated with acute DIC, although the exact mechanism or mechanisms remain unclear. One of the first organisms found to be associated with DIC was *Meningococcus*. Later, other gram-negative organisms were described in association with DIC. Thus it was thought that bacteremias triggered DIC by release of endotoxin, which induced both coagulation and the platelet release reaction. DIC has also been described with gram-positive organisms, so other mechanisms, in addition to endotoxin, must also be involved. Other potential mechanisms for initiation of DIC in gram-positive septicemia involve initiation of platelet release or "contact phase" activation of coagulation by materials from bacterial coats (mucopolysaccharides). Viremias may initiate DIC by antigen-antibody complex activation of platelet release or the coagulation system or both. In addition, antigen-antibody complexes may damage the endothelium,

which in turn may initiate platelet release and subsequent coagulation or may activate coagulation via endothelium/collagen-induced Factor XII_a generation.

Burns and crush injuries are associated with acute DIC. In burn patients, the microhemolysis (with subsequent release of red cell phospholipid or ADP or both) may provide the trigger for DIC. In patients suffering massive tissue necrosis from crush injuries, release of necrotic tissue or tissue enzymes with procoagulant (thromboplastin-like) activity may trigger the clotting sequence or the platelet release reaction.

Most patients with disseminated malignancy have laboratory evidence of DIC; however, many never develop clinical manifestations. Malignancy represents a special situation in that DIC may be acute, subacute, or chronic and may be manifest as local thromboses, diffuse thromboses, minor hemorrhage, diffuse hemorrhage, or any combination. The acute leukemias are also associated with DIC. This was first noted in acute promyelocytic leukemia. The release of procoagulants from promyelocytes appears responsible for triggering the clotting sequence. In many instances, the initiation of cytotoxic chemotherapy may initiate or significantly enhance the disseminated intravascular clotting process. For this reason, some have advocated the use of prophylactic heparin or miniheparin before initiating cytotoxic chemotherapy in patients with acute promyelocytic leukemia.

The malignancies most commonly associated with acute DIC are depicted in Table 24–21. However, acute DIC may also be seen in almost any type of solid tumor. There are numerous potential mechanisms by which malignancy may trigger DIC. The patient with malignancy and associated DIC presents a major problem in management, and thus a clear understanding and definition of possible triggering events are desirable and often necessary for efficacious management of the intravascular clotting process.

Pathophysiology. Figure 24–16 summarizes the manner by which numerous unrelated disease processes may trigger disseminated intravascular coagulation. The result of these mechanisms is the ultimate generation of systemic thrombin and systemic plasmin. Figure 24–17 depicts the pathophysiology of DIC once a trigger has been provided and generation of systemic thrombin and plasmin has occurred. As thrombin circulates, it enzymatically attacks fibrinogen, systemically rather than locally, creating fibrin monomer. Under physiologic conditions, fibrin monomer subsequently polymerizes into fibrin. However, in the face of plasmin generation, fibrinogen is simultaneously being degraded, creating fibrinogen/fibrin degradation products, the X, Y, D, and E fragments. Some of these fragments have a high affinity for fibrin monomer, and the two complex before much of the fibrin monomer can polymerize into fibrin.

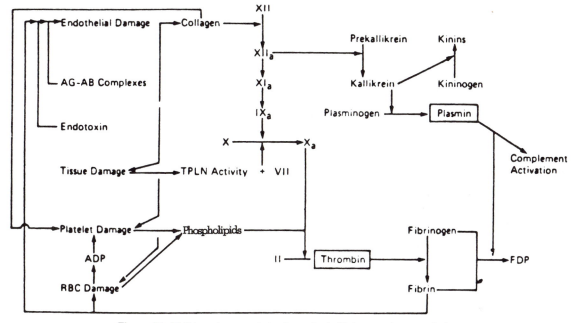

Figure 24–16 Triggering events in disseminated intravascular coagulation.

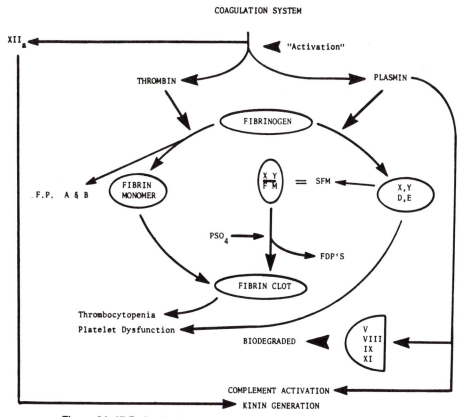

Figure 24–17 Pathophysiology of disseminated intravascular coagulation.

This combination of degradation products and fibrin monomer forms so-called "soluble fibrin monomer," the presence of which provides the basis of paracoagulation reactions (the protamine sulfate test and the ethanol gelation test), which are aids in diagnosing disseminated intravascular coagulation. When protamine sulfate is added to citrated plasma containing soluble fibrin monomer, it acts to dissociate degradation products, allowing fibrin monomer to polymerize, and resultant fibrin strands are observed in the test tube. While some fibrin monomer is complexing with degradation products to form soluble fibrin monomer, other fibrin polymerizes in the microvasculature, impeding blood flow, tissue hypoxia, and resultant ischemia and necrosis in multiple end-organs. In addition, polymerized fibrin deposited in the microvasculature leads to entrapment of platelets and attendant thrombocytopenia, and it may cause microangiopathic hemolytic anemia from fibrin-red cell contact. The microhemolysis can provide more triggering material for continued intravascular coagulation (ADP and red cell membrane phospholipid), thus creating a pathologic cycle (Fig. 24–18).

Plasmin is also capable of degradation and inactivation of Factor V, Factor VIII, Factor IX, Factor XI, ACTH, growth hormone, complement, insulin, and other plasma proteins. This may occur systemically in DIC. The syndrome of acute disseminated intravascular coagulation with hemorrhage might be more aptly referred to as *acute disseminated intravascular proteolysis,* as it is the systemic plasmin generation that appears to account for the majority of hemorrhage. This occurs through the creation of fibrinogen/fibrin degradation products that interfere with fibrin monomer polymerization, platelet dysfunction resulting from coating of platelet membranes with degradation products, and plasmin biodegradation of Factors V, VIII, and IX as well as other plasma proteins. By understanding the circular pathophysiology of DIC (thrombin plus plasmin generation), one can appreciate that if thrombin generation is moderate to maximum and the secondary fibrinolytic response (plasmin generation) is minimal, the same pathophysiology will be more commonly associated with polymerization of fibrin, minimal lysis, and diffuse thromboses (commonly seen in the patient with malignancy). Alternatively, if plasmin activity is dominant over thrombin activity, then hemorrhage, the more common expression of DIC, will result.

Another important consideration in appreciating the pathophysiology of DIC is the interrelationship between the intravascular clotting process and other plasma protein enzyme systems. During an intravascular clotting episode initiated by a variety of triggers (abnormal endothelium, exposed collagen, foreign surfaces, phospholipids, etc.), the activation of Factor XII often occurs. Factor XIIa, via the kallikrein system, indirectly activates the fibrinolytic system, which may be an alternate or major route of secondary fibrinolysis in DIC. Plasmin activates the first and third components of complement, thus initiating the complement sequence with subsequent cell lysis, immunoadherence, and other immune phenomena. Kallikrein generates kinins from kininogens, leading to hypotension, increased vascular permeability, pain, and other manifestations. This complex pathophysiology must be considered when dealing with, and trying to explain, many of the clinical and laboratory findings in patients with acute, subacute, and chronic DIC.

Diagnosis. The clinical diagnosis of disseminated intravascular coagulation need not be difficult. The key to a high index of suspicion is simply observation of the appropriate type of bleeding in the appropriate clinical setting. The usual settings associated with DIC are depicted in Table 24–21. If the patient has one of these clinical conditions with hemorrhage or thromboses, DIC should be suspected. The type of bleeding manifest by most patients with acute or subacute DIC is suggestive of multiple hemostatic compartment defects. Most patients with acute DIC will bleed from at least three unrelated sites. This may be manifest in a wide variety of ways and is commonly noted as melena and hematemesis, epistaxis, or hemoptysis, in association with oozing from intravascular sites, hematuria, and associated findings of petechiae and purpura. This type of bleeding suggests that multiple hemostatic compartments (i.e., plasma coagulation protein or platelets or the vasculature or any combination) are defective. Most patients also display shock, end-organ hypoxia, ischemic changes, or any combination of these findings. This may be manifest in a variety of ways, depending on end-organ involvement and degree of vascular occlusive changes. Renal failure, due to fibrin deposited in the renal microvasculature, is a usual manifestation. Additionally, one must recall the interplay among coagulation, fibrino(geno)lysis, kinin generation, and complement activation in these patients that accounts for

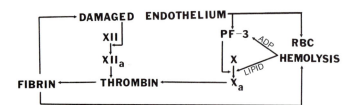

Figure 24–18 Selected "pathocybernetics" in disseminated intravascular coagulation.

many attendant signs and symptoms. Many patients with malignancy and subacute or chronic DIC will not display fulminant and multiple-site bleeding; more commonly, these patients have minor mucosal membrane bleeding, often manifest as excessive gingival bleeding with toothbrushing, minor hemoptysis, bothersome epistaxis, and, at times, hematuria. In addition, they will usually complain of easy and spontaneous bruising. Petechiae and purpura are usually present. Diffuse thrombosis in a patient with malignancy may be a manifestation of the opposite clinical spectrum of DIC, and the patient should be appropriately studied for confirmatory evidence.

Although observation of the appropriate type of bleeding in the appropriate clinical setting can virtually assure a diagnosis of DIC, laboratory confirmation is mandatory before a patient is committed to heparin or other anticoagulant type of therapy. In view of the pathophysiology of DIC, it is clear that patients will have numerous abnormal laboratory tests of hemostasis, particularly in acute DIC. In subacute or chronic DIC, especially when associated with malignancy, many laboratory parameters may be difficult to interpret or may be within normal limits. Table 24–22 depicts the laboratory tests that are typically abnormal in acute DIC. The most helpful tests are asterisked.

The prothrombin time is prolonged for several reasons: (1) Hypofibrinogenemia is usually present, (2) Factor V is often digested by plasmin, and (3) products of fibrino(geno)lysis (FDP) interfere with fibrin polymerization. Occasionally, the prothrombin time is normal or "super normal"; however, this does not rule out a diagnosis of acute DIC. The reason or reasons for a normal or shortened prothrombin time in DIC remain unclear, but may be linked to the presence of activated clotting factors, especially Factor Xa.

TABLE 24–22 LABORATORY TESTS THAT ARE TYPICALLY ABNORMAL IN DISSEMINATED INTRAVASCULAR COAGULATION (DIC)

Schistocytosis*
Leukocytosis
Reticulocytosis
Thrombocytopenia*
Hypofibrinogenemia*
Prolonged protime
Prolonged PTT
Prolonged thrombin time
Prlonged reptilase time
Elevated FDP*
Positive protamine sulfate test*
Decreased AT-III*
Decreased plasminogen
Increased plasmin
Hypocomplementemia
Elevated FP-A
Elevated PF-4/beta TGT

*Most useful tests at present.

Similarly, the partial thromboplastin time (PTT) is prolonged in approximately 50 per cent of patients with acute DIC, owing to plasmin digestion of Factors VIII, IX, and XI. As with the prothrombin time, the PTT may also be normal or "super normal."

The thrombin time is usually prolonged in acute DIC owing to hypofibrinogenemia and inhibition of the test system by FDP.

Like the prothrombin time and partial thromboplastin time, the thrombin time can also be normal or "super normal." Performance of a thrombin time and, alternatively or additionally, a reptilase time can add additional information if the resultant thrombin time clot (or reptilase time clot) is observed for evidence of lysis for 5 to 10 minutes. Observation of the clot incurs no additional expense, requires a minimum of laboratory time, is faster than plasminogen/plasmin assays, and provides evidence for significant fibrino-(geno)lysis. A reptilase time is often helpful as a baseline when one is diagnosing DIC, since it is one of the few laboratory modalities that can be used to follow the patient with acute DIC once heparin has been given.

In most instances of acute DIC, there is significant thrombocytopenia, which may be noted by careful observation of a peripheral smear or performance of a platelet count. Additional findings on a peripheral smear will often be a mild leukocytosis, usually between 12,000 and 15,000 per cubic millimeter, and a slight shift to the left. Furthermore, red cell fragments (schistocytes) are present in approximately 50 per cent of patients with acute DIC. The mechanism or mechanisms for these microangiopathic changes have been well described by Bull. Tests of platelet function will usually be abnormal in acute DIC because of thrombocytopenia and the coating of platelet membranes by fibrino(geno)lytic degradation products. Thus clot retraction, a tourniquet test, or template bleeding time will be abnormal. These last two tests should not be performed when acute DIC is suspected, as they will add little, if anything, to the diagnosis and may cause unnecessary bleeding. Platelet aggregation will usually be abnormal. Any combination of aggregation defects may be seen.

If factor assays are performed, low levels of Factors V, VIII, and IX will usually be noted owing to plasmin digestion. Factor assays are rarely, if ever, indicated or necessary for diagnosing acute DIC. In addition, meaningless factor assay results may occur, owing to the presence of activated clotting factors (Xa, thrombin). The vast majority of patients will have significantly elevated fibrinogen/fibrin degradation products (FDP). The actual titer may bear little relationship to the clinical course of the intravascular clotting process, since the titer of FDP will depend on an interplay between degree of procoagulant activity, degree of fibrino(geno)lytic response, and other factors such

TABLE 24–23 ANTITHROMBIN III IN ACUTE DISSEMINATED INTRAVASCULAR COAGULATION (DIC)

	Antithrombin III (Per Cent)	Abnormal Patients (Per Cent)
Pretreatment	63.1 ± 25	92
Posttreatment	106.7 ± 32	18
p Value	<0.001	—
Normal	89–125	—

as poor renal clearance (degree of renal failure) and activity of the reticuloendothelial system.

The paracoagulation reactions for detecting the presence of soluble fibrin monomer (protamine sulfate or ethanol gelation test) are simple to perform and are usually positive in the presence of acute DIC. Both tests are reported to have attendant advantages and disadvantages. These variables have been described, but the best test or methodology remains unclear. The protamine sulfate test, as described by Kidder and coworkers, detects soluble fibrin monomer, even after heparinization. As with all other laboratory modalities, paracoagulation reactions, especially the protamine sulfate test, must be interpreted in the appropriate clinical setting. Soluble fibrin monomer and elevated FDP titers may be seen in some instances of acute myocardial infarction, pulmonary embolism, and extensive deep vein thrombophlebitis as well as in contraceptive pill users.

A newer laboratory modality that is helpful in confirming a diagnosis of DIC is the antithrombin III (AT-III) determination by synthetic substrate (chromogenic, fluorogenic) method. Consumption of this inhibitor due to generation of thrombin and other serine proteases occurs early and, to a significant degree, in most instances of DIC. AT-III consumption may not be seen in some patients with malignancy and DIC, since this alpha$_2$-globulin may behave as an acute phase reactant and may be consumed only down to normal or near normal levels. The AT-III synthetic substrate assay is of additional benefit in monitoring the patient with DIC, as the system is unaffected by FDP or heparin. When one sees cessation of AT-III consumption, it can be assumed that therapy has been reasonably effective in either blunting or stopping the intravascular clotting process. Table 24–23 depicts AT-III levels before and after therapy in a series of patients with acute DIC. Another laboratory modality that is becoming available and may be quite useful for a diagnosis of DIC is the radioimmunoassay of fibrinopeptide A. From the clinical standpoint, the difficulty with this modality is the length of time required to perform the assay. The reliability of laboratory tests in aiding in a diagnosis of DIC is depicted in Table 24–24.

Therapy. In the past, acute DIC has been associated with a high mortality; efficacious therapy has been slow in developing, and many disease states associated with DIC are in themselves often fatal. However, many patients are now surviving as more rational and effective therapy is being developed. The therapy of acute DIC should be approached in a logical and sequential fashion. Clearly, the most important therapeutic modality that can be delivered to the patient is removal or treatment (blunting) of the triggering process. In many instances, this may not be possible, as in malignancy. However, in many diseases associated with DIC, some reasonable attempts can be made to treat the procoagulant triggering process effectively. This may in itself stop the intravascular clotting process, as is usually the case in obstetric accidents and sometimes the case in septicemia. If not, it will usually blunt the process and afford the patient a reasonable chance of responding to heparin or other therapy aimed at stopping intravascular clotting. However, if reasonable attempts are not directed to the triggering event or disease state, the patient often is unable to respond to heparin or other anticoagulant therapy. For example, obstetric accidents seldom, if ever, require heparinization. Evacuation of the uterus will almost always stop the intravascular clotting process within 3 to 4 hours. It is often difficult to persuade an obstetrician-gynecologist to take a bleeding patient to the operating room, but prompt cessation of hemorrhage after evacuation of the uterus is usually quite striking.

In sepsis and DIC, specific antimicrobial and usual supportive therapy should be instituted before therapy aimed specifically at DIC is considered. As in obstetric accidents, many patients with sepsis will also experience partial or complete correction of their intravascular clotting process with specific antimicrobial therapy. If antibiotic, supportive therapy alone does not stop the intravascular clotting process, it will usually blunt the

TABLE 24–24 RELIABILITY OF LABORATORY TESTS IN DIAGNOSING DISSEMINATED INTRAVASCULAR COAGULATION (DIC) AND IN MONITORING THERAPY*

Test	Abnormal Patients at Diagnosis (Per Cent)	Abnormal Patients After Therapy (Per Cent)
FDP	100	24
AT-III	97	16
Platelet count	97	34
PSO$_4$ test	92	18
Thrombin time	81	32
Fibrinogen level	79	16
Protime	76	58
PTT	63	24
Reptilase time	58	8

*Summary of reliability: FDP > AT-III = platelet count > PSO$_4$ > thrombin time > fibrinogen > protime > PTT > reptilase time.

process enough for the patient to have a chance of responding to heparin. In patients with shock and DIC, the infusion of fluids, stabilization of cardiac status, pH, electrolytes, and other measures to expand vascular volume and improve cardiac output may stop DIC, but more often will blunt the clotting process enough to allow response to heparin therapy.

In malignancy, removal of the triggering process or processes is often not possible. However, surgical, chemotherapeutic, or radiotherapeutic modalities to shrink the tumor mass may be of benefit in blunting or stopping the intravascular clotting process. In rarer instances, the initiation of chemotherapy or radiation therapy will cause further tissue necrosis and worsening of, or triggering of, a DIC process. Table 24–25 outlines the sequential therapy of DIC.

Following the first two sequential steps as outlined for the therapy of DIC (i.e., therapy aimed at the triggering disease state and the initiation of low-dose heparin or other therapeutic modalities to stop the intravascular clotting process) will cause cessation of DIC in the majority of patients. Occasionally, however, patients will continue to bleed. The most common reasons are failure to control the triggering disease or coagulation factor depletion due to plasmin digestion and, to a lesser extent, consumption of factors. In this situation, the third sequential step to be considered is blood component replacement. All reasonable attempts should be made to define which components are lacking and most likely contributing to continued hemorrhage. Only those thought necessary to control hemorrhage should be delivered. The patient may be treated with fresh frozen plasma, cryoprecipitate, prothrombin complex concentrates, plate-

lets, or any combination as indicated, but replacement should be as specific as possible. It should be emphasized at this point that component therapy should never be used (with the exception of packed red cells, AT-III, and platelets) until the patient has been heparinized and it is reasonably certain that the intravascular clotting process has been controlled. The addition of components in the face of continued DIC may "add fuel to the fire." If the patient is given fresh frozen plasma or clotting factor concentrates this may provide more fibrinogen/fibrin degradation products, further inhibition of fibrin monomer polymerization, further interference with platelet function, and further plasmin-induced biodegradation of clotting Factors V, VIII, and IX. This may exaggerate DIC, and clinical hemorrhage will often become much more pronounced.

Rarely, patients will continue to bleed after going through the three aforementioned steps. When this occurs, it is most often due to continued residual fibrino(geno)lysis. In this rare instance, antifibrinolytic therapy (usually aminocaproic acid) may be considered. This agent should always be given slowly, as it may be associated with hypokalemia, hypotension, ventricular arrhythmias, and diffuse intravascular thromboses, especially if the intravascular clotting process has not been arrested first. Monitoring of cardiac status, electrolytes, and renal output is essential. It must be re-emphasized that only in rare instances do patients with DIC require antifibrinolytic therapy (less than 5 per cent of patients, in our experience). As in the case of component therapy, antifibrinolytic therapy should never be used in acute DIC unless one is first assured that the intravascular clotting process has been successfully controlled with heparin or other therapy. If the intravascular clotting process is ongoing, the patient requires fibrinolysis for clearing of fibrin microthrombi. Thus, if antifibrinolytic therapy is used in the face of continuing clotting, the consequences are obviously catastrophic.

Related Syndromes. Appreciating the cybernetic nature of normal hemostasis (i.e., the numerous complex and delicate interplays between coagulation proteins, other plasma protein systems, the platelets, the vasculature, and all the attendant inhibitors to these various components), one cannot help but be impressed by similar, although exaggerated, interplays that must be occurring in a "pathocybernetic" manner in DIC. It is evident that numerous circular events are occurring in DIC. Thus, in many instances the point at which the process starts may not be necessarily relevant with respect to the end clinical results. For example, endothelial damage may occur via numerous mechanisms. Damaged endothelium may, in turn, activate coagulation or lead to red cell microangiopathic hemolysis, which may then lead to release of red cell ADP and membrane phospholipid, which may cause further triggering

TABLE 24–25 SEQUENTIAL THERAPY OF DISSEMINATED INTRAVASCULAR COAGULATION (DIC)

A. Remove/treat triggering event
1. Evacuate uterus
2. Treat shock
3. Fluids and electrolytes
4. Antineoplastics
B. Inhibit intravascular clotting process
1. Subcutaneous heparin
2. Intravenous heparin?
3. Antiplatelet agents (ASA/dipyridamole)
4. AT-III concentrates
C. Correct component depletion
1. Platelets
2. Packed red cells (washed)
3. Fresh frozen plasma
4. Prothrombin complex concentrates?
D. Inhibit residual fibrinolysis (rarely indicated)
1. EACA as 5.0 gm; slow IVP
2. Maintain at 2 gm q2h to cessation of hemorrhage
3. Beware of ventricular arrhythmias, hypotension, and hypokalemia with EACA

of coagulation or platelet release or both, with subsequent activation of coagulation. These singular isolated circular systems in DIC are depicted in Figure 24–18. Understanding these as well as numerous other potential circular events in DIC explains how many different starting points, via similar or related pathophysiology, can lead to similar clinical manifestations. The process may be local (organ-specific) or systemic. It may start with platelets, endothelium, or coagulation proteins, and it may represent dominant procoagulant activity with minimal or inadequate secondary fibrinolytic response (i.e., thrombosis) or minimal procoagulant activity and overwhelming secondary fibrino(geno)lysis (i.e., hemorrhage). Appreciating this wide spectrum of clinical manifestations allows for consideration of other syndromes that are probably related to what we label *classic DIC*. These potentially similar syndromes include microangiopathic hemolytic anemia, pediatric respiratory distress syndrome (hyaline membrane disease), hemolytic uremic syndrome, and adult shock lung syndrome.

Microangiopathic red cell changes (RBC fragments, schistocytes, Heilmeyer-helmet cells) may be seen in a variety of disorders, including DIC, TTP, hypertension, eclampsia, and hemolytic uremic syndrome. These changes may arise from RBC contact with fibrin or damaged endothelium. When fibrin or endothelium or both induce RBC fragmentation, a resultant release of RBC membrane phospholipids and RBC adenosine diphosphate (ADP) may initiate subsequent activation of the procoagulant system or platelets or both. This can result in further fibrin deposition and endothelial damage, thus recycling the pathophysiology. Alternatively, when RBC fragmentation occurs before the endothelial damage (cardiac valves, intravascular hemolysis, fibrin deposition), resultant RBC membrane phospholipids and ADP release may lead to platelet release, procoagulant drive, fibrin deposition, and subsequent resultant endothelial damage, with further RBC fragmentation and, again, a recycling of pathophysiology. Thus the starting points may differ, but the cycling pathophysiology is similar (i.e., endothelial damage, RBC fragmentation, procoagulant drive, fibrin deposition, resultant secondary fibrinolytic response, and back to endothelial damage).

It is obvious that any of the aforementioned events may be the starting point. However, the interplays and the balance between the endothelial damage, procoagulant drive, and secondary fibrinolytic response will determine whether the clinical manifestations will be hemorrhage or thrombosis or both. In addition, the DIC process may be systemic or localized to an individual organ system.

Renal vascular damage of any etiology may initiate microangiopathic hemolysis, with subsequent red cell ADP- and/or membrane phospholipid–induced platelet release and/or procoagulant activity. This leads to fibrin deposition, further endothelial damage, and a perpetuation of the cycle. The salient clinical manifestations are (1) uremia from renal vascular damage, and (2) RBC fragments from damaged endothelium or fibrin or both. More rarely, the cycle may start with procoagulant activity, fibrin deposition, and subsequent vascular endothelial damage to the kidney with resultant uremia. Hemolytic uremic syndromes, therefore, share similar if not identical pathophysiology with DIC, but in most instances the process begins with and is localized to the kidney. In some instances, the same pathophysiology may exist in the usual disseminated or systemic intravascular coagulation, with uremia (resulting from renal microvascular damage) being only one of the many systemic clinical manifestations of more classic DIC.

It has now become clear that the hyaline membrane of respiratory distress syndrome (RDS) represents excessive fibrin deposition. Triggers for the procoagulant drive in these infants at high risk for RDS (prematures and infants of diabetic mothers) remain unclear. However, it appears that the secondary fibrinolytic response that usually accompanies excessive fibrin deposition (such as in DIC) is lacking in these infants. Current evidence suggests that infants born of diabetic mothers have markedly elevated fibrinolytic inhibitors (alpha$_2$-macroglobulin) and premature infants have decreased plasminogen levels, thus explaining the lack of a fibrinolytic response to the procoagulant drive in RDS. Therefore, like HUS, RDS may be a DIC-like syndrome that is localized to the lungs rather than a systemic disease that is characterized by excessive procoagulant activity (fibrin deposition), without the usual fibrinolytic response (lysis and hemorrhage).

Summary. Current concepts of the etiology, pathophysiology, diagnosis, and management of DIC have been presented. Considerable attention has been devoted to interrelationships that have remained confusing for some time. Only by clearly understanding these interrelationships can one appreciate the divergent and wide spectrum of often confusing clinical and laboratory findings in these patients. This review has also pointed out that other syndromes, not clinically considered in the spectrum of DIC, may really represent similar or identical pathophysiology and, although organ-specific (as in HUS and RDS) may, in fact, be variants of DIC.

PRIMARY HYPERFIBRINO(GENO)LYTIC SYNDROMES

Until recently, primary activation of the fibrinolytic system was considered uncommon, and the only situations in which clinical fibrinolysis existed were assumed to be those secondary to disseminated intravascular coagulation (DIC).

However, these considerations were formulated in an era during which there were insufficient clinical laboratory tools to assess fibrinolytic activity in patients. Early work in clinical fibrinolysis was limited to the use of the euglobulin lysis time (EGLT), which is of questionable clinical significance in assessing fibrinolytic activity. With the advent of newer and more sophisticated techniques, such as synthetic substrate assays for plasminogen, plasmin, and alpha$_2$-antiplasmin, it is now recognized that primary activation of the fibrinolytic system is not uncommon. The conditions in which primary activation of the fibrinolytic system may occur are generally well defined and include cardiopulmonary bypass, chronic liver disease, and malignancy. Each of these clinical situations will be discussed subsequently.

Pathophysiology of Primary Hyperfibrino(geno)lysis. Primary hyperfibrino(geno)lysis usually occurs in well-defined clinical entities in which there is direct or indirect activation of plasminogen into systemically circulating plasmin. In most disorders, the precise mechanism by which this occurs is not known. In several types of malignancies, tumor extracts are capable of activating the fibrinolytic system either directly or indirectly. In other disorders, mechanisms that may be operative include poor hepatic clearance of plasminogen activators or a decrease or dysfunction of inhibitors such as alpha$_2$-antiplasmin or alpha$_2$-macroglobulin. In chronic liver disease, alpha$_2$-macroglobulin is often increased, but appears to lose significant biologic function in inhibiting the fibrinolytic system. Table 24–26 lists various mechanisms through which the fibrino-

TABLE 24–26 POTENTIAL MECHANISMS OF FIBRINOLYTIC SYSTEM ACTIVATION

A. Hyperplasminogenemia
  1. Reactive states
B. Decreased fibrinolytic system inhibitors
  1. Alpha$_2$-antiplasmin
  2. Alpha$_2$-macroglobulin
C. Increased plasminogen activators
  1. Poor hepatic clearance (cirrhosis)
  2. Reticuloendothelial blockade
D. Exposure of blood to foreign surfaces with plasminogen activator–like activity
  1. Cardiopulmonary bypass
  2. Hemodialysis
  3. LeVeen shunts?
E. Drug-induced fibrinolytic activation
  1. Anabolic steroids
  2. Nicotinic acid
  3. Adriamycin
  4. Daunomycin
F. Tumor-derived enzymes
  1. Sarcoma
  2. Prostate
  3. Gastric
G. Pathologic Hageman factor activation
H. Therapeutic activation
  1. Streptokinase
  2. Urokinase
  3. Nicotinic acid

lytic system could be activated. Figure 24–19 depicts the pathophysiology of primary hyperfibrino(geno)lysis.

As the fibrinolytic system becomes activated, there is systemic circulating plasmin (systemic proteolytic activity). Plasmin degrades fibrin(ogen)

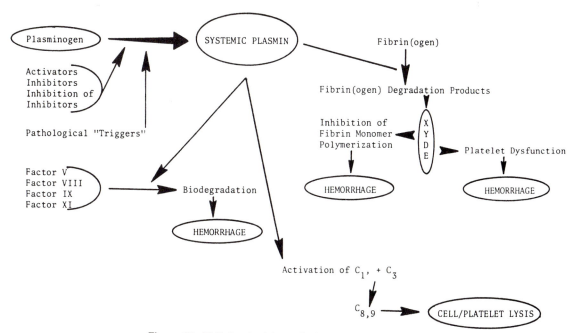

Figure 24–19 Pathophysiology of primary fibrino(geno)lysis.

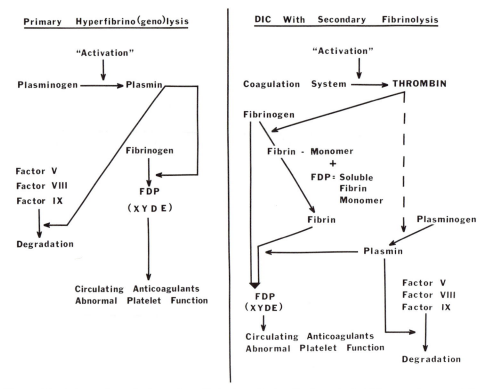

Figure 24–20 Comparison of primary hyperfibrino(geno)lysis with disseminated intravascular coagulation.

into the fibrinogen degradation products (FDP): X, Y, D, and E fragments. As in DIC, the presence of circulating plasmin and FDP results in compromised hemostatic function. Figure 24–20 compares and contrasts the salient features of DIC and primary hyperfibrino(geno)lysis. In primary hyperfibrino(geno)lysis there is no thrombin generated, there is no fibrin monomer for FDP to attach to, and thus there is no soluble fibrin monomer.

Since there has been little or no activation of the major serine proteases, there is little or no consumption of antithrombin III (AT-III), as is commonly seen in DIC. In addition, no fibrin is deposited in the microcirculation, and, consequently, there is no thrombocytopenia. However, the presence or absence of thrombocytopenia should not be used to establish a differential diagnosis because many disorders that are usually associated with a primary activation of the fibrinolytic system are often associated with thrombocytopenia via unrelated mechanisms. At present, an AT-III determination as well as a paracoagulation reaction test, such as the protamine sulfate test, appears to be a good differential diagnostic tool for distinguishing between primary hyperfibrino(geno)lytic syndromes and DIC with secondary fibrino(geno)lysis. The protamine sulfate test or ethanol gelation test may, on occasion, be negative in DIC. Thus, the careful interpretation of laboratory data in the appropriate clinical setting is the hallmark of making a differential diagnosis.

ALTERATIONS OF HEMOSTASIS IN CHRONIC LIVER DISEASE

Patients with chronic liver disease commonly experience significant hemorrhage, which presents a major challenge in clinical care, taxes the laboratory and local blood banking facilities, and is often the terminal event in the patient. The alterations of hemostasis that occur in these patients are complex and multifaceted.

Classically, it has been thought that hemorrhage in chronic liver disease is due to decreased synthesis of the vitamin K–dependent prothrombin complex factors, Factors II, VII, IX, and X. However, numerous additional hemostatic alterations must be appreciated before efficacious therapy can be instituted. The most common event in these patients is the development of localized bleeding, usually from a ruptured esophageal varix, peptic ulcers, or hemorrhagic gastritis. These bleeds tend to cascade into massive hemorrhage, which is generally poorly responsive to the usual therapeutic modalities of Sengstaken-Blakemore tamponade, massive transfusions with whole blood/fresh frozen plasma, and vasopressin infusion. Unsuccessful management is due to the fact that while some defects are treated and partially or completely corrected, other defects are left essentially unattended.

Etiology and Pathophysiology. The patient with chronic liver disease often demonstrates an early and significant decreased synthesis of the prothrombin complex Factors (II, VII, IX, and X). The decrease in Factor VII best correlates with the prothrombin time determination. However, the decreases in Factors IX and X best correlate with predisposition to clinical hemorrhage. The patient with chronic liver disease may also synthesize dysfunctional prothrombin complex factors, the so-called "PIVKA" derivatives (proteins induced by vitamin K absence/antagonism). These are prothrombin complex proteins rendered dysfunctional owing to absence of necessary calcium binding sites (gamma-carboxyglutamic residues).

Hypofibrinogenemia may occur. However, it rarely reaches a level of clinical significance. Normal or increased fibrinogen levels may also be seen in these patients, as fibrinogen may behave as an acute-phase reactant. In addition, many patients have an acquired dysfibrinogenemia, reflected by abnormal fibrin monomer polymerization or abnormal fibrinogen carbohydrate content or both.

As cirrhosis becomes terminal, there may also be decreased synthesis of Factors V and VIII. Early in the clinical course, these two factors may actually be elevated. The synthesis of prekallikrein is also decreased; however, the clinical significance of this defect remains unclear. Patients with chronic liver disease of any etiology usually demonstrate significantly decreased levels of AT-III. The pathophysiology of this remains unclear, as this may represent either a true decreased synthesis or synthesis of a dysfunctional AT-III molecule. Some patients may have normal or high AT-III levels, since this alpha$_2$-globulin, like fibrinogen, may behave as an acute-phase reactant. The clinical significance of this finding remains unclear with respect to developing hypercoagulability or thrombosis in cirrhosis.

The majority of patients with chronic liver disease experience a hyperfibrino(geno)lytic syndrome that is due to increased quantities of circulating plasmin. Primary hyperfibrino(geno)lysis (circulating plasmin) causes numerous hemostatic defects. Hypofibrinogenemia and "pseudodysfibrinogenemia" occur in the presence of fibrino(geno)lysis. Pseudodysfibrinogenemia is manifest in several forms; one is the creation of fibrinogen subspecies having high solubility (I-8, I-9 fractions) and low thrombin coagulability. This represents fibrinogen that has undergone minimal cleavage by plasmin. Because of fibrino(geno)lysis, patients with chronic liver disease usually demonstrate elevated FDP. The early degradation products also create a pseudodysfibrinogenemia by complexing with native fibrinogen and thus interfering with fibrin monomer polymerization. In addition, the latter degradation products coat the surfaces of platelets, rendering them dysfunctional. Circulating plasmin can also cause the proteolysis of Factors V, VIII, IX, and XI. These additional fibrino(geno)lytic insults to hemostasis

must always be borne in mind when clinical care is being rendered to the patient with chronic liver disease and hemorrhage.

About 35 per cent of patients with chronic liver disease develop thrombocytopenia via several mechanisms. The most pronounced of these is splenic sequestration secondary to congestive splenomegaly associated with portal hypertension. However, if the patient has disease that is due to alcoholism, ethanol itself is toxic to megakaryocytes and may suppress the bone marrow and bone marrow reserves, including megakaryopoiesis. Commonly unappreciated is the presence of significant platelet dysfunction in these patients. The precise reason or reasons for abnormal platelet function remain unclear. Decreased uptake of palmate and stearate in the platelet membrane in these individuals may be responsible. Abnormal platelet factor 3 release has also been noted. This may be a reflection of abnormal platelet membrane lipids or may be due to coating of platelet membranes by FDP. Thus, the patient with chronic liver disease may demonstrate thrombocytopenia as well as dysfunctional platelets. Both processes will contribute to clinical hemorrhage.

Patients with chronic liver disease often demonstrate poorly defined vascular defects. This has been ascribed to an estrogen effect on the vasculature, as these individuals do have abnormal metabolism and increased levels of estrogen. The vascular defect may reach clinical significance, especially in patients subjected to surgery or trauma. DIC rarely occurs de novo as a hemostatic defect in chronic liver disease until end-stage hepatic failure occurs. However, these patients are candidates for DIC if provided with one of the usual appropriate triggering events for this syndrome. Table 24–27 outlines the alterations of hemostasis associated with chronic liver disease.

Clinical Diagnosis. The clinical diagnosis of hemorrhage associated with chronic liver disease is usually obvious. Most often, the patient presents with or develops fulminant hemorrhage in the form of massive hemoptysis, hematochezia, and melena, often in association with epistaxis, in conjunction with ascites and other signs of portal hypertension. In addition, most patients presenting in this manner demonstrate petechiae, purpura, pulsating spider telangiectasia, and ecchymoses. The clinical bleeding often progresses into a more generalized disorder, with associated hematuria, oozing from intravascular catheter sites, and similar bleeding. More rarely, a patient who is clinically free of obvious hemorrhage when questioned will admit to spontaneous or easy bruising in association with periodic hematuria, periodic epistaxis, and gingival bleeding with toothbrushing.

Laboratory Diagnosis. Most tests of hemostasis will be abnormal in the face of the significant changes associated with chronic liver disease. The

TABLE 24–27 ALTERATIONS OF HEMOSTASIS ASSOCIATED WITH CHRONIC LIVER DISEASE

A. Defective hepatic synthesis
  1. Decreased synthesis of Factors II, VII, IX, and X
  2. PIVKA synthesis of Factors II, VII, IX, and X
  3. Hypofibrinogenemia
  4. Decreased synthesis of Factors V and VIII (end stage)
  5. Decreased synthesis of Fletcher factor
  6. Decreased/defective synthesis of AT-III
B. Increased destruction (hyperfibrinolysis)
  1. Abnormal fibrinolytic inhibitors (alpha$_2$-macroglobulin)
  2. Abnormal hepatic clearance of plasminogen activators
  3. Hypofibrinogenemia (lysis)
  4. Elevated FDP
  5. Proteolysis of Factors V, VIII, IX, and XI
C. Platelet defects
  1. Platelet function defects
    (a) Abnormal PF-3 availability
    (b) Elevated FDP
  2. Thrombocytopenia
    (a) Hypersplenism
    (b) Marrow suppression
D. Miscellaneous defects
  1. Vascular defects (hyperestrogenemia?)
  2. DIC? (requires independent trigger: hemolysis, sepsis, shock, etc.)

mainstay laboratory test for assessing the function of the prothrombin complex factors is the prothrombin time. In significantly decreased or dysfunctional synthesis of Factors II, VII, IX, and X, the prothrombin time will be abnormal. The decrease in Factor VII most closely correlates with prothrombin time prolongation, whereas the decreased synthesis of Factors IX and X most closely correlates with clinical bleeding. The prothrombin time may also be abnormal owing to elevated FDP or plasmin-induced degradation of Factor V.

The activated partial thromboplastin time is likewise often abnormal for reasons similar to those described for the prothrombin time. Specific factor assays will usually reveal low values. However, normal or elevated levels may also be noted. In particular, high levels of Factor VIII may be found unless significant plasmin is present.

Tests of fibrinolysis will be abnormal in about 75 per cent of patients. Plasmin and FDP will be found circulating at increased levels, and plasminogen will be decreased owing to depletion. Tests of platelet function will likewise be abnormal. The aggregation patterns are similar to those seen in DIC.

The template bleeding time will often be prolonged owing to a functional platelet defect, thrombocytopenia, the vascular defect present, or any combination of these factors. In fact, a template bleeding time should not be performed in the face of thrombocytopenia (platelets less than 100,000/mm^3), as it may cause undue bleeding and will render meaningless results. The use of a thrombin time and reptilase time will offer an indication of dysfibrinogenemia. However, both these laboratory modalities may also be prolonged in the face of elevated FDP.

It is clear that most tests of hemostasis may be abnormal in the patient with chronic liver disease. It is only with the use of a well-chosen hemostatic profile that each component of hemostasis can be assessed, the precise defect (or combination thereof) delineated, and a logical approach to treatment of hemorrhage planned.

Management. If the patient has significant fibrino(geno)lysis, the concomitant or subsequent use of antifibrinolytic agents, usually aminocaproic acid, may be indicated. If the patient is significantly thrombocytopenic, the use of platelet concentrates may be necessary. This will correct the thrombocytopenia and may alleviate bleeding from platelet dysfunction. The use of prothrombin complex concentrates in conjunction with other components, such as platelet concentrates, may have to be resorted to in patients failing to respond to the aforementioned modalities. An additional, although somewhat heroic, approach is the use of exchange transfusions. Exchange transfusion or the infusion of prothrombin complex concentrates should be considered investigational and probably not indicated in the patient with chronic liver disease and fulminant hemorrhage, unless a surgically correctable bleeding point is demonstrable.

Many patients with fulminant hemorrhage survive if they are approached in a logical manner (i.e., if the precise hemostatic defects present are diagnosed in the laboratory and treated individually). This approach usually allows for successful blunting or arrest of hemorrhage to the point at which the patient may become a reasonable candidate for surgical correction of the initiating event—usually peptic ulcer disease, a ruptured esophageal varix, or hemorrhagic gastritis.

Summary. Numerous hemostasis defects may occur in association with cirrhosis, and when significant or life-threatening hemorrhage develops, this may be due to any one or a combination of the defects previously defined. When approaching the patient with hemorrhage and chronic liver disease, the physician is challenged with the responsibilities of precisely defining those defects that are most likely at fault and then delivering specific and effective therapy.

ALTERATIONS OF HEMOSTASIS ASSOCIATED WITH CARDIOPULMONARY BYPASS

Cardiac surgery involving cardiopulmonary bypass (CPB) is now performed in many community hospitals. Catastrophic intraoperative or postoperative hemorrhage may be associated with this procedure and may place undue demands on local blood banks, lead to prolonged hospitalization, and significantly alter morbidity and mortality. The actual incidence of life-threatening hemorrhage associated with CPB varies between 5 and 25 per cent.

Many instances of CPB hemorrhage are clearly due to inadequate surgical technique. However, a significant number are also secondary to alterations in hemostasis created by CPB. When managing a hemorrhaging CPB patient, it is important to quickly distinguish between surgical and nonsurgical bleeding. This key question must be answered before the physician decides on whether to control hemorrhage surgically or medically.

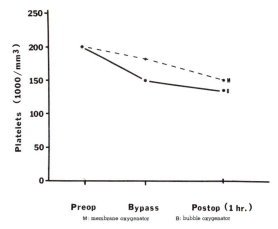

Figure 24–21 Platelet counts during cardiopulmonary bypass.

PATHOPHYSIOLOGY

Until recently, the pathophysiology of altered hemostasis created by CPB remained poorly understood. This has precluded the development of uniform concepts of successful prevention, adequate and rapid diagnosis, and efficacious control of hemorrhage. The abnormalities most frequently cited as factors in CPB hemorrhage include (1) inadequate heparin neutralization, (2) protamine excess, (3) heparin rebound, (4) thrombocytopenia, (5) hypofibrinogenemia, (6) primary hyperfibrinolysis, (7) disseminated intravascular coagulation (DIC), (8) isolated coagulation factor deficiencies, (9) transfusion reactions, and (10) hypocalcemia.

The suggestion that all these defects may contribute to CPB hemorrhage clearly demonstrates that the basic pathophysiology of hemostasis during CPB remains confusing to many.

Thrombocytopenia. Early studies of hemostasis during CPB demonstrated significant thrombocytopenia, in the range of 50,000 platelets per cubic millimeter. This was thought to be responsible for CPB hemorrhage. The degree of thrombocytopenia was related to time on bypass, becoming much more pronounced with perfusions lasting longer than 60 minutes. In 1968, Porter and Silver noted that the majority of patients undergoing CPB had platelet counts decreasing to 33 per cent of preoperative counts. In addition, the thrombocytopenia did not abate until several days after CPB. Some surgeons who discover thrombocytopenia during CPB have concluded that this finding may represent thrombocytopenia of DIC.

Others have failed to find significant thrombocytopenia during CPB. This wide variety in experience most likely represents different surgical and pumping techniques, such as flow rate, normothermic versus hypothermic perfusion, particular oxygenation mechanisms used, time on bypass, and priming solution used. Figure 24–21 demonstrates changes in platelet number during CPB. The particular type of oxygenation mecha-

nism used appears to play a minor causative role in thrombocytopenia. The mechanisms most commonly cited as factors in the development of CPB thrombocytopenia are (1) hemodilution, (2) formation of intravascular platelet thrombi, (3) platelet utilization in the pump or oxygenation system or both, and (4) peripheral utilization due to DIC. One study has failed to find a correlation between CPB hematocrit and platelet count, suggesting that hemodilution is not a major factor. Indeed, the role, if any, of these mechanisms in producing CPB thrombocytopenia remains unclear.

Platelet Function Defects. In spite of numerous investigations regarding platelet number during CPB, there has been a surprising lack of interest in assessing platelet function. Early investigators suspected development of abnormal platelet function by noting faulty clot retraction; however, other abnormal parameters known to effect clot retraction, such as hypofibrinogenemia and thrombocytopenia, were also present. Another early study by Holswade and coworkers assessed platelet adhesion before patients were placed on CPB but failed to evaluate platelet function during or after bypass. In this study, abnormal preoperative platelet adhesion was associated with increased postoperative bleeding. Salzman studied platelet adhesion before, during, and after CPB and noted abnormal adhesion in all patients during bypass. However, the significance of this defect was difficult to evaluate, since all patients were markedly thrombocytopenic. Further information obtained from this study was that heparin, in doses used during CPB, does not alter platelet adhesion. It was concluded that a circulating anticoagulant might be responsible for this platelet function defect, since the plasma from CPB patients altered adhesion when added to normal platelets. This "anticoagulant" probably represented FDP.

More recently, platelet function studies have been performed in patients without thrombocytopenia undergoing CPB. Platelet function becomes

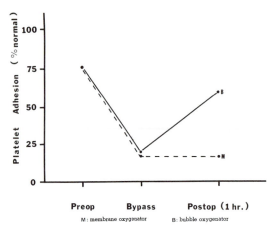

Figure 24–22 Platelet function during cardiopulmonary bypass.

profoundly abnormal in most patients at the initiation of bypass. Little correlation is noted between hematocrit, fibrinogen level, or FDP titer and abnormal platelet function. Figure 24–22 depicts platelet function changes during CPB. This degree of abnormal platelet function would be expected to compromise hemostasis significantly.

Many factors, some possibly altered by CPB, may affect platelet function as assessed by adhesion. These include (1) pH, (2) absolute platelet count, (3) hematocrit, (4) drugs, and (5) the presence of FDP. Although there are several studies that do not clearly define reasons for abnormal platelet function during CPB, they do suggest that several of the aforementioned mechanisms are most likely not involved. The finding of platelet counts greater than 100,000/mm^3 and hematocrits greater than 30 per cent in most patients with markedly abnormal platelet function at 1 hour after CPB suggests that these two parameters do not account for altered platelet function. In addition, patients have normal or near-normal pH at 1 hour following CPB. Heparin, in levels higher than those attained in patients undergoing CPB, has been shown not to alter platelet adhesion. Circulating FDP are known to interfere with platelet function, and these are often present during CPB. However, there has been poor correlation noted between levels of circulating FDP and degree of abnormal platelet function during CPB.

Other possible mechanisms for abnormal platelet function during CPB include (1) platelet membrane damage by shearing forces or contact with foreign material, resulting in partial release of platelet contents, (2) platelet membrane coating with nonspecific proteins, (3) incomplete platelet release, and (4) nonspecific platelet damage induced by fast flow rates. No studies done thus far allow conclusions to be drawn regarding the contribution of any of these mechanisms. One study by Harker has demonstrated selective alpha-granule release from platelets during CPB.

Regardless of mechanisms involved, studies to date clearly reveal a significant functional platelet defect in most patients undergoing CPB. The magnitude of this defect would certainly be expected to compromise hemostasis during and after CPB. In addition, patients ingesting drugs known to interfere with platelet function would be expected to have more blood loss than those not ingesting these agents.

Vascular Defects. Little attention has been devoted to vascular defects during CPB. A syndrome of mild to moderate nonthrombocytopenic purpura accompanied by splenomegaly and atypical lymphocytosis following CPB has been reported by Behrendt and coworkers. In this series, purpura was benign, self-limiting, and frequently only manifest after discharge from the hospital. Only one patient of seven suffered complications (glomerulonephritis of the type often seen with Schönlein-Henoch purpura) following development of purpura.

In addition, a case of fatal purpura fulminans was reported following extracorporeal circulation for coronary artery bypass. Massive purpura developed on the third postoperative day and was followed by development of progressive renal shutdown. High doses of steroids and low–molecular weight dextran afforded no improvement, and the patient died of renal failure on the eighteenth postoperative day. These two reports suggest the possibility of an inflammatory vasculitis associated with CPB.

Isolated Coagulation Factor Defects. Numerous investigators have examined and reported coagulation factor deficiencies during CPB. A wide variety of observations have been made and, like the finding of thrombocytopenia, may reflect only differences in surgical or pumping techniques (e.g., flow rate and priming solution). Most researchers have noted significant hypofibrinogenemia that does not seem to be correlated with pump time. Some investigators have found fibrinogen levels to be closely correlated with the degree of CPB fibrinolysis. Figure 24–23 depicts correlations noted among fibrinogen, plasminogen, plasmin, and FDP in patients undergoing CPB. Some authors have concluded that hypofibrinogenemia occurs primarily as a consequence of DIC; others have failed to find hypofibrinogenemia during CPB. It seems reasonable to conclude that hypofibrinogenemia, secondary to hyperfibrino(geno)lysis, is a frequent occurrence during CPB.

Other coagulation factors most often found decreased and reported to play a role in CPB hemorrhage are Factors II, V, and VIII. As with hypofibrinogenemia, some authors conclude that these changes are secondary to DIC, whereas others think that these decreases are secondary to a primary fibrino(geno)lytic syndrome. Others yet have failed to find significant decreases in most coagulation factors, and some have reported increased Factor VIII levels during CPB.

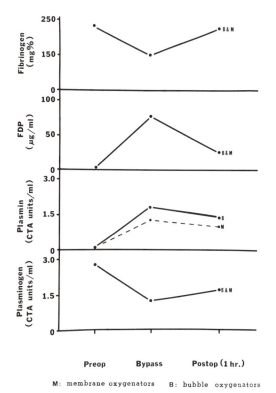

Figure 24–23 Activation of the fibrinolytic system during cardiopulmonary bypass.

Disseminated Intravascular Coagulation. The question of whether DIC develops during and after CPB has led to confusion regarding altered hemostasis. Numerous early studies concluded that DIC is present during CPB, based on the observations that coagulation factors were decreased. The findings of fibrinogen, Factor VIII, or prothrombin complex factor deficiencies were often assumed to be secondary to DIC, without appropriate confirmatory tests being performed. Current evidence suggests that, in view of massive heparinization and the absence of significant or uniform thrombocytopenia, DIC is not associated with CPB. Thus, although most early, and several more recent, studies have led to detection of primary hyperfibrino(geno)lysis in association with CPB, a few investigators have concluded that DIC is present. These conclusions most likely derive from the marked superficial similarities between primary hyperfibrino(geno)lysis and DIC with secondary lysis and from the difficulty in rendering a clear-cut differential diagnosis between these two states in the absence of sophisticated and complete coagulation studies.

Primary Hyperfibrino(geno)lysis. Fibrinolytic activity is generally decreased or inhibited during and following most general surgical procedures. However, most investigators, utilizing a variety of laboratory modalities, have found increased fibrinolysis during and after CPB. Many early studies

of hemostasis during CPB assessed the extent of fibrinolysis with the euglobulin lysis time (ELT), and thus the finding of fibrinolysis with CPB remained of unclear significance for a long period in view of recognized inadequacies of this technique. More recent studies, which have involved more specific methods for assessing fibrinolysis, have confirmed earlier reports of a primary hyperfibrino(geno)lytic syndrome in the majority of patients undergoing CPB. Figure 24–23 depicts changes in the fibrinolytic system in patients undergoing CPB.

Because of early reports of primary hyperfibrino(geno)lysis detected during CPB, the empiric use of antifibrinolytic agents, usually aminocaproic acid (ACA), has become commonplace despite attendant hazards of this agent, which include hypokalemia, hypotension, ventricular arrhythmias, and DIC. Controlled studies with and without antifibrinolytic agents have failed to reveal any clear-cut differences in CPB hemorrhage. Gomes and McGoon as well as Tsuji and coworkers have shown an increase in post-CPB hemorrhage with the empiric use of antifibrinolytics. Since primary hyperfibrino(geno)lysis occurs in the majority of patients subjected to CPB, it seems likely that activation of the fibrinolytic system may be occurring in the oxygenation mechanism or, alternatively, that pump-induced accelerated flow rates may activate the plasminogen-plasmin system or may alter endothelial plasminogen activator activity. In fact, the pathogenesis of fibrinolytic activation during CPB remains totally unclear. The degree of fibrinolysis appears to be equal between bubble and membrane oxygenation systems.

Other Defects. Heparin rebound and inadequate heparin neutralization are rarely, if ever, seen. In fact, heparin rebound, as well as inadequate heparin neutralization, has been poorly documented as a cause of CPB hemorrhage. Likewise, protamine excess has been occasionally incriminated in CPB hemorrhage. However, several carefully studied series have failed to demonstrate this phenomenon in a single patient undergoing CPB. In addition, although protamine sulfate is a well known in vitro anticoagulant, it is unlikely that it causes in vivo hemorrhage.

Several authors have reported both coagulation defects and significant CPB hemorrhage to be associated with hypothermic perfusion.

Many patients undergoing coronary artery bypass for coronary occlusive disease have been on warfarin. In their 1972 reports, Verska and associates noted that although the prothrombin time had returned to normal prior to CPB, these patients demonstrated more hemorrhage than patients not previously warfarinized. In one study, they noted increased hemorrhage to be associated with a repeat CPB procedure. Other investigators, however, have noted no increased hemorrhage to be associated with a second CPB procedure. Also, patients undergoing CPB for correction of cyanotic heart disease appear to have more severe derangements in hemostasis during perfusion than those with noncyanotic heart disease.

Predisposing factors that seem to be associated with enhanced CPB hemorrhage are (1) longer pump runs, (2) prior ingestion of warfarin drugs, (3) cyanotic heart disease, and (4) preoperative ingestion of drugs interfering with platelet function. More importantly, evidence suggests that the majority of patients undergoing CPB develop a primary hyperfibrino(geno)lytic syndrome. Although the exact triggering mechanism or mechanisms for this syndrome remain unclear, the resultant secondary alterations in hemostasis would certainly create a potential for hemorrhage. In addition, virtually all patients undergoing CPB develop a severe platelet function defect. It is not clear whether this defect is due to (1) coating of platelet surfaces by FDP, (2) membrane damage from the oxygenation mechanism, (3) platelet damage from fast flow rates, or (4) other unrecognized mechanisms. Whatever the triggering mechanisms, it is quite clear that the most significant alterations in hemostasis associated with CPB are primary hyperfibrino(geno)lysis and defective platelet function. These two defects, alone or in combination, account for the majority of nonsurgical and nontechnical hemorrhage in patients undergoing CPB. Preliminary studies suggest that the frequency and severity of functional platelet defects and primary hyperfibrino(geno)lysis are equal with membrane or bubble type oxygenators. However, thrombocytopenia appears to be less of a problem with the membrane oxygenation mechanism.

PREVENTION

Since hemorrhage associated with CPB is usually catastrophic and often life-threatening, caution must be emphasized in attending to differential diagnosis and rapid, efficacious therapy. Much attention must be given to prevention of CPB hemorrhage with respect to uncovering hereditary, acquired, or drug-induced bleeding diatheses before a patient is subjected to this procedure. The combination of an already existing bleeding diathesis, when coupled with alterations of CPB-induced hemostasis, may lead to disastrous results.

Many cases of CPB hemorrhage could be prevented by simply obtaining an adequate hemostasis history. Ideally, this should be obtained before hospital admission so that there is time for appropriate evaluation if a potential problem is uncovered.

The family history should always include inquiry about bleeding tendencies in parents, siblings, and offspring. Often neglected is a detailed drug history. Many cases of CPB hemorrhage have been attributed to the ingestion of drugs known to interfere with hemostasis. Figure 24–24 demonstrates the sequence of events in a patient ingesting aspirin before CPB. Many drugs interfere with hemostasis, and, in many instances, the bleeding is mild in nature. However, when drug-induced defects are combined with hemostatic defects induced during CPB, hemorrhage may reach alarming proportions. Drugs may interfere with hemostasis by many mechanisms, but most commonly ingested drugs interfere with platelet function. Aspirin, aspirin-containing compounds, antihista-

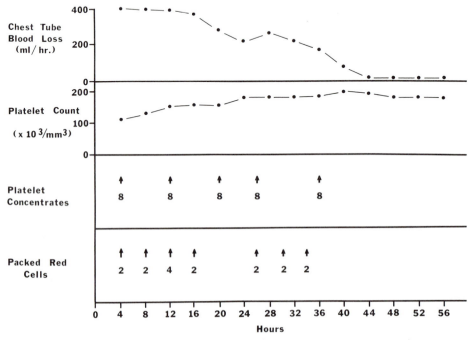

Figure 24–24 Bleeding due to aspirin ingestion prior to cardiopulmonary bypass.

mines, phenylbutazone, and papaverine-containing vasodilating drugs are the most common offenders in CPB patients.

If the drug history is positive and CPB is elective, surgery should be postponed for a full 14 days, since most drugs interfering with platelet function are generally effective for about 2 weeks, and this time period may be required for platelet function to return to normal. If the drug history is positive for antiplatelet agents and CPB is emergent, the patient should be given platelet concentrates (6 to 8 units for an adult) immediately prior to bypass, and the same quantity should be given immediately after the patient leaves the operating room and then each morning for 2 postoperative days. This approach is vigorous but certainly rewarding if life-threatening hemorrhage is avoided as a result.

The general appearance of the patient often provides hints of a bleeding tendency. Subtle hints of an occult bleeding tendency are uncovered by careful observation of the mucous membranes and skin. The finding of mucosal petechiae, purpura, or significant telangiectasia should be searched for and explained, if present. Likewise, petechiae, purpura, significant ecchymoses, and telangiectasia of the skin or nail beds are often suggestive of a vascular defect, a functional platelet defect, or significant thrombocytopenia. If any of these findings are present, they should be investigated and thoroughly explained before CPB is attempted. The usual physical findings of more common disorders associated with a significant hemorrhagic tendency, such as chronic liver disease, hypersplenism, chronic renal disease, rheumatoid arthritis, and systemic lupus, should also serve as an index of predisposition to hemorrhage. Prior laboratory screening will usually suggest the presence of any of these disorders if characteristic physical findings are absent. It should be emphasized that a bleeding disorder rarely, if ever, contraindicates CPB, provided the defect is first delineated and a sound approach to correcting hemostasis during CPB and during the postoperative period is designed.

Any preoperative laboratory screen should generally be simple and incur a minimal expense to the patient while providing adequate information. Usually, however, we tend to be too simple with respect to presurgical and, in particular, pre-CPB hemostasis screens.

The usually ordered biochemical survey, evaluation of electrolytes, and CBC will detect those common acquired disorders often associated with a bleeding tendency (e.g., chronic liver disease, chronic renal disease, and hypersplenism or bone marrow failure). Most commonly, a pre-CPB hemostasis screen consists of a prothrombin time, an activated partial thromboplastin time, and a platelet count. Although these tests will detect the majority of defects, they provide no information about vascular or platelet function and ignore fibrinolysis. Thus, two additional procedures should be performed as part of the routine preoperative screen. A standardized template bleeding time, as described by Mielke and coworkers, is performed on all patients. This provides a screen for adequate vascular and platelet function. In addition, a thrombin time is performed. The resultant clot is observed for 5 minutes after the test is run. A normal thrombin time and the absence of lysis after 5 minutes assures the absence of significant hypofibrinogenemia, dysfibrinogenemia, fibrinolysis, and FDP elevation. If hypothermic perfusion is to be performed, cryoglobulins should also be tested for.

CLINICAL AND LABORATORY DIAGNOSIS

When bleeding occurs during or after bypass, it is important for the surgeon to define the defect as quickly as possible. Many instances of CPB hemorrhage are due to inadequate surgical technique, but alterations of hemostasis may also be responsible or may accentuate surgical CPB bleeding. The reasons for bleeding occurring during CPB are limited and are depicted in Table 24–28 in their order of occurrence.

The primary distinction to be made immediately is between strictly surgical bleeding, defects in hemostasis, or a combination of the two. This distinction becomes more difficult and more important after the patient has left the operating room. During this period, a decision must be made regarding re-exploration and the adequacy of hemostasis for re-exploration. In distinguishing between surgical and nonsurgical bleeding, many physical findings are helpful. Is the bleeding localized or systemic? Hematuria, petechiae/purpura, and oozing from intravenous sites in conjunction with increased chest tube blood loss usually mean a hemostatic defect, whereas increased chest tube bleeding alone often signifies a surgical bleed.

As soon as CPB hemorrhage is seen or suspected, the following laboratory tests are ordered: PT, PTT, reptilase time, heparin assay, fibrin/fibrinogen degradation products, peripheral blood smear, platelet count, and plasminogen/plasmin levels. The physician obtains evidence for primary lysis by noting the FDP level hypoplasminogene-

TABLE 24–28 BLEEDING SYNDROMES
ASSOCIATED WITH
CARDIOPULMONARY BYPASS
(In Descending Order of Probability)

A. Platelet function defect
   1. CPB-induced
   2. Drug-induced
B. Primary fibrino(geno)lysis
C. Thrombocytopenia
D. Hyperheparinemia/heparin rebound?
E. Disseminated intravascular coagulation? (independent trigger required)

mia and by observing lysis of the reptilase clot. A smear and platelet count are essential to rapid evaluation of the potential of thrombocytopenic bleeding. The plasminogen and plasmin levels are time-consuming and are not used for an immediate diagnosis, but they are invaluable when the physician is making decisions regarding antifibrinolytic therapy at a later time.

If significant primary hyperfibrino(geno)lysis is present, FDP will be elevated, and plasminogen depletion and circulating plasmin will be noted.

All patients undergoing CPB display a platelet function defect. When bleeding occurs, it is wise to assume platelet dysfunction to be present, and, although this might not represent the primary reason for hemorrhage, platelet dysfunction will be additive to any other defect, regardless of whether it is surgical or due to altered hemostasis.

MANAGEMENT

When the physician first sees a patient with CPB hemorrhage, it is of prime importance for him to (1) note the type of bleeding (systemic vs. local), (2) order a laboratory screen as outlined previously, and (3) administer 6 to 8 units of platelet concentrates as quickly as possible. The administration of platelet concentrates while one is awaiting laboratory evaluation will often stop or significantly blunt most hemorrhages.

If a functional platelet defect, or thrombocytopenia, is found to be responsible for hemorrhage (with no laboratory evidence of significant fibrinolysis), hemorrhage should be controlled by platelet transfusions.

Hyperheparinemia and heparin rebound, if suspected to be a real clinical problem, are managed by administration of protamine. Once again, it should be emphasized that hyperheparinemia and heparin rebound are not likely to be responsible for bleeding and should not be dwelled upon unless concrete laboratory evidence of hyperheparinemia is present and evidence of primary lysis is clearly absent. Similarly, protamine excess is rarely, if ever, a clinical problem and should never require therapy.

Primary hyperfibrino(geno)lysis is commonly present and may or may not be responsible for hemorrhage. This syndrome should not be treated empirically, but antifibrinolytics should be considered if the patient has failed to respond to platelet concentrates and if there is reasonable laboratory evidence for hyperfibrino(geno)lysis.

Summary. The primary pathology of altered hemostasis during CPB appears to be twofold: (1) a functional platelet defect of unclear etiology, which occurs in virtually all patients, and (2) a primary hyperfibrino(geno)lytic defect, which oc-

curs in the majority of patients. Significant thrombocytopenia does not appear to be a consistent problem and is probably a function of perfusion techniques. This may, however, be an important source of hemorrhage in some instances. Although hyperheparinemia, heparin rebound, and protamine excess have occasionally been incriminated as sources of hemorrhage during CPB, no well-documented cases appear in the literature. Likewise, although DIC gained popularity in early reports of CPB hemorrhage, it appears that this syndrome rarely, if ever, arises as a consequence of CPB alone. It can be seen, however, in CPB patients who are provided with a trigger such as shock, sepsis, or hemolytic transfusion reactions. It is likely that many reported alterations of hemostasis during CPB that were thought to represent DIC actually were due to hyperfibrino(geno)lysis.

The vast majority of cases of nonsurgical hemorrhage during CPB are due to a functional platelet defect, primary hyperfibrino(geno)lysis, or a combination of the two. Prompt administration of platelet concentrates while one is awaiting laboratory evaluation will control or significantly blunt most CPB hemorrhages. If platelets fail to control bleeding and reasonable laboratory evidence of primary hyperfibrino(geno)lysis is present, antifibrinolytics should then be used.

CPB hemorrhage remains a very real problem in altering morbidity and mortality as well as in taxing blood banks. However, most instances of nonsurgical CPB hemorrhage are due to several well-defined defects in hemostasis, which should be readily controllable if approached in a logical manner and as a team effort among cardiac surgeons, pathologists, and hematologists.

HYPERFIBRINO(GENO)LYSIS IN MALIGNANCY

Solid tumors have been reported to be associated with a clinical hyperfibrino(geno)lytic syndrome. The spectrum of tumors involved is wide, but the most pronounced effect is seen in sarcomas. For the most part, the mechanism or mechanisms by which this occurs remain poorly understood. In several instances, tissue extracts from biopsy specimens, when purified, have demonstrated the ability to either directly or indirectly activate the fibrinolytic system. This has been noted especially with tissue homogenates from gastric carcinoma, sarcomas, and prostatic carcinoma. The initiation or primary fibrinolysis or a continuous "thrombolytic state" may be of benefit in impeding fibrin formation and tumor metastases. Doxorubicin and daunomycin have been shown to activate fibrinolysis. Doxorubicin is a commonly used antineoplastic agent, especially for breast carcinoma, and daunomycin is a mainstay form of therapy for the acute leukemias. Both agents are capable of inducing in vivo activation of the fibrinolytic system, which is not secondary to DIC. The precise mechanism or mechanisms of activation remain unclear. This fibrinolytic response may be of benefit to the patient with respect to tumor cell metastases and primary tumor growth, as these processes are thought to be facilitated by fibrin deposition. In addition, it has been noted that nicotinic acid is capable of fibrinolytic system activation by unclear mechanisms.

REFERENCES

Basic Physiology of Hemostasis
Mechanisms of Hemostasis
Murano, G.: A basic outline of blood coagulation. Semin. Thromb. Hemost. 6:140, 1980.
Ratnoff, O. D.: "Why do people bleed?" *In* Wintrobe, M. M. (Ed.): Blood, Pure and Eloquent. New York, McGraw-Hill Book Co., 1980, p. 601.

The Vasculature
Barnhart, M. I., and Baecher, C. A.: Endothelial cell physiology, perturbations, and response. Semin. Thromb. Hemost. 5:50, 1979.
Roberts, W. C., and Ferrans, V. J.: The role of platelets in the etiology of atherosclerosis (a positive one) and in precipitating fatal ischemic heart disease (a negative one). Semin. Thromb. Hemost. 2:123, 1976.
Santos de los, R. P., and Hoyer, L. W.: Antihemophilic factor in tissue; localization of immunofluorescence. Fed. Proc. 31:279, 1972.

The Platelets
Gerrard, J. M., and White, J. G.: Prostaglandins and thromboxanes: "middlemen" modulating platelet function in hemostasis and thrombosis. Prog. Hemost. Thromb. 4:87, 1978.
Henry, R. L.: Platelet function in hemostasis. *In* Murano, G., and Bick, R. L. (Eds.): Basic Concepts of Hemostasis and Thrombosis. Boca Raton, FL, CRC Press, 1980, p. 17.
McCoy, L. E.: Vascular function in hemostasis. *In* Murano, G., and Bick, R. L. (Eds.): Basic Concepts of Hemostasis and Thrombosis. Boca Raton, FL, CRC Press, 1980, p. 5.
Nalbandian, R. M., and Henry, R. L.: Platelet-endothelial interactions: metabolic maps of structures and actions of prostaglandins, prostacyclines, thromboxane, and cyclic AMP. Semin. Thromb. Hemost. 5:87, 1978.
Salzman, E. W.: Cyclic AMP and platelet function. N. Engl. J. Med. 286:358, 1972.

Blood Protein Function
Finlayson, J. S.: Crosslinking of fibrin. Sem. Thromb. Hemostas. 1:33, 1974.
Murano, G.: Plasma protein function in hemostasis. *In* Murano, G., and Bick, R. L. (Eds.): Basic Concepts of Hemostasis and Thrombosis. Boca Raton, FL, CRC Press, 1980, p. 43.
Ratnoff, O. D.: The molecular basis of hereditary clotting disorders. *In* Spaet, T. (Ed.): Progress in Hemostasis and Thrombosis 1:39, 1972.
Seegers, W. H.: Enzymes in blood clotting. J. Med. Enzymol. 2:68, 1972.
Seegers, W. H., Hassouna, H. I., Hewett-Emmett, D., et al.: Prothrombin and thrombin: selected topics of thrombin formation, properties, inhibition, and immunology. Semin. Thromb. Hemost. 1:211, 1975.
Walz, D. A., Seegers, W. H., Roeterby, J., and McCoy, L. E.: Proteolytic specificity of thrombin. Thromb. Res. 4:713, 1974.

Contact Activation
Griffin, J. H., and Cochran, C. H.: Recent advances in the understanding of contact activation reactions. Sem. Thromb. Hemostas. 5:254, 1979.

The Fibrinolytic System
Bang, N. U.: Physiology and biochemistry of the fibrinolytic system. *In* Bang, N. U., Beller, K. F., Deutsch, E., and Mammen, E. F. (Eds.): Thrombosis and Bleeding Disorders. New York, Academic Press, 1971, p. 292.
Bang, N., and Chang, M. L.: Soluble fibrin complexes. Semin. Thromb. Hemost. 1:91, 1974.
Barnhart, M. I., and Baecher, C. A.: Endothelial cell physiology, perturbations, and response. Semin. Thromb. Hemost. 5:50, 1979.
Barnhart, M. I., and Riddle, J. M.: Cellular localization of profibrinolysin (plasminogen). Blood 21:306, 1963.
Kaplan, M. H.: Nature and role of the lytic factor in hemolytic streptococcal fibrinolysis. Proc. Soc. Exp. Biol. Med. 57:40, 1944.
Kopec, M., Budzynski, A. Z., Stachurska, J., Wegrzynowicz, Z., and Kowalski, E.: Studies on the mechanism of interference by fibrinogen degradation products (FDP) with platelet function. Thromb. Diath. Haemorrh. 15:476, 1966.
Kopec, M., Wegrzynowicz, Z., Budzynski, A. Z., et al.: Interaction of fibrinogen degradation products (FDP) with platelets. Exp. Biol. Med. 3:73, 1968.
Kowalski, E.: Fibrinogen-derived inhibitors of blood coagulation. Thromb. Diath. Haemorrh. 4:211, 1960.
Kowalski, E.: Fibrinogen derivatives and their biological activities. Sem. Hematol. 5:45, 1968.
Marder, V. J., and Budzynski, A. Z.: The structure of fibrinogen degradation products. Prog. Hemost. Thromb. 2:141, 1974.
Mosesson, M.: Fibrinogen catabolic pathways. Semin. Thromb. Hemost. 1:63, 1974.
Murano, G.: The Hageman connection: interrelationships of blood coagulation, fibrino(geno)lysis, kinin generation, and complement activation. Am. J. Hematol. 4:303, 1978.
Murano, G.: Plasma protein function in hemostasis. *In* Murano, G., and Bick, R. L. (Eds.): Basic Concepts of Hemostasis and Thrombosis. Boca Raton, FL, CRC Press, 1980, p. 43.
Murano, G., and Bick, R. L.: Thrombolytic therapy. *In* Murano, G., and Bick, R. L. (Eds.): Basic Concepts of Hemostasis and Thrombosis. Boca Raton, FL, CRC Press, 1980, p. 259.
Reeve, E. N., and Franks, J. J.: Fibrinogen synthesis, distribution, and degradation. Sem. Thromb. Hemostas. 1:129, 1974.
Robbins, K. M.: Present status of the fibrinolytic system. *In* Fareed, J., Messmore, H. L., Fenton, J., and Brinkhous, K. M. (Eds.): Perspectives in Hemostasis. Elmsford, NY, Pergamon Press, 1981, p. 53.

Kinins, Complement, and Coagulation
Donaldson, V. H., Glueck, H. I., Miller, M. A., et al.: Kininogen deficiency in Fitzgerald trait: role of high molecular weight kininogen in clotting and fibrinolysis. J. Lab. Clin. Med. 87:327, 1976.
Eisen, V.: Kinin forming enzymes and substrates in human plasma. J. Physiol. (London) 186:133, 1966.
Frank, M. M.: Complement: current concepts. Kalamazoo, MI., Upjohn, 1975.
Guest, M., Murphy, R. C., Bodnar, S. R., et al.: Physiological effects of a plasma protein; blood pressure, leukocyte concentration, smooth and cardiac muscle activity. Am. J. Physiol. 150:471, 1947.

Kaplan, A. P., and Austen, K. F.: A prealbumin activator of prekallikrein. J. Immunol. *105*:802, 1970.

Kaplan, A. P., Meier, H. L., and Mandle, R.: The Hageman factor dependent pathways of coagulation, fibrinolysis, and kinin generation. Semin. Thromb. Hemost. *3*:1, 1976.

Margolis, J.: Activation of plasma by contact with glass, evidence for a common reaction which releases plasma kinin and initiates coagulation. J. Physiol. (London) *144*:1, 1958.

Muller-Eberhard, H. J.: Complement. Annu. Rev. Biochem. *44*:697, 1975.

Ratnoff, O. D.: The interrelationship of clotting and immunological mechanisms. *In* Good, R. A., and Fisher, D. W. (Eds.): Immunology. Sunderland, MA, Sinauer Association, 1971, p. 135.

Ratnoff, O. D., and Naff, G. B.: The conversion of C'1s to C'1 esterase by plasmin and trypsin. J. Exp. Med. *125*:337, 1967.

Rocha e Silva, M., Beraldo, W. T., and Rosenfeld, G.: Bradykinin, a hypotensive and smooth muscle stimulating factor released from plasma globulin by snake venoms and trypsin. Am. J. Physiol. *156*:261, 1949.

Ruddy, S., Gigli, I., and Austen, K. F.: The complement system of man. N. Engl. J. Med. *287*:489, 1972.

Schrieber, A. D., and Austen, F.: Interrelationships of the fibrinolytic, coagulation, kinin generating and complement system. Ser. Haematol. *6*:593, 1973.

Seidel, G.: Two functionally different kininogens in human plasma. Agents Actions *3*:12, 1973.

Taylor, F. B., and Ward, P. A.: Generation of chemotactic activity in rabbit serum by plasminogen-streptokinase mixtures. J. Exp. Med. *126*:149, 1967.

Ulutin, O. N.: The platelets: fundamentals and clinical applications. Istanbul, Turkey, Kagit Ve Basim Isleri, A. S., 1976.

Inhibitory Mechanisms

Bick, R. L., and Shanbrom, E.: A systemic approach to the diagnosis of bleeding disorders. Med. Counterpoint *6*:27, 1972.

Hatton, M. W. C., and Regoeczi, E.: The inactivation of thrombin and plasmin by antithrombin III in the presence of sepharose-heparin. Thromb. Res. *10*:645, 1977.

Murano, G.: Theory of blood coagulation in DIC. Folia Haematol. (Leipz.) *97*:5, 1972.

Pomerantz, M. W., and Owen, W. G.: A catalytic role for heparin: evidence for a ternary complex of heparin cofactor, thrombin, and heparin. Biochim. Biophys. Acta. *535*:66, 1978.

Rosenberg, R. D.: Biologic actions of heparin. Semin. Hematol. *14*:427, 1977.

Seegers, W. H.: Basic principles of blood coagulation. Semin. Thromb. Hemost. *7*:180, 1981.

Seegers, W. H.: Antithrombin III. Semin. Thromb. Hemostas. *7*:263, 1981.

Seegers, W. H.: Protein C and autoprothrombin II-A Sem. Thromb. Hemostas. *7*:257, 1981.

Seegers, W. H., Hassouna, H. I., Hewett-Emmett, D., et al.: Prothrombin and thrombin: selected topics of thrombin formation, properties, inhibition, and immunology. Sem. Thromb. Hemostas. *1*:211, 1975.

VASCULAR DISORDERS

Clinical Manifestations

Bick, R. L.: Vascular disorders associated with thrombohemorrhagic phenomena. Semin. Thromb. Hemost. *5*:167, 1979.

Bick, R. L.: Vascular disorders. *In* Murano, G., and Bick, R. L. (Eds.): Basic Concepts of Hemostasis and Thrombosis. Boca Raton, FL, CRC Press, 1980, p. 89.

Fairbairn, J. F.: An approach to the patient with peripheral vascular disease. *In* Fairbairn, J. F., Juergens, J. L., and Spittel, S. A. (Eds.): Vascular Diseases. Philadelphia, W. B. Saunders Co., 1972.

Ryan, T. J.: The Investigation of Vasculitis in Microvascular Injury. Philadelphia, W. B. Saunders Co., 1976, p. 333.

Hereditary Vascular Disorders

Anderson, M., and Pratt-Thomas, R. H.: Marfan's syndrome. Am. Heart J. *46*:911, 1953.

Bick, R. L.: Hereditary hemorrhagic telangiectasia and disseminated intravascular coagulation: a new clinical syndrome.

In Walz, D., and McCoy, L. E. (Eds.): Contributions to Hemostasis. Ann. N.Y. Acad. Sci. *370*:851, 1981.

Good, T. A., Carnazzo, S. F., and Good, R. A.: Thrombocytopenia and giant hemangiomata in infants. Am. J. Dis. Child. *90*:260, 1955.

Hans, F. M.: Multiple hereditary telangiectasia causing hemorrhage (hereditary hemorrhagic telangiectasia). Bull. Johns Hopkins Hosp. *20*:63, 1909.

Harrison, D. F. N.: Familial haemorrhagic telangiectasia. Quart. J. Med. *33*:25, 1964.

Hillman, R. S., and Phillips, L. L.: Clotting—fibrinolysis in a cavernous hemangiomata. Am. J. Dis. Child. *113*:649, 1967.

Inceman, S., and Tangun, Y.: Chronic defibrination syndrome due to a giant hemangioma associated with microangiopathic hemolytic anemia. Am. J. Med. *46*:997, 1969.

Johnson, S. A., and Falls, E. F.: Ehlers-Danlos syndrome: a clinical and genetic study. Arch. Derm. Suppl. *60*:82, 1949.

Pinnell, S. R., Krane, S. M., Kenzora, J., and Glincher, M. J.: A new heritable disorder of connective tissue with hydroxylysine-deficient collagen. N. Engl. J. Med. *286*:1013, 1972.

Polimer, I. J.: Pseudoxanthoma elasticum and gastrointestinal bleeding. J. Maine Med. Assoc. *58*:76, 1967.

Roberts, H. R., and Kroncke, F. G.: Tests of platelet activity: application to clinical diagnosis. *In* Brinkhous, K. M., Shermer, R. W., and Mostofi, F. K. (Eds.): The Platelet. Baltimore, Williams and Wilkins, 1971, p. 365.

Seibel, B. M., Briedman, I. A., and Schwartz, S. O.: Hemorrhagic disease in osteogenesis imperfecta: studies of platelet function defect. Am. J. Med. *22*:315, 1957.

Acquired Vascular Disorders

Behrendt, P. M., Epstein, S. E., and Marrow, A. G.: Postperfusion nonthrombocytopenic purpura: an uncommon sequel of open heart surgery. Am. J. Cardiol. *22*:631, 1968.

Bick, R. L., Comer, T. P., and Arbegast, N. R.: Fatal purpura fulminans following total cardiopulmonary bypass. J. Cardiovasc. Surg. (Torino) *14*:569, 1973.

Dixon, F. J., Vazquez, J. J., Wrigle, W. D., and Cochrane, C. G.: Pathogenesis of serum sickness. Arch. Pathol. *65*:18, 1958.

Farber, E. M., Hines, E. A., Montgomery, H., and Craig, W.: Arterioles of skin in essential hypertension. J. Invest. Dermatol. *9*:215, 1947.

Furie, B., Greene, E., and Furie, B. C.: Syndrome of acquired Factor X deficiency and systemic amyloidosis. N. Engl. J. Med. *297*:81, 1977.

Galbraith, P. A., Sharma, N., Parker, W. L., and Kilgour, J. M.: Acquired Factor X deficiency. Altered plasma antithrombin activity and association with amyloidosis. J.A.M.A. *230*:1658, 1974.

Glenner, G. G.: Factor X deficiency and systemic amyloidosis. N. Engl. J. Med. *297*:108, 1977.

Haim, S., Sabel, J. D., and Friedman-Birnbaum, R.: Thrombophlebitis and a cardinal symptom of Behçet's syndrome. Acta Derm. Venereol. *54*:299, 1974.

Kazmier, F. J., Didisheim, P., Fairbanks, V. F., et al.: Intravascular coagulation and arterial disease. Thromb. Diath. Haemorrh. Suppl. *36*:296, 1969.

Markowitz, A. S., and Lang, C. F.: Streptococcal related glomerulonephritis. J. Immunol. *92*:565, 1964.

Nalbandian, R. M., Mader, I. J., Barrett, J. L., et al.: Petechiae, ecchymoses, and necrosis of skin induced by coumarin cogeners. J.A.M.A. *192*:603, 1965.

Stefanini, M., and Mednicoff, I. B.: Demonstration of antivessel agents in serum of patients with anaphylactoid purpura and polyarteritis nodosa. J. Clin. Invest. *33*:967, 1954.

PLATELET DEFECTS

Qualitative Platelet Defects

Adams, T., Schultz, L., and Goldberg, L. S.: Platelet function abnormalities in the myeloproliferative disorders. Scand. J. Haematol. *13*:215, 1974.

Bernard, J., and Soulier, J. P.: Sur une nouvelle variété de dystrophic thrombocytaire hemorragipare congénitale. Semin. Hosp. Paris *24*:3217, 1948.

Bick, R. L.: Acquired circulating anticoagulants and defective hemostasis in malignant paraprotein disorders. *In* Murano,

G., and Bick, R. L. (Eds.): Basic Concepts of Hemostasis and Thrombosis. Boca Raton, FL, CRC Press, 1980, p. 205.

Bick, R. L., Adams, T., and Schamlhorst, W. R.: Bleeding times, platelet adhesion, and aspirin. Am. J. Clin. Pathol. 65:65, 1976.

Braunsteiner, H., and Pakesch, F.: Thrombocytoasthenia and thrombocytopathia: old names and new diseases. Blood 11:965, 1956.

Castaldi, P. A., Rosenberg, M. C., and Stewart, J. H.: The bleeding disorder of uremia. Lancet 2:66, 1966.

Deykin, D.: Hemorrhagic complications of drugs. In Coleman, R. W., Hirsh, J., Marder, V. J., and Salzman, E. W. (Eds.): Hemostasis and Thrombosis, Philadelphia, J. B. Lippincott, 1982, p. 602.

Hirsh, J.: Laboratory diagnosis of thrombosis. In Coleman, R. W., Hirsh, J., Marder, V. J., and Salzman, E. W. (Eds.): Hemostasis and Thrombosis. Philadelphia, J. B. Lippincott, 1982, p. 798.

Inceman, S., and Tangun, Y.: Essential athrombia. Thromb. Diath. Haemorrh. 33:278, 1975.

Kopec, M., Wegrzynowicz, Z., Budzynski, A. Z., et al.: Interaction of fibrinogen degradation products (FDP) with platelets. Exp. Biol. Med. 3:73, 1968.

Kowalski, E.: Fibrinogen derivatives and their biological activities. Semin. Hematol. 5:45, 1968.

Malmsten, C., Hamberg, M., Svenson, J., and Sammuelsson, B.: Physiological role of an endoperoxide in human platelets: hemostatic defect due to platelet cyclo-oxygenase deficiency. Proc. Natl. Acad. Sci. U.S.A. 72:1446, 1975.

Triplett, D.: Platelet function: laboratory evaluation and clinical application. Chicago, Am. Soc. Clin. Path. 1978, p. 123.

Triplett, D. A.: Platelet disorders. In Murano, G., and Bick, R. L. (Eds.): Basic Concepts of Hemostasis and Thrombosis. Boca Raton, FL, CRC Press, 1980, p. 95.

Weiss, H. J.: The pharmacology of platelet inhibition. Prog. Hemost. Thromb. 1:199, 1974.

Weiss, H. J., Chervenick, P. A., Zahiski, R., and Factor, A.: A familial defect in platelet function associated with impaired release of adenosine diphosphate. N. Engl. J. Med. 281:1264, 1969.

Weiss, H. J., and Lages, B. A.: Possible congenital defect in platelet thromboxane synthetase. Lancet 1:760, 1977.

Zucker, S., Mielke, C. H., Durocher, J. R., and Crosby, W. H.: Oozing and bruising due to abnormal platelet function (thrombocytopathia). Ann. Intern. Med. 76:725, 1972.

Quantitative Platelet Defects

Aster, R. H.: Pooling of platelets in the spleen: role in pathogenesis of "hypersplenic" thrombocytopenia. J. Clin. Invest. 45:645, 1966.

Aster, R. H.: Thrombocytopenia due to enhanced platelet destruction. In Williams, W. J., Beutler, E., Erslev, A. J., and Rundles R. W. (Eds.): Hematology. New York, McGraw-Hill, 1977, p. 1326.

Aster, R. H., and Jandl, J. H.: Platelet sequestration in man. J. Clin. Invest. 43:843, 1964.

Baldini, M.: Idiopathic thrombocytopenic purpura. N. Engl. J. Med. 274:1245, 1969.

Bottinger, L. E., and Westerholm, B.: Drug-induced thrombocytopenia. Acta. Med. Scand. 191:541, 1972.

Cooper, B. A., and Bigelow, F. S.: Thrombocytopenia associated with the administration of diethylstilbestrol in man. Ann. Intern. Med. 52:907, 1960.

Davidson, C. S.: Liver Pathophysiology: Its Relevance to Human Disease. Boston, Little, Brown and Co., 1970, p. 169.

Davis, W. M., and Ross, A. O. M.: Thrombocytosis and thrombocythemia. Am. J. Clin. Pathol. 59:243, 1973.

Finch, S. C., Castro, O., Cooper, M., et al.: Immunosuppressive therapy of chronic idiopathic thrombocytopenic purpura. Am. J. Med. 56:4, 1974.

Gunz, F. W.: Hemorrhagic thrombocythemia: a critical review. Blood 15:706, 1960.

Harker, L. A.: Kinetics of thrombopoiesis. J. Clin. Invest. 48:963, 1968.

Hirsh, J., and Dacie, J. V.: Persistent post-splenectomy thrombocytosis and thromboembolism: a consequence of continuing anemia. Br. J. Haematol. 12:44, 1966.

Karpatkin, S., Strick, N., Karpatkin, M. B., and Siskind, G. W.: Accumulative experience in the detection of antiplatelet antibody in 234 patients with idiopathic thrombocytopenic purpura, systemic lupus erythematosus, and other clinical disorders. Am. J. Med. 52:776, 1972.

Kass, G.: Bone Marrow Interpretation. Philadelphia, J. B. Lippincott, 1979, p. 263.

Kutti, J., and Linefield, A.: The frequency of thrombocytopenia in patients with heart disease treated with oral diuretics. Acta Med. Scand. 183:245, 1968.

Nalbandian, R. M., Henry, R. L., and Bick, R. L.: Thrombotic thrombocytopenic purpura. Semin. Thromb. Hemostas. 5:216, 1979.

Petter, H., and Lindsay, S.: Responses of platelets, eosinophils, and total leukocytes during and following surgical procedures. Surg. Gynecol. Obstet. 110:319, 1960.

Poley, J. R., and Stickler, G. B.: Petechiae in the newborn infant. Am. J. Dis. Child. 102:365, 1961.

Rodriquez, S. U., Leiken, S., and Hiller, N. P.: Neonatal thrombocytopenia associated with antepartum administration of thiazide drugs. N. Engl. J. Med. 270:881, 1964.

Thiery, J. P., and Bessis, M.: Mécanisme de la plaquettogenese: étude in vitro par la microtinemategraphie. Rev. Hematol. 11:162, 1956.

Zucker, S., and Mielke, C. N.: Classification of thrombocytosis based on platelet function tests: correlation with hemorrhagic and thrombotic complications. J. Lab. Clin. Med. 80:385, 1972.

HEREDITARY COAGULATION PROTEIN DEFECTS
Hemophilia

Abildgaard, C. F., Simone, J. V., Corrigan, J. J., et al.: Treatment of hemophilia with glycine-precipitated Factor VIII. N. Engl. J. Med. 275:471, 1966.

Aggelar, P. M., White, S. G., Glendening, M. B., et al.: Plasma thromboplastin components (PTC) deficiency: a new disease resembling hemophilia. Proc. Soc. Exp. Biol. Med. 79:692, 1952.

Bick, R. L.: Hereditary plasma protein disorders. In Murano, G., and Bick, R. L. (Eds.): Basic Concepts of Hemostasis and Thrombosis. Boca Raton, FL, CRC Press, 1980, p. 149.

Bick, R. L., Adams, T., and Radack, K.: Surgical hemostasis with a Factor XI–containing concentrate. J.A.M.A. 229:163, 1974.

Blatt, P. M., Lundblad, R. L., Kingdon, H. S., et al.: Thrombogenic materials in prothrombin complex concentrates. Ann. Int. Med. 81:766, 1974.

Breen, F. A., and Tullis, J. L.: Prothrombin concentrate in treatment of Christmas disease and allied disorders. J.A.M.A. 208:1848, 1969.

Brinkhous, K. M.: Clotting defect in hemophilia: deficiency in plasma factor required for platelet utilization. Proc. Soc. Exp. Biol. Med. 66:117, 1947.

Elodi, S., and Puskas, E.: Variants of hemophilia B. Thromb. Diath. Haemorrh. 28:489, 1972.

Fekete, L. F.: The partial thromboplastin time and related assays. In Bick, R. L. (Ed.): Modern Concepts of Hemostasis and Thrombosis, Manual #548. Chicago, Am. Soc. Clin. Pathol., 1978, Chap. 6.

Klein, H. G., Aledort, L. M., Bouman, B. H., et al.: A cooperative study for the detection of the carrier state of classic hemophilia. N. Engl. J. Med. 296:959, 1977.

Kruczynski, E. M., and Penner, J. A.: Activated prothrombin concentrate for patients with Factor VIII inhibitors. N. Engl. J. Med. 291:164, 1974.

Nilsson, I. M., Blomback, M., and Wichel, B.: Inhibitors in hemophilia. Tehran, Proc. 7th Cong. World Fed. Hemophilia, 1971.

Penner, J. A., and Kelly, P. E.: Management of patients with Factor VIII or IX inhibitors. Semin. Thromb. Hemost. 1:386, 1975.

Rosenthal, R. L.: Factor XI: general review. Bibl. Haematologica 23:1350, 1965.

Rosenthal, R. L., Dreskin, O. H., and Rosenthal, N.: New hemophilia-like disease caused by deficiency of a third plasma thromboplastin factor. Proc. Soc. Exp. Biol. Med. 82:171, 1953.

Rosher, F.: Hemophilia in the Talmud and Rabbinic writings. Ann. Int. Med. 70:833, 1969.

Tullis, J. L., Melin, M., and Jurigan, P.: Clinical use of human prothrombin complexes. N. Engl. J. Med. 273:667, 1965.

White, G. C., Roberts, H. R., Kingdon, H. S., and Lundblad, R. L.: Prothrombin complex concentrates: potentially thrombogenic materials and clues to the mechanism of thrombosis in vivo. Blood 49:159, 1977.

von Willebrand's Syndrome

Abildgaard, C. F., Suzuki, Z., Harrison, J., et al.: Serial studies in von Willebrand's disease: variability versus "variants." Blood 56:712, 1980.

Cornu, P., Larrieu, M. J., Caen, J., and Bernard, J.: Transfusion studies in von Willebrand's disease: effect on bleeding time and Factor VIII. Br. J. Haematol. 9:189, 1963.

Hirsh, J.: Laboratory diagnosis of thrombosis. In Coleman, R. W., Hirsh, J., Marder, V. J., and Salzman, E. W. (Eds.): Hemostasis and Thrombosis. Philadelphia, J. B. Lippincott, 1982, p. 798.

Howard, M. A., and Firkin, B. G.: Ristocetin: a new tool in the investigation of platelet aggregation. Thrombo. Diath. Haemorrh. 26:362, 1971.

Meyer, D., Frommel, D., Larrieu, M. J., and Zimmerman, T. S.: Selective absence of large forms of Factor VIII–von Willebrand factor in acquired von Willebrand syndrome: response to transfusion. Blood 54:600, 1979.

Reisner, H. ·M., Price, W. A., Blatt, P. M., et al.: Factor VIII coagulant antigen in hemophilic plasma: a comparison of five alloantibodies. Blood 56:615, 1980.

Salzman, E. W.: Measurement of platelet adhesiveness: a simple in vitro technique demonstrating an abnormality in von Willebrand's disease. J. Lab. Clin. Med. 62:724, 1963.

von Willebrand, E. A., and Jurgens, R.: Uber ein neues vererbbares blutingube: die konstitutionelle thrombopathie. Dtsch. Arch. Klin. Med. 175:453, 1933.

Rare Congenital Coagulation Protein Defects

Bick, R. L., Adams, T., and Goldberg, L. S.: Evidence for a new activation phase clotting abnormality in a patient with the Hughes-Stoven syndrome. Beitr. Pathol. 153:310, 1974.

Duckert, F.: Documentation of the plasma Factor XIII deficiency in man. Ann. N.Y. Acad. Sci. 202:190, 1972.

Hathaway, W. E., Belhasen, L. P., and Hathaway, H. S.: Evidence for a new plasma thromboplastin factor. I. Coagulation studies and physicochemical studies. (Case report). Blood 26:521, 1965.

Hougie, C.: Hemophilia and hemophilioid diseases. In Fundamentals of Blood Coagulation in Clinical Medicine. New York, McGraw-Hill Book Co., 1963.

Jackson, D. P., Beck, E. A., and Charache, P.: Congenital disorders of fibrinogen. Fed. Proc. 24:816, 1965.

Kazmier, F. J., Didisheim, P., Fairbanks, V. F., et al.: Intravascular coagulation and arterial disease. Thromb. Diath. Haemorrh. Suppl. 36:296, 1969.

Mammen, E. F.: Congenital abnormalities of the fibrinogen molecule. Semin. Thromb. Hemost. 1:184, 1974.

Mammen, E. F., Prasad, A. S., Bernhart, M. I., and Au, C. C. : Congenital dysfibrinogenemia: fibrinogen Detroit. J. Clin. Invest. 48:235, 1969.

McPherson, R. A.: Thromboembolism in Hageman trait. Am. J. Clin. Pathol. 68:470, 1977.

Owren, P. A.: Parahemophilia: hemorrhagic diathesis due to absence of a previously unknown clotting factor. Lancet 2:446, 1947.

Saito, H., Ratnoff, O. D., Waldmann, R., and Abraham, J. P.: Fitzgerald trait: deficiency of a hitherto unrecognized agent, Fitzgerald factor, participating in surface-mediated reactions of clotting, fibrinolysis, generation of kinins, and the property of diluted plasma enhancing vascular permeability (PF/DIL). J. Clin. Invest. 55:1082, 1975.

Van Crevald, S., and Veder, H. A.: Congenital hypoproconvertinemia. Ann. Paedriat. 190:316, 1958.

ACQUIRED HEMOSTASIS DEFECTS

Disseminated Intravascular Coagulation (DIC) and Related Syndromes

Ambrus, C. M., Weintraub, D. H., Durphy, D., et al.: Studies on hyaline membrane disease. I. The fibrinolytic system in pathogenesis and therapy. Pediatrics 32:10, 1963.

Bick, R. L.: Alterations of hemostasis associated with malignancy: etiology, pathophysiology, diagnosis, and management. Semin. Thromb. Hemost. 5:1, 1978.

Bick, R. L.: Disseminated intravascular coagulation and related syndromes. Am. J. Hematol. 5:265, 1978.

Bick, R. L.: Disseminated intravascular coagulation. Pract. Cardiol. 7:145, 1981.

Bick, R. L.: Disseminated intravascular coagulation: a clinical/laboratory study of 48 patients. In Walz, D. A., and McCoy, L. E. (Eds.): Contributions to Hemostasis. Ann. N.Y. Acad. Sci. 370:843, 1981.

Bick, R. L., and Adams, T.: Disseminated intravascular coagulation: etiology, pathophysiology, diagnosis, and management. Med. Counterpoint 6:38, 1974.

Bick, R. L., Bick, M. D., and Fekete, L. F.: Antithrombin III patterns in disseminated intravascular coagulation. Am. J. Clin. Pathol. 73:577, 1980.

Bick, R. L., Dukes, M., Wilson, W. L., and Fekete, L. F.: Antithrombin III (AT-III) as a diagnostic aid in disseminated intravascular coagulation. Thromb. Res. 10:721, 1977.

Bick, R. L., Fekete, L. F., and Wilson, W. L.: Treatment of disseminated intravascular coagulation with antithrombin III. Trans. Am. Soc. Hematol. p. 177, 1976.

Bick, R. L., Schmalhorst, W. R., and Fekete, L. F.: Disseminated intravascular coagulation and blood component therapy. Transfusion 16:361, 1976.

Bull, B., Rubenberg, M., Dacie, J., and Brain, M. C.: Microangiopathic hemolytic anemia: mechanisms of red-cell fragmentation. Br. J. Haematol. 14:643, 1968.

Gralnick, H. R., and Tan, H. K.: Acute promyelocytic leukemia: a model for understanding the role of the malignant cell in hemostasis. Hum. Pathol. 5:661, 1974.

Kidder, W. R., Logan, L. J., Rapaport, S. I., and Patch, M. J.: The plasma protamine paracoagulation reaction: clinical and laboratory evaluation. Am. J. Clin. Pathol. 58:675, 1972.

McGehee, W. H., Rapaport, S. I., and Hjort, P. F.: Intravascular coagulation in fulminant meningococcemia. Ann. Intern. Med. 67:250, 1967.

Primary Hyperfibrino(geno)lytic Syndrome

Bick, R. L.: Clinical significance of fibrin(ogen) degradation products. Semin. Thromb. Hemost. 8:302, 1982.

Bick, R. L., and Murano, G.: Primary hyperfibrino(geno)lytic syndromes. In Murano, G., and Bick, R. L. (Eds.): Basic Concepts of Hemostasis and Thrombosis. Boca Raton, FL, CRC Press, 1980, p. 181.

Fareed, J.: New methods in hemostatic testing. In Fareed, J., Messmore, H., Fenton, J., and Brinkhous, K. M. (Eds.): Perspectives in Hemostasis. New York, Pergamon Press, 1980, p. 310.

Huseby, R., and Smith, R. E.: Synthetic oligopeptide substrates. Their diagnostic application in blood coagulation, fibrinolysis, and other pathologic states. Sem. Thromb. Hemostas. 6:173, 1980.

Menon, I. S.: A study of the possible correlation of euglobulin lysis time and dilute blood clot lysis time in the determination of fibrinolytic activity. Lab. Pract. 17:334, 1968.

Alterations of Hemostasis in Chronic Liver Disease

Amir-Ahmadi, H., McGray, R. S., Martin, F., et al.: Re-assessment of massive upper gastrointestinal hemorrhage on the wards of the Boston City Hospital. Surg. Clin. North Am. 49:715, 1969.

Braunstein, K. M., and Evrenius, K.: Minimal heparin cofactor activity in disseminated intravascular coagulation and cirrhosis. Am. J. Clin. Pathol. 66:48, 1976.

Denson, K. W. R.: The levels of Factors II, VIII, IX, and X by antibody neutralization techniques in the plasma of patients receiving phenindione therapy. Br. J. Haematol. 20:643, 1971.

Donaldson, G. W. K., Davies, S. R., Darg, S., and Richmond, J.: Coagulation factors in chronic liver disease. J. Clin. Pathol. 22:109, 1969.

Kupfer, H. J., and Ewald, T.: Statistical correlation of liver function tests with coagulation factor deficiencies in Laennec's cirrhosis. Thromb. Diath. Haemorrh. 10:317, 1964.

Lane, D. A., Scully, M. F., Thomas, D. P., Kakkar, V. V., and Williams, R.: Acquired dysfibrinogenemia in acute and chronic liver disease. Br. J. Haematol. 35:301, 1977.

Lechner, K., Niessner, H., and Thaler, E.: Coagulation abnormalities in liver disease. Semin. Thromb. Hemost. 4:40, 1977.

Penny, R., Rosenberg, F. C., and Firkin, B. G.: The splenic platelet pool. Blood 17:1, 1966.

Pises, P., Bick, R. L., and Siegal, B.: Hyperfibrinolysis in cirrhosis. Am. J. Gastroenterol. 60:280, 1973.

Stenflo, J.: Vitamin K, prothrombin, and gamma-carboxyglutamic acid. N. Engl. J. Med. 296:624, 1977.

Thomas, D. P., Ream, V. J., and Stuart, R. K.: Platelet aggregation in patients with cirrhosis of the liver. N. Engl. J. Med. 276:1344, 1967.

ALTERATIONS OF HEMOSTASIS ASSOCIATED WITH CARDIOPULMONARY BYPASS

Pathophysiology

Bachmann, F., McKenna, R., Cole, E. R., and Maiafi, H. J.: The hemostasis mechanism after open-heart surgery. I. Studies on plasma coagulation factors and fibrinolysis in 512 patients after extracorporeal circulation. J. Thorac. Cardiovasc. Surg. 70:76, 1975.

Behrendt, P. M., Epstein, S. E., and Marrow, A. G.: Postperfusion nonthrombocytopenic purpura: an uncommon sequel of open heart surgery. Am. J. Cardiol. 22:631, 1968.

Bick, R. L.: Alterations of hemostasis associated with cardiopulmonary bypass: etiology, pathophysiology, diagnosis, and management. Semin. Thromb. Hemost. 3:59, 1976.

Bick, R. L.: Disseminated intravascular coagulation. Pract. Cardiol. 7:145, 1981.

Bick, R. L., and Adams, T.: Disseminated intravascular coagulation: etiology, pathophysiology, diagnosis, and management. Med. Counterpoint 6:38, 1974.

Bick, R. L., Arbegast, N. R., Holtermann, M., et al.: Platelet function abnormalities in cardiopulmonary bypass. Circulation 50(suppl. 3):301, 1974.

Bick, R. L., Arbegast, N. R., Holtermann, M., et al.: Hemostasis defects induced by cardiopulmonary bypass. Vasc. Surg. 9:228, 1975.

Bick, R. L., Arbegast, N. R., and Schmalhorst, W. R.: Alterations of hemostasis during cardiopulmonary bypass: a comparison between membrane and bubble oxygenators. Thrombos. Haemostas. 46:392, 1981.

Bick, R. L., Bishop, R. C., Warren, M., and Stemmer, E.: Changes in fibrinolysis and fibrinolytic enzymes during extracorporeal circulation. Trans. Am. Soc. Hematol., 1971, p. 109.

Bick, R. L., Comer, T. P., and Arbegast, N. R.: Fatal purpura fulminans following total cardiopulmonary bypass. J. Cardiovas. Surg. (Torino) 14:569, 1973.

Bick, R. L., Schmalhorst, W. R., and Arbegast, N. R.: Alterations of hemostasis associated with cardiopulmonary bypass. Thromb. Res. 8:285, 1976.

Bick, R. L., and Warren, M.: Personal observations.

de Vries, S. E., von Creveld, S., Groen, P., et al.: Studies on the coagulation of the blood in patients treated with extracorporeal circulation. Thromb. Diath. Haemorrh. 5:426, 1961.

Gomes, M. M., and McGoon, D.: Bleeding patterns after open heart surgery. J. Thorac. Cardiovasc. Surg. 60:87, 1970.

Harker, L. A., Malpass, T. W., Branson, H. E., et al.: Mechanism of abnormal bleeding in patients undergoing cardiopulmonary bypass: acquired transient platelet dysfunction associated with selective α-granule release. Blood 56:824, 1980.

Holswade, G. R., Machman, R. L., and Killip, T.: Thrombocytopathies in patients with open heart surgery. Preoperative treatment with corticosteroids. Arch. Surg. 94:365, 1967.

Penick, G. D., Averette, H. E., Peters, R. M., and Brinkhous, K. M.: The hemorrhagic syndrome complicating extracorporeal shunting of blood: a study of its pathogenesis. Thromb. Diath. Haemorrh. 2:212, 1968.

Porter, J. M., and Silver, D.: Alterations in fibrinolysis and coagulation associated with cardiopulmonary bypass. J. Thorac. Cardiovasc. Surg. 56:869, 1968.

Salzman, E. W.: Blood platelets and extracorporeal circulation. Transfusion 3:274, 1963.

Schmidt, P. L. J., Peden, J. C., Brecher, A., and Beravnowsky, A.: Thrombocytopenia and bleeding tendency after extracorporeal circulation. N. Engl. J. Med. 265:1181, 1961.

Signori, E. E., Penner, J. A., and Kahn, D. R.: Coagulation defects and bleeding in open heart surgery. Ann. Thorac. Surg. 8:521, 1969.

Tsitouris, G., Bellet, S., Eilberg, R., et al.: Effect of major surgery on plasma-plasminogen inhibitors. Ann. Intern. Med. 108:98, 1961.

Tsuji, H. R., Redington, J. V., Kay, J. H., and Goesswald, R. K.: The study of fibrinolytic and coagulation factors during open heart surgery. Ann. Thorac. Surg. 13:87, 1972.

Verska, J. J.: Letter to Editor. Ann. Thorac. Surg. 13:87, 1972.

Verska, J. J., Lonser, E. R., and Brewer, L. A.: Predisposing factors and management of hemorrhage following open heart surgery. J. Cardiovasc. Surg. 13:311, 1972.

HYPERFIBRINO(GENO)LYSIS IN MALIGNANCY

Bick, R. L.: Alterations of hemostasis associated with malignancy. In Murano, G., and Bick, R. L. (Eds.): Basic Concepts of Hemostasis and Thrombosis. Boca Raton, FL., CRC Press, 1980, Ch. 11, p. 213.

Bick, R. L., Fekete, L. F., Murano, G., and Wilson, W. L.: Daunomycin and fibrinolysis. Thromb. Res. 9:201, 1976.

Bick, R. L., Fekete, L. F., and Wilson, W. L.: Adriamycin and fibrinolysis. Thromb. Res. 8:467, 1976.

Bick, R. L., Schmalhorst, W. R., and Arbegast, N. R.: Alterations of hemostasis associated with cardiopulmonary bypass. Thromb. Res. 8:285, 1976.

Clifton, E. E., and Grossi, C. E.: Fibrinolytic activity of human tumors as measured by the fibrin plate technique. Cancer 8:1146, 1955.

Omar, J. B., Saxena, N., and Mitel, H. S.: Fibrinolytic activity in malignant disease. J. Assoc. Physicians India 19:293, 1971.

Soong, B. C. F., and Miller, J. P.: Coagulation disorders in cancer: fibrinolysis and inhibitors. Cancer 25:867, 1970.

Wilson, W. L., and Fostiropoulos, G.: Observations on the use of nicotinic acid to induce in vivo fibrinolytic activity. Am. J. Med. Sci. 238:591, 1959.

25 Pathophysiology of Neoplastic Disease*

Bart Barlogie and Martin N. Raber

INTRODUCTION

Traditionally, pathophysiology has been concerned with the etiologies, or mechanisms, of human disease, which are studied in an effort to understand the clinical manifestations and course of illness and the basis for success or failure of therapy. The etiologies of most human neoplasms, including the mechanisms underlying the growth and spread of human cancer, are still not completely understood. Despite these deficiencies, the results of therapy have been quite encouraging, particularly in the area of chemotherapy for metastatic disease. This chapter will review some of the fundamental advances in laboratory and clinical research that have helped elucidate the differences between normal and neoplastic growth and that have contributed to rational therapy.

DIFFERENTIATION OF MALIGNANT CELLS FROM NORMAL CELLS

Pathologists can diagnose neoplastic disease with confidence in most cases using classic histopathologic criteria (e.g., abnormal nuclear and cytoplasmic characteristics of the cells composing the lesions, frequently increased mitotic activity, ill-preserved normal tissue architecture, and evidence of metastatic spread). The specific tissue diagnosis of human cancer is generally made with regard to the most likely normal tissue histogenesis, although this may not be possible in the case of highly undifferentiated tumors. The diagnostic information provided by cytologic specimens is not as accurate as that obtained from tissue sections. The problems inherent in cytopathology stem from the lack of objective and quantitative neoplastic disease markers in traditional pathology.

The strongest single evidence of the neoplastic nature of a cell population comes from cytogenic studies demonstrating chromosomal abnormalities. Cytogenic abnormalities are almost ubiquitous in human neoplastic disease, and modern banding studies have identified specific aberrations in various forms of leukemia and lymphoma (t9:22 in chronic myelogenous leukemia; t15:17 in

acute promyelocytic leukemia; t8:14 in B-cell acute lymphoblastic leukemia and undifferentiated disease, including Burkitt's lymphoma, as well as in follicular center cell lymphomas). Cytogenetic studies have been extended to the study of pre- and semimalignant conditions and to family members of patients with hereditary forms of cancer. For example, Hsu and colleagues demonstrated chromosomal abnormalities in mitogen-stimulated lymphocytes in relatives of patients with medullary carcinoma of the thyroid in the absence of malignant disease. There has been much discussion regarding the role of such cytogenetic abnormalities in the inception of tumor growth. Studies using G-6-PDH isoenzyme patterns in patients with chronic myelogenous leukemia suggest clonal enzymatic patterns antedating the occurrence of the marker Philadelphia chromosome.

Although chromosomal studies have become routine in the assessment of hematologic malignancies, similar investigations of solid tumors are fraught with technical problems associated with in-vitro growth. In this context, the observation of an abnormal DNA content stemline by DNA flow cytometry permits objective and expedient quantitative analysis of tumor ploidy, regardless of proliferative activity. Although all tissues may express an abnormal DNA content in a small subpopulation of cells, the demonstration of cells with one or a few distinct DNA stemlines is unique to the neoplastic process. With such techniques, an 80 to 90 per cent incidence of aneuploidy in human solid tumors has been demonstrated; the relative incidence in hematologic malignancies has been shown to be 80 per cent for multiple myeloma, 50 to 60 per cent for large cell lymphoma, 25 to 30 per cent for lymphoblastic leukemia and indolent lymphoma, and 15 to 20 per cent for myeloid leukemia. Of interest is the role of abnormal DNA content as a neoplastic marker in certain conditions considered benign by most clinicians (e.g., benign monoclonal gammopathy, angioimmunoblastic lymphadenopathy, and preleukemia). These diseases provide an excellent opportunity for studying differences in tumor features or host cell characteristics or both in patients with either rapidly aggressive or relatively indolent disease courses.

The introduction of monoclonal antibodies has allowed detailed studies of tumor phenotype in lymphoma and leukemia. Thus, it has become possible to classify the predominant tumor cell

*Original work by the authors described in this section was supported in part by Grants CA 28153, CA 16672, and CA 28771 from the National Cancer Institute, National Institutes of Health, Bethesda, Maryland, 20205.

population with respect to specific evolutionary stages of the normal cell differentiation pathway. This permits speculation and, it is hoped, clarification regarding the stage of neoplastic transformation and maturation potential of the malignant cell population. The clonal expansion of cells with a homogeneous phenotype, however, is not in itself indicative of the neoplastic nature of a disease process. Thus, profound disregulation of the immune system has been found to be associated with clonal phenotypic abnormalities in both the presence and the absence of cancer. For example, circulating idiotype-bearing lymphocytes are found in multiple myeloma, and lymphocytes with monoclonal light chain excess are demonstrated in malignant lymphoma; however, peripheral blood lymphocytes with monoclonal light chain excess may also be observed in homosexual men who have acquired immunodeficiency syndrome *without* evidence of Kaposi's sarcoma, which may represent a premalignant alteration in such patients. Although usually associated with benign diseases, polyclonal immunoglobin production has been associated with some malignancies, particularly lymphomas. This may well represent nonspecific stimulation of lymphopoiesis by the malignancy.

Study of the microenvironmental genotypic and phenotypic tumor and host cell markers is useful in the delineation of the stages of transition from normal to cancerous growth. Lymph nodes from patients with malignant lymphoma are of particular interest in this regard. Of similar importance are studies of genotypic and phenotypic heterogeneity of tumor cells in metastatic versus primary lesions that are undertaken in an effort to clarify the differences in propensity for early hematogenous spread and preference of metastatic site.

ETIOLOGY OF HUMAN NEOPLASIA

In experimental animals, malignancies have been induced by chemical carcinogens, ionizing radiation, and a variety of viruses. In human cancer epidemiologic studies as well, the carcinogenic potential of a variety of different chemicals and ionizing radiation has been demonstrated (Table 25–1).

Although it would appear that susceptibility to some malignancies such as breast cancer is influenced by a genetic defect, it is difficult in most cases to demonstrate a specific Mendelian inheritance pattern and to separate possible environmental factors from the genetic ones. Nevertheless, there is a small number of familial neoplasms that follow an autosomal dominant transmission pattern. The best known example of this group is the multiple endocrine adenomatosis syndrome. Other syndromes involve the transmission not of the neoplasm itself but rather of an abnormality

TABLE 25–1 PRESUMED ETIOLOGY OF NEOPLASIA

I. *Genetic factors*
  A. Inherited neoplasms (dominant transmission, variable penetrance): multiple endocrine adenomatosis, polyposis coli, Gardner's syndrome, retinoblastoma
  B. Conditions predisposing to malignant degeneration
    1. Benign tumors: neurofibromatosis, tuberous sclerosis, Peutz-Jeghers syndrome, von Hippel-Lindau syndrome, multiple exostosis
    2. Cytogenic abnormality or instability (usually recessive): xeroderma pigmentosum (defective DNA repair), Fanconi's anemia, Bloom's syndrome, Down's syndrome
    3. Hereditary immunologic defects: ataxia teleangiectasia, Wiskott-Aldrich syndrome, X-linked agammaglobulinemia, combined immunodeficiency
  C. Conditions in which heredity plays a suspected but unproven role: breast, colon, stomach, lung, and endometrial carcinomas
II. *Environmental factors*
  A. Chemical carcinogens
    1. Drugs
      a. Chemotherapeutic agents: alkylating agents, procarbazine
      b. Hormones: estrogen, testosterone
      c. Other drugs: phenacetin, phenytoin, immunosuppressive agents
    2. Industrial exposures
      a. Organic compounds: vinyl chloride, amines, benzine, benzidine, soot, coal tar, asbestos
      b. Inorganic compounds: As, Cd, Cr, Ni
    3. Life-style–related: smoking, nitrites, alcohol, low-fiber diet (?)
  B. Radiation
    1. High-level exposure: atomic bomb, therapeutic radiation
    2. Low-level exposure: ultraviolet light, diagnostic radiation
  C. Infectious agents
    1. Viral (epidemiologic associations)
      a. EBV: Burkitt's lymphoma, nasopharygeal carcinoma
      b. Hepatitis B: hepatocellular cancer
      c. HTLV: T-cell acute leukemia, lymphoma
    2. Parasitic: schistosomiasis (bladder carcinoma)
    3. Fungal: aflatoxin
  D. Unknown etiology: acquired immunodeficiency

that predisposes the individual to the development of tumors. In some cases, this involves initially benign tumors that have a high potential for malignant transformation (e.g., von Recklinghausen's neurofibromatosis and the Peutz-Jeghers syndrome). In other cases, a known genetic defect or instability may be transmitted that directly increases the patient's risk of developing a neoplasm. Examples of this include xeroderma pigmentosum, in which ineffective DNA repair is transmitted in a recessive fashion and predisposes the patient to skin cancer after exposure to ultraviolet light, and Bloom's syndrome and Fanconi's anemia, in which chromosomal abnormalities and instability contribute to the high incidence of acute leukemia. Through a different mechanism that will be discussed later, a number of inherited immune deficiency states such as Wiskott-Aldrich syndrome, combined immunodeficiency, and ataxia-telangiectasia also predispose to neoplasia.

The devastating experience of the first nuclear bomb in Japan has taught us important lessons about the inducibility of many different types of cancers occurring with various latencies. Thus, the earliest neoplastic sequelae concern several types of acute leukemia, generally of the myeloid type, followed by chronic myeloid leukemias and, according to several surveys reported by Upton, succeeded by an increased incidence of various solid tumors. When one analyzes the frequency of neoplasms in a population by its distance from the epicenter of the nuclear bomb, the incidence appears to have a radiation-dose dependence.

Immunosuppression has been regarded both as an accommodating circumstance for development of human neoplastic disease and as the consequence of established cancer. Primary immunosuppression may be an important factor in the increased susceptibility of homosexual men to Kaposi's sarcoma and malignant lymphoma. In a murine plasmacytoma model, Ullrich and Zolla-Pazner demonstrated evidence of complex cellular and humoral circuitries between host and tumor cells. These may be operating in human cancer as well, but the "chicken-or-egg question" remains unanswered.

The history of experimental viral oncology should warn against hasty conclusions regarding more recent findings in human tumors. Virus particles and even viral footprints may be absent in virus-induced tumors. In DNA virus–transformed cells, the viral cycle is switched off, and the viral genome may be undetectable in the absence of suitable probes. Transformation of non-permissive cells by RNA viruses may be equally elusive. However, the presence of viruses or viral footprints in tumors does not necessarily indicate a causal relationship. In trying to distinguish between passenger viruses and etiologically important agents, the consistency of a given virus-tumor association and its independence of geographic and ethnic variation are particularly important. Along these lines, a few comments are in order both on Epstein-Barr virus (EBV) and its relevance to Burkitt's lymphoma and nasopharyngeal carcinoma and on hepatitis B virus (HBV) and its role in hepatocellular carcinoma.

Originally isolated from Burkitt's lymphoma, EBV is a lymphotropic herpesvirus that can infect and transform (immortalize) B-lymphocytes of human and some nonhuman primates. Transformed cells grow indefinitely as established lines. Under certain conditions, they can also grow in immunosuppressed animals. Primary infection of humans can pass without detectable symptoms or may lead to a self-limiting lymphoproliferative disease, infectious mononucleosis. The endemic African form of Burkitt's lymphoma contains the EBV genome in 97 per cent of cases, and all cells carry multiple copies of the viral genome and express the EBV nuclear antigen. Whereas the self-limited proliferation of EBV-infected B cells is polyclonal in mononucleosis, Burkitt's lymphoma is always monoclonal. Both EBV-carrying and EBV-negative forms of Burkitt's lymphoma have the same chromosomal anomaly (8:14 translocation). In immunodeficiency, as occurs regularly in renal transplant patients, unchecked proliferation of EBV-carrying cells appears to be responsible for the lymphoproliferative syndrome. However, these are polyclonal proliferations and as such are quite different from the monoclonal, cytogenetically altered Burkitt's lymphoma. Klein and coworkers have suggested that at least three conditions predispose one to EBV-carrying African Burkitt's lymphoma, including (1) immortalization of some B cells; (2) a geographic area or climate in which chronic malaria, an important stimulator of lymphoid proliferation and a possible tumor promoter, is common; and ultimately (3) the genetic risk of 8:14 translocation, which is the decisive event in the generation of autonomous lymphoma. Nasopharyngeal carcinoma is also linked to EBV infection, but the situation is less well understood.

There is mounting evidence of the association of HBV and hepatocellular carcinoma. There are, however, hepatoma-derived cell lines lacking HBV-DNA, and primary hepatocellular carcinoma also occurs in HBV-negative individuals.

Recently, a human T-cell leukemia virus has been described by Baxt and Spiegelman. This agent has been seroepidemiologically linked to T-cell leukemia and can provoke clonal evolution of T cells in-vitro.

Advances in molecular genetics have led to the demonstration of transforming genes in human cancer cells that may be identical to oncogenes of animal tumor viruses. Gene transfer methods (transfection experiments) have provided evidence that even normal cells contain latent transforming genes that may be exposed when their usual environment is disrupted. Furthermore, specific transforming genes may be activated in neoplasms of specific differentiated cell types.

Thus, although the etiology of some human cancers is being unraveled, the specific cause of an individual patient's cancer remains elusive. The aforementioned observations, however, provide impetus for both basic and clinical investigations of cancer prevention programs. Drastic reduction in cancer, particularly in that of the lung, should be expected to result from programs aimed at encouraging individuals to decrease or stop smoking. More cautious use of combined antitumor treatment modalities in the form of alkylating agents and radiation should lead to a lower incidence of treatment-induced second neoplasms, especially acute leukemia. Thus, investigators who conduct clinical trials for the treatment of Hodgkin's disease must consider the risk of inducing leukemia, particularly when dealing with early stage disease in young patients. Likewise, programs employing immunosuppressive medication for renal transplant recipients are undergoing scrutiny, in order to reduce the risk in such patients of developing lymphoma.

BIOLOGY OF TUMOR GROWTH

The growth rates of human cancers vary considerably, both among various cancer types and among different patients with the same type of tumor. Typical examples of slowly growing neoplasms are chronic lymphocytic leukemia and its related tissue form, diffuse well-differentiated lymphocytic lymphoma, and nodular poorly differentiated lymphocytic lymphoma. Carcinoid tumors and well-differentiated thyroid cancers also have a prolonged indolent disease course. Tumors of intermediate growth propensity include the more common solid tissue adenocarcinomas arising in the colon, prostate, breast, and lung. Rapidly growing tumors demanding prompt therapy include acute leukemia, oat cell lung cancer, large cell lymphomas, and undifferentiated lymphomas.

A net increase in tumor burden results from concomitant processes of cell production and cell loss. Cell production occurs in a well-defined fashion, sequentially along the stages of the division cycle as follows: pre-DNA synthesis (the G_1 phase), DNA synthesis (the S phase), premitosis (the G_2 phase), and the various substages of mitosis. Although the durations of S, G_2, and mitotic phases are fairly constant, differences in intermitotic, or cell cycle, times is largely accounted for by variation in the duration of G_1 phase. It is not clear whether those cells, remote from nutritional supply, are in a truly nonproliferating G_0 or Q (quiescent) state, or whether they instead have a protracted G_1 phase. Cell loss is believed to occur during any phase of the cell cycle but more frequently during the G_2 and mitotic phases.

Most of the current knowledge about human tumor cell kinetics has come from autoradiographic studies in which tritiated thymidine has been used as a DNA precursor molecule for both in-vivo and in-vitro investigations. Analysis of growth fraction and cell cycle time parameters has been accomplished in a small number of generally hematologic malignancies. One of the major observations that has been reported is that neoplastic cells do not necessarily proliferate faster than their normal tissue counterparts. Thus, the cytokinetic properties of human tumors do not necessarily favor preferential tumor cell kill by chemotherapy or radiation. As demonstrated by extensive in-vitro investigations in experimental systems, favorable cytokinetic properties for increased cell kill include high growth fraction, rapid cell cycle traverse, and, for phase-specific agents, the presence of tumor cells in the most sensitive cell cycle stage.

A number of strategies have been advanced by cell kineticists to enhance tumor cell kill by tumor cell synchronization and recruitment or by normal tissue protection, all of which have found limited clinical application. This is due primarily to the impracticality of currently available methods. However, the use of flow cytometry has greatly facilitated in-depth analysis of cell cycle stage distribution based on the measurement of cellular DNA content. From a practical point of view, preferential cell cycle arrest of normal host cells to protect against subsequently administered cytotoxic drugs appears most promising, as the required technology involves only DNA content analysis by flow cytometry and measurement of DNA synthetic activity by scintillation spectrophotometry.

If one accepts current evidence that human tumor growth is not necessarily due to more active proliferation of tumor in comparison with that of normal host cells, an increase in tumor burden in part results from a lack of differentiation or decreased cell loss or both. There is evidence that initiation of cell proliferation and increase in cell size as well as terminal differentiation are controlled by different genes. The delineation of the relationship among cell growth, proliferation, and differentiation processes will open exciting new areas of therapeutic intervention.

Neoplastic cell growth has classically been defined by the lack of control mechanisms operating in normal tissue. There is increasing evidence of the effect of both cellular and humoral factors on the regulation of tumor growth, which are exerted both spontaneously and during treatment. A number of tumors have been shown to carry hormone receptors, most notably breast cancer. The presence of estrogen and progesterone receptors in breast cancer seems to be inversely related to its proliferative activity, which in turn results in a longer disease-free interval following curative surgery. Thus, the presence of hormone receptors seems to provide some intrinsic growth control and can be exploited by administration of pharmacologic doses of hormonal therapy. In leukemia, there is evidence of differentiation occurring both spontaneously and during therapy, and the availability of tumor and differentiation markers will help in unraveling the biologic role of leukemic cell differentiation.

There is also evidence of interaction between tumor and normal cell growth. Thus, suppressed normal hemopoiesis in leukemia and in metastatic disease even without macroscopic marrow involvement is mediated by cellular and humoral (e.g., leukemia inhibitory activity) factors. Conversely, tumor-associated hypercoagulability may provide additional stimulation of tumor growth. Hematologic alterations associated with neoplastic disease are multifold and may concern different mechanisms in different diagnoses. In a murine plasmacytoma, for example, plasma cell tumors produce a number of effector and regulatory molecules, including osteoclast-activating factor, interferon, and immunoglobulin. In addition, malignant plasma cells release lymphokine, which induces macrophages to release a plasmacytoma-induced macrophage substance that interferes with humoral antibody response. This cascade of events results in the immunosuppression seen in plasmacytoma-bearing mice.

Efforts to take therapeutic advantage of tumor growth characteristics have been limited by cumbersome and often inappropriate technology. Clinical investigations of pretreatment tumor cell kinetics in leukemia, lymphoma, and breast cancer indicate that tumors with a higher proportion of cells in S phase respond more frequently, but the duration of disease control is generally short, unless effective tumor eradication has been accomplished. The lack of a simple correlation between tumor growth kinetics and responsiveness to therapy stresses the need to account for genotypic and phenotypic cellular heterogeneity.

GENERAL PATHOPHYSIOLOGY OF SIGNS AND SYMPTOMS OF MALIGNANT DISEASE

The clinical presentation of a tumor is determined by mass effects from both primary and metastatic tumor lesions and by indirect systemic effects from identifiable or yet unidentified humoral components or cellular factors or both (Table 25–2). The latter include ectopic hormone production, coagulation abnormalities, and immune abnormalities with immune complex or autoimmune phenomena as well as asthenia, anorexia,

TABLE 25–2 MANIFESTATIONS OF NEOPLASIA

A. *Local (mechanical) manifestations:* obstruction, compression of vital organs—bronchus, intestine, biliary tree, urinary system, blood vessel, lymphatic, heart or great vessels (pericardial tamponade), brain/spinal cord.

B. *Systemic manifestations*
  1. Metabolic: hypercalcemia, hyperuricemia, electrolyte imbalance, hypoglycemia
  2. Hormonal (ectopic): ADH, ACTH, PTH, OAF, HCG, calcitonin
  3. Hematologic: disseminated intravascular coagulation, hyperviscosity, blood cell dyscrasia (leukocytosis, leukopenia, thrombocytosis, thrombopenia, secondary polycythemia, anemia)
  4. Immunologic: immunosuppression, autoimmunity (myasthenia gravis, Eaton-Lambert syndrome (?), dermatomyositis), immune complexes (nephrotic syndrome)
  5. Constitutional: anorexia, asthenia, cachexia, fever

and weight loss, which are common in patients with malignant disease. These paraneoplastic manifestations may antecede or follow the development of overt neoplastic disease and offer unique opportunities to investigate the tumor-host relationship.

Knowledge of the natural history of tumors is important for the diagnostic evaluation of both regional and distant metastases. Although there may be considerable variation among patients with the same histopathologic tumor diagnosis, there are common patterns of tumor spread facilitating a more directed diagnostic work-up. To date, our understanding of cancer metastases is limited. Elegant studies in experimental systems, however, have demonstrated that serial intravenous passages from the same metastatic organ site result in progressive selection of cells with metastatic preference for this organ site. These studies lend support to the hypothesis that there is an intrinsic tumor cell heterogeneity that determines the ultimate sites of metastatic settlement. Investigations of human tumors have not yet revealed that genotypic or phenotypic tumor cell characteristics confer such metastatic preference. Ongoing work in several laboratories is aimed at the elucidation of cell surface characteristics associated with different patterns of metastatic spread.

BIOLOGICAL IMPORTANCE OF DIAGNOSIS AND STAGING OF MALIGNANT DISEASE

The purpose of establishing a specific tumor diagnosis and determining the extent of organ spread is to provide optimal treatment for the individual patient. In this regard, the fundamental question concerns whether or not a disease is curable with currently available means. Thus, demonstration of regionally invasive or metastatic organ spread in the case of a solid tissue neoplasm generally abrogates curative surgery. However, the recognition of tumors with systemic presentation at an early disease stage has fundamentally changed our approach to the treatment of malignant lymphomas and oat cell lung cancer. In the case of undifferentiated neoplasms without information as to the primary site of tumor origin, special laboratory investigations with electron microscopy and immunoperoxidase techniques may help determine whether the disease under question is chemotherapy-sensitive and potentially curable (e.g., lymphoma and oat cell carcinoma) or whether the physician is dealing with a neoplasm for which intensive treatment is generally ineffective (e.g., malignant melanoma). These examples point out the need for precise tissue diagnosis. At times, a repeat biopsy may be necessary to secure samples for electronmicroscopy or other specialized laboratory tests, including the rapidly propagated human tumor stem cell assay. Once the tissue diagnosis has been made with confidence, clinical or surgical staging should follow in order to determine the appropriate therapy. In circumstances of rapidly progressing metastatic disease, an extensive staging work-up can be deferred until the patient's clinical condition has stabilized.

In the following paragraphs, several examples of diagnostic work-up in common tumors will be discussed. The approach presented reflects our current understanding and should not be regarded as dogmatic in any way.

Lung Cancer. The management of a patient with lung cancer depends on whether or not a small cell (oat cell) carcinoma is present, since small cell lung cancer is now recognized as a widely disseminated disease from the outset; thus, as in leukemia, combination chemotherapy is the initial treatment of choice. Through vigorous restaging at the time of maximum antitumor effect, the heterogeneity of small cell lung cancer has been recognized, which accounts for the demonstration of non–small cell disease in residual tumor lesions. The coexistence of small cell and non–small cell tumors suggests a closer relationship between formerly distinct disease entities, either in the sense of initial heterogeneity with eventual clonal overgrowth of the non–small cell variety or by chemotherapy-induced differentiation of the more primitive small cell population. This observation of a different histology in patients with persistent disease after otherwise successful cytoreduction of small cell lung cancer has prompted investigations of adjunctive surgery after initial chemotherapy, producing complete remissions in 75 to 80 per cent of treated patients.

Thus, the management of small cell carcinoma of the lung has radically changed since the late 1960s. The major objective in the staging work-up of patients with non–small cell carcinoma, however, is the determination of resectability of the primary tumor, as it offers patients the best chance for long-term survival.

Breast Cancer. The approach to the patient with breast cancer has undergone a fundamental change with the recognition by Fisher that the frequent occurrence of metastatic disease after radical mastectomy is due to primary hematogenous spread as an early route of dissemination of breast cancer and, possibly, of other tumors. This clinical observation has led to the use of adjuvant chemotherapy to eradicate micrometastatic disease when, from a clinical standpoint, radical mastectomy has resulted in a disease-free state in the patient. Because not every woman with early-stage breast cancer will develop metastatic disease, the relative risk factors must be appreciated in order to spare patients with a high chance for cure the side effects of systemically administered chemotherapy. Studies conducted at the Southern Research Institute have provided important guidelines for the clinical conduct of adjuvant chemotherapy trials. According to these studies, the

degree of micrometastatic disease present at the time of resection of the primary tumor increases with increasing size of the primary lesion and increasing degree of lymphatic spread. Following resection of the primary tumor, increased growth rates of micrometastatic lung lesions have been demonstrated, resulting in increased sensitivity to chemotherapy and thus providing a rationale for the sequence of initial surgical resection followed by adjuvant chemotherapy for residual micrometastatic disease. Because there is evidence that adjuvant chemotherapy provides as good a local disease control as does adjunctive radiotherapy, the role of postoperative radiation has been questioned by many investigators. As a result of our understanding that breast cancer is a systemic disease from the outset, the surgical management of primary breast cancer has become more conservative, even to the point of breast-preserving resection with adjunctive local radiotherapy and systemic chemotherapy.

With the introduction of hormone receptor analysis, an additional biologic feature of breast cancer has been the subject of many clinical investigations. We now recognize that the prognosis of women with breast cancer is adversely affected by increasing local tumor burden at diagnosis, the absence of hormone receptor expression, and high proliferative activity of the primary tumor. It has been established that both hormone receptor expression and cytokinetic characteristics have prognostic implications that are independent of tumor stage. Therefore, the primary management of human breast cancer must include careful evaluation of local disease, of hormone receptor status with regard to both estrogen and progesterone receptor expression, and of proliferative activity by either tritiated thymidine autoradiography or DNA flow cytometry.

Malignant Lymphoma. The malignant lymphomas have been the subject of fascinating research and treatment. There is compelling evidence that the malignant cell in Hodgkin's disease is monocyte-derived, as demonstrated by the presence of esterase and phagocytic activity as well as the nucleolar antigen as a tumor cell marker in Sternberg cells. Treatment of stages I and IIA Hodgkin's disease generally consists of radiation therapy, whereas in patients with more advanced disease stages chemotherapy has become the predominant treatment. The role of staging laparotomy is undergoing continued discussion, based on treatment preferences for patients presenting with stage IIB or IIIA disease, in which a consensus regarding the need for exclusive use of chemotherapy is not established. Staging laparotomy does provide guidelines for an approach aimed at minimal but optimal therapy (i.e., radiotherapy for stage II and chemotherapy for stage III disease). Unfortunately, neither lymphangiography nor computed axial tomography provides adequate information concerning lymph node involvement in the splenic hilum, the porta hepatis, or the sub-diaphragmatic region. Patients with advanced Hodgkin's disease seem to benefit most from the use of two mutually non–cross resistant chemotherapy combinations that are employed in a rotating fashion. A delayed effect of treatment for Hodgkin's disease is the development of acute leukemia, generally of the myeloid type with a smoldering presentation. Controversy remains with regard to the relative contributions of radiation and chemotherapy.

The histogenesis of non-Hodgkin's lymphoma has been delineated with the armamentarium of modern immunology. This has led to the recognition that most non-Hodgkin's lymphomas are of the B cell type, originating in the follicular center of the lymph node. Lymphomas of T cell origin occur with an incidence of less than 30 per cent, and true histiocytic lymphomas are extremely rare. Despite the confusion with regard to the histopathologic classification of lymphomas, the consensus is that the majority of tumors are of either small cell or large cell type, with either nodular or diffuse patterns of lymph node involvement. Small cell lymphomas follow a more benign clinical course, whereas large cell lymphomas require the prompt institution of intensive combination chemotherapy. This is further underscored by the proliferative characteristics of these two major lymphoma types: Small cell lymphomas demonstrate little proliferation, with less than 5 per cent of cells in S phase, whereas large cell lymphomas are characterized by a higher S phase proportion. In addition, small cell lymphomas are generally diploid, whereas large cell lymphomas are aneuploid according to DNA flow cytometric analysis in 60 to 80 per cent of cases. The use of modern biologic tools should help clarify the microarchitecture of lymph nodes in lymphoma and thus elucidate the tumor–host cell interaction with regard to phenotypic and cytokinetic characteristics. To this end, the presence of an unambiguous neoplastic marker, such as abnormal DNA content or the nucleolar antigen, should prove extremely helpful.

One of the major changes in the treatment of non-Hodgkin's lymphoma has resulted from the observation that currently available cytotoxic combination chemotherapy promotes higher cure rates in patients with aggressive rather than indolent histologies. Thus, although there is still a 30 to 50 per cent early failure rate, the prospect for long-term disease control and eventual cure is considerably higher in large cell than in small cell lymphoma. Another relevant finding is that monoclonal light chain excess persists in the peripheral blood of patients who have small cell lymphoma but disappears in patients who have large cell lymphoma and who experience long-term, disease-free survival. Since there is evidence of malignant transformation from small to large cell lymphoma in a yet probably underestimated fraction of patients with favorable histologies, some institutions are evaluating both palliative therapy for patients with lymphomas of favorable histology and introduction of intensive combination chemotherapy when the tumor develops into an aggressive and potentially curable disease. Results of such trials are not yet available. The aforementioned considerations, however, stress the importance of detailed histopathologic diagnosis and staging in the determination of therapeutic intervention.

Leukemia. Acute myeloblastic leukemia is another disease that can be discussed with regard to important biologic concepts of therapy. The traditional belief that complete remission can be accomplished only by aggressive combination chemotherapy leading to a phase of marrow aplasia still holds; however, there are notable albeit not widely published exceptions. The observation of persistent hypercellularity and gradually increasing differentiation under the influence of intensive chemotherapy supports the experimental finding of chemotherapy-induced differentiation. Additional evidence of the existence of differentiated leukemia is the presence of the nucleolar antigen marker in mature granulocytes and in CFU_c from patients in remission. Also, abnormal DNA content and chemotaxis have been demonstrated in apparently morphologically normal granulocytes from patients with oligoleukemia. In this respect, acute leukemia may be analogous to teratocarcinoma and neuroblastoma, in which intensive chemotherapy provokes differentiation. Thus, although only anecdotal at the moment, the therapeutic alternative to cytoeradication, i.e., terminal tumor cell differentiation, deserves extensive laboratory and clinical research. It is conceivable that there are considerable differences in the susceptibility of tumors to terminal differentiation and, conversely, that for a given tumor, the potential of certain agents to induce differentiation may also vary considerably. In this regard, the availability of neoplastic markers such as abnormal DNA content, double-stranded RNA, and nucleolar antigen is invaluable. The concept of tumor cell differentiation has provided us with a new perspective in cancer therapy, namely, the long-term disease control of a patient still harboring neoplastic disease.

PRINCIPLES OF TREATMENT

Traditionally, *surgery* has been the mainstay of curative cancer therapy, supported by *ionizing radiation* for better control of bulky primary tumors and, more recently, by *adjuvant chemotherapy* when there is a high likelihood of micrometastatic disease leading to the patient's demise in a relatively short period of time. *Immunotherapy* traditionally has been conducted mainly in the form of active nonspecific therapy with various agents (e.g., BCG, *Corynebacterium parvum*, etc.)

in an attempt to boost the host defense mechanisms in a nonspecific fashion. More recently, immunotherapy has assumed the role of biologic therapy with agents now generally referred to as *biologic response modifiers,* including interferon and interferon inducers, removal of immune complexes by protein A–coated charcoal columns, and defined cell subpopulations of monocytes or lymphocytes. Monoclonal antibodies, initially developed for diagnosis, have already been employed for in-vivo therapeutic trials in lymphoma and for in-vitro purging of autologous bone marrow in acute leukemia. *Hyperthermia,* finally, has regained interest as a treatment modality that, in contrast to chemotherapy and ionizing radiation, seems to be highly effective in experimental systems against hypoxic and slowly cycling or noncycling cells.

More recently, the *sequence* of application of different antitumor *treatment modalities* has been modified for a number of tumors, most notably for small cell lung cancer and male germ cell tumors, for which combination chemotherapy has been established as the initial treatment of choice, as it has been for the treatment of certain hematologic malignancies (e.g., leukemias, multiple myeloma, and large cell lymphomas). With few exceptions, the specific drugs employed in combination therapy programs for disseminated disease cannot be considered established. The exceptions include childhood acute lymphoblastic leukemia in which a combination of vinca alkaloids, corticosteroids, L-asparaginase and anthracyclines has produced complete remissions in almost all patients treated, which are generally long-term, with 50 per cent of children alive and free of disease after 10 years. The treatment of advanced Hodgkin's disease has been conducted successfully with MOPP combination chemotherapy, as pioneered by DeVita and co-workers. However, even this solid backbone has been questioned, as equally effective non–cross resistant programs have been introduced for patients relapsing on MOPP chemotherapy. Thus, the concept of rotating two highly effective, mutually non–cross resistant chemotherapy programs has evolved and seems to be highly beneficial in the control of lymphomas and small cell lung cancer. Radiotherapy still maintains a role in the treatment of early stage Hodgkin's disease and some non–Hodgkin's lymphomas as well as in the treatment of both primary and metastatic brain tumors.

The successful treatment of tumors with chemotherapy has been shown to depend on a number of determinants relating to *drug pharmacology* and *tumor cell kinetics* (Table 25–3). Pharmacologic considerations concern the mode of drug administration, serum pharmacokinetics, degree of tissue distribution, presence and distribution of activating and deactivating enzymes, and primary route of drug excretion and metabolism. A typical pharmacologic sanctuary is the brain, and the

TABLE 25–3 CAUSES OF FAILURE OF CANCER THERAPY

Inadequate therapy
Incorrect diagnosis
Inadequate staging
Severe toxicity of therapy
Tumor cell resistance
Sanctuaries
Pharmacologic (brain, testicle)
Cytokinetic (nondividing cells)
Persistence of the etiologic agent

blood-brain barrier may still be intact in the presence of micrometastatic disease and account for CNS recurrence of leukemia and other tumors in the case of sustained disease control in other sites. Once the drug is within the tumor target tissue, the degree of inflicted lethal injury may depend, for example, on a favorable ratio of activating and deactivating enzymes (e.g., kinase and deaminase in the case of ara-C), on the presence of metabolites competing for the same target enzyme (e.g., dCTP for DNA polymerase-alpha in the case of ara-CTP), or on varying concentrations of target enzyme (e.g., dihydrofolate reductase in the case of methotrexate). Intracellular pharmacologic determinants are intimately linked to cytokinetic mechanisms, as the latter are merely cellular expressions of more complex biochemical interactions. In cytokinetic terminology, agents can be distinguished according to their preferential exertion of lethal injury (1) in a particular phase of the cell cycle (phase-specific), (2) during active cell division (cycle-active), or (3) independent of the degree of cell proliferation (non–cycle active). All chemotherapeutic and other tumor-active substances generally exert, besides their lethal or cytotoxic injury, a perturbation of cell cycle progression, which can be utilized for the design of combination chemotherapy programs employing strategies of cell synchronization, recruitment, and normal tissue protection. There are only a few studies in which pharmacologic and cytokinetic principles have been successfully utilized. Thus, very large doses of methotrexate can be safely administered in conjunction with citrovorum factor rescue. Application of adriamycin by continuous infusion is associated with lower peak plasma levels and has been shown to reduce the cardiotoxic side effects for a given integral dose. Cytokinetic strategies of cell synchronization and recruitment have long suffered from lack of appropriate technology to verify such events. Timed sequential chemotherapy programs for acute leukemia and other malignancies successfully exploit tumor cell recruitment.

One of the most significant observations in clinical oncology is that *combination chemotherapy* is superior to the use of single agents because the different biologic modes of action of multidrug regimens produce synergistic antitumor effects, thus increasing fractional cell kill and delaying the development of drug-resistant cell subpopulations. Although the current practice of combination chemotherapy employs agents that are active when given alone, it is conceivable that inactive drugs or ineffective schedules of agents may augment tumor cell inactivation or reduce host toxicity inflicted by other agents. Tumor cell kill by chemotherapeutic agents and ionizing radiation follows first-order kinetics, that is, for a given dose of treatment, there is a constant fraction of cell kill, so that complete tumor sterilization is theoretically not possible and requires host defense mechanisms. As mentioned earlier, cytotoxic agents not only exert lethal cell injury and perturbation of cell cycle progression but can also induce terminal tumor cell differentiation, the extent of which is currently unknown, as unequivocal neoplastic markers such as abnormal DNA content have only recently become available.

The development of effective treatment programs for the various forms of cancer have evolved empirically. This is also true for considerations of dosing and scheduling. Extensive experimental studies suggest that alkylating agents and DNA binders are best administered on an intermittent high-dose schedule in order to reach tissue concentrations well beyond the shoulder portion on the exponential part of the dose-response survival curve, thus minimizing the opportunity for cellular repair of sublethal damage. Antimetabolites, exerting a phase-specific cytotoxic action, are administered by continuous infusion in order to permit effective exposure of all potentially cycling cells.

For any treatment to be effective in an individual patient's tumor, the intrinsic tumor cell sensitivity should be high, and the host tissue susceptibility to damage should be low. Most of the presently conducted treatments of neoplastic disease subject patients to empirically selected agents with unpredictable antineoplastic and host cell toxicities. The development of the human tumor (and host) stem cell assay to test the individual patient's cells against an entire panel of potentially active agents appears to be a promising strategy for individualized chemotherapy.

DESIGN OF CLINICAL THERAPEUTIC TRIALS

Progress in cancer therapy has come about through the discovery and vigorous testing of potentially more effective cytotoxic agents that exhibit a higher degree of selectivity toward tumor versus normal cells. Initiation of new drug trials requires the identification of a patient population that is most likely to benefit from such new drug investigation. Such patients should have a poor prognosis when treated with standard therapy. Thus, recognition of *prognostic factors* is an extremely important and powerful tool for therapeutic research in cancer. In general, both short- and long-term prognosis are adversely influenced by the degree of tumor burden present at diagnosis. Prognostic implication of tumor load has been amply demonstrated in breast, lung, and colon cancer and in malignant lymphomas and myeloma. The quantitative assessment of tumor burden is often facilitated by the presence of humoral tumor markers, such as carcinoembryonic antigen, alpha-1-fetoprotein, and human chorionic gonadotropin. There remains, however, a considerable variation in the clinical course of patients with comparable tumor mass stage of the same disease. Such heterogeneity can be explained by differences in both tumor and host characteristics. The importance of host factors is readily apparent from the profound differences in prognosis among patients of different age groups. The often better prognosis in younger patients may be related both to age-determined differences in tumor phenotypic properties and to a greater capacity of host cells to absorb and repair cytotoxic damage. Efforts to account for tumor heterogeneity of the same histopathologic type and stage are directed toward the assessment of the phenotypic and cytokinetic characteristics of the tumor. In breast cancer, the presence and degree of hormone receptor expression and tumor cell proliferation both have been shown to affect prognosis: Patients with receptor-negative, highly proliferative breast cancer have a poor prognosis, even when they present with an early disease stage.

There are two fundamentally different strategies in clinical therapeutic trials in cancer and in other diseases: *randomization* and *historical controls*. Despite the known controversy between advocates of either approach, each of these methods has its respective role in clinical investigation. In diseases with a predictably poor outcome, such as cancer, many investigators prefer the use of historical controls, especially when prognostic features are well documented, in order to judge the superiority of the new treatment. This approach requires a profound knowledge of prognostic factors in both historical and current study groups for appropriate conclusions to be derived.

PROSPECTS OF CANCER RESEARCH AND THERAPY

The demonstration of curability of neoplastic disease, including acute leukemia, lymphoma, and germ cell tumors, lends testimony to the validity of empirical clinical investigation of new antitumor agents in the traditional vein of phase I, II, and III investigations. At the same time, the availability of supportive care with powerful antibiotics and defined cytopheresis, including bone marrow transplantation, has made it possible for investigators to take full advantage of effective anticancer agents with limited selectivity toward tumor cells. Strategies designed to augment the selectivity of cytotoxic agents toward tumor cells include the coupling of drugs to monoclonal antibodies against tumor cells and to liposomes, thereby providing higher drug concentrations in tumor tissue than in normal tissue. Relatively new forms of therapy include the so-called "biologic response modifiers," such as interferon and tumor-differentiating agents as well as cytotoxic monoclonal antibodies. In-depth study of the genotypic and phenotypic characteristics of tumors, aided by advances in instrumentation (flow cytometry) and immunologic research (hybridoma-generated monoclonal antibodies), should result in a better appreciation of the individual patient's prognosis so that treatment can be tailored according to risk factors. A better understanding of indolent forms of neoplastic disease may provide new directions for therapeutic research. Elucidation of oncogenes and their products may lead to novel forms of therapeutic intervention directed toward restoration of normal growth control. Ultimately, the recognition of those agents that actually induce and promote human neoplasia will permit treatment to be directed against the cause of malignancy rather than against its symptoms. Once the causal mechanisms have been identified, effective cancer prevention should greatly reduce the still-increasing morbidity and mortality that result from neoplastic disease.

REFERENCES

INTRODUCTION

DeVita. V. T., Henney, J. E., and Hubbard, S. M.: Estimation of the numerical and economic impact of chemotherapy in the treatment of cancer. In Burchenal, J. H., and Oettgen, H. T. (Eds.): Cancer. Achievements, Challenges and Prospects for the 1980's. New York, Grune & Stratton, 1981, pp. 859–880.

DIFFERENTIATION OF MALIGNANT CELLS FROM NORMAL CELLS

Ault, K.: Detection of small numbers of monoclonal B lymphocytes in the blood of patients with lymphoma. N. Engl. J. Med. 300:1401, 1979.

Barlogie, B., Hittleman, W., Spitzer, G., et al.: Correlation of DNA distribution abnormalities with cytogenetic findings in human adult leukemia and lymphoma. Cancer Res. 37:4400, 1977.

Barlogie, B., Gohde, W., Johnston, D. A., et al.: Determination of ploidy and proliferative characteristics of human solid tumors by pulse cytophotometry. Cancer Res. 38:3333, 1978.

Barlogie, B., Drewinko, B., Schumann, W. et al.: Cellular DNA content as a marker of neoplasia in man. Am. J. Med. 69:195, 1980.

Barlogie, B., Johnston, D. A., Smallwood, L., et al.: Prognostic implications of ploidy and proliferative activity in human solid tumors. Cancer Genet. Cytogenet. 6:17, 1982.

Blumberg, B. S., and London, W. T.: Hepatitis B virus and the prevention of primary hepatocellular carcinoma. N. Engl. J. Med. 304:782, 1981.

Fialkow, P. J., Dewman, A. M., Singe, J., et al.: Human myeloproliferative disorders: clonal origin in pluripotent stem cells. In Clarkson, B., Marks, P. A., and Till, J. E. (Eds.): Differentiation of Normal and Neoplastic Hematopoietic Cells. Vol. 5. New York, Spring Harbor Laboratory, 1978, pp. 131–144.

Fidler, I. J., and Hart, I. R.: Biologic diversity in metastatic neoplasma: origins and implications. Science 217:998, 1982.

Foon, K. A., Schroff, R. W., and Gale, R. P.: Surface markers on leukemia and lymphoma cells: recent advances. Blood 61:1, 1982.

Gallagher, H. S., and Martin, J. E.: The study of mammary carcinoma by mammogram and whole organ sectioning. Cancer 23:855, 1969.

Hecht, F., and Kaiser-McCaw, B.: Chromosome 14: a step in the development of lymphoid malignancies. In Burchenal, J. H., and Oettgen, H. F. (Eds.): Cancer. Achievements, Challenges and Prospects for the 1980's. Vol. 2. New York, Grune & Stratton, 1981, pp. 433–444.

Hecht, F., Koler, R. D., Rigas, D. A., et al.: Leukemia and lymphocytes in ataxia telangiectasia. Lancet 2:1195, 1966.

Hsu, T. C., Pathak, S., Samaan, N., and Hickey, R. C.: Chromosome instability with medullary carcinoma of the thyroid. J.A.M.A. 246:2046, 1981.

Kanhouwa, S. B., and Matthews, J. H.: Reliability of cytologic typing in lung cancer. Acta Cytol. 20:226, 1976.

Laszlo, J.: Hematologic effects of cancer. In Holland, J., and Frei, E. F. (Eds.): Cancer Medicine. Philadelphia, Lea & Febiger, 1982, pp. 1275–1288.

Latreille, J., Barlogie, B., Dosik, G., et al.: Cellular DNA content as a marker of human multiple myeloma. Blood 55:403, 1980.

Latreille, J., Barlogie, B., Johnston, D. A., et al.: Ploidy and proliferative characteristics in monoclonal gammopathies. Blood 59:43, 1982.

Mellstedt, H., Holm, G., Pettersson, D., and Peest, D.: Idiotype-bearing lymphoid cells in plasma cell neoplasia. Clin. Haematol. 11:65, 1982.

Nowell, P. C.: Chormosome changes and clonal evolution of cancer. In German, J., (Ed.): Chromosomes and Cancer, New York, John Wiley and Sons, 1974, pp. 267–285.

Reinherz, E. L., King, P. C., Goldstein, G., et al.: Discrete stages of human intrathymic differentiation: analysis of normal thymocytic and leukemic lymphoblasts of T-cell lineage. Proc. Natl. Acad. Sci. U.S.A. 77:1588, 1980.

Ritz, J., and Schlossman, S. F.: Review: utilization of monoclonal antibodies in the treatment of leukemia and lymphoma. Blood 59:1, 1982.

Sandberg, A. A.: The Chromosome in Human Cancer and Leukemia. New York, Elsevier-North Holland, Inc., 1980, pp. 387–393.

Yunis, J. J., Oken, M. M., Kaplan, M. E., et al.: Theologides A. Distinctive chromosomal abnormalities in histologic subtypes of non-Hodgkin's lymphoma. N. Engl. J. Med. 307:1231, 1982.

ETIOLOGY OF HUMAN NEOPLASIA

Baxt, N. G., and Spiegelman, S.: Leukemia specific DNA sequences in leukocytes of the leukemic member of identical twins. Proc. Natl. Acad. Sci. U.S.A. 70:1629, 1973.

Gallo, R. C., and Wong-Staal, F.: Review: retroviruses as etiologic agents of some animal and human leukemias and lymphomas and as tools for elucidating the molecular mechanisms of leukemogenesis. Blood 60:545, 1982.

Good, R. A., and Finstad, J.: Essential relationship between the lymphoid system, immunity and malignancy. Natl. Cancer Inst. Monogr. 31:41, 1969.

Hecht, F., and McCaw, B. K.: Chromosome instability syndromes. In Mulvihill, J. J., Miller, R. W., Fraumeni, J. F. (Eds.): Genetics of Human Cancer. Progress in Cancer Research and Therapy. Vol. 3. New York, Raven Press, 1977, pp. 105–123.

Henle, W., and Henle, G.: The Epstein Barr Virus: its relation to Burkitt's lymphoma and nasopharyngeal carcinoma. In Burchenal, J. H., and Ottegen, H. F. (Eds.): Cancer. Achievements, Challenges and Prospects for the 1980's. New York, Grune & Stratton, 1981, pp. 149–159.

Hersh, E. M., Gutterman, J. V., Mavligit, G. M., et al.: Immunocompetence, immunodeficiency and prognosis in cancer. Ann. N.Y. Acad. Sci. 276:386, 1976.

Klein, G.: Viruses in cancer. *In* Burchenal, J. H., and Oettegen, H. F. (Eds.): Cancer. Achievements, Challenges and Prospects for the 1980's. New York, Grune & Stratton, 1981, pp. 859–880.

Marx, J. L.: Cancer cell genes linked to viral onc Genes. Science *216*:724, 1981.

Marx, J. L.: Change in cancer gene pin-pointed. Science *218*:667, 1982.

Pedersen-Bjergaard, J., and Larsen, S. O.: Incidence of acute non-lymphocytic leukemia, preleukemia and acute myeloproliferative syndrome up to 10 years after treatment of Hodgkin's disease. N. Engl. J. Med. *307*:965, 1982.

Penn, I: The incidence of malignancy in transplant recipients. Transplant. Proc. 7:323, 1975.

Stahl, R. E., Friedman-Klein, A., Dubin, R., et al.: Immunologic abnormalities in homosexual men. Relationship to Kaposi's sarcoma. Am. J. Med. *73*:171, 1982.

Ullrich, S. E., and Zolla-Pazner, S.: Immunoregulatory circuits in myeloma. Clin. Hematol. *11*:87, 1982.

Upton, A. C.: Radiation hazards. *In* Burchenal, J. H., and Oettgen, H. F. (Eds.): Cancer. Achievements, Challenges and Prospects for the 1980's. New York, Grune & Stratton, 1981, pp. 185–198.

Upton, A. C.: Physical carcinogenesis: radiation history and sources. *In* Becker, F. F. (Ed.): Cancer, A Comprehensive Treatise. New York, Plenum Publishing Corp. 1975, pp. 387–403.

Wynder, E. L., and Gori, G. B.: Contribution of the environment to cancer incidence: An epidemiologic exercise. J. Natl. Cancer Inst. *58*:825, 1977.

BIOLOGY OF TUMOR GROWTH

Barlogie, B., Johnston, D. A., Smallwood, L., et al.: Prognostic implications of ploidy and proliferative activity in human solid tumors. Cancer Genet. Cytogenet. *6*:17, 1982.

Baserga, R.: The cell cycle. N. Engl. J. Med. *304*:453, 1981.

Baserga, R., and Kisieleski, W.: Comparative studies of the kinetics of cell proliferation of normal and tumorous tissue with the use of tritiated thymidine. I. Dilution of the label and migration of labeled cells. J. Natl. Cancer Inst. *128*:331, 1962.

Broxmeyer, H. E., Jacobson, N., Kurland, J., et. al.: In vitro suppression of normal granulocytic stem cells by inhibitory activity derived from human leukemia cells. J. Natl. Cancer Inst. *60*:497, 1978.

Diamond, L. W., Nathwani, B. N., and Rappaport, H.: Flow cytometry in the diagnosis and classification of malignant lymphoma and leukemia. Cancer *50*:1122, 1982.

Dosik, G., Barlogie, B., Smith, T. L., et al.: Pre-treatment flow cytometry of DNA content in adult acute leukemia. Blood *55*:474, 1980.

Ettinger, D. S., Karp, J. E., Abeloff, M. D., et al.: Intermittent high dose cyclophosphamide chemotherapy for small cell carcinoma of the lung. Cancer Treat. Rep. *62*:413, 1978.

Hill, B. T.: Cancer chemotherapy: the relevance of certain concepts of cell cycle kinetics. Biochim. Biophys. Acta *516*:389, 1978.

Jensen, E. V., and Jacobson, H. I.: Basic guides to the mechanism of estrogen action. Recent Prog. Horm. Res. *18*:387, 1962.

Kamentski, L. A., Melamed, M. R. and Derman, H.: Spectrophotometer: new instrument for ultra rapid cell analysis. Science *150*:630, 1965.

Marx, J. L.: Coagulation as a common thread in disease. Science *218*:145, 1982.

Mendelsohn, M. L.: The growth fraction: a new concept applied to tumors. Science *132*:1499, 1960.

Meyer, J. S.: Cell kinetic measurements of human tumors. Hum. Pathol. *13*:874, 1982.

Pardee, A., and James, L. J.: Selective killing of transformed baby hamster kidney (BHK) cells. Proc. Natl. Sci. U.S.A. *72*:4994, 1974.

Quastler, H., and Sherman, F. G.: Cell population kinetics in the intestinal epithelium of the mouse. Exp. Cell Res. *17*:420, 1959.

Steel, G.: Growth Kinetics of Tumors. New York, Oxford University Press, 1977.

Sulkes, A., Livingston, R. B., and Murphy, W. K.: Tritiated thymidine labeling index and respone in human breast cancer. J. Natl. Cancer Inst. *62*:513, 1979.

Ullrich, S. E., and Zolla-Pazner, S.: Immunoregulatory circuits in myeloma. Clin. Hematol. *11*:87, 1982.

Van Putten, C. M.: Are cell kinetics data relevant for the design of tumor chemotherapy schedules. Cell Tissue Kinet. 7:493, 1974.

GENERAL PATHOPHYSIOLOGY OF SIGNS AND SYMPTOMS OF MALIGNANT DISEASE

Laszlo, J.: Hematologic effects of cancer: *In* Holland, J., and Frei, E. F. (Eds.): Cancer Medicine. Philadelphia, Lea & Febiger, 1982, pp. 1275–1288.

Biologic Importance of Diagnosis and Staging of Malignant Disease

Ault, K.: Detection of small numbers of monoclonal B lymphocytes in the blood of patients with lymphoma. N. Engl. J. Med. *300*:1401, 1979.

Barlogie, B., Raber, M. N., Schumann, J., et al.: Flow cytometry in clinical cancer research. Cancer Res. *43*:3982, 1983.

Bonadonna, G.: Chemotherapy strategies to improve the control of Hodgkin's disease: The Richard and Hilda Rosenthal Foundation Award Lecture. Cancer Res. *42*:4309, 1982.

Bonadonna, G., Brusamoline, E., Rossi, A., et al.: Combination chemotherapy as an adjuvant treatment in operable breast cancer. N. Engl. J. Med. *294*:405, 1976.

Borella, L., Casper, J. R., and Laver, S. J.: Shifts in expression of cell membrane phenotypes in childhood lymphoid malignancies at relapse. Blood *64*:56, 1979.

Busch, H., Gyorkey, F., Busch, R. K., et al.: A nucleolar antigen found in a broad range of tumor specimens. Cancer Res. *39*:3024, 1979.

Cossman, J., Neckeds, L. M., Arnold, A., and Korsmeyer, S. J.: Induction of differentiation in a case of common acute lymphoblastic leukemia. N. Engl. J. Med. *30*:1251, 1982.

Davis, F. M., Gyorkey, F., Busch, R. K., and Busch, H.: Nucleolar antigen found in several human tumors but not in nontumor tissues studies. Proc. Natl. Acad. Sci. U.S.A. *76*:892, 1979.

Davis, F. M., Hittleman, W. N., McCredie, K. B., and Rao, P. N.: Estimation of tumor burden in leukemia patients using antibodies to neoplastic nucleoli. Proc. Am. Assoc. Cancer Res. *33*:229, 1980.

DeVita, V. T., Glatstein, E. J., Young, R. C., et al.: Changing concepts: the lymphomas. *In* Jones, S. E., and Salmon, S. E. (Eds.): Adjuvant Therapy of Cancer. II. New York, Grune & Stratton, 1979, pp. 173–190.

Fisher, B., Slack, N., Katrych, D., and Wolmarken, N.: Ten year follow up of breast cancer patients in a cooperative clinical trial evaluating surgical adjuvant chemotherapy. Surg. Gynecol. Obstet. *140*:528, 1975.

Hansen, H. H., Dombernowsky, P., and Hansen, M.: Chemotherapy of advanced small cell anplastic carcinoma. Ann. Intern. Med. *89*:177, 1978.

Kaplan, H. S.: Hodgkin's disease. Cambridge, Harvard University Press, 1980, pp. 52–116.

Lukes, R. J., and Collins, R. D.: Immunologic characterization of human malignant lymphomas. Cancer *34*:1488, 1974.

McKelvey, E., Wilson, H., Haut, A., et al.: Hydroxy daunorubicin combination chemotherapy in malignant lymphoma. Cancer *38*:1484, 1976.

Meyer, J. S.: Cell kinetic measurements of human tumors. Hum. Pathol. *13*:874, 1982.

Pederson-Bjergaard, J., Vindeloy, L., Philip, P., et al.: Varying involvement of peripheral granulocytes in the clonal abnormality-7 in bone marrow cells in preleukemia secondary to treatment of other malignant tumors: cytogenetic results compared with results of flow cytometric DNA, analysis and neutrophil chemotaxis. Blood *60*:173, 1982.

Pedersen-Bjergaard, J., and Larsen, S. O.: Incidence of acute nonlymphocytic leukemia, preleukemia and acute myeloproliferative syndrome up to 10 years after treatment of Hodgkin's disease. N. Engl. J. Med. *307*:965, 1982.

Schabel, R.: Concepts for systemic treatment of micrometastasis. Cancer *35*:15, 1975.

Seeger, R. C., Siegel, S., and Sidell, N.: Neuroblastoma: clinical perspectives, monoclonal antibodies and retinoic acid. Ann. Intern. Med. *97*:873, 1982.

Simpson-Herren, L., and Lloyd, H. H.: Kinetic parameters and growth curves for experimental tumor systems. Cancer Chemother. Rep. *54*:143, 1970.

Stjernsward, J.: Decreased survival related to irradiation postoperatively in early operable breast cancer. Lancet *2*:1285, 1974.

Zubrod, G. C.: Historic milestones in curative chemotherapy. Semin. Oncol. *6*:490, 1979.

PRINCIPLES OF TREATMENT

Barlogie, B., Corry, P. M., Yip, E., et al.: Total body hyperthermia with and without chemotherapy for advanced human neoplasms. Cancer Res. *39*:1481, 1979.

DeVita, V. T., and Schein, P. S.: The use of drugs in combination for the treatment of cancer. Rationale and results. N. Engl. J. Med. *288*:988, 1973.

DeVita, V. T., Simon, R. M., and Hubbard, S. M.: Curability of advanced Hodgkin's disease with chemotherapy: long-term follow up of MOPP treated patients at NCI. Ann. Intern. Med. *92*:587, 1980.

Djerassi, I., Rayer, G., Treat, C., and Carim, H.: Management of childhood lymphosarcoma and reticulum cell sarcoma with high dose intermittent methotrexate and citrovorum factor. Proc. Am. Assoc. Cancer Res. *9*:18, 1968.

Freidreich, E. J., Gehan, E. A., Frei, E. III, et al.: The effect of 6-mercaptopurine on the duration of steroid-induced remissions in acute leukemia: A model for evaluation of other potentially useful therapy. Blood *21*:699, 1963.

George, S. L., Aur, R. J. A., Mauer, A. M., and Simone, J. V.: A reappraisal of the results of stopping therapy in childhood acute leukemia. N. Engl. J. Med. *300*:269, 1979.

Hamburger, A. W., and Salmon, S. E.: Primary bioassay of human tumor stem cells. Science *197*:461, 1977.

Legha, S. D., Benjamin, R. S., Mackay, B., et al.: Reduction of doxorubicin cardiotoxicity by prolonged continuous intravenous infusion. Ann. Intern. Med. *96*:133, 1982.

Ritz, J., Sallan, S. E., Bast, R. C., et al.: Autologous bone marrow transplantation in CALLA positive ALL following *in vitro* treatment with J5 monoclonal antibody and complement. Blood *58*:175a, 1981.

Sachs, L.: The differentiation of myeloid leukemia cells. New possibilities for therapy. Br. J. Haematol. *40*:409, 1978.

Schabel, F. M., Jr.: The use of tumor growth kinetics in planning "curative" chemotherapy of advanced solid tumors. Cancer Res. *29*:2384, 1969.

Skipper, H. E., Schabel, F. M., and Wilcox, W. S.: Experimental evaluation of potential anti-cancer agents. XIII. On the criteria and kinetics associated with curability of experimental leukemia. Cancer Chemother. Rep. *35*:1, 1964.

Terman, D. S., Young, J. B., Shearer, W. T., et al.: Preliminary observation of the effects on breast adenocarcinoma of plasma perfused over immobilized protein A. N. Engl. J. Med. *305*:1195, 1981.

Vaughan, W. P., Karp, J. E., and Burke, P.: Long chemotherapy free remission after single cycle timed–sequential chemotherapy for acute myelocytic leukemia. Cancer *45*:859, 1980.

DESIGN OF CLINICAL THERAPEUTIC TRIALS

Armitage, P., and Gehan, E. A.: Statistical methods for the identification and use of prognostic factors. Int. J. Cancer *13*:16, 1974.

Gehan, E., and Freireich, E. J.: Non-randomized controls in cancer clinical trials. N. Engl. J. Med. *290*:198, 1974.

Meyer, J. S.: Cell kinetic measurements of human tumors. Hum. Pathol. *13*:874, 1982.

PROSPECTS OF CANCER RESEARCH AND THERAPY

Thomas, E. D., Storb, R., Clift, R. A., et al.: Bone marrow transplantation. N. Engl. J. Med. *292*:832, 895, 1975.

Section IV

GASTROENTEROLOGY, ENDOCRINOLOGY, AND METABOLISM

The Esophagus

26

David B. Skinner

INTRODUCTION

The primary function of the esophagus is the transportation of ingested material from the pharynx to the stomach. A second function is the prevention of involuntary regurgitation of stomach contents. Abnormalities of the esophagus can be considered in relation to the four major components contributing to normal esophageal function. These components are the cricopharyngeal sphincter at the upper end, the muscular layers of the esophagus, the mucosal lining of the esophagus, and the sphincter mechanism at the cardia. The esophagus plays no important role in the digestion or absorption of food, although the initial breakdown of starches by salivary gland secretions may occur during the transportation of food through the length of the esophagus.

STRUCTURE

The cricopharyngeal sphincter consists of skeletal muscle fibers, which are arranged obliquely in its upper portion and blend into those of the inferior pharyngeal constrictor muscle. In the lower portion of the sphincter the fibers are arranged transversely and are continuous with the muscle layers of the esophagus. The muscle bundles composing the sphincter arise and insert from the back and sides of the cricoid cartilage. The sphincter has no posterior fibrous raphe comparable to the inferior constrictor. In the resting state the sphincter is contracted, maintaining a mean pressure of approximately 30 mm Hg. During swallowing, relaxation occurs. When studied by intraluminal pressure recordings, the sphincter ranges from 3 to 5 cm in length, but appears somewhat shorter in radiographic examinations. It is located at the level of the sixth cervical vertebra.

Esophageal muscle fibers are of the striated or skeletal type in the upper one third of the esophagus and are of smooth muscle in the lower esophagus. The transition between skeletal and smooth muscle is indistinct and somewhat variable in location. Esophageal muscle is arranged in two layers, the outer layer running longitudinally, and the inner layer positioned transversely or obliquely around the lumen. There is no true serosal layer on the surface of the esophagus, but the outer longitudinal muscle fibers blend into the overlying fibrous tissue of the pleura and pericardium and the fibrofatty tissue of the mediastinum.

The mucosa of the esophagus is squamous epithelium continuous with that of the pharynx at the upper end. At the distal esophagus there is a sharp transition to simple columnar epithelium that may be visible during esophagoscopy as the ora serrata, or "Z" line. Scattered unevenly throughout the esophageal submucosa are glands. These produce mucus that reaches the lumen through small excretory ducts and provides lubrication for the passage of ingested material. Simple tubular glands similar to those at the cardia of the stomach may be located at the upper and lower ends of the esophagus and are confined to the lamina propria mucosae. In some individuals, there may be islands of gastric epithelium replacing squamous epithelium. These are more commonly encountered in the upper esophagus. Occasionally, acid-secreting or oxyntic cells are encountered in these patches of columnar epithelium. The esophageal mucosa is separated from the muscle layers by a submucosal layer that permits considerable movement of the mucosa in relation to the muscle.

In humans, a lower esophageal sphincter cannot be identified by anatomic dissection. However, functionally, the distal esophagus behaves as a sphincter, in that the resting luminal pressure at the gastroesophageal junction is greater than in the esophagus above or the stomach below. This contracted segment relaxes in response to a swallow. The characteristics of this sphincter are described by manometric studies. Normally, the sphincter straddles the gastroesophageal mucosal junction and ranges in length from 2 to 4 cm. Resting pressure is generally 8 or more mm Hg greater than gastric pressure. The reversal of pressure deflections caused by respiration occurs in the cephalad portion of this high pressure zone. Below the pressure reversal point, inspiration causes an increase in pressure similar to that in the abdomen, whereas proximal to this level inspiration causes a decrease in pressure similar to the intrathoracic pattern. When manometric studies and cineradiography are performed together, the lower portion of the distal esophageal sphincter corresponds to the submerged or closed segment within the diaphragmatic hiatus and upper abdomen, whereas the upper portion of the sphincter zone corresponds to the distal half of the phrenic ampulla radiographically.

The junction of the esophageal and gastric mucosa is located at the level of the tenth thoracic vertebra within the esophageal hiatus of the diaphragm. The hiatus is a muscular tunnel, 2 to 3 cm long, through which pass the esophagus, vagus nerves, and extensions of endoabdominal fascia. The endoabdominal fascia and endothoracic fascia join together to form the phrenoesophageal membrane. This sheet of fibrous and elastic tissue extends from the muscular margins of the hiatus to the esophagus circumferentially and inserts into the esophageal submucosa slightly above the upper margins of the hiatus and above the mucosal junction.

Disease of the esophagus may be classified and understood by considering its effect upon the two primary functions of the esophagus—transportation of ingested material and the prevention of reflux—and the four aforementioned major components that contribute to normal function: the cricopharyngeal sphincter, the muscle layers, the mucosal lining, and the lower esophageal sphincter. Since dysphagia, or difficulty in swallowing, is almost a universal complaint in patients with any disease interfering with esophageal function, this symptom must be regarded as nonspecific. However, dysphagia must be regarded as a strong indication for complete diagnostic evaluation of esophageal structure and function. Only in this way will a precise diagnosis of the individual pathologic condition be made at a time when therapy can be instituted to restore esophageal function to normal.

TRANSPORTATION OF INGESTED MATERIAL

NORMAL SWALLOWING

When food or liquid is swallowed, the bolus is transmitted from the pharynx to the stomach by the coordinated action of all four esophageal components. Instantaneously, with the onset of swallowing, the cricopharyngeal sphincter relaxes, and luminal pressure level falls to that in the body of the esophagus. This sphincter relaxation lasts for a short time, often 1 second or less, and is followed by a contraction of the sphincter that may produce a luminal pressure of up to 80 mm Hg.

The arrangement of circular and longitudinal esophageal muscle fibers allows both constriction of the lumen and shortening of the esophagus, which are essential for effective peristalsis. A primary peristaltic wave triggered by a swallow is characterized by a progressive contraction that moves down the body of the esophagus at the rate of 2 to 4 cm per second and generates intraluminal pressures that generally range between 30 and 60 mm Hg above resting pressure. Preceding the peristaltic contraction, relaxation occurs. The arrangement of mucosal folds, their loose adherence to the muscle, and the marked ability of the relaxed muscle to stretch permit distention of the esophagus to several centimeters without disruption. A single swallow generates a peristaltic contraction that progresses completely down the full length of the esophagus. However, if a second swallow is performed immediately, the initial peristaltic wave is interrupted, and a second wave begins in the upper esophagus and progresses downward. In older persons, the proportion of swallows followed by a primary progressive peristaltic contraction is diminished when compared with that of younger individuals.

Other types of esophageal contractions are observed. Secondary peristalsis is a progressive peristaltic wave that occurs without initiation by a swallow. These may be triggered by a bolus in the esophagus or may occur spontaneously. Tertiary or segmental contractions are nonperistaltic and may follow a swallow in an older patient with disordered esophageal function, may result from stimulation by an oversized bolus, or may be initiated by irritants such as regurgitated acid in the lumen. High-amplitude tertiary contractions are considered spastic and may persist for prolonged periods.

In response to a swallow, the lower esophageal sphincter segment relaxes promptly, permitting intraluminal pressure to drop to gastric level. This relaxation lasts until the peristaltic wave reaches the lower esophagus. As the peristaltic wave reaches the upper portion of the sphincter, it participates in the contraction with a marked increase in pressure, whereas the lower portion of the sphincter simply regains its resting tone of approximately 8 mm Hg above intragastric pressure. The concentric contraction of the distal esophagus is useful in differentiating between esophagus and stomach radiographically, since the latter does not contract in coordination with esophageal peristalsis. The termination of the peristaltic contraction can be employed to locate the muscular junction between esophagus and stomach.

The entire action of the esophagus in response to a swallow is coordinated by vagal or parasympathetic nerve fibers that provide the major innervation of the esophagus. Both central and local neural pathways appear to be involved in the peristaltic contraction. Administration of anticholinergic drugs or a proximal vagotomy causes a decrease in the strength of the peristaltic contraction and diminishes the resting pressure in the lower esophageal sphincter. Sympathetic innervation has been demonstrated anatomically, but the function of these nerve fibers is not completely understood.

DISORDERS OF THE CRICOPHARYNGEAL SPHINCTER

Failure to Relax. Precise neuromuscular coordination of swallowing is most critical at the level of the cricopharyngeal sphincter. Since this sphincter normally remains in the tonic or contracted state, it must relax to permit a swallowed bolus to enter the esophagus. The time of relaxation is short and must precede and overlap the time of pharyngeal contraction. Relaxation is controlled by branches from the vagus and glossopharyngeal nerves. A number of neurologic disorders may interfere with this coordinated function and cause faulty timing or failure of sphincter relaxation, which in turn prevents passage of the bolus into the esophagus and favors the likelihood of aspiration of swallowed material through the larynx into the tracheobronchial tree. Failure of the sphincter to open may cause symptoms of obstruction in the throat, with periodic choking or frequent cough accompanying swallowing. In some patients the symptoms are not very dramatic and the disorder may lead to chronic pulmonary damage from aspiration of small quantities without the patient being aware of difficulty in swallowing. Underlying diseases that may interfere with neuromuscular coordination include minor or major vascular occlusions in the brain stem, myasthenia gravis, amyotrophic lateral sclerosis, peripheral neuropathies involving the vagus or glossopharyngeal nerve, and skeletal abnormalities such as cervical osteoarthritis.

Spasm. A second source of failure of the cricopharyngeal sphincter to relax is spasm of this muscle. Radiographic studies have demonstrated that patients with disorders lower in the esophagus, such as severe gastroesophageal reflux, may have regurgitation or retention of material in the upper esophagus. This in turn irritates the sphincter and causes spasm. In addition to aspiration during swallowing, such patients may be aware of a chronic irritation in the throat and may develop a fear of swallowing that has been previously categorized as "globus hystericus." Some patients with neurologic or muscular dysfunction of the cricopharyngeal sphincter will develop secondary laryngeal changes, causing symptoms of hoarseness and chronic pharyngitis. Inflammatory polyps of the vocal cords and trachea may be found.

Cricopharyngeal (Zenker's) Diverticulum. Zenker's diverticulum is the most common type encountered in the esophagus. It is a false or acquired diverticulum characterized by pouching of the mucosal or submucosal layers through a defect in the muscular wall. The defect is located just proximal to the cricopharyngeal sphincter in the posterior wall of the inferior pharynx. Recent studies suggest that the pouch is secondary to dysfunction of the cricopharyngeal sphincter. When a bolus is forced into the lower pharynx against a closed sphincter, high pressures build up just above the sphincter. There is a weak place posteriorly in the musculature of the inferior pharynx where the oblique muscle fibers of the inferior constrictor blend into the transverse fibers of the sphincter. At this point, a blowout of mucosa or diverticulum may develop.

In patients with a fully developed cricopharyngeal diverticulum it is common to elicit a history of swallowing difficulty dating back several years prior to awareness of the pouch. Initially, the symptoms are cervical dysphagia and occasional bouts of aspiration or choking. As the pouch enlarges, solid particles and fluid become trapped and later regurgitate into the pharynx. When the patient lies down or stoops forward he may notice undigested food eaten hours earlier now regurgitating back into the mouth. The swallowing of large solid particles such as pills, capsules, or pieces of meat may be particularly difficult, as these routinely lodge in the pouch. A patient with a fully developed pouch finds that he must eat slowly and carefully to avoid aspiration. Friends and family frequently notice gurgling noises when the patient eats or swallows.

Complications of this disorder include chronic or acute aspiration, the risk of a large solid bolus lodging in the larynx that may cause asphyxiation, an increased risk of perforation from foreign bodies, and the development of ulcerations in the pouch from retained irritating particles. Carcinomas have developed within such pouches. There is a particular risk of perforation during endoscopic or intubation procedures for patients with this disorder.

DISORDERS OF ESOPHAGEAL MUSCLE

Esophageal muscular disorders may interfere with transmission of a swallowed bolus in several ways.

Other Esophageal Diverticula. Pulsion diverticula may occur at levels in the esophagus other than the cricopharyngeal region. The next most common site is the lower esophagus. These epiphrenic diverticula also consist of mucosal protrusions through the muscular layer that develop just proximal to the lower esophageal sphincter or just proximal to a segment of spastic esophageal muscle. The mechanism for development of such a diverticulum appears similar to that for the cricopharyngeal diverticulum. Although aspiration and laryngeal irritation do not occur, other symptoms from retention of swallowed material are similar.

When studied manometrically, the esophagus distal to the pulsion diverticulum characteristically demonstrates spastic or tertiary contractions, or failure to relax as the peristaltic wave progresses down the esophagus. When viewed radiographically, the usual finding is a segment of tonic or contracted muscle just beyond the opening of the pouch. Dysphagia frequently accompanies pulsion diverticulum. This has been attributed to the large size of the pouch hanging in a dependent position and compressing the adjacent lower esophagus. However, dysphagia may accompany a small diverticulum, in which case such a mechanical explanation cannot be invoked. It is now thought that the dysphagia represents a primary disorder in the esophageal muscle rather than a secondary effect of the diverticulum.

More rare are true diverticula that may occur at any level and in which the body of the esophagus appears to be normal above and below the opening of the pouch. The wall of the true diverticulum consists of both mucosal and muscular layers. Distinction is sometimes made between those diverticula that appear rounded and have a narrow orifice similar to that of pulsion diverticula and are considered of congenital origin and those with broad openings, generally in the midesophagus, which are commonly called *traction diverticula*. This latter term derives from the theory that the esophagus is pulled out of its normal course by contractions of adhesions to adjacent inflammatory lymph nodes or chronic mediastinal infection; however, clear evidence of this is frequently not demonstrable. These diverticula cause no or few symptoms unless they reach a large size.

Systemic Sclerosis. Systemic sclerosis or scleroderma is a generalized disease involving smooth muscle and connective tissues throughout the body. Esophageal involvement is the most common alimentary tract manifestation and may precede other clinical evidence of the disease. The esophageal changes consist of atrophy of the smooth muscle in the lower two thirds of the organ distal to the segment of skeletal muscle. The smooth muscle is gradually replaced by fibrosis. The muscle atrophy causes a failure of the peristaltic wave to progress into the lower esophagus and causes weakness or obliteration of the lower esophageal sphincter mechanism. This in turn permits increased gastroesophageal reflux, which may lead to secondary esophagitis. The fibrosis of the muscle may lead to a stricture of the distal esophagus, or stricture may develop owing to the severity of the esophagitis accompanying gastroesophageal reflux. The effects of reflux in such patients may be particularly severe because of the inability of the esophagus to respond by secondary peristalsis and empty itself of regurgitated gastric contents. Either aperistalsis or stricture may cause the symptom of dysphagia.

The absence of peristalsis when observed manometrically or by radiographic techniques and systemic manifestations of the disease differentiate this disorder from abnormal gastroesophageal reflux due to an incompetent lower esophageal sphincter in an otherwise healthy patient. The common radiographic finding is failure of ingested barium to pass the level of the carina when the patient is in a supine position. When the patient sits upright, the barium falls under the influence of gravity. When a stricture develops in such patients the esophageal disease may become the most prominent feature of systemic sclerosis and lead to progressive weight loss and starvation. Because of the atrophic esophageal wall and frequent secondary esophagitis, attempts to treat this disorder by dilatation may be difficult, and the risks of esophageal perforation are high.

Esophageal Spasm. When esophageal spasm is encountered, it is generally secondary to another esophageal disorder. The majority of patients who demonstrate spasm will be found to have either abnormal gastroesophageal reflux that appears to trigger spasm, particulary in the lower esophagus, or a partial obstruction such as a ring, web, hypertensive lower esophageal sphincter, or tumor. Occasionally, patients are encountered in whom none of these disorders can be identified, and spasm on a primary neurogenic or functional basis must be diagnosed. Whenever this diagnosis is made, careful search for an underlying cause should be undertaken.

Characteristically, spasm is localized or segmental in distribution, with the most prominent spastic contractions occurring repeatedly at the same level. Complete or partial obstruction to the passage of ingested food may result from spasm. A prominent feature of this disorder is severe substernal pain that may suggest the symptoms accompanying ischemic heart disease. Since the spasm may be reduced by the use of nitrites, response to nitroglycerin is not a useful way to differentiate between this disease and coronary heart disease. The diagnosis of esophageal spasm is made by the characteristic radiographic appearance of a corkscrew esophagus or multiple constrictive rings that do not dilate during fluoroscopic observation. Another useful diagnostic technique is manometry, which shows high-pressure contractions occurring spontaneously or in response to a swallow and located at the same level in the esophagus on repeated studies.

Leiomyoma. Benign tumors of smooth muscle in the esophagus are occasionally encountered. Normally, these are incidental findings in the course of barium swallow radiography, but occasionally these tumors may reach sufficient size to interfere with the passage of ingested food and cause dysphagia. They are not normally fixed to the esophageal mucosa and cannot be diagnosed endoscopically. When a leiomyoma is suspected from radiographic findings, a biopsy should not be attempted through the esophagoscope because of the dangers of introducing infection and causing inflammatory adhesion of the tumor to the mucosa, which interferes with later surgical removal.

DISORDERS OF MUCOSA

Neoplasm. Benign neoplasms of the esophageal mucosa are infrequent and generally of little clinical importance. Occasionally, squamous polyps or papillomas may be encountered. Adenomas arising in the esophageal glands are rare. The most common esophageal neoplasm is carcinoma. This most frequently causes the symptom of dysphagia and occurs with sufficient frequency that any patient complaining of persistent dysphagia should be thoroughly investigated for the possibility of this disease.

Carcinoma of the esophagus is a virulent neoplasm causing approximately five deaths per 100,000 population in the United States each year. The disease is more frequent in males than in females, and in nonwhite than in white Americans. It occurs more commonly in the sixth, seventh, and eighth decades of life. Carcinoma may develop in association with conditions contributing to esophageal retention or irritation such as excessive use of alcohol or tobacco, and among patients having achalasia or lye strictures. Patients with the Plummer-Vinson syndrome (see further on) are susceptible to squamous cell carcinoma of the cervical esophagus and hypopharynx.

Carcinoma may present a variety of appearances (e.g., ulceration, fungating tumor, or diffuse scirrhous strictures). The most common site of origin appears to be in the middle third of the esophagus. Microscopically, squamous cell carcinoma is by far the most common type. Adenocarcinoma truly arising in the esophagus separated from the stomach is rare. Adenocarcinoma at the cardia is more common and arises from columnar mucosa lining the distal 2 to 3 cm of esophagus. The incidence of esophageal adenocarcinoma is especially high in patients with columnar epithelium lining the distal esophagus (Barrett's esophagus). Carcinomatous change in esophageal mucosa may be multifocal. The disease spreads by direct extension, lymphatic invasion, and blood-borne metastases. The rich lymphatic network of the esophageal submucosa permits early and extensive spread of the tumor up and down the length of the esophagus. It is not uncommon to encounter malignant cells 5 cm or more from the visible margins of a tumor. Direct invasion of adjacent structures such as the trachea or aorta is common and a frequent cause of life-threatening complications. One reason for the poor prognosis of these tumors is the advanced state that they reach before causing symptoms. Because of the ability of smooth muscle to stretch, involvement of the esophageal lumen must be nearly circumferential before dysphagia and obstruction develop.

Although the patient may recall a sensation of substernal fullness or poorly localized chest pain, the usual presenting complaint is dysphagia, or difficulty in swallowing. Rapid weight loss and emaciation accompany the dysphagia. As the obstruction becomes more complete, regurgitation of swallowed food, vomiting, or choking and aspiration are noted. Hoarseness may develop from recurrent nerve involvement by the primary tumor or lymph node metastases. Horner's syndrome,

hematemesis, or melena may occur. When the tumor invades the trachea or bronchus, cough, hemoptysis, or dyspnea results. Complications of the tumor may be heralded by the presence of lymph nodes in the neck, bone pain from metastases, hemorrhage from invasion of mediastinal vessels, fever from perforation or abscess, and severe cough from tracheobronchial involvement. Tracheoesophageal fistula may develop in advanced cases and be the terminal event.

Because the obvious symptoms from carcinoma of the esophagus represent complications of the disease at an advanced stage, it is especially important that the diagnosis be made whenever possible at any earlier stage, when treatment is more favorable and symptoms are less apparent. Any patient complaining of symptoms that might arise from the esophagus should undergo radiographic examination and have specimens of esophageal brushings submitted for cytologic examination. In addition to the standard barium swallow observed fluoroscopically and recorded on permanent radiographs, it is often helpful to examine the esophagus by cineradiographic techniques, so that the course of the barium may be examined repeatedly if questionable regions in the esophagus are observed. Just as the pathologic presentation of esophageal carcinoma is variable, the radiographic manifestations may take many forms such as a fungating mass, ulcerations, stricture, or polypoid tumor. In some patients the radiographic appearances may be more suggestive of benign disease.

Cytologic examination of cells obtained from esophageal brushings offers a high diagnostic yield in patients with this disease. In addition to the patients whose symptoms or radiographs suggest a possible neoplasm, those who may have a high risk of the disease such as individuals with longstanding lye stricture, achalasia, Barrett's esophagus lined with columnar epithelium, or the Plummer-Vinson syndrome are good candidates for repeated cytologic examinations at 6- or 12-month intervals.

For confirmation of the diagnosis of carcinoma in patients whose symptoms or radiographs are suggestive, esophagoscopy is an essential diagnostic procedure. A biopsy will provide confirmatory evidence of the diagnosis and indicate the cell type. Because of the tendency for esophageal neoplasms to spread up and down the mucosa, biopsies are generally taken above the level of the tumor to ascertain whether submucosal spread has occurred. This has great importance in planning treatment for the disease. In patients whose neoplasm is located in the middle third of the esophagus, bronchoscopy should also be performed to detect evidence of tracheal or left main bronchial invasion or vocal cord paralysis.

Web or Ring. Benign rings or webs of the

esophageal mucosa may cause symptoms by obstructing the passage of solid food through the lumen. Although these mucosal constrictions may occur at any level in the esophagus, there are two specific clinical forms in which this lesion is more frequently encountered.

The Plummer-Vinson syndrome, when fully developed, includes a hypochromic microcytic anemia, spoon-shaped fingernails, atrophy of the tongue and of the pharyngeal and esophageal mucosa, fissures at the corners of the mouth, and dysphagia. This syndrome occurs most frequently in fair-complexioned females of Northern European descent. The dysphagia may result from a hypopharyngeal or upper esophageal mucosal web. These patients have a higher than normal incidence of carcinoma of the upper esophagus and must be carefully observed for a change in symptoms suggesting the development of a neoplasm. Such patients are candidates for periodic cytologic examination of esophageal brushings.

In 1953, Schatzki and Gary as well as Ingelfinger and Kramer independently described the condition of lower esophageal ring causing dysphagia. This clinical syndrome often occurs in older male patients and is manifested by sudden severe dysphagia after ingestion of a large bolus of solid food. The sensation of food sticking under the lower sternum and severe pain are prominent symptoms. As the food digests or is gradually propelled through the narrow segment, the symptoms subside and may not recur for prolonged periods until a large bolus is once again ingested. The symptoms of severe pain that may accompany this disorder are due to spasm of the esophageal muscle above the ring as the esophagus contracts upon the impacted bolus. In this regard, the symptoms of pain come from a mechanism similar to that which causes pain lower in the intestinal tract, namely, vigorous contraction of gut muscle above an obstructing point.

Pathologically, the "Schatzki" ring is found to have esophageal squamous mucosa on the superior surface and columnar mucosa on the inferior surface. A thin layer of fibrous tissue may be seen in the submucosa between the two layers of mucosa. Deeper layers of the esophagus are normal. The effect of the ring is to limit esophageal distention. Thus, when the esophagus is empty, no ring is visible. It is only when the lumen of the esophagus is distended beyond the diameter of the ring that it becomes noticeable. For this reason, the ring may be missed in radiographic examinations unless the lower esophagus is studied in the dilated condition. The diameter of the ring has a strong correlation with the presence of symptoms. Patients whose rings measure less than 13 mm in diameter almost always have symptoms of dysphagia, whereas those whose rings are larger than 13 mm may be asymptomatic. Rings of large diameter are frequent findings in routine barium swallow examinations, but those that progress to a narrow aperture and cause symptoms are uncommon. Because the ring represents a zone of restricted distensibility rather than a constant weblike defect in the esophagus, it may be easily missed by esophagoscopy. The diagnosis is generally made only on radiographic study.

Stricture. Stricture or abnormal narrowing of the esophagus may occur from a variety of causes. Malignant neoplasms may present as a stricture. The ingestion of corrosive substances such as lye may cause destruction of the esophageal wall, with stricture formation. The most common type of benign esophageal stricture is caused by reflux esophagitis. The diagnosis of a stricture is made on the basis of a persistent narrowing or contraction of the esophagus demonstrated radiographically. However, the specific type of stricture generally cannot be diagnosed solely with radiographs; it is determined by the clinical history and esophagoscopic findings.

Strictures secondary to gastroesophageal reflux are thought to occur through the following mechanisms: An incompetent lower esophageal sphincter permits free reflux of upper gastrointestinal secretions, including acid, pepsin, bile, and pancreatic secretions, into the lower esophagus. Prolonged contact of these substances with the esophageal mucosa causes penetration and breakdown of the mucosa, superficial ulceration, submucosal inflammation, edema, and muscle spasm. The damage is repaired by deposition of inflammatory tissue followed by collagen deposition and fibrosis, just as injured tissue heals elsewhere in the body. If the reflux decreases, the mucosa may be restored by migration and regeneration of columnar epithelial cells rather than the squamous epithelium that normally lines the lower esophagus. Continuous or repeated insults to the mucosa lead to increasing amounts of tissue destruction and fibrosis. Initially this occurs in the superficial layers, but as the condition becomes more severe the muscle fibers are damaged and replaced by fibrous tissue as well. As the collagen matures, it contracts, causing rigidity, narrowing, and shortening of the esophageal wall until a tight stricture develops. As the lumen is gradually occluded by the contracting fibrous tissue, the amount of reflux diminishes, and the mucosa and esophagus above the level of the stricture are spared from further insult and appear normal. The development of a stricture through these steps has been documented sequentially in individual patients and has been seen in various stages in many others, providing evidence for this theory of stricture development.

At the time when a stricture is apparent radiographically, the fibrosis may still be limited to the submucosal layers, with edema and spasm causing much of the narrowing, or the appearance of a stricture on the radiograph may represent far advanced disease, with total breakdown and replacement of the esophageal wall by fibrosis and granulation tissue. Thus, the clinical and radiographic diagnosis of esophageal stricture may represent pathologic conditions of varying degrees of severity. This must be taken into account when therapy is planned and the results of treatment are assessed.

The physiologic effects of reflux esophagitis and stricture are initially those of disordered peristalsis. Partial esophageal narrowing as well as esophageal reflux can disrupt or alter progression of the peristaltic wave and cause synchronous or tertiary contractions. Inability of the esophagus to empty permits prolonged contact of refluxed material with the mucosa and aggravates the esophagitis. It is only when the stricture becomes far advanced that the bolus of food is mechanically obstructed by the narrowing. By this time, the patient's intake of solid food is markedly restricted. As the stricture tightens, the reflux may be less, so that the symptoms of heartburn and regurgitation are diminished. Dysphagia may be the only complaint. This leads to a paradox in which the most severe stages of esophagitis may be associated with few symptoms of reflux, although this is thought to be the underlying cause of the inflammation and stricture. In patients whose esophagus is relatively insensitive to reflux or in whom reflux occurs mainly while the individual is supine and asleep, dysphagia may be the earliest complaint leading the patient to the physician.

In addition to symptoms of reflux, dysphagia, and inanition, the patient with a stricture is likely to have pulmonary complaints of nocturnal cough, or choking or coughing when eating, and may develop pulmonary infection secondary to aspiration. Other complications of a stricture include hemorrhage, usually from ulceration in areas of ectopic columnar mucosa, and perforation of the esophagus, again usually due to ulceration in areas of ectopic gastric epithelium.

Between the two common types of benign esophageal strictures—those due to reflux esophagitis and those secondary to ingestion of caustic materials—important differences exist. The stricture secondary to reflux is almost always rather short and localized to the region just above columnar epithelium, whether this be at the gastroesophageal junction or high in the esophagus in patients whose esophagus is lined with columnar or gastric epithelium (Barrett's esophagus). Thus, the patient with a short stricture in the midesophagus caused by reflux will have columnar epithelium below the stricture. However, a patient whose stricture is due to ingestion of lye or other corrosives will often have long segments of esophagus damaged by the chemicals and replaced with fibrous tissue. Damage may be particularly severe at the levels of the esophagus where there is a shelf or transient holdup of the bolus, such as the cricopharyngeal region, the level of the aortic arch, and just above the diaphragm.

A second distinction between the reflux and corrosive strictures is that the cause of the reflux stricture persists, so that the condition continues to worsen rather than improve with time. Methods of therapy that do not prevent the underlying reflux may fail to provide relief from further stricture development. However, the stricture secondary to ingestion of corrosives is caused by a single injury. Taking this into account, one may employ methods of therapy that differ from those used in treatment of a reflux stricture.

Malignant strictures of the esophagus are considered in a preceding section and are not discussed further here. The secondary effects and complications of the malignant stricture may be similar to those of the benign stricture.

DISORDERS AT THE CARDIA INTERFERING WITH TRANSPORTATION OF INGESTED MATERIAL

Achalasia. Achalasia is an uncommon disease of unknown etiology in which the lower esophageal sphincter fails to relax in response to a swallow, and there is an absence of peristalsis in the body of the esophagus. Findings on visual or radiographic examination include a normally contracted distal esophageal segment of approximately 2 to 4 cm in length composed of normal muscle. The body of the esophagus is generally dilated and may distend to a very large size sufficient to contain a quart or more of fluid. Generally, the muscle of the esophageal wall in its midportion is thickened, but in far advanced cases it may become atrophic and fibrotic. Microscopically, the distinctive feature of achalasia is the absence or decrease in number of the ganglion cells in Auerbach's plexus. Fibrosis of the plexus may be noted. These changes are found throughout the esophagus but are more conspicuous in the lower portion. The inner circular muscle layer may be hypertrophied or sclerotic, and scarring of the muscle cells may be noticed microscopically. Although several reports have suggested that there may be abnormalities of the vagus nerves or the central nervous system in patients with achalasia, these findings have not been thoroughly substantiated or generally accepted.

While the etiology of achalasia is unknown, a similar type of megaesophagus with similar pathologic changes in the muscle and Auerbach's plexus may be seen in Chagas' disease. This disease occurs in South America and is caused by *Trypanosoma cruzi*. Evidence suggests that the organism secretes a neurotoxin that affects the ganglion cells. Although this disease is clinically similar to achalasia, the organism has not been found in the vast majority of patients suffering from typical achalasia in North America or Europe.

The physiologic disorder of achalasia may best be studied by esophageal manometry. The characteristics of the lower esophageal sphincter segment in the resting state are the same as in normal individuals. However, in the body of the esophagus the resting intraluminal pressures are generally high and may exceed the pressures of the gastric fundus. The manometric abnormalities of achalasia are most striking when the response to a swallow is studied. The lower esophageal sphincter fails to relax following a swallow, and contraction may occur prematurely in the upper portion of the sphincter, so that the sphincter is effectively closed when the peristaltic wave would normally reach the lower esophagus. In addition to the failure of the sphincter to relax, absence of peristalsis in the body of the esophagus impedes passage of the bolus. Following the swallow, a simultaneous contraction generally occurs throughout the length of the esophagus with no progression of the pressure waves. In far advanced cases in which the muscle has become sclerotic, atrophic, and fibrotic, no contraction at all may be observed.

A further physiologic abnormality in the patient with achalasia is the response to methacholine. In the normal subject, injection of this drug generally causes no change in pressure in the body of the esophagus. In a patient with achalasia, subcutaneous injection of 5 to 10 mg of methacholine chloride may cause an increase in resting esophageal pressure of 20 cm of water or more. This may be associated with severe substernal pain, similar to that in patients with esophageal spasm. The methacholine response may be abolished by administration of atropine sulfate.

The symptoms caused by these specific pathologic and physiologic changes are sufficiently distinctive to separate this disease from other esophageal disorders. Initially, the patient will notice intermittent obstruction to swallowing localized to the lower substernal region. The obstruction is generally less when a meal is taken slowly and the food is warm. The obstruction may be intermittent and may be more severe when the patient is tense or nervous. As the symptoms become more pronounced, the patient becomes aware of regurgitation whenever he stoops forward. Unlike gastroesophageal reflux, the regurgitated material is not acid or sour, and undigested food can often be identified. Pain is generally not associated with the regurgitation. The pain that occurs with achalasia, if any, is usually of the spastic type, rather than heartburn. It may be quite severe, is located substernally, and persists for a long time.

When esophageal retention becomes marked, pulmonary symptoms secondary to aspiration become prominent. The patient may awaken to find ingested food material regurgitated onto the pillow. Secondary pulmonary complications including lung abscess may occur. Nutrition may be impaired, and the patient suffers weight loss and vitamin deficiency. Although bleeding is quite uncommon in these cases, a retention esophagitis may develop and cause chronic anemia from blood loss. In addition to these complications from obstructed swallowing, patients with achalasia are thought to have a higher than normal incidence of squamous cell carcinoma in the midportion of the esophagus.

Hypertensive Lower Esophageal Sphincter. A rare variation of the spastic esophageal motor disorders may be increased tone in the lower esophageal sphincter, causing dysphagia and severe pain. Generally, retention of ingested food in the esophagus is not prominent in these patients. This finding differentiates it from achalasia, as does the finding of increased sphincter pressure during manometric studies. In other respects, this syndrome is similar to that of esophageal spasm. Whether the hypertensive sphincter syndrome occurs as secondary manifestation of a gastroesophageal reflux remains uncertain.

OTHER DISEASES AFFECTING TRANSPORTATION OF INGESTED MATERIAL

A variety of diseases that involve the esophagus may have a secondary effect of blocking transportation of ingested material. Extrinsic conditions such as neoplasm metastatic to the mediastinum or esophageal wall may interfere with swallowing in a manner similar to that of primary carcinoma of the esophagus. An enlarging thoracic aortic aneurysm may compress the esophagus and cause secondary dysphagia. Primary bronchogenic carcinoma adjacent to the esophagus may involve the esophageal wall and block ingestion of food. A foreign body lodged in the esophagus generally interrupts swallowing, owing to both its physical presence and the edema and inflammation it causes in the wall of the esophagus.

Esophageal atresia with tracheoesophageal fistula is a fairly common abnormality of the newborn that obviously interferes with transportation of ingested food. Following surgical correction of the atresia and fistula, function of the distal esophagus generally remains abnormal with disordered peristalsis. Acquired tracheoesophageal fistulas may occur from malignant disease in the mediastinum or rarely from inflammatory diseases such as tuberculosis and histoplasmosis. Such fistulas permit transportation of food material from the esophagus directly into the lungs, with resulting severe cough and pulmonary infection.

Rupture of the esophagus may occur spontaneously, from penetrating wounds or external trauma, from foreign bodies, or during the course of esophageal intubation. This catastrophic event occurs most commonly during esophagoscopy or gastroscopy. When perforation accompanies endoscopy, the common sites are just distal to the cricopharyngeal sphincter and in the lower esophagus. Spontaneous rupture of the esophagus is almost always caused by vomiting and occurs most frequently along the left lateral aspect of the lower esophagus. During vomiting, the antrum of the stomach contracts and the upper stomach and esophagus relax, permitting increased intra-abdominal pressure to force the gastric contents cephalad. The distal esophagus may increase dramatically in diameter fivefold or more. The left lower esophageal wall is the weakest point of the organ and can be ruptured by pressures of 5 lbs per square inch or less, providing the setting for spontaneous rupture during vomiting.

Following esophageal rupture, the patient experiences a sudden severe substernal or epigastric pain. If the rupture occurs when the patient is anesthetized or sedated for endoscopy, this initial symptom may be absent. Following rupture, mediastinal dissection of air or pneumothorax develops. This is manifested by crepitus felt in the neck or a mediastinal crunching sound heard on auscultation over the back. If the rupture does not penetrate the pleura, an effusion secondary to the mediastinitis develops in the pleura within the course of several hours. Free perforation into the pleura causes a hydropneumothorax and empyema. A tension pneumothorax may occur. The patient rapidly becomes gravely ill, with signs of shock. This illness may be mistaken for perforated duodenal or gastric ulcer, acute pancreatitis, acute myocardial infarction, or dissecting aortic aneurysm. The diagnosis can be resolved by abdominal and thoracic radiographs, serum amylase levels, electrocardiogram, and x-ray visualization of the esophagus by a swallow of radiopaque water-soluble substance.

PREVENTION OF GASTROESOPHAGEAL REFLUX

The second major function of the esophagus is the prevention of involuntary regurgitation of stomach contents. The responsibility for this function is vested in the esophagogastric junction, or cardia.

MECHANISMS FOR COMPETENCY OF THE CARDIA

In normal individuals the mechanism that permits unimpeded passage of swallowed material into the stomach while preventing regurgitation of gastric contents back through the esophageal orifice is remarkably effective. Withdrawal of a pH electrode across the cardia often reveals a 5-unit change in pH over a distance of approximately 0.5 cm. This represents a 100,000-fold difference in hydrogen ion concentration across this short distance. In spite of a great deal of investigation as to the structure and function of the esophagogastric junction, precise understanding of the mechanism that prevents reflux remains incomplete.

A number of factors are suggested as contributing to competency of the cardia. The strength or resting pressure of the lower esophageal sphincter has a statistical correlation with the control of reflux. Yet, in individual patients a high pressure in the sphincter may be present, and free reflux occurs. Conversely, a low sphincter pressure may be found in a patient without reflux. Since no anatomic sphincter can be demonstrated in humans, the source of the pressures recorded in the distal esophagus remains uncertain. The high-pressure zone probably represents a summation of intrinsic pressure generated from the lower esophageal muscle, extrinsic pressure resulting from the diaphragmatic hiatus, and positive abdominal pressure exerted against the distal esophageal segment below the insertion of the phrenoesophageal membrane (endoabdominal fascia). An active role of the distal esophageal muscle in generating the measured sphincter pressure and in the prevention of reflux is suggested by the observation that pressures in the lower esophageal segment rise when the hormone gastrin is administered in pharmacologic doses. In some animal species such as the opossum, the distal esophageal muscle responds to chemical stimulation differently from other esophageal muscle, suggesting a specialized sphincter-like function. Most investigators accept the lower esophageal muscle as being at least partially responsible for competency of the cardia.

The esophageal hiatus of the diaphragm may play a role in the normal control of reflux, but it is not essential. Some patients with a hiatal hernia have a competent cardia, whereas others in whom a hiatal hernia cannot be demonstrated may have an incompetent cardia.

The location of a portion of the lower esophageal sphincter within the positive pressure abdominal environment appears to be important in the prevention of reflux. The pressure gradient across the diaphragm is usually 10 mm Hg or more and increases during inspiration. The compressing effect of abdominal pressure during all phases of respiration supplements the intrinsic pressure generated by the lower esophageal muscle segment. In humans, both the pressure recorded in the distal esophagus and length of esophagus exposed to abdominal pressure correlate independently with the control of reflux. Intra-abdominal pressure may remain effective even in patients with hiatal hernia if the extension of endoabdominal fascia through the hiatus inserts into the esophagus several centimeters above the esophagogastric junction. Compression by the right crus of the diaphragm or muscular contraction of the diaphragm does not appear important, but an intra-abdominal location of the distal esophageal segment does contribute to competency of the cardia. Other suggested factors for which there is less evidence of effectiveness include an acute esophagogastric angle of entry and the plugging of the esophageal orifice by redundant gastric folds.

Hiatal Hernia. Hiatal hernia is one of the most common disorders of the alimentary tract. Its significance varies greatly, depending on type, size, and associated complications. It is necessary to understand that gastroesophageal reflux and hiatal hernia, which often appear together, are separate entities, each of which may occur without the other. For this reason, it is important to differentiate the symptoms, diagnosis, and complications for each of the two conditions.

Hiatal hernia is defined as stomach passing through the esophageal hiatus of the diaphragm. There are two basic types of hiatal hernia that can be differentiated by the anatomic and physiologic abnormalities of each. Combinations of the two types constitute a third group of hiatal hernias, and the presence of other organs in addition to the stomach passing through the esophageal hiatus makes up a fourth category of hiatal hernia.

In type I, the axial or sliding hiatal hernia, the esophagogastric junction is displaced through the diaphragm as the leading point of the hernia. In type II, the paraesophageal (rolling) hernia, the esophagogastric junction remains fixed at the level of the hiatus, but a portion of the gastric fundus advances above the cardia into a hernial sac. It is the type I hiatal hernia that may be accompanied by gastroesophageal reflux and its distinctive symptoms and complications. Type II hiatal hernia is rarely associated with abnormal reflux. The combined type III hiatal hernia, in which the esophagogastric junction is herniated through the diaphragm but a portion of the gastric fundus is more cephalad than the cardia, may be associated with the symptoms and complications of both type I and type II hernias.

The diagnosis of a hiatal hernia is established primarily by radiographic study and is confirmed by surgical dissection. Diagnostic methods such as manometry, mucosal potential difference measurements, and pH recordings are more useful in diagnosing gastroesophageal reflux and its complications than in establishing the presence of a hiatal hernia.

Generally, the common small type I hiatal hernia is asymptomatic and causes no complications unless abnormal gastroesophageal reflux is present. The symptoms and complications often attributed to this hernia are really those of reflux and will be described in the next section.

The type II hiatal hernia may be asymptomatic, even though quite large, or it may cause symptoms related to the abnormal position of the stomach in the hernial sac. These symptoms are most commonly mild discomfort or fullness in the epigastrium or chest after eating. This may be relieved by belching or vomiting. Dysphagia may occur because of extrinsic compression of the esophagus by the adjacent large hernial pouch. This type of hernia is associated with a substantial incidence of serious mechanical complications involving the gastric pouch. Complications include hemorrhage from ulcers or gastritis in the supra-

diaphragmatic stomach, gastric obstruction, volvulus, which may lead to strangulation and gastric infarction. Very large type II hernias are commonly combined with displacement of the cardia proximally and may be associated with reflux and its complications. Large hernias introduce a risk of intrathoracic gastric dilatation with respiratory embarrassment. When the sac is sizable, other organs such as colon, small intestine, or spleen may herniate and provide a further source of complications.

Gastroesophageal Reflux. Regurgitation of gastric contents through the esophagogastric junction probably occurs at times in everyone, usually after a meal. Manometric study has shown that newborn infants lack a lower esophageal high pressure zone, and they frequently regurgitate. During the first year of life, competency of the cardia is acquired, and regurgitation ceases. Although occasional postprandial reflux occurs as a normal event in older patients, frequent reflux into an esophagus sensitive to the irritating gastrointestinal secretions may cause symptoms and complications. When this occurs, the clinical condition of abnormal gastroesophageal reflux results. This rarely develops in the interval between infancy and late adolescence. Thereafter, the incidence of abnormal reflux rises, and the problem is most common in patients over 40 years of age. There seems to be an increased tendency for reflux to occur in obese individuals.

Although abnormal reflux commonly is associated with type I, or sliding, hiatal hernia, a causal relationship between these two conditions is not established. Individuals without a hiatal hernia demonstrated radiographically or at surgery may experience reflux through an incompetent cardia, and patients having a hiatal hernia do not necessarily experience abnormal reflux.

In the typical patient with gastroesophageal reflux, manometric studies often demonstrate a decreased resting pressure in the lower esophageal segment. Generally, the sphincter segment will be of normal length unless a large hiatal hernia is present that distorts the pressure recordings. However, the length of sphincter reflecting abdominal pressure is usually decreased. Relaxation to swallowing is normal. There is not a precise one-to-one relationship between sphincter pressure and competency of the cardia, so that manometric studies alone are not acceptable as diagnostic evidence of abnormal reflux.

Radiography is the most useful technique for detecting a hiatal hernia, but it is less successful in demonstrating reflux. The diagnosis of abnormal reflux can be made by the radiologist if he sees reflux at a time other than when the patient swallows. If reflux is suspected as the cause of the patient's complaint but cannot be demonstrated radiographically, the use of pH recordings is a more sensitive and reliable diagnostic method. In patients with severe reflux there may be a disorder of esophageal motor function manifested by an increased proportion of simultaneous contractions rather than progressive peristalsis. A bolus of acid placed in the esophagus in such subjects may not be cleared normally.

The typical symptoms caused by gastroesophageal reflux are pain and regurgitation aggravated by postural positions such as stooping or lying down. Discomfort is usually felt beneath the sternum and in the subxiphoid region, with occasional radiation to one side. The pain may radiate to the shoulders, neck, arms, ears, or between the scapulae, but it nearly always includes the substernal region. The nature of the pain is a burning sensation and is frequently called "heartburn" by the patient. Regurgitation may be noted as a sour or bilious taste in the mouth or as the "repeating" of food. Effortless vomiting after meals may occur in severe cases. Aggravation of the symptoms by bending over or lying flat permits the diagnosis of reflux clinically. If the patient's complaints are not related to posture, heartburn or regurgitation may be the result of other causes and cannot be attributed to abnormal reflux on the basis of symptoms alone.

Other symptoms that may be caused by reflux include vague epigastric or substernal discomfort, a foreign sensation, fullness or tightness in the neck, hoarseness, change in voice, chronic pharyngitis from reflux through the cricopharyngeal sphincter, or symptoms that mimic those of angina pectoris. When atypical symptoms are noted, the diagnosis cannot be made on clinical grounds and must depend on objective evidence of reflux and exclusion of other causes. Recordings of pH in the esophagus to document reflux may be especially helpful. In patients with atypical symptoms, the perfusion of acid and saline alternately into the esophagus may be useful in determining whether the symptoms are of esophageal origin. Reproduction of the patient's spontaneous symptoms by infusion of acid and not with saline represents a positive acid perfusion test.

The complications of gastroesophageal reflux include esophagitis, stricture, bleeding, ulceration, spasm, and aspiration of regurgitated material into the lungs. Esophagitis is the most common complication of reflux. Since the severity of the patient's symptoms correlate poorly with esophagitis, this diagnosis can be made with certainty only by esophagoscopy. Patients who present with advanced esophagitis and stricture may have minimal or no symptoms of reflux prior to the onset of obstruction, whereas some who complain most bitterly of heartburn and regurgitation are found on esophagoscopy and biopsy to have no or minimal esophagitis. The reason for such variability is the different pattern that reflux may take in individual patients. Some reflux mainly while supine during sleep and may be unaware of symptomatic reflux. Clearing of acid is diminished during sleep, so advanced esophagitis may develop without many symptoms. Those who reflux mainly in the upright position during the day may clear acid well and avoid esophagitis but still be highly symptomatic. One symptom that does suggest the presence of esophagitis and mediastinal inflammation is soreness between the scapulae following ingestion of hot or alcoholic liquids. When dysphagia develops, esophagitis is more likely to be present. However, reflux alone may trigger esophageal muscle spasm, causing dysphagia in the absence of esophagitis, and therefore this symptom is not diagnostic.

Because of the lack of specific symptoms for reflux esophagitis, esophagoscopy is essential to diagnosing this condition. The esophagoscopic findings may be categorized based upon severity. These include no visible esophagitis and grade I esophagitis, when the mucosa is reddened but not ulcerated. In such cases, biopsy may show only thinning of the mucosa and perhaps dilatation of epithelial vessels without other change. Grade II esophagitis is recorded when superficial erosions and ulcerations are noted. When the wall of the esophagus becomes somewhat stiffened and fibrotic in addition to being ulcerated, grade III esophagitis is present. When the fibrosis and contraction has caused a stricture, grade IV esophagitis is observed. Stricture is discussed in detail in a preceding section. Ulceration of the esophageal mucosa commonly takes the form of circumferential destruction of the squamous epithelium just above the columnar epithelial border. Localized penetrating ulcers into the wall of the esophagus, particularly in islands of ectopic gastric mucosa, may occur and cause rapid hemorrhage. Bleeding may also be severe in milder forms of esophagitis when diffuse oozing of blood from the mucosal surface is encountered.

Another common complication of an incompetent cardia is aspiration. Mild degrees manifested by nocturnal cough and occasional hoarseness are frequently noted in the histories of patients who prove to have reflux. When aspiration becomes more severe, pulmonary complications such as recurring pneumonitis or lung abscess may occur.

REFERENCES

Allen, T. H., and Clagett, O. T.: Changing concepts in the surgical treatment of pulsion diverticula of the lower esophagus. J. Thorac. Cardiovasc. Surg. 50:455, 1962.

Belsey, R.: The pulmonary complications of oesophageal disease. Br. J. Dis. Chest. 54:342, 1960.

Belsey, R.: Functional disease of the esophagus. J. Thorac. Cardiovasc. Surg. 52:164, 1966.

Bennett, J. R., and Hendrix, T. R.: Diffuse esophageal spasm: A disorder with more than one cause. Gastroenterology 59:273, 1970.

Berenson, M. M., Riddell, R. H., Skinner, D. B., and Freston, J. W.: Malignant transformation of esophageal columnar epithelium. Cancer 41:544, 1978.

Bernstein, L. M., Fruin, R. C., and Pacini, R.: Differentiation of esophageal pain from angina pectoris: role of the esophageal acid perfusion test. Medicine (Baltimore) 41:143, 1962.

Bombeck, C. T., Dillard, D. H., and Nyhus, L. M.: Muscular anatomy of the gastroesophageal junction and role of phrenoesophageal ligament. Autopsy study of sphincter mechanism. Ann. Surg. 164:643, 1966.

Castell, D. O., and Harris, L. D.: Hormonal control of gastroesophageal sphincter strength. N. Engl. J. Med. 282:866, 1970.

Cauthorne, R. T., VanHoutte, J. J., Donner, M. W., and Hendrix, T. R.: Study of patients with lower esophageal ring by simultaneous cineradiography and manometry. Gastroenterology 49:632, 1965.

Christensen, J., Freeman, B. W., Miller, J. K.: Some physiologic characteristics of the esophagogastric junction of the opossum. Gastroenterology 64:1119, 1973.

Cohen, S., and Lipshutz, W.: Hormonal control of lower esophageal sphincter competence: interaction of gastrin and secretin. Gastroenterology 58:937, 1970.

Cohen, B. R., and Wolfe, B. S.: Roentgen localization of the physiologically determined esophageal hiatus. Gastroenterology 43:43, 1962.

Delahunty, J. E., Alonso, W. A., Margulies, S. I., and Knudson, D. H.: Relationship of reflux esophagitis to pharyngeal pouch (Zenker's diverticulum) formation. Laryngoscope 81:570, 1971.

DeMeester, T. R., Johnson, L. F., Joseph, G. J., et al.: Patterns of gastroesophageal reflux in health and disease. Ann. Surg. 184:459, 1976.

Dowlatshahi, K., Daneshbod, A., and Mobarhan, S.: Early detection of cancer of the esophagus along the Caspian Littoral. Lancet 1:125, 1978.

Ellis, F. H., Jr., and Olsen, A. M.: Achalasia of the Esophagus. Philadelphia, W. B. Saunders Co., 1969.

Foster, J. H., Jolly, P. C., Sawyers, J. D., and Daniel, R. A.: Esophageal perforation: diagnosis and treatment. Ann. Surg. 161:701, 1965.

Fyke, F. E., Jr., Code, C. F., and Schlegel, J. G.: The gastroesophageal sphincter in healthy human beings. Gastroenterologia (Basel) 86:135, 1956.

Gryboski, J. D., Thayer, W. R., Jr., and Spiro, H. M.: Esophageal motility in infants and children. Pediatrics 31:382, 1963.

Harris, L. D., and Pope, C. E., II: "Squeeze" vs. resistance: an evaluation of the mechanism of sphincter competence. J. Clin. Invest. 43:2272, 1964.

Hayward, J.: The lower end of the oesophagus. Thorax 16:36, 1961.

Hiebert, C. A., and Belsey, R.: Incompetency of the gastric cardia without radiologic evidence of hiatal hernia. J. Thorac. Cardiovasc. Surg. 42:352, 1961.

Holder, T. M., and Ashcraft, D. W.: Esophageal atresia and tracheoesophageal fistula. Curr. Probl. Surg., August, 1966.

Hunt, P. S., Connell, A. M., and Smiley, T. B.: The cricopharyngeal sphincter in gastric reflux. Gut 11:308, 1970.

Ingelfinger, F. J.: Esophageal motility. Physiol. Rev. 38:533, 1958.

Ingelfinger, F. J., and Kramer, P.: Dysphagia produced by contractile ring in lower esophagus. Gastroenterology 23:419, 1953.

Ismail-Beigi, F., Horton, P. F., and Pope, C. E., II: Histological consequences of gastroesophageal reflux in man. Gastroenterology 58:163, 1970.

Just-Viera, J. O., Morris, J. D., and Haight, C.: Achalasia and esophageal carcinoma. Ann. Thorac. Surg. 3:526, 1967.

Katz, D., and Hoffman, F. (Eds.): The Esophagogastric Junction. Amsterdam, Excerpta Medica, 1971.

Mackler, S. A.: Spontaneous rupture of the esophagus, an experimental and clinical study. Surg. Gynecol. Obstet. 95:345, 1952.

Mossberg, S. M.: The columnar lined esophagus (Barrett syndrome): an acquired condition? Gastroenterology 50:671, 1966.

Olsen, A. M., and Schlegel, J. F.: Motility disturbances caused by esophagitis. J. Thorac. Cardiovasc. Surg. 50:607, 1965.

O'Sullivan, G. C., DeMeester, T. R., Smith, R. B., et al.: Twenty-four-hour pH monitoring of esophageal function. Arch. Surg. 116:581, 1981.

Schatzki, R.: The lower esophageal ring: Long-term followup of symptomatic and asymptomatic rings. Am. J. Roentgenol. 90:805, 1963.

Schatzki, R., and Gary, J. E.: Dysphagia due to diaphragm-like localized narrowing in lower esophagus ("lower esophageal ring"). Am. J. Roentgenol. 70:911, 1953.

Skinner, D. B., and Booth, D. J.: Assessment of distal esophageal function in patients with hiatal hernia and/or gastroesophageal reflux. Ann. Surg. 172:627, 1970.

Skinner, D. B., and DeMeester, T. R.: Gastroesophageal reflux. Current Problems in Surgery, Vol. 13, 1976.

Skinner, D. B., Belsey, R. H. R., Hendrix, T. R., and Zuidema, G. D. (Eds.): Gastroesophageal Reflux and Hiatal Hernia. Boston, Little, Brown and Co., 1972.

Sutherland, H. E.: Cricopharyngeal achalasia. J. Thorac. Cardiovasc. Surg. 43:114, 1962.

Wilkins, E. W., Jr., and Skinner, D. B.: Recent progress in surgery of the esophagus: I. Pathophysiology and gastroesophageal reflux. II. Clinical entities. J. Surg. Res. 8:41, 90, 1968.

Wynder, E. L., and Fryer, J. H.: Etiologic considerations of Plummer-Vinson (Paterson-Kelly) syndrome. Ann. Intern. Med. 49:1106, November, 1958.

The Stomach* **27**

H. Juergen Nord and William A. Sodeman, Jr.

ANATOMIC VARIATIONS

The form and position of the stomach vary in different persons and in the same person at various times, depending on the degree of filling, the size and position of the adjacent organs, the condition of the anterior abdominal musculature, and the physical habitus. In the relatively short, obese person with a tense abdominal wall, the stomach often lies high in the upper left quadrant of the abdomen and is steer-horn in shape, whereas in the tall, thin person the greater curvature may extend to the brim of the true pelvis and the stomach is in the shape of the letter J. Such variations in the position of the stomach are of no clinical significance; they do not produce symptoms. The important consideration is not the location but rather the structure and the physiologic activity of the stomach.

CONGENITAL ANOMALIES

HYPERTROPHIC STENOSIS OF THE PYLORUS

Obstructive narrowing of the pylorus by hypertrophy of the pyloric muscle is most common in infants 2 or 3 weeks old, although it may be observed at any time between the ages of 10 days and 3 or 4 months. Males are involved four times as often as females, and first-born children more frequently than later-born siblings. A genetic predisposition is suggested by the fact that hypertrophic pyloric stenosis is 10 times as common among first-degree relatives of male index patients and 25 times as common among first-degree relatives of female index patients as in the general population. The condition is attributed to congenital hypertrophy, with or without spasm. The stenotic pylorus is represented by an oval tumor of muscular tissue approximately 3 cm long and 1.5 cm in diameter, with hypertrophy, especially of the circular layer of the muscularis propria, and fibrotic thickening of the submucosa. Microscopically, the hypertrophic muscular layer may be edematous and infiltrated with leukocytes. Decreased numbers of myenteric plexus ganglion cells, sometimes appearing immature or degener-

ated, have been described, suggesting that the primary defect is in the innervation of the muscle. Symptoms usually begin during the second to fourth weeks after birth, and consist of nonbilious projectile vomiting after feeding, constipation or obstipation, and rapid loss of weight. The nutritional depletion may be pronounced. Dehydration and alkalosis develop as a consequence of the loss of fluid and electrolytes in the gastric content.

Rarely, primary hypertrophic pyloric stenosis becomes symptomatic only in adulthood. The congenital origin of such cases is less certain, although similar histologic patterns and the occurrence of both infantile and adult-onset cases in some families support this possibility. More commonly, however, pyloric stenosis in adults is secondary, acquired in association with peptic ulcer disease of the duodenum or pyloric channel, extrinsic adhesions, or infiltrative neoplasms and inflammatory disorders. In such instances there is little or no true circular muscle hypertrophy and the increase in pyloric mass is due to fibrosis, inflammation, or tumor.

DIVERTICULA

Diverticula of the stomach are rare in man. Seventy-five per cent of gastric diverticula are located near the cardia, high on the posterior wall of the stomach. Such diverticula are usually congenital in origin. Many, however, have little or no muscular coat, suggesting the possibility that they are of the acquired, "pulsion" type. The characteristic juxtacardiac location in a weakened area where the longitudinal muscle fibers are divided and the muscular wall is formed mainly of circular and oblique fibers is consistent with this possibility. The next most common location for gastric diverticula is the prepyloric area, where about 15 per cent are found. Most of these probably are acquired as a result of gastric or extragastric disease. Some antral diverticula, especially the "partial" or intramural diverticula, are associated with ectopic pancreatic tissue, implying a congenital origin. Gastric diverticula are not more common in individuals with diverticula of other portions of the digestive tract. They do not often cause symptoms except, unusually, in the presence of inflammation or ulceration, or unless they are huge and so situated as to fill readily with food and secretions.

---

*This current revision incorporates the structure and presentation of material established by Dr. Joseph B. Kirsner and by Dr. Kirsner and Dr. Charles S. Winans in prior editions of this text.

GASTRIC TORSION AND VOLVULUS

The stomach may rotate about its long axis so that the greater curvature turns upward or at 90° to this axis, the pylorus turns forward to the left, and the cardia passes backward. Torsion is present when the degree of rotation is less than 180° and obstruction is not complete. Some degree of rotation of the stomach is a common radiologic finding and probably of little clinical significance. Volvulus is an extension of torsion in which the degree of rotation is more than 180° so that obstruction occurs at each end of the twisted segment. Volvulus may develop as an exacerbation of torsion, or it may occur in a previously normally situated stomach. Diaphragmatic anomalies, including large paraesophageal hernias, contribute to the development of volvulus. The onset of acute gastric volvulus is sudden and painful. The precipitating cause may be a large meal, a minor injury, or a sudden movement. Pain is severe and continuous and is experienced chiefly in the epigastric and left subcostal regions. It then may radiate through to the back or remain retrosternal in site. There may be repeated attempts at vomiting but with the emission of only small amounts of mucoid material. These symptoms are accompanied by the rapid development of very severe epigastric distention. Perhaps the most important clinical observation is inability to pass a nasogastric tube to relieve the gastric distention.

SENSORY DISTURBANCES

APPETITE AND HUNGER

The sensations of appetite and hunger are closely related. Appetite is a pleasant sensation, conditioned by previous agreeable experiences with the smell, taste, and appearance of food. Hunger is an unpleasant sensation of abdominal emptiness, epigastric discomfort, or pangs of dull pain produced by the intermittent contractions of the empty stomach or intestine or both and arising from the physiologic need for food. The distinction between hunger and appetite is not always sharp, and accentuation of the appetite often is interpreted as a part of the total complex of hunger. The following sensory components may be enumerated:

1. Pleasant olfactory and gustatory sensations with their associated pleasant memories of the taste and smell of food are the classic features of appetite.

2. Painful hunger pangs result from contractions of the empty stomach and intestines.

3. An indefinite, unpleasant, generalized, steady, and continuous sensation is interpreted as hunger and is vaguely referred to the abdomen.

4. Accessory phenomena such as lassitude, weakness, drowsiness, faintness, irritability, restlessness, and headache may occur concomitantly.

As summarized by Janowitz:

At the physiologic level of regulation of intake, deficits of the body's stores of calorically significant nutrients activate feeding reflexes which are facilitated by areas in the lateral hypothalamus and are inhibited by the ventromedial hypothalamus. These deficits concomitantly give rise to hunger sensations which may be cues for food intake. These hypothalamic centers are sensitive to local temperature and appear to be influenced by body stores of water. Day-to-day regulation of the amount of food consumed is regulated in part by oropharyngeal receptors; and the size of an individual meal is controlled by gastric and upper intestinal receptors responding to distention, probably mediated by the vagus nerve. The hypothalamic areas also are believed to be influenced by the metabolic consequences of food absorbed and assimilated. The specific dynamic action of food, the utilizable blood glucose, and concentration of other metabolites in the blood, the level of protein in the diet and depot fat, all have been proposed as cues to the central nervous system, but none has been firmly established as governing short or long-term control.

Excessive appetite and hunger occur in various conditions, as in convalescence from an acute infectious disease, but the mechanism is unexplained. A similar situation obtains in thyrotoxicosis, in which the requirement for food is maintained at a high level because of the excessive metabolism. In diabetes mellitus the glucose in the blood is not available to the tissues; hunger and polyphagia result. Excessive appetite may also be a characteristic of the emotionally disturbed individual. In peptic ulcer the distress may be interpreted as hunger because the patient fails to differentiate it from a hunger pang or because it occurs when the stomach is thought to be empty and is relieved by eating.

Anorexia is a loss of appetite or lack of desire for food. Loss of appetite is a variable but common symptom in many diseases, including hepatitis, gastric or pancreatic neoplasm, advanced renal disease, congestive heart failure, alcoholism, and endocrine disorders such as Addison's disease and panhypopituitarism. Loss of appetite may also be a manifestation of an emotional disturbance, usually depression. *Anorexia nervosa* and the related condition *bulimia* represent unusual emotional disturbances of food intake. They occur chiefly in adolescent girls and young women and much less commonly in males. In a few patients *anorexia nervosa* has been described in association with extreme levels of exercise. The clinical features include cachexia, amenorrhea, constipation, and hypothermia. Laboratory findings include hypoproteinemia, anemia, and a number of abnormalities of endocrine function. The disease is chronic and progressive. Fatalities occur in 6 per cent of cases. The problem is thought to be psychosocial, although a physiologic predisposition may play a role. Hunger is a feature, and the word *anorexia* in the title may be inappropriate. The hunger is suppressed to the point of progressive starvation. *Bulimia* is a variant in which eating, often gorging, is followed by induced vomiting. This may alternate with periods of anorexia. Weight loss is more gradual than with *anorexia nervosa,* but electrolyte abnormalities and alkalosis can occur with loss of secretion, and acid erosion of the teeth is also common.

NAUSEA

Nausea denotes an unpleasant sensation, ordinarily referred to the back of the throat, the epigastrium, or both, and often culminates in vomiting. It may be accompanied by vasomotor manifestations of autonomic stimulation, such as salivation, sweating, faintness, vertigo, and tachycardia. The clinical significance of nausea is identified with that of vomiting. It may be produced by gastric or pancreatic disease, by pyloric or intestinal obstruction, by emotional disturbances, by unpleasant visual or olfactory or gustatory stimuli, by various biochemical abnormalities associated with metabolic disorders, or by intense pain from any source. Nausea (and anorexia) often are associated with gastric hypofunction: hypotonicity, hypoperistalsis, and hyposecretion.

VOMITING

Vomiting is defined as the forceful explusion of gastric and intestinal contents through the mouth. Immediately preceding vomiting are tachypnea, copious salivation, dilatation of the pupils, sweating, pallor, and rapid heartbeat—all signs of widespread autonomic stimulation. Vomiting begins with deep inspiration. The glottis is closed and the nasopharynx is shut off partly or completely. Inspiration is converted to an expiratory effort, with simultaneous contraction of the abdominal muscles. Because the glottis is closed, the increase in intrathoracic and intra-abdominal pressure is transmitted to the stomach and esophagus. The body of the stomach and the muscle of the esophagus relax. At the same time a strong annular contraction at approximately the angulus of the stomach nearly divides the body from the antrum. While the body of the stomach remains flaccid, peristaltic waves sweep aborally over the antrum. The positive intrathoracic and intra-abdominal pressures force expulsion of the gastric contents through the mouth. Finally the voluntary muscles relax and respiration resumes.

The vomiting center is located in the dorsolateral border of the lateral reticular formation, immediately ventral to the tractus solitarius and its nucleus, near the sensory nucleus of the vagus nerve. It may be excited directly by mechanical stimuli such as increased intracranial pressure; by impulses mediated by the chemoreceptor trigger zone (lying superficially in the floor of the fourth ventricle) as in emesis from motion sickness or irradiation or such emetic drugs as apomorphine, morphine, and digitalis; by afferent impulses produced by distention of the stomach and duodenum; or by impulses from any region of the body. The diversity of the causes of vomiting is reflected in its association with such metabolic problems as renal failure, hyperparathyroidism, and alkalosis and in situations such as migraine and labyrinthine disorders. Vomiting may be produced in susceptible persons by impulses from the higher cerebral centers, as when unpleasant subjects are discussed or when offensive odors are encountered. The afferent impulses reach the center along many routes, the chief ones being the vagal and sympathetic nerves from the stomach and other abdominal viscera. The efferent fibers are contained chiefly in the phrenic, vagus, and sympathetic nerves.

BELCHING

Belching is the eructation of swallowed air. Normally a small amount of air is swallowed in the process of eating, swallowing food rapidly, chewing gum, or smoking excessively. Most of the swallowed air does not reach the stomach, but is regurgitated immediately from the lower esophagus as a part of the act of belching. Some of the gas passes into the stomach and accumulates in the gastric air bubble until it is eliminated in a more or less spontaneous belch. The chronic belcher then renews the cycle by swallowing more air, most of which he regurgitates with each belch, but some of which passes on into the stomach, until once more a spontaneous belch occurs. In time, the act becomes almost involuntary. The consumption of carbonated beverages, especially in large volume, increases belching. Fatty foods likewise lead to eructations in some patients. A possible explanation is the resulting delayed gastric emptying, which does not allow escape of some of the gastric air into the duodenum and small bowel. Belching is not related specifically to disease of the gallbladder, stomach, or any other organ. It is primarily a functional event, often induced by a sensation of abdominal fullness or discomfort, which the patient attempts to relieve by the gastroesophageal expulsion of air.

MOTOR DISTURBANCES

PHYSIOLOGIC CONSIDERATIONS

Although structurally a single organ, functionally the stomach must be viewed as having two distinct portions. Proximally, the fundus and body of the stomach serve primarily as a reservoir, increasing in volume as it fills with food and secretions in such a fashion as to maintain intragastric pressure unchanged. This process has been termed *receptive relaxation*. Vasoactive intestinal polypeptide (VIP) is the hormone at present considered responsible for mediating this effect, which is controlled by the vagus nerve. Distally, the antrum of the stomach subserves the process of mixing, triturating, and emptying. Contraction waves originating in the midportion of the stomach proceed peristaltically toward the pylorus, creating an "antral pump" mechanism, the efficiency of which in emptying the stomach presumably is determined not only by the frequency and strength of peristaltic contractions but also by the dimensions of the antrum.

Electromyography of gastric muscle has allowed the beginning of an understanding of antral motor activity. Arising from a pacemaker high on the greater curvature, electrical *slow waves* are propagated through the longitudinal muscle layer toward the pylorus. The electrical slow wave (also termed gastric pacesetter potential) is a cylical wave of partial depolarization and repolarization of the muscle membrane that, in humans, occurs at a frequency of three per minute. Under physiologic circumstances this frequency is extremely constant, and the slow waves are generated continuously regardless of the presence or absence of muscular contractions. At times, presumably under appropriate conditions of stimulation, bursts of *fast-wave* depolarizations are superimposed upon the nadir of slow-wave depolarization. These depolarization spikes initiate muscular contractions that, being phase-linked to the moving slow waves, move peristaltically through the antrum.

The precise mechanisms for the control of fast-wave activity, and thereby gastric peristalsis, are not known. The stomach may be viewed, however, as a pump that is constantly under varying degrees of restraint. Indeed, with the exception of gastric distention, which speeds emptying, all other influences on gastric motor activity are inhibitory. Receptors within the duodenal mucosa sensitive to osmolarity, acidity, and fat concentration of the duodenal content initiate enterogastric nerve reflexes that inhibit gastric emptying. Additionally, secretin, cholecystokinin, enterogastrone, perhaps other hormones liberated from the duodenum, and gastrin, released from the antral mucosa, delay gastric emptying. Thus, in a complex fashion gastric motor activity and emptying are the integrated result of central nerve impulses, local and central nerve impulses, local and central nerve reflexes, and hormonal influences acting upon the intrinsic gastric neuromuscular apparatus.

Although the muscular thickening that characterizes the pylorus strongly suggests a sphincteric function that might influence the rate of gastric emptying, such a function for the pylorus has been difficult to establish. Indeed, evidence suggests that the pyloric sphincter functions mainly to prevent retrograde flow of intestinal content. Thus, in health, the pyloric high-pressure zone, as determined by intraluminal manometry, is increased by the presence of acid or fat within the duodenum, presumably by the action of endogenously released regulatory peptides. If marker substances are infused into the duodenum together with acid, a reduction in recovery of the marker from the stomach accompanies the increased pyloric sphincter pressure, suggesting that pyloric contraction indeed slows duodenogastric reflux. Gastrin antagonizes the effect of the duodenal hormones on the pyloric sphincter. Failure of secretin and cholecystokinin to augment pyloric sphincter pressure in gastric ulcer patients has been suggested as an important pathophysiologic defect in that disorder.

Liquids and solids are handled in a totally different fashion by the stomach. Liquids are primarily accommodated by the fundus and proximal body of the stomach, where slow contractions produce a pressure gradient between stomach and duodenum. The rate of emptying is quite rapid and occurs in an exponential fashion, slowing down later as relaxation occurs. Water is emptied at the rate of 50 per cent in 20 minutes. As calories, acidity, fat, or hypertonicity are added to the liquid the emptying rate decreases.

Solids empty quite differently. Particles must be broken down to less than 1 mm in diameter before they can pass the contracted pyloric sphincter. The circular contractions beginning in the body become stronger in the antrum and sweep down toward the pylorus at a maximal rate of three or four per minute. They push food toward the contracted pylorus, where it is retropulsed into the stomach, the result being a grinding action. Ultimately this process produces a chyme of adequate particle size and consistency to allow passage through the pylorus.

Between meals there is an interesting change in gastric motility patterns, which are divided into three phases. In Phase I, which occurs 1½ to 2 hours after meals, gastric contractions decrease markedly from three per minute to only one every 4 or 5 minutes. In Phase II, during a 30-minute time span, there are irregular contractions that lead to Phase III, in which over a 5- to 15-minute period intense sweeping contractions occur that travel from the stomach all the way to the cecum. Secretions, indigestible food fiber, and larger particles are emptied into the intestine during this phase, which is then followed again by the relatively quiescent motor activity of Phase I. Ingestion of a meal disrupts this interdigestive gastric motor pattern.

PATHOPHYSIOLOGIC STATES

Delayed gastric emptying in the absence of mechanical obstruction occurs in a variety of conditions such as diabetic ketoacidosis, electrolyte abnormalities, progressive systemic sclerosis, myotonic dystrophy, progressive muscular dystrophy, and others. It is a common problem in the stomach after operations such as vagotomy and pyloroplasty and partial gastric resection. After vagotomy the receptive gastric function is compromised and the pressure/volume ratio is impaired, resulting in a more rapid emptying of liquids (dumping). Emptying of solids is usually markedly delayed. In diabetic gastroparesis liquids do not empty rapidly as in the postvagotomy state. In both conditions gastric motor activity is decreased and Phase III ("housekeeper") interdigestive contractions are usually absent in the stomach but exist in the upper small bowel. This may explain the frequent occurrence of "bezoars" in these conditions. Metoclopramide (a dopamine antagonist) and bethanechol (a cholinergic agent) can restore gastric motor activity, suggesting a neural regulatory disorder rather than a primary smooth muscle failure.

Delayed gastric emptying has been observed in asymptomatic patients, in whom it has been termed "idiopathic." It may be a significant contributing factor in gastroesophageal reflux disease and gastric ulcer.

Spasm of the entire stomach or of a portion of the stomach has been described in lesions of the central nervous system and also in the presence of cholelithiasis or pancreatic disease. The relationship of such spasm to abdominal pain is questionable. Painful gastric spasms are noted occasionally in the apparently normal stomach. Localized muscular spasm occurs not infrequently with gastric lesions, as in hourglass contracture with a benign ulcer, the contracture disappearing when the ulcer heals. Contraction of the stomach along the greater curvature also has been observed in emotionally disturbed patients who ruminate. The incisura-type indentation is presumably spastic in nature, but it is not accompanied by pain. Painless spasm of the pylorus, as evidenced by rather persistent closure, occurs with intrapyloric peptic ulcer, with gastric and duodenal lesions adjacent to the pylorus, and occasionally with gastric ulcers located proximal to the pylorus on the lesser curvature.

GASTRIC SECRETION

PHYSIOLOGIC CONSIDERATIONS

The secretion of hydrochloric acid physiologically is a composite of three interrelated phases: neurogenic (vagal), gastric (gastrin), and to an extent less well understood, intestinal. The neurogenic phase is initiated by stimuli such as the sight, smell, or taste of food acting upon receptors in the cerebral cortex and the subsequent stimulation of the vagal nucleus. The process presumably is mediated chemically by acetylcholine from postganglionic parasympathetic nerve endings acting upon gastric parietal cells. Vagal excitation also releases gastrin from the antrum and sensitizes the parietal cells to stimulation by gastrin. Chief cell secretion is also augmented by vagus nerve stimulation, which elicits a copious secretion of gastric juice rich in acid and pepsin. Truncal division of the vagi is followed by a pronounced reduction in the volume and acidity of the gastric secretion in all patients but it is quantitatively most impressive in hypersecreting duodenal ulcer patients. The parietal cell retains the ability to produce hydrochloric acid with direct stimulation as by gastrin or histamine. Stimulation of the splanchnic nerves evokes an alkaline secretion, chiefly from the pyloric glands, rich in mucus and poor in peptic activity. Emotional disturbances exert an important influence upon the secretory and motor functions of the stomach. Prolonged anxiety, hostility, and resentment can cause engorgement of the gastric mucosa and increased secretion, whereas depression and fear induce pallor of the mucosa and a reduction in acid output. These changes are related, respectively, to increased and decreased rates of blood flow through the gastric vasculature.

The gastric phase of secretion is mediated primarily by the hormone gastrin. Gastrin release may be neurogenic, through vagal stimulation, mechanical by distention with food or fluid, chemical by the action of peptides or certain amino acids or calcium, or systemically mediated by parenteral calcium or epinephrine or bombesin. Inhibition of gastrin release may likewise be neurogenic through vagal inhibitory fibers, humoral as a result of low pH, or chemical. At least six regulatory peptides, including secretin, VIP, gastric inhibitory peptide (GIP), somatostatin, calcitonin and glucagon are inhibitors. Multiple molecular species of gastrin now have been identified (Fig. 27–1). Three are biologically active as stimulators of acid secretion. The heptadecapeptide (G-17) was the first identified and is joined by "big gastrin" (G-34) and "minigastrin" (G-14). Each exists in forms with and without the sulfated tyrosine in position 12. The C-terminal four amino acids of the gastrin molecule (TRP-MET-ASP-PHE-NH$_2$) possess the full physiologic range of actions of the parent molecule. This material, with 4-butyloxycarbonyl-beta-alanine attached to the N-terminus, now is available commercially as the gastrin-like pentapeptide, pentagastrin. It is noteworthy that cholecystokinin, which shares many physiologic actions with gastrin, possesses five C-terminal amino acids in common with gastrin.

The other major circulating form of gastrin is "big gastrin" or G-34. Amino acid sequencing indicates it to have 34 amino acids, the C-terminal heptadecapeptide sequence of which is identical with that of G-17. Like G-17, G-34 exists in sulfated and nonsulfated forms. An even larger gastrin molecule ("big-big gastrin"), and a smaller gastrin ("minigastrin," G-14) have been isolated

	Molecular Weight	Amino Acid Sequence

"Big Gastrin"
G-34   3,839

```
  1   2   3   4   5   6   7   8   9  10  11  12  13  14  15  16  17
Glu-Leu-Gly-Pro-Gln-Gly-His-Pro-Ser-Leu-Val-Ala-Asp-Pro-Ser-Lys-Lys-

 18  19  20  21  22  23  24  25  26  27  28  29  30  31  32  33  34
Glu-Gly-Pro-Trp-Leu-Glu-Glu-Glu-Glu-Glu-Ala-Tyr-Gly-Trp-Met-Asp-Phe-NH2
                                            |
                                            R
```

"Little Gastrin"
G-17
Heptadecapeptide Gastrin   2,098

```
  1   2   3   4   5   6   7   8   9  10  11  12  13  14  15  16  17
Glu-Gly-Pro-Trp-Leu-Glu-Glu-Glu-Glu-Glu-Ala-Tyr-Gly-Trp-Met-Asp-Phe-NH2
                                            |
                                            R
```

Gastrin I: R = H   Gastrin II: R = SO3H

Figure 27–1 The molecular species of gastrin.

by chromatographic techniques. G-17 has a greater molar potency for acid secretion, but a shorter half-life in serum than G-34. The immunologic methods commonly employed for the quantitation of gastrin in serum specimens do not distinguish between these two major molecular forms. The longer and shorter forms of gastrin do not appear to have any major function in gastric acid secretion. Antral extract contains predominantly G-17, while the duodenal mucosa contains 60 per cent G-34 and 40 per cent G-17. Fasting human serum contains more G-34, while postprandial serum contains equal amounts of G-17 and G-34.

Gastrin performs a wide spectrum of motor and secretory actions affecting multiple target organs. These include strong stimulation of acid gastric secretion from parietal cells, weak to moderate stimulation of pepsin secretion, increased gastric intrinsic factor secretion, increased blood flow in the stomach, stimulation of gastric motor activity, and a trophic action upon the gastric fundal mucosa. Gastrin also has important extragastric actions. Thus, it stimulates water and electrolyte secretion by the pancreas, liver, and small intestine and enzyme secretion by the pancreas. Gastrin stimulates release of insulin and calcitonin, and stimulates smooth muscle contraction in the lower esophageal sphincter, small intestine, colon, and gallbladder. Absorption of glucose, electrolytes, and water by the small intestine is inhibited by gastrin, as is contraction of smooth muscle of the pyloric sphincter, ileocecal sphincter, and the sphincter of Oddi.

By use of fluoresceinated antibodies to human gastrin I, investigators have localized gastrin in greatest concentration within special mucosal cells in the gastric antrum. These cells, termed "G cells," are most abundant in the midportion of the pyloric glands. They have a flasklike shape with a broad base and narrow apex that extends to the mucosal surface. Electron microscopy reveals characteristic secretory granules 150 to 250 nm in diameter within the G cells as well as microvilli at the mucosal surface that may contain receptors for inhibition and stimulation of the G cells by stomach contents. Gastrin also can be extracted from the mucosa of the proximal duodenum. Indeed, although its concentration here is much less than that in the antrum, because of the larger mass of duodenal mucosa, the duodenum contains nearly as much gastrin as the antrum. Tiny amounts of gastrin also have been found by some investigators in the delta cells of the pancreas. The identity of the G cells, the factors that control their proliferation, and their possible relationship to the pancreatic delta cells remain to be determined.

Radioimmunoassay techniques for the measurement of serum gastrin content indicate normal fasting levels to be from 20 to 200 pg per ml. It must be recognized, however, that the gastrin antibodies used in this measurement detect not only G-17 but also other of the various molecular subtypes of gastrin, in some cases with varying affinities. Specimens containing the same measured level of "gastrin" may differ markedly in gastrin subtype composition. Although potentially important, the actual significance of such gastrin heterogeneity is uncertain. The fasting serum gastrin concentration of duodenal ulcer patients in the majority of studies has not differed significantly from that of normal control subjects, whereas the fasting level of serum gastrin of gastric ulcer patients usually is moderately elevated. In general, an inverse relationship between gastric acid output and serum gastrin has been recognized, although this relationship appears to pertain only to subjects with relatively low levels of maximal gastric acid output below 10 mEq per hour. The higher serum gastrin levels in patients with low levels of acid secretion presumably reflect the absence of inhibition of antral gastrin release by acid antral content in the hyposecretors. Elevation of serum gastrin, often to levels in excess of 1000 pg per ml, is seen in certain clinical situations. The hypergastrinemia of the Zollinger-Ellison syndrome arises not from the antral G cells but from the hyperfunctioning, gastrin-secreting pancreatic tumor cells. In contrast, in the other diseases in which hypergastrinemia is associated with acid hypersecretion the gastrin arises from the antrum itself. For example, in a few duodenal ulcer patients, study of antral mucosal biopsy tissue with fluoresceinated antibody to gastrin has revealed a marked increase in the number of antral G cells, a condition termed antral G-cell hyperplasia. The cause of this hyperplasia remains obscure, but marked elevation of serum gastrin is seen following a protein meal. Acute gastric distention causes a rise in serum gastrin to a lesser degree. Rarely, surgical error will leave a portion of the antrum attached to the afferent duodenal loop when partial gastrectomy with Billroth II gastroenterostomy is performed. Distention of the retained antrum with highly alkaline biliary and pancreatic secretions will lead to hypergastrinemia. These latter two conditions can be distinguished from the Zollinger-Ellison syndrome because antral gastrin release is inhibited following the intravenous injection of secretin, resulting in a fall in serum gastrin, whereas gastrin release from gastrin-secreting pancreatic tumors is augmented by secretin. Hypergastrinemia without acid hypersection is seen in pernicious anemia and atrophic gastritis. About one third of pernicious anemia patients develop hypergastrinemia in the range characteristic of the Zollinger-Ellison syndrome, apparently because chronic achlorhydria leads to hyperplasia of the antral G cells. Increased serum gastrin levels also are demonstrable in atrophic gastritis associated with antibodies to parietal cells but with adequate absorption of vitamin B_{12}, but not in simple atrophic gastritis without parietal cell antibodies. Hypergastrinemia thus may be characteristic only of gastritis associated with autoimmune reactions to gastric antigens. Simple atrophic gastritis appears to be a different disease and the unelevated serum gastrin levels may reflect disease of the antral mucosa with loss of G cells, whereas "autoimmune gastritis" selectively affects the parietal cell–bearing mucosa, and the antral mucosa is spared. Anephric patients, those with advanced renal failure, and patients with extensive resection of small intestine may demonstrate gastric hypersecretion or hypergastrinemia or both. As the kidneys and small intestine are both active sites of gastrin removal, the hypergastrinemia in these conditions results from delay in gastrin metabolism. Hypergastrinemia is sometimes seen in hyperparathyroidism, particularly when a gastrinoma is present, as in the multiple endocrine adenoma, type I, syndrome. In this instance, the elevated level of serum calcium appears to stimulate gastrin release. Epinephrine-induced gastrin release presumably is the mechanism for the hypergastrinemia observed with pheochromocytoma.

In addition to acetylcholine and gastrin, it has been known for more than 50 years that histamine elicits from parietal cells a large amount of hydrochloric acid secretion. Paradoxically, the conventional antihistamine drugs (now termed H_1-receptor antagonists), although capable of blocking many of the actions of histamine on smooth muscle and vascular permeability, are ineffective in reducing gastric acid secretion. Recently, however, it has been determined that the parietal cell possesses a special H_2-receptor and that blocking this receptor with a specific antagonist markedly reduces parietal cell acid secretion as stimulated by all known stimulants of human gastric acid secretion. It is currently believed most likely that receptors for gastrin and acetylcholine as well as histamine exist, but that blocking one receptor type modifies the interaction between the other receptors and their agonists in a way that makes the parietal cell less responsive to all stimulants. The gastric acid hypersecretion sometimes seen in patients with systemic mast cell disease is associated with hyperhistaminemia. Similarly, the gastric hypersecretion seen following portacaval anastomosis involves the effect of a secretory stimulant, produced in the alimentary canal and not inactivated within the liver as a consequence of the shunt. High blood levels of histamine, in fact, have been reported in one such patient with intractable peptic ulcer disease.

The physiologic activity of the gastric chief and parietal cells appears to depend also upon adequate circulating quantities of pituitary, adrenal, thyroid, and parathyroid hormones. In their insufficiency or absence, gastric secretory activity is greatly diminished. The growth of the gastric mucosa probably depends upon growth hormone from the pituitary gland and a normal pituitary gland is essential to the structural integrity of the gastric mucosa and to the normal secretory function.

The third or intestinal phase of gastric secretion begins with the entrance of partly acidified or neutralized food into the small intestine, initiating a humoral mechanism, with the release of gastrin and other hormones. The resting serum gastrin concentration of partial gastrectomy patients with Billroth I gastroduodenostomies is about half that of duodenal ulcer patients who have not been operated on, presumably owing to the loss of antral gastrin. Following an oral homogenized beef meal, a slow increase in serum gastrin occurs in Billroth I patients, with peak values at about two hours —strikingly later than the peak serum gastrin level in normal subjects, which is seen between 30 and 45 minutes after the meal—suggesting that the rise in the serum gastrin level in the former group is of small intestinal origin. If the beef meal is instilled directly into the duodenum, the increase in serum gastrin is identical in magnitude and duration in both Billroth I and normal subjects. When serum gastrin and gastric acid secretion are measured simultaneously following intraduodenal administration of the test meal to duodenal ulcer patients, a significant rise in acid output with peak secretion coinciding with peak gastrin level occurs, suggesting that intestinal gastrin release may be of physiologic significance. In addition to gastrin, there may be other intestinal mechanisms for stimulation of gastric acid secretion, and there are also a number of hormonal and neural intestinal mechanisms for the inhibition of acid secretion, making the intestinal phase of gastric secretion quite complex.

Gastric secretion may be inhibited under various circumstances, such as emotional disturbances, presumably via inhibitory fibers in the vagus and splanchnic nerves. Gastric secretion also is influenced by at least two major autoregulatory mechanisms. All stimulants for gastrin release are inhibited by acid in contact with the antral mucosa, presumably by a direct effect on the G cell. A pH of about 1.0 produces maximal suppression, with lesser degrees of inhibition resulting from the presence of less acid gastric content. Additionally, the presence of acid or fat in the upper small intestine releases inhibitory hormones, termed enterogastrones, which inhibit both the release of gastrin from the G cells and the action of gastrin upon the acid-secreting parietal cells. The best known is secretin, which is capable of inhibiting gastrin-stimulated acid secretion. Other peptide hormones, including glucagon, vasoactive intestinal peptide, gastric inhibitory peptide, somatostatin, and calcitonin, similarly inhibit the action of gastrin, although their possible physiologic significance in the inhibition of acid secretion has not been determined. A depressant of gastric secretion, gastrone, has been identified in the mucous secretion of the stomach, particularly in patients with achlorhydria. Its physiologic role, if any, is undetermined.

The volume of gastric juice secreted under fasting conditions in the average normal adult ranges from 1000 to 1500 ml per day. The principal components of this gastric secretion are hydrochloric acid; various mucosubstances (acid amino polysaccharides, fucomucins, sialomucins); proteolytic enzymes, including at least seven pepsins; rennin, cathepsins, gastric intrinsic factor, water-soluble blood group substances, and other biologically active materials; nonproteolytic enzymes; the anions chloride, phosphate, and sulfate; and the cations sodium, potassium, calcium, and magnesium. The alkaline component of gastric secretion is a mixture of various constituents, including mucus from the surface mucous cells, cytoplasm of desquamated cells, and a transudate of interstitial fluid. The known sources of various gastric secretory products are listed in Figure 27–2.

Pepsin is the major proteolytic enzyme found in human gastric juice. It is synthesized and stored within the chief cells of the oxyntic gland area in an inactive form, pepsinogen. Following secretion into the gastric lumen it is converted autocatalytically in the presence of acid to pepsin by the cleavage of several small basic peptides. In general, pepsinogen secretion is stimulated by the same factors that augment gastric acid secretion, with the exception that secretin, which inhibits acid secretion, is a strong stimulant of pepsinogen. Immunochemical studies of pepsinogen have revealed that there are, in fact, at least seven electrophoretically distinct pepsinogens that can be divided immunologically into two unrelated groups. Group I includes pepsinogens 1 to 5, which are limited to the oxyntic gland mucosa, where they are identified by immunofluorescent studies within the chief and mucous neck cells. Group II pepsinogens 6 and 7 are found in the fundal (oxyntic), pyloric, and duodenal mucosa. Whether quantitative or qualitative differences in pepsinogen secretion are seen in disease states remains to be determined, although the relative proportions of the different pepsinogens in human gastric mucosa apparently vary from person to person.

Hydrochloric acid is secreted by the parietal cell, found in the oxyntic gland mucosa just below the mucous neck area. Parietal cells are pyramidal in shape, with the apex extending toward the lumen of the gland and the broader base placed against the basement membrane of the gland. Electron microscopy demonstrates numerous intracellular mitochondria, an extensive secretory canalicular system lined with microvilli, and numerous tubulovesicular structures. With secretory stimulation, the tubulovesicles are transformed into a microvillous membrane, resulting in a marked increase in the area of the parietal cell's secretory surface. The peak acid output following maximal acid stimulation is directly related to the total number of parietal cells, which in adult human males, averages about one billion cells. The parietal cell mass in duodenal ulcer patients is 1.5 to 2 times as great. Whereas the trophic effect of chronic hypergastrinemia may explain the parietal cell hyperplasia in the Zollinger-Elli-

Cells	Products
Fundic gland area:	
Parietal	acid, intrinsic factor
Chief	Group I and II pepsinogens
Mucous	Group I and II pepsinogens, mucus
Argentaffin	Serotonin, histamine
Antral gland area:	
Mucous	Mucus
Gastrin (G)	Gastrin
Pyloric gland mucous	Group II pepsinogens, mucus

Figure 27–2 Gastric cells and their secretory products (after Isenberg, 1975).

son syndrome, the cause of the increased parietal cell mass in duodenal ulcer patients is not known.

The biochemical events leading to acid secretion are not fully understood. There is some evidence, however, to suggest that acetylcholine, histamine, or gastrin acts upon cell membrane receptors to stimulate guanylate cyclase, resulting in the production of cyclic GMP, which in turn stimulates intracellular activity. The hydrogen ion presumably results from the hydrolysis of water in the presence of carbonic anhydrase. The hydroxyl reacts with carbon dioxide, producing bicarbonate, which leaves the basal portion of the cell. The resulting increase in venous pH has been termed the "alkaline tide." The hydrogen ions are secreted into the secretory canaliculi in a process involving at least two types of ATPase. The secretion of the parietal cell contains hydrochloric acid in an initial acid concentration of 160 to 170 mEq per liter, has a pH of slightly less than 1.0, and is isosmotic or slightly hyperosmotic in relation to the blood. Because gastric juice is a mixture of both parietal and nonparietal secretions, the actual hydrogen ion concentration of gastric juice is much lower, averaging about 40 mEq per liter in fasting normal humans. Variations in the acid concentration of gastric juice presumably are due to changes in the ratio of the acid and nonacid components (Hollander's 2-component hypothesis).

DISTURBANCES IN GASTRIC SECRETION

Pathologic alterations in gastric secretion involve changes in total volume, acid concentration, or both. Consequently gastric acid secretion is most commonly expressed as acid output (mEq per unit time), the product of volume and concentration (Table 27–1). Variations in acid output do not correspond exactly with anatomic changes in the mucosa, although true anacidity occurs most frequently in association with atrophy of the stomach. Normal persons with apparently normal mucosa exhibit a wide variety of secretory responses, ranging from achlorhydria with a pH of approximately 8.0 to a highly acid juice with a pH of 1.0. These differing secretory rates are not correlated with specific symptoms or disease, except that chronic peptic ulcer does not occur in the continued absence of acid gastric juice. The complete absence of all gastric juice (achylia gastrica) is rare, for some secretion containing enzymes in small amounts is almost always present. The terms "achlorhydria" and "anacidity" therefore may be preferable. Anacidity may be defined as a decrease in pH of gastric content of less than one unit or a pH above 6.0 following maximal stimulation of the gastric secretory mechanism with pentagastrin. The pH of the gastric secretion in pernicious anemia usually ranges between 7.0 and 8.0; the pH in atrophy of the gastric mucosa unaccompanied by other disease is similar, although more

TABLE 27–1 REPRESENTATIVE OUTPUTS OF HYDROCHLORIC ACID IN DIFFERENT CLINICAL STATES

	Basal (mEq/hr)	Maximal after Histamine or Pentagastrin Stimulation (mEq/hr)	Nocturnal (mEq/12 hr)
Normal	2–3	16–20	18
Gastric ulcer	2–4	16–20	8
Duodenal ulcer	4–10	25–40	60
Zollinger-Ellison syndrome	30	45	120

variable; values between 3.5 and 7.0 may be observed in gastric carcinoma. Anacidity is not a normal variant, since it is associated with an almost total loss of functioning parietal cells, as in severe gastric atrophy. The gastric content in "true" gastric atrophy is characterized by progressive secretory failure involving initially hydrochloric acid, then pepsin, and, finally, intrinsic factor. Maximal stimulation tests indicate that anacidity occurs in no more than 20 per cent of patients with gastric carcinoma and with gastric polyps. Patients with true anacidity who do not have pernicious anemia require careful observation for the later development of pernicious anemia or gastric carcinoma. In gastric carcinoma the stomach content is characterized by reduced acid secretion and by elevated levels of certain enzyme constituents, including beta glucuronidase, lactic dehydrogenase, glutamic oxaloacetic transaminase, and phosphohexose isomerase. Whether these alterations precede as a reflection of a vulnerable mucosa or accompany the neoplasm remains unclear. Histologic studies indicate that the number of parietal cells in the fundus of the stomach is relatively high in patients with duodenal ulcer and decreases progressively in benign gastric ulcer and in gastric cancer, especially in patients without acid; parietal cells are virtually absent in pernicious anemia.

The clinical conditions associated with gastric hypersecretion are duodenal ulcer, stomal ulceration after partial gastrectomy, the Zollinger-Ellison syndrome, antral G-cell hyperplasia and the retained-excluded antrum after gastric surgery.

MECHANISM OF PAIN

The normal gastric mucosa is insensitive to touch, cutting, pinching, tearing, and exposure to solutions of varying hydrogen ion concentration. Heat and cold are experienced as such. Vigorous pressure on the gastric wall elicits a steady, dull, gnawing pain, experienced approximately in the region of the stimulus. This pain, like that produced by distention or by powerful contractions, arises from stretching of the muscular and peritoneal layers of the stomach. Its mechanism involves a local rise in smooth muscle tension produced by spasm, obstruction, or rapid distention and subsequent contraction or stretching of the nerve terminals lying between the circular muscle fibers. The intensity of the distress is proportional to the state of contraction of the stomach at the time and to the rapidity of the stimulus. The entire reflex involved in the transmission of such impulses may be via the afferent visceral fibers accompanying the sympathetic pathways; the cerebrospinal nerves need not participate. The threshold for pain in the stomach and, therefore, for the development of symptoms is influenced by the condition of the gastric mucosa at the time. Vascular engorgement and acute inflammation diminish the threshold for pain, and in their presence stimuli such as hydrochloric acid or gastric contractions not causing discomfort when the mucosa is normal can elicit painful sensations. Vascular ischemia causes pain presumably by altering the motor activity of the stomach. The stomach is in proximity to numerous other organs with differing nerve supplies; their involvement contributes additional components to the symptomatology of gastric disease.

The pain of peptic ulcer is caused primarily by the hydrochloric acid in the gastric content. The acid evokes a chemical inflammation and thereby lowers the pain threshold of the nerve endings present in the base and in the edges of the ulcer. The pain is a true visceral sensation, arising directly at the site of the lesion. It is not dependent on hyperperistalsis, gross spasm of the musculature, pylorospasm, or distention of the antrum. The acid may, however, activate not only the pain mechanism but also gastric motor activity; under these circumstances, ulcer pain originating in a sensitive ulcer may be increased by motility or muscle spasm. The importance of acid in the development of ulcer pain is further indicated by the occurrence of the distress only when the gastric content is acid. The concentration of hydrochloric acid at the time of distress is not necessarily excessive, nor does it exceed that present in the same stomach without pain when the ulcer is healed or in the healing phase. The threshold of acidity necessary to evoke pain varies from one patient to another and in the same patient from time to time. The presence of pain is dependent, therefore, on the presence of both an inflamed lesion lowering the pain threshold and an adequate stimulus, acid gastric juice. The pain is relieved by emesis or aspiration of the stomach, which removes the acid, or by the ingestion of food or alkali, which neutralizes hydrochloric acid. When the stomach is sensitive, pain may be induced by the introduction of hydrochloric acid in physiologic concentrations (0.1N) or by acid gastric

juice and is alleviated by withdrawal or neutralization of the acid. The pain induced by the hydrochloric acid is not prevented by prior parenteral or oral administration of anticholinergic compounds. Pain sensitivity disappears quickly with treatment, presumably as the acute inflammatory process in the ulcer subsides and long before appreciable healing of the ulcer could occur. Furthermore, gastroscopic studies demonstrate that many peptic ulcers occur in the absence of symptoms. In at least a quarter of patients whose ulcers are complicated by hemorrhage or perforation, no history of antecedent ulcer pain can be elicited. The absence of pain in these instances is difficult to explain, except on the vague basis of an individually high pain threshold, protection of the ulcer crater from the hydrochloric acid by blood during the course of hemorrhage, and the very rapid formation of an acute perforating ulcer encompassing development and penetration into a blood vessel within hours.

LOCATION OF PAIN

The pain of peptic ulcer is almost always located in the epigastrium and usually is limited to an area several centimeters in diameter. With gastric ulcer, pain is most likely to be experienced in the midline high in the epigastrium below the xiphoid process, or sometimes to the left of the midline. When the ulcer is in the upper portion of the stomach, pain occasionally is perceived in the anterior or left lateral portion of the chest. Such shifts of pain usually occur with progressive deepening of the ulcer. So long as gastric ulcers remain shallow and do not actively penetrate or perforate, the distress usually is indistinguishable from that of duodenal ulcer. In duodenal ulcer, the pain ordinarily is located in the midepigastrium or slightly to the right of the midline. In jejunal ulcer, it is located periumbilically, but may be in the left midabdomen and also in the left lower abdominal quadrant. The pain may be referred laterally to the left side of the chest in the area supplied by the sixth and seventh thoracic nerves or may extend through to the back at the level of the eighth to tenth dorsal vertebrae. This latter radiation is more common in duodenal ulcer located on the posterior wall of the duodenum. Sudden, severe abdominal pain frequently indicates an acute perforation. Perforation of an ulcer on the posteror wall of the duodenum causes pain in the location characteristic of pancreatic pain, i.e., in the region between the twelfth thoracic and second lumbar vertebrae. The pain is characteristic in its occurrence at night, aggravation by the supine position, partial relief by sitting or by lying with the trunk flexed, or by pressure over the midabdomen while the patient leans forward over folded arms or a pillow. Perforation of an ulcer on the anterior wall of the duodenum may cause pain in the right lower abdominal quadrant, where the lesion may be confused with acute appendicitis, or it may produce pain in the right groin or testis, simulating right ureteral pain. Its distribution also depends partly on the course taken by the escaping gastric contents. Gravitation of the contents to the right paracolic gutter produces pain in the right lower abdominal quadrant. Pain in front, behind, or on top of the shoulder and at the base of the neck denotes involvement of the diaphragm and irritation of the phrenic innervation. When an ulcer on the lesser curvature of the stomach perforates into the lesser omental tissues, lesser omental sac, undersurface of the liver, anterior aspect of the pancreas, or the diaphragmatic crura, there may develop an upward and left shift of pain into the anterior part of the thorax and left hypochondrium, and a referred or somatic pain often is present in the interscapular region, usually at about the level of the sixth thoracic vertebra. If pain is transmitted to the left shoulder cap, the lesion usually is located high in the stomach. If perforation occurs into the peritoneal aspect of the pancreas and into the anterior surface of the pancreas, the pain usually is at the umbilical level anteriorly and at the level of the twelfth thoracic vertebra to the second lumbar vertebra posteriorly.

PAIN IN GASTRIC CARCINOMA

The pain originating from gastric carcinoma may be of several types. In the presence of hydrochloric acid, it is often indistinguishable from that produced by benign peptic ulcer, because the mechanism is the same: acid irritation. An ulcerating carcinoma perforating the greater curvature may simulate a benign ulcer and also may cause pain in the left shoulder cap, pancreatic pain, and pain in the left lower abdominal quadrant, secondary to involvement of the left transverse mesocolon, perisplenitis, and parietal involvement of peritoneum in the eleventh or twelfth thoracic segment. In the absence of acid and peptic activity, gastric cancer is painless until the tumor progresses beyond the confines of the stomach and involves somatic tissue. The pain then becomes constant, is unrelated to the nature of the gastric content, and is relieved only by opiates. This pain is attributable to malignant infiltration of both the somatic and splanchnic nerves. Benign gastric tumors, e.g., polyps and leiomyomas, do not produce pain unless they obstruct the pylorus or the cardioesophageal orifice.

TRANSMISSION OF PAIN

At least three distinct mechanisms may be involved in pain originating within the abdomen: true visceral pain with impulses transmitted over afferent visceral fibers accompanying the sympathetic trunks; referred pain, with impulses carried over both afferent visceral and cerebrospinal nerve fibers; and the peritoneocutaneous reflex of Morley, with impulses transmitted only via cerebrospinal nerves. True visceral pain alone may be present, or all three mechanisms may participate, as in the perforation of peptic ulcer with peritonitis.

Pain impulses arising in the stomach and duodenum are conducted along sensory fibers in the splanchnic branches of the sympathetic nerves. The splanchnic nerves enter first the celiac ganglion, travel via the greater splanchnic nerves to the spinal cord, probably to the corresponding posterior roots of the eighth through thirteenth thoracic spinal nerves, and thence to the higher centers by way of the spinal thalamic tract. The parasympathetic supply of the stomach and duodenum arises in the dorsal vagal nucleus in the floor of the fourth ventricle, and the afferent fibers end in the same nucleus, which is a mixture of visceral efferent and afferent cells. The fibers are conveyed to and from the abdomen through the vagus nerves, esophageal plexus, and vagal trunks. The reproduction of ulcer pain after complete section of the vagi by introducing hydrochloric acid into the stomach of a patient with a sensitive ulcer demonstrates that pain impulses travel via the splanchnics. The skin area to which visceral pain is referred is determined by the segment of the cord receiving the visceral afferent (sympathetic) fibers. Ulcer distress arising from lesions not penetrating to the serosa has a cutaneous reference, indicating that visceral nerves are capable of mediating pain referred to somatic segments.

GASTRITIS

In health, the mucosa of the gastric fundus and body consists of the gastric pits or foveolae, constituting the superficial 25 per cent of mucosal thickness, and the deeper, glandular portion forming the remaining 75 per cent. The surface and pits are lined with columnar mucus-producing cells that originate at the base of the pits and eventually are extruded into the gastric lumen after migrating upward along the epithelial basement membrane. These surface mucous cells have a relatively rapid turnover time of about four to six days. Into each pit enter three to seven gastric glands, which are more or less straight tubular structures extending downward to the muscularis mucosa. In the superficial portions of the glands are found the parietal cells, while the chief cells are located predominantly in the deeper portions of the glands. A lamina propria extends throughout the mucosa and contains capillaries, collagenous fibers, and cellular elements, predominantly mononuclear cells. An absolutely normal mucosa is found only during infancy or in the first decade of life. Subsequently, there is a progressive interstitial infiltration with lymphocytes, plasma cells, and eosinophils accompanied by metaplasia of the glandular epithelium in virtually every adult stomach. These changes, which probably reflect local inflammatory and possibly immunologic influences, are descriptively termed "gastritis."

The diagnosis of gastritis is based most satisfactorily on the objective histologic criteria outlined as follows. Indeed, much confusion has arisen in the medical literature about the diagnosis and classification of gastritis based on gross endoscopic appearance. Even worse, the term "gastritis" also has been used loosely to describe vague dyspeptic symptoms of uncertain cause with the implication that these symptoms are attributable to gastric mucosal inflammation. Such an implication often is without foundation and many times cannot be verified objectively in patients with such nonspecific complaints. Indeed, the majority of patients whose gastric mucosal biopsies evidence objective changes of gastritis are asymptomatic or suffer from gastrointestinal hemorrhage.

Acute gastritis is said to be present when histologic examination of the gastric mucosa reveals a patchy, superficial, local cell necrosis, often with small areas of cellular exfoliation. Associated features include vascular congestion, sometimes with extravasation of blood into the lamina propria, acute inflammatory cell infiltration, and edema. The changes are generally superficial and the deeper layers of the mucosa are not involved. Although the mucosal appearance may be normal endoscopically, frequently the endoscopist notes erythema, petechial or confluent intramucosal hemorrhage, multiple small erosions or acute ulcerations, and increased amounts of surface mucus. Some special terms, for instance "acute hemorrhagic gastritis" and "acute erosive gastritis," are occasionally used when one or another of the aforementioned pathologic features is especially prominent. All the changes, however, presumably represent the acute mucosal reaction to a wide variety of endogenous or exogenous injurious factors. Examples of such agents include alcohol, salicylates and a variety of other medications, bile acids, bacterial and fungal infections, and metabolic states such as uremia. Again, descriptive terms such as "acute alcoholic gastritis," "caustic gastritis," and "phlegmonous gastritis" are sometimes used to emphasize a presumed cause.

Current concepts suggest that most causes of acute gastritis have in common the breakdown of the gastric mucosal barrier. In health, gastric acid secreted into the lumen of the stomach stays there, and very little diffuses back through the mucosal surface cells, which are protected by their lipid-protein surface membrane and tight intercellular junctions, and by the thin surface layer of gastric mucin. According to Davenport, hydrogen ion diffuses rapidly back into the mucosa when this barrier is broken. There it releases histamine from

mast cells, which stimulates additional acid secretion and causes dilatation of mucosal capillaries with an increase in their permeability. There ensues transudation of plasma and red cells into the interstitial spaces, producing edema and increased interstitial pressure. The interstitial fluid containing electrolytes, proteins, and glucose is filtered across the mucosa surface and, as modified by the filtration process, enters the gastric lumen. The back-diffusion of hydrogen ions may also cause rapid release of vasoactive substances, including, in addition to histamine, serotonin, kinins, and other products of cellular injury.

Among agents that may potentially injure the mucosal barrier, aspirin has been studied in greatest detail. At a pH of 2.0, aspirin is more than 95 per cent in the nonionized, fat-soluble form that can diffuse readily across the lipid mucosal membrane. In this circumstance, it breaks the tight junctions between cells, leading to their exfoliation and enhancing the back-diffusion of hydrogen ions. In addition to salicylates, other potentially injurious substances include alcohol, bile salts, steroids, indomethacin, antibiotics, digitalis preparations, xanthine derivatives, potassium chloride, and thiazides. The breakdown of the normal gastric mucosal barrier also has been demonstrated in critically ill human patients and in dogs subjected to experimental hemorrhagic shock. An alteration in gastric mucosal blood flow may be of importance in these situations.

Acute gastritis often develops suddenly in a previously healthy gastric mucosa and is capable of healing completely within the short period of a few days. Clinically, acute gastritis is of greatest importance when the mucosal injury includes extensive erosions and is complicated by severe hemorrhage.

Gastric mucosal erosions are the leading cause of upper gastrointestinal hemorrhage and occur in up to 30 per cent of patients with significant bleeding. While salicylates and to a lesser degree nonsteroidal anti-inflammatory drugs can break the gastric mucosal barrier, induce hydrogen ion back-diffusion and ultimately bleeding, drugs are the cause of bleeding in only a small percentage of patients. The majority of lesions occur in patients with severe underlying abnormalities like burns, sepsis, multiple trauma, respiratory insufficiency, coma, and others. The mortality rate from bleeding in these conditions is 25 per cent, while that from gastric irritants is low (5 per cent) even if bleeding is substantial. Therapy is usually medical because surgery short of total or subtotal gastrectomy carries a substantial potential for rebleeding and the mortality rate for all surgical procedures is unacceptably high. Gastric lavage and intravenous infusion of vasopressin can temporize the bleeding. Antacids in large doses with an attempt to control the intragastric pH close to 7.0 can stop bleeding but data are uncontrolled. H_2-receptor antagonists are ineffective in active bleeding but like antacids have been shown to be effective if used prophylactically in patients at risk. The key again appears to be control of the gastric pH as nearly as possible to the neutral point. Antacids that can be given in large doses and as a continuous intragastric drip appear to be superior to cimetidine. Somatostatin and prostaglandin analogues appear attractive, but data are inconclusive.

Chronic *gastritis* is also best defined and classified on the basis of mucosal histologic examination. Although the literature again is confused by classifications of chronic gastritis based on gastroscopic or clinical features, Morson recognizes three basic histologic patterns: chronic superficial gastritis, atrophic gastritis, and gastric atrophy.

The major features of *chronic superficial gastritis* include a mucosa of normal thickness with abnormalities of the mucus-producing cells lining the surface and pits and preservation of the deeper tubular structures without loss of glandular elements. The surface cells may be decreased in number and may assume a cuboidal rather than a columnar appearance. Their mucin content is decreased and their nuclei hyperchromatic. The lamina propria is infiltrated by increased numbers of lymphocytes and plasma cells. There is variable edema and vascular congestion. The clinical significance of chronic superficial gastritis is uncertain, although it is sometimes seen in association with peptic ulcer and gastric carcinoma. The relationship, if any, to acute gastritis also is unclear. Although chronic superficial gastritis may regress, long-term follow-up of such patients indicates that the majority progress to the stage of *atrophic gastritis*. In this condition the overall mucosal thickness may or may not be decreased, but in addition to changes in the superficial epithelial cells, there is damage to the gastric glands, with loss of greater or lesser numbers of chief and parietal cells, which are replaced by mucus-secreting cells. In the superficial mucosa, and sometimes also in the deeper zones, a metaplastic change toward an intestinal type of epithelium is seen. This includes the appearance of mucus-containing goblet cells, not normally found in the stomach. In addition, the columnar cells of the metaplastic epithelium may have a prominent brush border, and Paneth cells may be found in large numbers. Mitotic activity is increased. Histochemically, alkaline phosphatase and aminopeptidase are found in the superficial columnar cells, together with a marked increase in thiamine pyrophosphatase and beta-glucuronidase. Finally, in atrophic gastritis an infiltrate of lymphocytes and plasma cells, often marked, is found within the lamina propria. *Gastric atrophy* may be the end result of chronic gastritis and usually involves extensive areas of the gastric mucosal surface. The mucosal thickness is greatly decreased, and chief and parietal cells are virtually absent from the mucosa of the body and fundus; in the antrum only a few pyloric gland elements may remain. The changes of intestinal metaplasia are extensive. The inflammatory cell infiltrate in the lamina propria usually is minimal.

The cause of chronic gastritis and of gastric atrophy is not well understood, although these conditions are more common with increasing age. In general, there is little evidence that the exogenous agents associated with acute gastritis are responsible for the chronic disorders. All types of chronic gastritis are observed in association with gastric ulcer, while atrophy of the gastric mucosa is invariably present in pernicious anemia and gastric polyposis and not infrequently in patients with sprue, pellagra, and iron-deficiency anemia.

There is growing evidence that in some instances chronic atrophic gastritis may be the consequence of chronic mucosal injury by bile salts and other components of intestinal juice regurgitated through the pylorus, perhaps by disruption of the gastric mucosal barrier as outlined earlier. Extensive chronic gastritis is seen in the distal portion of the stomach of patients with gastric ulcers, a group in whom duodenogastric bile reflux is known to be unusually frequent and severe. Following partial gastrectomy with Billroth II gastrojejunostomy, there ensues both extensive bile reflux into the gastric remnant and a severe and progressive chronic gastritis extending proximally from the stoma, where it is most severe. Experimentally, atrophic gastritis develops in tubes of canine gastric mucosa exposed to constant bile flow. Although these facts suggest a relationship between bile reflux and chronic gastritis, the hypothesis remains to be proved.

A possible immune mechanism in the development of gastric atrophy has been suggested on the basis of a series of interesting observations in patients with pernicious anemia: resemblance of the gastric mucosal lesion in pernicious anemia to that of the thyroid in autoimmune thyroiditis; the frequent clinical interrelations of pernicious anemia with autoimmune disease of the thyroid (thyroiditis, myxedema, Hashimoto's disease), the high incidence of circulating thyroid antibodies in patients with pernicious anemia, and, conversely, the high incidence of gastric antibodies in serum from patients with these thyroid diseases; the infiltration of the atrophic mucosa by lymphocytes and plasma cells that contain immunoglobulins reactive with gastric antigens; the frequent presence of circulating antibodies reacting specifically with parietal cell cytoplasmic antigen, gastric intrinsic factor, or both in patients with pernicious anemia; and the presence of the same parietal cell antibody in serum from patients with atrophic gastritis without pernicious anemia, who are presumably candidates for the later development of that disease. Treatment with corticosteroids may permit regeneration of gastric mucosa glands, with recovery of acid and intrinsic factor secretion and normal absorption of vitamin B_{12}. Those who respond tend to have the highest titers of circulating parietal cell antibodies. There is no correlation in this regard with the presence of antibodies to intrinsic factor. Patients with extensive intestinal metaplasia of the gastric mucosa are least likely to benefit from steroid therapy.

Parietal cell antibodies are circulating antibodies of the IgG variety with an affinity for the cytoplasm of parietal cells. They are demonstrable in 80 to 90 per cent of patients with pernicious anemia and in 60 per cent of patients with other forms of gastritis without hematologic abnormality. Parietal cell antibodies also are more common in older patients. Their presence, however, is not necessarily correlated wih the severity of the gastritis. The presence of parietal cell antibodies suggests that such patients have a genetically determined ability to form antibodies, but there is no evidence in such patients that the gastritis is the result of these antibodies or that antibodies predispose to the severity and the chronicity of the gastritis. Interestingly, gastric antibodies are not found in patients with postgastrectomy gastritis, and damage to the gastric mucosa by chemical or physical agents does not stimulate the appearance of these immunologic phenomena. Although these facts are all consistent with the hypothesis that in at least some patients immunologic mechanisms are of etiologic importance in atrophic gastritis, this possibility remains unproved and must be confirmed by additional evidence.

The evaluation of symptoms in patients with chronic gastritis is difficult. Experimentally, acute inflammation and sustained hyperemia of the gastric mucosa lower the threshold for pain. Chronic inflammation, therefore, may be expected to provoke the occurrence of gastric symptoms. Clinically, however, chronic gastritis is noted gastroscopically quite often in the absence of abdominal distress. In other patients with chronic gastritis, the symptoms are varied and vague; their incidence, type, or severity cannot be correlated with the character or degree of gastritis. The most frequent complaints of such patients are loss of appetite, fullness, belching, vague epigastric pain, nausea, and vomiting. These are also the symptoms of functional gastrointestinal distress.

The consequences of chronic gastritis are not completely known. Although minor surface alterations, such as erosions and hemorrhages, usually heal completely, severe and complete atrophy of the stomach generally tends to persist unchanged. The association of chronic atrophic gastritis and gastric ulcer, and the fact that the gastritis persists even after the ulcer heals, suggest that the gastritic mucosa is more vulnerable to chronic peptic ulceration.

Benign gastric polyps of the hyperplastic or adenomatous type are generally rare but occur more commonly in patients with chronic atrophic gastritis. Adenomas are true neoplasms and their malignant potential is significant. It increases with the polyp size especially if it is over 2 cm.

Focal carcinoma in these larger polyps has been reported as from 6 to 75 per cent. Benign gastric polyps are further found in association with gastric carcinoma arising in a chronic atrophic gastritis. Gastric polyps are therefore considered an important marker of gastric carcinoma.

Initially, a higher incidence of gastric carcinoma in patients with gastric atrophy and pernicious anemia was suggested. Recent studies, however, show the incidence to be only slightly increased over that in other patients with gastric mucosal atrophy. Routine screening for cancer by endoscopy is therefore no longer indicated in asymptomatic patients with pernicious anemia.

Finally, a number of gastritis syndromes not included in the preceding classification have been described. *Giant hypertrophic gastritis* (Menetrier's disease) is a disorder of unknown cause, characterized by conspicuous increases in the height and thickness of the gastric folds, especially along the greater curvature of the body of the stomach. The hypertrophy is limited to the mucosa, the submucosa and the muscle layers of the stomach remaining normal. The disorder is restricted to the body and fundus of the stomach and usually stops abruptly at the margin of the antrum. Microscopically, there is marked hyperplasia of the surface epithelial cells that line elongated, tortuous, and cystic gastric pits that may extend to or even through the muscularis mucosae. An intense inflammatory cell infiltrate may be present in the lamina propria. The gastric mucosa is abnormally permeable, and the pronounced exudation of serum proteins into the gastric content and their subsequent digestion may lead to hypoproteinemia. The clinical manifestations in addition to the edema associated with the protein loss include vague, nonspecific gastrointestinal complaints. Gastric bleeding may be the sole manifestation. While gastric secretion may be normal, low, or even increased, many patients have achlorhydria.

The gross appearance of the mucosa in *hypertrophic glandular gastritis* (hypertrophic hypersecretory gastritis) is somewhat similar. The mucosa in this condition is greatly thickened because of the glandular hyperplasia, with great increases in the numbers of parietal and chief cells. Inflammatory changes may be present, together with cysts and collections of lymphocytes. Both types of hypertrophic gastritis must be differentiated from the mucosal hypertrophy of the Zollinger-Ellison syndrome and from infiltrating adenocarcinoma or lymphoma. *Eosinophilic gastroenteritis* is a disorder of the intestinal tract characterized by infiltration of one or more layers of the gut wall by large numbers of eosinophilic leukocytes accompanied by a striking increase in the number of eosinophils in the peripheral blood. Most commonly the gastric antrum is involved. Symptoms are nonspecific and include early satiety, intermittent nausea, vomiting, and abdominal pain. Although the pathogenesis of eosinophilic gastroenteritis is not clearly understood, its frequent occurrence in patients with a history of asthma, allergic rhinitis, and atopic eczema, and its dramatic relief by corticosteroid therapy suggest an allergic or immunologic etiology. *Granulomatous gastritis* may occur as a manifestation of tuberculosis, sarcoidosis, late syphilis, histoplasmosis or Crohn's disease. Crohn's disease of the stomach usually involves the gastric antrum and in many cases extends into the duodenum. It occurs in about 5 per cent of patients with Crohn's disease, and usually other parts of the intestinal tract are involved. The x-ray appearance may be confused with scarring after peptic ulcer disease, corrosive gastritis, and linitis plastica. Endoscopically the aphthous and serpiginous erosions are characteristic. On biopsy, granulomata are found in slightly more than 50 per cent of patients.

PEPTIC ULCER

PATHOPHYSIOLOGY

A peptic ulcer develops as a result of a localized area of necrosis and digestion of the lining of the digestive tract. The process is a penetrating one, beginning in the mucosa and gradually extending through the muscularis mucosae into or through the muscularis propria. In some cases the ulcer penetrates into blood vessels, resulting in hemorrhage, or completely through the gut wall into adjacent organs or as a free perforation into the peritoneal cavity. Regenerative activity is almost always present and at any time may lead to the healing of the ulcer, especially if it is protected from gastric juice. Healing occurs from below upward with the growth of granulation tissue and fibroblasts. In small superficial lesions, healing is complete. In large, chronic ulcers, healing is slower; new glands are not formed, and tissue is replaced by fibrous and elastic tissue.

Clinically, chronic peptic ulcer occurs only in those portions of the digestive tract exposed to the action of acid juice: the lower portion of the esophagus, the stomach, the upper portion of the small intestine, or the small bowel adjacent to a patent gastroenterostomy or a Meckel's diverticulum containing ectopic gastric glands. The majority of peptic ulcers, however, occur along the lesser curvature of the stomach and in the first 3 or 4 cm of the duodenum, including the duodenal bulb.

Although a common disorder, the exact incidence of peptic ulcer has been difficult to establish because of inaccuracies in diagnosis and the failure to distinguish between gastric and duodenal ulcer in many reports. It has been generally believed, however, that 1 of every 10 American males will suffer from duodenal ulcer during his lifetime, whereas the peak prevalence of duodenal ulcer in females is about 40 per cent that of males. The frequency of gastric ulcer is only about 25 per cent

that of duodenal ulcer, and again males predominate over females with a ratio of about three to one. Interestingly, over the past several decades there has been a substantial decrease in the frequency with which duodenal ulcer is diagnosed, with a decline in incidence of 40 to 50 per cent, particularly among the younger members of the population. The cause of this important change is unknown, although it has been suggested that the data are consistent with the effect of an environmental factor, maximal around the turn of the century and now disappearing. Peptic ulcer disease is more common in patients with rheumatoid arthritis, chronic obstructive lung disease, and patients with hepatic cirrhosis who have been treated by portacaval shunt. Both gastric and duodenal ulcer are significantly more common in cigarette smokers than in nonsmokers, and gastric ulcer appears to be more prevalent among habitual users of aspirin. Although it is commonly believed that corticosteroids, alcohol, coffee, indomethacin, phenylbutazone, and reserpine predispose to peptic ulcerations by virtue of their ability to alter the characteristics of gastric mucus, interfere with epithelial cell replication, or increase gastric acid secretion, critical evaluation of available data has failed to substantiate this belief. A significant relationship is present between blood group status and peptic ulcer. Duodenal ulcer appears to be 35 per cent more common in individuals of blood group O than among individuals of groups A, B, and AB. Patients who fail to secrete blood group substances into their gastric juice are 50 per cent more liable to duodenal ulceration, while those of blood group O who are also nonsecretors are most susceptible, with a liability of abut 2.5 times that of secretors of groups A and B. Gastric ulcers, on the other hand, are significantly more common in individuals of blood group A. Contrary to popular opinion, studies have failed to demonstrate that any particular personality type is common to ulcer patients. The psychosomatic theory of peptic ulcer proposes that long-standing psychic conflict or anxiety predisposes to peptic ulceration by increasing gastric secretion or damaging mechanisms of mucosal homeostasis. Presumably, these effects are mediated via the vagus nerve and render the individual vulnerable to acute ulceration shortly after some stressful emotional event. Although gastric secretory studies as well as direct observation of the gastric mucosa in patients with gastrostomies have confirmed the assumption that emotional events can alter mucosal function, studies designed to test the assumption of the psychosomatic theory have in general been poorly controlled and, therefore, inconclusive.

The term "peptic ulcer" carries the implication that the lesion is the result of the action of the acid peptic juice. Pure gastric secretion is capable of destroying and digesting all living tissues, including the stomach. Current concepts emphasize the importance of the destructive effect of the peptic juice in the development of peptic ulcers, particularly in the many duodenal ulcer patients who are acid-hypersecretors. Indeed, peptic ulcer does not occur in patients whose gastric glands are incapable of secreting acid. Conversely, especially severe peptic ulcer disease is frequently seen in patients with extreme hypersecretion, such as those with the Zollinger-Ellison sydrome. Experimentally, peptic ulcer may be produced by various operations that interfere with the neutralization of acid by the intestinal content, by the administration of acid, or by the continuous stimulation of highly acid gastric secretion.

Also of presumably great importance in the development of peptic ulcer is the vulnerability of the mucosa to digestion by the acid peptic juice. Tissue resistance depends on multiple factors, including the integrity of the gastric and duodenal mucosal cells, the rapid and continuous regeneration of epithelial cells to replace those lost by exfoliation, the quality of the mucus layer overlying the epithelial cells, the tight junctions linking each cell to its neighbor, and the mucosal vascular supply. Failure of one or more of these aspects of mucosal resistance may explain the development of gastric ulcers, which characteristically occur in patients with normal or reduced acid secretory capacity, and may be of importance in the development of duodenal ulcer in patients without gastric acid hypersecretion. Because little can be done to bolster weakened mucosal defenses beyond the removal of harmful exogenous substances such as aspirin, most current medical and surgical therapy for peptic ulcer is directed toward preventing the secretion of gastric acid or removing it by intraluminal neutralization after it has been secreted.

During the past decade detailed investigations have led to a better understanding of physiologic abnormalities found in ulcer patients that might be of importance in the development of their lesions. For *duodenal ulcer* the outstanding characteristic is the increase in parietal cell mass accompanied by augmented secretory capacity. Although the cause of this hyperplasia of the acid-secreting mucosa is really unknown, it often has been assumed that increased stimulation by the vagus nerve mechanism is responsible. Because "vagal tone" is impossible to measure, this concept is difficult to substantiate. Furthermore, because the percentage reduction in acid secretion following vagotomy is no greater in duodenal ulcer patients than in normosecretors, some other as yet undiscovered mechanism may be important. The parietal cell in duodenal ulcer patients seems to be stimulated by an enhanced vagal response and is abnormally sensitive to gastrin. Thus, the dose of pentagastrin required to produce half the maximal secretion in such patients is only about one third that needed in patients without duodenal ulcer. Although the fasting serum gastrin level in duodenal ulcer is, if anything, slightly lower than normal, following a meal an abnormally large rise in serum gastrin ("integrated gastrin response") characterizes the duodenal ulcer patient. A possible explanation for this is the failure of normal mechanisms to inhibit release of gastrin from the antrum of patients with duodenal ulcer. For example, similar degrees of antral acidification inhibit gastrin release much less in duodenal ulcer patients than in normal subjects. The most important buffer in food is found in its protein content. The rate of gastric emptying is increased in duodenal ulcer patients and this leads to an increased duodenal acid load, particularly during the second half-hour after the meal when much of the protein buffer has been consumed or emptied from the stomach. It often has been postulated that duodenal ulcer subjects have a defect in secretin release from the duodenal mucosa or diminished pancreatic bicarbonate output following entry of acid into the duodenum. Recent studies have, however, failed to substantiate these hypotheses. Although the abnormalities of gastroduodenal function just catalogued are interesting, it has not been possible to combine them into a logical pathophysiologic sequence for the development of duodenal ulcer disease.

Patients with *gastric ulcer* are perhaps best characterized by their lack of gastric acid hypersecretion and by the almost universal presence of chronic superficial or atrophic gastritis around and distal to the location of the ulcer in the stomach. Indeed, a gastric ulcer most often occurs in the gastritic mucosa adjacent to the more normal parietal cell–bearing, acid-secreting mucosa. The presence of excessive duodenogastric reflux and an increased bile acid concentration within the gastric content are also typical of gastric ulcer. These latter abnormalities are possibly explained by malfunction of the pyloric sphincter, which fails to tighten in a normal fashion following entry of acid, protein, or fat into the duodenum. Because all these abnormalities persist after healing of the gastric ulcer, it is unlikely that they are merely secondary phenomena. These observations can be interpreted to suggest that the pyloric sphincter abnormality is a major factor in the pathogenesis of gastric ulcer in that it permits harmful duodenogastric bile reflux. This may result in damage to the gastric mucosa, rendering it more susceptible to ulceration by even reduced amounts of gastric acid secretion. The strength of this argument is somewhat weakened by the fact that the addition of acid to the stomach is reported to restore pyloric sphincter function in gastric ulcer patients to normal. Thus, hyposecretion may somehow be responsible for the pyloric malfunction. Clarification of these relationships and their importance, if any, in the pathogenesis of gastric ulcer awaits further study.

Although ulcerative lesions of the gastrointestinal tract in regions exposed to acid are grouped together under the term "peptic ulcer," it is quite probable that not all ulcers, even those in a similar location, originate from a single cause. For example, there is considerable evidence that, although a hereditary predisposition exists for both, gastric and duodenal ulcers represent separate diseases. Relatives of gastric ulcer patients have a threefold increased prevalence of gastric ulcer as compared with the population at large, but a normal prevalence of duodenal ulcer. Similarly, relatives of duodenal ulcer patients experience a threefold increase in risk for development of duodenal ulcer, but no increased risk of gastric ulcer. Differences in blood group distribution mentioned earlier between the two types of ulcer patients also suggest that the disorders are separate but both have a hereditary predisposition. It is also likely that duodenal ulcer is merely the common clinical result of a variety of separate diseases arising from different causes, both genetic and nongenetic. For example, duodenal ulcer associated with the multiple endocrine adenoma syndrome, type 1 (Wermer syndrome), appears to be inherited as a distinct autosomal dominant disorder, whereas such simple Mendelian inheritance patterns cannot explain the familial aggregation in ordinary duodenal ulcer disease. Clinically, duodenal ulcer patients can be separated into at least two groups on the basis of the degree of acid secretion and certain clinical characteristics. A bimodal distribution of serum pepsinogen concentrations among duodenal ulcer patients also suggests the presence of at least two distinct disorders. These observations are consistent with the hypothesis that peptic ulcer disease in fact represents a heterogeneous group of diseases that result from a variety of genetic and environmental causes. The failure to recognize such heterogeneity may explain the failure of investigations to identify a likely cause for "peptic ulcer." Future studies of clinically and biochemically well-defined homogeneous groups of ulcer subjects may be more fruitful.

ENDOCRINE RELATIONSHIPS

There is no known etiologic relationship between the ordinary peptic ulcer and primary endocrine disorders. Certain endocrine (humoral) abnormalities may, however, be associated with refractory peptic ulcer and gastric hypersecretion. The *Zollinger-Ellison (Z-E) syndrome* is characterized by single or multiple non–beta islet cell adenomas of the pancreas; enormous outputs of hydrochloric acid and pepsin; single or multiple ulcers in the esophagus, the second, third, and fourth portions of the duodenum, and the jejunum, in addition to the stomach and duodenal bulb; and refractoriness to medical or to surgical treatment short of total gastric resection. The parietal cell mass is sixfold larger than normal and threefold larger than in patients with the usual duodenal ulcer. Gastric rugae and the mucosal folds in the

small intestine often are enlarged. The Z-E syndrome is relatively uncommon but not rare, and is more common in men, the ratio being six males to four females. It occurs in all age groups, but especially during the third to fifth decades.

Ulcer pain is present in approximately 95 per cent of patients. Symptoms exceed one year in duration in more than 80 per cent, and range from 5 to 10 years in duration in 30 per cent. Atypically located and multiple peptic ulcers strongly suggest the disorder. Three fourths of the ulcers in the syndrome are not located atypically, however, and they are not multiple, at least as determined by conventional barium x-ray examination. While case reports often describe the severe, occasionally dramatic complications of atypically located peptic ulceration, the symptoms often are indistinguishable from those of ordinary peptic ulcer until operation removes the anatomic integrity of the stomach and duodenum and disrupts normal homeostatic mechanisms controlling acid gastric secretion. The course then usually, although not invariably, is more complicated, with severe recurrent ulcer pain, bleeding, and perforation, the entire sequence occasionally developing very rapidly after ulcer surgery.

Diarrhea occurs in approximately one third of patients with the Z-E syndrome and can be regarded as the consequence of gastric acid hypersecretion and the presence of large amounts of acid within the upper small intestine, for removal of gastric acid by nasogastric suction markedly alleviates or eliminates the diarrhea. Steatorrhea is not uncommon and is attributable to multiple factors: acid inactivation of pancreatic lipase, precipitation of bile salts leading to defective micelle formation, direct injury to the intestinal mucosa by the excessive hydrochloric acid, and acid injury to the vitamin B_{12}–intrinsic factor complex.

Aside from the damage to the gastrointestinal tract, the most striking anatomic finding in the syndrome is the presence of the adenomas within the pancreas. They may occur anywhere within the pancreas, but especially in the body and tail. Aberrant adenomas may be found in the hilus of the spleen, in the gastric wall, and along the curvature of the second portion of the duodenum. In about 10 per cent of patients no distinct adenoma is discovered, but rather an increased number of pancreatic islets containing a higher than usual proportion of non-beta cells is found. Despite the frequently benign histologic characteristics of the adenoma cells, approximately 60 per cent are malignant, as evidenced by the presence of metastases. Extracts of pancreatic adenoma in the Z-E syndrome contain large quantities of gastrin, and ultrastructural studies indicate that the secretory granules within the adenoma cells generally resemble those of the G cells of the gastric antrum. Because immunofluorescence studies have shown the delta cells of normal pancreatic islet to contain gastrin, it is believed that the pancreatic "gastrinomas" of the Z-E syndrome originate from the delta cells.

The fasting serum from the majority of patients with the Z-E syndrome contains gastrin levels in excess of 300 pg per ml and usually tenfold or more higher than the normal mean serum gastrin level of 100 pg per ml. In contrast, the fasting serum gastrin of patients with ordinary duodenal ulcer disease averages less than 100 pg per ml. Thus, measurement of serum gastrin provides a useful technique for the detection of the Z-E syndrome when it is suspected. As physicians have become more alert in recognizing patients with the Z-E syndrome, it has become apparent that some patients have only moderately elevated serum gastrin levels. These cases can be differentiated from others in which hypergastrinemia arises from other causes (such as atrophic gastritis, retained gastric antrum, renal insufficiency, and massive small bowel resection) by testing with intravenous injection of secretin or calcium infusion.

The other characteristic laboratory finding in the Z-E syndrome is the enormous "basal" secretion of hydrochloric acid by the fasting stomach. Volumes in excess of 200 ml per hour are common; half the patients have a basal acid output of more than 15 mEq per hour and two thirds have a basal acid output of greater than 10 mEq per hour. This basal hypersecretion results from the constant near-maximal stimulation of the parietal cells by the elevated levels of circulating serum gastrin. In fact, additional stimulation of the parietal cells by exogenous histamine or pentagastrin produces relatively little augmentation of gastric acid secretion, so the ratio of basal to maximal (poststimulation) acid output is usually 0.6 or greater.

Although frequently metastatic, the pancreatic tumors of the Z-E syndrome, like many carcinoid tumors, are quite indolent and progress very slowly. Death seldom results from the neoplasm itself, but rather from complications of the severe peptic ulcer disease it produces. Thus, treatment is directed toward the peptic ulcer disease rather than directly toward the tumor. Unfortunately, the severe ulcer diathesis is not controlled by the usual antacid and anticholinergic therapy; by gastric irradiation; or by conventional peptic ulcer surgery, including vagotomy with pyloroplasty, gastroenterostomy, or resection of the antrum. The surgical therapy is total gastrectomy with ablation of the parietal cell mass. Preoperatively a careful search should be made to identify that 10 per cent of patients with a localized tumor that may be resected. Gastrectomy may not be necessary in these select patients or in those in whom careful surgical exploration identifies a resectable lesion. H_2-receptor antagonists (cimetidine, ranitidine) have been shown to be effective for control in most patients with the Z-E syndrome. Larger than usual doses are necessary, however, and continuous long-term medication is necessary.

H_2-receptor antagonists do not alter serum gastrin levels or change the biologic tumor behavior. Anticholinergics can allow reduction in the cimetidine dose. Possible side effects are always a concern when a drug has to be taken over years, but these medications represent a true alternative to total gastrectomy.

Multiple endocrine adenomatosis, type I, (Wermer's syndrome) is a familial disorder characterized by the concomitant presence of multiple tumors or hyperplasia of several endocrine glands. The parathyroid glands are most frequently involved, and next most frequently are the pancreatic islets, pituitary, adrenals, and thyroid glands. Bronchial and intestinal carcinoid tumors, pheochromocytomas and lipomas are included in the syndrome. The adenomas may or may not be hormonally active in one or more glands and in any combination. Peptic ulcer is present in more than 50 per cent of cases; the sexes are affected equally; and the disease has been described in all age groups after the first decade, with the peak occurrence in the third and fourth decades. Multiple endocrine adenomatosis appears to have a genetic basis attributable to the action of an autosomal dominant gene of high penetrance. Approximately half the ulcers are multiple and in atypical locations. The most common presenting feature of the syndrome is peptic ulcer and its complications. Symptoms of hypoglycemia are next in frequency. Acromegaly, pituitary dwarfism, hypogonadism, Cushing's syndrome, hyperaldosteronism, and hyperthyroidism may occur alone or in any combination. Complications of perforation, obstruction, and hemorrhage are common. Diarrhea and steatorrhea occur in 10 per cent of patients in association with ulcer. Although gastrin has been extracted from the pancreatic adenomas, all attempts to isolate gastrin or a gastric secretagogue from adenomas of other endocrine glands have failed. The peptic ulcer associated with multiple endocrine adenomatosis seems identical in all respects to that of the Zollinger-Ellison syndrome. On the basis of present information, therefore, it perhaps is justifiable to regard the Z-E syndrome as the "gastrin-secreting, pancreatic islet-cell tumor component" of multiple endocrine adenomatosis. Treatment of each endocrine abnormality follows the usual measures; management of the ulcer in multiple endocrine adenomatosis is the same as for the Z-E syndrome.

Peptic ulcers are not more frequent in patients with adrenocortical hyperfunction. An association between duodenal ulcer and hyperparathyroidism, however, especially among men, has been frequently suspected. This suspicion is based on the simultaneous presence of hyperparathyroidism in 4 (1.3 per cent) of one series of 300 duodenal ulcer patients, a prevalence somewhat higher than one would expect from chance alone. Similarly, in some reported series as many as 30 per cent of patients with hyperparathyroidism have been noted to suffer from peptic ulcer disease. In other reports, however, the prevalence of peptic ulcer disease has not been greater among patients with hyperparathyroidism, and the matter must still be regarded as uncertain and controversial. If such a relationship exists, the mechanism is unclear. Although gastric hypersecretion has been noted to decrease to normal following removal of parathyroid tumors in a few patients, in the majority of patients with hyperparathyroidism the rates of both basal and maximal acid secretion are normal.

There are, however, a number of observations that might lead one to suspect an association between hyperparathyroidism and hypercalcemia and peptic ulcer disease. Calcium has an important influence on gastric acid secretion. In hypoparathyroid patients with serum calcium values under 7.0 mg/dl, the stomach is usually achlorhydric. Conversely, as little as 2 gm of oral calcium carbonate or an intravenous infusion of calcium will increase the rate of gastric acid secretion temporarily. Indeed, the calcium-containing antacids, although potent neutralizers of acid, enjoy little current use clinically because of the "rebound" gastric hypersecretion that follows their use. The mechanism of this calcium-associated hypersecretion appears to be the release of gastrin by calcium. The situations cited, however, are acute ones; with chronic hypercalcemia, gastric acid secretion usually appears to adapt and become normal.

One special relationship between hyperparathyroidism and peptic ulcer disease has been well documented. Patients whose hyperparathyroidism is part of the multiple endocrine adenomatosis, type I, syndrome who also have pancreatic gastrinomas have a particularly severe ulcer diathesis. In such patients the hypercalcemia stimulates marked release of gastrin from the pancreatic tumor and extreme hypersecretion of acid by the stomach, in contrast to normal subjects or ordinary duodenal ulcer patients in whom calcium infusions result in relatively modest rises in serum gastrin and gastric acid secretion.

MECHANISMS OF SYMPTOM PRODUCTION

The outstanding symptom of peptic ulcer is pain, characterized by its chronicity, periodicity, and relation to the ingestion of food. The average duration by the time the patient is first seen by the physician is 6 or 7 years; in occasional cases the symptoms have been present for 40 or 50 years. The periodicity of the distress is striking, the symptoms lasting from a few days to a few months, followed by periods of remission of similar duration. The explanation for this intermittent pattern remains unknown, but presumably it is the symptomatic reflection of spontaneous cycles of ulcera-

tion and healing. Exacerbations of peptic ulcer occur at all times of the year, but in some patients they may be confined to the spring and fall seasons. In some patients the tendency is for the periods of distress to become more frequent and of longer duration while the remissions are less frequent and shorter. On the other hand, progression is not inevitable; in many individuals recurrences may heal completely.

The pain is usually a gnawing or aching sensation, sometimes described as burning, boring, "heartburn," pressure in the upper abdomen, cramplike, or indeed hunger. It differs from the intermittent pangs of true hunger in that ulcer distress is almost always steady and continuous for 15 minutes to an hour or more unless relieved, whereas the hunger pang lasts for only a minute or so. The rhythm of pain in peptic ulcer is related to the digestive cycle; it is the same for both gastric and duodenal ulcer. Pain attributable to peptic ulcer usually is absent before breakfast, appears 1 to 4 hours after breakfast, and lasts 30 minutes or more, perhaps until relief is obtained at the noon meal. The distress recurs 1 to 4 hours later and usually is more severe than in the forenoon. The afternoon pain likewise may disappear spontaneously, but more often food or alkali is required to obtain relief. In the evening, the pain may recur 1 to 4 hours after eating; it may be less severe than in the afternoon. The patient may be awakened with pain, usually between midnight and 3:00 in the morning. Rarely does nocturnal pain appear unless pain has been present in the evening, and rarely does pain attributable to ulcer develop in the night unless it has been present earlier. The presence of nocturnal pain often is interpreted as evidence of pyloric obstruction or high-grade stenosis, but it occurs also in nonobstructive, acutely inflamed, or penetrating lesions. In young children with peptic ulcer the distress may lack the usual rhythmicity and periodicity; the pain is vague, and vomiting is common. In older children, the symptoms resemble those of adults. Nausea, vomiting, anorexia, and weight loss in older patients with gastric ulcer initially may suggest the presence of malignant disease.

Nausea is not a common symptom. Vomiting may result from severe pain, but usually indicates pyloric obstruction. Painless vomiting may occur with nonobstructive ulcer, and is more common with gastric than with duodenal ulcer. The appetite and weight usually are well preserved, but severe loss of weight may result from continued vomiting or the patient's fear of eating. The frequent ingestion of food to relieve pain, on the other hand, more often produces a gain of weight. Constipation and flatulence reflect an associated irritable colon. Diarrhea may result from various causes: the excessive use of laxative antacids; gastric hypersecretion, the acid inactivating intestinal and pancreatic enzymes and thus interfering with normal digestive processes; and a gastrojejunocolic fistula, short-circuiting the gastrointestinal content.

COMPLICATIONS

Bleeding occurs in the life history of at least 25 per cent of patients with peptic ulcer; the ulcers associated with bleeding vary in size and duration, with all gradations from superficial erosions to huge penetrating lesions. They may be located in the esophagus, stomach, duodenum, or the jejunal stoma after a gastroenterostomy. The anterior surface of the stomach and duodenum do not contain major vessels, and the vascular channels are smaller than on the posterior wall. The associated symptoms are determined by the rapidity and severity of the blood loss. The manifestations of severe hemorrhage include sudden weakness, faintness, perspiration, dizziness, headache, palpitation, chilliness, abdominal cramps, thirst, dyspnea, syncope, and collapse as a consequence of the pronounced decrease in blood volume and diminished cardiac output. These symptoms respond promptly to the transfusion of whole blood and other supportive measures. Ulcer pain may be absent or infrequent.

In the absence of a definite diagnosis of peptic ulcer, upper gastrointestinal bleeding requires differentiation from a variety of other conditions associated with bleeding. These include erosive gastritis, esophageal varices, carcinoma of the stomach, vascular abnormalities, and the Mallory-Weiss syndrome. The latter condition is characterized by longitudinal lacerations in the cardioesophageal region varying from 3 to 20 mm in length and from 2 to 3 mm in width. They occur during the retching and straining associated with intense vomiting. The mucosal tears are attributed to unequal distensibility of the mucosa and musculature and severe pressure in the cardioesophageal area. Duodenal and gastric ulcers are each responsible for a quarter of all bleeding episodes. While the overall mortality rate for patients with upper gastrointestinal bleeding from all causes is 10 per cent, the mortality rates for duodenal and gastric ulcer bleeding are 7 and 8 per cent. A third of these patients rebleed, with a fivefold increase in death rate. Major risk factors in these patients are associated conditions such as congestive heart failure, respiratory insufficiency, and hepatic and renal disease, which may increase the overall mortality rate two- to sevenfold.

Pyloric or duodenal obstruction results from spasm, edema, and inflammation in an active pyloric or duodenal ulcer, from cicatricial stenosis, or from a combination of these changes. The obstruction in the majority of patients is temporary and disappears during medical treatment as the inflammation and edema subside. Permanent narrowing may result from frequent recurrences of ulcer. Each episode produces proliferation of connective tissue, followed eventually by cicatricial contraction. The end result is a firmly contracted scar narrowing the lumen. Obstruction in gastric ulcer may result from inflammation and narrowing of the gastric antrum, and from shortening of the lesser curvature of the stomach, with upward retraction of the antrum and distortion of the pylorus. The most significant symptoms of obstruction are the vomiting of retained food and gastric content, loss of weight, and weakness. In addition, the pain may become continuous rather than periodic, and the usual pain relief from food and alkali may be absent.

The loss of large quantities of chloride ion and a smaller but significant amount of sodium, as well as of potassium and fluid, in the vomitus produces an alkalosis characterized by an increase in the carbon dioxide content and pH and a decrease in the concentration of chloride, potassium, and sodium ions in the plasma. The consequent diminution in blood volume, reduction in the flow of blood through the kidneys, and tissue dehydration lead to a temporary impairment of renal function. The symptoms of the electrolyte imbalance (alkalosis) include loss of appetite, distaste for food, increased nausea, weakness, lassitude, headache, nervous irritability, and occasionally coma. Tetany is rare, since the carbon dioxide tension of the blood usually is maintained above the critical level, but muscular twitchings and hyperirritability of the reflexes may be present. These manifestations disappear rapidly with correction of the biochemical disturbance by the intravenous administration of appropriate amounts of chloride, sodium, potassium, and water.

Perforation complicates 1 to 2 per cent of all ulcers, and perforations recur in 1 to 2 per cent of these cases. Pyloroduodenal perforations exceed gastric perforations in a proportion of 20:1 for men and 5:1 for women. Perforations in males exceed those in females by a ratio of 50:1. The ulcers usually are on the anterior wall of the stomach or duodenum, unsupported by contiguous structures. Ulcers on the posterior wall tend to penetrate rather than perforate, and their further extension is limited to adjacent solid organs. Perforations occur more often after eating and during the latter part of the afternoon or evening. Ulcers perforate at all times of the year, but probably less often during the summer and more frequently during the winter. The symptoms begin with sudden, extremely severe pain in the upper abdomen, extending rapidly throughout the abdomen as a consequence of the escape of the irritating gastric and intestinal contents and the development of a chemical peritonitis. The pain may be referred to one or both shoulders because of irritation of the diaphragm, which is innervated by the phrenic nerves. The sudden severe pain is replaced within 6 to 12 hours by a dull discomfort, and may disappear within 24 hours. The subsequent development of a bacterial peritonitis produces fever, tachycardia, increasing abdominal distention, and toxemia. Death occurs within 5 to 7 days if surgical and medical management prove inadequate.

Jejunal ulcer is a complication of the surgical treatment of peptic ulcer developing under circumstances of ineffective control of gastric secretion and exposure of the vulnerable jejunal mucosa to the acid-pepsin gastric content. Jejunal ulcers are most frequent in the efferent loop, approximately 1 cm beyond the anastomosis. Jejunal ulcer also may develop in the absence of surgery in patients with the Zollinger-Ellison syndrome. Males predominate 10:1. The pain of jejunal ulcer may be in the left lower quadrant or in the lower abdomen. It often is more severe than the presurgical pain and less responsive to treatment. The characteristic relationship to the intake of food may disappear, and nocturnal distress is frequent. Nausea and vomiting may signify an associated malfunction or obstruction of the stoma. Loss of weight is common but is not pronounced unless a jejunocolic fistula develops.

A gastrojejunocolic fistula may develop from penetration of an ulcer at the anastomosis between the stomach and jejunum into the adjacent transverse colon, or a gastrocolic fistula may complicate a penetrating gastric ulcer. The principal symptoms are the pain of peptic ulceration and diarrhea of varying intensity. The diarrhea and the bypass of the small intestine result in rapid and severe loss of weight, electrolytes, and water. Regurgitation of colonic contents into the stomach produces fecal vomiting. The associated malnutrition often is pronounced. Rarely, duodenal ulcer may cause an obstructive jaundice as a consequence of ulceration into the common bile duct, inflammatory obstruction of the duct, penetration into the head of the pancreas that causes pancreatitis, or penetration into the gastrohepatic ligament that obstructs the common bile duct proximally.

Various surgical procedures are available for the management of peptic ulcer. These are designed to limit the acid-secreting capacity of the stomach by severing its vagal connections with the central nervous system and limiting antral gastrin release by antral resection or drainage. They include partial gastric resection; truncal or "selective" vagotomy combined with pyloroplasty, antral resection, or gastrojejunostomy; and the so-called "super selective" vagotomy wherein only the vagal innervation of the acid-secreting mucosa is severed. Important postsurgical problems, both gastrointestinal and metabolic, follow gastric resection. These include the mechanical difficulties of reduced gastric capacity, stomal dysfunction, jejunogastric intussusception, uncovering of a latent malabsorption (gluten-sensitive enteropathy), chronic obstruction of the afferent loop, recurrent ulcer formation, and the dumping syndrome. Diarhea is a common occurrence and usually of multifactorial origin. Alterations in gastric emptying usually result in inadequate mixing of food with

digestive juices leading to steatorrhea; a malabsorption syndrome may be unmasked. The changes in small bowel motility as a result of truncal vagotomy may lead to a bacterial overgrowth syndrome with resulting deconjugation of bile salts leading to steatorrhea. Because of the loss of the gastric acid barrier there is a higher degree of bacterial colonization of the upper intestinal tract, which can also lead to diarrhea. The nutritional and metabolic problems after gastric secretion occur later, sometimes many years later, as in the disordered calcium metabolism with demineralization of bone, associated with deficiency of vitamin D, resulting from the combination of diminished oral intake and impaired absorption. The late difficulties also include deficiencies of vitamin B_{12} and folic acid, decreased absorption of iron, intestinal leakage of albumin, increased susceptibility to infections including pulmonary tuberculosis, and in emotionally vulnerable patients, addiction to alcohol or drugs or psychotic episodes. Late gastrointestinal problems may include the development of gastric carcinoma involving the gastric stump, bezoar formation, and milk intolerance. The evidence for an increased incidence of cholelithiasis after gastric resection or vagotomy is inconclusive.

The dumping syndrome is caused by accelerated gastric emptying following gastric surgery, especially partial gastric resection but also gastroenterostomy, pyloroplasty, vagotomy, and rarely without surgical modification of the stomach. Two pathophysiologic mechanisms may be involved. With the rapid entrance of large amounts of gastric content into the proximal jejunum, the hyperosmolar intestinal content initiates the movement of extracellular fluid from the plasma to the bowel lumen to achieve isotonicity, decreasing the circulating blood volume and inducing compensatory vasoconstriction. The distention of the jejunum and the presence of a hypertonic solution also activate a humoral mechanism that stimulates the release of regulatory peptides and other compounds, including serotonin. Bradykinin, enteroglucagon, neurotensin, and substance P have all been implicated. The early manifestations, within 5 to 30 minutes after eating, include such vasomotor phenomena as a sense of warmth, sweating, weakness, palpitation, vertigo, desire to lie down, and such digestive complaints as abdominal discomfort, nausea, and explosive diarrhea. The late manifestations relate to the rapid entrance of glucose into the blood, producing hyperglycemia before sufficient insulin has been mobilized to metabolize it. The hyperglycemia elicits an overproduction of insulin, causing hypoglycemia 2 to 3 hours after a meal. Studies suggest that postgastrectomy hypoglycemia is caused by an inducible gastrointestinal insulin-secretory factor, possibly related to glucagon, potentiating glucose-mediated insulin release. Dumping may be precipitated by any food but especially by those rich in glucose and disaccharides when fluids are taken simultaneously, and by nervous tension. Dumping is more frequent after surgery for duodenal ulcer in women and among emotionally labile patients.

BENIGN GASTRIC TUMORS

Gastric neoplasms may be classified pathologically as of epithelial, mesenchymal, or endothelial origin. Their clinical differentiation, however, is difficult. The benign epithelial tumors include tubular adenomas and villous adenomas, which appear grossly as sessile or pedunculated mucosal polyps. The mesenchymal tumors include leiomyoma, leiomyoblastoma, lipoma, osteoma, and osteochondroma. Endothelial tumors include hemangioma, lymphadenoma, and endothelioma. Gastric teratomas arise from the visceral wall, the embryonic splanchnopleure, and are composed of tissues representing all three embryonic germ layers. They apparently occur exclusively among males. Tumors originating in the neural tissue, such as neurofibroma, neuroepithelioma, and neurilemoma, also may occur. Gastric polyps are a feature of the familial polyposis syndromes. The pathogenesis of most benign gastric tumors is as obscure as that of carcinoma of the stomach.

Tubular adenomas are most commonly associated with chronic atrophic gastritis or gastric mucosal atrophy. They may be single or multiple; they vary in size from a few millimeters to 7 cm in diameter. Their surface is smooth and lobulated, or the epithelium may be thrown into frondlike processes if the lesion is a villous adenoma. Histologically, the proliferating epithelial tubulae are packed closely together, and there may be crowding of the nuclei with variable degrees of hyperchromatism and increased numbers of mitotic figures—all features of a neoplastic process. There is some liability to malignant change, which is uncommon in growths less than 1.5 cm in diameter and becomes increasingly frequent with polypoid lesions of larger size.

Leiomyomas are the most frequently seen tumors of mesenchymal origin, constituting about 2 per cent of all gastric tumors. They originate from the smooth muscle of the gastric wall and may remain for some time as an intramural structure. As the tumor enlarges, it may grow either into the gastric mucosa toward the lumen or outward toward the serosa, sometimes taking both directions to assume an hourglass appearance. About one third present as an ulcerated intragastric polypoid tumor and one fourth as a polypoid lesion covered by intact mucosa. The risk of evolution to leiomyosarcoma is slight. Because of their tendency to remain silent, leiomyomas may grow to very large size. They may outgrow their blood supply, leading to central necrosis and large cavities in the tumor connected by fistulous tracts to the gastric lumen. The most common symptom is

hemorrhage, either acute or chronic. Abdominal discomfort, partially suggestive of peptic ulcer, may be present. Leiomyomas situated close to the pylorus induce symptoms of obstruction.

A variety of non-neoplastic disorders may simulate benign or malignant neoplasms of the stomach. Heterotopias, most frequently consisting of aberrant pancreatic tissue, are not uncommon in the distal antrum and pyloric canal. Rarely polypoid hamartomas, including the genetically transmitted polyps of the Peutz-Jeghers syndrome and "juvenile" polyps, are seen in the stomach, although such hamartomas are more frequently present in the small intestine and colon. Occasionally, inflammatory pseudotumors consisting of collections of lymphocytes, lymphoblasts, histiocytes, or plasma cells together with a mixed inflammatory infiltrate and reactive changes are found within the gastric mucosa. In the past these have sometimes been erroneously diagnosed as malignant lymphoma and so are commonly termed "pseudolymphomas." The most important feature distinguishing pseudolymphomas from true malignant lymphomas is the presence of follicle formation with true germinal centers. Pseudolymphomas are commonly associated with chronic gastritis and with peptic ulcer. Also arising in stomachs with chronic atrophic gastritis are "regenerative" or "hyperplastic" polyps. Microscopically, there is overgrowth of the tubules of the superficial epithelium, sometimes with a degree of cystic change. The lamina propria is edematous and infiltrated with inflammatory cells.

CARCINOMA OF THE STOMACH

PATHOGENESIS OF GASTRIC NEOPLASIA

Malignant neoplasms of the stomach may be squamous cell carcinomas, carcinoid tumors, lymphomas, leiomyosarcomas, or other sarcomas, but approximately 95 per cent are adenocarcinomas. Gastric cancer afflicts primarily the older segment of the population, with the average being in his mid-50s at the time of diagnosis. Males develop gastric cancer slightly more frequently than females, and there is an inverse relationship between cancer risk and socioeconomic status. Between 1930 and 1979, the age-adjusted mortality rate from gastric cancer in the United States decreased from 28 to 8 per 100,000 in men and from 19 to 5 per 100,000 in women. This appears to be a true decrease in incidence as, despite the increasing application of surgical treatment, the overall 5 year survival rate for patients with gastric cancer remains stable at about 12 per cent. No reasonable explanation for this fortunate trend in the gastric cancer mortality rate is apparent. Similar trends have been noted in Canada and Australia, but not in other major countries. For example, in Japan, Finland, and Chile, gastric carcinoma has been and remains the most common gastrointestinal carcinoma and one of the major causes of death.

The cause of adenocarcinoma of the stomach is unknown. It is certainly not directly inherited, although a hereditary predisposition to its development is suggested by a clear familial aggregation of gastric cancer cases demonstrated in many studies and by the fact that individuals of blood group A appear to be slightly, but significantly, at greater risk. Furthermore, there seems to be some ethnic relationship in that the incidence of gastric cancer is unusually high in Japan, Chile, Finland, and Iceland. In Sumatra, the incidence is high among the Chinese population, but rare among the Japanese; in Israel, gastric carcinoma appears to be more common among Jews of Northern European ancestry than among Jews of Mediterranean or Asian origin.

These ethnic and geographic differences in gastric cancer incidence also suggest the possibility of an environmental influence. Indeed, the death rate from gastric carcinoma among Japanese-born immigrants to the United States is lower than that in Japan, while among Japanese born in the United States the risk of gastric cancer is essentially the same as that for other native-born Americans. Although one study suggests a relationship between gastric cancer and air pollution, in that gastric cancer rates correlated well with levels of suspended particulate matter in the air, the search for carcinogenic environmental factors has centered primarily on dietary factors and other ingested substances. The use of alcohol, tobacco, coffee, and condiments apparently is of no etiologic significance. In Japan smoked meats, sake, and rice treated with talc contaminated with asbestos have been suggested as possible carcinogenic influences. In other geographic areas, fish, cabbage, potatoes, superheated fats, soybean products, and rye bread have been suggested. Most recently the ingestion of nitrites and nitrates as water contaminants or food additives has been investigated as a possible carcinogenic factor, as these substances are easily converted to nitrosamines, which are potent carcinogens. In Colombia, a positive correlation has been found between the risk of gastric cancer and the nitrate concentration in well water. Nitrates and nitrites also are used as preservatives in bacon, cured meats, and fish preparations and may react with amines to produce nitrosamine in the process of cooking. There is an inverse relationship between the hydrogen ion concentration of the gastric content and its nitrite content, and achlorhydric gastric juice contains metabolically active bacteria capable of generating nitrites from nitrate and of nitrosating amines. Of particular interest in this context is the widespread use of H_2-receptor antagonists and the prolonged marked reduction in gastric acidity in a significant number of patients and possible proliferation of nitrite-forming bacteria. Furthermore, cimetidine when nitrosated may be transformed into a mutagenic compound. Evidence to date does not, however, suggest an association between gastric cancer and the use of cimetidine. Thus, the characteristic hypochlorhydric or achlorhydric intragastric environment of the gastric ulcer patient is most suitable for the formation of carcinogenic nitrosamines. Despite this intriguing circumstantial evidence, it must be stressed that no single substance has yet been identified with certainty as an important gastric carcinogen.

The relationship of atrophic gastritis to carcinoma is obscure. Some degree of atrophy is observed in almost all cancer-bearing stomachs. Extensive atrophy of the gastric mucosa is invariably present in pernicious anemia and gastric polyposis, diseases in which the incidence of gastric carcinoma is distinctly higher than among similar age groups in the general population. In pernicious anemia the severe gastric atrophy affects the mucosa of the body of the stomach. Yet when cancer develops, it may be in either the body or the antrum, suggesting that some factor other than the gastritis may be responsible for predisposing to the development of the tumor. The transitional changes from atrophic gastritis with small areas of hyperplasia to papilloma and to carcinoma have been demonstrated. On the other hand, atrophic gastritis occurs in association with gastric disease other than carcinoma and in the absence of any other apparent disorder. Perhaps the associated intestinal metaplasia of the gastric epithelium is more significant than the atrophy as a vulnerable substrate for gastric neoplasia. Possibly the gastritis is associated with a high cell turnover, creating an unstable cellular situation and increasing the vulnerability to neoplasia.

The possible role of achlorhydria in the development of gastric carcinoma is closely related to that of atrophic gastritis. Complete anacidity is present in only a very small proportion of patients with carcinoma; in many, the output of hydrochloric acid is reduced; but in some instances the acidity is great. Neither the atrophy nor the anacidity appears to be of direct etiologic significance; rather, they represent detectable abnormalities produced by some as yet undefined defect in the cells of the gastric mucosa. The apparently increased incidence of gastric carcinoma in the residual stomach after operations (especially gastrojejunostomy) for peptic ulcer, especially among males with blood group A, represents still another clinical situation reflecting an increased tissue vulnerability to neoplasia. Gastric carcinoma thus may be regarded as an acquired disease, developing in an abnormal gastric mucosa and probably arising on the basis of cellular reaction to continued injury, presumably from unknown chemical carcinogens.

Carcinoma may involve any part of the stomach but most frequently develops from the mucus-secreting cells of the antrum and pylorus, especially along the lesser curvature, an area probably more exposed to carcinogenic influences. As noted, the majority of gastric cancers are adenocarcinomas, and these originate in the mucus-secreting cells of the mucosa. The tumor does not necessarily begin with a single cell, but many cells throughout an area of variable size may undergo neoplasia, as in multiple polyposis and frank multicentric carcinoma. Gastric carcinoma, like other neoplasms, varies enormously in its rate of growth, from "acute" rapidly metastasizing tumors to "subacute" and "chronic" neoplasms. Nothing is known of the factors that accelerate its progress in some instances and retard it in others, nor of the conditions that inhibit growth in some directions and favor it in others. Some cancers project into the lumen with little penetration into the wall, others extend directly through the gastric wall, and still others spread chiefly along the wall, primarily along the mucosa, the so-called superficial spreading carcinoma. This latter neoplasm extends no deeper than the muscularis mucosae, and surgical removal offers an excellent prognosis for long-term survival. Acid gastric juice can digest neoplastic as well as non-neoplastic mucosa, submucosa, and muscularis, producing a lesion closely resembling a benign ulcer. Metastatic spread occurs by direct extension through the stomach to involve adjacent organs. Lymphatic spread involves the regional nodes along the lesser curvature, in the greater omentum, and in the hilum of the spleen and the subpyloric and suprapancreatic nodes.

The resistance of the body to cancer is not well understood, but it exists, as indicated in part by the sharp circumscription of some tumors, with atrophy and pyknosis of cancer cells at the margins of the lesion and the proliferation of fibrosis tissues. Other histologic features associated with a favorable prognosis include the presence of an inflammatory reaction around the tumor, good cellular differentiation, and of course, the absence of lymph node metastases. Some lesions are associated with early ulceration; in others it is a late manifestation, and in some never occurs. The immunologic aspects of gastric (and other) carcinoma only now are attracting attention.

MECHANISMS OF SYMPTOM PRODUCTION

There are no symptoms pathognomonic of early gastric carcinoma. The onset of the disease usually is so insidious and its course so latent that it is seldom suspected by the patient or the physician until it is advanced. An interval of 6 to 12 months usually elaspses between the initial manifestations and establishment of the diagnosis. The development and nature of the symptoms depend chiefly on the location of the growth, the presence of hydrochloric acid, the size and extent of the carcinoma, and its tendency to ulcerate, bleed, or

metastasize. A tumor at the cardiac end of the stomach, sufficiently large to narrow the lumen of the esophagus, causes the progressive difficulty in swallowing characteristic of an esophageal neoplasm. Severe vomiting often is the first indication of neoplasm obstructing the pylorus. On the other hand, a carcinoma on the lesser or greater curvature of the stomach, or the body, may not cause symptoms until ulceration, bleeding, secondary infection, or metastases develop.

Symptoms include some type of indigestion, such as vague upper abdominal discomfort, a sense of fullness, ulcerlike distress but without the usual relief obtained by taking food or antacid, or continuous epigastric pain. Anorexia is common, although in many instances the appetite initially may be unimpaired. The patient experiences a sense of fullness after eating less than the customary amount of food. The cause of the anorexia is not known. Loss of appetite in later stages is attributed generally to a diminution of gastric tone and peristalsis secondary to neoplastic infiltration, but this explanation is not entirely satisfactory. The decreased desire for food reduces the total caloric intake and results in progressive loss of weight. The inadequate diet and the loss of nutrient substances by vomiting or diarrhea may lead to protein and vitamin deficiencies; in patients with pyloric obstruction, the malnutrition may become extreme.

Pain may occur early or late in the disease, or occasionally not at all. It seldom is severe until the carcinoma has ulcerated or invaded the wall of the stomach. The distress may be only a vague sensation of fullness or burning in the epigastrium. When hydrochloric acid is present, the pain often if indistinguishable from that of benign peptic ulcer. In general the pain tends to appear earlier and to be more severe in patients with acid gastric secretion than in those with anacidity, presumably because of peptic ulceration. In many cases, however, the distress of carcinoma differs from that of peptic ulcer in that it is aggravated by the ingestion of food and relieved partially or not at all by alkali or emesis. With progression and extension of the carcinoma to involve the celiac plexus and the spinal nerves, the pain may become severe and constant and be relieved only by opiates.

Nausea and vomiting may occur relatively early in the disease, regardless of the location of the lesion, but are much more frequent when the tumor obstructs the pylorus. The vomitus may or may not contain food, bile, or blood, but the so-called coffee-ground emesis is common. Dysphagia and substernal distress are characteristic of a tumor involving the cardiac orifice of the stomach and the lower end of the esophagus. Ulceration of a comparatively small tumor located in a "silent" area, with penetration into the wall of a blood vessel, may cause hematemesis or melena before other symptoms appear. Anemia is frequent, usually hypochromic and microcytic in type, and is caused by the occult loss of blood. The hematologic picture may be that of a true pernicious anemia, however, owing probably to coexistence of the two diseases. The anemia very occasionally results from carcinomatous infiltration of the bone marrow and displacement of the hematopoietic cells. Weakness, increasing fatigue, and lack of energy are related usually to the loss of weight and anemia, but they may precede these latter manifestations. Diarrhea is not uncommon, and in patients with diffusely infiltrating linitis plastica of the stomach, may be ascribed to rapid gastric emptying in addition to increased bacterial invasion of the upper gastrointestinal tract as a consequence of the diminished acid secretion. Infrequently, the "initial" manifestations are those of metastatic lesions such as carcinomatosis of the peritoneum, massive enlargement of the liver, or severe backache caused by extension of the neoplasm into the celiac plexus or the spine. Severe progressive dyspnea results from diffuse pulmonary lymphatic spread of gastric carcinoma.

REFERENCES

Anton, A. H., and Woodward, E. R.: High levels of blood histamine and peptic ulcer in a patient with portacaval shunt. Arch. Surg. 92:96, 1966.

Ballard, H. S., Frame, B., and Hartsock, R. J.: Familial multiple endocrine adenoma-peptic ulcer complex. Medicine 43:481, 1964.

Beaven, M. A.: Histamine. N. Engl. J. Med. 294:30, 320, 1976.

Berenson, M. M., Sannella, J., and Freston, J. W.: Menetrier's disease. Serial morphological, secretory, and serological observations. Gastroenterology, 70:257–263, 1976.

Code, C. F.: Reflections of histamine, gastric secretion and the H_2-receptor. N. Engl. J. Med. 296:1459, 1977.

Davenport, H. W.: Salicylate damage to the gastric mucosal barrier. N. Engl. J. Med. 276:1307, 1967.

Davenport, H. W.: Back diffusion of acid through the gastric mucosa and its physiological consequences. In Jerzy-Glass, G. (ed.): Progress in Gastroenterology, Vol. II. New York, Grune & Stratton, 1970.

Davenport, H. W.: Physiology of the digestive tract, 5th ed. Chicago, Yearbook Medical Publishers Inc., 1982.

Deering, T. B., and Malagelada, J. R.: Comparison of an H_2-receptor antagonist and a neutralizing antacid on postprandial acid delivery into the duodenum in patients with duodenal ulcer. Gastroenterology 73:11, 1977.

Dragstedt, L. R., Woodward, E. R., Seito, T., Isaza, J., Rodriguez, J. R., and Samijan, R.: The question of bile regurgitation as a cause of gastric ulcer. Ann. Surg. 174:548, 1971.

Edward, F. C., and Coghill, N. F.: Aetiological factors in chronic atrophic gastritis. Br. Med. J. 2:1409, 1966.

Elder, J. B., Ganguli, P. C., and Gillespie, L. E.: Cimetidine and gastric cancer. Lancet 1:1005, 1979.

Ellison, E. H., and Wilson, S. D.: The Zollinger-Ellison syndrome: reappraisal and evaluation of 260 registered cases. Ann. Surg. 160:512, 1964.

Fritsch, W. P., Hausamen, T. U., and Rick, W.: Gastric and extragastric gastrin release in normal subjects, in duodenal ulcer patients and in patients with partial gastrectomy (Billroth I). Gastroenterology 71:522, 1976.

Gershon, M. D., and Erde, S. M.: The nervous system of the gut. Gastroenterology 80:1571–1594, 1981.

Gilbert, D. A., Silverstein, F. E., Tedesco, F. J., et al.: Symposium: The National ASGE Survey on upper gastrointestinal bleeding. III. Endoscopy in upper gastrointestinal bleeding. Gastrointest. Endosc. 27:94, 1981.

Grossman, M. I., Guth, P. H., Isenberg, J. I., Passaro, E. P., Roth, B. E., Sturdevant, R. A. L., and Walsh, J. H.: A new look at peptic ulcer. Ann. Int. Med 84:57, 1976.

Grossman, M. I., Kirsner, J. B., Gillespie, I. E., and Ford, H.: Basal and histalog-stimulated gastric secretion in control subjects and in patients with peptic ulcer or gastric cancer. Gastroenterology 45:14, 1963.

Hoffman, N. R.: The relationship between pernicious anemia and cancer of the stomach. Geriatrics 25:90, 1970.

Holmes, K. D.: Mallory-Weiss syndrome. Review of 20 cases and literature review. Ann. Surg. 164:810, 1966.

Isenberg, J. I.: The parietal cell. Viewpoints on Digestive Diseases 7: No. 2, 1975.

Ivey, K. J.: Gastric mucosal barrier. Gastroenterology 61:247, 1971.

Janowitz, H. D.: Hunger and appetite—physiologic regulation of food intake. Am. J. Med. 25:327, 1958.

Keller, R. T., and Roth, H. P.; Hyperchlorhydria and hyperhistaminemia in a patient with systematic mastocytosis. N. Engl. J. Med. 283:1449, 1970.

Kirsner, J. B: Peptic ulcer. In Beeson, P. B., and McDermott, W. (eds.): Cecil-Loeb Textbook of Medicine, 13th ed. Philadelphia, W. B. Saunders Co., 1971, p. 1259.

Kirsner, J. B., Levin, E., and Palmer, W. L.: Observations on the excessive nocturnal gastric secretion in patients with duodenal ulcer. Gastroenterology 11:598, 1948.

Lipkin, M.: The development of gastrointestinal cancer. Viewpoints on Digestive Diseases 4: No. 4, 1972.

Longstreth, G. F., Go, V. L. W., and Malagelada, J. R.: Cimetidine suppression of nocturnal gastric secretion in active duodenal ulcer. N. Engl. J. Med. 294:801, 1976.

McCarthy, D. M.: Report on the United States experience with cimetidine in Zollinger-Ellison syndrome and other hypersecretory states. Gastroenterology 74:453, 1978.

McCarthy, D. M.: The place of surgery in the Zollinger-Ellison syndrome. N. Engl. J. Med. 302:1344, 1980.

Mendeloff, A. I.: What has been happening to duodenal ulcer? Gastroenterology 67:1020, 1974.

Ming, S.: The classification and significance of gastric polyps. International Academy of Pathology Monograph: The gastrointestinal tract, 1977: pp. 615–647.

Morson, B. C., and Dawson, I. M. P.: Gastrointestinal Pathology. London, Blackwell Scientific Publications, 1972.

Overholt, B. F., and Jeffries, G. H.: Hypertrophic, hypersecretory protein-losing gastropathy. Gastroenterology 58:80, 1970.

Palmer, W. L.: The mechanism of pain in gastric and duodenal ulcers. II. The production of pain by means of chemical irritants. Arch. Int. Med. 38:694, 1926.

Paulino, F., and Roselli, A.: Carcinoma of the stomach; with special reference to total gastrectomy. Curr. Probl. Surg., 1973, pp. 2–72.

Pearse, A. G. E., and Bussolati, G.: Immunofluorescence studies of the distribution of gastrin cells in different clinical states. Gut 11:646, 1970.

Prolla, J. C., Kobayashi, S., and Kirsner, J. B.: Gastric cancer. Arch. Int. Med., 124:238, 1969.

Rotter, J. I., and Rimoin, D. L.: Peptic ulcer disease—a heterogeneous group of disorders? Gastroenterology 73:604, 1977.

Rovelstad, R.: The incompetent pyloric sphincter bile and mucosal ulceration. Am. J. Dig. Dis. 21:165, 1976.

Silverstein, F. E., Gilbert, D. A., Tedesco, F. J., et al.: Symposium: The National ASGE Survey on upper gastrointestinal bleeding. I. Study design and baseline data. Gastrointest. Endosc. 27:73, 1981.

Silverstein, F. E., Gilbert, D. A., Tedesco, F. J., et al.: Symposium: The National ASGE Survey on upper gastrointestinal bleeding. II. Clinical prognostic factors. Gastrointest. Endosc. *28*:80, 1981.

Smith, B. M., Skillman, J. J., Edwards, B. G., and Silen, W.: Permeability of the human gastric mucosa. N. Engl. J. Med. *285*:716, 1971.

Snyder, N., III, Scurry, M. T., and Deiss, W. P., Jr.: Five families with multiple endocrine adenomatosis. Ann. Int. Med. *76*:53, 1972.

Soll, A. H.: Physiology of isolated canine parietal cells: Receptors and effectors regulating function. *In* Johnson, L. R. (ed.): Physiology of the Gastrointestinal Tract, New York, Raven Press, 1981, pp. 673–691.

Strickland, R. G., and McKay, I. R.: A reappraisal of the nature and significance of chronic atrophic gastritis. Am. J. Dig. Dis. *18*:426, 1973.

Tatsuta, M., and Okuda, S.: Location, healing and recurrence of gastric ulcers in relation to fundal gastritis. Gastroenterology *69*:897, 1975.

Taylor, I. L., Duckray, G. J., Calam, J., et al.: Big and little gastrin response to food in normal and ulcer subjects. Gut *20*:957, 1979.

Taylor, K. B.: Gastritis. N. Engl. J. Med. *280*:818, 1970.

Te Velde, K., Hoedemaekerm, P. J., Anders, G. J. P. A., Arenda, A., and Nieweg, H. O.: A comparative morphological and functional study of gastritis with and without autoantibodies. Gastroenterology *51*:138, 1966.

Twomey, J. J., Jordan, P. H., Jr., Laughter, A. H., Mauwissen, H. J., and Good, R. A.: The gastric disorder in immunoglobulin-deficient patients. Ann. Int. Med. *72*:499, 1970.

Van Wayjen, R. G. A., and Linschoten, H.: Distribution of ABO and Rhesus blood groups in patients with gastric carcinoma, with reference to its site of origin. Gastroenterology *65*:877, 1973.

Walker, I. R., Strickland, R. G., Ungar, B., and MacKay, I. R.: Simple atrophic gastritis and gastric carcinoma. Gut *12*:906, 1971.

Walsh, J. H., and Grossman, M. I.: Gastrin. N. Engl. J. Med. *292*:1324, 1975.

Walsh, J. H., and Lam, S. K.: Physiology and pathology of gastrin. Clin. Gastroenterol. *9*:567, 1980.

Walsh, J. H., Trout, H. H., II, Debas, H. T., and Grossman, M. I.: Immunochemical and biological properties of gastrins obtained from different species and of different molecular species of gastrins. *In* Chey, W. Y., and Brooks, F. P. (eds.): Endocrinology of the Gut. Thorofare, N. J., Charles B. Slack, Inc., 1974, pp. 277–289.

Weiner, H. (ed.): Duodenal Ulcer. Advances in Psychosomatic Medicine, Vol. 6. Basel, London, New York, S. Karger, 1971.

Wellmann, K. F., Kagan, A., and Fang, H.: Hypertrophic pyloric stenosis in adults. Gastroenterology *46*:601, 1964.

Wermer, P.: Endocrine adenomatosis and peptic ulcer in a larger kindred. Am. J. Med. *35*:205, 1963.

Wright, L. F., and Hirschowitz, B. I.: Gastric acid secretion. Am. J. Dig. Dis. *21*:409, 1976.

Yalow, R. S.: Gastrins: Small, big, and big-big. *In* Chey, W. Y., and Brooks, F. P. (eds.): Endocrinology of the Gut. Thorofare, N. J., Charles B. Slack, Inc., 1974, pp. 261–276.

Zollinger, R. M., and Ellison, E. H.: Primary peptic ulceration of the jejunum associated with islet cell tumors of the pancreas. Ann. Surg. *142*:709, 1955.

The Small Intestine

28

David W. Watson and William A. Sodeman, Jr.

The small intestine is a complex tube whose structure is well designed to subserve such seemingly diverse but related functions as the aboral transport of luminal contents, the secretion of enzymes and hormones, the digestion and absorption of ingested materials, and the mounting of an immune response. These functions are modified by neurohumoral influences and are materially aided by contributions from the pancreas and hepatobiliary system. The primary function of the small bowel, however, is digestion and absorption. All other activities either regulate or facilitate this process.

In the small intestine, as elsewhere, structure and function are intimately although not always obviously related, and the greater our knowledge of how this relationship operates to ensure the gut's contribution to health the easier it will be to understand the consequences of changes induced by disease.

Although our understanding of small intestinal pathophysiology has increased, many unanswered questions remain. This discussion is based on information that is firmly established for the human small intestine and does not present concepts based solely upon presumably parallel animal models, however applicable they may appear. Sufficient species differences in small bowel structure and function exist so as to make such carte blanche applications hazardous.

We will present an outline of normal structure from the gross to the electron microscopic level and discuss normal function and abnormal structure-function relationships as they apply to motor function, digestion and absorption, secretion, and immune responses. Circulatory disturbances have wide-ranging effects involving several of the aforementioned functions and will be discussed separately.

NORMAL STRUCTURE

Postmortem measurements of the length of the small intestine yield estimates of 6.5 to 7.0 meters. In life, however, tubes only 3 meters long may pass into the cecum. Its caliber diminishes slightly from duodenum to terminal ileum, in part accounting for the fact that foreign bodies such as gallstones more frequently obstruct the lower ileum. The division of the small bowel into duodenum (20 to 30 cm), jejunum (2.5 meters), and ileum (3.5 meters) is imprecise and based upon rather slight modifications of structure and rela-

tively more important differences in function. Certain of the latter, such as the absorption of monosaccharides, amino acids, and β-monoglycerides, occur mainly in the jejunum, but other portions of the small intestine can to a large extent compensate for loss of this segment. However, the physiologic absorption of vitamin B_{12} and the active transport of bile salts are exclusive functions of the terminal ileum.

The wall of the small bowel is composed of four basic layers: the mucosa, submucosa, muscularis externa, and serosa. The mucosa is composed of an epithelial cell layer with its filamentous basement membrane, a lamina propria containing blood vessels, lymphatics, smooth muscle cells, nerve fibers, plasma cells, lymphocytes, fibroblasts, eosinophils, macrophages, reticular cells, mast cells, collagen, and reticular fibrils, and it is separated from the submucosa by the muscularis mucosa. The submucosa contains larger blood vessels and lymphatics and more connective tissue, nerves, ganglia, and lymphoid elements. The muscularis externa is divided into an inner circular layer and an outer longitudinal layer of smooth muscle, with the myenteric plexus interspersed between the two. In the past, the longitudinal muscle was described as a long, drawn-out spiral and the circular layer as a tight spiral. Later studies indicate that fibers in both layers deviate, at random, both to the right and to the left, from a strictly longitudinal or circular orientation, so that the net direction in the two layers is axial and circumferential.

The small intestine is distinguished by four structural features that together enormously increase its luminal surface area. The valvulae conniventes are circumferential folds of mucosa and submucosa absent from the duodenal bulb, but prominent in the duodenum and jejunum, that disappear in the midileum. They are responsible for the feathery appearance of the small bowel on barium studies and constitute the transverse folds seen in plain radiographs of air-filled intestine. The villi are projections of mucosa, readily discernible with a hand lens, that are usually finger-like or leaflike but under some conditions appear as ridges or convolutions. Figure 28–1 is an illustration of villi as viewed with the scanning electron microscope. The individual cells of the villi and, to a lesser extent, the crypts possess filamentous microvilli, which in turn are coated with a finely filamentous material, or "fuzz." The surface area of the adult small intestine has been estimated to be from 5100 to 5900 cm².

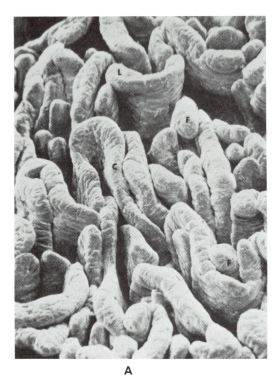

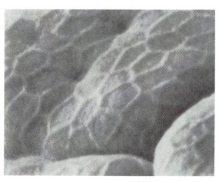

Figure 28–1 *A,* Human jejunal biopsy. Scanning electron micrograph (SEM) showing a leaf-shaped villus, *L;* finger-shaped villi, *F;* and a convolution, *C.* Surface creases can be distinguished (× 110). *B,* Human jejunal biopsy. SEM of part of the surface of a single villus. The mouths of two goblet cells are prominent, and the hexagonal cell outlines are clearly seen (× 2300). (From Toner, P. G., and Carr, K. E.: J. Pathol. 97:611, 1969.)

A   B

The mucosal crypts lie between the villi and extend basally to the muscularis mucosa. This relationship is depicted in Figure 28–2. In normal Americans and Europeans, the villi constitute two thirds to three fifths of the mucosal thickness, and the crypts account for two fifths to one third. As many as 20 crypts surround each villus, but a

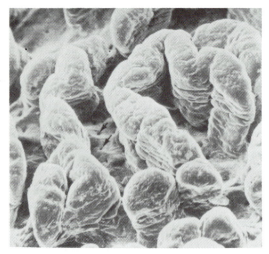

Figure 28–2 Human duodenal biopsy. SEM showing various shapes of villi. The mouths of intestinal crypts opening into the circumvillar basin are arrowed (× 210). (From Toner, P. G., and Carr, K. E.: J. Pathol. 97:611, 1969.)

functional ratio of 3:1 seems likely. It also has been appreciated that the intestine is coated with a relatively thick layer of water molecules through which other molecules move by diffusion. This is a stagnant layer wherein bulk mixing caused by intestinal motility is unimportant. This "unstirred layer" constitutes an important determinant of the kinetics of absorption.

The surfaces of the villi and the linings of the crypts are covered by a continuous single layer of five different types of columnar cells: goblet cells, Paneth cells, enterochromaffin cells, undifferentiated crypt cells, and the differentiated villous epithelial cells (enterocytes, or absorptive cells).

The majority of cells in the crypts are undifferentiated cells that have a high mitotic index. They have numerous ribosomes and polysomes but little endoplasmic reticulum, scant microvilli, and undeveloped terminal webs. Although they contain what appear to be secretory granules, no secretory function has been established, and their main purpose is to serve as a source of the differentiated epithelial cell types. Newly formed cells migrate up the crypts, and as they reach the junction of the crypt and villus they undergo morphologic, biochemical, and functional maturation to become villous absorptive cells, goblet cells, or Paneth cells. The origin of the enterochromaffin cells is less certain. During this migration-maturation process, the differentiating cells demonstrate larger and more numerous microvilli, a well-demarcated terminal web, more numerous mitochondria and rough endoplasmic reticulum, a decrease in free ribosomes and polysomes, loss of secretory granules, and the formation of large apical dense bodies that represent lysosomal derivatives. As these cells differentiate into villous absorptive cells, they acquire enzymes, receptors, and carriers essential to the final phases of digestion and the processes of absorption. Cells migrating up the villus continually push the older, more differentiated cells toward the villous tip, from which they are eventually extruded into the lumen. This renewal process is accomplished in a period of 3 to 7 days.

The absorptive cells are the most numerous and functionally most important cells on the villous surface. They are simple columnar cells in which the luminal surface is specialized to form a striated, or brush, border. This brush border is composed of microvilli ranging in length from 0.75 to 1.5 μ and in width from 0.10 to 0.20 μ. They number 3000 to 6500 per cell and are closely and regularly spaced with an intervillous distance of 0.01 to 0.05 μ. They are enclosed by an extension of the same trilaminar-appearing plasma membrane that surrounds the remainder of the cell. The microvillous core contains a central zone of 10 to 50 closely packed parallel filaments, or tubules, that extend from the microvillous tip to the terminal web, which is the area just basal to the microvilli. It contains no organelles but only nonparallel tubular filaments similar to those in the microvilli and a few structures termed *apical vesicles,* thought to represent lysosomes. These tubular filaments are smaller and quite distinct from the cytoplasmic microtubules that lie roughly parallel to the long axis of the absorptive cell in the supranuclear cytoplasm. The microvillous plasma membrane is coated with a strongly adherent overlying surface coat composed of a complex mixture of mucoproteins, glycoproteins, and glycolipids. The fuzzy coat, or glycocalyx, that is seen on electron microscopy makes up only a small fraction of this layer. The glycocalyx is composed of a sulfated, weakly acidic mucopolysaccharide that appears to be continuously synthesized by the Golgi apparatus of the epithelial cell, transported to the microvillous surface, and eventually shed into the lumen. The glycocalyx is most prominent on the absorptive cells, especially at the villous tips. Figure 28–3 illustrates the fine structural relationships of these cells.

The microvillous plasma membrane and its glycocalyx constitute a digestive-absorptive unit. Several enzymes have been localized to this structure, including alkaline phosphatase, the disaccharidases, aminopeptidases, dipeptidases, adenosine triphosphatase, thiamine triphosphatase, and folic acid conjugase. The active transport of glucose, galactose, and amino acids as well as the uptake of the vitamin B_{12}-intrinsic factor complex is mediated by receptors and carriers localized to this region.

The epithelial cells covering the villi and lining the crypts are joined at their lateral margins by a junctional complex composed of three parts. Just basal to the origin of the microvilli the outer leaflets of the lateral plasma membranes fuse to form the tight junction (zonula occludens). Just basal to this lies the intermediate junction (zonula adherens), and beneath it is the desmosome (macula adherens), so named because the cytoplasm underlying the plasma membrane at this point is condensed. These latter two structures represent only close approximations of the plasma membranes, not fusion. The epithelial cells with their junctional complexes form a tight unbroken membrane lining the luminal surface of the small intestine

This epithelial membrane is a complex dynamic "organ" regulating the flux of materials between the lumen and the lamina propria. Its integrity depends on the continual replication, maturation, and metabolism of its cells. Interruption of any of these vital processes will lead to a failure of this organ, which will usually be expressed as a malabsorption syndrome.

ABNORMAL STRUCTURE

Most structural abnormalities affecting the small intestine, whether gross or microscopic, are acquired as the result of many different disease entities, the pathophysiologies of which are discussed in subsequent sections of this chapter. It is convenient at this point, however, to mention briefly congenital abnormalities, even though their clinical manifestations depend upon pathophysiologic mechanisms similar to those that produce acquired abnormalities.

Developmental abnormalities of the small intestine include atresia and stenosis, duplication, persistence of vestigial structures and heterotopia, errors of rotation, and defective innervation. For a discussion of small intestinal embryology, the reader is referred to the article by Trier and Krone.

CONGENITAL ATRESIA AND STENOSIS

Intestinal atresia consists of either complete separation of two segments with a wedge-shaped defect of the mesentery or two segments joined by a fibrous cord. Stenosis implies an incomplete interruption or narrowing with preservation of luminal continuity. Pathogenesis may involve persistence or failure of resolution of the epithelial proliferative phase during the fifth through eighth weeks of development or an acquired defect caused by ischemia. Twenty-five per cent of cases of intestinal atresia may be due to meconium ileus, and the frequency of mucoviscidosis in atresia is about 9 per cent. Congenital rubella and genetic factors have also been implicated. Patients with atresia present with intestinal obstruction within

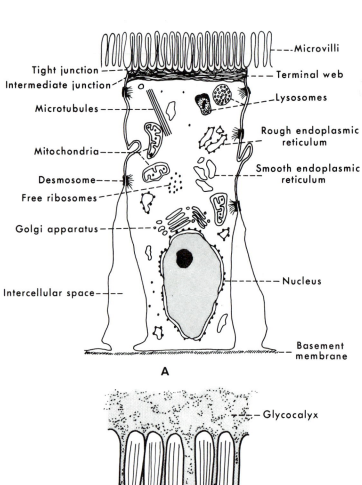

A

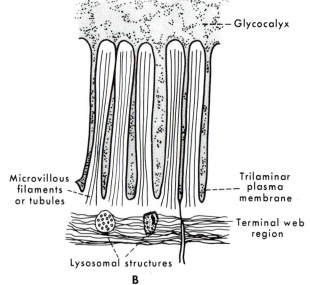

B

Figure 28–3 Schematic representation of differentiated villous absorptive cell (A) and the glycocalyx-microvillus structure (B).

the first 2 weeks of life, whereas stenosis may become manifest somewhat later. Treatment is surgical.

DUPLICATIONS

A duplication is a spherical or tubular cyst intimately attached to the intestine and located on the mesenteric side. Most are located in the ileum and may or may not communicate with the intestinal lumen. Communicating duplications are generally lined by gastric mucosa, and peptic ulceration with its complications may occur. The adjacent intestine may also become obstructed as the result of compression or intussusception. Pathogenesis remains unknown, and presentation may be in early life or adulthood. Diagnosis and treatment are accomplished by laparotomy.

MECKEL'S DIVERTICULUM

This is the most frequent congenital anomaly of the intestinal tract. At birth the vitelline duct normally is completely obliterated, but if this process is incomplete the intestinal end persists as a sac arising from the antimesenteric border of the ileum, usually within 100 cm of the ileocecal valve. Ectopic gastric mucosa is often present near the mouth of the diverticulum. Complications include hemorrhage, diverticulitis, perforation with peritonitis, and intestinal obstruction due to intussusception or volvulus around a fibrous remnant of the vitelline duct.

The demonstration of a Meckel's diverticulum is often possible by pertechnitate imaging following cimetidine administration if the lesion contains gastric mucosa. Forty percent of intravenous ^{99m}Tc sodium pertechnitate is excreted via the gastrointestinal tract, initially by mucus and parietal cells. Pretreatment with cimetidine does not block uptake by these cells but does inhibit secretion, thereby enhancing isotopic imaging. Most diverticula remain asymptomatic throughout life, but for those with complications treatment is surgical.

ANOMALIES OF ROTATION AND FIXATION

Abnormalities of intestinal rotation result in an anomalous position of the small intestine and colon and abnormal fixations and bands that may result in internal herniation and volvulus. Classification of these abnormalities is usually based on the stage of rotation in which they occur. Therefore, the intestine may be contained within an omphalocele, fail to rotate at all, malrotate (incomplete rotation), or undergo reverse rotation. Abnormalities of mesenteric attachment also may

occur. Clinical manifestations are due to acute or chronic intestinal obstruction. Radiographic examinations may demonstrate rotational anomalies, but final diagnosis and treatment remain surgical.

MOTOR FUNCTION

NORMAL MOTOR FUNCTION

The overall concept of small intestinal motor activity becomes more meaningful when it is not viewed as the primary function of the small bowel but rather as complementary to the organ's major activity. To facilitate the digestive-absorptive process, small intestinal movements must do two things: mix ingested materials with pancreatic and hepatobiliary secretions and propel luminal contents from one end to the other at a rate suitable for both optimal absorption and the continuing entry of gastric contents. Normally, this rate is approximately 1 cm per minute, and as a result the residue from the previous meal leaves the ileum at about the same time the next meal enters the stomach. An understanding of how these two activities are accomplished requires a consideration of the electrical and contractile events taking place in the small intestine.

Intestinal smooth muscle exhibits spontaneous contractions, can be stimulated by stretch, and will conduct impulses independently of nerves. Its resting membrane potential is unstable and varies irregularly with basal tension and the general level of contractile activity, but it also fluctuates in two consistent patterns. The first is a rhythmically occurring, omnipresent fluctuation arising in the longitudinal muscle and is identified as either the *slow wave*, the *basic electrical rhythm (BER)*, or the *pacesetter potential*. As visualized by Code and coworkers, if at any one instant the electrical activity of the small bowel could be stopped or frozen in place, each slow wave or pacesetter potential would be fixed in the wall and would extend over a distance that may be termed its *cycle length (wavelength)* for that particular segment. The bowel beneath each cycle would then represent a physiologic motor unit, with the slow wave prescribing its dimensions and controlling the nature of motor activity occurring within it at any one instant. These pacesetter potentials evoke no muscular contractions themselves but instead govern the rate at which the second type of electrical activity may take place. These are termed *spike potentials* and are responsible for the contractions of the circular muscle. Spike potentials can occur only during the periods of maximal depolarization of the pacesetter potentials. This relationship between pacesetter potentials, spike potentials, and circular muscle contraction is presented in Figure 28–4.

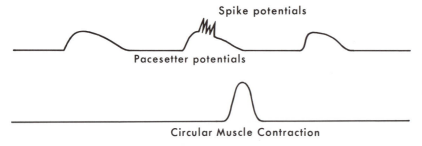

Figure 28–4 Diagrammatic presentation of the relationship between pacesetter potentials, spike potentials, and circular muscle contraction.

The pacesetter potential passes caudally as a sheath, or ring, whose front constitutes a rapid depolarization reaching all circumferential points simultaneously. An intact intrinsic nerve plexus is required for this to occur. Its frequency is rather constant with time but displays a declining gradient over the small bowel from 11.8 cycles per minute in the duodenum and first 10 cm of the jejunum to 9.0 cycles per minute in the ileum. This decline may be stepwise through a sequence of frequency plateaus, each representing the distance traversed by the pacesetter potentials originating in that segment, but there is no agreement on this point. Since pacesetter potentials of a given frequency pass over relatively long segments and exhibit this declining frequency, they serve to integrate the activity of the whole organ.

The conduction of either pacesetter or spike potentials is made possible by tight side-to-side or end-to-end junctions between the individual muscle cells. These nexuses represent a partial fusion of the outer leaflets of the trilaminar plasma membranes and provide low resistance electrical shunts between cells.

The pacesetter potential therefore sets the frequency but not the magnitude of circular muscle contraction. An alteration in frequency of the pacesetter potential may be brought about in several ways. Duodenal compression or transection causes a decrease in frequency distal to the injury. A decrease in frequency is also seen with hypothermia, hypothyroidism, hypoglycemia, malabsorption syndromes, substances interfering with active membrane transport, and damage to the intrinsic nerve plexuses. Serotonin, posterior pituitary, hormone, and vasopressin also cause a decrease in frequency, the latter two by reducing blood supply to the longitudinal muscle. An increase in frequency occurs with pyrexia, hyperthyroidism, adrenergic stimulation, and morphine administration. Pacesetter potentials are relatively insensitive to cholinergics, anticholinergics, and topical anesthetics. Extrinsic nerve stimulation, the ingestion of food, and changes in electrolyte concentrations also have little or no effect on the frequency of pacesetter potentials.

Spike potentials are the electrical counterparts of circular muscle contraction and therefore are associated with luminal pressure changes. They are not propagated, and their sequential occurrence in successive segments (peristalsis?) is due rather to propagation of the pacesetter potentials to which they are coupled. Not every pacesetter potential need evoke a spike potential, but the frequency of spike potentials can never exceed the frequency of pacesetter potentials. The latter are conducted from their origin in the longitudinal muscle to the circular muscle, probably via the nexuses.

The electrical response, if any, of the circular muscle to a given pacesetter potential is governed by an interplay of influences provided by the activity of the intrinsic nerve plexuses acting as part of local or central reflexes and various circulating or locally produced hormones. The amplitude of circular muscle contraction is proportional to the number, duration, and amplitude of the spike potentials. The factors that influence the generation of spike potentials are somewhat different from those that alter the frequency of pacesetter potentials. Spike potentials are initiated by rapid radial stretch or distention of the bowel wall, vagal stimulation, and ingestion of food. In contrast to pacesetter potentials, spike potentials are relatively sensitive to the effects of drugs, hormones, and other pharmacologically active substances. They are initiated by cholinergic drugs, hydrochloric acid, serotonin, and morphine and are eliminated by anticholinergics, ganglionic blocking agents, barbiturates, and sympathomimetics. Mechanical obstruction at first results in an increase in spike potentials proximal to the obstruction and a decrease distally. Anoxia causes an initial stimulation but eventually results in their disappearance.

Although coordinated intestinal motor activity may occur in the absence of extrinsic autonomic innervation, this system is important in modifying motor activity in relationship to other physiologic responses within the body. Unfortunately, its structure and function are still not completely understood. The vagi contain motor preganglionic parasympathetic fibers that make synaptic connections with secondary parasympathetic motor neurons in the subserosal, myenteric, and submucosal plexuses. Postganglionic sympathetics also traverse the vagi, but their termination is unclear. Motor fibers in the splanchnic nerves are preganglionic sympathetic fibers terminating in the abdominal sympathetic ganglia and postganglionic sympathetic fibers arising in the paravertebral ganglia. Postganglionic sympathetic fibers are then distributed to the gut with branches of the associated arteries. Their sites of termination are not known, although some catecholamine-containing fibers form meshes around cholinergic ganglion cells and others enter the muscle layers. Sensory nerves travel in both systems, with vagal fibers originating in the unipolar cells of the nodose ganglion. The nerve cells lying within the gut are postganglionic, parasympathetic, or internuncial neurons and perhaps cells with sensory function, although no specialized neural structures have been identified as sensory. The enteric plexuses appear to be interconnected, but the anatomic relationship between fibers originating in them and secretory and smooth muscle cells is unknown.

The influence of extrinsic nerve stimulation on spike potentials is imperfectly understood, and for the present only the following generalization can be made. In the absence of significant small intestinal activity, both parasympathetic and sympathetic stimulation initiate spike potentials, whereas an actively contracting bowel tends to be inhibited. The small intestine contains both alpha- and beta-adrenergic receptors. Alpha receptors have an affinity for epinephrine and act to eliminate spike potentials. Beta receptors bind isoproterenol, and, in the duodenum at least, their stimulation tends to elicit spike potentials, but the remainder of the intact human small intestine has not been adequately studied. Alpha receptors predominate in the small bowel, and the net effect of either alpha or beta stimulation is an inhibition of small intestinal smooth muscle activity. How this is mediated in the case of beta receptors is not clear.

Apart from serving as a source of pacesetter potentials, the contribution of the longitudinal muscle layer to small intestinal motor function is not well understood. No electrical events corresponding to its contraction have been recorded. Current views suggest that it serves largely to regulate the overall "tone" of the bowel wall and the caliber of its lumen. Its contraction produces a net increase in luminal diameter and thereby a decrease in pressure.

Little is known about the electrochemical events involved in the contractile process. It appears that the release of calcium ions from a site of storage triggers contraction. The term "smooth" is not strictly apt, however, since faint striations are in fact present as uniform small filaments of actin. Myosin has also been identified in "smooth" muscle, but its location is unknown.

The interaction of these electrical and contractile events under the direction of various local and systemic neurohumeral influences results in intestinal *motility*. This is an ambiguous term at best, however, and may refer to movements of the bowel wall, smooth muscle contraction, luminal pressure changes, or propulsion of luminal contents. Since circular muscle contraction and the rate of flow of luminal contents may have an inverse relationship, the term is self-contradictory. The ambiguity is further compounded by adding the prefixes *hyper* and *hypo*. From the standpoint of small intestinal function, only two types of motor activity are important—mixing and propulsion.

Mixing is accomplished predominantly by isolated stationary "standing ring" contractions of circular muscle involving a 1- to 2-cm segment of bowel or as a series of such contractions, referred to as *rhythmic segmentation*. This latter type of motor pattern is represented diagrammatically in Figure 28–5. Segmenting activity decreases in frequency from the duodenum to the ileum, and although it is the predominant type of activity recordable, it is present only 2 per cent of the time in the resting small intestine. Segmenting contractions are more frequent after a meal or following morphine administration and have the effect of slowing transit. In patients with rapid transit, segmenting activity is decreased.

Flow through the alimentary canal can be thought of as analogous to flow through the vascular system, albeit more complex and less well understood. Both systems possess pacemakers, pressure receptors, and osmoreceptors, and flow is enhanced as viscosity decreases. The rate at which intestinal contents move through the small intestines depends on a pressure gradient generated by the bowel wall and the peripheral resistance of the gut. The resistance varies with the diameter of the lumen and the contractility, or tone, of the intestinal wall. The prime regulator of transit, however, is peripheral resistance. Precisely how this resistance is varied and in what manner contractile activity is ordered to bring about the required pressure differential for transit to occur is still largely undefined. Peristalsis, a moving ring contraction, is controversial. It must occur infrequently and over short distances, if at all, since normally it takes several hours for contents to traverse the small bowel. There is no quantitative information about the frequency, velocity, or range of movement of peristalsis in the human small intestine. The so-called "peristaltic rush" connotes a vigorous ring contraction progressing rapidly from the duodenum to the ileum. Its existence is debated, and if it does occur it is probably always pathologic. Some aboral movement of contents will occur with isolated or rhythmic segmenting contractions. As viewed by Texter, the aboral transport of luminal contents is more closely related to the pressure gradient between proximal and distal segments than to the activity of any single type of contraction. With the probable exception of waves that progress over a considerable distance (peristalsis) and of rhythmic sequences, pressure waves contribute more to the increase of peripheral resistance than to the promotion of propulsion. Since there is a progressive

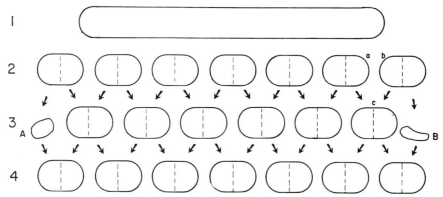

Figure 28–5 Diagram representing process of rhythmic segmentation. Rows 1, 2, 3, and 4 indicate sequence of appearances in loop. Dotted lines mark regions of division. Arrows show relation of particles to segments they subsequently form. (From Hightower, N. C., Jr.: In Code, C. F. [Ed.]: Handbook of Physiology. Vol. IV. Washington, D.C., American Physiological Society, 1968.)

decrease in the level of activity in sequentially more distal segments of the small intestine, the resulting gradient probably constitutes the most important mechanism for transit. It is therefore the total motor pattern of the entire small bowel that underlies transit rather than any specific kind of contractile activity. Because this pattern moves slowly from the stomach down to the terminal ileum, it has been termed the *migrating myoelectric (motor) complex (MMC)*. The types of contractions and wave forms making up this motor complex are the subject of considerable debate and bewildering terminology. As pointed out by Asher, the coinage of scientific terminology confers a sense of reality that may be spurious. A generalized increase in activity will retard transit just as effectively as complete atony will, since in neither case will a pressure gradient be produced.

ABNORMAL MOTOR FUNCTION

Without a satisfactory knowledge of normal motor function, an understanding of pathologic processes must also be incomplete. Furthermore, the definition of abnormal motor function depends on one's point of view. To the physiologist it is an alteration of smooth muscle contractility; the radiologist finds it reflected in some abnormality of the distribution and movement of barium; those interested in "motility" patterns will be impressed by unusual fluctuations in intraluminal pressures; and the physician at the bedside wonders about the origin of abdominal pain, constipation, and diarrhea. Unfortunately, it is not possible to describe any consistent or reproducible relationship between these different kinds of measurements, and in many instances signs and symptoms of altered function remain largely unexplained.

On the clinical level, disturbed motor function will be manifest primarily as abdominal pain or

some alteration in transit perceived as constipation or diarrhea. The only known stimulus for pain production in the small bowel is an increase in intramural tension. Distention therefore will produce pain only when accompanied by significant tone in the intestinal wall or a strong contraction involving a relatively broad segment. The intensity of pain is proportional to the rapidity with which the tension develops and its magnitude. Any stimulus capable of eliciting such increases in tension may produce pain. Most commonly they arise as a result of luminal obstruction, vascular insufficiency, ulceration, increased levels of certain pharmacologically active substances, or the administration of drugs such as parasympathomimetics or codeine. Whether ulceration and ischemia produce pain by causing secondary intramural tension changes or by some other mechanism is not clear. Like other visceral forms of pain, that arising in the small intestine is not sharply localized. The sensory innervation of the small intestine derives largely from the tenth thoracic spinal segment, and small bowel pain is perceived in the corresponding somatic dermatome. Since pain originating in midline-derived structures tends to be referred to the midline, small bowel pain is characteristically periumbilical, with some spillover into the adjacent supra- and infra-umbilical areas. The increased intramural tension, regardless of cause, tends to wax and wane episodically, and therefore the pain is usually described as cramping or colicky. In the presence of a pain-causing lesion, the superimposition of factors contributing to increased motor activity will lead to intensification; for example, the pain of intestinal obstruction or mesenteric vascular insufficiency is more prominent after eating. This classic description is often modified, however, by individual variations in pain threshold, prior abdominal surgical procedures, and the presence of concurrent disease. Although bilateral vagotomy has no effect on pain perception, it appears that bilateral abdominal sympathectomy, like midthoracic cord lesions, may reduce or abolish it.

Diarrhea and constipation as expressions of altered motor function cannot be as readily interpreted in terms of small intestinal disease or transit times. They are described by events occurring or not occurring at the anal opening, and interposed between this point of awareness and the small bowel are the colon and rectum. Transit times through the small bowel vary within a wide range under presumably normal conditions, and only extremes will be manifest as an alteration in bowel habit. Complete obstruction of the small bowel eventually will lead to constipation. Partial obstruction may do so as well, but not infrequently the process causing the partial obstruction leads to more rapid emptying of the small bowel and colon distal to the obstruction, causing diarrhea.

The small intestine may initiate diarrhea in two ways: by exposing the colon to intestinal contents at a rate-volume relationship that exceeds its absorptive capacity or by allowing the entry into the colon of substances stimulating rapid emptying, as may occur in the malabsorption syndromes. Small intestinal causes of diarrhea that are the result of abnormalities involving secretion (e.g., cholera) or malabsorption (e.g., nontropical sprue) will be discussed in relationship to the pathophysiology of those disorders.

Lesions that do reflect primarily, although not exclusively, abnormal motor function include obstruction, ileus, and humoral influences provided by the products of certain tumors and endocrine disorders.

Obstruction and Ileus. The term *obstruction* should be reserved for partial or complete occlusion of the intestinal lumen, regardless of cause. *Simple obstruction* implies luminal occlusion only, whereas *strangulating obstruction* involves both luminal occlusion and interference with blood supply. Closed loop obstruction implies a segment of intestine with its lumen occluded at both ends. Ileus, however, refers to an adynamic state of the intestine occurring either segmentally or throughout its entire length.

Small intestinal obstruction may follow external compression from tumors or abscesses, torsion or volvulus (usually in relationship to a fibrous adhesion), herniation, intussusception, intramural fibrosis (as in Crohn's disease), intramural hemorrhage or edema, and intraluminal tumors or foreign bodies such as gallstones. The manifestations of an obstruction depend on its site, degree, duration, rapidity of development, and whether or not it is a simple, closed loop, or strangulating obstruction.

When the obstruction is in the duodenum or proximal jejunum, distention is slight and there is early vomiting of large amounts of bile-stained fluid. With lesions of the lower jejunum and ileum, distention is often marked by the time vomiting of fecal-appearing material occurs. Periumbilical, cramping pain is the most prominent symptom. With complete obstruction, constipation is usual, but with partial obstruction, diarrhea or constipation may be present. Bowel sounds are more frequent and often of higher pitch in partial obstructions and early in complete obstruction, with increases in intensity often coinciding with crescendos of pain. Abdominal examination in the patient with early simple obstruction usually discloses only distention, occasional visible contractile activity, and the auscultatory findings mentioned. Percussion may reveal increased resonance, but this will depend on the relative amounts of fluid and gas within the bowel lumen. Signs of peritonitis appear rapidly with strangulating obstructions, somewhat later in untreated closed loop obstructions, and relatively late in untreated simple obstructions. Although rigidity of the abdominal wall signifies peritonitis, rebound tenderness may be elicited with a distended, inflamed bowel in the absence of actual peritoneal inflammation.

Acute obstructions are usually the result of torsion or volvulus, intussusception, or herniation. Chronic obstructions are more often due to inflammatory strictures or tumors. The more slowly the obstruction develops, the more indolent and less pronounced the symptoms will be. As distention progresses in acute, high-grade obstruction, the initial intestinal hyperactivity is replaced by generalized ileus, even in a localized segment. This is due to the activation of alpha- and beta-adrenergic receptors by a sympathoadrenal discharge, with inhibition of contractile activity.

Chronic partial obstruction leads to generalized protein-calorie malnutrition, but acute obstruction causes marked abnormalities of fluid and electrolyte balance.

In contrast to obstruction, ileus represents inadequate or absent propulsive motor activity. It occurs with such regularity following abdominal operations that postoperative ileus has been referred to as *physiologic ileus*, even though at times it may represent a mortal complication. More severe and protracted ileus results from bacterial and chemical peritonitis or sudden and usually painful distention of other hollow structures such as the bile ducts, ureters, and urinary bladder. It may also be a sequel to complete or near complete luminal occlusion, intestinal ischemia, or hypokalemia. Ileus under these circumstances has been termed *paralytic* as opposed to physiologic, but the difference is in degree rather than kind. All true ileus can properly be described as adynamic. Reference has occasionally been made to something called "dynamic ileus," supposedly representing functional obstruction due to intestinal spasm. This is a contradiction in terms, and it is doubtful that such a condition exists, at least within the small intestine.

In the case of postoperative ileus, the stomach

may remain atonic for several days, but the small intestine usually exhibits activity within a few hours. If the ileus persists, the bowel becomes progressively distended with gas and fluid. The gas is largely swallowed air, but colonic bacteria may contribute significant amounts, especially if the small bowel has become colonized.

The most prominent findings in the patient with ileus are those related to the postoperative abdomen or the underlying disease process, usually peritonitis. There is abdominal distention, and bowel sounds are minimal or absent. Signs of dehydration and evidence of ineffective circulating plasma volume may also be present.

It has been known for some time that the gut is not intrinsically paralyzed but is capable of contraction when properly stimulated. Neely and Catchpole have redrawn attention to this fact and have proposed that ileus is due to inhibition of contractile activity by sympathetic overactivity brought about by increased levels of circulating adrenal catecholamines or sympathetic nerve stimulation or both. As previously pointed out, this reaction is mediated by adrenergic stimulation. The experimental observation that postoperative or paralytic ileus can be prevented by abdominal sympathectomy or splanchnic anesthesia has strengthened this view.

Such a mechanism readily suggests a rational approach to management. First one must administer drugs that will cause blocking of the sympathetic overactivity, followed by parasympathetic stimulation of the "liberated" intestine. Guanethidine and bethanechol, guanethidine and prostigmine, or phentolamine and prostigmine have been utilized with good results. Since guanethidine blocks the release of norepinephrine rather than causing alpha blockade, phentolamine, an alpha blocker, may be required if there are already increased circulating levels of epinephrine and norepinephrine. Since alpha receptors predominate in the small intestine, beta blockers appear not to be required. Patients selected for this therapy must fulfill certain criteria. Hypovolemia must be corrected first to prevent hypotension from sympathetic blockade; electrolyte balance, especially hypokalemia, must be managed and intestinal obstruction carefully excluded. Nasogastric suction also remains a useful adjunct for minimization of distention. Long Miller-Abbott tubes have been employed, but it is often difficult to obtain passage through an adynamic gut.

Radiologic examinations utilizing plain films of the abdomen may be of help in substantiating the presence of obstruction or ileus and occasionally, in differentiating the two. Dilated air-filled loops of bowel with air-fluid levels are characteristic of both. In ileus, the air-filled bowel may not be as dilated as in obstruction, but many exceptions will be found. Perhaps most helpful is the distribution pattern of intestinal gas. With ileus, gas is characteristically found throughout the small and large bowel, although not necessarily in a continuous column, whereas in obstruction, gas may not be present distal to the occlusion. A localized ileus may mimic obstruction, however, and it must be remembered that as the fluid-gas ratio increases, little of note may be seen radiologically.

Examination with soluble contrast agents such as Gastrograffin may aid in differentiating obstruction and ileus in the acutely ill patient. Small-bowel follow through examinations utilizing barium in patients with less acute manifestations may be helpful in identifying obstructing lesions and suggesting their cause. As conventionally performed, however, such examinations are seldom helpful. It is only by means of intubation and the direct instillation of contrast material into the small bowel that the accelerated transit, lumen distention, and proper transradiancy necessary for accurate diagnosis can be attained. This technique, referred to as *enteroclysis (small bowel enema)*, is associated with a high degree of diagnostic accuracy when used with double contrast methods in which air or methyl cellulose is employed.

The consequences of acute obstruction or ileus are reflected in marked alterations of fluid and electrolyte distribution. The severity of fluid loss and the extent of acid-base derangement depend not only on the anatomic portion and extent of bowel involved but also on the duration of the process. In proximal obstruction there is external loss through vomiting of large amounts of gastric, pancreatic, biliary, and duodenal secretions, with a lesser amount remaining sequestered within the gastrointestinal lumen. As much as 5 liters may be lost within a 24-hour period. Most commonly a metabolic acidosis develops, since the amount of bicarbonate loss usually exceeds the loss of hydrogen ion. With lower obstructions or generalized ileus, as much as 40 per cent of the circulating blood volume may accumulate within the gut without evidence of external fluid loss. As the bowel distends, there is increasing fluid and electrolyte accumulation within its lumen, representing a shift from the extracellular compartment. This loss is nearly isosmotic with plasma with regard to the concentrations of major ions. It represents both a decrease in insorption and an increase in exsorption. Elevations of intraluminal pressure up to 20 cm of water increase insorption, but above this level insorption falls off while exsorption continues to increase. The mechanism underlying this effect is unknown. Initially, the serum sodium concentration remains relatively normal, but hyponatremia gradually develops as sodium loss exceeds that of water. The reason for this also is not clear. Both clinical and experimental observations indicate that hypotonic dehydration leads to more profound circulatory abnormalities than does isotonic dehydration. The resulting decrease in plasma volume is at first compensated for by generalized vasoconstriction, so that blood pressure and pulse rate remain normal for a time. When these homeostatic mechanisms are interfered with by generalized anesthesia, precipitous drops in blood pressure may occur, underscoring the need for preoperative fluid replacement in all patients. Depending on the stage of the process and the rapidity of its development, various degrees of dehydration and circulatory collapse will be observed. Because of starvation, dehydration, ketosis, loss of alkaline secretions, and declining renal function, a metabolic acidosis develops. If ischemia is present, as in a strangulating obstruction, a profound and often fatal lactic acidosis may occur. Losses of potassium are high and the resulting hypokalemia may contribute to atonicity and distention. The fully developed clinical picture is one of an acutely ill patient exhibiting signs of dehydration, abdominal distention, tachycardia, hypotension, diaphoresis, hemoconcentration, normal or low serum concentrations of sodium and potassium, normal or elevated BUN and serum creatinine, and metabolic acidosis.

Strangulating obstructions develop the same pattern of fluid and electrolyte abnormalities but because of the associated intestinal ischemia also exhibit signs of tissue necrosis. Closed loop obstructions also commonly result in ischemia of the bowel wall, as do simple obstructions if they remain untreated for a sufficient length of time. As noted by Bynum and Jacobson, however, it is doubtful that increased intraluminal pressure per se can cause ischemic necrosis of the intestine. Decreased blood flow, mainly involving the mucosa, occurs at pressures above 30 mm Hg, but marked anoxia is prevented by the phenomena of autoregulation and autoregulatory escape (see section on mesenteric vascular disease). Additional factors such as decreases in plasma volume and reflex vasoconstriction probably are of material importance in the production of ischemia in untreated simple obstruction. In simple and closed loop obstructions, venous outflow is usually impeded first, whereas in strangulating obstructions, both arterial and venous occlusion occur early. The results are tissue anoxia, increased capillary permeability, and intramural and mucosal hemorrhage. Intramural edema and marked losses of protein develop and the integrity of the epithelial membrane is disrupted, resulting in bacterial invasion with peritonitis and bacteremia. Progressive ischemia, gangrene, and peritonitis rapidly ensue. This stage is accompanied by fever and leukocytosis in addition to the previously discussed fluid and electrolyte disturbances. With tissue necrosis and compromised renal function, hypokalemia may be replaced by hyperkalemia. Materials produced by tissue necrosis, hemorrhage, and infection accumulate in the peritoneal cavity, and their absorption is a major factor in the profound cardiovascular collapse that too often characterizes the terminal phase of this condition.

Management of patients with intestinal obstruction or ileus requires early recognition of the problem, prompt differentiation of various forms of obstruction and ileus, replacement of fluid and electrolyte losses, correction of acidosis, nasogastric suction to minimize distention, and prompt surgical correction in the case of obstruction. Therapy with adrenergic blocking agents and parasympathomimetics may prove helpful adjuncts to the successful management of the patient with simple ileus.

Patients who are receiving increasing attention are those with intestinal pseudo-obstruction. These individuals exhibit features of both obstruction and ileus. Intestinal pseudo-obstruction is a clinical syndrome caused by ineffective propulsive activity and characterized by symptoms and signs suggesting obstruction in the absence of a mechanical cause. Although any part of the gastrointestinal tract may be involved, including the esophagus, the major manifestations are usually related to the small intestine and colon. The disorder may be acute and transient but is usually recurrent or chronic. Primary and secondary forms are recognized. Intestinal pseudo-obstruction may be secondary to many different disorders, including collagen vascular disease, primary muscle disease (e.g., progressive muscular dystrophy), hypothyroidism, diabetes mellitus, Chagas' disease, various drugs (e.g., phenothiazines, anticholinergics, and tricyclic antidepressants), jejunoileal bypass, and mesenteric vascular insufficiency. The primary form is referred to as *chronic idiopathic intestinal pseudo-obstruction (CIIP)*. These patients fall into three groups: (1) those with hollow visceral myopathy in which there is vacuolar degeneration of smooth muscle with fibrosis and a familial incidence; (2) those with hollow visceral neuropathy in which there are neuronal abnormalities throughout the body; and (3) those in whom no clearly defined abnormality can be demonstrated. This last group includes some patients who have demonstrated increased levels of prostaglandins, abnormalities of platelet aggregation, and a response to indomethacin. Since intestinal pseudo-obstruction is another cause of stasis and bacterial overgrowth, steatorrhea may occur. Treatment is directed toward correction of electrolyte abnormalities (especially those of calcium, magnesium, and potassium), tube decompression, nutritional support, stimulation of intestinal activity through administration of drugs such as urecholine, metoclopramide, and, possibly, indomethacin.

Motor Dysfunction Due to Humoral Mechanisms. The electrical and contractile processes that underlie normal intestinal motor function are integrated and modified by various humoral substances, the concentrations of which under certain circumstances may be markedly altered. Hyperthyroidism, hypoparathyroidism, adrenal insufficiency, carcinoid tumors, medullary carcinomas of the thyroid, gastrin-producing tumors of the pancreas (Zollinger-Ellison syndrome), certain non-gastrin-producing pancreatic tumors (Verner-Morrison syndrome), and neural crest tumors may be associated with crampy abdominal discomfort and diarrhea, whereas hypothyroidism and hyperparathyroidism are often characterized by constipation. Carcinoid tumors and medullary carcinomas of the thyroid may be regarded as examples of this type of abnormality. It is to be emphasized, however, that most of the aforementioned conditions affect small bowel secretion as well as motor activity, so that the clinical expression observed is a net effect of the two processes.

Carcinoids may appear in any entodermally derived tissue or teratomas. In the small intestine, they arise from enterochromaffin cells (Kulchitsky cells, or argentaffin cells). The appendix is the most frequent site of origin (53 per cent), but carcinoids are the most common neoplasm of the small intestine, most arising in the ileum. They also may develop in other portions of the gastrointestinal tract, biliary tree, pancreas, ovary, and bronchi. They are generally small, 95 per cent being less than 2 cm in diameter. Most appear cytologically benign, and the only reliable criteria of malignancy are invasion and metastasis. The majority are asymptomatic, being discovered in the course of investigating and treating other conditions such as appendicitis.

Clinical manifestations may be due to ulceration or obstruction or to the carcinoid syndrome. This syndrome occurs most commonly with tumors of the jejunum or ileum that have metastasized to the liver. The pharmacologically active principles of these tumors are inactivated by hepatic enzyme systems, and therefore no systemic symptoms will be produced unless they are released into the systemic circulation. Systemic manifestations include characteristic attacks of flushing involving the head, neck, and upper trunk, at times precipitated by food, alcohol, emotion, or pressure on the tumor; abdominal cramping pain and diarrhea; bronchoconstriction; right-sided heart failure; pellagra-like skin lesions; and ascites. Usually, only a few of these features are present intermittently in any one patient.

The tumors are known to contain serotonin, 5-hydroxytryptophan, kallikreins, histamine, and ACTH. Increased serotonin levels probably are responsible for the increased intestinal motor activity and diarrhea as well as the endocardial fibrosis leading to pulmonary and tricuspid valve deformity. The metabolic pathway of serotonin is presented in Figure 28–6. Serotonin lowers the excitation threshold of intestinal smooth muscle, resulting in increased responsiveness to otherwise inadequate stimuli. In keeping with this mechanism is the sometimes beneficial effect of serotonin antagonists such as methysergide and cyproheptadine and the deleterious response to monoamine oxidase inhibitors. Improvement may also occur with *p*-chlorophenylalanine, which inhibits the

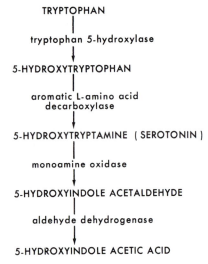

TRYPTOPHAN

tryptophan 5-hydroxylase

5-HYDROXYTRYPTOPHAN

aromatic L-amino acid decarboxylase

5-HYDROXYTRYPTAMINE (SEROTONIN)

monoamine oxidase

5-HYDROXYINDOLE ACETALDEHYDE

aldehyde dehydrogenase

5-HYDROXYINDOLE ACETIC ACID

Figure 28–6 Outline of tryptophan metabolism.

hydroxylation of tryptophan, the rate-limiting step in serotonin synthesis, or with methyldopa, a decarboxylase inhibitor. Serotonin is known to produce fibroblastic proliferation, and its administration to experimental animals has resulted in endocardial lesions similar to those encountered in humans. Serotonin is metabolized primarily in the liver and lungs to 5-hydroxyindoleacetic acid, and increased urinary excretion of the latter is presumptive evidence of the presence of a functioning carcinoid. Slight increases in urinary 5-hydroxyindoleacetic acid, however, may be found after the ingestion of foods high in serotonin such as bananas, tomatoes, avocados, red plums, walnuts, and eggplant. Cough syrups containing glyceryl guaiacolate may cause false-positive reactions for 5-hydroxyindoleacetic acid, and patients with nontropical sprue may exhibit slight elevations. The pellagra-like syndrome seen in some patients results from the diversion of large amounts of tryptophan to serotonin synthesis.

The substances responsible for the attacks of flushing and bronchoconstriction are less certain. Serotonin appears to be a less likely cause than histamine or bradykinin. Since epinephrine may provoke flushing as well as release kallikreins from tumor tissue, alpha-adrenergic blocking agents may ameliorate flushing by blocking their release.

Efforts to treat the various components of the syndrome are worthwhile even if only partially successful, since the average duration of life from the onset of symptoms to death is 8 years, with a 21 per cent 5-year survival for patients with liver metastases.

The most recent substances to be incriminated in disturbances of intestinal motor activity are the prostaglandins. They are derivatives of prostanoic acid and occur in four forms, designated *E, F, A,* and *B*, that differ in the structure of the attached five-membered carbon ring. Although no clear role for prostaglandins in normal gut motor physiology has been demonstrated, types E and F do affect intestinal smooth muscle function. Prostaglandins $F_{1\alpha}$ and $F_{2\alpha}$ generally cause contraction of both longitudinal and circular muscle, and prostaglandins E_1 and E_2 produce contraction of longitudinal muscle and inhibition of circular muscle. The intravenous infusion of E_1 in humans causes abdominal cramps, and administration of $F_{2\alpha}$ results in diarrhea. The F series act via a direct effect on circular muscle, whereas the E compounds affect longitudinal muscle directly and stimulate cholinergic nerve fibers within the small intestine. The resulting net effect is smooth muscle contraction. Some medullary carcinomas of the thyroid and neural crest tumors contain large amounts of prostaglandins E_1 and $F_{2\alpha}$, and patients often exhibit increased blood levels of these substances and have diarrhea. Since the prostaglandins probably also augment intestinal secretion via cyclic AMP, this may further contribute to the diarrhea in such patients.

Some conditions, such as scleroderma, appear to interfere with normal intestinal motor responses by structurally altering smooth muscle. Others, like diabetes mellitus, may affect function by way of lesions involving the autonomic nerve supply.

DIGESTIVE-ABSORPTIVE FUNCTION

Advances in our knowledge of normal digestive and absorptive mechanisms have enabled physicians to understand more clearly the pathophysiology of the different malabsorption syndromes. The terms *digestion* and *absorption* merely emphasize different phases of a single continuing process initiated by events taking place within the small intestinal lumen and completed by the specialized functions of the villous absorptive cell. Its plasma membrane maintains differences in composition and electrical charge between the luminal and intracellular environment by influencing the rates at which molecules enter the cell. The differences between the function of this membrane at the cell's apical and basal surfaces result in a net movement of molecules through the cell that we call *absorption*.

Substances traverse this membrane by processes having different kinetics and energy requirements. These transport mechanisms include passive diffusion, nonionic diffusion, carrier-mediated transport, facilitated transport, and exchange diffusion. The term *active (uphill) transport* is best used in a general sense to refer to a process requiring energy and coupled directly with cellular metabolism. Net movement is usually but not invariably against a concentration gradient and electrochemical potential difference. In this sense,

only carrier-mediated processes constitute true active transport. Carrier-mediated transport is coupled with cell metabolism and exhibits substrate specificity, saturation kinetics, competitive inhibition, and counter transport. The transported substance binds reversibly to a carrier on one side of the membrane and is released on the opposite side. Solutes such as hexoses, amino acids, and pyrimidines are absorbed by this mechanism. Passive diffusion is movement due solely to the kinetic energy and electrical charge of molecules and the electrical field in which they exist. Free fatty acids and beta-monoglycerides are examples of substances absorbed by this mechanism. Nonionic diffusion involves the association between an anion and cation on one side of a membrane, with the complex then crossing the membrane and dissociating on the side opposite to the original anion and cation. The net effect is the transfer of ionized compounds. In contrast to passive diffusion, nonionic diffusion accounts for the movement of a charged species independent of the electrical potential difference. Such processes are, however, highly dependent on the H^+ concentration. This type of transport characterizes the absorption of unconjugated bile salts and many drugs. *Facilitated transport* refers to a process that also exhibits substrate specificity, saturation kinetics, competitive inhibition, and counter transport and results in net movement of substrate but is not directly coupled with cell metabolism and cannot produce net transport against an electrochemical potential difference. Fructose absorption is in part accomplished in this way. Exchange diffusion implies the obligatory exchange of a molecule on one side of a membrane for a molecule of the same species on the opposite side. It is not directly coupled with cell metabolism and cannot produce net transport but may result in substantial fluxes across membranes. Sodium transport under certain conditions may constitute an example of exchange diffusion.

NORMAL DIGESTION AND ABSORPTION

The digestion of dietary lipids, carbohydrates, and proteins is initiated in the lumen of the duodenum and proximal jejunum and completed at the glycocalyx and microvillous plasma membrane of the jejunal absorptive cells. Normally, the resulting fatty acids, beta-monoglycerides, monosaccharides, and amino acids as well as water- and fat-soluble vitamins (with the exception of vitamin B_{12}) are absorbed predominantly in the jejunum. The ileum is capable of transporting these substances, but absorption is usually complete before this portion of the intestine is reached. Ileal absorption may become quantitatively important when the jejunum is abnormal or no longer present. Figure 28–7 outlines the basic steps involved in the digestion and absorption of fat, carbohydrate, and protein.

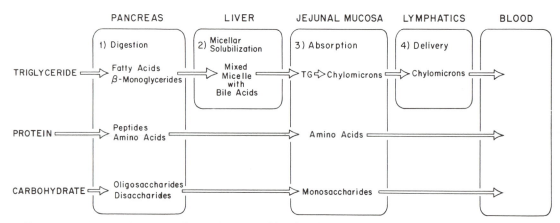

Figure 28–7 A comparison of the four major steps of fat digestion and absorption and the corresponding processes involved in the assimilation of protein and carbohydrates. This diagram emphasizes that the processes of micellar solubilization and delivery of chylomicrons through the intestinal lymphatics are not involved in the absorption of these latter two nutrients. Thus, diseases that cause dysfunction at level of step 2 or 4 result in malabsorption only of fat (i.e., isolated steatorrhea), whereas diseases that exert their effect at the level of step 1 or 3 may produce significant malabsorption of fat, protein, and carbohydrate. (From Wilson, F. A., and Dietschy, J. M.: Gastroenterology *61*:911, 1971.)

Fat Absorption. The average American and Northern European diet contains 60 to 100 gm of fat, the majority of which is in the form of neutral fat or triglyceride. Most is hydrolyzed in the proximal small intestine by pancreatic lipase, which preferentially splits the ester bonds in the α and α' positions, forming free long-chain fatty acids and beta-monoglycerides. Pancreatic juice also contains a protein, termed *colipase*, that helps the lipase adhere to the lipid droplets. The optimal pH of pancreatic lipase is between 6 and 7, and the protein is inactivated by higher H^+ concentrations. Cephalic stimulation via the vagus causes the release of cholecystokinin-pancreozymin from the duodenal and jejunal mucosa, which in turn increases the secretion of lipase and other enzymes from the pancreas. Fatty acids and especially essential amino acids augment this hormonal response, which also causes contraction of the gallbladder, increasing the delivery of bile salts and other biliary constituents to the intestinal lumen. Lipolysis does not directly alter dietary lipid solubility, but the resulting fatty acids and beta-monoglycerides differ from triglycerides in being amphipaths. The bile salts are detergent-like molecules that when present in a concentration greater than 1 to 2 mM per liter (the critical micellar concentration) aggregate into macromolecular complexes known as *micelles*. The fatty acids and beta-monoglycerides, being amphipaths, will dissolve into the micelle structure of the bile salts to form mixed micelles and so achieve aqueous solubilization. Micelle formation accelerates the diffusion of lipolytic products through the unstirred layer to the absorptive cells. It also indirectly increases the rate of lipid hydrolysis by removing the end products of the reaction. An important characteristic of the bile salts participating in this process is their conjugation with either taurine or glycine. Normally, there are no unconjugated bile salts in bile. Unconjugated bile salts are weaker detergents and less efficient contributors to micellar solubilization.

When the mixed micelle reaches the epithelial cell membrane, the fatty acids and beta-monoglycerides enter the cell by passive diffusion. There is then rapid re-esterification to triglyceride, which becomes associated with protein, cholesterol, cholesterol esters, and phospholipid to form a specific class of lipoproteins called *chylomicrons*. The chylomicrons are next released from the basal portion of the epithelial cell, and they then cross the interstitial space and enter the lacteal. The chylomicrons are coated with apoproteins that potentiate the action of lipoprotein lipase in the systemic circulation. The chylomicrons enter the systemic circulation via the thoracic duct and are hydrolyzed as they pass through capillaries by lipoprotein lipase coating the capillary surface. The resulting fatty acids are then solubilized by being bound to albumin and transported to sites of uptake. The important steps involved in the digestion and absorption of fat are outlined in Figure 28–8.

The lacteal has a blind distal end at the villous tip and proximally anastomoses with the submucosal lymphatics. The manner in which chylomicrons gain entry into the lacteal is still debated. Electron microscopy has demonstrated no pores in the lacteal wall, but pinocytotic vesicles appear to occupy approximately 15 per cent of the endothelial cell cytoplasm, suggesting to some that this is a major pathway of chylomicron uptake. Others, however, maintain that these macromolecular aggregates enter the lacteal through gaps at the endothelial cell junctions.

The flow of lymph through the lacteal appears to be dependent on the "pumping" action of the villus, which occurs independently of intestinal

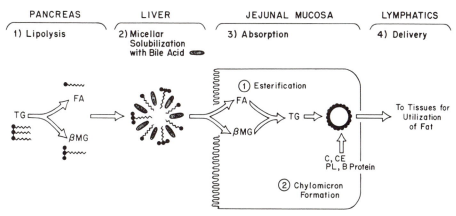

Figure 28–8 Diagrammatic representation of the major steps in the digestion and absorption of dietery fat. These include (1) the lipolysis of dietary triglyceride (TG) by pancreatic enzymes; (2) micellar solubilization of the resulting long-chain fatty acids (FA) and beta-monoglycerides (βMG) by bile acids secreted into the intestinal lumen by the liver; (3) absorption of the fatty acids and beta-monoglyceride into the mucosal cell, with subsequent re-esterification and formation of chylomicrons; and finally (4) movement of the chylomicrons from the mucosal cell into the intestinal lymphatic system. During the process of chylomicron formation, small amounts of cholesterol (C), cholesterol ester (CE), and phospholipid (PL) as well as triglyceride are incorporated into this specific lipoprotein class. (From Wilson, F. A., and Dietschy, J. M.: Gastroenterology 61:911, 1971.)

motor activity. The smooth muscle fibers of the villus are responsible for this movement and may be under the control of a hormone, villikinin, found only in small intestinal mucosa and released in response to mechanical and chemical stimuli.

Some deconjugation of bile salt molecules occurs normally in the intestinal lumen, and the unconjugated bile salts are absorbed largely by nonionic diffusion throughout the small bowel. Conjugated bile salts are taken up by an active transport mechanism in the terminal ileum. Approximately 96 per cent of the bile salt pool is reabsorbed during each cycle of the enterohepatic circulation, and each day the pool is cycled 6 to 10 times. This results in a normal daily loss of only 500 mg of bile salts in the feces. This loss is compensated for by hepatic synthesis, and, to an extent, increased losses can be balanced by increased production. Active ileal absorption is crucial, however, to maintaining the integrity of the total bile salt pool and normal micellar solubilization.

In contrast to dietary fat, the medium-chain triglycerides now widely used as dietary supplements in certain gastrointestinal disorders are composed of fatty acids of 6 to 12 carbon atoms and are handled by the gut in a somewhat different manner. They are hydrolyzed largely by pancreatic lipase, which is more active against triglycerides composed of short-chain fatty acids. Effective hydrolysis appears to occur in the presence or absence of bile salts, and the hydrolytic products are mainly free fatty acids with little monoglyceride. They are not incorporated into chylomicrons but are transported by the portal venous system. Micelle formation is probably not necessary for their effective absorption, since bile diversion has little

effect on their uptake by the epithelial cells. Furthermore, a small but significant amount of medium-chain triglycerides is absorbed intact. In some patients with defective lipolysis or inadequate fat absorption or both, they may constitute important forms of diet therapy because they are more efficiently handled by the gut.

Carbohydrate Absorption. Western diets contain approximately 350 gm of carbohydrate, with an average composition of 60 per cent starch, 30 per cent sucrose, and 10 per cent lactose. The conversion of these substances to monosaccharides is a necessary process for normal absorption. Salivary and, to a greater extent, pancreatic α-amylase attack the interior 1,4 α-linkage of amylase (starch), producing maltose and maltotriose. Amylopectin, a branched-chain carbohydrate having similar 1,4 α-linkages but also 1,6 α-linkages at the branching points, yields maltose, maltotriose, and branched saccharides called α-*dextrins* containing an average of eight glucose molecules. Isomaltose, the disaccharide with 1,6 α-linkages, is not a physiologic substrate in the small intestine. Since amylase has little or no activity for the outer 1,4 α-linkages in these molecules, no glucose is formed in the intestinal lumen under physiologic conditions. Although the intestinal mucosa is the site of some intrinsic and adsorbed amylase activity, most hydrolysis takes place within the lumen. The resulting maltose, maltotriose, and α-dextrins as well as ingested lactose and sucrose are then presented to the brush border, where they are converted to their component monosaccharides by enzymes (maltase, sucrase, lactase, and α-dextrinase), located in the glycocalyx-plasma membrane structure. From a pathophysiologic point of view, lactase is the most important of these enzymes.

Lactase activity has been demonstrated to reside in three different beta galactosidases: enzyme I, a neutral lactase with a pH optimum of 5.5 to 6.0, located in the brush border and active against lactose and synthetic beta-galactosides; enzyme II, an acid beta-galactosidase with a pH optimum of 4.5, located in the cellular lysosomal fraction and active against lactose and synthetic beta-galactosides; and enzyme III, a cytoplasmic neutral hetero-beta-galactosidase, having a pH optimum of 5.5 to 6.0 and hydrolyzing only synthetic beta galactosides. Enzyme I is responsible for most normal intestinal lactase activity.

Some monosaccharides diffuse back into the lumen, but most of the glucose, galactose, and fructose is absorbed. Existing data are compatible with the hypothesis that glucose and galactose are transported from the intestinal lumen across the brush border into the epithelial cell by a shared carrier-mediated process and that the rate and direction of movement depend on the distribution ratio of Na^+ and possibly K^+ across this membrane. Sodium is therefore required for absorption, and this asymmetric distribution of cations depends directly on energy production. Fructose, however, appears to be absorbed to a large extent by facilitated transport, since it does not accumulate against its own concentration gradient, but the mechanism is saturable and its absorption is more rapid than that of pentoses although slower than that of glucose or galactose. Fructose is becoming an increasingly important commercial sweetener, and some individuals have experienced cramping and diarrhea after ingesting fructose-containing foods. Various studies of the completeness of fructose absorption in which breath hydrogen analysis has been used have shown that approximately 35 per cent of individuals do not absorb fructose completely. Although fructose malabsorption appears to be both dose- and concentration-related, the cause remains to be defined. The events involved in the digestion and absorption of carbohydrates are schematically summarized in Figure 28–9.

An important concept not yet fully developed, involves the dietary regulation of small intestinal enzyme activity. Rosensweig and coworkers have studied the adaptive responses of disaccharidase and glycolytic enzymes (common to all cells) in humans following dietary manipulation. Sucrose- or fructose-feeding increases the activities of sucrase and maltase but not lactase, whereas glucose and galactose also enhance glycolytic enzyme activity, although the increase is less than that observed after feeding isocaloric amounts of noncarbohydrate calories. In the case of disaccharidases, the adaptive response occurs within a 2- to 5-day period (the time required for intestinal cell renewal), suggesting an action on the undifferentiated crypt cells. In experimental animals, lactase activity adapts in a period of 8 to 10 weeks, but short-term experiments in humans have failed to show lactase adaptation.

The full implication of this phenomenon is not yet apparent, but it is obvious that dietary habits must be taken into considerations when abnor-

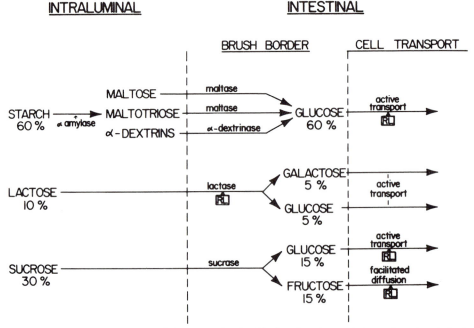

Figure 28–9 Schematic representation of the events involved in the digestion and absorption of carbohydrates. RL is the rate-limiting step in the particuar reaction. (From Gray, G. M.: Gastroenterology *58*:96, 1970.)

malities of epithelial enzyme activity are present.

Protein Absorption. The usual dietary intake of 70 to 90 gm of protein presents the digestive-absorptive mechanism with a more complex task than that presented by fat or carbohydrate. A much larger group of enzymes is required to reduce native proteins to their amino acid components. This process is initiated in the gastrointestinal lumen by pepsin, which is dispensable for adequate protein assimilation, and the numerous pancreatic proteases, including trypsinogen, chymotrypsinogen, procarboxypeptidase A, procarboxypeptidase B, leucine aminopeptidase, proelastase, and nucleases. They are released largely in response to vagal influences and the action of cholecystokinin-pancreozymin. These mechanisms are described more fully in Chapter 32 and in the portion of this section in which the endocrine function of the small intestine is discussed. The inactive trypsinogen is converted to active trypsin by enterokinase, and the trypsin then acts to complete the conversion of the other proenzymes to their active forms. Trypsin and chymotrypsin are endopeptidases that split the peptide bonds within the protein molecule, whereas the carboxypeptidases are exopeptidases that act only on the terminal peptide bonds. These various enzymes differ in both topographic activity and amino acid specificity, and, because of their restricted sites of action, protein digestion occurs only by virtue of their sequential activity.

A large proportion of the pancreatic proteases are adsorbed onto the epithelial cell surface, and whether their activity is exerted mainly within the lumen or in the region of the microvilli is uncertain. In either case, peptides that are 3 to 6 amino acid residues long are released and presented to the brush border and intracellular enzyme systems, where three groups of peptidases complete the process of amino acid liberation. The amino-oligopeptidases have been partially localized to the brush border and hydrolyze the longer peptides, probably to amino acids, dipeptides, and tripeptides. The aminotripeptidases, also partially localized to the brush border, split the N-terminal residues from tripeptides. Lastly, there are several dipeptidases, including glycylglycine peptidase, leucylglycine peptidase, glycylleucine peptidase and imino- and imidopeptidases that hydrolyze proline-containing peptides. Their location is not known.

From studies comparing normal and cystinuric patients, it is clear that both free amino acids and dipeptides can enter the epithelial cell and that significant dipeptidase activity probably takes place within the cytoplasm. Only certain amino acids are in fact readily released within the lumen in free form. Appreciable amounts of the basic amino acids (arginine and lysine) and neutral amino acids (valine, phenylalanine, tyrosine, methionine, and leucine) are released and transported by the epithelial cell membrane. In contrast, gly-

cine, the imino acids (proline and hydroxyproline), the hydroxyl-substituted amino acids (serine and threonine), and the dicarboxylic amino acids (aspartic and glutamic) remain about 90 per cent peptide-linked until their disappearance from the lumen, and they presumably enter the cell as constituents of small peptides. It is clear that glycine is more rapidly and efficiently absorbed as the di- and tripeptide than as the free amino acid. The physiologic importance of oligopeptide absorption, however, remains unclear. Most peptides are hydrolyzed by several electrophoretically distinct enzymes and, conversely, each enzyme hydrolyzes several different peptides. The specificity and localization of the many intestinal peptidases are still uncertain, and their role in protein digestion is obviously more complex than that of the brush border disaccharidase system.

The manner in which peptides cross the plasma membrane is unknown. It has been proposed that amino acids are transported via a carrier-mediated process that, like hexose absorption, is stimulated by Na^+. Amino acid influx is not tightly coupled to Na^+ influx, however, and in the absence of Na^+, amino acid transport still exhibits saturation kinetics and competitive inhibition. Sodium does not affect the maximum velocity of amino acid influx but does increase the apparent affinity of the carrier system. Hereditary defects of amino acid transport have provided evidence for several different transport systems, each having different affinities for different groups of amino acids. These are presented in Table 28–1.

Somewhat analogous to carbohydrate digestion, it is apparent that the absorption rates of essential amino acids at least can be influenced by dietary, caloric, or protein deprivation in humans. Adibi and Allen subjected patients to a 14-day period of either protein or protein-calorie deprivation and found a decreased rate of jejunal amino acid transport with a corresponding increase in fecal nitrogen, which could not be correlated with any light or electron microscopic changes. This sort of observation again emphasizes the potential modifications in intestinal absorptive function that may follow dietary manipulation.

Folic Acid and Cobalamin (Vitamin B$_{12}$) Absorption. Folic acid is 2-amino,4-hydroxypteridine joined to a *p*-aminobenzoic acid residue and linked to one molecule of L-glutamic acid. Naturally occurring folates contain additional L-glutamic acid molecules linked by the unusual γ-peptide bond, with pteroylheptaglutamic acid being the principal species in most plant and animal tissues. This conjugated form is converted in the small intestine to the free monoglutamate by γ-glutamyl carboxypeptidase ("conjugase"), an enzyme associated with the mucosal cell but of which the precise site of action is unknown. Absorption of pteroylmonoglutamic acid occurs largely in the proximal small intestine, but its transport mechanism has not been defined. Within the intestinal cell, the mon-

TABLE 28–1 INTESTINAL AMINO ACID TRANSPORT MECHANISMS

Type	Amino Acids Transported	Type of Transport	Rate
Neutral (monoamino-monocarboxylic)	Aromatic (tyrosine, tryptophan, phenylalanine) Aliphatic (glycine,* alanine, serine, threonine, valine, leucine, isoleucine) Methionine, histidine, glutamine, asparagine, cysteine	Active, Na$^+$-dependent	Very rapid
Dibasic (diamino)	Lysine, arginine, ornithine, cystine	Active, partially Na$^+$-dependent	Rapid (10% of neutral)
Dicarboxylic (acidic)	Glutamic acid, aspartic acid	Carrier-mediated, ?active, partially Na$^+$-dependent	Rapid
Imino acids and glycine	Proline, hydroxyproline, glycine*	Active, ?Na$^+$-dependent	Slow

*Shares both the neutral and imino mechanism with low affinity for the neutral.
(From Gray, G. M., and Cooper, H. L.: Protein digestion and absorption. Gastroenterology *61*:535, 1971.)

oglutamate is converted by dihydrofolate reductase and a methylating mechanism to reduced methyl folate (largely 5-methyltetrahydrofolate) prior to entry into the portal circulation. Tetrahydrofolic acid functions as a cofactor in various important enzyme systems.

Vitamin B$_{12}$ (cobalamin) is not present in plants, and that found in animal sources is tightly bound to proteins. It is released in the stomach by the action of hydrochloric acid and pepsin, making it available for binding by two proteins in gastric juice, intrinsic factor and R protein. The former is secreted by the parietal cells in response to the same stimuli causing hydrochloric acid secretion. The source of R protein is not known. R protein demonstrates a much greater affinity for cobalamin than intrinsic factor does and has a pH range of 2 to 8. Thus, cobalamin entering the small intestine is bound exclusively to R protein. Pancreatic proteases do not alter intrinsic factor but do degrade R protein, decreasing its affinity for cobalamin with the result that the latter is transferred to intrinsic factor. Cobalamin is also secreted into the bile bound to R protein; therefore, the absorption of dietary cobalamin and the reabsorption of biliary cobalamin both depend on pancreatic proteases.

The free vitamin can be absorbed by passive diffusion throughout the small intestine, but only 1 per cent is handled in this way. The absorption of physiologic amounts (>2 mg) is intrinsic factor–mediated and takes place only in the terminal ileum, where 60 to 80 per cent is absorbed. The cobalamin intrinsic factor complex attaches to receptors located in the glycocalyx-plasma membrane complex of the terminal ileal absorptive cells. This attachment requires the presence of Ca^{++} or Mg^{++} or both and a pH above 5.6. Cobalamin is released from intrinsic factor in or on the ileal absorptive cell and is transported to the portal blood bound to a carrier, transcobalamin II. The optimal absorption of cobalamin therefore depends on adequate intake, acid-peptic activity in the stomach, the availability of intrinsic factor, pancreatic proteases, and an intact ileal absorptive mechanism.

The absorption of other water-soluble vitamins has been little studied, and the manner in which ascorbic acid, riboflavin, and other members of the B group are handled by the small intestine is largely unknown. Absorption of the fat-soluble vitamins A, D, E, and K in general parallels that of lipid absorption. Vitamin A deserves special comment here, since its absorption has been utilized as a form of lipid tolerance test. It is ingested largely in an esterified form that requires hydrolysis by pancreatic and brush border enzymes prior to micellar solubilization. After entering the epithelial cell it is re-esterified with long-chain fatty acids and transported via the lymph in association with the chylomicrons. It has recently been appreciated, however, that significant absorption occurs by way of the portal vein. Consequently, vitamin A transport is a more general index of absorption and is not strictly equatable with lipid tolerance. The absorption of the other fat-soluble vitamins as well as that of iron and calcium is discussed in those sections dealing with their overall metabolism and pathophysiology.

The digestive-absorptive process therefore involves not only the handling of a wide range of ingested materials but numerous enzymes and hormones, each requiring its own optimal environment, as well as highly specialized cellular structure-function relationships. Although such physiologic complexity quite naturally predisposes to pathophysiologic diversity, it is in most instances possible to understand the different malabsorption syndromes in terms of one or more alterations in this overall process.

ABNORMALITIES OF DIGESTION AND ABSORPTION

Many disease processes directly or indirectly alter gastrointestinal physiology in such a manner that normal absorptive mechanisms are compromised and maldigestion or malabsorption of one or more dietary constituents occurs. There may be malabsorption of fat alone or of protein and carbohydrate as well. A defect may be so severe and widespread that it precludes the normal absorption of any ingested nutrient or so circumscribed that only single substances are affected. Furthermore, some disorders cause malabsorption by more than one pathophysiologic mechanism.

A large number of tests have been utilized in the differential diagnosis of malabsorption syndromes. However, many are of little value despite their continued use. The physician who has a sound understanding of the normal mechanisms of digestion and absorption as well as the tests useful in their investigation will be able to arrive at a correct diagnosis in the vast majority of cases by correlating clinical information with the following diagnostic procedures: the quantitative determination of stool fat, the quantitative determination of stool nitrogen, the xylose absorption test, the lactose tolerance test, the vitamin B_{12} absorption test, and peroral intestinal biopsy. Hemoglobin concentrations and red cell morphology as well as serum levels of albumin, cholesterol, carotene, prothrombin activity, iron, calcium, phosphorus, and alkaline phosphatase are *nutritional indices* and not tests of absorption. Abnormalities may reflect not only malabsorption but also inadequate intake and increased utilization or loss by other routes.

The quantitative chemical determination of fecal fat is the most reliable measure of steatorrhea. The amount of fat appearing in the stool of normal individuals usually accounts for less than 7 per cent of the dietary intake. With the usual intake of 60 to 100 gm, this will result in the excretion of less than 6 gm per 24 hours. Even with intakes as high as 200 gm, only 8.7 plus or minus 0.7 gm will appear in the stool. With zero fat intake, approximately 3 gm will still be present, presumably from sloughed epithelial cells and bacterial lipids. In the patient with compromised digestive or absorptive capacity, the amount of fat excreted in the stool is more directly related to the amount ingested. The van de Kamer method is most commonly employed for quantitating fecal fat, but this procedure must be modified for the patient receiving medium-chain triglycerides, since medium-chain fatty acids will otherwise be underestimated.

The normal fecal nitrogen excretion is in the range of 2.0 to 2.5 gm in persons with intakes between 80 and 100 gm. Desquamation of epithelial cells, secretory proteins, and leakage of plasma proteins contribute to the intraluminal nitrogen pool, and, provided that significant protein-losing enteropathy is not present, fecal nitrogen determinations are a useful measure of protein malabsorption.

Xylose, a 5-carbon monosaccharide, is absorbed primarily by passive means in the proximal small intestine. The amount excreted in the urine during the first 5 hours following an oral dose of 25 gm should be greater than 4.5 gm. Artifactually low values may be due to vomiting, delayed gastric emptying, dehydration, impaired renal function, or the presence of massive ascites. The mean normal excretory rate also decreases with advancing age and probably reflects declining renal function. Values less than 2.5 to 3.0 gm are encountered in disease states in which there is significant loss of the functional integrity of the jejunum or massive bacterial overgrowth in the proximal small intestine, resulting in bacterial utilization. The administration of antibiotics may correct abnormal values due to the latter condition.

The serum cobalamin level is currently the most important test in establishing the diagnosis of cobalamin *deficiency*. The Schilling test, on the other hand, assesses the ability of the individual to *absorb* cobalamin and with certain modifications may aid in determining the cause of malabsorption. This test involves the ingestion of a physiologic amount (0.1 to 2.0 micrograms) of radioactive crystalline cobalamin and the administration of a large (1000 micrograms) amount of nonradioactive cobalamin. The latter saturates all of the plasma cobalamin-binding protein and results in the urinary excretion of most of the absorbed radioactive cobalamin. A low value indicates cobalamin malabsorption. Provided the patient has or has been given an adequate amount of intrinsic factor, low excretory rates are found in three situations: 1) in the presence of bacterial overgrowth or parasitic infection; 2) disease states or surgical procedures that lead to loss of the functional integrity of the terminal ileum; and 3) pancreatic exocrine insufficiency. Correction of cobalamin malabsorption by the administration of intrinsic factor, trypsin, or antibiotics will aid in the differentiation of gastric mucosal atrophy with or without pernicious anemia, pancreatic insufficiency, or a bacterial overgrowth syndrome.

Peroral intestinal biopsy has considerably facilitated the diagnosis of certain malabsorption syndromes. Knowledge of normal histology at various levels of the intestine as well as variations encountered in different populations is a definite requisite for making comparisons with diseased tissues. In at least five specific disorders, the histologic findings are sufficiently unique to be diagnostic: nontropical sprue, Whipple's disease, abetalipoproteinemia, amyloidosis, and mastocytosis. In radiation enteritis, lymphangiectasia, tropical sprue, nongranulomatous ulcerative jejunitis, scleroderma, eosinophilic gastroenteritis, dermatitis herpetiformis, hypogammaglobulinemia, and some

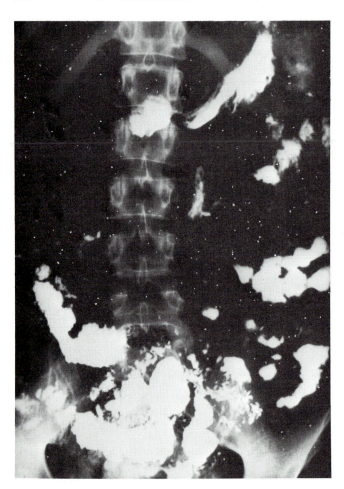

Figure 28–10 Barium meal demonstrating a typical malabsorption pattern consisting of segmentation, localized dilatation, and moulage formation.

parasitic infestations the changes are usually compatible with but not diagnostic of the particular disorder. In most other conditions leading to maldigestion and malabsorption small intestinal histology is normal, at least to light microscopy.

The signs and symptoms exhibited by the patient with a malabsorption syndrome quite naturally will vary with the disease responsible. The manifestations of the malabsorption itself will depend on the nature and amount of the substances involved and the duration of the process. Weight loss, muscle wasting, anemia, tetany, edema, bleeding tendencies, osteomalacia, osteoporosis, fatigue, abdominal distention, multiple vitamin deficiencies, steatorrhea, and diarrhea are commonly observed in various combinations. Classically, with steatorrhea the stools are described as voluminous or bulky, foul smelling, greasy, frothy, pale yellow, and floating. Unfortunately, not all such descriptions by the patient will be associated with an increase in fecal fat, and significant steatorrhea may exist in the absence of any of these characteristics. True diarrhea may be produced by disorders causing a decrease in transit time, the malabsorption of water and electrolytes,

the malabsorption of bile salts, or the cathartic action of hydroxylated fatty acids. Hypocalcemia and hypophosphatemia result from the formation of insoluble calcium soaps with unabsorbed fatty acids, vitamin D deficiency, and loss of calcium-binding protein normally located in the glycocalyx.

It is also now well established that patients with steatorrhea have an increased risk of nephrolithiasis as the result of hyperoxaluria. Unabsorbed fatty acids bind to dietary calcium, preventing the formation of insoluble calcium oxalate, which occurs normally in the absence of fat malabsorption. Thus, dietary oxalate remains in solution and available for absorption. Oxalate absorption takes place primarily from the colon, and both unabsorbed fatty acids and bile acids increase the permeability of the colon to oxalate. Treatment involves some combination of a low-oxalate diet, restriction of fat intake and substitution of medium-chain triglycerides, which do not bind calcium or alter colonic permeability, and administration of calcium salts. Cholestyramine can be used to bind bile acids but usually aggravates the steatorrhea.

Radiographic examination of the small intestine with a barium meal may be helpful in disclosing a "malabsorption pattern" but is rarely capable of providing an etiologic diagnosis. The characteristic features are illustrated in Figure 28–10 and include localized dilatations, segmentation of the barium column, loss of mucosal detail (moulage), flocculation of the barium due to the presence of increased amounts of water and mucus in the intestinal lumen, and thickening of the valvulae conniventes.

The presence of a malabsorption syndrome therefore must be suspected under a variety of clinical circumstances. An understanding of the pathophysiologic mechanisms that may be responsible is essential to the proper interpretation of clinical signs and symptoms as well as abnormalities reported by the clinical laboratory. A classification of malabsorption syndromes based on the type of defect responsible is presented in Table 28–2. The normal digestive-absorptive process may be disrupted by abnormalities occurring within the intestinal lumen, at the level of the mucosa (involving the absorptive cells or the lamina propria) or the intestinal lymphatics.

Intraluminal Abnormalities. The intraluminal phase of the digestive-absorptive process is concerned with the digestion of fats, carbohydrates, and proteins, and the micellar solubilization of free fatty acids and beta-monoglycerides. Maldigestion will result from any disorder interfering with *effective* pancreatic enzyme activity. This may be due to abnormalities of pancreatic exocrine function secondary to chronic pancreatitis, carcinoma of the pancreas, mucoviscidosis, or pancreatic resection, which reduce the absolute amount of enzyme available, or to acid hypersecretion and gastric resection, which result in ineffective activity of otherwise adequate amounts of enzyme.

Several factors appear to play a role in the malabsorption associated with the acid hypersecretion of the Zollinger-Ellison syndrome. The low intraluminal pH denatures or inactivates pancreatic enzymes, especially lipase, and conjugated bile salts may be precipitated from solution. It is also possible that the absorptive capacity of the mucosal cells may be impaired by acid injury. Pancreatic exocrine insufficiency results in severe steatorrhea and nitrogen loss, but xylose absorption and jejunal histology are normal. Mild, variable decreases in vitamin B_{12} absorption may occur. The cause is unknown. Since micelles are present in most instances, the absorption of fat-soluble vitamins is less affected. Patients with the Zollinger-Ellison syndrome exhibit moderate increases in fecal fat and slight impairment of xylose absorption. B_{12} absorption and jejunal histologic findings are normal. No values for fecal nitrogen have been reported.

Following gastric resection, particularly with a Billroth II anastomosis, malabsorption may involve interference with absorptive processes at

TABLE 28–2 A PATHOPHYSIOLOGIC CLASSIFICATION OF DISORDERS ASSOCIATED WITH MALABSORPTION

Abnormalities of intraluminal events
    Inadequate digestion
        Pancreatic insufficiency
        Acid hypersecretion
        Gastric resection
    Altered bile salt metabolism
        Intraluminal binding of bile salts
        Hepatobiliary disease
        Ileal resection or disease
        Bacterial overgrowth
Abnormalities of mucosal transport
    Generalized defects
        Nontropical sprue (celiac disease, gluten
          enteropathy)
        Tropical sprue
        Crohn's disease
        Intestinal resection or bypass
        Nongranulomatous ulcerative jejunitis
        Radiation enteritis
        Whipple's disease
        Drug-induced malabsorption
        Hypothyroidism
        Addison's disease
        Hyperthyroidism
        Hypoparathyroidism
        Parasitic disease
        Mast cell disease
        Dermatitis herpetiformis
        Intestinal ischemia
        Intestinal lymphoma
        Protein malnutrition
        Amyloidosis
    Selective defects
        Abetalipoproteinemia
        Disaccharidase deficiency
        Monosaccharide malabsorption
        Amino acid malabsorption
        Vitamin B_{12} malabsorption
Abnormalities of lymphatic transport
        Primary intestinal lymphangiectasia
        Whipple's disease
        Crohn's disease
        Radiation enteritis
        Intestinal lymphoma
        Constrictive pericarditis
        Congestive heart failure
Unclassified abnormalities
        Carcinoid syndrome
        Dysgammaglobulinemias
        Diabetic gastroenteropathy
        Scleroderma

several steps. Duodenal bypass leads to a poor secretory response of the pancreas and inadequate mixing of food with bile salts and pancreatic enzymes. Rapid intestinal transit also may occur, with a reduction of contact time between the intestinal contents and the mucosal absorptive cells. The reasons for the abnormal transit time are essentially unknown. An additional factor in certain patients is massive bacterial overgrowth in the afferent loop, giving rise to an intestinal stasis syndrome (see further on). Steatorrhea is generally mild, and nitrogen excretion and xylose absorption are usually normal, although the latter may be reduced in the presence of a stasis syndrome. Jejunal biopsy usually is normal but occasionally reveals mild villous atrophy of doubtful functional significance. Vitamin B_{12} absorption may be reduced for three possible reasons: (1) inadequate intrinsic factor secretion by the gastric remnant; (2) rapid passage of B_{12} through the gastric remnant, preventing the formation of the B_{12}-intrinsic factor complex; or (3) the presence of an afferent loop stasis syndrome. Correction of an abnormal Schilling test with exogenous intrinsic factor or antibiotics will help in determining the precise cause. Although many inconsistencies are encountered, malabsorption tends to occur with a decreasing order of severity subsequent to the following surgical procedures: total gastrectomy with esophagojejunostomy, subtotal gastrectomy with gastrojejunostomy, subtotal gastrectomy with gastroduodenostomy, and vagotomy and pyloroplasty.

Altered bile salt metabolism with failure to achieve adequate micellar solubilization may result from one or more different mechanisms. Intraluminal binding of bile salts occurs with the administration of cholestyramine, a nonabsorbable anion exchange resin used in the management of intractable pruritus due to increased tissue levels of bile salts. In general, steatorrhea is present only in patients receiving in excess of 12 gm per day and fecal fat losses are relatively mild. Portal-systemic shunts that lower the extraction of bile salts from portal venous blood, hepatocellular disease that reduces bile acid synthesis, and intra- or extrahepatic cholestasis with or without jaundice that limits biliary excretion all may contribute to a micellar defect. The result is an isolated, mild steatorrhea. The steatorrhea is not more severe because the two most important steps in fat absorption remain intact: lipolysis and epithelial cell uptake. Furthermore, the ileum, which does not normally participate significantly in fat absorption, in part compensates for decreased jejunal uptake. In patients with an external biliary fistula, for example, fat absorption is little impaired on a low-fat diet, and as much as 75 per cent of an intake of 120 gm may be absorbed. With increasing intake, however, there is increasing steatorrhea. More severe disturbances in the absorption of the fat-soluble vitamins occur, since they are not detectably absorbed in the absence of micelles.

Blind loop or intestinal stasis syndromes may be due to a variety of anatomic or motor disturbances of the intestine, including afferent loops following gastric resection, enteroenterostomy or internal fistulas with bypass of a segment of small bowel, multiple strictures, jejunal diverticulosis, scleroderma, diabetic enteropathy, and gastrocolic fistula. The common denominator consists of stasis and bacterial colonization of the small intestine with a more fecal type of flora. Bacterial counts in luminal fluid from the duodenum, jejunum, and proximal ileum normally are low, in the range of less than 10^4 per ml and consist primarily of streptococci, aerobic lactobacilli, and diphtheroids as well as fungi. The distal ileum represents a transitional zone, with bacterial counts between 10^5 and 10^8 per ml. In two thirds of cases there are appreciable numbers of gram-negative organisms, largely aerobic coliforms with very few anaerobic bacteria, such as bacteroides. The two most important factors controlling the "relative sterility" of the proximal small intestine are gastric acid secretion and the cleansing action of propulsive motor activity. It is also probably important that bacterial generation times are much longer in the intestinal lumen than under in-vitro conditions. An alteration in these protective mechanisms may permit the establishment of a colonic type of flora containing large numbers of bacteroides, coliforms, and clostridia. This bacterial overgrowth has several important metabolic effects. First, and most important, there is deconjugation and dehydroxylation of bile salts resulting in decreased micelle formation. Second, the bacteria are capable of binding the B_{12}-intrinsic factor complex, preventing its absorption, and of metabolizing xylose. The characteristic findings in patients with an intestinal stasis syndrome therefore include mild steatorrhea and abnormal B_{12} absorption. Fecal nitrogen values and jejunal histologic findings usually are normal, while xylose absorption may be normal or decreased. The abnormal values for fecal fat and the diminished B_{12} and xylose absorption most often return to normal after several days of antibiotic therapy.

The bacterial catabolism of D-xylose and the deconjugation of bile salts form the basis of several breath tests designed to demonstrate small intestinal bacterial overgrowth. An increased breath $^{14}CO_2$ after the administration of either D-[^{14}C]xylose or cholyl[1-^{14}C]glycine occurs in the presence of bacterial colonization of the small bowel. One limitation has been the inability to distinguish this situation clearly from that in which these substrates are malabsorbed for other reasons with bacterial degradation in the colon. The one-gram D-[^{14}C]xylose test has been reported to obviate this problem, but further experience is necessary.

Bacterial stasis syndromes may result in some additional effects unrelated to malabsorption: (1) increased serum folate levels due to bacterial synthesis and release of folic acid; (2) increased urinary indican excretion from the conversion of tryptophan to indole, which is hydroxylated and sulfated in the liver to indoxysulfate or indican; and (3) increased ammonia production by the deamination of dietary protein to form urea, with subsequent conversion to ammonia by intestinal ureases.

Abnormalities of Mucosal Transport. Most disorders affecting the small intestinal mucosa result in widespread defects characterized by malabsorption of most normally transported materials. Any process causing structural or functional abnormalities of the glycocalyx-plasma membrane digestive-absorptive unit, the remainder of the epithelial cell proper, or the surrounding lamina propria may produce a generalized malabsorption syndrome. Most, if not all, tests of absorption will be abnormal, and the fecal losses of fat and nitrogen are often severe. However, highly specific defects may occur with only single substances exhibiting abnormal transport.

Nontropical sprue (celiac disease, gluten-sensitive enteropathy) provides a good example of generalized primary intestinal malabsorption. Jejunal biopsies of patients with untreated celiac disease almost always show total or near total villous atrophy. In order for this to be apparent, it is important that the sections be properly oriented so that they are cut perpendicular to the luminal surface. The total mucosal thickness is relatively normal, and as a result the crypts appear elongated. The surface epithelial cells exhibit several abnormalities: (1) their vertical height is decreased, and they assume a more cuboidal shape; (2) the simple columnar orientation is replaced by a stratified configuration; (3) cytoplasmic degenerative changes are apparent; (4) the brush border structure is attenuated or even inapparent; (5) there is a relative decrease in goblet cells; and (6) there is infiltration of the epithelial cell layer by lymphocytes. The crypt cells generally appear normal by both light and electron microscopy but there is a relative increase in the number of Paneth and enterochromaffin cells, and the undifferentiated cells at the bases of the crypts exhibit increased mitoses. In fact, Trier and Browning, using tissue cultures of intestinal epithelium from untreated patients, observed an increased proliferation and migration of crypt cells, findings similar to those seen during the recovery phase of sublethal ionizing radiation. The cells also reverted to a more normal appearance after only 24 hours in a gluten-free medium. The lamina propria contains increased numbers of plasma cells and eosinophils, and the interstitial spaces appear to be filled with a lightly staining amorphous material. Morphologic changes are most marked in the duodenum and jejunum and tend to be less prominent in the ileum.

Although the cereal protein gluten (wheat, rye, barley, and oats) is firmly established as the offending agent, the mechanism of its noxious effect remains unknown. Gluten is the starch-free portion of the cereal grain, and the toxic factor is contained in its 70 per cent alcohol-soluble fraction (gliadin). This consists of a complex mixture of several electrophoretically and chromatographically separable proteins of varying molecular weight. Clinical challenge with peptic-tryptic digests suggests that the toxic factor is a polypeptide of molecular weight less than 1000. Efforts to demonstrate abnormal peptidase activity in treated patients, however, have failed. Antibodies to gluten fractions are present in the serum and intestinal secretions of untreated individuals and, to a lesser extent, of treated patients, but their significance is debated. No antibodies in the diseased tissue itself react with gluten fractions, and no complement-fixing immune complexes have been demonstrated. Interestingly enough, however, the celiac jejunal epithelial cells uniquely bind gluten fractions in vitro. Whatever the reason, the basic problem appears to be an inadequately compensated, shortened life span of the villous absorptive cells.

The net result is a decrease in intestinal surface area, a loss of enzymes and carriers, and compromised absorptive cell function. The main physiologic defect is a failure of transport by the epithelial cell. The result is malabsorption of most dietary constituents, including fat, carbohydrate, protein, vitamins, iron, and calcium. The fecal losses of fat and nitrogen tend to be relatively severe, and the absorption of xylose is markedly impaired. Jejunal histology in the untreated case is essentially diagnostic. Vitamin B_{12} absorption may be normal or low, depending on the severity of the ileal abnormality. The anemia that develops is most commonly due to iron deficiency, but macrocytic anemias due to folic acid and less often to B_{12} deficiency are also frequent. With the loss of brush border enzymes, disaccharidase deficiencies occur, of which lactose intolerance is clinically the most prominent. Water and electrolyte transport also are affected, and perfusion of the jejunum with isotonic electrolyte solutions results in a net secretion of water, sodium, and potassium instead of absorption.

Improvement of absorption coincides with the removal of gluten-containing cereals and cereal products from the diet. Cytologic abnormalities begin to disappear within a matter of days, whereas villous architecture reverts toward normal over a period of weeks and months. It is doubtful, however, whether villi ever achieve a totally normal appearance.

Other clinical entities that are characterized by abnormal villous architecture and distorted morphology of intestinal absorptive cells include tropical sprue, dermatitis herpetiformis, and nongranulomatous ulcerative jejunitis. The absorptive defect therefore is qualitatively similar to that of celiac disease.

In contrast, the morphologic changes in Whipple's disease are most striking in the lamina propria, where the normal cellular elements are replaced by macrophages that contain glycoprotein within their cytoplasm, as demonstrated by the periodic acid–Schiff test. In addition, rod-shaped structures can be seen in the lamina propria that under the electron microscope have the features of bacteria. The villous absorptive cells and mucosal surface area, however, are relatively well preserved. Nonetheless, in-vitro studies of tissue biopsy specimens have demonstrated impaired amino acid transport and fatty acid esterification. There is also morphologic evidence suggesting an impaired delivery of triglyceride to the lymphatics. Precisely how the observed structural abnormalities are translated into functional defects is not clear. Characteristically, patients with Whipple's disease exhibit severe malabsorption of fat and protein but very little alteration of xylose or B_{12} absorption.

The malabsorption associated with intestinal resection can be divided into three essentially distinct syndromes: massive resection or bypass, removal of the jejunum, and ileectomy. It is patently obvious why the first of these conditions results in severe malabsorption of fat and protein and of xylose and vitamin B_{12}. However, removal of the jejunum causes only a mild defect in fat absorption, presumably because the ileum can almost totally compensate for its loss. This may simply represent the expression of functions not normally called upon in the presence of an intact jejunum. The jejunum, however, is selectively important for the absorption of iron, calcium, and folic acid, and extensive jejunal resection commonly results in severe deficiencies of these nutrients. Conversely, loss of the ileum leads to a more severe malabsorption of fat and B_{12}. This occurs because disruption of the enterohepatic circulation of bile salts results in ineffective micellar solubilization. Ordinarily, this would produce only a modest steatorrhea, because the ileum would partially compensate for the resulting reduced jejunal absorption. When the ileum is missing or diseased, however, this cannot occur. Furthermore, the coexisting B_{12} deficiency itself appears to affect the maturation of villous absorptive cells, thereby contributing to the absorptive defect. Loss of the ileum is also frequently associated with watery diarrhea, which is due to the cathartic action of the large amount of unabsorbed bile salts entering the colon.

The functional integrity of the terminal ileum can be assessed by the Schilling test and the bile acid breath test. The bile acid breath test involves the measurement of exhaled $^{14}CO_2$ after the ingestion of ^{14}C-labeled bile salts. With loss of ileal function, these conjugated bile salts enter the colon and are metabolized to $^{14}CO_2$ by colonic bacteria. As discussed elsewhere, bacterial overgrowth syndromes will also produce abnormal Schilling and bile acid breath tests.

The frequent failure of nonoperative efforts to manage morbid obesity led to the surgical development of a method of creating generalized malabsorption, accomplished by bypassing all but 45 cm of the small intestine. This technique is known as *jejunoileal bypass*. The pathophysiologic consequences of the procedure are obvious:

1. The exclusion of most of the small bowel results in malabsorption of carbohydrate, protein, lipid, minerals, and vitamins.

2. Bypassing the major site of bile acid reabsorption further reduces fat and fat-soluble vitamin absorption.

3. The huge amounts of fatty acids and bile acids entering the colon cause the secretion of an excessive volume of water and electrolytes, especially sodium and potassium.

Despite these results, most patients plateau 20 to 50 lbs above their ideal weight, probably because of increased dietary intake and adaptation of the unbypassed intestine. Intestinal adaptation is a well-established phenomenon involving increased villous height and greater absorptive capacity.

The complications that result from jejunoileal bypass are listed in Table 28–3. Abnormalities of hepatic function occur in at least 30 per cent of patients. Although steatosis is uniformly present, histologic changes similar to those seen in alcoholic hepatitis develop in 5 per cent of bypass patients, with progression to cirrhosis and death in 1 to 2 per cent. A combination of protein depletion and the influence of toxic products from the bypassed intestine are thought to be responsible. Renal insufficiency may occur for several reasons: obstruction by oxalate stones, parenchymal deposition of oxalate, immune complex nephritis, and so-called "functional renal failure,"

TABLE 28–3 COMPLICATIONS OF JEJUNOILEAL BYPASS

Mineral and electrolyte imbalance
  Decreased serum potassium, magnesium, calcium, and bicarbonate
  Increased serum chloride
  Osteoporosis and osteomalacia secondary to protein depletion, calcium and vitamin D loss, and acidosis
Protein-calorie malnutrition
  Hair loss, anemia, edema, and vitamin depletion
Cholelithiasis
Enteric complications
  Abdominal distention, irregular diarrhea, increased flatus, pneumatosis intestinalis, colonic pseudo-obstruction, bypass enteropathy, volvulus with mechanical small bowel obstruction
Extraintestinal manifestations
  Arthritis
  Liver disease
    Steatosis, "alcoholic" type hepatitis, cirrhosis
  Erythema nodosum, nonspecific pustular dermatosis
  Weber-Christian syndrome
  Renal disease
    Hyperoxaluria with oxalate stones or interstitial oxalate deposits, immune complex nephritis, "functional" renal failure
  Miscellaneous
    Peripheral neuropathy, pericarditis, pleuritis, hemolytic anemia, neutropenia, and thrombocytopenia

similar to the hepatorenal syndrome. Bypass enteropathy is characterized by abdominal bloating, cramping, air-fluid levels on abdominal radiographs, an inflammatory response in the bypassed bowel (sometimes with ulceration), and frequently fever. Severe liver disease, non–oxalate-related renal failure, and bypass enteropathy all appear to be related to anaerobic bacterial overgrowth in the defunctionalized intestine. Although antimicrobial therapy with agents such as metronidazole has been successful in some cases, definitive treatment usually involves taking down the bypass.

The rationale for this approach to the treatment of morbid obesity cannot be questioned. The pathophysiologic consequences, however, have combined to discourage its further use. Still, morbidly obese patients continue to present themselves to physicians for surgical management of complications.

Adaptive changes in the remaining intestine leading to increased absorption are well documented in experimental animals but have been little studied in humans. It has been shown in humans that a gradual improvement in fat, carbohydrate, and nitrogen absorption occurs after extensive small bowel resection, and intestinal biopsies have revealed an increase in the number of epithelial cells per unit length of the villus, suggesting mucosal cell hyperplasia.

A number of drugs have been implicated in the production of mucosal transport defects primarily involving fat. Cholestyramine has been discussed in relation to its effect on micelle formation. Colchicine produces a diffuse alteration of absorptive function, manifested by slightly increased fecal losses of fat and nitrogen and decreased xylose absorption. It probably exerts this effect by disturbing epithelial cell function and inhibiting cell renewal. A variety of cathartic agents may also cause slight steatorrhea, hypokalemia, and protein-losing enteropathy, but no satisfactory explanation of their effect has been proposed. Neomycin, the most widely studied of the drugs producing malabsorption, has been shown to produce morphologic changes in intestinal villi, to inhibit the intraluminal hydrolysis of triglycerides, and to precipitate bile salts. Neomycin is a polybasic aminoglucoside, and it has been suggested that an interaction between its cationic amino groups and the anionic fatty acids and bile acids leads to precipitation of the whole micellar complex. Triparanol produces an intestinal lesion indistinguishable from celiac disease and results in mild fat and nitrogen losses. High doses of para-aminosalicylic acid also have induced a reversible defect in fat and xylose absorption.

The remainder of the mucosal transport defects listed in Table 28–2 lead to malabsorption by even less well understood mechanisms. Some disorders such as amyloidosis, radiation enteritis, parasitic infection, and mast cell disease are associated with morphologic abnormalities, whereas the various endocrinopathies appear to represent mucosal cell dysfunction induced by metabolic influences.

In contrast to these generalized absorptive defects, a few conditions represent defective transport of a single substance. Except for abetalipoproteinemia, they are not characterized by any morphologic abnormalities, and only lactase deficiency and pernicious anemia occur with any frequency.

Abetalipoproteinemia is a rare disorder involving partial or total absence of plasma betalipoprotein. It is probably inherited as an autosomal recessive trait, and total deficiency is associated with lipid malabsorption, acanthocytosis, peripheral neuropathy, and retinal lesions. The defect in lipid absorption and the absence of beta-lipoproteins appear to be due to an inability of the epithelial cell to synthesize the protein moiety of chylomicrons. Jejunal biopsies reveal a normal villous architecture, but in the fasting state numerous cytoplasmic fat droplets are found in the absorptive cells. Mild steatorrhea is the only absorptive abnormality observed.

Isolated cobalamin deficiency may occur for several reasons. Strict vegans who ingest neither animal products nor multivitamins may become deficient on a dietary basis. Achlorhydria and the loss of pepsin secretion secondary to aging or partial gastrectomy lead to an inability to liberate cobalamin from its protein-bound form. However, sufficient intrinsic factor usually remains for the reabsorption of biliary R-protein–bound cobalamin, which is independent of acid-peptic activity, and vitamin deficiency may either never occur or supervene only after a period of 15 years. A complete lack of intrinsic factor is found in patients who have undergone total gastrectomy or who have developed pernicious anemia involving an idiopathic and complete atrophy of the gastric mucosa. These individuals malabsorb both dietary and biliary cobalamin. As would be expected, cobalamin malabsorption occurs in the presence of severe pancreatic exocrine insufficiency but rarely leads to clinically evident insufficiency. Bacterial overgrowth syndromes or infestation with parasites such as fish tapeworm or Giardia lamblia may also result in cobalamin malabsorption, but the mechanism remains unknown. Finally, any process interfering with ileal absorption will result in malabsorption of cobalamin. This may be due to resection, ileal disease, marked acid hypersecretion, or congenital defects involving absence of ileal receptors for the intrinsic factor–cobalamin complex.

Abnormalities of hexose transport may also involve a single substance. Congenital glucose-galactose malabsorption presents in infancy as intractable diarrhea until these monosaccharides or their disaccharide precursors are excluded from the diet. In some, there is an associated glycosuria, suggesting a coexisting renal tubule transport defect. It seems likely that the specific carrier involved in glucose-galactose transport is lacking or defective, since sodium flux and other sodium-dependent processes such as amino acid absorption are normal.

Spontaneously occurring defects of amino acid transport have contributed important information to our understanding of the different types of carrier systems involved in normal amino acid transport. They have also emphasized the great similarity between intestinal and renal tubule transport systems. Cystinuria, an inherited disorder of basic amino acid transport, is perhaps the best studied of such defects. These patients have defective renal and intestinal transport systems for cystine, arginine, ornithine, and lysine. Three forms have been described, defined by the type of intestinal transport defect: type I, in which there is absent intestinal transport of both cystine and the dibasic amino acids; type II, in which (a) there is absent intestinal transport of both cystine and the dibasic amino acids or (b) only dibasic amino acids are improperly absorbed; and type III, in which there is abnormal transport only by the renal tubule. Patients with Hartnup's disease have defective renal tubule transport systems for neutral amino acids, but only tryptophan malabsorption has thus far been demonstrated in the small intestine. This accounts for the increased urine indican characteristic of such patients. Joseph's syndrome (prolinuria, iminoglycinuria) involves the urinary loss of proline and glycine, with a variable defect present in the intestine; some individuals demonstrate transport defects for both amino acids, some for proline alone, and others have no intestinal transport defect. Patients with Lowe's syndrome (oculocerebrorenal syndrome) have a renal tubule defect involving neutral and dibasic amino acids, but apparently only dibasic amino acids are handled abnormally by the intestine.

Isolated deficiencies of the various disaccharidases have also been described, lactase deficiency being the most frequent and best understood. Its prevalence remains disputed, but it may appear as a congenital or presumably acquired abnormality affecting Negroes, Orientals, and Cypriot Greeks somewhat more frequently than Caucasians. Its more frequent occurrence in patients with ulcerative colitis, Crohn's disease (uninvolved intestine), and even viral hepatitis has been alleged by some and denied by others. A previously asymptomatic lactase deficiency may become manifest when combined with other gastrointestinal disease, however, because of (1) an increased lactose load contained in a diet prescribed for patients with ulcers, (2) an increased rate of gastric emptying following gastric resection, or (3) the concurrent development of intestinal disease. Several criteria have been proposed for diagnosis of lactase deficiency: (1) diarrhea, cramping abdominal pain, and flatulence upon ingesting lactose; (2) absent or diminished lactase activity in mucosal biopsy specimens; (3) a flat lactose tolerance curve after the oral administration of 50 gm of lactose, with normal tolerance curves for glucose and galactose; (4) a fall in the stool pH after ingestion of lactose due to the conversion of the unabsorbed lactose to lactic acid by the colonic bacteria; and (5) disappearance of symptoms upon the removal of lactose from the diet. Two kinds of breath tests have also been developed. When trace quantities of ^{14}C-labeled lactose are administered with 50 gm of unlabeled lactose, normal subjects excrete about 25 per cent of the labeled CO_2 in their breath in 4 hours, whereas lactase-deficient individuals excrete 10 per cent or less. Measurement of breath hydrogen after ingestion of a lactose load has also been utilized. In lactase-deficient patients, there is an increase in breath hydrogen when unabsorbed lactose reaches the colon and is metabolized by the bacterial flora. Measurement of either labeled CO_2 or hydrogen in the breath provides more accurate information than does measurement of blood glucose with the standard lactose tolerance test. The severity of the defect varies widely, and since there is a gradient of lactase activity in the small bowel with peak levels in the jejunum and proximal ileum, it is not possible to measure total intestinal lactase activity with biopsy specimens, and this information therefore may be misleading. Spuriously flat lactose tolerance curves may occur in the presence of delayed gastric emptying or a rapid rise and fall of the blood glucose during the first 30 minutes of the test. Direct instillation of lactose into the duodenum will resolve the first problem, and the measurement of capillary rather than venous blood glucose will obviate the latter.

Abnormalities of Lymphatic Transport. Any condition interfering with the normal flow of lymph from the lacteal through the abdominal lymphatic systems to the thoracic duct and thence to the general circulation may result in increased losses of lymph constituents, namely, plasma proteins, chylomicron fat, and small lymphocytes. From a pathophysiologic point of view, such conditions are not, strictly speaking, absorptive defects as much as they are disorders of lymph flow. However, fat does tend to accumulate in the villous absorptive cells, in the intercellular spaces between absorptive cells, in the extracellular space of the lamina propria, and in the endothelial cells of the lacteals; from the standpoint of lipid absorption, these conditions can be considered exit blocks.

Disorders of lymphatic transport may be congenital, as in the case of primary intestinal lymphangiectasia, or acquired secondary either to structural abnormalities that occur as part of other primary intestinal disease or to an increase in lymphatic pressure due to increases in central venous pressure. Because of the associated loss of plasma proteins, lymphatic abnormalities also represent one type of protein-losing gastroenteropathy. Pure lymphatic abnormalities result in mild steatorrhea, modest elevations of fecal nitrogen, hypoalbuminemia, hypogammaglobulinemia, and, not infrequently, lymphocytopenia. Circulating immunoglobulins may therefore be low, and cellular immune responses may be impaired. Clinical manifestations related to the lymphatic abnormality may include diarrhea, edema, and sometimes repeated infections and cutaneous anergy, including the ability to accept homografts. The edema in patients with primary intestinal lymphangiectasia may be asymmetric because there is often an asymmetric hypoplasia of peripheral lymphatics as well. Small intestinal radiographs show thickening of the mucosal folds and sometimes features that suggest a mild malabsorption pattern. Lymphangiography will demonstrate the structural lymphatic defect and occasionally puddling of the dye in the intestinal lumen. Mucosal biopsy reveals the dilated mucosal lymphatics but cannot provide an etiologic diagnosis. Ideally, therapy should be directed toward relief of the responsible lymphatic obstruction; however, this may be possible in only a few situations, such as constrictive pericarditis or congestive heart failure. In the other conditions, especially primary intestinal lymphangiectasia, a reduction in lymph flow and pressure can be achieved by reducing the dietary intake of long-chain triglycerides and replacing them with medium-chain triglycerides, which are absorbed by the portal vein.

It is evident that management of a patient with a malabsorption syndrome must proceed from a definition of the mechanism or mechanisms involved whenever possible. In many instances, treatment of the responsible disease process, such as nontropical sprue or Whipple's disease, will restore adequate absorption. When specific therapy is not possible, alternative measures must be employed. In some cases, simply providing more nutrients may suffice, unless increasingly severe diarrhea develops as steatorrhea becomes more extreme. Simple bile acid deficiency probably is best treated with a low-fat diet for this reason. Bile acid replacement is not practical; the amount required (4 to 8 gm per meal) leads to diarrhea, since dihydroxy bile acids are potent cathartics. When indicated, pancreatic enzyme replacement is helpful but inefficient owing to inactivation by gastric acid. In both situations, medium-chain triglycerides may be useful. They are more rapidly and efficiently hydrolyzed by lipase, and the principal resulting fatty acid, octanoic acid, is fully water soluble. It is absorbed via the portal circulation and does not form chylomicrons. When bacterial overgrowth is present, long-term continuous or intermittent therapy with antibiotics may be beneficial. Total parenteral nutrition is also an important adjunct in many patients, providing nutritional support while more definitive and lasting treatment is being developed. Finally, some patients, especially those with extensive intestinal resection, may require permanent home parenteral nutrition.

Protein-Losing Gastroenteropathies. Although not strictly disorders of absorption, other aspects of the protein-losing gastroenteropathies merit discussion at this point, since they do represent states of increased intestinal nitrogen loss. A classification of the major protein-losing states is presented in Table 28–4. Over 40 disorders have been associated with abnormal protein loss, many representing only single case reports, and the reader is referred to the review by Waldmann for a more complete listing of these conditions. Generally, protein-losing states fall into one of the following categories: (1) benign or malignant tumors, largely of the stomach or colon; (2) any condition associated with gastrointestinal inflammation with loss of epithelial cell integrity; (3) primary or secondary structural abnormalities of lymphatic channels from the lacteal to the terminal of the thoracic duct; and (4) a sustained and significant increase in central venous pressure, which is then transmitted to the thoracic duct. Fecal nitrogen is often mildly elevated but is not diagnostically helpful because of the digestion and absorption of variable amounts of the protein lost and the inability to distinguish between increased loss and malabsorption. Therefore, techniques using radiolabeled macromolecules are employed in an attempt to document and quantitate gastrointestinal protein loss.

An ideal substance should fulfill the following requirements: (1) The labeled substance should have a normal metabolic behavior; (2) there should be no excretion of the label into the gastrointestinal tract unless it is bound to protein; and (3) there should be no absorption of the label from the gastrointestinal tract after its catabolism. None of the readily available substances completely fulfills these requirements.

Using intravenously administered ^{131}I-labeled

TABLE 28–4 CLASSIFICATION OF PROTEIN-LOSING GASTROENTEROPATHIES

Loss of epithelial integrity
    Menetrier's giant hypertrophic gastritis
    Gastric carcinoma
    Carcinoma of the colon
    Nontropical sprue
    Crohn's disease
    Gastrointestinal lymphoma
    Acute gastroenteritis
    Ulcerative colitis
    Gastrointestinal polyposis syndromes
Lymphatic hypertension
    Primary intestinal lymphangiectasia
    Retroperitoneal tumors
    Retroperitoneal fibrosis
    Constrictive pericarditis
    Congestive heart failure
    Whipple's disease
    Crohn's disease
    Gastrointestinal lymphomas

albumin, one may determine the plasma volume, the total albumin pool, the rate of albumin degradation, and, in the steady state, the rate of albumin synthesis. Patients with protein loss, regardless of the mechanism involved, have reduced circulating and total body pools of albumin, a normal or slightly increased rate of albumin synthesis, and a markedly shortened albumin survival. Data obtained from serum and urinary radioactivity curves, however, indicate only that hypercatabolism or increased loss is the cause of the hypoproteinemia but do not necessarily implicate the gastrointestinal tract. The fecal output of ^{131}I cannot be used as an estimate of protein loss, since most of the label entering the intestinal tract is removed, reabsorbed, and excreted in the urine. Also, there is active secretion of ^{131}I into the gastrointestinal tract, regardless of where in the body it is removed. Amberlite IRA-400, an ion exchange resin, has been utilized in an effort to trap the ^{131}I in the lumen but with only partial success. The half-life of ^{131}I-albumin is 14 to 22 days.

[131]I-labeled polyvinylpyrrolidone is a synthetic polymer with an average molecular weight of 40,000 that is unaffected by digestive enzymes and is poorly absorbed. Normal subjects excrete 0 to 1.5 per cent of an intravenous dose, whereas patients with protein loss excrete 2.9 to 32.5 per cent. Variable but significant amounts of the label are removed and absorbed; nevertheless, it can be of great value as a screening test.

[51]Cr-labeled albumin is perhaps the most useful of the readily available substances, since the label is neither significantly absorbed from nor secreted into the gastrointestinal tract. Normals excrete 0.1 to 0.7 per cent of an intravenous dose, whereas patients with protein loss excrete 2 to 40 per cent of the radioactive substance. A disadvantage is its short apparent half-life of 3 to 10 days, which is due to the elution of the label from the protein. For this reason, ^{51}Cr-albumin cannot be used to determine pool sizes or rates of protein synthesis and catabolism.

A more complete analysis of protein metabolism can be achieved by the simultaneous use of ^{51}Cr-albumin and ^{125}I-albumin. The size of the albumin pool and rates of albumin catabolism and synthesis can be determined from the ^{125}I data and the magnitude of gastrointestinal protein loss estimated by ^{51}Cr-albumin.

WATER AND SOLUTE TRANSPORT

The usual concentrations of electrolytes in small intestinal fluid vary somewhat between the jejunum and the ileum. Sodium and potassium concentrations are similar in the two areas, the former being approximately 140 mEq per liter and the latter 7 mEq per liter. Jejunal chloride concentrations, however, are higher than ileal concentrations (129 mEq per liter as compared with 81 mEq

per liter), whereas the reverse is true for bicarbonate (17 mEq per liter versus 63 mEq per liter). The manner in which water and ion fluxes are regulated to maintain these differences as well as to accomplish the efficient absorption of large volumes of fluid and electrolytes is imperfectly understood. The following general principles, although lacking incontrovertible experimental support, are consistent with present information. For a more detailed discussion and reference to the literature, the reader is referred to the excellent discussion by Krejs and Fordtran.

It is generally accepted that crypt cells secrete and villous cells absorb, but it must be appreciated that what is measured in most instances is net transport, not unidirectional fluxes. Since cell membranes are lipoidal structures, solutes such as glucose and electrolytes must pass the epithelial layer via either pores or some carrier-mediated mechanism. Pores appear to exist at the tight junctions and are larger in the jejunum than in the ileum. They are more permeable for cations than anions, and approximately 80 per cent of sodium, potassium, and chloride is transported by this route in the jejunum and ileum. The brush border contains a mobile carrier binding both sodium and glucose, and each increases the affinity of the carrier for the other. Thus, in the presence of intraluminal glucose, sodium is actively absorbed. Amino acids have a similar but weaker effect mediated by a different carrier. The most important specialized activity of the brush border membrane, however, is the neutral sodium chloride entry mechanism. This double ion exchange mechanism allows sodium to be absorbed in exchange for hydrogen and chloride in exchange for bicarbonate.

In both the jejunum and ileum the basolateral membrane of the absorptive cells contains a sodium pump that actively secretes sodium into the intercellular space. In the jejunum, bicarbonate exits with sodium; in the ileum, chloride accompanies the sodium ions. This sodium pumping generates a potential difference (PD), especially in the jejunum, so that the intercellular and subserosal spaces are positive compared with the luminal surface and intracellular compartment. This PD causes intercellular sodium to diffuse to some extent back into the lumen, resulting in a final PD near zero. A portion of this intercellular sodium also enters the plasma, accompanied by an anion.

In the jejunum, active sodium transport is achieved by both the glucose-sodium carrier mechanism and sodium-hydrogen exchange. No chloride-bicarbonate exchange mechanism appears to operate here, and chloride absorption is passive, being absorbed with sodium via pores.

In the ileum, the same mechanisms plus the chloride-bicarbonate exchange mechanism are operative. The secreted hydrogen and bicarbonate form CO_2 and water in the lumen and are absorbed. In the ileum the luminal contents equilibrate at about pH 7.8. Often there is net bicarbonate secretion due to more rapid anion than cation exchange.

All water transport is passive secondary to osmotic or hydrostatic forces. The active ion transport mechanisms discussed increase the concentration of solute in the intercellular space, and as a result water moves across the basolateral membrane and through the tight junctions. The hydrostatic pressure in this space increases, forcing fluid into the capillaries. The fluid finally absorbed is isotonic, but the combined activities of the ion transport and hydrostatic mechanisms make possible the absorption of water against a concentration gradient (lumen to plasma).

An important observation is that increases in hydrostatic pressure at the mucosal surface have relatively little effect on water and solute transport. At the serosal surface, however, such elevations may result in increased secretion and decreased absorption. This effect becomes significant at venous pressures more than 15 cm of water above normal.

Water absorption in turn has an effect on solute transport that is termed *solvent drag*. Small solutes may be caught in the moving stream of water and absorbed, especially in the jejunum because of its larger pore size. Movement of water out of one compartment also may increase the concentration of some solutes and, therefore, their electrochemical potential.

Present evidence indicates that potassium movement in the small intestine is passive and dependent on concentration and electrochemical differences generated by the mechanisms already discussed.

The fasting intestine contains little fluid. After a meal, between 2 and 3 liters of exogenous and endogenous fluid are presented to it, with the daily load amounting to about 8.5 liters. It is truly remarkable that humans can ingest a diet that varies markedly in its water and solute content without causing osmotic disequilibrium. This is prevented largely because (1) the gastric mucosa is relatively impermeable to bulk water flow; (2) gastric emptying is controlled by osmoreceptors; (3) nutrients in the small bowel lumen are largely macromolecules with relatively lower osmotic activity; (4) these nutrients are rapidly broken down and absorbed; and (5) ingested fat, a significant component of most diets, is not osmotically active.

The diarrhea of cholera, almost entirely of small bowel origin, offers an impressive demonstration of abnormal fluid and electrolyte fluxes in this organ. In the adult with acute cholera, the secretory capacity amounts to 1 to 2 liters per hour. The fluid is approximately isosmotic with plasma and is nearly protein-free. The predominant cation is sodium and the predominant anions are chloride and bicarbonate, the latter two exhibiting the same relationships in the jejunum and ileum as under normal circumstances. The *Vibrio cholerae* does not invade the intestinal wall, and as a result there is no disruption of the epithelium or significant inflammation. Consistent with the absence of epithelial cell damage is the fact that glucose absorption and glucose-coupled sodium transport remain normal. Once investigators recognized this, the oral administration of glucose to stimulate fluid absorption became an important adjunct to therapy. The epithelium of the small intestine can be triggered to secrete chloride actively by both cholera exotoxin and cyclic AMP. Furthermore, the exotoxin results in an increase in the cyclic AMP concentration in the intestinal mucosa. Despite its gradual development, secretion is difficult to reverse once the toxin has come into contact with the epithelium. The fluid loss results from an active secretory process. The massive diarrhea characteristic of acute cholera ensues because the absorptive capacity of the colon is readily overwhelmed by the large quantity of water and electrolytes presented to it.

The products of several other bacteria also elicit small intestinal fluid secretion, including *Escherichia coli, Shigella,* and *Clostridium perfringens.* The massive diarrhea occasionally occurring in association with several hormone-secreting tumors such as malignant carcinoids, medullary carcinomas of the thyroid, and some non–beta cell tumors of the pancreatic islets may also be due in part to an enhancement of cyclic AMP activity. This possibility rests on the concept of a two-messenger system of hormone action. The first messenger is a hormone stimulating adenylate cyclase activity within the target cell. This results in the formation of increased amounts of cyclic AMP (the second messenger) from ATP. In view of the large number of agents that increase cyclic AMP concentrations in this way, it is likely that this secretory mechanism plays an important part not only in cholera but also in other disorders associated with diarrhea.

THE SECRETION OF HORMONES AND ENZYMES

The gut has been known for some time to contain a large number of endocrine cells. Immunocytochemical and ultrastructural techniques have permitted the localization of several peptide hormones to these cells. Table 28–5 lists the cell types as presently designated, their location, and the hormones they contain. Physiologic roles have so far been demonstrated only for gastrin, cholecystokinin-pancreozymin, and secretin. Several of the remainder are of sufficient interest, however, to warrant some discussion.

Although most small bowel enzymes are fixed in that they function at sites in the glycocalyx-plasma membrane structure or epithelial cell cy-

TABLE 28–5 ANATOMIC AND CELLULAR LOCALIZATION OF SMALL INTESTINAL HORMONES

Hormone	Cell	Distribution
Gastrin	G	Upper duodenum
	G1	Duodenum and jejunum
GIP	K	Duodenum and jejunum
Motilin	EC2	Duodenum and jejunum
Somatostatin	D	Duodenum and jejunum
Enteroglucagon	L	Duodenum and jejunum
		Ileum and colon
Secretin	S	Duodenum
CCK-PZ	I	Duodenum and jejunum
VIP	D1(H)	Duodenum and jejunum
		Ileum and colon

(Modified from the Revised Wiesbaden Classification of Human Endocrine Cells. Solcia, E., Pearse, A. G. E., Grube, D., et al.: Revised Wiesbaden classification of gut endocrine cells. Rendic. Gastroenterol. 5:13, 1973.)

toplasm, one enzyme is released into the lumen in physiologic concentrations (enterokinase).

SECRETIN AND CHOLECYSTOKININ-PANCREOZYMIN

Secretin is released from the duodenum and probably the proximal jejunum in response to H^+, the magnitude of response being proportional to the amount rather than to the concentration of the H^+. It shares a 14 amino acid sequence with glucagon, but no fragment with superior biologic activity has been identified. Cholecystokinin-pancreozymin is secreted from the duodenum and jejunum following vagal stimulation, but especially in response to free fatty acids and essential amino acids in the intestinal lumen. It contains the same C-terminal pentapeptide as gastrin, but most of its activity is contained in the C-terminal heptapeptide. The activities of these two hormones are summarized in Table 28–6. Their function in coordinating the various phases of the digestive-absorptive process is related to their effects on gastric emptying, gastroduodenal motor responses, and the secretion of acid, bile, and pancreatic juice.

No primary disorders of their secretion have been reported. In diffuse mucosal lesions of the small intestine such as nontropical sprue, however, their activities may be reduced. These patients often exhibit delayed emptying of the gallbladder; decreased luminal concentrations of pancreatic lipase, bile acids, and micellar lipid; and decreased intestinal motor activity. Further-

more, the secretion of bicarbonate by the pancreas is impaired following duodenal acidification.

The physiology and pathophysiology of gastrin are discussed elsewhere. As yet, no physiologic role for duodenal gastrin has been determined.

GASTRIC INHIBITORY PEPTIDE (GIP)

GIP shares structural similarities with secretin and glucagon, and the highest concentrations are found in the jejunum, with significant amounts in the duodenum and upper ileum. It inhibits gastric acid secretion, pepsin secretion, and antral and fundic motility and stimulates small intestinal secretion. Plasma concentrations rise rapidly after a meal, and fat, glucose, and amino acids appear to be effective stimuli for its release. It is of interest that acidification of the duodenum has no effect on GIP release, thus eliminating it from a negative feedback role. The most significant physiologic action of GIP, however, probably is the postprandial enhancement of insulin release. This most likely accounts for the greater insulin release following oral as compared with intravenous glucose. Its most potent insulin-releasing action is seen in conditions of hyperglycemia. A role for GIP in reactive hypoglycemia at present is undefined.

MOTILIN

Motilin is confined to a distinct population of enterochromaffin cells of the duodenum and upper

TABLE 28–6 PHYSIOLOGIC EFFECTS OF SECRETIN AND CHOLECYSTOKININ-PANCREOZYMIN

	Cholecystokinin-Pancreozymin (CCK-PZ)	Secretin
Gallbladder contraction	S	0
Stomach		
H^+	Sw	I
Pepsin	Sw	S
Motility	S	I
Exocrine pancreas		
HCO_3^-	Sw	S
Enzymes	S	Sw
Endocrine pancreas		
Insulin	S	S
Glucagon	S	0
Intestine		
Brunner's glands	S	S
Motility	S	I
Hepatic bile		
HCO_3^-	Sw	Sw

S = stimulates; Sw = stimulates weakly; I = inhibits; 0 = no effect. (Modified from Go, V.L.W., and Summerskill, W.H.J.: Am. J. Clin. Nutr. 24:160, 1971.)

jejunum. Levels rise after acidification of the duodenum and after fat ingestion. It causes marked contractions in isolated gastric and upper small intestinal tissue, an increase in lower esophageal sphincter pressure, and delayed gastric emptying. No physiologic role has been established.

ENTEROGLUCAGON (EG)

Enteroglucagon appears to be chemically and biologically different from pancreatic glucagon but shares immunoreactivity. It is found in highest concentrations in the lower ileum and colon. Plasma EG rises after a meal, and its release is stimulated primarily by carbohydrate and long-chain triglycerides. Owing to its distal localization its release is enhanced by rapid transit, and it is greatly increased in the dumping syndrome. Little is known of its physiology but one patient with an EG-producing tumor exhibited intestinal stasis and increased mucosal growth.

VASOACTIVE INTESTINAL PEPTIDE (VIP)

VIP is structurally related to secretin, glucagon, and GIP. It is not only produced by an endocrine cell in the gut but also is found in fine nerve fibers in the lamina propria and in the cell bodies of the myenteric plexus. VIP inhibits gastric acid production, stimulates insulin release, has a glucagon-like action, and stimulates both pancreatic and small intestinal secretion. It is not significantly released after a meal and probably functions as a local hormone. Its production by pancreatic islet cell tumors and ganglioneuromas has implicated it in the clinical expression of the Verner-Morrison, or watery diarrhea, syndrome.

SOMATOSTATIN

Most somatostatin-containing cells are located in the gastric antrum, with fewer cells in the duodenum and jejunum. Somatostatin exhibits a wide range of inhibitory activities, including growth hormone and TSH release, insulin and glucagon release, gastrin release, gastric acid production, gallbladder contraction, and pancreatic enzyme production. It also suppresses motilin and VIP production. For this reason, it has been suggested that it functions as a local rather than a circulating hormone.

Several other poorly characterized peptides have been collectively referred to as *candidate hormones*. These include such designated substances as urogastrone, gastrone, bulbogastrone, and substance P. Little or nothing is known of their precise localization or biologic activity.

ENTEROKINASE

As previously discussed, enterokinase is concerned with the conversion of pancreatic proenzymes to their active forms. The enzyme is located in the proximal duodenum in relationship to the microvilli, but its mechanism of release into the duodenal lumen has not been established. Bile salts appear to constitute one effective stimulus, and in their presence enterokinase activity is increased. Recently, several cases of enterokinase deficiency have been recognized in infants presenting with diarrhea from birth, showing failure to thrive, and exhibiting a good clinical response to pancreatic extracts.

IMMUNOLOGIC FUNCTION

NORMAL STRUCTURE AND FUNCTION

Unlike most other organs such as the heart or kidney, the gastrointestinal tract is replete with immunologically competent tissue. It is capable not only of experiencing but also of mounting an immune response. In this respect, it maintains functional identity with other peripheral lymphoid tissues such as the lymph nodes and spleen. Little is known, however, regarding either the qualitative or quantitative contributions of the gut to the body's immune responses. Of further importance is the realization that all the currently recognized, so-called "central lymphoid tissues" such as the thymus and avian bursa of Fabricius, which determine the immunologic capabilities of the whole organism, are lymphoepithelial derivatives of the gut. The small intestine, therefore, assumes a position of considerable importance to the immunologist as well as to those who seek an understanding of its more classic functions. Any attempt to relate abnormalities of the small bowel to concurrently observed immunologic changes must proceed from an awareness of the potential of the small intestine as both a central and peripheral lymphoid organ as well as an immunologic target.

The lymphoid elements of the small bowel are arranged in different ways, but the functional implications of these structural variations are unknown. The Peyer's patches lie in the lamina propria and submucosa and consist of lymphoid follicles containing germinal centers. The lymphocytes in the follicular cortex appear to represent a separate population when compared with similar areas of spleen and lymph nodes. Small lymphocytes from thoracic duct lymph preferentially "home" to the Peyer's patches as well as lymph nodes and spleen. These structures are well developed by the fifth month of fetal life, increase in size and number until 10 to 12 years of age, and gradually atrophy thereafter. Although Peyer's patch cells are capable of antibody synthesis and probably of both primary and secondary immune responses, the importance of this function in relation to their location is unclear. The means of antigen uptake by the small intestine is unknown. The epithelium over the dome area of Peyer's patches differs in being cuboidal. This specialized epithelial cell has been termed an *M cell* and may play a role in antigen transport. The lamina propria also contains a second population of lymphoid cells differing in certain respects from the Peyer's patches. Its lymphocytes and plasma cells also contain various immunoglobulins, but they are not arranged in any structured fashion. Large lymphocytes from the thoracic duct lymph preferentially seed the lamina propria as do lymphoblasts formed in lymph nodes following antigenic stimulation. It is not known, however, whether primary or secondary immune responses occur in situ within this nonaggregated lymphoid tissue of the lamina propria. Peyer's patches and the lamina propria both contain T and B lymphocytes. B lymphocytes are responsible for local antibody production, but the role of T cells in this location is not firmly established. Some probably are helper T cells, modulating B-cell function, and others are engaged in cell-mediated immune reactions. The presence of F_c-receptor cells and C'-receptor lymphocytes in the normal small intestine remains controversial. The third type of lymphoid elements found in the small intestine are the theliolymphocytes. They lie within and between the mucosal epithelial cells and have been identified as activated T cells. Their source, function, and fate, however, are unknown.

The lymphoid tissues of the Peyer's patches and lamina propria are sparse and appear undeveloped prior to birth and in the germ-free state. With the development of an intestinal flora, lymphocytes and plasma cells become more numerous and germinal centers develop.

It is apparent that all three of these lymphoid "structures" maintain a lymphoepithelial relationship that is similar to that of the thymus and the avian bursa of Fabricius. The former is responsible for the development of the cellular immune system, and the latter, in avian species at least, regulates the development of the humoral immune system. This has led to considerable speculation concerning which, if any, of the small intestinal lymphoid elements constitute a human bursal equivalent.

The gut-associated lymphoid tissue as well as the spleen and lymph node is on the route of recirculating lymphocytes. Present evidence suggests that only activated T and B cells (immunoblasts) gain access to this compartment. Although these cells may originate in any of the organized peripheral lymphoid tissues, it seems clear that a significant number arise within the aggregated lymphoid tissue of the gut as a result of the interaction of lymphocytes with intraluminal antigen. This accounts for most of the immunoblasts in thoracic duct lymph, and a high proportion of these migrate back to the large and small intestine. Indeed, thoracic duct lymphocytes activated by histocompatability antigens migrate preferentially to the gut and have been traced to Peyer's patches, the lamina propria, and intraepithelial sites. It has been postulated that immunoblasts cross the capillaries in the intestinal mucosa in a random fashion, and, under the influence of intraluminal antigen, appropriately primed effector cells are inhibited from returning to the general circulation as a consequence of antigen-driven stimulation to final differentiation or multiplication. An important consequence of this recirculating and homing mechanism is the propagation throughout the gut and the dissemination throughout the body of a local immune response by means of mobile effector cells.

Most immunoglobulin-containing cells in the small intestine are mature plasma cells, although some immunoglobulins are found within immature plasma cells and lymphocytes. It is well established that IgA is the predominant immunoglobulin in the lymphoid cells and secretions of the small intestine. IgM, IgG, and IgD are also present in that order. Recently, IgE has been identified in the small intestine, but its relative amount has yet to be established. The IgA found in the small intestine and its secretions differs from 7S serum IgA in that it is an 11S globulin with a molecular weight of 390,000. This secretory IgA appears to represent a dimer of the 7S serum IgA coupled to a nonimmunoglobulin glycoprotein, referred to as *secretory piece* or *T (transport) component*. This secretory component has been identified as a product of the epithelial cells. Its precise function is not known, although it no doubt confers some biologic advantage on IgA in the external secretions. The J piece, which interconnects these molecules, is also produced in the mucosal cells. There are two subclasses of IgA—IgA_1 and IgA_2. IgA_2 appears to predominate in the intestinal secretions and differs from IgA_1 in that it contains no disulfide bonds linking the light and heavy chains and contains a genetic marker, Am_2, within its heavy chain structure.

The human infant is born totally lacking IgA in serum and external secretions, and secretory IgA appears sooner and reaches adult levels more quickly than serum IgA does. The small intestine therefore has been regarded as a potentially important source not only of secretory but also of serum IgA. Secretory IgA has been demonstrated to possess antiviral and antibacterial activity as well as the properties of isohemagglutinins. Although the precise role played by secretory IgA in the external secretions remains unsettled, it probably constitutes an important defense against certain microorganisms and perhaps other potentially harmful substances.

ABNORMAL STRUCTURE AND FUNCTION

Gastrointestinal symptoms consisting usually of diarrhea, malabsorption, and malnutrition are found in patients with primary immunodeficiency syndromes, occurring in 20 to 50 per cent of those with adult onset but rarely in the congenital disorders. Table 28–7 presents a classification of these syndromes developed by a group of the World Health Organization. Although the syndromes are not discussed in the following chapter, the colon and rectum also participate in many of the histologic and functional alterations described here.

Two distinctive histologic patterns have been described in the small intestine of patients with immunodeficiency syndromes and gastrointestinal symptoms. The first, nodular lymphoid hyperplasia of the small intestine, has been so named

TABLE 28–7 CLASSIFICATION OF PRIMARY IMMUNODEFICIENCY SYNDROMES AND INCIDENCE OF GASTROINTESTINAL (GI) DISEASE

Type of Immunodeficiency	Incidence of GI Disease	Characteristic GI Syndromes, Findings, and Morphologic Abnormalities
B-cell defects		
Infantile X-linked agammaglobulinemia	(+)	*Giardia lamblia* (rare), absence of plasma cells in mucosa, early crypt abscesses
X-linked immunodeficiency with hyper-IgM	–	–
Selective IgA deficiency	+ +	Celiac sprue, nodular lymphoid hyperplasia, *Giardia lamblia,* malignancy
Transient hypogammaglobulinemia of infancy	–	–
Immunodeficiency syndrome with normal serum immunoglobulin levels	(+)	Diarrhea, malabsorption
Variable immunodeficiency (acquired hypogammaglobulinemia)	+ + +	Nodular lymphoid hyperplasia, celiac sprue, severe B_{12} malabsorption, *Giardia lamblia,* colitis, malignancy
T-cell defect		
DiGeorge's syndrome (thymic hypoplasia)	(+)	Recurrent diarrhea, failure to thrive
B- and T-cell defects		
Immunodeficiency with ataxia-telangiectasia	(+)	Vitamin B_{12} malabsorption, carcinoma of stomach
Immunodeficiency with thrombocytopenia and eczema (Wiscott-Aldrich syndrome)	+ + +	Severe recurrent bloody diarrhea, malabsorption
Immunodeficiency with short-limbed dwarfism	+	Diarrhea, crypt abscesses
Cartilage-hair hypoplasia	+	Recurrent diarrhea, failure to thrive, steatorrhea, vacuolated and lipid-laden macrophages
Immunodeficiency with thymoma	(+)	Diarrhea (frequently)
Severe combined immunodeficiency Autosomal recessive (with or without red blood cell adenosine deaminase deficiency; with reticuloendotheliosis) X-linked Sporadic	+ + +	Severe diarrhea, malabsorption, absence of plasma cells, vacuolated and lipid-containing macrophages
Nezelof's syndrome	+ +	Recurrent infection, lymphadenopathy, hepatosplenomegaly, malabsorption, candidiasis, enterocolitis

(Modified from Ochs, H. D., and Ament, M. E.: Gastrointestinal tract and immunodeficiency. *In* Ferguson, A., and MacSween, R. N. M. (Eds.): Immunological Aspects of the Liver and GI Tract. Lancaster, England, MTP Press, Ltd., 1976, p. 85.)

because of the multiple small lymphoid nodules present within the mucosa. These nodules contain hyperplastic germinal centers but plasma cells are sparse throughout the intestine, and the epithelial and villous architecture usually remains well preserved. The second pattern has been referred to as "hypogammaglobulinemic sprue" because there is villus atrophy, and the mucosa often presents a flat appearance. These patients differ, however, from those with gluten-sensitive enteropathy not only in the presence of the immunodeficiency but also in failing to respond in many instances to a gluten-free diet. Plasma cells are also nearly completely absent in the small intestine of patients with this type of pattern.

In their initial report, Hermans and his associates described five characteristic features of patients with nodular lymphoid hyperplasia: (1) dysgammaglobulinemia, consisting of the virtual absence of IgA and IgM, with a moderate reduction in IgG; (2) susceptibility to sinopulmonary infections; (3) diarrhea; (4) *Giardia lamblia* in the stools; and (5) nodular lymphoid hyperplasia of the small intestine. Additional cases have been described with idiopathic acquired hypogammaglobulinemia, and two subjects have been reported with a selective absence of IgA. In those patients studied, cellular immune mechanisms appear to be intact. Mild steatorrhea is often present, and in many instances both the diarrhea and steatorrhea respond favorably to treatment of the *Giardia* infection. The radiographic findings in nodular lymphoid hyperplasia are characteristic, demonstrating innumerable small filling defects that measure only a few millimeters in diameter and that are uniform in size and smooth in contour. Segmental involvement of the small intestine and colon may be present, or the entire small bowel may be involved, and a mild malabsorption pattern is at times superimposed.

In so-called "hypogammaglobulinemic sprue," steatorrhea is often more marked. These patients also frequently harbor *Giardia lamblia* in the small intestinal secretions, and in many instances the associated diarrhea and steatorrhea are improved after treatment of the giardiasis. These patients generally exhibit an acquired type of hypogammaglobulinemia, although again selective IgA deficiency has been encountered.

The relationship between the immunodeficiency and the structural and functional abnormalities present in the small intestine is unknown. It should be noted that selective IgA deficiency is not uncommon in the general population, occurring in approximately one of every 700 individuals. Many of these patients are without any intestinal symptoms, and many patients with acquired hypogammaglobulinemia fail to demonstrate structural abnormalities or symptoms related to the small intestine. At the present time, therefore, these various structural and functional changes cannot be understood in pathophysiologic terms.

Of perhaps greater practical importance is the relationship between IgE, allergy, and the gut. It is known that ingestion of foods may provoke immediate systemic anaphylactic reactions manifested by angioedema, urticaria, and shock as well as more subtle allergic reactions resulting in various types of gastrointestinal dysfunction. This latter group, often associated with chronic, vague, and diverse symptoms, is presently not well understood. One study has demonstrated an increase in both serum and intestinal fluid IgE levels in patients with various manifestations of allergy but without food intolerance and in patients with atopic sensitivity to foods. The relationship of such observations to eosinophilic gastroenteritis is of considerable interest. Eosinophilic gastroenteritis is a disorder of the stomach or small intestine or both that is characterized by infiltration of some part of the gut wall with eosinophils, peripheral eosinophilia, and the development of clinical manifestations often but not invariably following the ingestion of specific foods. Three clinical patterns have been identified: (1) primary mucosal disease with enteric protein loss and malabsorption; (2) predominant muscle layer disease with obstructive symptoms; and (3) subserosal involvement with eosinophilic ascites. The strongest evidence of gastrointestinal allergy is found in the predominantly mucosal form. In such patients, clinical manifestations are often reproduced by food challenge and accompanied by an increase in serum IgE.

It is likely that further investigations will place gastrointestinal food allergy and eosinophilic gastroenteritis on the same level of immunologic respectability as allergic rhinitis and asthma.

VASCULAR DISORDERS OF THE SMALL INTESTINE

NORMAL PHYSIOLOGY

The splanchnic circulation receives 28 per cent of the cardiac output and contains 20 per cent of the total blood volume, with 65 per cent distributed to the mucosa. There is also a gradient in blood flow over the length of the intestine, with the highest mean flows in the jejunum and the lowest in the colon. Blood flow in the small intestine is determined by both intrinsic and extrinsic mechanisms. Intrinsic mechanisms consist of myogenic and metabolic factors, whereas extrinsic regulation is provided by the sympathetic nervous system and circulating vasoactive agents. Of these, myogenic and metabolic factors are believed to play a major role in the regulation of intestinal blood flow. Any condition that produces a discrepancy between tissue oxygen supply and demand, or an abnormality of interstitial P_{O_2}, will cause an increase of metabolites in the interstitial fluid, resulting in relaxation of arteriolar or precapillary sphincter smooth muscle or both. The result is the maintenance of intracellular P_{O_2} above the level necessary to ensure adequate energy metabolism. The myogenic regulation of local blood flow is based on the fact that vascular resistance is directly proportional to transmural pressure at the arteriolar level. An increase in transmural pressure results in arteriolar vasoconstriction and an increase in vascular resistance. From a homeostatic viewpoint, the myogenic mechanism is directed primarily toward maintaining intestinal capillary pressure and transcapillary fluid exchange, whereas the metabolic mechanism subserves adequate blood flow and oxygen delivery.

Intestinal blood flow is regulated primarily by the sympathetic nervous system via alpha-receptor activity. Stimulation can virtually interrupt flow, especially to the mucosa, whereas the elimination of normal constrictor activity results in a 20 to 40 per cent increase. The vagal parasympathetic nerves appear to have no effect on blood flow through the small intestine. After eating, there is a 30 per cent increase in splanchnic flow that correlates with the processes of secretion and absorption. This effect is probably mediated in part by the release of gastrin, secretin, cholecystokinin-pancreozymin, and serotonin, all of which act to increase superior mesenteric artery flow. When all factors capable of augmenting blood flow are operative, the maximal possible increase is in the range of 500 per cent. A decrease in splanchnic flow may result from a number of influences, including exercise, standing, intraluminal pressures above 30 mm Hg, and increased sympathetic neurohumoral activity. Although muscle contraction leads to a decrease in flow, the net effect of intestinal motor activity is to produce a greater flow, probably as a result of the release of various metabolites.

Intestinal blood flow also exhibits autoregulation and autoregulatory escape. Autoregulation involves the coordination of physiologic mechanisms to maintain blood flow in the face of a decrease in arterial pressure, whereas autoregulatory escape is the intrinsic ability of the intestinal vasculature to "escape" from persistent vasoconstrictor activity imposed by alpha-adrenergic stimulation. It therefore represents a protective mechanism within the intestinal circulation to counter ischemia during prolonged sympathetic activity.

An additional concept important to an understanding of intestinal ischemia is that of countercurrent exchange (Fig. 28–11). The effect of such an arrangement is that arterial substances (e.g., oxygen) entering at the base of the villus will progressively decrease in concentration toward the villous tip, whereas absorbed materials entering at the villous tip will leave the villus more slowly. Countercurrent exchange operates at low perfusion rates and aggravates mucosal ischemia.

INTESTINAL ISCHEMIA AND INFARCTION

A compromise in the arterial supply of the small intestine may result in either chronic intestinal ischemia or infarction. Approximately 60 per cent of infarctions result from nonocclusive disease, and 30 per cent are due to either thrombosis or embolism, the former probably being more frequent. The remaining 10 per cent follow venous occlusion.

Chronic intestinal ischemia is best understood as a series of recurring attacks of acute ischemia that do not result in infarction. Although any disease process that results in a decrease in arterial flow may be responsible, the vast majority of cases are a result of atherosclerotic narrowing of the celiac axis and superior or inferior mesenteric arteries. The constriction is asymmetric and most

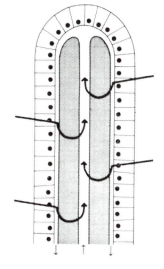
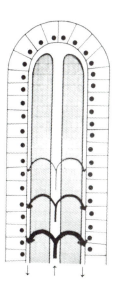

Figure 28–11 The functional implications of the mucosal countercurrent exchanger schematically illustrated. *A,* Absorbed materials are delayed in their egress from the villus, and *B,* arterial O_2 achieves a progressively lower concentration at the villous tip.

evident in the first centimeter of the involved vessel. The most prominent manifestation is cramping, periumbilical pain (intestinal angina), which characteristically occurs 10 to 15 minutes after eating and lasts 2 to 3 hours. Larger meals produce more pain, and there is a tendency for it to become worse with the passage of time. As noted previously, ischemia causes increased contractility of smooth muscle, and the mechanism responsible for pain production is probably smooth muscle spasm. Patients tend to restrict their food intake in an effort to avoid these episodes of pain, and as a result weight loss may be marked. Not uncommonly, mild diarrhea with or without a slight increase in stool fat and nitrogen occurs, probably as a result of impaired epithelial cell function and an increase in propulsive motor activity.

It must be recognized, however, that symptom production cannot always be correlated with anatomic abnormalities demonstrated by arteriography. Even occlusion of all three major arterial branches of the abdominal aorta has been encountered in the absence of apparent symptoms. Granting such inconsistencies, the general view is that a patient who has characteristic abdominal pain and weight loss not explained by a primary disorder of the gut, pancreas, or hepatobiliary system and who has significant (>50 per cent of the lumen) narrowing in two of the three mesenteric arteries should be regarded as having a clinical disturbance of the mesenteric arterial circulation. If a gradient of >35mm Hg is present at the time of operation, this assumption is strengthened. Surgical correction will result in relief of pain in 90 per cent of such patients and reversal of the malabsorption in 75 per cent. Protection from future fatal infarction, however, is less well established.

Main stem occlusion of the superior mesenteric artery is characterized by two phases: first, mucosal ischemia, necrosis, and hemorrhage, with associated intestinal muscle spasm; and second, paralysis of smooth muscle, intestinal dilatation, and necrosis of the entire bowel wall, with peritonitis and major fluid and blood loss into the gut. Significant inflammatory changes are characteristically absent, with hemorrhage and edema being the predominant features. Patients at first complain of colicky periumbilical pain that gradually becomes continuous, severe, and poorly localized. Initially, there is a disproportionate lack of physical findings followed by signs of sympathetic overactivity, peritonitis, and cardiovascular collapse. Occlusion by an embolus may occur at different levels. In the presence of significant atheromatous disease, the main stem of the superior mesenteric artery may be involved (18 per cent), but 55 per cent of emboli lodge at the origin of the middle colic artery.

Nonocclusive infarction results from an interplay of several factors. The common denominator is a decrease in splanchnic flow resulting in a reduced perfusion pressure. This may be due to a reduced cardiac output or a decrease in the fraction entering the mesenteric circulation. A further decrease in flow, especially to the mucosa, is brought about by the activation of alpha-adrenergic receptors and the renin-angiotensin mechanism. The gut is therefore placed in an impossible situation. Autoregulatory escape will not maintain flow, and continued sympathetic activity reduces flow, especially to the mucosa. An increase in blood viscosity and the collapse of small vessels at low perfusion pressure no doubt provide aggravating factors. Furthermore, many of these patients are taking digitalis, which has a mesenteric constrictor effect, and this may be a contributing influence. The result is mucosal necrosis and hemorrhage and, if the process is severe enough, transmural infarction.

In patients suspected of having acute intestinal ischemia, the role of early arteriography is controversial. Its proponents point out that it offers the only means of establishing the presence of arterial embolization or thrombosis—conditions often amenable to prompt surgical correction. Also, although of unproved benefit, the intraarterial administration of vasodilators (e.g., papaverine, isoproterenol, sodium nitroprusside, and dopamine) has some theoretical basis. The prognosis of nonocclusive acute intestinal ischemia is poor, the mortality rate approaching 100 per cent. This is true because extensive amounts of bowel are usually involved, the patients are poor surgical risks, and no correctable lesion is present.

Venous occlusion affects the superior mesenteric vein 20 times more frequently than it affects the inferior mesenteric vein, but it is doubtful that occlusion of the latter leads to symptoms. Venous occlusion is associated with the gradual onset of vague abdominal discomfort, anorexia, and a change in bowel habits associated with slight abdominal tenderness and diminished bowel sounds. Intramural edema is marked, and the sequence of events described previously takes place, albeit more slowly. Most often, it represents a complication of hypercoagulable states, polycythemia, carcinomas, portal hypertension, sepsis, or surgical injury.

REFERENCES

Adibi, S. A., and Allen, E. R.: Impaired jejunal absorption rates of essential amino acids induced by either dietary caloric or protein deprivation in man. Gastroenterology 59:404, 1970.

Allen, R. H.: Cobalamin (Vitamin B$_{12}$) Absorption and malabsorption. Viewpoints on Digestive Diseases 14:17, 1982.

Ament, M. E.: Immunodeficiency syndromes and the gastrointestinal tract. Pract. Gastroenterol. 6:17, 1982.

Asher, R. A. J.: Sense and sensibility. Trans. Med. Soc. Lond. 75:66, 1959.

Asp, N. G., and Dahlqvist, A.: Multiplicity of intestinal beta-galactosidases. Contribution of each enzyme to the total lactase activity in normal and lactose intolerant patients. Acta Paediatr. Scand. 60:364, 1971.

Asp, N. G., Dahlqvist, A., and Koldovsky, O.: Small intestinal beta-galactosidase activity. Gastroenterology 58:591, 1970.

Balcerzak, S. P., Lane, W. C., and Bullard, J. W.: Surface structure of intestinal epithelium. Gastroenterology 58:49, 1970.

Bass, P.: In vivo electrical activity of the small bowel. In Code, C. F. (Ed.): Handbook of Physiology. Vol. IV. American Physiological Society, Washington, 1968, p. 2051.

Baum, S.: Pertechnitate imaging following cimetidine administration in Meckel's diverticulum of the ileum. Am. J. Gastroenterol. 76:464, 1981.

Bayless, T. M., Swanson, V. L., and Wheby, M. S.: Jejunal histology and clinical status in tropical sprue and other chronic diarrheal disorders. Am. J. Clin. Nutr. 24:112, 1971.

Belut, D., Moneret-Vautrin, D. A., Nicolas, J. P., et al.: IgE levels in intestinal juice. Dig. Dis. Sci. 25:323, 1980.

Bennett, A., and Fleshler, B.: Prostaglandins and the gastrointestinal tract. Gastroenterology 59:790, 1970.

Bentley, D. W., Nichols, R. L., Condon, R. E., et al.: The microflora of the human ileum and intra-abdominal colon: results of direct needle aspiration at surgery and evaluation of the technique. J. Lab. Clin. Med. 79:421, 1972.

Binder, H. J.: A comparison of intestinal and renal transport systems. Am. J. Clin. Nutr. 23:330, 1970.

Bloom, S. R., and Polak, J. M.: The new peptide hormones of the gut. In Glass, G. B. (Ed.): Progress in Gastroenterology, Vol. III. New York, Grune and Stratton, 1977, p. 109.

Braddock, L. E., Fleisher, D. R., and Barbero, G. J.: A physical chemical study of the van de Kamer method for fecal fat analysis. Gastroenterology 55:165, 1968.

Brandborg, L. L.: Structure and function of the small intestine in some parasite diseases. Am. J. Clin. Nutr. 24:124, 1971.

Brooks, F. P.: Absorption. In Control of Gastrointestinal Function. London, The Macmillan Co., 1970.

Bynum, T. E., and Jacobson, E. D.: Blood flow and gastrointestinal disease. Digestion 4:109, 1971.

Bynum, T. E., and Jacobson, E. D.: Blood flow and gastrointestinal function. Gastroenterology 60:325, 1971.

Christensen, J.: The control of gastrointestinal movements: some old and new views. N. Engl. J. Med. 285:85, 1971.

Code, C. F., Szurszewski, J. H., and Kelly, K. A.: A concept of motor control by the pacesetter potential in the stomach and small bowel. Am. J. Dig. Dis. 16:601, 1971.

Corcino, J. J., Waxman, S., and Herbert, V.: Absorption and malabsorption of vitamin B_{12}. Am. J. Med. 48:562, 1970.

Cornes, J. S.: Number, size and distribution of Peyer's patches in the human small intestine. I. The development of Peyer's patches. Gut 6:225, 1965.

Daniel, E. E., Robinson, K., Duchon, G., et al.: The possible role of close contacts (nexuses) in the propagation of control electrical activity in the stomach and small intestine. Am. J. Dig. Dis. 16:611, 1971.

Demling, L.: The motility of the gastrointestinal tract. Digestion 2:362, 1969.

Dharmsathaphorn, K., Freeman, D. H., Binder, H. J., et al.: Increased risk of nephrolithiasis in patients with steatorrhea. Dig. Dis. Sci. 27:401, 1982.

Dixon, J. A., Harman, C. G., Nichols, R. L., et al.: Intestinal motility following luminal and vascular occlusion of the small intestine. Gastroenterology 58:673, 1970.

Dobbins, W. O., III: Morphologic and functional correlates of intestinal brush borders. Am. J. Med. Sci. 258:150, 1969.

Dobbins, W. O., III: Intestinal mucosal lacteal in transport of macromolecules and chylomicrons. Am. J. Clin. Nutr. 24:77, 1971.

Donaldson, R. M., Jr.: Small bowel bacterial overgrowth. Adv. Intern. Med. 16:191, 1970.

Dowling, R. H.: The enterohepatic circulation. Gastroenterology 62:122, 1972.

Editorial: "Enterogastrone(s)." Lancet 1:1224, 1971.

Editorial: Ileus: paralytic or sympathetic? Lancet 1:329, 1971.

Eggermont, E., Molla, A. M., Rutgeerts, L., et al.: The source of human enterokinase. Lancet 2:369, 1971.

Elsas, L. J., Hillman, R. E., Patterson, J. H., et al.: Renal and intestinal hexose transport in familial glucose-galactose malabsorption. J. Clin. Invest. 49:576, 1970.

Farrar, J. T., and Zfass, A. M.: Small intestinal motility. Gastroenterology 52:1019, 1967.

Fasel, J., Hadjikhani, H., and Felber, J. P.: The insulin secretory effect of the human duodenal mucosa. Gastroenterology 59:109, 1970.

Fichtelius, K. E.: The gut epithelium—a first level lymphoid organ? Exp. Cell Res. 49:87, 1968.

Field, M.: Intestinal secretion: effect of cyclic AMP and its role in cholera. N. Engl. J. Med. 284:1137, 1971.

French, A. B.: Protein-losing gastroenteropathies. Am. J. Dig. Dis. 16:661, 1971.

Freter, R.: Locally produced and serum derived antibodies in "local immunity." N. Engl. J. Med., 285:1375, 1971.

Ginsburg, A. L.: The azathioprine controversy: J. E. Lennard-Jones versus John W. Singleton. Dig. Dis. Sci. 26:364, 1981.

Gleich, G. J.: IgE, allergy and the gut. Dig. Dis. Sci. 25:321, 1980.

Go, V. L. W., and Summerskill, W. H. J.: Digestion, maldigestion, and the gastrointestinal hormones. Am. J. Clin. Nutr. 24:160, 1971.

Gorbach, S. L.: Intestinal microflora. Gastroenterology 60:1110, 1971.

Granger, D. N., Richardson, P. D. I., Kvietys, P. R., et al.: Intestinal Blood Flow. Gastroenterology 78:837, 1980.

Gray, G. M.: Carbohydrate digestion and absorption. Gastroenterology 58:96, 1970.

Gray, G. M., and Cooper, H. L.: Protein digestion and absorption. Gastroenterology 61:535, 1971.

Greenberger, N. J.: The intestinal brush border as a digestive and absorptive surface. Am. J. Med. Sci. 258:144, 1969.

Hall, J. G., and Smith, M. E.: Homing of lymph-borne immunoblasts to the gut. Nature 226:262, 1970.

Harrison, L. A., and Jacobson, E. D.: Gastrointestinal hormones. J. Okla. Med. Assoc. 63:157, 1970.

Hellier, M. D., Perrett, D., and Holdsworth, C. D.: Dipeptide absorption in cystinuria. Br. Med. J. 4:782, 1970.

Hellier, M. D., Perrett, D., Holdsworth, C. D., et al.: Absorption of dipeptides in normal and cystinuric subjects. Gut 12:496, 1971.

Hendrix, R. T., and Bayless, T. M.: Digestion: intestinal secretion. Ann. Rev. Physiol. 32:139, 1970.

Henry, C., Faulk, W. P., Kuhn, L., et al.: Peyer's patches: immunologic studies. J. Exp. Med. 131:1200, 1970.

Herlinger, H.: Why not enteroclysis? J. Clin. Gastroenterol. 4:277, 1982.

Hermans, P. E., Huizenga, K. A., Hoffman, H. N., et al.: Dysgammaglobulinemia associated with nodular lymphoid hyperplasia of the small intestine. Am. J. Med. 40:78, 1966.

Hightower, N. C., Jr.: Motor action of the small bowel. In Code, C. F. (Ed.): Handbook of Physiology. Vol. IV. American Physiological Society, Washington, 1968, p. 2001.

Hirsh, E. H., Brandenburg, D., Hersh, T., et al.: Chronic intestinal pseudo-obstruction. J. Clin. Gastroenterol. 3:247, 1981.

Hofmann, A. F.: Fat absorption and malabsorption: physiology, diagnosis and treatment. In Isenberg, J. I. (Ed.): Viewpoints on Digestive Diseases. Vol. 9, Number 4, 1977.

Holt, P. R.: Medium chain triglycerides: their absorption, metabolism and clinical applications. In Glass, G. B. J. (Ed.): Progress in Gastroenterology. New York, Grune and Stratton, 1968, p. 277.

Hughes, W. S., Cerda, J. J., Holtzapple, P., et al.: Primary hypogammaglobulinemia and malabsorption. Ann. Intern. Med. 74:903, 1971.

Jacobson, E. D., Brobmann, G. F., and Brecher, G. A.: Intestinal motor activity and blood flow. Gastroenterology 58:575, 1970.

Jeffries, G. Y. H., Weser, E., and Sleisenger, M. H.: Malabsorption. Gastroenterology 56:777, 1969.

Jordan, P. H., Jr., Boulafendis, D., and Guinn, G. A.: Factors other than major vascular occlusion that contribute to intestinal infarction. Ann. Surg. 171:189, 1970.

King, C. E., Toskes, P. P., Guilarte, T. R., et al.: Comparison of the one-gram d-[^{14}C]xylose breath test to the [^{14}C]bile acid breath test in patients with small intestine bacterial overgrowth. Dig. Dis. Sci. 25:53, 1980.

Kraft, S. C., and Kirsner, J. B.: Immunological apparatus of the gut and inflammatory bowel disease. Gastroenterology 60:922, 1971.

Krejs, G. T., and Fordtran, J. S.: Physiology and pathophysiology of ion and water movement in the human intestine. In Sleisenger, M. H., and Fordtran, J. S. (Eds.): Gastrointestinal Disease. Philadelphia, W. B. Saunders Co., 1978, p. 297.

Kriebel, G. W., Jr., Kraft, S. C., and Rothberg, R. M.: Locally produced antibody in human gastrointestinal secretions. J. Immunol. 103:1268, 1969.

Lenz, H., Blomer, A., and Dux, A.: Analysis of the propulsive movements of the small intestine. Cineradiographic and experimental studies. Am. J. Dig. Dis. 16:1107, 1971.

Leung, F. W., Drenick, E. J., and Stanley, T. M.: Intestinal bypass complications involving the excluded small bowel segment. Am. J. Gastroenterol. 77:67, 1982.

Lucak, B. K., Sansaricq, C., Snyderman, S. E., et al.: Disseminated ulcerations in allergic eosinophilic gastroenteritis. Am. J. Gastroenterol. 77:248, 1982.

Lundgren, O.: Countercurrent exchange in the small intestine. Am. Heart J. 79:285, 1970.

Marsh, M. N., and Swift, J. A.: A study of the small intestinal mucosa using the scanning electron microscope. Gut 10:940, 1969.

Neeley, J., and Catchpole, B.: Ileus: the restoration of alimentary tract motility by pharmacologic means. Br. J. Surg. 58:21, 1971.

Nordstrom, C., and Dahlqvist, A.: Intestinal enterokinase. Lancet 1:1185, 1971.

Ochs, H. D., and Ament, M. E.: Gastrointestinal tract and immunodeficiency. In Ferguson, A., and MacSween, R. N. M. (Eds.): Immunological Aspects of the Liver and Gastrointestinal Tract. Lancaster, England, MTP Press Ltd., 1976, p. 83.

Parrott, D. M. V.: The gut associated lymphoid tissues and gastrointestinal immunity. In Ferguson, A., and MacSween, R. N. M. (Eds.): Immunological Aspects of the Liver and Gastrointestinal Tract. Lancaster, England, MTP Press Ltd., 1976, p. 1.

Pearse, A. G. E., Coulling, I., Weavers, B., et al.: The endocrine polypeptide cells of the human stomach, duodenum, and jejunum. Gut 11:649, 1970.

Peters, T. J.: Intestinal peptidases. Gut 11:720, 1970.

Pettersson, T., and Wegelius, O.: Biopsy diagnosis of amyloidosis in rheumatoid arthritis. Malabsorption caused by intestinal amyloid deposits. Gastroenterology 62:22, 1972.

Phillips, S. F., and Gaginella, T. S.: Intestinal secretion as a mechanism in diarrheal disease. In Glass, G. B. J. (Ed.): Progress in Gastroenterology. Vol. III. New York, Grune and Stratton, 1977, p. 481.

Porter, H. P., Saunders, D. R., Tytgat, G., et al.: Fat absorption in bile fistula in man. A morphological and biochemical study. Gastroenterology 60:1008, 1971.

Ravich, W. J., Bayless, T. M., and Thomas, M.: Fructose: incomplete intestinal absorption in humans. Gastroenterology 84:26, 1983.

Reynolds, D. G., Gurll, N. J., Swan, K. G., et al.: The clinical significance of gastrointestinal blood flow. J. Clin. Gastroenterol. 1:353, 1979.

Rosenberg, I. H., and Godwin, H. A.: The digestion and absorption of dietary folate. Gastroenterology 60:445, 1971.

Rosensweig, N. S., Herman, R. H., and Stifel, F. B: Dietary regulation of small intestinal enzyme activity in man. Am. J. Clin. Nutr. 24:65, 1971.

Rubin, W.: Celiac disease. Am. J. Clin. Nutr. 24:91, 1971.

Rubin, W.: The epithelial "membrane" of the small intestine. Am. J. Clin. Nutr. 24:45, 1971.

Sadikali, F.: Dipeptidase deficiency and malabsorption of glycylglycine in disease states. Gut 12:276, 1971.

Sarva, R., Farivar, S., Fromm, H., et al.: Comparative sensitivity of 8 and 24 hour bile acid breath tests and schilling test in ileopathies. Am. J. Gastroenterol. 76:432, 1981.

Savilahti, E., Visakorpi, J. K., and Pelkonen, P.: Morphological and immunohistochemical findings in small intestinal biopsy in children with IgA deficiency. Acta Paediatr. Scand. 60:363, 1971.

Schiff, E. R., and Dietschy, J. M.: Steatorrhea associated with disordered bile acid metabolism. Am. J. Dig. Dis. 14:432, 1969.

Scratcherd, T., and Case, R. M.: The role of cyclic adenosine-3′,5′-monophosphate (AMP) in gastrointestinal secretion. Gut 10:957, 1969.

Sessions, J. T., Jr., de Andrade, S. R. V., and Kokas, E.: Intestinal villi: form and motility in relation to function. In Glass, G. B. J. (Ed.): Progress in Gastroenterology. New York, Grune and Stratton, 1968, p. 248.

Shanbour, L. L., and Jacobson, E. D.: Autoregulatory escape in the gut. Gastroenterology 60:145, 1971.

Shih, V. E., Bixby, E. M., Alpers, C. S., et al.: Studies of intestinal transport defect in Hartnup disease. Gastroenterology 61:445, 1971.

Storer, E. H.: The pharmacologic and biochemical nature of carcinoid tumors. Curr. Probl. Surg., November, 1970, p. 41.

Summers, R. W., Switz, D. M., Sessions, J. T., et al.: National Cooperative Crohn's Disease Study: results of drug treatment. Gastroenterology 77:847, 1979.

Tarlow, M. J., Hadorn, B., Arthurton, M. W., et al.: Intestinal enterokinase deficiency. A newly recognized disorder of protein digestion. Arch. Dis. Child. 45:651, 1970.

Texter, E. C., Jr.: Pressure and transit in the small intestine. The concept of propulsion and peripheral resistance in the alimentary canal. Am. J. Dig. Dis. 13:443, 1968.

Thompson, D. G., and Malagelada, J. R.: Guts and their motions (gastrointestinal motility in health and disease). J. Clin. Gastroenterol. 3(suppl. 1):81, 1981.

Thompson, G. R., Barrowman, J., Guterrez, L., et al.: Action of neomycin on the intraluminal phase of lipid absorption. J. Clin. Invest. 50:319, 1971.

Tidball, C. S.: The nature of the intestinal epithelial barrier. Am. J. Dig. Dis. 16:745, 1971.

Tomasi, T. B., Jr., Tan, E. M., Solomon, A., et al.: Characteristics of an immune system common to certain external secretions. J. Exp. Med. 121:101, 1965.

Toner, P. G., and Carr, K. E.: The use of scanning electron microscopy in the study of the intestinal villi. J. Pathol. 97:611, 1969.

Toner, P. G., Carr, K. E., Ferguson, A., et al.: Scanning and transmission electron microscopic studies of human intestinal mucosa. Gut 11:471, 1970.

Toner, P. G., and Ferguson, A.: Intraepithelial cells in the human intestinal mucosa. J. Ultrastruct. Res. 34:329, 1971.

Trier, J. S., and Browning, T. H.: Epithelial-cell renewal in cultured duodenal biopsies in celiac sprue. N. Engl. J. Med. 283:1245, 1970.

Trier, J. S., and Krone, C. L.: Anatomy, embryology, and congenital abnormalities of the small intestine. In Sleisenger, M. H., and Fordtran, J. S. (Eds.): Gastrointestinal Disease. Philadelphia, W. B. Saunders Co., 1978, p. 979.

Trier, J. S., Phelps, P. C., Eidelman, S., et al.: Whipple's disease: light and electron microscope correlation of jejunal mucosal histology with antibiotic treatment and clinical status. Gastroenterology 48:684, 1965.

Ursing, B., Alm, T., Barany, F., et al.: A comparative study of metronidazole and sulfasalazine for active Crohn's disease: the Cooperative Crohn's Disease Study in Sweden. Gastroenterology 83:550, 1982.

van de Kamer, J. H., ten Bokkel, H., and Weyers, H. A.: Rapid method for determination of fat in feces. J. Biol. Chem. 177:347, 1949.

Waldmann, T. A.: Protein-losing enteropathy. Gastroenterology 50:422, 1966.

Watson, D. W.: Immune responses and the gut. Gastroenterology 56:944, 1969.

Welsh, J. D., Payne, D. L., Manion, C., et al.: Interval sampling of breath hydrogen (H_2) as an index of lactose malabsorption in lactase-deficient subjects. Dig. Dis. Sci. 26:681, 1981.

Weser, E.: Intestinal adaptation to small bowel resection. Am. J. Clin. Nutr. 24:133, 1971.

Weser, E.: Intestinal adaptation after small bowel resection. In Isenberg, J. I (Ed.): Viewpoints on Digestive Diseases. Vol. 10, Number 2. American Gastroenterological Association, Thorofare, New Jersey, 1978.

Weser, E., and Sleisenger, M. H.: Pathophysiology of sprue syndromes. Adv. Intern. Med. *15*:253, 1969.

Williams, L. F., Jr.: Vascular insufficiency of the bowels. D. M., August, 1970.

Williams, L. F., Jr.: Vascular insufficiency of the intestines. Gastroenterology *61*:757, 1971.

Williams, L. F., Jr., and Wittenberg, J.: Vascular insufficiency of the intestine. *In* Isenberg, J. I. (Ed.): Viewpoints on Digestive Diseases. Vol. 5, Number, 2, 1973.

Wilson, F. A., and Dietschy, J. M.: Differential diagnostic approach to clinical problems of malabsorption. Gastroenterology *61*:911, 1971.

Wilson, H.: Carcinoid syndrome. Curr. Probl. Surg. November, 1970, p. 36.

Wilson, H., Cheek, R. C., Sherman, R. T., et al.: Carcinoid tumors. Curr. Probl. Surg., November, 1970, p. 4.

Wingate, D. L.: Backwards and forwards with the migrating complex. Dig. Dis. Sci. *26*:641, 1981.

29

The Large Intestine

William A. Sodeman, Jr., and David W. Watson

INTRODUCTION

The colon, including the rectum, forms the multifunctional termination of the gastrointestinal tract. Its anatomy is substantially differentiated from the relatively uniform muscular tube of the small intestine. The colon is approximately 150 cm long, although its functional length and mucosal surface area are difficult to estimate. It is highly variable in diameter, although as a general rule the cecum is the widest part and the angulation at the rectosigmoid juncture forms its narrowest constriction. The cecum, ascending colon, and proximal one half of the transverse colon are derived from the midgut and share innervation and vascular supply with the small intestine. The distal colon is a hindgut derivative and utilizes the inferior mesenteric artery and sacral parasympathetic innervation. There is substantial anastomosis between the two vascular beds and considerable overlap of innervation, so that these embryonic divisions become indistinct.

The wall of the colon has four layers: mucosa, submucosa, muscularis externa, and serosa. The mucous membrane is not thrown into villous extensions. Scanning electron microscopy (Fig. 29–1) shows a flat epithelial surface broken into polygonal units by clefts. Openings of the numerous goblet cells are apparent, and the center of each polygonal unit is perforated by a crypt of Lieberkühn that is lined with goblet cells and penetrates down to the muscularis mucosa. Cells lining the crypt have been observed to be oriented in spiraling lines. A second larger structural unit consisting of 20 to 100 crypts has been identified under the scanning electron microscope and suggested by cell turnover studies. Both the small and the large units seem to be defined by mucosal vascular patterns. On conventional microscopic examination, the surface epithelial cells present a striated border similar to that of small intestinal cells. Under the electron microscope, the striated border resolves into microvilli complete with a fuzzy coat. There are scattered argentaffin cells. Cell renewal is initiated in the crypts, and cells migrate upward to the surface and are extruded at the midpoint between crypts. The cell renewal time, based on cultured biopsy specimens of the rectum, averages 90 hours. Crypts disappear in the anal canal, and the mucosa is replaced by stratified squamous cell epithelium. The lamina propria is represented by a thin layer of connective tissue that extends between the crypts. The submucosa resembles that of the small intestine, and it contains nerves, plexuses, larger blood vessels, and scattered lymphoid follicles.

The muscular wall of the colon consists of two layers: an inner circular and outer longitudinal layer. Muscle fibers of the inner circular layer deviate from a strict circular orientation; however, because of close attachment to the taeniae it has, thus far, been impossible to identify a helical orientation. The longitudinal layer is gathered into three strips or bundles, the taeniae coli. The taeniae are spaced approximately equally around the circumference of the bowel. One taenia follows the mesenteric attachment. A thin layer of longitudinal muscle bridges the gap between the taeniae. The colon wall presents the appearance of being drawn into multiple loose sacculations, the haustra. Haustrations are most apparent in the transverse colon and may be absent from the descending colon and sigmoid. The haustral folding is a dynamic process that is a result of circular muscle contraction, not puckering by taenial shortening. Each individual apparently has some points of regular haustral folding that are marked histologically by a concentration of muscular tissue and bridging by the serosa; however, intrahaustral folding can occur, so that the radiographic appearance of haustration may seem to vary from time to time (Fig. 29–2).

The mesenteric attachments permit substantial mobility of the colon. Only the descending colon and rectum are relatively fixed structures. The colon is supplied with external sympathetic and parasympathetic innervation and an extensive ganglionic plexus that permits intrinsic reflex innervation. Motor nerves include both excitatory cholinergic and noncholinergic and inhibitory cholinergic and noncholinergic fibers. Classic teaching holds that sympathetic stimulation is inhibitory and parasympathetic activity is stimulatory toward colonic musculature. It must be remembered that the final expression of any sort of stimulation in terms of motility will depend on the state of the intrinsic innervation and that paradoxic responses may occur. From the anatomic standpoint, parasympathetic fibers to the right colon are carried in the vagus, and those that arrive at the left colon come from the second through fourth sacral segments by way of the pelvic nerves. Sympathetic innervation is derived from cord segments thoracic 11 through lumbar 2 and arrives from the mesenteric ganglia in mesenteric and hypogastric nerves.

Integration of motility is the responsibility of the myenteric and submucosal plexuses. When

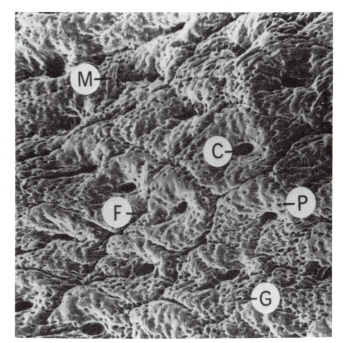

Figure 29–1 Scanning electron micrography of normal rectal mucosa. Each polygonal unit is surrounded by a furrow *(F)*, with the crypt lumen *(C)* opening centrally. Filled *(P)* and empty *(G)* goblet cells and a mucous thread *(M)* can be identified (× 240). (From Kavin, H., et al.: Gastroenterology *59*:426, 1970.)

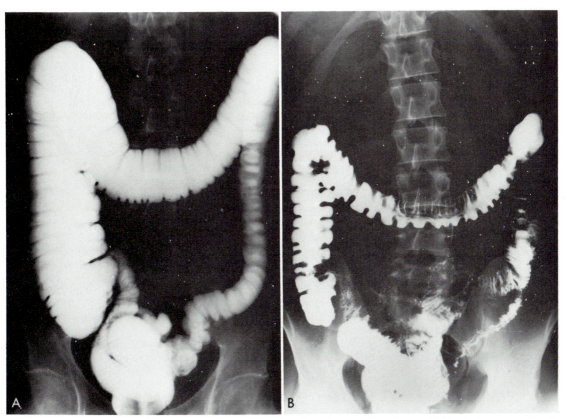

Figure 29–2 *A,* Normal barium enema examination showing both inter- and intrahaustral folds. *B,* Postevacuation film of the same patient showing the position of interhaustral folds.

they are absent, as in megacolon, contractions may continue in the aganglionic segment, but integrated motility is absent. As in the small intestine, the colon contains α- and β-receptors, with β-receptors predominating; however, their function remains poorly elucidated. Central innervation may modify the ganglia activity but it cannot substitute for it. Mechanisms for extrinsic influence on colonic activity originating in the CNS do exist but are poorly understood. There also is substantial evidence for some degree of humoral modification of intestinal activity. This clearly implies further difficulty in assigning roles to the various components of intestinal innervation.

The normal function of the colon encompasses controlled transit, absorption, and, to a limited degree, secretion. These culminate in defecation, a mechanism for elimination of metabolic wastes and dietary residue. It is customary to speak in relatively laudatory terms of the colon's ability to desiccate and evacuate fecal contents, but it seems to us that the task, relative to the magnitude of small intestinal function, is unimpressive. The degree of mixing of intestinal content in the colon makes transit time only a relative approximation. Material ingested as a bolus will become dispersed over a substantial length of bowel and aliquots may appear over several days. When glass beads are ingested, a different color at each of the three meals, their appearance in the stool, including their distribution in the fecal pellet, is completely mixed and it is impossible to tell which color was ingested first. This mixing seems to occur in the cecum and ascending colon. The colonic lumen may contain, alone or in a mixture, material behaving as a solid, liquid, or gas. Transit times do vary with the differing phases. Intestinal gas may transit, mouth to anus, in 1 to 2 hours, with liquids and solids lagging hours to days behind. Actual transit intervals in individuals are affected by a variety of factors, with the quantity of nonabsorbable residue in intestinal contents as a primary factor.

NORMAL MOTOR FUNCTION

ELECTRICAL ACTIVITY

All evidence suggests that the membrane electrical properties of colonic smooth muscle, including the rectum and anal sphincter, resemble those of the remainder of the gastrointestinal tract. Innervation, both extrinsic and intrinsic, plus circulating humoral substances must combine to provide integrated function in the colon. The pacesetter potential, or basic electric rhythm (BER), in the small intestine seemingly acts as a governor initiating and integrating its function. The decreasing aboral gradient of the rhythm of slow-wave depolarization integrates the pattern of flow of small intestinal content, resulting in transit

down the intestine. Net flow down the colon is slower than in the small intestine and is modified by a degree of voluntary control. A simple gradient of BER has not been established in the colon; rather, there is the suggestion that the colon may be divided into several functionally distinct segments. There have been few studies in humans, largely because of technical difficulties. Slow waves have been recorded throughout the colon, in the rectum and anal sphincter in humans. The BER arising in the transverse colon proceeds aborally toward the cecum and adorally toward the rectum. The slow waves are irregular in occurrence. A BER of 9 to 16 cycles per minute has been identified in the transverse and descending colon. No gradient has been identified. Results in the sigmoid have been variable. A rhythm ranging from 8.4 to 10.6 cycles per minute has been recorded; however, such rhythmic activity has been present for only brief intervals in one study, averaging 5 per cent of the total observation time. BER in the rectum has been recorded with a major component of 6 cycles per minute and a minor component of 3 cycles per minute. Spike waves have also been recorded, frequently appearing in bursts. In the small intestine, spikes appear related to circular muscle contraction and can result in intraluminal pressure changes. A relationship among slow waves, spike bursts, contractions, and flow is assumed to prevail in the colon. The internal anal sphincter claims a BER with the highest frequency thus far identified in the intestinal tract, averaging 17 cycles per minute. This has been correlated with high resting tone and active closure of the sphincter. Sphincter relaxation correlates with inhibition of the BER. Curiously, the internal anal sphincter represents the only identification of BER in circular muscle thus far. Our sketchy knowlege of BER in the colon provides us little insight concerning integration of colonic motor activity.

MOTILITY MECHANISMS

Bayless and Starling initiated manometric studies of colonic motility in 1899. Cannon performed contrast studies of the colon in cats in 1902. Holzknecht described mass movement in humans in 1909. To the present, no completely satisfactory description of motility mechanisms in the colon has been forthcoming. A number of technical problems remain. Access to proximal colon has been difficult, and the lumen size plus the character of its contents make motility recording either by a balloon or by open-tip manometry difficult. Radiologic study utilizing contrast material has been hampered by the intermittent nature of colonic mechanisms. Transit is regularly measured in days, yet motility events may be of short duration, separated by long quiet intervals. It is difficult to identify a decisive moment. The few definitive combined radiologic and manometric studies have been burdened with both sets of technical difficulties.

It is important for the interpretation of available information concerning colonic motility to identify the strengths and weaknesses of the methods utilized in its study. The classic approach to motility study utilizes liquid-filled open-tipped tubes or liquid-filled balloon-tipped tubes that are connected to strain gauge manometers. Balloon-tipped tubes not only introduce the artifactual stimulus of the balloon itself but also seem to vary in their response, depending on the proximity of the balloon to the wall of the colon. Open-tipped tubes, even if perfused, face artifactual hazards from the semisolid colonic contents. Finally, in the saccular colon it is clear that pressure changes do not necessarily always reflect contraction of muscle immediately adjacent to the sensor tip. A series of wave patterns of the classic types I, II, III, and IV have been described but they have been difficult to translate into motility events. Colonic activity is best separated into segmentation or kneading by alternate formation and relaxation of haustral-like folds, and transportation, which implies peristalsislike movement over longer segments of bowel. From the clinical standpoint, manometry's most significant contribution has been the identification of the negative relationship between colonic activity and motility. Segmenting activity produces in the colon a state of high resistance to flow. Normal (i.e., slow or controlled) transit is associated with a substantial degree of manometric activity, much of which is segmenting. Peristalsis and mass transit, which can sweep colonic contents over distances of 10 to 100 cm, are found only in the absence of segmenting activity. When mechanisms of mass movement are employed, colons are manometrically quiet except at the instant when the wave of mass movement passes down the bowel. For this reason, anticholinergics that quiet the bowel and reduce segmenting activity are likely to worsen simple diarrhea. Drugs that increase tone and thus trigger spike activity will retard transit, reducing stool frequency in simple diarrhea.

Radiologic assessment of motility likewise has its strengths and weaknesses. Radiographs of hollow viscera all produce negative shadows that depend on the use of contrast material. Both the physical and chemical qualities of the contrast can modify motility. Most contrast media will form a diffuse nonparticulate shadow and one must be satisfied with several assumptions to interpret changes in size, shape, and density of the opacified masses in terms of motility. Changes in density may as easily be the result of dilution by nonopacified material as of the loss of material by transit. Finally, colonic movements are slow and ill-suited to cine recording. Static films are poor records of dynamic events. Several groups of investigators, most notably Ritchie and coworkers, have utilized time-lapse radiography to identify motility mechanisms. They administered a suspension of barium orally, and on the following day performed a time-lapse radiographic study, taking films at intervals of one a minute for a period of 1 to 3 hours. Both control observations and a variety of stimuli have been utilized.

Ritchie's analysis has demonstrated two separate classes of activity (Table 29–1). The first is produced by haustral systole. It may involve one or several haustra. It may or may not result in transit, and transit may be in either direction. The second is progressive contraction of the bowel, a ringlike wave of activity that is propulsive and may go in either direction. These are not the exact equivalents of manometric segmentation and transit. These two broad classes of activity have been further subdivided on the basis of their apparent mechanical effect. The simplest activity is haustral shuttling. This consists of successive formation of a constriction at the midpoint of the haustrum, with relaxation of the immediately preceding and following folds. Colonic content in effect shuttles back and forth from haustrum to haustrum, with mixing but without a net aboral or adoral transit. Ritchie's observations were based on studies of 190 individuals. This sort of activity was observed in 38 per cent of individuals at rest but in only 13 per cent after a meal. As an extension of this simple activity, there is haustral

TABLE 29–1 COLONIC MOTILITY: TYPES OF CONTRACTIONS

Type of Movement	Frequency of Occurrence		Distance Traveled	Rate
	At Rest (%)	Postprandial (%)		
Haustral shuttling	38	13	0	0
Haustral propulsion	36	57	5 to 10 cm	2.5 cm/min
Haustral retropulsion	30	52	5 to 20 cm	2.5 cm/min
Multihaustral propulsion				
Systolic	9	17	Variable	5 cm/min
Serial				2.5 cm/min
Peristaltic ripples	Not Reported	Not Reported	5 to 10 cm	0.1 to 2.0 cm/min
Peristalsis	6	8	18 to 20 cm	1 to 2 cm/min
Mass propulsion	Rare	12	30 cm +	5 to 35 cm/min

(Data taken from Ritchie, J. A.: Gut 9:442, 1968.)

propulsion and retropulsion. This is simple, successive, sequential contraction of individual haustra that does result in movement in one or the other direction. This occurred in 36 per cent of fasting individuals as aboral movement and in 30 per cent as adoral movement. After a meal, aboral movement occurred in 57 per cent of individuals, and adoral movement was experienced by 52 per cent. In some individuals, there was movement in both directions during the period of observation. The distances covered ranged from 5 to 20 cm. A more complex variety of movement was termed *multihaustral propulsion*. This could be systolic or serial. Systolic movement occurred when three or more haustra merged. Transit occurred by the addition of single haustra to the head of the mass, with formation of empty haustra at the tail. Multihaustral propulsion was termed *serial* when three haustra joined. The contents merged, and subsequently one empty haustrum reformed, with the net transfer of its contents to the remaining two.

Activity involving either of these mechanisms was observed in 9 per cent of these individuals at rest and 17 per cent postprandially. Transit could be in either direction and at rates up to 5 cm per minute. Systolic activity appeared best suited to moving fluid contents either alone or around more solid contents without displacement of the solid stool.

Progressive contractions appeared to occur with several degrees of magnitude. Peristaltic ripples are ring contractions that are progressive and that do move contents over 5 to 10 cm lengths. They move at a rate that is usually less than 1 cm a minute. At their maximum, they merge with peristalsis proper, which is a propagated ring contraction carried over a distance of 18 to 20 cm. It is preceded by relaxation and often followed by tonic contraction of the bowel. Some sort of peristalsis was noted to occur in 6 per cent of colons at rest and in 8 per cent postprandially. Contractions of this sort have been noted to move both aborally and adorally. Finally, there is mass propulsion, which is thought to be a peristaltic movement of the colon contents that may empty up to one half the length of the large bowel. This sort of activity was observed in only a few of the individuals studied. Mass propulsion seemed rare in the resting state and in most cases was observed postprandially. Mass propulsion has been noted to move aborally only and at a rapid rate of progression, in the range of 5 to 35 cm per minute. Progressive waves depend on relaxation of interhaustral folds. If the relaxation fails, progressive waves are aborted. Progressive waves move the entire intestinal content, solid or liquid.

There are two other components in motility, the significance of which is not clearly defined. The first is colonic shortening by taenial contraction. This does occur in combination with many of the aforementioned activities, but its role in transit is not clear. Secondly, there are the postural or gravity effects. In an organ in which the lumen is partially open, such as the colon, and which is filled with gaseous, liquid, and semisolid contents, gravity and postural changes have observable effects, but these have been difficult to define, and their significance remains unclear. They are important, however, in pathologic states. Those individuals suffering from diarrhea may achieve some control over their bowel action by simple bed rest. The constipation that plagues many patients upon admission to the hospital with enforced bed rest probably has its origin in the same mechanism.

TRANSIT

Contractile mechanisms not only are complex but also have segmental, or regional, expression. It is rare to observe a completely inactive colon. It is similarly rare to observe a normal colon that is active throughout its entire length. There are nearly always inactive portions. In general, the right colon is responsible for the largest absorption of water and solute. Haustral shuttling and systolic propulsion yield the maximum mucosal contact necessary to make this process efficient.

The left colon is faced with semisolid colonic contents, which it stores and evacuates. This is carried out most economically in terms of effort by serial propulsion and peristalsis. While this is generally true if viewed as a net response, all varieties of activity have been observed throughout the colon. Again, the clearest documentation of the spectrum of segmental activity has come from the work of Ritchie (Table 29–2). He noted marked changes in activity postprandially, with haustral activity most notable in the right colon. Other investigators have suggested that the activity of the distal colon, as measured by the motility index, is enhanced by eating. Stimulation of motor activity in the human sigmoid colon by exogenous cholecystokinin and inhibition of activity by exogenous secretin have been reported. A similar effect has been observed with endogenous release of cholecystokinin. This supports the suggestion that at least some of the integration of colonic activity may rest on hormonal basis though the hormone responsible remains unclear.

In Western man with normal bowel habits, colonic activity is punctuated three times a day by a change in colonic activity that follows eating. Activity as a general rule is enhanced in the postprandial state, but transit down the colon as a whole remains unchanged. Retropulsion apparently balances increased propulsion. Following the ingestion of a meal, there is an increase in ileal activity, with resultant slow filling of the cecum and ascending colon. The ileal influx is shuttled and propelled by systolic haustral contractions. Movement is adoral, resulting in mixing of con-

TABLE 29–2 COLONIC MOTILITY: DISTRIBUTION OF ACTIVITY

	Proportion of Section Remaining Inactive		Proportion of Colon Showing (Nonpropulsive Segmentation)	
	At Rest (%)	Postprandial (%)	At Rest (%)	Postprandial (%)
Cecum and ascending colon	42	16	38	45
Transverse colon	8	5	44	20
Descending colon	25	19	31	18
Pelvic colon	34	26	22	28
Rectum	60	59	20	22
Whole colon (mean)	32	21	35	25

(Data taken from Ritchie, J. A.: Gut 9:502, 1968.)

tents. Peristaltic movements may occur. Gradually, as the prandial stimulus subsides, areas of inactive bowel re-emerge. Retropulsive movements occur in the right colon under the stimulus of a meal but are uncommon at rest. In this fashion the fluid contents of the right colon are rocked back and forth over the absorptive epithelium with each fresh surge of ileal influx. At rest, the net propulsion amounts to about 1 cm per hour. The contents are desiccated, and, as the left colon is approached, the character of the colonic activity changes. At 18 to 24 hours, some portion of the ileal influx will have entered the rectum, but because of mixing, the colon clearance times for the entire bolus will be much longer. Retropulsion increases as the sigmoid region is approached. Gradually the sigmoid fills and periodically material passes on into the rectum. This distention initiates a defecatory urge. Response to this is governed, as will be discussed, by a number of physiologic and environmental variables. Defecation may result in simply local rectal emptying or it may lead to mass propulsion emptying the entire distal colon.

Variations of this normal sequence result not only from changes in the stimulus in the muscle, as by inflammation or distention, but also from changes in the character of the colonic content. This explains why a response to a barium enema bears so little relationship to normal function. The rapid propulsion of gas through the colon and its passage reflect its relatively unaltered state during its passage down the large intestine.

DEFECATION

The rectum constitutes the distal 15 cm of the large intestine. The rectosigmoid junction is indistinct, but the caudal level is well marked by the junction of mucous membrane with the anal canal's transitional epithelium. The rectum below its junction with the sigmoid enlarges to form the rectal ampulla. Above the peritoneal reflection, the rectum is bound to the pelvis by a fibrous sheath, and below the support is provided by the muscles of the pelvic diaphragm. The musculature of the rectum is formed by a continuation of the

colonic muscular coats. The outer longitudinal layer spreads from the taeniae of the sigmoid to form a continuous even coat. The superficial fibers insert into the perineal body and merge with the levator. The deep fibers insert into the perianal skin. The circular muscle differentiates into the internal sphincter surrounding the anal canal. The anus forms the terminal 2 to 4 cm of the intestinal tract. The pectinate line marks the boundary between the anal canal and the rectum. The anus is lined with stratified squamous epithelium.

The external sphincter is made up of striated muscle that lies outside the internal sphincter and extends down below it to encircle the terminal portion of the anal canal. This muscle arises in the central perineum and inserts into the coccyx. The integrated function of the colon, rectum, and sphincters depends on both sensory and motor innervation. Sensory endings are provided with both somatic and autonomic pathways. Sensory pathways for the anal canal and the perianal skin ascend through the somatic nerves to segments S2, S3, and S4. Proprioceptive spindles are present in the striated muscles of the external sphincter. Autonomic sensory innervation for the rectum passes to the same segments, although it does so along parasympathetic pathways. A wide variety of sensory endings are present in both the rectum and anal canal. Motor fibers to the striated external sphincter arrive through the pudendal nerve and the coccygeal plexus and originate in segments S2 to S5. Parasympathetic motor nerves to the internal sphincter descend from L5 and S1 to S3 through the pelvic nerves. These stimuli are inhibitory. Sympathetic fibers arrive via the hypogastric nerve and are excitatory motor stimuli. Sympathetic innervation of the rectum is drawn from L2 to L4, and parasympathetic fibers arrive from S2 to S4.

A variety of mechanisms combine to maintain fecal continence. These include mechanical factors resulting from rectosigmoid angulations and the valves of Houston and reflex sphincter responses. None is as important as the variety of reflex responses that are capable of operating without central control. A degree of basal tone is the feature of both rectum and sphincter. Flow of feces into the rectum gives rise to increase in intraluminal pressure. Sufficient distention stimulates rectal contraction and produces an urge to defecate. If this is denied, the rectum will relax and accommodate the feces, as evidenced by a fall in pressure. When defecation is denied, some feces may be returned to the sigmoid or a higher portion of the colon. When the rectum is distended with volumes of 300 to 400 ml at pressures of 50 mm Hg, defecation becomes imperative. Both sphincters are in a continuous state of contraction. BER identified in the internal sphincter is inhibited by sphincter relaxation. Of the two, the internal sphincter seems to contribute the largest share (85 per cent) of the squeeze closing the anal canal. The external sphincter is variably contracted with posture and other activities that stress continence. Distention of the rectum results in short-lived relaxation of the internal sphincter. That will allow rectal contents to descend into the anal canal far enough to permit their identification by sensory receptors. Voluntary contraction of the external sphincter can maintain continence during the short interval of internal sphincter relaxation. There is a prompt (but poorly understood) increase in external sphincter squeeze that defends continence against increases in intra-abdominal pressure from straining and other activity. Micturition results in reflex relaxation of the external sphincter.

With such a wide variety of reflex controls, anorectal function is susceptible to many sorts of neurologic lesions. These may be grouped into three broad categories:

1. Loss of central innervation with intact sensation. This results in defecatory urge, which, although it cannot be denied, does remain under some local voluntary control.

2. Loss of both sensory and motor control above the sacral outflow, which results in a reflex colon.

3. Loss of the sacral cord or peripheral nerves, which results in an absence of reflex control.

Defecation is initiated in a continent human when the central nervous system accepts the information that the left colon and rectum are primed for defecation and when the environment is deemed acceptable for this activity. Intra-abdominal pressure increases, the sphincters relax, the pelvic floor tenses, and the colon contracts. Evacuation of the distal rectum may be coupled with mass peristalsis, which can empty the colon as high as the splenic flexure, but as often as not it seems to be related to multihaustral movement that empties only the distal end of the colon. Edwards and Beck obtained pre- and postdefecation films of individuals with radiopacified feces. They noted that small quantities of feces moved in and out of the rectum regularly and that a "call to stool" is initiated only when a critical volume to which the individual person is habituated is reached. This differs from the established teaching that the rectum remains empty until immediately prior to defecation, but it confirms the regular clinical observation of feces palpable at the rectal examination. Some individuals empty the rectum only partially, but others empty it completely. A number of factors remain to be defined to understand completely the controls of normal defecation.

NORMAL ABSORPTION AND SECRETION

In addition to regulating transportation and elimination of dietary and metabolic waste, the colon is charged with the task of defending fluid and electrolyte homeostasis in the gastrointestinal tract. Fine regulation of electrolyte and fluid balance belongs to the renal and respiratory systems, yet the flux of liquid and electrolytes across the gastrointestinal mucosa is of such a magnitude that highly developed gastrointestinal regulation is essential.

WATER AND ELECTROLYTES

Under ordinary circumstances, the gastrointestinal tract is presented with a volume of 8 to 9 liters of combined secreted and ingested fluid daily. Absorption by the small intestine will reduce this to a volume of 500 to 600 ml. This daily volume will pass the ileocecal valve carrying an electrolyte load of 40 to 70 mEq of sodium, 3 to 6 mEq of potassium, 20 to 40 mEq of chloride, and 30 to 35 mEq of bicarbonate. Passage through the colon will reduce the volume to 100 ml. Average electrolyte concentrations, based on fecal dialysis studies by Wrong and colleagues, will be as follows: sodium, 30 mEq per liter; potassium, 75 mEq per liter; chloride, 15 mEq per liter; and bicarbonate, 30 mEq per liter. Approximately 50 per cent of the anion in fecal water will be made up of organic anion that results from bacterial action on carbohydrates. The resultant stool will be hyperosmolar (376 mOsm).

The absorptive work is not uniformly distributed down the colon, and there is evidence of regional specialization. The greatest fluid volume and electrolyte absorption occurs in the right colon. The rectum is apparently impermeable to electrolytes and water in short-term studies; however, it is regularly observed clinically that fecal impactions gradually dry to an almost rock-hard consistency. These values for absorption and secretion represent the net result, underlying which may be a substantial effort in terms of flux of electrolytes in both directions across the mucosa (Table 29–3).

In terms of mechanisms, the absorption of water seems to be passive following the osmotic gradient produced by the absorption of sodium. The absorption of sodium is an active process. Absorption may be accomplished against a signif-

TABLE 29–3 COLONIC ABSORPTION AND SECRETION FROM THE COLON

| | | Flux | | Maximum Capacity/24 Hr |
	Average Capacity/24 Hr	Absorbed	Secreted	Net
Water	400 ml	10,800 ml	7800 ml	3000 ml +
Na$^+$	66 mEq +	878	418	460 +
K$^+$	3 mEq −	26	58	32 −

(Data taken from Shields, R., and Miles, J. B.: Postgrad. Med. J. *41*:435, 1965.)

icant concentration gradient. Absorption has been noted from colonic luminal concentrations as low as 25 mM sodium. Sodium is absorbed along an electrical gradient of 30 to 40 mv, mucosa-negative.

Potassium can be secreted into the colon. Several mechanisms may be involved in the entry of potassium into the lumen. Mucus secreted by goblet cells in the colon may contain extraordinary quantities of potassium. Concentrations of up to 140 mEq per liter have been noted. The potassium is not bound and may be reabsorbed, so that the contribution of mucus to potassium secretion will vary with the rapidity of transit and the total quantity of mucus secreted. The majority of potassium passing into the colon does go passively down an electronegative gradient. When luminal potassium concentrations rise above 15 mEq per liter, the flux of potassium changes to absorption rather than excretion. There is no apparent interaction between the transfer of sodium and potassium.

The colon is sensitive to aldosterone and other mineralocorticoids. The effect, increased sodium absorption and potassium secretion, resembles the steroid action on the kidney. A cyclic AMP–dependent mechanism for Na secretion similar to small intestinal response has been suggested.

Chloride has a net absorption that exceeds that of sodium. Chloride transport itself is not active, and it seems to be absorbed as a paired ion with sodium. The absorption of chloride and the secretion of bicarbonate are coupled. In the absence of chloride, bicarbonate will be absorbed as a paired ion with sodium. When chloride is present, bicarbonate will be secreted, apparently in exchange for chloride. Some secreted bicarbonate will combine with organic acids produced by bacteria in the feces. The absorptive capacity of the colon is limited. Calculations based on extrapolations of perfusion results are indicated in Table 29–3, along with the magnitude of the flux and the usual daily load.

NUTRIENTS AND METABOLIC PRODUCTS

The large intestine also has a meager digestive and synthetic role that only rarely may achieve clinical significance. Bacterial digestion does break down some cellulose and hemicellulose, but lignin remains undigested. In constipated individuals with markedly prolonged transit times, colonic digestion of cellulose and absorption can become a significant factor in the diet. In addition to breaking down cellulose, colonic bacteria can synthesize a number of vitamins, most notably folic acid but also including riboflavin, biotin, vitamin K, and nicotinic acid. Failure to produce these compounds can occasionally result in a clinical deficiency. An enterohepatic circulation involving the colon has been identified for several compounds. A urea-ammonia cycle is apparently limited to the colon. The colon also participates in the enterohepatic circulation of bile acids. Urea is synthesized by the liver and enters the systemic circulation. The small intestinal mucosa is permeable to urea, which may diffuse into the lumen, but quantitatively the amount involved is small, less than 500 mg of the 7 gm normally degraded by the gut daily. The colonic mucosa is relatively impermeable to the diffusion of urea in either direction. Circulating blood urea is hydrolyzed in the colonic epithelial wall by bacterial ureases that either penetrate or are closely applied to the mucosa. Most of the ammonia that is produced is absorbed by the circulation. The alkaline pH in the lumen favors the dissociation of any ammonium that may diffuse into it. Free ammonia readily penetrates the mucosa, and the nitrogen is returned to the liver for resynthesis of urea or use in protein synthesis. This colonic conservation of nitrogen may achieve clinical importance in the face of protein malnutrition. The apparent involvement of blood urea rather than luminal urea helps explain the success of systemic urease inhibitors such as acetohydroxamic acid in treatment of hepatic encephalopathy.

Synthesis of bile acids by the liver is limited. The bile acid pool, which varies from 1.2 to 6.0 gm, is conserved by cycling through the enterohepatic circulation. In the course of 6 to 10 cycles a day, a small amount escapes the small intestinal absorption mechanism. The daily fecal excretion amounts to an average of 500 mg of bile acid. Chenodeoxycholic acid escaping into the colon is dehydroxylated by bacteria to form lithocholic acid, which is nonabsorbable and is excreted. It accounts for 300 mg of the 500 mg of bile acid lost daily. Cholic acid is dehydroxylated to desoxycholic acid, and about half of this will be reabsorbed by the colon. Since 200 mg is lost in the feces, there must be addition to the bile acid pool of approximately 200 mg of this secondary bile acid daily from the colon.

DRUGS

A wide variety of drugs are regularly administered by enema or suppositories. Salicylates, sedatives, antiemetics, opiates, bronchodilators, tranquilizers, and selected antibiotics all have significant absorption and systemic effect. A number of agents administered for local action, such as corticosteroids and neomycin, may have significant systemic absorption that will limit their use.

A seemingly endless number of drugs have been administered rectally without successful systemic absorption. Chloramphenicol, tetracycline, and sulfonamides are erratically absorbed by the rectal mucosa, although they may be well absorbed by the oral route. There are no identified carrier mechanisms in the colonic mucosa. Absorption depends on several factors. Small molecules may diffuse through the pores in the colonic epithelium. They could be carried in by water during its passive absorption. Rectal absorption of water and electrolytes is markedly restricted if it occurs at all, and hence the absorption of a drug by diffusion will depend on the level to which the preparation is carried in the colon. Its retention time will also be a critical factor that determines absorption. This may well account for the erratic absorption of many of the antibiotic compounds. As a general rule, compounds that remain in a lipid-soluble state at colonic pH are better absorbed. They presumably dissolve through the lipid-containing cell membrane. Some drugs such as neomycin are as well absorbed rectally as they are orally, and the absorption appears completely unaffected by retention time or other identifiable factors. The mechanism of their absorption remains to be defined. An additional avenue for absorption may be available for those agents that are used topically in the treatment of inflammatory bowel disease. The ulcer bed and denuded mucosa expose deeper, perhaps barrier-free areas that may permit absorption.

GAS

The gastrointestinal tract contains an average of 100 ml of gas, and daily elimination as flatus amounts to 1 liter. This may be subject to wide variation with changes in diet. Although gas may be distributed down the entire length of the intestinal tract, a substantial percentage of it accumulates in the colon. Gas passed rectally is made up of swallowed air, gas diffusing across the mucosa from the circulation, and gas produced by bacteria in the small intestine and colon. Its final

composition will obviously reflect the activity of these various sources. In addition to oxygen, nitrogen, and carbon dioxide, methane and hydrogen may be major components of flatus. A number of gaseous components are present in trace amounts. Swallowed air contains small quantities of the rare gases, and a number of volatile metabolic products may be present. These can include ammonia, hydrogen sulfide, skatole, indole, and fatty acids. Ordinarily, these represent less than 1 per cent of flatus.

Hydrogen is produced by bacteria, and in the absence of bacterial overgrowth of the small intestine it is derived primarily from the colon. There is no other source for production of gaseous hydrogen in the human body. Methane is similarly produced by bacterial fermentation in the intestine. Bacteria utilize only substrate found within the lumen, and production of gas is related to the numbers of gas-forming bacilli and the dietary availability of suitable substrate. Carbon dioxide may be swallowed, but more significant amounts are produced in the intestinal tract as a consequence of neutralization of acid by bicarbonate. Free carbon dioxide is in equilibrium with bicarbonate and with circulating carbon dioxide. It can diffuse across the mucosa. A similar equilibrium exists for nitrogen and oxygen. In the colon, bacterial utilization of oxygen may result in extremely low or negligible concentrations of oxygen. In this fashion, an anaerobic environment may be maintained within the colon.

Passage of gas through the colon may be far more rapid than liquid or semisolid feces. Resistance to flow by haustration is substantially less effective for gases than it is for liquids. Also, colonic activity is usually sufficient to prevent layering of fluid and solid fecal contents into separate phases, but it is insufficient to prevent the separation of a gaseous phase. This makes possible the differential motility of gas in the colon.

DISORDERS OF MOTOR AND ABSORPTIVE FUNCTIONS

DIARRHEA WITH NORMAL-APPEARING COLON

Diarrhea may be a result of a wide variety of stimuli. The final common path resulting in frequent stools lies with an increase in the volume load, a decrease in the absorptive capacity, or in rapid transit. Occasionally, stimulation of colonic secretion may be a factor. The number of pathophysiologic mechanisms that may lead through one or several of these pathways is huge, and a comprehensive discussion is beyond the limits of this chapter. In this and subsequent sections, examples utilizing each of the pathways will be presented, and it should be remembered that these are illustrative and not a complete portrayal. It is rare to find only a single mechanism operative, and even in an apparently pure disorder, there may be secondary involvements of several mechanisms ultimately producing the diarrhea. This feature has important therapeutic implications. Without this concept clearly in mind, one may find the use of some agents (and their success) in the treatment of diarrhea paradoxic. This is particularly true with regard to the use of hydroscopic, bulk-producing materials in the treatment of diverticulosis and irritable bowel syndrome.

The primary causes of most diarrheal disease without structural abnormality remain either hidden (i.e., idiopathic) or beyond any reasonable hope of control, and one relies on a number of nonspecific agents to obtain symptomatic relief. There are a few circumstances in which the primary pathologic condition is identifiable and susceptible to modification. Diarrhea associated with hyperthyroidism presumably represents an extension of the general hypermetabolic state. Control of excess circulating thyroid hormone, medically or surgically, offers primary control of diarrhea. Similarly, epinephrine-producing neurogenic tumors offer an identifiable mechanism. In addition, the case for an excitatory role for sympathetic innervation is strengthened by the clinical observation of the result of these tumors. Although resection of the tumor may not always be feasible, the use of epinephrine-blocking agents offers a therapeutic avenue. Diarrhea may be associated with certain medullary tumors of the thyroid. This is thought to be related to release of a prostaglandin. Some non-β islet cell tumors of the pancreas produce vasoactive intestinal peptide (VIP), which stimulates both small and large intestinal secretion. The syndrome of watery diarrhea and hypokalemia has occurred in individuals with the Zollinger-Ellison syndrome when multiple mechanisms have been thought to be active. The gastric hypersecretion constitutes a fluid load. The acid overload can damage small intestinal mucosa as well as precipitate bile acids and interfere with micelle formation and fat digestion. Pancreatic enzymes may be denatured by the acid, adding a component of pancreatic insufficiency. Primary mechanisms of this sort deserve specific therapy. However, in absolute numbers they form a relatively insignificant proportion of the diarrheal disease. One identifiable primary mechanism that is significant is lactose malabsorption. Many individuals on a constitutional or acquired basis will have a decline in lactase activity in the small intestine following weaning. The final level of lactase activity seems to vary from individual to individual. When the small intestinal mucosa is stressed with a lactose load beyond its metabolic capacity, the unsplit disaccharide will be carried down the small intestine and discharged into the colon. In the colon, lactose can serve as a substrate, and it will be fermented by a variety of bacteria. The fermentation process produces lactic acid and gas. The combination of volume and the acid stimulus pro-

duces intestinal hyperactivity that may be manifested by audible intestinal sounds, cramping abdominal pain, and occasionally diarrhea. Small intestinal lactase does appear to be an inducible enzyme in some animals. However, it remains to be demonstrated that the enzyme level is inducible in humans. The only effective therapy at this time is either the elimination of lactose from the diet or use of exogenous lactase to produce a reduction to levels that an individual may tolerate.

Simple Diarrhea

Volume overload of the colon resulting in frequent stools probably represents the commonest of gastrointestinal afflictions. The colonic overload in simple diarrhea is a product of disturbed small intestinal function. Cholera is a classic example. Exposure of small intestinal mucosa to cholera toxin results in activation of the adenylate cyclase system regulating sodium secretion. Massive flux of sodium and fluid into the bowel lumen is the result. This secretion exceeds the reabsorptive capacity of the small intestine and the colon. The colon simply fills to capacity, and watery diarrhea ensues. The radiologists can ordinarily fill a colon at the time of barium enema with 1500 ml of barium suspension. Patients with full-blown cholera ordinarily produce watery stools at the rate of 500 ml per hour. Cholera as a clinical entity is exotic. The diarrhea of travelers (enteropathogenic *Escherichia coli* infection), viral gastroenteritis, clostridial and staphylococcal enterotoxin food poisoning, and the use of saline cathartics represent more practical clinical extensions of the concept of simple volume overload of the colon. Although the colon is capable of absorbing up to 3000 ml of fluid daily (Table 29–3), this represents a relatively meager absorption capacity of 125 ml per hour, or slightly more than 2 ml a minute. It is not difficult for a volume load to exceed these limits over a short time. One effect of the volume load is a change in the ionic composition of the stool. As the volume increases, so does the sodium concentration, and the potassium content of the stool decreases. Gradually, at a volume of approximately 3000 ml of stool a day, the ionic composition approaches that of normal plasma. Clearly, there must also be some alteration in intestinal motility; however, this is less impressive in simple diarrhea than in the irritable colon syndrome and inflammatory bowel disease. Perhaps the absence of the motility components is more apparent than real, since, as will be discussed, the motility alterations associated with diarrhea produce a quiet colon.

Irritable Colon Syndrome

A great deal of human emotion is expressed by conscious voluntary activity such as a smile, clearing of the throat, or a nod of the head. Often, the translation of the emotional content into activity, such as applause, will vary from culture to culture. There is a similar body of reflex emotional expression, such as blushing or weeping, over which voluntary control has never been remarkably effective. Some reflex emotional responses cross the rather indistinct boundary that separate physiologic from pathologic response. It is not uncommon to identify individuals who respond to stress with urticaria, asthma, or emesis. When the emotional expression alters intestinal motility and absorption, producing pain or diarrhea or both, often alternating with constipation, the condition is described as the *irritable colon syndrome.*

The stringent limits that we as individuals set to identify as our normal bowel habits are more often culturally than physiologically inspired. Much, but not all, of what is diagnosed as irritable bowel syndrome is hardly disease, yet patients can be effectively disabled.

Three other factors seem to have a strong impact on the expression of irritable colon. One is a poorly understood constitutional or familial factor, about which little more can be said than that it exists. Second, the observation has been made that individuals with irritable bowel syndrome have a preponderance of a fast BER (3 cycles per minute) in the distal colon when contrasted with normal individuals. Hormonal stimuli such as CCK produce a contractile response that matches the 3 cycles per minute BER. The last factor is related to irritants. These may be infections, respiratory as well as gastrointestinal, or, more commonly, food irritants. Food as an irritant seems as often as not to represent an idiosyncratic response of an individual rather than the expression of a toxic food. The kind of food that precipitates symptoms varies widely from individual to individual. This brings the full circle back to emotional factors.

There is, to be sure, an element of emotional overlay that will accompany any of the colonic afflictions discussed in this chapter. Also, there is great individual variation in terms of colonic response to emotional stress. The various appellations applied to the irritable colon syndrome (i.e., *spastic gut, psychophysiologic gastrointestinal reaction, functional bowel syndrome, and mucous colitis*) indicate that in many people the emotional disturbance predominates. When irritable colon syndrome is seemingly not an extension of organic disease, that is, when it is truly idiopathic, it poses a challenge to physicians to achieve symptomatic control in the patient. It is true that patients with irritable colon syndrome must once have included those individuals with lactose intolerance, amebiasis, *Campylobacter* enteritis, and a wide variety of other identifiable colonic diseases, and there probably remain some primary mechanisms yet to be identified and extracted. However, this does not make it a "wastebasket" diagnosis. Clearly, an

exaggerated response to stress can, alone and unaided, be responsible for both the spastic and diarrheal varieties of irritable colon syndrome.

From the standpoint of pathologic physiology, irritable colon syndrome may be separated into two varieties—spastic and diarrheal. The spastic variety presents clinically with an alteration in bowel habits and abdominal pain. Diarrhea may alternate with constipation. The cramping abdominal pain seems to be the key clinical feature in determining the pathophysiology. Individuals with this illness experience a stimulation of haustral contractions. Vigorous segmental contractions produce closed chambers containing trapped fluid and gas. Further contractions result in increased tension in the colonic wall and cramping abdominal pain. Increased segmentation yields a high resistance state within the colon, and there will be little effective transit. As the increased segmentation subsides, haustral transit may occur and peristaltic activity may be stimulated; thus, the cramping abdominal pain may terminate in a diarrheal rush.

The diarrheal form of the syndrome is relatively more simple in clinical appearance. Patients do not have cramping abdominal discomfort, although there may be ample audible intestinal activity. The call to stool may be precipitated and result in passage of a liquid stool. A sequence of response with a number of watery stools in progressively smaller volume, beginning on rising and terminating with the patient remaining relatively symptom-free for the remainder of the day, is not uncommon.

With this variety, the mechanism seems to be related to a quiet colon. Manometrically, there is an absence of the phasic contractions that are usually identified with segmentation. In this case, small changes in pressure may result in substantial flow down the lower resistance colon. Absence of haustral activity sets the stage for peristalsis and mass movement. The response by the sigmoid colon to the ingestion of food may be a normal increase in phasic contraction, but this quickly fades at the termination of the meal, and the colon returns to its basic hypotonic state.

Either variety of irritable colon syndrome may be associated with increased mucus secretion. Occasionally, this may present as spectacular ropy strands of mucus passed in the stool without apparent associated feces. More often, small amounts of mucus will collect in the rectum, just above the sphincter. The quantity will be too small to act as a stimulus, but the patient quickly learns that the passage of flatus may prove embarrassing. This additional anxiety and the necessity to retreat to the toilet to pass flatus further compound the irritable colon syndrome.

Each mechanism implies specific therapy. In the spastic variety, anticholinergics, which have been noted manometrically to inhibit phasic activity, may give a measure of control over the cramping abdominal pain. For this to occur, the dose must be carried to a critical level. The inhibition of phasic activity carried to completion may exacerbate the diarrheal component as the colon is reduced to a low-resistance state. It takes great patience to direct anticholinergic therapy in this situation. Irritable bowel of the diarrheal variety obviously responds poorly to anticholinergics. The addition of opiates, which enhance tone and may stimulate phasic activity, and the use of hydroscopic bulk agents, which act to increase resistance to fluid flow, constitute a better and more effective regimen. In either case, the thoughtful selection of sedatives and tranquilizers may support the regimen.

Bile Acid Diarrhea

Bile acid diarrhea illustrates a third general response to the development of diarrhea in a normal-appearing colon. Suitable concentrations of conjugated and unconjugated dihydroxy bile acids in the colon stimulate secretion of sodium and water. This produces diarrhea by a volume overload that has its primary genesis within the colon itself.

Disorders of the enterohepatic circulation of bile acids may lead to diarrhea by a number of mechanisms. When the bile acid circulation is broken and the pool size falls, the concentration of bile entering the duodenum may be insufficient to permit complete fat absorption. Steatorrhea, often with diarrhea, may result. In small intestinal stasis syndrome, bacterial deconjugation of bile acids may lead to similarly insufficient levels of bile acid for the formation of micelles and fat absorption. The diarrhea under these circumstances is a result of hepatic and small intestinal failure. When the enterohepatic circulation is broken because of ileal dysfunction and failure of active ileal absorption of bile acids, larger than normal quantities of bile acids may pass into the colon. Experimentally, perfusion of the human colon with deconjugated dihydroxy bile acids in a concentration of 3 to 5 mM produces a marked secretion of sodium and water. A cyclic AMP–dependent Na secretory mechanism has been suggested. Equimolar mixtures of conjugated bile acids cause similar secretion of sodium and water plus additional secretion of potassium and bicarbonate. The magnitude of secretion is sufficient to explain diarrhea associated with an enterohepatic circulation broken at the ileal level. Inhibition of absorption of water and electrolyte by bile acid has also been observed. Successful therapy of bile acid diarrhea has been described using cholestyramine, a resin that binds bile acid. Successful application of cholestyramine requires a careful selection, for although it reduces bile acid effects, it increases steatorrhea. There is a relatively limited zone in which the net result is an effective reduction of diarrhea.

DIARRHEA WITH STRUCTURAL CHANGES IN THE COLON: INFLAMMATORY BOWEL DISEASE

Inflammatory disease of the wall of the colon results in diarrhea by one or a combination of several mechanisms. Mucosal erosion and ulceration destroy the epithelial barrier and leave a raw exuding surface. When the stool content is primarily exudate, blood, and necrotic epithelium, the clinical diagnosis of dysentery is appropriate, and widespread colonic disease may be suspected. Amebae, *Shigella, Campylobacter jejuni* and *Clostridium difficile* toxin that produces pseudomembranous enterocolitis are perhaps the commonest specific agents producing dysenteric symptoms. Pathologic changes are not limited to the mucosal inflammation. Inflammatory cell infiltration and ulceration may extend into the submucosa and the muscularis. Rarely, septic perforation will occur. The extension of inflammatory disease to deeper levels, with resultant infiltration and edema, changes the physical characteristics of the wall, particularly the stiffness, and, because of irritation of nerve plexuses, it may alter motility mechanisms. In the presence of active inflammation, it is common to see absence of haustration, with resultant low resistance to flow down the colonic lumen. As inflammation subsides and healing occurs, several varieties of derangement are possible, depending on the pattern of fibrosis that evolves. If the fibrotic reaction is diffuse, the pattern of absent haustration may solidify. This is best exemplified in the hosepipe appearance of the colon in burnt-out chronic ulcerative colitis and is a less frequent but not unheard of sequela of specific infectious colitis. Changes of this sort require rather massive involvement of the colon or prolonged repetitive bouts of inflammation. When fibrosis is localized, a partial or complete stricture may result. Complete obstruction in the large intestine, whether by stricture or volvulus or whatever mechanism, results in changes similar to those described in the small intestine. In individuals with a competent ileocecal valve, the added complication of closed loop obstruction with toxic dilatation can occur. When stricture produces only partial obstruction, the distention may result in an irritable focus with a distal increase in transit, producing diarrhea.

Several agents that produce inflammatory bowel changes do not ordinarily present with widespread colonic disease. Amebic, tuberculous, and fungal infections typically present with a regional involvement. The usual involvement is cecal and is thought to be related to stasis in the cecal segment. For most organisms, this location represents the first point of slowing of the intestinal stream, affording an opportunity for prolonged contact by multiple organisms that is necessary for penetration of the epithelial barrier. It is also possible that the relative fluidity and concentration of nutrients plus the favorable redox potential in the cecum play an important role in the establishment of infection in this area. Regional infection is also common in the rectosigmoid, the other point of relative stasis of the fecal stream. In addition to an ulcerative inflammatory response, a proliferative granulomatous response to most of these agents may occur. These infectious pseudotumors can disorder motility and result in diarrhea. Several of the parasites, particularly schistosomes, produce colonic lesions by embolization or deposition of ova in the intestinal wall. With the development of delayed immune sensitivity, a granulomatous reaction surrounds these lesions, which may ulcerate through the mucosa or may produce proliferative granulomatous polyps. In all these cases, specific and effective chemotherapy can halt progression of these lesions. However, their resolution may lead to significant structural changes and to the production of additional symptoms.

Diverticular Disease of the Colon

Diverticula in the colon represent outpouchings or herniations of mucosa and submucosa between fasciculi of the circular muscle of the colonic wall. True diverticula contain all coats of the colon wall, similar to Meckel's diverticula in the small intestine. These do occur, but they are extremely rare. The usual diverticula form in response to two sets of circumstances. In the colon there are, in effect, two kinds of diverticular disease: simple diverticulosis and spastic diverticulosis. Both may eventuate in inflammatory bowel disease; however, in both the inflammation is a late phenomenon complicating the end stage of the disease. In the absence of inflammation, simple diverticula are silent and usually unassociated with any symptoms. Some workers have felt that they are the sequelae of the diarrheal variety of irritable bowel syndrome. The diverticula of spastic diverticulosis are not asymptomatic. Here the disease is felt to be an extension of the spastic variety of irritable bowel syndrome. Thus, pain and alteration of bowel habits will precede the development of diverticula.

Simple diverticula are outpouchings through weakened portions of an otherwise normal circular muscle. They increase in frequency with age, and after age 40 years, 5 per cent or more of the population of the United States will have demonstrable diverticula. Constitutional and environmental factors are thought to be major factors in their occurrence. Diverticula are rare among African and Asian populations. Simple diverticula represent herniations at points of anatomic weakness, often at points of penetration of the musculature by arteries. While single scattered diverticula are common, occasional individuals may present with massed simple diverticula. With massed diverticula, each herniation is thought to be the result of increased pressure pushing the

mucosa through the muscular defect. The result is an apparent shortening of the colon, because the total area of the mucosa remaining to line the lumen is smaller. This apparent shortening is unassociated with inflammation and is a simple mechanical phenomenon. Simple diverticula may become inflamed, just as any outpouching of the gut may in a fashion similar to the appendix develop intraluminal inflammation. This sort of inflammation seems to be a rare occurrence. However, rupture of inflamed simple diverticula with peritonitis, abscess, and fistula have been reported. Inspissated contents may produce ulceration of the diverticulum neck. Because of the close association of many simple diverticula with small arteries, the ulceration can lead to spectacular lower gastrointestinal bleeding. Right-sided diverticula may bleed for this reason as readily as those on the left. Selective angiography is apparently the most reliable method of identifying the bleeding diverticula. Bleeding diverticula are notoriously inapparent at surgery and may require multiple colostomies for their identification. Selective infusion of epinephrine or vasopressin through arterial catheters offers some hope for medical therapy of massive bleeding from this source. Evidence suggests that many colonic bleeds in elderly patients are secondary to the development of submucosal vascular ectasias. These are degenerative lesions that increase in frequency with aging. Commonly they are multiple.

Spastic diverticulosis, which is limited in distribution to the sigmoid and distal descending colon, is an entirely different entity in terms of its pathologic physiology. The circular muscle in the distal colon is organized into fasciculi or rings. There are fibers that bridge from one ring to another ring, but the general structural orientation remains and is visible in a longitudinal cross section of the bowel. In certain individuals with a spastic variety of irritable colon syndrome, these rings of sigmoid musculature begin to undergo remarkable muscular hypertrophy with a crowding together of the muscle fibers. This hypertrophy usually is eccentric and will involve only a portion of the circumference of a ring. The portion of the colonic wall running between the mesenteric taenia and the two antimesenteric taeniae is involved. The remaining one third of the circumference of the wall lying between the two antimesenteric taeniae is relatively spared. The muscular hypertrophy permits the formation of multiple closed chambers from the lumen of the sigmoid, and within these chambers there may be significant increase in intraluminal pressure as a result of contraction of the hypertrophied circular muscle (Fig. 29–3). This increase in tension results in cramping abdominal pain. The muscular thickening and crowding of the circular muscle yields a characteristic pattern on radiographic examination, often termed a *sawtooth deformity* (Fig. 29–4). The wall thickening may also present as a palpable mass. All these features—the pain, the

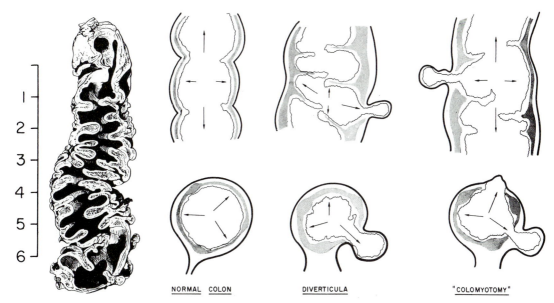

Figure 29–3 Figure on left is a drawing of a gross specimen of a sigmoid colon that is involved in sigmoid diverticulitis. The hypertrophied rings of circular muscle that give rise to the saw-tooth deformity on radiographs are clearly apparent. The remainder of the illustration indicates the mechanism of formation of diverticula and their relief by colomyotomy (see also Fig. 29–4). (From Ranson, J. H. C., et al.: Am. J. Surg. *123*:185, 1972.)

NORMAL COLON   DIVERTICULA   "COLOMYOTOMY"

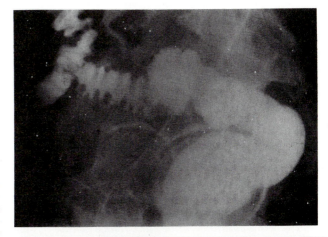

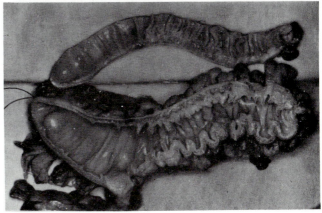

Figure 29–4 Photograph of a gross specimen of sigmoid colon *(bottom)* and a preoperative barium enema of this colon *(top)* showing the abrupt change from normal sigmoid to that involved with hypertrophy of the circular muscle. The saw-tooth, or serrated, deformity is easily visualized on radiographs. (From Arfwidsson, S.: Acta Chir. Scand. Supplement *342*:40, 1964.)

mass, and the radiologic abnormality—may present in the absence of inflammation and have been reported in the absence of diverticula. Diverticula form in a fashion similar to that of simple diverticula as herniations of mucosa blown out through weakened areas between the hypertrophied fasciculi of the circular muscle. Occasionally, the increased pressure generated in the closed chamber will cause a perforation of the tip of the diverticulum. This can give rise to the formation of pericolitis, abscess, peritonitis, and fistula formation. This then represents true diverticulitis and will also give rise to a palpable mass and pain. It may be distinguished from the noninflammatory "diverticulitis" by the presence of fever, leukocytosis, and the finding of extravasated barium at the time of enema. Treatment will vary with the stage of the disease. When perforation and pericolitis occur, the patient must be treated as any perforated viscus is treated. Recurrent diverticulitis may be a management problem. Connell treats recurrent pericolitis with intermittent courses of nonabsorbable sulfa for periods of 4 to 5 days each month. In the absence of inflammation, two courses are currently open. Long sigmoid myotomy dividing the hypertrophied rings of muscle but without penetrating the mucosa has been reported to give symptomatic relief (Fig. 29–3). The use of high-residue diets based largely on bran content has been reported to yield relief of symptoms that is maintained indefinitely. If the relationship between spastic irritable bowel and spastic diverticulitis is verified, earlier and more aggressive therapy of the former may be preventative.

Idiopathic Chronic Inflammatory Bowel Disease

On the basis of clinical and histopathologic features, two distinct forms of chronic inflammatory bowel disease are currently recognized. The utility of this separation derives from differences in histologic appearances and clinical events that reflect different patterns of morbidity and mortality. The terms *ulcerative colitis* and *Crohn's disease* have been most frequently applied to these disorders, but in the colon the latter has also been frequently referred to as *granulomatous colitis, transmural colitis,* or *ileocolitis* when disease is present in both the small and the large bowel. The differential features of the two conditions are summarized in Table 29–4. This separation into two seemingly distinct conditions, however, should not obscure their obvious interrelationship, which is expressed most fully in the colon, in which the distinction between ulcerative and granulomatous colitis at times may not be possible. If the morbid anatomy characteristic of each form is kept in mind, the clinical differences between the two are more readily appreciated. In classic Crohn's disease, the submucosal edema and fibrosis and the

deep fissure ulcers often lead to partial intestinal obstruction and fistulae, whereas the mucosal ulceration characteristic of ulcerative colitis more commonly results in hemorrhage and perforation. In the colon, however, chronic inflammatory bowel disease often presents a mixed histologic appearance, with a corresponding overlapping of clinical manifestations.

Ulcerative Colitis

Although occurring most frequently in Great Britain, North America, New Zealand, and Australia, ulcerative colitis has a worldwide distribution, as evidenced by reports from Costa Rica, Africa, and India. The peak incidence occurs in the second and third decades, with a smaller peak observed after 60 years of age. A genetic predisposition appears likely for the following reasons: (1) the higher incidence in Jews and the less common occurrence among blacks; (2) a familial occurrence ranging between 5 and 12 per cent that is interdependent with Crohn's disease; (3) an association with ankylosing spondylitis, which itself has genetic determinants; and (4) the presence of anticolon antibodies in healthy relatives. With respect to ankylosing spondylitis, it should be noted that the prevalence of the histocompatibility antigen HLA-B27 found in that disorder does not occur in ulcerative colitis except in association with spondylitis.

Efforts to determine the cause of ulcerative colitis have emphasized infectious, psychogenic, and immunologic factors. An infectious origin appears highly unlikely, and the potential influence of psychogenic factors probably has been overemphasized. It has been widely held that patients with ulcerative colitis exhibit a characteristic personality type, but the few controlled studies available fail to demonstrate a relationship between ulcerative colitis and various psychologic parameters. Some type of immune reaction involving small lymphocytes and bacterial or colonic antigens appears most likely, but present evidence is inconclusive. Circulating lymphocytes have been demonstrated to be cytotoxic for colon epithelial cells, and this effect can be modified by bacterial extracts. Recent evidence suggests these may be Fc-receptor cells "armed" by antigen-antibody complexes containing colonic or bacterial antigens.

Although primarily a disorder of the colon, it is clear that ulcerative colitis is often a systemic disease exhibiting a wide range of extracolonic manifestations. These are listed in Table 29–5.

The colon's contribution to the clinical picture is in the form of some combination of diarrhea, hematochezia, and cramping lower abdominal pain. The intensity of these symptoms varies widely between patients and from time to time in the same patient. Onset may be gradual or fulminant, and the course may be chronic and contin-

TABLE 29–4 PATHOLOGIC FEATURES OF CROHN'S DISEASE AND ULCERATIVE COLITIS

	Crohn's Disease	Ulcerative Colitis
Gross Features		
Anal and perianal lesions	Major and common	Minor and uncommon
Bowel wall	Thickened	Normal to slight increase
Strictures	Common	Uncommon
Fistulas	Common	Rare
Pseudopolyps	Rare	Common
Ulcers	"Fissure"	Punctate to troughlike
Distribution	More proximal	More distal
Continuity	Often "skip" areas	Always contiguous
Toxic megacolon	Uncommon	More common
Carcinoma	Rare	Increased
Microscopic Features		
Primary impact	Submucosa	Mucosa
Type of reaction	Productive	Exudative
Lymphoreticular hyperplasia	Marked and transmural	Minimal and superficial
Granulomas	40 to 80%	Occasional
Crypt abscesses	Occasional	Usual
Vascular ectasia and edema	Marked	Related to acute inflammation
Epithelial regeneration	Rare	Common

(Watson, D. W.: Calif. Med. *117*:25, 1972.)

uous or remittent and relapsing. Asymptomatic intervals vary from a few weeks to many years, but eventual relapse is the rule, the rate varying between 27 and 50 per cent per year. Fever and leukocytosis may occur with acute attacks, and hypoalbuminemia and anemia are common. The latter is most often due to blood loss, but other causes include malabsorption of iron, autoimmune hemolytic anemia, microangiopathic hemolytic anemia, G6PD deficiency, and Heinz body anemia related to sulfasalazine therapy.

Diagnosis depends on observation of characteristic features of the disease by proctosigmoidoscopy or barium enema. Since both gross and microscopic features are nonspecific, it is also important to exclude bacterial and parasitic infections, especially in patients with acute disease of recent onset. Classically, the mucosa appears hyperemic, edematous, granular, and friable, often with fine ulcerations and active bleeding. Involvement is always continuous over the length involved. Rectal biopsy may reveal characteristic but nonspecific changes and will always be abnormal in the presence of active disease or demonstrable disease elsewhere in the colon. A histologically normal rectum in the presence of more proximal disease is highly unlikely in ulcerative colitis and favors a diagnosis of Crohn's disease. The radiographic appearance of ulcerative colitis is well known, and only a few comments are appropriate here. In more acute phases, there will be rather broad-based mucosal ulcerations, edema of the mucosa, and often loss of haustrations. More chronic involvement is manifested by loss of mucosal detail, loss of haustrations, shortening of the colon, widening of the retrorectal space, pseudopolyps, and occasionally rectovaginal or rectovesical fistulae. The terminal ileum may be involved with a superficial "backwash" ileitis in about 10 per cent of cases. Involvement begins distally and proceeds proximally always in a continuous fashion without skip areas. There is little or no fibrosis even with long-standing disease, and the majority of radiographic findings, including shortening and loss of haustrations, are potentially reversible.

TABLE 29–5 EXTRACOLONIC MANIFESTATIONS OF ULCERATIVE COLITIS

Skin lesions
  Erythema nodosum
  Erythema multiforme
  Pyoderma gangrenosum
  Nonspecific pustular dermatosis
Mucous membrane lesions
  Aphthous stomatitis
  Ulcerative esophagitis
Eye lesions
  Episcleritis
  Uveitis
  Iritis
  Conjunctivitis
  Marginal corneal ulceration
Bone and joint lesions
  Arthralgias
  Sacroiliitis
  Arthritis of ulcerative colitis
  Ankylosing spondylitis
  Rheumatoid arthritis
Hepatobiliary lesions
  Active chronic hepatitis
  Pericholangitis
  Unclassified inflammatory changes
  Cirrhosis (postnecrotic and biliary)
  Carcinoma of extrahepatic bile ducts
  Primary sclerosing cholangitis
Pericarditis
Renal calculi

Complications include severe hemorrhage, perforation, toxic megacolon, malnutrition, carcinoma of the colon, and, in children, growth retardation and failure of sexual development. Three high-risk factors have been identified with respect to the development of carcinoma of the colon: (1) onset in childhood, (2) total or near total colonic involvement, and (3) duration of disease longer than 10 years. Obstruction and fistulization are seldom encountered in patients with ulcerative colitis.

All nonsurgical treatment is empirical and symptomatic. Emphasis has been placed upon the administration of sulfasalazine (salicylazosulfapyridine), measures to control diarrhea, and the use of systemic or topical steroids. Both sulfasalazine and corticosteroids may suppress active disease, but only the former has demonstrated prophylactic value in continuing remissions. The aforementioned complications are frequent indications for colectomy, but the most frequent reason for surgical intervention in patients with ulcerative colitis continues to be intractability and failure of medical management. Although some physicians continue to employ subtotal colectomy, there is a growing emphasis upon one-stage total proctocolectomy and permanent ileostomy.

The outcome of the disease is most dependent on the age of the patient, the extent of the involvement, and the severity of the current attack. Mortality is highest in those above the age of 60 years, those with total involvement and the severest attacks. The single most important factor governing prognosis is the severity of a given attack. The reported mortality for severe attacks varies between 11 and 26 per cent, and that for mild or moderate attacks is less than 1 per cent. The late-outcome or long-term mortality remains inadequately defined, since most studies are based on projected values involving relatively small numbers of patients.

Crohn's Disease

Crohn's disease most frequently is confined to the small intestine with 90 per cent of cases involving the terminal ileum. It may occur, however, in a segmental distribution anywhere in the small bowel and has been described in the esophagus and stomach. The colon may be the only site of involvement in some 10 to 17 per cent of patients or may be involved as part of an enterocolitis in 17 to 40 per cent. It has ethnic and age distributions similar to those of ulcerative colitis except for the lack of a secondary peak in the older age group. Reliable data concerning its incidence and prevalence in the general population and its geographic distribution are not available, however, owing to the uncertain frequency of granulomatous colitis, since a firm diagnosis of the latter often requires surgical material. Again, a genetic predisposition seems probable, but hypotheses concerning etiology are even less well formulated than in the case of ulcerative colitis. Similar to the latter, these patients frequently possess anticolon antibodies and circulating lymphocytes that are cytotoxic for allogenic colon epithelial cells. The presence of anergy in a significant proportion of patients has been found by some but not by others, and this question remains unsettled.

The proclivity to transmural involvement with edema and fibrosis often results in chronic partial intestinal obstruction. The mucosa may become secondarily involved to a lesser extent, so that hemorrhagic ulceration is not as frequently encountered as in patients with ulcerative colitis. Similarly, the thickened bowel wall rarely is the site of a free perforation. Instead, the deep cleftlike fissure ulcers, characteristic of this disease, lead to fistulization and abscess formation. The relative sparing of the mucosal layer probably also accounts for the less frequent development of carcinoma in these patients compared with those with ulcerative colitis.

Sigmoidoscopic examination presents a variable appearance. Fully one half of patients with large bowel involvement and all the patients with disease limited to the small bowel will have a normal rectum, both grossly and histologically. In the known presence of more proximal inflammatory disease, this in itself strongly favors a diagnosis of Crohn's disease as compared with ulcerative colitis. A small proportion of patients have rectal involvement that will be grossly or microscopically indistinguishable from ulcerative colitis. The remainder exhibit features suggesting the presence of Crohn's disease. These include skip areas, large ulcerations and various anal and perianal lesions. The latter may present as indolent, undermined anal fissures, sometimes extending to involve the perineum and even to the inguinal regions; enterocutaneous fistulae; solitary ulcers; and edematous anal tags. These anal lesions at times are the initial manifestation of disease, and biopsy of an ulcer, fissure, or fistulous tract may demonstrate granulomas and greatly assist in diagnosis. The point of demarcation between normal and abnormal bowel is relatively sharp in contrast to ulcerative colitis. Opinions differ regarding the usefulness of rectal biopsy in establishing a diagnosis, since the major thrust of the disease is in the submucosa and therefore a biopsy, to be helpful, must be deep enough to include a substantial portion of this area. This is often safe only on the rectal valves or the margin of an ulcer, and if characteristic changes are observed, including marked submucosal fibrosis and inflammation with granulomas, a diagnosis of Crohn's disease may be possible.

Radiographically, the presence of certain features strongly suggests a diagnosis of Crohn's disease as opposed to ulcerative colitis. These include strictures, asymmetric involvement of the

bowel wall, fissure ulcers, enteric or enterocutaneous fistulae, disease limited to the more proximal portions of the colon, skip areas, and the
presence of similar abnormalities within the small
intestine. Many cases, however, will be indistinguishable from ulcerative colitis on radiographic
grounds, and many of these will exhibit overlapping histologic features. The spectrum of extraintestinal manifestations seen in patients with ulcerative colitis is also encountered in patients with
Crohn's disease, although they are seen somewhat
less frequently. Nonsurgical therapy in Crohn's
disease follows the same general pattern of that
utilized in patients with ulcerative colitis. Sulfasalazine has proved beneficial in patients with
Crohn's disease involving the colon and in those
with ileocolitis but not in disease limited to the
small intestine. Corticosteroids, however, are of
value in patients with small bowel disease and in
those with ileocolitis but not in patients with
disease confined to the colon. Azathioprine may be
a useful adjunct in patients who have responded
to steroids, permitting a decrease in dose or at
times discontinuance of therapy. Attention has
been drawn to the use of metronidazole. This agent
is active against anaerobes and appears to interfere with some aspects of cell-mediated immunity.
Although further study is needed, it offers promise
in patients with colonic disease and in treating
perineal and perianal complications. The surgical
management of Crohn's disease is less satisfactory
than in the case of ulcerative colitis. This is due
to the frequent necessity for resection of physiologically important amounts or areas of bowel and
the relatively high recurrence rate. Recurrence
rates vary from 30 to 65 per cent, depending on
the distribution of disease at the time of surgery.
Recurrence is least frequent with disease limited
to small bowel, especially terminal ileum, is somewhat more frequent with colon involvement, and
is most likely in the presence of ileocolitis. Some
30 per cent of patients will require more than one
operation, with the risk of recurrence rising somewhat with each successive procedure. Resection is
preferable to bypass procedures, the latter being
carried out only when resection is technically
unfeasible.

The prognosis of Crohn's disease has been
difficult to define, since it often depends on confirmation of the diagnosis by surgical means and the
length of observation. It has generally been considered to be a chronic disease of high morbidity
and low mortality, with physicians often trying to
recall when they had last witnessed an autopsy on
a patient with the disorder. Chronic and recurrent
intestinal obstruction and malnutrition dominate
the clinical picture. Malnutrition may be due to
inadequate intake or malabsorption. The latter
may result from loss of absorptive surface due to
disease or resection (short bowel syndrome), loss
of bile salts with defective micellar solubilization,
bacterial overgrowth, or stasis secondary to blind

loops or strictures. The underlying mechanisms
are discussed in Chapter 28. Total parenteral nutrition is often required to correct nutritional defects prior to surgical therapy, and in patients in
whom surgery is not possible long-term management may include home hyperalimentation. The
overall mortality is probably in the range of 15
per cent. In a study by Prior and coworkers, of 295
patients followed for 1 to 38 years there were 53
deaths, more than twice the number expected for
either sex. There was also a tendency for mortality
to be higher in those with onset before age 40
years and when corticosteroids had been employed.

It is obvious from the foregoing discussion
that in many, probably most, instances ulcerative
colitis and Crohn's disease appear to be distinct
and separable entities, clinically, radiographically,
and histopathologically. It is also true that they
share many familial, ethnic, and immunologic
similarities, and as many as 20 per cent of cases
of large bowel disease cannot be fitted into one of
the two available types. Whether we are dealing
with distinct entities having overlapping manifestations or a spectrum of a single disease remains
unclear. In either case, differences exist that have
prognostic and therapeutic relevance. Although
the clinical course and complications encountered
in the classic forms of the two extremes of chronic
inflammatory bowel disease are readily understood
in terms of histopathologic events characteristic of
each, the latter cannot at present be understood
in etiologic or pathogenic terms.

CONSTIPATION

There is remarkably wide variation in human
bowel habits. Diarrhea is present when stool frequency increases to the point at which formed
stools are no longer produced. The end-point for
constipation is less easy to define. Davenport reports human tolerance for fecaliths of up to 100
lbs and intervals between defecation as long as 1
year. Under normal circumstances, failure to defecate regularly at intervals of at least 7 days
probably requires investigation. Many individuals
may be appropriately diagnosed as constipated
with smaller changes in bowel habit. Except for
the emotional turmoil, the only pathologic changes
that may regularly be associated with constipation
are the development of hemorrhoids, anal fissure,
and the consequences of straining at stool.

Constipation may occur by several mechanisms. Congenital failure in the formation of intramural ganglia will result in a constricted colonic segment. Failure of integrated contraction
causes a functional obstruction, with the backup
of feces and the presentation of megacolon. Excision of the offending segment results in return of
transit and a resumption of bowel function. The
pathophysiology of simple constipation is much

less clear. Two varieties are recognized: spastic, or colic, constipation, and sensory constipation.

In spastic, or colic, constipation, individuals demonstrate a motility abnormality of the sigmoid and descending colon. In the resting state, there is a substantial increase in segmentation and nonpropulsive activity, and there is delay of transfer of feces into the rectum. Rectal examination reveals a relatively empty rectum containing at best a few small lumps of hard feces. The underlying cause of the motility abnormality remains unclear. There has been a demonstration of the failure of normal physiologic mechanisms, such as the effect of eating to stimulate a change of activity in the sigmoid colon. Stool softeners and thoughtful use of contact laxatives orally or in suppository form and the use of bulk agents may effect a return to normal bowel habits.

Sensory constipation is an extension of the normal social inhibition of bowel action necessary to control defecation. When the rectum is distended to a critical volume, the urge to defecate is initiated. If it is denied, the rectum will relax and distend to accommodate the feces. The addition of larger quantities of feces will be required to reactivate the reflex. When voluntary denial is frequent, the rectum may become desensitized and a failure of call to stool by rectal distention results. On examination, these individuals will be found to have a rectum full of soft feces. This resembles the circumstances that result from cord transection with sensory failure. Therapy is more difficult with sensory constipation and requires reeducation of the patient to achieve normal bowel habits.

Local pain and fear of its recurrence can inhibit defecation. Careful evaluation for rectal inflammatory lesions is an essential part of the therapy of constipation.

DISORDERS OF SECRETORY FUNCTION

Normal function of the colon includes net absorption of sodium and chloride and absorption of water. Potassium and bicarbonate may be absorbed or secreted. Because there is a substantial flux of sodium and potassium into and out of the lumen, it often is difficult to identify a disorder that is the result of enhanced secretion. The net secretion of sodium and water when the colon is exposed to conjugated bile acids may as well be the result of decreased active sodium absorption as an increase in secretion. There are two disorders in which abnormal electrolyte secretion seems to be a primary defect—chloridorrhea and the hypokalemia associated with villous adenoma of the rectum. In addition, the colon shares with the small intestine a role in the immune system. The colon may mount its own immune response, secreting coproantibodies into the lumen.

CHLORIDORRHEA

Chloridorrhea occurs in both a congenital and an acquired form. Normal handling of chloride in the colon results in passive absorption as a paired ion with sodium. In the absence of chloride in the lumen, bicarbonate is absorbed. When chloride is present in the lumen, the chloride absorption seems to be coupled with an exchange for bicarbonate. The acquired form of chloridorrhea occurs in individuals who suffer from both diarrhea, due to some primary colonic disease, and severe hypokalemia. It is thought that the potassium deficiency affects the permeability of the mucosa, and the chloride-bicarbonate exchange is interrupted. Increased delivery of chloride into the gut is postulated. Although the chloride secretion may be reabsorbed in individuals with normal colons, in individuals with some primary colonic disease absorptive failure due to mucosal abnormality or increased transit results in chloridorrhea. In congenital chloridorrhea, a similar mechanism exists. The primary colonic lesion is the congenital inability to absorb chloride adequately through the colonic mucosa. The excess fecal chloride acts as an osmotic cathartic. With development of hypokalemia, additional chloride loss by secretion results. Fecal chloride concentrations regularly exceed the sum of fecal sodium and potassium concentrations. Correction of potassium defect by supplementation and by limiting dietary chloride results in a significant improvement in diarrhea and electrolyte balance. Similar therapy should prove effective in acquired chloridorrhea.

VILLOUS ADENOMA

Villous adenomas are benign tumors of the colon. They may occur throughout the colon, although they are most common in the rectosigmoid. Their gross and microscopic appearance is that of multiple frondlike extensions. The folds are lined with numerous goblet cells and may produce truly astounding quantities of mucus secretion. Villous adenomas are distinguished clinically by a well-established potential for malignant transformation and for the production of mucus diarrhea that may occasionally lead to severe hypokalemia. Although the frequency of carcinomatous change has been reported to be as high as 50 per cent, the biologic activity of this tumor is low, and successful secondary resections are reported. Mucus secretion is a result of the large number of goblet cells contained in the tumor. The occasional villous adenoma that is found in the colon higher than the rectosigmoid does not result in diarrhea, since reabsorption of electrolytes secreted in the mucus may occur. There is little reabsorption from the rectum, and therefore tumors in the rectal segment are the prime offenders. Colonic mucus generally contains concentrations of sodium that are isotonic with plasma, 140 mEq per liter. Concentrations of potassium are very much higher than serum concentrations. Concentrations as high as 140 mEq per liter have been reported. However, the potassium concentration in mucous diarrhea usually remains only 3 to 10 times the serum level. The resultant loss of potassium will involve not only electrolyte changes but can precipitate kaliopenic nephropathy, digitalis toxicity, muscle weakness, and fatigue. Losses of a magnitude sufficient to cause death have been reported. The proper treatment is surgical removal of the tumor.

TUMORS OF THE COLON

The colon may play host to a full range of neoplasms, both benign and malignant. By far the most common benign tumor is the adenomatous polyp, and the most common malignant tumor is adenocarcinoma. Villous adenomas have been presented under disorders of secretion. The benign adenoma, whether sessile or pedunculated, rarely produces significant symptoms. Occasionally, a benign tumor will bleed significantly or a low-lying polypoid adenoma will cause enough rectal irritation to produce diarrhea, but for the most part they are silent lesions. Extensive discussion of polyps would be unrewarding were it not for the controversy over whether benign adenomatous polyps are inclined to develop into adenocarcinoma. Hyperplastic polyps frequently occur in the colon. The simple adenomatous polyp is a neoplasm.

Studies of small polyps by Lane and coworkers reveal distinct changes in glands with absence of papillary infolding and increase in cellularity. Mitotic figures may be found well above their normal zone of occurrence in the crypts, and there are distinct changes in nuclei and distribution of cell types. In addition, there are changes in the pattern of secretion and the basement membrane. Studies suggest that hyperplastic polyps are a result of hypermaturation of an area of colonic epithelium. Cell turnover and invagination are delayed, but the features just mentioned serve to distinguish adenomatous polyps from them. The question of whether they are prone to undergo malignant transformation is controversial. There are two groups with views on this subject. The first consists of individuals who believe that adenomatous polyps have no greater potential for becoming carcinomatous than any of the remaining colonic epithelium; the second is composed of those who suggest that such polyps actually do have malignant potential. The first group states that although polyps may develop the cytologic appearance of cellular atypia, their biologic behavior remains that of a benign tumor. Although these researchers admit the presence of polypoid carci-

nomas, they believe that these lesions represent cancers from the time of their origin and not malignant degeneration in a polyp. Generally, all cancers are felt to be larger than 1.5 cm in diameter. Thus, risk of operation has been felt to be greater than the risk that a polypoid lesion less than 1.5 cm in diameter is a carcinoma. Long pedicles tend to favor slow-growing tumors of longer duration (Fig. 29–5). Both groups agree that villous adenomas can undergo malignant degeneration, but the group believing in malignant potential of an adenomatous polyp has yet to demonstrate unequivocally that a metastasizing carcinoma has developed from a benign adenomatous polyp in any individual. The group favoring no malignant potential appears to have the balance in their favor; however, a barium enema never permits one to make a cytologic differentiation between villous adenoma, polypoid carcinoma, and adenomatous polyp. The resolution of the problem at this time lies with the endoscopist. Flexible fiberoptic colonoscopes are available in lengths suitable to permit examination of the entire colon from the cecum to the anus. It is technically feasible to reach the cecum in 75 to 85 per cent of cases. Snares with electrocoagulation and forceps are available to permit removal or biopsy at any level. The safety of the procedure contrasts favorably with the alternative direct surgical approach. Overholt has collected figures for 3793 polypectomies. Perforations occurred in 0.23 per cent of patients, bleeding in 0.9 per cent, and death in less than 0.03 per cent. The estimated economic savings of colonoscopic polypectomy over surgery are significant. At the present time, colonoscopy represents the most reasonable approach to the diagnosis and therapy of small polypoid lesions. If one accepts the suggestion that adenomatous polyps remain benign, even fragmentary biopsy will provide the necessary differentiation of the polypoid lesions. There will of course always be individuals for whom colonoscopy, for medical, technical, or emotional reasons, cannot be performed. A like group for similar reasons will not be operable. With regard to carcinoma proper, several additional points bearing on the pathologic physiology of their presentation should be mentioned. Carcinomatous lesions remain silent until they encroach on the lumen, bleed, or present with metastasis. The fluid contents in the right colon make obstruction a late occurrence. Right-sided lesions characteristically come to attention because of blood loss from the ulcerated and friable tumor surface or because of distant metastasis. The semisolid contents of the left colon, particularly the rectum and sigmoid, permit obstruction with smaller, earlier tumors. The critical feature of the colonic cancer and practically any cancer is not its size or location as much as its biologic activity. Cancers of low biologic activity may remain resectable after long intervals and after

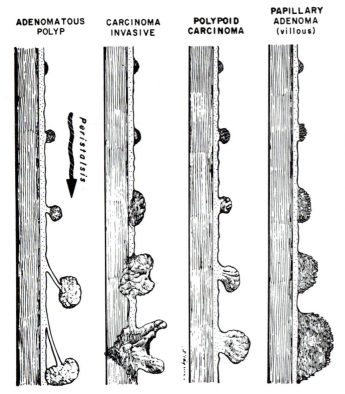

ADENOMATOUS POLYP   CARCINOMA INVASIVE   POLYPOID CARCINOMA   PAPILLARY ADENOMA (villous)

Peristalsis

Figure 29–5 Castleman's conception of pedicle formation. With papillary adenomas, the broad base prevents prolapse, so pedicles are rare. Polypoid cancer may develop with a short pedicle. Invasive cancer rapidly fixes mucosa to the muscularis, and thus pedicle formation becomes impossible. Simple adenomas, by proliferation at the tip, develop large heads, so that the underlying mucosa is soon pulled into a pedicle by peristalsis. (From Welch, C. E., and Hedberg, S. E.: Polypoid Lesions of the Gastrointestinal Tract. Philadelphia, W. B. Saunders Co., 1975.)

reaching large size. Tumors of high biologic activity will metastasize before any hope of identification is present. There is no practical measure of biologic activity that may be used clinically at this time. Some hope exists for the use of quantitative determination of fetal intestinal tract proteins and other endogenous substances produced by cancer. Apparently gastrointestinal tumors, particularly colonic cancer plus a number of nongastrointestinal tumors, undergo regression to an embryonic cellular activity at the time of malignant transformation. Gold and coworkers have described a radioimmunoassay for carcinoembryonic antigen (CEA), one of these fetal intestinal tract proteins. LoGerfo and coworkers have utilized a similar assay for a tumor-associated antigen (TAA) that may be different from CEA. CEA and TAA testing remain the current hope for any increase in sensitivity for the diagnosis and management of colon carcinoma.

COLONIC MICROFLORA

The colon is best known for the lush growth of bacteria that inhabits the lumen. The difference in numbers of microorganisms in samples aspirated from the distal ileum in the cecum may be in the order of 4 to 6 $\log_{10}$. The bacterial flora of the large intestine does not represent an uncontrolled growth of a mass of organisms, for there appear to be a variety of mechanisms for qualitative and quantitative control of the flora. Normal flora performs several "functions." The digestion of cellulose and hemicellulose and the production of a variety of vitamins have been discussed. Balanced normal flora may inhibit the overgrowth of pathogenic organisms, particularly staphylococci. The risk of bacterial overgrowth with enterocolitis is always present when normal flora is rendered unstable by antibiotic therapy. There also is an apparent necessity for specific bacterial flora to be present for full clinical expression of ameba infection. Normal flora may contribute to local and systemic pathologic changes in a number of other ways. Fermentation of lactose produces symptoms in lactase deficiency, and bacterial metabolism of bile acids may alter the enterohepatic circulation. The urea-ammonia cycle also depends on bacterial action and may achieve significance in protein malnutrition and hepatic encephalopathy. Specific infections with organisms such as *Shigella* have been discussed. The colon may also harbor a range of other pathogenic organisms, particularly *Vibrio cholerae* and *Salmonella*, contributing to the carrier state. The full significance in terms of the pathologic physiology of colonic disease of alterations of controls over bacterial flora remains to be identified.

REFERENCES

Allen, F. D.: Essentials of Human Embryology. 2nd ed. New York, Oxford University Press, 1969.

Ammon, A. V., and Phillips, S. F.: Inhibition of colonic water and electrolyte absorption by fatty acids in man. Gastroenterology 65:744-749, 1973.

Bentley, D. W., Nicols, R. L., Condon, R. E., and Gorbach, S. L.: The microflora of the human ileum and intraabdominal colon: results of direct needle aspiration at surgery and evaluation of the technique. J. Lab. Clin. Med. 79:421, 1972.

Blaser, M. J., and Reller, L. B.: *Campylobacter enteritis.* N. Engl. J. Med. 305:1444, 1981.

Bleiberg, H., Mainguet, P., Galand, P., et al.: Cell renewal in the human rectum. In vitro autoradiographic study on active ulcerative colitis, Gastroenterology 58:851, 1970.

Bloom, A. A., LoPresti, P., and Farrar, J. T.: Motility of the intact human colon. Gastroenterology 54:232, 1968.

Boley, S. J., Sammartano, R., Adams, A., et al.: On the nature and etiology of vascular ectasias of the colon. Degenerative lesions of aging. Gastroenterology 72:650, 1977.

Breen, K. J., Bryant, R. C., Levinson, J. D., and Schenker, S.: Neomycin absorption in man. Studies of oral and enema administration and effect of intestinal ulceration. Ann. Intern. Med. 76:211, 1972.

Casarella, W. J., Kanter, I. E., and Seaman, W. B.: Right-sided colonic diverticula as a cause of acute rectal hemorrhage. N. Engl. J. Med. 286:450, 1972.

Castleman, B., and Krickstein, H. I.: Do adenomatous polyps of the colon become malignant? N. Engl. J. Med. 267:469, 1962.

Castleman, B., and Krickstein, H. I.: Current approach to the polyp-cancer controversy. Gastroenterology 51:108, 1966.

Chaudhary, N. A., and Truelove, S. C.: The irritable colon syndrome. A study of the clinical features, predisposing causes, and prognosis in 130 cases. Quart. J. Med. 31:307, 1962.

Christensen, J.: The controls of gastrointestinal movements: some old and new views. N. Engl. J. Med. 285:85, 1971.

Christensen, J.: Myoelectric control of the colon. Gastroenterology 68:601. 1975.

Christensen, J.: Colonic motility. Viewpoints Dig. Dis. 13:9, 1981.

Connell, A. M.: The motility of the pelvic colon. Part II. Paradoxical motility in diarrhoea and constipation. Gut 3:342, 1962.

Connell, A. M.: Motor action of the large bowel. In Code, C. F. (Ed.): Handbook of Physiology. Vol. IV. Washington, D.C., American Physiological Society, 1968.

Couturier, D., Roze, C., Couturier-Turpin, M. H., and Debray, C.: Electromyography of the colon in situ. An experimental study in man and in the rabbit. Gastroenterology 56:317, 1969.

Crane, C. W.: Observations on the sodium and potassium content of mucus from the large intestine. Gut 6:439, 1965.

Cudmore, M. A., Silve, J., Fekety, R., et al.: *Clostridium difficile* colitis associated with cancer chemotherapy. Arch. Intern. Med. 142:333, 1982.

Davenport, H. W.: Physiology of the Digestive Tract. 5th ed. Chicago, Year Book Medical Publishers, Inc., 1982.

deDombal, F. T.: Ulcerative colitis. Epidemiology and aetiology, course and prognosis. Br. Med. J. 1:649, 1971.

Derjanecz, J. J., and Clarke, C. W.: Papillary adenomas of the colon and rectum: clinical and pathological behavior. A plea for more conservative treatment. Can. J. Surg. 7:389, 1964.

Devroede, G. J., and Phillips, S. F.: Conservation of sodium, chloride and water by the human colon. Gastroenterology 56:101, 1969.

Devroede, G. J., and Phillips, S. F.: Failure of the human rectum to absorb electrolytes and water. Gut 11:438, 1970.

Dinoso, V. P., Jr., Meskinpour, H., Lorbin, S. H., et al.: Motor responses of the sigmoid colon and rectum to exogenous cholecystokinin and secretin. Gastroenterology 65:438-444, 1973.

Dowling, R. H.: The enterohepatic circulation. Gastroenterology 62:122, 1972.

Edwards, D. A. W., and Beck, E. R.: Fecal flow, mixing and consistency. Am. J. Dig. Dis. 16:706, 1971.

Edwards, D. A. W., and Beck, E. R.: Movement of radiopacified feces during defecation. Am. J. Dig. Dis. 16:709, 1971.

Elsen, J., and Arey, L. B.: On spirality in the intestinal wall. Am. J. Anat. 118:11, 1966.

Evanson, J. M., and Stanbury, S. W.: Congenital chloridorrhoea or so-called congenital alkalosis with diarrhoea. Gut 6:29, 1965.

Feldman, F., Cantor, D., Soll, S., and Bachrach, W.: Psychiatric study of a consecutive series of 34 patients with ulcerative colitis. Br. Med. J. 3:14, 1967.

Fenogilio, C. M., Richart, R. M., and Kaye, G. I.: Comparative electron-microscopic features of normal, hyperplastic and adenomatous human colonic epithelium II. Gastroenterology, 69:100, 1975.

Field, M.: Intestinal secretion: Effect of cyclic AMP and its role in cholera. N. Engl. J. Med. 284:1137, 1971.

Field, M.: Intestinal secretion. Gastroenterology 66:1063, 1976.

Fleischner, F. G.: Diverticular disease of the colon; new observations and revised concepts. Gastroenterology 60:316, 1971.

Fordtran, J. S., and Ingelfinger, F. J.: Absorption of water, electrolytes and sugars from the human gut. In Code, C. F. (Ed.): Handbook of Physiology. Vol. III. Washington, D.C., American Physiological Society, 1968.

Goligher, J. C., deDombal, F. T., Watts, J. M., and Watkinson, G.: Ulcerative Colitis. Baltimore, Williams and Wilkins Co., 1968.

Gorbach, S. L.: Intestinal microflora. Gastroenterology 60:1110, 1971.

Hayashi, T., Yatami, R., Apostol, J., and Stemmermann, G. N.: Pathogenesis of hyperplastic polyps of the colon: a hypothesis based on ultrastructure and in vitro cell kinetics. Gastroenterology 66:347, 1974.

Hellmans, J., Vantrappen, G., Valembois, P., et al.: Electrical activity of striated and smooth muscle of the esophagus. Am. J. Dig. Dis. 13:320, 1968.

Hofmann, A. F.: The syndrome of ileal disease and the broken enterohepatic circulation: cholerheic enteropathy. Gastroenterology 52:752, 1967.

Hofmann, A. F., and Poley, J. R.: Cholestyramine treatment of diarrhea associated with ileal resection. N. Engl. J. Med. 281:397, 1969.

Holzknecht, G.: Die normale Peristaltick der Kolon. Muench Med. Wschr. 56:2401, 1909.

Ivey, K. J.: Are anticholinergics of use in the irritable colon syndrome? Gastroenterology 68:1300, 1975.

Kingham, J. G., Levison, D. A., and Fairclough, P. D.: Diarrhoea and reversible enteropathy in Zollinger-Ellison syndrome. Lancet 2:610, 1981.

Kirsner, J. B.: The irritable bowel syndrome. Arch. Intern. Med. 141:635, 1981.

Kirsner J. B., and Shorter, R. G.: Recent developments in "nonspecific" inflammatory bowel disease. N. Engl. J. Med. 306:775, 1982.

Kirsner, J. B., and Shorter, R. G.: Recent developments in nonspecific inflammatory bowel disease (second of two parts). N. Engl. J. Med. 306:837, 1982.

Lane, N., Kaplan, H., and Pascal, R. R.: Minute adenomatous and hyperplastic polyps of the colon: divergent patterns of epithelial growth with specific associated mesenchymal changes. Contrasting roles in the pathogenesis of carcinoma. Gastroenterology 60:537, 1971.

Levitan, R., and Ingelfinger, F. J.: Effect of *d*-aldosterone on salt and water absorption from the intact human colon. J. Clin. Invest. 44:801, 1965.

Levitt, M. D., and Bond, J. H., Jr.: Volume, composition, and source of intestinal gas. Gastroenterology 59:921, 1970.

LoGerfo, P., Herter, F., and Hansen, H. J.: Tumor associated antigen in patients with carcinoma of the colon. Am. J. Surg. 123:127, 1972.

Matsumoto, K. K., Peter, J. B., Schultze, R. G., et al: Watery diarrhea and hypokalemia associated with pancreatic islet cell adenoma. Gastroenterology 50:231, 1966.

Mekhjian, H. S., Phillips, S. F., and Hofmann, A. F.: Colonic secretion of water and electrolytes induced by bile acids: perfusion studies in man. J. Clin. Invest. 50:1569, 1971.

Mendeloff, A. I., Monk, M., Siegel, C. I., and Lilienfeld, A.: Illness experience and life stresses in patients with irritable colon and with ulcerative colitis. N. Engl. J. Med. 282:14, 1970.

Meshkinpour, H., Dinoso, V. P., and Lorber, S. H.: Effect of intraduodenal administration of essential amino acids and sodium oleate on motor activity of the sigmoid colon. Gastroenterology 66:373, 1974.

Morson, B. C.: The muscle abnormality in diverticular disease of the sigmoid colon. Br. J. Radiol. 36:385, 1963.

Morson, B. C.: Current concepts of colitis. Trans. Med. Soc. London 86:159, 1970.

Overholt, B. F.: Colonoscopy. Gastroenterology 68:1308, 1975.

Painter, N. S., Almeida, A. Z., and Colebourne, K. W.: Unprocessed bran in treatment of diverticular disease of the colon. Br. Med. J. 2:137, 1972.

Phillips, R. A.: Cholera in the perspective of 1966. Ann. Intern. Med. 65:922, 1966.

Phillips, S. F.: Absorption and secretion by the colon. Gastroenterology 56:966, 1969.

Phillips, S. F., and Edwards, D. A. W.: Some aspects of anal continence and defecation. Gut 6:396, 1965.

Prior, P., Waterhouse, J. A., Fielding, J. F., and Cooke, W. T.: Mortality in Crohn's disease. Lancet 1:1135, 1970.

Provenzale, L., and Pisano, M.: Methods for recording electrical activity of the human colon in vivo. Am. J. Dig. Dis. 16:712; 1971.

Reilly, M.: Sigmoid myotomy—interim report. Proc. Roy. Soc. Med. 62:715, 1969.

Ritchie, J. A.: Colonic motor activity and bowel function. Part I. Normal movement of contents. Gut 9:442, 1968.

Ritchie, J. A.: Colonic motor activity and bowel function. Part II. Distribution and incidence of motor activity at rest and after food and carbachol. Gut 9:502, 1968.

Ritchie, J. A.: Movement of segmental constrictions in the human colon. Gut 12:350, 1971.

Ritchie, J. A., Truelove, S. C., Ardran, G. M., and Tuckey, M. S.: Propulsion and retropulsion of normal colonic contents. Am. J. Dig. Dis. 16:697, 1971.

Rosch, J., Gray, R. K., Grollman, J. H., Jr., et al.: Selective arterial drug infusions in the treatment of acute gastrointestinal bleeding. A preliminary report. Gastroenterology 59:341, 1970.

Samuel, P., Saypol, G. M., Meilman, E., et al.: Absorption of bile acids from the large bowel in man. J. Clin. Invest. 47:2070, 1968.

Schanker, L. S.: Absorption of drugs from the rat colon. J. Pharmacol. Exp. Ther. 126:283, 1959.

Schultz, S. G., and Curran, P. F.: Intestinal absorption of sodium chloride and water. In Code, C. F. (Ed.): Handbook of Physiology. Vol. IV. Washington, D.C., American Physiological Society, 1968.

Schuster, M. M.: The riddle of the sphincters. Gastroenterology, 69:249, 1975.

Shields, R., and Miles, J. B.: Absorption and secretion in the large intestine. Postgrad. Med. 41:435, 1965.

Shorter, R. G., Huizenga, K. A., Spencer, R. J., et al.: Cytophilic antibody and the cytotoxicity of lymphocytes for colonic cells in vitro. Am. J. Dig. Dis. 16:673, 1971.

Snape, W. J., Jr., Carlson, G. M., and Cohen, S.: Colonic myoelectric activity in the irritable bowel syndrome. Gastroenterology 70:326, 1976.

Snape, W. J., Jr., Carlson, G. M., Matuango, S. A., and Cohen, S.: Evidence that abnormal myoelectrical activity produces colonic motor dysfunction in the irritable bowel syndrome. Gastroenterology 72:383, 1967.

Solomon, S. S., Moran, J. M., and Nabseth, D. C.: Villous adenoma of rectosigmoid accompanied by electrolyte depletion. J.A.M.A. 194:5, 1965.

Stobo, J. D., Tomasi, T. B., Huizenga, K. A., and Shorter, R. G.: In vitro studies of inflammatory bowel disease: surface receptors of the mononuclear cell required to lyse allogeneic colonic epithelial cells. Gastroenterology 70:171, 1976.

Thompson, D. M. P., Murphy, J., Freedman, S. O., and Gold, P.: The radioimmunoassay of circulating carcinoembryonic antigen of the human digestive system. Proc. Nat. Acad. Sci. 64:161, 1969.

Torsoli, A., Ramorino, M. L., and Crucioli, V.: The relationships between anatomy and motor activity of the colon. Am. J. Dig. Dis. 13:462, 1968.

Ustach, T. J., Tobon, F., Hambrecht, T., et al.: Electrophysiological aspects of human sphincter function. J. Clin. Invest. 49:41, 1970.

Waller, S. L., and Misiewica, J. J.: Colonic motility in constipation or diarrhoea. Scand. J. Gastroenterol. 7:93, 1972.

Watson, D. W.: The problem of chronic inflammatory bowel disease. Calif. Med. 117:25, 1972.

Williams, I.: Changing emphasis in diverticular disease of the colon. Br. J. Radiol. 36:393, 1963.

Wolpert, E., Phillips, S. F., and Summerskill, W. H. J.: Transport of urea and ammonia production in the human colon. Lancet 4:1387, 1971.

Wrong, O., Metcalfe-Gibson, A., Morrison, R. B. I., et al.: In vivo dialysis of faeces as a method of stool analysis. I. Technique and results in normal subjects. Clin. Sci. 28:357, 1965.

Zamcheck, N., Moore, T. L., Dhar, P., and Kupchik, H.: Immunologic diagnosis and prognosis of human digestive-tract cancer: carcinoembryonic antigens. N. Engl. J. Med. 286:83, 1972.

Zetzel, L.: Granulomatous (ileo) colitis. N. Engl. J. Med. 288:600, 1970.

Normal and Pathologic Physiology of the Liver

30

Frank L. Iber and Patricia S. Latham*

HEPATIC ARCHITECTURE: CORRELATION OF STRUCTURE TO FUNCTION

The liver is uniquely designed and situated in the vascular system of the body to modulate the nutrients presented to it from the intestinal tract. The portal vein is the conduit from gastrointestinal absorption to the capillary network of the liver. The total blood flow in the liver is the same as the hepatic venous blood flow or the sum of the hepatic arterial and portal venous flow. About 20 per cent (1 to 2 liters per minute) of the resting cardiac output reaches the liver, with one third traveling via the hepatic artery and two thirds transported via the portal vein. The portal venous flow varies markedly during the day because the arterial flow to the stomach and intestines varies. Stimulation of gastric or pancreatic secretion enhances their arterial flow and the portal venous drainage. Similarly, food in the intestine stimulates motility and blood flow. Inflammation of these organs or of the spleen also increases blood flow.

The hepatic artery seems more responsive to the needs of the liver. Hepatic anoxia lowers intrahepatic resistance and increases arterial flow. Hepatic inflammation also increases hepatic arterial flow. The hepatic, splenic, and superior mesenteric arteries are similarly responsive to many regulatory agents. Bradykinin, low doses of epinephrine, and some prostaglandins are arterial vasodilators, whereas serotonin, pitressin, high doses of epinephrine, norepinephrine, and other prostaglandins diminish arterial flow. In the resting state, blood actively flows in only about one fifth of the sinusoids. The remaining four fifths are temporarily static, but the actual flow into the sinusoids can change from moment to moment. A higher proportion of the total number of sinusoids is conducting blood when the total liver blood flow increases. The liver resistance changes with flow, so that a doubling of portal venous flow is associated with only a slight rise of pressure in the portal vein.

The hepatic artery, the portal vein, and the bile duct join together at the hilus of the liver and then, surrounded by loose fibrous tissue, progressively branch to each lobe of the liver from the porta hepatis to the portal triad of the functional acinar complex at the level of the sinusoids (Figs. 30–1 and 30–2). The arterial and portal venous circulation join in the capillary network of the sinusoids. The hepatocytes form plates of cells, one and occasionally two cells in thickness, between the sinusoids such that each hepatocyte has multiple surfaces exposed to sinusoids in order to maximize the direct interchange with the circulation.

The sinusoidal space is lined by a wall of endothelial cells that are separated from the hepatocytes by a distinct space (Disse's space) (Figs. 30–3 to 30–5). Fingerlike projections of the hepatocyte membrane are abundant in Disse's space. The endothelial cells themselves are unusual in being fenestrated, creating a "sieve-plate" between the sinusoids and hepatocytes. The endothelial lining, unlike other capillaries, has a basement membrane that is indefinite and discontinuous. These features make the sinusoidal wall the most permeable capillary in the body. The unique structure of the sinusoidal wall protects the hepatocytes from intravascular pressure and creates an "undisturbed layer" at the surface of the hepatocytes, yet allows the liver cell access to the sinusoidal space for interchange with blood (Figs. 30–3 to 30–5).

The hepatocyte is rich in organelles, reflecting an active metabolism. The tight junctions (zonula occludens) between hepatocytes define the limitations of the bile canaliculus and provide a relatively impermeable barrier between that space and the sinusoid (Figs. 30–3 to 30–5). The tight junction also prevents the migration of membrane surface proteins from the basolateral surface of the hepatocyte to the bile canalicular surface. Thus, two distinct surfaces of hepatocytes exist, one connected to adjacent hepatocytes with a bile canaliculus between them, and the other surrounded by Disse's space with a sinusoid immediately adjacent. This structure allows the hepatocyte to establish a polarity of transport between the sinusoidal space and the bile canaliculus.

Kupffer's cells lie loosely between the endothelial cells or on top of them, clearly in contact with the circulation in the sinusoidal space (Fig. 30–2 to 30-4). These cells, resting macrophages,

*The authors wish to thank Mr. Barry O'Neill of Boston, Mass., who did the original art work; Ms. Arline Caliger, VAMC, Baltimore, Md., for photography and reproductions; and Ms. Marge Rodgers, Ms. Pamela Miller, and Ms. Beverly Vance from University of Maryland School of Medicine/VAMC, Baltimore, for their intense administrative participation.

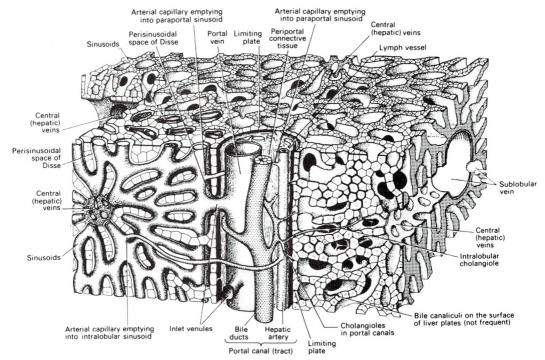

Figure 30–1 Drawing of the liver cell plates. Note that most of the plates are one or two cells thick, with one or more sinusoidal surfaces touching each cell. Between every two liver cells there are bile ducts that coalesce into larger ducts. Hepatic artery twigs supply only a few of the sinusoids. Surrounding the portal triad is loose connective tissue and a limiting plate. Lymphatic vessels that are direct extensions of the space of Disse also are present in the portal vein. (From Sherlock, S.: Diseases of the Liver and Biliary System. 6th ed. Oxford, Blackwell Scientific Publications, 1982.)

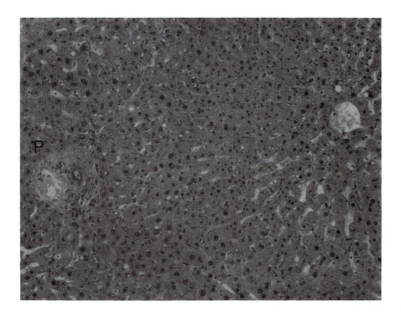

Figure 30–2 Light microscopy of human liver (×63). Contrast this illustration with Figure 30–1. A portal triad (P) shows artery, vein, bile duct, and loose connective tissue. The open space to the right is the central hepatic vein; the plates of liver cells oriented between these two structures can be seen. The plates of liver cells are one or two cells thick.

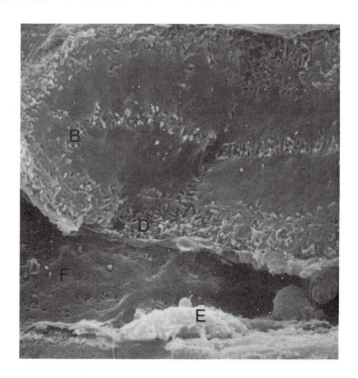

Figure 30–3 Scanning electron micrograph of rat liver. A prominent sinusoid (F) lined by endothelial cells (E) with clear fenestrations should be noted. Two adjacent hepatocytes with a bile canaliculus (B) coursing along their intercellular surface are evident. The canalicular membrane has many villous extensions. The surface of the hepatocytes protruding into the space of Disse (D) have many microvilli that increase surface area. (Dr. K. Kim and Ms. N. Trump assisted in producing this photograph.)

phagocytose particulate matter, specifically ingest soluble materials for which they have receptors, and participate in the immune system of the body. The blood comes into sufficient contact with the reticuloendothelial cells (Kupffer's cells) and liver cells to assure that more than 99 per cent of substances taken up by either cell will be removed in a single passage through the liver.

Two other cell types (Table 30–1) in the liver have less clear roles in metabolism. The Ito cell, or adipocyte, resides between hepatocytes within Disse's space. The cell is identified by its position and content of lipid vacuoles. It is believed to function as a storage site of fat-soluble vitamins because the number of these cells increases in vitamin-A overload. It may also play a role in fibrogenesis, since an increase in cell number has been noted in some conditions of fibrosis.

"Pit cells" have been identified in electron micrographs. Neuroendocrine granules are present in these cells, but their significance in liver tissue is unknown.

The liver cells are normally undergoing constant repair, and it is estimated that hepatocyte renewal occurs each 50 to 75 days. A newly formed liver cell is less enzymatically mature than an older one and cannot perform many liver functions efficiently.

In all forms of hepatic damage, the bile ducts and large blood vessels seem to emerge more intact than the other hepatic elements. Mesenchymal elements (connective tissue) grow predominantly following certain types of liver damage (e.g., alcoholic). New blood vessel formation is far more prominent in cancer nodules than in regenerative liver nodules. There is no evidence that regeneration is impaired in liver disease; in fact, often there is a pattern of increased regeneration to compensate for increased necrosis.

The mammalian liver possesses a remarkable capacity both to regenerate its polygonal cells when portions are damaged and to cease regeneration when the proper mass is eventually reached. (Regeneration occurs in areas receiving portal blood.) Any form of dietary deficiency, particularly of folic acid, B_{12}, and protein, will restrict regeneration. Animal perfusion studies clearly indicate that a humoral factor stimulates hepatic mitosis—perhaps arginine, pituitary hormones, insulin, or glucagon may be such a substance. Regeneration is much more striking in the young than in the old.

EVALUATIONS OF HEPATIC ANATOMY AND ARCHITECTURE

Excellent means exist to provide an image of the outer boundaries of the liver and the presence of 2-cm or larger nodules of tissue that are not liver and to demonstrate the vasculature and biliary duct systems. These modalities are listed in Table 30–2 and are discussed in the following sections.

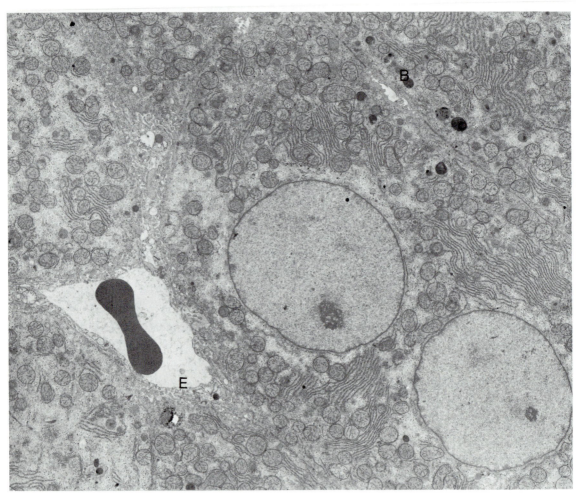

Figure 30–4 Transmission electron microscopic view of rat liver. Portions of four hepatocytes surround a sinusoid with a biconcave erythrocyte prominently displayed. Endothelial cells (E) make up the lining of the sinusoid, and the many microvilli from the surface of the hepatocytes are clearly seen. A bile canaliculus (B) is identified in the upper right, and a second unmarked one is present in the top center of the photograph. Tight junctions are clearly seen as electron-dense areas of the membrane between the two liver cells on either side of B. The hepatocytes are rich in organelles, with numerous round to oval mitochondria and parallel arrays of rough endoplasmic reticulum. Two nuclei are prominent in a single hepatocyte, a frequent finding in normal liver tissue.

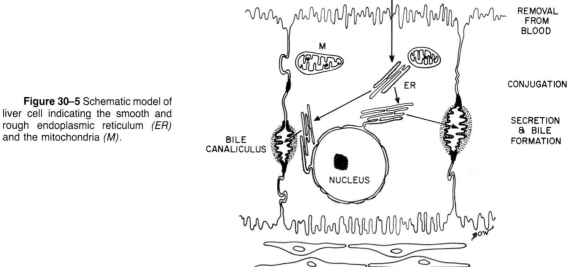

Figure 30–5 Schematic model of liver cell indicating the smooth and rough endoplasmic reticulum *(ER)* and the mitochondria *(M)*.

TABLE 30–1 CELLS WITHIN THE LIVER AND POSSIBLE FUNCTION

Name of Cell	Approximate Frequency	Function	Comment
Hepatocyte	50% of nuclei	All liver cell functions	Renewed each 50 days
Kupffer's cells	20% of nuclei	Phagocytosis; specific uptake	Part of RE system
Endothelial cells	20% of nuclei	Line sinusoid	
Ito cells (lipocytes)	2% of nuclei	Store excess fat-soluble vitamins	Possibly make collagen
Bile duct cells	7% of nuclei	Reabsorb sugar; adjust bile, water, and electrolytes	Actively secrete bicarbonate
Lymphocytes	2% of nuclei	As in other locations	
"Pit cells"	1% of nuclei	Endocrine function	

TABLE 30–2 APPRAISAL OF LIVER ANATOMIC
STATUS

1. Outline and position
   a. Palpation
   b. Sonography
   c. CT scans
   d. Isotopic scans (^{99m}Tc-labeled sulfur colloid)
   e. Peritoneoscopy
2. Lobular anatomy
   a. Biopsy
   b. Biochemistry specific to organelles
3. Circulatory condition
   a. Arteriography (inject hepatic artery)
   b. Portal venography
      (1) Inject through spleen or umbilical vein
      (2) Inject splenic artery and wait for portal filling
   c. Hepatic vein injection (retrograde)
4. Portal hypertension
   a. Measure pressure in spleen, umbilical vein
   b. Indirectly measure in hepatic vein or liver parenchyma
   c. Demonstrate collateral flow by angiography
5. Bile ducts
   a. Oral and I.V. cholangiography, cholecystography
   b. Sonography
   c. Transhepatic cholangiography (when ducts are dilated)
   d. Retrograde endoscopic cholangiography (normal ducts)

Ultrasonography

Bursts of sound of specific wavelength may be released into the abdomen through sensitive transducers and the reflected echo recorded to provide information on the reflectivity and absorbance of various structures. The normal liver is homogeneous to echoes, except that fluid-filled spaces such as the gallbladder do not reflect sound. Fibrosis reflects sound, calcification stops the transmissions, and fluid-filled spaces have no echo. The gallbladder, enlarged bile ducts, and normal portal veins are observed. Gallstones, increased fibrosis, or calcium within the liver may also be seen. Abscesses or tumor nodules are often demonstrated by the contrast they provide against the background of homogeneous liver parenchyma. Ultrasonography has no adverse effects on the patient and is currently the best way to image the gallbladder, gallstones, or dilated bile ducts. Table 30–3 contrasts various methods of imaging.

Liver-Spleen Scan (Scintiscan)

Sulfur colloid labeled with ^{99m}Tc is taken up by reticuloendothelial cells (mostly in the liver) and allows liver imaging with a camera sensitive to gamma irradiation, even when liver cells are diseased. The colloid must be administered intravenously, and the outline of the liver and usually the spleen is obtained. The method is sensitive to liver blood flow; in cirrhosis, irregular blood flow from one portion to another will result in patchiness in the image. Space-occupying lesions that displace Kupffer's cells will also appear as zones of decreased uptake.

Computerized Axial Tomography (CT Scan) (Fig. 30–6)

A CT scan is a computer-constructed image of the information obtained from many tomograms taken of the body. The machine may be adjusted to take more cuts of a given organ or fewer, but each cut requires 5 to 30 seconds, depending on the apparatus. Usual images are taken at 2-cm intervals in the abdomen, thus requiring an aberration of 2 cm or more to be identified with

TABLE 30–3 COMPARATIVE VALUE OF ISOTOPIC, ULTRASONIC, AND CT SCANS

	Isotope*	Ultrasonography	CT
Ease of interpretation	Easy	Difficult	Easy
Approximate cost (dollars)	100	100	300
Size, shape, and position of liver	Good	Good	Best
Presence of nonliver nodules in liver	Good (4 cm)	Best (cystic 1 cm)	Good (2 cm)
Showing impaired vascularity (cirrhosis)	Good	0	0
Budd-Chiari syndrome	Fair	0	0
Size and shape of gallbladder	0 (†Very good)	Best	Fair
Presence of gallstones	0	Best	0
Dilated intrahepatic ducts	Poor	Best	Good
Dilated common duct	Fair	Excellent	Excellent
Obstruction of cystic duct	Good†	0 unless stimulated	0 unless stimulated
Abscess	Possible‡	Mass	Mass
Complete cholestasis	Good†	0	0
Support diagnosis of cirrhosis	Positive	0	0

*^{99m}Tc labeled sulfur colloid unless indicated otherwise
†^{99m}Tc PIPIDA
‡Gallium

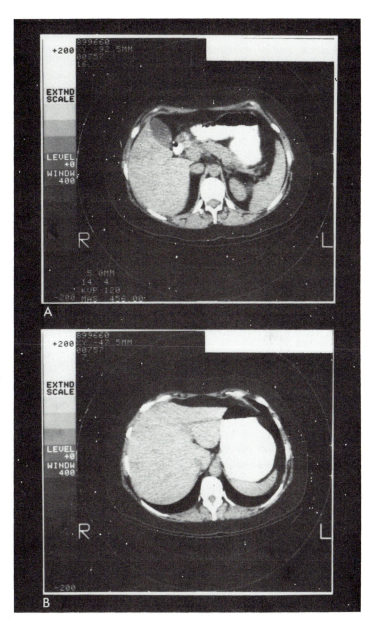

Figure 30–6 Two views taken from 36 cuts of a CT scan of a normal liver. All 36 views are the products of transverse reconstructions by the computer. For enhancement of contrast, the subject was given radiopaque barium sulfate to drink. The dense white areas indicate the stomach, duodenum, ribs, and vertebrae, reflecting the increased absorption of x-rays in these structures. *B* illustrates the area above the insertion of the diaphragm; the view shown in *A* is about 4 cm more caudad. In *A*, the barium-filled stomach and a small portion of the duodenum adjacent to the liver, rounded and white, are demonstrated. The aorta is in front of the vertebrae, and the rounded inferior vena cava is to the patient's right. The tip of the right kidney can be seen posteriorly on the patient's left. The liver is smaller at this level, and the rounded dent produced by the gallbladder is seen anteriorly. The elongated structure behind the stomach and in front of the great vessels is the pancreas. In *B*, the vertebrae are seen posteriorly, and the radiolucent lung is behind them. The dense white stomach is on the right, and a portion of spleen extends behind it. The rounded aorta is seen just in front of the vertebrae, and the large organ on the left is the liver. The vague radiolucent areas in the liver are blood vessels and bile ducts. (Films provided by Dr. Ann Tipton.)

certainty. Contrasts between structures may be enhanced with a dye that is taken into the blood vessels, the gallbladder, or the liver parenchyma. CT scanning is more sensitive than ultrasonography for visualization of tumor metastases, but it is less sensitive for fluid-filled bile ducts. CT scans are usually more costly, and in most institutions the method is more tightly scheduled than ultrasonography.

Liver Biopsy and Peritoneoscopy

Some centers frequently examine the surface of the liver by peritoneoscopy. In this procedure, the peritoneal cavity is distended with air, and a lighted instrument is inserted to inspect the surfaces of the anterior organs. The liver, a portion of the gallbladder, some of the mesenteric circulation, and portions of the intestine are nearly always seen, as well as a great expanse of both parietal and visceral peritoneum. Nodular lesions may be biopsied directly.

In liver biopsy, 10 to 20 mg of a 1500-gm organ is sampled by the insertion of an aspiration needle into the liver, usually between the right lower ribs and through the diaphragm. In the absence of coagulation problems, the procedure is remarkably safe; hemorrhage is the major complication. The sample is representative of the entire liver about 85 per cent of the time in those conditions that influence all lobules of the liver (e.g., cirrhosis, hepatitis, and metabolic diseases), but it is of limited value *if negative* in those conditions that are usually irregular in distribution (e.g., metastatic or primary cancer and abscess).

A great deal of information is obtained from the sample, which will usually consist of portions of 8 to 15 lobules. In a general way, information concerning the hepatocytes themselves, including necrosis, inflammation, and metabolic diseases, may be seen. Information regarding portions of the lobule showing injury or collapse or scarring of the entire lobule is often seen. The presence of foreign tissue such as cancer may also be identified.

A number of features obtained on liver biopsy are of great value in understanding the effect of disease on the overall function of the liver. Thus, in conditions such as chronic hepatitis and cirrhosis, large portions of the liver may be damaged. The bile ducts and blood vessels collapse together as the dead liver cells are removed. Eventually, scar tissue forms around many bile ducts and blood vessels. Such scars allow the portal venous and arterial blood to reach hepatic veins directly without perfusing hepatocytes (portal shunting). An increase in collagen bundles may also be seen in Disse's space. When the normal reticulin architecture of the hepatic lobule is lost by necrosis, hepatocytes regenerate to form plates, two or more cells in thickness. Both changes make the efficient contact with the liver circulation no longer possible. Sometimes bile ducts are destroyed and are not present in all portal spaces; other times, fibrosis of portal or hepatic vein branches are seen in biopsy. These changes clearly predict problems with the appropriate supply or drainage to the liver. Occasionally, increased fat and inflammation in the liver cells and sinusoids combined with scarring suggests that the ability of blood to reach the liver cells is diminished, and this is impressively verified when tested. Thus, the histologic examination of the liver, to the extent that the small sample is representative, is of great value in estimating the microscopic environment of the liver cells.

Enzymes Specific to Organelles

Several organelles in the liver release substances into the blood when they are injured or hypertrophied. Acid phosphatase for lysosome stimulation, gamma glutamyl transpeptidase for smooth endoplasmic reticulin injury, and neuraminidase for formation of granulomas are three fairly well-established markers, and many more have been proposed. Such markers may be expected to increase in prominence in diagnosis.

Liver Circulatory Status

Arteriovenography is accomplished by direct cannulation of the splenic or hepatic artery, usually introduced into the femoral artery. In the early phase, arteriograms will outline the arterial vessels of the liver or spleen and in the late phase will demonstrate the portal or hepatic veins. This technique permits one to determine the patency and anatomic course of all groups of blood vessels. Nodularity, erosion, new blood vessel formation, tumor blush, and collateral circulation may also be indicated. Portovenograms are made either by injecting radiopaque dye into the spleen (the dye is subsequently picked up and returned via the splenic and portal veins) or by cannulating the vestigial umbilical vein or a branch of the mesenteric vein.

Crude estimates of liver blood flow may be made from scintillation scans of the liver after ^{99m}Tc-labeled sulfur colloid is administered. If the intrahepatic circulation bypasses large areas of parenchyma, the colloid will not be taken up by these bypassed areas, and a patchy, or nonhomogeneous, uptake is apparent on the scan. The colloid that is not taken up by the liver becomes available for uptake by reticuloendothelial cells of the marrow and the spleen with the result that areas over the spine and spleen will be much more strongly visualized on the scan. The removal rate of these colloid particles is a function of how much of the cardiac output is actually reaching the liver. Isotopic techniques have been sufficiently refined to permit estimation of liver flow from external counting.

Liver blood flow can be directly measured following the intravenous infusion of a material such as indocyanine green (ICG), which is removed from the body solely by the liver. After 30 minutes of constant infusion, the blood level of ICG reaches a plateau as the liver removal of the dye parallels the rate of infusion. If simultaneous samples of mixed hepatic venous blood (via a catheter guided into a large hepatic vein) and arterial blood are obtained, the blood flow can be calculated. All blood entering the liver (portal vein and hepatic artery) has the same concentration of ICG as any other artery, since only the liver can remove this material. The hepatic vein sample reflects the liver removal, and the milligrams of ICG removed from each milliliter of arterial blood passing through the liver is divided into the total ICG infused per minute. This method is valuable when liver function is normal or only mildly diminished, but it does not work in severe liver disease or in conditions of severe obstruction to biliary excretion. In practice, liver blood flow is of limited value in diagnosis. All forms of stable chronic liver disease seem to alter blood flow. Any form of splenic disease and most forms of pancreatic, small intestinal, gastric, and colonic inflammatory disease are associated with enhanced portal blood flow. Inflammatory liver diseases increase liver blood flow, but diseases associated with loss of total numbers of liver cells are associated with diminished blood flow.

Portal Pressure

The pressure measured in the portal vein or its feeding veins fluctuates not only with each respiration but also with intra-abdominal pressure, and it modestly increases following each meal. Knowledge of the pressure at only one point in time may be misleading or unrepresentative; one desires to know whether the pressure is persistently above normal levels.

The pressure may be persistently elevated because of an obstruction in the portal vein or at any point retarding flow of blood from the portal vein to the heart. In the presence of a totally normal liver, increased liver blood flow usually will not result in an elevated pressure because more sinusoids are recruited at very little increase in pressure. Minor abnormalities of the liver, however, along with an increased portal blood flow, may be responsible for some forms of portal hypertension.

Measurement of portal pressure is complicated and requires complex apparatus (Table 30–2). One accurate procedure is to dissect out the occluded umbilical vein in the umbilicus under local anesthesia and pass a catheter into the portal vein for direct measurement. Less directly, a needle may be passed into the pulp of the spleen, and the pressure in the splenic sinusoids will indicate a close approximation of the portal pressure. Still more indirect is measurement of the pressure recorded when a straight catheter it passed retrograde into a hepatic vein until is occludes the lumen. The pressure in the occluded vein will rise until blood is forced through available collateral channels proximal to this blockage; these are at the level of hepatic sinusoids. If such a recorded pressure is normal, this indicates that the resistance to flow from sinusoids is normal. In some diseases, the pressure recorded in this manner is much elevated, indicating an increased resistance to the escape of blood from the sinusoids. This pressure, called the *wedged hepatic venous pressure,* is a measurement of postsinusoidal resistance; a similar value is the pressure recorded by

a thin needle in the pulp of the liver. Injection of radiocontrast dye under fluoroscopic control verifies that the needle is not in a large vessel—the pressure recorded is sinusoidal or postsinusoidal.

The detailed evaluation of portal pressure requires the measurement of pressure in the portal vein or one of its branches. If it is elevated, the site of increased resistance must be determined. Wedged hepatic venous pressure may be measured to determine whether the elevation arises between that point and the heart or on the portal vein side of the sinusoid. Peripheral venous pressure may sometimes indicate a cardiac or peripheral localization of the resistance producing portal hypertension. Table 30–4 indicates some forms of portal pressure elevation and the anatomic localization of the increased resistance. Figure 30–7 emphasizes possible anatomic blockages found in disease.

There are many abnormalities that result from portal hypertension regardless of the basic cause. The severity and duration of portal hypertension seem more important determinants than the exact level of obstruction. The level of obstruction is of greatest importance in the mode of treatment and prognosis.

The sequelae of portal hypertension are conveniently divided into four groups: (1) splanchnic sequestration of blood, (2) congestion of viscera, (3) high pressure, and (4) development of collaterals (Table 30–5). It is apparent that the portal pressure rises in order to permit blood to leave the splanchnic bed (all blood vessels that normally drain into the portal system). If for any reason there is an increased entry of blood into the portal system (e.g., following a meal or any temporary boost in the cardiac output), this blood cannot promptly return to the heart. It must pool in the splanchnic bed and raise the pressure slightly to allow the flow to return to the heart. This increase in portal volume and pressure occurs concomitantly with a diminution in the blood volume available to the remainder of the body. As a result, the renal mechanisms for increasing the blood volume become operative, and a portion of the sodium retention is a direct result of this maldis-

TABLE 30–4 CAUSES OF PORTAL PRESSURE ELEVATION AND ANATOMIC LOCATION

Cause	Frequency	Anatomic Level Block	Comment
Extrahepatic portal vein occlusion	Rare	Portal vein	
Schistosomiasis	Common	Tiny portal veins	Endemic areas
Cancer nodules	Common	Portal	
Extramedullary hematopoiesis	Common	Presinusoidal	
Fat, lipid, amyloid accumulation	Common	Sinusoids	
Hypertrophy of endoplasmic reticulum	Rare	Sinusoids	
Cirrhosis	Common	Postsinusoid	
Budd-Chiari syndrome	Rare	Hepatic veins	
Veno-occlusive disease	Rare	Hepatic veins	Endemic areas
Inferior vena cava	Rare	Hepatic veins	
Constrictive pericarditis	Rare	Hepatic veins	
Heart failure	Common	Right auricle	

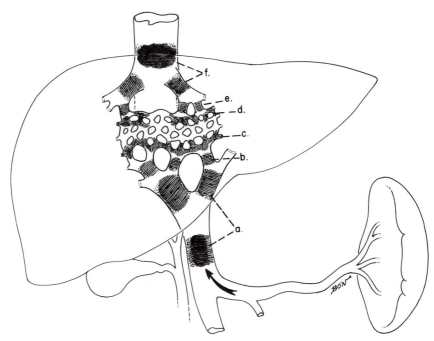

Figure 30–7 Schematic representation of the levels of obstruction of the portal vein producing portal hypertension. *a,* Blockage of the extrahepatic or large intrahepatic branches of the portal vein. *b,* Blockage of the tiny portal veins, such as is found in noncirrhotic portal hypertension of India. *c,* Blockage immediately presinusoidal, as produced by embolism and granuloma with schistosomiasis. *d,* Postsinusoidal block common in alcoholic cirrhosis. *e,* Block as in veno-occlusive disease. *f,* Hepatic vein, subhepatic vein, and inferior vena cava blockage.

tribution of the blood volume. Because of this, blood volume in every patient with portal hypertension rises above normal. The increase is entirely sequestered behind the obstructed portal circulation. No matter how large the volume, each

TABLE 30–5 SEQUELAE OF PORTAL HYPERTENSION

1. Splanchnic sequestration of blood
   a. Increased portal pressure after meal
   b. Diminished nonsplanchnic blood volume
   c. Increased renal retention of sodium
   d. Increased overall plasma volume
   e. Impaired maintenance of renal-brain-heart circulation during hemorrhage
2. Congestion of viscera
   a. Splenomegaly, hypersplenism
      (1) Increased contact time between spleen and blood cells
   b. Impaired intestinal and stomach motility
   c. Thrombosis of splenic and mesenteric veins
   d. Enhanced liver and mesenteric lymph formation
   e. Ascites
3. High portal pressure
   a. Development of collaterals promoted
      (1) Esophageal varices most common
      (2) Intra-abdominal varices second most common
      (3) Abdominal wall varices third most common
   b. Hemorrhage from varices promoted
4. Shunting of portal blood to systemic circulation
   a. Major cause of liver encephalopathy
   b. Altered insulin and glucagon regulation
   c. Altered "first pass" effect of many drugs and foods
   d. Altered kinetics of enterohepatic circulation

time more blood enters the splanchnic circulation, there is a temporary maladjustment. Should hemorrhage occur, this portion of the blood volume is only slowly available to the heart because of the high resistance before entry into the systemic circulation.

The elevated pressure promotes, over weeks or months, formation of collaterals to permit blood to return to the heart through other channels. Rarely, if ever, do these collateral channels restore the pressure to normal. Collaterals prevent pressure from reaching levels that would rupture vessels. Wherever the inferior vena cava and portal vessels have a common distribution, significant anastomoses may occur. The more important clinical areas are (1) directly from the portal vein along the stomach, up the esophagus, and anastomosing with the intercostal veins; (2) the section of the spleen between the diaphragm and the posterior abdominal wall; (3) along the umbilical vein or the mesentery through adhesions with the anterior abdominal wall; (4) posterior from branches in the area of the pancreas to the lumbar veins; and (5) around the rectum in the area of the hemorrhoidal vessels. These various collateral channels may be seen by various techniques. Sometimes they are visually prominent (abdominal, periumbilical, hemorrhoidal areas), or loud bruits (over the umbilicus) are detectable. They often produce large protrusions into the esophagus (opacified by a barium swallow) or, similarly, into the stomach. They are sometimes seen in the esophagus (esophagoscopy) or in the peritoneum (peritoneoscopy) and may also be demonstrated radiographically by the injection of a radiocontrast medium into the portal vein or its branches. The same techniques may be used to measure portal pressure directly, or large quantities of radiopaque media may be injected into the splanchnic arteries and thus opacify the portal vein and its branches (Table 30–2).

Finally, the presence of collateral channels may sometimes be suspected when divergence of large amounts of materials normally limited to the portal circulation appear in the systemic circulation. Extremely high levels of glucose (postprandially), high levels of ammonia and amino acids, and extremely high levels of urinary urobilinogen may be produced by large quantities of portal blood bypassing the liver and directly reaching the systemic circulation. The role of ammonia in liver coma is discussed in a later section.

Enlarged submucosal veins of the esophagus, known as *esophageal varices,* serve as collateral vessels between the portal venous system and the superior vena cava. These vessels are tortuous and distended up to 8 mm in diameter. The submucosa of the esophagus has little or no supportive-connective tissue. Esophageal varices are produced when portal pressure of more than 20 mm Hg above right heart pressure persists for months. At pressures above 35 mm, the varices tend to rupture and bleed profusely. Bleeding almost always occurs in the vicinity of the transition from intra-abdominal pressure to intrathoracic and is mainly caused by a temporary elevation in portal pressure. Surface irritation in the esophagus occasionally plays a role. Once bleeding begins, it is kept active by the sustained pressure, and the consequences of such hemorrhage are serious in that at least one sixth of such episodes produce death. Significant bleeding from other collateral beds in portal hypertension is infrequent. The surgical construction of a large low-resistance communication between the portal bed and the vena cava

(portacaval shunt) will eliminate portal hypertension. Shunting, if adequate, is effective in removing the hazard of variceal bleeding and may facilitate disappearance of varices (Fig. 30–8). The amount of portal blood shunted to the systemic circulation increases markedly. Shunts are most widely used to prevent subsequent hemorrhage from esophageal varices in patients in whom this has occurred at least once. Shunts do, however, produce some additional morbidity, largely from the increased shunting of blood to the systemic circulation (liver encephalopathy).

Congestion of viscera is prominent in portal hypertension. Over many months, it is rare for a patient with portal hypertension not to have an enlarged spleen, usually apparent on palpation but invariably demonstrated by scanning. Infarction, a common occurrence in portal hypertension, may develop owing to an enlarged, congested spleen and the slow turnover of blood. The congested sinusoids of the spleen and the prolonged contact of the active reticuloendothelial cells of the spleen with the formed elements of the blood (platelets, erythrocytes, leukocytes) may injure and destroy some or all three of these. The loss of any of these formed elements due to enlarged spleen is sometimes called *hypersplenism.* This is most apparent in the lowering of the peripheral counts. Platelet count is often lowered from a normal of 250,000 to half that level or less; the number of leukocytes is lowered to less than 4000, mostly owing to loss of polymorphonuclear leukocytes. Decrease in the red blood cells is less frequent. Despite the frequent occurrence of these lowered levels, they are rarely of clinical consequence in producing bleeding (due to platelet lack), increased infection (due to leukocyte lack), or symptoms of anemia; complete reversal requires both splenectomy and a portacaval shunt.

Congestion of the mesenteric vessels may lead to mesenteric infarction. Small thromboses of the mesenteric veins seem frequent in portal hyper-

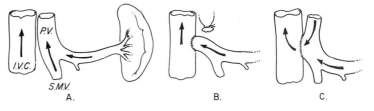
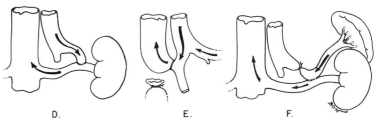

Figure 30–8 Types of portal systemic shunts constructed surgically. *A,* Normal. *I.V.C.,* inferior vena cava; *P.V.,* portal vein; *S.M.V.,* superior mesenteric vein.

B, End-to-side portacaval shunt—the portal vein is transected and the intestinal side anastomosed to I.V.C.

C, Side-to-side portacaval shunt.

D, Splenorenal shunt—the spleen is usually resected.

E, Mesocaval shunt. The I.V.C. is transected, and the proximal portion is anastomosed to the S.M.V. A prosthesis is often used and is called an "H graft."

F, Reverse splenorenal shunt, used to preserve S.M.V. blood flow to liver but decompress varices by permitting splenic venous flow and the variceal collaterals to drain through the renal circulation.

tension. They produce altered motility of the small intestine and occasionally damage the wall, producing peritonitis and septicemia, but they are difficult to recognize unless they are major. Whenever there are abrupt changes in congestion, intestinal function and motility may be temporarily impaired, and edema of the gut and impaired absorption may result. This congestion is one of the factors contributing to ascites, which is discussed in a later section. These consequences of portal hypertension are summarized in Table 30–5.

Lymph Flow

The hepatic sinusoid is possibly the most permeable capillary in the body; it is estimated that normally 0.3 per cent of the blood flow through the liver passes through the walls of the sinusoid and appears as liver lymph (compared with approximately 0.01 per cent for muscle). This lymph mainly follows the bile channels in lymphatic vessels, exits from the liver in the porta hepatis, and joins the cisterna chyli along with the mesenteric and large leg lymphatics. Any process that increases sinusoidal pressure (such as cirrhosis) may markedly increase liver lymph formation. In patients with cirrhosis, this increased lymph may exude from the surface of the liver and flow into the peritoneal cavity as ascites. This happens only when the rate of production exceeds the ability of the lymphatics to convey it back into the circulation. Protein elevation in lymph content reflects protein production by the liver (above 3.0 gm per 100 ml). Any interruption of hepatic lymphatics, such as may occur in biliary tract surgery or during surgery on the portal veins, may lead to large lymph fistulas into the peritoneal cavity.

In a similar fashion, any form of portal hypertension will increase the forces forming intestinal lymph in all parts of the bowel. If the increase is only slight, the lymphatics can convey it at about the same rate that it is formed. If the formation is acute or extremely rapid, it will produce edema of the cells of the bowel and may cross into the peritoneum and appear as ascites. Intestinal lymph is lower in protein content but may contain large amounts of lipid (chyle), particularly after fatty meals. Chylous ascites may result in patients with portal hypertension, although it is more frequent in patients with blockage of the lymphatics from obstruction. It has been observed that in all forms of portal hypertension, the flow of lymph in the thoracic duct is markedly increased from 3 to 60 times the normal level.

Biliary Tract

The biliary tree must provide adequate bile drainage for hepatocyte function to occur. Bile flow begins at the level of the canaliculus where he-

patocytes directly excrete the fluid volume and molecular elements that compose bile (Figs. 30–1, 30–3, and 30–5). The canaliculi enter together into the canals of Hering, which are formed from hepatocytes and bile duct epithelial cells at the fibrous edge of the portal triad. The canals of Hering then drain into bile ducts lined by cuboidal epithelial cells, which are functional in absorbing and secreting, in addition to conveying, the bile.

Bile flow may be hindered at any point along its course from the canaliculi to the ampulla at the duodenal outlet. Hepatocyte disease might result in decreased bile formation, the canaliculus may be injured or damaged, or obstructing lesions may occur at the hilum of the liver or along the extrahepatic bile duct. Pathologic processes at the level of the hepatocyte or canaliculus tend to decrease the volume of bile entering the large ducts, which results in a decrease in diameter of these ducts. Hilar or extrahepatic obstructions do not impair bile formation but impede its flow such that the bile ducts become dilated. The cystic duct leading to the gallbladder may be obstructed independently of the common bile duct; this is the most frequent antecedent to acute cholecystitis and is commonly caused by gallstones.

Bile continues to form and increase in volume following obstruction of the biliary tract until the pressure reaches about 25 cm of water. Such pressure allows the back diffusion of bile salts out of the biliary tree. Inflammation, edema, ischemia, and sometimes infection may also occur and lead to sepsis, which is often fatal if not surgically relieved.

Cholangiography. Gross dilatation of the bile ducts might be evident on ultrasonographic or CT scans. A more direct means of evaluating the biliary tree, however, is by cholangiography using radiopaque dyes and radiographs or using radioiodine-labeled dyes and scintiscan.

Three methods exist to fill the bile ducts and gallbladder with radiopaque dyes in order to permit radiographic examination and identification of the ducts and their branches. Oral cholecystography usually demonstrates the gallbladder. When ingested orally, several iodinated anionic dyes are absorbed, excreted by the liver, and concentrated by the gallbladder sufficiently to permit the gallbladder to be seen radiographically. Intravenous dyes of similar properties but not undergoing absorption are given to provide even more opacification of the ducts, and usually the ducts and gallbladder may be visualized. Neither process is adequate in the patient with disease of either the liver or major biliary passages. The accumulation of bile salts and bilirubin (anions) interfere with excretion of anionic dyes (Table 30–8).

Transhepatic cholangiography is useful when the ducts are blocked and dilated following continued secretion by the liver. A long, very thin needle is inserted blindly into the liver, and a duct is entered by chance. Radiopaque dye is injected under fluoroscopic control until sufficient dye is present to demonstrate the blocked portion. An alternative means of placing dye into the biliary tree is via an orally inserted endoscope. A trained operator can cannulate the ampulla of Vater directly and in retrograde fashion fill the biliary passages via a flexible endoscope inserted into the duodenum. This process is called *endoscopic retrograde cholangiography.*

Cationic dyes labeled with ^{99m}Tc have been developed for scanning agents that allow a gamma camera image of the liver, biliary passages, and bile duct, even in the presence of jaundice or elevated bile acids. Such agents can usually demonstrate the gallbladder if the cystic duct is patent—the only common diseases in which it is not patent are acute cholecystitis and empyema of the gallbladder. Excretion of the dye into the duodenum will occur within 1 to 2 hours if the liver is normal and the bile duct patent and within 24 hours if there is abnormal liver disease and a patent common bile duct. Obstruction to the extrahepatic bile duct by gallstone, tumor, or stenosis will prevent the normal pattern or time course for visualization of the dye in the intestinal tract.

CLINICALLY IMPORTANT BIOCHEMICAL FUNCTIONS OF THE LIVER

If one looks at the emergence of the liver by means of comparative physiology, it is apparent that processing of food, conversion of food from one form to another, food storage, and formation of an important digestive fluid are activities common to nearly all species. Removal of noxious substances, both those in the environment and those produced metabolically, is another major function. Finally, most species use the liver to make substances used elsewhere in the body.

DETOXIFICATION OF ENDOGENOUS PRODUCTS—PORPHYRINS, AMMONIA, AND PURINES

Three substances are produced in quantity each day in the human body, and all seem to be toxic, since they are excreted. These are ammonia, porphyrins, and purines. The body has developed complex mechanisms that involve the liver and the kidney working in conjunction to remove these substances, without producing harm and with a great deal of energy expenditure. Thus, ammonia is converted to urea, porphyrins are converted to bilirubin, and purines are converted to uric acid. The liver has a major role in the removal of all these substances from the body. Many other molecules are modified and removed by the liver. Ammonia and purine metabolism will be briefly considered in this section.

Ammonia arises metabolically from the breakdown of amino acids when they are used for energy production and as a by-product of renal production of ammonia to conserve base. Additional ammonia arises from the intestinal tract. The intestinal production is usually the most important. Intestinal ammonia is predominantly the result of action of intestinal bacteria on dietary nitrogen-containing food and of metabolically produced urea. The portal blood contains from four to 50 times the ammonia content of other blood of the body, yet the liver so successfully removes it that hepatic venous blood is the lowest in content of any in the body. The liver cell contains the enzyme machinery that condenses ammonia with bicarbonate in the presence of mitochondrial carbamyl phosphate synthetase as the first step in the formation of urea. Impairment of ammonia uptake is more prominent in liver disease than is impairment of overall urea synthesis, although urea formation is significantly impaired in cirrhosis of the liver. Increased peripheral blood ammonia is frequently found in liver disease. It arises most notably from the shunting of portal blood directly to the systemic circulation. Increased production of ammonia is also due to the increased small intestinal flora in liver disease and to the diminished uptake of ammonia by damaged liver cells.

Purines are progressively oxidized to uric acid in primates, and the final enzyme in this oxidation, xanthine oxidase, is contained solely in the liver. As far as can be determined, there seem to be no clinical consequences of mild impairment of this system in liver cell disease.

BILIRUBIN METABOLISM

The liver plays a varied and intimate role in bilirubin metabolism. The prominent and unique yellow color of the patient with liver disease (jaundice) invites attention to those factors basic to an understanding of liver physiology.

All bilirubin in the body results from the breakdown of cyclic tetrapyrroles, functioning as electron transport pigments. Hemoglobin is the most significant of these pigments in the production of bilirubin; however, myoglobin, P-450, and various cytochromes may all contribute cyclic tetrapyrroles that are catabolized and eliminated via the bilirubin pathway. These pigments are engulfed by reticuloendothelial cells, particularly in the spleen and bone marrow, to be converted into free bilirubin. Although the hemoglobin resulting from the breakdown of aged red blood cells is the most important source of bilirubin, significant amounts of the tetrapyrrole may also occur from ineffective erythropoiesis in the bone marrow. Once within the tissue macrophage, heme oxygenase acts on hemoglobin to produce biliverdin, which is subsequently converted to free bilirubin for release from the cell. For each molecule of cyclic tetrapyrrole converted to bilirubin, a molecule of CO is released and eventually eliminated through the lungs. A precise measure of the rate of formation of CO is an exact measure of bilirubin formation.

Although free bilirubin contains several polar groups, it is highly insoluble in water and body fluids owing to a tight intramolecular arrangement that renders the active groups unavailable. Free bilirubin is tightly bound to serum albumin to be soluble in blood; the binding constant is about the same as that between albumin and free fatty acids. The nearly total association of bilirubin with albumin leads to a volume of distribution identical with that of albumin. Free bilirubin is lipid-soluble and over several days is extracted into body fat. This extraction and subsequent tissue staining are responsible for jaundice; bilirubin confined to the blood is not apparent to an observer, regardless of the level.

Functions of the Hepatocyte in Bilirubin Metabolism

Three separate functions of the liver cell are commonly distinguished in bilirubin metabolism: (1) uptake of albumin-bound free bilirubin, (2) combination of free bilirubin with glucuronide into conjugated bilirubin, and (3) active secretion of conjugated bilirubin into the bile. Each of these operations illustrates important liver physiologic characteristics, and abnormalities of each occur that result in disease.

Uptake. Specific binding sites for albumin-bound bilirubin exist on the cell surface. The liver contains a protein of about 30,000 MW (ligandin) that binds bilirubin in the liver cell and seems responsible for the transfer of albumin-bound bilirubin into the liver cell. This process occurs at the cell surface, the albumin does not enter the liver cell, and no energy is required in this transfer. It seems to maintain an equilibrium in which bilirubin moves from tightly bound to albumin to slightly tighter binding on this intrahepatic transport and storage protein, called *ligandin;* movement continues from blood to liver because the ligandin in the liver cell is constantly divested of its bilirubin load.

The ligandin has a short half-life, and its rate of restoration is impaired by protein starvation. Thus, any form of free hyperbilirubinemia is exaggerated by a 24-hour fast. This also is seen in normals who are chronically starved. The same transport system is utilized by a number of albumin-bound organic acids. Sulfobromophthalein, bile salts, fatty acids, and many acidic drugs removed by the liver initially enter the cell bound to ligandin.

Normal albumin is saturated with 2 moles of free bilirubin per mole of albumin; thus, each gram of albumin can convey about 8 mg of free bilirubin, a state seldom reached in disease. Many molecules share the same binding sites on albumin as bilirubin and if present in sufficient concentration may displace bilirubin. Synthetic vitamin K and certain salicylates are examples. The rate of transfer of free bilirubin into the liver cell depends on (1) the concentration of bilirubin in the blood, (2) the concentration of albumin in the blood, (3) the blood flow to the liver, (4) the concentration of ligandin in the liver cell, (5) the concentration of bilirubin on the ligandin in the liver cell, and (6) the binding sites on the liver cell. Two- or threefold increases in this transport may be achieved over a period of time, probably by increasing the last two of the aforementioned variables, but abrupt lesser increases or chronic increases exceeding this range can be accomplished only by increasing the level of bilirubin in the blood. At bilirubin levels of 6 or 7 mg per 100 ml, any achievable amount of free bilirubin may be transported. If serum free bilirubin level is above this, the transport machinery is defective.

Conjugation. Conjugation occurs inside the liver cell. This process combines two proprionic acid side chains on the bilirubin molecule with glucuronide molecules. In this fashion, the tight intramolecular arrangement of bilirubin is destroyed, and a water-soluble molecule called *conjugated bilirubin* is produced. Conjugation occurs on the smooth endoplasmic reticulum (ER) and requires activated glucuronic acid to combine with bilirubin through the intervention of an enzyme called *glucuronyl transferase.* There is evidence that portions of the ER adjacent to the bile canaliculus are principally responsible for this enzyme activity.

Conjugation enzymes mature late in the development of the fetus and are not fully developed until the tenth month after conception. Thus, premature infants have impaired conjugation, and varying degrees of impairment may be commonly found in underweight newborns. This is emphasized by the abrupt destruction of erythrocytes that occurs at the time of birth (hemoglobin decreases from about 19 to 14 gm per 100 ml) and its concomitant pigment load. Under this circumstance, free bilirubin accumulates in the blood in large amounts. When the level exceeds 20 mg per 100 ml, the possible entry of free bilirubin into central nervous tissues with subsequent brain damage is quite high. Anoxic brain damage occurring at birth makes this possibility a likelihood. Such brain damage resulting from free bilirubin is called *kernicterus* after the yellow staining of basal ganglia of the brain. The abnormal hemolysis produced by maternal Rh antiserum reaching the Rh-positive fetus most often produces such damage. If the hazard arises after birth, the level of bilirubin may be monitored; if the level is above 20 mg per 100 ml, it may be lowered by removing about one fifth of the patient's blood and replacing it with normal blood. This exchange transfusion is highly effective in lowering the circulating free bilirubin. Alternatively, intense ultraviolet irradiation of the child destroys bilirubin in the skin and prevents it from reaching the brain. A series of circumstances combine to make bilirubin brain damage feasible in childhood but nearly impossible later in life. These are as follows:

1. Physiologic or abnormal breakdown of red cells in large amounts.

2. Conjugation impairment due to prematurity.

3. Failure of immature blood-brain barrier to exclude bilirubin.

4. Anoxic birth injury.

Secretion. Conjugated bilirubin is produced in proximity to the bile canaliculus and is rapidly secreted into the bile. Under normal conditions it does not escape from the hepatic cell. However, if there is necrosis of liver cells, conjugated bilirubin in the bile ducts may reach Disse's space. Accumulation of conjugated bilirubin in the liver cells for any reason may also lead to conjugated bilirubin in the blood and in the urine. Conjugated bilirubin passes freely into all the fluids of the body; it is partially bound to albumin, so that its distribution is influenced by the protein content. Conjugated bilirubin stains most protein-containing subcutaneous fluids and is readily observed in the sclerae of the eye and in the loose connective tissue beneath the tongue. It enters urine, spinal fluid, ascites, and most edema fluid. The most clinically useful difference between free and conjugated bilirubin is the regular appearance of conjugated bilirubin in the urine, whereas free bilirubin, which is not water-soluble, cannot be excreted in urine. Conjugated bilirubin is the only form in the bile.

Enterohepatic Circulation

Once excreted into bile, bilirubin is carried to the intestinal tract, where bacteria reduce conjugated bilirubin progressively to compounds called *stercobilin* or *urobilinogen*. These products, which number approximately 20 different substances, account for the color of stool. If intestinal bacterial reduction occurs normally, no bilirubin is found in the stool. Several of these products undergo extensive enterohepatic circulation, i.e., the reabsorption of the compounds in the intestine with hepatic uptake and subsequent re-excretion in the bile. The determination of urobilinogen in the urine is a useful means of assessing overall pigment metabolism.

Normally, the urine contains 0.5 to 4 mg urobilinogen in 24 hours. This represents approximately 5 per cent of about 70 mg of urobilinogen absorbed via the portal vein and excreted almost entirely via the liver. Urobilinogen is a weak acid and as such is more concentrated in alkaline than

in acid urine. Normally, fresh urine with a pH of 5.5 or more contains urobilinogen, demonstrating that conjugated bilirubin is reaching the gut and normal bacterial reduction and intestinal absorption of the urobilinogen are occurring. The total absence of urobilinogen in fresh urine of pH 5.5 or higher indicates that this cycle is broken. Most commonly, total obstruction of the biliary passages is present; less commonly, bacterial reduction (such as after extensive antibiotic use) is interrupted. Marked increase in urine urobilinogen suggests an increased production of urobilinogen, inefficient hepatic cell removal (such as in liver cell disease), or abnormal vascular communications between the portal and systemic circulation, bypassing the liver.

Tests of Bilirubin Metabolism
(Table 30–6)

Total bilirubin in the blood and urine may be accurately measured. However, differentiation of free and conjugated may be only crudely approximated by the "direct-reacting" and "indirect-reacting" bilirubin. Pure free bilirubin will almost always be less than 20 per cent direct-reacting. Conjugated bilirubin, however, may be as much as 50 per cent indirect-reacting. In clinical situations, if less than 25 per cent of the bilirubin is direct-reacting, it may be presumed that essentially all the bilirubin is free. If 50 per cent or more of the bilirubin is direct-reacting, it should be assumed that essentially all is conjugated. Determination of bilirubin in a fresh urine sample is the most precise method of determining whether or not bilirubin is entirely in the free form; in such cases, the dipstick test will show it to be absent from the urine.

Urine Urobilinogen. A fresh urine sample should be used and the pH determined; only if the pH is 5.5 or higher should urobilinogen be measured. The serial dilution that contains detectable material should be ascertained or the level estimated from a dip stick. The important questions concern (1) whether there is some urobilinogen present, and (2) whether it is present in a dilution of 1 to 50 or greater. Absence of urobilinogen indicates either (1) that conjugated bilirubin is not reaching the intestine, or (2) that bacterial conversion to urobilinogen is not occurring, usually owing to antibiotics but occasionally because of colectomy or rapid diarrhea preventing sufficient numbers of the correct bacteria. An excess of urobilinogen indicates one of the following: (1) increased production of bilirubin, (2) impaired removal of urobilinogen from portal blood due to damaged liver cells, or (3) increased shunting of portal blood into the systemic circulation.

Sulfobromophthalein (BSP) and Indocyanine Green (ICG) Tests. These materials behave similarly in assessing liver metabolism. Both are in-

TABLE 30–6 ABNORMALITIES OF BILIRUBIN METABOLISM AND TESTS OF FUNCTION

Tests	Liver Biopsy	Specific Evaluation
1. Increased production (> 75% bilirubin indirect-reacting)		
a. Increased RBC breakdown		Hemolytic evaluation
b. Ineffective erythropoiesis with marrow breakdown		Hbg electrophoresis, folate B_{12}
2. Impaired uptake/conjugation (> 75% bilirubin indirect-reacting)		
a. Prematurity		
b. Gilbert's syndrome		Fasting → ↑ unconjugated bilirubin ± ↓ glucuronyl transferase with response to phenobarbital
c. Crigler-Najjar syndrome I		Absent glucuronyl transferase
d. Crigler-Najjar syndrome II		↓ Glucuronyl transferase
3. Impaired bilirubin excretion (> 75% bilirubin direct-reacting)		
a. Dubin-Johnson syndrome	+	Secondary rise of injected BSP at 90 minutes
b. Drugs/toxins	+	↑ Drug levels
4. Obstruction to bile flow (> 75% bilirubin direct-reacting)		
a. Canaliculus	+	
(1) Hepatitis		↑ AST, ALT, HBsAg, IgM-hepatitis A-SMA, ANF
(2) Infiltrative processes/tumor		↑ Alkaline phosphatase
b. Intrahepatic bile ducts	+	
(1) PBC		Antimitochondrial antibody
(2) Intrahepatic biliary atresia/hypoplasia		
c. Extrahepatic bile ducts	+	
(1) Secondary obstruction		Sonography, cholangiography,
(2) Inflammation (sclerosing cholangitis, pancreatitis)		T_c-HIDA scan,
(3) Extrahepatic biliary atresia		↓ urobilinogen

travenously administered anionic dyes. Both travel tightly adherent to albumin, both are taken up by the ligandin of the liver (in direct competition with bilirubin), and BSP but not ICG is conjugated by an enzyme on the endoplasmic reticulum with glutathione. Conjugated BSP and ICG are then secreted by the anion pump into the bile. In clinical use, a fixed dose of the dye is administered intravenously (5 mg per kg BSP; 0.5 mg per kg ICG), and a blood sample is taken 45 minutes later for BSP (20 minutes for ICG) to determine how much dye has persisted in the blood. If more than 6 per cent is found, liver cell uptake is considered defective. Any form of jaundice competes with the removal of both dyes, but in the nonjaundiced patient the removal from blood is mainly a measurement of the uptake and storage of the liver cell.

Pathophysiology of Bilirubin Metabolism

Disease states resulting in abnormal bilirubin metabolism may be categorized into four main groups (Table 30–6): (1) increased production, (2) impaired hepatic uptake and conjugation, (3) impaired excretion into bile, and (4) impaired excre-

tion of bile and bilirubin from the liver into the duodenum.

Increased bilirubin production may be the product of excess hemoglobin resulting from hemolysis, ineffective erythropoiesis, enhanced red blood cell breakdown following transfusions of stored blood (aged RBCs), or reabsorption of massive hematomas. The unconjugated fraction of free bilirubin produced temporarily overwhelms the ability of hepatocytes to bind it and clear it from the circulation.

Impairment of hepatic uptake or conjugation or both after the newborn period is most frequently the result of inherited deficiencies in the hepatocellular binding proteins or the conjugation of bilirubin and thereby interrupts bilirubin transport prior to adequate conjugation of bilirubin with glucuronide. These conditions, like those associated with increased bilirubin production, will result in an increase in the serum level of unconjugated bilirubin. Impaired hepatic uptake occurs in the benign condition known as *Gilbert's syndrome*. This disorder affects up to 5 per cent of the normal population, particularly males, and is characterized by intermittent mild increase in unconjugated bilirubin during times of stress, fasting, or infection. It is presumed that binding proteins and, possibly, glucuronyl transferase are mildly deficient in these patients. The normal decrease of binding protein that occurs in fasting, for example, will be exacerbated and may result in clinically apparent hyperbilirubinemia.

Conjugation of bilirubin is impaired by several experimental drugs, by a steroid occasionally occurring in maternal milk, and by certain plant toxins. Two inborn errors of metabolism are associated with impairment of bilirubin conjugation due to deficiency in glucuronyl transferase. The first of these, the Crigler-Najjar syndrome, is present at birth, is associated with a high degree of brain damage (two thirds of cases), and is unresponsive to any known treatment; glucuronyl transferase is absent, and there is no bilirubin in bile. The second, the Arias type of the Crigler-Najjar syndrome, appears shortly after birth and does not result in brain damage. One can control it by inducing microsomal enzymes with phenobarbital, thereby stimulating a deficient glucuronyl transferase and lowering the bilirubin to normal. The diagnostic features of both forms are very high levels of free bilirubin (more than 10 mg per 100 ml), present early and throughout life, and absence of any apparent bilirubin conjugation in liver biopsy specimens. In type I, there is no bilirubin in bile; in type II, large amounts appear. In acquired disease, conjugation impairment almost never accounts for jaundice.

Impaired excretion of bilirubin into bile most commonly occurs with injury to the canalicular network and the hepatocytes themselves. Inflammatory processes such as hepatitis and residual scarring are the usual etiologic factors. Inherited disorders of bilirubin excretion from the cell into bile are the Dubin-Johnson and Rotor syndromes.

Impaired excretion of bile and bilirubin from liver to duodenum most commonly results from obstruction. The obstruction may occur at any level of the biliary tree (Fig. 30–9). At the level of the canaliculus, cholestasis may result from drugs such as estrogens or in altered hormonal states such as pregnancy.

At the level of the intrahepatic bile ducts, inflammation and subsequent sclerosis of the bile ducts themselves are the most common pathologic findings. Primary biliary cirrhosis is a common etiologic factor in the adult. Infiltrative diseases might also produce cholestasis by compression of intrahepatic bile ducts. In the obstructive cholangiopathy of infancy, however, pathology specifically involving the intrahepatic bile ducts is usually secondary to a congenital (and frequently familial) syndrome of atresia or hypoplasia of the ducts.

At the level of the extrahepatic bile ducts, obstruction in adults most commonly occurs by an intraluminal gallstone or by compression and stenosis secondary to tumor or inflammation. As for the intrahepatic biliary tree, obstruction of the extrahepatic biliary tree in infancy is more commonly the result of atresia from birth or congenital

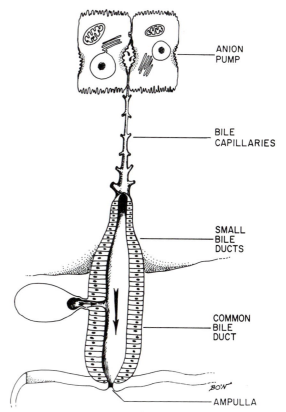

Figure 30–9 Schematic outline of bile formation starting with the anion pump and the canaliculus. Bile arises as bile-salt–independent flow (possibly from the hepatocytes, more likely from the bile ducts) and bile-salt–dependent flow (certainly from the hepatocyte, anion pump). The small bile ducts clearly have absorptive and secretory functions, and ducts at this level dilate markedly with distal obstruction. Interference with the process of bile formation or with bile flow at any level produces cholestasis.

abnormalities of the biliary tree such as the choledochal cyst.

BILE FORMATION AND BILE FLOW

Integral to the successful removal of bilirubin from the body is the ability of the liver to form and excrete bile. Bile contains water and electrolytes in amounts approximately equal to those found in plasma. In addition, it contains four major organic components (bile salts, lecithin, cholesterol, bilirubin) and many others. Bile is formed initially at the level of the bile canaliculus (Fig. 30–9). Water diffuses passively to maintain isotonicity. The thick epithelium of intermediate-sized bile ducts may add or remove water or electrolytes or both, and about two thirds of the initially formed bile is absorbed in the small bile ducts. The gallbladder markedly concentrates hepatic bile by removal of water and electrolytes. Remarkably, the contents of the biliary tree remain nearly isotonic throughout all these alterations, largely owing to the propensity of the organic molecules to form loose molecular complexes called *micelles*. These micelles serve principally to keep the more insoluble components (cholesterol) in solution. Many substances are secreted by the liver into bile for excretion; almost any organic acid may be so excreted. The normal composition of the major components of bile are indicated in Table 30–7.

Composition of Bile

Bile salts are the principal component of bile, constituting 90 per cent of the nonelectrolyte solutes. They are synthesized exclusively by the liver from cholesterol.

Bile salts have two, three, or four polar groups all on one surface; the remainder of the molecule is water-insoluble but lipid-soluble. This amphoteric property provides a major function in forming micelles, which keep insoluble materials in contact with a water surface in the biliary passages and in the intestine. Bile salts facilitate the excretion of cholesterol and phospholipid from the liver in bile and facilitate the absorption in the intestine of long-chain fatty acids and lipid-soluble materials, especially the fat soluble vitamins A, D, E, and K.

Figure 30–10 illustrates the relationship among the molar ratios of cholesterol, lecithin, and bile salts. Cholesterol is essentially insoluble in aqueous solutions such as bile, but both lecithin and bile salt contribute to the formation of micelles, which permit the cholesterol to be dissolved. The small area at the bottom of the illustration is the soluble region; the shaded area is the metastable region. Whenever the cholesterol concentration, relative to the other components of bile, is outside this region, two phases occur and the cholesterol precipitates out of solution. Although this usually happens once or twice each 24 hours

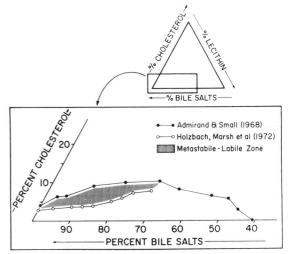

Figure 30–10 The relationship between the major components of bile that determine whether cholesterol remains in solution or precipitates out. The molar percentage of each component is plotted on the triangular coordinates, and the sum is always 100 per cent. Only for values in the small, clear section in the lower left corner of the triangle (see enlargement) is cholesterol soluble. The molar percentage of bile salt must exceed 40 per cent. Lecithin at concentrations from very little to 50 per cent also enhances cholesterol solubility. At values in the area above the upper dotted line, cholesterol will rapidly form crystals, since the solution is highly unsaturated; at values in the shaded area, cholesterol will slowly precipitate. Patients forming cholesterol gallstones (the most common type) have supersaturated bile throughout most of the day; normal subjects have this only intermittently, a few times each day. (From Carey, M.C.: Principles of Internal Medicine. 8th ed. New York, McGraw-Hill Book Co., 1977.)

in normal persons, those who form cholesterol gallstones (the most common type) have this abnormality almost half of the day and night. Sometimes drugs are given that work to increase the solubility of cholesterol and may even cause cholesterol gallstones to dissolve.

Cholic acid and chenodeoxycholic acid are the two bile salts made by the human liver (Fig. 30–11). Adults form about 200 to 300 mg of cholic acid per day and a similar amount of chenodeoxycholic. Under stimulation, cholic acid synthesis can increase seven- to tenfold, and chenodeoxycholic acid synthesis can increase two- or threefold. Bile salts are conjugated in the acid group with either glycine or taurine, with two thirds of the total as glycine. Conjugation of bile salts is important for both hepatic excretion and distal ileal reabsorption. If intestinal bacteria deconjugate large quantities of bile salts in the intestine, and reabsorption becomes inefficient, they are lost via the stool. The human adult body contains 3 to 4 gm of bile salts, and these are completely excreted into the intestine and reabsorbed 6 to 10 times each day. This excretion and reabsorption are so remarkably complete that only about 0.1 gm of

TABLE 30–7 COMPOSITION OF HUMAN HEPATIC BILE

Component	mg/100 ml	Total Solids (per cent)	mEq/L
Bile salts	140–2230	8–53	3–45*
Lecithin	140–810	9–21	2–8*
Cholesterol	97–320	3–11	2–6*
Bilirubin	12–70	0.4–2.0	<1
Urobilinogen	5–45	0.2–1.5	<1
Sodium			146–165
Potassium			2.7–4.9
Bicarbonate			27–55

*Variability due to micelle formation.
(After Thureborn, E: Acta Chir. Scand. *303*(suppl.):1, 1962.)

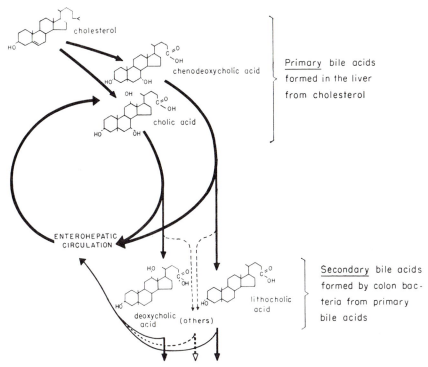

Figure 30–11 Formation of primary and secondary bile acids from cholesterol. (Reproduced from Carey, J.: *In* Schiff, L. [Ed.]: Diseases of the Liver. 3rd ed. Philadelphia, J.B. Lippincott Co., 1969.)

bile salt or less is lost from the body during each "enterohepatic circulation." Disorders of liver cell function retard the rate at which the bile salts are cleared from the enterohepatic circulation and peripheral blood and thus decrease the amount returned to the intestine. However, disorders of terminal ileal function or disorders of bacterial overgrowth that cause deconjugation of bile salts increase the amounts lost from the body. About 0.5 gm of bile salt is normally lost from the body each day. The liver synthesizes and replaces this amount. Intestinal bacteria reduce bile acids (Fig. 30–11) to new ones called *secondary bile acids*. The product of cholic acid reduction, deoxycholic acid, acts as a normal bile salt and undergoes enterohepatic circulation. The product of chenodeoxycholic acid reduction, lithocholic acid, is reabsorbed once but is then sulfated by the liver and can no longer be reabsorbed.

Assessment of Bile Salt Serum Levels and Metabolism. Since the liver manufactures bile acids and salts, abnormalities due to liver cell disease might be anticipated. The most common disorders in liver disease are related to control of the blood level. The diseased liver cannot rapidly clear bile salts from the portal flow because of impaired liver function and shunting of portal blood. This results in higher fasting levels of bile salts. This defect is particularly marked 2 hours after a meal, when the blood levels are high from the reabsorbed load recently poured into the intes-

tine. The 2-hour postprandial bile acid level is among the most sensitive of tests known for detecting mild liver cell damage.

In severe liver disease, a diminution in cholic acid and an increase in deoxycholic acid as primary bile acids are noted. Although conjugation may be impaired in liver disease, the defect is less pronounced than the increased production of dehydroxy acids.

Other tests of bile formation are essentially those measuring bile flow as a function of bilirubin metabolism, as already discussed. Tests evaluating the biliary tree itself include cholangiography and scanning techniques as reviewed previously.

Bile Flow

Bile acids play a significant role in the flow of bile out of the liver parenchyma at the level of the canaliculus, referred to as *bile salt–dependent flow* *(BSDF)*.

The wall of the bile canaliculus, with the likely participation of adjacent endoplasmic reticulum and Golgi apparatus, is capable of actively secreting a variety of materials into the lumen. The most active transport system excretes a number of organic anions; as noted in Table 30–8, bile salts are by far the most important single material secreted by this system, called the *anion pump*. There is some support for different specific trans-

TABLE 30–8 REPRESENTATIVE COMPOUNDS ACTIVELY EXCRETED BY HEPATIC CELLS

Organic acids

Naturally occurring:	Used diagnostically:
Bile salts*	Sulfobromophthalein†
Bilirubin	Indocyanine green
Urobilinogen*	Iopanoic acid†
Lecithin†	Iodipamide
Therapeutic agents:	
Sulfonamides†	
Penicillin†	
Ampicillin†	
Chlorthiazide†	
Streptomycin†	
Tetracycline*	

Bases

Procaine amide	HIDA
ethobromide	
Xylocaine	PIPIDA

Neutral

Adrenal and sex
sterols
Cholesterol*
Digitalis glycosides†

*Highly active enterohepatic circulation.
†Mildly active enterohepatic circulation.

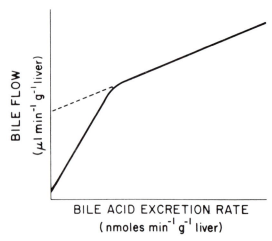

Figure 30–12 Relationship of bile flow to bile-acid excretion rate. Studies in the rat and rhesus monkey suggest that bile flow varies with bile-acid excretion rate in a curvilinear fashion (solid line). The slope of the line relating bile flow to bile-acid excretion is steeper at lower rates of bile-acid excretion than at higher excretion rates. Traditional estimates of bile-acid–independent flow were obtained by extrapolating the terminal portion of the curve back to the ordinate (dashed line). (From Blitzer, B.L., and Boyer, J.L.: Gastroenterology 82:346, 1982.)

port systems for different anions. The wall of the bile canaliculus seems freely permeable to water and uncharged molecules up to a molecular weight of about 900, but charged molecules seem retarded in their passage. As a result of the active secretion of bile salt and other molecules, water moves to preserve isotonicity. Bile volume is highly dependent on total bile salt secretion; normal flow is 450 to 700 ml per 24 hours.

A portion of canalicular bile flow independent of bile salt excretion is commonly called *bile salt–independent flow (BSIF)*. This aspect of bile flow is demonstrated in Fig. 30–12, in which bile flow is plotted over a wide range of excreted bile salts. It is noted that over much of the range, bile flow increases linearly with bile salt excretion, but even when bile salt excretion is zero there remains appreciable bile flow. In humans, this equals approximately 30 per cent of the maximal flow.

Although the precise mechanism of the BSIF is unknown, several hypotheses have been suggested. Na^+, K^+-ATPase is one enzyme that has been linked to BSIF, since agents that alter Na^+, K^+-ATPase alter BSIF in rodents. However, this enzyme is so widespread and germane to many transport systems that the mechanism is not established by these experiments.

Structural components of the canaliculus itself have also been proposed as mechanically important in BSIF. The tight junctions between hepatocytes at either end of the bile canaliculus may be semipermeable to ion secretion and water movement, creating a paracellular pathway for BSIF.

Finally, bile ducts are clearly able to both absorb and secrete into the bile, providing still

another important mechanism in bile flow. The bile duct epithelium responds to secretin with a 20 per cent increase in bile volume and a change in ionic composition with an increase in bicarbonate ion. This epithelium also responds to somatostatin.

Many of the organic molecules contained in the bile are reabsorbed by the intestine into the portal venous blood and are transported to the liver, where they are re-excreted. Intestinal reabsorption may be highly efficient (95 per cent for bile salts), of intermediate efficiency (30 to 50 per cent for urobilinogen), or very slight (bilirubin). The process of liver bile excretion, gut absorption, and liver re-excretion is called *enterohepatic circulation*. The hepatic extraction of the reabsorbed material may be so efficient that little reaches the peripheral venous blood. This recycling of substances through the biliary tree is employed in the treatment of biliary tract infections. An antibiotic that is recycled through the biliary tract many times is chosen. Enterohepatic circulation assumes substantial importance when interrupted. In intestinal disease, bile salt conservation is impossible, and depletion occurs. When inefficient liver cell extraction occurs, products normally removed by the liver appear in the urine (e.g., urobilinogen). If portal blood is shunted to the periphery, higher peripheral blood levels may occur. Cholestyramine, an insoluble resin taken orally, binds certain materials undergoing enterohepatic circulation (bile salts, digitalis glycosides, cholesterol) in the intestine and can deplete the body of them.

Cholestasis. Cholestasis is the usual manifestation of abnormal bile flow. Whenever there is evidence that adequate amounts of both bile salt and bilirubin have failed to reach the intestinal tract and have accumulated in the blood, the condition is designated *cholestasis*. This concept is useful, since there are marked similarities in patients with jaundice from the extremes of disease of the liver cell to mechanical obstruction at the level of the ampulla of Vater.

Cholestasis is ordinarily diagnosed with evidence from three different sources (Table 30–9). Lack of bilirubin and bile salts in the stool produces steatorrhea, vitamin K deficiency and associated prolongation of the prothrombin time, light stools, and lack of urobilinogen in the urine. Accumulation of bilirubin and bile salts in the blood produces pruritus and jaundice. If the cholestasis is severe and prolonged for months, the blood cholesterol and phospholipid levels will rise markedly. The cholesterol may deposit in the skin as xanthomas. The high cholesterol is caused by increased rate of hepatic and intestinal manufacture. Bile salts reaching the gut normally repress hepatic and intestinal synthesis of cholesterol. Finally, in cholestasis some evidence of stimulation or injury to the hepatic and biliary epithelial cells is present. This is demonstrated most prominently by marked elevation of the enzyme alkaline phosphatase due to induction of hepatic production. The result of bile salt injury of liver cell membranes is a modest elevation to serum transaminase. Injury and mild inflammation are also apparent on liver biopsy. This takes the form of distorted bile canaliculi, bile lakes (lysed cells due to bile accumulation), and occasional inflammatory cells.

TABLE 30–9 FINDINGS SOMETIMES PRESENT IN CHOLESTASIS

Clinical	Laboratory
	Due to accumulation in blood:
Jaundice	Elevated bilirubin
Itching	Elevated bile salts
	Due to lack in intestine:
Bulky, loose stools	Increased stool fat and weight
Ecchymoses	Prolonged prothrombin time
White or light stools	No bile pigment, no urobilinogen
	Decreased urine urobilinogen
Xanthoma	Elevated serum cholesterol (after prolonged cholestasis)
	Injurious effects on liver:
Mild hepatomegaly	Elevated serum alkaline phosphatase
	Elevated ALT, AST
	Liver biopsy changes

In practice, cholestasis is diagnosed when there is jaundice, elevation of the serum alkaline phosphatase, and little or no evidence of major hepatocellular damage. If the stools are light (owing to both increased fat content and reduced pigment) and there is no urine urobilinogen, the syndrome is even more firmly established.

The practical problem of cholestasis is to determine at what level from the liver cell to the ampulla the block has occurred (Fig. 30–9). Studies of bile salt and bilirubin metabolism are usually not helpful in this determination. From the level of the bifurcation of the hepatic ducts distally, surgical removal or bypass of the lesion producing cholestasis is indicated; at higher levels, surgical intervention is not practical and often exaggerates the underlying condition.

Two little-known factors about the common causes of cholestasis often permit one to suspect correctly the proper cause: 1. Bile ducts larger than 1 mm in diameter are capable of tremendous dilatation with the secretory pressure of the liver and are thus seen clearly with sonography after 12 to 14 days. 2. Cholestasis at the level of the anion pump or the bile capillaries rarely is complete for more than a few days. Each factor is useful in several ways. If cholestasis is caused by a surgical lesion, dilatation of the many ducts and moderate to marked enlargement of the liver must be present. If a patient with cholestasis has a normal-sized liver, a surgical lesion is very unlikely. The most common cause of surgical cholestasis is a gallstone impacted in the common bile duct. This most often lodges in the narrowest and least distensible portion of the common bile duct, which is the portion of the duct traversing the wall of the duodenum. Dilatation proximal to such an obstruction will usually produce a 2- to 4-cm turgid tube resembling a garden hose and passing beneath the duodenal bulb. A standard barium meal will usually reveal this mass, producing a silhouette as it passes posteriorly. Sonograms and CT scans readily identify such a mass as a dilated common bile duct. Occasionally, the ducts in the hilum are sufficiently enlarged to produce a defect on colloid scan of the liver. Sometimes, the turgid distended gallbladder is clearly and diagnostically palpable, indicating this problem. Visualization of the ducts by direct or radiologic means (direct laparotomy or peritoneoscopy; transhepatic or direct cholangiography) should indicate substantial dilatation beyond the normal 8 to 10 mm in diameter. Ultrasonography, or sonography, has become sufficiently precise to detect the fluid-filled and enlarged bile ducts within the hepatic parenchyma and to provide an excellent measure of the size of the gallbladder. This technique, of no harm to the patient, has markedly enhanced the ability to detect a dilated gallbladder and the bile ducts. Computer assisted tomography (CT scan) of the liver area provides information of a similar nature.

The lack of complete obstruction in medical cholestasis is best appreciated by serial observations over several days. If small amounts of pigment appear in the stools or if urobilinogen is seen in the urine, incomplete obstruction is present. The newer radiopharmaceuticals excreted by the liver into the bile may also be used both for scans and for demonstrating the patency of the common bile duct. A trace of these given intravenously is completely taken up by the normal liver in 30 to 60 minutes and completely excreted into the bile within 2 hours. In cholestasis, the uptake by the liver is normal, but the subsequent excretion is retarded. However, in surgical cholestasis the obstruction is usually complete, so that scans done 1 hour and 24 hours after a single dose of TcHIDA are essentially identical; in contrast, in the less complete intrahepatic cholestasis the scan at 24 hours is decreased in intensity, usually by 50 per cent or more, and often all the dye has passed into the gut. Newer radioactive molecules make this differentiation even more precise. If the cause of the jaundice is not clear by this time, some procedure must be initiated to demonstrate the intrahepatic and extrahepatic bile ducts directly. Either percutaneous cholangiography or endoscopic retrograde cholangiography may be used.

CHOLESTEROL SYNTHESIS

Cholesterol, a major component of bile, is also the biochemical precursor of bile salts and steroid hormones. It is an integral component of phospholipid/protein cell membranes. Hepatocytes, more than other cell types, make cholesterol in large amounts for use in liver cells themselves, for synthesis of bile salts, and for export into the blood stream as part of very low density lipoprotein (VLDL). The excess cholesterol in the system is returned to the liver for use in synthesis there or for excretion into bile. Serum levels are determined in large part by the rate of synthesis in the liver and intestines and excretion in the liver.

Serum Cholesterol. Profound liver dysfunction is associated with a normal to low cholesterol level, whereas chronic biliary tract obstruction is associated with an increased serum level, the latter caused by intestinal activity.

Pathophysiology of Cholesterol Synthesis. Increased serum levels of cholesterol seen in chronic biliary obstruction, such as primary biliary cirrhosis, are associated with the appearance of xanthomata and xanthelasma in the skin. Prolonged elevation of circulatory lipids may be associated with an increased incidence of atherosclerosis.

The formation of cholesterol gallstones is the result of an imbalance between the amount of cholesterol in the bile and the amount of bile salt, producing a bile supersaturated with cholesterol (Fig. 30–10). This condition over many years may result in gallstone formation. Treatment with one of two bile salts, chenodeoxycholic acid or ursodeoxycholic acid, seems to correct the imbalance by altering hepatic synthesis and excretion so that less cholesterol comes into the bile and more bile salt is present, causing the stones to dissolve slowly.

PROTEIN SYNTHESIS

Table 30–10 indicates the wide variety of proteins that are made almost exclusively by the liver in the ribosomal network and rough endoplasmic reticulum. Supporting this extensive synthetic factory is a rich array of systems in the liver cell that store amino acids, convert an amino acid present in excess to one present to a lesser degree, and are sources of energy. Protein synthesis will be completely normal only when there are adequate numbers of completely normal liver cells, few or no inhibitors of protein synthesis, and an adequate supply of dietary protein to provide essential amino acids.

The blood level of a given protein is a function of both its rate of synthesis and its rate of removal. Some proteins persist a very short time in the blood after release. Factors operative in disease may hasten the removal of the protein from blood (such as loss of albumin into the intestinal tract or urine or depletion of serum fibrinogen due to accelerated coagulation).

Under normal circumstances, serum proteins synthesized in the liver vary widely in removal rates. Thus, albumin persists in the serum with a half-life of approximately 30 days; fibrinogen with a half-life of approximately 4 days; and prothrombin with a half-life of approximately 12 hours. This means that total cessation of hepatic manufacture and release would result in a fall of prothrombin to 5 per cent, of fibrinogen to 60 per cent, and of albumin to 92 per cent of initial level in 2 days. The serum half-life of these several proteins is helpful in dating the onset of severe liver cell failure.

The wide variety of proteins made by the liver and present in the serum is less useful in diagnos-

TABLE 30–10 PROTEINS MADE PREDOMINANTLY BY THE LIVER

1. Albumin
2. Coagulation proteins
   a. Fibrinogen (Factor I)
   b. Prothrombin (Factor II)
   c. Factors III, V, VII, IX, X, and XI
3. Transport proteins
   a. Haptoglobin
   b. Transferrin
   c. Ceruloplasmin
   d. Hormone transport proteins
   e. α-Lipoprotein (VLDL)
4. Reaction to injury
   a. α-Globulin
   b. β-Globulin

ing than in comprehending the many changes present in long-standing liver cell disease.

The liver is responsible for the synthesis of many proteins important in the intravascular space for maintenance of osmotic balance, transport, and coagulation (Table 30–10). The synthesis of these proteins may be depressed when liver function is depressed. The altered levels of albumin and the clotting factors, in particular, frequently have clinically significant manifestations.

Albumin Synthesis

The liver is the only site of synthesis for this key protein. Albumin is the major protein responsible for osmotic regulation and the maintenance of plasma volume. It is also an important transport protein for compounds in the circulation that are relatively water-insoluble, such as bilirubin. The liver is capable of synthesizing 10 to 20 mg per hour of this crucial protein. The half-life of the protein is approximately 15 to 30 days.

Serum Albumin. Serum levels will be depressed in liver disease of sufficient severity to result in decreased synthesis and of sufficient duration to exceed the half-life of the protein.

Pathophysiology of Albumin Synthesis. Chronic liver disease is frequently associated with a decrease in serum albumin. Since albumin is responsible for greater than 75 per cent of plasma osmotic balance, a decrease in the serum level is associated with a decrease in intravascular oncotic pressure. This results in a tendency for the vessels to lose fluid into the interstitial space, contributing to the development of edema and ascites.

The physiologic substances and drugs that are tightly bound to albumin will also be altered in their effective blood levels and in their hepatic and renal transport by a decrease in this protein.

Synthesis of Clotting Factors

The liver is solely responsible for the synthesis of fibrinogen (Factor I) and primarily responsible for the synthesis of prothrombin (Factor II) as well as Factors VII, IX, and X. These four factors all require vitamin K as a cofactor for their synthesis. The liver is capable of synthesizing factors V, XI, and XIII along with other tissues. Should synthesis cease, Factor VII has the shortest half-life, about 5 hours. The other factors have half-lives of 1 to 5 days. Inadequate levels of clotting factors result in an increased tendency to bleed.

The coagulation process consists of the sequential activation of many clotting factors, usually starting with thromboplastin (which is released by the inciting injury), and finishing with fibrinogen in the serum and fibrin at the site of injury. It is not commonly appreciated that each of the activated steps in this cascade depends on serum factors that are inactivated predominantly

by the liver. Thus, when coagulation is initiated in liver disease, it continues beyond that in normal persons because of the persistence of activated factors in the circulation. Activated coagulation or "intravascular coagulation" is almost always present to some degree in chronic liver disease and may be impressive. Since the coagulation process consumes fibrinogen, prothrombin complex (Factors II, VII, IX, X) and platelets, coagulation as well as failure in synthesis may contribute to depletions of these components. In coagulopathy, serum enzymes degrade fibrin, and the "fibrin split" products appear and are measurable in serum. The level generally correlates with the rate of formation of new fibrin and sometimes reveals the cause of prolonged prothrombin times as being increased coagulation rather than diminished synthesis in liver disease.

Prothrombin Time (PT) and Partial Thromboplastin Time (PTT). The prothrombin time is prolonged in liver disease when any combination of Factors II, VII, IX, and X is reduced by about one third. Since all depend on vitamin K and vitamin K absorption is defective when inadequate amounts of bile reach the digestive tract, it is always of value to administer vitamin K intravenously or intramuscularly and to remeasure the PT after 12 hours. The one-stage PT measures the extrinsic pathway of prothrombin formation but not the overall coagulability of blood or the intrinsic pathway; therefore, when making decisions about the safety of liver biopsy or replacement of missing coagulation factors in bleeding patients with hepatic disease, one should include the partial thromboplastin time. The PTT is prolonged if factors in the intrinsic pathway are deficient or qualitatively abnormal or if inhibitors are present.

Pathophysiology of Clotting Factors. Substantial hemorrhage due to a deficient clotting mechanism may be a complication of liver disease. Absorptive defects of vitamin K, increased activation of intravascular clotting with subsequent consumption of coagulation factors, and platelet defects due to persistence of products of fibrinolysis are additional commonplace problems of coagulation that require detailed evaluation.

The most frequent coagulation abnormality in cholestasis (with or without jaundice) results from inadequate absorption of vitamin K. Administration of vitamin K will correct the prothrombin time when malabsorption of vitamin K is at fault, but not when inadequate liver protein synthesis is the etiologic factor.

The most frequent coagulation abnormality in liver disease is an inability to manufacture coagulation proteins. Both the one-stage prothrombin time and the partial thromboplastin times are prolonged and respond little or not at all to parenteral vitamin K replacement.

An infrequent but treatable coagulation abnormality is excessive activation of the coagulation cascade with consumption of the platelets and coagulation proteins. This is best detected by a low platelet count (under 50,000) and a reduced level of total fibrinogen, and it is often associated with prolonged prothrombin time and partial thromboplastin time. Split products of fibrinogen breakdown can be detected if reliable methods are available, and a serum Factor VIII level may be helpful.

Synthesis of Transport Proteins and Proteases

The liver is also primarily responsible for the synthesis of specific binding proteins for various substances, especially transferrin (iron), ceruloplasmin (copper), haptoglobin (hemoglobin), and the apoproteins for lipid transport. Other proteins such as α_1-antitrypsin and C-reactive protein are also synthesized predominantly in the liver. Acute liver inflammation may stimulate release of these proteins ("reactive" proteins) and increase serum levels. Chronic liver disease usually results in depressed serum levels, since synthesis is decreased.

CARBOHYDRATE METABOLISM

The liver is a focal point for glucose metabolism because it is responsible for storage, release, and new synthesis of this sugar. A normal man after an overnight fast releases from the liver 150 to 200 mg/minute of glucose in order to maintain the blood level for tissues that require glucose (brain, blood cells, renal medulla). Seventy-five per cent of this serum glucose comes from the approximately 70 gm of stored glycogen in the liver, and 25 per cent comes from gluconeogenesis arising from recycled lactate, pyruvate, amino acids, and glycerol. The glycogen is totally gone by 24 hours, and fasts beyond this period require new synthesis of glucose, for which alanine is the major precursor. The minimum glucose consumption per day is about 150 gm. Dissolution of protein to provide this glucose results in about 10 to 12 gm/day of urinary nitrogen in the first week of starvation but eventually drops to about 5 gm/day.

During fasting, the portal levels of insulin and glucagon drop to the lowest levels of the day. With ingestion of carbohydrate, a rapid rise in blood sugar occurs that results in the outpouring of insulin. In normal persons who receive a 100-gm glucose meal, approximately 60 gm is stored in the liver on the first passage, and 40 gm enters the systemic circulation; of this 40 gm, only 15 per cent is above the basal glucose released by the liver.

The liver is extraordinarily sensitive to fluctuations in hepatic insulin. Marked momentary variations in the amount of insulin reaching liver cells occurs in liver disease owing to variations in the amount of vascular shunting and rates of blood flow. In patients with chronic liver disease, the peripheral insulin levels throughout the day average higher than those in normals. This results in an adaptive decrease in insulin receptors; consequently, peripheral tissue insulin insensitivity develops. Peripheral glucagon levels are usually elevated in chronic liver disease compared with those observed in the normal state. This results in increased protein catabolism and increased utilization of the released branched-chain amino acids.

Measurement of Blood Glucose and the Glucose Tolerance Test. In liver disease, the blood glucose is usually lower than normal, but only in severe hepatic necrosis is there symptomatic hypoglycemia (blood sugar less than 20 mg/dl).

Glucose intolerance with a diabetic pattern of blood sugar in response to a glucose load is the frequent finding in cirrhosis. Clear diabetes by criteria of serum glucose level is found in 12 to 32 per cent of patients with cirrhosis. Increased insulin (partly due to shunts and hepatic unresponsiveness) causes a down-regulation of peripheral insulin receptors, and increased glucagon is also frequently found.

Pathophysiology of Glucose Metabolism. Acute damage to large numbers of liver cells may result in substantial amounts of lactic, pyruvic, citric, and α-ketoglutaric acids in the serum; these acids may replace other anions and result in both acidosis and a 10 to 30 mEq/L increase in the undetermined anion (the numerical difference between the sum of the sodium and potassium and the sum of the bicarbonate and chloride).

Injury to liver cells usually results in elevated levels of circulating amino acids. All except valine and leucine are highly stimulatory to the release of glucagon, which in turn promotes gluconeogenesis. Both insulin and glucagon are released into the portal vein flow and therefore reach the liver in much higher concentrations than in the peripheral blood; both have different sensitivities on liver cells than on peripheral tissues. When portal hypertension develops and there is collateral flow, the peripheral levels of these hormones may be elevated and the liver levels diminished, resulting in hyperglycemia or hypoglycemia, depending on which hormone predominates. In acute liver disease, glycogen stores are decreased, there is diminished glucose response to glucagon, and failure of glycogen repletion following a high carbohydrate intake. Symptomatic hypoglycemia is occasional in severe hepatitis but almost unheard of in cirrhosis of the liver.

LIPID METABOLISM

The liver is active in lipid metabolism, particularly in the management of fatty acid synthesis, oxidation, and packaging for transport.

Fatty acids may appear in the hepatocyte as a result of synthesis in response to an excess in glucose metabolism, as just discussed, or synthesis from amino acids. The liver cell may also actively take up albumin-bound free fatty acids that enter the plasma. The fatty acids derived from the circulation by hepatocytes are released mainly from adipose cells. Lipolysis is regulated by a balance of hormones that are closely related to systemic energy requirements and that have an effect on glucose metabolism as well. Insulin inhibits the lipolytic lipase in adipose tissue, whereas glucagon, norepinephrine, steroids, and some pituitary hormones stimulate lipolysis through activation of the lipase.

Once fatty acids are increased in the liver cell, they may be re-esterified to the triglyceride for export. Esterification of free fatty acids is almost entirely a liver function. Triglycerides are packaged with protein and carbohydrate portions made by the rough endoplasmic reticulum into very low density lipoproteins (VLDL) that are extruded via the Golgi apparatus into Disse's space.

Alternatively, fatty acids may be oxidized in the hepatocyte. Mitochondrial oxidation proceeds with successive shortening of the carbon chain of the fatty acids and results in acetoacetyl CoA and acetyl-CoA. These products may enter the tricarboxylic acid cycle or may be converted to ketone bodies. Ketones may be released into the circulation to provide a substitute energy source for the central nervous system when glucose is deficient.

Serum Triglyceride and VLDL Levels. Triglyceride levels may be elevated in liver disease owing to a decrease in clearance, but more frequently they are normal. VLDL may be decreased in the compromised liver that is unable to add the necessary apoprotein to the triglyceride for hepatocellular export.

Pathophysiology of Lipid Metabolism. Fatty liver is the most dramatic consequence of abnormal lipid metabolism in liver disease. Triglyceride deposition in hepatocytes may occur when delivery or synthesis of fatty acids exceeds the ability of the cell to oxidize or export it. The mechanisms for lipid export and oxidation cannot keep pace with the input of fatty acid. Increased delivery of fatty acids to the liver occurs during lipolysis. Lipolysis in turn may be stimulated by hypoinsulinemic states such as diabetes, energy-requiring catabolic states such as starvation, or conditions in which the adipose lipase is hormonally activated, as by increased circulating levels of steroid, glucagon, or norepinephrine. A decrease in triglyceride export from the liver may occur when the necessary apoprotein is unavailable by fault of inadequate synthesis or when the completed lipoprotein molecule cannot be released. Protein-calorie imbalance with an excess of calories will stimulate fatty acid synthesis but provides inadequate protein for export. Drugs that inhibit protein synthesis (e.g., tetracycline and carbon tetrachloride) can also inhibit and prevent triglyceride release.

DETOXIFICATION OF DRUGS AND HORMONES

Large numbers of enzymes are bound to the smooth endoplasmic reticulum. Figure 30–13 illustrates a widely utilized electron transport scheme employed in the metabolism of many drugs. Each enzyme used is bound to the membranes of the endoplasmic reticulum so that an insoluble molecule can be sequentially acted on by enzymes attached adjacent to one another. The substrates are usually of limited solubility and are often combined by these enzymes with highly polar molecules (such as sulfate, glucuronide, glutathi-

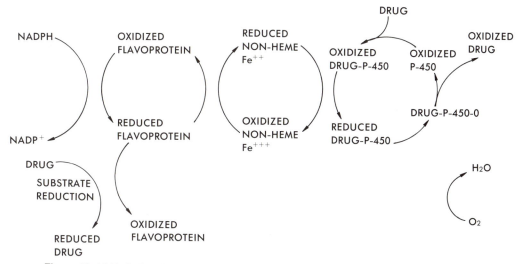

Figure 30–13 Endoplasmic reticulum electron transport used for drug oxidation and reduction.

one, glycine, acetate) to permit subsequent excretion by liver or renal tubular cells.

A few normal substances are metabolized using these membrane-bound enzymes. Most steroid hormones are made inactive by this system. The system is also important for many trace materials and particularly significant in drug metabolism. Many drugs are fairly insoluble in water and resist excretion. The liver is a major organ responsible for biotransformation—the chemical modification of a drug that usually alters its biologic activity and renders it more susceptible to excretion by both the kidney and the liver. Oxidation reactions such as N- and O-dealkylization, aromatic-ring and side-chain hydroxylation, N-oxidation, N-hydroxylation, and deamination of primary and secondary amines are common. Reduction of nitrogroups, reductive cleavage of azo- groups, and reduction of ring double bonds may occur. Conjugation of phenols, alcohols, carboxylic acids, and amines with glucuronides, sulfates, acetates, or glycine is a common mode of rendering molecules more polar for excretion. Specific enzymes for each reaction are usually necessary to activate the drug or to carry out portions of the chemistry. However, certain of the enzymes in the endoplasmic reticulum are used in common by many systems. NADPH and cytochrome P-450 are common requirements for most of these. Figure 30–13 indicates a common relationship between these enzymes.

Lipid solubility seems an important determinant of which drugs utilize the endoplasmic reticulum enzymes. The rates of reaction vary markedly, and, similarly, the effect of liver disease on these drug removal reactions varies.

An important and unique aspect of the endoplasmic reticulum is its near total hypertrophy (with all the contained enzymes) after treatment with certain agents that saturate one or more of its enzymes. Most substances (nearly all common drugs and many environmental trace elements) are type I inducers of endoplasmic reticulum and cause an increased activity of nearly all drug and steroid metabolizing enzymes. Type I inducers (e.g., phenobarbital) are best known and most widespread. Drug removal rates are accelerated for nearly all agents using enzyme on the endoplasmic reticulum. For this reason, many patients with hepatic disease may have increased rather than impaired endoplasmic reticulum enzymes. This may be from drugs they have received in the course of treatment or it may be from alcoholism.

A less frequent type of inducer (type II), exemplified by many carcinogenic molecules (e.g., methylcholanthrene), leads to hypertrophy only of the enzymes for type II molecules. There is some evidence that activation of the type II system renders a person more susceptible to carcinoma.

Abnormalities in detoxification can be anticipated either in patients with evidence of deranged liver metabolism or in patients who are receiving drugs known to induce the microsomal enzyme system as discussed. The clinical half-life of drug level or effect is the clinically pertinent test of this function.

Pathophysiology of Liver Function in Detoxification. Prolonged hormonal effect is frequently observed when microsomal function is compromised in severe liver disease. Steroid inactivation is usually slow in almost any form of liver disease, and sex hormone, adrenal cortical hormone, and aldosterone may persist in the circulation. Bilirubin conjugation is usually not altered in liver cell disease, bile salt conjugation is often impaired, and the normal threefold increase of glycine conjugations over taurine is reduced.

Antibiotics, hypnotics, and hypoglycemic agents all show unusual persistence in the presence of liver disease. One can best generalize by stating that any drug using the hepatic endoplasmic reticulum should be administered with caution and its blood level or biologic effects observed in the presence of liver disease.

An additional pathophysiologic manifestation of this system is seen with the occasional drug whose toxicity is actually enhanced by liver metabolism rather than reduced (e.g., isoniazide and acetaminophen). The metabolism of these drugs produces an intermediate that is more toxic than the parent compound and produces injury to surrounding membranes. Enhanced microsomal enzyme activity (e.g., that induced by phenobarbital or, perhaps, alcohol) tends to potentiate the toxicity of these drugs. Genetic determinants of metabolism may also play a key role, as demonstrated by the increased toxicity of isoniazid in patients who more rapidly acetylate the parent compound to the toxic intermediate. The amount of toxic intermediate produced correlates with the amount of tissue damage, which results in these "predictable" drug reactions. The liver can tolerate low levels of the toxic intermediates because of detoxificants in the cell (e.g., glutathione) that bind the toxin. When this naturally occurring protection is depleted, toxic effects will appear as hepatocellular necrosis and fatty infiltration. Administration of glutathione precursors (e.g., acetyl cysteine) in this case will ameliorate the hepatotoxicity.

APPROACH TO THE PROBLEM OF CLINICAL LIVER DISEASE

LIVER FUNCTION TESTS

A wide variety of tests assess aspects of the liver. Those tests listed in Tables 30–2, 30–3, and 30–6 are liver function tests. Usually, however, one restricts the term "liver function test" to those blood and urine tests indicated in Table 30–11. The meaning and method of performance of each of these will now be discussed. Of the several thousand known biochemical functions of the liver,

TABLE 30–11 TESTS OF LIVER CELL DAMAGE

A. Cell Necrosis
1. AST (SGOT)
2. ALT (SGPT)
3. Bile salts 2 hr post cibum
4. Bilirubinuria
5. Biopsy*
6. Serum Fe
7. Serum B_{12}
B. Liver cell function
1. Bilirubin
2. Albumin
3. Prothrombin
4. Urine urobilinogen
5. Indocyanine green
6. Fibrinogen
7. Amino acidemia and aciduria
8. Increased undetermined anion
C. Inflammation
1. α, δ immunoglobulin, IgM, IgG
2. Total globulin
3. Electrophoresis of proteins—wide base, δ elevation
4. IgM, IgG
5. Sed rate (reactive protein), rheumatoid factor, haptoglobin
D. Cholestasis
1. Alkaline phosphatase
2. δ-glutamyl transpeptidase (GGTP)
3. 5'-Nucleotidase
4. Fasting bile salts
E. Specific etiology
1. Hepatitis A, B antigen and antibody markers
2. Antimitochondrial antibody
3. Amebae, hydatid complement fixation
4. Epstein-Barr agent antibody
5. α-Antitrypsin
6. α-Fetoprotein
F. Intraheptic or extrahepatic shunts
1. Ammonia

*Increased risk

only a few are abnormal during the early stages of liver disease. Some tests have been abandoned because they give abnormal results too frequently, others because the patient must be close to death before an abnormality appears.

Tests of Cellular Necrosis

Intact hepatocytes contain a number of substances in the cytosol in concentrations much higher than those in the circulating blood. These substances may be released into the serum following damage to the cell wall. Persistence of each abnormal substance is determined by a balance between its rate of release and its duration of survival in the bloodstream. Serum alanine aminotransferase (ALT) is the most specific and widely used measure of hepatocellular necrosis. In a person in good nutritional state with good stores of intracellular enzyme, damage to as little as 1 per cent of the liver cells will raise the serum level.

Serum aspartate aminotransferase (AST) acts similarly but is less specific, for all forms of striate muscle contain this material. Serum iron and vitamin B_{12} behave similarly but remain elevated longer than the transferase.

In severe necrosis, amino acids are released from the liver cells and appear in high concentration in the blood; the more insoluble ones (tyrosine and cysteine) appear in the urine as crystals.

The liver biopsy may reveal damaged cells with pyknotic nuclei or feathery degeneration, but more commonly it reveals an inflammatory cell infiltrate surrounding the area in which a normal cell was or distorted liver cords due to loss of many cells or rapid regeneration, indicating their replacement. Very active necrosis may leave cellular debris in the form of acidophilic bodies, lipofuscin, or Councilman's bodies.

CLINICAL SYMPTOMS AND SIGNS OF LIVER DISEASE

Liver disease may start predominantly as a focal process; such processes use the rich blood supply of the liver but interfere little with the hepatocyte function. In contrast, liver disease may indicate diffuse involvement of the hepatocytes. These two types of initial disease are quite distinct in typical cases but may completely overlap as they advance. There is some value in having a clear understanding of each.

Focal Liver Disease and Its Typical Syndromes (Table 30–12)

Two prototypes of focal liver disease must be considered. One is a single abscess or metastasis within the liver that progressively grows but, even when massive, interferes only slightly with overall liver function. The other consists of myriad small foci (such as miliary tuberculosis or extramedullary hematopoiesis) that similarly may grow without affecting liver function.

Systemic symptoms are a function of the basic pathologic condition invading the liver. Abscesses, specific infectious agents (amebae, hydatid, tuberculosis), and cancer with necrosis may produce impressive systemic signs of fever and weight loss;

TABLE 30–12 SYNDROMES OF FOCAL LIVER DISEASE

1. Pain in right upper quadrant
2. Mass in upper abdomen
3. Hepatomegaly
4. Liver test abnormality, ALT, alkaline phosphatase
5. Scan defect in liver
6. Wasting, fever

however, these signs may not reveal themselves in the history, physical examination, or laboratory screening to indicate that the liver is the host to the problem. This is particularly true in the diseases mentioned and in some cases of lymphoma.

Modest hepatomegaly is most readily detected by scanning or sonography. Uniform distribution of an increased mass of 20 per cent throughout the liver would result in an average increase in each dimension of 1 cm, and this amount cannot be detected on ordinary physical examination. If the increase is not uniformly distributed or if it produces symptoms (fullness in the abdomen, pulling on the side), hepatomegaly might well be found. Tight clothing often reveals abdominal masses, and hepatomegaly may be found in this way. If the enlargement is rapid or if the underlying process is one that may hemorrhage into itself, pain may result.

Painful sensations in the liver seem to arise from receptors lying in the liver capsule and along the fibrous tissue following the portal veins and its branches. These sensations pass from the liver via the sympathetic nerves, through the celiac plexus, and on to the seventh through twelfth paravertebral ganglia. These nerve endings seem particularly sensitive to distention but are not affected by penetration, heat, or cold. Acute distention of the capsule, as produced by vascular or bile congestion or rapid infiltration of inflammation, produces exquisite pain and tenderness. Pain and tenderness will disappear after a few days of steady distention. Other innervated portions include the hepatic veins and bile ducts, which produce the sensation of pain when they are acutely distended or in spasm. The parietal peritoneum overlies much of the liver capsule and is particularly sensitive after inflammation or occurrence of fibrin deposits. Thus, focal processes may alter the capsule, vessels, or overlying peritoneum and produce pain and tenderness.

Slow-growing, usually benign tumors or infiltrations of the liver may remain indefinitely silent. Patients with moderate infiltrations of fat, amyloid, Gaucher's lipid, or hamartomas may remain asymptomatic throughout life. Sonograms, CT scans, and radioisotopic scans with specific substances (gallium localizing in abscesses or tumors) often specifically assist in identifying focal liver disease.

Generalized Liver Disease and Its Typical Syndromes (Table 30–13)

Jaundice. In liver cell disease, jaundice is due either to damage to the anion pump or to cholestasis. Both produce jaundice in which the serum bilirubin is more than half direct-reacting. If there is no increased production of bile pigments, the degree of jaundice is a general reflection of the severity of the disease, and the level of jaundice

TABLE 30–13 SYNDROMES OF GENERALIZED LIVER DISEASE

1. Jaundice, including cholestasis
2. Acute liver failure
3. Fluid retention
4. Portal hypertension
5. Confusion, including hepatic encephalopathy and hypoglycemia
6. Systemic wasting

may increase as its course progresses. Stable jaundice of liver cell origin is usually an indication of increased destruction of liver cells exceeding their replacement rate. If there is no evidence of liver cell destruction, cholestasis is usually prominent owing to the huge regenerative capacity of the liver.

Acute Liver Cell Failure. Destruction of about 90 per cent or more of liver cells within a few weeks or less results in a rapid, devastating, often fatal syndrome in which jaundice and confusion are nearly always present but often mild, and in which metabolic changes, hemorrhage, and cardiovascular collapse may be prominent enough to produce death. Many of the common manifestations of liver disease, such as jaundice, require time to occur while material accumulates in the blood, and the course, until death due to liver failure occurs, may be so rapid that these manifestations do not occur prominently.

The totally failing liver is unable to clear amino acids or the citric acid cycle intermediates from the blood (lactate, pyruvate, alphaketoglutarate), and these materials are acidic. Prominent acidosis and a marked increase in the undetermined anion may be observed. The undetermined anion is the numerical difference between the sum of the sodium and potassium minus the sum of the chloride and bicarbonate. It is usually less than 16 mEq/L but may be as high as 60 mEq/L in acute liver failure.

Increased plasma amino acids are a feature of liver failure. The total α-amino nitrogen in plasma may double, but specific elevations of methionine, tyrosine, and phenylalanine are prominent. In addition, levels of valine, leucine, isoleucine, and often threonine are lower than normal. The elevations reflect the inability of the liver to remove amino acids mobilized from the diet and the periphery; the lowered levels reflect the influence of glucagon, which increases the utilization of these in the periphery.

Coagulation is interfered with, as discussed in earlier sections. Hypoglycemia may occur; this too is considered in preceding discussions.

In animals it has been noted that when liver tissue is permitted to autolyze under sterile conditions and is then reinjected, peripheral vasodilatation and increased cardiac output result. It is likely that the sudden release of destroyed liver tissue is responsible for some cardiovascular changes. In addition, acute liver failure may have manifestations in all the other areas.

Fluid Retention. Any form of liver cell disease is associated with prominent fluid retention mediated via sodium retention by the kidney. Any experimental design leading to congestion within the liver results in profound sodium retention. It is possible that a portion of this is due to sequestration of an important proportion of the plasma volume behind the liver, but other factors may also be important. Sodium retention is mediated by the renin-angiotensin-aldosterone mechanisms, but after a few days a fundamental alteration in blood distribution occurs within the kidney and is probably hormonally mediated (third factor). The common pathway of sodium retention by the kidney is clearly understood. Most patients with liver cell failure have 6 to 30 lb. (3 to 15 L) of increased extracellular fluid and will secrete increasing amounts of sodium and water as the liver disease improves.

This increased extracellular fluid will distribute itself in a variety of places. It will be manifest as edema or ascites, dependent upon local factors. If there is mostly erect posture or venous stasis of the legs, the fluid will be most visible in the legs. If there is portal hypertension, the venous pressure in either the hepatic or mesenteric bed must exceed that in the legs, and ascites results. Fluid retention usually corrects itself when the disease improves. If this is unlikely or complications are feared, it is appropriate to stimulate sodium excretion by the kidney.

The important relationship between plasma volume and portal pressure was discussed earlier. An ambulatory patient with fluid is often put to bed, the result being redistribution of leg fluid, increased portal pressure, and finally hemorrhage. Patients exhibiting increased fluid stores should have the fluid gently controlled before bed rest is enforced.

Portal hypertension has been discussed in an earlier section, including its major complications (hypersplenism and esophageal varices with hemorrhage) and its indirect complications (ascites and increased collateral circulation).

Confusion, Including Hepatic Encephalopathy and Hypoglycemia. Hypoglycemia occurs so frequently that it should be the first problem suspected when a patient with liver disease becomes confused. Hypoglycemia usually arises from impaired gluconeogenesis in (1) severe liver cell damage; (2) congestive heart failure; and (3) alcoholism, particularly after a prolonged fast.

Liver encephalopathy is an altered metabolic state of the central nervous system. It is brought about by the direct shunting of some material from the intestinal tract bypassing the liver to the brain. This material, which may be ammonia, seems to be present in proteins in the intestinal tract. Once encephalopathy is present, a variety of noxious materials seem to affect the central nervous system adversely in a similar manner. The signs and symptoms of liver encephalopathy are aggravated by ammonia, hypokalemia (which stimulates urinary formation of ammonia), anoxia, sedative drugs, and central nervous system depressants (e.g., morphine).

The shunting of intestinal blood through or around the liver cells seems more important in the production of liver coma than does the presence of damaged liver cells. This syndrome is known to occur in the presence of a normal liver cell mass.

In the mildest form of liver encephalopathy, there is a slight disturbance of thought processes and a disturbance of the diurnal sleep rhythm, so that the patient is awake at night and dozes all day. At the next stage, there is mental-motor dissociation, which shows far more impairment than is revealed by any routine neurologic testing. Thus, if the patient is asked to copy a simple line drawing or to write his name, it cannot be done, even though the patient tries. Still later, the "flapping tremor," or asterixis, becomes apparent. The examiner elicits this tremor by asking the patient to hold the arms and hands extended maximally against gravity and encouraging him to hold them perfectly still. Periodically, the sustained stimulus to hold them against gravity will be relaxed owing to a temporary block in the signal, and against the will of the patient the hand will drop; the patient, in trying to comply, will quickly jerk the limb back into position, and a flapping effect is produced. Subsequently, there is progressive loss of memory, which is followed by unconsciousness. Finally, deep coma may intervene and death occurs. The level of consciousness has been raised by treatments aimed at interrupting the supply of ammonia reaching the brain. One achieves this by discontinuing oral administration of all protein- and nitrogen-containing materials. The gastrointestinal tract is purged to remove blood and other foodstuffs and to lessen the stasis that promotes accumulation of ammonia-forming bacteria. Nonabsorbed antibiotics, particularly neomycin, are highly effective in inhibiting the growth of urease-producing bacteria, which can act on urea (excreted into the gut with all secretions) to produce ammonia. Lactulose, a disaccharide that cannot be absorbed, produces lactate from bacterial action and osmotic diarrhea, which interferes with ammonia absorption and is useful in treating liver encephalopathy.

An alternative hypothesis of the cause of liver coma (and also the hepatorenal syndrome) is the false-transmitter hypothesis. Biologic amines, related structurally to norepinephrine, may accumulate in liver disease and make the usual neurotransmitter substance, norepinephrine, less effective owing to the accumulation of these false transmitters at the synapse. One could overcome such a problem by providing the nerve cells with more precursor for norepinephrine synthesis, such as dopa or dopamine. Animal and human data consistent with this hypothesis exist, but trials in man with these agents have not been of benefit. Mercaptans and 6- to 8-carbon fatty acids have also been suggested as possible contributory factors in the etiology of hepatic encephalopathy. Wasting of muscles due to inefficient nitrogen metabolism and loss of body weight is commonly seen.

REPRESENTATIVE HEPATIC DISEASES

Vascular Impairment

An example of vascular impairment is congestive heart failure due to myocardial disease. The liver has two vascular supplies, and either is sufficient to maintain a fully functioning liver. However, when the venous drainage is blocked from the liver owing to either intrahepatic or extrahepatic disorders, it produces a profound derangement of liver function that is largely due to damage from anoxia. Initially, there is vascular stasis throughout the liver without death of liver cells, but all metabolic function of the liver is inefficient. The liver becomes enlarged owing to vascular congestion and may become very tender. Fluid retention, a result of sodium retention, usually is present. After several weeks, liver cells die, with prominent transaminase elevation. Lack of liver cells is apparent from marked BSP retention, jaundice, hypoalbuminemia, and low prothrombin time. In order for blood to continue to flow through the liver, portal hypertension, splenomegaly, and in extreme cases even portal collateral circulation must develop. Healing following correction of the circulatory problem is rapid and dramatic.

Hepatitis

Viral hepatitis, alcoholic hepatitis, and allergic or idiosyncratic hepatitis (from drugs or other environmental agents) are the principal forms of hepatitis. Coincidental with the injury to liver cells are systemic symptoms such as fever, nausea, vomiting, and malaise. The exact cause of these symptoms is unclear. The liver soon becomes enlarged from edema of injury and by the infiltration of inflammatory and regenerative cells (they are larger than the destroyed cells). Tenderness may be prominent at this stage. Jaundice, a cumulative phenomenon, usually becomes most marked after healing has started. Transaminase elevation is most prominent during the maximal injury phase.

Self-limited hepatitis caused by the aforementioned factors is usually not associated with either hyperglobulinemia or hypoalbuminemia. The majority of all forms of hepatitis completely heal, and the liver is later completely normal. Among previously healthy young people who develop viral hepatitis, 95 per cent recover completely, and 85 percent of these patients do so within 3 months. Among patients with alcoholic hepatitis, about 50 per cent later develop cirrhosis; among patients with viral hepatitis, about 3 per cent have cirrhosis and about 2 per cent have a chronically active (destructive) form of the disease that may persist for years or until death.

There are hepatotoxic substances in nature and medicine; however, most of those in the latter group have been replaced by safer drugs. A hepatotoxic substance is an agent that, if given in a sufficient amount, will cause liver damage; the toxic pattern is readily reproduced in animals but not in all species. Idiosyncratic or allergic hepatitis is the most common and troublesome form of liver disease. It develops in only a small number of people, is not dose related, and cannot be predicted from animal testing. Nearly every drug and many environmental chemicals have produced this form of hepatitis. Some drugs, such as phenothiazine tranquilizers, isonicotinic acid hydrazide, and halothane, are very frequent causes.

Cirrhosis

The term *cirrhosis* as used in medicine has two definitions; occasionally they are synonymous, but very often they are quite different. The most precise description is a pathologic entity that has three features:

1. Present or deduced major hepatic necrosis sufficient to destroy total lobules in at least two thirds of the liver. This may occur in a single wave or many small waves of necrosis.

2. Major permanent scarring with the formation of complete fibrous bands encircling hepatic tissue (nodules).

3. Formation of new liver through the process of regeneration. As a result, the architecture of the liver is completely destroyed and is largely formed of scars and regenerative nodules.

To the clinician the term *cirrhosis* refers to any form of long-standing liver disease in which the features of portal hypertension are prominent. Although these conditions are usually presumed to be synonymous, only with some element of proof is this actually the case.

The cirrhotic liver (in pathologically confirmed cases) is strikingly different from the normal or precirrhotic liver in the following ways:

1. The necrosis usually continues and may be the most prominent feature.

2. The new liver cells have a very inefficient relationship to the blood supply. They are usually very deficient and much less subject to increase with need. There is little to no portal blood supply, and if a high perfusion pressure is not maintained, the blood supply, already marginal, will drop precipitously and may produce additional ischemic damage. A regenerative nodule grows concentrically like a berry, and the blood supply and drain-

age come in from the outside like fingers surrounding a ball. The growth of a nodule depends on its success in developing a blood supply. Soon, competition develops for space, and the growing nodule presses against the contracting scars. This pressure is detrimental to the veins. The nodule, if successful, becomes totally arterially dependent. Because the venous drainage is under high pressure, there is increased lymph flow from the sinusoids. This interferes with efficient cellular exchange and thus causes postsinusoidal resistance or outflow obstruction, found in cirrhosis.

3. Regeneration is rarely complete; there is always liver cell deficiency.

4. Major shunts of portal blood exist in vascularized scars, portal collaterals, and plexuses surrounding bile ducts.

5. Sequestration of additional portions of the plasma volume behind the liver due to portal hypertension impairs vascular homeostasis.

Despite the fact that on the average there is a 20 per cent increase in total blood volume, the blood volume available to perfuse the kidneys, heart, and brain is less than normal. These features explain many of the problems that patients with cirrhosis have in common, but in varying degrees. These features are as follows:

1. Liver destruction (activity) and liver cell insufficiency.

2. Inefficient metabolism of food—mild malabsorption (reflecting bile salt insufficiency), frequent glycosuria, and weight loss despite adequate calorie intake.

3. Portal hypertension, esophageal varices, and an enlarged spleen with hypersplenism. The collateral circulation is responsible for elevated urinary urobilinogen, extremely high postprandial blood sugar, and often hyperammonemia.

4. Poor tolerance to hemorrhage or electrolyte depletion resulting from impaired vascular homeostasis. The frequent postural hypotension and impaired renal function may be features of this problem.

5. Prominent ascites.

Patients with cirrhosis show a propensity for the complications of gastrointestinal hemorrhage (usually from esophageal varices), liver encephalopathy, liver cell failure, and renal insufficiency. It is likely that the poor vascular homeostasis and possibly a small hemorrhage are the principal precipitants of the additional liver cell failure and renal insufficiency.

In the cirrhotic liver, there is an increased tendency for a primary tumor called a *hepatoma* to form. This tumor often produces a primitive protein made in the fetus (fetoglobulin), which enters into the blood. This is found in about 50 per cent of the patients with hepatoma and seems to occur in no other tumor.

Cirrhosis may result from many different causes of liver damage. Viral hepatitis, alcoholic liver damage, biliary cirrhosis, and hemochroma-

tosis are the principal forms. In approximately one third of all cases a cause cannot be assigned. Prognosis is far more dependent on continuation of destructive activity and on the maximal functioning liver cell mass that can be attained than on any specific complication. Except for hepatoma and renal insufficiency, effective treatments exist for the other complications, including portal hypertension, hypersplenism, bleeding esophageal varices, liver coma, and ascites.

EFFECT OF LIVER DISEASE ON OTHER ORGANS

Cardiovascular Effects

Acute hepatic necrosis may release vasodilating substances into the blood. Wide pulse pressure, warm palms, and high cardiac output may be manifestations of this. An inflamed liver may have such a high blood flow that it creates cardiac overload by acting as an arterial venous shunt. Most forms of active liver disease cause a 20 to 50 per cent increase in cardiac output.

Plasma volume is usually increased by one third in chronic liver disease; this increased volume is entirely sequestered in the obstructed splanchnic circulation. It has no influence on cardiovascular function except that the return of blood to the systemic circulation is retarded and occasionally leads to hypovolemia and postural hypertension. Regulation of plasma volume following hemorrhage is limited.

Lowered arterial P_{O_2} commonly accompanies liver disease, particularly when associated with ascites. Many patients regain normal P_{O_2} by breathing high concentrations of oxygen. This suggests ventilatory perfusion abnormalities brought about by the large liver or the prominent ascites. Rarely, an unresponsive lowering of the P_{O_2} after oxygen inhalation is found and is caused by anatomic shunts within the substance of the lung. This is most likely to occur after 3 to 7 years of cirrhosis, and clubbing of the fingers is often seen at this stage.

Many hepatic alterations of pH are possible. Liver disease is often associated with nausea, vomiting, or diarrhea, and large depletions of potassium may occur. Depletion may be accompanied by an intracellular acidosis and an extracellular alkalosis. Severe impairment of renal acidification is often present in chronic hepatic disease and further accentuates potassium depletion. In any form of hepatocellular damage, acidic products of metabolism, amino acids, and carbohydrate intermediates may be released into the blood and produce acidosis. This is most commonly seen as a persistent lowering of the serum bicarbonate.

In liver encephalopathy, hyperventilation due

to an altered central threshold is common, and alkalosis results.

Renal Changes

Renal blood flow and glomerular filtration are well preserved in most cases of mild and moderately severe liver disease. Chronic sodium retention by the kidney in association with liver disease initially involves the aldosterone mechanism, but when severe or prolonged it involves a different system. A far higher proportion of the glomerular filtrate is reabsorbed by the proximal loop of Henle (as much as 99.6 per cent), thus limiting the amount of sodium that reaches the distal convoluted tubule. A hormone called *third factor* is postulated to be the cause. Severe limitation of sodium on the distal convoluted tubule impairs excretion of free water and impairs responsiveness to diuretics acting on the distal convoluted tubule (spironolactones, thiazides).

In cirrhosis, a higher than normal portion of renal blood flow goes to the medulla. This high flow cleanses the high concentration of medullary solutes, so that in the water-deprived person with cirrhosis there is only about a twofold increase in medullary osmolality compared with the three- or fourfold increase in the normal subject. This makes urine concentration more difficult for the patient with cirrhosis.

It may be concluded that the person with chronic hepatic disease excretes sodium poorly and is unable either to excrete large volumes of free water or to concentrate the urine as markedly as the normal person in order to conserve water.

Renal tubular acidosis is commonly observed in the presence of liver disease. This condition is simply an expression of the kidney's production of an inappropriately alkaline urine, even in the presence of a large acid load and systemic acidosis. This reflects the limited ability of the cirrhotic kidney to make and excrete hydrogen ion. In order to compensate for this defect, both excretion of potassium into the urine and formation of ammonia increase. Thus, if hydrogen ions cannot be excreted, an acid load is excreted that is largely neutralized with sodium, potassium, or ammonium. Since sodium cannot be easily excreted, potassium is the predominant ion, and losses of 150 mEq/day have been observed. Ammonia for the urine is manufactured in the renal tubular cells from glutamate. Increased ammonia due to an acid pH and rapid flow is diffused into both urine and blood. In patients with this disorder, approximately twice as much ammonia is delivered into the renal venous blood as into the urine, further increasing the load to be removed by the liver.

The hepatorenal syndrome is progressive oliguria and azotemia occurring without apparent cause in patients with liver disease. There is an abrupt increase in glomerular filtration resistance, with the maintenance of normal renal histology and overall blood flow. There is shunting of blood from the glomeruli, the cause of which is unknown but is probably a hormone. Studies of arteriography and of the washout curves of radioactive krypton indicate that glomerular flow to such kidneys is markedly reduced but that tubular and medullary flow is preserved. If the urine is carefully examined, one finds that its sediment is normal but that the sodium content is extremely low (less than 5 mEq/L). If the kidney from such a patient who has died is transplanted into a normal recipient, it functions normally, indicating that it was the original environment that caused the malfunction.

Since oliguria and azotemia are present in the hepatorenal syndrome, the principal differential diagnosis is shock kidney or necrosis of the tubule epithelium. In the hepatorenal syndrome, the amount of urinary sodium is less than 5 mEq/L, and the ratio of urine to blood creatinine or urea is greater than 1:3 and usually greater than 1:15. In contrast, in disease with renal tubular damage, the urinary sodium is rarely less than 30 mEq/L, and the ratio of urine to plasma creatinine or urea is 1:3 or less, indicating that there is little tubular function.

Endocrine Changes

The liver is not considered an endocrine organ, yet it plays a significant role in hormone metabolism because most nonpeptides are biotransformed by the liver into an inactive form. Most nonpeptide hormones are bound to a carrier protein in the plasma that limits the level of free hormone; the liver usually manufactures these carriers. These two functions may lead to increases in the circulating level of the free hormone that may persist longer than normal. If the production of the hormone is under careful feedback regulation (i.e., the rate of release of hormone is also controlled by the tissue level of the hormone), this will have no effect. However, if this regulatory mechanism is insensitive, the hormone levels may be altered in liver disease.

Peptide hormones may be inactivated by the liver. Careful study of blood hormone levels in patients with liver cell disease often reveals many abnormalities.

Immune Disorders in Liver Disease

The immune system has been thoroughly investigated in liver disease, and there are great numbers of abnormalities in circulating antibodies, cellular immune systems, and interactions between them and the liver. There is little agreement as to whether these are a result of liver damage (such as circulating antibodies to components of liver tissue) or a primary cause of the liver injury.

Hypergammaglobulinemia with specific elevations of IgM and, later, IgG immunoglobulins is common in most chronic destructive liver diseases. These have been attributed to shunting of blood past Kupffer's cells, B-cell hyperreactivity, increased autoantibodies, and synthesis of antiantibodies such as rheumatoid factor. Anticytoplasmic antibodies are present. Anti–smooth muscle antibody is elevated in chronic active hepatitis, but there is no clear comprehension of why it arises or any role in pathogenesis. Antimitochondrial antibodies are abundant in biliary cirrhosis and in some cases of chronic active hepatitis. Even though their presence is of diagnostic value, it is not clearly related to pathogenesis. Although there

are often antibodies to liver-specific antigens, there is no body of data supporting these in the pathogenesis of liver disease.

Chronic liver disease is associated with a general hypofunction of T cells, manifest by decreased numbers of these cells, reduced responsiveness to mitogens, relative anergy in cutaneous reactions, and depression of response to dinitrochlorobenzene. B-cell responsiveness is often enhanced.

Circulating immune complexes are found in many forms of chronic liver disease but are most prominent in biliary cirrhosis.

The myriad of abnormalities in cellular and circulating immunology in liver disease is the basis of great investigative interest, and many of the speculations that exist at the time of this writing shed little light on the pathogenesis and treatment of any form of liver disease.

REFERENCES

GENERAL
Several excellent texts, current monographs, and journals exist that provide up to date reviews of each item discussed in this chapter.

Texts
Arias, I. (Ed.): The Liver: Biology and Pathobiology. New York, Raven Press, 1982. The most comprehensive basic science of the texts.
Schiff, L., and Schiff, E. R.: Diseases of the Liver. 5th ed. Philadelphia, J. B. Lippincott Co., 1982. Most clinical of the texts.
Sherlock, S.: Diseases of the Liver and Biliary System. 6th ed. Oxford, Blackwell Scientific Publications, 1981. The most concise of the texts.
Zakim, D., and Boyer, T.: Hepatology: A Textbook of Liver Disease. Philadelphia, W. B. Saunders, 1982. A happy blend of basic science and clinical information.

Current Monograph Series
Berk, P. D. (Ed.): Seminars in Liver Disease. New York, Thieme-Stratton, Inc. Started in 1981; published four times yearly. Very practical.
Popper, H., and Schaffner, F. (Eds): Progress in Liver Diseases. New York, Grune and Stratton, Vol. I, 1961; Vol. II, 1965; Vol. III, 1970; Vol. IV, 1973; Vol. V, 1976; Vol. VI, 1979; Vol. VII, 1982. In depth, state of the art review articles that usually remain timely for 5 to 10 years after written.

Journals
The two following journals regularly have state of the art reviews on topics concerning the liver:
Gastroenterology, Elsevier, published monthly.
Hepatology, Williams and Wilkins, published bimonthly.

ANATOMY AND TESTING
Baum, S.: Hepatic angiography. *In* Popper, H., and Schaffner, F. (Eds): Progress in Liver Diseases. Vol. III. New York, Grune and Stratton, 1970, p. 444.
Castell, D. O., O'Brien, K. D., Muench, H., and Chalmers, T. C.: Estimation of liver size by percussion in normal individuals. Ann. Intern. Med. 70:1183, 1969.
Gumucio, J. J., and Miller D. L.: Functional implications of liver cell heterogeneity. Gastroenterology 80:393, 1981.
Motta, P. M.: Scanning electron microscopy of the liver. *In* Popper, H., and Schaffner, F. (Eds.): Progress in Liver

Diseases. Vol. VII. New York, Grune and Stratton, 1982, p. 1.
Rappaport, A. M.: Physioanatomic considerations. *In* Schiff, L., and Schiff, E. R. (Eds.): Diseases of the Liver. 5th ed. Philadelphia, J. B. Lippincott Co., 1982, p. 1.
Rogoff, T. M., and Lipsky, P. E.: Role of the Kupffer cells in local and systemic immune responses. Gastroenterology 80:854, 1981.
Taylor, K. J. W., Neumann, R. D., and Russo, R. D.: Ultrasonography, scintigraphy and computerized tomographic scanning of the hepatobiliary system. *In* Schiff, L., and Schiff, E. R. (Eds.): Diseases of the Liver. 5th ed. Philadelphia, J. B. Lippincott Co., 1982, p. 1349.
Wisse, E., Van't Noordende, J. M., Van de Meullen, J., et al.: The pit cell description of a new type of cell occurring in the rat liver sinusoids and peripheral blood. Cell Tissue Res. 173:423, 1976.

HEPATIC BLOOD FLOW, PORTAL HYPERTENSION
Chiandussi, L.: Umbilical-portal catherization in diagnosis of liver disease. *In* Popper, H., and Schaffner, F. (Eds.): Progress in Liver Diseases. Vol. III. New York, Grune and Stratton, 1970, p. 466.
Dumont, A. E., and Mulholland, J. H.: Hepatic lymph in cirrhosis. *In* Popper, H., and Schaffner, F. (Eds.): Progress in Liver Diseases. Vol. II. New York, Grune and Stratton, 1965, p. 427.
Kimber, C., Deller, D. J., Ibbotson, R. N., and Lander, H.: The mechanism of anemia in chronic liver disease. Q. J. Med. (new series) 34:33, 1965.
Reynolds, T. B.: Portal hypertension. *In* Schiff, L., and Schiff, E. R. (Eds.): Diseases of the Liver. 5th Ed. Philadelphia, J. B. Lippincott Co., 1982, p. 393.
Reynolds, T. B., and Redeker, A. G.: Hepatic hemodynamic and portal hypertensin. *In* Popper, H., and Schaffner, F. (Eds.): Progress in Liver Diseases. Vol. II. New York, Grune and Stratton, 1965, p. 457.
Richardson, P. D. I., and Withrington, P. G.: Liver blood flow I. Intrinsic and nervous control of liver blood flow. Gastroenterology 81:159, 1981.
Richardson, P. D. I., and Withrington, P. G.: Liver blood flow II. Effects of drugs and hormones on liver blood flow. Gastroenterology 81:356, 1981.
Sherlock, S.: Portal hypertension. *In* Berk, P. D., and Sherlock, S. (Eds.): Seminars in Liver Disease. Vol. 2, No. 3. New York, Thieme-Stratton, Inc., 1982, p. 177.

BIOCHEMISTRY

Bloomer, J. R., Berk, P. D., Howe, R. B., and Berlin, N. I.: Interpretation of plasma bilirubin levels based on studies with radioactive bilirubin. J.A.M.A. 218:216, 1971.

Bourke, E., Milne, M. D., and Stokes, G. S.: Mechanism of renal excretion of urobilinogen. Br. Med. J. 2:1510, 1965.

Combes, B., and Schenker, S.: Laboratory tests. In Schiff, L. (Ed.): Diseases of the Liver. 4th ed. Philadelphia, J. B. Lippincott Co., 1975, p. 204.

Felig, P., and Sherwin, R.: Carbohydrate homeostasis, liver and diabetes. In Popper, H., and Schaffner, F. (Eds.): Progress in Liver Diseases. Vol. V. New York, Grune and Stratton, 1976, p. 149.

Fingl, E., and Woodbury, D. M.: General principles. In Goodman, L. S., and Gilman, A. (Eds.): The Pharmacological Basis of Therapeutics. New York, The Macmillan Co., 1970, p. 1.

Fleischner, E. M., and Arias, I. M.: Structure and function of ligandin. (Y Protein, GSH Transferase B) and Z Protein in the Liver: a progress report. In Popper, H., and Schaffner, F. (Eds.): Progress in Liver Diseases. Vol. V. New York, Grune and Stratton, 1976, p. 172.

Goldman, M. A., Schwartz, C. C., Swell, L., and Vlahcevic, Z. R.: Bile acid metabolism in health and disease. In Popper, H., and Schaffner, F. (Eds.): Progress in Liver Diseases. Vol. VI. New York, Grune and Stratton, 1979, p. 225.

Gollan, J. L., and Schmid, R.: Bilirubin update formation, transport and metabolism. In Popper, H., and Schaffner, F. (Eds.): Progress in Liver Diseases. Vol. VII. New York, Grune and Stratton, 1982, p. 261.

Grace, N. D., and Powell, L. W.: Iron storage disease and the liver. Gastroenterology 67:1257, 1974.

Hecker, R., and Sherlock, S.: Electrolyte and circulatory changes in terminal liver failure. Lancet 2:1121, 1956.

McFadzean, A. J., and Yeung, R. T. T.: Further observations on hypoglycemia in hepatocellular carcinoma. Am. J. Med. 47:220, 1969.

Odell, G. B., Ryan, W. B., and Richmond, M. D.: Exchange transfusion. Pediatr. Clin. North Am. 9:605, 1962.

Powell, L. W., Hemingway, E., Billing, B. H., and Sherlock, S.: Idiopathic unconjugated hyperbilirubinemia (Gilbert's syndrome). N. Engl. J. Med. 277:1108, 1967.

Sabesin, S. M., Ragland, J. B., and Freeman, M. R.: Lipoprotein disturbances in liver disease. In Popper, H., and Schaffner, F. (Eds.): Progress in Liver Diseases. Vol. VI. New York, Grune and Stratton, 1979, p. 243.

Scharschmidt, B. F., and Gollan, J. L.: Current concepts of bilirubin metabolism and hereditary hyperbilirubinemia. In Popper, H., and Schaffner, F. (Eds.): Progress in Liver Diseases. Vol. VI. New York, Grune and Stratton, 1979, p. 187.

Schmidt, E., and Schmidt, F. W.: Fundamentals and evaluation of enzyme patterns in serum. In Popper, H., and Schaffner, F. (Eds.): Progress in Liver Diseases. Vol. VII. New York, Grune and Stratton, 1982, p. 411.

Wolkoff, A. W., Weisiger, R. A., and Jakoby, W. B.: The multiple roles of the glutathione transferases (ligandins). In Popper, H., and Schaffner, F. (Eds.): Progress in Liver Diseases. Vol. VI. New York, Grune and Stratton, 1979, p. 213.

BILE FORMATION, BILE FLOW, AND CHOLESTASIS

Blitzer, B. I., and Boyer, J. L.: Cellular mechanisms of bile formation. Gastroenterology 82:346, 1982.

Chapman, R. W. G., Arborgh, B. A. M., Rhodes, J. M., et al.: Primary sclerosing cholangitis. A review of its clinical features, cholangiography and hepatic histology. Gut 21:870, 1980.

Coyne, M. J., and Schoenfield, L. J.: Gallstone formation and dissolution. In Popper, H., and Schaffner, F. (Eds.): Progress in Liver Diseases. Vol. V. New York, Grune and Stratton, 1976, p. 622.

Danzinger, R. G., Hofmann, A. F., Schoenfield, L. J., and Thistle, J. L.: Dissolution of cholesterol gallstones by chenodeoxycholic acid. N. Engl. J. Med. 286:1, 1972.

Hanson, R. F., and Pries, J. M.: Synthesis and enterohepatic circulation of bile salts. Gastroenterology 73:611, 1977.

Javitt, N. B.: Bile acids and hepatobiliary disease. In Schiff, L. (Ed.): Diseases of the Liver. 4th ed. Philadelphia, J. B. Lippincott Co., 1975, p. 111.

Kaplan, M. M.: Alkaline phosphatase. Gastroenterology 62:452, 1972.

McIntyre, N.: Plasma lipids and lipoproteins in liver disease. Gut 19:526, 1978.

Mistilis, S. P., and Lam, K. C.: Extrahepatic biliary obstruction. In Schiff, L. (Ed.): Diseases of the Liver. 4th ed. Philadelphia, J. B. Lippincott Co., 1975, p. 1388.

Paumgartner, G., and Paumgartner, D.: Current concepts of bile formation. In Popper, H., and Schaffner, F. (Eds.): Progress in Liver Diseases. Vol. VII. New York, Grune and Stratton, 1982, p. 207.

Seidel, D.: The abnormal lipoprotein of cholestasis. N. Engl. J. Med. 285:1538, 1971.

Simon, F. R., and Reichen, J.: Bile secretory failure: recent concepts of the pathogenesis of intrahepatic cholestasis. In Popper, H., and Schaffner, F. (Eds.): Progress in Liver Diseases. Vol. VII. New York, Grune and Stratton, 1982, p. 195.

Thureborn, E.: Human hepatic bile. Composition changes due to altered enterohepatic circulation. Acta Chir. Scand. 303 (suppl.):1, 1962.

Wheeler, H. O.: Secretion of bile. In Schiff, L. (Ed.): Diseases of the Liver. 4th ed. Philadelphia, J. B. Lippincott Co., 1975, p. 87.

LIVER FUNCTION TESTS

Abdi, W., Millan, J. C., and Mezey, E.: Sampling variability on percutaneous liver biopsy. Arch. Intern. Med. 139:680, 1979.

Edmondson, H. A., and Schiff, L.: Needle biopsy of the liver. In Schiff, L. (Ed.): Diseases of the Liver. 4th ed. Philadelphia, J. B. Lippincott Co., 1975, p. 247.

Feizi, T.: Immunoglobulins in chronic liver disease. Gut 9:193, 1968.

Menghini, G.: One second biopsy of the liver. Problems of its clinical applications. N. Engl. J. Med. 283:582, 1970.

Moore, T. L., Kupchik, H. Z., Marcon, N., and Zamchek, N.: Carcino-embryonic antigen assay in cancer of the colon and pancreas and other digestive tract disorders. Am. J. Dig. Dis. 16:1, 1971.

Rachmilewitz, N., Stein, Y., Aronovitch, J., and Grossowicz, N.: The clinical significance of serum cyanocobalamine in liver disease. Arch. Intern. Med. 102:1118, 1958.

Ratnoff, O. D.: Disordered hemostasis in hepatic disease. In Schiff, L. (Ed.): Diseases of the Liver. 3rd ed. Philadelphia, J. B. Lippincott Co., 1969, p. 147.

Smith, J. B., and O'Neill, R. T.: Alphafetoprotein occurrence in germinal cell and liver malignancies. Am. J. Med. 41:767, 1971.

Zieve, L., Hill, E., Hanson, M., Falcone, A. B., and Watson, C. J.: Normal and abnormal variations and clinical significance of the one minute and total serum bilirubin determinations. J. Lab. Clin. Med. 38:446, 1951.

CLINICAL LIVER DISEASE

Dickson, E. R., Fleming, C. R., and Ludwig, J.: Primary biliary cirrhosis. In Popper, H., and Schaffner, F. (Eds.): Progress in Liver Diseases. Vol. VI. New York, Grune and Stratton, 1979, p. 487.

Ferrucci, J. T., Jr., and Mueller, P. R.: Interventional radiology of the biliary tract. Gastroenterology 82:974, 1982.

Leevy, C. M., Chen, T., Luisada-Opper, A., Kanagasundarum, N., and Lieber, C. S.: Alcohol, protein metabolism, and liver injury. Gastroenterology 79:373, 1980.

Losowsky, M. D., Jones, D. P., Lieber, C. S., and Davidson, C. S.: Local factors in ascites formation during sodium retention in cirrhosis. N. Engl. J. Med. 268:651, 1963.

Maddrey, W. C., and Boitnott, J. K.: Drug induced chronic hepatitis and cirrhosis. In Popper, H., and Schaffner, F. (Eds.): Progress in Liver Diseases. Vol. VI. New York, Grune and Stratton, 1979, p. 595.

Rake, M. O., Panneli, G., Flute, P. T., and Williams, R.: Intravascular coagulation in acute hepatic necrosis. Lancet 1:533, 1970.

Shear, L., Cheng, S., and Gabuzda, G. J.: Compartmentalization of ascites and edema in patients with hepatic cirrhosis. N. Engl. J. Med. 282:1391, 1970.

Sherlock, S. (Ed.): Virus hepatitis. Clin. Gastroenterol. 9:1, 1980.

Zetterman, R. K.: Liver disease of the alcoholic: role of immunologic abnormalities in pathogenesis, recognition, and treatment. *In* Popper, H., and Schaffner, F. (Eds.): Progress in Liver Diseases. Vol. V. New York, Grune and Stratton, 1976, p. 516.

Zetterman, R. K., and Sorrell, M. F.: Immunologic aspects of alcoholic liver disease. Gastroenterology *81*:616, 1981.

Zieve, L.: Hepatic encephalopathy: summary of present knowledge with an elaboration on recent developments. *In* Popper, H., and Schaffner, F. (Eds.): Progress in Liver Diseases. Vol. VI, New York, Grune and Stratton, 1979, p. 327.

Zimmerman, H. J., and Maddrey, W. C.: Toxic and drug induced hepatitis. *In* Schiff, L., and Schiff, E. R. (Eds.): Diseases of the Liver. 5th ed. Philadelphia, J. B. Lippincott Co., 1982, p. 621.

EFFECT OF LIVER DISEASE ON OTHER ORGANS

Abelmann, W. H., Kramer, G. E., Verstraete, J. M., et al.: Cirrhosis of the liver and decreased arterial oxygen saturation. Arch. Intern. Med. *108*:34, 1961.

Adlercreutz, H.: Hepatic metabolism of estrogens in health and disease. N. Engl. J. Med. *290*:1081, 1974.

Baldus, W. P., Summerskill, W. H. J., Hunt, J. C., and Maher, F. T.: Renal circulation in cirrhosis. Observations based on catheterization of the renal vein. J. Clin. Invest. *43*:1090, 1964.

Fischer, J. E., and Baldessarini, R. J.: Pathogenesis and therapy of hepatic coma. *In* Popper, H., and Schaffner, F. (Eds.): Progress in Liver Diseases. Vol. V. New York, Grune and Stratton, 1976, p. 363.

Maddrey, W. C., Sen Gupta, K. P., Basu Mallick, K. C., et al.: Extrahepatic obstruction of the portal venous system. Surg. Gynecol. Obstet. *127*:989, 1968.

Murray, J. F., Dawson, A. M., and Sherlock, S.: Circulatory changes in chronic liver disease. Am. J. Med. *24*:358, 1958.

Ratnoff, O. D.: Disordered hemostasis in hepatic disease. *In* Schiff, L. (Ed.): Diseases of the Liver. 4th ed. Philadelphia, J. B. Lippincott Co., 1975, p. 184.

Schenker, S., Breen, K. J., and Hoyumpa, A. M.: Hepatic encephalopathy: current status. Gastroenterology *66*:121, 1974.

Shear, L., Bonkowsky, H. L., and Gabuzda, G. J.: Renal tubular acidosis in cirrhosis. A determinant of susceptibility to recurrent hepatic precoma. N. Engl. J. Med. *280*:1, 1969.

Summerskill, W. H. J.: Hepatic failure and the kidney. Gastroenterology *51*:94, 1966.

Summerskill, W. H. J., and Baldus, W. P.: Ascites. *In* Schiff. L. (Ed.): Diseases of the Liver. 4th ed. Philadelphia, J. B. Lippincott Co., 1975, p. 424.

Pathophysiology of Gallbladder Disease

31

Robert J. Bolt

NORMAL STRUCTURE

The gallbladder is a pear-shaped distensible organ with an average length of 10 cm and a width of 3 to 5 cm. It is attached to the inferior surface of the liver, occupying a position between the right and quadrate lobes. It is joined to the rest of the biliary tree by the cystic duct at the point at which the common hepatic duct becomes the common bile duct. The common bile duct enters the second portion of the duodenum. In this region there is a neuromuscular sphincter, the sphincter of Oddi. The body of the gallbladder is normally in contact with both the duodenum and colon. Its impression on the duodenum often can be seen by the radiologist during barium contrast examinations. Its position is variable, and the tip may be below the level of the iliac crest, especially when the patient is erect. An inflamed gallbladder can thus be mistaken for an inflamed appendix. The mucosa of the gallbladder consists of an epithelial layer of tall columnar cells overlying a lamina propria. It is thrown into multiple irregular folds that increase its absorptive area. A fibromuscular layer lies deep to the mucosa and is surrounded by a subserous adventitia and a serosa continuous with the serosa of the liver.

The cystic artery arises from the right hepatic artery and passes posterior to the common bile duct before dividing into superior and inferior branches that supply the gallbladder and cystic duct. The venous drainage begins in capillary plexuses that drain into superficial veins on the surface of the liver and then directly into the liver.

The gallbladder has an extensive lymphatic network that communicates with lymphatic channels draining the adjacent liver. These join the lymphatics of the cystic duct and the proximal portions of the extrahepatic duct system and drain into the nodes at the porta hepatis.

The biliary tree is innervated by both the sympathetic and the parasympathetic systems. Preganglionic sympathetic fibers are derived from the seventh to the tenth thoracic segments, and postganglionic fibers originate chiefly from the celiac ganglia. The hepatic division of the anterior vagal trunk supplies parasympathetic preganglionic fibers that synapse with postganglionic fibers in the gallbladder wall. Afferent fibers course with the splanchnic nerve as the right phrenic nerve; the latter relationship explains the occurrence of right shoulder pain in some patients

with gallbladder disease. Parasympathetic stimulation causes gallbladder contraction.

NORMAL FUNCTION

Although the gallbladder concentrates and stores bile, the physiologic importance of this function is unknown. Hepatic bile (prior to entry into the gallbladder) has a specific gravity of 1.008 and a pH of 5.9 to 8.6 (usually 8 to 8.6). It is an isosmotic solution containing approximately 97 per cent water. Its solids consist largely of cholesterol, bile salts, phospholipids (especially lecithin), mucin, conjugated bilirubin, and electrolytes. The major electrolytes are sodium, potassium, chloride, and bicarbonate. Bile also contains significant amounts of calcium as well as many enzymes and drug metabolites (Table 31–1).

In adults, the liver secretes 250 to 1500 ml (average 700 ml) of bile per day. Bile is secreted continuously, but its flow (choleresis) is augmented after meals. The volume of bile secreted is determined largely by the amount of bile salts synthesized within the liver. This in turn depends on the integrity of their enterohepatic circulation. Conjugated bile salts are secreted by the hepatocytes, providing an osmotic driving force for the movement of water into bile. As bile flows through the biliary tree its volume increases because of the act of secretion by the biliary epithelium of an electrolyte solution rich in bicarbonate.

Choleresis is under the control of neural and humoral mechanisms. It is increased by vagal stimulation and the action of secretin, cholecystokinin-pancreozymin (CCK-PZ), gastrin, and glucagon. Other choleretic agents include exogenously administered bile salts, acetylsalicylic acid, cincophen, pilocarpine, acetylcholine, choline, insulin, and histamine. Most of these agents cause an increase in hepatic bile output and contraction of the gallbladder. Vagal stimulation and CCK-PZ also cause relaxation of the sphincter of Oddi.

The gallbladder is a reservoir and concentrates hepatic bile four- to tenfold by absorbing electrolytes and water. This concentrating mechanism proceeds rapidly and helps prevent large increases of pressure within the system. The bile salts, bile pigments, lecithin, and cholesterol, to which the gallbladder wall is essentially impermeable, become highly concentrated. Under fasting conditions, the gallbladder is relaxed and may contain 50 to 60 ml of bile. During this time the sphincter of Oddi is closed.

A knowledge of bile salt metabolism is important because bile salts are necessary for two significant functions: (1) micellar solubilization in the absorption of dietary lipids, and (2) maintenance of biliary cholesterol in solution. The latter function is essential to an understanding of cholesterol gallstone formation.

In humans, two "primary" bile acids, cholic (trihydroxy) acid and chenodeoxycholic (dihydroxy) acid, are synthesized in the liver from cholesterol and conjugated with glycine and, to a lesser extent, with taurine. They then form salts with sodium and potassium. Most of the primary bile salts reaching the gut are absorbed, a relatively small amount throughout the small intestine by nonionic diffusion but a more significant proportion by an active transport process in the terminal ileum. Bile salts not absorbed enter the colon, where bacterial enzymes deconjugate and dehydroxylate them to form the "secondary" bile acids. Thus, deoxycholic (dihydroxy) acid is derived from cholic acid, and lithocholic (monohydroxy) acid originates from chenodeoxycholic acid. Deoxycholic acid is absorbed, reconjugated in the liver, and secreted into bile. Lithocholic acid is poorly absorbed, and only minute quantities normally appear in bile.

Bile therefore contains sodium or potassium salts of six different conjugated bile acids. Cholic and chenodeoxycholic acids account for 80 per cent of the total bile salt pool, with deoxycholic acid making up most of the remaining 20 per cent. This pool contains approximately 4 to 5 gm of bile salts and has a half-life of 3 to 5 days. It is recirculated six to ten times each day, and the daily hepatic synthesis of new bile acids accounts for about 10 per cent of the total pool. This is roughly equivalent to the amount lost in the feces (200 to 500 mg daily).

TABLE 31-1

Composition of Normal Hepatic Bile

pH	5.7–8.6
Bile salts	30–50 mM
Phospholipids	10–15 mM
Cholesterol	2–4 mM
Bilirubin	0.25–1.25 mM
Electrolytes	Na^+, K^+, Ca^{++}, Mg^{++}, Fe^{++}, Cl^-, HCO_3^-, PO_4^-, SO^-
Organic anions, drugs, hormones, etc.	H_2O–97%

Concentration of Major Electrolytes

	mEq/L
Sodium	146–165
Potassium	2.7–4.9
Calcium	2.5–4.8
Magnesium	1.4–3.0
Chloride	88–115
Bicarbonate	27–55

DISEASES

CHOLELITHIASIS/CHOLECYSTITIS

Prevalence

In 1959, Wilbur and Bolt presented figures indicating that 14.6 per cent of "normal Caucasian men" with an average age of 46.8 years had evidence of gallbladder abnormalities, past or present. Previous reports based on autopsy evidence had placed the incidence in this age group at somewhat lower figures. However, it is now generally accepted that approximately 10 to 15 per cent of adults residing in the United States do indeed have cholelithiasis. If one were to accept previous studies that indicated that at least 50 per cent of patients harboring gallstones are asymptomatic, the true prevalence could be estimated on the basis of the clinical prevalence as reported in the Framingham study. Thus, there must be approximately 20 million or more individuals carrying gallstones in the United States. Approximately 800,000 new cases develop each year, and half the patients ultimately will have surgery. In a 1971 report, Small stated that gallstone disease accounts for 5000 to 8000 deaths per year and that the total cost of morbidity from this disease approaches one billion dollars.

Studies of population surveys reveal interesting trends and patterns of gallstone disease prevalence with geographic locations and race. Sampliner's startling epidemiologic survey of Pima Indians showed that 70 per cent of females over the age of 30 years and males over the age of 55 years harbored gallstones. Subsequent surveys have shown that native American Indians of other tribes have a similarly high prevalence of gallstones. Inhabitants of Sweden approach these astounding figures, with 57 per cent incidence in females and 32 per cent incidence in males over the age of 20 years. This compares with an incidence of under 5 per cent in Japan. The incidence in England and Wales is only slightly lower than that quoted for the United States: 6.2 per cent in males and 12.1 per cent in females aged 45 to 69 years. These figures are based on routine cholecystograms obtained on 1442 inhabitants. It is obvious that gallstones have both medical and financial significance throughout the world and reach epidemic proportions in certain populations.

Pathophysiology

Types of Stones. In discussing gallstones, one should clearly differentiate the bilirubin line from the cholesterol line. Not only is the basic pathophysiology different in these two groups but also clinical manifestations, including prognosis and management, are different. This statement should be modified by the clause that bilirubinate stones

TABLE 31–2 TYPES OF GALLSTONES

	Pigment Line	*Cholesterol Line*
Distribution	Asia	Europe, United States
Appearance	Jagged edge	Smooth surface
Color	Dark reddish-brown	Light
Formation	Intraductal	Intragallbladder
Postcholecystectomy	May recur	Seldom recur
Associated disease	Hemolytic states	See text
	Cirrhosis	
	Parasitic infestation	

on the one hand, and cholesterol stones on the other, are rarely, if ever, pure pigment or pure cholesterol. There are multiple variations in percentage composition embracing the entire spectrum from almost pure pigment to almost pure cholesterol. In the United States, approximately three fourths of patients with gallstones will prove to have cholesterol as the primary component, and approximately one fourth will be shown to have gallstones of the pigment type. Table 31-2 demonstrates the primary points of difference between the bilirubin line and the cholesterol line of stones.

Calcium bilirubinate stones are fragile, dark reddish-brown masses, and their surface areas are quite irregular. The cut surface is amorphous, and stones are frequently formed within the biliary tree as well as within the gallbladder. As a result, residual stones as well as recurrent stone formation is more common with the bilirubinate line than with the cholesterol line of gallstones. It has become increasingly important to differentiate these two types in view of newer methods for medical dissolution of the cholesterol line. It has been suggested that this differentiation can be made on the basis of radiolucency or radiopacity of the stone on plain films of the abdomen. Unfortunately, such differentiation is far from precise. In one study, Trotman and coworkers demonstrated that although 86 per cent of radiolucent stones were of the cholesterol line, 14 per cent were of the pigment line. On the contrary, 67 per cent of radiopaque stones were found to be primarily of the pigment line, and 33 per cent were shown to be of the cholesterol line. Radiopacity is related to calcium content, and bilirubinate stones generally contain more calcium than do cholesterol stones. Bilirubinate stones are found more commonly in Asian countries than in the United States or in European countries. In addition, they are associated with specific diseases—particularly hemolytic anemias (sickle cell, thalassemia major, congenital spherocytosis)—and are seen in infants with severe erythroblastosis fetalis. Of interest is the report of an apparent increase in pigment stones following insertion of prosthetic mitral valves. Gallbladders containing stones removed from patients with alcoholic cirrhosis have been reported to be primarily of the bilirubin line. Sex and age differences are also noted in that the average age for clinical presentation of pigmentary

stones is in the 50s, and the average age for cholesterol stones is in the 40s. Males are as commonly afflicted with pigment stones as females are. However, cholesterol stones occur more commonly in females than in males.

PIGMENT STONES. Maki undoubtedly has been the most authoritative investigator studying the pathogenesis of calcium bilirubinate stones. Figure 31–1 summarizes the factors involved in bilirubin precipitation in bile.

In stone formation of either type, the initial step is precipitation of a substance that is normally soluble in bile. Maki has postulated that β-glucuronidase, perhaps of bacterial origin, hydrolyzes bilirubin glucuronide to free bilirubin and glucuronic acid. Calcium, a normal constituent of bile, combines with the carboxyl radical of liberated bilirubin to form calcium bilirubinate. The excess unconjugated bilirubin forms columnar complexes that precipitate to form calculi that are opaque radiographically. This postulate is supported by studies that show that bile infected with *Escherichia coli* does indeed exhibit intense β-glucuronidase activity in vitro and that the addition of commercially prepared β-glucuronidase to normal bile results in precipitates similar to those of infected bile. Maki further postulates that the cause of cholangiohepatitis in southeast Asia is not *E. coli* reaching the liver by the portal vein but an "ascending infection," possibly occurring in association with duodenitis. Hypo- or achlorhydria, "common in Japan," may facilitate bacterial growth in the duodenum and result in ascending infection of the biliary system, thus accounting for the high incidence of both pigmentary stones and cholangiohepatitis in these population groups.

Maki's proposals have received further support as the result of studies by Boonyapisit and others at the University of Pennsylvania. Their data revealed that normal human gallbladder bile does indeed contain low concentrations of unconjugated bilirubin and no evidence of detectable hydrolysis of conjugated bilirubin. Further, they demonstrated that an abnormally increased concentration of unconjugated bilirubin in gallbladder bile is associated with formation of pigment calculi. Moreover, lithogenic biles with elevated concentrations of unconjugated bilirubin also exhibited abnormal hydrolysis of conjugated bilirubin. However, hydrolysis was unrelated to the presence

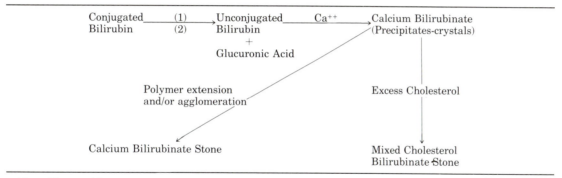

Conjugated Bilirubin →(1)/(2) Unconjugated Bilirubin + Glucuronic Acid →Ca++ Calcium Bilirubinate (Precipitates-crystals)

Polymer extension and/or agglomeration

Excess Cholesterol

Calcium Bilirubinate Stone

Mixed Cholesterol Bilirubinate Stone

(1). β-Glucuronidase
(2). Glucaro-1,4-lactone

Figure 31–1 Bilirubin stone formation.

of bacteria. This would support previous studies indicating that the gallbladder bile surrounding pigment gallstones is usually sterile. They suggest that β-glucuronidases produced by the gallbladder epithelium or secreted into bile by the liver may be the basic cause. An alternative explanation is that the inhibitor glucaro-1-4-lactone, normally present in bile, may be decreased, allowing the small amount of β-glucuronidase present to act. It has been shown that oral administration of glucaric acid inhibits β-glucuronidase activity. Once calcium bilirubin is precipitated in the form of bilirubin crystals, further aggregation, concretion, and related processes occur, resulting in the formation of stones. Although this stage is poorly understood, work by Sutor suggests that inhibitors of crystal growth play a role in radiopaque stone aggregation and stone formation.

CHOLESTEROL STONES. Cholesterol is normally maintained in clear solution by a remarkably precise control of the relative proportions of bile acids, phospholipids (lecithin), and cholesterol. Cholesterol is relatively insoluble in a solution of bile salts alone, but its solubility is greatly increased in the presence of appropriate concentrations of both bile acid and lecithin, at which point micelle formation occurs. The development of "critical micelle concentration" was elegantly summarized by Hofmann and Small in 1967. Subsequently, the method for presenting the three major components of bile on triangular coordinates has been widely accepted (Fig. 31–2).

When the molar concentrations are determined in vitro and when counter ion concentrations, pH, temperature, biliary solid content, and related factors are maintained under standard conditions, plotting the determinations in the triangle by lines parallel to sides of the triangle will differentiate bile that is supersaturated from bile in which cholesterol is fully solubilized. Supersaturated, or lithogenic, bile would be represented by all intercepts outside the ABC line. Metzger

and coworkers have proposed the use of a simple calculation, expressed as the lithogenic index, to denote the degree of saturation. Regardless of the manner of expression, the first step in cholesterol stone formation involves a change in bile acid/lecithin/cholesterol ratios sufficient to exceed the capability of bile to solubilize cholesterol. Thus, factors causing a decrease in total bile acid (quantitative or qualitative), a decrease in phospholipid

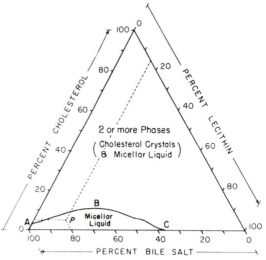

Figure 31–2 Method for presenting the three major components of bile (bile salts, lecithin, and cholesterol) on triangular coordinates. Each component expressed as percentage mole of total bile salt, lecithin, and cholesterol. Line ABC represents the maximum solubility of cholesterol and varying mixtures of bile salt and lecithin. Point represents bile composition containing 5% cholesterol, 15% lecithin, and 80% bile salt and falls within the zone of the single phase of micellar lipid. Expressed in other terms, the line ABC represents the metastable limit for cholesterol. (From Redinger, R. N., and Small, D. M., Arch. Int. Med. *130*:618, 1972. Reprinted by permission.)

concentration, or an increase in relative concentration of cholesterol will favor stone formation. Similarly, factors tending to increase the total pool of bile acids and phospholipids or tending to decrease the cholesterol in bile will favor dissolution of stones.

Evidence suggests that stone formation is not inevitable, even in the presence of lithogenic bile. Additional, albeit less clearly defined, factors favoring the initial step of nucleation (e.g., the presence of unconjugated bilirubin and/or absence of a nucleation inhibitor in bile) have been implicated (Hofmann et al., 1982; Carey and Small, 1978; Holan et al., 1979).

Bile Acids. Alteration of bile acid metabolism at any one of several points as indicated in Figure 31–3 could result in formation of lithogenic bile. Factors enhancing HMG CoA reductase activity or depressing 7-α-hydroxylase activity favors supersaturation of bile with cholesterol (Fig. 31–3, Points *1* and *2*). Under normal circumstances, gallbladder mucosa is virtually impermeable to conjugated bile acids, bilirubin, cholesterol, and cholecystographic contrast media. However, disturbance of the integrity of the gallbladder mucosa may result in absorption of bile acids in amounts inappropriate for cholesterol, leading to supersaturation (Fig. 31–3, Point *3*). Enterohepatic cycling of bile acid has been described earlier in this chapter. Certain conditions interfering with absorption and thus disrupting this cycle might be expected to reduce the effective total bile acid pool, resulting in formation of lithogenic bile (Fig. 31–3, Point *4*). These conditions include the following:

1. Impaired intestinal absorption from any cause.

2. Administration of bile acid–binding drugs such as cholestyramine.

3. Ileal inflammation or bypass surgery (since the majority of bile acids are actively absorbed in the terminal ileum).

4. Bacterial overgrowth in the proximal small bowel resulting in qualitative ineffectiveness of the bile acids.

5. Marked reduction of enterohepatic cycling, as in fasting.

It has been suggested that the decreased enterohepatic cycling associated with fasting may of itself result in greater inhibition of bile acid synthesis relative to cholesterol. Basing their theory on this supposition Redinger and coworkers proposed that bile acid synthesis is decreased for several weeks following surgery, leading to supersaturation.

Cholesterol Metabolism. Cholesterol synthesis and metabolism are depicted in Figure 31–4. The rate-limiting enzyme, as previously stated, is β-hydroxy-β-methyl, glutaryl CoA reductase (HMG CoA reductase). Factors stimulating HMG CoA reductase activity increase endogenous cholesterol synthesis. Endogenous cholesterol is believed to be the major precursor of bile acids, although the precise degree of compartmentalization (i.e., contribution to bile acid formation, excretion unchanged in bile, or transport in plasma to peripheral tissues) of endogenous versus exogenous (dietary) cholesterol remains controversial.

Phospholipids. The precise role of phospholipid metabolism in the alteration of nonlithogenic to lithogenic bile is unclear. The relative proportions of lecithin in bile of patients with cholesterol stones has been reported as normal. Moreover, direct measurements of phospholipid secretion in patients with cholesterol stones have failed to reveal significant abnormalities. Thus, the role of altered phospholipid metabolism in production of bile lithogenicity appears to be, at best, minimal.

Gallbladder Function. Elsewhere in this chapter, it is pointed out that cholesterol stones, in contrast to bilirubin (pigment) stones, form almost exclusively within the gallbladder. Moreover, recurrent cholesterol stones following cholecystectomy are the exception rather than the rule. On this basis, it would seem logical to conclude that gallbladder function or dysfunction might play a major role in promoting lithogenicity by one or more of the following methods:

1. Inappropriate absorption of bile acids as compared with cholesterol absorption. This alternative may be operative in an uncommon situation such as vascular insufficiency of the gallbladder associated with periarteritis nodosa or other instances of noncalculous cholecystitis. Certainly

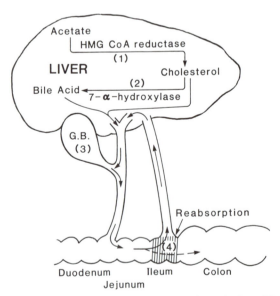

Figure 31–3 Bile acid synthesis and metabolism. (1) Hydroxymethylglutaryl CoA reductase (rate-limiting enzyme in cholesterol synthesis). Increase = lithogenicity. (2) Rate-limiting enzyme in conversion of cholesterol to bile acid. Decrease = lithogenicity. (3) Gallbladder mucosa inflammation = increased bile acid absorption = lithogenicity. (4) Malabsorption = bile acid loss = lithogenicity.

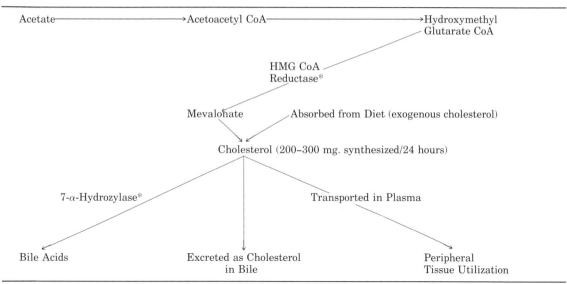

*Rate limiting enzymes

Figure 31-4 Cholesterol metabolism.

this factor does not appear to play a role in most situations.

2. Support of nucleation and growth as a result of stagnation.

3. Secretion of a substance inducing the liver to increase its synthesis of cholesterol or decrease its synthesis of bile acid or both.

Several investigators have confirmed the finding that bile secreted by the liver in patients with gallstones is already supersaturated with cholesterol. Whether cholecystectomy corrects this, as claimed by Shaffer and coworkers, or whether hepatic secretion of a supersaturated bile continues as suggested by McDougall's and Kimball's groups, remains controversial. Perhaps more than one factor is involved, that is, secretion of supersaturated bile by the liver aided by stagnation in the gallbladder whereby crystallization and growth of gallstones would more readily occur.

There are certain clinical situations favoring lithogenicity. Depression of bile acid synthesis or increased secretion of cholesterol in bile or both appear to play a role in the following situations:

1. Heredity (70 per cent lithogenic bile in Pima Indians; 0 per cent lithogenic bile in Masai).

2. Increasing age.

3. Obesity. Since obese patients are notoriously intermittent fasters, it has been suggested that stone formation may be associated with fasting rather than ascribed to obesity itself. Support for this concept comes from the demonstration that bile returns to a normal nonlithogenic state after weight reduction.

4. Increased cholesterol intake in the diet.

5. Pregnancy, oral contraceptives, and post-menopausal estrogen therapy.

6. Clofibrate therapy.

Literature concerning the effect of a polyunsaturated fat diet is confusing. In at least one retrospective study, the suggestion is made that there is an increased prevalence of stones in men on long-term polyunsaturated fat diets. This finding is not, as yet, confirmed by other studies. Finally, the increased prevalence of stones in patients with cirrhosis is associated with an increase in the number of pigment stones and is not related to cholesterol metabolism.

Dissolution

Much of the knowledge regarding stone formation has resulted from the discovery that administration of chenodeoxycholic acid will dissolve cholesterol stones. The concept of dissolving stones by medical means has been entertained ever since 1896, when Naunyn first demonstrated that gallstones dissolved when placed in dog bile. Substances used in attempts to dissolve gallstones include lecithin, plant sterols, medium-chain glycerides, phenobarbital, Zanchol, Bilron, wheat bran, and chenodeoxycholic acid. Table 31-3 summarizes these results. It should be emphasized that treatment with chenodeoxycholic acid poses the following potential problems:

1. Although it has been demonstrated to alter bile constituents so that super saturated is converted to unsaturated bile (lithogenic to nonlitho-

TABLE 31–3 GALLSTONE DISSOLUTION STUDIES

Investigator	Number of Patients	Agent and Dose (daily)	Length of Study (mo)	Number with Stones Unchanged	Number (%) Reduced	Number (%) Dissolved
Danzinger, 1972	7	CDCA* 0.75–4.5 gm	6–22	3(43)	3(43)	1(14)
Bell, 1972	12	CDCA 0.75–1.5 gm	6	6(50)	3(25)	3(25)
Thistle, 1973	18	CDCA 18 mg/kg	6	7(39)	11(61)	0
	17	Cholic 18 mg/kg	6	17(100)	—	—
	18	Placebo	6	18(100)	—	—
Dowling, 1974	26	CDCA 0.75–1.0 gm	6	11(42)	4(15)	11(42)
Coyne, 1975	10	CDCA 9 mg/kg	12	6(60)	4(40)	—
	8	Phenobarb 1.5 mg/kg	12	8(100)	—	—
	8	Placebo	12	8(100)	—	—
Iser, 1975	25	CDCA 0.25–12.5 gm	6–42	9(36)	6(24)	10(40)
Tompkins, 1976	7	Commercial Soybean Lecithin 48 gm	24	7(100)	—	—

*Chenodeoxycholic acid.

genic), this acid does not correct the basic defect underlying formation of supersaturated bile by the liver. Hence, it must be continued, in all probability, for the lifetime of the patient.

2. Its breakdown to lithocholic acid may cause liver damage. This has been reported to occur in baboons.

3. Its use during pregnancy (when bile tends to become supersaturated) may be dangerous to the fetus, since it has been shown that chenodeoxycholic acid can cross the placental barrier.

To minimize or eliminate these aforementioned undesirable side effects, ursodeoxycholic acid (chenodeoxycholic acid with the 7-hydroxy radical in the beta position rather than the alpha position) has been clinically evaluated. A retrospective comparative study of chenodeoxycholic acid and ursodeoxycholic acid by Meredith and coworkers demonstrated that the latter agent caused less diarrhea and was associated with only a 2.6 per cent incidence of "transaminitis." Diarrhea was a common side effect of chenodeoxycholic-acid therapy, and transaminitis occurred in 37 per cent of the cases. Rate of gallstone dissolution was similar. Bazzoli and coworkers have shown that the rate of lithocholic acid formation with chenodeoxycholic acid approximates that of ursodeoxycholic acid, suggesting that the risk of liver damage is also similar. However, Bazzoli's study revealed a small subgroup among the patients treated with chenodeoxycholic acid who appeared to be at higher risk owing to more rapid formation of lithocholic acid. Overall, it appears that urso-

deoxycholic acid is the preferred bile acid in stone dissolution. However, neither acid corrects the underlying metabolic defect, and recurrence, if not inevitable, is certainly common. Thus, the need for long-term therapy is apparent. Because treatment with these agents is neither inexpensive, short-term, nor curative, it cannot be recommended as routine treatment for cholesterol stone disease.

NEOPLASMS

Tumors of the gallbladder are rare. Most adenocarcinomas that do appear are solitary, hard, fibrous masses in the wall of the gallbladder. They spread by direct extension to the liver and by the lymphatics to cystic and periportal lymph nodes. They almost always develop in a gallbladder that contains stones. Their incidence is so low that this possibility is not an indication for prophylactic cholecystectomy in a patient with otherwise asymptomatic stones. The prognosis is poor (in large part because of late diagnosis), and survival is rare despite any form of therapy. Cholesterolosis and adenomyomatosis may be confused with benign or malignant polypoid lesions of the gallbladder. Most patients with either cholesterolosis or adenomyomatosis are asymptomatic. However, in the presence of symptoms compatible with biliary colic, surgical intervention is indicated in selected instances.

SCLEROSING CHOLANGITIS

Primary sclerosing cholangitis is a rare disease of unknown cause. It is frequently associated with ulcerative colitis or other chronic inflammatory bowel disease. It may simulate a very slowly growing bile duct carcinoma and is difficult to distinguish from other extrahepatic causes of biliary obstruction. Only the chronicity of the process militates against a diagnosis of neoplasm. Clinically, it manifests as a progressively obstructive jaundice, and the usual differential diagnostic procedures are necessary. If a localized sclerosis is found, resection or bypass procedures or both may be possible. Some investigators have recommended the use of corticosteroids and broad-spectrum antimicrobial agents, but results have been unpredictable. As with carcinoma of the biliary tree, the prognosis is poor, and death generally occurs within a few years after the appearance of symptoms.

CONGENITAL LESIONS

Congenital lesions of the gallbladder involving variations in size, shape, and location are of little or no clinical significance. The only clinically significant congenital lesions are those that involve the bile ducts themselves, including partial absence, or atresia, of one or both of the hepatic ducts or common bile ducts. Depending on the degree of absence, or atresia, jaundice usually is noted after the first week of life and is progressive. Surgical exploration and correction must be carried out relatively early, but the condition is amenable to relief in only about 15 per cent of patients.

CLINICAL EVALUATION

The gallbladder is studied primarily by the use of radiopaque substances given orally, intravenously, or, in selected patients, by percutaneous transhepatic injection of the bile ducts or retrograde cannulation of the common bile duct under endoscopic control. The latter two techniques are used when there is need to visualize the biliary duct system in the presence of jaundice.

The drugs presently used are all substituted triiodobenzoic acid compounds. Those excreted by the liver and used to evaluate the gallbladder are of high molecular weight and have at least one side chain at the five position of the benzene ring. They are moderately lipid-soluble and, when absorbed from the duodenum or administered intravenously, become tightly bound to plasma albumin and are transported to the liver. Within the liver, they are conjugated with glucuronic acid, rendering them water soluble, and then excreted into the biliary tree. When given orally, they are administered 12 hours before the radiographs are taken,

and fatty foods are prohibited to prevent emptying of the gallbladder. The gallbladder mucosa is normally impermeable to the drug, and absorption does not occur. Thus, visualization of the gallbladder is made possible.

There are four reasons for nonvisualization of the gallbladder by oral cystography:

1. The patient did not take the tablets, the tablets were vomited, or the drug was not absorbed.

2. The material was absorbed but could not be excreted owing to liver disease or obstruction of the biliary tree.

3. The drug was absorbed and excreted, but the gallbladder was inflamed, and absorption through the gallbladder wall occurred.

4. The cystic duct was blocked, and the drug could not enter the gallbladder.

It must be emphasized that if, for any reason, the liver is unable to excrete bilirubin it also will be unable to excrete contrast material. Thus, it is seldom worth attempting an oral examination when the serum bilirubin is above 2 mg per 100 ml. Complications of oral cholecystography include bowel irritation and, rarely, reaction to the drug itself.

Intravenous cholangiography presents the liver with a large amount of drug in a shorter period of time. It is rapidly excreted by the liver, filling the gallbladder and biliary ducts; therefore, the entire extrahepatic biliary tree can be visualized, especially when tomography is utilized. Since the gallbladder need not concentrate the drug, it will be visible even when its wall is damaged by inflammation. Cholangiography carries some risk; hepatic damage and acute renal failure due to tubular necrosis have been reported. Less serious reactions consist of nausea, vomiting, and a fall in blood pressure. Slow injection reduces the chances of such complications.

The failure of either oral or intravenous cholangiography to visualize the gallbladder in the presence of jaundice and occasional reactions to intravenous injection have stimulated a search for alternative, noninvasive methods of visualizing the gallbladder and biliary duct system. Labeling of pharmaceuticals with ^{99m}Tc for intravenous injection has proved to be a quite safe, effective, and rapid method for visualization of the biliary tree and gallbladder. Pyridoxylidene glutamate (^{99m}Tc-PG) was the initial radiopharmaceutical of proven clinical value. Subsequently, various N-substituted iminodiacetic acids (IDA) have been used. These compounds are structurally related to lidocaine and, when labeled with ^{99m}Tc, are efficiently extracted from the blood by the liver and rapidly excreted into the bile. Several IDA derivatives are now available; the most commonly used are HIDA (dimethyl IDA), PIPIDA (para-isopropyl IDA), and disofenin (diisopropylphenyl carbamoyl-methyl IDA). Blood clearance of these radiopharmaceuticals is almost complete by 3 to 5 minutes after intravenous injection of 5 to 10 mCi. Bile ducts are best visualized 10 to 20 minutes after injection, and the duodenum may be visualized in 20 to 30 minutes. Visualization of the gallbladder is optimal 15 to 30 minutes after injection. The only preparation required is that the patient be fasting. Although Stadalnik and colleagues have suggested that ^{99m}Tc IDA may be of value in the presence of jaundice, it is seldom helpful when serum bilirubin levels exceed 5 mg per cent. Visualization of the common duct without visualization of the gallbladder and cystic duct indicates cholecystitis or cystic duct stone or both in 90 per cent or more of the cases.

In the presence of jaundice, the major noninvasive method of demonstrating stones or ductile dilatation or, in some cases, both is ultrasonographic scanning. No preparation is needed except for a fat-free diet for some hours (an empty gallbladder cannot be located). Stones of any size can be demonstrated with ultrasonography with about the same accuracy as that achieved with radiography. Ultrasonography cannot localize the site nor define the nature of the obstruction. This requires invasive procedures such as percutaneous transhepatic or retrograde cholangiography.

MANAGEMENT

It must be remembered that for every patient presenting with an acute episode of cholecystitis/cholelithiasis there is one and possibly two patients whose gallbladders contain stones but who have no symptoms whatever. Thus, the average practitioner is dealing only with the "tip of the iceberg" when he is faced with the management of an individual patient suffering an acute episode of gallbladder disease. Moreover, this group of patients may present symptoms at any point on a severity spectrum—from very mild, right upper quadrant distress without fever and with minimal tenderness to severe, excruciating right upper quadrant pain accompanied by diaphoresis and shock. Chills, rigor, and fever frequently accompany this latter syndrome. Therefore, treatment must be individualized. Management of patients presenting with an acute episode is surgical, but controversy exists about whether operative treatment should be immediate or delayed. The great frequency of remission with conservative treatment suggests that surgery can be delayed until the patient is in the best possible state of health. Exceptions to this rule are made when the patient presents with a complication such as bile peritonitis or ascending cholangitis with septicemia. Routine medical management of an acute episode consists of the following:

1. Use of analgesics for relief of pain.
2. Attempts to decrease the rate of enterohe-

patic cycling by removing gallbladder and pancreatic stimuli. This involves intermittent suction and nothing by mouth.

3. Careful intravenous rehydration and electrolyte repletion.

Early relief of pain is desirable, and parenteral morphine sulfate (15 mg) continues to be an effective drug. Some have recommended the use of sublingual glyceryl trinitrate (0.5 mg) to reduce the spasmogenic effect of morphine. Other synthetic drugs such as meperidine (50 mg), believed by many to have less spasmogenic effects, may be substituted for morphine. The use of local heat to the abdomen in addition to the aforementioned measures often is helpful.

Patients in the early state have variable degrees of inflammatory change in the gallbladder. The importance of bacterial rather than chemical inflammatory change in the gallbladder wall is impossible for the clinician to measure. Fever and leukocytosis are, at best, crude indices of bacterial inflammation and may be quite misleading, particularly in the aged. In view of this, antibiotic coverage should not be routine but should be individualized.

Fluid replacement during the period of nasogastric suction is essential. In most situations alkalosis is relatively mild, and acidifying agents are rarely necessary. Sufficient fluid must be given to rehydrate the patient and keep up with both urinary and insensible water loss. Discretion must be used in fluid replacement, particularly in older individuals. Certainly a hypertonic glucose solution and physiologic saline will form the basis for replacement therapy. Calcium, sodium, potassium, and other electrolytes should be replaced as indicated by serum electrolyte values. The vast majority of patients will demonstrate gradual improvement with this regimen, permitting the removal of the nasogastric tube after approximately 48 hours and initiation of feeding by mouth. Repeated use of morphine sulfate or sublingual glyceryl trinitrate or both should be unnecessary.

As soon as removal of the nasogastric tube is indicated the patient may be started on clear liquids for the first few meals. Following this, progression to a low-fat diet, with no more than 20 gm of fat, relatively high carbohydrate levels, and average protein content, may be instituted. If the diagnosis of cholelithiasis or cholecystitis or both is firm, cholecystectomy should be advised. Certainly if rapid and complete recovery has occurred and the patient is in acceptable condition, cholecystectomy may be performed any time during the 2 weeks following the initial attack. If surgical contraindications exist, the patient should be discharged and continued on a low-fat, low-cholesterol diet, with cholecystectomy planned at the time optimal conditions exist.

Continued treatment is required for those patients in whom symptoms persist or progress after 48 hours of therapy. Nasogastric suction and intravenous fluid should be continued. If progression is marked by onset of fever or leukocytosis or both, antibiotic therapy should be started. Multiple choices exist, but one should choose a drug not only effective against a wide spectrum of bacteria but also specifically effective against coliform organisms. Ampicillin (1 gm) intravenously every 6 hours or tetracycline (250 mg) intravenously every 6 hours may be used. Some have recommended doxycycline; others have preferred to use a combination of penicillin and gentamicin. If progression is marked by increasing episodes of biliary colic, chills, and fever, emergency cholecystectomy may be necessary. A small percentage of patients under conservative treatment may progress or may develop a complication or both. Complications include the following:

1. Pancreatitis.
2. Empyema.
3. Emphysematous cholecystitis.
4. Fistula formation (gallbladder-bowel).
5. Ascending cholangitis.
6. Perforation, abscess, peritonitis.
7. Common duct obstruction.

Pancreatitis rarely has its onset while treatment is being carried out. However, this possibility should be entertained whenever a patient develops increasing abdominal pain despite treatment. It becomes more obvious if the location of the pain changes from the right upper quadrant or epigastric region to the back. Serum amylase and lipase determinations should be obtained in these patients to verify the diagnosis. The use of morphine sulfate can cause elevation of these enzymes and may be misleading. Failure to respond to the treatment just outlined may require emergency exploration.

Empyema of the gallbladder most often occurs in the older age group. Symptoms in this group may be inconspicuous and the diagnosis difficult. If the development of empyema is recognized, institution of intravenous penicillin G (20 million units daily) as well as an aminoglycoside is indicated. Emergency cholecystectomy is indicated.

A rare patient will manifest continued symptoms, and plain films of the abdomen may reveal collections of gas, either in the wall or within the gallbladder itself. With the patient in the erect position, a fluid level may be seen in the gallbladder. This is diagnostic of acute gaseous (emphysematous) cholecystitis. Colon bacilli, some forms of streptococci, and clostridia are the chief bacterial infections producing sufficient gas to be seen on radiographs. Again, emergency cholecystectomy is indicated.

An equally serious circumstance occurs when a patient suddenly develops spiking fever, chills, and rigor. This is usually associated with increasing jaundice, elevation of alkaline phosphatase, and leukocytosis. This triad of leukocytosis, increasing jaundice, and chills is strongly suggestive of ascending cholangitis. A shocklike state may ensue. Blood cultures must be obtained, since antibiotic therapy should be instituted and may be modified, depending on results of the blood cultures. Shock accompanying ascending cholangitis is distressing. When this occurs steroids should be instituted in high doses. Dexamethasone-21-phosphate in doses of 20 to 40 mg intravenously and 4 to 20 mg every 4 to 6 hours is recommended. The mortality rate is extremely high. Metaraminol or levarterenol bitartrate may be necessary to maintain blood pressure.

Rupture or perforation of the gallbladder is extremely rare when the patient is under treatment for an acute episode of cholecystitis. However, when it does occur, bile salts released in the abdominal cavity irritate the peritoneum. The result is an outpouring of fluid and in some instances hypovolemic shock. Bile is a good culture medium in which gram-negative and clostridia organisms are commonly found. The patient must be prepared for immediate surgery, and fluid loss into the peritoneal cavity may require replacement of as much as 2 to 8 L within a brief period. Electrolyte loss is usually uniform, so an imbalance is unusual. It is recommended that plasma and whole blood as well as intravenous saline and glucose be used. Antibiotics, nasogastric suction, narcotics, vasopressors, and steroids must be used as indicated. The prognosis is worse in those patients over 50 years of age, but the mortality rate is significant at any age.

Common duct obstruction can occur initially or any time during the course of an attack of cholecystitis. Its occurrence is a straightforward indication for surgical intervention.

Discussion thus far has concerned treatment of acute cholecystitis or acute episodes of chronic cholecystitis/cholelithiasis. When the diagnosis of chronic cholecystitis is unequivocal, the treatment of choice remains surgical. Conservative treatment is reserved for the debilitated and aged or for patients with associated conditions definitely contraindicating operation. Moreover, a few patients refusing surgery will require long-term treatment. In this group of patients, one of the stone-dissolving substances previously discussed can be tried. It should be re-emphasized that medical dissolution should be attempted only in those patients with cholesterol stones and is ineffective for pigment or bilirubin stones. Concomitant measures have been recommended regardless of the type of stones present. The degree of efficacy of these concomitant measures remains unproved. However, it seems reasonable that the diet should be low in fat with protein and carbohydrate dependent on the caloric requirements of the individual. Overeating at any one meal should be avoided. Protein supplements in the form of skim-milk powder, 120 gm in 1000 ml of skim milk taken in amounts of 120 to 240 ml with and between meals, are often helpful in the older patient. Hydrocholeretic drugs such as Zanchol have been recommended. As previously noted, this has been shown to have an effect on altering bile composition toward the nonlithogenic side. Evaluation of the effectiveness of drugs of this type on symptoms is difficult owing to the unpredictability of the disease process. Zanchol (florantyrone) is a gamma-oxy-gamma-(8-fluoranthene) butyric acid. It is supplied in tablets of 250 mg and can be given before each meal. Unfortunately, side effects of this drug include the very symptoms for which the drug is being used (i.e., nausea, vomiting, and diarrhea). Moreover, changes in liver profile have been reported. Because of these factors, the use of hydrocholeretic drugs of this type cannot be strongly recommended. Finally, an anticholinergic

sedative combination such as Donnatol or Butibel may be prescribed before each meal. Occasionally pharmacologic side effects such as sleepiness, tiredness, blurring of vision, or difficulty on urination may occur. Used in the usual dosage of one tablet before each meal, these side effects are mild. An occasional hypersensitivity reaction may be seen. This is manifested primarily as a mild dermatitis medicamentosa.

In summary, the treatment of proved acute or chronic cholecystitis continues to be surgical. Medical attempts at control of symptoms or dissolution of cholesterol gallstones or both, if present, should be reserved for those patients in whom surgery is strongly contraindicated or refused by the patient.

REFERENCES

Bainton, B., Davies, G. T., Evans, K. T., and Gravelle, I. H.: Gallbladder disease: prevalence in a South Wales industrial town. N. Engl. J. Med. 294:1147, 1976.

Balint, J. A., Beeler, D. A., Kyriakides, E. C., and Treble, D. H.: The effect of bile salts upon lecithin synthesis. J. Lab. Clin. Med. 77:122, 1971.

Bazzoli, F., Fromm, H., Sarva, R. P., et al.: Comparative formation of lithocholic acid from chenodeoxycholic and ursodeoxycholic acids in the colon. Gastroentenology 83:753, 1982.

Bell, C. C., Vlahcevic, Z. R., and Swell, L.: Alterations in the lipids of human hepatic bile after the oral administration of bile salts. Surg. Gynecol. Obstet. 132:36, 1971.

Bell, G. D., Whitney, B., and Dowling, R. H.: Gallstone dissolution in man using chenodeoxycholic acid. Lancet 2:1213, 1972.

Bennion, L. J., and Grundy, S. M.: Effects of obesity and caloric intake on biliary lipid metabolism in man. J. Clin. Invest. 56:996, 1975.

Biss, K., Ho, K. J., Mikkelson, B., Lewis, L., and Taylor, C. B.: Some unique biologic characteristics of the Masai of East Africa. N. Engl. J. Med. 284:694 1971.

Boonyapisit, S. T., Trotman, B. W., and Ostrow, J. D.: Unconjugated bilirubin and the hydrolysis of conjugated bilirubin in gallbladder bile of patients with cholelithiasis. Gastroenterology 74:70, 1978.

Boston Collaborative Drug Surveillance Program: Oral contraceptives and venous thromboembolic disease, surgically confirmed gallbladder disease and breast tumors. Lancet 1:1399, 1973.

Boston Collaborative Drug Surveillance Program: Surgically confirmed gallbladder disease, venous thromboembolisms, and breast tumors in relation to postmenopausal estrogen therapy. N. Engl. J. Med. 290:15, 1974.

Carey, M. G., and Small, D. M.: The physical chemistry of cholesterol solubility in bile. Relationship to gallstone formation and dissolution in man. J. Clin. Invest. 61:998, 1978.

Comfort, M. W., Gray, H. K., and Wilson, J. M.: The silent gallstone: ten to twenty year followup study of 112 cases. Ann. Surg. 128:931, 1948.

Cooper, J., Geizerova, H., and Oliver, M. F.: Clofibrate and gallstones. Lancet 1:1083, 1975.

Coyne, M. J., Bonorris, G. G., Chung, A., et al.: Treatment of gallstones with chenodeoxycholic acid and phenobarbital. N. Engl. J. Med. 292:604, 1975.

Coyne, M. J., Bonorris, G. G., Goldstein, L. I., and Schoenfield, L. J.: Effect of chenodeoxycholic acid and phenobarbital on the rate-limiting enzymes of hepatic cholesterol and bile acid synthesis in patients with gallstones. J. Lab. Clin. Med. 87:281, 1976.

Danzinger, R. G., Hofmann, A. F., Schoenfield, L. J., and Thistle, J. L.: Dissolution of cholesterol gallstones by chenodeoxycholic acid. N. Engl. J. Med. 286:1, 1972

Danzinger, R. G., Hofmann, A. F., Thistle, J. L., and Schoenfield,

L. J.: Effect of oral chenodeoxycholic acid on bile acid kinetics and biliary lipid composition in women with cholelithiasis. J. Clin. Invest. 52:2809, 1973.

DenBesten, L., Conner, W. E., and Bell, S.: The effect of dietary cholesterol on the composition of human bile. Surgery 73:266, 1973.

Dowling, R. H.: Chenodeoxycholic acid. The British experience. Hosp. Prac. 9:85, 1974.

Friedman, K. K., Kannel, W. B., and Dawler, T. R.: Epidemiology of gallbladder disease: observations in the Framingham study. J. Chron. Dis. 19:273, 1966.

Gerdes, M. M., and Boyden, E. A.: The rate of emptying of the human gallbladder in pregnancy. Surg. Gynecol. Obstet. 66:145, 1938.

Goswitz, J. T.:Bacteria and biliary tract disease. Am. J. Surg. 128:644, 1974.

Grundy, S. M., Duane, W. C., Adler, R. D., et al.: Biliary lipid outputs in young women with cholesterol gallstones. Metabolism 23:67, 1974.

Grundy, S. M., Metzger, A. L., and Adler, R. D.: Mechanisms of lithogenic bile formation in American Indian women with cholesterol gallstones. J. Clin. Invest. 51:3026, 1972.

Herman, A. H., Redinger, R. N., and Small, D. M.: The effects of surgery on bile secretion and composition. Surg. Forum 22:378, 1971.

Heywood, R., Palmer, A. K., Foll, C. V., and Lee, M. R.: Pathological changes in fetal Rhesus monkey induced by oral chenodeoxycholic acid. Lancet 2:1021, 1973.

Hofmann, A. F., Grundy, S. M., Lachin, J. M., et al.: Pretreatment biliary lipid composition in white patients with radiolucent gallstones in the National Cooperative Gallstone Study. Gastroenterology 83:738, 1982.

Hofmann, A., and Small, D. M.: Detergent properties of bile salts. Correlation with physiological function. Ann. Rev. Med. 18:333, 1967.

Holan, K. R., Holzbach, R. T., Hermann, R. E., et al.: Nucleation time: a key factor in the pathogenesis of cholesterol gallstone disease. Gastroenterology 77:611, 1979.

Iser, J. H., Dowling, R. H., Mok, H. Y. I., and Bell, G. D.: Chenodeoxycholic acid treatment of gallstones. A follow-up report and analysis of factors influencing response to therapy. N. Engl. J. Med. 293:378, 1975.

Kerner, M., Raicht, R. F., Mosbach, E. H., and Zimmon, D. S.: Zanchol, a potential litholytic agent in man. Gastroenterology 69:836, 1975.

Kimball, A., Pertsemlidis, D., and Panveliwalla, D.: Composition of biliary lipids and kinetics of bile acids after cholecystectomy in man. Am. J. Dig. Dis. 21:776, 1976.

Lewis, R., and Gorbach, S.: Modification of bile acids by intestinal bacteria. Arch. Int. Med. 130:545, 549, 1972.

Lieber, M. M.: Incidence of gallstones and their correlation with other diseases. Ann. Surg. 135:394, 1952.

Ludlow, A. I.: Autopsy incidence of cholelithiasis based on records of Institute of Pathology, Western Reserve University and University Hospital. Am. J. Med. Sci. *193*:481, 1937.

Mabee, T. M., Meyer, P., DenBesten, L., and Mason, E. E.: The mechanism of increased gallstone formation in obese human subjects. Surgery *79*:460, 1976.

Maki, T.: Pathogenesis of calcium bilirubinate gallstones: role of E. coli, β-glucuronidase and coagulation by inorganic ions, polyelectrolytes and agitation. Ann. Surg. *164*:90, 1966.

Matolo, N.: Gallbladder and biliary tract scanning with ^{99m}Tc-PG. West. J. Med. *126*:386, 1977.

McDougall, R. M., Walker, K., and Thurston, O. G.: Prolonged secretion of lithogenic bile after cholecystectomy. Ann. Surg. *182*:150, 1975.

McSherry, C. K., Morrissey, K. P., Swarm, R. L., et al.: Chenodeoxycholic acid induced liver injury in pregnant and neonatal baboons. Ann. Surg. *184*:490, 1976.

Meredith, T. J., Williams, G. V., Maton, P. N., et al.: Retrospective comparison of "cheno-" and "urso-" in the medical treatment of gallstones. Gut *23*:382, 1982.

Merendino, K. A. and Manhas, D. R.: Man-made gallstones: a new entity following cardiac valve replacement. Ann. Surg. *177*:694, 1973.

Metzger, A. L., Heymsfield, S., and Grundy, S. M.: The lithogenic index—a numerical expression for the relative lithogenicity of bile. Gastroenterology *62*:499, 1972.

Miettinen, T. A.: Cholesterol production in obesity. Circulation *44*:842, 1971.

Nakayama, F., and van der Linden, W.: Bile composition. Sweden versus Japan. Its possible significance in the difference in gallstone incidence. Am. J. Surg. *122*:8, 1971.

Naunyn, B.: A Treatise on Cholelithiasis. (Translated by A. E. Garrod.) The New Syndenham Society, London, 1896, p. 22.

Nicholas, P., Rinaudo, P. A., and Conn, H. O.: Increased incidence of cholelithiasis in Laennec's cirrhosis. Gastroenterology *63*:112, 1972.

Nicolau, G., Shefer, S., Salen, G., and Mosbach, E. H.: Determination of hepatic cholesterol 7α-hydroxylase activity in man. J. Lipid Res. *15*:146, 1974.

Nicolau, G., Shefer, S., Salen, G., and Mosbach, E. H.: Determination of 3-hydroxy-3-methylglutaryl CoA reductase. J. Lipid Res. *15*:94, 1974.

Nicolau, G., Shefer, S., Salen, G., and Mosbach, E. H.: Hepatic 3-hydroxy-3-methylglutaryl CoA (HMG CoA) reductase and cholesterol 7α-hydroxylase in man. Gastroenterology *64*:887 (abstr.), 1973.

Northfield, T. C., and Hofmann, A. F.: Biliary lipid output during three meals and an overnight fast. I. Relationship to bile acid pool size and cholesterol saturation of bile in gallstone and control subjects. Gut *16*:1, 1975.

Pertsemlidis, D., Panveliwalla, A., and Ahrens, E. H.: Effects of clofibrate and of an estrogen-progestin combination on fasting biliary lipids and cholic acid kinetics in man. Gastroenterology *66*:565, 1974.

Pomare, E. W., Low-Beer, T. S., and Heaton, K. W.: The effect of wheat-bran on bile salt metabolism and bile composition. In Advances in Bile Acid Research. Stuttgart, F. K. Schattauer Verlag, 1974, pp. 355–360.

Redinger, R. N., Herman, A. R., and Small, D. M.: The effects of surgery on hepatic physiology in the primate. Gastroenterology *60*:795 (abstr.), 1974.

Rosenak, B. D., and Kohlstaedt, K. S.: Bile salt therapy in liver and gallbladder disease. Am. J. Dig. Dis. Nutr. *3*:577, 580, 1936.

Sampliner, R. E., Bennett, P. H., Comess, L. J., et al.: Gallbladder disease in Pima Indians. N. Engl. J. Med. *283*:1358, 1970.

Schreibman, P. H., Pertsemlidis, D., Liu, G. C. K., and Ahrens,

E. H.: Lithogenic bile, a consequence of weight reduction. J. Clin. Invest. *53*:72a (abstr.), 1974.

Schwartz, C. C., Vlahcevic, Z. R., Halloran, L. G., et al.: Evidence for the existence of definitive hepatic cholesterol precursor compartments for bile acids and biliary cholesterol in man. Gastroenterology *69*:1379, 1975.

Scott, G. W., Smallwood, R. E., and Rowlands, S.: Flow through the bile duct after cholecystectomy. Surg. Gynecol. Obstet. *140*:912, 1975.

Shaffer, E. A., Braasch, J. W., and Small, D. M.: The influence of cholecystectomy and obesity on biliary lipid secretion in cholesterol gallstone disease. Gastroenterology *70*:A–78/936, 1976.

Small, D. M.: Gallstones 1971. Viewpoints Dig. Dis. *3*:3, 1971.

Stadalnik, R. C., Matolo, N. M., Jansholt, A., et al.: Clinical experience with ^{99m}Tc-disofenin as a cholecystographic agent. Radiology *140*:797, 1981.

Sturdevant, R. A. L., Pearce, M. L., and Dayton, S.: Increased prevalence of cholelithiasis in man ingesting a serum-cholesterol-lowering diet. N. Engl. J. Med. *288*:24, 1973.

Sutor, D. J., and Percival, J. M.: Presence or absence of inhibitors of crystal growth in bile. I. Effect of bile on the formation of calcium phosphate, a constituent of gallstones. Gut *17*:506, 1976.

Sutor, D. J., and Wooley, S. E.: The nature and incidence of gallstones containing calcium. Gut *14*:215, 1973.

Swell, L., Bell, C. C., and Vlahcevic, Z. R.: Relationship of bile acid pool size to biliary lipid excretion and the formation of lithogenic bile in man. Gastroenterology *61*:716, 1971.

Tangedahl, T. N., Matseshi, J. W., Thistle, J. L., and Hofmann, A. F.: Plant sterols increase effectiveness of chenodeoxycholic acid therapy in lowering cholesterol saturation of fasting state bile in patients with radiolucent gallstones. Gastroenterology *72*:2 (abstr.), 1977.

The Coronary Drug Project: Clofibrate and niacin in coronary heart disease. J.A.M.A. *231*:360, 1975.

Thistle, J. L., Carlson, G. L., Hofmann, A. F., and Babayan, V. K.: Medium chain glycerides rapidly dissolve cholesterol gallstones in vitro. Gastroenterology *72*:2 (abstr.), 1977.

Thistle, J. L., Eckhart, K. L., Nensel, R. E., et al.: Prevalence of gallbladder disease among Chippewa Indians. Mayo Clinic Proc. *46*:603, 1971.

Thistle, J. L., and Hofmann, A. F.: Efficacy and specificity of chenodeoxycholic acid therapy for dissolving gallstones. N. Engl. J. Med. *289*:655, 1973.

Tompkins, R. K.: The systemic treatment of gallstones. Adv. Surg. *10*:87, 1976.

Trotman, B. W., and Soloway, R. D.: Pigment vs. cholesterol cholelithiasis: clinical and epidemiological aspects. Am. J. Dig. Dis. *20*:735, 1975.

Trotman, B. W., Soloway, R. D., Sanchez, H. M., et al.: Evaluation of radiographic lucency or opaqueness of gallstones as a means of identifying cholesterol or pigment stones. Gastroenterology *68*:1563, 1975.

Wenckert, A., and Robertson, B.: The natural course of gallstone disease. Eleven-year review of 781 nonoperated cases. Gastroenterology *50*:376, 1966.

Wilbur, R. S., and Bolt, R. J.: Incidence of gallbladder disease in "normal" men. Gastroenterology *36*:251, 1959.

Winch, J., Burnett, W., Banks, M., and Cranvitch, B.: Factors concerned in the pathogenesis of gallstones. Gut *10*:954 (abstr.), 1969.

Yamaguchi, I., Sato, T., Sato, H., and Matsushiro, T.: Quantitative determination of D-glucaric acid in bile in relation to the inhibitory effect upon bacterial B glucuronidase. Tokyo J. Exp. Med. *87*:123, 1965.

INTRODUCTION

The key to understanding the pathophysiology of diseases of the human pancreas is a knowledge of its biochemistry and physiology. The mechanism of injury in acute pancreatitis is generally agreed to be *autodigestion*, which depends on factors that activate or inhibit within the gland the enzymes normally secreted into pancreatic juice. Diagnosis of diseases like acute pancreatitis, chronic pancreatitis, and cancer of the pancreas depends on study of these enzyme activities in serum, urine, or pancreatic juice and their responses to physiologic stimulants. Treatment of pancreatic disease also depends on knowledge of how enzymes can damage tissue and of the results of enzyme deficiency in the gut. More than in almost any other organ, diseases of the pancreas are manifestations of disordered physiology and biochemistry.

ENZYMES OF THE HUMAN PANCREAS

Electrophoretic studies on human pancreatic juice indicate that at least 19 different proteins can be detected. Table 32–1 reviews the proteins of human pancreatic juice. The key to the activation of the pancreatic zymogens is *enterokinase,* a proteolytic enzyme found in the mucosa of the duodenum, both bound to the brush border and present in the soluble fraction of the duodenal mucosa cells. The enzyme is released into the lumen of the duodenum by a number of stimuli, such as the polypeptide hormones cholecystokinin (CCK), secretin, gastrin, and glucagon, and by bile salts as well. As shown in Table 32–1, enterokinase converts both trypsinogens of human pancreatic juice to *trypsins 1 and 2*. Enterokinase cleaves the lysine-isoleucine bond of residues 6 and 7 of trypsinogen, splitting off the N-terminal activation peptide and allowing the generation of active trypsin. Enterokinase does this more efficiently than autocatalysis of trypsin. Enterokinase binds trypsinogen six times as strongly as trypsin does, and it produces trypsin 2000 times faster than trypsin acting on trypsinogen. Enterokinase recognizes the N-terminal sequence of trypsinogen and is tailored to act specifically on trypsinogen. However, it cannot activate chymotrypsinogen or other zymogens. Calcium stabilizes the trypsin molecule at alkaline pH and retards its autodigestion by trypsin and other proteases. Another reason for the effectiveness of enterokinase in the activation process is that it is not inhibited by the trypsin inhibitor of human pancreatic juice. Enterokinase synthesis may be induced by feeding trypsinogen to a mutant mouse (CBA/Jepi) that lacks pancreatic acinar cells. The essential nature of enterokinase is best demonstrated by congenital enterokinase deficiency, in which children afflicted with this disease develop severe protein maldigestion because they are not able to activate zymogens; hence, they maldigest proteins.

Trypsin rapidly activates chymotrypsinogen to two chymotrypsins, two proelastases to two elastases, two procarboxypeptidases to two carboxypeptidases, prophospholipase A_2 to phospholipase A_2, and a procolipase to colipase. In human pancreatic juice, two separate trypsinogens have been identified, and each gives rise to a separate trypsin: one that is cationic in its electrophoretic migration and one that is anionic. The anionic protein is much less stable than the cationic one, even in the presence of calcium. A third form of trypsinogen has been identified in human juice that is important because its corresponding trypsin shows no inhibition with bovine basic trypsin inhibitor (aprotinin). Elastolytic activity resides in two different proteins in human pancreatic juice. The first one, *proelastase I*, is classic elastase, which works primarily on the internal bonds of elastin and of other proteins. Another enzyme, called *proelastase II,* or *protease E*, splits elastin poorly and digests protein well. The two carboxypeptidases that act on different C-terminal amino acids are both zinc metalloenzymes and contain one mole of firmly bound zinc per mole of enzyme; the zinc is essential to catalytic activity.

From the point of view of digestion of calorically important foods, the key lipolytic enzyme is *lipase,* also called *glycerol-ester hydrolase.* This enzyme acts by splitting the primary (alpha) ester bonds of water-insoluble, emulsified carboxylic esters, particularly esters of glycerol. Thus, triglyceride is cleaved to yield fatty acids from the two alpha positions, leaving the 2-(beta) monoglyceride. Lipase functions by binding the hydrophobic side of the molecule to particles of triglyceride, which are water-insoluble. The activity is a direct function of the particle size: the more interface available for the enzyme to bind, the faster the activity. Emulsifying agents for water-insoluble substrates are therefore essential to this enzyme activity. These emulsifying agents exist in the duodenum, but their exact nature has not been defined. Bile salts are often said to be the duodenal emulsifying agents, but bile salts, rather than

TABLE 32–1 ENZYMES IN HUMAN PANCREATIC JUICE

Zymogen	Enzyme or Protein	Activator(s)	Cofactors, Stabilizers	Substrates, Products, Bonds Cleaved
	(PROTEOLYTIC)			
Trypsinogen 1	Trypsin 1 (cationic)	Enterokinase Trypsin	Ca^{++}	Internal peptide bonds of protein whose carbonyl group is contributed by arg or lys
Trypsinogen 2	Trypsin 2 (anionic)	Enterokinase Trypsin	Ca^{++}	Same as trypsin 1
Chymotrypsinogen	Chymotrypsin 1 Chymotrypsin 2	Trypsin	Ca^{++}	Internal peptide bonds of proteins whose carbamyl group is from try, phe, tyr, leu, met
Proelastase 1	Elastase 1 (cationic)	Trypsin		Internal bonds of elastin or other proteins formed from neutral amino acids, especially ala
Proelastase 2	Elastase 2 (anionic)	Trypsin		Same as elastase 2 but digests other proteins better than elastin
Procarboxypeptidase A	Carboxypeptidase A	Trypsin	Zn	All C-terminal amino acids except arg, lys, penultimate pro
Procarboxypeptidase B	Carboxypeptidase B	Trypsin	Zn	C-terminal arg, lys
	(LIPOLYTIC)			
	Lipase (Glyercol ester hydrolase; bile salt–inhibited lipase)	Colipase	Ca^{++}	Primary ester bonds of water-insoluble, aggregated carboxylic esters (triglyceride → fatty acids + 2-monoglyceride)
Procolipase	Colipase	Trypsin		Binds to phospholipid-tryglyceride emulsions and to lipase, forming active complex with lipase
	Carboxylic ester hydrolase (bile salt–dependent lipase; cholesterol esterase; lysophospholipase)		Bile salts with 3 α- and 7α-hydroxyl groups	Water-insoluble carboxyl esters of primary and secondary alcohols in micellar solution (vitamin A palmitate → vitamin A alcohol + palmitic acid). Also splits cholesterol esters, 2-monoglycerides, lysophospholipids, short-chain lecithins
Prophospholipase A_2	Phospholipase A_2	Trypsin	Bile salts, Ca^{++}	Fatty acid ester bond at 2 position of 1, 2 diacylphosphoglyceride (lecithin → fatty acid + 1-lysolecithin)
	(OTHER)			
	α-Amylase (α-1, 4 glucan-4-glucanohydrolase)		Cl' Ca^{++}	Endoamylase; cleaves α-1, 4 bonds of polyglyucosides (starch) to maltose, maltotriose, and limit dextrins; exists as 6 isoenzymes
	Ribonuclease		Phosphate Citrate	Endonuclease; cleaves ribonucleic acid adjacent to cytidine nucleotide phosphodiester bonds to produce oligonucleotides
	Deoxyribonuclease I		Mg^{++} plus Ca^{++} or Mn^{++}	Endonuclease; splits between purine and phosphate of pyrimidine nucleotide; products are oligonucleotides
	(INHIBITORS)			
	Pancreatic secretory trypsin inhibitor			Inhibits trypsin incompletely and reversibly as 1:1 complex (Kazal type)

being activators of lipase at the critical micellar concentration found in the duodenum, are actually inhibitors. Bile salts shift the pH optimum of lipase from between 8 and 9 to between 6 and 7, the pH found in the duodenum. Lipase requires for activity a 10,000 molecular weight protein activator, colipase, which is secreted in pancreatic juice. It binds to triglyceride substrates first, and then lipase binds 1:1 to colipase. Colipase protects lipase against inhibition by bile salts and against denaturation when it is spread out on an interfacial surface. A procolipase exists in the juice that is activated when trypsin cleaves an N-terminal pentapeptide. Calcium ions are also essential to lipase activity in the presence of bile salts and allow the enzyme to bind to water-insoluble substrates.

A nonspecific carboxylic-ester hydrolase has been purified from human pancreatic juice and found to serve many functions. It requires bile salts and substrates in micellar form. Among its important substrates are vitamin A, D_3, and E esters; cholesterol esters; 2-monoglycerides; short-chain phospholipids; and lysophospholipids. It incorporates the activity of what used to be called *cholesterol esterase*. At pH 7.4 it splits cholesterol esters, and at pH 5.3 it forms them. This enzyme is crucial in cholesterol absorption because ingested cholesterol is in the form of cholesterol esters, which cannot be absorbed by humans unless they are first cleaved to free cholesterol and then taken up out of micellar solution.

The next lipolytic enzyme is the only one known to exist as a proenzyme—*phospholipase A₂*. It cleaves fatty acids from the 2 position of a phospholipid such as lecithin, giving rise to a fatty acid and lysolecithin. Its zymogen is activated by trypsin, which cleaves off an N-terminal activation peptide to yield the active enzyme, which is activated by bile salts and stabilized by calcium.

The only enzyme in human pancreatic juice able to digest polysaccharides is *amylase*, which cleaves the α-1,4 bonds of polymers of glucose, such as starch. It is activated by chloride ions and contains one firmly bound mole of calcium per mole of enzyme, which is essential to activity. It produces a disaccharide (maltose), a trisaccharide (maltotriose), and a core of starch resistant to amylase, called a *limit dextrin*. Pancreatic amylase is the product of a gene located on human chromosome 1 and is closely linked to a locus on the same chromosome that produces the amylase found in salivary glands and many other human tissues. The most purified form of human pancreatic amylase has six bands on electrophoresis. These result from two families of amylases, with or without glycosyl groups. The families are further modified by loss of amide groups. Salivary amylase also exists as 6 to 8 isoenzymes, but the pancreatic and salivary isoenzyme families can be distinguished by electrophoresis or electrofocusing techniques.

Ribonuclease requires phosphate or citrate for activation and cleaves internal bonds of a ribonucleic acid molecule adjacent to cytidine to produce oligonucleotides. *Deoxyribonuclease I* is also an endonuclease, and it splits the phosphate diester bond joining the purine and pyrimidine nucleotide. The human enzyme requires divalent cations for optimal activity, either Mg^{++}, $Mg^{++} + Ca^{++}$, or Mn^{++}. It hydrolyzes double- as well as single-stranded DNA by single-strand breaks.

Lastly, a significant part of the protein content of human pancreatic juice is a low molecular weight pancreatic secretory trypsin inhibitor. This small molecule binds strongly to both cationic and anionic human trypsins and inhibits their activity. However, it does not completely inhibit trypsin, even when present in excess, and the inhibition is reversible, owing to digestion of the inhibitor by bound trypsin plus calcium ions. It does not inhibit enterokinase and cannot prevent the rapid release of excess trypsin, which reverses any inhibition in the intestinal lumen. Within the pancreatic cells and ducts, however, it acts as a major protective mechanism against inappropriate activation of trypsinogen molecules. There are actually 2 to 4 variants of this inhibitor in human pancreatic juice.

The pancreatic proteolytic enzymes represent a great danger to the organism should they be activated within the substance of the pancreas. Evidence accumulated over many years indicates that acute pancreatitis results from activation of these zymogens within the pancreas and that the disease is due to autodigestion. Different protective mechanisms have evolved to prevent such a catastrophe. The first is that the proteolytic enzymes are synthesized as zymogens and require activation before they can carry out their functions. Although the only lipolytic enzyme made as a zymogen is prophospholipase A₂, lipase is not active unless its activator, procolipase, is in turn activated by trypsin. Carboxylic esterase is not active unless bile salts are present, and phospholipase A₂ and lipase-colipase also require bile salts for activity. Bile salts normally do not gain access to the pancreatic ductal system.

Another protective mechanism is that these enzymes are not freely dispersed within the cell cytoplasm but are always contained within lipoprotein membranes. Attached to the N terminal of each enzyme is a hydrophobic signal peptide that penetrates the membrane of the endoplasmic reticulum when the ribosome is attached. The growing peptide enters the lumen of the tubules, where these signal peptides are removed and the proenzymes assume their tertiary structures. They migrate to the Golgi region of the cell, where they are invested in a membrane, glycosidic groups added to some, and condense as zymogen granules, which accumulate at the apex of the cell. With proper stimulation, the membrane of the zymogen granule fuses with the apical cell membrane of the acinar cell of the pancreas, and the enzymes are secreted into the lumen.

In addition to the secretory trypsin inhibitor in pancreatic juice, there are proteolytic enzyme inhibitors in many body fluids and tissues that probably play a role in protecting against the uncontrolled activity of these pancreatic enzymes within the gland or when the enzymes gain access to the blood stream and lymphatics (Table 32–2). In species other than primates, such as the cow, there is present in the acinar cell (but not in the juice) a trypsin inhibitor (Kunitz type) that is a very potent inhibitor of trypsin, chymotrypsin, kallikrein, plasmin, and thrombin. The human pancreas does not have this trypsin inhibitor. In the cow, this trypsin inhibitor has also been found in salivary gland, lung, and liver. If the human is found not to have this protein in his tissues, he lacks an important safety factor that protects against protease injury.

Circulating in human plasma are a number of protease inhibitors that are effective in inhibiting the activity of any pancreatic protease that might inadvertently gain entrance to the plasma or extracellular fluids. Alpha-1-antitrypsin is a glycoprotein molecule of 120,000 molecular weight that very potently inhibits both cationic and anionic trypsin, chymotrypsin, and elastase as well as plasmin and thrombin. Alpha-2-macroglobulin, an 800,000 molecular weight glycoprotein, binds both forms of trypsin and prevents it from digesting proteins. When this inhibitor is bound to the trypsin molecule, trypsin can still split small, synthetic peptide or ester substrates. Thus, a benzoyl arginine esterase activity is found in plasma even when added trypsin is bound to α_2-macroglobulin.

Finally, there is an inhibitor of the complement protein C1 esterase in plasma, and it also has the ability to inhibit chymotrypsin, kallikrein, and plasmin (Table 32–2). Other proteolytic inhibitors have been described but not well characterized in human plasma. The physiologic role of these plasma protease inhibitors is thought to be control of enzymatic processes such as clotting, fibrinolysis, and kinin production. They may play a secondary protective role when enzymes from the pancreas enter the extracellular fluids.

An important biochemical and clinical phenomenon concerning the pancreatic enzymes is the exocrine-endocrine partition. This term is used to describe the fact that although 99.9 per cent of the enzymes secreted by the acinar cells of the pancreas enter the ducts and pass down into the duodenum, a small fraction diffuses back into the extracellular fluid and then into the plasma. It has been known for many years that there is amylase activity in normal human plasma that is derived from the pancreatic form of amylase. There is also a normal or basal lipase, phospholipase, ribonuclease, and deoxyribonuclease activity in human plasma. Pancreatic proteases cannot be enzymatically assayed in plasma accurately because they are bound to inhibitors. However, radioimmunoassays can measure the amount of zymogens, or proteases, even when bound to inhibitors. Normal human plasma or serum contains unbound cationic and anionic trypsinogens and chymotrypsinogen. Normally, no free or bound trypsin is found; elastase 2 and chymotrypsin are present bound to α_1-antitrypsin, possibly generated in plasma from their zymogens. Trypsin released during pancreatitis is bound to α_2-macroglobulin and is still able to split small synthetic

TABLE 32–2 PROTEASE INHIBITORS IN HUMANS*

Human Proteases	Plasma Inhibitors†				Tissue Inhibitors†
	α_1AT	α_2MG	C1 INH	PSTI	Bovine Basic TI (Aprotinin)
Trypsin 1	+ + +	+ + +	+ + +	+ +	+ + +
Trypsin 2	+ + +	+ + +	+ + +	+ +	+ + +
Chymotrypsin	+ + +	+ + +	+	0	+
Elastase	+ + +	+ + +	?	0	+
Carboxypeptidase A	0	0	?	?	?
Carboxypeptidase B	0	0	?	?	?
Kallikreins	0	+ +	+ + +	0	+ + +
Plasmin	+ +	+ + +	+	0	+ + +
Thrombin	+ + +	+ +	0	+ + +	+ +
C1 esterase	?	?	+ + +	?	?
Factor XIIa	0	0	+ + +	?	?
Factor XIa	0	0	+ + +	?	?
Enterokinase				0	0

*Inhibition is defined as ability to prevent activity versus usual protein substrates. May not prevent cleavage of synthetic ester or peptide substrates. Relative inhibitory potency is given as a qualitative scale: 0 = none; + = slight; + + = moderate; + + + = strong.

†α_1AT = α_1-antitrypsin; α_2MG = α_2-macroglobulin; C1 INH = C1 esterase inhibitor; PSTI = pancreatic secretory typsin inhibitor.

substrates, accounting for trypsinlike activity of serum. More importantly, it can still cleave fibrinogen and protein hormones as well as trypsinogen and chymotrypsinogen to active proteases. One point that may be of importance clinically is that no protease inhibitors for carboxypeptidases A and B have been detected, and it is possible that in pathologic states these enzymes might be able to act uncontrolled by peptidase inhibitors.

FEEDBACK INHIBITION OF PANCREATIC SECRETION

Considerable evidence is available that if pancreatic enzymes, particularly trypsin and chymotrypsin, are not present in the intestinal lumen in their active form there is some form of feedback stimulation of pancreatic acinar cell function. In rats fed soybean trypsin inhibitor, which inactivates pancreatic trypsin, the animals develop marked hyperplasia and hypertrophy of the pancreas as well as excessive pancreatic secretion. In normal humans, acute and chronic feedback inhibition of pancreatic exocrine secretion by trypsin has been demonstrated. The mechanism is unknown. Removal of bile from the gut lumen also increases secretion in animals. It appears that bile prevents rapid degradation of trypsin and chymotrypsin in the lumen of the bowel and that any situation in which the concentration of active enzyme is maintained sustains the feedback. It is known that bile stabilizes human trypsin in vitro. The clinical significance of these findings, if they can be extended to humans, is that diseases in which there are decreased bile salts in the intestine may be associated with decreased pancreatic enzyme function and a hypersecretion of the pancreas.

STIMULUS-SECRETION COUPLING IN THE PANCREAS

As a result of studies of mice, rats, guinea pigs, rabbits, cats, and dogs including such model systems as dispersed acinar cells, isolated acini, lobules, slices, perfused isolated pancreas, and intact animals, a cohesive picture is emerging of the various stimuli and their secretion mechanisms in animal pancreatic acinar and ductal cells. We assume that much of this is true for human pancreas as well.

In acinar cells, secretagogues bind to specific receptors on the plasma membrane and via one of two secondary messengers elicit enzyme secretion. One mechanism involves the release of *calcium* from a "trigger pool" bound to the plasma membrane, increasing cytosolic free calcium activity and by a series of poorly defined steps triggering exocytosis of enzymes held in zymogen granules. The excess cytosolic Ca^{++} is then actively extruded

from the cell. When the secretagogue binds, the plasma membrane also becomes more permeable to Na, Cl, and K, leading to increased secretion of NaCl and water into the apical lumen. Continued enzyme secretion requires ATP-mediated uptake of external calcium and sequestration of the calcium in mitochondria and endoplasmic reticulum. After stimulation ceases, the storage pools are discharged externally, and the "trigger pool" refills to resume a resting state. Calcium appears to activate a cyclic-nucleotide–independent protein kinase that phosphorylates an endogenous protein that is somehow concerned with enzyme secretion. The four classes of secretagogues that trigger this calcium-dependent mechanism through their specific receptors are (1) CCK, gastrin, and caerulein, a CCK-like peptide from frog skin; (2) acetylcholine and muscarinic cholinergic agonists; (3) bombesin and related peptides; and (4) physalaemin, substance P, eledoisin, and related peptides.

The second mechanism involves the activation of a plasma membrane adenyl cyclase when the secretagogue binds, increased concentrations of *cyclic AMP* in the cytoplasm, and activation of a cyclic AMP–dependent protein kinase that probably phosphorylates the same protein as the calcium-dependent protein kinase. The three classes of cyclic AMP-related secretagogue receptors are those for secretin, for vasoactive intestinal peptide (VIP), and for cholera toxin. In the acinar cell, this cyclic AMP mechanism leads to protein and NaCl secretion, whereas in the ductal cells it causes secretion of bicarbonate and water. The two mechanisms interact in the acinar cell, presumably at the level of a common phosphorylated protein, so they potentiate each other's responses; that is, the output of amylase is greater with CCK plus secretin than the sum of their maximal responses.

The process of exocytosis involves fusion of the zymogen granule membrane to specific sites on the luminal membrane, discharge of the contents into the lumen, and recycling of granule membrane material by endocytosis back to the Golgi region or lysosomes to be reused. Exocytosis is accompanied by the cleavage of phosphatidylinositol, a minor membrane phospholipid, but its role is undefined. Microtubules and microfilaments probably play a role in the final steps of granule fusion and discharge.

In ductular cells, secretin and increased cytosolic cyclic AMP somehow stimulate bicarbonate secretion. A postulated sequence of events involves uptake of CO_2 from interstitial fluid, its hydration catalyzed by carbonic anhydrase to yield H_2CO_3, and dissociation into HCO_3^-, which enters the lumen partly by an unknown mechanism and partly by chloride-bicarbonate exchange. The H^+ ions are exchanged for Na^+ at an antiport on the plasma membrane, and the Na^+ is pumped out of the cell at the basolateral membrane in exchange with K^+ by a Na^+-K^+-ATPase. On the luminal membrane, a Mg^{++}-ATPase pumps Na^+ into the lumen in exchange for H^+. Between cells, and through rather leaky tight junctions, osmotic gradients draw Na^+, Cl^- and water from interstitium to lumen. Where cyclic AMP works in this sequence is not known.

The product of these secretory mechanisms during a meal is an isosmolar juice, with a sodium concentration of 160 mM, a potassium concentration equal to that in plasma, and a bicarbonate plus chloride concentration that is constant and equal to that of $Na^+ + K^+$. Bicarbonate increases with increasing flow rate, and chloride decreases reciprocally. Calcium is both bound to proteins and ionized, the former acinar and the latter ductular, stimulated by secretin. At high rates of flow it falls to 0.4 mM, and at low rates of flow it rises to 1.6 mM. Magnesium averages 1.4 mM. The daily output ranges from 1500 to 4000 ml per day and contains 6 to 12 gm of protein and 7 to 18 gm of bicarbonate. These are sufficient to neutralize gastric acid and to digest ingested proteins to dipeptides, tripeptides, and amino acids by the time they reach the upper jejunum.

HORMONAL CONTROL OF PANCREATIC SECRETION

In Table 32–3 are summarized the hormones that are known to play a role in stimulating human exocrine pancreatic secretion and those hormones that are postulated to play such a role. The first hormone ever described, *secretin*, is secreted by cells found in the duodenal mucosa, called *S cells*. Since the advent of reliable radioimmunoassays for secretin, it has been possible to prove what releases secretin into the plasma of humans. Hydrochloric acid and bile in the duodenum do this; amino acids, fatty acids, and hypertonic solutions do not. Studies in animals and humans indicate that the release of secretin is a function of the surface area of the duodenum that is titrated below a pH of 4.5. After a standard meal, intermittent drops in intraduodenal pH are each followed in 2- to 5-minute intervals by increments in plasma secretin concentration. Secretin is strongly potentiated by gastrin and CCK in secretion of bicarbonate and water.

Secretin release is also elicited by *ethanol:* Two ounces of 86-proof vodka will release secretin into the plasma of humans, presumably by its stimulation of gastric acid secretion. Secretin has a half-life in human plasma of 3 to 4 minutes. It is not removed significantly by the liver, but the kidneys remove both secretin and CCK.

When secretin stimulates the pancreas, there is an increased output of cAMP in pancreatic juice that correlates well with evidence in isolated pancreas fragments that secretin results in an increased cAMP level in pancreatic cells. Previously, secretin was thought to stimulate only centroaci-

nar and ductal cells to secrete bicarbonate, and the protein that poured out during early secretin stimulation was considered a "wash-out" phenomenon, a flushing out of proteins that had accumulated in the duct system. However, dose-response curves in humans show a linear increase of output as a function of the log dose of secretin for volume, bicarbonate, *and* for protein. Trypsin output also increases in a linear fashion as the secretin dose is increased logarithmically. The main evidence that bicarbonate comes from ductal cells is that carbonic anhydrase is present only in ductal cells, not in acinar cells. This enzyme is thought to play a role in bicarbonate secretion by forming bicarbonate from plasma CO_2, which diffuses into the cell and combines with OH^- groups. Acetazolamide, a carbonic anhydrase inhibitor, decreases volume and bicarbonate output by 50 per cent in humans.

Antidiuretic hormone in large doses can reduce the volume and bicarbonate concentration of secretin-stimulated juice; thus, the permeability to water is increased in pancreatic ductal cells as it is in renal collecting duct cells.

VIP is in parentheses in Table 32–3 because at the present time there is insufficient evidence that it plays a physiologic role in human pancreatic secretion. VIP has a predominantly neuronal origin in the gut, in specific peptidergic neurons in the myenteric and submucosal plexuses. It occurs in D_1 cells of the pancreas and in the cerebral cortex. Its stimulus for release is not known, and it is considered to be a paracrine agent (i.e., a hormone that diffuses through extracellular spaces to adjacent target cells). There is little evidence that it has endocrine functions (i.e., that it enters the blood stream). VIP and secretin are very similar in structure, and in both the biologic activity resides in the N terminal of their molecules. Acinar cells have high-affinity binding sites for each hormone, but either can bind with low affinity to the other's preferred receptor. VIP is assumed to bind to and stimulate ductal cells as does secretin, and it potentiates CCK or other calcium-mediated secretagogues in acinar cells.

Glucagon, which also resembles structurally both secretin and VIP, does not stimulate exocrine pancreatic secretion but inhibits enzyme secretion and volume output in the presence of secretin.

Insulin does not affect pancreatic secretion directly but increases the response of acinar cells to CCK by binding to specific cell membrane receptors. It also increases protein synthesis in general and increases glucose uptake as in many other tissues. *PHI* is a 27-amino acid peptide isolated by Jensen, Tatemoto and Mutt from intestinal extracts. It resembles secretin in structure and produces increased cyclic AMP levels in acinar cells. It increases amylase secretion and potentiates CCK but has not been shown to play a physiologic role in humans. *Neurotensin* is a 13-amino acid peptide originating in endocrine cells in ileal mu-

TABLE 32–3 HORMONAL CONTROL OF PANCREATIC SECRETION

Hormone*	Origin†	Stimuli for Release	Pancreas Target Cells	Second Messenger	Effects on Exocrine Pancreas
Secretin	S cells, duodenum	Duodenal pH<4.5 and length of gut acidified; bile in the duodenum	Acinar, centroacinar, ductal cells	cAMP	Bicarbonate and water secretion (+ + + +); protein secretion (+); potentiates CCK
(VIP)	Neuronal cells in plexuses of gut and pancreas	Unknown; local tissue hormone or paracrine agent	Acinar, ductal cells	cAMP	Bicarbonate and water secretion (+ +); protein secretion (+); potentiates CCK
(PHI)	Unknown	Unknown	Acinar cells	cAMP	Potentiates CCK, acetylcholine; releases insulin; increases glucagon response to arginine
(Neurotensin)	Endocrine cells in ileal mucosa	Mixed meal	Acinar and ductal cells	?	Potentiates bicarbonate response to secretin; releases pancreatic polypeptide
Glucagon	A cells, pancreas islets	Hypoglycemia; secretin, CCK, GIP, amino acids	Acinar and ductal cells	cAMP	Inhibits protein secretion, CCK release, volume output
Insulin	B cells, pancreas islets	Glucose, amino acids, glucagon	Acinar cells	?	Stimulates protein synthesis; potentiates CCK
CCK	Duodenum, jejunum, I cells	Essential amino acids, especially phe, met, val; HCl to duodenal pH<3; fatty acids; soaps; Ca^{++}, K^+, Mg^{++}; bile salts inhibit release	Acinar cells and ? ductal cells	Ca^{++}	Increases enzyme secretion (+ + +) and synthesis; potentiates secretin; stimulates acinar hyperplasia
Gastrin	Stomach antrum, duodenum, G cells	Antrum or duodenum >pH3; post-ganglionic vagal stimulation	Acinar cells and ? ductal cells	Ca^{++}	Increases enzyme secretion (+); potentiates secretin
Acetylcholine	Postganglionic cholinergic fibers	CNS stimulation to vagal nucleus, smell, taste, hypoglycemia; local reflexes like gastric distention	Acinar cells	Ca^{++}	Increases enzyme secretion (+ + +) and synthesis
Pancreatic polypeptide	Nonislet D$_2$ cells, acinar and ductal cells	Mixed meal, especially protein, fat; cholinergic and β-adrenergic stimuli; CCK and gastrin	Acinar cells and ? ductal cells	?	Suppresses protein secretion by CCK, bicarbonate secretion by secretin
(Substance P)	Neurones, endocrine cells of gut mucosa	Unknown	Acinar cells	Ca^{++}	Increases enzyme secretion
(Somatostatin)	D cells of islets, antrum, upper intestine	Unknown, paracrine agent	Endocrine cells	?	Inhibits CCK, secretin, acetylcholine, pancreatic polypeptide, insulin, and glucagon release

*VIP = vasoactive intestinal peptide; CCK = cholecystokinin; PHI = peptide-N-terminal histidine; GIP = gastrointestinal inhibitor peptide. Hormones in parentheses ( ) have not been proved to have a physiologic role in human pancreatic secretion.
†Revised Wiesbaden classification for endocrine cell types.

cosa. Its serum level rises after ingestion of a mixed meal. Infusions that give physiologic plasma levels increase bicarbonate output on a background of secretin and CCK infusions and increase plasma levels of pancreatic polypeptide. It has no proven physiologic function in humans.

Cholecystokinin, which has the same C-terminal pentapeptide sequence as gastrin (Fig. 32–1), is the most potent stimulus of pancreatic enzyme secretion, and on prolonged stimulation it also increases pancreatic enzyme synthesis. It

strongly potentiates secretin action, and secretin weakly potentiates enzyme secretion by CCK. There is also evidence that, on prolonged stimulation, CCK promotes DNA synthesis and acinar cell hyperplasia.

Immunofluorescent studies with an antibody to CCK in humans indicate that the hormone is found in cells scattered throughout the duodenum and jejunum in the crypts and occasionally in the villi. The cells are not found in the ileum, pancreas, stomach, or colon. The release of CCK from

PORCINE CHOLECYSTOKININ

$$\begin{array}{cccccccccc} 24 & 25 & 26 & 27 & 28 & 29 & 30 & 31 & 32 & 33 \end{array}$$

NH$_2$-Lys-(22 residues)-Glu-Glu-Asp-Tyr-Met-Gly-Try-Met-Asp-Phe-NH$_2$
$$\underline{\hspace{4cm}}$$
SO$_3$

LITTLE HUMAN GASTRIN I

$$\begin{array}{ccccc} 1 & 2 & 3 & 4 & 5 \end{array} \qquad \begin{array}{cccccccc} 10 & 11 & 12 & 13 & 14 & 15 & 16 & 17 \end{array}$$

pyroGlu-Gly-Pro-Try-Leu-(Glu)$_4$-Glu-Ala-Tyr-Gly-Try-Met-Asp-Phe-NH$_2$
$$\underline{\hspace{4cm}}$$
SO$_3$

CAERULEIN, from skin of Australian hylid frog, Hyla caerulae

$$\begin{array}{cccccccccc} 1 & 2 & 3 & 4 & 5 & 6 & 7 & 8 & 9 & 10 \end{array}$$

pyroGlu-Glu-Asp-Tyr-Thr-Gly-Try-Met-Asp-Phe-NH$_2$
$$\underline{\hspace{4cm}}$$
SO$_3$

Figure 32–1 The structural basis for the similar effects on the pancreas of cholecystokinin, gastrin II and caerulein.

these cells occurs with exposure to essential amino acids, fatty acids, or HCl below pH 3. Bile apparently does not stimulate but probably inhibits CCK release. Radioimmunoassays of CCK combined with chromatography show that intestinal CCK exists in multiple molecular forms, 60 per cent reacting like the C-terminal octapeptide and 18 per cent reacting like CCK$_{33}$, CCK$_{39}$, or larger. By one plasma radioimmunoassay, the normal level is 60 ± 17 pg/ml, but after meals there is a tremendous increase to nanogram levels. In chronic pancreatitis with exocrine insufficiency, there is a persistent fasting hypersecretion to levels as high as 8000 pg/ml. This finding suggests that CCK release is inhibited by some feedback mechanism that has not been defined.

The amino acids that are most potent in releasing CCK in humans are L-phenylalanine, tyrosine, valine, and tryptophan. Nonessential amino acids do not release CCK. Raising the serum calcium by calcium infusions increases fasting trypsin output in humans and increases the response to a low dose of CCK. CCK isolated from pork duodenum has an activity of 3000 Ivy dog units per mg in the purest preparation thus far available. On a molar basis, the C-terminal octapeptide of CCK has a threefold greater activity on the pancreas than does the whole molecule, and caerulein, which is a decapeptide, has 1.4 times the activity on a molar basis (Fig. 32–1). Gastrin-I is 1/34 as potent as CCK in stimulating pancreatic secretion, and gastrin II, which lacks the sulfate group on the tyrosine, is only 1/1000 as strong as CCK. The C-terminal pentapeptide of gastrin, which lacks a tyrosine sulfate, has only 1/3400 of CCK activity. Studies of a series of CCK fragments showed that the shortest one with CCK activity on the gallbladder and pancreas is the C-terminal tetrapeptide. Maximal activity is achieved with the decapeptide, and activity falls off thereafter with the entire CCK sequence. The active site as far as gallbladder contraction and pancreatic secretion are concerned must be the C-

terminal end of the molecule, and the N-terminal residues therefore must lend specificity to the CCK action. CCK also has effects on the endocrine pancreas: It releases insulin from isolated rat islet cells even without glucose in the medium. CCK release from the duodenum is prevented by atropine, suggesting that there is an intramucosal reflex susceptible to muscarinic receptor blockade. Essential amino acids and glyceryloleate, a product of triglyceride digestion, increase enzyme secretion and contract the gallbladder. Adding various bile salts to either acids or glyceryloleate decreases this CCK effect.

During the purification of CCK from porcine duodenal extracts, Jorpes and Mutt found that the activities on the gallbladder and on the pancreas increased in constant proportion and proved once and for all that cholecystokinin and pancreozymin are one hormone. All surface anesthetics such as cocaine or procaine will prevent release of secretin, CCK, or gastrin when stimulators of the mucosal lumen are used, suggesting that there is some kind of receptor site on the plasma membrane that must be triggered in order to release these hormones from their secretory granules.

Jorpes developed a hypothesis for the release of secretin and cholecystokinin based on their structure and charge. At physiologic pH, the net charge of the 27 amino acids of secretin is +4; that is, it is a very basic amino acid. Jorpes suggested that when hydrochloric acid enters the duodenum it titrates the ionized carboxyl groups of proteins that bind secretin by ionic bonds to the basic groups on the peptide. CCK is also a basic protein, having a net charge of +2, so its release by a pH <3 in the duodenum could be by the same mechanism. Gastrin, however, is a very acidic molecule and is released by titrating the contents of the stomach to a pH of 5.5 to 6.5, suggesting that basic groups on proteins bind the gastrin via the carboxyls of its aspartate groups. When these are neutralized and the carboxyl groups on the proteins are ionized, gastrin is released. The general theory has never been tested in an in-vitro system.

Inactivation of CCK or gastrin is minimal on transit through the liver, and only 25 per cent of secretin is inactivated. The short half-lives of these hormones in plasma may result from deamidation of the C-terminal phenylalanine amide of CCK and gastrin and of the valine amide of secretin, since the amide groups are essential to activity. As the dose of CCK is increased logarithmically, secretion of protein in humans increases in a sigmoid curve to a maximum. Although alkaline phosphatase activity increases in the juice after CCK or secretin stimulation, this may be a wash-out phenomenon from the duct cells, which are known to contain alkaline phosphatase in their luminal membranes. Secretin and vagal stimulation together increase the volume response synergistically. Similarly, CCK increases secretin bicarbonate output more than the sum of the two separate responses. All investigators find that secretin and CCK together give a greater volume and bicarbonate response than do the sum of secretin and CCK separately. Secretin and gastrin given simultaneously show only an additive effect.

Gastrin, given in pharmacologic doses, can produce enzyme secretion much as CCK does, but there is controversy concerning whether after normal meals serum gastrin rises high enough in humans to stimulate the pancreatic acinar cells. The weight of the evidence at present is that it does so, and gastrin should be considered a normal stimulant of pancreatic enzyme secretion. The C-terminal pentapeptide of gastrin (Pentavlon) also stimulates volume and bicarbonate and enzyme output when there is a secretin background infusion. The standard subcutaneous dose of pentagastrin, 6 μg/kg, which gives a maximum acid output, increases the volume and bicarbonate and lipase output of the pancreas as well. A linear log dose-response of protein, volume, and bicarbonate output occurs in the dog on stimulation with gastrin, caerulein, or CCK. The relative molar potencies as far as enzyme output is concerned are 1.0 for CCK, 2.8 for cerulein, and 0.25 for gastrin.

Pure gastrin II (17 amino acids) in humans gives a maximal trypsin output and empties the gallbladder at a dose of 60 picomoles/kg/hr, whereas it takes 540 picomoles/kg/hr to get a maximal acid output. Gastrin levels found after a meal are those that give a 50 per cent maximal acid response. All of this strongly supports the physiologic effect of gastrin on the human pancreas.

Acetylcholine released from the postganglionic cholinergic fibers plays a major role in pancreatic secretion via the pathways of the vagus nerve.

Somatostatin, a hormone widely dispersed in the central nervous system and intestinal tract, has been found to be an inhibitor of the release of many hormones including growth hormone, insulin, glucagon, secretin, CCK, acetylcholine, and

pancreatic polypeptide. When CCK is given intravenously, somatostatin in relatively large doses can block the effect of CCK on enzyme secretion. Its physiologic role in the function of the pancreas is still not defined, so it is shown in parentheses in Table 32–3.

Pancreatic polypeptide is composed in humans and other species of 36 amino-acid residues with a tryosine-amide on the C terminal that is essential to activity. The C-terminal hexapeptide can mimic the actions of the whole molecule on pancreatic secretion. In humans, all the peptide-secreting cells are in the pancreas. The hormone is released into the plasma by a mixed meal, with protein being the most potent food stimulant, followed closely by fat, whereas glucose is relatively ineffective. The plasma response curve to food is biphasic, with a peak at 5 minutes, a 30 to 60 minute shoulder, and a secondary response lasting 1 to 5 hours. The first response is due to acetylcholine and is blocked by atropine. Beta-adrenergic stimuli also release the peptide. The secondary response is due to synergistic vagal and hormonal (CCK, gastrin) actions. The physiologic role of this hormone is direct inhibition of pancreatic secretion elicited by CCK, gastrin, and secretin. It serves as a feedback mechanism to shut off pancreatic secretion after protein, fat, and HCl enter the duodenum.

Substance P is a peptide composed of 11 amino acids that is found in brain and gut mucosa. It releases Ca^{++} after binding to a class of acinar cell receptors also stimulated by eledoisin and another frog-skin peptide, physalaemin. It promotes enzyme secretion, but a physiologic role in humans has not been proved. Another frog-skin peptide, bombesin, also binds to specific acinar cell receptors, releases Ca^{++}, and stimulates enzyme secretion. Peptides resembling bombesin have been isolated from porcine intestinal mucosa and have been found to have gastrin-releasing action, but a role in human pancreas secretion has not been identified.

NEUROSTIMULATION

In humans, there is good evidence for a *cephalic phase* of pancreatic secretion mediated by the vagus nerve and triggered by the sight, smell, taste, and chewing of food. The main result is increase of enzyme output, and this may be achieved by both acetylcholine and vagally released gastrin acting on acinar cells. Surprisingly, volume and bicarbonate secretion also increase even when acid is excluded from the duodenum, suggesting that a low level of secretin release is present and is potentiated by acetylcholine and gastrin. Fasting duodenal bicarbonate concentrations are equal to those in plasma, whereas enzyme output is one tenth of the peak cephalic response, suggesting that resting vagal tone or hormone release is very low in fasting humans, accounting for the basal volume of 2 to 10 ml per hour. There is also a *gastric phase* that is twofold in origin. Secretion is stimulated by distention of the antrum of the stomach, which releases gastrin, and by distention of the fundus, which stimulates by a vagovagal reflex. This response is blocked by atropine or vagotomy. The pancreatic juice from vagal or gastrin stimulation is high in enzymes and low in volume and bicarbonate. When the HCl enters the duodenum, the release of secretin can be blocked by atropine, whereas atropine has no effect on the intravenous secretin response. Atropine does partially block the effect of exogenous CCK.

An important clinical question is whether operations for peptic ulcer disease involving a truncal vagotomy and drainage procedures influence pancreatic secretion. Vagotomy with a pyloroplasty or a gastroduodenostomy decreases basal enzyme output and also decreases the release of secretin by HCl or the release of CCK by amino and fatty acids. High-dose exogenous CCK or secretin gives a normal response, however. The output of enzymes after a test meal is decreased in vagotomized humans. In spite of these findings, there is little clinical evidence that truncal vagotomy causes a clinically significant impairment of digestion. Highly selective vagotomy, in which only the parietal-cell area of the stomach is denervated, does not impair pancreatic secretion, however. Truncal vagotomy also eliminates the early release and blunts the secondary release of pancreatic polypeptide after a meal in humans.

The vagus nerve has an influence on pancreatic acinar mass. Stimulation over a period of days by the cholinergic agent bethanechol chloride causes hypertrophy of the pancreas. In contrast, prolonged stimulation with CCK also causes hypertrophy and in addition increases DNA synthesis (i.e., causes hyperplasia).

DIAGNOSTIC TESTS IN PANCREATIC DISEASE

The exocrine-endocrine partition of pancreatic enzyme activity serves as the most important basis of diagnosis of pancreatic disease. Because the normal activities of amylase and of lipase were detected in human serum many years ago, these have become by tradition the mainstays of diagnosis of pancreatic inflammation or neoplasia. There is no intrinsic reason that these particular enzymes should have been selected, since plasma activity of phospholipase A, ribonuclease, and deoxyribonuclease also have been detected and found to be useful. The proteolytic enzymes cannot be assayed by enzymatic means in plasma with reliability because they are bound to the plasma protease inhibitors. Although the bound trypsin, chymotrypsin, or elastase may cleave small molecular weight synthetic substrates while bound to

α_2-macroglobulin, for example, the enzyme bound to α_1-antitrypsin is not active. Moreover, much of the cleavage of synthetic trypsin substrates in human serum is due to thrombin and plasmin bound to α_2-macroglobulin during the process of blood clotting. Therefore, arginine amidase activity does not represent serum trypsin activity, and during acute pancreatitis, the increase in arginine amidase activity is not a measure of pancreatic trypsin release into plasma. Radioimmunoassays for trypsin are now commercially available and circumvent these problems.

Serum amylase activity remains the most widely used diagnostic serum pancreatic enzyme assay, in spite of the fact that amylase is also found in the salivary glands and many other tissues and that there are many isoenzymes of amylase. Many methods are used to assay serum amylase. Each one must have its normal values defined and must be tested to make certain that it can accurately measure amylase activity in urine and in other body fluids in which inhibitors may be present. The classic amyloclastic method involves the cleavage of starch, which causes fading of the blue color of starch stained with iodine. The saccharogenic method involves the measurement of the reducing substance, maltose, which is produced when amylase cleaves starch. Another method uses a dye that is bound to the starch molecule and released during amylase digestion. Lastly, there are coupled enzyme reactions in which the maltose released is split to glucose by added maltase, and the glucose is converted by hexokinase to glucose-6-phosphate, which is used to reduce NAD to NADH by glucose-6-phosphate dehydrogenase. The differing normal ranges resulting from these various methods are confusing to the clinician.

The isoenzymes of amylase have also been separated in different ways (e.g., with polyacrylamide gel, agarose gel, cellulose acetate electrophoresis, DEAE-Sephadex column separation, and isoelectric focusing). The problem with these methods is that none is simple and rapid enough to use for emergency pancreatic isoamylase determinations. A promising technique uses an inhibitor protein from wheat that inhibits the human salivary isozyme 100 times more potently than the pancreatic isozyme. Using the Phadebas blue starch method and the inhibitor, one finds that of a total amylase activity in males of 132 ± 50 IU/L, pancreatic isozyme equals 82 ± 30 and salivary isozyme equals 50 ± 30.

One of the best methods available for simultaneous resolution of the various bands in body fluids is polyacrylamide gel slab electrophoresis. After the enzymes have been separated, they are incubated with a starch solution and the color is developed with iodine. This method of separation allows the two main bands of salivary amylase (2 and 4) and of pancreatic amylase (2 and 4) to be seen in normal serum and urine. Salivary isozyme band 2 overlaps pancreatic band 4, salivary band 4 overlaps pancreatic band 6, and genetic variants occur where a slowly moving salivary amylase overlaps pancreatic band 2, so complete separation of the total salivary from total pancreatic amylase activity is difficult. In disease states in which either the pancreatic or the salivary isoenzymes are increased in amount, more of the bands become visible in serum or urine so that qualitative judgment as to which type of amylase is increased becomes easier. The electrofocusing agarose gel and cellulose acetate electrophoretic methods allow the main pancreatic band to be separated from the salivary bands enough to be useful in the clinical chemistry laboratory.

The advantage derived from separating the isoenzymes is that one can tell whether changes in total serum amylase activity are due to the pancreas or to the salivary glands and other tissues that contain the salivary isoenzymes. Patients with mumps, carcinoma of the ovary or lung, or acute salpingitis have been found to have an increased salivary amylase activity. Patients with severe pancreatic exocrine insufficiency due to chronic pancreatitis or cystic fibrosis have a decreased pancreatic isoamylase activity, whereas the total activity remains normal because the salivary isoenzymes are increased.

All methods for measuring amylase in serum are interfered with when there is a lipemic serum due to a high concentration of chylomicrons or very low density lipoproteins, such as occurs in some patients with acute pancreatitis. The true activity is revealed by dilution of the serum. The serum inhibitor, which is not the triglyceride molecules themselves, also appears in urine.

A controversy existed as to whether there is a true α-amylase in liver and whether any of the serum amylase is from liver. An α-amylase has been clearly demonstrated in isolated rat liver cells and it is released by perfused rat liver. The enzyme isolated from rat liver has been found to differ greatly from pancreatic and salivary amylase in its structure, however. There is still no proof that an α-amylase exists in human liver or that a liver isozyme can be found in serum or urine.

EVOCATIVE SERUM ENZYME TESTS

When the serum enzymes are not elevated by a disease process at the time the patient is being studied, pancreatic disease may be revealed by stimulating the pancreas with CCK and secretin to cause maximal secretion. If areas of ductal obstruction exist, increased regurgitation of amylase or other enzymes into the plasma may occur, (i.e., the endocrine-exocrine partition ratio will be increased). Normal individuals given CCK plus secretin show no changes in serum amylase or lipase activities over a period of 4 to 6 hours, whereas patients who have functioning but obstructed pancreatic acinar tissue usually show a change in either the serum amylase or lipase from normal to abnormal levels and usually a twofold or greater rise above the basal activity. This so-called "evocative test" has been useful in patients who have early pancreatic disease with an obstructive component as in chronic pancreatitis and cancer.

When a patient has exocrine insufficiency, proved by an output of less than 10 per cent of normal lipase or bicarbonate into the duodenum on CCK-secretin stimulation, he rarely responds with any increase in serum enzyme activities because the acinar tissue is mostly destroyed. A similar negative response can be expected in a patient whose disease has led to islet damage and diabetes. In patients with functioning tissue and chronic pancreatitis, the test is positive about 75 per cent of the time. The test has been criticized because patients who have biliary tract disease and no known pancreatic disease occasionally have had positive tests, but this may be due to obstruction at the sphincter of Oddi by fibrosis. One of the most valuable corroborative techniques is to reproduce the patient's pain syndrome at the time that the pancreas is stimulated and to correlate that with an increase in enzyme activities.

Another kind of evocative serum enzyme test involves stimulation of the pancreas with a parasympathomimetic agent, such as neostigmine, while giving an agent that obstructs flow of pancreatic juice by causing spasm of the sphincter of Oddi, such as morphine. In this test, normal individuals show an increased serum amylase or lipase activity, whereas the test does not elevate the activity in patients who have no duct obstruction and advanced acinar destruction. The highest serum enzyme activities occur in normal subjects and in patients with moderate acute pancreatitis. This reflects competent secretory function in the presence of high-grade obstruction, but it is not of great differential diagnostic value. Surprisingly, none of these evocative tests has been reported to cause attacks of acute pancreatitis.

URINARY AMYLASE SECRETION

The molecular weight of amylase is 55,000. Proteins of this size are cleared by the glomerulus at a slow rate, and some of the proteins are reabsorbed by the renal tubules, resulting in an overall amylase renal clearance of 1 to 3 ml per minute. Some years ago it was found that urinary amylase excretion in acute pancreatitis increased as expected when the serum amylase rose, but, when the serum amylase returned to normal, urinary amylase excretion remained elevated for some days. Urinary amylase excretion proved a more sensitive index of pancreatitis than did the serum amylase test. When this was investigated by calculating urinary amylase clearance over a 2-hour period and comparing it with creatinine clearance, it was found that in acute pancreatitis the clearance of amylase rose on the average 3.8-fold, the clearance of creatinine 1.9-fold, and the amylase:creatinine clearance ratio rose 1.9-fold. Subsequent research has established the mechanism for this increased urinary amylase:creatinine clearance ratio. There is no increase in glomerular permeability nor in a serum isoenzyme that is more easily cleared during acute pancreatitis. The clearance ratio of pancreatic amylases is 3 per cent normally, and that of salivary amylases is 0.5 per cent. During acute pancreatitis, the clearance of pancreatic amylases goes to 7.3 per cent and that of salivary amylases rises to 4.6 per cent. When β_2-microglobulin, a small molecular weight protein, is infused, the clearance of this protein increases 80-fold in acute pancreatitis. This finding suggests that it is the reabsorption by the renal tubule cells of small molecular weight proteins that is impaired in acute pancreatitis. In other situations such as massive burns, diabetic ketoacidosis, or following open-heart surgery with bypass, the clearance of amylase also is increased, yet no pancreatitis is apparent. An increased amylase:creatinine clearance ratio can be produced in animals by poisoning the renal tubule cells with maleate. Thus the phenomenon can occur with various forms of renal tubule cell injury.

Although the mechanism of this increased clearance is reasonably well established, the clinical usefulness is still a matter of argument. Most investigators find that the clearance ratio is increased above the upper limits of normal in acute pancreatitis, but many find that it is not sufficiently increased in chronic pancreatitis or in carcinoma of the pancreas to be of diagnostic help. During evocative tests with CCK and secretin, amylase excretion into the urine and the amylase:creatinine clearance ratio are increased more than the serum activity. In acute and chronic renal failure, the clearance ratio should remain normal if the loss of renal function affects amylase proportionately to creatinine. The data are conflicting on this point, some giving normal and some elevated clearance ratios. In general, a serum amylase above 300 Somogyi units/dl is more consistent with acute pancreatitis than with renal failure. Another problem results from the fact that the amylase:creatinine clearance ratio varies with the method used to assay the amylase. With an iodometric method, the normal mean ratio is 1.5 per cent; with a saccharogenic method it is 2.2 per cent; and with a dyed-starch method it is 0.8 per cent. Therefore, every laboratory has to establish its own normal clearance ratios, using the method of the laboratory. When separate amylase and creatinine clearances are analyzed before the ratio is calculated, it is clear that the amylase clearance gives the same information as the ratio. The only reason that the ratio has become so popular is that it can be done on a random voided urine specimen and a simultaneous serum value. A timed urinary collection is not necessary. Since convenience reigns in clinical medicine, the clearance ratio seems to be with us.

Assay of serum lipase eliminates many of the problems that occur with the serum amylase. First, serum lipase activity is elevated in pancreatitis as often as is the serum amylase. Second, lipase activity is elevated in chronic renal failure only when the BUN is above 250 mg/dl. Third, the serum lipase is not elevated in burns or diabetic ketoacidosis. Fourth, lipase activity using long-chain triglycerides as substrates (triolein) is found only in the pancreas. Previous techniques were slow, but rapid methods have been developed using stabilized triglyceride emulsions at alkaline pH and titrating the mEq of hydrogen ion produced as the fatty acids are released. These tests can be performed as rapidly as the serum amylase assays. Urinary lipase measurements have been done only rarely, and little is known about their usefulness.

MACROAMYLASES

Patients have been found with elevated serum amylase activities, but normal-to-low activities in the urine. The clearance ratios calculated in these patients are low. When the amylase was studied by methods that allow measurements of molecular weight, it was found that instead of the amylase migrating as a protein with a molecular weight of 55,000, it was now migrating with proteins of molecular weights 200,000 to a million. These large molecular weight amylases are bound to immunoglobulins (IgG or IgA), or in some cases they are polymers of amylase. Because they cannot be filtered by the glomerulus, their renal clearance is decreased and they persist in plasma. The best way to detect macroamylases is to filter the serum over cross-linked dextrans to get approximate molecular weights. The polymers of amylase can be depolymerized under certain conditions by treating with guanidine hydrochloride or by incubating the material with starch, suggesting that the binding of the amylase to other proteins is via the polysaccharides of a glycoprotein. A simple and rapid test to screen for macroamylases makes use of the fact that 12 per cent polyethylene glycol 6000 precipitates 73 per cent or more of macroamylases, whereas less than 52 per cent of normal-sized amylases precipitate. Patients with macroamylasemia rarely have any significant diseases. It is a harmless curiosity unless the patient is erroneously treated for pancreatitis.

DIGESTION-ABSORPTION TESTS OF PANCREATIC FUNCTION

One of the standard approaches toward estimating pancreatic function is oral administration of a material that requires pancreatic enzymatic activity to make the products absorbable by the intestine. The appearance of the digested product is measured in either the plasma or the urine, and the undigested substrate can be measured in the stool. The most common manifestation of exocrine pancreatic insufficiency is steatorrhea, so the commonly used tests are those involving lipids. The secondary motive for these tests is to avoid if possible the unpleasant handling and analysis of fecal samples. Humans have such a great excess of lipase in pancreatic juice that when triglyceride is substituted for carbohydrate there is no increase in fecal fat excretion over an intake range of 90 to 170 gm per day. Lipid excretion is 2 gm per day on a lipid-free diet; this lipid probably is bacterial in origin. In an animal after total pancreatectomy, 60 per cent of oral fat is absorbed without pancreatic enzymes. In patients with severe pancreatic insufficiency, aspiration of ileal contents revealed that 75 per cent of the lipid was in the form of neutral fat and 25 per cent was fatty acids. Analysis of their stool fat indicated that 30 per cent of the fat was in the form of triglycerides and 70 per cent was split fat. The partial digestion of triglyceride in the colon was due to bacterial and fungal lipases.

The standard method for analyzing fecal fat involves saponification of the neutral fat to fatty acids, followed by titration of the fatty acids. The results are given as total fatty acids and not as neutral versus split fat, so the degree of digestion of the fat is not assessed quantitatively. Qualitative methods, to be described later, are necessary to estimate relative amounts of triglyceride and fatty acids. The total excretion of fat still remains the baseline against which all other fat tolerance or excretion tests are measured. In normal humans on a diet of approximately 100 gm of fat per day, fat excretion should not exceed 5 to 7 gm. As a general rule, stool fat should not exceed 7 per cent of intake.

One of the lipid absorption tests that has received the most evaluation is the comparison of absorption of a tracer dose of ^{131}I-labeled triolein with that of ^{131}I-labeled oleic acid. Blood samples are taken hourly for 8 hours, and the radioactivity of plasma determined. The stools are also collected for 72 hours until only trace levels of radioactivity are present, and one measures the percentage of the dose administered found in the stool rather than doing a fat analysis. The total radioactivity in stool should be less than 5 per cent in 72 hours, and the peak blood radioactivity should be greater than 10 per cent of the dose. The fate of absorbed long-chain fatty acids is complex. They are reesterified in the intestinal mucosal cell; the triglycerides are incorporated into chylomicrons, which are secreted into lymph; and the chylomicron triglycerides are removed by liver and peripheral tissues by lipoprotein lipase. The level of labeled triglyceride at any time is a function not only of

absorption but also of abnormalities that occur at any later step in metabolism.

In patients with severe exocrine pancreatic insufficiency, abnormal stool and blood levels are usually obtained, but the correlation between the chemical and radioactive fecal fat excretion is not close. When mild to severe cases of steatorrhea are evaluated, the incidence of false-positives plus false-negatives is about 25 per cent for both the blood and fecal measurements. The errors occur in the patients who have borderline pancreatic insufficiency. The oleic acid absorption in patients with pancreatic insufficiency is often abnormal and has been improved by pancreatic extracts, a finding that causes one to question whether the difference between the absorption of triolein and that of oleic acid is an adequate test for defects in digestion. Perhaps the 2-monoglycerides are required to form mixed micelles from which fatty acids are absorbed.

A recent extension of this approach is the administration of ^{14}C-labeled palmitic acid or glycerol tripalmitate. The excretion of ^{14}C-CO$_2$ in the breath is measured for 2-minute periods hourly for 8 hours. Palmitic acid is oxidized to CO$_2$ in mitochondria of tissues that take up triglyceride, but the rates vary with other substrate availability. The results of such tests indicate that normal individuals reach a specific radioactivity in their breath CO$_2$ that is at least 60 per cent of the activity of the label given. In a mucosal disease such as celiac disease, both palmitic acid and glyceryl tripalmitate give low results, but the ^{14}C-CO$_2$ levels in the breath after ingestion of ^{14}C-tripalmitate or palmitic acid are equally depressed, and the ratio remains normal. In severe pancreatic insufficiency, the ^{14}C-CO$_2$ excretion is low after tripalmitate and near normal with palmitic acid, so the ratio of the neutral fat over the split fat excretion is low. When correlations between chemical fecal fat excretion and the breath test with tripalmitate have been found, it turns out that there is a good correlation in the normal range, or above 20 gm per day, but between 7 and 20 grams per day there is a 20 per cent incidence of false-positives and false-negatives.

Another variation on this theme is to measure peak per cent dose per hour of ^{14}CO$_2$ after ingestion of a tracer dose of [^{14}C] triolein in corn oil with and without concomitant ingestion of pancreatic extracts. The average increase is 8-fold with oral pancreatin over the level without in patients with severe exocrine insufficiency. Other causes of fat malabsorption do not show a response to pancreatin.

One can use the same approach without radioactive material by administering vitamin A acetate or vitamin A alcohol orally and comparing the blood levels of vitamin A over the ensuing 6 hours. Vitamin A esters cannot be absorbed until a pancreatic esterase releases the vitamin A alcohol. In pancreatic insufficiency, the peak increment above the fasting level after the vitamin A alcohol is normal, whereas that after the acetate is low. In celiac disease both give low results. The correlation between fecal fat excretion and depression in vitamin A acetate absorption indicates that false-positives and false-negatives account for about 25 per cent of the results. The main conclusion from fat tolerance tests is that they lack the sensitivity to detect early pancreatic damage because more than 90 per cent of the lipase output of the pancreas must be absent before the tests become abnormal. They are accurate in gross steatorrhea and avoid the unpleasant chemical analysis of stools for fat, but they sacrifice accuracy for convenience. The major defect is their inability to tell reliably whether the steatorrhea is due to maldigestion or malabsorption.

Similar tests have been done to test protein digestion. The physiology that underlies these tests will be reviewed briefly. Digestion of bovine serum albumin when mixed with a normal mixed meal is much slower than previously thought, so that at 4 hours protein still remains undigested in the ileum, and amino acids, dipeptides, and tripeptides are still found throughout the jejunum and ileum. The peptides are more rapidly absorbed than the free amino acids, and they are split in the mucosal or liver cells to amino acids. Stool nitrogen content, which should not exceed 2 gm per day, does not become abnormal until more than 90 per cent of pancreatic protease secretion is lost. Thus, one approach has been to measure the enzyme activity in the stool assuming that it bears a constant relation to the duodenal protease secretion. The results are confused by the presence of bacterial proteases that have activities that mimic those of chymotrypsin, for example.

The best indirect approach to assessing pancreatic proteolytic activity has been the administration in the test meal of a synthetic substrate for chymotrypsin. Benzoyl-tyrosine-p-amino-benzoic acid (BT-PABA) is cleaved by chymotrypsin, releasing the PABA, which is absorbed through the intestinal mucosa and excreted in the urine. After administration of 1 gm of the compound, at least 50 per cent should be excreted in the urine in 6 hours. In advanced chronic pancreatitis, the excretion usually is low, and the percentage excreted correlates well with the degree of abnormality of the Lundh test. However, since this test requires not only digestion but also absorption, severe mucosal disease may give abnormal values. PABA must be excreted in the urine; therefore, renal disease invalidates the test. Patients with a serum creatinine above 2 mg/dl are usually excluded.

In one large study, the excretion of PABA correlated with total trypsin concentration in duodenal juice (Lundh test) with a correlation coefficient equal to 0.75. In patients without renal disease, the BT-PABA test had a sensitivity of 86 per cent in those with chronic pancreatitis and 76 per cent in those with pancreatic cancer. The specificity was 93 per cent in patients with no pancreatic disease. Others reported a lower sensitivity (50 per cent) but 100 per cent specificity when mild cases of chronic pancreatitis were included, as would be expected because chymotrypsin digestive capacity is not decreased until about 90 per cent of normal output is lost.

The pancreolauryl test is similar except that the substrate, fluorescein dilaurate, is split by pancreatic carboxylic ester hydrolase. The fluorescein is absorbed, partly conjugated in the liver, and excreted in the urine. Thus, mucosal disease or renal disease may impair fluorescein excretion in the urine. As a control to correct for these, an equal dose of pure fluorescein can be given another day, and a ratio of excretion of the ester/alcohol calculated (normal > 0.3). In the same group of patients in which the sensitivity of the BT-PABA test was 33 per cent, the sensitivity of the pancreolauryl test was 81 per cent using the ratio. Its specificity was 94 per cent. Both tubeless tests correlated poorly with the secretin-caerulein test owing to lack of sensitivity of the noninvasive tests. The role of these tests will be to confirm that patients with steatorrhea have pancreatic insufficiency. They will never show enough sensitivity to be screening tests in early exocrine insufficiency in which the duodenal enzyme activities are still able to hydrolyze these substrates.

A variant of the Schilling test for vitamin B_{12} absorption can also be used as a digestion-absorption test for exocrine insufficiency. One isotope of cobalamin is administered prebound to human intrinsic factor (IF), and a second isotope of cobalamin is given bound to hog R protein. R protein is a protein in human salivary and gastric juice that binds B_{12} and as such prevents it from being absorbed unless pancreatic proteases, especially trypsin, degrade R protein and allow IF to bind B_{12}. A large excess of a nonradioactive B_{12} analogue that binds to R protein but not to IF and human IF is administered orally so that labeled B_{12} will not be removed by hog R protein, and 1000 μg of B_{12} is given parenterally. Normal individuals who degrade R protein will have a ratio of isotopes in the urine close to one, whereas those with pancreatic insufficiency absorb only the isotope bound to IF and very little bound to hog R protein. The isotope ratio is less than one. Ileal disease suppresses both isotope absorptions, but their ratio remains one.

Figure 32–2 shows a simplified algorithm for the evaluation of patients with possible steatorrhea. The intent is to confirm steatorrhea if present and to differentiate that due to pancreatic insufficiency from other forms. If a patient's history or physical examination or the gross appearance of his stools suggests that he may have steatorrhea and this history indicates an adequate fat intake, the simplest and most direct test that can be done is to stain a fresh stool sample ob-

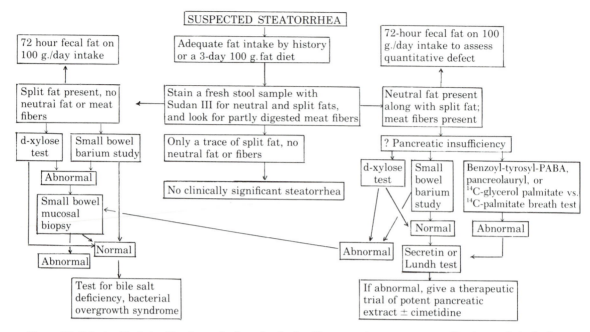

Figure 32–2 A simplified algorithm for evaluation of patients with pancreatogenous versus other forms of steatorrhea.

tained at rectal examination with a saturated solution of Sudan III dye in methanol, homogenized with the stool in water or saline. This should detect neutral fats (triglycerides). Emulsifying another fragment of stool with 33 per cent acetic acid and Sudan stain, covering the emulsion with a cover slip, and warming to the point at which bubbles appear (about 80° C) will change fatty acid soaps into undissociated fatty acids and melt them so that they can take up Sudan stain. As the slide cools, fatty acids will crystallize out in long colorless, needlelike sheaves. A qualitative Sudan stain is positive when more than 10 globules measuring 20 μ or more in diameter are seen per high-power field. A test showing 0-trace neutral or split fat contains less than 7 gm/day; one showing 4+ split fat or neutral fat usually contains more than 20 gm/day by analysis. A 1+ to 3+ grade may contain normal to elevated values. Thus, only the qualitative extremes are reliable guides to amounts of fat in the stool.

Both slides can be used to look for partially digested meat fibers that still contain cross striations and sharp edges. If neutral fat is present and partially digested meat fibers are apparent, it is very probable that a defect in digestion is present. Neutral fat is present in normal stool only as a few 5- to 10-μ particles. Undigested meat fibers are not seen in other situations unless the patient has very rapid peristalsis. Split fat, of course, is seen whenever neutral fat is present because of bacterial lipases in the colon. Such a patient has presumed pancreatic insufficiency and should be placed on 100 gm of fat a day for 3 days to assess

the quantitative severity of the steatorrhea. A D-xylose test and a small bowel barium study, looking for a malabsorption pattern, are screening tests that, when negative, point toward a diagnosis of pancreatic disease. If they are normal, there is unlikely to be a mucosal lesion, and a secretin or Lundh test is worth doing. If available, either a ^{14}C-glycerol palmitate breath test or a BT-PABA urine test would be a good screening test, justifying a duodenal intubation test if found abnormal. If the screening test is normal, it does not rule out pancreatic disease.

An abnormal secretin or Lundh test justifies a therapeutic trial of a potent pancreatic extract along with an agent that prevents gastric acid and pepsin inactivation of the enzymes, such as cimetidine, or an enzyme preparation that is encapsulated to be resistant to gastric acid but is released in the duodenum and jejunum at a neutral pH. If the patient has pancreatic insufficiency as the only cause of steatorrhea, he should cease to have diarrhea and should gain weight, and his stool should show no significant fat on Sudan stain. If no significant fat is seen on the initial examination, the patient should be given 100 gm of fat per day for 3 days and then return for another microscopic examination. A negative examination rules out clinically significant steatorrhea as a cause of diarrhea or weight loss.

The usefulness of the 72-hour fecal fat determination is to decide whether the fat losses can account for weight loss. They rarely do so if they are below 20 gm per day, but 7 to 20 gm of fat per day may contribute to diarrhea via the effect of fatty acids on colonic absorption of sodium and chloride. If the stool contains split fat in large amounts and no neutral fat or meat fibers, the patient's steatorrhea has either a mucosal or luminal cause. Here the D-xylose test and small bowel barium study should be abnormal, leading to small bowel biopsy. The biopsy may show evidence of villous atrophy, as seen in gluten enteropathy, or it may lead to a diagnosis of Whipple's disease and other rare diseases. If the pancreatic studies and small bowel biopsy are both normal, the patient probably has a bile salt deficiency that is due to liver disease, ileal disease, or bacterial overgrowth. Every physician should obtain experience with the Sudan examination of stool. It takes only 5 minutes and allows an efficient evaluation of steatorrhea if present.

RADIOLOGIC AND NUCLEAR METHODS OF DIAGNOSIS

The radiologic and nuclear medicine methods of diagnosis of pancreatic disease depend primarily on anatomic variations induced by disease states but in some situations also depend on pancreatic physiology and biochemistry. We will review briefly the conditions that control the effectiveness of these imaging methods.

The traditional *barium contrast* studies of the stomach and duodenum reflect pancreatic disease secondarily by a mass effect or by mucosal edema due to inflammation or lymphatic obstruction. Considering all pancreatic diseases, a prospective barium study had a sensitivity of 52 per cent and an overall accuracy of 57 per cent. The sensitivity of barium studies of the duodenum can be increased by paralyzing its motility with a large dose of anticholinergic agent and infusing barium and air by tube into the duodenum, the so-called *hypotonic duodenogram*. The sensitivity for all diseases of the pancreas in the aforementioned prospective study was 55 per cent, and overall accuracy was 56 per cent. The limitation here is that the disease must affect the head of the pancreas.

Because the pancreas avidly takes up amino acids and synthesizes them into pancreatic enzymes, attempts have been made to label the pancreas with radioactive amino acids, the most successful of which has been substituting ^{75}Se, a gamma-emitting isotope, for the sulfur of methionine. When this is administered intravenously after a meal, there is immediate uptake of the isotope into the pancreas, incorporation of the amino acid into pancreatic proteins, and eventual discharge of the radioisotope into the duodenum. Over a period of approximately 1 hour, repeated gamma camera scans usually allow a visualization of the normal pancreas, although it is often difficult to separate it from the overlying liver, which also takes up selenomethionine. The signal-to-

noise ratio for a *selenomethionine scan* of the pancreas is poor because of uptake of the amino acid in the blood stream and in other tissues, and the pancreatic image is less well defined than on hepatic scans. Eaton found that the scan in various pancreatic diseases had a sensitivity of 86 per cent and an accuracy of 72 per cent. It was most useful when it was normal. A prospective comparison of diagnostic tests in cancer of the pancreas from Mayo Clinic showed that the scan had a sensitivity of 90 per cent but a specificity of only 33 per cent.

Various workers have improved imaging of the pancreas by administering ^{11}C-labeled L-amino acids made in a cyclotron and using *positron emission tomography* to detect uptake by the pancreas. Positron emission occurs simultaneously at 180° angles and allows transverse images to be calculated for tomographic body slices. One large study reported for all pancreatic diseases a sensitivity of 85 per cent, a specificity of 98 per cent, and an accuracy of 92 per cent. Decreased uptake of ^{11}C-L-methionine occurred in chronic pancreatitis and in cancer of the pancreas, and they could not be distinguished. Uptake in the liver was 0.8 of that in the pancreas and interfered less than in ^{75}Se-methionine scans. The availability of a cyclotron and the half-life of 20.4 minutes for ^{11}C make this approach feasible in only a few centers.

Angiography of the pancreas is technically difficult because the splenic, gastroduodenal, and superior mesenteric arteries must be cannulated in order to visualize all the blood vessels. Subselective cannulation of either of the pancreaticoduodenal vessels or the dorsal pancreatic is sometimes necessary, and this is even more difficult to do. Vessels of the pancreas are not arranged in a constant order, and it is difficult to tell whether they have been displaced by a mass. Furthermore, cancer of the pancreas infiltrates tissue and does not push vessels aside. It is a hypovascular tumor and does not cause a tumor stain. Its major angiographic characteristics are encasement of an artery by a process of fibrosis or edema and occlusion of large veins, such as the splenic or superior mesenteric. A 25 per cent incidence of false-positives for cancer exists owing to atherosclerosis or chronic pancreatitis, and there is a 25 per cent false-negative rate because small lesions cannot be seen. A prospective study of patients with a normal pancreas, chronic pancreatitis, or pancreatic cancer yielded sensitivities of 97, 68, and 80 per cent and specificities of 77, 100, and 97 per cent, respectively, on blinded readings by three radiologists. The angiogram accurately predicted resectability of tumors. Once disease was detected by other means, the Mayo Clinic study showed that the sensitivity for the diagnosis of pancreatic cancer was 70 per cent but the specificity was 95 per cent. The usefulness of the angiogram is in confirming the diagnosis of cancer of the pancreas and predicting resectability.

Ultrasonography is a noninvasive and relatively inexpensive technique. State-of-the-art equipment includes both real-time and gray-scale instruments. B-scanners are used with the latter for static images. The effectiveness of pancreatic ultrasonography is limited by bowel air and extreme adiposity. The normal pancreas is characterized by relatively high-level echoes compared with the surrounding normal liver parenchyma. In addition, the echo pattern seen with a normal pancreas differs from that seen with pancreatitis and carcinoma. Ultrasonography is more effective than computed tomography (CT) in patients with little fat. The length and thickness of the gland have been well defined with ultrasonography in normal persons. Cysts can be clearly seen, and an edematous gland can usually be appreciated. Suboptimal, technically unsatisfactory examinations occurred in 8 to 24 per cent of patients in a prospective evaluation of ultrasonographic examination of the pancreas. When these suboptimal examinations were included (as they are in clinical diagnosis) at a true-positive ratio of 80 per cent, the false-positive rate associated with ultrasonography was 46 per cent. At this true-positive rate, CT was associated with only a 4 per cent false-positive rate. Sensitivities for detecting an abnormal pancreas when suboptimal examinations were included were 69 per cent for ultrasonography and 87 per cent for CT; specificities were 82 and 90 per cent, respectively. Ultrasonography was less successful than CT in identifying pancreatic disease and classifying it as neoplastic or inflammatory; the respective sensitivities were 56 and 84 per cent.

Computed tomography is now performed with instruments with 2- to 10-minute scan times for each 1-cm body section. Pancreatic scans are done with and without intravenous contrast material, which illuminates blood vessels and cysts. Pancreatic disease is detected by CT because of changes in size or contour and involvement of adjacent tissues. X-ray absorption coefficients of a normal pancreas differ little from those associated with a pancreas affected by cancer or pancreatitis. The major weakness of CT is an inability to detect small tumors that do not enlarge or deform the gland. In spite of this problem, CT remains the best noninvasive screening method for pancreatic cancer. The conclusion of a large prospective evaluation of CT versus ultrasonography was that CT is the method of choice for detecting pancreatic abnormalities and for defining their nature and extent. In one large clinic, CT alone was adequate in 75 per cent of patients; invasive studies such as angiograms were needed in only 10 per cent, and endoscopic pancreatography was required in only 20 per cent. CT may be as sensitive (70 to 80 per cent) and accurate as any other diagnostic method for acute pancreatitis. The abnormalities that can be visualized with CT include enlargement of the gland, phlegmons, cysts, hemorrhage, abscess, and calcium deposition. In chronic pancreatitis, 16 per

cent of patients have been reported to have a normal scan.

Nuclear magnetic resonance (NMR) imaging is achieving clinical applicability. The patient is placed in a strong magnetic field, and a microwave pulse is applied at the frequency of hydrogen protons to measure proton density and proton spin–lattice relaxation times. One instrument computed transverse sections of the body 17.5 mm thick and displayed relaxation times in 16 colors over a range of 50 to 450 milliseconds. In preliminary studies, the pancreas was not visualized without pancreatic disease. Pancreatitis, cysts, cancer, and abscess could be recognized and differentiated. This noninvasive method promises to give anatomic displays as detailed as those provided by CT and to distinguish one disease process from another more accurately.

Endoscopic retrograde cholangiopancreatography (ERCP) is a demanding procedure requiring an expert endoscopist, a radiologist, a radiologic suite, and technical help. It requires from 15 to 60 minutes, is very expensive, and gives the patient a moderate radiation exposure. In spite of these problems, in centers where this special expertise is available it has turned out to be one of the most reliable means of confirming pancreatic disease. For example, the success rate of this technique in the hands of experienced workers is 85 per cent, the complication rate is 3.5 per cent, and the mortality rate is 0.1 per cent. Because of overdistention of the ductal system, acute pancreatitis has been reported in about 1 per cent of total studies, although death rarely results. Cholangitic sepsis occurring behind an obstructed ductal system is the most lethal complication. It is seen in 0.8 per cent of patients and has caused death in 10 per cent of that group. Filling of a pseudocyst by ERCP is a serious error because it almost always results in infection and requires immediate drainage. The mortality rate is 20 per cent. Ultrasonography should always be performed before ERCP to avoid this complication. Some investigators give antibiotics in the contrast medium and intravenously when they feel that a risk may be present. The amount of filling of the pancreatic ductal system usually is monitored by fluoroscopy, but some investigators have used manometry and find that the main and second order ducts are visualized with 3 to 5 ml injected at a pressure of 110 mm Hg.

The overall sensitivity of ERCP was 88 per cent in a large series in the hands of experts, and the specificity was 96 per cent. In chronic pancreatitis, the diameter and tapering pattern of the main and secondary ducts can vary from normal to patterns demonstrating dilatation, stenosis, obstruction, cyst formation, calculi, and shortening of the main duct. It is occasionally difficult to differentiate cancer from pancreatitis by changes in the ductal system. Pancreatic cancer can also cause obstruction, stenosis, dilatation, and shortening. The Mayo Clinic study concluded that ERCP provided a sensitivity of 95 per cent in cancer detection and a specificity of 90 per cent. Results of cytologic studies on endoscopically obtained juice have been positive in about 50 per cent of proven cancer patients. After CT or pancreatic function testing indicates that pancreatic disease is present, ERCP is the best method of confirming it.

Although *transhepatic cholangiography* is technically not a study of the pancreas, it is often used to confirm or deny the presence of a tumor or stone obstructing the distal common duct. Its success rate and its complication rate are approximately equal to those of ERCP, although it is easier to perform than ERCP when the Chiba or skinny needle is used. With dilated hepatic ducts, the success rate is 98 per cent; with nondilated ducts, it is 70 per cent. The complication rate is about 5 per cent, with major problems being sepsis, bile leakage, and bleeding. It is ideally used when there are dilated ducts but no ampullary lesions for biopsy nor impacted stone to be removed.

In summary, the best application of these radiologic and nuclear medicine methods in detecting pancreatic disease is as follows: CT scanning should be performed first, with or without support from a pancreatic function test. If disease is thought to be present and cancer is possible, then retrograde pancreatography is the procedure of choice, adding cytology with its yield. If ERCP is technically unsuccessful or not available, angiography is the next step. An obstructing lesion of the common duct can be evaluated successfully by transhepatic cholangiography as well as by ERCP.

DUODENAL DRAINAGE TESTS OF PANCREATIC FUNCTION

The most reliable method for determining the functional capacity of the exocrine pancreas is to measure its ability to secrete water, bicarbonate, or enzymes into the duodenal lumen after an appropriate stimulus. Over the last 40 years, repeated attempts have been made to develop the perfect, or "best," duodenal drainage test, that is, the most sensitive and specific test of exocrine pancreatic secretion. This should be applicable on a routine clinical level and should show a high level of predictability in the diagnosis of exocrine insufficiency, chronic pancreatitis, or cancer of the pancreas. To the present time, this goal has not been achieved. The reason seems to be that the goal is not realistic. The reserve capacity of the exocrine pancreas is so great that early alcoholic pancreatitis may still give enzyme or bicarbonate outputs within the wide normal range. However, if only patients with advanced pancreatic insufficiency are studied, any test of secretion will give abnormal values in all such cases. Secretory tests

for cancer of the pancreas cannot be expected to be abnormal unless the main duct is blocked in the head or body of the gland, causing a measurable reduction in secretory mass. The pancreas may not function normally because it has lost secretory tissue or because it is not being stimulated normally by the gut hormones. In the latter case, a test meal that requires release of gastrin, CCK, and secretin, as well as vagal stimulation, provides a better approach than use of exogenous CCK and secretin. The "best test" may differ with the question being asked. If the question is whether a reduction in pancreatic acinar or ductal secretory mass has occurred, as in chronic pancreatitis, we can design an ideal test to answer this question, but it may not be applicable in every physician's hands.

First, a tube must be positioned in the duodenum to collect pancreatic juice, and a separate tube or another lumen of the same tube must be positioned in the stomach to remove gastric acid, which might destroy bicarbonate in the duodenum. Because no duodenal tube allows 100 per cent recovery of duodenal fluid, the duodenum must be perfused with physiologic saline containing a nonabsorbable marker, such as polyethylene glycol, that will allow correction for volume losses.

Next, one must decide what physiologic stimulus should be used and in what manner it should be delivered. The best stimulation would be one that permits an evaluation of the functioning secretory mass of the pancreas. Reasoning from studies undertaken to measure parietal cell mass in the stomach with histamine or gastrin, we should develop dose-response curves in normal males and females of varying ages. If a maximal response occurs, we will assume that it is proportional to the functioning mass of certain secretory cells, since we cannot count them or weigh the gland in normal humans. In the pancreas, the acinar cell secretion of enzymes could be assessed by a maximal stimulation by CCK or by a cholinergic stimulus, whereas the centroacinar and ductal cells of the pancreas could be maximally stimulated to produce bicarbonate by secretin. A measurement of maximum response is most easily accomplished if the stimulus is applied by a constant intravenous infusion, so that the output of the pancreas rises to a plateau response and remains there over a period of time. The maximum volume and bicarbonate outputs into the duodenum have resulted from intravenous infusion of pure secretin at a dose of 4 to 6 clinical units/kg/hr. The maximal enzyme response is obtained by a constant infusion of pure CCK at a rate of 4 to 8 Ivy dog units/kg/hr or, alternatively, the synthetic C-terminal octapeptide of CCK (Syncalide), which gives a maximal response at a dose of 20 ng/kg/hr. Caerulein, a decapeptide that has almost the same structure as the 10 C-terminal amino acids of CCK, stimulates enzyme secretion maximally at a dose of 75 ng/kg/hr. With polyethylene glycol used as a marker of water flux, it is apparent that some duodenal fluid is lost beyond the tube and that there is some reabsorption of water and bicarbonate in the duodenum, so that overall recovery by a duodenal tube is 85 per cent. Maximal stimulation of both the acinar and ductal tissues would mean that volume output, maximal bicarbonate concentration, or hourly bicarbonate output could be measured as well as the concentration or output of any of the pancreatic enzymes.

The enzymes that should be most accurately measured are trypsin and chymotrypsin. Lipase and amylase require careful control of assay conditions, and activities may not be linear on dilution. Collaborative studies of interlaboratory precision revealed disturbingly wide coefficients of variation with the same lyophilized duodenal juice and assay methods. The variances are 24 to 53 per cent for lipase, 16 to 58 per cent for amylase, 24 to 52 per cent for trypsin, and 28 to 63 per cent for chymotrypsin. These findings indicate clearly that results from different centers cannot be compared quantitatively. There is evidence that in the normal human the outputs of each of these enzymes are parallel, but in pancreatic disease the outputs of trypsin or chymotrypsin are reduced more than that of amylase. The output of lipase correlates most closely with the degree of steatorrhea. When less than 10 per cent of the normal lipase output is obtained, steatorrhea is always present. One of the problems in measuring proteolytic enzymes is that the activation of trypsinogen to trypsin relies on endogenous enterokinase, and this should be circumvented by addition of purified enterokinase to the collected juice. The assay of chymotrypsin is best accomplished by addition of bovine trypsin to ensure complete activation. Duodenal contents contain bile, which tends to inhibit lipase, so the assay should be carried out immediately in the presence of an optimal calcium concentration and after addition of a well-emulsified substrate, preferably triolein. The lipase activity will be a function not only of the amount of lipase but also of the amount of colipase present. This molecule reverses the inhibition by bile acids and stabilizes the lipase molecule. The assay should properly be called a *lipase-colipase activity*. True total lipase activity requires addition of colipase; in controls, the activity with endogenous colipase averaged only 68 per cent of that with added colipase. In juice from steatorrheic patients, the ratio of actual to potential lipase activity was even lower. Colipase appears to be the controlling factor of lipolysis. In exocrine insufficiency, a lipase activity is measurable in the duodenum that is not inhibited by bile salts or stimulated by colipase; this is probably lingual lipase. Measurements of amylase activity are accurate only if salivary amylase is excluded from the duodenum during the study.

It should now be apparent that the measurement of pancreatic secretory mass requires at least 2 hours, meticulous care in doing the test, and accurate enzyme assays. Each laboratory must perform its standard pancreatic function test on a series of normal individuals in order to establish normal ranges. Maximal pancreatic responses to these stimuli apparently do not decrease with age.

Different methods of collection will give different outputs and concentrations of bicarbonate and enzymes. If CCK and secretin are used, the sphincter of Oddi will remain open and bile will constantly dilute the pancreatic juice. Bile contains bicarbonate produced from biliary duct epithelium by the secretin stimulus. Brunner's gland secretion is said to be stimulated by secretin. Thus, the duodenal tube collects a mixture of at least three secretions, in which only the enzyme outputs are reliable markers of pancreatic function. This problem can be avoided by the more invasive and difficult procedure of cannulating the pancreatic duct through an endoscope. Secretin given alone leaves the sphincter of the bile duct closed, and bile goes into the gallbladder unless it is nonfunctional. Duodenal bile is minimal, so bicarbonate output more certainly reflects pancreatic function. Thus, normal values for a secretin test in individuals who have been cholecystectomized would have to be determined separately.

The endoscopic method has given us our first reliable data on pure pancreatic juice secretion in normal humans. Secretin infusions produce a maximal rate of secretion at a dose of 0.5 clinical units/kg/hr. The maximal bicarbonate concentration of this juice is 135 ± 9 mEq/L, and the bicarbonate output reaches a maximum of approximately 0.37 mEq/hr/kg body weight. Secretin leads to a constant protein output in pure pancreatic juice resulting from the rise in volume and a matched decrease in protein concentration, suggesting that secretin in humans does release enzyme. Cyclic AMP output also correlates closely with bicarbonate concentration, supporting the studies that show that secretin stimulates via cAMP. The technical problems involved with cannulating the pancreatic duct, however, make it unlikely that this will ever become a routine method of assessing human pancreatic function.

A major problem for all who wish to measure pancreatic exocrine function is the plethora of different units employed for standardizing the hormones. The purest preparation of secretin available is that from the GIH Laboratory of the Karolinska Institute in Sweden. This is calibrated in clinical units, one of which is equal to four Crick-Harper-Raper units, which is the way Boots Pure Drug Company in England assays its secretin. Over the years, as the manufacturers have changed their methods, their standards, and their assays, the relative potencies of clinical to C-H-R units also have changed. One clinical unit also equals, at the present time, 20 Hammersten cat units, an older method of expressing secretin potency. Synthetic secretin is now available; its potency has been compared with that of the GIH secretin. One μg of synthetic secretin is equivalent to about four clinical units; the vial of GIH secretin containing 75 clinical units contains 19 μg of secretin (four clinical units/μg). In duodenal juice, the maximal bicarbonate secretory rate is achieved at a dose of 4 to 6 clinical units/kg/hr, whereas the maximal concentration of bicarbonate is achieved at a lower dose, 1 clinical unit/kg/hr. Secretin has been given for years as a single bolus intravenously, which results in a rise and fall in rate of flow over a 60- to 80-minute period. This method of testing measures the total amount of bicarbonate put out in 60 or 80 minutes and, by short intervals of collection, looks for the maximal bicarbonate concentration. In one of the best of such studies, a dose of GIH secretin of 2 units/kg body weight was used, which gave a volume greater than 1.8 ml/kg/hr, a maximal bicarbonate concentration of 100 ± 10 (lower limit of normal, 82) mEq/L, and a bicarbonate output of 15 ± 7 (lower limit, 6.2) mEq/hr. For reasons given previously, these results do not apply to patients without a gallbladder.

There is evidence in animals for dietary adaptation of the enzymes in pancreatic juice. Thus, rats fed a high-carbohydrate, low-protein diet have an increase in amylase and a decrease in protease outputs. The reverse is true on a high-protein, low-carbohydrate diet. However, no adaptation occurs in humans for amylase, lipase, trypsin, chymotrypsin, or ribonuclease on isocaloric diets varying from 1 to 350 gm of protein per day over a period of 2 weeks.

For a routine evaluation of pancreatic ductal secretory mass, the simplest method is a secretin test. There should be a constant infusion of 4 clinical units/kg secretin over a period of an hour and the juice should be collected in 10-minute periods with a double-lumen duodenal tube in which polyethylene glycol is infused through the proximal orifice and 20 cm distally juice is collected. Volume and bicarbonate outputs should be corrected for PEG recovery. The reproducibility of such assays should be ± 10 per cent. Since enzyme output is weakly stimulated by secretin and enzyme activities are difficult to quantitate, bicarbonate should be the mainstay. Any hospital laboratory can accurately measure bicarbonate concentrations.

In cirrhosis of the liver, the volume output usually is increased on a secretin test, and the bicarbonate concentrations are therefore low, partly because of a great increase in volume output from the pancreas and from the biliary tree. Bicarbonate outputs are low when both the pancreas and the liver are diseased but are normal when only the liver is diseased. The information derived from measuring volume, bicarbonate concentration, and output after secretin gives as much useful clinical information in the diagnosis of chronic pancreatitis and carcinoma of the pancreas as do added measurements of enzyme activities or outputs.

In 1962, Lundh suggested another test of pancreatic secretion that evaluates the entire sequence of events that follows ingestion of a meal. A single-lumen tube is passed into the duodenum, and no attempt is made to remove gastric juice. The patient drinks a mixed liquid meal containing carbohydrate, protein, and fat. As the meal empties into the duodenum, endogenous CCK, secretin, gastrin, and other GI hormones are released and act on the exocrine pancreas. The variables that influence this test are (1) the rate of emptying of the test meal from the stomach; (2) the gastric acid output, which acidifies the meal and releases secretin; (3) the release of hormones from duodenal and jejunal mucosa; (4) the response of the acinar cells and ductal cells to gut hormones; (5) the dilution of pancreatic juice by bile and Brunner's gland secretion. Lundh chose to measure peak enzyme activity in the duodenal secretion over a period of 2 hours by collecting at 10-minute intervals in the first hour and at 20-minute intervals in the second hour. The enzyme outputs show a rise, a fall, and a second rise over the 2-hour period. Most investigators observe all the events that occur over the entire 2-hour period and measure average trypsin, amylase, or lipase activity. Although bicarbonate and volume are not measured, secretin plays a role by diluting the enzymes and reducing enzyme concentration. This tube leads to collections of only 20 to 50 per cent of the total duodenal secretion, so outputs of enzymes cannot be measured. The maximal enzyme activities are close to those obtained with maximal CCK stimulation.

Lundh's test has been compared with secretin and CCK function tests in a small number of patients. There are no significant differences in diagnostic sensitivity or specificity, except that abnormal results occur in Lundh's test when disease is present in small bowel mucosa, the liver, or the biliary tree—not just in the pancreas. In patients who have a gastrojejunostomy, there is good correlation in Lundh's test between the lipase activity in the efferent loop and the degree of fat malabsorption. In enterogenous malabsorption due to gluten enteropathy and other small bowel diseases, Lundh's test shows decreased concentrations of enzymes in about one third of patients. This is due to dilution with excessive fluid in the duodenum, to decreased CCK release, and to decreased acinar cell function. In a CCK test, protein malnutrition also interferes, as it does in the test meal. Thus, in patients with protein malnutrition the amylase output correlates very well with serum albumin, which is a good marker of protein malnutrition. In patients with gastrojejunostomies, it is difficult to study pancreatic secretion because the water and bicarbonate are reabsorbed as they travel down the duodenum and jejunum and falsely low values are obtained. Studies comparing output at the papilla of Vater with that at the efferent loop from the stomach indicate a loss of 65 per cent of volume, 70 per cent of the bicarbonate, and 50 per cent of the enzymes.

The sensitivity of the CCK-secretin test was evaluated by Sarles in 1963 in a small group of patients who underwent multiple biopsies of the pancreas at the time of surgery for chronic pancreatitis. In these patients, studied with a combination of secretin and CCK, the average maximal bicarbonate concentration in patients with minor damage on biopsy was 79 mEq/L. Those with diffuse and moderate damage had a mean value of 41 mEq/L, and in those with diffuse major damage it was 23 mEq/L. The average normal bicarbonate was 100, with a lower limit of normal of 75 mEq/L. Maximum fasting lipase activity also declined from 29 to 8.7 to 8.1 units/min/L as the degree of damage increased. Another study compared volume, bicarbonate, trypsin, and lipase outputs with length of opacified main ducts at ERCP. These parameters showed a linear correlation with duct length in cancer and chronic pancreatitis. A decrease could not be detected until more than 60 per cent of the length of the main duct was obstructed. Thus, either bicarbonate or enzyme output appears to reflect both diffuse parenchymal damage and obstruction when damage is moderate or severe.

In summary, then, an ideal exocrine pancreatic function test is difficult to carry out and probably never will be widely applied clinically. The two most reasonable compromises that have evolved are (1) the secretin test with measurement of bicarbonate and volume after constant infusion of maximal secretin; (2) a test meal with measurement of trypsin activity over a 2-hour period.

ACUTE PANCREATITIS

PATHOGENESIS AND ETIOLOGY

The major condition with which human acute pancreatitis occurs is stones in the gallbladder, usually with passage of stones through the common duct into the duodenum. Attempts to explain this association have led to an extensive literature testing the hypothesis that a common channel between the common bile duct and pancreatic duct of Wirsüng, combined with obstruction of the papilla of Vater by a stone, results in reflux of bile into the pancreatic ducts. The mixture of bile and pancreatic juice is postulated to cause acute pancreatitis by initiating autodigestion. The observation that triggered this theory was that of Eugene Opie, a pathologist at Johns Hopkins Hospital, who in 1901 performed an autopsy on a patient who had died with acute pancreatitis and found a gallstone impacted in the ampulla of Vater. Opie postulated that a common channel allowed bile to reflux into the pancreatic ducts and set off pancrea-

titis. He aspirated gallbladder bile and injected it under high pressure into the pancreatic duct of seven dogs and produced an acute hemorrhagic pancreatitis in all seven animals.

Over the years, investigators have tried to create various animal models to assess the role of bile reflux in human pancreatitis. We will summarize the important findings and indicate whether or not any animal model has reproduced a form of acute pancreatitis that closely resembles that occurring spontaneously in humans. One model in the dog allowed bile from the common duct to reflux into the pancreas by connecting the main pancreatic duct end-to-side to the common duct. Such animals tended to have spontaneous attacks of acute pancreatitis, but they were also triggered by morphine, which causes spasm of the sphincter of Oddi. In the Opie model, which involves a high-pressure injection of bile (above 40 to 50 cm of water), an immediate acute hemorrhagic pancreatitis resulted, but histologically it consisted primarily of a bile necrosis unlike that seen in human pancreatitis. If, however, purified pancreatic enzymes are injected into the pancreatic duct under low pressures (less than 40 cm of water), different histologic patterns occur. When trypsin is injected, a pancreatic edema with occasional areas of necrosis occurs that resembles human edematous pancreatitis. When elastase is injected, an acute hemorrhagic pancreatitis occurs in which the major damage involves blood vessel walls. Such hyaline necrosis of vessels is seen in human pancreatitis. If enterokinase is injected, acute pancreatitis can be produced, but again it is not severe and looks like that obtained with trypsin. A widely used dog model incubates sterile gallbladder bile and pancreatic juice together at room temperature for 24 hours; this mixture is then infused into the pancreatic duct under low pressure. Almost uniformly, a severe hemorrhagic pancreatitis occurs.

The two elements in bile that are critical for this incubation to be effective are bile salts and lecithin. The element in pancreatic juice that seems to be most crucial is phospholipase A. Activated by bile salts, phospholipase A cleaves a fatty acid from lecithin to produce *lysolecithin*. When lysolecithin itself is injected into the pancreatic duct, a necrotizing pancreatitis occurs that resembles the human lesion. The cell membranes of the pancreas, of course, contain lecithin and are an adequate substrate without the addition of lecithin from bile. Thus, the simplest model that closely mimics human pancreatitis is the infusion of trypsin and a single bile salt into the pancreatic duct at physiologic concentrations and at pressures below 40 cm of water for 30 minutes. Trypsin produces the phospholipase A, which is activated by the bile salt, and cell membrane lecithin serves as the substrate.

In confirmation of these experimental studies it has been found that a normal human pancreas at autopsy contains only a trace of lysolecithin, whereas in a patient with acute pancreatitis there is a high concentration of free lysolecithin. In addition, in the normal postmortem human pancreas there is usually found to be no free elastase activity, but there is some free chymotryptic and trypsin activity. In acute pancreatitis, all of the elastase is free and the chymotrypsin and the trypsin activities are increased. These findings support the hypothesis that acute pancreatitis in humans is associated with activation of trypsin, which activates the other zymogens, most importantly prophospholipase A to phospholipase A. This enzyme produces lysolecithin, which then lyses cell membranes, releasing more zymogens to be activated. A positive feedback process occurs that perpetuates the pancreatitis.

Another form of experimental pancreatitis also bears on the human situation. If the duodenum of a dog is ligated proximally and distally to the papilla of Vater and the lesser papilla of Santorini, stimulation of pancreatic secretion by feeding these animals results in severe hemorrhagic pancreatitis, the so-called "closed-loop" pancreatitis. There is good evidence that this is due to reflux of duodenal contents into the pancreatic duct. This process of duodenal reflux has been postulated to occur after the passage of a gallstone through the sphincter of Oddi, when there is temporary damage to the smooth muscle fibers.

One simple but effective approach toward understanding the pathogenesis of gallstone pancreatitis has been to filter the feces for 8 days after an attack of pain consistent with pancreatitis. In two series, 84 per cent of patients found to have acute pancreatitis and gallstones had gallstones recovered from their stools, whereas only 11 per cent of patients with gallstones and no evidence of pancreatitis had stones recovered. Operative cholangiograms showed reflux into the pancreatic duct in 67 per cent of those who had gallstone pancreatitis, whereas among the controls only 18 per cent refluxed. At surgery, gallstones in those with pancreatitis were found in the gallbladder, occasionally in the common duct, and rarely impacted in the ampulla. Patients who had gallstones without pancreatitis had few common duct stones. Therefore, gallstones and pancreatitis seem to be associated with the passage of stones through the cystic duct into the common duct and through the sphincter of Oddi. This finding strengthens the theory of those who postulate that acute pancreatitis is due to reflux into the pancreas, and it makes reflux of duodenal contents through a damaged sphincter a much more likely theory than simple reflux of bile. When enterokinase mixes with pancreatic juice, it is thought to lead to activation of trypsin from trypsinogen in amounts that overwhelm the available pancreatic secretory trypsin inhibitor, thus producing acute pancreati-

tis. Moreover, enterokinase is not inhibited by the trypsin inhibitor in pancreatic juice.

When cholangiograms are obtained at the time of gallbladder surgery, contrast medium injected into the common bile duct refluxes into the pancreatic duct 60 to 80 per cent of the time. In autopsy specimens in humans, 80 to 90 per cent of specimens show a common channel of 5 mm or less in length that allows reflux into the pancreas if the papilla is obstructed. Reflux from the common duct into the pancreatic duct is rarely seen on ambulatory intravenous cholangiograms, suggesting that anesthesia creates an abnormal relationship between the two ductal pressures.

The pressures in the pancreatic and common bile ducts and in their sphincters can be measured in unanesthetized humans during ERCP manometry. The absolute values vary widely, depending on either the rate of perfusion or compliance of small side-hole catheters or the use of microtransducer catheters. The conclusion derived from many studies is that the pressure in the pancreatic duct of controls is higher than that of the common duct, with duodenal pressure used as a baseline. A zone of phasic high pressure has been found in the distal common duct, the pancreatic duct, and the papilla, corresponding to the smooth-muscle sphincters found in dissections of human specimens.

Because the secretory pressure in the pancreatic duct is higher in the resting and secretory states than it is in the common duct, reflux does not occur in vivo unless a decreased resistance to pancreatic ductal filling occurs. Preincubation of pancreatic juice and bile in the gallbladder of dogs creates a condition in which the pancreas takes up bile at a normal bile-duct pressure. Pancreatic enzyme activity is detectable in 10 per cent of individuals in whom elective cholecystectomies are performed, so many patients have the anatomic and biochemical setting for reflux of activated bile to occur. When we consider the entire literature concerning pancreatic reflux, we must admit that it remains a plausible but unproved explanation for acute pancreatitis.

The other factor important in experimental pancreatitis in animals is *obstruction* of the ductal system. Intense stimulation of the pancreas produces no lesions, but in the presence of ductal obstruction pancreatic edema can be produced in most species. Obstruction of the ductal system combined with feeding of mice results in the appearance of zymogen granules in the extracellular fluid and lymphatics at the basal portion of the cells and the appearance of the enzymes in plasma. Whether the granules pass through the basement membranes or through tight junctions from acinar lumina is not known. Occasionally, some fat necrosis is seen, but hemorrhagic pancreatitis is rare in uncomplicated ductal obstruction in animals. The lesion can be changed from edema to necrosis by decreasing blood flow to the pancreas via 15 minutes of occlusion of the pancreaticoduodenal artery or by venous occlusion. How does impaired blood flow convert edema to necrosis? The lesion is not simply ischemic necrosis but also autodigestion, so it may be that the plasma protease inhibitors are the critical missing items. When the α_2-macroglobulin in pancreatic exudate and in ascitic fluid of a dog with experimental pancreatitis becomes saturated with proteolytic enzymes, there is a sudden worsening of the animal's condition and it dies rapidly. In human pancreatitis, pancreatic edema often leads to severe plasma loss, hypotension, and impaired pancreatic perfusion, which may help transform edematous into necrotic pancreatitis as in the animal model.

When the large or small pancreatic ducts are obstructed, enzymes reach the blood stream by absorption into the lymphatics. These channels also carry enzymes throughout the retroperitoneum, through the posterior parietal peritoneum into the ascitic fluid, and across the diaphragm into the pleural spaces. In dogs there are connections of the lymphatics between the gallbladder, cystic duct, common duct, lymph nodes of the duodenum, and the pancreatic lymphatic system. Thus, India ink injected into the lymphatics of the gallbladder can be found in the interstitium of the pancreas, particularly if there is any obstruction to main lymph flow via the thoracic duct. Acute cholecystitis produced in a dog can result in associated local areas of acute pancreatitis, and injection of lipase into the obstructed pancreatic duct has produced acute cholecystitis. These lymphatic connections are postulated as being another mechanism for the occurrence of acute pancreatitis in patients with a single large gallstone that does not enter the common duct. In addition, acute cholecystitis has been seen as a complication of acute pancreatitis in humans.

Evidence for the appearance of pancreatic proteases in blood is now available with the advent of radioimmunoassays for trypsin, chymotrypsin, and elastase. In pancreatitis these are present, bound primarily to α_1-antitrypsin and α_2-macroglobulin. When α_2-macroglobulin binds to these enzymes, small synthetic peptide or ester substrates can still reach the active site of trypsin, chymotrypsin, or elastase, which can hydrolyze such synthetic substrates at a rate close to that seen in the free state. Moreover, trypsin bound to α_2-macroglobulin is still able to digest intact or denatured proteins slowly, and, in particular, it is able to activate trypsinogen or chymotrypsinogen quite rapidly. Trypsinogen in plasma and ascitic fluid decreases and trypsin bound to α_2-macroglobulin and α_1-antitrypsin increases as the severity of human pancreatitis increases. Trypsin also can act on fibrinogen to produce clot formation and eventual lysis by digestion of the fibrin clot. Alpha$_1$-antitrypsin is a more important inhibitor in plasma because it binds strongly and irrevers-

ibly to the active site of these three proteases. During acute pancreatitis in humans, free trypsin, chymotrypsin, and elastase have been measured in the juice. After recovery only the zymogens are present, raising the possibility that acute pancreatitis is associated with a relative decrease in the synthesis or release of the secretory trypsin inhibitor.

The conclusion from studies of animal models for acute pancreatitis is that the critical factor seems to be activation of trypsinogen to trypsin, which leads to subsequent activation of prophospholipase A and the other zymogens. Bile salts are necessary for phospholipase activity. Trypsin and bile salts alone are enough to initiate intraductal pancreatic digestion, but the process is circumscribed unless there is impaired blood flow to the pancreas or impaired delivery of the plasma protease inhibitors, particularly α_1-antitrypsin. Ductal obstruction resulting from edema may intensify the process, as can venous thrombosis in and about the pancreas. The key factor still remains activation of trypsinogen to trypsin.

For some reason, the idea has been accepted that hypercalcemia itself is able to activate trypsinogen to trypsin. This theory is used to explain why patients with hyperparathyroidism have a marked increase in the incidence of acute and chronic pancreatitis. In hospital controls, about 0.3 per cent of patients have had acute or chronic pancreatitis, whereas 6 per cent of patients with hyperparathyroidism have had pancreatitis. Acute pancreatitis is also seen in other diseases in which hypercalcemia occurs, such as multiple myeloma and sarcoidosis. It is true that calcium is necessary to stabilize trypsin and prevent autodigestion of the enzyme, but calcium itself is not able to activate trypsinogen to trypsin. Thus, the reason that pancreatitis is more frequent in hypercalcemic states is still unknown. There is no question that the concentration of ionized calcium in pancreatic juice increases in proportion to the increase in ionized calcium in the plasma, and pancreatic secretion is stimulated by hypercalcemia both directly and indirectly by the release of gastrin. Yet there is no reason that stimulation of secretion in a normal gland should lead to pancreatitis. Another theory states that the high ionized calcium concentration in the pancreatic juice leads to precipitation of proteins in the ducts, leading to obstruction. How obstruction leads to activation of trypsin or to more than pancreatic edema is not explained.

Another hypothesis that has been proposed to explain the formation of trypsin within the gland is the autoactivation of trypsinogen by trypsinogen. This hypothesis is based on the fact that highly concentrated solutions of trypsinogen, completely free of trypsin, incubated over a period of time, result in a slow generation of trypsin molecules. It is known that the active center of trypsin is present in an incomplete state in the trypsinogen molecule, requiring a folding process that brings a serine and histidine into apposition to create the active site. When the concentration of trypsinogen is high enough, as exists in the zymogen granules or in the small pancreatic ducts, this theory predicts that two molecules of trypsinogen become apposed to one another and that the serine of one and the histidine of the other complete an active site of trypsin, which will split the activation peptide off the N terminal of trypsinogen. This is only speculation at present, but at least it is based on experimental fact and implies that within the pancreas a constant, slow rate of activation of trypsinogen to trypsin goes on and that the secretory trypsin inhibitor is the key to protecting against the accumulation of free trypsin. A transient impairment in synthesis or secretion of the inhibitor or digestion of the inhibitor such as occurs in the presence of calcium ions could set the stage for autodigestion.

SPECIFIC CAUSES OF ACUTE PANCREATITIS

Listed in approximate order of frequency in Table 32–4 are the generally accepted causes of acute pancreatitis. In most of these, the mechanisms for the pancreatitis are not understood. The controversies about the mechanism for *gallstone pancreatitis* do not diminish its paramount importance in the etiology of the disease. *Trauma* due to blunt or penetrating injuries appears to be a simple mechanism, but *how* trauma activates the zymogens is unexplained. One hypothesis incriminates release of lysosomal proteases. Often the

TABLE 32–4 CAUSES OF ACUTE PANCREATITIS

Gallstone disease, with or without common duct stones
Trauma, blunt or penetrating
Postoperative
Peptic ulcer, penetrating into the pancreas
Hyperlipemia, types 1 or 5
Hypercalcemia, especially hyperparathyroidism
Hereditary, with or without aminoaciduria
Drugs (see Table 32–5)
Mumps
Infectious hepatitis
Coxsackievirus B
Mycoplasma pneumoniae
Atheromatous embolism
Vasculitis (systemic lupus, periarteritis nodosa)
Thrombotic thrombocytopenic purpura
Behçet's disease
Primary tumors
Metastatic tumors
Ascariasis of the biliary tree
Scorpion bite
Hypothermia
Idiopathic

pancreatitis is minimal and the patient ends with a pancreatic fistula that drains externally or into a gut lumen.

Pancreatitis after *surgery* usually follows procedures in the region of the gland such as a gastrectomy, but it may occur without obvious trauma to the pancreas or interference with its blood supply. It is a particularly lethal form of pancreatitis. A *peptic ulcer* that penetrates into the pancreas usually causes no more than a localized pancreatitis in the region of the ulcer bed.

Hyperlipoproteinemias types I and V are associated with acute attacks of pancreatitis. Both forms are associated with grossly elevated levels of chylomicrons and very low density lipoproteins. The current hypothesis states that the chylomicrons lodge in the capillaries of the pancreas, where they are digested by pancreatic lipase or by endothelial lipoprotein lipase, releasing fatty acids at such a rapid rate that they exceed the capacity of circulating serum albumin to bind them. Unbound fatty acids somehow damage cell membranes and release enzymes. This theory needs better experimental verification, but it is empirically true that reducing the chylomicron level with a low-fat diet in type I or with insulin in a diabetic with type V hyperlipemia prevents attacks of pancreatitis.

Hyperchylomicronemia may play a role in the pathogenesis of pancreatitis in other patients. As many as 40 per cent of patients with acute pancreatitis have elevated triglyceride levels, and 10 to 20 per cent have grossly milky serum. No relationships with postheparin lipolytic activity (lipoprotein lipase activity) or a circulating inhibitor of liproprotein lipase have been found with the triglyceride levels. All hyperlipemic patients during the acute disease have been found to have lipoprotein electrophoretic patterns that resemble type I or V.

After these patients have recovered and are asymptomatic, they have been studied again, and at this time their fasting triglyceride patterns show type IV or V, occasionally normal patterns, and, rarely, type I or III. Their postheparin lipolytic activities are the same as those in controls. A single load of ethanol or carbohydrate does not increase their serum lipids, but feeding of a meal containing 250 gm of corn oil along with a small amount of carbohydrate and protein shows in almost all these patients a marked increase in plasma triglycerides, and the free fatty acid levels are much higher than normal between 6 and 10 hours after the meal. In two such patients, ingesting the high lipid meal precipitated another attack of pancreatic pain—one in an alcoholic patient, the other in a patient with type V hyperlipemia.

Three criteria must be fulfilled in order to ascertain that an individual has *hereditary pancreatitis:* (1) At least three members of his family must have the disease; (2) painful attacks must be traceable back to childhood; and (3) there should

TABLE 32–5 DRUGS IMPLICATED IN THE ETIOLOGY OF ACUTE PANCREATITIS

Drug	Level of Confidence	Presumed Mechanism
Corticosteroids, ACTH	+ + +	? ductular obstruction by secretions
Synthetic or natural estrogens	+ + +	Hypertrygglyceridemia in type I or V hyperlipemics
Azathioprine	+ + +	?
Thiazide diuretics	+ +	Toxic to mouse acini
Furosemide	+ +	Pancreatic hypersecretion
Ethacrynic acid	+	?
Tetracycline	+ +	Toxic to rat acini
Rifampin	+ +	?
Phenformin	+ +	Only with lactic acidosis
L-asparaginase	+ +	
Cytosine arabinoside	+ +	Follows pancreas injury by L-asparaginase
Pentachlorophenol	+	Mitochondrial injury, many tissues
Organophosphates	+	?
Paracetamol	+	?
Beta-blockers	+	Impair triglyceride clearance
Propoxyphene	+	?
Clonidine	+	?
Salicylate	+	?
Indomethacin	+	?
Warfarin	+	?
Salicylazosulfapyridine	+	?

+ + +   many good cases reports ± animal models
+ +   some fair case reports
+   one or two case reports

be no other definable etiologic factors. It is usual to delete from this classification types I and V hyperlipemia. The renal tubule abnormality that has been associated with a minority of cases of hereditary pancreatitis results in the loss of lysine, cystine, ornithine, and arginine in the urine. The renal tubule absorption of lysine is normally about 99 per cent, but it falls to 90 per cent in patients with this syndrome. There is no evidence in these patients of a basic amino acid absorption defect in the gut as there is in genetic cystinuria. It is postulated that the basic defect in hereditary pancreatitis is some anatomic defect in the ductal system of the pancreas or in the sphincter of Oddi. The occurrence of the aminoaciduria in a few of these patients is not thought to have an etiologic role in the pancreatitis, but simply to be a linked genetic defect to whatever the defect is that results in the pancreatitis.

Many *drugs* (Table 32–5) have been reported as causing acute pancreatitis, but often they have been implicated on the basis of case reports confused by the presence of other drugs. When the case reports are multiple and involve only one drug and when drug challenges are positive, we grade the level of confidence as 3+. When there are more than one or two case reports of reasonable quality, the grade is 2+, and when there are only isolated case reports, the grade is only 1+.

Certain specific *infections* such as mumps and infectious hepatitis as well as those caused by Coxsackie virus B and *Mycoplasma* can involve the pancreas and cause an inflammatory process.

The pancreas receives *atheromatous emboli* from the aorta with a frequency secondary only to that of the kidney. When they lodge in small pancreatic vessels they may elicit localized areas of pancreatitis about them, but they rarely cause diffuse pancreatitis. The end-result is usually pancreatic atrophy and fibrosis. In a similar way, localized pancreatitis can occur with any form of *vasculitis* that obstructs blood flow, such as periarteritis nodosa, systemic lupus erythematosus, Behçet's disease, and thrombotic thrombocytopenic purpura. *Primary tumors,* such as adenocarcinoma of the pancreas, or metastatic tumors such as oat cell carcinoma of the lung can obstruct pancreatic ducts and lead to localized pancreatitis behind the obstruction. *Ascaris lumbricoides,* the roundworm, may migrate up into the biliary radicals from the duodenum and has been associated with acute pancreatitis in adults and children. *Scorpion bite* is a fairly common cause of pancreatitis in Jamaica. The toxin of this arachnid produces an increased pancreatic volume and enzyme secretion and at the same time causes spasm of the sphincter of Oddi. It might be the form of pancreatitis that best supports the obstruction and secretion theory. Lastly, patients have been reported to develop pancreatitis after accidental *hypothermia.* After all possible causes have been considered, 10 to 20 per cent of patients in every series must be called *idiopathic* at our present state of knowledge. There is still room for astute bedside observation to help uncover the causes of these cases.

Conspicuously absent from Table 32–4 is *al-*

coholism as a cause of acute pancreatitis. As we will discuss in greater detail in the section on chronic pancreatitis, alcohol seems to play its role by creating a chronic obstructive disease of the pancreas that eventually results in acute symptoms. The first attack should not be called "acute pancreatitis," but should be called the "first symptomatic episode of chronic pancreatitis." There is little clinical evidence that a human with a normal pancreas who indulges in an alcoholic debauch can suffer acute pancreatitis. The effect of acute alcohol ingestion on a normal individual is to produce transient increases in volume, bicarbonate, and enzyme secretion and then to inhibit pancreatic secretion as the blood alcohol level rises above 100 to 150 mg/dl. There is no evidence that alcohol produces spasm of the sphincter of Oddi.

THE PATHOGENESIS OF CLINICAL FINDINGS IN ACUTE PANCREATITIS

The natural history of acute pancreatitis varies with its etiology. Patients who have chronic alcoholic pancreatitis tend to have severe first episodes and less severe episodes thereafter. The mortality rate associated with alcoholic pancreatitis in most countries is less than that related to gallstone pancreatitis.

Since typical acute pancreatitis is associated with gallstones, we will use this as the model for the natural history of acute pancreatitis. The pathologic forms are (1) pancreatic edema; (2) edema and disseminated foci of necrosis; (3) widespread necrosis, hemorrhage, fat necrosis but intact capsule and a relatively intact central core of tissue; and (4) total necrosis and capsular rupture, with necrosis spreading outside the gland. As a general rule, the pathologic changes in the pancreas are a function of the duration of the acute pancreatitis. For example, patients who die within the first week usually show pancreatic edema and some fat necrosis. During the second week, the gland shows an increase in the amount of necrosis, hemorrhage, and fat necrosis. Severe necrosis and autodigestion of the gland and its surrounding tissues usually are not seen until the third week, and by then (or later) abscess formation is common. All of this is consistent with an ongoing autodigestive process that progresses until a complication develops that finally kills the patient. Those who die within the first 14 days of the disease (75 per cent) usually die with irreversible shock, yet the changes in the gland may be quite minimal, showing only pancreatic edema. This suggests that even though fluid replacement is adequate, shock persists, causing many observers to believe that some hypotensive factors are produced in acute pancreatitis. The late deaths (25 per cent) occur because of complications of the pancreatitis and deterioration of the patient's nutrition.

The risk factors that make pancreatitis more

lethal are older age (over 60 years), coincident cardiovascular disease, and pre-existing diabetes mellitus. The physical findings with the worst prognostic import are persisting lack of peristalsis (ileus), the appearance of a mass, and Grey Turner's sign. The latter is the appearance of bluish-brown discoloration in the flanks due to retroperitoneal hemorrhage dissecting out subcutaneously between the muscle layers.

The complications of this disease that lead to late death are pseudocyst formation, abscess formation, duodenal obstruction due to ileus, gastroduodenal ulcerations, and pulmonary failure.

Evidence that persisting autodigestion leads to the late complications and mortality in this disease has come from autopsy findings in patients in the fourth to fourteenth week after onset of illness in which areas of relatively normal pancreas have been found in a sea of necrotic material, the normal tissue being connected with large areas of autodigestion retroperitoneally. This suggests that the remaining functioning pancreas is now a source of great danger to the patient. The patient theoretically would be better off if all functioning and necrotic pancreas could be removed at the time the collections of debris are drained. Studies are underway to evaluate this surgical approach. Generally speaking, surgery is avoided in acute pancreatitis unless the diagnosis is in doubt. If the patient has an acute abdominal syndrome with an elevated amylase, it may be due to acute cholecystitis, a perforated ulcer of the anterior duodenal wall, or intestinal obstruction with strangulation, all of which can lead to increased serum amylase activities. To allow a patient to go untreated surgically with a perforated or ischemic gut may be fatal. Therefore, any patient in whom the diagnosis of acute pancreatitis is not secure should undergo a diagnostic laparotomy to settle the diagnosis and to repair other lesions. The mortality in a simple exploration of a patient was not greater than that of no laparotomy in some rather poorly controlled studies.

It should also be remembered that in acute pancreatitis about 25 per cent of the patients develop *jaundice*, but only 10 per cent have their jaundice on the basis of obstruction of the common duct. Only 2 to 3 per cent have obstruction due to stones. The rest are obstructed by swelling of the head of the pancreas, compressing the common duct. The 15 per cent who have nonobstructive jaundice have some cholestatic form of liver disease, usually alcoholic. In these latter two situations surgical drainage would not be helpful. Abscesses that arise within or outside the pancreas are usually infected by bowel organisms, commonly *Escherichia coli,* other gram-negative organisms, sometimes anaerobic bacteria, and occasionally *Staphylococcus aureus.* There is no evidence from controlled studies that treatment with antibiotics from the beginning improves survival or reduces morbidity, but once infection is established aggressive treatment with antibiotics is important. Unfortunately, proof of secondary infection often requires positive blood cultures or radiographic signs showing evidence of gas formation in the retroperitoneal area by gas-forming organisms. The only effective treatment for an abscess is surgical drainage.

Follow-up studies in patients with acute pancreatitis due to gallstone disease indicate that if they do not have the gallstones removed they are likely to have recurrences of acute pancreatitis. Those whose gallstones are removed, leaving none behind in the common duct, are cured of recurrent attacks of pancreatitis in 95 per cent of cases. Recurrence of pancreatitis after gallstone surgery is a good indication that stones have been left behind in the common duct. There is very little evidence in follow-up studies that patients with acute gallstone pancreatitis, even after a number of attacks, develop chronic pancreatitis. The pancreas, although severely damaged by an attack of acute pancreatitis, has the ability to regenerate by hypertrophy and hyperplasia. Many patients with abnormal pancreatic function in the post-acute stage have returned to normal function after 1 to 3 months. It is therefore extremely important that any patient with acute pancreatitis have gallstone disease ruled in or out and treated definitively. It is a medical tragedy to suffer recurrent and possibly lethal pancreatitis because of neglect to remove gallstones.

The mechanism of *disseminated fat necrosis* has never been defined. The usual hypothesis states that lipase or phospholipase is released into the blood stream and travels to the peripheral tissues, where it digests triglycerides and phospholipids. However, the bile salts necessary to activate phospholipase A or the emulsifying agents required to break up triglycerides into tiny droplets so that lipase can act are not present in the periphery. One possible mechanism by which the enzymes reach the periphery is that they may be carried by white cells inside their granules, the enzymes having been taken up into granules by endocytosis. Another hypothesis suggests that the lipase of the adipose tissue is being activated by something released during acute pancreatitis, since glucose plus insulin will prevent disseminated fat necrosis in the epididymal fat pad of a rat with acute pancreatitis.

Another complication of acute pancreatitis is *pancreatic ascites*. This occurs in both acute and chronic pancreatitis and is almost always due to a rupture in the substance of the pancreas so that pancreatic secretions escape into the peritoneal cavity. This results in 85 per cent of cases from leakage from a pancreatic pseudocyst that still connects to the ductal system. Most of the patients in whom this has been described have had chronic pancreatitis due to alcoholism. Pancreatic ascites can occur after an attack of pancreatitis or as a presenting symptom, coming on insidiously. The patient is plagued with increasing abdominal girth, weight loss, and varying amounts of abdominal pain. The ascites usually is massive. Such patients often have erythema nodosa or other signs of subcutaneous fat necrosis. The ascitic fluid contains very high levels of amylase and lipase, averaging 20,000 Somogyi units/dl of amylase. The protein content is usually greater than 3 gm/100 dl. The clinical picture is such that many patients are thought to have cirrhosis of the liver with ascites. At laparotomy, fat necrosis is infrequent; in most cases only chronic inflammation is found in the peritoneum. The fluid usually is serous or serosanguinous, occasionally turbid, and rarely chylous. Other causes of ascites must be excluded, including cancer, cirrhosis, and tuberculous peritonitis. In none of these is the amylase or lipase activity as high as in pancreatic ascites. One way of determining preoperatively the source of the leak is to perform ERCP, which often demonstrates the area of the leak and allows the surgeon to plan his procedure. Since ERCP may cause sepsis when an obstructed pancreatic ductal system or pseudocyst is entered, the surgeon should be ready to perform immediate surgery when ERCP is done in a patient with pancreatic ascites. The cause of the fluid accumulation is not understood. The fluid is not all pancreatic exocrine secretion; it is partly an exudate due to the action of the pancreatic enzymes on the peritoneal surface. Sometimes with parenteral hyperalimentation, resting of the pancreas, and removal of the ascitic fluid the problem will resolve on its own. When this does not occur, surgical correction of the problem is necessary. The ascitic fluid contains no bilirubin unless jaundice occurs and shows no bacteria on Gram stain. The differential points between this fluid and that in a perforated ulcer, mesenteric vascular obstruction, or strangulation-obstruction is that in these cases bacteria can often be seen on Gram stain, and in a perforated ulcer bilirubin appears in the fluid. The amylase activity of ascites can be elevated in infarcted or perforated bowel, so this is not a diagnostic differential point. Flecks of digested fat sometimes can be seen in the ascites of acute pancreatitis. The finding of an elevated amylase activity in pleural fluid is, however, much more specific for acute pancreatitis. It apparently reaches the pleural cavity via lymphatic connections.

The possibility that vasoactive peptides are being released into the peritoneal cavity in acute pancreatitis led to therapy by peritoneal dialysis. In various partly controlled studies, blood pressure returned to normal and noncardiac pulmonary edema and renal failure improved with this type of treatment. Bovine glandular trypsin-kallikrein inhibitor (aprotinin, Trasylol) has been given intravenously to treat severe cases of pancreatitis, but without consistent effects on survival rates or other signs of improvement. This small peptide is excreted very rapidly by the kidneys, and high plasma levels are difficult to achieve. Glucagon, which suppresses pancreatic function, has failed to help in controlled trials. Although autodigestion seems to be critical in the pathogenesis of pancreatitis, at the present time we have no therapy capable of blocking either the proteases or the lipases once they become active within the pancreas and surrounding tissues.

In an American series of pancreatitis cases, primarily alcoholic, 60 per cent of patients developed respiratory problems, with 20 per cent having acute respiratory failure; 20 per cent developed renal failure; and 20 per cent developed other complications. Studies of patients with shock and acute pancreatitis indicate that it is primarily due to a critical reduction in plasma volume. Large volumes of colloid and crystalloid restored hemodynamic findings to normal in most patients. It is in those who are resistant to volume that bradykinin or other hypotensive peptides may be playing a role. The volume needs may be as great as 6 liters in the first 24 hours. There is good evidence for activation of the complement system by trypsin bound to α_2-macroglobulin, with low C_3 levels found in the plasma of one third of patients. In ascitic fluid, complete C_3 cleavage is the rule. The products of further complement protein cleavages by C_{3a} release anaphylatoxins, which in turn release histamine and chemotactic factors.

Another problem rarely encountered in acute pancreatitis is that of excessive *bleeding* and *clotting*. During the acute attack it is not unusual for thrombosis to occur in the large veins about the pancreas, such as in the splenic vein. Occasionally, diffuse clotting occurs, and in a rare number of patients disseminated intravascular coagulation (DIC) results in diffuse bleeding. When patients have been followed serially with a number of clotting parameters during acute pancreatitis, DIC is actually rare. Some patients show an increase in fibrin split products or show a positive ethanol gel test for fibrinolysis, but rarely does full-blown DIC occur with decreased platelet counts, decreased fibrinogen levels, and prolonged prothrombin or thrombin times. In spite of the fact that trypsin can activate factors 2 and 11 and can digest fibrinogen and fibrin, thereby precipitating clotting or bleeding, the problem of DIC is surprisingly infrequent clinically. As a model of blood clotting problems in pancreatitis, low concentrations of trypsin given intravenously to animals led to clotting, and high concentrations led to uncoagulable blood. Thrombin is formed at low doses of trypsin, and fibrinogen is degraded at high doses. The prothrombin activation cannot be blocked by the plasma trypsin inhibitors. Trypsin can activate factor 11 (PTA) directly without the mediation of factor 12.

The adult *respiratory distress syndrome*, also called *noncardiac pulmonary edema*, is one of the most serious complications of acute pancreatitis. It is associated with a decreased compliance and a

decreasing arterial P_{O_2}. It is due to accumulation of interstitial edema fluid, which eventually breaks out into the alveoli. The factors in acute pancreatitis that cause increased permeability of the pulmonary capillaries are not known. The usual speculation is that pancreatic lipases and proteases enter the blood and digest the membranes of the pulmonary capillaries, but there is no proof for these theories. The end result is a severe pulmonary edema, which results in decreased gas exchange, shunting of blood to unventilated segments, and a decreased P_{O_2} with a normal P_{CO_2}. In addition, there is almost always atelectasis, which is postulated as being due to decreased surfactant in the alveoli. The surfactant, a phospholipid, is thought to be destroyed by phospholipase A. Finally, pleural effusions occur on both sides as a result of the subdiaphragmatic inflammatory process.

Another major complication of acute pancreatitis is *pseudocysts*. A pseudocyst is defined as a collection of fluid and necrotic debris surrounded or walled-off by peritoneal membranes or by a fibrous pseudocapsule. It results from active enzymes escaping into surrounding tissues, usually through breaks in the capsule of the pancreas. These can occur in the lesser sac, anywhere in the retroperitoneum, or between the leaves of the mesentery. When the ductal system dilates within the substance of the pancreas, it is a true or retention cyst. When these retention cysts or pseudocysts become infected, they then are described as abscesses. Since the advent of ultrasonography, it has been apparent that many patients with acute pancreatitis develop pseudocysts. Eighty per cent of these cystic collections resolve in 2 weeks, according to ultrasonographic evaluation. Those that do not resolve may cause complications. As they expand they press on adjacent tissues, resulting in pain, compression of the common bile duct and jaundice, thrombosis of the portal or splenic vein, or even gastric outlet obstruction. If a pseudocyst ruptures suddenly into the peritoneal cavity, it causes a shocklike state in the patient. In one series, the mortality rate associated with rupture was 14 per cent. Chronic leakage usually results in pancreatic ascites. Cysts may erode through the diaphragm and rupture into the thorax, leading to pleural effusion, chylothorax, or a pleural abscess. One of the most severe complications is hemorrhage into the cyst due to erosion of an arterial vessel in the wall. Management of hemorrhage is most difficult. Some have been treated by infusion of vasopressin into the surrounding vessels. Surgical drainage is often unsuccessful in the acute stage when the wall is friable. After 6 weeks, pseudocysts develop a thick fibrous capsule that allows an anastomosis with the intestinal tract for internal drainage. If they are drained after 6 weeks when a good capsule is formed, the mortality rate is 9 per cent. If attempts are made to drain them in the acute stage, the mortality rate is quite high—as great as 60 per cent. According to controlled studies, there is no evidence that prophylactic antibiotics prevent infection of necrotic collections, nor do they prevent the infection of pseudocysts. Once infection does occur, early drainage of the infected cyst or abscess is critical to the patient's survival.

The pancreas often is injured during upper abdominal trauma, such as penetrating wounds due to a knife, a bullet, or shotgun pellets or blunt injury due to forceful contact with a steering wheel. The pancreas is especially susceptible to crushing injury against the unyielding vertebral bodies. The mortality rate with trauma to the upper abdomen varies with the mode of injury. In one series, the mortality rate associated with stab wounds was 8 per cent; with gunshot wounds, 25 per cent; with shotgun injuries, 60 per cent; and with steering wheel injuries, 50 per cent. Injuries involving the head of the pancreas are more severe than those in the body or tail (i.e., 28 per cent versus 16 per cent mortality, respectively) because injuries to the head often involve the liver, duodenum, bile duct, major vessels, and colon. Penetrating trauma usually damages other organs, whereas in blunt trauma one third of cases involve isolated damage to the pancreas. Injury to the pancreas alone rarely kills, but it often results in complications and morbidity. For example, in blunt injury to the pancreas, pseudocysts appear in 33 per cent of cases. When this occurs, the mortality is 20 per cent, and the complication rate is 37 per cent. The major complications are a fistula, which results from the opening up of the ductal system, and abscess formation, which occurs later. After blunt injury, there may be a delay in development of symptoms of hours to days. One way of detecting damage early is peritoneal lavage and assay of pancreatic enzymes. A decision not to explore such patients surgically requires a radiologic study with swallowed contrast material (Gastrografin) to prove that there has not been a breach in the integrity of the intestinal lumen. The optimal management at the present time seems to be immediate surgery and removal, not drainage, of the damaged pancreas and anastomosis of the remaining functioning pancreas to a small bowel loop. This allows the pancreatic juice to drain into the intestine, where it belongs, and removes the contused, damaged gland, which often is the site of pancreatitis and fistula or cyst formation. When first operating after blunt trauma, the surgeon sees an edematous pancreas with patchy hemorrhage. It is difficult to decide whether to resect injured areas. Postoperatively, 30 per cent of these patients will develop a fistula, acute pancreatitis, or a pseudocyst. It is interesting that, in spite of a severe crushing injury to the pancreas, diffuse acute pancreatitis is relatively uncommon, testifying to the effective protective mechanisms against autodigestion in a normal gland.

Ranson has identified 11 early prognostic findings that predict an increased risk of death or complications in acute pancreatitis. At admission, patients are over 55 years of age, and they have a white blood cell count over 16,000/mm³, blood glucose over 200 mg/dl, serum lactic dehydrogenase (LDH) over 350 IU/L, or serum glutamic oxaloacetic transaminase (GOT) over 250 Sigma U/dl. During the initial 48 hours, the following findings are serious: hematocrit fall greater than 10 per cent, blood urea nitrogen increase greater than 5 mg/dl, serum calcium below 8 mg/dl, arterial Po_2 below 60 mm Hg, base deficit above 4 mEq/L, or estimated fluid sequestration above 6000 ml. The fewer previous episodes, the worse the prognosis. The mortality rate with fewer than three of these 11 findings was 1 per cent; with 3 to 4, 18 per cent; with 5 to 6, 50 per cent; and with 7 to 9, 90 per cent. The white cell count reflects extent of inflammation; the serum enzymes, extent of tissue damage; blood glucose, extent of islet cell damage plus stress hormones; and Po_2, extent of pulmonary complications. The rise in BUN reflects the blood volume deficit as do the acidosis and fluid replacement needs. The other findings are discussed subsequently. Discriminant analysis of these variables in 300 cases showed that the aforementioned admission variables plus the number of previous episodes predicted severity in 89 per cent of cases. Nine variables at 48 hours (age, glucose, LDH, GOT, previous episodes, hematocrit increase, serum calcium Po_2, and fluid sequestration) predicted severity in 96 per cent of cases.

PATHOGENESIS OF LABORATORY FINDINGS IN PANCREATITIS

The laboratory findings are characteristic in most surviving patients, and not finding the usual pattern may have serious prognostic implications. For example, the serum amylase, which is elevated at the onset, falls rapidly within the first few days, regardless of whether the disease process is mild or severe. The serum and urinary amylase tests are useful as diagnostic tools but have no relation to prognosis unless a late rise or a persistent elevation of the amylase occurs, suggesting pseudocyst formation. The use of serum amylase assays can be made much more specific by doing a pancreatic isoamylase determination on every elevated total amylase activity. This will eliminate the false-positive results due to salivary amylase elevations.

The hematocrit is usually elevated on admission because of loss of plasma from the intravascular space. When the plasma volume is repleted and the hematocrit falls below normal, it means that bleeding has occurred within or around the pancreas or into the gastrointestinal tract from erosions. The white count is usually elevated between 10,000 and 20,000 on admission and falls slowly as the patient improves. A white count that remains elevated or rises again is evidence that severe pancreatitis or a septic complication has occurred.

The appearance in serum of methemalbumin has been proposed as a test for digestion of blood and therefore a clue to the transition from edematous to hemorrhagic pancreatitis. When hemorrhage occurs in or around the pancreas, blood is digested, ferroheme is split from the globin by pancreatic enzymes, and the heme is oxidized to ferriheme or metheme. Metheme binds both to albumin to form methemalbumin and to a protein called *hemopexin*. Methemalbumin can be measured in serum by a number of methods, and its presence is always abnormal. It is not specific for pancreatitis, however, as it is seen in other situations in which blood is being digested by enzymes of white cells or macrophages, as in a large hematoma, or in which blood is being digested in the wall of the bowel, as in strangulation-obstruction, or in which hemoglobin is being released in large amounts by hemolysis. The differentiation between hemolysis and pancreatitis as a source of methemalbumin can be made because in hemolysis the hemoglobin released binds to the serum protein, haptoglobin, and the complex is removed, leading to a low serum haptoglobin level. In acute pancreatitis, the haptoglobin usually is elevated as an acute phase reactant. Experience with this test over a period of years has indicated that it is not reliable for hemorrhagic pancreatitis, as it has provided false-negative results in proved cases. The most important false-positive situation is in gut necrosis, in which the finding of methemalbumin may mislead the physician away from exploratory surgery.

Hyperglycemia is observed commonly in patients undergoing their first attack of pancreatitis, and they may develop or present with diabetic ketoacidosis. The serum insulin levels are inappropriately low for the level of blood sugar. Plasma glucagon levels are markedly elevated compared with those of patients undergoing stress for other reasons. This low insulin:glucagon ratio, plus elevated blood catecholamine and cortisol levels, appears to account for the hyperglycemia. Almost always the diabetes of acute pancreatitis is transient, unless chronic alcoholic pancreatitis has permanently damaged the islets.

Among patients with severe acute pancreatitis, up to 30 per cent have a serum calcium that falls below 8.5 mg/dl, the lower limits of normal. The calcium begins to fall within 1 or 2 days of onset, reaches its nadir at about 5 to 7 days, and then usually returns to normal. A number of studies have indicated that a low total calcium is a bad prognostic sign associated with high mortality. One of the problems in the interpretation of the low serum calcium is that approximately 50 per cent of calcium is protein bound in the plasma and there is frequently a decrease in serum albu-

min during the course of acute pancreatitis. In addition, many of these patients never show signs of tetany or of a decreased *ionized* calcium. Therefore, the crucial question has been whether there is a decrease in serum ionized calcium, and, if so, what the mechanism for this might be. When the pancreatic and peripancreatic tissues were analyzed in patients dying of acute pancreatitis, a considerable amount of calcium was present as calcium soaps in the areas of fat necrosis. The total calcium in fat was 1 to 2 gm and was considered to be the explanation for the early fall in serum calcium. However, other states associated with a falling ionized calcium set off parathyroid hormone secretion and mobilization of calcium from bone. Why does this not happen in acute pancreatitis and why does a prolonged period of low ionized calcium occur in some patients?

Glucagon levels are increased in severe acute pancreatitis, and glucagon can increase serum urinary calcium excretion and decrease serum calcium in animals to a small extent after large doses. Glucagon might be releasing calcitonin, although calcitonin's role in reducing serum calcium in humans is not clear. Glucagon in large doses decreased the serum calcium in dogs only about 0.4 mg/dl. Parathyroid extract increased both the serum calcium and magnesium in humans and dogs with acute pancreatitis. Understanding of the problem had to await the development of radioimmunoassays for many of these hormones. In 1976, Robertson at the Medical College of Virginia studied patients with severe relapses of chronic alcoholic pancreatitis. In these patients, the serum glucose, radioimmunogastrin, serum magnesium, and tubular reabsorption of phosphate all were normal. The albumin concentration fell from a normal average of 4.5 to 3.6 gm/dl, and the serum phosphate fell from a normal of 3.6 to 2.4 mg/dl. The ionized calcium measured with an ion electrode fell from a normal range of 1.10 to 1.22 mM to 0.9 to 1.05 mM in all the patients, even though the total serum calcium was still normal in two of these patients. In many of these patients the glucagon and calcitonin levels were increased, but there was no correlation between the ionized calcium and the calcitonin levels. Glucagon given in a large dose of 1 mg parenterally to these patients caused no change in the serum calcium. Parathyroid hormone levels were measured with a radioimmunoassay sensitive to the carboxyl-terminal end of the peptide and might have reacted with biologically inactive fragments. All but one of the patients had low parathormone levels, whereas in a group of patients with chronic hypocalcemia due to other conditions, most had an elevated parathormone level. The administration of a large dose of parathormone increased the serum calcium in these patients and increased urinary cAMP secretion; moreover, basal cAMP activity was higher than normal. This study shows that there was an inappropriately low parathyroid hormone response for the reduction in serum ionized calcium, that there was no evidence of failure of the kidney to respond to PTH, and there was no evidence that bone was responding to the PTH available. Other studies have shown that the parathormone level by a different assay was elevated in six of 11 patients; calcitonin was low in seven of 11; ionized calcium was low to low-normal; the total calcium, magnesium, and phosphorus were low to low-normal; gastrin levels were normal; and glucagon levels usually were increased two- to fourfold.

Studies from England with another parathormone assay in a large number of patients showed that some with severe pancreatitis have a markedly elevated parathormone level, which falls to the normal range in 4 or 5 days, whereas another group of patients with severe cases showed a low PTH level throughout. The tubular reabsorption of phosphate and the serum phosphate were low, suggesting renal responsiveness to parathormone. The albumin usually was low, but the ionized calcium in this series was rarely decreased. The best conclusion from these conflicting studies seems to be that parathormone secretion in some patients with acute pancreatitis is inappropriately low considering the decrease in serum ionized calcium. The initial decrease in serum calcium probably does relate to sequestration of calcium as soaps in and about the pancreas, but thereafter the persistent hypocalcemia in some patients is not explained. Probably the problem has been overemphasized, since ionized calcium is rarely measured and total calcium depends greatly on the albumin concentration. Lack of bone response to parathormone could be due to resistance to parathormone resulting from magnesium deficiency or vitamin D deficiency, but there is little evidence for either. One source of confusion is that different antisera to parathormone measure different parts of the molecule and do not necessarily correlate with biologic activity. From a clinical point of view, the important fact is that patients who develop a low serum ionized calcium have a poor prognosis, but there is no evidence that treating the calcium, which is relatively easy to do, is going to restore these patients to a good prognosis. It is mostly an index of severity of the disease process.

CHRONIC PANCREATITIS

The different clinical types of pancreatic inflammatory disease were delimited as follows by a panel of experts in Marseilles, France in 1962: (1) acute pancreatitis; (2) recurrent acute pancreatitis; (3) chronic relapsing pancreatitis; and (4) chronic (persistent) pancreatitis. The clinical differentiation between acute and chronic disease was based on the presence of continuing pancreatic dysfunction after the acute attack was over. After recovery, pancreatic function tests in patients with acute or recurrent acute pancreatitis return to normal, whereas patients who have chronic pancreatitis have persisting abnormalities of function. Chronic relapsing pancreatitis is the familiar syndrome in which recurrent attacks of pain are experienced at weekly to monthly intervals. The term *chronic pancreatitis* describes the condition seen in patients who experience daily episodes or constant pain; it also describes the disease in a small group of patients, 10 per cent of the total, who have no pain but who show progressive loss of function that eventually results in exocrine pancreatic insufficiency. This latter type is more precisely called *chronic persistent pancreatitis* to contrast with the relapsing form.

PATHOLOGY OF CHRONIC PANCREATITIS

Classification of pancreatitis can also be done on the basis of gross and microscopic pathology. The commonest type of chronic pancreatitis is calcifying pancreatitis, which is quite distinct from the pancreatitis that occurs secondary to obstruction of the main pancreatic duct by a slowly growing cancer. The first characteristic of calcific pancreatitis is patchy lobular distribution of lesions. An affected lobule can be surrounded by normal ones, and even at advanced stages of the disease some more or less intact lobules persist. Within the affected lobule, the following features are seen: (1) dilatation of the acini, leading to the formation of rounded cavities surrounded by atrophic cuboidal epithelium; (2) atrophy of the ductal epithelium; (3) eosinophilic protein plugs within the ductal lumina that subsequently calcify; these plugs consist of precipitated pancreatic zymogens and enzymes, often with calcium coprecipitated; (4) perilobular and intralobular fibrosis; and (5) perineural inflammation and fibrosis. In the beginning, the main pancreatic duct of Wirsung is normal, but later it may become dilated if calculi accumulate in the head of the gland or stenosis occurs near the ampulla of Vater, leading to generalized ductal dilatation. Part of the dilatation also may result from loss of surrounding parenchymal tissue and fibrotic retraction. The protein plugs or stones that occur in the small ducts precede the large ductal calculi. This pathology of calcifying pancreatitis is found associated with certain conditions: (1) chronic alcoholic pancreatitis, (2) idiopathic chronic pancreatitis, (3) familial pancreatitis, (4) chronic pancreatitis in regions in which protein-calorie malnutrition is prevalent, and (5) chronic pancreatitis in cases of hyperparathyroidism. On a cellular basis, in early calcifying pancreatitis there is an increase in the number of prozymogen granules and a decrease in the number of mature zymogen granules. The rough endoplasmic reticulum and Golgi apparatus are dilated. These findings are consistent with hyperfunction of the acinar cells.

During an acute attack of relapsing pancreatitis, the gross findings at surgery are pancreatic and peripancreatic edema, variable amounts of fat necrosis, and, rarely, some hemorrhage and necrosis. The lesion usually is patchy at the beginning. As the disease progresses, the normal elasticity of the gland is lost and it becomes hard, even woody, to palpation. The lobular architecture is lost in affected areas. On section, the tissue is firm and pale and does not bleed much, reflecting the increased fibrosis. Healthy areas of parenchyma can be seen surrounded by fibrosis. The surface is marked by the presence of sacculations, which are dilated ducts. The disease can be quite severe and yet show little effect on the main ductal system. Large ductal cysts may develop that contain proteinaceous or calcified precipitates identical with those seen in the small ducts. The calculi consist primarily of protein and calcium carbonate and may grow to be as large as 200 gm. Retention cysts are ductal sacs containing cloudy or bloody fluid. They communicate with the ductal system and usually are found in the head or neck of the pancreas, where they may obstruct the main duct. These rarely become infected.

The pathology of chronic pancreatitis involves the common bile duct secondarily and leads to stenosis of the intrapancreatic course of the bile duct. Other pathologic consequences are compression and, sometimes, thrombosis of the splenic vein with splenic enlargement. Rarely, migratory thrombophlebitis in peripheral veins is present in chronic pancreatitis. Pleural effusions and ascites are also rare complications. The ascites may be chylous owing to obstruction of lymphatics in the retroperitoneum. Disseminated fat necrosis is a rare but puzzling complication of chronic pancreatitis. Subcutaneous fat necrosis resembles erythema nodosum or Weber-Christian disease. The joints may be involved by a periarticular inflammation, mimicking gout or rheumatoid arthritis. Punched-out areas of bone loss or linear calcifications in the medullary cavities of the long bones may be seen. The frequency of cancer of the pancreas is increased in chronic pancreatitis; in some series, as high an incidence as 2 per cent has been recorded, whereas the overall incidence in white males is 0.01 per cent.

In areas involved with acute exacerbations, edema, necrosis, hemorrhage, and fat necrosis can be seen microscopically. Polymorphonuclear leukocytes and plasma cells are not seen frequently; lymphocytes and fibroblasts predominate. The nerves become involved in this chronic inflammatory, sclerosing process, and this may account for the severe pain. The islets of Langerhans tend to be spared, appearing as islands in a sea of fibrosis without any exocrine cells remaining.

There are two patterns of calculus deposits in the pancreas. One is associated with heavy alcohol ingestion, and the calculi are small, diffuse, and spread throughout the gland, with some larger calculi in the ductal systems. Another group of patients who do not have alcohol as an etiologic factor have large calculi that usually are found in the head and body of the gland. These larger calculi are frequent in females, sometimes with a familial incidence. They may be related in some cases to malnutrition or primary hyperparathyroidism. Therefore, chronic calcifying pancreatitis is not always a sign of alcoholism.

Nonspecific ductular ectasia is seen in a number of chronic wasting diseases, such as uremia, and is not a specific lesion for the pancreas. The initial change is proliferation, or hyperplasia, of centroacinar and intercalated ductal cells. Later, there is swelling of these hyperplastic cells, some necrosis, and atrophy leading to ductular dilatation. It is a common, nonspecific lesion that is possibly due to inspissation of secretory protein.

Another form of chronic pancreatic degeneration not related to alcoholism is that due to atheromatous embolization. The pancreas is often involved by emboli of cholesterol and lipid material from an atheromatous aorta or other large vessels, third only in frequency to involvement of the kidney and spleen. It is characterized by cholesterol clefts in the thrombosed vessels. As a result, focal atrophy and fibrosis can result in the areas of ischemia. Rarely, an inflammatory process of pancreatitis may be generated. Some individuals have been found to have enough destruction of the pancreas to result in pancreatic exocrine insufficiency. Hemochromatosis also leads to fibrosis and atrophy of the exocrine pancreas as well as the islets of Langerhans.

EFFECTS OF ETHANOL ON PANCREATIC SECRETION OF NORMAL INDIVIDUALS AND OF PATIENTS WITH CHRONIC PANCREATITIS

Because the commonest etiology of chronic pancreatitis world-wide is alcohol abuse, the effects of alcohol on the pancreas of humans and animals deserve review. The major contributor to these studies is Henri Sarles and his group from Marseilles, France. The general conclusions that have emerged from these studies are as follows:

(1) Intravenous ethanol sufficient to elevate the blood alcohol level to 100 mg/dl or above causes a decrease in the *outputs* of bicarbonate, enzymes, and bile salts into the duodenum. This inhibition occurs in normal controls and in patients with chronic alcoholic pancreatitis. Since volume of juice is not reduced much, the concentrations of solutes are also decreased, enzymes more than bicarbonate. A jejunal infusion that raises the blood alcohol to this level accomplishes the same effect. Inhibition by intravenous alcohol can be

blocked by atropine, suggesting that it is mediated by the vagus.

(2) An intragastric ethanol meal stimulates secretion of gastric acid by a cholinergic mechanism and by release of gastrin. Radioimmunoassays of secretin confirm the rise after *oral* ethanol, but there is no secretin release when the ethanol is placed in the duodenum, confirming that it is the HCl that releases the secretin. Oral ethanol also increases plasma radioimmunogastrin levels by a small amount, but duodenal alcohol does not increase gastrin release.

THE PATHOGENESIS OF ALCOHOLIC PANCREATITIS

The clinical history underlying chronic alcoholic pancreatitis in humans is similar to the conditions required to produce lesions in the animal models. First, the intake of alcohol must be at a moderate level for a long period of time. The diagnosis of chronic pancreatitis occurs at an average age of 38 years in subjects with an average daily consumption of 200 ml/day, which equals a pint of 80 proof liquor, 2 liters of wine, or 4 quarts of beer. In Marseilles, surveys of chronic pancreatitis patients showed that prior to onset of pain they ingested an average of 180 gm of alcohol per day compared with controls without the disease who drank an average of 70 gm/day. There are strong differences in individual susceptibility, however. Some develop the disease on 50 gm/day, and some escape it on 300 gm/day. Duration of ingestion is an important variable: The average duration before the first symptom appeared was 11 ± 18 years for men and 8 ± 11 for women in Marseilles, with a minimum of 1 year. Thus, heavy social drinkers who do not meet current definitions of alcohol addiction can develop chronic pancreatitis. Only 7 per cent had a painless course. The first attack was similar to acute pancreatitis, although autopsy studies in patients who died showed established lesions of chronic pancreatitis as well as acute autodigestion. The average age of onset of acute pancreatitis due to gallstones and other causes was 51 years, which is evidence against recurrent acute attacks causing chronic pancreatitis.

Protein plugs similar to those seen in animals appear in the pancreatic juice of the patients with chronic alcoholic pancreatitis when at surgery a polyvinyl drainage tube is left in the main pancreatic duct. In humans, these plugs are also made up of precipitated pancreatic enzymes. The hypothesis has therefore been proposed by Sarles that chronic alcohol ingestion superimposed on a diet rich in proteins and lipids results in secretion of a pancreatic juice high in protein and that the enzymes tend to precipitate out in the ductal system.

Lactoferrin is an iron-containing protein present in human milk, in a wide variety of exocrine secretions, and in specific granules of neutrophilic leukocytes. It resembles transferrin and binds two atoms of iron per molecule. Its physiologic role is not known. Lactoferrin has been identified in a very low concentration in normal human pancreatic juice by radioimmunoassay, but its concentration is much higher in patients with chronic pancreatitis. The lactoferrin in pancreatic juice probably is not derived from the plasma, where it is also found, but seems to be secreted by acinar cells of the pancreas. The concentration in the juice rises after injection of cholecystokinin. Lactoferrin is regarded as a rather specific marker of chronic pancreatitis.

When the protein precipitates are dissolved and analyzed, besides the usual pancreatic juice proteins, two or three other proteins are found in the citrate-solubilized fraction. One of these "stone proteins" has a molecular weight of 13,500 and a high content of aspartic and glutamic acids, which give it four binding sites for calcium. This secretory glycoprotein has been named *pancreolithin* and seems to serve as the matrix of pancreatic ductal calculi.

About 10 per cent of patients with relapses of alcoholic pancreatitis are found to have lactescent serum (i.e., serum with triglyceride concentrations above 300 to 400 mg/dl). Feeding these patients a high-fat meal elevated their serum triglycerides above 500 mg/dl and occasionally precipitated an attack of pain. Cameron postulates that certain alcoholics have an underlying hyperlipemic trait and that a fatty meal or alcohol can acutely increase the triglyceride level. Infusing an isolated dog pancreas with triglyceride caused it to swell and release enzymes into the blood. The pancreas of an alcoholic already has many areas of ductal obstruction and regurgitates lipase and procolipase during fat ingestion. This theory attributes cell membrane damage to fatty acid release, but how trypsinogen is activated to trypsin, which is necessary to release colipase, is unexplained.

OTHER CAUSES OF CHRONIC PANCREATITIS

Hypercalcemia, as occurs in hyperparathyroidism, vitamin D intoxication, multiple myeloma, sarcoidosis, and milk-alkali syndrome, has been associated with calcifying chronic pancreatitis. Total calcium in pancreatic juice is the sum of ionized Ca^{++}, protein-bound calcium, and complexes of $CaHCO_3{}^+$ and $CaCO_3$. Basal secretion in dogs is usually supersaturated. In patients with chronic alcoholic pancreatitis, the basal concentration of calcium in the juice is higher than normal, and after secretin stimulation the concentration increases even further. It appears likely that the solubility of $CaCO_3$ can be exceeded in human juice and lead to coprecipitation with proteins.

Hereditary pancreatitis can present over an age range of 11 months to 61 years. The average age of onset is 11 years, and the average age at the time of diagnosis is 31 years. Most patients have an Anglo-Saxon background, but some cases have been reported from Japan. The mode of inheritance is autosomal dominant with incomplete penetrance. An increased incidence of pancreatic calcification and pancreatic carcinoma among affected individuals has been reported. The incidence of carcinoma in one series was 21 per cent within these kindred.

Malnutrition also can result in a form of pancreatic exocrine failure, but not a true inflammatory lesion. Studies on the pathology of kwashiorkor indicate that patients who die with the disease show atrophy of the acinar cells, dilatation of the ducts, fine bands of fibrosis, little inflammation, and, rarely, loss of islets. This seems to be primarily an atrophic lesion that is due to protein malnutrition. Early in the course of the disease, these patients can be treated with a normal protein diet, and the lesion is reversible and secretory protein output returns to normal. In the acute stage, when essential amino acids are absent, protein output in the juice is decreased and the pancreas contains few zymogen granules. Volume and bicarbonate output are normal. Thus, kwashiorkor is not a cause of chronic pancreatitis as much as a cause of chronic pancreatic atrophy.

There is also a syndrome in countries in which kwashiorkor exists wherein patients have calcifying pancreatitis with inflammation resembling that seen with alcoholism. Some of these patients have alcoholism and malnutrition, but some do not drink alcohol. For example, in Indonesia, a chronic pancreatitis is seen that is associated with calcification of the gland, usually with diabetes, but is not associated with ethanol ingestion. The patients often have a painless course. The only etiologic factor recognized is chronic poor nutrition, yet protein deficiency alone does not cause this lesion. The macronutrients or micronutrients important in the development of this disease are unknown.

Many surgeons believe that *obstruction of the sphincter of Oddi* by chronic inflammation can cause chronic pancreatitis. But is there such an entity as "Odditis"? Histology of biopsies of the papilla of Vater and the sphincter of Oddi does show mucosal proliferation, chronic inflammation, and submucosal fibrosis in a few patients with pancreatitis. Usually, this is seen in patients who have passed common duct stones, not in those with chronic alcoholic pancreatitis. The same histology also can be seen in patients with no pancreatic or biliary disease. Studies of the sphincter's resistance to passage of probes or of infused saline are suspect because they are done under anesthesia. Often, a tight sphincter relaxes with a physiologic stimulus such as CCK. The conclusion drawn from reviewing a large and poorly controlled series of reports in the literature is that obstructive lesions of the sphincter of Oddi are rare as a primary lesion. The evidence that chronic Odditis, or sphincter fibrosis, causes chronic pancreatitis is unconvincing. Perfusion studies of sphincter function during endoscopic cannulation of the ducts do not suggest that papillary stenosis is associated with idiopathic recurrent pancreatitis.

CLINICAL ASSOCIATIONS OF CHRONIC PANCREATITIS

Chronic pancreatitis is not associated with severe calcium malabsorption or osteomalacia as it is in diseases in which the intestinal mucosa is diseased (celiac sprue) or in which the small bowel is resected. The nutritional defect of pancreatic insufficiency rarely results in a hemoglobin below 10 gm. The albumin is reduced in only 16 per cent of cases, the serum calcium in 9 per cent, and the prothrombin time in 34 per cent, whereas low values for these are seen in 60 to 89 per cent of patients with sprue. The key to the mild nutritional deficiency in patients with chronic pancreatitis is that (1) they have a normal small bowel mucosa and can absorb many nutrients in spite of poor digestion; (2) they have an increased food intake compared with patients with malabsorption; and (3) they have less accumulation of fatty acids in their small intestine that tend to bind calcium and magnesium and lead to losses in the stool. *Iron absorption* was originally thought to be increased in certain patients with chronic pancreatitis, but studies with radioactive isotopes of iron indicate that there is no correlation between iron absorption or storage pools and the degree of pancreatic insufficiency.

Vitamin B malabsorption occurs in a minority of patients with pancreatic insufficiency. This can be improved by feeding pancreatic extract, the active principle of which is trypsin and the other proteases. Vitamin B_{12} is bound in the stomach to salivary proteins, so-called "R proteins," which prevent intrinsic factor from competing for B_{12} in the acid pH of the stomach. It is not until these R proteins are digested in the small bowel lumen by pancreatic proteases that the B_{12} is released and intrinsic factor can bind it, thereby allowing it to be absorbed in the ileum.

Patients with acute gallstone pancreatitis or first attacks of alcoholic pancreatitis have an increased plasma glucagon, averaging ninefold above control patients, but at the same time only a twofold increase in insulin. This is a diabetogenic ratio of glucagon to insulin and helps explain their transient diabetes. In patients with chronic pancreatitis, however, the glucagon level is not elevated during relapses. Patients with pancreatic insufficiency show no glucagon response to alanine, whereas the genetic diabetic shows a brisk response to alanine infusion. The clinical significance of this is that the brittleness of diabetes in chronic pancreatitis may be due to an inability to secrete glucagon under stress and thus to increase gluconeogenesis. Chronic pancreatitis patients show an increased blood glucose during intravenous glucose testing, combined with a delayed and poor insulin output. Their diabetes is therefore due to impaired insulin secretion and requires insulin administration.

Pancreatic ascites is almost inevitably due to a leak from a pancreatic duct. If this occurs in the anterior wall of the pancreas, it drains into the peritoneal cavity via the lesser sac or greater peritoneal surface. If this leak is walled off, a pseudocyst is formed. If the leak occurs posteriorly from the pancreas and enters the retroperitoneum, juice moves by least resistance into the mediastinum and sometimes breaks through into the pleura. The fluid contains very high amylase activity and a high albumin concentration owing to a low-grade enzymatic inflammation of the peritoneal membranes.

Only about one half of the patients in a series of pancreatic ascites cases have acute pancreatitis. The other half have chronic pancreatitis, where pain is not frequently a part of the syndrome. Massive distention is the main complaint. Occasionally, subcutaneous fat necrosis occurs. The fluid is clear, yellow, occasionally chylous, and rarely bloody. The localization of the leak can be found by endoscopic retrograde pancreatography, and, once the site is apparent, it is possible to close it surgically when conservative drainage of the ascitic fluid or effusions has not been successful in allowing the leak to close spontaneously.

In some patients with chronic pancreatitis, *stenosis of the distal common duct* occurs. During relapses, these patients are prone to become jaundiced, and infection of the partially obstructed common duct can occur with ascending cholangitis.

The correlations of ductal changes on ERCP with pancreatic secretion tests indicate that defects of secretion with CCK-secretin or Lundh tests can be found when the main and secondary ducts are normal or slightly dilated. However, advanced dilatation, strictures, and stones in the ducts almost always predict impaired secretory function. Diagnosis of early exocrine insufficiency has also proved impossible with noninvasive tests, such as the benzoyl-tyrosine-PABA, fluorescein dilaurate, and ^{14}C-triglyceride breath tests, owing to impaired sensitivity and lack of specificity. Low plasma concentrations of pancreatic isoamylase or cationic trypsin are seen in advanced pancreatic damage, but they lack the sensitivity to detect early damage. The plasma pancreatic polypeptide concentration by radioimmunoassay increases after CCK or secretin administration, and the response is impaired in moderate to severe chronic pancreatitis. Again, this test lacks the sensitivity to detect early pancreatitis. The only available method for detection of early chronic pancreatitis

then remains duodenal intubation tests with CCK-secretin or meal stimulation.

Exocrine function has been studied repeatedly in patients with diabetes, and the consensus is that some patients who have no evidence of exocrine insufficiency may show impaired responses to secretin or cholecystokinin. It is juvenile-onset diabetics who have impaired pancreatic function, not adult-onset diabetics. Age-matched controls were compared with juvenile-onset diabetics who had had the disease from 1 to 10 years. There was a decrease in bicarbonate output after cholecystokinin and secretin proportional to the duration of diabetes and to the insulin dosage.

Patients with chronic pancreatitis and diabetes had the expected low bicarbonate values, whereas those with adult-onset diabetes had normal values. This suggests that the viral or autoimmune injury currently thought to be the etiology of juvenile-onset diabetes also damages the acini and ductal cells and that this is progressive with time. None of the patients showed a reduction in secretion greater than 90 per cent, so they did not exceed the exocrine reserve of the pancreas and did not show pancreatic insufficiency.

THE NATURAL HISTORY OF ALCOHOLIC PANCREATITIS

A series of 113 patients were followed for 4 years or more after the onset of their first symptoms of chronic alcoholic pancreatitis. The clinical course showed improvement in 42 per cent, remained stable in 32 per cent, and showed worsening of signs and symptoms in 26 per cent. The onset of diabetes and steatorrhea usually began 9 years after the onset of pain. Only two of these 113 patients died of their disease during the follow-up period. Four of every five continued to work. These results indicate that chronic pancreatitis is a painful but not life-threatening disease.

Figure 32–3 shows the sequence of events in a typical patient with chronic alcoholic pancreatitis. The graph includes a period of 15 years of drinking at a level of 150 to 180 gm/day. In those patients who are destined to develop the disease, the average time of onset of various symptoms is shown.

For 8 years after the onset of heavy drinking, pancreatic damage is asymptomatic and subclinical, but during that time functioning acinar and ductal mass is being destroyed by the process described previously. At the same time, the output of enzymes and bicarbonate after stimulation with CCK or secretin is also slowly declining, although there are few data on patients in this asymptomatic stage. At an average of 8 years, the patients begin to have acute painful episodes, the first being the most severe. It often results in transient diabetes. Thereafter, the episodes are less severe, resembling pancreatic edema, and usually follow

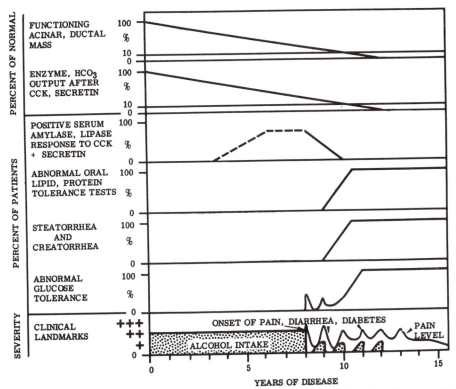

Figure 32–3 The natural history of a typical patient with chronic relapsing alcoholic pancreatitis.

resumption of alcohol intake. Somewhere in the middle of the course of the disease stimulation of the patient with CCK and secretin in 50 to 80 per cent of patients will elicit an elevation in the serum amylase or lipase. It is not until functioning pancreatic mass is reduced to about 10 per cent and the enzyme and bicarbonate output to about 10 per cent that symptoms and signs of exocrine insufficiency develop. The onset of diarrhea is due to steatorrhea; then, shortly thereafter or at the same time, clinical diabetes becomes permanent. Tolerance tests begin to become abnormal once less than 10 per cent of functioning mass is left, and steatorrhea and creatorrhea make their appearance.

CYSTS OF THE PANCREAS

Two types of cysts are associated with pancreatic disease. The first is the true *retention cyst* of the pancreas, which is lined with an epithelial layer derived from the pancreas and presumably is a result of the dilatation of the ductal system. These retention cysts usually are in the head of the gland and communicate with the ductal system, and they usually are small and therefore cannot be palpated externally or cannot be detected by barium contrast studies of the duodenum or by angiography. They are best detected by endoscopic retrograde pancreatography or by ultrasonography. Occasionally, these true retention cysts can be massive and may develop as a congenital abnormality.

The so-called *pseudocyst* is lined with a fibrous capsule or with the peritoneal membranes of adjacent peripancreatic structures. The pseudocyst may or may not communicate with the ductal system. These cysts usually are large and therefore can be detected either by palpation externally or by barium contrast studies or angiography. They can occur anywhere in the gland. The best screening test for a pseudocyst is ultrasonography. The pseudocysts enlarge and spread into almost any area surrounding the pancreas. By far the most common site is the lesser sac. If they perforate posteriorly, they enter the retroperitoneum and can go up into the mediastinum or can dissect down over the kidneys all the way to the groin. Occasionally, they have dissected up the mediastinum as far as the neck. They have been known to rupture into the pericardium or into the pleural cavity. Some pseudocysts dissect between the leaves of the mesentery of the small bowel or the mesocolon. Occasionally, pseudocysts become secondarily infected with bacterial organisms, and this results in a sudden rise in temperature and white count, tenderness, and signs of sepsis. The bacteria found in infected pseudocysts are single organisms in about one half of the patients, and multiple organisms are found in the other half. The commonest organisms are staphylococcal species, *Eschericia coli*, streptococcal species, and *Proteus* species. The presence of gas within a cystic cavity on plain film of the abdomen is diagnostic of an infected pseudocyst. If the pseudocyst ruptures into the peritoneal cavity, mortality is high. If it merely leaks into the peritoneal cavity, massive pancreatic ascites usually is the sequela. Rarely, these pseudocysts have ruptured into vessels such as the portal vein, leading to generalized fat necrosis of the skin, bone marrow, and tissues throughout the body.

The serum amylase tends to be elevated in about 50 per cent of patients with a pseudocyst. Since many of them do not contain significant amounts of pancreatic enzymes, the elevation is thought to result from compression of the adjacent pancreas. Rarely, the course of pseudocysts is a wasting, downhill course. Spontaneous remission, sepsis, bleeding, and obstructive jaundice may all occur. Rarely, hematobilia may result from bleeding from a pancreatic pseudocyst into the pancreatic ductal system.

The causes of a pseudocyst vary from acute pancreatitis due to biliary disease to trauma to chronic pancreatitis. About 10 to 20 per cent of patients with alcoholic chronic pancreatitis will develop a pseudocyst; therefore, repeated ultrasonographic studies at the time of acute attacks pay dividends.

THE PATHOPHYSIOLOGY OF CARCINOMA OF THE PANCREAS

Carcinoma of the pancreas has become an increasingly serious problem in oncology. The age-adjusted death rate in males is approximately 11 per 100,000 and for females 7 per 100,000 ranking this disease fourth and sixth respectively among cancer causes of death. An estimated 25,000 deaths from cancer of the pancreas occurred in the United States in 1983. Between 1920 and 1965 the incidence increased from 2.9 to 8.2 per 100,000, a change not due to improved reporting of the disease. The average age of patients with cancer of the pancreas is approximately 64 years, but it can occur in people as young as 30 years, the rate increasing progressively with increasing age.

The etiologic factors for cancer of the pancreas are mostly unknown, and the candidate causes are poorly documented. For example, there is a 2.5-fold higher incidence of cancer of the pancreas in heavy smokers, and the onset is 10 years earlier on the average than in nonsmokers. However, there is some confusing evidence that heavy smoking actually results in a lower incidence, possibly because these patients die of cancer of the lung before they can die of cancer of the pancreas. The presumed mechanism by which smoking causes cancer of the pancreas is thought to be the absorption of carcinogens that are taken up by the pancreas. There is an increased incidence of pancreatic cancer and of lymphoma among chemists in the United States, and this fact has been interpreted to mean that industrial carcinogens may play a role in the disease. There is no question that tumors of the pancreas can be induced by feeding or injecting rodents with benzanthracene or methylcholanthrene analogs and, in particular, various forms of nitrosamines. The pancreas is only one of many organs in which these agents will cause an adenocarcinoma.

There appears to be an increased incidence of cancer of the pancreas in patients with diabetes mellitus, particularly in patients who have had diabetes for some years. The Joslin Clinic reported an incidence of 256 cases of cancer of the pancreas in 10,000 diabetic patients, an extremely high incidence compared with that reported in the normal population, which is approximately one per 10,000. Chronic pancreatitis is alleged to have a relationship to cancer of the pancreas, particularly if there are calcifications in the pancreas. One review of the literature suggests that 3.6 per cent of patients with calcified chronic pancreatitis developed cancer of the pancreas, but adequate controls are lacking. Patients with hereditary pancreatitis of the mendelian-dominant form that results in calcification of the pancreas appear to have an increased incidence of carcinoma of the pancreas. One third of the disease-related deaths in patients with hereditary pancreatitis are due to cancer of the pancreas.

A study carried out with age-matched controls indicated that a high intake of alcohol was related to an increased incidence of cancer of the pancreas. Sixty-five per cent of patients with cancer of the pancreas at a VA Hospital had a moderate to heavy ethanol intake for an average of 15 years, whereas only 14 per cent of the age-, sex-, and race-matched controls were moderate to heavy alcoholics, and these had been drinking an average of 10 years. Unfortunately, the incidence of chronic pancreatitis in these heavy drinkers was not established.

An association of pancreatic cancer with coffee consumption has been postulated. Even correcting for smoking, researchers have found that the correlation is only suggestive, not conclusive.

The clinical features of cancer of the pancreas are well described in textbooks and will not be reviewed here. One of the most discouraging aspects of cancer of the pancreas is its almost total resistance to therapy. Over the period ranging from 1960 to 1970, there was no increase in 1-year survival, which is only 14 per cent. There is no evidence that radical surgery, chemotherapy, radiation therapy, or any other form of therapy can cure or prolong life to a greater extent than palliative procedures. One of the reasons for this dismal mortality rate is the tendency of the tumor to spread before it becomes locally symptomatic.

By the time of surgery, 90 per cent of patients show spread to regional lymph nodes and to the liver. There is a hypothesis that if we could detect the tumor when it is smaller it might be possible to increase the cure rate, but this has not been proved. The 5-year survival, adjusted for normal life expectancy, remains at 1 per cent for males and 2 per cent for females.

The combination of ultrasonography as the initial screening test, a CCK pancreatic function test as the second screen, and ERCP as the confirming test will detect 90 per cent of patients with pancreatic disease and 80 per cent of those with cancer of the pancreas. Patients without pancreatic disease will be reliably shown not to have it. The usual secretin pancreatic function test cannot be considered to give similar results until this is demonstrated by a prospective study. The accuracy of cytologic examination of duodenal fluid has been investigated repeatedly in patients with pancreatic-biliary-duodenal cancers. Three large series that we have analyzed gave a positive predictive capacity of 90 per cent, a negative predictive capacity of 93 per cent, a sensitivity of 60 per cent, and a specificity of 99 per cent. Such success rates require expert cytologists. Obtaining fluid directly from the papilla of Vater has not improved sensitivity, but cytology has improved the sensitivity of ERCP for cancer from 73 to 85 per cent and has increased specificity in noncancer cases to 96 per cent.

Another approach to diagnosis is to test for circulating tumor antigens, such as carcinoembryonic antigen (CEA), α-fetoprotein, and pancreatic oncofetal antigen in patients with cancer of the pancreas. Of a large number of patients tested, none have shown specificity for the pancreas, and they have such low positive predictive capacity that they cannot be used as screening tests. However, a prospective study showed that assay of serum galactosyl transferase II was 67 per cent sensitive and 98 per cent specific for discriminating between benign and malignant disease. When combined with other tests for suspected pancreatic carcinoma, it increased the sensitivity of ultrasonography, CT, or ERCP.

Measurements of serum amylase, serum lipase, or urinary amylase excretion are not helpful in the diagnosis of cancer of the pancreas. Only 13 per cent of the serum amylases, 11 per cent of lipases, and 27 per cent of the hourly urinary amylase excretions were elevated in a large series from the Mayo Clinic. There is no evidence that the amylase:creatinine clearance ratio improves these statistics. The results of duodenal intubation and secretin tests by Dreiling indicated that the usual finding in cancer of the head of the pancreas is a decreased volume of pancreatic juice that contains a normal concentration of bicarbonate and enzymes. Enzyme output was decreased in 90 per cent of patients with cancer of the head of the pancreas and proportionately less as the tumor

blocked the duct in the body and in the tail of the gland. The ability of pancreatic function tests to discriminate between cancer and chronic pancreatitis unfortunately is low.

A more direct diagnostic procedure is percutaneous aspiration biopsy of the pancreas. The physician uses a long 23-gauge needle and vigorously aspirates with saline to obtain cells, which are then examined cytologically. The guiding of the needle into a mass in the pancreas is done by ultrasonography or CT. The sensitivity was 80 per cent in 10 series. The usefulness of fine-needle biopsy is that it helps one establish a diagnosis in unresectable patients, thus avoiding laparotomy.

Angiography has other advantages. It allows one to predict the size of the tumor, often permits one to predict whether it is resectable, and can help distinguish whether a positive ERCP is due to cancer or chronic pancreatitis.

CT has proved itself as useful as ultrasonography as the initial screening test for cancer of the pancreas. It relies almost entirely on alterations of pancreatic contour and thus cannot detect early lesions that do not do this. The sensitivity was 79 per cent and specificity 64 per cent in the Mayo Clinic series compared with 92 and 89 per cent in the Mason Clinic series. The sensitivity of ultrasonography in pancreatic cancer diagnosis was 74 per cent, and the specificity was 84 per cent. The Mason Clinic results were 71 and 75 per cent, respectively. As a confirmatory test, ERCP had a sensitivity of 94 per cent and a specificity of 96 per cent. Percutaneous transhepatic cholangiography is useful in confirming the presence of a cancer as a cause of common duct obstruction: its sensitivity was 100 per cent and its specificity was 96 per cent in one series. Thus, we have the tools to detect and confirm pancreatic cancer once the suspicion is present. None of these methods has allowed us to detect cancers early enough to improve the resectability or cure rate. Until we find a screening test for the high-risk age groups that has acceptable positive and negative predictive capacities, we will not be able to make an impact on the mortality of this common and lethal cancer.

CYSTIC FIBROSIS

This is the commonest lethal *genetic* disease of white populations, in which it occurs in one in 2000 live births. Cystic fibrosis is inherited as an autosomal recessive trait, which means that about 5 per cent of the population are carriers. It is characterized clinically by chronic pulmonary disease, pancreatic achylia, and abnormally high sweat electrolytes. Other symptoms that can complicate the picture are meconium ileus, hepatic cirrhosis, and rectal prolapse. Cystic fibrosis is a generalized disorder that involves the pancreas seriously in 80 to 90 per cent of patients.

Two main defects lead to the pathologic damage. The first is an abnormality in the glycoprotein-rich secretions of most exocrine glands that leads to precipitation of secretions in the ductal system of these glands. The cause of the precipitation has never been explained. As a result, the pancreas, the lungs, the biliary tree, and the crypts of the gastrointestinal tract suffer primarily from this abnormality. The second major abnormality is an electrolyte defect of the eccrine sweat glands that results in high sodium and chloride concentrations in the sweat. Its clinical significance is that salt depletion may occur in hot weather. The diagnosis rests on the demonstration of an elevated sweat chloride concentration in a patient who either has a history of cystic fibrosis in the family or has chronic pulmonary disease, malabsorption, or failure to grow. The standard method of measuring sweat sodium and chloride is now pilocarpine iontophoresis with collection of the sweat in a cellulose sponge. Values of sweat chloride above 70 mEq/L are diagnostic, and values between 50 and 60 mEq/L are suggestive of cystic fibrosis. The upper normal value for sweat sodium is 70 mEq/L.

After the age of 20 years, sweat sodium and chloride values are not much different than in the younger age group. The upper limits of normal (i.e., two standard deviations above the mean) are 52 mEq/L for chloride and 70 mEq/L for sodium. Potassium concentrations are also slightly elevated in cystic fibrosis. An abnormal sweat test alone is not sufficient for a diagnosis of cystic fibrosis because there are other conditions in pediatrics in which these sweat electrolytes may be elevated. In these cases, duodenal drainage to assess pancreatic function is useful.

At the present time, there is no method by which heterozygotes can be identified by any chemical tests, including sweat electrolytes. Adult patients with chronic obstructive pulmonary disease have been repeatedly studied to see if some of them represent subclinical or primarily pulmonary forms of cystic fibrosis. The evidence at the present time is that this is a rare occurrence and that most patients with chronic obstructive pulmonary disease have normal sweat electrolytes. Those who have slight elevations return promptly to normal with the stimulus of salt restriction in the diet or a salt-retaining hormone. Patients with cystic fibrosis are not able to reduce their sweat electrolytes by either form of stress.

Pancreatic insufficiency is not the major clinical problem in cystic fibrosis because it can be treated adequately. Progressive lung disease determines the fate of the patient. At the present time, about 50 per cent of patients live to their tenth birthday, 30 per cent to their twentieth birthday, and few beyond the age of 30 years. An increasing number of patients are coming into adult medicine and require the treatment of internists.

Pancreatic achylia is present in 80 to 90 per cent of patients. The pancreatic ducts are obstructed by inspissated pancreatic secretions, leading to distention and dilatation of the ducts, atrophy and degeneration of the acini, and severe fibrosis that eventually results in almost total destruction of acinar tissue, fatty replacement of pancreatic parenchyma, and persistence of the islets of Langerhans surrounded by fibrous tissue. Meconium ileus is due to the accumulation of thick, sticky material in the lumen of the bowel. This material is predominately sloughed mucosa and precipitated protein. Previously, this was thought to accumulate because of lack of pancreatic enzyme digestion, but pathologic studies indicate that meconium ileus can occur in the newborn when the pancreas is still normal or mildly affected, whereas the crypts of Lieberkühn are always severely affected in the intestinal mucosa of patients with meconium ileus.

The pancreatic secretory abnormality has been studied with CCK-secretin tests in children with early pancreatic insufficiency. These children produce a small volume of juice containing high enzyme concentrations but a low bicarbonate content, suggesting that the initial damage is much more severe to the ductal cells than to the acinar cells. Eventually, acinar function is lost as well.

Pancreatic achylia produces the expected syndrome of maldigestion, but there is some evidence of malabsorption as well. Although the D-xylose test is normal and peroral biopsies of the small intestine have shown normal histologic patterns in the majority of cases, disaccharidase activities are sometimes decreased, usually lactase. Moreover, a fascinating abnormality in bile acid metabolism has been reported in which patients with cystic fibrosis and pancreatic insufficiency are found to excrete excessive amounts of bile acids into the stool, with losses as large as those seen in patients with ileal resection. Patients without steatorrhea do not excrete excessive bile acids. Administration of pancreatic enzymes in large amounts eventually will correct both the bile acid loss and the fat loss. This puzzling situation has been further investigated in cystic fibrosis patients who have normal intestinal function, biopsies, disaccharidase levels, and functioning gallbladders. It was found that such patients have a low bile acid pool, which doubles on administration of pancreatic enzymes. The secondary bile acids are reduced somewhat by treatment, from 57 per cent of the total to 40 per cent. Surprisingly, total bile acid synthesis remains the same before and after treatment. The fractional turnover rate of the untreated patients is very high, 0.6 or 0.7 per day for cholic and chenodeoxycholic acid; this turnover is reduced by treatment with pancreatic enzymes to 0.2 or 0.4 per day. The data are consistent with rapid cycling of the bile acid pool through the intestine, as is seen in patients who have a nonfunctioning gallbladder or who have had their gallbladder removed. There is no correlation between fat loss and bile acid loss in these patients. Bile acid concentrations in the duodenum, either during fasting or after stimulation of gallbladder contraction, are normal both before and after pancreatic enzyme treatment. Several studies in adults with exocrine insufficiency showed that their bile acid malabsorption was due to precipitation of bile acids by the acid pH in the duodenum and upper jejunum, secondary to lack of pancreatic bicarbonate. Addition of cimetidine to pancreatin corrected this defect and restored normal micellar concentrations of bile acids and fatty acids. The upper small bowel has an acid pH in cystic fibrosis, so this mechanism probably contributes to the bile acid losses and malabsorption in this disease. Enteric-coated, pH-sensitive enzyme preparations that dissolve at neutral pH are more effective in cystic fibrosis than an equipotent dose of a standard pancreatin.

The gallbladder also can be involved in cystic fibrosis, leading to atrophy and obstruction in up to 25 per cent of patients. This would lead to increased cycling of bile salts but would not explain the loss in the stool.

Oral glucose tolerance tests in patients with cystic fibrosis show abnormal findings in 40 per cent of patients. As the glucose intolerance becomes more severe, the release of insulin into the peripheral plasma is more delayed and blunted. A small number of these patients eventually end with true diabetes. The striking fact is that when these patients are stimulated with glucagon or tolbutamide they show a sudden increase in release of insulin, suggesting that there is not a deficiency in number of beta cells or in stored insulin but an abnormality in stimulation or release by the normal stimulus, elevated blood glucose. Further studies have indicated that both insulin and glucagon release are impaired after a standard stimulation, such as intravenous arginine infusion. As long as the patients maintain a normal glucagon:insulin ratio, they do not show much glucose intolerance. In addition, cystic fibrosis patients are not insulin-resistant as are adult-onset obese diabetics. Therefore, the conclusion has been that the islet cells encased in their fibrotic pancreas may not receive stimuli such as glucose normally or that the release of glucagon or insulin may be impaired because of the anatomic situation. Fortunately, clinical diabetes is an unusual complication in this disease.

The pathogenesis of cystic fibrosis has not been explained—either the precipitation of exocrine secretions or the impairment in sodium and chloride loss from eccrine glands. At present, it is important to differentiate a few rare disease entities from cystic fibrosis in children. There is a condition called *aplasia of the exocrine pancreas* in which there is complete replacement of the exocrine parenchyma by fat, normal islets of Langerhans, and no fibrosis or dilatation of the ducts. There is also a syndrome of pancreatic deficiency and bone marrow dysfunction in which the patients have pancreatic achylia, shortness of stature, a normal sweat test, no pulmonary involvement, and a variety of hematologic abnormalities including thrombocytopenia, neutropenia, and anemia. Fecal fat is only slightly increased, and malabsorption is not marked.

REFERENCES

GENERAL REVIEWS

Howat, H. T. (Ed.): Clinics in Gastroenterology. Vol. 1. Philadelphia, W. B. Saunders Co., 1972.

Howat, H. T., and Sarles, H. (Eds.): The Exocrine Pancreas. Philadelphia, W. B. Saunders Co., 1979.

BIOCHEMISTRY, PHYSIOLOGY

Bieger, W., and Scheele, G. A.: Two-dimensional isoelectric focusing/sodium dodecylsulfate gel electrophoresis of protein mixtures containing active or potentially active proteases: analysis of human exocrine pancreatic proteins. Anal. Biochem. 109:222, 1980.

Boden, G., Wilson, R. M., Essa-Koumar, N., and Owen, O. E.: Effects of a protein meal, intraduodenal HCl, and oleic acid on portal and peripheral venous secretin and on pancreatic bicarbonate secretion. Gut 19:277, 1978.

Brodrick, J. W., Geokas, M. C., and Largman, C.: Human carboxypeptidase B. II. Purification of the enzyme from pancreatic tissue and comparison with enzymes present in pancreatic secretion. Biochim. Biophys. Acta 452:468, 1976.

Brodrick, J. W., Geokas, M. C., Largman, C., et al.: Molecular forms of immunoreactive pancreatic cationic trypsin in pancreatitis patient sera. Am. J. Physiol. 237:E474, 1979.

DeCaro, A., Bonicel, J., Pieroni, G., and Guy, O.: Comparative studies of human and porcine pancreatic lipases. Biochimie 63:799, 1981.

Feinstein, G., Hofstein, R., Koifmann, J., and Sokolovsky, M.: Human pancreatic proteolytic enzymes and protein inhibitors. Eur. J. Biochem. 43:569, 1974.

Funakoshi, A., Tsubota, Y., Wakasugi, H., et al.: Purification and properties of human pancreatic deoxyribonuclease I. J. Biochem. (Tokyo) 82:1771, 1977.

Gaskin, K. J., Durie, P. R., Hill, R. E., et al.: Colipase and maximally activated pancreatic lipase in normal subjects and patients with steatorrhea. J. Clin. Invest. 69:427, 1982.

Grataroli, R., Dijkman, R., Dutilh, C. E., et al.: Studies on prophospholipase A₂ and its enzyme from human pancreatic juice. Eur. J. Biochem. 122:111, 1982.

Guy, O., Lombardo, D., Bartelt, D. C., et al.: Two human trypsinogens. Purification, molecular properties, and N-terminal sequences. Biochemistry 17:1669, 1978.

Herzog, V.: Endocytosis in secretory cells. Philos. Trans. R. Soc. Lond. (Biol.) 296:67, 1981.

Hildebrand, H., Borgstrom, B., Békássy, A., et al.: Isolated colipase deficiency in two brothers. Gut 23:243, 1982.

Jensen, R. T., and Gardner, J. D.: Identification and characterization of receptors for secretagogues on pancreatic acinar cells. Fed. Proc. 40:2486, 1981.

Jensen, R. T., Tatemoto, K., Mutt, V., et al.: Actions of a newly isolated intestinal peptide PHI on pancreatic acini. Am. J. Physiol. 241:G498, 1981.

Jorpes, E., and Mutt, V.: Cholecystokinin and pancreozymin, one single hormone? Acta Physiol. Scand. 66:196, 1966.

Lombardo, D.: Catalytic properties of modified human pancreatic carboxylic-ester hydrolase. Biochim. Biophys. Acta 700:75, 1982.

Lonovics, J., Devitt, P., Watson, L. C., et al.: Pancreatic polypeptide. Arch. Surg. 116:1256, 1981.

Maroux, S., Baratti, J., and Desnuelle, P.: Purification and specificity of porcine enterokinase. J. Biol. Chem. 246:5031, 1971.

Meldolesi, J., and Ceccarelli, B.: Exocytosis and membrane recycling. Philos. Trans. R. Soc. Lond. (Biol.) 296:55, 1981.

Merritt, A. D., and Karn, R. C.: The human α-amylases. Adv. Hum. Genet. 8:135, 1977.

Patton, J. S., Albertsson, P.-A., Erlanson, C., and Borgström, B.: Binding of porcine pancreatic lipase and colipase in the absence of substrate studied by two-phase partition and affinity chromatography. J. Biol. Chem. 253:4195, 1978.

Pearse, A. G. F., Polak, J. M., and Bloom, S. R.: The newer gut hormones. Cellular sources, physiology, pathology, and clinical aspects. Gastroenterology 72:746, 1977.

Petersen, O. H.: Stimulus-secretion coupling in plasma membranes of pancreatic acinar cells. Biochim. Biophys. Acta 694:163, 1982.

Peterson, L. M., Sokolovsky, M., and Vallee, B. L.: Purification and crystallization of human carboxypeptidase A. Biochemistry 15:2501, 1976.

Pubols, M. H., Bartelt, D. C., and Green, L. J.: Trypsin inhibitor from human pancreas and pancreatic juice. J. Biol. Chem. 249:2235, 1974.

Rehfeld, J. F.: Immunochemical studies on cholecystokinin. II. Distribution and molecular heterogeneity in the central nervous system and small intestine of man and hog. J. Biol. Chem. 253:4022, 1978.

Schaffalitzky de Muckadell, O. B., and Fahrenkrug, J.: Secretion pattern of secretin in man: regulation by gastric acid. Gut 19:812, 1978.

Schmitz, J., Preiser, H., Maestracci, D., et al.: Subcellular localization of enterokinase in human small intestine. Biochim. Biophys. Acta 343:435, 1974.

Schulz, I., Wakasugi, H., Stolze, H., et al.: Analysis of Ca^{++} fluxes and their relation to enzyme secretion in dispersed pancreatic acinar cells. Fed. Proc. 40:2503, 1981.

Scratcherd, T., Hutson, D., and Case, R. M.: Ionic transport mechanisms underlying fluid secretion by the pancreas. Philos. Trans. R. Soc. Lond. (Biol.) 296:167, 1981.

Singh, M., and Webster, P. D. III: Neurohumoral control of pancreatic secretion. Gastroenterology 74:294, 1978.

Sternby, B., and Erlanson-Albertsson, C.: Measurement of the binding of human colipase to human lipase and lipase substrates. Biochim. Biophys. Acta 711:193, 1982.

Stiefel, D. J., and Keller, P. J.: Preparation and some properties of human pancreatic amylase, including a comparison with human parotid amylase. Biochim. Biophys. Acta 302:345, 1973.

Taylor, I. L., Feldman, M., Richardson, C. T., and Walsh, J. H.: Gastric and cephalic stimulation of human pancreatic polypeptide release. Gastroenterology 75:432, 1978.

Weickman, J. L., Elson, M., and Glitz, D. G.: Human pancreatic ribonuclease. Biochemistry 20:1272, 1981.

Williams, J. A., Sankaran, H., Korc, M., and Goldfine, I. D.: Receptors for cholecystokinin and insulin in isolated pancreatic acini: hormonal control of secretion and metabolism. Fed. Proc. 40:2497, 1981.

DIAGNOSTIC TESTS IN PANCREATIC DISEASE

Burton, P., Hammond, E. M., Harper, A. A., et al.: Serum amylase and serum lipsase levels in man after administration of secretion and pancreozymin. Gut 1:125, 1960.

Cotton, P. B.: Progress report. ERCP. Gut 18:316, 1977.

Eaton, S. B., Fleischli, D. J., Pollard, J. J., et al.: Comparison of current radiologic approaches to the diagnosis of pancreatic disease. N. Engl. J. Med. 279:389, 1968.

Johnson, S. G., and Levitt, M. D.: Relation between serum pancreatic isoamylase concentration and pancreatic exocrine function. Dig. Dis. 23:914, 1978.

Lankish, P. G.: Exocrine pancreatic function tests. Gut 23:777, 1982.

Largman, C., Brodrick, J. W., and Geokas, M. C.: Radioimmu-

noassay determination of circulating pancreatic endopeptidases. Methods Enzymol. 74:272, 1981.

Levitt, M. D., and Ellis, C.: A rapid and simple assay to determine if macroamylase is the cause of hyperamylasemia. Gastroenterology 83:378, 1982.

O'Donnell, M. D., FitzGerald, O., and McGeeney, K. F.: Differential serum amylase determination by use of an inhibitor, and design of a routine procedure. Clin. Chem. 23:560, 1977.

Rammeloo, T., van Haard, P. M. M., and Beunis, M. H.: Two serum pancreatic isoamylase determinations compared. Clin. Chem. 28:145, 1982.

Sigstedt, B., Boijsen, E., Lunderquist, A., and Tylen, U.: Angiography in pancreatic disease re-evaluation: a prospective and blind evaluation. Acta Radiol. 22:235, 1981.

Syrota, A., Duquesnoy, N., Paraf, A., and Kellershohn, D.: The role of positron emission tomography in the detection of pancreatic disease. Nucl. Med. 143:249, 1982.

ACUTE PANCREATITIS

Acosta, J. M., and Ledesma, C. L.: Gallstone migration as a cause of acute pancreatitis. N. Engl. J. Med. 290:484, 1974.

Becker, V.: Pathological anatomy and pathogenesis of acute pancreatitis. World J. Surg. 5:303, 1981.

Creutzfeldt, W., and Schmidt, H.: Aetiology and pathogenesis of pancreatitis (current concepts). Scand. J. Gastroenterol. 6 (suppl.):47, 1970.

Drew, S. I., Joffe, B., Vinik, A., et al.: The first 24 hours of acute pancreatitis. Changes in biochemical and endocrine homeostasis in patients with pancreatitis compared to those in control subjects undergoing stress for reasons other than pancreatitis. Am. J. Med. 64:795, 1978.

Elliott, D. W.: Appraisal of the usefulness of various experimental models for the study of acute pancreatitis. In Beck, I. T., and Sinclair, D. B. (Eds.): The Exocrine Pancreas. Baltimore, Williams & Wilkins Co., 1971, p. 86.

Koehler, D. F., Eckfeldt, J. H., and Levitt, M. D.: Diagnostic value of routine isoamylase assay of hyperamylasemic serum. Gastroenterology 82:887, 1982.

Opie, E. L.: The etiology of acute hemorrhagic pancreatitis. Bull. J. Hopkins Hosp. 12:182, 1901.

Popper, H. L., Necheles, H., and Russell, K. C.: Transition of pancreatic edema into pancreatic necrosis. Surg. Gynecol. Obstet. 87:79, 1948.

Ranson, J. H. C.: Conservative surgical treatment of acute pancreatitis. World J. Surg. 5:351, 1981.

Ranson, J. H. C., and Pasternack, B. S.: Statistical methods for quantifying the severity of clinical acute pancreatitis. J. Surg. Res. 22:79, 1977.

Robertson, G. M., Moore, E. W., Switz, D. M., et al.: Inadequate parathyroid response in acute pancreatitis. N. Engl. J. Med. 294:512, 1976.

Trapnell, J. E.: Pathophysiology of acute pancreatitis. World J. Surg. 5:319, 1981.

Weir, G. C., Lesser, P. B., Drop, L. J., et al.: The hypocalcemia of acute pancreatitis. Ann. Int. Med. 83:185, 1975.

CHRONIC PANCREATITIS

Allen, R. H., Seetharam, B., Podell, E., and Alpers, D. H.: Effect of proteolytic enzymes on the binding of cobalamin to R protein and intrinsic factor. J. Clin. Invest. 61:47, 1978.

Braganza, J. M., Hunt, L. P., and Warwick, F.: Relationship between pancreatic exocrine function and ductal morphology in chronic pancreatitis. Gastroenterology 82:1341, 1982.

Cameron, J. L.: Chronic pancreatic ascites and pancreatic pleural effusions. Gastroenterology 74:134, 1978.

Cameron, J. L., Capuzzi, D. M., Zuidema, G. D., and Margolis, S.: Acute pancreatitis with hyperlipemia. Evidence for a persistent defect in lipid metabolism. Am. J. Med. 56:482, 1974.

DiMagno, E. P.: Diagnosis of chronic pancreatitis: are noninvasive tests of exocrine pancreatic function sensitive and specific? Gastroenterology 83:143, 1982.

DiMagno, E. P., Go, V. L. W., and Summerskill, W. H. J.: Relations between pancreatic enzyme outputs and malabsorption in severe pancreatic insufficiency. N. Engl. J. Med. 288:813, 1973.

Frier, B. M., Saunders, J. H. B., Wormsley, K. G., and Bouchier, I. A. D.: Exocrine pancreatic function in juvenile-onset diabetes mellitus. Gut *17*:685, 1976.

Gross, J. B., and Jones, J. D.: Hereditary pancreatitis: analysis of experience to May 1969. *In* Beck, I. T., and Sinclair, D. G. (Eds.): The Exocrine Pancreas. Baltimore, Williams & Wilkins Co., 1971, p. 247.

Guy, O., Robles-Diaz, G., Adrich, Z., et al.: Protein content of precipitates present in pancreatic juice of alcoholic subjects and patients with chronic calcifying pancreatitis. Gastroenterology *84*:102, 1983.

Levrat, M., Descos, L., Moulinier, B., and Pasquier, J.: Evolution au long cours des pancréatites chroniques. Arch. Fr. Mal. App. Dig. *59*:5, 1970.

Multigner, L., Figarella, C., Sahel, J., and Sarles, H.: Lactoferrin and albumin in human pancreatic juice. A valuable test for diagnosis of pancreatic diseases. Digest. Dis. Sci. *25*:173, 1980.

Sarles, H.: Chronic calcifying pancreatitis—chronic alcoholic pancreatitis. Gastroenterology *66*:604, 1974.

Sarles, H., Sarles, J.-C., Camatte, R., et al.: Observations of 205 confirmed cases of acute pancreatitis, recurring pancreatitis, and chronic pancreatitis. Gut *6*:545, 1965.

CANCER OF THE PANCREAS

DiMagno, E. P., Malagelada, J.-R., Taylor, W. F., and Go, V. L. W.: A prospective comparison of current diagnostic tests for pancreatic cancer. N. Engl. J. Med. *297*:737, 1977.

Moosa, A. R., and Levin, B.: The diagnosis of "early" pancreatic cancer: the University of Chicago experience. Cancer *47*:1688, 1981.

CYSTIC FIBROSIS

di Sant'Agnese, P. A.: Cystic fibrosis and other genetic pancreatic diseases in childhood. *In* Beck, I. T., and Sinclair, D. G. (Eds.): The Exocrine Pancreas. Baltimore, Williams & Wilkins Co., 1971, p. 227.

Handwerger, S., Roth, J., Gorden, P., et al.: Glucose intolerance in cystic fibrosis. N. Engl. J. Med. *281*:451, 1969.

Seber, A. M., Roy, C. C., Chartrand, L., et al.: Relationship between bile acid malabsorption and pancreatic insufficiency in cystic fibrosis. Gut *17*:295, 1976.

33 Nutritional Factors in Disease

George A. Bray

The nutritional disorders that result from the interaction of diet with the human body are numerous. This chapter will review certain aspects of biochemistry and physiology as they relate to the mechanisms by which deviations from normal nutrition produce their pathologic consequences.

An overall view of the interaction of nutrition and metabolism is presented in Figure 33–1. In this figure, the dietary, or storage, forms of triglycerides, polysaccharides, and proteins are shown at the top, their circulating forms in the middle, and the final common pathway for metabolism at the bottom. Dietary intake of macro- and micronutrients varies considerably among individuals in a given population. They also change from day to day in the same individual and even more strikingly among cultural and population groups. In spite of this, the requirements for operation of the "human machine" are essentially the same. The body is thus confronted with a series of metabolic problems: (1) ingestion and digestion of diverse nutrients, (2) absorption of the simple products for storage, (3) utilization of nutrients for body needs, (4) disposal or storage of excesses, and (5) attempts to remedy deficiencies by interconversion of nutrients.

The essential nature of vitamins and minerals has been clearly established, and these will be discussed in detail subsequently. There is no clearly established requirement for carbohydrates, since in their absence glucose can be obtained from amino acids, provided that sufficient quantities of protein are available. Most diets provide a mixture of polysaccharides and simple carbohydrates, which are usually the major dietary source of calories. The polyunsaturated fatty acids (i.e., linoleic and linolenic acids) cannot be synthesized in the body. A requirement of approximately 1 to 3 per cent of total caloric intake as essential fatty acids is necessary for maintenance of health. When essential fatty acids are absent, changes in the skin are seen clinically. Deficiencies in essential fatty acids are most easily demonstrated in growing children but can also be manifested in adults if they are fed a diet deficient in these acids for several weeks. A number of amino acids are also required in the diet because they cannot be synthesized in the body. These nine essential amino acids are lysine, methionine, valine, leucine, isoleucine, tryptophan, phenylalanine, threonine, and histidine. Deficiency of essential amino acids impairs protein synthesis. There is great variability in the amino acid composition of dietary proteins. For example, vegetable proteins, compared with human proteins, tend to be relatively deficient in one or another amino acid. Thus, wheat is deficient in lysine, whereas corn is deficient in tryptophan. Of the vegetable proteins, soy beans and other beans provide the highest quantities of essential amino acids.

ASSESSMENT OF OBESITY

Obesity is appropriately defined in terms of body fatness. In its extreme forms, obesity can be recognized at a glance. The round-jowled, puffing, often red-faced individual weighing in excess of 300 pounds is a familiar sight. However, quantitative assessment of the degree of obesity in these individuals and in lesser degrees of obesity may be difficult. Neither the usual recording of body weight nor the criteria based on weight in relation to height are sufficiently accurate in many instances. For example, above average muscle development or an unusually large skeleton could be mistaken for obesity. It is fair to say, however, that when weight exceeds the norm by more than 30 per cent in any but the most athletic male, there is almost certainly obesity, that is, an above-normal percentage of fat.

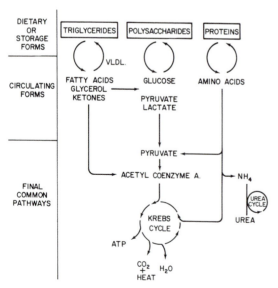

Figure 33–1 An overview of metabolism. This figure provides a view of the flow of nutrients from their dietary sources and their stored forms into the final common pathway of acetyl-CoA formation and metabolism through the tricarboxylic acid cycle.

Chemical Structure: $CH_3 - (CH_2)_{14} - COOH + 23\ O_2 \rightarrow 16\ CO_2 + 16\ H_2O$

(palmitic acid)

Molecular Weights: 256   736   704   288

Figure 33–2 Oxidation, or complete combustion, of palmitic acid to CO_2 and water. During this oxidation, a compound weighing 256 gm/mole is burned. Since the CO_2 and O_2 will equilibrate with the environment, 288 gm of water remain after the combustion of only 256 gm of fatty acid. This explains how the oxidation of fat can lead to the temporary accumulation of weight in individual patients.

Measurement of body weight on a scale does not differentiate mass occurring as fat, as bone, as muscle, and as water, and this lack of distinction can have significant clinical implications. Obese patients often fail to lose weight and may even gain weight when put on a diet. This is usually attributed to "cheating" by the patient when it may, in fact, be the result of the wrong measurement. This can happen even when caloric intake is severely restricted and careful measurements show that food intake is less than that required to maintain weight. This paradox is explained in terms of the oxidation of fatty acids (Fig. 33–2). This equation shows that when 256 gm of palmitic acid are completely oxidized, 288 gm of water are produced. When gaseous exchange of O_2 and CO_2 is completed, the body is left with a net gain in weight of 32 gm of water for every mole of palmitic acid that is oxidized. Until this excess water is excreted, a patient may gain weight when fatty acids are the principal metabolic fuel. Such a phenomenon has been observed frequently and has been known to persist for more than 30 days, even when patients have been hospitalized under strictly controlled conditions. Measuring body weight on a scale would be misleading under these circumstances, since the scale could not assess changes in the various components of the body weight. For this reason, more sophisticated techniques are necessary to understand the nature of the weight in obesity and its relation to the normal composition of the human body.

ANALYSIS OF HUMAN BODY COMPONENTS

Several techniques have been used to assess the components of the human body (Table 33–1). The most direct method is analysis of individual cadavers for lipid, water, protein, and ash components. Because of technical difficulty in such analyses and the scarcity of cadavers for this purpose, only seven complete studies on the subject have been published. The data from five of these analyses of total body composition are shown in Figure 33–3. Water represented just under two thirds of the total body weight. Fat and protein were at least 15 per cent of body weight. Since direct analyses cannot be performed on the living subject, alternative methods have been used. Measurement

of density of the human being is one approach. This can be accomplished by weighing the subject in and out of water, a principle that Archimedes discovered centuries ago. It allows an assessment of the fractions of body weight that are fat and nonfat. Measurement of body density has been widely applied, since it is simple and highly accurate.

Another method is measurement of body composition in vivo by isotopic dilution. When a known quantity of isotope is injected into the bloodstream and its concentration is measured after allowing for equilibration with the body stores of that compound, the ratio of radioactivity in plasma to the quantity injected will give a measure of the apparent volume of distribution for the substance. Radioactively labeled water (^3H_2O), potassium (^{42}K or ^{40}K), and sodium (^{22}Na or ^{24}Na) have been among the most widely used substances for obtaining measurements of body composition by this technique. The data from the measurements obtained by isotopic dilution are similar to those obtained through body-density and direct-carcass analysis. However, measurements by isotopic dilution provide additional information, since they allow for an estimate of intra- and extracellular fluid compartments.

Studies on humans during gain and loss of weight have provided important insights into the nature of the components that are accumulated or lost. In normal volunteers gaining 10 to 20 kg over a period of 6 months, nearly two thirds of the increase in weight is fat; the remainder is extracellular fluid and cellular components. Direct

TABLE 33–1 TECHNIQUES FOR MEASURING "FATNESS"

A. Direct carcass analysis
B. Indirect methods
   1. Densitometry
   2. Dilution
      a. Radioactive labeling (^3H_2O, ^{40}K)
      b. Chemical analysis (cyclopropane)
   3. Anthropometry
      a. Height and weight
      b. Skin folds
      c. Ultrasonography
      d. Soft-tissue radiographs
   4. Computerized tomographic (CT) scan
   5. Electromagnetic scan

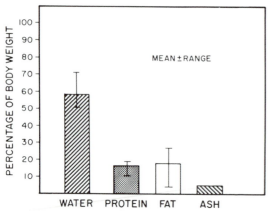

Figure 33–3 Analysis of body composition in five cadavers. The heights of individual bars are the mean for five patients, and the vertical lines represent the range. Body components are plotted as per cent of total body weight. (Adapted from Widdowson, E. M.: In Brozek, J. [Ed.]: Human Body Composition: Approaches and Application. New York, Pergamon Press, 1965.)

measurements of the size of fat cells from such individuals have shown that the size of the fat cells has increased with weight gain. Conversely, when obese patients lose weight in a hospital, the initial weight loss is predominantly water and protein, but with prolonged caloric restriction the largest fraction of the loss is fat. These data therefore illustrate the complexity of body composition and the difficulties in assigning a diagnosis of obesity based on body weight alone.

Measurement of the thickness of skin folds is another approach to assessing the amount of body fat. Criteria have been developed for assessing fatness by measuring the triceps skinfold, the combined triceps and subscapular skinfold, or a group of skinfolds in four regions including biceps, triceps, subscapular, and suprailiac. A midtriceps skinfold greater than 25 mm in females and more than 18 mm in males is defined in some studies as obesity, and a combined triceps plus subscapular measurement of 37 mm signifies obesity in other studies. Criteria for other skinfolds and their relationships to body fat can be obtained by consulting the 1976 monograph by Bray.

Despite all its limitations, the scale is still the best tool available for patients and most physicians to use in determining the degree of excess weight. When this overweight is sufficiently great (i.e., 30 per cent or more above values in standard tables for height and weight; Table 33–2), one can assume that the patient is obese.

An even more adequate way to relate height and weight for assessing the magnitude of overweight is with the body mass index. This index is the ratio of the body weight in kilograms divided by the square of the height in meters (Wt/[Ht]²). When the body mass index (BMI) is 27, this is usually defined as overweight, and when the body mass index is 30 or more, it is in a range associated

with excess risk of disease. A table for obtaining body mass index from measurements of height and weight can be obtained in the 1976 report by Bray, Jordan, and Sims.

IMBALANCE BETWEEN CALORIC INTAKE AND EXPENDITURE

There is little argument at present that obesity results from an excess intake of food in rela-

TABLE 33–2 GUIDELINES FOR BODY WEIGHT

	Metric				
Height* (m)	Men Weight (kg)*		Women Weight (kg)*		
	AVERAGE	ACCEPTABLE		AVERAGE	ACCEPTABLE
1.45				4.60	42 53
1.48				46.5	42 54
1.50				47.0	43 55
1.52				48.5	44 57
1.54				49.5	44 58
1.56				50.4	45 58
1.58	55.8	51 64		51.3	46 59
1.60	57.6	52 65		52.6	48 61
1.62	58.6	53 66		54.0	49 62
1.64	59.6	54 67		55.4	50 64
1.66	60.6	55 69		56.8	51 65
1.68	61.7	56 71		58.1	52 66
1.70	63.5	58 73		60.0	53 67
1.72	65.0	59 74		61.3	55 69
1.74	66.5	60 75		62.6	56 70
1.76	68.0	62 77		64.0	58 72
1.78	69.4	64 79		65.3	59 74
1.80	71.0	65 80			
1.82	72.6	66 82			
1.84	74.2	67 84			
1.86	75.8	69 86			
1.88	77.6	71 88			
1.90	79.3	73 90			
1.92	81.0	75 93			

	Nonmetric				
Height* (ft, in)	Men Weight (lb)*		Women Weight (lb)*		
	AVERAGE	ACCEPTABLE		AVERAGE	ACCEPTABLE
4 10				102	92 119
4 11				104	94 122
5 0				107	96 125
5 1				110	99 128
5 2	123	112 141		113	131
5 3	127	115 144		116	105 134
5 4	130	118 148		120	108 138
5 5	133	121 152		123	111 142
5 6	136	124 156		128	114 146
5 7	140	128 161		132	118 150
5 8	145	132 166		136	122 154
5 9	149	136 170		140	126 158
5 10	153	140 174		144	130 163
5 11	158	144 179		148	134 168
6 0	162	148 184		152	138 173
6 1	166	152 189			
6 2	171	156 194			
6 3	176	160 199			
6 4	181	164 204			

*Height without shoes, weight without clothes.
(Adapted from the recommendations of the Fogarty Center Conference on Obesity, 1973.)

tion to body needs. The basis for this proposition resides in the work published in 1783 by Lavoisier and Laplace, who studied this subject using the guinea pig. The "law of the conservation of energy" gave this early work a theoretical basis. This law applies to all species. In classic experiments, Rubner found that the amount of heat produced by a dog in the absence of food equals the heat from combustion of the fat and protein that were metabolized during starvation minus the heat from combustion in the urine. Atwater and Benedict made similar observations in humans and concluded that "for practical purposes we are, therefore, warranted in assuming that the law of conservation of energy obtains in general in the living organism as indeed there is every a priori reason to believe that it must." A demonstration that this law applied to the obese subject was delayed until the twentieth century. It has been convincingly shown that obese subjects, like their lean counterparts and all other known living systems, obey the law of conservation of energy.

Measurements of the energy contained in food are expressed in calories or joules (joule = 4.18 kcal). A calorie measures the quantity of heat required to raise the temperature of 1 gm of water from 15° to 16° C. As already noted, the quantity of heat obtained by the combustion of a foodstuff outside the body is equal to the quantity of heat obtained by combustion inside the body of the same foodstuff to the same end products. In the case of carbohydrate and lipid, the end products are carbon dioxide and water, and the heat produced during their combustion in vitro is directly related to the heat produced in vivo. Since protein is incompletely oxidized in the living organism, a correction is required. The end products of protein catabolism are carbon dioxide, water, and urea. The urea excreted in the urine represents a significant number of calories. Thus, to obtain an accurate assessment of total caloric utilization, one must know the quantity of urea.

Measurement of O_2 consumption and CO_2 production with a correction for urinary nitrogen allows an indirect quantitation of energy expenditure. This technique of indirect calorimetry (measurement of oxygen consumption and carbon dioxide production) has been widely used in assessing the caloric needs of the human organism. Figure 33–4 is a presentation of the energy expenditure for a reference man and a reference woman as estimated by the National Research Council in 1980. The male, aged 22 and weighing 70 kg, required 2800 calories; the female, aged 22 and weighing 58 kg, required 2000 calories. The total requirements for the reference subjects are about 10 per cent lower than those reported a decade earlier. Yet, even these current estimates are probably too high. The increased use of the automobile and decreased amount of physical activity have accounted for a steady reduction in total caloric requirements of men and women.

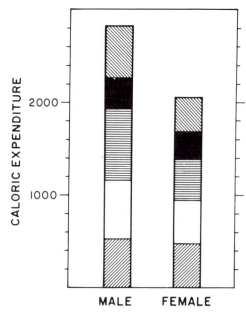

Figure 33–4 Estimated average energy expenditure of men and women. The lower hatched bars represent the energy expended during sleep and reclining (1.0 to 1.1 kcal/min). The unshaded open portion represents the average energy expended during sitting (1.1 to 1.5 kcal/min). The horizontally shaded section represents the energy expenditure during standing (1.5 to 2.5 kcal/min). The solid segment represents the energy expended during walking (2.5 to 3 kcal/min). The top portion of each bar represents other activities (3 to 4.5 kcal/min). The lower value within each preceding set of parentheses represents the average value for females and the upper value the average for males. (Adapted from Recommended Dietary Allowances.)

Since these are "reference" figures, they must be modified before being applied to a given individual. Factors such as age, the degree of activity, pregnancy, and the presence of certain diseases all serve to modify energy requirements. There are convincing data that the caloric needs decline with age at approximately 5 per cent per decade. Since activity also declines, the actual caloric need declines even more rapidly. Pregnancy, as well as several hormones, can increase the body's oxygen consumption. Thyroid hormone was the first hormone shown to have a calorigenic action. In conditions of thyroid hormone excess, total energy requirements are increased, and in the absence of this hormone, total caloric requirements drop sharply. Other hormones that have a calorigenic action include the catecholamines (epinephrine and norepinephrine), human growth hormone, and the androgenic steroids.

REGULATION OF ENERGY BALANCE

As noted earlier, obesity represents an imbalance between caloric intake and caloric expenditure. It now appears that both the regulation of food intake and the utilization of calories are defective in the obese individual. This net effect appears as an increase in the efficiency for food utilization. Efficiency may be defined in a number of ways. We will consider efficiency from the point of view of food storage. The more weight gained for a given food intake, the greater the efficiency. Thus, a more efficient animal or human being will store a greater fraction of total calories ingested. For every 1000 calories ingested, the efficient animal might store 3 to 5 per cent, whereas the inefficient animal would store only 0.5 to 2 per cent. This means that for the same caloric intake, it is possible for one animal to become considerably heavier and more obese than another. Such considerations have obvious commercial significance. Animals bred for obesity will store a larger fraction of their calories in their carcass than will lean animals. Differences in efficiency have also been noted in laboratory animals in which obesity is inherited as a recessive trait. In these obese animals, more fat will accumulate per gram of food ingested than in lean littermates. Although few measurements are available, the current data would suggest that this form of efficiency results from inactivity of the fat animal. Thus, for any given food intake, fewer calories are used for activity than in the lean animal. We must conclude that the efficiency of the fat animal may be substantially greater than for lean animals.

REGULATION OF FOOD INTAKE

Control of food intake is integrated in the central nervous system which is influenced by the metabolic state of the organism as well as the external environment.

Central Nervous System. The classic experiment of Hetherington and Ranson demonstrated that injury to a portion of the ventromedial hypothalamus near the "ventromedial nucleus" would consistently induce increased food intake and obesity in laboratory animals. This syndrome in experimental animals is analogous to the development of obesity noted by Fröhlich in his classic 1901 report of a young boy with a hypothalamic tumor. Hypothalamic obesity resulting from injury to the ventromedial hypothalamus is accompanied by a number of alterations. The animals are consistently and uniformly hyperphagic and prefer a high-fat diet rather than a high-carbohydrate or a high-protein diet. They will avoid eating food that tastes bad or that has an unpalatable consistency. They show increased levels of insulin and enlargement of the pancreatic islets of Langerhans. Finally, these animals, though initially hyperactive following introduction of these lesions, become hypoactive, although they can easily be aroused to rage. Injury to this region of the brain is followed by a period of rapid weight gain (dynamic phase) and then by a plateau weight (static phase),

at which they will again regulate their food intake and body weight.

Lateral to this ventromedial nucleus is a second hypothalamic area, destruction of which leads to total, but temporary, aphagia. If animals are tube-fed following this initial injury, eventually they will begin eating again but will maintain weight at a level lower than normal. Animals with this lateral hypothalamic lesion will no longer eat in response to insulin-induced hypoglycemia but will eat in response to cold or to other metabolic stimuli. Thus, there appear to be two hypothalamic centers involved in the regulation of food intake: a ventromedial system, which is involved in controlling signals for satiety, and a lateral system, which is involved in regulating the drive for food intake.

Studies on the distribution of adrenergic fibers in the brain stem have added significantly to our understanding of the relationship between the ventromedial and lateral regions of the hypothalamus. The ventromedial region of the hypothalamus is rich in dopaminergic fibers and also contains significant fibers from the ventral noradrenergic bundle. Destruction of the ventral noradrenergic bundle can reproduce many of the symptoms of the syndrome of hypothalamic obesity, suggesting that the noradrenergic fibers may mediate many of the phenomena associated with the ventromedial hypothalamus. The lateral hypothalamic area is traversed by the dopaminergic fibers that pass through this region from the brain stem. An injury to the lateral hypothalamus that causes a substantial reduction in dopamine will produce total aphagia (cessation of eating). Smaller reductions will produce graded decreases in food intake and loss of weight. It thus appears that the ventromedial and lateral hypothalamic regions are associated with bundles of adrenergic nerve fibers that have a predominantly anterior, posterior, or rostral caudal orientation, with little or no direct medial-lateral connection. Further evidence for the importance of adrenergic control of the hypothalamic centers in feeding has been provided by the injection of small quantities of norepinephrine into these regions. Norepinephrine will elicit feeding behavior in satiated animals, whereas the injection of isoproterenol into the hypothalamus will lead to inhibition of food intake. Currently, the regulation of food intake is considered to be controlled by an "alpha-adrenergic" feeding center and "beta-adrenergic" satiety center.

The cellular nuclei and fiber tract in the hypothalamus exert significant influences on food intake and on regulation of peripheral metabolism. For example, injury to the ventromedial hypothalamus that produces obesity is associated with increased activity of the vagus nerve, manifested experimentally by increased acid secretion in the stomach and increased insulin secretion from the pancreas. Such hypothalamic injury may also re

$$2800 \text{ cal/d} \times 365 \text{ days/year} \times 20 \text{ yrs.} = 20.5 \times 10^6 \text{ cal}$$

$$\text{Gained 20 lbs.} \times 3500 \text{ cal/lb.} = 70 \times 10^3 \text{ cal}$$

or 0.3% of ingested calories stored

Figure 33–5 Caloric intake and expenditure to accumulate 20 pounds. This figure assumes the average caloric intake of the standard male to be 2800 kcal/day and calculates the total number of calories expended during a period of 20 years. If 20 pounds are gained and if each pound is assumed to have 3500 calories, only 70,000 calories, or less than 0.34 per cent of the total calories, are stored. This shows the high efficiency of the human body in regulating energy intake and expenditure over prolonged periods of time.

duce the activity of the sympathetic nervous system and these reciprocal changes in the autonomic nervous system can explain many of the manifestations of this syndrome. These findings also provide a mechanism by which treatment of certain selected types of obesity might be developed. If alterations in the autonomic nervous system play an important role, drugs that modulate the activity of this system might be of value in directing the design of new pharmacologic agents.

Metabolic Factors. Metabolic factors are a second group of regulatory mechanisms for food intake. In most animals, body fat is a fairly constant fraction of total body weight. Although there is a tendency for the human being to gain weight with increasing age, the number of calories stored in fat in relation to the total calories eaten is very small. This is illustrated in Figure 33–5. No more than 0.34 per cent of calories need be stored to gain 1 pound per year. The nature of the mechanism involved in providing information about the quantity of metabolic energy is unknown. Several theories have been put forward, but they are as yet too limited to provide a sufficient explanation. That the body does regulate its food intake based on metabolic stores is, however, clearly shown by two kinds of experiments. In the first, the available food is diluted with various indigestible substances such as cellulose. In normal animals, the total amount of nutritional value is maintained constant, although the quantities of diluted food that are ingested vary. A similar result has been obtained by giving part of the food by stomach tube. As the quantity of food provided through a tube is increased, the amount ingested orally is decreased. Thus, there are mechanisms by which the feeding centers discern the metabolic needs of the organism and respond by food-seeking behavior.

The External Environment. The external environment provides a third category of information that regulates food intake. As already noted, animals with injury to the hypothalamus become finicky about what they will eat. A similar observation has been made in obese human subjects. When exposed to ice cream adulterated with small amounts of quinine, the obese will eat less than the lean, although they eat much more normal ice cream. Other factors in the external environment similarly influence food intake. The experiments

of Schachter and his colleagues have shown that the obese individual eats more when food is readily available. It appears from these and other experiments that the obese subject is more responsive to external cues than he is to metabolic cues. In contrast, the lean subject eats largely in response to metabolic needs, with external cues from taste, smell, and sight playing a much smaller role.

Adipose Tissue and Caloric Storage

Triglycerides represent the primary form of energy storage in most mammalian species (Table 33–3). Whether the excess caloric intake occurs as protein, fat, or carbohydrate seems to be of little importance. The storage form is primarily triglyceride. This has obvious advantages. One gram of triglyceride contains 9 calories. The adipocyte has about 7 to 7.5 calories per gram, with the aqueous components making up the difference. The caloric value of 1 gram of lean body mass, in contrast, is in the range of 1.5 calories, since approximately two thirds of this weight is fluid. Storage of carbohydrate as glycogen, though of importance as an immediate source of glucose, has the disadvantage of requiring a substantial addition of water and therefore a substantial addition of total weight relative to caloric storage. The rapid storage and subsequent utilization of large stores of triglyceride are of prime importance in two situations—the migratory bird and the hibernating mammal. Prior to flight across the Gulf of Mexico, birds will

TABLE 33–3 METABOLIC FUELS

Fuel Supply	Normal Man (70 kg)		Obese Man (140 kg)	
Fat	15.00 kg	141,000 kcal	80.00 kg	752,000 kcal
Protein	6.00 kg	24,000	8.000 kg	32,000
Glycogen				
Muscle	0.12 kg	480	0.160 kg	640
Liver	0.07 kg	280	0.700 kg	280
Glucose	0.02 kg	80	0.025 kg	100
		165,840 kcal		785,020 kcal

(Adapted from Cahill, G. F., and Owen, O. E.: *In* Rowland, C. V., Jr.: Anorexia and Obesity. Boston, Little, Brown & Co., 1970.)

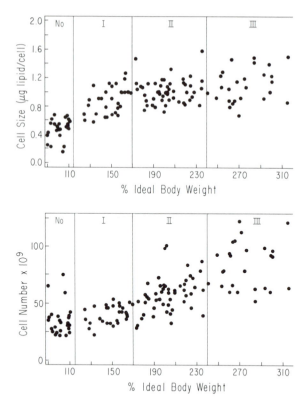

Figure 33–6 Body weight and fat cell size and number. The top panel displays data obtained by Dr. Hirsch on the relation of fat cell size to body weight. Essentially all overweight individuals showed an increase in the size of fat cells. The lower panel shows the relation of fat cell number to body weight. An increase in number of fat cells was more common among the more obese individuals. However, there were some with childhood-onset obesity who had a normal number of fat cells and others with adult-onset obesity who had an increased number of fat cells. (From Hirsch, J., and Batchelor, B.: Clin. Endocrinol. Metab. 5:2, 1976. Reproduced by permission of the author and publisher.)

eat enormous quantities of food and store it as fat that can be released and burned during the long-distance flight. A similar mechanism is involved in energy storage for the hibernating animal.

Three mechanisms are available for the storage of excess calories as triglycerides. The triglyceride can be stored by an increase in the size of the existing fat cells. It is also possible for the number of fat cells to increase, with little or no change in the size of individual cells. Finally, it is possible for both the size and number of adipocytes to increase. The adipocyte is a highly differentiated cell that arises from the adipoblast, a mesenchymal precursor. During the process of growth and development, a number of these precursor cells differentiate into fat cells. The mature fat cell does not divide but may dedifferentiate into fat-free cells. Thus once developed, the fat cell appears to remain throughout the life of the organism. Almost all forms of obesity are accompanied by an increased size of fat cells. This form of adaptation to glyceride storage is probably the principal mechanism when obesity develops in adult life (Fig. 33–6, top panel). In the forms of obesity that develop in early years of life, however, an increase in the total number of fat cells appears to be a major mechanism for adapting to the increased demands for triglyceride storage. Thus, individuals with gross obesity that begins in the early years of life show an increased mass of fat cells

that do not subsequently dedifferentiate (Fig. 33–6, bottom panel).

A series of biochemical reactions are involved in the formation of fatty acids and their conjugation with α-glycerophosphate (sn-glycerol-3-phosphate) to form triacylglycerols. Lipogenesis, the formation of fatty acids, appears to be controlled by nutritional state, by the presence of hormones, and by the size of the adipocyte. There is now substantial evidence in studies of human fat that incorporation of radioactivity into long-chain fatty acids can occur and that this process depends on the nutritional state of the individual from whom the fat is obtained. De novo synthesis of fatty acids is observed in adipose tissue taken from overfed patients. With caloric restriction, the rate of lipogenesis is severely depressed. Of the hormonal factors, insulin is of primary importance in controlling the rate of lipogenesis both in vivo and in vitro. The size of the adipose cell is also a determining factor in the rate of lipogenesis. With large fat cells, the rate of fatty acid synthesis is reduced. However, overfeeding for a short period of time will increase lipogenesis in large fat cells to a striking degree. The frequency with which food is ingested is a final factor that seems to be of importance in controlling lipogenesis. In experimental animals and in humans, the ingestion of food in one or two large meals produces significant changes in the metabolic and biochemical function.

When an individual eats a few large meals, he tends to have an impaired ability to metabolize glucose, to have a higher level of plasma cholesterol, to be more obese, and to show a greater rate of fatty acid formation in adipose tissue than is observed in individuals eating more frequent meals, but of smaller size.

The triglyceride stores in adipose tissue generally serve the body's needs during the intermeal periods. Thus, storage of carbohydrate as fatty acids in adipose tissue represents a storage form for fatty acids that are produced following food ingestion. After eating, there is an increased secretion of insulin that is stimulated by ingestion of glucose and amino acids, and there is also a stimulation of gastrointestinal hormones, which facilitate the release of insulin. As the nutrients absorbed from the gastrointestinal tract enter the blood, the concentration of insulin is rising, and this augments the storage of glucose in the liver as glycogen and of fatty acids and glucose in adipose tissue as triglycerides. As the concentration of glucose returns toward normal, there is a concomitant decline in the concentration of insulin and a return of the concentration of fatty acids toward their initial levels. This transition from the fed to the fasting state is facilitated by a reduction in insulin and may also be facilitated by the rise in growth hormone that is frequently observed 4 to 5 hours after eating. The release of fatty acids from adipose tissue is essential to fulfillment of the metabolic needs of peripheral tissues during the intermeal period. Measurement of the turnover and metabolism of fatty acids has shown that obese patients release and metabolize fatty acids more rapidly than lean subjects do. Moreover, the breakdown of triglycerides with the formation of free fatty acids and glycerol in vitro occurs at a higher rate with large adipose cells of the kind obtained from obese subjects, as compared with adipocytes from normal-weight subjects. Present evidence would thus suggest that the utilization of adipocyte triglycerides is normal or supernormal in obese individuals.

ENDOCRINE CONSEQUENCES OF OBESITY

The consequences of obesity can be divided into several groups, but we will consider only those of hormonal or metabolic origin. The most frequent endocrine change is hyperinsulinemia. Figure 33–7 shows that the level of insulin in the fasting state has a highly significant, positive correlation with the degree of obesity. The more obese an individual, the higher his fasting insulin. Similarly, the release of insulin in response to such stimuli as glucose, leucine, and tolbutamide is greater in obese individuals than in lean subjects. Thus, not only are their basal levels of insulin elevated but also their output of insulin in response to several stimuli is increased. Moreover, when glucose utilization and insulin are related, the obese individual requires more insulin to stimulate the utilization of glucose than normal. This implies that obese people are resistant to insulin. Studies by Salans and his collaborators have suggested that the adipocyte may be one site for this resistance. Other studies have shown, however, that muscle is also resistant to insulin. With a technique for perfusing the human forearm, it is possible to examine the response of muscle and adipose tissue together. The muscle of the obese individual behaves as the muscle of a normal individual does after exposure to high concentrations of insulin. Thus, the obese individual has an induced resistance to insulin in muscle, adipose tissue, and probably liver.

The initial step in the response of tissues to insulin is the interaction of circulating insulin with receptors for insulin located on the cell surface. Measurement of the binding of insulin to

Figure 33–7 Relation of immunoreactive insulin to body weight. Fasting levels of immunoreactive insulin have been plotted against the percentage of ideal body weight. Thus, body weight is a primary factor in determining the fasting serum insulin. (Reproduced with permission from Bagdade, J. D., et al.: J. Clin. Invest. 46:1549, 1967.)

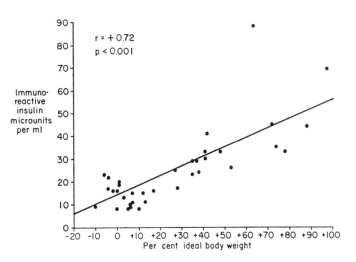

insulin receptors on monocytes, in adipose tissue, and liver membrane from obese and normal humans and experimental animals has shown that the number of insulin-binding receptors on the plasma membranes from obese humans are significantly reduced when compared with those from normal weight subjects. Evidence from tissue culture studies suggests that the number of receptors that bind insulin on a cell surface can be reduced by incubating the tissue in a high concentration of insulin. This type of feedback reduction in the number of receptors in the presence of high concentrations of insulin has important value in preventing excessive response to insulin in peripheral tissues. In addition to demonstrating changes in the binding of insulin to the cell membrane, many obese subjects show an impaired effect of insulin on biochemical events occurring later in the metabolism of glucose.

A second consistent alteration in obesity is an impaired output of growth hormone. Basal concentrations of growth hormone are normal or slightly reduced. Most striking is the impaired response to stimuli that usually increase growth hormone. The concentration of this hormone can usually be increased 4 to 5 hours after the oral administration of glucose, by the induction of hypoglycemia with insulin, or by the intravenous administration of arginine. In the obese individual, the output of growth hormone is impaired to all these stimuli.

The third consistent alteration in endocrine function of obese subjects is the increased production rate of adrenocortical steroids. Although the concentrations of plasma cortisol remain normal, the production rate of cortisol by the adrenal gland and the excretion of its metabolites in the urine are increased in obesity.

Fasting and very-low-calorie diets as well as overfeeding have significant effects on the concentration of thyroid hormone. With starvation, the concentrations of thyroxine and thyrotropin usually remain normal, but the concentrations of triiodothyronine $(T_3)(T_3 = 3,5,3'$-triiodothyronine) and reverse triiodothyronine ($rT_3 = 3,3',5'$-triiodothyronine) change in opposite directions. Both T_3 and reverse T_3 are generated by deiodination of thyroxine. Starvation significantly reduces the 3'-deiiodination of thyroxine, and the circulating levels of this hormone consequently fall. Because the substrate T_4 is available, the concentration of reverse triiodothyronine is usually increased during starvation. With overfeeding, reciprocal changes are observed. That is, with overfeeding the concentration of triiodothyronine increases, whereas the concentration of reverse triiodothyronine (rT_3) falls.

Changes in the reproductive hormones also occur in obesity. In both males and females, the concentration of the sex hormone-binding globulin (SFBG) is decreased, a change that is associated with a reduction in the concentration of total testosterone and estradiol. The production of es-

trone, however, is significantly increased. One mechanism for the increased production of estrone is the peripheral conversion of adrenal androgenic steroid, such as $\triangle^4$-androstenedione, to estrone in peripheral tissue. In-vitro incubations have demonstrated that stromal components of adipose tissue can convert androstenedione to estrone by aromatization of the A ring. One mechanism that heightens the risk for developing endometrial carcinoma in obese women is thought to be the increased estrogenic exposure of this tissue due to increased peripheral formation of estrone.

These endocrine adaptations are ones that would be expected from an internal milieu that favored the synthesis of fatty acid and deposition of triglycerides. It might be supposed that these endocrine alterations were causally related to obesity. However, it is possible that they are the consequence of overeating rather than a cause of corpulence. To gain insight into this question, Sims and his collaborators induced a weight gain of 30 to 40 pounds in a group of normal volunteers and studied their endocrine and metabolic responses. In all cases, the pattern of endocrine adaptation was similar to that observed in the patients with spontaneous obesity. That is, normal volunteers who gained weight by overeating demonstrated hyperinsulinemia, a reduced output of growth hormone in response to arginine, and increased production of cortisol by the adrenal gland. They also demonstrated insulin resistance of the muscle in the forearm similar to that observed in patients with spontaneous obesity. It would thus seem that the endocrine alterations in obesity are probably a consequence rather than a cause of the disease.

Figure 33–8 presents a diagram of the metabolic consequences of ingesting excess calories. On the right side, this diagram shows the effects on fat tissue; in the middle, the effects on carbohydrate; on the left, the effect on protein metabolism; and at the top, the effect on energy metabolism. Increased caloric ingestion from whatever cause leads to increased storage of fat, enlarged fat cells, increased basal lipolysis, and increased turnover of free fatty acids. This sequence of events may be responsible for the increased secretion of cholesterol that occurs in obesity and thus in turn makes obese patients more susceptible to the development of gallstones. The increased turnover of glucose and secretion of insulin may be related to the tendency of obesity to be the precipitating factor for diabetes mellitus. The increased circulating concentrations of the branch-chain amino acids may be a factor in stimulating insulin secretion.

PROTEIN AND/OR CALORIE DEFICIENCY

Several clinical syndromes result from the deficiency of proteins or calories or both. These

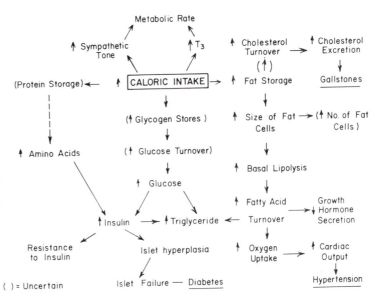

Figure 33–8 Consequences of ingesting an excess number of calories. An increased intake of calories will increase the size of the storage forms of protein, glycogen, and fat. However, since triglyceride can expand far more than the others, it is the principal storage site for extra calories. The ingestion of a surfeit of calories is associated with a number of metabolic changes, increasing lipolysis and re-esterification, increased insulin secretion, and increased concentration of five amino acids. It will also increase the formation of T_3 and the activity of the sympathetic nervous system.

conditions can occur when there is an insufficient supply of food, as in times of war or famine, or when the quality of the available food is inadequate for human needs. The presence of severe disease of the gastrointestinal tract may also impair absorption of nutrients. Finally, voluntary reduction in or abstinence from food has been used as a treatment of obesity. Our knowledge of the consequences of starvation increased rapidly during the first and second World Wars and more recently with the introduction of fasting as a treatment for obesity. Several clinical and pathologic features of the syndromes with caloric or protein deprivation are presented in Table 33–4. Three of these—starvation, anorexia nervosa, and marasmus in children—represent deficiencies of both protein and calories and may more appropriately be named protein-calorie malnutrition, although there are some features unique to each.

Kwashiorkor develops when protein is deficient in the diet.

STARVATION

Death is the ultimate consequence of total starvation and is frequently observed during periods of acute famine or in concentration camps during international conflagrations. The duration of survival following restriction of intake depends on the severity of the deprivation, on the quantity of reserve energy (i.e., fat), and on the adaptive mechanisms of the body. The presence of concurrent diseases accelerates deterioration. In classic studies on animals, Howe showed that dogs could be trained to starve. After 45 days during an early fast, his champion dog was near death. After a period of recovery with refeeding, the same animal

TABLE 33–4 A COMPARISON OF SOME FORMS OF MALNUTRITION

	Starvation	Anorexia Nervosa	Kwashiorkor	Marasmus
Primary deficiency	Calories	Calories	Protein	Calories
Age	Any age	10 to 30 yrs	At weaning	Children
Sex	Both	90% Female	Both	Both
Growth retardation	—	—	Slight	Significant
Body water	Decreased	Decreased	Increased	Decreased
Subcutaneous fat	Decreased	Decreased	May be normal	Decreased
Skin and hair lesions	—	—	Increased	Absent
Edema	Late	Late	Present	Absent
Diarrhea	Late	Absent	Present	Marked
Weight loss	Marked	Marked	Mild or absent	Marked
Serum albumin	Normal	Normal	Decreased	Normal
Hemoglobin	Normal	Normal	Decreased	Normal
Mg	Decreased	Decreased		Decreased
Liver	Normal	Normal	Enlarged and fatty	Normal
Pancreatic enzyme	—	—	Decreased	Normal

was able to "learn" to starve for more than 117 consecutive days. In each case the nutritional needs during this period were supplied by the stores in the body. The distribution of calories in fat, protein, and carbohydrate in a normal and an obese individual is shown in Table 33–3. Carbohydrates stored in the form of glycogen in liver and muscle or as circulating glucose represent only a small fraction of total body calories. The mechanisms by which the body adapts to the deficiency of carbohydrate intake are examined in detail subsequently. Although the maintenance of blood glucose is essential to survival, it is clear that the triglycerides in adipose tissue are the principal source of calories. These represent nearly 80 per cent of the total caloric stores of the normal individual and well over 95 per cent in an obese subject. With a caloric requirement of 2000 calories daily, a normal man would be expected to survive between 30 and 60 days of starvation. In contrast, the obese subject exemplified in Table 33–3 could survive for nearly a year. Indeed, obese individuals have been starved for therapeutic purposes in excess of 250 days without apparent ill effects.

The supply of glucose is clearly limited, yet it is an obligatory substrate for the brain under normal circumstances and is the primary fuel used by nervous tissue, red cells, leukocytes, and the renal medulla. If glycogen were supplying total caloric needs, the available supply would provide for the body for only 10 hours. In the absence of carbohydrate intake, therefore, protein or fat must provide for most of the caloric needs. In addition, glucose must be formed from one of these substances. There is no net conversion of fatty acids or acetate to carbohydrate, and, therefore, essentially all the new glucose formed during starvation comes from alanine, lactate, or pyruvate. This process of gluconeogenesis occurs primarily in the liver, with the kidney participating to a small extent. The oxidation of fatty acids activates the conversion of amino acids to glucose. In the short-term fast, lasting several hours to 2 or 3 days, the needs of the body for glucose are supplied from protein and Cori-cycle intermediates (lactate) and are stimulated by the release of free fatty acids from the adipose tissue. Evidence from studies of Cahill and his collaborators suggest that insulin is the principal hormone concerned with regulating the initial process of adaptation to fasting. This is most clearly seen by comparing the period of food ingestion with the intermeal period. Following the ingestion of food, insulin is released from the pancreas and serves to increase the uptake of glucose into muscle and adipose tissue and to enhance the conversion of glucose to glycogen in the liver. Insulin similarly diminishes the release of free fatty acids from adipose tissue by inhibiting lipolysis while accelerating the conversion of glucose into long-chain fatty acids within the adipocytes. Thus, the outpouring of insulin

following the ingestion of foods containing carbohydrate or amino acids accelerates the storage of fuels for the coming period without food. With fasting, the concentration of insulin declines, and the entry of glucose into tissues falls. Triglycerides are hydrolyzed and the fatty acids are released into the circulation to be metabolized in liver and peripheral tissues. The low levels of insulin similarly reduce the conversion of carbohydrate to glycogen in muscle. Thus, in a short-term fast, reduction in the concentration of insulin increases the release of free fatty acids from adipose tissue and of amino acids from muscle. In this way the substrates for gluconeogenesis and energy metabolism in peripheral tissues are supplied. This is shown schematically in Figure 33–7.

As fasting is continued, the excretion of nitrogen falls, indicating that mobilization of amino acids has diminished. In time, the supply of carbon precursors for the formation of glucose from amino acids falls below the metabolic requirements of the brain, red cells, and renal medulla. Two possibilities exist to permit survival. One is that the glucose-requiring tissue can adapt to utilize other substrates; the other is that glucose could be formed from long-chain fatty acids. With prolonged fasting the brain can adapt to utilize ketone bodies to provide a significant fraction of the total caloric needs. In addition, ketones can be converted to glucose by formation of acetone, which is then oxidized to form pyruvate. Thus, after a prolonged period of fasting (i.e., 5 to 6 weeks), a number of adaptations have occurred in fuel consumption by the organism. The brain that was previously consuming 140 gm of glucose has decreased its consumption to 80 gm, the remainder being derived by oxidation of ketone bodies. The release of amino acids is significantly reduced, partly through the inhibitory effects of circulating ketones. With prolonged fasting, gluconeogenesis from the liver is decreased, and the kidney becomes a more significant source of new glucose (Fig. 33–9). Indeed, during prolonged fasting the kidney provides as much or more glucose than the liver primarily because of the renal ammonia production. With fasting, there is also a reduction in total caloric requirements by 15 to 20 per cent. Finally, up to 20 per cent of glucose comes from adaptive oxidation of acetone to pyruvate.

One mechanism for the decreased metabolism in starvation may be the reduced concentration of triiodothyronine. Approximately 75 per cent of the circulating triiodothyronine is formed from thyroxine in peripheral tissues. As mentioned earlier, in starvation, the production of triiodothyronine falls significantly. Reverse triiodothyronine (i.e., 3,3',5'-triiodothyronine) is increased in reciprocal fashion to the reduction in triiodothyronine. Since triiodothyronine is the most potent calorigenic hormone, reduction in the concentration of this hormone during starvation might account for the lower consumption of oxygen.

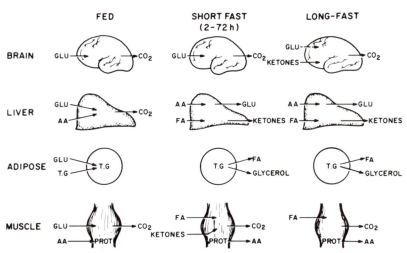

Figure 33–9 Effect of fasting on substrate utilization. Effects of substrate utilization by brain, liver, adipose tissue, and muscle in the fed state after short fast of 2 to 72 hours and following a prolonged fast. In the fed state and during a short fast, glucose is the principal substrate for the brain. With prolonged fasting, however, the brain adapts to the use of ketones for a significant fraction of its total energy requirements. With fasting, the liver adapts from burning glucose and amino acids to converting amino acids to glucose and converting free fatty acids to ketones, which are then used in the peripheral tissues. In the fed state, adipose tissue stores fatty acids as triglyceride, and in the short- and long-term fast it releases these triglycerides as their fatty acid and glycerol moieties. Muscle during the fed state utilizes glucose and amino acids, but with fasting muscle uses free fatty acids or ketones. (Adapted from Cahill, G. F., Jr., and Owen, O. E.: *In* Rowland, C. V., Jr. [Ed.]: Anorexia and Obesity. Boston, Little, Brown and Co., 1970.)

The decreased concentration of insulin appears to provide the principal signal for the early responses to fasting. Insulin, however, remains low during prolonged fasting and does not seem to be a signal for the adaptive processes observed primarily in the brain and liver. Human growth hormone, glucocorticoids, and glucagon have also been explored as possible agents in the adaptation of fasting but do not appear to provide the needed hormonal signal. The major differences between the fed state and short- or long-term fasts are shown in Figure 33–9.

In addition to causing the endocrine and metabolic changes already described, fasting produces a number of other alterations that warrant brief comment. The decrease in circulating levels of insulin and glucose already has been noted. Changes in the concentration of growth hormone are variable, but it is frequently increased. The excretion of 17-hydroxycorticosteroids and 17-ketosteroids is decreased. Concentrations of gonadotropins and testosterone show no change with fasting. Plasma levels of amino acids undergo a variety of changes. Alanine, which is an important precursor for gluconeogenesis, falls to one third of its normal level. Valine, leucine, and isoleucine initially increase in concentration but subsequently decline. Glycine, however, rises significantly with continued fasting. In addition to these changes in amino acids, there are significant losses of sodium, potassium, and magnesium from the body. Plasma magnesium remains normal, yet magnesium depletion of up to 20 per cent can

occur. A mild ketoacidosis is uniformly found along with hyperuricemia. The increased concentrations of uric acid probably result from an increase in the concentrations of β-hydroxybutyrate. This has been supported by the fact that the excretion of uric acid is reduced by the infusion of lactate or β-hydroxybutyrate. Riboflavin is decreased most rapidly, but there is also a delayed fall in pantothenic acid, pyridoxine, and thiamine.

Some of the consequences of starvation are diagrammed in Figure 33–10. It shows the decreased fat content, decreased fat cell size, and increased fatty acid and ketone production that result from the mobilization of triglycerides in adipose tissue. The changes in metabolism of glucose and insulin, whose concentrations decline, and of glucagon, whose concentration goes up, are also depicted. The hyperuricemia observed during starvation can be largely accounted for by the increased concentration of β-hydroxybutyrate, which competes at the renal tubule for secretion of uric acid. One hypothesis for the increased sodium excretion is that increased concentrations of glucagon stimulate sodium loss during fasting. The alterations in protein and amino acid metabolism have been described earlier.

Several significant consequences can occur during fasting. Postural hypotension and collapse have been observed. Gouty arthritis and precipitation of uric acid stones have been reported and can be prevented by treatment with the appropriate drugs. The most serious consequence, death, has been reported in several patients undergoing

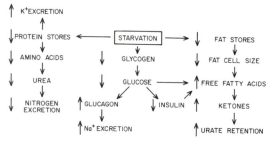

Figure 33–10 Effects of starvation on body function. This diagram shows the effects of starvation on body stores of fat, carbohydrate, and protein. There is a reduction in fat stores and fat cell size and an increase in free fatty acids as the primary energy source. This increased ketone concentration impairs uric acid excretion by the kidney, with urate retention in the blood and the occasional precipitation of gouty arthritis. Starvation also depletes glycogen and glucose and, through the increase in glucagon, may lead to a rise in sodium excretion. Protein stores that initially are mobilized to provide glucose are conserved as the body adapts to using more fatty acids and to conserving protein stores.

therapeutic starvation. These cases indicate that such treatment should be undertaken only with careful medical supervision.

ANOREXIA NERVOSA

Anorexia nervosa represents a second form of protein-calorie deficiency with loss of tissue. Although this is a clinically defined entity, it represents a physiologic pattern of change similar to that observed with caloric restriction or total starvation. This disease primarily affects females in the age range of 10 to 30 years. Not infrequently, these individuals have been modestly overweight and suddenly go into a catabolic phase. Patients with anorexia nervosa show little concern about their relatively cachectic state. Weight loss is marked, and subcutaneous fat is often nearly absent. Adipocytes can be expected to be very small indeed. Breast development remains little changed, and there is no loss of axillary or pubic hair and no development of skin lesions. The concentration of adrenocortical hormones in the plasma remains normal, but it is reduced in the urine. Menstrual cycles are absent in these individuals. Plasma growth hormone is elevated.

MARASMUS AND KWASHIORKOR

The findings in the various forms of starvation are to be contrasted with those observed when protein deficiency is the principal defect. This illness, known as kwashiorkor, is occasionally seen in its relatively pure form but is more frequently observed with various degrees of simultaneous caloric deficiency. In its relatively pure form, kwashiorkor begins at the time of weaning if the infant receives a very low protein supply but is given an adequate number of calories. Growth retardation is slight in this illness in comparison with the significant growth retardation observed with caloric restriction. Subcutaneous fat may be normal in the individual with kwashiorkor but is uniformly reduced in patients with marasmus. This is readily explained in terms of the alterations in the ingested fuel mixture. When protein is deficient but calories are adequate, these calories must be either carbohydrate or fat. The ingestion of carbohydrate as just noted stimulates the release of insulin and serves as a stimulus for the production and storage of triglyceride and glycogen. It is thus not surprising that body fat stores are relatively well preserved in kwashiorkor.

A second consequence is that body weight loss is mild or absent in contrast to starvation, in which marked weight loss occurs. Edema, however, is a common feature in kwashiorkor and can be attributed largely to the striking reduction in serum albumin. Since the intake of protein is reduced, the supply of amino acids to the liver from the gastrointestinal tract is inadequate. In the presence of normal carbohydrate intake, the release of amino acids from muscle tissue is low, and consequently the supplies of amino acids to the liver are insufficient for the synthesis of normal amounts of serum albumin. With the reduction in serum albumin to levels of 1 to 2 gm per 100 ml of blood (20 to 30 per cent of normal), the oncotic pressure in plasma is reduced. Plasma osmotic pressure becomes insufficient to counterbalance the hydrostatic and osmotic forces in the extracellular fluid, and there is a tendency for fluid to accumulate in the extravascular compartment. This has been confirmed by the measurements of increased quantities of total body water and of extracellular fluid in patients with kwashiorkor. The deficiency in protein is also accompanied by an enlarged, fatty liver that is usually not seen when both calories and protein are deficient. The appearance of skin and hair lesions in kwashiorkor may be a reflection of vitamin deficiencies, which are often observed when protein is deficient. Diarrhea, a late event in starvation, is less common in patients with kwashiorkor. It is thus possible to distinguish between the various forms of protein-calorie malnutrition on clinical grounds and with laboratory measurements. Particularly prominent in the patient with protein depletion but adequate caloric intake are the marked reduction in albumin, the enlarged fatty liver, and the nearly normal amounts of subcutaneous fat. With starvation, however, adipose stores are mobilized to provide energy for body stores and to spare protein and carbohydrate.

ACCELERATED STARVATION

There are important differences between the physiologic adaptation to starvation alone and the sequence of food deprivation when it is associated with trauma, injury, or infection. First, stressful situations associated with injury, burns, or infection activate the autonomic nervous system. Many of the differences between starvation and injury can be attributed to enhanced activity of the sympathetic nervous system. Among these are enhanced glucagon secretion, impaired insulin secretion, and increased epinephrine release. This sequence of events leads to a relative decline in insulin and a rise in glucose resulting from enhanced glycogen mobilization and accelerated gluconeogenesis. The inhibition of insulin secretion and increased concentrations of catecholamines would also be associated with increased release of free fatty acids. In addition to the marked hyperglycemia, there is an increase in vasopressin and corticosteroid secretion, which are responsible for decreased water excretion by the kidneys and increased sodium reabsorption by the renal tubule. In addition, elevated levels of corticosteroids may be responsible for the accelerated rates of protein breakdown that have been observed in stress. These metabolic differences resulting from neural and endocrine disturbances associated with stress are important when one is considering the use of nutrient replacement during stress and starvation. This field of parenteral nutrition is of growing importance as the availability of solutions containing amino acids and lipids becomes widespread. For additional discussions of parenteral nutrition, the reader is referred to Chapter 28.

LIPIDS

Interest in the role of lipids in human disease has been continually reinforced by the observation that cardiovascular disease, particularly acute myocardial infarction, occurs with significantly higher frequency in individuals with high serum cholesterol. The major lipid components of blood are listed in Table 33–5. Cholesterol is a 25-carbon molecule with four rings and is a normal constituent of animal and plant fats. Triglycerides are esters of fatty acids and glycerol. Phospholipids are a class of diglycerides with a phosphate ester on the third hydroxyl of glycerol. Fats or lipids account for approximately 40 per cent of the calories available for consumption in the retail market of the United States. Since the late 1950s, there has been a gradual decrease in the sources of

TABLE 33–5 LIPID COMPONENTS OF BLOOD

Serum Lipids		Concentration
Total cholesterol	mg/100 ml	230 ± 35*
Phospholipids	mg/100 ml	220 ± 30
Triglycerides	mg/100 ml	105 ± 25
Free fatty acids	μEq/L	400 to 800

*Mean ± S.D.

animal fat from 75 to 66 per cent, whereas the fraction of fats available from vegetable sources has increased from 25 to 34 per cent. This transition has been accelerated by observations that the quality of fats in the diet, as well as their total quantity, may play a role in the development of human cardiovascular disease. A relationship between changes in serum cholesterol and the intake of fats and cholesterol has been demonstrated by many investigators. From the formula shown on page 980, it can be seen that a reduction in saturated fats in the diet would have a more significant effect on serum cholesterol than increasing unsaturated fats. The effect of dietary cholesterol is small, since it appears as the square root of its concentration.

FAT INGESTION AND METABOLISM

The ingestion of fats is followed by their cleavage into smaller moieties prior to absorption. Considerable interest has been focused on the mechanism for hydrolysis, absorption, and transport of dietary lipids. Triglycerides are cleaved by a pancreatic lipase into monoglycerides or glycerol and fatty acids. In the presence of bile acids and phospholipids, water-soluble micelles composed of fatty acids and monoglycerides are formed. These micellar aggregates are then absorbed into the mucosal cells. The bile acids are recycled into the portal circulation, taken up by the liver, and secreted into the bile again. The fate of the fatty acids depends on their chain length. For fatty acids with less than 12 carbon atoms, the triglycerides formed in the intestinal epithelium are released into the portal circulation and transported directly to the liver. With the long-chain fatty acids of more than 12 carbon atoms, however, transport is more complex. These fatty acids, after conversion to triglycerides, are surrounded by a protein coat to form chylomicrons. Although chylomicrons consist predominantly of triglycerides, they also contain small amounts of cholesterol and phospholipid. These aggregates are secreted into the lacteals of the intestinal villi and enter the general circulation through the thoracic duct. In high concentration, they give the serum a creamy appearance. Chylomicrons are removed from the circulation after hydrolysis of the triglyceride by lipoprotein lipase, which is present in many tissues. This enzyme is increased by insulin and glucose and is activated by heparin and apoprotein CII. The fatty acids and glycerol thus formed enter adipose or muscle cells for metabolism or storage.

In addition to the chylomicrons formed in the gastrointestinal tract, very-low-density lipoproteins (VLDL) can be assembled in the liver and secreted into the circulation. The fatty acids in these lipoproteins can be synthesized from glucose in the liver or from fatty acids taken up from the blood. The fate of the lipoproteins is similar to that of the chylomicrons; that is, the triglycerides are hydrolyzed by lipoprotein lipase. The cholesterol and phospholipid remaining after cleavage of the triglycerides are partly transferred to higher density lipoproteins, with the remainder becoming β-lipoproteins. There are thus two sources of the large triglyceride-rich lipoproteins: (1) chylomicrons formed from dietary lipid, and (2) hepatic lipoproteins formed from fatty acids synthesized in the liver or taken up from the circulation.

Our understanding of lipid metabolism was greatly expanded by the introduction of techniques for separating the various serum lipoproteins by ultracentrifugation or electrophoresis. By using the latter technique along with measurements of triglyceride and cholesterol and, in some instances, by using flotation methods in the ultracentrifuge, one can distinguish chylomicrons from alpha-, beta-, and prebetalipoproteins. A typical electrophoretic pattern of normal serum is shown in Figure 33–11. When analyzed quantitatively, the components of these various lipoproteins differ. The cholesterol content is highest in the α-lipoprotein and lowest in chylomicrons and pre–β-lipoproteins, with the β-lipoprotein being intermediate. In contrast, the triglyceride concentration is highest in chylomicrons and lowest in the α-lipoproteins.

Defects in Fat Metabolism and Their Determination by Electrophoretic Techniques

Several proteins make up the envelope for these circulating lipoproteins. The apoprotein A is associated in highest concentration with the α-lipoproteins. The apoprotein B is associated in highest concentration with the β-lipoproteins. The very-low-density lipoproteins and the chylomicrons also contain apoproteins B, CI, CII, and CIII. Deficiency of the B protein presents a characteristic clinical picture. As might be expected, the concentrations of chylomicrons and β-lipoproteins are very low, since the protein that provides the principal coating is absent. Indeed, some patients have no detectable β-lipoproteins. Serum cholesterol is also strikingly reduced. Patients with this disorder also demonstrate neurologic abnormalities and an irregularity of the red blood cells, called *acanthocytosis*. Persons lacking the B protein manifest their disease in infancy as a failure to grow and the appearance of fat in the stools. The basic pathophysiology is failure to form the protein coat by which triglycerides of long-chain fatty acids can be transported. Since triglycerides formed from short- and medium-chain fatty acids do not require a protein coat for transport, they have proved useful in treating patients with a β-lipoproteinemia.

A second defect in transport of lipoproteins is observed with absence of the A protein. This disease was originally found on Tangier Island in Chesapeake Bay and has since been called *Tangier disease*. The defect is an absence of A protein associated with a reduction in the concentration of cholesterol and phospholipid in the plasma, but triglyceride shows only mild changes. The most striking abnormality in individuals with this disease is the large orange-colored tonsils that result from the deposition of cholesterol esters in this tissue. Similar esters are also deposited in the reticuloendothelial cells of liver and spleen. In the absence of α-lipoprotein, lipid is carried primarily by the β-lipoproteins, which appear normal by immunoelectrophoresis.

Absence of lipoprotein lipase from peripheral tissues produces a third defect in lipid metabolism and is inherited as an autosomal recessive trait. This enzyme is essential to the hydrolysis of triglycerides carried on chylomicrons and pre–β-lipoproteins prior to their entry and storage in adipose cells and other peripheral tissues. Absence of this enzyme would lead to an accumulation of these lipoproteins in the serum. On visual examination the serum from such patients is creamy. The marked elevation in serum triglycerides and chylomicrons results from the dietary intake of triglyceride. If fat is excluded from the diet, the chylomicrons disappear and lipid levels return almost to normal. Thus, exclusion of fat from the diet represents the principal mode of treatment for individuals with this disease. The symptom complex observed is also susceptible to treatment by dietary restriction of fat and therefore probably results from the high levels of chylomicrons. These symptoms include abdominal pain, a creamy color to the retinal vessels, and the appearance of reddish-yellow lipid-containing plaques in the skin.

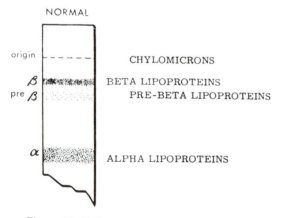

Figure 33–11 Electrophoretic pattern for lipoproteins. This schematic diagram shows the pattern obtained during electrophoresis of normal serum. The sample applied at the origin undergoes electrophoresis in the albumin buffer. Chylomicrons, if present, remain at the origin. The first band contains β-lipoproteins, and the faint band running just in front of the β-lipoproteins contains the pre–β-lipoproteins. The high-density α-lipoproteins migrate farthest on paper electrophoresis.

TABLE 33–6 CLASSIFICATION OF HYPERLIPOPROTEINEMIA BASED ON LIPOPROTEIN PATTERN

	Lipoprotein					Lipids		
Type	Chylo-microns	LDL β	VLDL pre-β	Floating β	Appearance of Standing Plasma	Cholesterol	Tri-glyceride	Chol/TG
I	+				Creamy	N or ↑	↑↑↑	< 0.2
IIa		+			Clear	↑↑	N	> 15.0
IIb		+	+		Clear or faintly turbid	↑↑	↑	Variable
III				+	Turbid	↑	↑↑	Frequently > 1.0
IV			+		Clear or turbid	N or ↑	↑↑	Variable
V			+		Creamy	↑	↑↑↑	> 0.15; < 0.06

Key: + = Present
↑ = Increased
↑↑ = Modestly increased
↑↑↑ = Greatly increased
N = Normal

Using the technique illustrated in Figure 33–11 along with measurement of cholesterol and triglyceride, one can segregate the lipoprotein patterns into six groups, as illustrated in Table 33–6, which is adapted from the currently recommended international classification.

Type I results from deficiency of lipoprotein lipase and was already described. As would be expected with a deficiency of this enzyme, the pattern on electrophoresis shows a marked increase in concentration of chylomicrons.

The second type of pattern observed with this technique is a marked increase in the β-lipoprotein fraction without elevation of triglycerides (IIa) or when this moiety is also elevated (IIb). This protein carries a significant fraction of the total cholesterol and is accompanied by significant elevations in concentration of plasma cholesterol. The familial form is inherited as an autosomal dominant, and types IIa and IIb appear in the same families. The defect in removal of low-density lipoproteins that characterizes this disease was described earlier. This disease is often associated with accumulations of lipid (xanthomas) in tendons. Early cardiovascular death has often been associated with this syndrome. Evidence indicates that high levels of cholesterol can be detected in up to 0.5 per cent of newborns, making it an easily detectable and optimistically treatable affliction.

The third abnormality in the electrophoretic pattern (type III) is known as broad beta disease. This is observed when the β-band is increased in width and streaks over into the pre-β region but without a separate band. This is a rare disease and must be distinguished from IIb by showing that the lipoprotein floats at a density of 1.006. The familial form of this disease is inherited as an autosomal recessive trait and is manifested mainly in adult life. The increased amounts of triglyceride and cholesterol often result in lipid deposition in the skin. Such individuals are also plagued by coronary artery disease at an early age. Glucose metabolism is often abnormal in patients with this disease.

The fourth type of electrophoretic abnormality (type IV) shows a striking increase in the concentration of pre–β-lipoproteins and is among the two most common types. This disease is inducible by a high-carbohydrate diet and is often termed endogenous, or carbohydrate-inducible, hyperlipoproteinemia. This abnormality and that of type II are frequently seen as complications of other diseases including diabetes, hypothyroidism, and the nephrotic syndrome. The serum from patients is usually cloudy. Glucose tolerance is often abnormal, and afflicted individuals are frequently obese.

The final syndrome (type V) is manifested by an elevation in both chylomicrons and pre–β-lipoproteins. The activity of lipoprotein lipase is frequently low in patients with type V disease and may account for their increased level of chylomicrons. As with type I, patients suffering from type V abnormalities frequently have abdominal pain and usually show abnormal metabolism of glucose. Progestational and anabolic steroids have been found to enhance the activity of lipoprotein lipase and to lower levels of triglyceride.

With the technique of lipoprotein electrophoresis and measurements of cholesterol and triglyceride, sophisticated genetic studies have been performed on the prevalence of lipoprotein types in

TABLE 33–7 GENETIC CLASSIFICATION OF HYPERLIPIDEMIA

	Prevalence in Population (Per Cent)
Monogenic hyperlipidemia*	
Familial hypercholesterolemia	~0.1 – 0.2
Familial hypertriglyceridemia	~0.2 – 0.3
Combined hyperlipidemia	~0.3 – 0.5
Polygenic hypercholesterolemia	
Sporadic hypertriglyceridemia	

*Inherited as an autosomal dominant.
(Adapted from Goldstein, J. L., et al.: J. Clin. Invest. 52:1544, 1973.)

$$\Delta \text{ Cholesterol } = 1.2[2(\Delta S) - \Delta U] + 1.5\Delta \left(\sqrt{\text{Chol} \frac{\text{mg}}{1000 \text{ cal}}} \right)$$

ΔS = Glycerides of saturated fatty acids (C_{12} to C_{16}) as a percentage of total calories.

ΔU = Glycerides of polyunsaturated fatty acids in the diet as a percentage of total calories.

---

the population, and a new classification based on this information has been introduced (Table 33–7). This classification is based on a study of 157 survivors of myocardial infarction and their relatives. The monogenic hyperlipidemia that is transmitted as an autosomal dominant trait can be subdivided into three genetic groups: familial hypercholesterolemia, familial hypertriglyceridemia, and a combined hyperlipidemia. Polygenic inheritance of hypercholesterolemia and the sporadic appearance of hypertriglyceridemia have also been noted.

Studies by Brown and Goldstein have provided new insight into the pathogenic sequence involved in the manifestation of hypercholesterolemia (Fig. 33–12). Using tissue culture of fibroblasts from normal and hypercholesterolemic individuals, they found that cells from heterozygotes had a reduction and cells from homozygotes had a nearly complete absence of receptors that bind low-density lipoprotein. The mechanism for increased hypercholesterolemia can thus be explained by the loss of inhibition of cholesterol synthesis because the circulating cholesterol was unable to enter the cell and inhibit the key regulatory enzyme, HMG CoA^{+1} reductase. In the normal individual, the low density of lipoprotein binds to a receptor on the cell surface, and the receptor and LDL are incorporated into the cell. The cholesterol is then released and serves to inhibit further cholesterol synthesis within that cell. When these low-density lipoprotein receptors are reduced or absent, the quantity of LDL entering the cell is reduced, and intracellular cholesterol synthesis is enhanced. The sites of abnormalities in this scheme for pro-

duction of cholesterol are shown in Figure 33–12.

In summary, the absorption, digestion, transport, and storage of the lipid components of the diet represent a complex and well-integrated system. Lipoproteins represent the principal form of transporting lipids in plasma. The introduction of electrophoretic techniques for separating the lipoproteins in plasma has provided significant new insights into the pathogenesis of a number of disease states. The two principal lipoproteins, α- and β-lipoproteins, are associated primarily with A and B proteins in their coats. Disease syndromes have been described that result from the deficiency of one or the other of these proteins. Elevated chylomicrons result from a deficiency of lipoprotein lipase, the enzyme that hydrolyzes circulating triglycerides, so that they can be absorbed and stored in adipose tissue. Four other types of abnormality in lipoprotein patterns have also been described that can occur as genetically transmitted forms or in association with other diseases.

VITAMINS

Vitamins may be defined as small chemical molecules that are essential to maintenance of normal metabolic processes but that cannot be synthesized within the body. These substances must therefore be provided in adequate amounts from dietary sources. Since the early 1900s, a number of vitamins have been elucidated and their clinical correlates put into focus. A listing of these vitamins is presented in Table 33–8. They can be divided into two groups: the water-soluble vita-

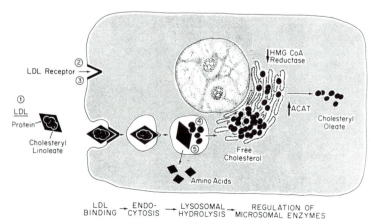

Figure 33–12 A diagram of the metabolism of cholesterol. This figure illustrates the entry of low-density lipoproteins into the cell after interaction with cell receptors. The cholesterol esters are then broken down, and the cholesterol that is released inhibits the synthesis of new cholesterol and increases the rate of esterification of cholesterol. States of hypercholesterolemia can occur when the receptors for lipoproteins are reduced. (From Brown, M. S., and Goldstein, J. L.: N. Engl. J. Med. 294:1387.)

mins, including the B-complex vitamins and vitamin C, and the fat-soluble vitamins, A, D, E, and K. The precise metabolic role of some vitamins has been clearly described, but the role of others is less well understood. The B-complex vitamins as a group are involved in the metabolism of carbohydrate as cofactors either for the transfer of hydrogen or for decarboxylation or transamination. Pyridoxine is involved in transfer of amino groups and biotin in the fixation of CO_2 during fatty acid synthesis and gluconeogenesis. Folic acid and vitamin B_{12} are involved in nucleic acid synthesis. The precise role of vitamin C is unclear. Vitamin A has several functions, but its role in the visual cycle has been most clearly defined. Vitamin D has an essential role in bone metabolism. Vitamin K is dealt with in more detail in Chapter 24.

Defining the requirements for these nutritional factors has occupied considerable research effort. Since most of them are intimately involved in intermediary metabolism, their requirements in general vary with the overall rate of metabolism. It would thus be expected that diseases that alter metabolism would also alter the rates at which the vitamins are metabolized and thus increase or decrease their requirements. Hyperthyroidism, which increases oxygen consumption, enhances the need for thiamine and riboflavin. When thyroid function is decreased, the requirements for these vitamins fall. The definition of requirements for many vitamins must, therefore, be stated in terms of total caloric requirement. In general, however, the minimum daily requirements are high enough to allow a reasonable margin of safety for individual variation.

TABLE 33–8 RECOMMENDED DAILY ALLOWANCES FOR VITAMINS

Vitamins	Recommended Daily Allowance
Water-soluble vitamins	
Thiamine (B_1)	0.3 to 1.5 mg
Riboflavin (B_2)	0.4 to 1.7 mg
Pyridoxine (B_6)	0.3 to 2.2 mg
Niacin	6.0 to 19.0 mg
Panthothenic acid*	2.0 to 7 mg
Folacin (folic acid)	0.03 to 0.4 mg
Cyanocobalamin (B_{12})	0.5 to 3.0 μg
Biotin*	35 to 200 μg
Ascorbic acid (C)	35 to 60 mg
Fat-soluble vitamins	
Vitamin A	420 to 1000 μg
Vitamin D	5 to 10 μg
Vitamin E	3 to 10 μg
Vitamin K*	12 to 140 μg
Electrolytes	
Sodium	115 to 3300 mg
Potassium	350 to 5625 mg

*Safe and adequate (infants and adults).

WATER-SOLUBLE VITAMINS

Thiamine (Vitamin B_1). Thiamine was among the first of the B-complex vitamins to be chemically identified and serves as an important cofactor in the decarboxylation of pyruvic and α-ketoglutaric acids. Deficiency of this vitamin is manifested by defective metabolism of carbohydrates. One of the cardinal biochemical alterations accompanying the clinical states of thiamine deficiency is an increase in circulating levels of pyruvic acid. The inability to utilize pyruvate in thiamine deficiency is accompanied by the development of two clinical syndromes, one involving the peripheral nervous system and the other the cardiovascular system. Peripheral involvement of the nervous system, known as *peripheral neuritis*, is manifested as increased pain, a loss of sensation, or an aching or burning sensation. Significant alterations in the central nervous system also occur and are most commonly observed in patients ingesting large quantities of alcohol. The cardiovascular manifestations are primarily those of inadequate energy supply to the myocardium and the periphery with an increase in cardiac output. Arterioles are dilated, leading to an increased flow of blood between the arterial and venous circulation. As a result of the high cardiac output and defective carbohydrate metabolism, heart failure occurs associated with shortness of breath, increased heart rate, subjective feelings of palpitation, and objective findings of irregular rhythms. The heart is usually enlarged, and, as might be expected in a heart that is unable to pump blood at a sufficient rate, there is an increase in venous pressure. These neurologic and cardiovascular symptoms are most prominent in severe deficiencies, but careful studies of hospitalized patients have revealed significantly reduced levels of thiamine in approximately one third of such patients. Since the requirements for thiamine are related to the metabolic rate, both deficient food intake and hypermetabolism can produce symptoms of disease. Patients with prolonged alcoholic intake or people eating hypocaloric diets can suffer from mild symptoms of thiamine deficiency, whereas individuals with hypermetabolism (usually hyperthyroidism) will suffer from similar symptoms even though thiamine intake may be adequate normally.

Riboflavin (Vitamin B_2). Although riboflavin was chemically identified for the first time in 1879, its role in the production of disease was not appreciated for some years thereafter. Normal subjects on a riboflavin-deficient diet developed characteristic lesions within 3 months. Among the pathologic changes were vascularization of the cornea and cheilosis. Riboflavin and its two active nucleotides, flavin mononucleotide (FMN) and flavin-adeninedinucleotide (FAD), are the hydrogen-accepting cofactors for several enzymes, including xanthine oxidase, succinate dehydrogenase, and mitochondrial glycerophosphate oxidase. Like thiamine requirements, those for riboflavin depend on overall metabolic activity and have been defined as 0.25 to 0.30 mg per 1000 kcal of food oxidized. Thyroid hormones play a major role in the control of flavoprotein metabolism. Hyperthyroidism clearly produces an increased metabolic rate and enhances the metabolism of riboflavin. This latter effect is manifested as an increase in the enzymes that convert riboflavin to its active form, flavin mononucleotide. Hypothyroidism, however, produces a decrease in hepatic flavin-containing enzymes that are similar to those produced by riboflavin deficiency. The metabolic rate is reduced in riboflavin-deficient animals as it is in hypothyroidism. Similarly, α-glycerophosphate dehydrogenase, a mitochondrial enzyme, is decreased in hypothyroidism and in riboflavin deficiency. These observations suggest that certain clinical features of hypothyroidism may be attributable to the inability to metabolize riboflavin in a normal manner.

Niacin (Nicotinamide). Deficiency of niacin produces pellagra, or black tongue. This illness is characterized by symptoms referable to the skin, gastrointestinal tract, and central nervous system. In experimentally induced deficiency in humans, the earliest manifestations are a red eruption on the skin resembling sunburn that first appears on the back of the hand. Other areas that are exposed to light are subsequently involved. The lesions, which are symmetric, may darken, shed skin, and eventually scar. Sores on the mucocutaneous membranes, a swelling of the tongue, nausea, and vomiting are present in a significant number of individuals. Symptoms referable to the central nervous system include headache, insomnia, depression, dizziness, and difficulty with memory. The presence of a nutritional factor that could cure these symptoms was demonstrated in the classic work of Goldberger and his colleagues, and this substance was subsequently found to be nicotinamide, or niacin. This vitamin is a critical part of two cofactors, NAD and NADP, which are involved in the transfer of hydrogen in most biologic oxidations. Although the roles of NAD and NADP in biologic oxidations and biochemical synthesis are well known, the mechanism by which the symptoms observed with deficiency of niacin relate to the levels of these cofactors remains unclear. One thing is known, however—the administration of nicotinic acid to patients suffering from pellagra produces dramatic alterations within 24 hours.

Pyridoxine (Vitamin B₆). After the identification of thiamine, riboflavin, and niacin, it became clear that other water-soluble nutritional factors were also necessary for normal metabolic function. In the period between 1930 and 1935, several groups of workers described an additional factor, vitamin B_6, subsequently called *pyridoxine*. This compound is activated by conversion to pyridoxal phosphate and is involved in a number of metabolic reactions with amino acids, including decarboxylation and transamination. Pyridoxine deprivation can produce symptoms in humans and other species. These include changes in the skin and central nervous system and production of red blood cells. In humans, the skin lesions consist of seborrheic changes around the eyes, nose, and mouth and of swelling and redness of the tongue. With prolonged deficiency, convulsive activity in the central nervous system has been demonstrated. The anemia that accompanies pyridoxine deficiency is microcytic and hypochromic in type. All these symptoms can be promptly relieved by the administration of small doses of pyridoxine. The recommended dose of pyridoxine is related to protein intake, since its principal role is in the metabolism of amino acids. The range is between 1.25 and 2.00 mg with protein intakes of 100 gm or less. With high protein intake, more pyridoxine may be needed.

In addition to the symptoms of deficiency that are cured by low doses of pyridoxine, there are a group of clinical states in which symptoms can be cured by much higher doses of this vitamin. These include some forms of convulsions, particularly in children; vitamin B_6-dependent anemia; xanthinuric aciduria; cystathionuria; and homocystinuria. The doses of vitamin B_6 required for control or amelioration of these conditions are in the range of 200 to 600 mg daily, as compared with a range of 1.5 to 2.0 mg per day for normal maintenance. The convulsive activity in the brain appears to be related to altered levels of gamma-amino butyric acid (GABA). This amino acid is produced by decarboxylation of glutamate, a process involving transamination and requiring pyridoxal phosphate. A reduction in the level of GABA increases the tendency for convulsive activity and probably accounts for the convulsions observed in such patients. The physiologic basis for the effect of pyridoxine in the other conditions is unknown at present.

Pantothenic Acid and Biotin. These two water-soluble agents are important cofactors in the metabolism of fats. Pantothenic acid was first identified in 1933 and was clearly associated with a nutritional deficiency disease in fowl by Wooley and his collaborators in 1939. Pantothenic acid is an essential component of coenzyme A, which is of prime importance in both synthesis and degradation of fatty acids. The presence of biotin was demonstrated from studies showing the production of a disease by feeding egg white. It is now known that raw egg white contains avidin, a glycoprotein of high molecular weight that irreversibly binds biotin. The structure of biotin was established in 1942. It is an important cofactor in the fixation of CO_2 during synthesis of fatty acids and during gluconeogenesis. Although specific syndromes can be produced in humans by feeding synthetic diets deficient in pantothenic acid or biotin, these are almost unknown under natural conditions because of the wide availability of these two substances in foods.

Folic Acid and Vitamin B$_{12}$ (Cobamide). These two vitamins are essential to the maintenance of normal hematopoiesis. Because of their integral relationship with the blood, discussion of vitamin B$_{12}$ and folic acid is included in Chapter 23.

Vitamin C (Ascorbic Acid). Vitamin C, the last water-soluble vitamin, is essential to the prevention of scurvy. The existence of a nutritional factor that would prevent scurvy was recognized in 1753 by Lind, who demonstrated that oranges, lemons, and limes could prevent and cure scurvy among sailors, hence the nickname "limey" for British sailors. The chemical identification of this antiscurvy, or antiscorbutic, factor was not made for nearly 200 years. Progress was greatly aided by the demonstration that guinea pigs could be made scorbutic (i.e., could be induced to develop scurvy). With this bioassay, several groups of workers demonstrated the essential nature of ascorbic acid. It was a hexuronic acid present in high concentrations in the adrenal gland as well as in citrus fruits and cabbages.

The physiologic and biologic functions for ascorbic acid are far less clearly defined than for the other water-soluble vitamins. Most of the other vitamins function as cofactors for a specific enzymatic step in a chain of biochemical reactions. No such enzymatic step has been defined that requires ascorbic acid as a cofactor. The vitamin rather appears to function in its reduced form, dehydroascorbic acid, in oxidation-reduction reactions. Its role in the metabolism of tyrosine has been studied in some detail. The first step in metabolism is the transamination of tyrosine to p-hydroxyphenylpyruvic acid. The next step is conversion to homogentisic acid by parahydroxyphenylpyruvic acid oxidase, an enzyme that is inhibited by its substrate unless ascorbic acid is present. This effect occurs when the quantities of tyrosine are large. The functional role of the high concentrations of ascorbic acid found in the adrenal gland and in the ovary are unclear at present.

When vitamin C deficiency is produced, two groups of symptoms occur: those involving growth of bones and those involving blood vessels. During periods of rapid growth, a separation of the periosteum from the cortex occurs, and subperiosteal hemorrhages may result. When growth is less rapid, the lesions in the epiphyseal-diaphyseal junction may lead to disunion or fragmentation or both. Changes in the capillary walls are also prominent, and hemorrhages into the space around hair follicles are common. All these symptoms are rapidly reversed by the administration of ascorbic acid, which is required in the range of 50 to 75 mg per day. It is of interest that only humans, certain primates, and the guinea pig have a requirement for vitamin C; other mammals are able to synthesize the vitamin by a series of reactions involving the glucuronic acid pathway. The correlation between the clinical symptoms and the biochemical reactions is unclear. Definition of this area again awaits further understanding of the biochemical mechanisms by which ascorbic acid acts at the cellular level.

FAT-SOLUBLE VITAMINS

The vitamins A, D, E, and K differ from the group discussed previously because they are soluble in fat. Toxicity from overdosage has been reported for vitamins A and D because body fat serves as a storage depot. Toxicity is not observed with the water-soluble vitamins because any excess is excreted in the urine.

Vitamin A. The discovery of vitamin A stemmed from studies on the skin lesions and xerophthalmia in rats fed artificial diets containing lard. The chemical factor that prevented this deficiency was identified in 1929 as β-carotene, and its structure was proved in 1931. Subsequent work on the physiologic role of β-carotene and other carotenoid pigments has taken two lines: (1) studies on its effect on vision, and (2) studies on growth and development. The actions in the visual cycle have been clearly elucidated by work from several laboratories. Deficiency of vitamin A impairs adaptation of the retina to the dark. It also impedes growth. The mechanism for the stimulation of growth by vitamin A has not yet been clearly established. Retinoic acid, an oxidation product of retinal, is a potent promoter of growth in the vitamin A–deficient animal, yet it is ineffective in restoring visual function. It may thus be that the components of vitamin A that are essential to growth may not be those that are involved in maintenance of the visual response to dark. The nature of this growth-promoting component of vitamin A awaits further investigation.

Induction of vitamin A deficiency requires prolonged periods of a deficient intake owing to the fat solubility of this vitamin. The clinical symptoms that eventually appear involve desiccation and ulceration of the cornea and conjunctiva in the eye, increased frequency of respiratory infection, and keratinization and drying of the skin, with an occasional papular eruption. Kidney stones and alterations in the pancreatic ducts are frequently found. These symptoms of vitamin A deficiency are most commonly seen in patients suffering from impaired intestinal fat absorption. Thus, pancreatic disease, disease of the biliary tract, sprue, and ulcerative colitis are the primary causes of vitamin A deficiency; only rarely does dietary deficiency alone produce symptoms.

Overzealous treatment with preparations containing vitamin A can, however, induce symptoms of toxicity. These symptoms, which usually take 6 months or more to develop, require doses in excess of 50,000 units of vitamin A per day and consist of irritability, loss of appetite, and itching of the skin. Fatigue, myalgia, changes in body hair, and enlargement of the liver and spleen have also been observed. Withdrawal of the vitamin leads to rapid regression of most of the symptoms. The one exception is the bony hyperostoses that develop in the extremities and in the occipital region of the skull.

Vitamin D, Calcium, Magnesium, and Their Control. Vitamin D is a fat-soluble sterol that can prevent rickets. Much of the early work on this disease was prompted by the significant numbers of afflicted children in urban areas of the temperate zones. By 1920, it had been established that the disease was the result of a dietary deficiency and lack of sunlight. Irradiation of dietary rations and the skin was effective in preventing the disease. Demonstration of an antirachitic factor in various fish oils was followed by intensive chemical studies, leading to the identification and elucidation of the structure of vitamin D_2 by 1937. The next major advance in the physiology of vitamin D was the synthesis of radioactively labeled vitamin D_2 of high specific activity. With radioactive vitamin D_2, it was shown that orally administered vitamin D_2 is converted to a metabolite now known to be 25-hydroxycholecalciferol. This metabolite is active in vitro, whereas the native vitamins D_2 and D_3 require conversion. In the presence of parathyroid hormone, renal tissue converts 25-hydroxylcholecalciferol to 1,25-dihydroxycholecalciferol, which is much more potent than its precursor. The dihydroxy derivative may thus be the "active" form of vitamin D.

Figure 33–13 shows a diagram of the pathways involving metabolism of vitamin D. Absorption of this hormone from the gut is followed by transport to the liver and hydroxylation at the 25 position (Fig. 33–13, middle). This hydroxylation can be modified by drugs that influence the micro-

somal drug metabolizing enzyme system in liver, such as phenytoin (diphenylhydantoin). Such an effect is probably the basis for the development of osteomalacia (i.e., reduced calcification of bone matrix) in some individuals treated with this drug. The 25-hydroxylated vitamin D is then transported from the liver to the kidney, where further hydroxylation occurs, producing the active 1,25-dihydroxylated vitamin D_3 or the inactive 24,25-dihydroxylated vitamin D_3. These processes are influenced by the concentration of parathyroid hormone, serum phosphorus, and calcium, as indicated in the accompanying figure.

Vitamin D has two principal actions: (1) to increase the absorption of calcium from the intestine, and (2) to facilitate the reabsorption of calcium from bone in the presence of parathyroid hormone. The effects of vitamin D on the absorption of calcium from the gastrointestinal tract depend on the formation of a transport protein in the gastrointestinal mucosa. When isolated intestine is perfused with solutions of vitamin D, it takes 4 hours or more to increase calcium absorption. The active metabolite 1,25-dihydroxycholecalciferol produces an increase in calcium transport in less than 1½ hours. This effect is blocked by actinomycin D, an inhibitor of RNA synthesis, suggesting that the synthesis of new protein is involved. Parathyroid hormone also plays a role in calcium absorption from the gut. In the hypoparathyroid animal, normal intake of vitamin D does not produce a normal rate of calcium absorption, although increased intake of vitamin C can restore calcium absorption to normal. Injections of parathyroid hormone lead to normal calcium absorption in the presence of normal intake of vitamin D. Similarly, in vitamin D–deficient animals, absorption of calcium is deficient, although there is excess secretion of parathyroid hormone. In the mechanisms of calcium absorption from the gut,

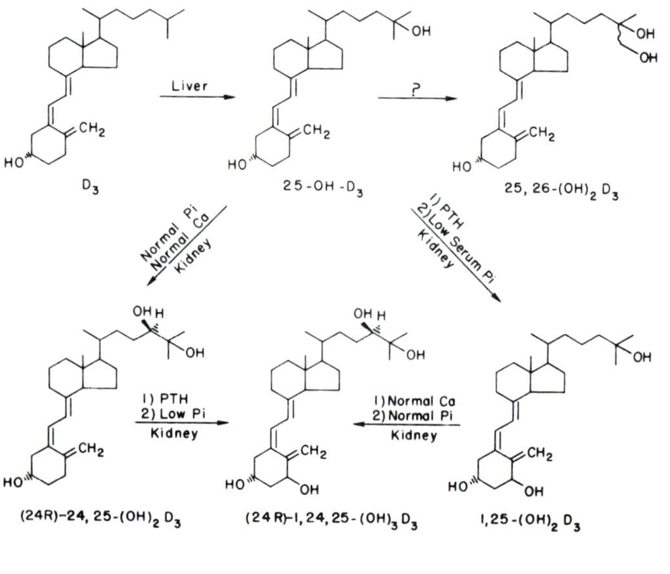

Figure 33–13 Metabolism of vitamin D. The initial hydroxylation of vitamin D occurs in the liver. Subsequent metabolism in the kidney is modulated by the levels of serum phosphorus and calcium and the concentrations of parathyroid hormone (PTH). The active metabolite is primarily the 25-$(OH)_2$-vitamin D_3. (Reproduced from DeLuca, H. F.: Ann. Intern. Med. *88*:369, 1976, with permission of the author and publisher.)

vitamin D appears to have the primary role, with parathyroid hormones making a secondary, or minor, contribution.

The actions of vitamin D on bone have been less extensively studied, but an essential interaction with parathyroid hormone is again evident. In tissue cultures of bone, the addition of 25-hydroxycholecalciferol will stimulate bone reabsorption in a manner similar to that observed with parathyroid hormone. Moreover, this metabolite of vitamin D acts synergistically with parathyroid hormone. Although evidence suggests that parathyroid hormone acts on the kidney and bone to increase the production of cyclic AMP, vitamin D does not influence this system. Thus, the synergism of parathyroid hormone and vitamin D on the reabsorption of bone appears to occur at different sites. This synergism could be explained if parathyroid hormone controlled entry of calcium into the nucleus and thus controlled the nuclear events of transcription and cellular transformation.

The maintenance of normal levels of circulating calcium is of prime importance for both neuromuscular transmission and cellular transport. The control mechanisms involved in maintaining the normal levels of serum calcium are determined not only by vitamin D but also by parathyroid hormone, phosphorus, magnesium, and calcitonin. It is beyond the scope of this chapter to review these interactions in detail, but certain effects of pathologic derangements are worthy of note. Osteomalacia and rickets are the consequences of vitamin D deficiency that result from lack of sunlight, deficiency of this vitamin in the diet, resistance at the cellular level, or malabsorption in the gastrointestinal tract. Pathologic consequences also occur with increased amounts of vitamin D. When parathyroid hormone is present, the ingestion of markedly increased amounts of vitamin D can induce a pathologic state similar to that observed with an excess excretion of parathyroid hormone. The state of vitamin D intoxication increases the concentrations of serum calcium and reduces the level of circulating phosphate. Calcium absorption from the gastrointestinal tract is increased, and bony abnormalities can be induced by increased absorption of calcium from bones. The consequences of hypercalcemia on the electrocardiogram and on neuromuscular conduction can be observed. Finally, persistent hypercalcemia can produce renal failure by damaging the kidney.

In the metabolism of *magnesium*, increased concentrations of parathyroid hormone can increase magnesium excretion and induce a state of magnesium deficiency. Such a change tends to reduce the effects of parathyroid hormone. Magnesium deficiency can also be induced by dietary means and by alcoholism, and such a state is usually associated with hypocalcemia. The pathologic mechanism by which magnesium deficiency leads to hypocalcemia is unclear, although it has been attributed to resistance of the skeleton to the action of parathyroid hormone. One would expect that with hypomagnesemia the output of parathyroid hormone would be increased, as observed under in-vitro and in-vivo conditions, yet serum calcium is usually below normal. Support for diminished effectiveness of parathyroid hormone with magnesium depletion has been shown in studies with bone cultures and in measurements of cyclic-AMP excretion in the urine. By use of the technique of bone culture, it was shown that the effect of parathyroid hormone on calcium mobilization was reduced when the concentration of magnesium was low. Similarly, magnesium-deficient patients failed to excrete normal amounts of cyclic AMP after the administration of parathyroid hormone. Since the action of parathyroid hormone on bone and kidney appears to involve cyclic AMP, this may be the essential biochemical defect in this interaction. It is known from other studies on this membrane-bound enzyme complex that magnesium is essential to the conversion of ATP to $3',5'$-AMP (cyclic AMP). Thus, in magnesium deficiency the impaired response of parathyroid hormone might be due to the slowed rate of conversion of ATP to cyclic AMP in the absence of this divalent cation.

Vitamin E. The place of vitamin E, or α-tocopherol, in human nutrition is still unsettled. It was originally discovered as an essential factor in the maintenance of pregnancy in rats. Because this is a fat-soluble vitamin, depletion of the body stores occurs very slowly. Prolonged feeding of diets deficient in vitamin E to adults failed to produce clear-cut evidence of a deficiency state. However, in infants with protein-calorie malnutrition, vitamin E can reverse the hemolytic anemia that is often present. A similar hemolytic anemia occurs in monkeys fed a diet free of α-tocopherol, suggesting that this vitamin may play a role in hematopoiesis.

Vitamin K. Vitamin K is a fat-soluble vitamin essential to hepatic synthesis of clotting factors II, VII, IX, and X (see Chapter 24). Because it is a fat-soluble quinone, it is often deficient in states of malabsorption. Indeed, this is one of the observations that led to its discovery. Although the quinone structure was rapidly elucidated, it is still not known how the vitamin acts to enhance the synthesis of clotting factors. Of pathophysiologic importance is that this vitamin is competitively antagonized by such drugs as aspirin. Thus, bleeding disorders from deficiency of vitamin K can occur with hepatic disease or malabsorption or by use of drugs that are competitive antagonists.

PATHOPHYSIOLOGIC MECHANISMS OF DISEASE STATES RESULTING FROM VITAMIN DEFICIENCIES

Several pathogenic mechanisms can lead to deficiencies of one vitamin or another and thus to the production of clinical or subclinical syndromes.

Deficient dietary intake is the first such mechanism. This can result from selective absence of one or more vitamins or its precursor in the diet or from a generalized deficiency of all vitamins as observed in malnutrition or during total starvation. In other diseases such as alcoholism, dietary intake is frequently reduced, but loss of vitamins is also accelerated. Absence of vitamin D in the diet or inadequate exposure to sunlight is associated with rickets. Failure to calcify bony matrix, which characterizes this disease, is now rare in this country because vitamin D is added to most milk supplies and because most infants receive supplements of vitamins. However, rickets is still seen occasionally when vitamin D is insufficient or when the response is impaired by genetic defects. Although relatively rare, it must be pointed out that cases of rickets due to vitamin deficiency are still seen even in the major metropolitan centers of the United States.

Generalized malnutrition and *therapeutic starvation* are also mechanisms for producing vitamin deficiency. During the late 1960s and through most of the 1970s, the use of starvation as therapy for human obesity was widespread. During starvation there is a marked reduction in the circulating concentration of many vitamins. Thiamine, niacin, biotin, pantothenic acid, folate, riboflavin, and pyridoxine are among the vitamins that are lost. The decline in pyridoxine is progressive with the duration of starvation and reaches very low levels by 5 to 6 months. With starvation, riboflavin also drops progressively but rises promptly when food is returned to the diet. Thiamine is also reduced. In one particular patient with hypotension, vomiting, and weakness occurring after 3 weeks of fasting, the symptoms disappeared following the intravenous administration of thiamine. Other vitamin supplements had no effect.

Total absence of food, however, is not the only mechanism for nutritional reduction in vitamin levels. Surveys of hospitalized patients, particularly children, have shown that up to 45 per cent had lowered serum concentrations of one or more vitamins. This reduction varied with the ethnic origin of the patients. For example, Puerto Rican children in New York City showed lower circulating levels of thiamine, niacin, vitamin B_{12}, and folate than children from other ethnic groups in that city. In contrast, Chinese children showed many instances of higher levels than other groups. Protein intake was of primary importance in determining the levels of many vitamins. When less than 38 gm of protein were ingested daily, there were marked reductions in the levels of biotin, thiamine, and ascorbic acid. Supplements with oral vitamins did not raise the serum levels to normal until protein intake was increased. Thus, protein deficiency per se influences the circulating levels of vitamins in a manner that is as yet poorly understood.

Alcoholism is a third pathologic state associated with reduced serum levels of some vitamins. These individuals frequently have a deficiency of folic acid, and they are often deficient in thiamine. The deficiency in folic acid probably accounts for the frequent association of hematologic abnormalities and megaloblastic anemia. However, folic acid deficiency may also impair the ability of the liver to regenerate, since it is necessary for both synthesis of DNA and cell replication. The deficiency of thiamine in alcoholics is associated with a characteristic group of symptoms that include a wobbling gait, inability to move the eye muscles appropriately, and confusion. This symptom complex can be rapidly reversed by the intravenous administration of thiamine.

Malabsorption is another pathologic mechanism that induces vitamin deficiency. A number of disease states are associated with ineffective absorption of one or more vitamins and/or minerals from the gastrointestinal tract. Thus, food intake may be normal, but body supplies of essential elements may be deficient. This is more often seen when the pathologic alteration leads to increased loss of fat in the stools. As might be expected with increased fat excretion, the amount of fat-soluble vitamins A, D, and K is most frequently affected.

Similarly, calcium, which complexes with fatty acids formed during hydrolysis of triglyceride, is also lost with fatty acids. Thus, deficiencies of vitamin D and calcium lead to impaired formation of bone, with decreased circulating levels of calcium. This complex of symptoms in adults is known clinically as *osteomalacia* and is analogous to rickets in children. It is characterized by a loss of mineral from the skeleton with ensuing deformities of the weight-bearing bones. Pseudofractures may be detected on radiographs as symmetric lines at areas of bony reabsorption where nutrient arteries penetrate the bone. There is relative impairment of normal bone reabsorption and histologically defective mineralization of the newly formed bony matrix. The hypocalcemia that is usually present is relatively unresponsive to the injection of parathyroid hormone. Urinary excretion of calcium and increased secretion of phosphate from the kidney are observed. As a result of the lowered levels of circulating calcium, parathyroid hormone is secreted from the parathyroid gland in increased amounts but appears to be relatively less active than normal in improving calcium reabsorption from bone.

In addition to osteomalacia that results from loss of vitamin D and calcium, a loss of vitamin A occurs as a result of malabsorption. As noted earlier, vitamin A affects visual function and growth. Impaired adaptation of the retina to the dark is the principal effect of vitamin A deficiency. The chemical process of dark adaptation requires the synthesis of rhodopsin, a combination of a protein opsin and a prosthetic group, 11-cis-retinal, which is derived from vitamin A. After exposure to light, this pigment undergoes a number of changes which lead to initiation of the nerve impulse. When vitamin A is deficient, the essential prosthetic group 11-cis-retinal is reduced, and the production of rhodopsin, the photosensitive pigment, is impaired. Thus, malabsorption of fat can impair both bone formation and visual adaptation to darkness.

The third effect of malabsorption is the loss of vitamin K. This vitamin is essential to the synthesis of prothrombin. In its absence, prothrombin levels are reduced and coagulation of blood is impaired, with a tendency to hemorrhage. In contrast to the other two fat-soluble vitamins, water-soluble forms of vitamin K can be administered and overcome this defect in formation of prothrombin.

Specific forms of malabsorption can also influence vitamin absorption. Pernicious anemia is a case in point in which vitamin B_{12} is not absorbed because intrinsic factor is lacking from the gastrointestinal mucosa. Injections of vitamin B_{12} will bypass this abnormality.

Although vitamin ingestion and absorption are normal, the *administration of antimetabolites or drugs* that compete directly or indirectly with vitamins for their active sites on enzymes may lead to symptoms of vitamin deficiency. Antimetabolites of folic acid are among the best known examples of this type of induced vitamin deficiency. Megaloblastic anemia responsive to folate therapy can be produced by two classes of drugs. The first class includes the anticonvulsants such as phenytoin (Dilantin) or phenobarbital. Both these drugs induce folate deficiency, presumably by interfering with its reduction to dihydrofolic acid or by interfering with its role in the formation of DNA. A second group of antifolic acid metabolites includes those used in the treatment of certain cancers. These drugs interfere directly with folic acid metabolism.

Aspirin is an example of the second group of drugs that will inhibit the effects of a vitamin. Salicylates compete with vitamin K and thus lower the production of prothrombin. Hypoprothrombinemia is frequently observed in patients treated with high doses of aspirin, and this effect can be overcome by administering supplements of vitamin K.

Isoniazid (INH) is the final example of a drug that inhibits vitamin metabolism. This drug is widely used for the treatment of tuberculosis and has been observed to increase the excretion of pyridoxine (vitamin B_6). With high doses of isoniazid, a peripheral neuropathy, convulsions, and anemia have been observed. All three of these untoward effects resulting from the administration of isoniazid can be prevented or treated by supplements of pyridoxine.

Increased vitamin utilization in the presence of a normal dietary intake is another mechanism by which the effects of vitamin deficiency can be produced. This can occur in hypermetabolic states, such as those due to prolonged fever or other causes. There are three such common clinical states: (1) increased levels of thyroid hormone (hyperthyroidism or administration of exogenous thyroid hormone), (2) pregnancy, and (3) childhood. In hyperthyroidism, the metabolic rate is significantly increased. As noted earlier, the requirements for thiamine, riboflavin, niacin, and possibly the other water-soluble B-complex vitamins are a function of the total caloric expenditure. As caloric expenditure rises in hyperthyroidism, the daily requirements for each of these vitamins increases. To avoid induction of nutritional deficiency, it is often wise to treat patients who have hyperthyroidism with supplements of B vitamins when their disease is being controlled. A second physiologic state of hypermetabolism is observed during pregnancy, and a third is seen in the growing child. Caloric requirements per kilogram body weight are increased in children, and vitamin requirements for this age group are similarly higher than for adults. Many illnesses in children are accompanied by vitamin deficiencies as shown by low circulating levels of vitamins. Vitamin requirements are also increased in pregnancy. During gestation, a second body is formed and the increased metabolism required by this procedure demands more vitamins. It is customary to give vitamin supplements during this period to prevent depletion of maternal supplies, with potential pathologic consequences for the developing infant.

TRACE ELEMENTS

Improvements in analytical methods have expanded our understanding of the role of trace elements in human nutrition and disease. In this section, some of these elements and their role in the production of disease will be examined. The ability to induce pathologic changes by selective removal of one element from the diet provides one of the best examples of the correlation between pathologic and physiologic alterations. We will illustrate, when possible, the biochemical basis of these changes. In many instances, however, such a fundamental understanding is not yet possible because our knowledge of the role of these trace elements is as yet incomplete. A summary of the data concerning body content, plasma concentration, functional role, and deficiency appears in Table 33–9. Calcium, magnesium, iron, and zinc are quantitatively the largest, present in gram quantities. Copper, chromium, manganese, iodine, and fluoride, however, are found only in milligram quantities.

ZINC

The content of zinc is approximately 1.4 to 2.3 gm in a 70-kg man, with 20 per cent of this amount

TABLE 33–9 TRACE ELEMENTS

Element	Body Content	Concentration		Average Intake	Absorption
		Whole Blood	Plasma or Serum		
Calcium	1000 gm	9–10.5 mg/100 ml	9–10.5 mg/100 ml	0.2–1.5 gm/day	0.1–0.5 gm
Magnesium	25 gm	3.0 mEq/L	1.8–2.5 mEq/L	400 mg/day	100 mg
Iron	5 gm	43 mg/100 ml*	70–180 µg/100 ml	12–15 mg/day	0.6–1.5 mg
Zinc	2 gm	800 µg/100 ml	120 µg/100 ml†	10–15 mg/day	1 mg
Copper	100–150 mg	98 µg/100 ml	109 µg/100 ml	2.5–5 mg/day	0.6–1.6 mg
Iodine	10–20 mg	—	4–8 µg/100 ml	50–1000 µg/day	50–1000 µg
Manganese	12–20 mg	9.8 µg/100 ml	1.4 µg/100 ml	2–8 mg/day	
Molybdenum	10–20 mg	15 µg/100 ml	1.4 µg/100 ml	100 µg/day	90 µg
Chromium	6 mg	15 µg/100 ml	1–6 µg/100 ml	50 µg/day	0.5 µg
Cobalt	1 mg	53 µg/100 ml	4.3 µg/100 ml	300 µg/day	30–60 µg/day

*As iron in hemoglobin (0.34% × 12.7 gm/100 ml).
†Serum 16% higher than plasma (lysis of platelets releases zinc).

in the skin. Circulating concentrations can be readily measured and average 121 µg per 100 ml in serum and somewhat more than ten times this concentration in red blood cells. Although intake is between 10 and 15 mg per day, absorption is usually low, representing less than 10 per cent, and is decreased by certain binding agents, particularly phytates, which are present in various cereals. Zinc is a factor in a number of enzymes, including alkaline phosphatase (found in liver and bone), carbonic anhydrase, carboxypeptidase (from the pancreas), and lactate, malate, and alcohol dehydrogenase. Zinc is also of importance in the β cells of the pancreas and may be involved in the crystallization of insulin in the granules within these cells. This element also has an important role in the synthesis of DNA and protein, as shown by the reduced incorporation of radioactivity from thymidine into nuclear DNA in zinc deficiency. This impairment can be overcome by injecting zinc a short time before giving thymidine. The effects of zinc on the activity of ribonuclease offer one explanation for these effects on nucleic acid synthesis. Zinc is an inhibitor of this enzyme, and in the deficient state the activity of ribonuclease might be enhanced.

Experimental zinc deficiency has been produced in several laboratory animals and has been documented with reasonable certainty in human beings. Zinc deficiency in humans is characterized by dwarfism and hypogonadism. Most patients have come from certain villages in Egypt and Iran in which the ingestion of clay and diets high in cereal might impair the absorption of zinc. The subjects in question are usually males and show a marked delay in onset of sexual development. Pubic hairs are sparse or absent, and the testes are small. Facial hair is sparse, and hepatosplenomegaly is frequent. Administration of zinc accelerated growth of these boys and led to an enhanced rate of sexual development. On this basis, it appears that zinc deficiency can be a causative factor in human disease.

The mechanism by which zinc impairs growth is unclear. It is known to be an essential part of the enzyme alkaline phosphatase, which is found in bone, but its role in bone growth and development is still unsettled. Zinc deficiency is also accompanied by slow rates of growth in experimental animals, an effect that is independent of growth hormone. Although reproductive function is impaired in zinc-deficient dwarfs, the mechanism has not been established. Pituitary function, as indicated by thyroid status, is normal, and adrenal function is only slightly impaired. Failure of sexual development suggests that the output of gonadotropins is deficient.

Zinc deficiency also impairs the healing of wounds. Over 20 per cent of the total zinc stores are located in skin. Zinc supplements were shown to accelerate the rate of wound healing in groups of apparently normal men. Detailed studies of this phenomenon, however, showed that the effects of zinc were detectable only in those individuals with mild degrees of zinc deficiency. Little or no effect was present in individuals with normal levels of this element. A mild zinc deficiency occurs in a significant number of people. Among the groups in which the levels of zinc are reduced are cirrhotics, who show enhanced urinary zinc levels, and patients with the nephrotic syndrome.

COPPER

Although copper has been a known element for centuries, its importance in nutrition has been appreciated only since 1930. At that time, an anemia in rats due to copper deficiency was clearly demonstrated. Since that time, it has been possible to show that patients with protein-calorie malnutrition have copper deficiency. The body stores approximately 80 mg of copper. The largest fraction of this is in the liver, and significant abnormalities in liver and brain occur in Wilson's disease, in which the transport protein for copper is markedly reduced. In this disease, the copper content of both the liver and the brain is increased, with the development of neurologic symptoms and hepatic failure. Copper is part of several enzymes, including cytochrome oxidase, tyrosinase, and uricase. Deficiency of copper produces three changes. The first is a hypochromic, microcytic anemia. Although copper is not known to be an important element in the production of the enzymes involved in hemoglobin synthesis, it appears to play a critical role in the overall process for utilization of iron. Copper-deficient infants recovering from protein-calorie malnutrition develop an anemia that is cured by administration of copper. These infants also have brittle bones. Leukopenia is the second principal manifestation of copper deficiency. Induction of this state in adults is difficult because of the ubiquity of copper. However, in severe malnutrition in which initial replacement is with milk for sustained periods, a deficiency in copper can be observed.

CHROMIUM

Interest in the element chromium was stimulated by the work of Mertz and his collaborators, who demonstrated that chromium deficiency in experimental animals was accompanied by abnormalities in the metabolism of glucose. This diabetes-like syndrome could be reversed by the administration of chromium. The body contains only 6 mg of chromium. It is transported in blood by a specific protein known as *siderophilin*. Most, if not all, chromium is present with a valence of $+3$. This element appears to be an integral part of membranes and is contained in the enzyme phosphoglucomutase. The induction of experimental chromium deficiency impairs glucose tolerance in rats in addition to lowering the sensitivity to the effects of insulin in vitro. The suggestion that chromium acts at the cell membrane is supported by the observation that the addition of certain chromium-containing compounds restores the response to insulin in vitro. These observations in experimental animals may be relevant to diabetes in humans. It has been established that the concentration of chromium declines with age, paralleling reduced metabolism of glucose. There is suggestive evidence that in some individuals with impaired glucose tolerance, supplements of chromium can restore the metabolism of glucose toward normal. The possibility thus exists, presenting a fascinating challenge to medical science, that chromium deficiency may play a significant role in certain types of human diabetes.

FLUORIDE METABOLISM

Fluoride is widely distributed in nature and is present in small concentrations in most supplies of soil and water. Whether this element is essential to nutrition, however, has not yet been established. Animals fed diets with very low levels of fluoride are not significantly different in growth rate and metabolic characteristics from animals fed diets supplemented with this element. The principal interest in fluoride has come from its inhibition of dental decay and the toxic state of fluorosis (i.e., the disease of excess fluoride intake). The initial studies demonstrating that fluoride had an effect on dental caries were conducted in the 1930s. The results of one such experiment are shown in Table 33–10. It is clear from this table that in a 5-year period, there was a significant reduction in the number of carious teeth in children receiving fluoride supplements but no significant change in the control groups. This effect of fluoride was most striking in younger children and decreased with age. These data and many other controlled experiments clearly demonstrate that fluoride supplements at a level of 1 part per million (ppm) in drinking water are capable of reducing dental caries. The mechanism by which this occurs, however, is unclear. Fluoride is found in its highest concentrations in bone and teeth and appears to be involved in the formation of bone matrix. An intake of water of 1 to 2 L per day with a fluoride concentration of 1 ppm will provide an intake of 1 to 2 mg of fluoride. This appears to be optimal for reducing dental caries. At higher levels, fluoride poisoning or fluorosis occurs. This is primarily observed in animals but can be seen in humans following industrial accidents. The symptoms develop after the compensatory mechanisms for disposition of fluoride have been exhausted. When the intake of fluoride increases sharply, the urinary excretion also rises until the maximum is achieved. Bone uptake also increases but has a finite capacity. When the capacities of the kidney and bone have been saturated, the extra fluoride is stored in tissue and induces the symptoms of fluorosis, which consist of a loss of appetite and a loss of body weight. Symptoms referable to the

TABLE 33–10 EFFECT OF FLUORIDE ON DENTAL CARIES IN CHILDREN*

Age in Years	Control Areas		Areas with Fluoride Added in 1956		Per Cent Reduction with Fluoride
	1956	1961	1956	1961	
3	3.53	3.32	3.80	1.29	66
4	5.18	4.83	5.39	2.31	57
5	5.66	5.39	5.81	2.91	50
6	6.32	6.22	6.49	4.81	26
7	7.08	6.89	7.06	6.05	14

*Fluoride added to drinking water of one area in 1956 at 1 part per millon.
(Adapted from British Ministry of Health: Roy. Soc. Health J. *82*:173, 1962.)

gastrointestinal and neuromuscular systems also occur, as do pulmonary congestion and respiratory and cardiac failure. It must be noted, however, that such levels of fluoride are hardly ever reached in humans.

One of the principal sources of fluoride in the human diet is tea. This plant absorbs large quantities of fluoride from the soil and is in this sense unique. For most other foods, concentrations of 1 to 2 ppm of fluoride are maximal. Fluoride concentrations in tea, however, can be up to 100 ppm or 100 times that usually seen in almost all other sources of food.

IODINE

The importance of iodine in human metabolism has been known since the 1920s. This element, discovered in the early part of the nineteenth century, was studied extensively by Chatin, who correlated the prevalence of goiter with availability of iodine supplies in the soil, food, and water. His work in the middle of the nineteenth century strongly suggested that the regions in which there was a high incidence of thyroid enlargement (goiter) were those regions in which there were low iodine levels in food and water. Chatin's analytical methods were relatively crude by present standards, and his work went largely unnoticed. Revival of interest in iodine came from the observations by Baumann that the thyroid gland contained iodine. In 1915, thyroxine was isolated and the synthesis of this hormone was reported in 1927 by Harrington. At the same time, studies by Marine and his collaborators demonstrated the efficacy of iodine supplements as a treatment for thyroid enlargement. In a series of studies carried out in the school system of Akron, Ohio from 1916 to 1920, these investigators showed that supplements of iodine significantly reduced the incidence of goiter among school children. From their work and the observations of many since that time, the essential nature of iodine intake for prevention of goiter and the need to supplement iodine intake in regions in which there is low iodine content in food and water have become clear. The principal supplementary sources of iodine in diet have come by the addition of iodide to salt in the form of iodized salt and more recently by the use of iodates in bread.

The iodide ingested in the diet is absorbed and circulates at a concentration of 0.06 to 0.80 µg per ml of serum. This iodide has two principal exit routes from the serum: (1) into the thyroid gland, and (2) into the urine by filtration at the glomerulus. The fraction of iodide concentrated by the thyroid gland and converted to hormone is related to the total quantity of iodine already present in the thyroid. In areas in which there is iodine deficiency (i.e., those areas in which intake is less than 75 µg per day on the average), the iodine stores in the thyroid become deficient, since the daily requirements for hormone synthesis are approximately 80 µg. Thus, as deficiency develops, compensatory mechanisms increase the fraction of circulating iodine that is trapped by the thyroid gland and decrease the fraction that is excreted in the urine. Conversely, when iodine intake is high, the thyroid stores become saturated, further uptake of iodine is inhibited, and the relative fraction concentrated by the gland falls as the fraction appearing in the urine increases. This reciprocal relationship between uptake of iodine by the thyroid gland and its excretion in the urine has been used by Oddie and collaborators to evaluate levels of iodine intake in various parts of the United States. Regional differences in dietary intake are clearly apparent (Fig. 33–14). The incidence of endemic goiter is highest in those regions in which intake of iodine is low.

Severe iodine deficiency occurs in several regions of the world. One of the earliest studies of the pathophysiologic consequences of iodine deficiency was carried out by Stanbury and collaborators in the Mendoza region of Argentina. More recent studies have been conducted in the Congo, in New Guinea, and in portions of South America and the Middle East. The more severe the lack of iodine, the greater the frequency of enlarged thyroid glands. However, even in the most severely deficient areas, enlargement of the thyroid gland does not occur in all persons. This observation suggests significant variability among individuals in their ability to compensate for severe iodine deficiency. Several mechanisms are involved in this compensation. The first of these is an increase in the fraction of ingested iodine that is trapped by the thyroid gland. In many areas, iodine uptake is frequently above 70 per cent and may reach 100 per cent of an administered dose. The iodine that is trapped by the thyroid is attached to tyrosine to form mono- and diiodotyrosine, which are in turn coupled to form thyroxine and triiodothyronine. As iodine becomes scarce, the percentage of monoiodotyrosine is increased in the thyroid gland relative to diiodotyrosine. Similarly, the proportion of 3,5,3'-triiodothyronine increases relative to thyroxine. Thus, the quantities of monoiodotyrosine and triiodothyronine are increased, and the concentrations of diiodotyrosine and thyroxine are reduced in areas of iodine deficiency. Because the iodine stores are low, the turnover rate of thyroid iodine increases. Thus, triiodothyronine becomes a larger fraction of the circulating thyroactive hormone in iodine deficiency than when iodine stores are adequate. Finally, the thyroid gland itself enlarges in an attempt to compensate for the low iodine intake. Two underlying mechanisms are thus involved in the adaptation to iodine deficiency. The first is the intrathyroidal mechanism of autoregulation. By this term, one means that the responsiveness of the thyroid to the thyroid-stimulating hormone from the pituitary gland

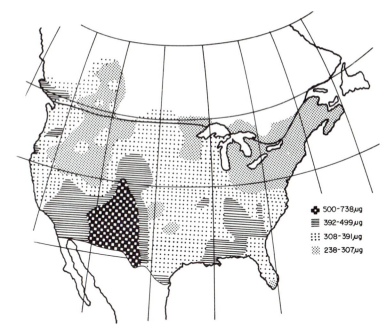

Figure 33–14 Iodine intake in the United States. These data on iodine intake in the United States were calculated from data on the regional uptake of radioactive iodine. The areas of highest iodine intake are in the southwest United States, and the regions of lowest intake are in the midwest, along the east coast, and in some sections of the upper Rocky Mountains. (Reproduced with permission from Oddie, T. H., et al.: J. Clin. Endocrinol. *30*:659, 1970.)

500–738μg
392–499μg
308–391μg
238–307μg

is increased in iodine deficiency. Thus, the uptake of iodide, the conversion to hormone, the release of hormone, and enlargement of the thyroid gland are all increased in an iodine-deficient thyroid. The second mechanism for regulating thyroidal iodine stores is the increase in the concentrations of thyroid-stimulating hormone (TSH). This mechanism presumably is activated by a reduction in the concentration of circulating thyroxine and triiodothyronine detected by the hypothalamic receptors that control the output of thyrotropin-releasing hormone from the pituitary.

The enlarged thyroid that occurs in iodine-deficient populations can be reduced in size in many individuals given iodine supplementation, as repeatedly shown by administration of iodine supplements to deficient groups. Thus, iodine is essential to human nutrition, and in its absence compensatory processes occur that lead to thyroid enlargement. Failure of the compensatory mechanism to provide a reasonable circulating level of thyroid hormone is accompanied by hypothyroidism and failure to grow normally. Areas in which there is severe iodine deficiency show an increase in the number of such goiterous cretins suffering from deficiency of thyroid hormones.

In some regions of the world, iodine supplies occur in excess. In these regions, thyroid glands tend to be smaller than normal, but in some individuals, thyroid enlargement occurs. This consequence of high intake of iodine has been termed *iodide myxedema*. The mechanism for this effect appears to be suppression of thyroid function by high iodide intake resulting in a drop in circulating thyroid hormone and compensatory increase in the output of thyrotropin by the pituitary. This, in turn, stimulates the thyroid gland to enlarge. A comparable effect of high iodide intake was observed in animals by Wolff and Chaikoff, and the mechanism of this effect is still not understood.

REFERENCES

Obesity

Bagdade, J. D., Bierman, E. L. and Porte, D., Jr.: The significance of basal insulin levels in the evaluation of the insulin response to glucose in diabetic and nondiabetic subjects. J. Clin. Invest. *46*:1549, 1967.

Bray, G. A.: The Obese Patient. (Vol. IX in the series Major Problems in Internal Medicine.) Philadelphia, W. B. Saunders Co., 1976.

Bray, G. A.: Obesity. Disease-a-Month. *26*:1, 1979.

Bray, G. A. (Chm. and Ed.), Cahill, G., Jordan, H. A., Horton, E. S., Salans, L. B., and Sims, E. A. H. (Editorial Board): Obesity in Perspective. Fogarty Int. Ctr. Series on Preventive Med. Vol. 2, Parts 1 and 2. Washington, D.C., U.S. Government Printing Office, 1976.

Bray, G. A., Jordan, H. A., and Sims, E. A. H.: Evaluation of the obese patient. 1. An algorithm. J.A.M.A. *235*:2008, 1976.

Bray, G. A., and York, D. A.: Hypothalamic and genetic obesity in experimental animals: an autonomic and endocrine hypothesis. Physiol. Rev. *59*:718, 1979.

Cioffi, L. A., James, W. P. T., and van Itallie, T. B.: The Body Weight Regulatory System: Normal and Disturbed Mechanisms. New York, Raven Press, 1981.

Garrow, J. S.: Energy Balance and Obesity in Man. 2nd ed. New York, American Elsevier Publishing Company, Inc., 1978.

Goldman, R. F., Haisman, M. F., Bynum, G., et al.: Experimental obesity in man. Metabolic rate in relation to dietary intake. *In* Bray, G. A. (Ed.): Obesity in Perspective. Fogarty Int. Ctr. Series on Preventive Med. Vol. 2, Part 2. Washington, D.C., U.S. Government Printing Office, 1976, p. 165.

Hetherington, A. W., and Ranson, S. W.: Hypothalamic lesions and adiposity in the rat. Anat. Rec. 78:149, 1940.

Hirsch, J., and Batchelor, B.: Adipose tissue cellularity in human obesity. Clin. Endocrinol. Metab. 5:299, 1976.

Horton, E. S., Danforth, E., Jr., Sims, E. A. H., and Salans, L. B.: Endocrine and metabolic alterations in spontaneous and experimental obesity. *In* Bray, G. A. (Ed.): Obesity in Perspective. Fogarty Int. Ctr. Series on Preventive Med. Vol. 2, Part 2. Washington, D.C., U.S. Government Printing Office, 1976, p. 323.

Lusk, B: The Elements of the Science of Nutrition. Philadelphia, W. B. Saunders Co., 1928.

Moore, F. D., Olesen, K. H., McMurrey, J. D., et al.: The Body Cell Mass and Its Supporting Environment. Philadelphia, W. B. Saunders Co., 1963.

Novin, D., Wyrwicka, W., and Bray, G. A.: Hunger: Basic Mechanisms and Clinical Implications. Raven Press, New York, 1976.

Recommended Dietary Allowances, 9th ed. Washington, D.C., National Academy of Sciences, 1980.

Salans, L. W., Horton, E. S., and Sims, E. A. H.: Experimental obesity in man: cellular character of the adipose tissue. J. Clin. Invest. 50:1005, 1971.

Schachter, S., and Rodin, J.: In Festinger, L., and Schachter, S. (Ed.): Obese Humans and Rats. Washington, D.C., Lawrence Erlbaum Associates, 1974.

Sims, E. A. H., Danforth, E., Jr., Horton, E. S., et al.: Endocrine and metabolic factors of experimental obesity in man. Recent. Progr. Horm. Res. 29:457, 1973.

Smith, Y., and Sjostrom, L. (Eds): Adipose tissue. Int. J. Obesity 5:445, 1981.

Stock, M., and Rothwell, N.: Obesity and Leanness. Basic aspects. London, John Libbey, 1982.

Stunkard, A. J. (Ed.): Obesity. W. B. Saunders Co., Philadelphia, 1980.

PROTEIN AND/OR CALORIE DEFICIENCY

Cahill, G. F., Jr., Herrera, M. G., Morgan, A. P., et al.: Hormone-fuel interrelationships during fasting. J. Clin. Invest. 45:1751, 1966.

Cahill, G. F., Jr., and Owen, O. E.: Body fuels and starvation. *In* Rowland, C. V., Jr. (Ed): Anorexia and Obesity. Boston, Little, Brown and Company, 1970, pp. 25–36.

Latham, M. C.: Protein-calorie malnutrition in children and its relation to psychological development and behavior. Physiol. Rev. 54:541, 1974.

Meguid, M. M.: Uncomplicated and stressed starvation. Surg. Clin. North Am. 61:529, 43, 1981.

Owen, O. E.: Energy metabolism in feasting and fasting. Adv. Exp. Biol. Med. 111:169, 1979.

Vigersky, R. A., Loriaux, D. L., Anderson, A. E., and Lipsett, M. B.: Anorexia nervosa: behavioral and hypothalamic aspects. Clin. Endocrinol. Metab. 5:517, 1976.

Young, V. R., and Scrimshaw, N. S.: The physiology of starvation. Sci. Am. 225:14, 1971.

LIPIDS

Brown, M. S., and Goldstein, J. L.: Regulation of plasma cholesterol by lipoprotein receptors. Science 212:628, 1981.

Cuthbertson, W. F. J.: Essential fatty acid requirements in infancy. Am. J. Clin. Nutr. 29:559, 1976.

Friedman, H. I.: Intestinal fat digestion absorption and transport: a review. Am. J. Clin. Nutr. 33:1108, 1980.

Glueck, C. J., and Connor, W. E.: Dietary coronary heart disase relationships reconnoitered. Am. J. Clin. Nutr. 31:727, 1978.

Goldstein, J. L., Schrott, H. G., Hazzard, W. R., et al.: Hyperlipidemia in coronary heart disease. II. Genetic analysis of lipid levels in 176 families and delineation of a new inherited disorder, combined hyperlipidemia. J. Clin. Invest. 52:1544, 1973.

Levy, R. I.: The structure function and metabolism of high density lipoproteins. A status report. Circulation 62:4, 1981.

Silberman, H., and Eisenberg, D.: Parenteral and Enteral Nutrition for the Hospitalized Patient. Norwalk, Connecticut, Appleton, Century and Crofts, 1982.

VITAMINS

Combs, G. F.: Assessment of vitamin E status in man and animals. Proc. Nutr. Soc. 40:187, 1981.

Darby, W. J., McNutt, K. W., and Todhunter, E. N.: Niacin. Nutr. Rev. 33:289, 1975.

DeLuca, H. F.: Vitamin D: revisited 1980. Clin. Endocrinol. Metab. 9:1, 1980.

Frimpter, G. W., Andelman, R. J., and George, W. F.: Vitamin B_6 dependency syndromes. Am. J. Clin. Nutr. 22:794, 1969.

Gallop, D. M.: Carboxylated calcium binding proteins and vitamin K. N. Engl. J. Med. 302:1460, 1980.

Gubler, C. J.: Thiamine. New York, Wiley Press, 1976.

Horwitt, M. K.: Vitamin E: a reexamination. Am. J. Clin. Nutr. 29:569, 1976.

Irwin, M. L.: A conspectus of research on vitamin C requirements in man. J. Nutr. 106:821, 1976.

Stewart, C. P., and Guthrie, D.: Lind's Treatise on Scurvy. Edinburgh, The Edinburgh University Press, 1953.

Terris, M.: Goldberger on Pellagra. Baton Rouge, Louisianna State University Press, 1964.

TRACE ELEMENTS

British Ministry of Health: Report on the five year fluoridation studies in the United Kingdom, July 3, 1962. Roy Soc. Health J. 82:173, 1962.

Mertz, W., Toepfer, E. W., Roginski, E. R., and Polansky, M. M.: Present knowledge of the role of chromium. Fed. Proc. 33:2275, 1974.

Oddie, T. H., Fisher, D. A., McConahey, W. M., and Thompson, C. S.: Iodine intake in the United States: a reassessment. J. Clin. Endocrinol. 30:659, 1970.

Richard, J. R.: Current concepts in the metabolic response to injury. Infection and starvation. Proc. Nutr. Soc. 39:113, 1980.

Sandstead, H. H.: Zinc nutrition in the United States. Am. J. Clin. Nutr. 26:1251, 1973.

Stanbury, J. B., Brownell, G. L., Riggs, D. S., Perinettia, H., Itiuz, J., and Del Castillo, E. B.: Endemic Goiter. The Adaptation of Man to Iodine Deficiency. Cambridge, Harvard University Press, 1954.

Underwood, E. J.: Trace elements in human and animal nutrition. New York, Academic Press, 1977.

Wolff, J., and Chaikoff, I. L.: Plasma inorganic iodide, a chemical regulator of normal thyroid function. Endocrinology 42:468, 1948.

Endocrinology

34

Thomas W. Burns and Harold E. Carlson

INTRODUCTION

The endocrine system is composed of glands that secrete one or more hormones directly into the bloodstream. The ductless glands of the endocrine system are in contrast to the exocrine glands, the secretions of which pass into the lumen of the gastrointestinal tract or onto the skin. More than 100 years ago, Claude Bernard introduced a fundamental concept of biology—homeostasis of the internal milieu. Survival of mammalian species has required mechanisms to maintain the constancy of the internal environment despite wide fluctuations in the physical environment and the availability of essential nutrients. The endocrine system provides many of these mechanisms.

If a principal function of the endocrine system is the preservation of homeostasis, its method of accomplishing this is communication. Increasingly it appears that the nervous system and the endocrine system form a complementary "wire" and "wireless" communications network regulating a broad array of metabolic processes. Neural transmitters from higher centers impinge on the hypothalamus, thereby modulating the synthesis and secretion of neurohumoral substances that either regulate the release of anterior pituitary hormones or pass directly to the posterior pituitary. Once these hormones are released into the circulation, they in turn stimulate the secretion of hormones by specific target glands or act directly on other tissues of the body. At the distal end of the communications circuit, these hormones powerfully affect intracellular events. At the proximal end, many of these hormones, including those secreted by the thyroid, gonads, parathyroids, and pancreas, are essential to the proper development and function of the central nervous system. Although in no instance has the precise mechanism of action of the hormone on a tissue been elucidated, recent work suggests that hormone action commences with the interaction of the hormone with a specific receptor protein in either the cell membrane or cytosol. The hormone-receptor protein complex then activates the first of a series of enzymatic steps leading to the overt expression of the hormone's biologic activity. Thus, the central nervous system, the endocrine system, and the intracellular enzymatic systems form an interlocking triad of regulation, each element capable of directing and responding to appropriate signals that allow the transfer of information from the integrated center of the organism to its smallest operating unit.

BASIC PHYSIOLOGIC CONCEPTS

ELEMENTS OF THE ENDOCRINE SYSTEM

The principal components of the endocrine system are the hypothalamus, the anterior and posterior pituitary, the thyroid, the parathyroids, the endocrine pancreas, the adrenal cortex, the adrenal medulla, and the gonads (ovaries and testes). The endocrine function of the human pineal gland has not been established and will not be considered here. The placenta produces several hormones, but there are few data implicating the endocrine placenta in human disease and it will not be commented upon further here. Another endocrine "organ" that will not be discussed is the gastrointestinal tract. The so-called "gut hormones" are of historical interest (see further on) as well as the subject of intensive current investigation; however, the physiologic role of these factors has yet to be determined. Several others substances that have hormone-like qualities (e.g., erythropoietin and the prostaglandins) are not discussed in this chapter.

The secretory activity of the adrenal cortex, the thyroid, and the gonads is subservient to the trophic hormones of the anterior pituitary. The secretion of parathyroid hormone is regulated by the level of plasma ionized calcium and that of insulin principally by the serum glucose concentration. The secretion of epinephrine by the adrenal medulla is controlled by the sympathetic nervous system.

HORMONES: DEFINITION AND BASIC CHARACTERIZATION

The term "hormone" was first used by Starling and Bayliss in 1906 to describe secretin and gastrin. They defined hormones as chemical substances that are released into the circulation by one group of cells and that affect one or more different groups of cells. A more useful definition, proposed by Huxley in 1935, emphasizes the biologic function of hormones rather than their means of transport. According to Huxley, hormones are molecules whose essential purpose is the transfer of information from one set of cells to another to meet the needs of the total organism.

At the present time, it is possible to distinguish at least two groups of hormones. Those in the first group clearly subserve the transfer of information role of Huxley's definition. Examples include epinephrine, parathyroid hormone, insulin, and most of the hormones of the anterior pituitary. In general, the response of the body to these hormones is rapid and proportionate to the quantity of hormone present. The response promptly ceases when the concentration of hormone falls below a critical level. These hormones appear to act through the adenylate cyclase-cyclic AMP system, to be described later. The second group of hormones is exemplified by the steroids, thyroxine, growth hormone, and possibly vitamin D. The response of cells to these hormones is slow and may persist after the plasma concentration of the hormone has fallen below a physiologically effective level. Their primary function appears to be growth and maintenance. Because, in their absence, cells may not be able to respond to the first group of hormones, hormones of the second group have been termed permissive. Their mechanism of action appears to involve modification of protein synthesis. Thus far, there has been no demonstration that they activate the cyclic AMP system. Insulin, discussed in detail in Chapter 35, represents a special case, not fitting satisfactorily into either group.

The terms *neurocrine* and *paracrine* are used to indicate cells that release a humoral substance capable of modifying the function of adjacent cells. Neurocrine cells release neutrotransmitters. Examples of paracrine cells are the alpha cells of the pancreatic islets of Langerhans. These cells release glucagon, which, in addition to its systemic effects, may act locally to influence the secretion of insulin and somatostatin by beta and delta cells.

FEEDBACK CONTROL IN THE REGULATION OF HORMONE SECRETORY ACTIVITY

The concept of negative and positive feedback control is basic to a clear understanding of the normal and pathologic physiology of the endocrine system. The interrelations between the anterior pituitary and the thyroid, which will be given in detail further on, exemplify the principles involved. The secretory rate of thyroid hormone is increased by plasma thyroid-stimulating hormone (TSH) which is secreted by the anterior pituitary. (*Note:* Throughout this chapter, the term "thyroid hormone" is intended to include thyroxine [T_4] and triiodothyronine [T_3]). As the level of thyroid hormone in the plasma increases, it reaches a concentration called the "set point," which causes the cessation of TSH secretion and hence of the secretion of thyroid hormone itself. The plasma concentration of thyroid hormone then falls, and when it declines below the set point, TSH secretion resumes. An analogy may be drawn between this process and the control of room temperature by the interaction of a thermostat and a furnace. The thermostat setting, for example 70°, is similar to the set point. Heat from the furnace will be delivered until the room temperature exceeds 70°. At that point, the thermostat signals the furnace to shut off and delivery of heat ceases. When the temperature falls below the set point, the thermostat is activated and signals the furnace to turn on. In this analogy, the furnace represents the thyroid gland, the heat represents plasma thyroid hormone, the thermostat represents the anterior pituitary, and the electrical signal between the thermostat and the furnace is analogous to TSH. As will be seen subsequently, the regulation of thyroid hormone secretion is more complicated than this analogy suggests; it involves a third hormone, thyrotropin-releasing hormone (TRH), secreted by the hypothalamus.

The control of parathyroid hormone secretion is based on a simpler negative feedback system. The principal stimulus to its secretion is a fall in plasma calcium concentration below a set point of approximately 10 mg/dl. The increase in plasma parathyroid hormone, by its action on kidney and bone, increases serum calcium until the set point is reached. The relationship between insulin secretion by the pancreas and the plasma concentration of glucose exemplifies a positive feedback system. When glucose concentration exceeds the normal fasting level of about 80 mg/dl, insulin secretion increases and diverts glucose into the liver and peripheral tissues, thus reducing the blood glucose. The advantages of these feedback systems, which have many counterparts in the servomechanisms in industry, are obvious. They permit maintenance of closely controlled concentrations of hormones, metabolites, and nutrients in the plasma, and thus preserve the homeostasis of the internal milieu. As will repeatedly be emphasized, the diagnosis of an endocrine disease frequently is based on the interpretation of laboratory data in light of the feedback concept.

CHEMICAL NATURE, ELABORATION, SECRETION, AND TRANSPORT OF HORMONES

If hormones are classified on the basis of chemical structure, the following four broad categories emerge:

1. Small peptides
2. Large polypeptides
3. Steroids
4. Derivatives of amino acids

The structures of some neurohumoral substances elaborated by the hypothalamus are only now being elucidated. Some appear to be peptides with only a few amino acid residues; others are much larger. For example, corticotropin releasing factor (CRF) has 41 amino acid residues. Vasopressin, also formed in hypothalamic nuclei, has eight amino acids. The hormones of the anterior pituitary are large polypeptides, as are insulin, glucagon, and parathyroid hormone. The steroid hormones include secretions of the adrenal cortex, the ovaries, the testes, and the metabolites of vitamin D. Both thyroxine and epinephrine are amino acid derivatives.

Much information is being accrued regarding the molecular events involved in the biosynthesis, storage, and release of hormones, especially thyroid hormone, insulin, and the steroid hormones. The fabrication of a hormone requires several enzymatic steps, and many diseases are now recognized that are due to a deficiency of a biosynthetic enzyme. This leads either to the absence of hormone production by the involved gland or to the synthesis of a defective hormone. It should be recalled that many hormones have the secondary fuction of interacting with either the hypothalamus or the pituitary to assist in the regulation of their own secretion. The structural requirements for both these hormonal functions are thought to be the same. The consequences of a target endocrine gland that secretes a biologically inactive hormone are predictable according to the negative feedback concept. An individual in whom this occurs will display not only the effects of hormonal deficiency but also enlargement of the affected gland because of an increase in the specific circulating tropic hormone. Examples of this phenomenon, involving deficiencies in the biosynthesis of thyroid hormone, will be discussed later.

After their release into the circulation, many of the small hormones quickly combine with a carrier protein. In general, the structure of the carrier protein is highly specific for its client hormone. Because only the free hormone is metabolically active, the binding of hormone to a specific protein provides another means of regulating its activity. The concentrations of carrier proteins are influenced by various factors, including sex hormones, drugs, and certain diseases. Instances of both genetically induced deficiency and excess of the thyroid-hormone–binding protein (thyroxine-binding globulin or TBG) have been observed. Carrier proteins have been used as reagents in the laboratory for the measurement of the specific hormones that they bind.

MECHANISM OF ACTION OF HORMONES

Students of biology are gratified when a unifying concept becomes established as fact. Such was the case when the nucleotide adenosine-triphosphate (ATP) was identified as the final donor of energy in almost all biologic reactions. A similar event has occurred concerning the mechanism of hormone action, since most if not all hormones appear to act through one of two pathways.

Adenylate Cyclase–Cyclic AMP System

Mostly through the patient and creative investigations of Sutherland and coworkers during the 1960s, the nucleotide cyclic AMP was recognized as a key mediator of the action of epinephrine on liver glycogen. Since then, research on the role of cyclic AMP has proliferated at a fantastic rate. A long list of hormone-tissue interactions in which cyclic AMP has been implicated has accumulated. Not only has cyclic AMP been found in cells of all animal species studied, but Pastan demonstrated its necessity for the induction of certain enzymes in the bacterium E. coli. Cyclic AMP has also been identified as the attractant substance that signals individual cells of the social ameba, the slime mold, to aggregate. Thus, the significance of cyclic AMP in biology rivals that of ATP.

The manner in which cyclic AMP mediates hormonal action appears to be generally the same for all hormones and animal species thus far studied. It is depicted schematically in Figure 34–1. The hormone circulating in plasma interacts with a receptor in the plasma membrane of the cell. The receptor appears not to be directly linked to the enzyme but to a large macromolecule, the guanine nucleotide regulatory protein (N). Interaction between the hormone (H)-receptor (R) complex and N activates the latter, which in turn converts the catalytic unit (C) of adenylate cyclase to its active state (Fig. 34–2). This enzyme catalyzes the formation of cyclic AMP from ATP. Cyclic AMP then triggers the response that is recognized as the hormone's biologic action. In this scheme, the hormone is frequently designated as the "first

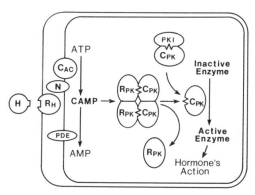

Figure 34–1 Cyclic AMP–mediated hormone action. Circulating hormone (H) binds to specific receptor sites (R_H) on the plasma membrane, leading to activation of the catalytic unit (C_{AC}) of the adenylate cyclase system. This process is shown in more detail in Figure 34–2. Cyclic AMP is formed and interacts with the receptor of protein kinase (R_{PK}), thus freeing the catalytic unit (C_{PK}) of the enzyme. C_{PK} activates the target enzyme, leading to expression of the hormone's biological action. Cyclic AMP is degraded to AMP by phosphodiesterase, while protein kinase is inactivated by a PK inhibitor (PKI).

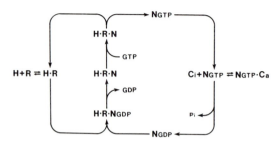

Figure 34–2 This figure is a hypothetical model of the membrane hormone-receptor-adenylate cyclase system. In it, the system is viewed as having three principal macromolecular components: the receptor (R), the guanine nucleotide regulatory protein (N), and the catalytic unit, or enzyme, itself (C). In the resting state, the N protein is bound to the inhibitory nucleotide GDP. When an agonist or hormone (H) binds to R, the resulting H•R combination associates with N to form a ternary complex H•R•N. In this reaction, GDP is lost, permitting GTP to attach to N. In the latter interaction, H and R are released, leaving the regulatory protein as N_{GTP}, which is believed to be its active form. N_{GTP} extends to the inner surface of the membrane, where it is linked to the previously inactive catalytic unit, C. N_{GTP} C is thought to be the form of the enzyme that catalyzes the formation of cyclic AMP from ATP. The existence of N_{GTP} C is terminated when GTP is converted to GDP by a GTPase. The presence of GDP causes the complex to dissociate rapidly to C and N_{GDP}.

While this model (modified from one described by Lefkowitz and coworkers) is tentative, it is consistent with a large body of experimental data. An N protein has been isolated and characterized, and, as described later, a deficiency of N protein has been discovered in the clinical disorder *pseudohypoparathyroidism*. Experimentally, the action of a hormone can be prolonged by substituting a GTP analogue resistant to hydrolysis in place of GTP itself or by including cholera toxin in the in vitro system. Cholera toxin inhibits GTPase, preventing the disruption of the N_{GTP} C complex.

messenger" and cyclic AMP as the "second messenger." The intracellular level of cyclic AMP is decreased by the activity of a potent, specific esterase, phosphodiesterase. This enzyme is inhibited by xanthine derivatives such as theophylline and caffeine. These agents cause an increase in cyclic AMP and tend to mimic hormonal action in in-vitro systems. Additional details are now known regarding the mechanism by which cyclic AMP initiates the cellular response to a hormone. The nucleotide interacts with protein kinase. This enzyme has two components: a receptor and a catalytic unit. In its unstimulated state, the receptor component prevents action by the catalytic unit. Interaction of the receptor with cyclic AMP removes the former from the complex, allowing the catalytic unit to act. This active form of protein kinase stimulates another enzyme or enzymes, presumably by phosphorylation, and this secondary enzyme (or enzymes) catalyzes the final step leading to the hormonal action and is thought to be inactivated by a phosphatase.

Sutherland and coworkers have suggested that the following four criteria be met if cyclic AMP is to be considered the "second messenger" for a given hormone:

1. The hormone should be capable of stimulating adenylate cyclase in broken cell preparations from appropriate tissue.

2. A physiologic concentration of hormone should be able to increase the cyclic AMP concentration of intact cells, and this increase in cyclic AMP should precede the physiologic response.

3. Phosphodiesterase inhibitors such as theophylline should potentiate the response to the hormone.

4. The activity of the hormone should be mimicked by cyclic AMP or its more soluble dibutyryl derivative.

A question that naturally arises when one considers the large number of hormone-tissue interactions that involve cyclic AMP concerns how this one compound can mediate the highly specific responses of such a diverse array of hormone. There are at least two sites at which specificity could be determined. It is presumed that all cells of the body (exclusive of those in the central nervous system) are equally exposed to a hormone circulating in the plasma. However, only the cells of responsive tissue have receptor sites that "recognize" the hormone. The receptor site has a conformational structure complementary to that of the hormone, permitting the latter to bind to the former with high affinity. Additional specificity is imparted by the nature of the substance or substances available to serve as substrates for the cyclic AMP protein kinase catalytic unit. In adipose tissue, the substance is a lipase; in liver, it is a phosphorylase. Specificity could also result if cyclic AMP were compartmentalized within the cell, but this has not, as yet, been demonstrated.

Cyclic AMP is not the only "second messenger" that has been identified; calcium ion has been shown to be involved in the mediation of the actions of some hormones. For example, stimulation of alpha-adrenergic receptors of hepatocyte membranes by epinephrine prompts an influx of calcium ion that is quickly bound to a specific protein, calmodulin. The calmodulin-Ca^{++} complex activates phosphorylase kinase, which in turn activates phosphorylase, with a resultant increase in glycogenolysis.

Interaction of Hormones with Cytoplasmic Receptor Protein and Nuclear Acceptors

At present, it appears that all the steroid hormones (testosterone, estradiol, progesterone, aldosterone, and cortisol) exert their metabolic effects in a similar fashion (Fig. 34–3). Each appears to combine with a specific receptor protein located in the cytoplasm; the steroid-receptor com-

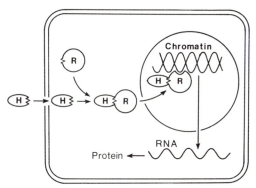

Figure 34–3 Mechanism of action of steroid hormones. Unbound steroid hormone (H) penetrates the cell membrane and combines with a highly specific receptor molecule (R) in the cytosol. The H·R complex enters the nucleus and binds to specific chromatin sites, resulting in the transcription of information into RNA. In the cytosol, mRNA translates the coded message via ribosomes, with resultant synthesis of new protein.

plex is translocated to the nucleus, where it combines with specific acceptors located on chromatin. The steroid-receptor-acceptor complex causes the nuclear genetic material to produce messenger RNA, which in turn signals the fabrication of the enzyme, which is more directly responsible for the biologic expression of the hormone's activity. Specificity results from the conformational structure of the receptor protein and the nuclear acceptor sites.

Thyroid hormones also appear to act by activating RNA transcription and subsequent translation of the mRNA message into protein products in the cytoplasm. The thyroid hormones bind directly to nuclear chromatin, however, without the mediation of a cytoplasmic receptor.

The Role of Receptor Abnormalities in the Pathophysiology of Endocrine Disease

Many years ago, one of the great pioneers in endocrinology, Fuller Albright, predicted the existence of endocrinopathies in which the relevant endocrine gland and its secretion are normal but in which the tissues normally responsive to the hormone are, in fact, resistant to it. Albright cited the Seabright bantam as an animal model of his hypothesis. The Seabright rooster shows normal androgen effects in every respect except for an underdeveloped comb. The comb tissue in this species is insensitive to androgen. The first clinical example of end-organ resistance, pseudohypoparathyroidism, was described by Albright and colleagues in 1942.

Mechanisms underlying the resistant state in some of these disorders are beginning to be clarified. From the work of Roth and colleagues and several other workers, it appears that both the

number of receptors and their affinity for hormone may be altered in disease. In the case of insulin, both in-vivo and in-vitro studies suggest that a major determinant of the number of receptors on insulin-sensitive cells is the ambient concentration of insulin itself. Thus, in type II (maturity onset) diabetes, one may find the combination of obesity, hyperglycemia, increased levels of circulating insulin, and a *decrease* in insulin receptors on the cells of peripheral tissues. Rarely, autoantibodies to insulin receptors may develop, producing a profound state of insulin resistance.

MANIFESTATIONS OF ENDOCRINE DISORDERS

Most endocrine diseases are secondary to either an excess or a deficiency of one or more hormones. Commonly, the clinical description of an endocrine disorder has antedated by many years an appreciation of the gland and hormone involved. Progress in relating clinical syndromes to deficient or excessive hormone was relatively slow until techniques became available for the measurement of hormones and their metabolites in blood and urine. The protean modes of presentation of endocrine disease are best appreciated by considering the specific examples given in the following sections. However, it is important to appreciate the close symbiosis that exists between bedside medicine and laboratory physiology in endocrinology. Perhaps in no other field of medicine has clinical observation been more important in shaping the direction of physiologic experimentation, and similarly, there is no area in which the physician is more dependent on an understanding of physiologic principles in diagnosing and treating patients.

Generally, the clinical manifestations of hormone excess and deficiency are extremely slow in evolving. With few exceptions, even the abrupt loss of a given hormone causes no immediate distress. Thus, when one recognizes clear-cut evidence of excessive or deficient endocrine function, one can usually conclude that the patient's condition began many months or even years earlier. Before he becomes critically ill, the patient passes through a prolonged period of increasing disability. Unfortunately, the early symptoms of the underlying disease are often vague and not very convincing to either the patient or the physician. Efforts at early diagnosis are further handicapped by the not infrequent occurrence of predominantly psychiatric symptoms, which distract the physician from the organic basis of the patient's illness.

LABORATORY PROCEDURES

Although the presence of an endocrine problem is frequently suggested by symptoms, signs, or an abnormal finding among screening laboratory tests, establishing the diagnosis usually requires one or more relatively specific laboratory procedures. Increasingly, the latter include direct measurement of the hormone under suspicion.

Capability in this area has been greatly enhanced by the development of radiobinding assay methods. All these methods use a binding reagent (i.e., antibody, binding protein, or cellular receptor) that is highly specific for the substance to be measured. In the radioimmunoassay, the reagent is an antibody generated by a laboratory animal in response to injections of the foreign human hormone to be measured. In the competitive protein-binding procedure, the binding reagent is a protein that in most cases normally transports in plasma the hormone to be measured. Similarly, the binding reagent can be membrane or cytosol receptor material, as in the radioreceptor assay.

Radioimmunoassay was first applied to the measurement of insulin in human serum by Berson and Yalow in 1960. At the present time, satisfactory procedures for most of the polypeptide hormones and many of the steroid hormones have been developed. The technique requires not only a specific antiserum of high affinity but also a small supply of pure hormone to serve as a standard. In addition, a small quantity of pure hormone is labeled with a radioactive tracer. To perform an assay, a fixed quantity of antiserum and a fixed amount of tracer are added to a series of tubes. The amount of tracer is selected to provide a statistically significant number of counts; a titer of antiserum is chosen that will bind 30 to 60 per cent of the total radioactivity. For the definition of a dose-response relationship or standard curve, known quantities of highly purified, *unlabeled* hormone are added to a portion of the tubes (equation 1). Aliquots of unknown serum are added to the remaining tubes (equation 2). All tubes are incubated, during which time there is a partitioning of tracer between the bound (i.e., attached to antibody) and free state. The quantitative aspects of this partitioning are determined by the amount of unlabeled hormone (either standard or that contained in the unknown specimen) present in the tube. The kinetics are illustrated by the following equations:

Free (F)   *Bound (B)*

$$H_s + H^* + Ab \rightleftharpoons H^* Ab + H_s Ab \text{ (equation 1)}$$

$$H_u + H^* + Ab \rightleftharpoons H^* Ab + H_u Ab \text{ (equation 2)}$$

H^* = Radioactive labeled hormone
H_s = Pure hormone standard
H_u = Hormone in unknown
Ab = Antibody

Because both unlabeled and labeled hormones compete for a fixed number of antibody binding sites, an increase in the amount of unlabeled

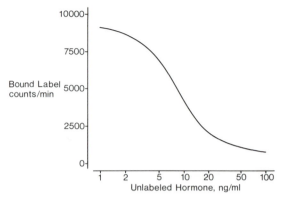

Figure 34–4 Radioimmunoassay standard curve showing the amount of radioactively labeled hormone bound to antibody on the vertical axis and the concentration of unlabeled hormone present on the horizontal axis. As the amount of unlabeled hormone in the reaction mixture is increased, there is a progressive decrease in the binding of radioactively labeled hormone to antibody.

hormone results in fewer sites available to bind the tracer, consequently more tracer remains unbound or free. For quantitation, it is necessary to separate antibody-bound hormone from free hormone. A number of satisfactory methods (physical, chemical, and immunologic) have been developed. Following the separation, the radioactivity of either the bound or free fraction of each tube is counted. The relationship of response versus dose for the standards is plotted, for example, as counts bound versus log dose, and the response of the unknown specimens is calculated from this standard curve (Fig. 34–4). The procedure outlined for radioimmunoassay is also applicable to competitive protein-binding (CPB), to assays using carrier proteins and radioreceptor techniques.

Radioreceptor techniques to measure the serum concentration of hormones such as insulin and growth hormone are currently being performed in select research laboratories; others are in the developmental stages. These assays utilize the hormone receptors found either on cell membranes or in the cytosol, and consequently they are potentially more representative procedures. However, these assays are demanding in regard to both material preparation and technologic skill.

In summary, the advantages of radioimmunoassay and competitive protein-binding assays include the following:

1. *Sensitivity.* The ability to measure the microgram, nanogram, and even picogram quantities of hormone that normally are present in the plasma.

2. *Simplicity.* After the assay has been established, hundreds of samples per week can be processed.

3. *Specificity.* Because of the high binding affinity of the reagent (be it antibody or transport protein) specificity is inherent in these methods.

One potential disadvantage of radioimmunoassays is that they measure the immunologically active portion of the hormone rather than the biologically active portion. Some peptide hormones undergo fragmentation after they are secreted into the circulation. Because these fragments may have different rates of disposal, it is theoretically possible to have a high level of a fragment measurable by radioimmunoassay concomitantly with a normal concentration of fragments that have biologic activity. Radioreceptor assays may ultimately prove more desirable because of their ability to identify biologically active hormone.

THE HYPOTHALAMUS

One of the most exciting advances in endocrinology in recent years has been the discovery that the secretory activity of the anterior pituitary, which, for a long time, was thought of as the "master gland" of the endocrine system, is subservient to humoral substances elaborated by the hypothalamus. The concept that neurosecretory cells could function both as neurons and hormone-secreting cells was not new. For some time, it has been appreciated that the hypothalamic supraoptic and paraventricular neurons elaborated vasopressin and oxytocin, which are transmitted down the axons of the cells to the posterior pituitary. Comparable neural connections between the hypothalamus and the anterior pituitary were searched for but not found. However, it has now been established that there are vascular connections between the hypothalamus and the anterior pituitary. The median eminence of the hypothalamus contains a capillary network that drains into the hypophyseal portal veins. The latter enter the anterior pituitary and subdivide into a second capillary network. Thus, substances produced by neurosecretory cells of the median eminence and adjacent areas have ready access to the cells of the anterior pituitary via the hypophyseal portal system.

In 1969, two groups that were working independently established the identity of the first hypothalamic factor, thyrotropin releasing hormone (TRH). The leaders of these two groups, Dr. Roger Guillemin and Dr. Andrew Schally, were the recipients of the 1977 Nobel Prize in physiology and medicine. TRH is a tripeptide, pyroglutamyl histidylproline amide, which has been synthesized and is now being applied in the diagnosis of thyroid and pituitary disease in humans. It is generally accepted that the secretion of each of the anterior pituitary hormones is controlled by a specific hypothalamic releasing hormone or an inhibiting factor or both. A 10-amino acid peptide (LHRH) that prompts release of luteinizing hormone (LH) has been identified and is available on a limited basis for clinical use. This substance stimulates the release of follicle-stimulating hormone (FSH) as well as LH and hence is often referred to as gonadotropin-releasing hormone (GnRH). Inhibitory substances appear to be involved in the control of prolactin and growth hormone secretion. Dopamine is the principal physiologic inhibitor of prolactin; in the absence of hypothalamic influences, pituitary prolactin release increases. A 14-amino acid peptide that suppresses the release of growth hormone has been isolated and identified by Guillemin. This substance, termed *somatostatin,* not only affects growth hormone secretion but also, when injected intravenously into normal humans, drastically curtails the secretion of insulin and glucagon as well as thyroid-stimulating hormone (TSH).

Recently, a 44-amino acid peptide with growth hormone–releasing activity has been isolated, providing a firm basis for the dual regulatory control of growth hormone secretion. CRF, a 41-amino acid peptide, also has recently been purified from hypothalamic extracts.

If one assumes that anterior pituitary secretion is regulated by humoral substances from the hypothalamus, the question arises as to what, in turn, regulates the release of the latter. It has long been known that the hypothalamus is a major relay station within the central nervous system. Presumably, neural signals from many parts of the brain could activate the neurosecretory cells of the hypothalamus. Using neuropharmacologic agents known either to stimulate or to block specific neurotransmitters, investigators have shown that the monoamines norepinephrine, dopamine, serotonin, acetylcholine, and histamine have important influences on the secretion of the hypothalamic releasing and inhibiting factors. Obviously, much remains to be learned concerning the interactions among the higher centers of the brain, the hypothalamus, and the pituitary.

Another question that arises is how the hypothalamic factors interact with the target gland hormones that inhibit anterior pituitary secretion in a negative feedback fashion. The mode of interaction may be unique for each pituitary hormone. For example, thyroid hormone appears to oppose TRH at the level of the TSH-producing cells of the anterior pituitary. Cortisol, however, may act by inhibiting the production or release or both of CRF at the level of the median eminence as well as inhibiting the effect of CRF on the anterior pituitary.

Thus, it is clear that the central nervous system has a profound influence on the endocrine glands, the interface being the hypothalamus. Although less well documented, the converse may also be true; that is, the endocrine system may have profound influences on the central nervous system. For example, if newborn male rats are castrated and if male hormone is withheld for only 4 or 5 days, they will subsequently fail to exhibit normal male mating behavior as adult animals, even though they are given androgen replacement therapy. Impaired testicular function during a critical perinatal period conceivably could prevent the induction of the normal male behavior pattern in the central nervous system. Consistent with such a hypothesis is the fact that the testes of the newborn male are normally adult-like histologically; later in infancy, the testes regress to the prepubertal pattern and remain so until adolescence. Perhaps in men, as in the rat, male hormone is required in the neonatal period to induce modification in the central nervous system that is necessary for the development of male behavior in later life.

NEUROENDOCRINE DISORDERS

From knowledge recently attained regarding the role of the hypothalamus in regulating pituitary function, it seems likely that some diseases previously attributed to malfunction of the pituitary may actually be due to disordered function of the hypothalamus. For example, Cushing's syndrome results from prolonged excessive secretion of cortisol by the adrenal cortex. In many cases, the abnormal secretion of cortisol is associated with adrenal hyperplasia secondary to excessive secretion of ACTH. In some patients, it may be that the latter is also a secondary phenomenon (i.e., that the anterior pituitary is being subjected to excessive stimulation by CRF). With this possibility in mind, one might consider adrenal hyperplasia a disease of the hypothalamus or of even higher loci in the central nervous system. Later evidence, however, indicates that this is probably not the case; in most instances, an ACTH-secreting pituitary tumor is found, functioning independent of hypothalamic influences.

However, in some states of hormonal deficiency, the problem clearly resides at the level of the hypothalamus rather than at the target gland or the pituitary. Kallman's syndrome is a form of hypogonadism, without evidence of other endocrine problems, that illustrates the phenomenon of hypothalamic deficiency. In this disorder, young males fail to undergo puberty. They enter adulthood with a eunuchoid habitus and other evidences of androgen lack, such as immature genitalia, absence of facial hair, feminine body contour, female escutcheon, and the absence of libido and potentia. As expected, the plasma level of testosterone is very low; however, the gonadotropins are also very low in these patients, and the administration of LHRH results in increases in both LH and FSH, indicating that the pituitary is intact. Treatment of these individuals with LH in the form of human chorionic gonadotropin (HCG) and FSH (human menopausal gonadotropin, HMG) stimulates both Leydig cell function (as reflected by a dramatic increase in plasma testosterone) and the germinal epithelium of the testes (as indicated by the appearance of spermatozoa in the seminal fluid). Thus, therapy can result in normal sexual functioning, including normal fertility. Interestingly, in the classic form of the syndrome, the patient has an impaired sense of smell, either hyposmia or anosmia, due to hypoplasia of the olfactory bulbs. Less commonly, these patients may have other congenital anomalies such as cleft lip or palate and deafness. These features, as well as the hypogonadism, reflect a failure of development of certain midline structures in embryonic life.

ANTERIOR PITUITARY

PHYSIOLOGY

The pituitary is a small gland, weighing approximately 0.6 gm and measuring about 1 cm in diameter. It is contained in a bony socket, the sella turcica ("Turkish saddle"), situated at the base of the brain above the sphenoid sinus. The anterior lobe, derived from ectodermal tissue embryologically, makes up about 75 per cent of the gland by weight. In the human fetus and in lower species of animals, a distinct intermediate lobe is present; such a structure may reappear during pregnancy but is otherwise absent in normal adult humans.

The anterior pituitary produces several peptide hormones, of which six have clearly defined functions in humans. ACTH stimulates the biosynthesis and release of cortisol by the adrenal cortex. Thyroid-stimulating hormone (thyrotropin, TSH) stimulates the uptake of iodide and the synthesis and release of thyroid hormone by the thyroid. Follicle-stimulating hormone (FSH) stimulates the development of the graafian follicle and secretion of estrogen in the ovary and spermatogenesis in the testes. Luteinizing hormone (LH) prompts ovulation and the luteinization of the mature follicle in the ovary. In the male, this hormone, formerly called the *interstitial cell-stimulating hormone (ICSH),* stimulates the production and release of testosterone by the Leydig cells of the testes. Prolactin (PRL) stimulates the secretion of milk by the breast of the postpartum female. Human growth hormone (HGH, somatotropin) promotes growth of all tissues in the immature subject. Its physiologic function in the adult, if any, is not clear. Although distinct melanocyte-stimulating hormones (MSH) derived from the intermediate lobe promote pigmentation in many species, such substances may not be important or even present in humans. At present, it is believed that ACTH is the primary human pigmentary hormone.

In addition to these six hormones with defined functions, there are others whose role is less clearcut. One of these is beta-lipotropin (β-LPH). This substance, which has been isolated and purified, stimulates lipolysis in rats but not in humans. Both β-LPH and ACTH are synthesized in the anterior and intermediate lobes of corticotrophs as part of a larger precursor molecule, pro-opiomelan-ocortin. This substance, when cleaved, may also yield melanotropic hormones (in nonhuman species) and endorphins. The latter peptides have potent morphine-like properties of great interest.

On the basis of their staining characteristics, the cells of the anterior pituitary have classically been characterized as *chromophobic* (without granules), *eosinophilic,* and *basophilic.* In the traditional view, chromophobe cells were believed to be either precursor or supportive cells without secretory activity; eosinophilic cells were considered responsible for the secretion of growth hormone and prolactin; and basophilic cells were thought to be responsible for the secretion of ACTH, TSH, LH, and FSH. Such a schema is undoubtedly greatly oversimplified. For example, some pituitary tumors that produce excessive quantities of ACTH, growth hormone, or prolactin have consisted of chromophobe cells. It should be remembered that stained granules represent stored hormone. Tumor cells may release hormone as rapidly as it is formed and thus be agranular when stained. With the electron microscope, it is often possible to relate the hormone secreted to granule size. Additionally, immunohistochemical techniques in which highly specific antibodies directed against pituitary hormones are applied to the tissue and visualized using fluorescent or colored labels usually permit a precise characterization of a cell's secretory activity.

Control of Anterior Pituitary Secretion

The dual system that controls anterior pituitary hormone secretion has previously been described. These control mechanisms are (1) negative feedback, in which the target gland hormone, acting at the level of the pituitary or hypothalamus, inhibits secretion of its tropic hormone; and (2) control by hypothalamic hormones that arise from neuronal cells in or near the median eminence and that are secreted into the hypophyseal portal circulation.

These mechanisms are so important, both from conceptual and pragmatic points of view, that their repeated emphasis is warranted. The interaction among the hormonal elements that control thyroid hormone secretion is the most firmly established and illustrates the principles involved.

Evidence suggests that the normal pituitary can secrete TSH at a low level *independent* of influences from higher centers. It is presumed that TRH tonically maintains the secretory rate of TSH at a basal level that constitutes the set point. The rate of TRH release is thought to be determined by neural signals, but the source of such signals and their relationship to physiologic phenomena such as temperature regulation is poorly understood. There is a small diurnal variation in circulating TSH levels.

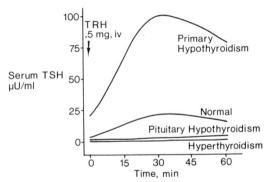

Figure 34–5 Serum thyrotropin (TSH) responses to intravenous TRH in normal subjects and in patients with various thyroid disorders. Patients with primary hypothyroidism have elevated baseline serum levels of TSH with an exaggerated response to TRH, whereas patients with secondary hypothyroidism due to pituitary destruction have low baseline levels that fail to increase following TRH administration. Patients with *hyper*thyroidism also show suppressed baseline TSH levels with no response to TRH, owing to the negative feedback effects of elevated circulating thyroid hormones on the pituitary.

TRH stimulates both the synthesis and the release of TSH; these two actions can be dissociated. The latter is very prompt; in humans, an increase in plasma TSH is detectable within minutes of an intravenous infusion of TRH (Fig. 34–5). This release process appears to be mediated by the adenylate cyclase–cyclic AMP system. Thyroid hormone blocks the releasing action of TRH on the pituitary *if* the thyroid hormone is administered some time before TRH is given. If the two hormones are administered at the same time or if thyroid hormone is administered just a few minutes before TRH, no block occurs. There is evidence that thyroid hormone stimulates the synthesis of a protein within the pituitary that inhibits TRH action. Whether thyroid hormone also acts on the hypothalamus or higher in the central nervous system to inhibit the formation or secretion of TRH is not known. These interrelations are illustrated in Figure 34–6. TRH also stimulates the secretion of prolactin from the pituitary.

The very marked biologic activity of TRH illustrates the phenomenon of amplification, in which a relatively minute amount of hormone that is acting as a primary signal stimulates the secretion of a much larger amount of a second hormone. It has been estimated that this amplification factor is about 100,000 in the case of the TRH-TSH interaction (i.e., 10 ng of TRH will cause the secretion of 1 mg of its tropic hormone).

CLINICAL ENTITIES

Pituitary Tumors

The pathophysiology of pituitary tumors involves two basic considerations: (1) the pressure

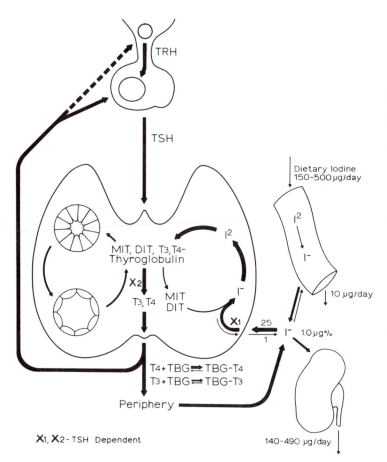

Figure 34–6 Pathways of iodine metabolism and the relationships among the hypothalamus, pituitary, and thyroid. Ingested iodine is assimilated as iodine ion that is selectively taken up, or "trapped," by the thyroid. Normally, the gradient between intrathyroidal and plasma iodide is about 25:1. Once in the thyroid, iodide is rapidly oxidized and combined with tyrosyl residues in a series of steps collectively termed "organification." This process occurs in thyroglobulin molecules. Thyroglobulin is stored as colloid in the lumina of follicles. Iodine from the thyroid hormone precursors—diiodotyrosine (DIT) and monoiodotyrosine (MIT)—is recycled. Thyroid hormone (T_4 and T_3) is released from thyroglobulin by enzymatic cleavage. Both thyroid hormone release (X_2) and iodide "trapping" (X_1) are TSH-dependent. Nearly all circulating T_4 and most T_3 are bound to proteins such as thyroxine-binding globulin (TBG). Thyroid hormone interferes with the action of TRH on the TSH-secreting cells of the anterior pituitary. Whether thyroid hormone has a direct action on the hypothalamus is not known (see text).

effects of a space-occupying mass in the strategic area above and lateral to the sella turcica, and (2) the effects of excess or deficiency of one or more pituitary hormones.

From the standpoint of the first consideration all pituitary tumors are similar in that presenting symptoms may be headache and visual impairment. The latter manifestation usually results from pressure of the tumor on the decussating fibers of the optic chiasma. Characteristically, the first pattern of visual field loss is the upper outer quadrant, followed by the lower outer quadrant. The resulting defect, bitemporal hemianopsia, may be apparent when the visual fields are assessed by gross confrontation at the bedside.

From the standpoint of the second consideration, pituitary tumors may be divided into five groups: (1) craniopharyngiomas, which never elaborate hormones; (2) prolactin-secreting tumors; (3) growth hormone–secreting tumors; (4) ACTH-secreting tumors, in Cushing's and Nelson's syndromes (tumors that secrete TSH, LH, or FSH are rare); and (5) nonsecretory pituitary adenomas. Hormonal deficiencies may arise in any of these five groups because of (1) the pressure of the tumor on normal cells; (2) the consequence of treatment; or, rarely, (3) apoplexy or hemorrhage into the

tumor. When hypopituitarism does occur, growth hormone is typically the first hormone affected, followed, in sequence, by deficiency of gonadotropins, TSH, and ACTH. Thus, declining sexual function is an early clinical clue that suggests the presence of a pituitary tumor. However, any single hormonal loss or combination of hormonal losses may occur. The consequences of deficiencies of anterior pituitary hormones and the manifestations of excessive hormone production by a pituitary tumor will be discussed.

Prolactin-Secreting Tumors. Pituitary tumors that secrete prolactin cause hyperprolactinemia, with serum PRL levels above the upper limits of normal, about 20 ng/ml for women and 15 ng/ml for men. Large tumors (macroadenomas, greater than 1 cm in diameter) often produce great amounts of PRL; a serum PRL level over 200 ng/ml is highly suggestive of a pituitary tumor. Smaller tumors (microadenomas, less than 1 cm in diameter) may produce lesser elevations in serum PRL. Galactorrhea (inappropriate lactation) is frequently seen in women who have hyperprolactinemia and is caused by the stimulatory effects of PRL on the estrogen-primed breast. Additionally, hyperprolactinemia usually results in amenorrhea in women and in decreased libido and potency in men because of the inhibition of gonado-tropin secretion by PRL, probably mediated by a decrease in GnRH.

Acromegaly and Gigantism. Acromegaly (excessive size of the distal parts of the body) results from sustained, excessive secretion of growth hormone in adults. The source of the growth hormone is an eosinophilic, or less often a chromophobic, tumor of the anterior pituitary. When such a tumor develops in childhood or adolescence prior to closure of the epiphyses, growth in height is greatly accelerated, with resulting gigantism. In this circumstance, the disease process usually continues into adult life, so that the typical patient with gigantism also has the striking features of acromegaly. Massive enlargement of the hands, feet, and skull, particularly the mandible, occurs. The broadened nose and the large head have suggested the term *leonine facies* to describe some acromegalic patients (Fig. 34–7). Acromegaly is an outstanding example of an endocrine disorder that was recognized decades before the hormone involved was discovered. The classic features of

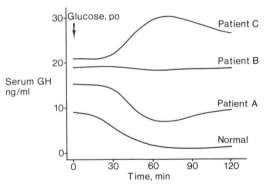

Figure 34–8 In normal subjects, serum growth hormone (GH) is suppressed by oral glucose ingestion (50 to 100 gm) to levels less than 5 ng/ml; patients with acromegaly may show partial suppression, no change, or a rise in serum GH after glucose administration.

acromegaly were first described in 1886 by Pierre Marie. The metabolic effects of long-standing excess of growth hormone are often surprisingly mild. Impairment of glucose tolerance is commonly seen, and frank diabetes mellitus, due to antagonism of insulin action by human growth hormone (HGH), occurs in perhaps 15 per cent of the cases. Other clinical features of acromegaly include degenerative arthritis, due to bony and cartilaginous overgrowth around joints; hypertension, due perhaps to the salt-retaining properties of HGH; excessive sweating, due to enlarged sweat glands and to a hypermetabolic state; and pain, numbness, and weakness in the hand, due to compression of the median nerve at the wrist by overgrown soft tissue (carpal tunnel syndrome). Increased mortality in acromegaly is principally caused by cardiovascular and cerebrovascular disease, which are in turn accelerated by the presence of hypertension and diabetes mellitus; a few patients may suffer from an unexplained cardiomyopathy.

The normal hypothalamic-pituitary-target tissue interrelations of HGH are poorly understood. It is known that there is a hypothalamic HGH-releasing factor that stimulates the growth hormone–producing cells of the anterior pituitary. Perhaps some of the tumors in acromegalics arise from chronic overstimulation of the pituitary by this HGH-releasing factor. As will be discussed, several stimuli that are capable of increasing plasma growth hormone have been identified, but relatively few inhibitors are known. One of these, hyperglycemia, is of practical value in the diagnosis of acromegaly. When a glucose load is administered to people who do not have acromegaly, the ensuing hyperglycemia is associated with a decline in HGH to low or to undetectable levels. The basal HGH level of the acromegalic individual not only is typically elevated but also cannot be suppressed to within normal limits by hyperglycemia (Fig. 34–8).

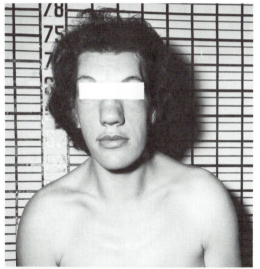

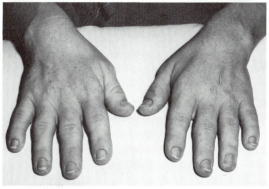

Figure 34–7 Coarse facial features *(A)* and large, fleshy hands *(B)* of a typical patient with acromegaly.

Nelson's Syndrome. Because of the underlying mechanisms that are characteristic of them, ACTH-secreting tumors deserve additional explanation. In 1960, Nelson and coworkers reported the occurrence of intense pigmentation in patients who were previously subjected to bilateral adrenalectomy for Cushing's disease. Each patient was found to have a pituitary adenoma and a very high level of plasma ACTH. Since Nelson's original report, clinical experience indicates that as many as 20 per cent of all patients who undergo adrenalectomy for adrenal hyperplasia due to Cushing's disease develop this complication. The pituitary tumor in these patients is more aggressive than is the usual variety. Complications caused by pressure on the surrounding structures are frequent, as is pituitary apoplexy. According to one hypothesis, one can best explain the syndrome by assuming that the initial pathologic event is the development of an ACTH-secreting pituitary tumor that is inadequately suppressed by the resultant abnormally high levels of plasma cortisol. During a period of many months, the latter leads to Cushing's disease, which can be treated by removal of the hyperplastic adrenal glands and by providing a replacement dosage of exogenous glucocorticoid in physiologic amounts. The manifestations of Cushing's disease regress with time. Unfortunately, the diminished, now normal, levels of plasma cortisol permit a further increase in ACTH secretion and encourage further growth of the pituitary tumor. It is ACTH hypersecretion that leads to pigmentation, which may be so intense that a white person may be mistaken for a black. It has been established that ACTH has pigmenting capability, which is very likely a result of the similarity of its N-terminal amino acid sequence to that of other melanocyte-stimulating hormones. Thus, despite receiving appropriate therapy for Cushing's disease, these unfortunate patients may trade the severe disabilities of Cushing's disease for those of a pituitary tumor.

Multiple Endocrine Neoplasia (MEN 1; Wermer's Syndrome). In a few patients who have pituitary tumors, there is also a tumor or hyperplasia of the parathyroids or an islet cell tumor of the pancreas or both. In 1954, Wermer described such tumors in four siblings and a parent; several similar reports have followed, and there is general agreement that neoplasia that arises from two or more endocrine glands is a distinct entity. Although isolated cases have been reported, more often, when appropriate studies are carried out, it is found to be familial, with an autosomal dominant mode of inheritance. The combination of pituitary, parathyroid, and pancreatic neoplasia has been labeled *MEN type I,* to distinguish it from a second condition, *MEN type IIa,* or *Sipple's syndrome,* in which medullary carcinoma of the thyroid is found in association with pheochromocytoma and hyperplasia or adenoma of the parathyroids, and from *MEN type IIb,* in which medullary carcinoma of the thyroid, pheochromocytoma, and multiple ganglioneuromas occur. Needless to say, the dramatic presentation of three endocrine tumors occurring in the same individual has invited much speculation as to the pathogenesis of the syndrome. Practically speaking, a patient who has any one of the three tumors should be assessed for the other two, and his close relatives should also be screened. Because the second or third tumor can emerge years after the first, appropriate screening tests should be done periodically.

The Empty Sella Syndrome. The empty sella syndrome is an interesting condition in which there is entry of cerebrospinal fluid into the sella turcica, usually seen by cranial computed tomography or by the older technique of pneumoencephalography. In living patients, the diagnosis can be made with certainty only with these procedures. The sella is often enlarged, suggesting the presence of a pituitary tumor and leading to the performance of radiologic studies. Although several exceptions have been noted, in general, patients who have empty sella syndrome do not have deficiencies of pituitary hormones. The question that immediately comes to mind is, "If the sella is empty, why doesn't the patient manifest hypopituitarism?" The answer is that the sella is not completely empty; a shell-like remnant of tissue, sufficient to permit normal secretory activity, remains. The pathophysiologic basis for the development of the empty sella syndrome is not clear. One plausible hypothesis is that cerebral spinal fluid pressure is transmitted into the sella through a defect in the diaphragma sella. Probably in only a small percentage of the affected individuals is the condition recognized. In one postmortem study, 40 cases were found in 788 consecutive autopsies. The clinical and radiographic features of many patients with the disorder were reviewed by Neelon and coworkers in 1975. The possibility that the empty sella syndrome might be present should be kept in mind during the evaluation of patients who have enlarged sella turcicas. Unfortunately, empty sellas have been discovered in patients who have undergone surgery directed at a misdiagnosed pituitary tumor. Preoperative computed tomography scans or pneumoencephalograms should obviate these tragic errors. Occasionally, an "empty sella" may develop following spontaneous infarction of a pituitary tumor and often follows successful treatment of pituitary neoplasms.

Growth Failure. The most outstanding manifestation of pituitary deficiency that develops prior to puberty is failure to grow. This is true whether the deficiency is restricted to HGH alone or includes deficiencies of other tropic hormones. The term *pituitary infantilism* implies dwarfism, in addition to immaturity of the secondary sexual characteristics. The latter finding, of course, can be appreciated clinically only in the postadolescent patient. The most common cause of pituitary infantilism is a craniopharyngioma; frequently, however, no organic lesion can be shown (idiopathic hypopituitarism). In pituitary infantilism, impaired secretion of tropic hormones other than HGH can almost always be shown. In contrast, Merimee and researchers have described a variety of dwarfism that is caused by a selective inability of the pituitary to secrete growth hormone; in these patients, all other anterior pituitary hormones are secreted normally. The term *sexual ateliotic (ateliosis* means imperfect development) *dwarfism* has been applied to this disorder to denote normal sexual development in an individual with short stature. McKusick, Merimee, and collaborators extensively studied uncommon types of pituitary dwarfism in which only peripheral responsiveness to HGH is deficient.

Before discussing these types, one should briefly consider what is known about the mechanism of the action of growth hormone. In terms of promoting growth, the hormone acts in the intact, immature animal to stimulate cartilage formation. One can study this process in vitro by incubating cartilage from immature rats with isotopically labeled sulfate and by measuring the incorporation of the label, as chondroitin sulfate, into cartilage. When one adds growth hormone itself to such a system, no increase in sulfate incorporation occurs. Similarly, serum from an animal that has undergone hypophysectomy has little activity. However, serum from such an animal that was treated with growth hormone is very active.

These findings led Daughaday to speculate that growth hormone does not affect growth directly; rather, it interacts with hepatic receptors that in turn generate the "sulfation factor" (now called *somatomedins*), which actually stimulate cartilaginous growth. The somatomedins appear to be a group of peptides with molecular weights of around 7000 daltons. They have insulinlike actions in vitro and show considerable structural similarity to proinsulin; hence, they also have been termed *insulinlike growth factors (IGF)*. Although the nomenclature for these peptides is still in a state of flux, it appears that one of the major somatomedin peptides, somatomedin C, is identical with IGF-I. In attempting to explain the possible value of the somatomedin mechanism, Daughaday has pointed out that growth hormone is secreted in bursts throughout the day in response to a host of metabolic and neurogenic stimuli. This irregular and intermittent pattern of secretion would seem inappropriate for the gradual progressive processes involved in orderly cell growth. The interaction of growth hormone with a system generating the actual growth substance (e.g., somatomedin) would provide an attractive mechanism to explain the normal smooth regulation of skeletal growth.

Relevant to the somatomedin hypothesis are findings from patients who have a rare form of

dwarfism that was first described in oriental Jews in Israel by Laron. By their physical characteristics, these individuals resemble pituitary dwarfs. However, there is abundant growth hormone in their sera, as determined by radioimmunoassay. Like true pituitary dwarfs, they have very low serum levels of somatomedins. Unlike pituitary dwarfs, however, these dwarfs fail to achieve an increase in somatomedins and experience relatively little increase in stature following administration of therapeutic amounts of growth hormone. One explanation for these findings is that these patients have a defect in somatomedin generation that cannot be overcome by the administration of even large amounts of growth hormone. Alternatively, their pituitary glands could be elaborating an abnormal growth hormone that lacks biologic activity but is antigenically normal and thus measurable by radioimmunoassay. It is conceivable that such a molecule could interfere with exogenous growth hormonal action by competitive inhibition. There is now evidence that both phenomena occur. Dwarfism related to the release of biologically inactive HGH is known as *Laron dwarfism, type I*; when the defect is in the production of somatomedins (HGH being normal), it is called *Laron dwarfism, type II*.

Theoretically, many mechanisms that involve growth hormone synthesis, secretion, and tissue interaction that would interfere with normal growth might occur, including the following:

1. An absence or reduction in the hypothalamic growth hormone–releasing factor.

2. An absence or abnormality of the growth hormone–producing cells of the anterior pituitary.

3. Defects in the mechanisms required for the release of stored growth hormone.

4. Production of a biologically abnormal growth hormone molecule, that is, one that is without metabolic activity but that is antigenically intact and thus measurable by immunoassay (Laron type I dwarfism).

5. Production of an abnormal growth hormone molecule with partial biologic activity that may or may not be measurable by immunoassay.

6. Circulating antagonist or antagonists to growth hormone in the bloodstream.

7. Increased destruction of normally secreted growth hormone.

8. A defect in the somatomedin generation system (resistance to HGH; Laron type II dwarfism and African pygmies).

9. End-organ resistance to somatomedin.

Obviously, several of these proposed mechanisms could overlap, and it should be emphasized that most of them are hypothetical.

To evaluate the ability of the anterior pituitary to secrete growth hormone, three stimuli are commonly used. The first stimulus is hypoglycemia, induced by the intravenous administration of 0.1 to 0.2 units of regular insulin per kg of body weight to a fasting patient. The second stimulus is the infusion of 30 gm of the amino acid *arginine monohydrochloride*. In these tests, blood samples are obtained every 15 to 30 minutes over a 1- to 2-hour period for growth hormone and blood sugar determinations. Most normal individuals respond to these stimuli with a maximum plasma HGH of 7 ng/ml or more. The third stimulating agent is L-dopa, which has the advantage that it can be used orally.

It should be emphasized that most of the current information concerning growth hormone has been obtained since the early 1960s, following the development of a highly sensitive radioimmunoassay and the availability of purified growth hormone suitable for administration to humans. Unfortunately, growth hormone is highly species-specific. Preparations from domestic animals do not elicit metabolic effects in humans. Because human growth hormone has necessarily been prepared from pituitary glands obtained at autopsy, the available supply has obviously been limited. The recent identification of the amino acid sequence of growth hormone and its subsequent synthesis by recombinant DNA techniques will greatly expand the availability of HGH for therapeutic purposes.

Panhypopituitarism (Postpubertal). The term *panhypopituitarism* signifies a deficiency of all anterior pituitary hormones. The most common cause in the adult is an expanding pituitary adenoma. In females, it may also occur as a sequel of hemorrhagic shock at the time of delivery. For reasons that are not entirely clear, the pituitary of the pregnant female at term is highly vulnerable to hypotension. When excessive blood loss occurs during delivery, there is a definite risk of pituitary necrosis. The resulting panhypopituitarism bears the eponym *Sheehan's syndrome*. Less common causes of adult hypopituitarism include craniopharyngioma and granulomas that involve the pituitary or hypothalamus (e.g., sarcoidosis and histiocytosis X).

The peripheral manifestations of panhypopituitarism in the adult are mostly the consequence of deficiencies of four hormones: the gonadotropins (LH and FSH), TSH, and ACTH. Characteristically, evidence of target gland deficits appear in that order (i.e., gonadal, thyroidal, and cortical). Thus, loss of libido in the male and amenorrhea in the female are early symptoms. Loss of thyroid function causes dry skin, cold intolerance, somnolence, bradycardia, and constipation. Decrease in adrenal cortical function causes symptoms of hypovolemia and hypoglycemia and, in the female, loss of axillary and pubic hair. Typically, the patient who has panhypopituitarism has pale skin and premature, fine wrinkles around the eyes and mouth. The loss of pigment has been attributed to ACTH deficiency.

As is often the case in endocrinology, the definitive diagnosis of panhypopituitarism requires the judicious selection of certain laboratory procedures. The traditional approach has been the demonstration of hypofunction of the adrenal cortex and thyroid which is reversed by the administration of ACTH and TSH, respectively. The advent of radioimmunoassays for several anterior pituitary hormones has permitted a more direct approach to the diagnosis. The use of arginine infusion, insulin-induced hypoglycemia, or L-dopa to provoke growth hormone secretion has already been mentioned, as has the use of TRH to stimulate TSH and prolactin release. In panhypopituitarism, the responses of HGH, TSH, and prolactin to these stimuli are severely impaired or absent.

Much less common than panhypopituitarism are instances of isolated deficiency of a single pituitary hormone, so-called "monotropic hypopituitarism." Monotropic growth hormone deficiencies (sexual ateliotic dwarfism) have already been mentioned, as has familial hypogonadotropic hypogonadism (Kallmann's syndrome), a deficiency of both pituitary gonadotropins. Kallmann's syndrome is a relatively common cause of hypogonadism in males and may also afflict females. Selective deficiencies of LH, TSH, ACTH, and prolactin have also been well documented.

POSTERIOR PITUITARY

PHYSIOLOGY

Vasopressin (antidiuretic hormone, ADH), the octapeptide that is the principal secretion of the posterior pituitary, has a major physiologic role in regulating water metabolism. Unlike anterior pituitary hormones, this hormone is actually produced in the hypothalamus by the supraoptic and paraventricular nuclei. It is transported down the axons of the hypothalamic-hypophyseal tracts to the stalk and the posterior pituitary, where it is stored until secreted. It has been established, however, that the storage of ADH in the posterior pituitary is not essential to normal function. Normal water metabolism can persist after complete destruction of the posterior pituitary *if* the hypothalamus and proximal pituitary stalk are not damaged.

The usual stimulus to ADH secretion is an increase in plasma osmolality. Normally, the latter is closely maintained at 280 mOsm/kg plasma. When extracellular water is lost, plasma osmolality increases, causing the activation of osmoreceptors, which signal the release of ADH. The precise location of the osmoreceptors and the manner in which they stimulate the release of ADH are not known. Increased plasma osmolality also stimulates the thirst center, which is anatomically adjacent to or connected with the supraoptic nuclei.

The action of ADH to conserve water is exerted primarily on the cells of renal collecting ducts. At this site, ADH exerts its unique ability to change permeability of the epithelial cell mem-

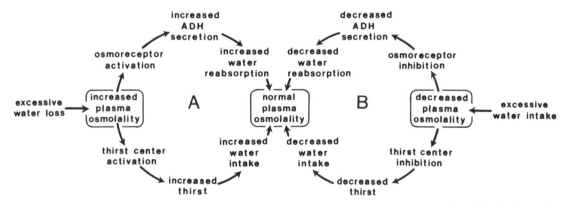

Figure 34–9 Regulation of plasma osmolality. Maintenance of plasma osmolality at or near 285 mOsm/kg depends on a close balance between water intake and water loss. When excessive water loss occurs *(A)*, as in fulminant diarrhea, the resultant increase in plasma osmolality triggers activation of the hypothalamic osmoreceptors and thirst center. Alteration in ADH secretion and thirst tends to restore osmolality to normal as shown. When excessive water intake occurs *(B)*, as in compulsive water drinking, plasma osmolality is diluted, leading to inhibition of the osmoreceptors and thirst center. The resultant increase in water excretion and decrease in fluid intake (assuming the patient is now under supervision) will lead to a normal osmolality.

branes to enhance the egress of water from the tubules to the hypertonic fluid of the peritubular or interstitial space. This action of ADH is mediated by the adenylate cyclase–cyclic AMP system. The consequent shift of water reduces urine volume and increases its concentration. Thus, an increased serum osmolality tends to correct itself by reducing water loss and increasing water intake as depicted in Figure 34–9.

The integrated activity of ADH and thirst is highly effective in maintaining the osmolality of the body fluids within very narrow limits. These interrelations provide an ideal example of the precision with which the endocrine system normally functions to maintain the constancy of the internal milieu. Although plasma osmolality is the most important regulator of ADH secretion, other factors also influence it. For example, an abrupt decrease in plasma volume due to acute blood loss stimulates ADH secretion. Neural signals triggered by painful stimuli may also prompt ADH release, as do certain drugs, such as nicotine. The posterior pituitary also secretes oxytocin. Although large doses of this substance will induce contractions of the gravid uterus, its physiologic importance in humans has not yet been established.

CLINICAL ENTITIES

Diabetes Insipidus

Diabetes insipidus is the clinical condition that results from an impaired or absent capacity to secrete ADH. The term *diabetes* (from the Greek word meaning *siphon*) signifies copious amounts of urine. The causes of diabetes insipidus are numerous. In one large series, one third of the cases were due to tumor, one third were of unknown origin, and one third were caused by a variety of conditions, including trauma, inflammation, and granuloma (Thomas, 1957). The principal manifestation of diabetes insipidus is the excretion of large volumes of urine (5 to 15 L or more daily) of low specific gravity (1.007 or less). To compensate for this prodigious water loss, the patient must drink large volumes of fluid. These two symptoms are particularly troublesome during the sleeping hours. Frequent urination and the need to satisfy thirst substantially encroach on the patient's rest, and loss of sleep is frequently the presenting complaint. For reasons that are not clear, the onset of symptoms is often dramatically abrupt. The patient may recall the precise day or hour when polyuria and thirst began. Another peculiar feature of the disease is the patient's marked preference for chilled fluids. He will go to considerable trouble to relieve his thirst with ice water.

Several other disorders associated with the passage of large volumes of urine may simulate diabetes insipidus. An abbreviated differential diagnosis of polyuria is summarized in Table 34–1.

The presence of diabetes mellitus, chronic renal failure, or disturbances in calcium and potassium metabolism is easily established. Patients who have psychogenic thirst should theoretically respond to water deprivation in a normal manner, that is, by decreasing urine volume and increasing urine concentration. Thus, after water is withheld from the patient who is an obsessive water drinker, the specific gravity of his urine should rise above 1.012 within a few hours and reach 1.020 or more after 12 hours. Unfortunately, the value of this procedure may be compromised by the patient's

TABLE 34–1 DIFFERENTIAL DIAGNOSIS OF POLYURIA

Cause		Mechanism
Diabetes insipidus	=	Decreased ADH secretion
Diabetes mellitus	=	Osmotic diuresis
Nephrogenic diabetes insipidus	=	End-organ resistance to ADH
Hypercalcemia	=	Impaired concentrating ability
Hypokalemia	=	Impaired concentrating ability
Psychogenic thirst	=	Obsessive water drinking

ability to obtain water surreptitiously and, conversely, by the ability of some patients with *partial* diabetes insipidus to concentrate urine to a specific gravity of 1.012 or 1.014. Lastly, water deprivation in a patient who has unequivocal, total diabetes insipidus is potentially dangerous.

A second method of diagnosing diabetes insipidus involves the use of hypertonic saline and vasopressin. After the patient is well hydrated and has a urine flow rate of at least 5 ml/min, a 3 per cent sodium chloride solution is infused for 45 minutes. If no antidiuresis occurs within the first 30 minutes, aqueous vasopressin (ADH) is given and urine collection is continued for another 30 minutes. If both kidney function and neurohypophyseal function are normal, the hypertonic saline infusion should cause a prompt fall in urinary flow and an increase in urinary specific gravity and osmolality. If ADH secretion is impaired, the saline infusion will be ineffective, but there will be a prompt decline in urine volume in response to vasopressin. If the defect is caused by inability of the renal tubules to respond to ADH (i.e., nephrogenic diabetes insipidus), neither hypertonic saline nor vasopressin infusion will influence the rate of urine flow. Lastly, although not readily available, there is a radioimmunoassay for ADH that can be helpful in the diagnosis of diabetes insipidus. In a normal well-hydrated adult (serum osmolality less than 285 mOsm/kg), plasma ADH is less than 2 pg/ml. With dehydration (serum osmolality greater than 290 mOsm/kg), plasma ADH increases to a range of 2 to 15 pg/ml. Patients who have diabetes insipidus fail to show the expected increase in ADH following water deprivation.

The Syndrome of Inappropriate Antidiuretic Hormone Secretion (SIADH)

This syndrome was first described by Schwartz in 1957 in patients who had cancer of the lung. It has subsequently been noted as a complication of various underlying conditions, including head trauma, myxedema, tuberculosis, and meningitis. Several drugs have also been found to cause SIADH. In all instances, the manifestations are those that would be expected from the inappropriate release of ADH into the circulatory system. (In some instances—for example, cancer of the lung—presumably the tumor does indeed elaborate and release autonomously an ADH-like peptide. In contrast to the anterior pituitary, no example of a hormone-producing tumor of the posterior pituitary or hypothalamus has been described. In SIADH, there is retention of water and consequently dilution of body fluids. The increase in plasma volume leads to an increase in glomerular filtration and a decrease in aldosterone secretion, both factors causing an increase in the loss of sodium into the urine. Thus, the concentration of serum sodium is decreased by at least two mechanisms: (1) dilution by inappropriate water retention, and (2) failure to reduce urinary sodium excretion.

When evaluating a patient for SIADH, one should carefully rule out conditions that would *appropriately* lead to an increase in ADH secretion or to sodium wasting, such as absolute or relative intravascular volume depletion (e.g., congestive heart failure) and adrenal cortical insufficiency. The symptoms of SIADH, essentially those of water retention that lead to water intoxication, vary depending on how low the serum sodium is and how fast it has fallen. As sodium falls below 120 mEq/L, there is the insidious appearance of headache, apathy, somnolence, and muscle weakness. With a rapid fall in sodium, nausea and vomiting may be the first symptoms. When the sodium concentration falls below 110 mEq/L, changes in the patient's sensorium occur. With further reduction, delirium, convulsions, coma, and death may occur. Unlike patients who suffer from hyponatremia from other causes such as congestive heart failure, individuals who have SIADH do not have peripheral edema. Although the diagnosis is usually made on clinical grounds, it can be substantiated by finding a high concentration of plasma ADH (greater than 5 pg/ml) associated wtih a reduced serum osmolality (less than 285 mOsm/kg). Besides removing the underlying cause, therapy consists of reducing the intake of free water.

THYROID

PHYSIOLOGY

Essential to the understanding of thyroid disorders is an appreciation of normal iodine metabolism and the normal interrelations between the thyroid and the pituitary-hypothalamic unit (Fig. 34–6). The latter was discussed on pages 1000 to 1001.

Iodine Metabolism

A daily absorption of approximately 100 to 200 μg of dietary iodine is required to ensure adequate thyroid hormone synthesis. Because of the use of iodine compounds in the production of flour in some parts of the United States, the daily ingestion of iodine may be 500 to 600 μg. With the exception of that contained in organic compounds, ingested iodine is reduced to ionic iodide (I^-) before being assimilated into the bloodstream. During the first hour after absorption, iodide is distributed in a space that is approximately 35 per cent of one's body weight, or about 25 L in a human who weighs 70 kg. The concentration of circulating iodide has been estimated at about 1.0 μg/100 ml of plasma.

Uptake (Trapping). Normally, the thyroid has an iodide clearance rate of between 10 and 35 ml/min of plasma. This uptake by the thyroid is an active, energy-requiring process, sometimes referred to as the "iodide pump." It is stimulated by TSH and is blocked by several anions such as thiocyanate and perchlorate. Normally, a concentration gradient of 1 to 25 exists between the plasma and thyroidal I^-. This gradient may be increased tenfold or more in toxic goiter. Iodide ion constitutes approximately 10 per cent of the total intrathyroidal iodine, which normally amounts to 5000 to 7000 μg. The iodide pool may be increased when organification is impaired by drug action, inflammation, or genetically determined enzyme defects. Careful studies have revealed that there are in fact two independent iodide pools within the thyroid gland. The first, normally about 10 μg, is composed of newly trapped iodide. Its uptake can be blocked by perchlorate or thiocyanate. The second pool, estimated at about 490 μg, consists of iodide released by enzymatic dehalogenation of monoiodotyrosine (MIT) and diiodotyrosine (DIT). This pool, apparently part of an internal recycling process that conserves iodide, is not directly affected by agents that block trapping. One can view the action of perchlorate or thiocyanate in "discharging" iodide as one of inhibition of the inward transport of iodide while the outward diffusion is unaffected.

Oxidation and Organification. After being trapped, iodide ions are rapidly transported into the luminal space of follicles and either are incorporated into an organic molecule or diffuse out of the follicles unchanged. Oxidation of iodide to molecular iodine (I_2) occurs prior to its displacement of hydrogen at the C_3 position of tyrosine. These reactions, which lead to the formation of MIT and DIT, occur rapidly, and their exact sequence has not been established. The oxidation step is probably catalyzed by a perioxidase. MIT is then iodinated at the C_5 position to form DIT. Probably the tyrosyl residues are attached to thyroglobulin or to other iodoproteins during these

reactions. The oxidation-organification steps can be blocked by thiourea drugs such as propylthiouracil and are stimulated by TSH. The formation of the iodothyronines, thyroxine (T_4), and triiodothyronine (T_3), probably results from the condensation of iodotyrosines, either two DIT molecules or one DIT and one MIT molecule, with the extrusion of one side chain. DIT and MIT molecules that are not utilized in the formation of T_4 and T_3 undergo catalytic deiodination by a dehalogenase. The regenerated iodide (the second iodide pool) is subsequently reutilized in hormone synthesis in the thyroid, as previously mentioned.

Storage and Release. Most of the iodinated compounds of the thyroid are contained in thyroglobulin, a 650,000 MW protein, which is the principal iodoprotein in thyroidal colloid. Analysis of the globulin-bound iodinated compounds reveals the following relative amounts: MIT, 17 to 28 per cent; DIT, 25 to 42 per cent; T_3, 5 to 8 per cent; and T_4, 35 per cent. The quantity of these stored compounds is sufficient to maintain normal metabolism in an adult for several months. The large size of the thyroglobulin molecule precludes its escape from the intraluminal colloid under normal circumstances. The secretion of thyroid hormones (T_3 and T_4) requires that they first be cleaved from thyroglobulin by proteolytic enzymes. T_3 and T_4, being freely diffusible, then readily enter the circulation. This process is stimulated by TSH and may be inhibited by large amounts of iodine. Although the principal secretion of the thyroid is thyroxine (90 per cent or more), there is a small amount of T_3 in the venous effluent of the thyroid. It is estimated that approximately 80 to 90 μg of thyroxine is secreted every day.

Transport of Thyroid Hormones. Once released, free thyroxine and triiodothyronine quickly bind with one of several carrier proteins. The protein with the strongest affinity for T_4 and T_3 is thyroxine-binding globulin (TBG), an interalpha (α_1-α_2) glycoprotein. The normal concentration of TBG is about 1 mg/100 ml of serum, a quantity sufficient to bind 10 to 26 μg of T_4. A second protein, thyroxine-binding prealbumin (TBPA), also effectively binds thyroxine. Lastly, serum albumin binds T_4 but with less affinity than either TBG or TBPA. The equilibrium between TBG and bound and free T_4 is reversible, as illustrated by the following equation:

$$TBG \cdot T_4 \rightleftarrows TBG + T_4$$

The total concentration of T_4 in serum (bound and free) is 4.5 to 13 μg/100 ml, whereas the concentration of free T_4 is normally about 1.0 to 2.0 ng/100 ml (less than 1.0×10^{-10} Molar), representing about 0.05 per cent of the total T_4. The total serum T_3 concentration is approximately 80 to 200 ng/100 ml, whereas the free T_3 concentration is about 200 to 600 pg/100 ml, reflecting the fact that the binding affinity of T_3 for the protein carriers is substantially less than that of T_4. Because it is the free hormone that penetrates cells to regulate metabolism, the metabolic contribution of T_3 is in fact important. Despite an absolute concentration, which is small compared with that of total T_4, the amount of free T_3 approaches that of free T_4 because of the weaker affinity of T_3 for its carrier proteins.

There are numerous drugs that affect either the binding capacity or the amount of circulating thyroid-binding proteins. For example, diphenylhydantoin competes with T_4 for TBG binding sites, and salicylates displace T_4 from TBPA. Estrogenic compounds increase the amount of carrier protein. Familial deficiencies and excesses of TBG have been well documented. However, the concentration of *free* thyroxine is normal in these patients; hence, they are euthyroid.

It is estimated that the total extrathyroidal content of thyroxine-iodine in the normal adult is about 500 µg. Assuming a normal plasma volume and a T_4-iodine concentration of 5 µg/100 ml of plasma, only 150 µg can be accounted for in the bloodstream. The large amount of remaining thyroxine-iodine is presumed to be bound to tissue protein. According to various studies, the liver is the major storage organ, containing up to 30 per cent of total body thyroxine-iodine. Normally, the fractional turnover of thyroxine-iodine is about 10 per cent per day, reflecting a biologic half-life of 6.7 days. The fractional turnover rate is increased in hyperthyroidism and decreased in hypothyroidism.

Thyroid Hormone Metabolism. Evidence indicates that T_4 can be converted to T_3 in peripheral tissues. In fact, approximately 80 per cent of circulating T_3 is derived from the peripheral deiodination of T_4. Monodeiodination of T_4 leads to biologically active T_3 (3,5,3'-triiodothyronine) *and* to the biologically inactive compound, reverse T_3 (3,3',5'-triiodothyronine, rT_3). Normally, approximately equal quantities of T_3 and reverse T_3 are produced. However, the rT_3 pathway is favored in certain circumstances, such as during starvation and in the presence of systemic disease, whereas the T_3 pathway is favored in others, such as in the presence of a high carbohydrate diet. From the work of Chopra and others, the details of the peripheral deiodination of T_4 are emerging; it appears to be an important regulatory process in overall metabolism. Recognition that a large proportion of secreted thyroxine is converted to T_3 peripherally has increased speculation that T_4 is a prohormone.

Cell Entry, Intracellular Metabolism, and Fate of Thyroxine. *Free* thyroxine and triiodothyronine appear to cross most cellular membranes; however, thyroxine is not present in cerebral spinal fluid, and it crosses the human placenta slowly and in small amounts. Factors that control the entry of thyroxine into cells are poorly understood. The presence within the cell membrane of one or more proteins that have a high binding affinity for T_4 is one possibility. After it is in the cell, the manner in which thyroxine or an active derivative acts to increase cellular metabolism is another enigma. A previously well-established hypothesis implicates the stimulation of uncoupling of oxidative phosphorylation. In contradiction to this possibility is the failure of other uncoupling agents such as 2,4-dinitrophenol to mimic the full spectrum of physiologic actions of T_4. Currently, studies are being conducted to test the hypothesis that changes in mitochondrial membrane function and alterations in nuclear RNA, RNA polymerase, and protein synthesis represent the initial manifestations of T_4 action within the cell. Three principal pathways for disposal of T_4 have been described: (1) conjugation of the phenolic portion of the molecule with formation of the glucuronide or sulfate; (2) degradation of the alanine side chain; and (3) deiodination.

Excretion of Iodide. Almost all the iodide that circulates through the kidneys is filtered by the glomeruli. However, much of the filtered iodide is reabsorbed, so that the renal iodide clearance rate is about 40 ml/min. In humans, iodide reabsorption appears to be a passive, unregulated process. As indicated in Figure 34–6, urinary loss of iodine normally almost balances iodine ingestion, with only small quantities of iodine being excreted in the feces.

TESTS OF THYROID FUNCTION

In recent years, radioimmunoassays for serum TSH and T_3 as well as for T_4 have become available. The first biochemical marker of a failing thyroid is elevation of the serum TSH. The serum T_4 may be maintained in the normal range (and the patient eumetabolic) because of an increase in TSH. The determination of TSH is valuable in assessing the significance of a borderline T_4 determination and in ruling out pituitary deficiency when the T_4 is definitely low. Infrequently, serum T_3 elevation precedes an increase in T_4 in hyperthyroidism. Measurement of T_3 by radioimmunoassay confirms the diagnosis in such cases. The resin T_3 uptake (RT_3U) reflects the level of circulating thyroxine-binding globulin (TBG). When TBG is elevated, as in pregnancy, the patient usually has a high level of T_4 but is not hyperthyroid because *free* T_4 is not elevated. Determination of the RT_3U will show an increase in TBG and allow for the correction of the T_4 value. This corrected serum T_4 value, called the *free T_4 index (FT_4I)*, is generally proportional to the absolute free T_4 concentration. To calculate the FT_4I, the RT_3U is first expressed as the ratio of the patient's RT_3U to the RT_3U of a normal serum pool. The FT_4I is then equal to the patient's total serum T_4 multiplied by this RT_3U ratio. For example, a pregnant euthyroid women might have the following values:

$$T_4 = 15 \ \mu g/dl$$
$$RT_3U = 20 \text{ per cent (mean normal } = 30 \text{ per cent)}$$
$$FT_4I = T_4 \times RT_3U \text{ ratio}$$
$$FT_4I = 15 \times \frac{20}{30} = 10$$

Because the corrected T_4 or FT_4I has the same range as the total serum T_4 (4.5 to 13), the patient is seen to be chemically euthyroid.

To discuss the pathophysiology of thyroid disease in a meaningful fashion, it is useful to refer to other tests that are used in assessing thyroid function. In general, these tests fit into one of two categories: (1) those that depend on thyroidal iodine kinetics, and (2) those that reflect the impact of thyroid hormone on body metabolism.

The first group of tests is illustrated by the 24-hour uptake of radioactive iodine by the thyroid gland. In this procedure, a small amount (approximately 300 μCi) of radioactive iodine (^{123}I) is administered orally, and radioactivity over the thyroid gland is determined 24 hours later. As previously mentioned, both the normal uptake of iodine and the discharge of thyroid hormone require TSH and a functioning thyroid gland. The second category is exemplified by the basal metabolic rate (BMR). In this procedure, the patient's rate of oxygen consumption is measured and compared with normal values based on the patient's age, size, and gender. Although the BMR is not in use now, it is conceptually useful because it reflects the overall metabolic status of the patient.

The value of these procedures in defining the pathophysiology of thyroid disease is best conveyed by citing examples of their application (Table 34–2).

In the first two examples, the results are straightforward and require no comment. In the third example, goitrous cretinism due to either a severe dietary deficiency of iodine or to an abnormality in the biosynthesis of thyroid hormone, the patient is unable to secrete an adequate amount of thyroid hormone. As a result, the level of circulating hormone is low and the patient is hypothyroid. The low concentration of hormone stimulates an increase in TSH release from the pituitary, which, in turn, causes an increase in iodine uptake and, over a period of time, thyroid enlargement or goiter. In the fourth example, a patient who has normal thyroid function has been placed on a therapeutic dose of thyroxine. Because of the negative feedback relation between the thyroid and anterior pituitary, this exogenous thyroid is not additive; rather, it suppresses TSH release as reflected by a low to absent uptake of radioactive iodine, and endogenous thyroid hormone secretion virtually ceases. The normal metabolic rate (BMR) and T_4 (RIA) reflect the euthyroid condition associated with the ingestion of physiologic quantities of thyroxine. The fifth example is similar, except that the serum T_4 is low because thyroidal secretion is suppressed and the eumetabolic state is maintained by exogenous T_3.

CLINICAL ENTITIES

Primary Adult Hypothyroidism (Myxedema)

The cause of adult hypothyroidism is often unknown. The pathologic findings are quite nonspecific, the thyroid being atrophic and replaced by fibrous tissue. In many cases, the presence of high titers of serum antithyroglobulin or antithyroid microsomal antibodies suggests that the disease was a result of autoimmune thyroiditis. Not infrequently, hypothyroidism follows either radioactive iodine treatment or surgery for Graves' disease. The onset of the clinical disease in the idiopathic variety is extremely gradual. Thus, one can be reasonably confident that the manifestation of florid myxedema is the result of a condition that has slowly been developing for many years. Because all cells of the body are affected by the deficiency of thyroid hormone, the physician may encounter manifestations of the disease that arise from any major organ or system. As one might expect, these manifestations are often the opposite of those seen in hyperthyroidism (Table 34–3). The term "myxedema" refers to the infiltration of the dermis by a mucinous substance that contains a mucopolysaccharide. The hypothyroid patient may

TABLE 34–2 ILLUSTRATIVE APPLICATIONS OF THYROID FUNCTION TESTS

Example	Serum T_4	RAI Uptake	BMR	Serum TSH
Hyperthyroidism	Increased	Increased	Increased	Decreased
Primary hypothyroidism	Decreased	Decreased	Decreased	Increased
Goitrous cretinism	Decreased	Increased	Decreased	Increased
Normal subject on 0.15 mg thyroxine	Normal	Decreased	Normal	Decreased
Normal subject on 75 μg T_3	Decreased	Decreased	Normal	Decreased

TABLE 34–3 CONTRASTING FEATURES OF HYPERTHYROIDISM AND HYPOTHYROIDISM

	Hyperthyroidism	Hypothyroidism
Appetite	Increased	Decreased or no change
Weight	Decreased	No change
Cold tolerance	Increased	Decreased
Perspiration	Excessive	Absent
Menses	Amenorrhea	Menorrhagia
Skin	Satin smooth	Coarse, dry
Pulse	Rapid	Slow
Mentation	Rapid	Sluggish
Reflexes	Brisk	Slow

be hypothermic, and his skin is usually dry and cold. He is comfortable during the hot days of summer and is distressed by cool weather. His slow mentation and poor memory are often erroneously attributed to aging. The generalized decline in metabolic activity is reflected in the cardiovascular system by bradycardia and in the gastrointestinal tract by constipation.

The biochemical consequences of myxedema are formidable. Although cholesterol synthesis is decreased, its disposal rate is slowed to an even greater extent, resulting in a high level of cholesterol in the plasma. It is likely that chronic hypercholesterolemia is responsible, at least in part, for the increase in coronary artery disease encountered in patients who have hypothyroidism. These patients are also extremely sensitive to most drugs and anesthetic agents, presumably because of marked slowing of the metabolic pathways involved in drug disposal.

Cretinism and Juvenile Hypothyroidism

Because both the skeletal and nervous systems are profoundly dependent on thyroid hormone for normal development, it is predictable that the consequences of thyroid hormone deficiency in childhood are more severe with early onset. Hypothyroidism in the infant may result from congenital absence of the thyroid (athyreotic cretinism) or from abnormal biosynthesis of thyroid hormone. In the latter circumstance, there is compensatory goiter formation. Occasionally, thyroid function is normal during infancy but then fails owing to less severe developmental defects or to Hashimoto's thyroiditis during childhood or adolescence. As in the infant, a marked retardation in skeletal and mental development is observed. The importance of making an *early* diagnosis of hypothyroidism at any age cannot be overly stressed. An intriguing exception to the overall impairment of growth and development in juvenile hypothyroidism is the occurrence of sexual precocity, manifested by menstruation and

breast development in the female and by penile and testicular enlargement in the male, first described by Van Wyk and Grumbach in 1960. A popular hypothesis used to explain this manifestation is that in children there is normally an "overlap" in the suppressive effect of thyroid hormone on the anterior pituitary and hypothalamus (i.e., thyroid hormone suppresses not only TSH but also pituitary gonadotropin release). Thus, when there is a deficiency of circulating thyroid hormone, not only TSH but also the gonadotropins are secreted in increased quantities, the latter leading to the premature development of secondary sexual characteristics. Alternatively, others have suggested that greatly elevated serum levels of TSH may result in gonadal stimulation because of the structural similarity of the TSH molecule to the other glycoprotein hormones, LH and FSH.

Hyperthyroidism

Toxic Diffuse Goiter (Graves' Disease). The most common cause of thyrotoxicosis, or hyperthyroidism, (85 per cent of the cases) is Graves' disease, a syndrome in which there is diffuse enlargement of the thyroid gland associated with excessive secretion of thyroid hormone. Exophthalmos is a common but not invariable feature of the syndrome. However, the eye signs may appear before thyrotoxicosis is evident or not until after the thyrotoxicosis has been treated and the patient is euthyroid. The degree of enlargement of the gland is highly variable. It may be so slight that no goiter is evident. Thus, the three major components of the syndrome—diffuse thyroid enlargement, thyrotoxicosis, and exophthalmos—need not be present concurrently. A possible fourth component of Graves' disease, pretibial dermopathy (pretibial myxedema), in which the skin is red, shiny, and thickened, is uncommon; on microscopic examination the skin is infiltrated with mucopolysaccharide and chronic inflammatory cells.

Although its cause is unknown, Graves' disease is characterized by certain features that may be clues to the underlying cause. It is a common disease, and as in most thyroid diseases, women are afflicted much more commonly than are men; among patients with Graves' disease, the ratio of women to men is approximately 9:1. There often is family history of thyroid disease; close relatives have a high incidence of nontoxic goiter, chronic lymphocytic thyroiditis, or Graves' disease itself. It was once believed that the diffuse enlargement and increased function of the thyroid might be due to an excessive secretion by the pituitary of TSH. If this were so, Graves' disease would be analogous to Cushing's disease, in which an excessive secretion of ACTH leads to adrenal hyperplasia and elevation in plasma cortisol. With the availability of a highly sensitive radioimmunoassay for TSH, it is now clear that the serum concentrations of

TSH in patients who have Graves' disease are decreased or undetectable; thus, the anterior pituitary and hypothalamus are eliminated as the primary pathogenic sites.

The diffuse hyperplasia of the gland in Graves' disease does suggest that it is being stimulated by some extrathyroidal substance. Some years ago, Adams and Purves reported that sera from patients who have Graves' disease contained a factor with TSH-like activity. This substance was capable of discharging thyroid hormone from the glands of experimental animals. Unlike the response to TSH, which was evident within 1 hour, the serum factor did not cause detectable changes until 4 to 6 hrs after administration. Because of this characteristic it was labeled *long-acting thyroid stimulator,* or *LATS.* Subsequent investigations have revealed that LATS is a 7S gamma globulin antibody that is capable of interacting with thyroid cells. It has the capability of stimulating protein synthesis and glucose metabolism of thyroid tissue and effecting the release of thyroid hormone. Although LATS cannot be detected in the sera of many patients who have Graves' disease, it is now believed that the sera of all patients who have this disease contain an abnormal IgG of one kind or another. These IgG moieties are collectively termed *human thyroid stimulators (HTS).* These immunoglobulins are antibodies directed against the TSH receptor of thyroid follicular cells. Binding of the antibody to the receptor stimulates the cell, leading to hypertrophy of the gland and an increase in hormone production. In-vitro studies indicate that both TSH and HTS act via adenylate cyclase and cyclic AMP. The autoimmune hypothesis of the pathogenesis of Graves' disease just decribed leaves the cause of the abnormal autoantibody production unexplained.

Other Causes of Hyperthyroidism. Painful subacute thyroiditis as well as "painless thyroiditis" may result in hyperthyroidism owing to the leakage of thyroid hormone from damaged follicles. "Painless thyroiditis" may account for as much as 15 per cent of all the cases of hyperthyroidism; the histologic findings of this condition have led to its also being called *"lymphocytic thyroiditis* with spontaneously resolving hyperthyroidism." As the name implies, the disease process runs its course in a few weeks or months, which is also true of the painful variety. These conditions can be distinguished from Graves' disease by the presence of a very low thyroidal radioiodine uptake, resulting from the suppression of TSH and the inability of the damaged thyroid to concentrate iodine. In toxic multinodular goiter and toxic adenoma, autonomously functioning thyroid tissue secretes excessive amounts of thyroid hormone. If one administers radioactive iodine to a patient with toxic adenoma and then scans over the neck, radioactivity is found only over the adenoma. This occurs because the excessive thyroid hormone secreted by the adenoma has suppressed TSH secre-

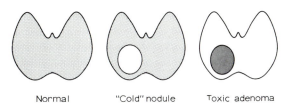

Figure 34–10 Thyroid scans. The *normal thyroid gland* picks up radioactive iodine (RAI) uniformly, resulting in a homogeneous distribution of radioactivity as shown. *"Cold" nodule:* Lesions such as cysts or tumors that occupy space but lack normal biologic activity appear as deficits on scan. *Toxic adenomas ("hot" nodule):* Occasionally, adenomas develop that produce thyroid hormone autonomously; when the production of thyroid hormone from this source exceeds physiologic quantities, the patient becomes mildly toxic, TSH production is curtailed, and uptake of iodide by the surrounding normal thyroid virtually ceases.

tion and hence iodine uptake by the normal tissue that surrounds the adenoma (Fig. 34–10).

Because all cells of the body are influenced by thyroid hormone, it is not surprising that, as in hypothyroidism, manifestations of thyroid hormone excess may involve all systems of the body. The clinical picture of florid thyrotoxicosis is distinctive. Typically, the patient is thin, hyperkinetic, and impatient with the relatively slow pace of those around him. Palpitation, heat intolerance, sweating, and hyperdefecation are common symptoms. On physical examination, a goiter is usually present, in addition to characteristic eye signs such as lid retraction and lid lag (distinguished from true exophthalmos and extraocular muscle palsies, which are specific features of Graves' disease that are not found in other causes of hyperthyroidism). The skin is satiny smooth and warm, the pulse rate is elevated, and the pulse pressure is widened. The latter is a result of mild systolic hypertension and a decrease in diastolic pressure due in part to dilatation of peripheral vessels. These alterations in pulse rate and blood pressure, as well as lid retraction and lid lag that were previously mentioned, appear to result from a thyroid hormone–induced increase in the number of β-adrenergic receptors in certain tissues, in addition to a decrease in α-adrenergic receptor number. There is often evidence of muscle weakness and wasting, particularly of the temporalis, shoulder girdle, and quadriceps. The deep tendon reflexes are very brisk. Infrequently, the manifestations of hyperthyroidism are markedly exaggerated. In this condition, termed *thyroid storm,* the patient becomes agitated, delirious, and febrile and has a sustained tachycardia. Such an occurrence is a true medical emergency that often terminates fatally, despite prompt and appropriate therapy.

The description of thyrotoxicosis as presented in the foregoing paragraphs is applicable to patients who are middle-aged or younger. When patients who are older than 60 years develop the disease, the clinical picture is often not so clear-cut. Frequently, a second disease such as congestive heart failure obscures the underlying thyrotoxicosis. The older person may not respond to excessive thyroid with the marked increase in energy and physical activity that is characteristic of the younger patient. The terms *masked hyperthyroidism* and *apathetic hyperthyroidism* are thus frequently appropriate for the disease as it manifests in the older patient.

Usually, the determination of serum T_4 confirms the presence of hyperthyroidism suspected on clinical grounds. There are circumstances in which additional laboratory data are helpful in establishing the diagnosis. Two such situations will be described because they illustrate facets of the pathophysiology that underlies thyrotoxicosis.

The first circumstance is exemplified by a young woman who experienced weight loss, nervousness, palpitations, and a small goiter. Laboratory examinations revealed a serum T_4 of 15 μg/dl (normal, 5.0 to 13) and a radioactive iodine uptake (RAI) of 20 per cent in 24 hours, a normal value. The question then concerns whether the patient's thyroid function is within the normal range, albeit near the upper limit or whether it is definitely but minimally elevated. To answer this question, the physician can make use of the thyroid suppression test in which the radioactive iodine uptake is repeated after administering physiologic amounts of thyroid hormone for 10 days (e.g., 75 μg of triiodothyronine daily). If the patient is normal, the second radioactive iodine uptake should be significantly reduced compared with the first; if the patient has early hyperthyroidism, the radioactive iodine (RAI) uptake will be virtually unchanged because the gland is no longer being normally regulated by TSH. The availability of TRH has provided an alternate approach to this problem. In thyrotoxicosis, the level of serum TSH not only is suppressed but also fails to rise in response to intravenously administered TRH.

The second circumstance concerns the finding of a normal serum T_4 in a patient who by clinical appearance is clearly thyrotoxic and in whom the RAI uptake is abnormally high. When the sera of such patients have been analyzed for triiodothyronine as well as thyroxine, abnormally high concentrations of the former thyroid hormone have been found to be coexistent with normal levels of thyroxine. In hyperthyroidism, usually both triiodothyronine and thyroxine are increased. In this variant, which has been termed *T_3 toxicosis,* only triiodothyronine is elevated. If left untreated, the patient who has T_3 toxicosis will eventually manifest an increase in serum T_4. As in the more usual varieties of thyrotoxicosis, patients who have T_3 toxicosis also have a suppressed TSH response to exogenous TRH, providing further confirmation of the diagnosis.

Thyroiditis

Several varieties of thyroiditis exist and are discussed in the following paragraphs.

Acute suppurative thyroiditis, due to bacterial infection of the gland, is a very rare condition that is characterized by fever, leukocytosis, pain, swelling, and other signs of acute inflammation. Abscess formation often occurs.

Subacute thyroiditis, also called *deQuervain's, giant-cell,* or *granulomatous thyroiditis,* has a longer course. Pain, firm swelling of the gland, and tenderness are present for several weeks or months; release of thyroid hormones from damaged follicles may produce thyrotoxicosis. Thyroidal radioiodine uptake is very low, fever may be present, and the erythrocyte sedimentation rate is increased. Histologically, the gland shows infiltration with polymorphonuclear leukocytes and destruction of colloid and follicular cells; histiocytes and foreign-body giant cells are abundant. The disease process spontaneously resolves in 1 to 3 months, usually with a short hypothyroid phase followed by complete recovery of normal thyroid function. The etiology of subacute thyroiditis is unclear, but its common occurrence following an upper respiratory illness suggests that it may be viral in origin. Serum antithyroid antibodies are absent or present in only low titer, making autoimmune processes unlikely.

Chronic lymphocytic thyroiditis, also known as *Hashimoto's thyroiditis*, is a common disorder that afflicts perhaps 5 to 10 per cent of women; the disease is nine times more common in women than in men. It tends to be familial, as is Graves' disease. This disorder is probably autoimmune in nature, as is reflected by the presence of high-titer circulating antibodies to thyroglobulin and thyroid microsomes, as well as circulating lymphocytes that are sensitized to thyroid antigens. On pathologic examination, the gland is diffusely infiltrated with lymphocytes and plasma cells, often forming germinal centers. The thyroid follicles are small, and there may be considerable fibrosis. Clinically, patients usually present either with a firm, painless, asymptomatic goiter, which may be either diffuse or nodular, or with hypothyroidism. Serum TSH is increased in the presence of hypothyroidism and in patients who have milder thyroid impairment ("compensated thyroid failure"). The course is often prolonged, and hypothyroidism may develop only after chronic thyroiditis has been present for many years.

It is believed by some investigators that one cause of hyperthyroidism, "painless thyroiditis," is a variant of chronic lymphocytic thyroiditis.

Thyroid Carcinoma

Although a detailed discussion of thyroid cancer is beyond the scope of this chapter, the pathophysiologic aspects of two varieties of malignancy are of sufficient interest and importance to warrant brief comment.

Postirradiation Thyroid Carcinoma. For several years, it was common medical practice to use irradiation to treat a number of benign conditions in infants and young children. Thus, until about the late 1950s, radiation therapy was applied to children who had breathing difficulties, enlarged lymphoid tissue in the nasopharynx (adenoids), enlarged thymus, acne, and other conditions. Recently, it has been discovered that several of these patients have developed carcinoma of the thyroid. It is now understood that the low levels of ionizing irradiation applied in the area of the head, neck, and shoulders, particularly to the very young, are carcinogenic to the thyroid. Individuals who have a history of such irradiation should be carefully evaluated for the presence of thyroid tumor. The use of radioiodine imaging may disclose "cold nodules" that are not evident on physical examination (Fig. 34–10).

Medullary Carcinoma of the Thyroid. This malignancy arises from the parafollicular cells (C cells) of the thyroid. These cells are responsible for the elaboration of the calcium-lowering hormone, calcitonin; individuals who have medullary carcinoma characteristically have high serum levels of calcitonin. Medullary carcinoma tends to be familial and may be associated with neoplasia of the adrenal medulla (pheochromocytoma) and parathyroid hyperplasia or adenoma (multiple endocrine neoplasia, type IIa), or with pheochromocytoma and ganglioneuromatosis (multiple endocrine neoplasia, type IIb).

ADRENAL CORTEX

PHYSIOLOGY

The classic description by Addison in 1849 of the disease caused by the destruction of the adrenal cortex first attracted attention to the critical importance of this gland in the maintenance of life. Many years later, cortisol and aldosterone, the principal secretions of the adrenal cortex, were identified as steroid molecules of basically similar structure. It is of interest that the other endocrine glands of mesodermal origin, the testes and ovaries, also elaborate steroidal hormones that have structures and modes of action similar to those of the adrenal cortex.

Regulation of Cortisol Secretion
(Fig. 34–11)

The negative feedback control of cortisol secretion has already been alluded to (see earlier discussion). Normally, a rising level of plasma cortisol inhibits the release of ACTH from the anterior pituitary; this effect is probably achieved by interference with the stimulatory action of CRF on the pituitary rather than inhibition of CRF release from the hypothalamus. The reduction in plasma ACTH leads to a decline in cortisol secretion by the adrenal glands and, hence, a corresponding reduction in its plasma concentration, completing the negative feedback loop. This mechanism is modulated by several additional factors. There is evidence that elevations of ACTH in the plasma that perfuses the median eminence of the hypothalamus suppress CRF release, creating a "short loop" negative feedback control. Because the plasma concentration of cortisol required to inhibit CRF release (the so-called "set point") varies diurnally, presumably on the basis of neural signals reaching the CRF-synthesizing neurons, ACTH and, in turn, cortisol are secreted in a cyclic fashion. Thus, the peak level of cortisol in the plasma normally occurs between 6:00 and 8:00 AM. By 5:00 PM the concentration has decreased by about 50 per cent, and the fall continues until the nadir is reached around 12:00 AM, following which plasma cortisol increases. This normal circadian rhythm is blunted in Cushing's syndrome. Other neural signals such as those triggered by various forms of "stress" can also override the normal feedback control and transiently increase cortisol secretion. CRF, which causes ACTH release within minutes, has been found to be a large peptide with 41 amino acid residues. ACTH is a 39-amino acid peptide with all biologic activity, including MSH-like activity, residing in the first 24 amino acids. This sequence has been synthesized and is available commercially. The amino acids from 25 to 39 vary from one species to another and account for the molecule's immunologic specificity.

ACTH exerts its action through the adenylate cyclase–cyclic AMP system. The interaction of ACTH with receptors linked to the adenylate cyclase of adrenal cortical cell membranes leads to an increase in intracellular cyclic AMP, which then promotes the synthesis of a protein capable of catalyzing the conversion of cholesterol to 20-α-hydroxycholesterol. The latter compound in turn is converted to pregnenolone, the precursor of all steroidal hormones of the adrenal cortex. A simplified schema for the biosynthesis of cortisol, aldosterone, testosterone, and estradiol from cholesterol is shown in Figure 34–12.

Regulation of Aldosterone Secretion
(Fig. 34–13)

The principal regulator of aldosterone secretion is the renin-angiotensin system. Renin, a proteolytic enzyme of approximately 40,000 MW, is produced in the kidney by specialized cells of the juxtaglomerular apparatus. Although the complete details regarding its synthesis and release are not yet clear, it is known that a decrease in

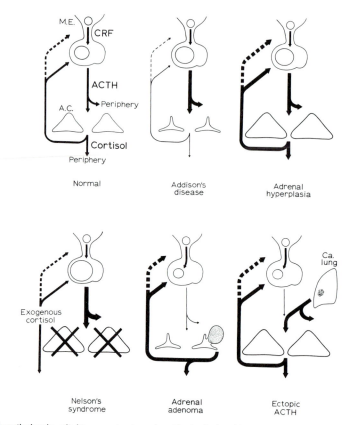

Figure 34–11 Hypothalamic, pituitary, and adrenal cortical relationships.

Normal: CRF elaborated by the median eminence (M.E.) stimulates the secretion of ACTH by the anterior pituitary (A.P.). ACTH triggers the synthesis and release of cortisol, the principal glucocorticoid of the adrenal cortex (A.C.); a rising level of cortisol inhibits the stimulatory action of CRF on ACTH release (or, as shown by the interrupted arrow, cortisol may inhibit CRF release), completing the negative feedback loop.

Addison's disease: In primary destructive disease of the adrenal cortex, the level of plasma cortisol is drastically low, and the effect of CRF on the anterior pituitary proceeds without inhibition, causing a marked increase in the secretion of ACTH. High levels of the latter hormone promote the pigmentary changes characteristic of Addison's disease.

Adrenal hyperplasia: The primary lesion may be at the level of the pituitary or hypothalamus. In either case, production of ACTH and cortisol is excessive. The latter causes the peripheral manifestations of the disorder Cushing's disease. Cells of the pituitary are relatively resistant to the high levels of circulating cortisol.

Nelson's syndrome: When Cushing's disease is treated by bilateral adrenalectomy, the physiologic quantity of cortisol subsequently used to treat the patient is a relatively weak "break" on CRF production or on CRF's effect on the anterior pituitary. ACTH-secreting cells of the pituitary may undergo tumor formation, or a pre-existing microadenoma may become aggressive. In either case, the production of ACTH is markedly increased, leading to extreme pigmentation, a characteristic feature of the syndrome.

Adrenal adenoma: An adenoma or carcinoma of the adrenal may produce cortisol autonomously. When the rate of production exceeds physiologic quantities, Cushing's syndrome results; the effect of CRF on the anterior pituitary is inhibited by the high levels of circulating cortisol, with resultant diminished ACTH secretion and atrophy of normal adrenal tissue.

Ectopic ACTH: In this syndrome, an ACTH-like peptide is elaborated by a tumor such as carcinoma of the lung. The adrenals are stimulated, circulating cortisol is increased, and ACTH secretion inhibited. Tumors elaborating CRF have also been reported.

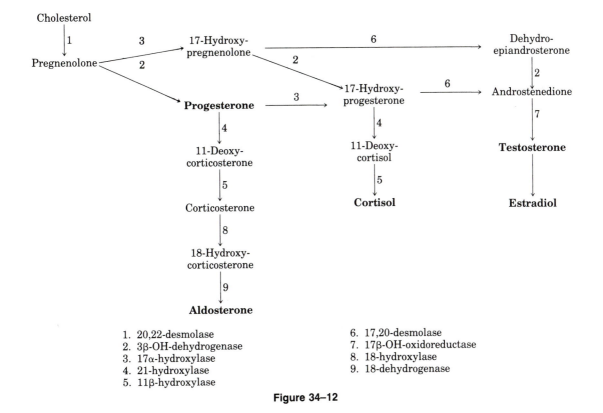

1. 20,22-desmolase
2. 3β-OH-dehydrogenase
3. 17α-hydroxylase
4. 21-hydroxylase
5. 11β-hydroxylase

6. 17,20-desmolase
7. 17β-OH-oxidoreductase
8. 18-hydroxylase
9. 18-dehydrogenase

Figure 34–12

plasma volume causes an increase in renin release and that conversely, an increase in plasma volume inhibits its release. Apparently, the juxtaglomerular apparatus contains specialized cells capable of reacting to changes in renal perfusion pressure.

Once in the plasma, renin interacts with a substrate produced in the liver, angiotensinogen, to form angiotensin I, a decapeptide. In the lung, angiotensin I is converted to angiotensin II, an octapeptide that stimulates aldosterone secretion. Aldosterone, by promoting sodium retention, causes plasma volume expansion, which then shuts off renin release, and the feedback loop is completed.

Aldosterone release is also influenced by potassium. An increase in plasma potassium promptly increases aldosterone secretion. Conversely, depletion of body potassium inhibits aldosterone release. ACTH administration also increases aldosterone secretion, but this effect is transient; aldosterone production declines to normal within 48 hours, despite continued ACTH administration.

Biologic Actions

In humans, cortisol and aldosterone are the principal representatives of glucocorticoids and mineralocorticoids, two of the main classes of adrenal cortical steroids. The biologic activities of these steroids can be inferred from the descriptions of the classic clinical entities in which they are either deficient or in excess. An important action of cortisol is promotion of the conversion of protein into glucose by induction of the enzymes of gluconeogenesis. In its role in regulation of glucose homeostasis, cortisol frequently acts in opposition to insulin. The primary functions of aldosterone are interlinked: regulation of extracellular fluid volume and potassium metabolism. Unlike cortisol, which affects all cells of the body, the action of aldosterone appears limited to the kidney and the sweat and salivary glands. In the kidney, aldosterone acts on the distal tubule to promote the absorption of sodium ions in exchange for potassium and hydrogen ions. In excess, aldosterone initially stimulates sodium reabsorption by the proximal renal tubules, but after a short time "escape" from this effect occurs. Escape from the action of aldosterone on the distal tubule does not occur. Thus, in chronic aldosterone excess (primary aldosteronism) there is expansion of the extracellular fluid volume and profound potassium depletion, but no edema. The androgenic steroids constitute a third functional group of steroids elaborated by the adrenal cortex. The androgenic steroids have anabolic effects and are thought to

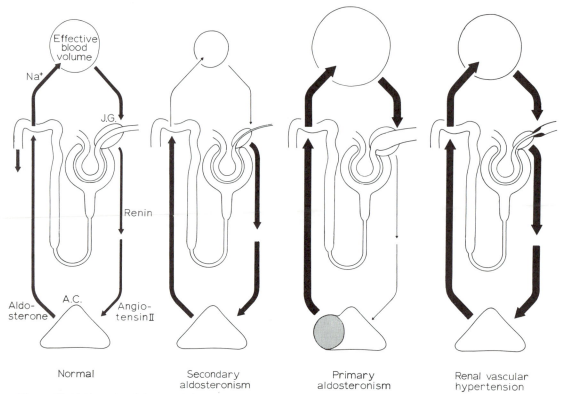

Figure 34–13 Normal and deranged aldosterone-renin-angiotensin relationships.

Normal: An increase in blood volume suppresses renin release by the juxtaglomerular apparatus (JGA) of the kidney, whereas a decrease in volume stimulates its release. In the plasma, renin reacts with renin substrate to form angiotensin I; the latter is converted to angiotensin II in the lung. Angiotensin II stimulates aldosterone release from the adrenal cortex (A.C.) and (not shown in the diagram) causes vasoconstriction by direct action on the arterial bed. Changes in angiotensin II and aldosterone reflect those of plasma renin activity (PRA). Alterations in plasma aldosterone cause changes in sodium reabsorption and, in turn, in blood volume, completing the feedback loop. (See text for details.)

Secondary aldosteronism caused by restriction of dietary sodium: In the face of chronic inadequate dietary sodium, hypovolemia gradually ensues, leading to increased blood levels of PRA, angiotensin II, and aldosterone. Because of sodium deficiency, the increased aldosterone is ineffective in restoring plasma volume. Congestive heart failure is another cause of secondary aldosteronism on a different basis. Because of a decrease in cardiac output, there is a relative decrease in effective blood volume that is refractory to re-expansion by increased sodium reabsorption.

Primary aldosteronism: Here the initial pathologic event is the excessive, unregulated secretion of aldosterone from an adenoma or from hyperplastic adrenal glands. The high level of aldosterone causes hypervolemia and suppressed PRA.

Renal vascular hypertension: Significant narrowing of the renal arteries from any cause results in activation of the juxtaglomerular baroreceptors and an increase in PRA, angiotensin, and aldosterone. The hypertension in these disorders is due not only to an increase in sodium reabsorption but also to the direct vasopressor effect of angiotensin.

be required for the maintenance of libido and the capacity to achieve orgasm in the female. At least part of their effect on female sexuality depends on their tropic action on the clitoris. The mechanism of action of all steroid hormones probably involves interaction with specific protein receptors in the cytosol and nucleus, leading to modification of a portion of the genome, transcription of messenger RNA, and protein synthesis.

Biosynthesis, Transport, and Metabolism of the Adrenal Steroids
(Fig. 34–12)

Cholesterol is the basic precursor of steroid biosynthesis. It is initially converted to its 20-α

hydroxyl derivative in a reaction stimulated by ACTH via the adenylate cyclase–cyclic AMP system. There is then cleavage of the terminal, 6-carbon side chain of cholesterol, yielding pregnenolone. Pregnenolone is transformed to progesterone by the action of a 3-β-hydroxysteroid dehydrogenase and an isomerase. Thereafter, a series of hydroxylations occur, each catalyzed by a specific hydroxylase and requiring NADH to form compounds successively with a hydroxyl group at C_{17}, C_{21}, and finally C_{11}, the last being cortisol. As will be discussed, inborn errors of metabolism exist in which these enzymes are deficient.

In the mineralocorticoid pathway, progesterone is hydroxylated at the C_{21} position to form 11-desoxycorticosterone. There is then hydroxyla-

TABLE 34–4 SECRETORY RATES AND CONCENTRATIONS IN BODY FLUIDS OF THE ADRENAL CORTICAL HORMONES

	Plasma Level (μg/dl)		Secretion Rate (mg/day)	Urinary Metabolites (mg/day)
	Total	Free		
Cortisol	15	1	15–30	4–8
Aldosterone	0.003–0.015	0.003	0.050–0.250	0.025–0.035
Dehydroepiandrosterone	65	65	15–30	4–8

(Modified from Catt, K. J.: Lancet *1*:1279, 1970.)

tion at the 11 position to form corticosterone, followed by hydroxylation at the 18 position to form 18-hydroxycorticosterone. Oxidation of this C_{18} hydroxyl group yields the final product, aldosterone. Another principal pathway involves the formation of dehydroepiandrosterone, a major metabolite of the adrenal cortex. This compound is formed by dehydroxylation of pregnenolone and cleavage of the C_{20}, C_{21} side chain to form the C_{19} steroid. Dehydroepiandrosterone is converted to androstenedione by a 3-β-hydroxysteroid-dehydrogenase and an isomerase. The latter steroid is the immediate precursor of testosterone in the testes. In females, circulating testosterone is derived from the peripheral conversion of androstenedione and from ovarian secretion, rather than from direct secretion by the adrenal gland.

Following its secretion, cortisol is transported and bound to an alpha-2-globulin called *transcortin*, or *cortisol-binding globulin (CBG)*. It is estimated that approximately 90 per cent of circulating unconjugated cortisol is thus bound and that only 10 per cent is in the biologically active, free form. Aldosterone circulates loosely bound to albumin. Both hormones are metabolized in the liver by the reduction of ring A to tetrahydro derivatives, which are conjugated with glucuronide. These water-soluble biologically inactive derivatives are excreted by the kidneys. The plasma half-life of cortisol, normally about two hours, is prolonged in liver disease and decreased in thyrotoxicosis; the half-life of aldosterone is 30 minutes. Adrenal steroid secretory rates and concentrations in body fluids are listed in Table 34–4.

CLINICAL ENTITIES

Addison's Disease

As previously mentioned, the clinical features of chronic adrenal insufficiency were first described by Addison over one hundred years ago. The underlying pathologic process may be tuberculosis or other granulomatous disease such as histoplasmosis, metastatic carcinoma, or, most commonly, simple atrophy. Although the cause of the latter is unknown, there is reason to believe that it may be the consequence of an autoimmune

reaction. Typically, the clinical manifestations of primary adrenal insufficiency are extremely insidious; rare exceptions are the acute adrenal insufficiency associated with meningococcemia (the Waterhouse-Friderichsen syndrome) and that due to adrenal hemorrhage secondary to anticoagulation therapy.

The manifestations of chronic adrenal insufficiency, regardless of the cause, are attributable to deficiencies of cortisol and aldosterone and, in the female, androgenic steroids. Cortisol deficiency results in loss of appetite, weight loss, severe weakness, gastrointestinal disturbances, and emotional instability. Because of impaired gluconeogenesis, patients may become hypoglycemic after an overnight fast. The persistently low or absent plasma concentrations of cortisol cause marked hypersecretion of ACTH. Because the ACTH molecule has intrinsic melanocyte-stimulating activity, a variety of pigmentary changes can occur, such as diffuse darkening of the skin, increased pigmentation of scars, creases, pressure points, and pigmentary lesions of the mucous membranes. Aldosterone deficiency results in unregulated loss of body sodium and retention of potassium, with consequent reduction in plasma volume and hyperkalemia. The hypovolemia leads to prerenal azotemia, orthostatic hypotension, and, if untreated, to shock. Because of its deleterious effect on cardiac rhythm, hyperkalemia is potentially a lethal complication of Addison's disease. In female patients, the absence of adrenal androgens may result in the loss of pubic and axillary hair. Although the course of Addison's disease is typically prolonged, it may abruptly worsen if the patient is stressed by trauma or infection. Under these conditions, acute adrenal crisis may develop, manifested by vomiting, shock, high fever, and coma.

The laboratory findings in Addison's disease include a reduction in serum sodium, elevation in serum potassium, a reduced fasting blood glucose, and mild azotemia. These findings are of course not diagnostic of Addison's disease. In order to establish the diagnosis, one must show a low level of plasma cortisol (<3 μg/dl) and the inability of the adrenal glands to respond normally to ACTH stimulation. This may be done by obtaining an 8:00 AM plasma sample for cortisol estimation, injecting 250 μg of synthetic ACTH (cosyntropin or Cortrosyn) intravenously or intramuscularly, and obtaining plasma cortisols at 60 and 120 min. In Addison's disease, there is virtually no increase in plasma cortisol following Cortrosyn; normal subjects usually have a twofold or greater increase, and patients who have secondary adrenocortical insufficiency show responses intermediate between the Addisonian and normal groups. Because the management of Addison's disease entails lifelong replacement therapy, one may wish to corroborate the diagnosis with more prolonged stimulation. This can be done by assessing the response of the urinary 17-hydroxycorticoids to ACTH that is administered daily over a 3- to 5-day period.

One particularly common form of secondary adrenal insufficiency deserves special comment. Large doses of cortisone and related glucocorticoids are often used in the chronic treatment of a variety of diseases, such as asthma and rheumatoid arthritis. When such treatment is extended beyond 4 or 5 weeks, prolonged suppression of CRF and ACTH secretion ensues. If the steroid is then abruptly discontinued, the hypothalamic-pituitary axis is unable to respond normally to the reduction in circulating cortisol. The result is a mild degree of hypoadrenocorticism, which can become particularly significant if the patient is subjected to stress. This potential problem is minimized by using alternate day steroid therapy whenever possible.

Cushing's Syndrome

Cushing's syndrome is the clinical condition that results from chronic exposure to excessive circulating levels of glucocorticoids. Four etiologic subsets of the disorder have been identified. First, the primary lesion may be either an adenoma or a carcinoma within the adrenal cortex that elaborates cortisol autonomously. Alternatively, the disease may be due to disordered hypothalamic-pituitary function, with a persistent overproduction of ACTH, resulting in hyperplasia and hyperfunction of both adrenal glands. Characteristic of this disorder is a blunting of the diurnal, or circadian, rhythm of ACTH secretion and a relative inability of cortisol to suppress ACTH secretion. The pituitary itself may be normal morphologically or it may contain a small tumor, as did the pituitary glands of the patients originally described by Cushing. This variety of Cushing's syndrome is often called *Cushing's disease*. The role of CRF in the pathogenesis of this form of Cushing's syndrome remains unclear. Third, the adrenal cortex may be stimulated excessively by ACTH or by an ACTH-like peptide elaborated by a nonpituitary tumor. This variety of Cushing's syndrome has been called the *ectopic ACTH syndrome*. Carcinoma of the lung is the most frequent responsible neoplasm. Fourth, the most common form of Cushing's syndrome is that resulting from long-term therapy with pharmacologic doses of glucocorticoids for an illness such as rheumatoid arthritis, asthma, or ulcerative colitis.

The clinical manifestations of Cushing's syndrome are explicable on the basis of known effects of cortisol. Principal actions of cortisol include the promotion of protein catabolism and the diversion of amino acids into gluconeogenesis. When these physiologic processes are exaggerated by chronic cortisol excess, marked loss of protein occurs. The clinical consequences are muscle wasting, thinning of the skin, easy bruisability, abdominal striae, and osteoporosis. Cortisol, in addition to promoting glucose formation in the liver, also antagonizes the action of insulin in transporting glucose into cells. Predictably, diabetes mellitus is a common complication of Cushing's syndrome. In several ways, cortisol alters the normal response to infection and injury. Antibody formation is suppressed, and the accumulation and migration of polymorphonuclear cells at inflammatory sites are inhibited. Some manifestations of the disease are not well understood; for example, the characteristic redistribution of adipose tissue that causes moon facies, buffalo hump, supraclavicular fat pads, and truncal obesity. Also obscure is the basis of the mental aberrations commonly seen in Cushing's syndrome.

Because cortisol has some mineralocorticoid activity, a few patients who have Cushing's syndrome have elevations in blood pressure and hypokalemia, findings typical of primary aldosteronism.

Although clinical findings may strongly suggest the diagnosis of Cushing's syndrome, supporting laboratory data are essential. Very useful for screening purposes is the overnight dexamethasone suppression test in which 1.0 mg of dexamethasone is given at 11:00 PM, and a plasma sample is taken for cortisol estimation at 8:00 AM the following morning. In normal subjects, the early morning surge in cortisol is suppressed, resulting in steroid values of less than 5 μg/dl; in Cushing's syndrome, the cortisol secretion is not suppressed, and one finds steroid values that are greater than 10 μg/dl. A positive result should be followed by more extensive testing to confirm the diagnosis. One approach entails the estimation of the 17-OHC content of 24-hour urine samples collected in the basal state and then during the sequential adminstration of intravenous ACTH and oral dexamethasone, 2 mg/day for 3 days, followed by 8 mg/day for 3 days. The results of these procedures should establish the presence of Cushing's syndrome and, moreover, provide information regarding its cause. Illustrative data are summarized in Table 34–5 and shown graphically in Figure 34–11. It should be noted that the basal urinary excretion of 17-OHC in Cushing's syndrome due to hyperplasia may be normal (15 per cent of cases) or only slightly elevated. However, usually the hyperplastic glands respond very briskly to ACTH stimulation. In contrast to 17-

TABLE 34–5 TYPICAL LABORATORY FINDINGS IN CUSHING'S SYNDROME DUE TO HYPERPLASIA, ADENOMA, CARCINOMA, AND ECTOPIC ACTH PRODUCTION

	Normal	Hyperplasia	Adenoma	Carcinoma	Ectopic ACTH
Plasma					
Cortisol (µg/dl, AM/PM)	17/8	30/25	35/35	50/50	35/35
ACTH (pg/ml)	<100	50 to 500	<10	<10	200 to 10,000
Urine					
17-hydroxycorticoids (mg/24 hr)					
Basal	2 to 10	15	30	50	30
After ACTH stimulation	2 to 5× ↑ *	3 to 5× ↑	↑ /↔†	↔	2×/↔
Dexamethasone suppression (2 mg/day)	<3	>4	30	50	30
Dexamethasone suppression (8 mg/day)	<3	<3	30	50	30
Free cortisol (µg/24 hr)					
Basal	<100	200	300	500	300
Dexamethasone suppression (2 mg/day)	<20	125	300	500	300
Dexamethasone suppression (8 mg/day)	<20	50	300	500	300

* ↑ = increase
† ↔ = no change

OHC levels, urinary free cortisol values are rarely normal in Cushing's syndrome, and the determination of urinary free cortisol is the procedure of choice of many clinical endocrinologists.

Congenital Adrenal Hyperplasia (CAH)

The term *CAH* embraces a fascinating spectrum of disorders, each of which results from an inherited deficiency of a specific enzyme involved in the biosynthesis of adrenal steroids (Fig. 34–12). In considering the pathophysiology of CAH, one must remember that (1) of the various steroids elaborated by the adrenal cortex at physiologic concentrations, cortisol, *and only cortisol,* suppresses ACTH secretion; and (2) the rate-limiting step in cortisol biosynthesis is the ACTH-dependent conversion of cholesterol to pregnenolone. If a block exists between cholesterol and cortisol, excess pregnenolone will be produced because of increased plasma ACTH and the large amount of available cholesterol. Pregnenolone then flows down the pathway or pathways that are available to it. Thus, we can anticipate the possibility of overproduction of intermediaries (with or without biologic activity). Excess of one hormone may coexist with deficiency of cortisol and possibly other hormones. In general, the clinical presentation is predictable if the site of the block is known; conversely, the clinical picture provides reliable clues as to the locus of the enzymatic defect.

C₂₁ Hydroxylase Deficiency. Deficiency of C_{21} hydroxylase is by far the most common cause of CAH, constituting approximately 90 per cent of

the cases. The deficiency of this enzyme results in impaired cortisol production and an increase in 17-OH progesterone, androstenedione, and testosterone. When the enzymatic deficiency is partial, as it is in about 70 per cent of the cases, impaired cortisol production is corrected to a normal or near-normal rate by a compensatory increase in pituitary secretion of ACTH, prompted by the initially low level of plasma cortisol. This increase in stimulation of the adrenals leads to hyperplasia and an increase in production of androgens. When the defect is more severe, this compensatory mechanism is inadequate, and adrenal insufficiency ensues. Marked salt wasting is the most significant charactertistic of such patients. Besides cortisol deficiency, these individuals also produce inadequate amounts of aldosterone and other mineralocorticoids such as DOC.

C_{21} hydroxylase deficiency is perhaps the most common cause of female pseudohermaphroditism (a term denoting the presence of male or ambiguous external genitalia in an individual who has female karyotype and gonads). All newborn infants who have ambiguous genitalia should be suspected of having CAH, and karyotypes should be done to determine genetic sex. The sex chromatin pattern, using buccal mucosal scrapings, is unreliable in early infancy. The presence of a phallus-like clitoris and a partially fused labial fold in a genetic female strongly suggests a C_{21} defect. Urinary 17-ketosteroids and pregnanetriol (the principal metabolite of 17-OH progesterone) are both elevated in C_{21} hydroxylase deficiency; however, urinary collections are difficult in the newborn. It is now possible to determine plasma 17-OH progesterone, and a marked elevation in this intermediary provides biochemical confirmation of the diagnosis. The diagnosis may be missed in infancy. The youngster who has unrecognized CAH due to C_{21} hydroxylase deficiency has an accelerated growth rate and an advanced bone age. Young girls who have this deficiency will fail to menstruate or to develop feminine secondary sexual characteristics. Very mild degrees of deficiency probably account for the presence of hirsutism in some adult females.

In the minority of newborn patients, the defect is severe. Virilization, present in females, is overshadowed by life-threatening salt wasting. Such patients have reduced plasma sodium concentrations and elevated levels of plasma potassium: Blood volume is reduced, and blood pressure is difficult to maintain.

C_{21} hydroxylase deficiency appears to be inherited as an autosomal recessive trait with variable penetrance. Parents of affected patients are presumably heterozygous for that trait. In one study, when individuals were infused with ACTH, and when 17-OH progesterone was measured at frequent intervals thereafter, the rise noted in heterozygotes was substantially greater than that seen in control subjects, suggesting some limitation of the C_{21} hydroxylation step in the former.

Once the diagnosis is established, the management of CAH is usually straightforward, if not always gratifying. A glucocorticoid such as cortisone acetate is given orally in physiologic doses. This exogenous replacement supplies the need of the peripheral tissues for cortisol. At the same time, ACTH secretion is suppressed, adrenal hyperplasia regresses, and the excessive production of androgens ceases. If salt-wasting is present, an aldosterone-like mineralocorticoid such as fluorohydrocortisone must be included in the therapeutic regimen.

Other Defects in Adrenal Steroidogenesis. In addition to 21-hydroxylase deficiency, CAH may arise from lack of 11-β-hydroxylase, 17-hydroxylase, 3-β-hydroxysteroid dehydrogenase, or cholesterol desmolase. The latter two conditions are extremely rare. Deficiency of 11-hydroxylase constitutes about 10 per cent of the cases of CAH. In this form of the disease, hypertension is a prominent clinical feature. Impairment of hydroxylation of C_{11} leads to the accumulation of both 11-desoxycortisol and desoxycorticosterone. Whereas 11-desoxycortisol is biologically inactive, excessive serum levels of desoxycorticosterone cause hypertension by mechanisms presumably comparable to those involved in the action of aldosterone. Confirmation of a clinical diagnosis of 11-hydroxylase deficiency requires the demonstration of excessive quantities of tetrahydrodesoxycortisol (the excretory product of 11-desoxycortisol) in the urine or of increased serum levels of 11-desoxycortisol. It is of interest that the pharmacologic agent metyrapone, used to test for pituitary ACTH reserve, acts by inhibiting 11-hydroxylase, thus transiently

simulating the inborn error of metabolism under discussion. CAH due to 11-β-hydroxylase deficiency also responds to physiologic doses of glucocorticoid.

Primary Aldosteronism (Conn's Syndrome)

Primary aldosteronism is the clinical condition caused by excessive, unregulated secretion by the adrenal cortex of the potent, salt-retaining steroid, aldosterone. The underlying pathologic lesion is a small adenoma in about two thirds of the cases or bilateral hyperplasia in the remaining cases. The history of both the clinical entity and the hormone is brief but instructive. By 1950, the research of many investigators had indicated that certain known actions of the adrenal cortex could not be attributed to cortisol alone. Greep and Deane were among those who postulated that there was an unidentified substance responsible for the powerful effect exerted by the adrenal cortex on mineral metabolism. In search of this missing "mineralocorticoid," Tait and coworkers isolated a factor they termed *electrocortin*. This substance was soon characterized chemically and named *aldosterone* because of the aldehyde group on C_{18}. In 1955, the first case of primary aldosteronism was reported by Conn, who stated: "When in April, 1954, I was confronted with a patient who exhibited a most fascinating disturbance in electrolyte metabolism similar to a few cases which had been reported as potassium-losing nephritis, it could not have been presented to anyone more conscious of the possibility of aldosteronism in man than I was at that moment." Dr. Conn modestly goes on to say, "It actually required little imagination."

Chronic excessive secretion of aldosterone leads to hypertension and hypokalemia, the two characteristic findings in primary aldosteronism. Although the hypertension is usually mild or moderate in severity, it may result in manifestations of sustained hypertension, such as left ventricular hypertrophy and narrowing of the retinal arterioles. The hypokalemia causes muscle weakness that may be so severe that an ascending neuritis such as that found in the Guillain-Barré syndrome is suggested. The electrolyte disturbance also leads to other symptoms such as polyuria, muscle cramps, intestinal atony, and paresthesias. On laboratory examination, the serum potassium is typically below 3.6 mEq/L, serum sodium is normal or slightly elevated, bicarbonate is increased, and chloride is decreased (hypokalemic, hypochloremic alkalosis). There are inappropriately large amounts of potassium in the urine. The electrocardiogram reflects reduction in serum potassium (flattening of T waves and the appearance of U waves).

Although the occurrence of hypokalemia in a

hypertensive patient should suggest the diagnosis, confirmation requires the demonstration of both increased aldosterone secretion and low plasma renin activity. Plasma aldosterone is usually greater than 90 pg/ml, and urinary aldosterone should exceed 20 µg/day in a patient who has primary aldosteronism and who is receiving ample dietary sodium (e.g., greater than 120 mEq/day). In addition, the plasma renin activity should be low and remain suppressed, despite a low sodium diet and several hours of ambulation. Patients who have malignant hypertension or hypertension due to chronic renal disease or renal artery stenosis will also excrete large amounts of aldosterone, but in contrast the plasma renin activity will be elevated. The most common form of hypertension is termed *essential,* since no specific etiologic factor can currently be identified. Although these patients have normal urinary aldosterone levels, approximately one third of them will display suppressed plasma-renin values for reasons that are not yet clear. Although abbreviated protocols are now commonly used for the evaluation of primary aldosteronism, the following one that is described by Conn and coworkers illustrates the pathophysiology of this disorder.

Procedures

1. Two weeks: Unrestricted diet, no diuretics
2. Day 1: 120 mEq Na diet.
   Day 2: 120 mEq Na diet.
   Day 3: 120 mEq Na diet; collect 24-hour urine for aldosterone; take fasting blood for plasma renin activity (PRA) after 2-hour ambulation.
3. Day 4: 10 mEq Na diet.
   Day 5: 10 mEq Na diet.
   Day 6: 10 mEq Na diet; collect 24-hour urine for aldosterone; take fasting blood for plasma renin activity (PRA) after 2-hour ambulation.

Typical Results		*120 mEq Na diet*	*10 mEq Na diet*
Plasma aldosterone (pg/ml)	Normals:	20–110	175–500
	Patients:	inc.	inc.
Urinary aldosterone (µg/24 hr)	Normals:	9–12	32–48
	Patients:	21–72	16–75
Plasma renin activity (ng/ml/hr)	Normals:	3–4.5	9.5–14
	Patients:	0–3.7	0–4.5

Although aldosterone antagonists such as spironolactone have been used, the usual treatment of primary aldosteronism consists of surgical extirpation of the adenoma. Preoperative localization of the tumor may be made by the use of isotopically labeled cholesterol, which concentrates in the involved adrenal, arteriography, or by CT scanning. The prognosis is variable; if the process has been

going on for many years, the cardiovascular complications of long-standing hypertension are usually irreversible and the hypertension itself tends to be fixed.

PARATHYROIDS

PHYSIOLOGY: BONE METABOLISM AND CALCIUM HOMEOSTASIS

The maintenance of the integrity of bone and calcium metabolism is dependent in large part on the interaction of three substances—parathyroid hormone, vitamin D, and calcitonin—on three tissues: bone, the kidney and the gastrointestinal tract.

Hormones

Parathyroid Hormone. The parathyroid glands are minute, with a total mass of only 200 mg; they are of endodermal origin, being derived from the third and fourth branchial pouches. In the adult, although they are usually located either in close proximity to or within the thyroid gland, their location, particularly that of the inferior pair, is quite variable. The glands secrete parathyroid hormone, a polypeptide with a molecular weight of approximately 8500, which has the principal function of maintaining calcium homeostasis. The narrow range within which the serum calcium concentration is normally maintained attests to the importance of calcium homeostasis in higher life forms. Calcium plays an important role in such vital processes as neuromuscular excitability, muscular contraction, membrane permeability, and coagulation of blood. Furthermore, it is required for the activation of many critical enzymes and provides the major structural support for the organism. In the plasma, calcium circulates in three forms: bound to protein, complexed with anions such as citrate, and free or ionized. Only the latter, normally about 4 mg/dl, is metabolically active. In the skeleton and in the plasma, calcium is chemically linked to phosphate. Like calcium, phosphate has great importance outside the skeleton. Phosphorylated compounds (e.g., ATP) are the currency of energy in cellular metabolism. Although parathyroid hormone is important in the regulation of plasma phosphate, there is no evidence that plasma phosphate has any direct effect on parathyroid hormone secretion. Apparently, the release of parathyroid hormone in normal humans is determined by one factor only—the level of ionized calcium that perfuses parathyroid tissue.

Vitamin D. A second substance, vitamin D, has a major role in the maintenance of calcium homeostasis. A naturally occurring vitamin D is produced by the conversion of 7-dihydrocholesterol to cholecalciferol (CC, vitamin D_3). This reaction takes place in the skin and requires ultraviolet light. A second form of the vitamin, D$_2$, is produced commercially by the irradiation of the plant sterol, ergosterol. Apparently, neither vitamin D$_3$ nor D$_2$ is itself metabolically active. Through the patient efforts of several workers, particularly DeLuca and his colleagues, the fascinating and complex metabolism of vitamin D has been greatly illuminated. The first step takes place in the liver; it is the hydroxylation of vitamin D$_3$ to 25-hydroxycholecalciferol (25 HCC). The latter metabolite is transported to the kidney, bound to a specific carrier protein. In the kidney, 25 HCC is hydroxylated to 24,25 dihydroxycholecalciferol (DHCC) and 1,25 DHCC. It is 1,25 DHCC that is now believed to be the active metabolite. It also requires a specific carrier protein for transportation to its target tissues, bone and gut, where it stimulates calcium mobilization and absorption, respectively. The synthesis of 1,25 DHCC in the kidney appears to be a closely regulated process, the details of which are beginning to emerge. Both low calcium and low phosphate stimulate the synthesis, whereas elevated calcium and high phosphate depress it. Interestingly, PTH enhances the production of 1,25 DHCC. Whether this is a direct or an indirect effect involving, for example, phosphate, remains to be seen.

On the basis of these recent developments, it seems appropriate to consider 1,25 DHCC a hormone rather than a vitamin. A vitamin is traditionally defined as a substance that is required in trace amounts for one or more vital metabolic processes. Except for those deprived of sunshine, 1,25 DHCC fails to fit this definition. However, it does have several hormonal attributes. Its synthesis is tightly controlled to prevent overproduction, and its sites of action are remote from its site of production.

Calcitonin. In addition to PTH and vitamin D, a third hormone, calcitonin, has been implicated in calcium metabolism. Calcitonin, first described by Copp in 1962, is elaborated by the parafollicular cells, or C cells, of the thyroid. Calcitonin lowers plasma calcium by inhibiting calcium mobilization from bone. Although calcitonin may be critical in lower species, its importance in human physiology is doubtful. The fact that patients who have undergone total thyroidectomy (and are thus without a source of calcitonin) have normal plasma calcium concentrations is an argument against a significant role for calcitonin in humans.

Gastrointestinal Tract

The gastrointestinal tract is a critical site in the regulation of calcium metabolism. Intestinal absorption of calcium occurs either from the duodenum by active transport or at any point along the entire small bowel by simple diffusion. The latter movement of calcium across the intestinal mucosa is bidirectional; hence, fecal calcium consists of calcium excreted into the gut, as well as nonabsorbed dietary calcium. Although vitamin D has effects on other tissues, its primary action is to promote calcium absorption from the gastrointestinal tract by stimulation of its active transport. The absorption of intestinal phosphate is probably linked to that of calcium. The optimal ratio of intestinal calcium to phosphate for calcium absorption is 2:1. Absorption of calcium is impaired by diseases of the small bowel, such as sprue and celiac disease, and by hepatic disease, such as biliary cirrhosis. It is also influenced by the acidity of the intestinal content and by dietary factors, such as acetic acid, phytic acid, and oxalates.

Calcium absorbed from the gastrointestinal tract enters the extracellular pool of calcium, estimated at about 950 mg in the adult. Extracellular calcium is in dynamic equilibrium with calcium in the intracellular component of soft tissue (about 11,000 mg) and with the so-called "exchangeable calcium pool of the skeleton." The latter pool is estimated to turn over 40 to 50 times each day. The precise quantity and even the location of this exchangeable pool of bone calcium are not known. Some believe that it is contained within partially calcified bone, and others contend that it is calcium released from bone undergoing active resorption.

Bone

In the calcium balance of normal adults, approximately 300 mg of calcium per day is resorbed from bone, and the same amount is deposited each day. This turnover largely reflects the continuous process of bone remodeling. Although several factors (e.g., age, bone disease and deficiency of calcium or phosphate) influence bone remodeling, the principal controlling factors are (1) parathyroid hormone and vitamin D, and (2) the effects of mechanical stress on the skeleton. The actions of parathyroid hormone and vitamin D on bone resorption subserve calcium homeostasis. Thus, when a conflict arises between maintenance of a normal serum calcium and skeletal integrity, bone is sacrificed to provide the needed calcium. Mechanical stress, the second factor, causes a remodeling of bone to meet changing requirements for structural strength. Within physiologic limits, it appears that parathyroid hormone is the principal determinant of the magnitude of remodeling, whereas mechanical stresses are the principal determinants of the location in which remodeling occurs.

The mechanism of action of parathyroid hormone on bone at the cellular level has not been determined. One line of evidence suggests that parathyroid hormone stimulates both the osteolytic activity of osteocytes, causing an early rise in plasma calcium, and the differentiation of mesenchymal cells into osteoclasts, the cells responsible for bone resorption.

The Kidneys

The normal kidney is extraordinarily efficient in its conservation of calcium. Despite filtration by the glomeruli of an estimated 10,000 mg of calcium daily, no more than 300 mg of this is normally excreted in the urine. Calcium virtually disappears from the urine when plasma calcium falls below 7 mg/dl. Tubular reabsorption of calcium is enhanced by parathyroid hormone, but this effect is small compared with hypercalcemia caused by the action of parathyroid hormone on bone. Vitamin D has a weak calciuric effect. The efficiency of the kidney in conserving calcium is not matched by an equal ability to excrete it when the need arises. Even with continued severe hypercalcemia, the 24-hour urinary excretion of calcium will rarely exceed 500 mg. This limitation is detrimental if calcium is being absorbed from the gut or mobilized from bone in an excessive and unregulated fashion as occurs, for example, in vitamin D intoxication or metastatic bone disease. A major renal action of parathyroid hormone is to inhibit the reabsorption of phosphate by the tubule. In the absence of parathyroid hormone, about 90 per cent or more of filtered phosphate is reabsorbed, whereas in hyperparathyroidism this value usually is less than 70 per cent. Parathyroid hormone may also stimulate the secretion of phosphate by the tubules as well as decrease its reabsorption. The mechanism of action of parathyroid hormone on the renal tubules involves the adenylate cyclase–cyclic AMP system. Following the injection of parathyroid hormone, the urinary excretion of cyclic AMP is markedly increased.

CLINICAL ENTITIES

Hypoparathyroidism

By far the leading cause of parathyroid hormone deficiency is inadvertent removal or damage to the parathyroids during thyroid surgery. Permanent hypoparathyroidism is a serious complication of thyroidectomy, occurring with a frequency of about 1 per cent. Idiopathic hypoparathyroidism, a rare disorder, is noteworthy in several respects. It may be familial and be associated with generalized moniliasis and deficiencies of other endocrine glands. The sera of some patients who have idiopathic hypoparathyroidism have high titers of antibody to human parathyroid tissue, suggesting an autoimmune cause.

The manifestations of hypoparathyroidism are directly attributable to impaired calcium homeostasis due to parathyroid hormone deficiency. Both total and ionized serum calcium are low, and

serum phosphate is high. Hypocalcemia causes an increase in neuromuscular irritability. When the total serum calcium falls below 7 to 8 mg/dl, the patient develops symptoms such as numbness, tingling, formication, and muscle cramping. With a further depression is serum calcium, the physical manifestations of hypocalcemia, termed *tetany,* ensue. These include carpopedal spasm, laryngeal spasm and stridor, muscle twitching, and generalized convulsions. The latter occasionally lead to the erroneous diagnosis of epilepsy. This tragic mistake can be avoided by routinely determining the serum calcium in all patients undergoing their initial evaluation for a seizure disorder. The altered myocardial contractility due to hypocalcemia is reflected in the electrocardiogram by prolongation of the Q–T interval. Such a finding on a routine electrocardiogram should always arouse suspicion of occult hypocalcemia. Factors that alter the protein binding of calcium in the serum can either enhance or diminish the symptoms of hypocalcemia. For example, alkalosis will increase the quantity of calcium bound to protein with a corresponding reduction in ionized calcium; thus, hyperventilation can cause mild symptoms in the presence of a normal total serum calcium. Conversely, acidemia increases the dissociation of bound calcium and thus may prevent tetany, even when the total calcium is 5 or 6 mg/dl.

Chronic hypocalcemia can result in cataract formation and calcification within the central nervous system. The basal ganglia and cerebellum appear to be especially vulnerable. It has been thought that such calcification is the result of supersaturation of body fluids with calcium phosphate. Although the calcium × phosphate product may indeed be elevated in hypoparathyroidism, this fails to explain the peculiar distribution of calcification in hypoparathyroidism, which differs strikingly from that found in other diseases with a high calcium × phosphate product.

Pseudohypoparathyroidism

In 1942, Albright and colleagues introduced the term *pseudohypoparathyroidism* to describe a 28-year-old female of short stature who had a seizure disorder and serum calcium and phosphate findings of hypoparathyroidism. Large quantities of parathyroid hormone administered to this patient failed to correct the serum chemical abnormalities and did not cause an increase in phosphate excretion. These findings suggested that the basic problem was an inability to respond to parathyroid hormone rather than a deficiency of the hormone. Subsequently, patients of similar descriptions have been reported and have manifested, in addition to hypocalcemia and an elevated serum phosphate, short stature and a short neck, a rounded face, short metacarpal and metatarsal bones, extraosseous calcification, and mental retardation. The syndrome appears to be inherited as an X-linked dominant trait with partial penetrance. In patients who demonstrate the characteristic physiognomy but who do not have serum chemistry abnormalities, the disease is rather awkwardly termed *pseudopseudohypoparathyroidism*.

Considerable evidence supports Albright's thesis that pseudohypoparathyroidism is a disorder involving end-organ unresponsiveness to parathyroid hormone rather than a deficiency of the hormone. Hyperplastic parathyroid glands have been shown in these patients at surgery, and their sera have been shown to contain abnormally high levels of immunoassayable parathyroid hormone. As mentioned previously, the action of parathyroid hormone on the renal tubular cells is mediated by the adenylate cyclase–cyclic AMP system. When parathyroid hormone is administered to normal subjects or to patients who have hypoparathyroidism or pseudopseudohypoparathyroidism, the urinary content of cyclic AMP is greatly increased; contrariwise, no increase in cyclic AMP occurs in most patients who have pseudohypoparathyroidism. Thus, unresponsiveness of the renal tubule cells to parathyroid hormone is clearly implicated in the pathogenesis of the hypocalcemia and hyperphosphatemia of pseudohypoparathyroidism. This observation also tends to localize the biochemical defect in the kidneys to the interaction of either parathyroid hormone with adenylate cyclase or adenylate cyclase with cyclic AMP. Two groups of investigators have found that in the cell membranes of many patients who have this disorder there is a 50 per cent reduction in the guanine nucleotide regulatory protein that couples the hormone receptor to the catalytic component of the adenylate cyclase system (Fig. 34–2). This finding raises the possibility that at least partial states of hormone resistance are present in other organs. Indeed, hypothyroidism occurs frequently in these patients.

An additional question of importance in pseudohypoparathyroidism concerns the responsiveness of the other parathyroid hormone–sensitive tissues, especially bone. Because a few patients who have pseudohypoparathyroidism have developed osteitis fibrosa cystica, it would appear that bone is at least partially responsive to parathyroid hormone in some patients with this disorder. As is so often true in endocrinology, studies undertaken to clarify the nature of a relatively obscure disorder, pseudohypoparathyroidism, have yielded information of basic importance to an understanding of hormone action.

Primary Hyperparathyroidism

Primary hyperparathyroidism refers to the disorder in which parathyroid hormone is secreted autonomously and excessively by one or more of the parathyroid glands. It is to be distinguished from secondary hyperparathyroidism, which occurs in response to chronic renal disease, malabsorption, and other disorders characterized by long-standing hypocalcemia. The underlying pathologic disorder in primary hyperparathyroidism is either one or more adenomas (about 90 per cent of the cases), hyperplasia of all four glands (about 10 per cent of the cases), or carcinoma (less than 1 per cent of the cases). Infrequently, when hyperparathyroidism is familial, there is a high incidence of neoplasms that involve other endocrine glands, especially the pituitary and the pancreas or the thyroid and the adrenal medulla. As mentioned previously, these pluriglandular syndromes are termed *multiple endocrine neoplasia*, or *MEN*. Certain neoplasms that arise in other organs, especially the lung, liver, and genitourinary tract, occasionally elaborate a peptide with parathyroid hormone–like activity. The resulting biochemical disturbance may closely mimic primary hyperparathyroidism.

The major manifestations of primary hyperparathyroidism are due to the effects of hypercalcemia on several organs, including the kidneys, gastrointestinal tract, and nervous system. Hypercalcemia per se impairs the concentrating ability of the kidney, and polyuria is an early symptom of hyperparathyroidism. Precipitation of fine crystals of calcium salts in the renal tubules (nephrocalcinosis) impairs both glomerular and tubular function. Renal stone formation occurs commonly in patients who have hyperparathyroidism. A vicious cycle in which renal calculi predispose to infection may ensue, and alkalinization of the urine by infecting organisms in turn leads to further stone formation. If uninterrupted, this sequence of events may progress to uremia and death. Clearly, any patient who has or has had a renal stone should be investigated for hyperparathyroidism.

For reasons that are not yet clear, bone involvement in hyperparathyroidism sufficient to cause symptoms or to be detected on radiographs is becoming increasingly rare.

Peptic ulcer disease may be more common in patients who have primary hyperparathyroidism, probably as a consequence of hypercalcemia. It has been shown experimentally that increasing the level of serum calcium stimulates an increase in circulating gastrin and an increased rate of secretion of hydrochloric acid by the stomach. Hypertension is also a frequent finding in hyperparathyroidism and may not disappear after correction of the primary disorder.

Metabolic Bone Disease

The concept of metabolic bone disease was introduced more than 30 years ago by Albright. The term applies to those disorders of bone in

TABLE 34–6 COMPARISON OF THE MAJOR METABOLIC BONE DISEASES

	Osteitis Fibrosa Cystica	Osteoporosis	Osteomalacia
Etiology	Excessive PTH	Varied but usually unknown	Vitamin D deficiency; malabsorption
Serum			
Calcium	Increased	Normal	Decreased or normal
Phosphate	Normal or decreased	Normal	Decreased
Alkaline phosphatase	Normal or increased	Normal	Increased
Pathophysiology	Increased bone resorption	Decreased bone mass (resorp. > accret.)	Decreased mineralization
Histopathology	Cysts; fibrosis; "brown" tumor	Normal histology	Increased osteoid tissue
Radiology	Subperiosteal resorption; cysts	Rarefaction of axial skeleton; "codfish" vertebrae; compression fractures	Rarefaction of appendicular skeleton; pseudofractures (Looser's zones)

which—at the molecular level—all parts of the skeleton are involved. The qualification "at the molecular level" is important because clinically, radiographically, and even histologically, the disease may appear to be limited to only one or to several sites. As might be predicted from its generalized nature, the identified causes of metabolic bone disease are usually hormonal or nutritional. Features of the three "classic" examples of metabolic bone disease—osteitis fibrosa cystica, osteoporosis, and osteomalacia—are shown in Table 34–6. Other forms of bone disease may be widely disseminated, as for example in metastatic cancer, but between metastatic sites the bone will be normal, and thus the process is not considered under the aforementioned classification.

Renal Osteodystrophy. Although it has long been appreciated that chronic hypocalcemia can lead to hyperplasia of the parathyroids, the full implications of this phenomenon as it applies to chronic renal disease are just beginning to emerge. The term *renal osteodystrophy* embraces a syndrome in uremic patients that includes profound disturbances in divalent ion metabolism, metabolic bone disease (e.g., osteomalacia, osteitis fibrosa cystica, and osteosclerosis), hyperplasia of the parathyroids, and soft-tissue calcification. In the past, the brief life span of a patient who had severe renal failure precluded the development of advanced metabolic bone disease. With the advent of chronic dialysis and renal transplantation, the patient who has uremia may survive for extended periods, providing the time required to develop severe renal osteodystrophy. It is estimated that 25 per cent of the patients who have uremia who are treated with conventional therapy and 80 per cent of those in chronic dialysis programs have this bone disease.

The pathophysiology of renal osteodystrophy is complex; at least three independent factors are involved: (1) phosphate retention; (2) a decrease

in responsiveness of bone to the calcium mobilizing action of PTH; and (3) an acquired defect in vitamin D metabolism, wherein formation of the active metabolite, 1,25 DHCC, is diminished. These factors have in common the propensity to reduce plasma calcium and to cause parathyroid hyperplasia. Probably the earliest event in the pathogenic sequence leading to renal osteodystrophy is phosphate retention, commencing when the creatinine clearance falls to approximately 75 ml/min. The inverse relationship between the concentrations of calcium and phosphate in the plasma, emphasized many years ago by Albright, appears valid today. Thus, an elevation in phosphate causes a decrease in calcium so that the product of the two remains unchanged. The slight decline in calcium, however, causes an increase in PTH secretion; the latter prompts an increase in urinary phosphate excretion and a return of phosphate and calcium to normal. Thus, normal plasma levels of calcium and phosphate are achieved at the expense of an increase in PTH secretion. With advancing renal failure, plasma PTH continues to rise (as calcium and phosphate remain normal). However, when the creatinine clearance falls below 20 ml/min, few nephrons remain to respond to PTH; phosphate excretion decreases, plasma phosphate rises and calcium falls. At this point, hypocalcemia may be worsened by the relative resistance of the skeleton to PTH and by diminished intestinal absorption of calcium secondary to impaired synthesis of 1,25 DHCC. The latter events lead to a diminished miscible pool of calcium and reduced calcification of osteoid tissue (osteomalacia). The chronic state of hypocalcemia prompts an extraordinary degree of parathyroid hyperplasia and extremely high levels of plasma PTH. The combined weight of glands may be several grams, and the PTH concentrations are considerably higher than those seen in primary hyperparathyroidism. Whether hyperparathyroidism can become truly autonomous in renal failure (so-called tertiary hyperparathyroidism) is controversial. There have been reports of hypercalcemia that persists after renal failure has been corrected by successful renal transplant. In any event, levels of plasma PTH sufficient to overcome resistance to its calcemic action on bone are reached. The bone pathology that results from prolonged exposure to very high levels of PTH is osteitis fibrosa cystica. Typically, bone pain occurs in renal failure in patients whose lives have been prolonged by repeated dialysis. In fact, it may be the patient's major complaint, other manifestations of uremia being controlled by dialysis. Not surprisingly, the skeleton of these patients, weakened by the overlapping processes of osteomalacia and osteitis fibrosa cystica, is subject to fracture with little or no trauma. Calcium that is mobilized from the bone in late renal failure tends to normalize the plasma calcium; however, the high levels of phosphate remain unchanged. As a result, the product of the two rises, increasing the likelihood of deposition of calcium precipitates in nonosseous tissues. Soft-tissue calcification is often widespread, involving the subcutaneous tissue of the skin, the conjunctivae, joints, and blood vessels. Treatment of renal osteodystrophy is directed at reducing the amount of phosphate available for absorption by the gut and at increasing intestinal absorption of calcium. To meet the first objective, dietary phosphate is reduced, and nonabsorbable phosphate binding agents such as aluminum hydroxide are prescribed. Calcium as gluconate or carbonate is given to supplement dietary calcium. The highly potent vitamin D metabolite 1,25 DHCC is being used successfully in patients who have severe bone disease and hypocalcemia. The principal difficulty encountered with this agent has been hypercalcemia, which, fortunately, has persisted for only a few days after therapy has been discontinued. Lastly, total parathyroidectomy has been carried out in patients who have hypercalcemia unassociated with prior vitamin D therapy. It is particularly important to correct hypercalcemia before implanting a new kidney. To simplify postparathyroidectomy management, all four glands are removed from the neck and the substance of one of the four is cut into small fragments. These fragments are implanted beneath the skin of the forearm, where they are readily accessible if hypercalcemia develops in the future.

Osteoporosis. Osteoporosis is by far the most frequently encountered form of metabolic bone disease. It occurs most commonly in postmenopausal white females and in white males older than 60 years of age. Blacks are infrequently affected. The basic abnormality is loss of bone substance, which is seen radiographically as demineralization (osteopenia). The principal symptom is low back pain. Serum calcium, phosphate, and alkaline phosphatase are normal, as is the histologic and biochemical examination of biopsy samples of the bone itself.

The cause of primary or idiopathic osteoporosis is not known. As discussed previously, maintenance of normal skeletal integrity requires a balance between bone formation and bone resorption. In osteoporosis, the latter exceeds the former. Whether resorption is pathologically increased or formation is abnormally decreased or both is not clear. In recent years, sophisticated methodology has been applied to the problem. Calcium kinetics, using ^{45}Ca, have been evaluated in patients who have osteoporosis; in addition, their bones have been analyzed by microradiographic examination and by morphometric techniques with tetracycline labeling. Unfortunately, these different approaches have not yielded consistent results, and the cause or causes of primary osteoporosis remain unknown. Deficiency in dietary calcium may cause osteoporosis experimentally, but its role in the development of the disease in humans is uncertain. Deficiencies of estrogenic and androgenic hormones have long been considered to play important roles in the development of this disease. This view is supported by the high incidence of osteoporosis in postmenopausal women, in young women who have ovarian agenesis, and in older men. Although long-term treatment with estrogens may not cause a detectable increase in bone mass in women who have postmenopausal osteoporosis, it apparently prevents further bone loss. At the present time, it seems likely that primary osteoporosis may be the result of several coexistent factors.

Several specific conditions that lead to osteoporosis have been recognized, including Cushing's syndrome, prolonged treatment with glucocorticoids, immobilization, thyrotoxicosis, and pregnancy. In hyperparathyroidism, there may be osteoporosis coexistent with the more specific lesions of subperiosteal bone resorption and cyst formation.

Low back pain is the most frequent symptom of osteoporosis. Typically, it is insidious in its onset. Occasionally, the onset is acute, or there is an acute exacerbation of pain superimposed on the chronic discomfort. These latter events are associated with compression fracture of a vertebral body. Not infrequently, advanced osteoporosis is discovered on radiographs taken for an unrelated condition in a patient who is free of back pain. Progressive shortening of stature due to collapsed vertebrae may occur with little or no pain. Hip and wrist fractures are also common complications of this disorder.

The diagnosis depends on finding characteristic changes on the radiographs of the skeleton, particularly the spine. The end-plates of the vertebrae are less rarefied than the bodies, causing an increased contrast between the two. The end-plates may be depressed centrally, leading to the so-called codfish appearance of the spine. With further advance in the disease, the nucleus pulposus herniates through the end-plate, producing an irregular area of decreased density in the central portion of the vertebral body, a finding known as the *Schmorl node*. When a compression fracture occurs, typically the anterior portion of the body gives way, producing a wedgelike deformity of the vertebral body. Cortical bone is less affected than cancellous bone in osteoporosis. One can grossly assess the long bones by comparing the combined thickness of the bone's cortices with its total thickness. Normally, the former accounts for approximately 45 per cent of the latter.

ADRENAL MEDULLA

PHYSIOLOGY

The primary function of the adrenal medulla is to secrete catecholamines, which are substances that have diverse effects on intermediary metabolism, contractility of cardiac and smooth muscle, and neurotransmission. To accomplish these effects, the catecholamines reach target cells by two different routes: Epinephrine is secreted by the adrenal medulla into the circulation to perfuse peripheral tissues, and norepinephrine is released by nerve endings of the sympathetic nervous system to act on neighboring cells. Strictly speaking, only the first route fulfills the criteria for a hormone; however, from an operational point of view, it is helpful to discuss metabolic responses to catecholamines regardless of their origin. In the following sections, the biosynthesis, metabolic actions, and degradation of the catecholamines will be discussed.

Biosynthesis

The primary precursor in the biosynthesis of the catecholamines is phenylalanine. Successive hydroxylations, decarboxylation, and methylation yield norepinephrine and epinephrine as follows:

phenylalanine → tyrosine → dihydroxyphenylalanine (Dopa) → dopamine → norepinephrine → epinephrine

Epinephrine is the principal circulating catecholamine secreted by the adrenal medullary cells, but they also elaborate small quantities of norepinephrine. Norepinephrine is the principal neurotransmitter of the sympathetic nervous system as well as being one of the principal neurotransmitters of the central nervous system.

Mechanism of Action

As mentioned in the introduction to this chapter, the response to a hormone begins when it combines with a specific receptor in either the cell membrane or the cytosol. No example of this phenomenon has been studied more thoroughly than the interaction of catecholamines with their receptor sites.

The characterization of adrenergic receptors as *alpha* and *beta* originated with the classic pharmacologic studies of Ahlquist, which were designed to measure the relative potencies of epinephrine, norepinephrine, and synthetic catecholamines such as isoproterenol on selected responses, including myocardial and smooth muscle contractility. Isoproterenol possessed the greatest potential for stimulating the myocardium, and norepinephrine had the least ability; contrariwise, norepinephrine was the most effective vasoconstrictor, and isoproterenol was the least effective. It was postulated that the stimulatory effects of these agents on myocardial contractility was mediated by beta sites. The significance of this hypothesis was strengthened following the discovery of phentolamine, an agent that blocks alpha-site activity, and propranolol, a beta-site blocker. Extensive studies in which these and similar drugs were used showed that epinephrine and norepinephrine are agonists for both alpha and beta sites, whereas isoproterenol is essentially a beta agonist.

Since the early 1970s, a wide array of compounds that have either agonist or antagonist properties have become available. Moreover, several of these agents have been labeled with a radioactive isotope, usually tritium, thus providing the ingredients for highly sensitive and specific radioligand binding studies. With this newer methodology, both beta and alpha receptors have been further subdivided. Beta receptors in the myocardium and adipose tissue have common characteristics and are termed B_1 *sites*. Beta receptors in vasculature and bronchial smooth muscle behave in the same way and are known as B_2 *sites*. Similarly, alpha sites have been divided into A_1 and A_2 subtypes. The development of highly selective adrenergic agents has therapeutic as well as investigational value. For example, the beta blocker atenolol has 5- to 100-fold greater affinity for B_1 sites than for B_2 receptors. When used as a drug, the cardioselectivity of atenolol permits the heart rate and inotropy to be decreased via B_1 receptor blockade while sparing the bronchoconstrictive effects of B_2 receptor antagonism.

Epinephrine has long been known to stimulate lipolysis via the adenylate cyclase–cyclic AMP system. Recent studies using isolated human fat cells that were incubated with epinephrine alone, or with epinephrine plus phentolamine or propranolol indicate that both alpha- and beta-adrenergic sites are present on the adipocyte and that they mediate divergent effects on lipolysis. Epinephrine alone stimulates lipolysis and causes an increase in cyclic AMP, effects that are greatly enhanced if phentolamine is also present. Contrariwise, the addition of propranolol to epinephrine causes a sharp fall in both intracellular cyclic AMP and lipolysis. Thus, stimulation of beta sites increases the lipolytic response, whereas the activation of alpha sites has the opposite effect. The beta effect predominates because epinephrine alone causes an increase in lipolysis.

Similar in-vitro studies have been performed with isolated pancreatic islets of the rat. Epinephrine alone sharply decreases insulin release by the islets, and a further reduction occurs when the cells are exposed to both epinephrine and propranolol. Conversely, the addition of phentolamine to epinephrine causes a marked increase in insulin release. Thus, islet cells appear to have both alpha and beta sites that mediate divergent effects on insulin release. In contrast to adipose tissue, the alpha effect predominates because epinephrine alone decreases insulin release.

The major actions of the catecholamines include:

1. Inotropic and chronotropic action on the myocardium.

2. Blood vessel constriction and dilatation.

3. Bronchodilatation and constriction.

4. Contraction and relaxation of smooth muscle of the gastrointestinal system and uterus.

5. Neurotransmission in the central nervous system.

6. Metabolic effects, including those on lipolysis, insulin secretion, and hepatic glycogenolysis.

The major metabolic effects of epinephrine result from its action on four major tissues: adipose tissue, pancreas, liver, and muscle. Catecholamine interactions with the first two have already been mentioned. In the liver, epinephrine promotes glycogenolysis and an increase in gluconeogenesis. In muscle, epinephrine stimulates glycogenolysis by beta-site activation. Unlike liver, muscle does not have a phosphatase capable of dephosphorylating glucose-6-phosphate. Hence, the products of glycogenolysis are either CO_2 and water or, in the presence of hypoxemia, lactate.

The principal metabolic effects of epinephrine in humans are hyperglycemia and an increase in plasma free fatty acids. Hyperglycemia results from the release of glucose by the liver, the suppression of insulin release, and the stimulation of muscle glycogenolysis, resulting in a release of lactic acid into the circulation. The latter serves as substrate for gluconeogenesis by the liver. Lipolysis is increased by direct stimulation of adipose tissue by epinephrine and, indirectly, by the decline in plasma insulin. Thus, the responses of these four tissues to epinephrine are complementary in that each promotes an increase in the available supply of circulating free fatty acids and glucose. The increased levels of these two metabolic fuels ensure that the nervous system and muscle will have ample substrate during physiologic stress. The catecholamines have thus been characterized as the hormones of "flight or fight," because they are discharged most conspicuously at times of great threat to the animal's survival. Similarly, the cardiovascular and smooth muscle responses to catecholamines assist the organism in meeting such an emergency successfully. It is likely that the changes that occur during stress are only exaggerations of responses that take place continuously as the sympathetic nervous system and adrenal medulla act to modulate the flow of nutrients to and from the liver, adipose tissue, and muscle.

Degradation of the Catecholamines

The two principal pathways for the biochemical disposal of epinephrine and norepinephrine involve methylation and oxidation.

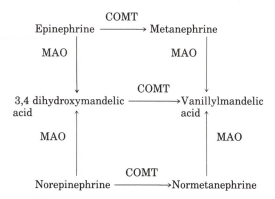

COMT (catechol-O-methyltransferase) is widely distributed throughout the body and acts rapidly to inactivate circulating catecholamines. MAO (monoamine oxidase) catalyzes the oxidative deamination of the catecholamines: It is located within nerve endings and acts to prevent excessive storage of norepinephrine. The enzyme COMT is now widely used as a reagent in highly sensitive and specific assays for plasma epinephrine and norepinephrine. Extracts of plasma are incubated with COMT and a labeled methyl donor ([3]H S-adenosyl-l-methionine, or ^{3}H SAM). The epinephrine and norepinephrine present are converted quantitatively to radioactive metanephrine and normetanephrine, which are separated by thin layer chromatography and oxidized with periodate, and their radioactivity is determined by a scintillation counter.

CLINICAL ENTITIES

States of Catecholamine Deficiency

Loss of adrenal medullary function appears to cause little or no disability. Thus, patients who have undergone bilateral adrenalectomy respond satisfactorily to replacement with only adrenal cortical hormones. Such a procedure, of course, leaves the sympathetic nervous system intact. However, the function of the latter has been reduced both surgically and pharmacologically in the treatment of hypertension. Although patients who undergo such treatment are subject to orthostatic hypotension, impaired metabolism among such patients has not been reported. A much more common cause of orthostatic hypotension is the sympathetic nervous system neuropathy of diabetes mellitus. Cryer and colleagues found that in some patients who have this disorder there is blunting in the usual rise of norepinephrine that occurs with standing.

Pheochromocytoma

Pheochromocytomas (Greek, *darkly staining cells*) are tumors that arise from chromaffin cells that secrete excessive amounts of epinephrine or both epinephrine and norepinephrine. Although usually located in the adrenal medulla, they may develop anywhere in the body where nests of chromaffin cells are found. The pre-eminent manifestation of pheochromocytoma is hypertension. In a series of 507 cases reviewed by Hermann and Mornex, 26 per cent of the patients had paroxysmal hypertension, 61 per cent showed sustained hypertension, and 4 per cent were found to be hypertensive during pregnancy. In 9 per cent of the cases, hypertension was not present. Among all patients who have hypertension, however, pheochromocytoma is extremely rare, probably found in less than 0.1 per cent of the cases. Nevertheless, in most cases pheochromocytomas are benign, accessible to the surgeon, and an important cause of curable hypertension.

Most of the manifestations of pheochromocytoma can be anticipated from the known actions of epinephrine and norepinephrine. Often, they occur in paroxysmal fashion, as in the patient who has had normal or moderately elevated blood pressure but who suddenly becomes severely hypertensive, blanches, and complains of headache, chest pain, and palpitation. The metabolic effects of excessive circulating catecholamines, hyperglycemia, and an increase in free fatty acids, can usually be shown. In most patients, however, the presentation of pheochromocytoma is less dramatic, consisting of sustained hypertension and nonspecific symptoms such as weakness, tremor, palpitation, and anxiety. In either event, a firm diagnosis can be established only by appropriate laboratory testing.

In the past, reliance was placed on pharmacologic tests. For example, the prompt attenuation of severe hypertension by the administration of the alpha blocker phentolamine was highly suggestive of pheochromocytoma. The usefulness of phentolamine has now shifted from the sphere of diagnosis to that of therapy. Diagnosis is dependent on the demonstration of abnormally high concentrations of epinephrine or norepinephrine or their metabolites in the urine or plasma. Radioenzymatic methods such as the one just mentioned have emerged as the procedures of choice to identify patients who have pheochromocytomas. Bravo and colleagues evaluated 24 patients who had proven tumors and 40 patients who were suspected of having tumors on clinical grounds but who had no evidence of the disease. They found that the estimation of plasma catecholamines (measured from samples obtained while the patient was supine) was more useful than either 24-hour urinary VMAs or metanephrines or both. Bravo and colleagues have devised a suppression test to distinguish those patients who have essential hypertension and borderline elevation of plasma catecholamines from individuals who have catecholamine secreting tumors. In the test, 0.3 mg of clonidine hydrochloride, a potent A_2 agonist, is administered orally; blood pressure, blood samples, and catecholamine determinations are taken periodically over the next 3 hours. The drug has little or no effect on the plasma catecholamine levels of patients who have pheochromocytomas because these tumors behave autonomously. Contrariwise, in patients who have essential hypertension dependent on centrally mediated catecholamine release, clonidine hydrochloride substantially lowers plasma norepinephrine by stimulating alpha receptors in the brain, with resultant reduction in sympathetic outflow. Clonidine hydrochloride is also used on a long-term basis in the therapy of patients who have essential hypertension. Apparently, with the doses used, the peripheral vasoconstrictive effects of the drug are negligible.

In the laboratory of Bravo and colleagues, the mean value of total plasma catecholamines was 260 ng/L, and the upper limit of normal (expressed as 2 SD of the mean) was 620 ng/L (n = 26). The daily excretion of catecholamines and metabolites in the normal adult are as follows:

1. Epinephrine—20 μg.
2. Norepinephrine—80 μg.
3. Metanephrines—1.3 mg.
4. Vanillylmandelic acid (VMA)—6.5 mg.

However, to be meaningful, these tests must be performed by competent laboratory personnel on specimens that are free of interfering drugs or dietary constituents. If the patient has paroxysmal hypertension, urine must be collected during such an episode, and the amount of catecholamine present must be expressed per gram of urinary creatinine.

TESTES

PHYSIOLOGY

The dual role of the testes in procreation and maintenance of male attributes has been appreciated from antiquity. Through history, castration has been practiced in many societies, usually with the goal of rendering the victim devoid of both the desire and capability of sexual activity. Thus, in contrast to pituitary, thyroid, or adrenal deficiencies, which occurred as the result of various diseases, one form of male gonadal deficiency, eunuchism, was deliberately induced. If the history of the involvement of the testes in reproduction is an old one, it is far from complete. In the following paragraphs, the current status of our knowledge of testicular physiology will be briefly reviewed.

In 1949, Barr and Bertram described a darkly staining chromatin material located at or very near the inner side of the nuclear membrane of neural tissue from female cats. This clump was conspicuously absent in tissue from males. In the ensuing years, comparable findings were obtained from human tissues. Properly stained material obtained from the buccal mucosa of the female was found to contain nuclear sex chromatin in 50 to 60 per cent of the cells examined. Cells derived from males contained nuclear sex chromatin, presumably artefactual, in 1 to 2 per cent of the cells counted. In 1954, while studying smears of human blood cells, Davidson and Smith found several clumps of chromatin lying beyond the main mass of nuclear material of the polymorphonuclear leukocytes of females but not of males. The ovoid clump was attached to the nucleus by a fine strand, producing a characteristic "drumstick" form. It is now generally accepted that the female nuclear sex chromatin of buccal mucosal cells (the "Barr" body) and the "drumstick" of the polymorphonuclear leukocyte represent the same phenomenon, presumably an inactivated X chromosome. The Lyon hypothesis, which attempts to explain the presence of female chromatin material, is discussed in Chapter 3.

Each human somatic cell (i.e., all cells other than germ cells) normally contains 46 chromosomes, 22 pairs of autosomes, and 2 sex chromosomes. This number is double (or diploid) the basic complement (termed the *haploid number*) contained in mature germ cells. In the normal female, the sex chromosomes are both X; in the normal male, there is one X and one Y chromosome.

Fetal Development of the Gonads, Genital Ducts, and External Genitalia

Until about the seventh week of fetal life, the primitive gonads have no histologic features that would permit them to be identified as male or female. If the genotype of the fetus is XY, a testis-determining gene is present, causing the gonad to transform into a testis; if the genotype is XX, the gonad continues to grow but remains undifferentiated until about the tenth or eleventh week, when primordial germ cells become transformed into oogonia. By the eighth week, the fetal testis contains functioning Leydig cells, which secrete testosterone. The presence of the latter hormone stimulates the development of the wolffian genital ducts, precursors of the epididymis, vas deferens,

and seminal vesicles. Somewhat later, at about the eleventh week, the primordial structures of the external genitalia (the genital tubercle, urethral folds, labial swellings, and urogenital sinus) begin to mature. Current evidence suggests that these latter structures are relatively insensitive to testosterone per se but are responsive to dihydrotestosterone (DHT). These target tissues contain a 5-α reductase that converts testosterone to DHT. Normal sexual development in the fetal male requires not only maturation of the male genital ducts and external genitalia but also regression of the female or müllerian ducts (precursors of the fallopian tubes, uterus, and upper vagina). This process begins at about the eighth week and appears to be prompted by a nonsteroidal, high molecular weight substance, müllerian duct regression factor, elaborated by the Sertoli cells of the testes.

Apparently, ovarian function plays little or no role in the fetal sexual development of the female. In the absence of testicular influences, the fetal internal and external genitalia mature into female structures. Patients who have Turner's syndrome, in which the karyotype is XO and gonads are primitive clusters of cells, invariably have a female phenotype.

The presence of testosterone in fetal life not only is required for normal male sexual development but also has an important influence on the developing central nervous system. Results of animal studies have shown that testicular deficiency at a critical time in fetal life results in impaired male sexual behavior in adult life.

Postnatal Testicular Function

The secretory activity of the testes in utero is probably stimulated by the high levels of placental chorionic gonadotropin. Not surprisingly, the fetal testis resembles the adult gonad histologically.

Following delivery, the testes become quiescent but probably not completely inactive. Recent careful studies indicate that there are measurable levels of both gonadotropins and androgens beginning in early childhood. The mechanisms that initiate pubescence are poorly understood. Presumably, the primary signal arises from the hypothalamus or higher sites in the central nervous system. In any event, at an average age of between 11 and 12 years plasma LH levels increase (FSH increases occur at an earlier age) and the testes enlarge, mainly owing to an increase in the volume of the seminiferous tubules. Leydig cell function is stimulated by LH, resulting in a marked increase in plasma testosterone. The latter is responsible for the development of male secondary sexual characteristics, including changes in external genitalia, body hair, voice, musculature, libido, and potentia. Eventually, this surge of androgens causes closure of the epiphyses of the long bones and growth ceases, but only after a pubescent growth spurt of 6 or more inches. If the sex steroid is deficient, epiphyseal closure is delayed and growth of the long bones continues. The result is the eunuchoid habitus characteristic of hypogonadism. In normal adults, span is approximately equal to height, and the lower segment of the body (measured from the top of the symphysis to the floor) equals the upper segment. In the eunuchoid subject, span and the lower segment exceed height and the upper segment, respectively.

The Adult Testis: Biosynthesis, Transport, and Action of Testosterone

The adult testis is approximately 4.5 cm by 2.5 cm and weighs between 15 and 20 gm. It is composed of two major elements: (1) Leydig or interstitial cells, which make up approximately 10 per cent of testicular volume, and (2) the seminiferous tubules, lined with the spermatogonia and Sertoli cells, composing about 75 per cent of the volume of the testes. Each day, the Leydig cells elaborate approximately 7 mg of testosterone and 2 mg of its immediate precursor, androstenedione, and the seminiferous tubules release about 150,000,000 spermatozoa.

The biosynthesis of testosterone follows the same basic pathway as that of the adrenal cortical steroids (Fig. 34–12). Either acetate or cholesterol can serve as the basic precursor; pregnenolone and 17-alpha-hydroxyprogesterone are important intermediaries. Once secreted, 98 per cent of the testosterone circulates in the plasma bound to a specific beta globulin, sex-steroid binding globulin (SSBG), and albumin. The normal range of testosterone in young adults is 300 to 1000 ng/100 ml. There may be a progressive decline in serum testosterone after middle age. In females, the normal range for serum testosterone is 34 to 90 ng/100 ml. In the peripheral tissues, testosterone is converted to dihydrotestosterone. The relative roles of these two androgens in the development and maintenance of the sexual characteristics of the male has been clarified by studies of patients who have familial 5 α-reductase deficiency (see page 1036). The proposed mechanism of action of the sex steroids including testosterone was mentioned previously.

Regulation of Testicular Function
(Fig. 34–14)

The evidence for a negative feedback relationship between the Leydig cells and the hypothalamic-pituitary axis is quite convincing. Kastin and colleagues have identified the hypothalamic substances capable of initiating the LH release from the anterior pituitary; this factor has been termed *gonadotropin-releasing hormone (GnRH)*.

LH acts on the testes to increase the conversion rate of cholesterol to pregnenolone, the rate-limiting step in the formation of testosterone. Cyclic AMP appears to function as an intermediary or second messenger in this action of LH. Above a critical concentration (the set point), plasma testosterone interferes with the release of LH. It is not clear whether this is accomplished by inhibition of LHRH secretion or by a direct inhibitory effect of testosterone on the anterior pituitary. In either event, the decline in plasma LH results in a decrease in testosterone secretion, completing the negative feedback loop.

The relationship between the anterior pituitary and the seminiferous tubules is not as clear-cut. It appears certain that FSH is required for spermatogenesis. In the absence of FSH, the germinal epithelium desquamates and the seminiferous tubules become fibrotic or remain infantile. Contrariwise, in those circumstances in which there is primary injury to the germinal epithelium, there is an increase in FSH secretion. This occurs even when Leydig cell function (and hence testosterone production) remains normal, as, for example, in primary seminiferous tubule failure. Such observations suggest that a substance capable of retarding FSH secretion is elaborated by the germinal epithelium. Indeed, several investigators have labeled this material *inhibin*. Current evidence suggests that inhibin is a protein secreted by the Sertoli cells.

CLINICAL ENTITIES

Klinefelter's Syndrome (Seminiferous Tubule Dysgenesis)

Klinefelter's syndrome is among the most common causes of male infertility and hypogonadism. Although reports of this entity had been published earlier, in 1942 Klinefelter, Reifenstein, and Albright emphasized the features of the syndrome in a paper significantly entitled "A Syndrome Characterized by Gynecomastia, Aspermatogenesis without A-Leydigism and Increased Excretion of Follicle-Stimulating Hormone." This report described nine patients who had small testes, gynecomastia, and increased FSH titers. The stature of the patients varied from normal to slightly eunuchoid, but all had good muscular development and masculine secondary sexual characteristics. The histologic alterations in the testes consisted of hyalinization of the seminiferous tubules, with loss of Sertoli cells and spermatogonia elements; the interstitial cells appeared normal. Subsequent experience with many patients has revealed that impaired Leydig cell function, reflected by subnormal levels of circulating testosterone, eunuchoid habitus, and underdeveloped secondary sexual characteristics, is a common feature of the syndrome.

	Father	Mother	Offspring, genotype	Offspring, phenotype
I. Nondisjunction in the father	(a) 22 + O	22 + X	45 + XO	Turner's syndrome
	(b) 22 + XY	22 + X	47 + XXY	Klinefelter's syndrome
II. Nondisjunction in the mother	(c) 22 + X	22 + XX	47 + XXX	"Super female"
	(d) 22 + X	22 + O	45 + XO	Turner's syndrome
	(e) 22 + Y	22 + XX	47 + XXY	Klinefelter's syndrome
	(f) 22 + Y	22 + O	45 + YO	Nonviable

The realization of the etiologic role of chromosomal abnormalities in the manifestations of Klinefelter's syndrome is one of the most exciting events in the history of endocrinology. Plunkett and Barr reported chromatin-positive cells in patients who had Klinefelter's syndrome. The disparity between the chromatin sex pattern ("female") and the physiognomy of the patients (male) was clarified when the chromosomal constitution of patients with classic Klinefelter's syndrome was identified as 47, XXY. Thus, it now appears certain that the pathogenesis of Klinefelter's syndrome begins with an abnormal meiotic phase in one of the parents. The most common abnormality consists of failure of the sex chromosomes of the dividing cell to move away from one another and is termed *nondisjunction*. In the male parent, the gamete that results from nondisjunction has a chromosomal constitution of either 22 + XY or 22 + O; in the female, it is 22 + XX or 22 + O. The possible chromosomal constitutions of the fertilized ova, resulting from union of an abnormal with a normal gamete, are summarized in the preceding chart. Thus, Klinefelter's syndrome can

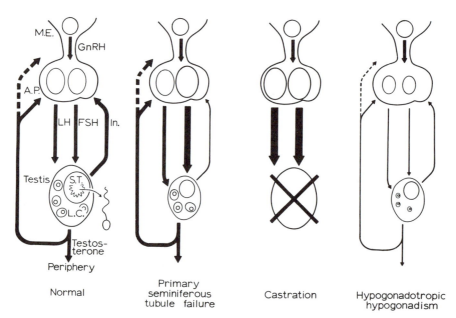

Figure 34–14 Anterior pituitary-testicular relationships.
Normal: The anterior pituitary (A.P.) secretes LH, which stimulates the Leydig cells (L.C.) to secrete testosterone. Rising levels of testosterone inhibit further LH secretion, completing the negative feedback loop. The anterior pituitary also secretes FSH, which stimulates the seminiferous tubules (S.T.) and spermatogenesis. The release of an FSH-suppressing humoral substance, termed *inhibin* (In.), by the seminiferous tubules has recently been established. The release of gonadotropin-releasing hormone (GnRH) by the median eminence (M.E.) of the hypothalamus is necessary for pituitary secretion of LH and FSH; the negative feedback effects of testosterone and inhibin may take place at the pituitary, the hypothalamus, or both. Although the drawing shows LH and FSH being produced in separate pituitary cells, evidence suggests that they may be produced in the same gonadotropic cell.
Primary seminiferous tubule failure: For unknown causes, the seminiferous tubules undergo atrophy, and spermatogenesis ceases; pituitary secretion of FSH is high. Leydig cell function remains intact.
Castration: When both Leydig cell and seminiferous tubular elements of the testes are lost, pituitary secretion of both LH and FSH is markedly increased.
Hypogonadotropic hypogonadism: Isolated loss of gonadotropin secretion by the pituitary in the pubescent male results in both sterility and underdeveloped male secondary sexual characteristics. Some of these cases may be due to GnRH deficiency.

arise from abnormal meiosis in either the father, as in (b), or the mother, as in (e).

Although classic Klinefelter's syndrome is usually associated with a karyotype 47,XXY, several variants of the syndrome have been reported (see Chapter 3). For example, if there is mosaicism (more than one stem line) of the sex chromosomes (e.g., XXY/XY), there may be few clinical abnormalities. However, when there is more than one abnormality of chromosomal division, as rarely occurs, there may be more than one supernumerary X chromosome, such as 48,XXXY and 49,XXXXY. In general, patients who have such chromosomes have more profound disturbances of gonadal function. The spectrum of Klinefelter's syndrome from both clinical and chromosomal standpoints was reviewed by Paulsen and coworkers in 1968.

The "Fertile Eunuch" Syndrome

Some patients have been reported to have eunuchoid habitus and decreased libido but to have normal fertility and to be of normal or near normal height. Histologic examination of testicular biopsy specimens has revealed normal seminiferous tubules but greatly reduced numbers of Leydig cells. The presumed pathogenesis of this uncommon condition—an isolated deficiency of pituitary LH, with normal FSH secretion—has recently been confirmed by radioimmunoassay determinations of plasma gonadotropins.

Hypogonadotropic Hypogonadism

When the gonadotropins FSH and LH, which are required to maintain normal testicular function in the male, are deficient or absent, as frequently occurs in patients who have pituitary tumors, both the germinal and Leydig cell elements of the testes become atrophic. Spermatogenesis ceases, and the level of circulating testosterone falls dramatically. The consequences of the latter event evolve slowly; the patient's libido falters, and there is loss of muscle mass and eventually loss of facial and body hair. For a time, the testicular changes are reversible, as shown by their response to the administration of replacement therapy such as human chorionic gonadotropin (HCG). However, after a period estimated at between 1 and 5 years, the testes become unresponsive to hormonal stimulation.

If the gonadotropins are deficient at the time of pubescence, the changes characteristic of that period do not take place. The external genitalia remain infantile; body form, hair distribution, and voice remain feminine; and the epiphyses of the long bones remain open, permitting an increase in eventual height.

An interesting familial variety of prepubertal hypogonadotropin deficiency in which the affected patients have a greatly impaired or absent sense of smell (hyposmia or anosmia), Kallmann's syndrome, was described earlier in this chapter.

Hereditary Male Pseudohermaphroditism (MPH)

The term *male pseudohermaphroditism* is used to refer to the condition of individuals who have male karyotypes and gonadal tissue but ambiguous or feminine external genitalia. This is a rare condition, but the elucidation of the mechanisms that underlie this problem has done much to clarify the normal sexual differentiation and the mode of action of testosterone. From the known sequence of events in normal male sex development in the fetus, one can predict the loci of defects that could lead to male pseudohermaphroditism. First, failure of elaboration of müllerian duct regression factor by the Sertoli cells could result in the development of female internal genitalia. Uteri and fallopian tubes have unexpectedly been found in male patients who undergo surgery for cryptorchidism or inguinal hernia. Because the external genitalia of these patients are essentially those of normal males, they are not, strictly speaking, examples of male pseudohermaphroditism. Further, there could be failure of androgen-mediated virilization of the wolffian ducts or the external genitalia analagen or both. Abnormalities in this sequence can be divided into two categories: (1) defects in testosterone biosynthesis, and (2) target tissue resistance to testosterone. In the first category, 5 distinct enzymatic deficiencies have been described, including cholesterol 20,22-desmolase, 3-β-OH dehydrogenase, 17 hydroxylase, 17,20-desmolase, and 17-β-OH oxidoreductase. The reactions catalyzed by these enzymes are shown in Figure 34–12.

In the second category, androgen resistance, three entities have been delineated: (1) androgen receptor disorders, (2) postreceptor disorders, and (3) defective conversion of testosterone to dihydrotestosterone (5α-reductase deficiency). In all three of these conditions, plasma testosterone levels are increased. The pathophysiologies of these entities are reasonably well established and are of sufficient interest to warrant a brief description.

Androgen Receptor Disorders. These X-linked recessive disorders have in common a quantitative or qualitative abnormality of the cytosolic androgen receptor in androgen-responsive tissues, leading to incomplete virilization. The most severe form of androgen resistance is known as *complete testicular feminization*. In this syndrome, the testes are usually located in the abdomen or the inguinal canals. Müllerian-regression factor is produced and acts normally, leading to absence of the fallopian tubes, uterus, and upper vagina. Testosterone is also secreted in normal amounts, but the androgen receptor defect leads to a failure of development of normal male internal (prostate, seminal vesicles, vas deferens) and external genitalia. At puberty, breast development and feminization of body contours occur, but there is minimal growth of axillary and pubic hair. Thus, patients who have this disorder have an external female phenotype in the presence of normal male gonads and a 46,XY karyotype. Circulating testosterone fails to suppress LH secretion, leading to elevated serum levels of both hormones. The elevated serum LH stimulates excessive estradiol secretion from the testes, and additionally, some of the testosterone is converted to estrogens in peripheral tissues; these elevated levels of circulating estrogens are responsible for both the feminization and the eventual feedback regulation of LH. Patients who have *incomplete testicular feminization* have a less severe receptor disorder; these individuals have a female phenotype but also manifest clitoromegaly and labioscrotal fusion and may undergo additional virilization at puberty.

Patients who have milder degrees of androgen resistance present with a male phenotype, broadly termed *Reifenstein's syndrome.* Clinical abnormalities may range from minimal (gynecomastia and azoospermia) to extensive (gynecomastia, sterility, severe perineoscrotal hypospadias, and incomplete labioscrotal fusion). As in testicular feminization, serum LH, testosterone, and estradiol levels are elevated.

Postreceptor Disorders. Some patients who have androgen resistance phenotypes will be found to have normal binding of androgen to cytosolic receptors. In these subjects, there may be abnormalities in translocation of the hormone-receptor complex to the nucleus, defects in the nuclear acceptor protein that interacts with the DHT-receptor complex, or even more distal abnormalities that affect the generation of messenger RNA. Nevertheless, clinical and laboratory findings in such patients are similar to those seen in receptor disorders.

5α-reductase Deficiency. This disorder, inherited in an autosomal recessive fashion, has as its basis the defective conversion of testosterone to dihydrotestosterone, a process normally accomplished by the cytosolic enzyme 5α-reductase. In individuals who are affected by this disorder, tissues that require dihydrotestosterone (DHT) for androgen action will remain unvirilized, whereas tissues that are capable of responding to testosterone will be normally virilized. Thus, at birth, male children who have 5α-reductase deficiency have a small phallus resembling a clitoris, a bifid scrotum, and a urogenital sinus that contains urethral and vaginal orifices. The vagina ends in a blind pouch. Internally, the wolffian structures are normally differentiated, and no müllerian structures are present. At puberty, partial virilization occurs, with deepening of the voice, increase in muscle mass, and growth of the external genitalia. The phallus grows to between 4 and 6 cm, the scrotum enlarges, and the testes enlarge and descend into the scrotum. Postpubertal males have little or no beard, no temporal hairline recession, no acne, and a smaller than normal prostate but normal muscle mass. Erection and ejaculation occur, and sperm counts are normal, although insemination usually does not occur because of the location of the urethral opening. The serum testosterone levels of affected subjects are greater and DHT levels are lower than those found in normal subjects. Thus, it appears that DHT is required for complete development of the fetal male external genitalia and for the pubertal effects of androgen on the prostate, sebaceous glands, and hair follicles. In contrast, testosterone itself appears sufficient to produce enlargement of the vocal cords and skeletal muscle at puberty, as well as to promote the development of wolffian duct structures in fetal life and the growth of the male external genitalia at puberty. Most remarkably, several patients who have this condition have undergone a spontaneous change in gender identity at puberty, assuming a normal male psychosexual role after having been raised as a female until that time.

OVARIES

PHYSIOLOGY

Follicle Development

The human ovaries are nodular bodies whose morphology and function are dynamically interwoven. Each weighs about 4 gm and measures 4 cm long by 2 cm wide. The adult ovary is estimated to contain 400,000 primordial follicles: oocytes encased in an avascular envelope of granulosa cells. At the onset of each menstrual cycle, several follicles migrate from the periphery of the ovary toward its center; concomitantly, there is proliferation of both the granulosa cells to form a multilayer band and the cells of the theca, which develop as an outer vascular mantle. As these processes progress, indentation of each follicle occurs, producing a cavity or antrum. Although these early events apparently do not require gonadotropins, FSH is required for the subsequent development of the mature graafian follicle. Of the several follicles that have undergone the changes just described, only one continues to develop; the remaining follicles regress into atretic forms. Under FSH stimulation, the chosen follicle accumulates fluid in its antrum, the cells of the granulosa and theca proliferate, and the whole mass migrates to the periphery. The ripened follicle comes to lie just beneath the outer covering of the ovary, creating a detectable bulge in its surface. As the follicle matures, the theca differentiates into the vascular theca interna and a theca externa, made up of stroma-like cells. The theca interna is composed of large glandular cells, which under FSH stimulation elaborate estrogen. Their secretory activity accelerates throughout the preovulatory stage, reaching a peak just before ovulation.

Ovulation

There is evidence that the rising level of estrogen (estradiol) triggers the release of LH, a positive feedback phenomenon, and that the high concentration of plasma LH acts on the theca cells to effect the release of the ovum from the ripened follicle. Following the extrusion of the ovum, the graafian follicle is transformed into the corpus luteum under the continued influence of LH. This complex process of luteinization includes cellular hypertrophy of both the granulosa and theca interna and their development into tissues that are capable of progesterone synthesis. If pregnancy does not occur, the corpus luteum continues to secrete progesterone and estrogen for 2 weeks, and as this function ceases, the levels of plasma estrogen and progesterone fall abruptly and menstruation occurs. The morphologic and functional changes that the ovary undergoes during the menstrual cycle have been lucidly described by Franchi.

Endometrial Changes

During the preovulatory or follicular phase of the cycle, proliferation of the endometrium occurs under the stimulation of estrogen. During the postovulatory or luteal phase of the cycle, both progesterone and estrogen act to slow down endometrial growth and to alter its structure in such a way that it is prepared for the nidation of a fertilized ovum. Glandular elements become engorged with secretions, and there is a substantial increase in vascularization. These uterine phases, corresponding to the follicular and luteal periods of ovarian function, are termed *proliferative* and *secretory,* respectively.

Pregnancy

There is evidence that the ovum is susceptible to fertilization for only a brief time following its release. When spermatozoa are present, fertilization usually occurs within 6 hours of ovulation in the distal third of the fallopian tube. The fertilized ovum then slowly migrates to the uterine cavity and becomes implanted in the secretory endometrium about 8 days after conception. Almost immediately, the implanted blastocyst or trophoblast begins to secrete chorionic gonadotropin, which stimulates the continued secretion of progesterone and estrogen by the corpus luteum. The latter hormones cause a continuing buildup of the endometrium, forming the decidua. Very early in pregnancy, the ovaries are the principal source of the necessary sex steroids; later, the feto-placental unit assumes this responsibility, and pregnancy proceeds without further assistance from the ovaries. It should be noted that the function of the corpus luteum becomes nearly autonomous following ovulation, secreting estrogen and progesterone with little stimulation from pituitary gonadotropins. Thus, the pituitary is not necessary for the maintenance of pregnancy, and only a very low level of circulating gonadotropins is required for corpus luteum function. This conclusion is substantiated by reports that describe the induction of ovulation by the administration of human menopausal and chorionic gonadotropins in women who had undergone hypophysectomy. The patients conceived, and the pregnancies proceeded uneventfully to a normal spontaneous delivery at term. Plasma levels of estrogen, pregnanediol (a metabolite of progesterone), and chorionic gonadotropin were normal throughout gestation.

Hypothalamic-Pituitary-Ovarian Interactions

Current evidence, albeit incomplete, indicates that the secretion of FSH and LH by the anterior pituitary is subservient to regulation by hypothalamic releasing factors, as mentioned earlier in this chapter. These, in turn, are influenced by plasma levels of estrogen, progesterone, and, undoubtedly, neural signals from higher centers. An understanding of the interactions among hypothalamic, pituitary, and ovarian factors in regulating the complex sequence of events of the menstrual cycle is gradually emerging. FSH stimulates follicle growth during the first (follicular) phase of the cycle; ovulation has been attributed to a rapid increase in plasma LH. Actually, both FSH and LH increase sharply just before ovulation. As previously mentioned, most investigators believe that the surge in LH is stimulated by the rapidly rising concentration of estrogen. Although FSH appears to be the principal factor that stimulates estrogen formation by the follicle, it is probable that both FSH and LH are necessary for optimal estrogen synthesis and release. Little if any progesterone is secreted by the developing follicle, a finding that is inconsistent with the thesis that progesterone stimulates the preovulatory surge of LH. It is generally agreed that following ovulation the corpus luteum secretes the sex steroids with relatively little stimulation from the pituitary for about 14 days. The abrupt fall in plasma estrogen and progesterone at the end of this time is responsible not only for initiating menstruation but also, in all likelihood, for the reinstitution of FSH secretion. Thus, the first day of menstruation signifies both the end and the beginning of the cycle.

Biosynthesis, Transport, Mechanism of Action, and Disposal of Estrogen and Progesterone

The formation of both estrogens and progesterone follows the basic pathway already described for cortisol synthesis (Fig. 34–12). In this sequence, cholesterol is converted to pregnenolone, the intermediate common to all the steroid hormones. Conversion of pregnenolone to progesterone requires two enzymes: an isomerase to shift the double bond in ring B to ring A, and a dehydrogenase to oxidize the hydroxy- at the 3 position to a keto- structure. Cleavage of the $C_{20,21}$ side chain yields an androgen, androstenedione, the major precursor of estrogen. Removal of C_{19} and aromatization of ring A yields estrone. Estrone and 17-beta-estradiol, the most potent estrogen, are interconvertible.

The ovarian hormones circulate bound to carrier proteins, sex-steroid binding globulin, and albumin. The plasma levels of estrone and estradiol in normal females range from 20 to 500 pg/ml, depending on the time of the cycle. Plasma progesterone concentrations average about 140 ng/100 ml during the follicular phase and about 1000 ng/100 ml during the luteal phase. These steroid hormones are inactivated primarily in the liver by conversion to water-soluble glucuronide and sulfate derivatives. Pregnanediol is the chief excretory metabolite of progesterone, and its content in a 24-hour urine collection provides another index of progesterone activity.

The principal functions of the ovarian hormones are to interact with both the hypothalamic-pituitary unit and the uterus to orchestrate the tightly integrated sequence of follicular development, ovulation, corpus luteum formation, and either menstruation or pregnancy. Beyond their direct effects on reproduction, the ovarian hormones, especially estrogen, are necessary for the development and maintenance of secondary sexual characteristics in the female. Estrogens also appear to promote epiphyseal closure and thus the termination of longitudinal growth, a role comparable to that of testosterone in the male. Estrogen deficiency in the adult female is associated with osteoporosis.

CLINICAL ENTITIES

Ovarian Failure

Insufficient ovarian function is manifested by amenorrhea and other evidence of estrogen deficiency. Such a state may arise as a consequence of hypothalamic or pituitary disease, as previously mentioned, or may be due to a disorder of the ovary itself. These two broad categories may be readily distinguished by measuring serum gonado-tropins. In the presence of estrogen deficiency due to ovarian disease (termed *ovarian failure*), normal feedback mechanisms lead to hypersecretion of LH and FSH with elevated serum levels of both these hormones. Conversely, ovarian hypofunction due to hypothalamic or pituitary disorders is characterized by low or low-normal serum gonadotropin levels with low serum estrogens. Two common examples of ovarian failure, menopause and Turner's syndrome, are discussed subsequently in greater detail.

Gonadal Dysgenesis (Turner's Syndrome)

In 1938, Turner described 7 females who had distinctive phenotypic abnormalities, including sexual infantilism, short stature, webbed neck, and an increased carrying angle of the upper extremities. Surgical explorations revealed gonadal tissue that consisted of only a primitive streak in the broad ligaments. On histologic examination, this tissue was sufficiently undifferentiated that it could not definitely be identified as ovarian. Because of the scanty amount and primitive nature of the gonadal tissue, the term *gonadal dysgenesis* was introduced and is currently the accepted, noneponymic designation of the syndrome.

Although uncommon (1 in 2000 live female births), the syndrome has been a focal point for the elucidation of sex determination. The determination of nuclear chromatin revealed that most patients who have Turner's syndrome have negative patterns. This finding, coupled with the high incidence of color blindness found by Polani and coworkers, led to the hypothesis that a deficient X chromosome was a basic factor in the pathogenesis of the syndrome. When it became possible to characterize the chromosomal constitution of individuals, the validity of the hypothesis was proved. Patients who had gonadal dysgenesis and a negative nuclear chromatin pattern were found to have a karyotype of 45,XO. Without the protection of a normal X chromosome, these individuals are subject to color blindness, a sex-linked recessive defect, with the same frequency as males. The 45, XO karytoype can be explained on the basis of nondisjunction occurring during gametogenesis in either parent. It is of academic interest that the site of abnormal meiosis can be determined in some instances by the pattern of red-green color blindness in the patient and her family. For instance, if both the patient and her father were color blind, one would suspect that nondisjunction occurred in oogenesis, depriving the patient of a maternal X chromosome.

The principal clinical features of Turner's syndrome are (1) primary amenorrhea, underdevelopment of secondary sexual characteristics, and infantile female internal genitalia; (2) short stature, usually less than 5 feet; (3) increased carrying angle of the arm (cubitus valgus); (4) webbed neck (pterygium colli); (5) shield chest; (6) coarctation of the aorta; (7) unexplained hypertension; and (8) skeletal defects. Of these, the first two are the most consistently seen. As with Klinefelter's syndrome, a spectrum of variants has been reported. Some of these result from mosaicism, in which some clonal lines have the deficiency of a sex chromosome (XO), whereas others are normal. Partial forms of the syndrome may also be due to deletion of a portion of an X chromosome. If the deletion is of the short arm of the X chromosome, the patient has short stature and the somatic features of the syndrome but may experience normal sexual development. If the deletion is of the long arm, the patient manifests sexual infantilism but is of normal stature and has few if any of the somatic anomalies.

The disorder does not seem to be familial. Only a few instances have been reported in which more than one member of a family has been affected. Neither does maternal age seem to be a causative factor; in a series of 27 cases, the mean maternal age was 24 years, the same as in a control group. Although theoretically one might expect Turner's syndrome to occur with the same frequency as Klinefelter's syndrome, this is not the case. The latter is considerably more common, occurring in about 1 of 500 newborn males.

The occurrence of short stature in an individual who has severe gonadal deficiency is at first glance inconsistent with the observation that castration in the prepubescent youth leads to a tall eunuchoid individual. The latter event is presumably related to delayed closure of epiphyses of long bones due to the absence of the gonadal hormones. If the basic abnormality in Turner's syndrome was limited to gonadal dysgenesis (i.e., equivalent to castration in infancy or youth), one would not expect short stature. Actually, Turner's syndrome is a multiple system disease, and short stature is

but one of several defects that are associated with, but not caused by, gonadal dysgenesis.

The typical patient who has Turner's syndrome seeks medical advice during the early adolescent years because of a delay in menarche and in the development of secondary sexual characteristics. The differential diagnosis of the triad of short stature, sexual infantilism, and primary amenorrhea involves Turner's syndrome and hypopituitarism. Often, additional clinical findings point to the correct diagnosis with near certainty. A webbed neck, coarctation of the aorta, or other stigmata of Turner's syndrome in a patient who has this triad would be virtually diagnostic. On the other hand, findings such as bitemporal hemianopsia would implicate a primary disease of the pituitary. When such features are absent or equivocal, the diagnosis can be established by appropriate laboratory studies. Examination of buccal mucosal scrapings reveals a negative chromatin pattern in 60 per cent of the cases of Turner's syndrome. Karyotypes prepared from leukocytes reveal a modal chromosomal constitution of 45, XO in most cases. Determination of serum gonadotropins usually provides a clear separation between the two entities, the concentrations being very low or absent in hypopituitarism and higher than normal in Turner's syndrome. The latter finding reflects the absence of feedback inhibition of the anterior pituitary by sex steroids. Another test of pituitary function, determination of growth hormone secretory capacity, is almost always abnormal in pituitary infantilism. The clinical and laboratory findings in these two conditions are contrasted in Table 34–7.

Menopause

Between the ages of 40 and 60 years, normal women experience the gradual loss of ovarian

TABLE 34–7 DIFFERENTIAL DIAGNOSIS OF PITUITARY INFANTILISM AND GONADAL DYSGENESIS (TURNER'S SYNDROME) IN THE ADOLESCENT OR YOUNG ADULT FEMALE

	Turner's Syndrome	Pituitary Infantilism
Stature	<5 feet	<5 feet
Bone age	Delayed-normal*	Marked delay
Secondary sexual characteristics: breasts, vagina, uterus, tubes, sexual hair	Infantile Delayed	Infantile Absent
Serum gonadotropins	Elevated	Low
Nuclear chromatin pattern	Negative	Positive
Sex chromosomal constitution	XO, XX/XO, or XX	XX
Hypertension	Frequent (even in absence of coarctation)	Absent
Other findings	Webbed neck, cubitus valgus, coarctation of aorta, skeletal defects	Headaches, visual field defects

*Because of delay in epiphyseal closures, bone age appears retarded in the adolescent. By early adulthood (e.g., 25 years), bone age is normal, adult.

function. Over the course of months or years, menses become less frequent and eventually cease entirely. Concomitantly, evidence of estrogen deficiency may appear, with some degree of breast atrophy and thinning of the vaginal epithelium. Bone mineral loss accelerates after menopause, with symptomatic osteoporosis often developing after several years of lack of estrogen. Many women are troubled by "hot flashes," brief episodes of flushing followed by profuse perspiration, during menopause. These uncomfortable occurrences have recently been shown to coincide with pulses of gonadotropin secretion, suggesting that both events originate in the central nervous system. Estrogen treatment, which suppresses the elevated serum gonadotropins, also abolishes the hot flashes and reverses the findings of estrogen deficiency; in addition, bone mineral content is stabilized.

Androgens in the Female

In women, as in men, the adrenal gland produces a large amount of weak androgens and androgen precursors (principally androstenedione and dehydroepiandrosterone sulfate), which are responsible for the development of pubic and axillary hair at the time of puberty. In addition, the normal ovary directly secretes small amounts of testosterone and androstenedione. A mild excess of circulating androgens often leads to hirsutism, with growth of coarse, dark terminal hairs on the face, chest, abdomen, and extremities. Such a condition may result from a variety of disorders, the two most important being polycystic ovary syndrome and so-called idiopathic hirsutism; perhaps 10 per cent of the women who have hirsutism may have a mild form of congenital adrenal hyperplasia. Serum androgens are often mildly elevated in women who have hirsutism.

Androgen excess more severe than that seen in simple hirsutism may produce virilization, with temporal hairline recession, deepening of the voice, increased muscle mass, and clitoromegaly, in addition to hirsutism. The underlying condition is often a steroid-secreting neoplasm of the adrenal glands or ovaries. Serum androgens are greatly elevated, often to the normal male range.

REFERENCES

GENERAL

Bondy, P. K., and Rosenberg, L. E. (Eds.): Metabolic Control and Disease. 8th ed. Philadelphia, W. B. Saunders Co., 1980.

Hershman, J. M. (Ed.): Endocrine Pathophysiology: A Patient-oriented Approach. 2nd ed. Philadelphia, Lea and Febiger, 1982.

Stanbury, J. B., Wyngaarden, J. B., Fredrickson, D. S., et al.: The Metabolic Basis of Inherited Disease. 5th ed. New York, McGraw-Hill, Inc., 1983.

Williams, R. H. (Ed.): Textbook of Endocrinology. 6th ed. Philadelphia, W. B. Saunders Co., 1981.

INTRODUCTION, PATHOPHYSIOLOGY OF ENDOCRINE DISEASE

Baxter, J. D., and Funder, J. W.: Hormone receptors (Medical Progress). N. Engl. J. Med. 301:1149, 1979.

Flier, J. S., Kahn, C. R., Roth, J., and Bar, R. S.: Antibodies that impair receptor binding in an unusual diabetic syndrome with severe insulin resistance. Science 190:63, 1975.

Grody, W. W., Schrader, W. T., and O'Malley, B. W.: Activation, transformation, and subunit structure of steroid hormone receptors. Endocr. Rev. 3:141, 1982.

Heinsimer, J. A., and Lefkowitz, R. J.: Adrenergic receptors: biochemistry, regulation, molecular mechanism, and clinical implication. J. Lab. Clin. Med. 100:641, 1982.

Huxley, J. S.: Chemical regulation and the hormone concept. Biol. Rev. 10:427, 1935.

Kahn, C. R. (Moderator): NIH Conference. Receptors for peptide hormones; new insights into the pathophysiology of disease states in man. Ann. Intern. Med. 86:205, 1977.

Liddle, G. W., et al.: Clinical and laboratory studies of ectopic humoral syndromes. Recent Prog. Horm. Res. 25:283, 1969.

Malbon, C. C.: Avenues of adrenergic research (editorial). J. Lab. Clin. Med. 94:381, 1979.

McEwen, B. S.: Interactions between hormones and nerve tissues. Sci. Am., 235:48, July, 1976.

Odell, W. D., and Moyer, D. L.: Hormone measurement. In Physiology of Reproduction. St. Louis, The C. V. Mosby Co., 1971, pp. 1–13.

O'Malley, B. W., and Schrader, W. T.: The receptors of steroid hormones. Sci. Am. 234:32, 1976.

Oppenheimer, J. H.: Thyroid hormone action at the cellular level. Science 203:971, 1979.

Pastan, I., and Pearlman, R. L.: Regulation of gene transcription in Escherichia coli by cyclic AMP. In Greengard, P., Paoletti, R., and Robison, G. A. (Eds.): Advances in Cyclic Nucleotide Research. Vol. 1. New York, Raven Press, 1972.

Pollet, R. J., and Levey, G. S.: Principles of membrane receptor physiology and their application to clinical medicine. Ann. Intern. Med. 92:663, 1980.

Robison, G. A., Butcher, R. W., and Sutherland, E. W.: Cyclic AMP. New York, Academic Press, 1971.

Roth, J., Neville, D. M., Kahn, C. R., and Gorden, P.: Hormone resistance and hormone sensitivity. N. Engl. J. Med. 296:277, 1977.

Roth, J., and Taylor, S. I.: Receptors for peptide hormones: alterations in diseases of humans. Annu. Rev. Physiol. 44:639, 1982.

THE HYPOTHALAMUS

Anderson, M. S., et al.: Synthetic thyrotropin-releasing hormone. N. Engl. J. Med. 285:1279, 1971.

Besser, G. M.: Hypothalamus as an endocrine organ-I. Br. Med. J. 3:560, 613, 1974.

Goldstein, A.: Opioid peptides (endorphins) in pituitary and brain. Science 193:1081, 1976.

Guillemin, R., et al.: Growth hormone–releasing factor from a human pancreatic tumor that caused acromegaly. Science 218:585, 1982.

Jackson, I. M. D.: Thyrotropin-releasing hormone. N. Engl. J. Med. 306:145, 1982.

Kastin, A. J., et al.: Release of LH and FSH after administration of synthetic LH-releasing hormone. J. Clin. Endocrinol. Metab. 34:735, 1972.

Krieger, D. T., and Martin, J. B.: Brain peptides. N. Engl. J. Med. 304:876, 944, 1981.

Lieblich, J. M., et al.: Syndrome of anosmia with hypogonadotropic hypogonadism (Kallmann's syndrome). Clinical and laboratory studies in 23 cases. Am. J. Med. 73:506, 1982.

McCann, S. M.: Physiology and pharmacology of LHRH and somatostatin. Annu. Rev. Pharmacol. Toxicol. 22:491, 1982.

Meites, J., and Sonntag, W. E.: Hypothalamic hypophysiotropic hormones and neurotransmitter regulation: current views. Annu. Rev. Pharmacol. Toxicol. 21:295, 1981.

Morley, J. E.: The endocrinology of the opiates and opioid peptides. Metabolism 30:195, 1981.

Pittman, J. A., Jr., Haigler, E. D., Jr., Hershman, J. M., and Pittman, C. S.: Hypothalamic hypothyroidism. N. Engl. J. Med. 285:844, 1971.

Vale, W., et al.: Characterization of a 41-residue ovine hypothalamic peptide that stimulates secretion of corticotropin and β-endorphin. Science 213:1394, 1981.

ANTERIOR PITUITARY

Archer, D. E.: Current concepts of prolactin physiology in normal and abnormal conditions. Fertil. Steril. 28:125, 1977.

Daughaday, W. H.: Sulfation factor regulation of skeletal growth: a stable mechanism dependent on intermittent growth hormone secretion. Am. J. Med. 50:277, 1971.

Eipper, B. A., and Mains, R. E.: Structure and biosynthesis of Pro-ACTH/endorphin and related peptides. Endocr. Rev. 1:1, 1980.

Frantz, A. G.: Prolactin. N. Engl. J. Med. 298:201, 1978.

Gill, G. N.: Mechanism of ACTH action. Metabolism 21:571, 1972.

Goodman, H. G., Grumbach, M. M., and Kaplan, S. L.: Growth and growth hormone II. A comparison of isolated growth-hormone deficiency and multiple pituitary-hormone deficiencies in 35 patients with idiopathic hypopituitary dwarfism. N. Engl. J. Med. 278:57, 1968.

Jadresic, A., et al.: The acromegaly syndrome. Q. J. Med. 51:189, 1982.

Lanes, R., Plotnick, L. P., Spencer, E. M., et al.: Dwarfism associated with normal serum growth hormone and increased bioassayable, receptorassayable, and immunoassayable somatomedin. J. Clin. Endocrinol. Metab. 50:485, 1980.

Laron, Z., Pertzelan, A., and Mannheimer, S.: Genetic pituitary dwarfism with high serum concentration of growth hormone. A new inborn error of metabolism? Isr. J. Med. Sci. 2:162, 1966.

Merimee, T. J., Zapf, J., and Froesch, E. R.: Dwarfism in the pygmy. An isolated deficiency of insulin-like growth factor I. N. Engl. J. Med. 305:965, 1981.

Molitch, M. E., and Reichlin, S.: Hyperprolactinemic disorders. D. M. 28:number 9, June 1982.

Neelon, F. A., Goree, J. A., and Lebovitz, H. E.: The primary empty sella: clinical and radiographic characteristics and endocrine function. Medicine 52:73, 1973.

Nelson, D. H., Meakin, J. W., and Thorn, G. W.: ACTH-producing pituitary tumors following adrenalectomy for Cushing's syndrome. Ann. Intern. Med. 52:560, 1960.

Phillips, L. S., and Vassilopoulou-Sellin, R.: Somatomedins. N. Engl. J. Med. 302:371, 438, 1980.

Post, K. D., Jackson, I. M. D., and Reichlin, S.: The pituitary adenoma. New York, Plenum Publishing Corp., 1980.

Purnell, D. C., Randall, R. V., and Rynearson, E. H.: Postpartum pituitary insufficiency (Sheehan's syndrome): review of 18 cases. Mayo Clin. Proc. 39:321, 1964.

Raisz, L. G., and Kream, B. E.: Hormonal control of skeletal growth. Ann. Rev. Physiol. 43:225, 1981.

Ridgway, E. C., et al.: Thyrotropin and prolactin pituitary reserve in the "empty sella syndrome." J. Clin. Endocrinol. Metab. 41:968, 1975.

Sheehan, H. L., and Summers, V. K.: The syndrome of hypopituitarism. Q. J. Med. 18:319, 1949.

Snyder, P. J., et al.: Diagnostic value of thyrotropin-releasing hormone in pituitary and hypothalamic diseases. Ann. Intern. Med. 81:751, 1974.

Tyrrell, J. B., et al.: Cushing's disease: selective transphenoidal resection of pituitary microadenomas. N. Engl. J. Med. 298:753, 1978.

Wright, A. D., et al.: Mortality in acromegaly. Q. J. Med. 39:1, 1970.

POSTERIOR PITUITARY

Bartter, F. C.: The syndrome of inappropriate anti-diuretic hormone secretion (SIADH). D. M. November 1, 1973.

Coggins, C. H., and Leaf, A.: Diabetes insipidus. Am. J. Med. 42:807, 1967.

Martin, F. I. R.: Familial diabetes insipidus. Q. J. Med. 28:573, 1959.

Moses, A. M.: Diabetes insipidus and ADH regulation. Hosp. Pract. 12:37, 1977.

Robertson, G. L.: Thirst and vasopressin function in normal and disordered states of water balance. J. Lab. Clin. Med. 101:351, 1983.

Robison, G. A.: Isolation, assay, and secretion of individual human neurophysins. J. Clin. Invest. 55:360, 1975.

Thomas, W. C.: Diabetes insipidus (teaching clinic). J. Clin. Endocrinol. 17:565, 1957.

Whitesman, R., and Kleeman, C. R.: Water metabolism and the neurohypophyseal hormones. In Maxwell, M. H., and Kleeman, C. R. (Eds.): Clinical Disorders of Fluid and Electrolyte Metabolism. 3rd ed. New York, McGraw-Hill, Inc., 1980, pp. 591–607.

THYROID

Adams, D. D., and Purves, H. D.: Abnormal responses in the assay of thyrotropin. Proc. Otago. Med. Sch. 34:11, 1956.

Brown, J. S., and Steiner, A. L.: Medullary thyroid carcinoma and the syndromes of multiple endocrine adenomas. D. M. 28:number 11, August 1982.

Burke, G.: The triiodothyronine suppression test. Am. J. Med. 42:600, 1967.

Chopra, I. J., et al.: Pathways of metabolism of thyroid hormones. Recent Prog. Horm. Res. 34:531, 1978.

Favus, M. J., et al.: Thyroid cancer occurring as a late consequence of head-and-neck irradiation: evaluation of 1056 patients. N. Engl. J. Med. 294:1019, 1976.

Gavin, L., et al.: Extrathyroidal conversion of thyroxine to triiodothyronine and reverse triiodothyronine in humans. J. Clin. Endocrinol. Metab. 44:733, 1977.

Hershman, J. M., and Bray, G. A. (Eds.): The Thyroid: Physiology And Treatment. Oxford, Pergamon Press, 1979.

Larsen, P. R.: Tests of thyroid function. Med. Clin. North Am. 59:1063, 1975.

Larsen, P. R.: Hyperthyroidism. D. M. 22:number 10, July 1976.

Larsen, P. R.: Thyroid-pituitary interaction. N. Engl. J. Med. 306:23, 1982.

Robbins, J., et al.: Thyroxine transport properties of plasma, molecular properties and biosynthesis. Recent Prog. Horm. Res. 34:477, 1978.

Schimmel, M., and Utiger, R. D.: Thyroid and peripheral production of thyroid hormones. Ann. Intern. Med. 87:760, 1977.

Strakosch, C. R., et al.: Immunology of autoimmune thyroid diseases. N. Engl. J. Med. 307:1499, 1982.

Tunbridge, W. M. D., et al.: The spectrum of thyroid disease in a community: the Whickham survey. Clin. Endocrinol. 7:481, 1977.

Van Herle, A. J., et al.: The thyroid nodule. Ann. Intern. Med. 96:221, 1982.

Werner, S. C., and Ingbar, S. H. (Eds.): The Thyroid. 4th ed. New York, Harper and Row Publishers, Inc., 1978.

Woolf, P. D.: Transient painless thyroiditis with hyperthyroidism: a variant of lymphocytic thyroiditis? Endocr. Rev. 1:411, 1980.

ADRENAL CORTEX

Aron, D. C., et al.: Cushing's syndrome: problems in diagnosis. Medicine (Baltimore) 60:25, 1981.

Besser, G. M., and Edwards, C. R. W.: Cushing's syndrome. Clin. Endocrinol. Metab. 1:45, 1972.

Burke, C. W., and Beardwell, C. G.: Cushing's syndrome. Q. J. Med. 42:175, 1973.

Conn, J. W.: Primary aldosteronism, a new clinical syndrome. J. Lab. Clin. Med. 45:6, 1955.

Crapo, L.: Cushing's syndrome: a review of diagnostic tests. Metabolism 28:955, 1979.

Frawley, T. F.: Adrenal cortical insufficiency. In Eisenstein, A. B. (Ed.): The Adrenal Cortex. Boston, Little, Brown and Co., 1967, p. 439.

Gold, E. M.: The Cushing's syndromes: changing view of diagnosis and treatment. Ann. Intern. Med. 90:829, 1979.

Horton, R.: Aldosterone: a review of its physiology and diagnostic aspects of primary aldosteronism. Metabolism 22:1525, 1973.

Kotchen, T. A., and Guthrie, G. P., Jr.: Renin-angiotensin-aldosterone and hypertension. Endocr. Rev. 1:78, 1980.

Krieger, D. T.: Physiopathology of Cushing's disease. Endocr. Rev. 4:22, 1983.

Laragh, J. H.: Modern system for treating high blood pressure based on renin profiling and vasoconstriction-volume analysis. Am. J. Med. *61*:797, 1976.

Lee, P. A., et al.: Congenital Adrenal Hyperplasia. Baltimore, University Park Press, 1977.

Liddle, G. W.: Cushing's syndrome. *In* Eisenstein, A. B. (Ed.): The Adrenal Cortex. Boston, Little, Brown and Co., 1967, p. 523.

Mitchell, J. R. (Moderator), et al.: Renin-aldosterone profiling in hypertension. Ann. Intern. Med. *87*:596, 1977.

Mulrow, P. J.: Glucocorticoid-suppressible hyperaldosteronism. N. Engl. J. Med. *305*:1012, 1981.

Nerup, J.: Addison's disease. Acta Endocrinol. *76*:127, 1974.

New, M. I., DuPont, B., Grumbach, K., and Levine, L. S.: Congenital adrenal hyperplasia and related conditions. *In* Stanbury, J. B., et al. (Eds.): The Metabolic Basis of Inherited Disease. 5th ed. New York, McGraw-Hill, Inc., 1983, pp. 973–1000.

Thorn, G. W.: The adrenal cortex. I. Historical aspects. II. Clinical considerations. Johns Hopkins Med. J. *123*:49, 1968.

Urbanic, R. C., and George, J. M.: Cushing's disease—18 years experience. Medicine *60*:14, 1981.

Weinberger, M. H., et al.: Primary aldosteronism. Ann. Intern. Med. *90*:386, 1979.

PARATHYROIDS

Albright, F., Burnett, C. H., Smith, P. H., and Parson, W.: Pseudohypoparathyroidism: an example of the "Seabright-Bantam syndrome." Report of three cases. Endocrinology *30*:922, 1942.

Albright, F., and Reifenstein, E. C., Jr.: The Parathyroid Glands and Metabolic Bone Disease. Baltimore, Williams and Wilkins, 1948.

Auerbach, G. D., et al.: Structure, synthesis and mechanisms of action of PTH. Recent Prog. Horm. Res. *28*:353, 1972.

Austin, L. A., and Heath, H.: Calcitonin physiology and pathophysiology. N. Engl. J. Med. *304*:269, 1981.

Broadus, A. E., et al.: The importance of circulating 1,25-dihydroxyvitamin D in the pathogenesis of hypercalciuria and renal-stone formation in primary hyperparathyroidism. N. Engl. J. Med. *302*:421, 1980.

Copp, D. H., et al.: Evidence for calcitonin—a new hormone from the parathyroid that lowers blood calcium. Endocrinology *70*:638, 1962.

DeLuca, H. F., and Schnoes, H. K.: Metabolism and mechanism of action of vitamin D. Ann. Rev. Biochem. *45*:631, 1976.

Farfel, Z., et al.: Defect of receptor-cyclase coupling protein in pseudohypoparathyroidism. N. Engl. J. Med. *303*:237, 1980.

Greenberg, S. R., Karabell, S., and Saade, G. A.: Pseudohypoparathyroidism: a disease of the second messenger (3'5'-cyclic AMP). Arch. Intern. Med. *129*:633, 1972.

Habener, J. E., and Schillor, A. L.: Pathogenesis of renal osteodystrophy—a role for calcitonin? N. Engl. J. Med. *296*:1112, 1977.

Harris, W. H., and Heaney, R. P.: Skeletal renewal and metabolic bone disease. N. Engl. J. Med. *280*:193, 1969.

Hermans, P. E., Gorman, C. A., Martin, W. J., and Kelly, P. J.: Pseudopseudohypoparathyroidism (Albright's hereditary osteodystrophy): a family study. Mayo Clin. Proc. *39*:81, 1964.

Kleeman, C. R., Massry, S. G., Coburn, J. W., and Popovtzer, M. M.: The problem and unanswered questions: renal osteodystrophy, soft-tissue calcification and disturbed divalent ion metabolism in chronic renal failure. Arch. Intern. Med. *124*:262, 1969.

Krane, S. M.: Selected features of the clinical course of hypoparathyroidism. J.A.M.A. *178*:472, 1961.

Lafferty, F. W.: Pseudohyperparathyroidism. Medicine *45*:247, 1966.

Norman, A. G., and Henry, H.: 1,25 Dihydroxycholecalciferol—a hormonally active form of vitamin D. Recent Prog. Horm. Res. *30*:431, 1974.

Rasmussen, H.: Ionic and hormonal control of calcium homeostasis. Am. J. Med. *59*:567, 1971.

Sinha, T. K., Deluca, H. G., and Bell, N. H.: Evidence for a defect of 1, 25-dihydroxyvitamin D in pseudohypoparathyroidism. Metabolism *26*:731, 1977.

Spiegel, A. M., et al.: Pseudohypoparathyroidism: the molecular basis for hormone resistance—a retrospective (editorial). N. Engl. J. Med. *307*:679, 1982.

Stanbury, S. W., Lumb, G. A., and Mawer, E. B.: Osteodystrophy developing spontaneously in the course of chronic renal failure. Arch. Intern. Med. *124*:274, 1969.

Van Dop, C., and Bourne, H. R.: Pseudohypoparathyroidism. Annu. Rev. Med. *34*:259, 1983.

ADRENAL MEDULLA

Bravo, E. L., et al.: Circulating and urinary catecholamines in pheochromocytoma. N. Engl. J. Med. *301*:682, 1979.

Bravo, E. L.: Clonidine suppression test. N. Engl. J. Med. *305*:623, 1981.

Cryer, P. E.: Physiology and pathophysiology of the human sympathoadrenal neuroendocrine system. N. Engl. J. Med. *303*:436, 1980.

Engelman, K.: Pheochromocytoma. Clin. Endocrinol. Metab. *6*:779, 1977. Philadelphia, W. B. Saunders Co.

Page, L. B., and Copeland, R. B.: Pheochromocytoma. D. M. January 1968.

TESTES

Baker, H. W. G., et al.: Testicular control of follicle stimulating hormone secretion. Recent Prog. Horm. Res. *32*:429, 1976.

Barr, M. L., and Bertram, E. G.: A morphological distinction between neurons of the male and female, and the behavior of the nucleolar satellite during accelerated nucleoprotein synthesis. Nature *163*:676, 1949.

Burger, H., and deKretser, D. (Eds.): The Testis. New York, Raven Press, 1981.

Davidson, W. M., and Smith, D. R.: A morphological sex difference in the polymorphonuclear neutrophil leukocytes. Br. Med. J. *2*:6, 1954.

Griffin, J. E., and Wilson, J. D.: The syndromes of androgen resistance. N. Engl. J. Med. *302*:198, 1980.

Hecht, F., Wyandt, H. E., and Erbe, R. W.: Revolutionary cytogenetics. N. Engl. J. Med. *285*:1482, 1971.

Hsueh, W. A., Hsu, T. H., and Federman, D. D.: Endocrine features of Klinefelter's syndrome. Medicine *57*:447, 1978.

Imperato-McGinley, J., et al.: Androgens and the evolution of male gender identity among male pseudohermaphrodites with 5α-reductase deficiency. N. Engl. J. Med. *300*:1233, 1979.

Kallman, F. J., Schoenfeld, W. A., and Barrera, S. E.: The genetic aspects of primary eunuchoidism. Am. J. Ment. Defic. *48*:203, 1944.

Klinefelter, H. F., Jr., Reifenstein, E. C., Jr., and Albright, F.: Syndrome characterized by gynecomastia, aspermatogenesis without A-Leydigism, and increased excretion of follicle stimulating hormone. J. Clin. Endocrinol. *2*:615, 1942.

Lippe, B. M.: Ambiguous genitalia and pseudohermaphroditism. Pediatr. Clin. North Am. 26:91, 1979.

Odell, W. D., and Swerdloff, R. S.: Abnormalities of gonadal function in men. Clin. Endocrinol. *8*:149, 1978.

Park, I. J., et al.: An etiologic and pathogenic classification of male hermaphroditism. Am. J. Obstet. Gynecol. *123*:505, 1975.

Parvinen, M.: Regulation of the seminiferous epithelium. Endocrine Rev. *3*:404, 1982.

Paulsen, C. A., et al.: Klinefelter's syndrome and its variants: a hormonal and chromosomal study. Recent Prog. Horm. Res. *24*:321, 1968.

Peterson, R. E., et al.: Male pseudohermaphroditism due to steroid 5α-reductase deficiency. Am. J. Med. *62*:170, 1977.

Plunkett, E. R., and Barr, M. L.: Cytologic test of sex in congenital testicular hypoplasia. J. Clin. Endocrinol. Metab. *16*:829, 1956.

OVARIES

Corral, J., Calderon, J., and Goldzieher, J. W.: Induction of ovulation and term pregnancy in a hypophysectomized woman. Obstet. Gynecol. *39*:397, 1972.

Ferguson-Smith, M. A.: Karyotype-phenotype correlations in gonadal dysgenesis and their bearing on the pathogenesis of malformations. J. Med. Genet. *2*:142, 1965.

Gerald, P. S.: Sex chromosome disorders. N. Engl. J. Med. *294*:706, 1976.

Ginsburg, J., and White, M. C.: Hirsutism and virilisation. Br. Med. J. *280*:369, 1980.

Goldberg, M. B., et al.: Gonadal dysgenesis in phenotypic female subjects. A review of eighty-seven cases, with cytogenetic studies in fifty-three. Am. J. Med. *44*:135, 1968.

Judd, H. L., et al.: Estrogen replacement therapy: indications and complications. Ann. Intern. Med. *98*:195, 1983.

Knobil, E.: The neuroendocrine control of the menstrual cycle. Recent Prog. Horm. Res. *36*:53, 1980.

McDonough, P. G., et al.: Phenotypic and cytogenetic findings in eighty-two patients with ovarian failure—changing trends. Fertil. Steril. *26*:638, 1977.

Means, A. R., and O'Malley, B. W.: Mechanism of estrogen action: early transcriptional and translational events. Metabolism *21*:357, 1972.

Penny, R., et al.: Correlation of serum follicular stimulating hormone (FSH) and luteinizing hormone (LH) as measured by radioimmunoassay in disorders of sexual development. J. Clin. Invest. *49*:1847, 1970.

Penny, R., Foley, T. P., Jr., and Blizzard, R. M.: Serum follicle-stimulating hormone and luteinizing hormone as measured by radioimmunoassay correlated with sexual development in hypopituitary subject. J. Clin. Invest. *51*:74, 1972.

Richards, J. S.: Hormonal control of ovarian follicular development: a 1978 perspective. Recent Prog. Horm. Res. *35*:343, 1979.

Sherman, B. M., and Korenman, S. G.: Hormonal characteristics of the human menstrual cycle throughout reproductive life. J. Clin. Invest. *55*:699, 1975.

Turner, H. H.: A syndrome of infantilism, congenital webbed neck and cubitus valgus. Endocrinology *23*:566, 1938.

Yen, S. S. C., and Jaffe, R. B. (Eds.): Reproductive Endocrinology: Physiology, Pathophysiology and Clinical Management. Philadelphia, W. B. Saunders Co., 1978.

35

The Endocrine Pancreas

Thomas W. Burns and David M. Klachko

INTRODUCTION

The endocrine pancreas consists of the islets of Langerhans, which are scattered throughout the gland. It has been estimated that the human pancreas contains about 1.5 million islets with a total weight of about 1 gm. Although the traditional view that islets are derived from endoderm has been challenged, recent evidence supports it. Approximately 75 per cent of the cells in each islet are the insulin-secreting beta (B) cells which tend to cluster centrally (Fig. 35–1A). Around the periphery lie the alpha (A), delta (D), and F (or PP) cells, which secrete glucagon, somatostatin, and pancreatic polypeptide, respectively. Of these, glucagon-secreting cells predominate, except in the posterior part of the head of the pancreas, which is rich in pancreatic polypeptide-secreting cells. Functional coupling between cells is suggested by the presence of gap junctions, not only between B cells but also between different types of cells such as A and B cells. Each islet is supplied by one or two afferent arterioles that branch into numerous capillaries; from this network, comparable to a renal glomerulus, efferent capillaries emerge to coalesce into venules outside the islet. The islets also are richly supplied with autonomic nerves. Thus, islet function may be modulated by neural control, by circulating metabolites and hormones, by intercellular communication via gap junctions, and by secretion of hormones into the surrounding interstitium (paracrine effects). The latter interactions have not yet been confirmed.

A brief review of the normal physiology of the endocrine pancreas will facilitate an understanding of the pathophysiology of the clinical entities that are described later in this chapter. The principal function of the endocrine pancreas is the secretion of insulin and other polypeptide hormones necessary for the orderly intracellular storage and retrieval of dietary nutrients such as glucose, amino acids, and triglyceride. It is not difficult to perceive the importance that insulin has in survival. Because food supply can be erratic, the animal capable of storing nutrient fuel during times of plenty had a great advantage over a species that could not. Furthermore, muscle and adipose tissue require insulin for glucose transport, but nervous tissue does not. Without the insulin mechanism, glucose would flow into muscle and adipose tissue cells in an unregulated fashion, resulting in recurrent hypoglycemia and impaired nervous system development and function.

INSULIN

BIOSYNTHESIS AND RELEASE

Insulin, elaborated by the B cells of the islets of Langerhans, has a molecular weight of 6000 and is composed of two chains (the alpha chain has 21 amino acids, the beta chain 30) linked by two sulfhydryl bonds. Steiner and coworkers demonstrated that insulin is derived from a larger molecule termed *proinsulin*. Proinsulin is relatively inactive, and normally little of it is secreted. It contains a connecting peptide composed of 33 amino acids, the C chain, which joins the N terminal of the alpha chain to the carboxyl end of the beta chain and which is cleaved off before insulin release. Although C peptide and insulin enter the circulation in equimolar quantities, the rate of disposal of C peptide is slower than that of insulin; thus, its plasma concentration tends to be greater than that of insulin. Diabetic patients receiving insulin therapeutically develop antibodies that interfere with the measurement of plasma insulin by radioimmunoassay but not with the radioimmunoassy for the C peptide. When first discovered, insulin-dependent diabetics have demonstrable levels of C peptide in their serum, indicating the presence of residual islet cell function. In most diabetics, circulating C peptide eventually declines over a period of years to zero or near zero levels. Typically, the pancreas of a normal adult contains approximately 200 units of insulin (equivalent to 8 mg); the average daily secretion of insulin ranges between 35 and 50 units. Although a number of physiologic events can alter insulin secretion, the most important regulatory factor is the concentration of glucose in the plasma perfusing the pancreas. When the plasma glucose level exceeds approximately 100 mg/dl, insulin release is stimulated; as plasma glucose falls, so does the rate of insulin secretion. However, even during prolonged fasting, when the plasma level of glucose remains low, a continuing basal secretion of insulin can be demonstrated. Other nutrients such as leucine and arginine also stimulate insulin release. Following oral ingestion of glucose, insulin secretion is greater than that induced by the same quantity of glucose given intravenously. This "incretin" phenomenon is due to the release of gastrointestinal hormones in response to food intake. These hormones include gastrin, secretin, pancreozymin, and a glucagon-like peptide. The one most important for potentia-

A

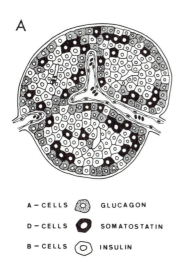

A – CELLS   GLUCAGON

D – CELLS   SOMATOSTATIN

B – CELLS   INSULIN

B

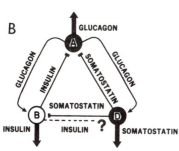

Figure 35–1 Postulated morphofunctional relations in the islets of Langerhans. Panel *a* shows a cross section of a normal islet. A heterocellular cortex, consisting of an outer rim of glucagon-containing A cells, surrounds the insulin-containing B cells and intervening somatostatin-containing D cells. The cortex often appears to penetrate the islet along the blood vessels. Panel *b* shows possible "paracrine" cell-cell interactions within the islet. The stimulatory actions of the peptides on neighboring cells are represented by thin arrows, and their inhibitory actions are indicated by short double bars near the A cell. Endocrine secretion of the polypeptides into the circulation is indicated by thick arrows. (Reproduced with permission from Unger, R. H., and Orci, L.: N. Engl. J. Med. *304*:1518, 1981.)

tion of insulin secretion appears to be GIP (gastric inhibitory polypeptide, or glucose-induced insulinotropic peptide). Insulin secretion is also influenced by catecholamines interacting with islet cell adrenergic receptor sites. Depending on the method of analysis, the fasting level of insulin ranges from 10 to 20 μU/ml and increases to 50 to 150 μU/ml following a meal or a glucose load. Insulin's half-life in plasma is less than 10 minutes, as it is rapidly cleared from the circulation by the liver and kidneys. The peak effect of intravenously administered insulin occurs between 30 and 60 minutes after infusion.

ACTIONS OF INSULIN

Investigators have not yet clarified the primary mechanism or mechanisms by which insulin exerts its metabolic effects, despite intensive efforts aimed at answering this question. A great deal is known about *what* insulin does, but relatively little is known regarding *how* it does it. There is good evidence that circulating insulin binds to specific receptors on the plasma membrane of cells and may then trigger the formation of a "second messenger" released from the membrane into the cytosol. Research suggests that this is an oligoglycopeptide that mediates the intracellular actions of insulin. These actions work in concert to promote anabolism by (1) the facilitation of the entry into cells of glucose, amino acids, and fatty acids; (2) the stimulation of anabolic pathways and suppression of catabolic pathways by phosphorylation or dephosphorylation of enzymes; and (3) the stimulation of production of energy donors necessary for anabolism (e.g., UTP).

The action of insulin on three metabolically important tissues—adipose tissue, muscle, and liver—is summarized as follows and illustrated more graphically in subsequent paragraphs in which the consequences of insulin deficiency are discussed.

Adipose Tissue. Insulin has profound effects on lipid metabolism. It stimulates lipogenesis, facilitates removal of triglyceride from the circulation, and inhibits lipolysis.

EFFECTS ON LIPOGENESIS. Insulin stimulates the transport of glucose into the fat cell and probably promotes the initial phosphorylation of glucose into glucose-6-phosphate. The ensuing metabolism of glucose-6-phosphate to acetyl-CoA stimulates lipogenesis in several ways:

1. Metabolism of glucose via the hexose monophosphate shunt generates NADH, the coenzyme required for fatty acid synthesis.

2. The metabolism of glucose provides two carbon fragments needed for fatty acid synthesis.

3. Metabolism of glucose via the Emden-Meyerhof pathway generates alpha glycerol-phosphate, which is necessary for the esterification of fatty acids to form triglycerides. Unphosphorylated glycerol is not reactive; accordingly, the glycerol derived from hydrolysis of triglyceride cannot be used in re-esterification, since adipose tissue does not contain a glycerol kinase.

Insulin has additional effects on fat metabolism in the periphery that are unrelated to its effect on glucose metabolism.

REGULATION OF PLASMA TRIGLYCERIDE. Circulating triglyceride does not enter the fat cell as such. It is hydrolyzed by a lipoprotein lipase present between the basement membrane of the capillary and the plasma membrane of the adipocyte. Fatty acids derived from this hydrolysis enter the adipocyte and are re-esterified. This lipase, necessary for the clearing of exogenous and endogenous triglyceride-bearing particles from the plasma, is insulin-dependent.

REGULATION OF LIPOLYSIS. The regulation of fat mobilization, or lipolysis, is complex and incompletely understood. In humans, catecholamines and insulin are the only hormones that have been shown to be physiologically important in controlling lipolysis. Epinephrine and norepinephrine interact with beta$_1$ and alpha$_2$ adrenergic receptors in the plasma membrane of fat cells. These receptors are linked to the adenylate cyclase–cyclic AMP system and mediate divergent effects on lipolysis: beta activation stimulates fatty acid release, whereas alpha stimulation inhibits it. In the fed state, the beta effect predominates, and epinephrine and norepinephrine cause an increase in lipolysis. During fasting, the balance shifts; the alpha effect predominates and the catecholamines cause a reduction in fatty acid release. Insulin is a potent inhibitor of lipolysis, and a fall in plasma insulin prompts an increase in lipolysis. The mechanism of action of insulin in altering lipolysis is not clear, although a stimulatory effect on the phosphodiesterase enzyme has been demonstrated.

In summary, the overall effect of insulin in adipose tissue is to promote the storage of nutrient energy by, on the one hand, facilitating the conversion of glucose to triglyceride and the passage of fatty acids derived from plasma glyceride into adipocytes while, on the other hand, inhibiting the release of stored triglyceride.

Muscle. Insulin is necessary for the transport of glucose into muscle cells and for repletion of intracellular glycogen stores. However, during physical activity, glucose uptake by muscle increases despite a fall in circulating insulin levels. With muscle contraction, glucose is oxidized to CO_2 or, if the availability of oxygen is limited, to lactic acid. Lactic acid then diffuses into the circulation, from which it is extracted by the liver and used as a substrate for glucose formation. The movement of carbon from the liver to the muscle in the form of glucose and its return as lactic acid is known as the *Cori cycle*. It should be emphasized that muscle metabolizes ketones and fatty acids in preference to glucose, and fatty acids are the principal fuel of muscle. In the process, both fatty acids and ketones are oxidized to CO_2 and water. Muscle serves as a major reservoir of amino acids for the body. Insulin stimulates transport of amino acids into muscle cells and their conversion into protein. This action is opposed by cortisol. During fasting, the cortisol influence predominates, and alanine and glutamine are released from muscle and circulate to the liver, where they serve as substrates for gluconeogenesis.

Liver. Insulin is not necessary for the transport of glucose into the liver, but the hormone powerfully influences glucose metabolism within hepatic cells. Insulin promotes the formation of glycogen, stimulates the disposal of glucose via glycolytic pathways, and suppresses those enzymes necessary for gluconeogenesis and glycogenolysis. Thus, insulin antagonizes the hepatic effects of cortisol, epinephrine, and glucagon on glucose metabolism. The overall effect of insulin is to increase glucose utilization and storage by the liver. During the fed state, because of the high concentration of insulin in the portal circulation, almost all of an ingested glucose load is extracted by the liver. During fasting, the concentration of plasma insulin falls, the influence of the gluconeogenic hormone cortisol and the glycogenolytic hormone glucagon predominate, and the liver releases the glucose required for the metabolism in the central nervous system.

With prolonged fasting and in insulinopenic diabetes mellitus, the release of fatty acids from adipose tissue is greatly accelerated. Fatty acids reaching the liver are metabolized by one of two major pathways. They may be converted to triglycerides, phospholipids, and cholesterol in the cytosol of the hepatocyte, or they may be transported into the mitochondria by carnitine acyltransferase and oxidized to acetyl-CoA. This then may undergo oxidization to CO_2 via the Krebs cycle or condense to form acetoacetate. Acetoacetate, the primary ketone body, is converted to beta-hydroxybutyrate and acetone, the other ketone bodies, by reduction and decarboxylation, respectively. In diabetic ketoacidosis, the "metabolic set" of the liver favors the mitochondrial pathway, and huge quantities of ketones are formed. Some investigators believe that the change in "set" in ketoacidosis favoring the shunting of fatty acids into mitochondria is caused by an elevation in glucagon. Such a premise is consistent with the thesis that diabetes mellitus is a bihormonal disease characterized not only by deficiency of insulin, but also by an excess of glucagon.

Two important differences between the liver on the one hand and muscle and adipose tissue on the other deserve emphasis. Insulin is not required for glucose transport into the liver, and hepatic cells have a phosphatase capable of cleaving glucose-6-phosphate to produce free glucose that readily diffuses into the plasma.

GLUCAGON

Glucagon is elaborated by the alpha cells of the pancreas. In addition, there is evidence that glucagon is secreted by cells scattered throughout the gastrointestinal tract. A large number of immunoreactive varieties of glucagon have been found; the biologically active form appears to contain 29 amino acids with a molecular weight of 3500. Currently available radioimmunoassays can distinguish between pancreatic glucagon and the similar peptides from the gut. Circulating glucagon levels are high in the fasting state. Secretion is stimulated by amino acids and gastrointestinal peptide hormones. Normally, ingested glucose is a potent suppressor of glucagon release, an effect that is probably mediated by an increase in circulating insulin. Secretion of glucagon is also inhibited by free fatty acids and by somatostatin, and it appears to be modulated by the autonomic nervous system. The hormone is removed from the circulation and metabolized mainly by the liver and kidneys.

Circulating glucagon binds to specific receptors on the hepatocyte membrane. Binding leads to stimulation of adenylate cyclase, formation of cyclic AMP, glycogenolysis, and an acute rise in blood glucose. The hormone causes activation of pyruvate kinase and increases the activity of phosphoenolpyruvate carboxykinase, leading to an increase in gluconeogenesis. Glucagon is estimated to be responsible for two thirds of the hepatic glucose production after an overnight fast. As mentioned earlier, glucagon probably promotes ketone formation in the hepatic mitochondria.

SOMATOSTATIN

This tetradecapeptide, elaborated by the D cells of the islets, was discovered in the hypothalamus and received its name because of its action in suppressing growth hormone secretion. It also has been found in other parts of the brain and the gastrointestinal tract. Somatostatin has a number of effects on digestion. It inhibits gastrointestinal motility, splanchnic blood flow, gastric acid secretion, pancreatic exocrine secretion, and the absorption of triglyceride. Following a fat meal, circulating levels of somatostatin rise, which may lead to the modulation of the release of other hormones. It has been shown to curtail the secretion of glucagon, insulin, gastrin, secretin, thyrotropin, and growth hormone. In vitro, the addition of serum containing antibodies to somatostatin to cultured pancreatic cells increases glucagon and insulin secretion.

Unger has suggested that the hormones, insulin, glucagon, and somatostatin act in concert to control the flow of nutrients into and out of the circulation. The relative concentrations of these hormones regulate the rates of absorption and peripheral disposal of substances such as glucose, amino acids, and fatty acids. The possible significance of the anatomic proximity of the B, A, and D cells in the islets is intriguing. Somatostatin and glucagon appear to have a paracrine relationship whereby they influence the secretion of each other, and both affect the rate of insulin release (Fig. 35–1B).

PANCREATIC POLYPEPTIDE

This polypeptide, secreted by the F, or PP, cells, contains 36 amino acids. Circulating levels rise following ingestion of a meal or cholinergic stimulation and during hypoglycemia. Elevation of plasma free fatty acids suppresses its secretion. Pancreatic polypeptide can inhibit gallbladder contraction and pancreatic exocrine secretion, but its biologic role is unknown.

GLUCOSE HOMEOSTASIS IN THE FED AND FASTED STATES

Following the ingestion of a meal containing carbohydrates, a rise in glucose concentration in the arterial blood perfusing the pancreas triggers the release of insulin into the portal circulation. In the peripheral venous blood, the level of hormone may be 50 to 100 μU/ml; in the portal circulation, it is 8 to 10 times higher. Thus, after a meal, the liver quickly becomes highly "insulinized," and, consequently, most of the absorbed glucose is removed by the liver. The insulin passing into the peripheral circulation promotes transport of glucose into muscle cells and adipose tissue. Thus, peripheral venous blood glucose shows only a modest increase to 140 mg/dl or less. Often there is no detectable increase at all (the so-called "flat" glucose tolerance curve). By about 3 hours after a meal, the plasma glucose level has returned to, or, frequently, has declined below, the fasting level. There are a number of mechanisms counteracting potential or actual hypoglycemia. Cryer and coworkers have studied those hormones that participate in the recovery from hypoglycemia. Plasma epinephrine, norepinephrine, glucagon, growth hormone, and cortisol levels all rose substantially when hypoglycemia was induced with intravenous insulin in normal subjects. In order to determine which of these hormones were most important in the correction of hypoglycemia, the investigators repeated the experiments while selectively blocking one or more of the hormones. For example, the alpha- and beta-adrenergic receptor antagonists phentolamine and propranolol were used to block the action of epinephrine and norepinephrine in one series of experiments. Later, somatostatin was used to block secretion of growth hormone and glucagon. The results of these studies indicate that glucagon is necessary for normal recovery from hypoglycemia, whereas the catecholamines become important only if glucagon secretion is deficient. Although levels of cortisol and growth hormone were markedly elevated during the hypoglycemia, they did not appear to influence the rate of correction of the low blood glucose during the acute phase of recovery.

When absorption of glucose is completed and plasma glucose levels decline, insulin secretion also decreases until the basal rate is reached. By 4 to 5 hours after a meal, the liver becomes a producer of glucose as rising glucagon levels stimulate glycogenolysis and gluconeogenesis. The declining insulin levels permit an increased rate of fatty acid release from adipose tissue, providing nutrient fuel for muscle cells. After 12 to 24 hours, liver glycogen stores are depleted. During prolonged fasting, blood glucose levels decline relatively little, glucose homeostasis being maintained by a combination of sustained gluconeogenesis and adaptation to alternate fuels. Lipolysis increases further, and much of the released fatty acids are converted to ketones by the liver. These are readily metabolized by muscle. During the fed state and the early stages of fasting, glucose is the obligatory substrate for cerebral metabolism, which requires 150 gm or more each day. Since gluconeogenesis depends in large part on precursors from muscle catabolism, continued dependence of the brain on glucose supply would be costly indeed. Instead, brain cells adapt to the rising levels of ketones in the blood so that, by the third or fourth day of fasting, about one third of the energy needs of the brain are met by the ketones. With more prolonged fasting, ketone utilization by the brain increases further until the ketones supply two thirds or more of the energy required for cerebral metabolism. As a consequence, there is a marked reduction in the need for muscle breakdown and nitrogen-loss decreases. This pattern of substrate utilization by the brain during fasting was dramatically demonstrated by the studies of Drenick and colleagues. These workers induced hypoglycemia in obese young men before and after a 50-day fast. Before the fast, moderate hypoglycemia induced by intravenous insulin injection caused moderate to marked symptoms. After 50 days of fasting, although insulin caused a greater degree of blood glucose fall, the subjects were free of symptoms. Glucose and beta-hydroxybutyric acid were measured in arterial and jugular venous blood; levels of beta-hydroxybutyric acid were very high in both vessels after the prolonged fast. During the hypoglycemic phase, the arteriovenous difference for glucose remained the same, indicating no change in glucose uptake by the brain. In contrast, although the arterial level of beta-hydroxybutyrate remained unchanged, the jugular venous blood concentration fell substantially, indicating that a marked increase in ketone extraction was occurring. Thus, the lack of symptoms in these hypoglycemic subjects could be explained by increased utilization by the brain of the readily available beta-hydroxybutyrate.

CLINICAL ENTITIES

DIABETES MELLITUS

A relative or absolute deficiency of insulin results in the disease diabetes mellitus. The term *diabetes*, from the Greek meaning "a syphon," denotes excessive urine formation, which characterizes this disorder; *mellitus* is derived from the Greek word "mel," meaning honey. Diabetes mellitus is by far the most common disease of the endocrine system in the United States, afflicting about 10 million people. Diabetic patients range from the elderly asymptomatic individual with modest fasting hyperglycemia to the youthful patient requiring daily exogenous insulin to avoid fatal ketoacidosis. Even more worrisome than its prevalence is the rate of increase of the disease. Epidemiologic studies indicate that the number of individuals with diabetes doubles every 15 years. While the discovery of insulin by Banting and Best in 1921 has prevented early demise from diabetic ketoacidosis, the use of insulin has not prevented the chronic complications of the disease. Public health statisticians list diabetes mellitus among the top 10 causes of death in the United States, and cite it as the leading cause of blindness and uremia in our country. The economic loss attributable to diabetes is estimated to be approximately 2 billion dollars annually. Diabetes is thus a national health problem of the first magnitude.

Classification and Criteria. In earlier years, diabetes was divisible into two forms, primary and secondary. The primary disease was further divided into juvenile and maturity-onset diabetes, with both diagnoses having a number of synonyms. Secondary diabetes included a number of miscellaneous disorders having in common either a deleterious effect on beta cell function or antagonism to the action of insulin. This classification had a number of shortcomings. For example, many patients developed "juvenile" diabetes when they were in the third or fourth decade of life or older. In contrast, glucose intolerance so mild as to not require insulin therapy was discovered in a few children and adolescents and labeled "maturity-onset diabetes of youth." Under the aegis of the National Institutes of Health, a committee of experts was formed to develop a new more workable classification. This committee, the National Diabetes Data Group, published its recommendations in 1979. The classification is shown in Table 35–1 with the description of the major classes summarized.

Type I, or Insulin-Dependent, Diabetes Mellitus (IDDM). Formerly termed *juvenile diabetes*, this variety of the disease can occur at any stage of life, including childhood and infancy. Individuals with this disease have insulinopenia due to islet cell loss and become ketonemic when exogenous insulin is withheld.

Type II, or Non–Insulin-Dependent, Diabetes Mellitus (NIDDM). This form of diabetes, previously called *maturity-onset diabetes*, also can occur at any age but is most common in adults. Affected individuals are not ketosis-prone except in the face of stress, although they often require insulin to control hyperglycemia. The majority are obese.

Other Types. This group is the miscellaneous one, formerly called *secondary diabetes*. It includes diseases attacking the pancreas (e.g., hemochromatosis, pancreatitis), syndromes characterized by insulin antagonism (e.g., Cushing's disease, acromegaly), and disorders of insulin receptors causing insulin resistance.

TABLE 35–1 CLASSIFICATION OF DIABETES MELLITUS AND OTHER CATEGORIES OF GLUCOSE INTOLERANCE

Clinical Classes
Diabetes mellitus (DM)
  Insulin-dependent type (IDDM), type I
  Non–insulin-dependent types (NIDDM), type II
    1. Nonobese NIDDM
    2. Obese NIDDM
  Other types, including diabetes mellitus associated
      with certain conditions and syndromes
    1. Pancreatic disease
    2. Hormonal abnormalities
    3. Drug- or chemical-induced
    4. Insulin receptor abnormalities
    5. Certain genetic syndromes
    6. Other types
Impaired glucose tolerance (IGT)
  Nonobese IGT
  Obese IGT
  IGT associated with certain conditions and
    syndromes (as above)
Gestational diabetes (GDM)

Statistical Risk Classes
Previous abnormality of glucose tolerance (Prev AGT)
Potential abnormality of glucose tolerance (Pot AGT)

Impaired Glucose Tolerance (IGT). Patients with this finding include those individuals who have oral glucose tolerance tests (OGTT) that fail to meet normal criteria but are not sufficiently abnormal to justify the diagnosis of diabetes mellitus. Formerly called *chemical diabetes*, most of these individuals do not progress to overt diabetes and do not develop the late complications of diabetes associated with microangiopathy.

Gestational Diabetes Mellitus (GDM). This term is reserved for diabetes or glucose intolerance that develops or is first recognized during pregnancy. Patients may revert to normal glucose tolerance following pregnancy.

In addition to reordering the classification of states of glucose intolerance, including diabetes mellitus, the National Diabetes Data Group has provided recommendations regarding diagnostic criteria. For example, in order to diagnose diabetes mellitus in an asymptomatic adult, one must observe either two fasting plasma glucose values greater than 140 mg/dl or any two values greater than 200 mg/dl following a 75-gm oral glucose load. Criteria for the diagnosis of glucose intolerance include a fasting plasma glucose value between 115 and 140 mg/dl, a 2-hour postprandial value between 140 and 200 mg/dl, and at least one value greater than 200 mg/dl during a standard oral glucose tolerance test.

Etiology. Although for many years it has conventionally been held that diabetes mellitus is principally a genetically determined disease, thus far no clear-cut pattern of inheritance has emerged. At the present time, it seems likely that two distinct pathogenic pathways account for type I and type II diabetes. A genetic factor appears to be more important in type II, since analysis of a large series of monozygotic twins has shown a concordance rate of more than 90 per cent for type II diabetes. However, in type I diabetes the rate of concordance among monozygotic twins was found to be about 50 per cent. This relatively low incidence of the disease among the identical twins of type I diabetics suggests that both intrinsic and extrinsic factors are involved. One such intrinsic factor may be immune-related. Among type I diabetics, there is a relatively high prevalence of certain patterns of the inherited histocompatibility antigens (HLA), principally DW3-DR3 and DW4-DR4. In type II diabetics, the prevalence of these HLA types is no different from that seen in the normal population. Since the HLA regions on chromosome 6 are close to the sites of immune response genes in humans, the high prevalence of certain HLA patterns among type I diabetics has been construed as evidence that immunologic mechanisms are important in this population of patients. Consistent with such a point of view are the high prevalence of autoantibodies to islet cells found in the sera of type I diabetics and the fact that there is often leukocytic infiltration of the islets of pancreases from type I diabetics.

There is evidence that the extrinsic factor may be related to viral infections. Notkins and coworkers isolated a coxsackievirus B4 from the pancreas of a child who died shortly after the onset of diabetes. This virus was maintained in culture and was found capable of producing beta cell necrosis when injected into mice. Further evidence supporting a viral role in the development of type I diabetes is the seasonal clustering of the disease and the occasional occurrence of multiple cases in association with viral epidemics among children. Similar extrinsic factors have not been implicated in the pathogenesis of type II diabetes.

Several intrinsic factors have been identified in type II diabetic patients. Studies of insulin dose-response curves have demonstrated varying types of insulin resistance. Some patients, with decreased numbers of insulin receptors, have shown a shift of the insulin-binding curve to the right, denoting a decrease in sensitivity to insulin. Other patients have shown a decrease in maximal response to insulin. This decrease in "responsivity" to insulin suggests a postreceptor defect in these patients. Loss of weight by the obese type II diabetic patient usually is associated with an increase in sensitivity to insulin and an improvement in the diabetic state. Many patients with type II diabetes have impaired insulin release in response to glucose. In a few non–insulin-dependent diabetics there may be synthesis of a flawed insulin molecule that does not have full biologic activity.

Manifestations. The manifestations of diabetes mellitus are predictable from the known actions of insulin discussed earlier. A relative or absolute deficiency of insulin results in hyperglycemia, the central biochemical feature of the disease. Hyperglycemia ensues because of impaired transport of glucose into muscle and adipose tissue and the release of glucose into the circulation by the liver. Above a glucose concentration of about 160 mg/dl, the renal tubules are unable to reabsorb all of the glucose filtered by the glomeruli. The renal excretion of glucose requires concomitant excretion of water and thus produces an osmotic diuresis. Loss of water causes an increase in the serum osmolality that stimulates the thirst center in the hypothalamus. The classic three "polys" of diabetes mellitus (polyuria, polydipsia, and polyphagia) are thus explicable in terms of the body's loss of large quantities of glucose and water, which leads to a compensatory increase in hunger and thirst.

Diabetic Ketoacidosis. When more severe insulin deficiency ensues, hyperglycemia and glycosuria intensify and ketonemia develops. The possible role of glucagon in the pathogenesis of ketoacidosis has already been mentioned. Both acetoacetic acid and beta-hydroxybutyric acid dissociate to yield hydrogen ions, depressing the plasma pH. At a pH level of about 7.2, the respiratory center is stimulated and the patient's breathing becomes deep and rapid (Kussmaul respirations). This hyperventilation is a compensatory effort to prevent a further decline in plasma pH. It will be recalled from the Henderson-Hasselbalch equation that pH is determined by the ratio of plasma bicarbonate to carbonic acid, $\frac{HCO_3^-}{H_2CO_3}$, which normally is about 20 to 1. With loss of bicarbonate (utilized to buffer hydrogen ions derived from ketone bodies), this ratio decreases, as does the pH. The increased loss of CO_2 from the lungs reduces plasma carbonic acid and tends to restore the ratio to normal. A further decline in the pH is associated with increasing

depression of cerebral function, eventually culminating in coma and death. The major components of the pathogenesis of ketoacidosis are depicted schematically in Figure 35–2.

Insulin deficiency permits excessive protein catabolism and release of nitrogen products into the circulation. The acidosis promotes the egress of potassium and phosphate from cells and their consequent loss into the urine. Later in the course of ketoacidosis, when dehydration and hypovolemia have occurred, renal perfusion falters. With the azotemia, hyperkalemia may occur despite the total body depletion. Appropriate fluid therapy leads to expansion of plasma volume and a return toward normal renal function. Both the administration of insulin and the correction of the acidosis cause potassium and phosphate to re-enter the cells. In the past, patients often did well during the first few hours of treatment and then developed profound muscle weakness and cardiac dysfunction without apparent cause. With the advent of frequent monitoring of plasma electrolytes, hypokalemia was soon identified as the cause of these complications. They are now readily prevented by the judicious administration of potassium and phosphate.

Although initially ketonemia is the only cause of acidosis, the subsequent occurrence of hypotension and tissue hypoxia leads to lactate accumulation and a further lowering of the plasma pH. Lactate accumulation sufficient to produce acidosis can also occur in nondiabetic patients severely ill from a variety of causes in whom tissue hypoxia is found.

Hyperosmolar Nonketotic Coma. A variant of diabetic coma has been recognized. In this syndrome, described as *hyperosmolar nonketotic coma,* hyperglycemia is usually extreme, between 900 and 3000 mg/dl, whereas ketonemia is mild or undetectable and acidosis is absent. It usually affects patients not known to be diabetic or those with mild diabetes not on insulin therapy. Char-

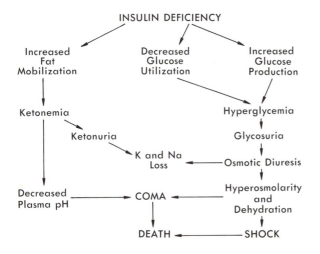

Figure 35–2 The pathogenesis of diabetic ketoacidosis (see text).

TABLE 35–2 HORMONAL AND METABOLIC DIFFERENCES BETWEEN DIABETIC KETOACIDOSIS AND HYPEROSMOLAR NONKETOTIC COMA

	Hyperosmolar Nonketotic Coma (9 Patients)	Diabetic Ketoacidosis (6 Patients)
Blood sugar (mg/100 ml)	1058	798
CO_2 (mEq/L)	22	9.6
Osmolality (mOsm/kg)	368	327
Free fatty acids (mEq/L)	880	2053
Immunoreactive Insulin (μU/ml)	0 to 15	0 to 15
Growth hormone (ng/ml)	2	12
Cortisol (μg/100 ml)	21	40

(Data adapted from Gerich, J. E., et al.: Diabetes *19*:354, 1970.)

acteristically, the diabetic state worsens insidiously, often associated with the stress of unrelated illness or trauma. Initially, the increasing fluid loss due to glycosuria is balanced by an increase in the patient's fluid intake. Ultimately, this intake becomes insufficient, and progressive dehydration, hypovolemia, and prerenal azotemia develop. With the consequent impairment of renal function, blood glucose rises precipitously, and the serum rapidly becomes hyperosmolar. Associated with this rise in serum osmolality, and probably because of it, the patient becomes increasingly obtunded and unable to respond to his thirst. Thus, a vicious cycle ensues and can quickly lead to coma and, if not treated, to death.

A puzzling feature of the syndrome is that the affected diabetic patients are severely hyperglycemic but not ketotic. This apparent paradox may be due to the relatively greater potency of insulin in inhibiting fat mobilization as compared with its effect on glucose transport. Thus, patients with hyperosmolar nonketotic coma seem to have had sufficient circulating insulin to retard the massive release of fatty acids that occurs in ketoacidosis but not enough insulin to promote the entry of glucose into peripheral tissues nor prevent the release of glucose by the liver. However, at the time of diagnosis, insulin levels are decreased (Table 35–2), perhaps as a consequence of the extreme hyperosmolality itself. Hyperosmolality per se may inhibit the release of fatty acids and may contribute to the absence of ketosis.

Hyperlipidemia. Although ketoacidosis and hyperosmolar nonketotic coma are the most dramatic, life-threatening manifestations of acute insulin deficiency, others deserve mention. Infrequently, the uncontrolled diabetic will present with evidence of hyperlipidemia as the major manifestation of this disease. On physical examination, there may be widespread skin lesions often of recent origin. These lesions, which are yellowish-orange in color, papular, and about 2 to 4 mm or

larger in diameter, are eruptive xanthomas. On funduscopic examination of the eye, the color of the venules may be startling. Instead of being deep red they may be white, grey, or light pink. This finding, lipemia retinalis, is directly related to the character of the patient's blood, which is pink when aspirated by venipuncture. The appearance of serum or plasma obtained from the fasted patient is indistinguishable from that of cream. Chemical analysis reveals a marked increase in triglycerides to several thousand mg/dl. Analysis by ultracentrifugation reveals that the increase in triglycerides is due largely to dietary chylomicra, although endogenous triglycerides carried by very low density lipoprotein particles are present as well. This buildup of triglyceride-bearing particles is due to impaired disposal that results from relative inactivity of the insulin-dependent lipoprotein lipase mentioned earlier. Treatment with insulin promptly increases the activity of this enzyme. The plasma triglyceride level falls to normal in a short time, the retinal changes promptly disappear, and the xanthomas gradually fade. It is curious that hyperlipidemia does not occur more often in untreated diabetics. Factors other than insulin, probably genetic or nutritional, must be important in influencing the activity of the lipoprotein lipase of peripheral tissues.

Chronic Complications. The prolonged survival of patients with diabetes has led to an increasing incidence of chronic complications involving all systems of the body. Some of the more common complications are listed in Table 35–3. Clinically, the three most important are retinopathy, nephropathy, and neuropathy. The pathogenesis of these abnormalities remains one of the major unanswered questions in diabetes, although some clues are emerging. Although interrelated,

TABLE 35–3 MAJOR CHRONIC COMPLICATIONS OF DIABETES MELLITUS

Ocular
  Retinopathy
    Background
    Proliferative
  Cataracts
Renal
  Diffuse intercapillary glomerulosclerosis
  Nodular intercapillary glomerulosclerosis
  Papillary necrosis
Neuromuscular
  Peripheral polyneuropathy
  Mononeuropathy
  Amyotrophy
  Autonomic nervous system neuropathy
    Atonic bladder, impotence, orthostatic hypotension, gastric paresis, diarrhea
Cardiovascular
  Myocardial infarction
  Peripheral vascular
    Indolent foot ulcers, gangrene

the chronic complications may be grouped into those that are predominantly vascular and those that are chiefly metabolic in origin.

VASCULAR COMPLICATIONS. In diabetes mellitus of long duration, there often is diffuse involvement of the vascular system with lesions in arteries, arterioles, and capillaries. Numerous studies have shown that diabetes is associated with abnormalities in metabolism of arterial smooth muscle cells and alterations in clotting factors, platelet function, and lipoprotein metabolism. The atherosclerosis associated with diabetes is indistinguishable from that affecting the general population; however, it tends to be more severe and occur at an earlier age. Premature atherosclerosis of the coronary arteries occurs commonly among insulin-dependent diabetics, and myocardial infarction is the leading cause of death among these patients. Diabetes is the most common cause of peripheral vascular disease of the lower extremities. Smaller arterioles may be involved to a greater degree than large arteries. Indolent ulcers of the foot and gangrene often complicate vascular disease and may necessitate amputation. Obstruction of nutrient vessels of nerves is considered the cause of isolated mononeuropathies. Their abrupt and painful onset with gradual resolution over weeks or months resembles the course seen with infarction in other organs.

The typical lesion of diabetic microangiopathy is characterized by abnormal· thickening of the basement membrane of capillaries. This thickening appears to increase both with the duration of the disease and with the severity of hyperglycemia. There is loss of pericytes in retinal capillaries, leading to microaneurysm formation. These show abnormal permeability demonstrable by fluorescein angiography and may bleed, forming "dot" and "blot" hemorrhages. Retinal ischemia leads to macular edema and probably is the stimulus for neovascularization. New, fragile capillaries may grow into the vitreous and cause recurrent hemorrhages, leading to vitreous opacities and retinal detachment. In the renal glomeruli, thickening of basement membranes also occurs, as well as accumulation of hyaline material in the mesangium. Abnormal glomerular permeability is detectable by microproteinuria. This often progresses in 15 to 20 years to clinically detectable or even severe proteinuria, the hallmark of diabetic nephropathy. Steady deterioration of renal function causes hypertension, progressive uremia, and death 3 to 5 years later. The availability of chronic dialysis and renal transplantation has modified this grim prognosis.

METABOLIC COMPLICATIONS. Some complications are not directly related to vascular disease. These include cataracts, autonomic neuropathy, and symmetric peripheral polyneuropathy. Mild dysfunction of the autonomic nervous system is common, but it may become severe and diffuse with impairment of both parasympathetic and sympathetic nerves. Manifestations of such involvement include postural hypotension, gastric atony, diarrhea, neurogenic bladder, and impotence. In contrast to the aforementioned isolated neuropathies, the peripheral polyneuropathies are gradual in onset and are symmetric. They cause paresthesias, numbness, and occasionally distressing pain in a "stocking and glove" distribution. Although motor function is usually intact clinically, both sensory and motor nerve conduction velocities are decreased. The nerves show axonal degeneration and segmental demyelinization. Biochemical abnormalities in nerve tissue include accumulation of sorbitol, loss of myo-inositol, and decreased protein synthesis. Accumulation of sorbitol in the crystalline lens of the eye is thought to contribute to cataract formation by causing osmotic swelling and membrane rupture of the cells.

The potential role of glycosylation in development of diabetic complications has received attention. It is now appreciated that proteins can undergo nonenzymatic glycosylation. Glucose attaches to amine groups in proteins, forming an aldimine (Schiff base). This sequence is rapid and reversible; it is followed by a slow Amadori rearrangement to a ketoamine configuration. This glycosylation lasts for the life of the protein, and the level of glycosylation is related to the average glucose concentration to which the protein has been exposed. Thus, the fraction of plasma albumin that is glycosylated reflects the mean plasma glucose over several days. Glycosylated hemoglobin (Hb A_1) or its subfraction (Hb A_{1c}) is a useful index of diabetic control, since it reflects the mean plasma glucose concentration during the life of the red cell (about 3 months). Glycosylation of the apoproteins of the low-density lipoproteins (LDL) reduces their uptake by cells and may contribute to the hypercholesterolemia seen in diabetes. Glycosylation of the crystallins, the transparent proteins of the lens, also may contribute to cataract formation. Repeated injections of glycosylated proteins into mice can cause lesions in the glomeruli resembling those caused by diabetes. Isolated microvessels will take up glycosylated albumin more avidly than normal albumin. These associations suggest that glycosylated proteins may play a role in the production of the microvascular complications of diabetes. Enzyme-mediated glycosylation is also accelerated in diabetes; the activity of glycosyltransferases in glomerular basement membrane is increased, as is the rate of basement membrane synthesis.

From a clinical point of view, the key question is whether or not the chronic complications of diabetes are due to long-standing hyperglycemia and insulin deficiency. Two conflicting views regarding the pathogenesis of the vascular complications of diabetes can be formulated as follows:

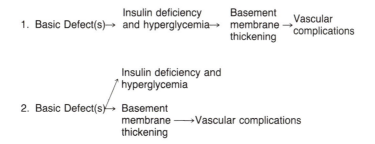

The question is of more than academic interest, since if the first hypothesis is correct, intensive efforts to minimize hyperglycemia would be justified, whereas if the second hypothesis is right, the argument for rigid control of the blood sugar would be considerably weakened. It is disappointing that, despite the years that have passed since the discovery of insulin, the answer to the question is not yet in hand. A number of animal studies have shown that typical diabetic lesions can be produced by hyperglycemia and that these lesions improve or disappear if the affected organ is transplanted into a nonhyperglycemic animal. A number of clinical studies have produced results suggesting that good control of the blood sugar favorably influences the rate of complications. That more definitive information has not been forthcoming relates to the fact that truly good control of the blood sugar (i.e., maintenance of the blood sugar within the normal range most of the time) has not been possible. Various developments may change this situation. Now available are highly purified insulins, including human insulin synthesized by recombinant DNA technology. Also available are insulin delivery systems of increasing sophistication and methods for monitoring blood glucose at home. The evidence so far indicates that strict control of the blood sugar causes a fall in Hb A_{1c} to near-normal levels. Whether such control will prevent complications is the focus of a long-term multicenter clinical study sponsored by the National Institutes of Health.

HYPOGLYCEMIA

Although a wide array of human ills are presently being attributed to hypoglycemia, well-documented significant hypoglycemia is not very common. Regardless of the underlying cause, the manifestations of hypoglycemia tend to evolve into a characteristic pattern. Mild hypoglycemia causes hunger, fatigue, tremor, perspiration, and weakness. These common symptoms can be attributed to hypoglycemia if Whipple's triad is found (i.e., a blood glucose level of less than 40 mg/dl, central nervous or vasomotor system symptoms, and prompt relief of symptoms by administration of glucose). More severe hypoglycemia leads to blurred vision, impaired mentation, and bizarre behavior, with the patient often becoming bellicose and resistant to help and manifesting impaired neuromuscular function. A staggering gait and irrational hostile behavior are frequently misinterpreted as drunkenness. Finally, the patient becomes comatose and may develop generalized seizures. If severe hypoglycemia remains untreated, permanent brain damage or death results. The sequence of events just described is typical, but the exact pattern varies among individuals and even in the same patient from one episode to another. For example, on one occasion, the patient may remain in a confused state for 2 or 3 hours; at another time, he might pass from an alert rational state into coma within one half hour or less.

The principal causes of hypoglycemia, listed in Table 35–4, can be grouped into two large categories: (1) fasting, and (2) fed, or "reactive." The time of day at which hypoglycemia occurs provides a clue to the underlying cause. Since hepatic production sustains the blood glucose level during periods of fasting, impairment in glycogen

TABLE 35–4 PRINCIPAL CAUSES OF HYPOGLYCEMIA

Underlying Condition	Mechanism
I. FASTING	
A. Addison's disease, panhypopituitarism	Impaired gluconeogenesis
B. Liver disease	Impaired gluconeogenesis, glycogen storage
C. Fasting + Alcohol	Impaired gluconeogenesis, depleted glycogen
D. Mesothelial tumors	Unknown
E. Insulin-dependent diabetes	Excessive insulin, iatrogenic
F. Islet cell adenoma	Excessive, unregulated insulin release
II. FED (Reactive)	
G. Postgastrectomy	Tachyalimentation of glucose
H. Functional	Tachyalimentation of glucose
I. Early ("chemical") diabetes	Abnormal "glucostat" ($\uparrow$ insulin secretion)

storage or gluconeogenesis will lead to fasting hypoglycemia. This typically occurs in the early morning after 8 or 9 hours of fasting. Such a pattern is seen with hypoglycemia due to insulin-secreting islet cell adenomas; hypoglycemia, prevented during the waking hours by near constant eating, occurs during hours of sleep. A level of serum insulin inappropriate to the blood glucose concentration helps confirm this diagnosis. In contrast to the fasting hypoglycemias are those that are reactive (i.e., they are triggered in reaction to the assimilation of glucose following a meal). Normally, the secretion of insulin is approximately commensurate with the degree of postprandial hyperglycemia. Following gastrectomy or other surgery that impairs the reservoir function of the stomach, ingested glucose is quickly dumped into the duodenum and upper jejunum, where it is very rapidly absorbed. The resulting excessive hyperglycemia stimulates a brisk release of insulin. The peak insulin action occurs within an hour of eating, by which time assimilation of glucose from the gastrointestinal tract has been completed in these patients. There is another group of patients who appear to assimilate glucose excessively fast in the absence of prior gastrointestinal surgery. These individuals with "functional" hypoglycemia typically become hypoglycemic 3 to 4 hours after a glucose load. The situation in patients with early diabetes mellitus is somewhat different. In these patients, glucose is assimilated at a normal rate, but the early phase of insulin secretion is deficient, as if the pancreatic sensing mechanism, or "glucostat," were not functioning properly. The resulting hyperglycemia stimulates an excessive sec-

ondary phase of insulin secretion, causing hypoglycemia about 4 to 5 hours after a meal. Symptomatic hypoglycemia can be avoided in each of these forms of reactive hypoglycemia by restricting the amount of free glucose in the diet.

The most frequent cause of clinically significant hypoglycemia is insulin self-administration by the diabetic patient. This may result from an excessive insulin dose or, more frequently, from dietary omission or excessive physical activity. Overnight hypoglycemia secondary to insulin overdose frequently is not recognized because the patient is asleep and unaware of the early symptoms of mild hypoglycemia. Furthermore, hypoglycemia occurring at 2:00 or 3:00 A.M. stimulates an increase in the counter regulatory hormones, glucagon and the catecholamines. As already discussed, these hormones cause the blood glucose to rise at an accelerated rate while the level of plasma insulin is falling. Consequently, the patient may find glucose and even ketones in the early morning urine test. This overshoot, or rebound, in glucose concentration that follows hypoglycemia, first emphasized by Somogyi, has great clinical significance. It is often interpreted as evidence of insufficient insulin effect rather than as a sign of too much insulin. Thus, as the dosage of insulin is increased, the overnight hypoglycemia becomes more marked and the rebound in blood glucose greater. The latter finding, of course, tends to perpetuate the mistake.

The correct diagnosis of coma in a diabetic patient is critical, since the two most common causes, too much or too little insulin, require diametrically opposite therapy. The major features

TABLE 35–5 DIFFERENTIAL DIAGNOSIS OF COMA DUE TO DIABETIC KETOACIDOSIS AND HYPOGLYCEMIA

	Acidosis	*Hypoglycemia*
Onset	Hours to days	Minutes
Background events	Intercurrent disease, omission of insulin	Exercise, omission of meal
Symptoms	Thirst, polyuria, headaches, nausea, vomiting, abdominal pain	Hunger, headache, perspiration, *confusion,* stupor
Physical findings	Kussmaul respirations, dehydration, flushed face, fast pulse; *appears ill*	Normal pulse, respirations: appears well
Typical laboratory findings *Urine*		
Glucose	5%	0 to 5%
Ketones	Strongly positive	0 to positive
Serum		
Glucose	400 mg/100 ml or more	Less than 40 mg/100 ml
Ketones	Positive, 1:8	Negative
HCO_3	Less than 10 mEq/L	26 mEq/L
Response to 50% glucose, I.V.	None	Dramatic

that distinguish the two disorders, listed in Table 35–5, are explicable in terms of the aforementioned pathophysiologic consequences of insulin deficiency and excess.

TUMORS OF THE ENDOCRINE PANCREAS

Inappropriate hypersecretion of pancreatic hormones may be due to diffuse hyperplasia of the secretory cells, adenoma, or carcinoma.

Hypersecretion of insulin is most frequently due to a single insulin-producing adenoma. Single or multiple insulinomas may occur as part of the syndrome of multiple endocrine neoplasia, type I (MEN 1, or Wermer's syndrome). Malignant insulinomas are less common. Diffuse hyperplasia of B cells (nesidioblastosis) may cause hypoglycemia in infants. The basis of diagnosis is fasting hypoglycemia associated with serum insulin concentrations inappropriate to the level of serum glucose. Serum levels of C peptide may also be elevated.

Glucagon-secreting tumors (glucagonomas) produce the "diabetes-dermatitis syndrome." Patients manifest mild diabetes, anemia, and a rash that has been characterized as a necrotizing migratory erythema. There is inhibition of intestinal motility causing ileus and constipation or, occa-sionally, diarrhea. Other clinical features include glossitis, angular cheilitis, and venous thrombosis. Patients have elevated plasma glucagon, but increased insulin secretion may ameliorate the diabetes.

Somatostatin-producing tumors (somatostatinomas) are difficult to diagnose clinically. Findings are nonspecific but may include diabetes mellitus, cholecystolithiasis, steatorrhea, indigestion, and hypochlorhydria. Plasma somatostatin levels are increased on radioimmunoassay, whereas both insulin and glucagon levels are suppressed.

Pancreatic polypeptide–secreting islet cell tumors have been found in patients with MEN 1. Increased plasma levels of pancreatic polypeptide in both the basal-fasting and food-stimulated states have led to identification of these tumors in patients before any symptoms have arisen. No clear-cut clinical picture has been associated with hypersecretion of pancreatic polypeptide.

Pancreatic tumors may also be the source of "ectopic" hormone secretions. These tumors may secrete ACTH or polypeptides with activity resembling that of parathyroid hormone. Gastrin-secreting islet cell tumors cause the Zollinger-Ellison syndrome, whereas the Verner-Morrison syndrome of "pancreatic cholera" has been ascribed to excessive secretion of vasoactive intestinal polypeptide (VIP).

REFERENCES

GENERAL

Ellenberg, M., and Rifkin, H. (Eds.): Diabetes Mellitus: Theory and Practice. 3rd ed. New York, McGraw-Hill, 1982.
Johnston, D. G., and Alberti, K. G. M. M. (Eds.): New aspects of diabetes. Clin. Endocrinol. Metab. 11:277, 1982.
Podolsky, S. (Ed.): Clinical Diabetes: Modern Management. New York, Appleton-Century-Crofts, 1980.
Raskin, P. (Ed.): Diabetes mellitus. Med. Clin. North Am. 66:1189, 1982.
Rifkin, H., and Raskin, P. (Eds.): Diabetes Mellitus. Vol. V. New York, American Diabetes Association, 1981.
Skyler, J. S., and Cahill, G. F., Jr. (Eds.): Symposium on diabetes mellitus. Am. J. Med. 70:101, 325, 579, 1981.

ISLETS OF LANGERHANS

Bonner-Weir, S., and Orci, L: New perspectives on the microvasculature of the islets of Langerhans in the rat. Diabetes 31:883, 1982.
Orci, L.: Macro- and microdomains in the endocrine pancreas. Diabetes 31:538, 1982.
Woods, S. C., and Porte, D., Jr.: Neural control of the endocrine pancreas. Physiol. Rev. 54:596, 1974.

INSULIN

Creutzfeldt, W.: The incretin concept today. Diabetologia 16:75, 1979.
Czech, M. P.: Insulin action. Am. J. Med. 70:142, 1981.
Johnston, D. G., and Alberti, K. G. M. M.: Hormonal control of ketone body metabolism in the normal and diabetic state. Clin. Endocrinol. Metab. 11:329, 1982.
Larner, J., Cheng, K., et al.: Chemical mechanism of insulin action via proteolytic formation of mediator peptides. Mol. Cell. Biochem. 40:155, 1981.
Pfeifer, M. A., Halter, J. B., and Porte, D., Jr.: Insulin secretion in diabetes mellitus. Am. J. Med. 70:579, 1981.
Steiner, D. F.: Insulin today. Diabetes 26:322, 1977.

OTHER HORMONES

Dobbs, R. E., and Unger, R. H.: Glucagon: secretion, function and clinical role. In Freinkel, N. (Ed.): Contemporary Metabolism. Vol. 2. New York, Plenum Press, 1982, P. 61.
Floyd, J. C., Fajans, S. S., et al.: A newly recognized pancreatic polypeptide; plasma levels in health and disease. Recent Prog. Horm. Res. 33:519, 1977.
Gerich, J., Raptis, S., and Rosenthal, J. (Eds.): Somatostatin symposium. Metabolism 27 (suppl. 1): 1129, 1978.

GLUCOSE HOMEOSTASIS

Cahill, G. F., Jr.: Starvation in man. Clin. Endocrinol. Metab. 5:397, 1976.

DIABETES MELLITUS

Banting, F. G., and Best, C. H.: The internal secretion of the pancreas. J. Lab. Clin. Med. 7:251, 1922.

Classification and Criteria

National Diabetes Data Group: Classification and diagnosis of diabetes mellitus and other categories of glucose intolerance. Diabetes 28:1039, 1979.

Etiology

Cahill, G. F., Jr., and McDevitt, H. O.: Insulin-dependent diabetes mellitus: the initial lesion. N. Engl. J. Med. 304:1454, 1981.
Cudworth, A. G., and Wolf, E.: The genetic susceptibility to Type I (insulin-dependent) diabetes mellitus. Clin. Endocrinol. Metab. 11:389, 1982.
Olefsky, J. M.: Insulin resistance and insulin action. An in vitro and in vivo perspective. Diabetes 30:148, 1981.
Yoon, J-W., Austin, M., Onodera, T., and Notkins, A. L.: Virus-induced diabetes mellitus: isolation of a virus from the pancreas of a child with diabetic ketoacidosis. N. Engl. J. Med. 300:1173, 1979.

Diabetic Ketoacidosis
Kreisberg, R. A.: Diabetic ketoacidosis: new concepts and trends in pathogenesis and treatment. Ann. Intern. Med. *88*:681, 1978.

Hyperosmolar Nonketotic Coma
Gerich, J. E., Martin, M. M., and Recant, L.: Clinical and metabolic characteristics of hyperosmolar nonketotic coma. Diabetes *20*:228, 1971.
Podolsky, S.: Hyperosmolar nonketotic coma in the elderly diabetic. Med. Clin. North Am. *62*:815, 1978.

Hyperlipidemia
Dunn, F. L.: Hyperlipidemia and diabetes. Med. Clin. North Am. *66*:1347, 1982.

Chronic Complications
Brownlee, M., and Cerami, A.: The biochemistry of the chronic complications of diabetes mellitus. Annu. Rev. Biochem. *50*:385, 1981.
Clements, R. S., Jr.: Pathogenesis of diabetic neuropathy. N. Y. State J. Med. *82*:864, 1982.
Kussman, M., Goldstein, H., and Gleason, R.: The clinical course of diabetic nephropathy. J.A.M.A., *236*:1861, 1976.
McVerry, B. A., Hopp, A., Fisher, G., and Huehns, E. R.: Production of pseudodiabetic glomerular changes in mice after repeated injections of glycosylated proteins. Lancet *1*:738, 1980.
Peterson, C. M. (Ed.): Conference on nonenzymatic glycosylation and browning reactions: their relevance to diabetes mellitus. Diabetes *31* (suppl. 3):1, 1982.
Rand, L. I.: Recent advances in diabetic retinopathy. Am. J. Med. *70*:595, 1981.

Siperstein, M. D., Unger, R. H., and Madison, L. L.: Studies of muscle capillary basement membranes in normal subjects, diabetic and pre-diabetic patients. J. Clin. Invest. *47*:1973, 1968.
Steiner, G.: Diabetes and atherosclerosis: an overview. Diabetes *30*(suppl. 2):1, 1981.
Williams, S. K., Devenny, J. J., and Bitensky, M. W.: Micropinocytotic ingestion of glycosylated albumin by isolated microvessels: possible role in pathogenesis of diabetic microangiopathy. Proc. Natl. Acad. Sci. USA *78*:2393, 1981.
Williamson, J. R., and Kilo, C.: Current status of capillary basement membrane disease in diabetes mellitus. Diabetes *26*:65, 1977.

HYPOGLYCEMIA
Cryer, P. E.: Hypoglycemic glucose counter-regulation in patients with insulin-dependent diabetes. J. Lab. Clin. Med. *99*:451, 1982.
Drenick, E. J., Alvarez, L. C., Tamasi, G. C., and Brickman, A. S.: Resistance to symptomatic insulin reactions after fasting. J. Clin. Invest. *51*:2757, 1972.
Fajans, S. S., and Floyd, J. A.: Fasting hypoglycemia in adults. N. Engl. J. Med. *294*:766, 1976.
Permutt, M. A.: Postprandial hypoglycemia. Diabetes *25*:7, 1976.
Somogyi, M.: Exacerbation of diabetes by excess insulin action. Am. J. Med. *26*:169, 1959.

TUMORS OF THE ENDOCRINE PANCREAS
Friesen, S. R.: Tumors of the endocrine pancreas. N. Engl. J. Med. *306*:580, 1982.
Oberg, K., Wälinder, O., Boström, H., et al.: Peptide hormone markers in screening for endocrine tumors in multiple endocrine adenomatosis Type 1. Am. J. Med. *73*:619, 1982.

Section V

TOXIC PHYSICAL AND CHEMICAL AGENTS

Effects of Physical Agents **36**

Charles E. Billings

INTRODUCTION

There exist within our physical environment a great number of stressors, or stimuli, nearly all of which in some dose over some time period are capable of causing dysfunction, disease, or death. These agents, however, are unique in that nearly all are essential to life and in that too little, as well as too much, of many of them may be injurious. It is the intent of this chapter to outline the tolerance envelope for each of these agents and to indicate what physiologic alterations occur when humans encounter unusual environments.

We may consider the physical environment as being made up of three parts, each necessary to life. One is the *gaseous* environment: the atmospheric envelope that surrounds our planet, exerting a pressure on every living thing on its surface and containing the oxygen, carbon dioxide, and nitrogen without which life, either animal or plant, could not have come to be.

Another facet of the environment is what we may call the *electromagnetic* environment: the sum of the electromagnetic waves and energetic particles that constantly bathe the earth. The infrared radiation upon which we depend for warmth, the light that allows us to visualize our surroundings and that triggers the photosynthetic reactions upon which we depend for food, the ultraviolet rays that produce vitamin D within our skin—all are necessary to life, yet each in insufficient or excessive amounts is harmful.

We may call the third part of our surroundings the *kinetic* environment—the accelerative forces that act upon us. Although many of the accelerations that we encounter are a consequence of our technology, gravity subjects us all to a constant acceleration toward the earth's center of mass. With our present dependence on machines for transportation, we must consider other linear and radial accelerations as well, and also the effects of rapid deceleration or impact. Vibration and noise are other products of our technology that evoke physiopathologic responses.

Life has been characterized as "the struggle of an organism to remain distinct from its environment." The attribute of biologic systems that allows them to carry on this struggle is adaptability—the ability to respond *actively* to imposed stresses. The sum of these responses is what we know as human physiology; it is this that allows us, for a time, to withstand the universe's inexorable march toward greater entropy. Humans can avoid toxic chemicals and microorganisms but not their physical environment; indeed, we depend on this environment for the oxygen, food, and energy necessary for survival. We must therefore learn to cope with naturally occurring alterations in the physical environment. It is the mechanisms of this coping behavior that will be examined here.

THE GASEOUS ENVIRONMENT

Under this heading, we must consider the human tolerance envelope for barometric pressure, our ability to withstand changes in pressure, and our tolerance limits for each of the gases found in the environment: oxygen, carbon dioxide, nitrogen, and the noble gases, argon, neon, helium, krypton, and xenon. We shall examine the lower end of the tolerance spectrum first, then attempt to define optimal levels for productive existence, and finally define the upper limits of tolerance as a time-dependent phenomenon.

First a word about units of measurement: Although the Système Internationale (S.I.) has been recommended for universal adoption, its unit of pressure being the Newton per square meter, nearly all texts on physiology still define pressures in millimeters of mercury. In order not to burden the reader unduly, we shall use mm Hg as our primary unit here, although we shall sometimes include in parentheses the equivalent in N/m^2 or in the more commonly used equivalent, millibars (mb). One additional pressure unit will also be used in discussing life at high pressures—atmospheres absolute (ATA). Since several systems of pressure measurement are in common use in Western countries, Figure 36–1 is provided as a convenient reference. It is a nomogram that shows the quantitative relationships among the various systems. It also shows barometric pressure as a function of pressure, altitude above mean sea level in meters and feet, and depth in sea water.

1 atmosphere absolute (ATA)
　　　= 1.0132×10^5 Newtons per square meter (N/m^2)
　　　= 1013.6 millibars (mb)
　　　= 760.0 millimeters of mercury (mm Hg)
　　　= 29.92 inches of mercury (in. Hg)
　　　= 14.70 pounds per square inch (psi)
　　　= 33.0 feet of sea water
　　　= 34.2 feet of fresh water

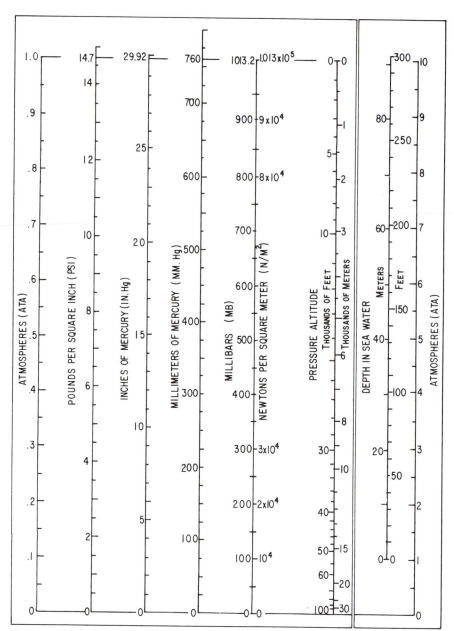

Figure 36–1 Nomogram showing relationship of barometric pressure, altitude or elevation, and depth in sea water. Several equivalent systems of pressure measurement are shown.

BAROMETRIC PRESSURE

Normal Range. Although 760 mm Hg (1.0132×10^5 N/m², 29.92 in. Hg) is the "standard" pressure exerted by the weight of the atmosphere upon the surface of the earth at mean sea level, the actual barometric pressure at any point on the earth's surface at a given time fluctuates with weather phenomena, with elevation, and with the acceleration due to gravity, which varies with latitude. Fluctuations caused by weather are gen-

erally in the range 745 to 785 mm Hg (980 to 1045 mb), although pressures at the center of severe thunderstorms or hurricanes may be as low as 956, and occasional readings as high as 1062 mb are reported. Pressures through the range of terrestrial elevations are shown in Figure 36–1.

Tolerance Limits for Low Barometric Pressure. The lowest barometric pressure at which a sea-level equivalent alveolar gas composition can be maintained if 100 per cent oxygen is breathed is about 187 mm Hg ($P_{A_{O_2}} = 100$, $P_{A_{CO_2}} = 40$, P_{H_2O}

= 47). This pressure is encountered at an altitude of 34,000 feet. At pressures below this, alveolar and therefore arterial oxygen tension decreases. A modest degree of hyperventilation occurs when the carotid sinus chemoreceptors sense a drop in arterial oxygen tension. The limit for continued consciousness occurs at an alveolar Po_2 of about 30 mm Hg; thus, at barometric pressures below about 100 mm Hg ($Po_2 = 30$, $Pco_2 = 25$, $Ph_2o = 47$), volitional human function ceases.

The ultimate limit for human tolerance of low barometric pressure is roughly 47 mm Hg (63,000 feet), the vapor pressure of water at body temperature. Sudden exposure to lower pressures causes rapid evolution of water-vapor bubbles within the blood and tissues, the condition known as *ebullism*. Central venous pressure rises as bubbles form in the more distensible venous reservoir and soon meets or exceeds mean arterial pressure. Circulation then ceases. Ventricular fibrillation may ensue within 90 seconds, although animals (dogs, primates) have sometimes recovered after exposure at 2 mm Hg absolute for as long as 180 seconds.

Humans breathing 100 per cent oxygen have survived and functioned for long periods of time at barometric pressures in the range 187 to 285 mm Hg (250 to 380 mb). The pressure suits used in lunar exploratory missions provided a total pressure of 187 mm Hg, 3.5 psi, and the Apollo spacecraft were pressurized at 285 mm Hg, 5.5 psi. There have been problems at these pressures (see discussion of inert gases), but they do not appear to have been caused by pressure as such. Newer U.S. and Soviet spacecraft are pressurized at approximately 1 ATA.

For humans breathing air, tolerance limits for low barometric pressures are related to hypoxia and will be discussed under that heading.

Effects of Pressure Fluctuations on Earth. A number of investigators have inferred from epidemiologic studies that psychological depression and suicide rates are more common during periods of weather that involve very low barometric pressures. Conclusive evidence is lacking. Patients with various forms of arthropathy commonly state that they can predict weather changes by observing changes in the pain and stiffness of their diseased joints. We are not aware of controlled studies of this phenomenon, but neither are we inclined to reject it outright.

Effects of High Barometric Pressure. We do not know what the ultimate tolerance limit for high pressures will be. Leaving aside the effects of high partial pressures of the various gases in the human breathing medium and the effects of relatively rapid changes in pressure, we know that normal humans can live and work at pressures of 37 to 50 ATA (equivalent to 1200 to 1600 feet depth in sea water) for substantial periods of time; briefer exposures at over 65 ATA (2200 ft) have been successfully tolerated, and studies at higher pressures are in the offing. A limiting factor in such exposures has been the type of central and peripheral nervous system hyperirritability that is now called the *high-pressure nervous syndrome*. The pathophysiology of this disorder is not fully understood, although it appears to be due to high hydrostatic pressure. Fenn has suggested that ultimate tolerance limits will occur at the point at which oxidative biochemical reactions, many of which involve increases in molecular volume, are inhibited by hydrostatic pressures. It seems more likely that limits will be imposed by impairment of distribution and mixing of inspired with alveolar air and by limitations in the ability to perform the work involved in breathing extremely dense gas mixtures, although Lambertsen has demonstrated that fit young men can perform moderate work while breathing gas with a density that approximates that which will be encountered at 150 ATA (5000 feet depth in sea water).

Effects of Rapid Changes in Barometric Pressure. Under this heading, we must consider the effects of both increases and decreases in total pressure as they act on gases within the various gas-containing cavities of the body (middle ear, paranasal sinuses, lungs, gut) and on gases dissolved in body fluids according to Henry's law. Dissolved gases can evolve as bubbles only when the total pressure on them is decreased, whereas trapped gas in body cavities will attempt to obey Boyle's law as the pressure on the body changes in either direction.

Increasing Barometric Pressures. Any increase in barometric pressure will cause a decrease in the volume of a given quantity of gas. If the gas is in free communication with a gaseous environment, more gas will flow into a rigid cavity of a given size. If such gas is not available from the environment (as in underwater swimming or breath-hold diving), a relative negative pressure will occur within the cavity.

The human middle ear is a cavity of relatively fixed volume that is ventilated only through the eustachian tube. The mucosal lining of the eustachian tube is so constructed that air within the middle ear can leave the cavity passively. Reentry of air, however, is impeded and in most people requires voluntary action (yawning, swallowing) to contract the pharyngeal muscles and open the tubal orifices. Attempts to ventilate the middle ear during a descent from altitude or a dive in shallow water may be impeded by swelling of the nasopharyngeal mucosa or lymphoid hypertrophy (as found in upper respiratory infections, allergic rhinitis, etc.).

If a substantial negative pressure differential is allowed to build up within the ear, voluntary attempts to reopen the eustachian tubes may become difficult or impossible. The Valsalva maneuver may help by forcing air into the ear. If the relative vacuum persists, however, fluid is drawn into the middle ear; it may be serous or hemorrhagic in character. Rarely, the tympanic membrane may rupture. Treatment of barotitis is physiologic: Air is introduced into the middle ear to neutralize the pressure differential across the eardrum. In refractory cases, a permanent tympanic ostium can be created surgically.

If the paranasal sinus ostia are occluded by mucosal swelling, a similar condition may arise in these cavities. This condition is called *aerosinusitis*, or *barosinusitis*. Unlike the middle ear, however, sinus pain may occur during either ascent or descent. The pain may be intense and incapacitating. It is caused by either a positive or negative differential pressure in the sinus cavities.

The lungs, unlike the middle ears and sinuses, are contained in a cavity of variable volume. The thoracic cavity is thus free to contract, within limits, even when air is not available from the environment (e.g., breath-hold diving). Limits are imposed on the contraction in volume, however; once the residual volume of the lungs is reached, further increases in barometric pressure cause a relative negative pressure to occur within the thorax (thoracic squeeze). This is compensated for in part by an increase in the volume of blood in the lesser circulation and the intrathoracic portion of the venous reservoir, but at high negative pressures, pulmonary parenchymal injury results. The world's record for a breath-hold dive is 231 feet, a 760 to 6080 mm Hg change.

If gas is available outside the body, very rapid increases in pressure are tolerated. Some people appear able to ventilate their eustachian tubes continuously; such subjects can tolerate pressure increases on the order of 60 mm Hg per sec (1 psi per sec) without difficulty. Entry of air into the lungs is not a limiting factor in these circumstances.

Blast waves in free air, however, may be a problem, since very high overpressures with very short rise times may occur. In these circumstances, air does not have time to enter the lungs, and very considerable differential pressures may occur across the chest wall, followed by marked underpressures in the environment during the rarefaction wave that follows the initial overpressure. These events occur so rapidly that the lung-chest system does not have time to adapt; it acts as a rigid system in which shear forces may cause tearing of delicate structures.

Decreasing Barometric Pressures. Relatively rapid decreases in barometric pressure occur during an ascent from depth to the surface in water, during decompression of a caisson, and during ascent to altitude in aircraft. The effects of such decreases in pressure are expansion of trapped gas and, when a substantial decrease in pressure is involved, evolution of gases from solution in the blood and body fluids.

Because of the peculiar structure of the eustachian tube, ear discomfort is almost never a problem when barometric pressure decreases.

Barosinusitis or barodontalgia, however, may occur owing to expansion of trapped gas. The latter disorder is due to pockets of gas in improperly filled or infected teeth.

Under normal circumstances, the gastrointestinal tract contains relatively small amounts of gas. As this gas expands, stretch receptors in the wall of the gut are stimulated, and peristalsis becomes more active. Relief from cramps is obtained by belching or passing flatus. During an extremely rapid decompression, however, massive expansion may occur before a muscular response is possible; the result may be vagovagal syncope. Rapid decompression can occur in the event of a window or door seal or wall failure in pressurized jet aircraft.

The foregoing comments suggest that the physician should be careful about allowing patients with hypomotile gut disorders to fly at high altitudes in unpressurized aircraft. Modern passenger aircraft are pressurized to keep cabin altitude at or below 8000 feet (564 mm Hg). Even at this moderate pressure, however, relative gas volume (saturated) is 38 per cent over sea-level values. In unpressurized light aircraft, altitudes of 12,000 feet (P_B = 483 mm Hg) are common.

The human lung-airway system at resting expiratory level has a time constant in the neighborhood of 0.05 to 0.10 second. During rapid decompression of an aircraft, if the time constant of the cabin (a function of its volume and the orifice through which air is escaping) is appreciably longer than that of the lungs and airway, no substantial overpressure will occur within the chest. If the reverse is true, however, overpressures will occur within the lungs. If the magnitude of the pressure drop is great enough, the lungs can become distended, and a further buildup of differential pressure within the lungs can cause parenchymal tears and possibly air embolism. Such rapid decompressions are very rare in civil aircraft but can occur in military jets that have small cabin volumes and large canopies.

It should be noted that during ascent from deep water to the surface, pressure decreases at the rate of 1 ATA per 33 feet. If a diver inspires from a breathing apparatus at depth, then attempts breath-holding during an ascent, he is in grave danger of lung rupture. It is necessary to expire actively throughout this maneuver and to limit the ascent rate. Naval divers are warned to "follow their bubbles" during such ascents, which gives them an ascent rate of about 60 feet per minute. This same precaution is necessary during emergency escape from submarines, which is accomplished through pressurized air locks.

Decompression Sickness. When the total pressure on a fluid containing dissolved gas is sharply decreased, the gases emerge from solution as bubbles (the phenomenon of effervescence observed when a bottle of soda or beer is uncapped). In the body, inert gas as well as oxygen and carbon dioxide are dissolved, both in water and in fat. The amount of inert gas in solution is a function of the alveolar partial pressure of the gas and its solubility coefficients in water and in oil.

Once bubbles of gas form in the tissues or the blood, they obey Boyle's law. If the pressure on the body is reduced further, they expand; if the pressure is increased, they contract, but they do not disappear until the pressure is increased considerably above the pressure at which they were formed.

During any ascent to high altitude or from depth, the amount of inert gas in solution in blood and various tissues is the limiting factor, since decompression at too rapid a rate will favor formation of bubbles. The rate at which inert gas is eliminated from any tissue is a function of the perfusion of that tissue and the partial pressure of inert gas in the perfusing blood. Since different tissues contain different proportions of lipid and water and have different rates of perfusion, some (such as depot fat) give up inert gas very slowly, whereas diffusion proceeds rapidly in muscle and liver.

The symptoms that occur when decompression occurs too rapidly are known collectively as *decompression sickness*. Although it is not certain that all the manifestations of decompression sickness are due to evolved gas, this is the most consistent explanation that has been offered to date. Regardless of the cause, however, the symptoms of decompression sickness are consistent. They fall into five distinct categories.

The most common and least ominous form of this disorder is called the *bends,* after the grotesque postures assumed in an effort to minimize the often excruciating joint and periarticular pain that characterizes the syndrome. Bends may come on suddenly or insidiously. Pain in or around a joint is the first symptom. It often afflicts a joint in use, or one which has previously been injured. The pain may remain localized, may migrate, or may affect several joints sequentially. A relatively small increase in barometric pressure may produce complete relief. If decompression continues, however, the pain may become incapacitating, or other forms of decompression sickness may supervene.

Localized paresthesias, itching, and rashes may also occur, presumably owing to bubbles in the skin or subcutaneous tissues. They are not dangerous. Much more ominous is a painless mottling of the skin that resembles patchy cyanosis. Its precise etiology is uncertain, but it is often seen in combination with or preceding the onset of the more severe forms of decompression sickness listed below.

A more serious form of decompression sickness is the symptom complex known as the *chokes.* This form is characterized by tachypnea, burning substernal pain that worsens on deep inspiration, and dry cough. It is believed that these symptoms, together with pulmonary hypertension, are caused by showers of bubbles arising in the venous circulation that lodge in pulmonary arterioles and capillaries. The chokes are a grave development, for they often precede the most serious forms of decompression sickness.

Central nervous system decompression sickness may occur in isolation or in combination with other forms of the disease. The symptoms may mimic virtually any acute discrete or disseminated CNS lesion. Hemianopsia, hemiparesis, aphasia, confusion, delirium, and other equally frightening symptoms and signs may be observed. These are thought to be caused by gas bubbles that either block or evoke severe spasm in cerebral arterioles. Despite the serious nature of this syndrome, dramatic relief is usually produced by immediate recompression to a pressure well above that at which the symptoms appeared. With effective treatment, permanent sequelae are rare although not unknown.

Syncope may be the first or a secondary symptom of decompression sickness. Particularly when recompression is prompt, the patient will usually return to consciousness rapidly. After some time, however, such a patient may quite suddenly begin to show signs of shock, which can progress rapidly to severe levels, with anuria, refractory peripheral vascular collapse, coma, and death.

The treatment of decompression sickness is relatively simple if, and only if, adequate facilities are at hand. Recompression is the specific treatment for this disorder. In the case of decompression sickness occurring at high altitude and persisting after return to sea level, overcompression in hyperbaric chambers has been remarkably successful. Although such treatment does not make gas bubbles dissolve immediately, it does make them smaller and probably promotes more rapid dissolution. Details as to the compression treatment of this disorder may be found in the U.S. Navy Diving Manual, the basic source document for anyone involved in situations in which decompression sickness can occur.

A late finding in caisson workers and divers who are repeatedly exposed to compression and marginally adequate decompression is aseptic bone necrosis, which often occurs in the heads of the long bones but may be seen elsewhere as well. This disorder may be serious and disabling. Once present, it does not differ appreciably from aseptic necrosis caused by other agents. It is probably due to compromise of the circulation to these areas.

OXYGEN

The oxygen concentration in the lower atmosphere (below 50,000 feet) is remarkably constant at about 20.9 per cent. Since barometric pressure changes geometrically with altitude (Fig. 36–1), the partial pressure of oxygen in air changes in the same manner. The reader will recall that humidification of air in the upper airways causes a decrease in the partial pressure of oxygen in the inspirate; another more marked drop in oxygen pressure or tension occurs in the alveoli owing to continuous extraction of oxygen from and addition of carbon dioxide to the alveolar air. A further drop is seen when pulmonary venous blood is examined (the alveolar-arterial gradient); there is another slight decrease in arterial oxygen tension due to admixture of venous with arterial blood. The relatively long diffusion pathway for oxygen in the tissues means that the oxygen tension at the mitochondria is usually remarkably low. This entire pathway must be considered when we deal with alterations in oxygen partial pressures in the environment or in the human.

Absence of Oxygen (Anoxia). True tissue anoxia probably occurs only when circulation ceases. With the exceptions of oxygen dissolved in tissue fluids and oxygen bound to myoglobin and hemoglobin, the body has no storage capacity for this vital substance. When circulation to the brain ceases completely, as in ventricular fibrillation or rapid decompressions to near-vacuum conditions, consciousness is lost within 5 to 10 seconds; in animals, anoxic brain damage is seen after 90 to 180 seconds. It is interesting that even after such extreme exposures, if consciousness is regained at all, signs of cerebral dysfunction may be transitory, and usually an apparently complete recovery follows. This may also be true following accidental electric shock.

Decreases in Oxygen (Hypoxia). As noted earlier, ultimate human tolerance for hypoxia of a duration longer than a few minutes is governed by the ability to maintain a state of consciousness. Consciousness is usually lost within 10 to 15 seconds after alveolar oxygen tension drops below 30 mm Hg. The arterial oxygen tension under these circumstances is generally below 20 mm Hg. The retina and brain have the highest oxygen uptakes per unit mass of any tissues in the body and thus are the tissues most rapidly and severely affected by hypoxia.

In persons breathing air, time of useful consciousness varies from hours at a barometric pressure of 350 to 380 mm Hg to about 10 to 20 seconds at a barometric pressure of 120 to 140 mm Hg.

At pressures greater than 380 mm Hg, indefinite survival on air is possible, although not without severe dysfunction. Impaired mentation and coordination are common during acute exposures to hypoxia of this degree. The symptoms of moderate hypoxia include dyspnea, difficulty in concentrating, and altered judgment and mood; euphoria or depression may be noted. The symptoms are due to impaired cerebral oxygenation, magnified by hypocapnia, which causes a degree of cerebral ischemia.

If exposure to alveolar oxygen tensions below about 50 mm Hg is prolonged for more than 6 to 12 hours, as in mountain climbing, symptoms of acute altitude sickness begin to appear. These symptoms include malaise, headaches (which may be severe), nausea, anorexia, and insomnia. They are made worse by strenuous physical activity or exposure to cold. Breathlessness and dyspnea may be extreme. The incidence of this syndrome reaches its height between 24 and 48 hours and usually subsides thereafter.

The cause of the disorder is not known, although it occurs during a period of multiple physiologic changes. In response to hyperventilation and hypocapnia, fixed base is excreted in the urine. Plasma and extracellular water decrease; the intracellular fluid space increases. A generalized stress response is observed. Roy and others have observed that diuresis usually occurs on the second or third day at altitude and that symptoms usually decline in severity at this time.

Nearly all persons going to high altitudes experience symptoms of acute altitude sickness. The severity of the symptoms may be lessened by taking acetazolamide for 24 hours prior to ascent.

A few people, instead of feeling better after an initial period of discomfort at altitude, may continue to have difficulty. If hypoxic exposure is continued, some will develop one or more symptoms of a more serious disorder known as *chronic altitude sickness*. The most ominous forms of this condition involve either cerebral edema or acute pulmonary edema or both. These are life-threatening if hypoxic exposure is not terminated. Again, the ultimate cause is not known. Some persons can endure repeated hypoxic exposures without showing these signs; others appear inordinately susceptible. The young are more affected; physical activity by susceptible persons hastens the onset of symptoms.

As exposure to hypoxia is prolonged past 3 to 5 days, hematologic changes begin to be evident. The hemoglobin, red cell count, and hematocrit all rise. The latter reaches values of 60 per cent or so after a month of exposure. Concomitant with these changes, heart rates at rest and during work decline; work tolerance increases, although not to sea-level values. Appetite improves and fluid intake increases.

The changes noted here, and others beyond the scope of this review, gradually revert toward sea-level values following cessation of exposure to hypoxia. Normal sea-level values are reached within 2 to 3 weeks after return from altitude.

Exposure to sustained hypoxia in the range of barometric pressures 640 to 520 mm Hg (5000 to 10,000 feet) normally evokes only mild to moderate exertional dyspnea, mild fatigue for a few days, and subtle psychomotor defects.

Oxygen Tensions at Sea Level (Normoxia). It can be shown that the oxygen tension of arterial blood at sea level (95 to 105 mm Hg) is still low enough to cause a mild tonic ventilatory stimulus in the carotid chemoreceptors. Nonetheless, persons with normal oxygen transport systems appear to have no other symptoms of hypoxia at rest at barometric pressures in the neighborhood of 760 mm Hg. During severe physical exercise, the administration of high concentrations of oxygen produces substantial reductions in minute ventilation and increases endurance and work capacity.

Increases in Oxygen (Hyperoxia). Since the arterial blood is virtually fully saturated with oxygen at an alveolar partial pressure of 100 mm Hg, an increase in alveolar oxygen tension above its normal sea-level value of 100 to 110 mm Hg results in an increase only in the quantity of oxygen dissolved in plasma, normally about 0.3 ml per 100 ml at an oxygen tension of 100 mm Hg. It is possible to attain alveolar oxygen tensions as high as 670 mm Hg by breathing 100 per cent oxygen at sea level for several hours. The gain in oxygen content of whole blood is only about 2 ml per 100 ml, however, in a normal person. If arterial desaturation is present owing to an increased A:a gradient, of course, the use of increased concentrations of oxygen can have much more substantial results. It should be emphasized, however, that the prolonged use of oxygen in persons who do not have either a ventilation or diffusion defect is not physiologic and may be harmful.

Oxygen at pressures above 200 to 250 mm Hg is toxic to humans. The toxicity is a time-dependent phenomenon. The most important manifestations of this toxicity at oxygen pressures up to 1 ATA are pulmonary inflammatory changes and, later, pulmonary edema. It also appears that high oxygen tensions interfere with surfactant formation or excretion, with the result that small areas of atelectasis are observed. One should note that all these pulmonary changes interfere with oxygenation of the blood, which is the reason oxygen is being administered. Such administration, therefore, is a two-edged sword. There is considerable evidence that intermittent administration of oxygen delays or prevents the appearance of pulmonary oxygen toxicity; this should be kept in mind when the gas is to be used for long periods of time.

At pressures of 2 to 3 ATA, oxygen begins to cause central nervous system dysfunction. Tremors, anxiety, and grand-mal convulsions are seen. Again, the effects are time- and pressure-dependent, an increase in either causing more severe signs. Oxygen at these pressures has been demonstrated to be useful in the treatment of acute carbon monoxide poisoning, gas gangrene, refractory osteomyelitis, radiation necrosis (as an adjunct to surgical reconstruction), and failing skin grafts. Other uses of oxygen at high pressure are speculative.

NITROGEN

There is no evidence that the human organism is able to "fix," or incorporate, molecular nitrogen into chemical compounds. In the absence of such evidence, we are unable to state with finality that gaseous nitrogen is an essential substance. It is necessary, in any discussion of this gas, to distinguish between its role as a unique element and its role as a diluent gas for oxygen, in which latter role any physiologically inert gas will serve as well.

The Role of Nitrogen. As we have said, there is no clear evidence that gaseous nitrogen is essential to human survival, although it has been shown that chick embryos fail to develop in environments free of the gas. Adult males have functioned effectively for up to 2 weeks in atmospheres virtually devoid of nitrogen in Gemini and some Apollo space flights.

There is absolutely no evidence that nitrogen at sea-level pressures of roughly 600 mm Hg is toxic. At substantially higher pressures, however, gaseous nitrogen begins to exert a narcotic effect. This effect limits the depth to which divers can descend breathing air. Nitrogen narcosis is pronounced at total pressures of 10 ATA (P_{N_2} of 6000 mm Hg), equivalent to a depth of about 270 feet of sea water.

This effect is not unique; we shall see that virtually all physiologically inert gases are narcotic at some pressure. The narcotic effect of nitrogen is enhanced by physical activity; it appears to be lessened by repeated exposure to narcotic pressures.

The Role of Inert Gases. Although nitrogen as such has not been shown to be essential, it has been shown that the absence of inert diluent gases has specific and predictable effects. Pure oxygen is absorbed rapidly in the lung, and even at pressures below toxic levels, patchy atelectasis has been demonstrated in subjects breathing 100 per cent oxygen. A similar phenomenon occurs in the middle ear if that cavity, after depressurization, is ventilated with pure oxygen. The gas is absorbed slowly, and the resulting pressure decrease within the ear causes symptoms of barotitis.

Inert diluent gases are necessary at sea level and higher barometric pressures, if only to prevent oxygen pressures from reaching toxic levels. At considerable depth, other inert gases must be substituted for nitrogen to avoid nitrogen narcosis. The most commonly used substitute is helium; neon is also used under special circumstances, although it is extremely expensive.

HELIUM

Effects of High Pressures of Helium. Helium is not an essential element and is normally present in air only in minute amounts. Helium-oxygen mixtures may be substituted for the usual nitrogen-oxygen mixture at sea level with predictable effects but without causing harm, even over extended periods of exposure.

Helium is much less dense than nitrogen,

although its viscosity is slightly higher than that of nitrogen. The work of breathing at rest at sea level is largely expended in producing laminar air flow and is a function of the viscosity of the gas mixture. Turbulent air flow, however, is a function of density; when the proportion of turbulent air flow is increased, either during intense work or in the presence of significant airway narrowing (as in bronchial asthma), the use of helium-oxygen mixtures appreciably reduces the work of breathing.

Also, helium has a very high thermal conductivity. Comfort temperatures in a helium-oxygen environment are several degrees higher than in air, as a result. The convective heat loss in helium environments is a serious problem in deep diving, particularly when hard work is being performed; respiratory heat loss under these circumstances may exceed the capacity of the diver to produce heat.

Only minimal narcotic effects of helium are seen even at the highest barometric pressures to which humans have thus far been exposed. The narcotic potency of all the noble gases is proportional to molecular weight, however; there is no reason to believe that helium will not be narcotic at some pressure, as yet undefined.

The relative insolubility of helium in body fluids and its low density and low narcotic potential have made it the diluent of choice in diving. Its disadvantages are its high thermal conductivity and its effects on speech; in the latter, the fundamental frequency is shifted upward, and the harmonic structure is sharply modified by altered gas density. At high helium pressure, human speech may become virtually unintelligible.

OTHER INERT GASES

Neon has been used in diving and in experimental sojourns at moderate depths. It is less narcotic than nitrogen and more dense than helium, so that speech is less altered; heat loss is sharply reduced compared with that seen with helium. Its major disadvantages are its expense and its narcotic action at pressures above 10 ATA, although research in this range is inadequate. *Argon* is more soluble in fat than nitrogen. Its use in diving therefore prolongs decompression time. *Krypton* and *xenon* are both potent narcotics at pressures near atmospheric. For these reasons, these gases have not been used in diving or as other than tracer gases at sea level.

THE ELECTROMAGNETIC ENVIRONMENT

Figure 36–2 is a schematic representation of the electromagnetic environment. It serves to re-

mind us of the reciprocal relation of frequency and wavelength, of the increasing energy of radiation as frequency increases, and of a few of the important effects of electromagnetic waves: molecular excitation at low frequencies, molecular interactions at higher frequencies, and molecular ionization and disruption at the highest frequencies.

In this section, we shall also consider briefly the effects of electric currents that may pass through the body, and we shall mention certain questions that have been raised about the effects of continuous and alternating magnetic fields on the human organism.

The reader will recall that electromagnetic waves are propagated at the speed of light. Since the speed of light varies in different materials, these waves, upon encountering matter, may be reflected, refracted, transmitted, or absorbed. When matter is truly transparent to waves, they transfer none of their energy to that matter. Only if matter is opaque or translucent to waves can energy transfer take place. The reader interested in pursuing this area in more detail should review briefly the thermodynamics of heat transfer.

MAGNETISM

Almost since the discovery of the lodestone, there has been speculation about the possible effects of magnetic fields upon physiologic function. Much medical quackery has been based on the supposed beneficial effects of magnetic fields.

Exposure to high-intensity magnetic fields causes the appearance of visual phosphenes, although whether these are due to the magnetic field or to an induced electrical field in the retina is uncertain. Growth disturbances have been observed in very high, nonuniform magnetic fields. Behavioral effects have also been reported. In theory, very high field strengths can cause migration of cell substances, although it should be noted that fields of several thousand gauss are not strong enough to overshadow the normal thermal movement of such molecules.

ELECTRICITY

Electricity is so much a part of our lives and is so easily kept under our control, that we tend to overlook its considerable dangers. Nearly everyone in a technologic society has been "bitten" by an electric current at some time; the overwhelming majority of such incidents cause nothing more than momentary annoyance. Yet electrical deaths are daily occurrences, and the difference between mere annoyance and a fatal outcome may be nothing more than fortuitous: a matter of whether one's hands are dry, whether shoes are being worn, and the like.

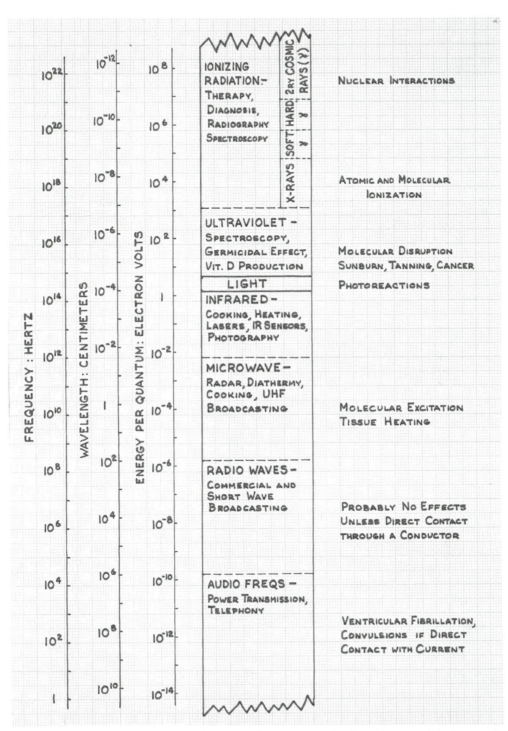

Figure 36–2 This chart shows the relationship between frequency, wavelength, and energy of electromagnetic waves, together with the commonly used division of the spectrum and comments on biologic effects.

In medicine, where biomedical sensors and monitors are increasingly useful, the hazards of inadvertent electrocution are compounded, since these devices are attached to the body in ways that minimize resistance to the passage of stray currents.

When the body is exposed to an electrical current, the electrical characteristics of the exposed part will determine how much current enters the body. Within the body, the conductivity of tissues between the entrance and exit points will determine the path taken by the current and the proportion of the total energy dissipated within the body as heat. Wide variations in individual responses are the rule.

In general, the threshold of perception for current entering the hand is about 5 mA for direct current, and less than 1 mA for 60 Hz alternating current. Little more than these amounts is generally reported as painful by some investigators; others report the range of 3 to 10 mA as the pain threshold.

With direct current, involuntary muscular contractions sufficient to prevent the exposed person from removing his hand from the source of current are produced by less than 60 mA in men, 40 mA in women. With alternating currents, corresponding values are 9 and 6 mA.

The most serious hazard in accidental contacts with electricity is ventricular fibrillation, since currents passing from a hand to any other extremity must traverse the chest. The heart is absolutely refractory to the induction of ventricular fibrillation except for a short period during the repolarization phase of the ventricles; thus, the timing of brief shocks is important.

Speaking generally, a 60 Hz alternating current of 100 mA crossing the chest for 1 second or more will often induce fibrillation. About five times this current, delivered during the sensitive phase of the cardiac cycle, is required with direct current. Much smaller currents are sufficient when they are delivered directly to the heart.

Electrical currents are used in electroconvulsive therapy of neurotic and psychotic depressive reactions. Currents of several hundred mA (60 Hz AC) passed transversely across the cerebrum produce momentary respiratory arrest and tonic, then clonic, convulsions, unconsciousness, and amnesia. Much smaller currents passed longitudinally through the brain stem produce severe physiologic respiratory arrest, often without other dysfunction or injury. It may be for this reason that recovery from accidental electric shock may occur after even protracted assisted ventilation. More severe shocks, as in legal electrocution, cause gross disruption of brain tissues and hemorrhage.

Electrical defibrillation of the heart can be life-saving in cases of "spontaneous" ventricular fibrillation. It is generally agreed that direct currents are safer than alternating currents for this purpose. Most defibrillators make use of a condenser discharge at controlled levels. The energy delivered to the chest wall can be varied from 25 to several hundred watt-seconds (joules).

When an electric current is delivered to a tissue the resistance of which is high, a considerable proportion of the energy appears as heat. The resistance of the skin is usually much higher than that of the interior of the body; this is the reason for the often serious electrical burns at entrance and exit points, even when the current through the body has not caused permanent injury. Use is made of this in electrocautery, which is also used to coagulate small blood vessels during surgery. Controlled electrical coagulation of portions of the central nervous system has also been used, both experimentally and therapeutically.

It should be noted that both the rate at which heat energy is generated in a tissue and the rate at which it can be dissipated by conduction or by convective transfer in blood are equally important in determining whether irreversible denaturation of tissue proteins will occur. Poorly vascularized tissues in the body, such as the lens of the eye, are particularly susceptible to injury by electricity or other radiation that can cause rapid energy transfer. Lenticular cataracts have been produced by electrical currents as well as by infrared and microwave radiation.

ELECTROMAGNETIC WAVES; RADIO FREQUENCIES

The human body is essentially transparent to low-frequency electromagnetic waves. Waves of frequencies above 200 MHz, however, are absorbed to an increasing degree by biologic tissues. The energy thus absorbed appears as heat (molecular excitation). Such waves are encountered in ultra–high-frequency radio and television broadcasting, in which they are usually propagated omnidirectionally, and in radar (radio detection and ranging), in which they are usually focused into a narrow beam by a parabolic antenna and reflector. Transmission may be continuous (CW) in broadcasting or pulsed (PW) in most radar applications. Microwave diathermy units, operating at about 2500 MHz, and microwave ovens, at similar frequencies, are usually CW devices, although some studies have suggested that PW devices may be more effective in diathermy.

A detailed description of this extremely broad band of radiation is beyond the scope of this chapter. Certain general principles can be stated, however. As frequency increases, penetration of these waves decreases in water or biologic tissues; the radiation is absorbed, therefore, by a smaller cone of tissue and the local heating increases. For example, 1 joule transferred through 1 cm² of skin and absorbed in a depth of 1 cm would yield the heat equivalent of 1 joule per cm³, whereas the same energy transfer at a higher frequency absorbed in the top 1 mm of skin would yield the heat equivalent of 10 joules per cm³.

Since the body has temperature receptors only at its surface, it has no way of sensing the presence of low-frequency microwave energy, which passes into the body core. High-intensity fields at high frequencies, however, may be sensed as warmth or a burning sensation.

Microwave radiation is reflected by metals and to a lesser extent by earth. Metal screens can be used to protect persons working in microwave fields.

Some investigators in this area have reported results of microwave radiation other than thermogenic effects. The most consistent findings have been in the hematopoietic system, although these reports are disputed by others. Interference with nerve conduction has also been reported.

There is little question that microwave radiation in large doses can cause cataracts. Reports of such lesions in industry have been rare, however, as have authentic reports of systemic injury caused by microwave radiation in general.

INFRARED (THERMAL) RADIATION

It is not possible to set a clear boundary between microwave and thermal, or infrared, radiation. As we have seen, tissue heating is produced by electromagnetic waves of much lower than infrared frequencies. Most authors place the boundary in the neighborhood of 10^6 MHz, or a wavelength of 3×10^7 Å.

Since thermal radiation is effectively absorbed by the body, and since metabolism results in endogenous heat production, we must consider in some detail the physiopathology evoked by both excessive and insufficient heat.

It will be recalled that humans must maintain rather precise internal temperature control in the face of widely varying environmental temperatures and levels of heat production. Thermal inputs to the body come by radiation, convection, or conduction from the environment and from metabolic heat production. Humans can lose heat to the environment by radiation, convection, conduction, and evaporation of water or sweat. The range of tolerance for heat is remarkably narrow: If we consider the individual purely as a container of heat, his total heat content is in the neighborhood of 9000 kcal, but his tolerance for alterations in heat content is only about ± 150 kcal.

We shall look first at the systemic effects of heat and then examine its local effects. Cold, or insufficient heat, will be considered in the same way.

Heat

Acute Systemic Effects. Whenever an individual is exposed to heat stress, a number of systems respond in an effort to rid the body of the thermal load. Peripheral vasodilatation occurs; as peripheral resistance falls, heart rate and cardiac output increase. If temperature gradients between the skin and the surrounding air are adequate, convective heat dissipation increases enough to restore balance. If not, or if the thermal load is large, sweating occurs. Evaporation is an extremely effective method of heat dissipation because of the high latent heat of vaporization of water. For evaporation to occur, however, the air surrounding the body must have a vapor pressure below the saturation vapor pressure at skin temperature.

If these mechanisms for heat loss are not adequate to keep pace with the rate of heat input to the body, heat storage must occur; the core temperature will rise. A number of symptom complexes are seen when an individual encounters heat stress beyond his capacities.

Heat stroke is the most serious of these syndromes. Its presence is made known by anxiety, irritability, visual disturbances, delirium, collapse, coma, and death if treatment is inadequate. The skin is dry, hot, and flushed. The rectal temperature is very high (40° to 43° C). Cessation of sweating in the presence of continued thermal stress, probably owing to failure of central thermoregulatory centers, allows a very rapid increase in the rate of heat storage.

Heat stroke constitutes a true medical emergency. Removal of the patient from the source of heat stress followed by vigorous attempts to cool the body are the first measures to be instituted. Rapid cooling should be used, although it must be realized that skin cooling induces peripheral vasoconstriction, which inhibits conduction of core heat to the surface.

As the rectal and core temperatures begin to fall, it becomes necessary to moderate treatment so that one does not induce hypothermia, for it must be realized that the thermoregulatory failure that allows heat to be retained will also fail to protect against excessive heat loss. In essence, the therapist must take over the task of maintaining thermal homeostasis until the patient recovers that capacity. Persons who have had heat stroke may tolerate intense heat poorly thereafter, because of permanent damage in the thermoregulatory centers.

Heat exhaustion is characterized by weakness, hypotension and elevated temperature. The skin is not dry, however; often the patient has been sweating vigorously. The condition is probably caused by moderate dehydration and salt imbalance. Removal from heat and treatment with fluid and electrolytes (the intravenous route may be necessary if the patient is nauseated) usually produce prompt recovery. There are no sequelae.

Heat cramps are seen in unacclimatized subjects doing strenuous work in hot environments. These cramps are attributed to salt depletion. The oral administration of dilute salt solution, or intravenous administration of physiologic saline, produces dramatic relief. These symptoms can be prevented by acclimatization (see later).

Thermogenic anhidrosis has been observed in healthy, acclimatized subjects after a considerable period of heat exposure. Profuse sweating for a prolonged period suddenly terminates except on the face and neck. Patients complain of malaise, warmth, fatigue, shakiness, and lightheadedness. The rectal temperature is usually normal. The skin is dry. Severe prickly heat is invariably present. The cause of the disorder appears to be either physical obstruction or physiologic exhaustion of sweat glands. Treatment consists of rest and return to a cooler environment.

Chronic Systemic Effects. Even physically fit people cannot work long or strenuously when they are first exposed to a very hot environment. If, however, they are allowed to perform work of gradually increasing intensity during the first 1 to 2 weeks of exposure, their work tolerance increases markedly. A number of physiologic changes are observed in the course of this acclimatization process. The volume of sweat increases; its electrolyte concentration decreases. Heart rates at given work loads decrease sharply. Postural hypotension no longer occurs. Work tolerance approaches values previously obtained in cool environments. Water intake increases sharply, although thirst still is not an adequate guide for fluid replacement.

Acclimatization is impeded or reversed, once present, by fatigue, ingestion of alcohol, restriction of water, systemic illness, or temporary removal from exposure.

Tolerance for work in hot environments has been studied by many authors. The data shown in Figure 36–3 are representative.

Local Effects. It has been noted repeatedly here that the radiant energy transferred to a volume of tissue, relative to the capacity of that tissue and its perfusing blood to remove heat, will determine whether heat storage and a temperature rise will occur. Most human proteins are easily denatured by heat; thus, the thermal capacity of living tissue is rather small.

If the rate of heat input to the skin is high, local heating occurs. Histamine and other vasodilator substances are released, producing erythema. If the temperature rises further, local vesiculation occurs. If the temperature continues to rise, coagulation necrosis of the germinal epithelium results, and the skin will slough. At still higher temperatures, charring is observed. This, in brief, is the sequence seen when the skin is burned. The relationship between the rate of energy input and duration of input is logarithmic.

The secondary and tertiary adjustments in fluid and electrolyte balance that occur following burns of considerable extent are beyond the scope of this survey. References to various reviews of the topic will be found at the end of this chapter.

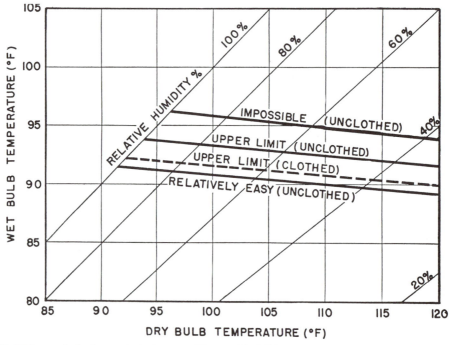

Figure 36–3 Diagram indicating equivalent zones of "impossible," difficult (upper limit), and relatively easy combinations of dry and wet bulb temperatures; the effect of relative humidity and of clothing on acclimatized men working for 4 hours at an energy expenditure of about 300 kcal/hr. (From Largent and Ashe, 1958.)

Infrared Radiation

Effects on the Eye. The cornea is virtually transparent to the highest portion of the IR spectrum (wavelengths shorter than 19,000 Å). The crystalline lens has a similar but not identical transmissibility characteristic; it becomes increasingly transparent at wavelengths shorter than 15,000 Å.

There is, therefore, a range of wavelengths in the high infrared portion of the spectrum for which the cornea and aqueous are more transparent than the lens. As a result, heating of the lens occurs, both directly and secondarily as a result of absorption of the same wavelengths by the iris.

The industrial phenomenon now known as "glass-blower's cataract" was described in the eighteenth century. Since that time, many workers have studied these lesions and have established conclusively that they are caused by thermal radiation rather than by light, as was first thought. Similar lesions would likely be produced by lasers radiating at appropriate wavelengths.

Normal Thermal Environments for Humans

Much research has been done on the limits of environmental comfort for humans under various conditions of activity. Since comfort is a subjective phenomenon, most of this research has necessarily made use of subjective indices. A unit of thermal insulation has been developed, the clo, which is "the amount of insulation necessary to maintain comfort in a seated, resting subject in a normally ventilated room (air movement 20 ft per min, or 10 cm per sec) at a temperature of 70° F (21° C) and a relative humidity of the air of less than 50 per cent." For American men and women wearing 1 clo of insulation, thermal comfort ranges are 70° to 85° F (21° to 29° C).

As environmental temperature falls, the individual's thermal environment begins to require him to cope with an inadequate thermal input. We call this *cold*.

Cold

Systemic Effects. In general, where an individual faces, lives with, and can acclimatize to heat, he tends to avoid or circumvent the effects of cold. Humans have only a limited number of ways of coping with lack of environmental heat; in the course of evolution, we have lost many of the mechanisms available to other mammals.

Humans can increase insulation somewhat by peripheral vasocontriction: Skin temperature drops and skin-environment gradients decrease. If cold air is flowing by the skin, however, convective losses are still considerable. The thick blanket of hair and the piloerector mechanisms of our mammalian cousins have long since been lost to us, as has the ability to vasoconstrict the rich blanket of scalp vessels in response to cold.

We do retain the ability to increase our rate of heat production, either by moving muscles in doing work or by shivering. We can also increase our effective insulation blanket by wearing clothing. The disadvantage of clothing is that the amount of insulation necessary to maintain comfort at rest is entirely too much when strenuous work is performed. Also, the insulating value of clothing is considerably reduced as it becomes wetted by sweat. It is thus necessary to maintain air flow over the skin to aid in evaporation while such work is being performed.

When a person is unable to maintain thermal balance, his core temperature begins to drop. Severe shivering and exhaustion induced by voluntary work give way to profound feelings of lassitude and an overwhelming desire to sleep. More prolonged exposure causes continued body cooling and usually death by ventricular fibrillation when the cardiac temperature drops to 27° C, although survival has been reported after rapid rewarming of humans whose core temperature was as low as 18° C.

Just as rapidly moving air removes heat from a warm object more rapidly than still air, water, with its high specific heat, removes heat from the body very much more rapidly than air. Immersion in water at near-freezing temperature renders a person incapable of helping himself within a very few minutes and is usually fatal in less than an hour, whereas he will survive in still air at this temperature for many hours.

Local Effects. When an extremity or other body part with the exception of the scalp is exposed to cold, piloerection ("goose pimples") and vasoconstriction occur. As the skin temperature approaches 0° C, metabolic needs are maintained for a time; pain in the area gives way to numbness. Thereafter, edema and blistering may appear. Gangrene, with or without infection, will occur if the part is allowed to remain cold; if rapid rewarming is instituted, permanent injury is minimized, although the part may be painful for a considerable time. If cell disruption due to formation of ice crystals has occurred, permanent disability of some degree is likely. This is the picture of *frostbite*.

Exposure of extremities (most often the feet) to cold, wet environments gives rise to related disorders known as *trench foot* and *shelter foot*. In this condition, actual tissue freezing is rare, but tissue maceration may be extreme, and permanent disability is not uncommon.

There is some evidence that local adaptation to cold may occur, especially in the hands. Massey's data suggest that such adaptation proceeds over a period of perhaps 7 weeks. Other studies indicate that there may be seasonal fluctuations in hand blood flow in cold climates, with larger flows being observed in the coldest seasons.

VISIBLE RADIATION: LIGHT

The narrow band of electromagnetic waves lying between 7.7 and 3.8 $\times$ 10[8] MHz (wavelengths between about 3900 and 7700 Å) has an importance to humans out of all proportion to its miniscule contribution to the total energy flux within the universe. It is important because our eyes can sense this band; visible radiation illuminates our world and thus gives us the mobility that has helped make us what we are. No less important, it is a portion of this band that provides the specific energy levels required for photosynthesis, the basic source of all our nutritive needs.

The physiology of the eye is adequately described in other textbooks; it will be alluded to only briefly here. More important in terms of pathologic physiology are the tolerable range of light intensities and human efforts to adapt to levels outside this range.

The human retina has two types of sensors: rods, or scotopic sensors, and cones, or photopic sensors. The rods are found in greatest numbers at distances of about 10° from the center of the fovea; their numbers remain relatively constant for a considerable distance toward the periphery. There are no rods at the center of the fovea, however, where cone cells are found in greatest density.

The rod cells in the completely dark-adapted eye have a threshold on the order of 5 $\times$ 10[-6] millilamberts (mL). Cones reach their maximum acuity at illumination intensities above 10[5] mL. The retina's visual range is thus at least 10 orders of magnitude.

After prolonged exposure to bright light, the retinal sensors require a finite time to become maximally adapted to low levels of light. It is presumed that this adaptation time reflects the time necessary for complete regeneration of the photosensitive pigments within the sensors. Cone cells reach maximum sensitivity (0.001 to 0.01 mL) within 6 to 8 minutes, whereas the more sensitive rods require about 30 minutes of darkness (or dim red light, to which they are insensitive) to reach maximum sensitivity (less than 0.00001 mL). Many environmental and endogenous factors influence these values.

At the other end of the range of light intensities, we must consider the effects of exceedingly intense levels of illumination. The luminance of a nuclear fireball viewed from 4 miles away may exceed 10[8] mL; the sun, viewed from earth, has a luminance of 4 $\times$ 10[8] mL. In evaluating the effects of those intensities, we must consider two factors peculiar to visible radiation and the eye. First, the cornea, aqueous, lens, and vitreous are all relatively transparent to electromagnetic waves in the visible band. Second, and perhaps more important, the eye is not merely a sensing system; it focuses a point source of light on the retina. For this reason, very intense light sources concentrate their energy on a very small area of the retina and choroid, where pigment absorbs nearly all visible radiation that reaches it. Thus, nearly all the energy incident upon this small area is converted to heat, in amounts that very rapidly produce irreversible changes in the affected cells.

Retinal burns from solar, nuclear, or laser radiation produce permanent visual field defects, or blind spots. If these are in the periphery, they represent no great problem. Unfortunately, it is also only natural to look directly toward the source of intense light, which focuses the radiation directly on the fovea. The central field defect thus produced severely limits the visual acuity of the eye—or of both eyes—thereafter, because acuity rapidly declines at angular distances of even a few degrees from the fovea. Eclipse blindness, caused by viewing solar eclipses through inadequate filters, is a form of this lesion. Even the image of the solar corona, still visible at the moment of total eclipse, is bright enough to cause such burns.

Lasers (*l*ight *a*mplification by *s*timulated *e*mission of *r*adiation) represent a special hazard. Because the energy emitted by these devices is coherent (all of one frequency), there is almost no beam divergence, and unbelievably energetic pulses of radiation can be generated. These can literally vaporize any matter not transparent to them. The increasing use of such devices in scientific, industrial, and military applications multiplies the hazards to which workers or troops may be subjected.

ULTRAVIOLET RADIATION

Visible radiation is energetic enough to trigger photosynthesis as well as a variety of oxidative reactions in inorganic chemicals. Since the energy content of radiation is directly proportional to its frequency, the ultraviolet band (wavelengths from roughly 3900 to 1000 Å) contains increasingly energetic radiation, whose energies are powerful enough to disrupt various types of intramolecular chemical bonds. Indeed, the considerable germicidal effectiveness of ultraviolet radiation is due to its ability to disrupt the helical structure of DNA.

Fortunately, earth's atmosphere absorbs nearly all the very considerable flux of ultraviolet radiation that reaches it. Wavelengths shorter than 2400 Å are strongly absorbed by molecular oxygen, with the production of ozone in the upper atmosphere. Ozone itself absorbs all ultraviolet rays shorter than 2900 Å and some of those between 2900 and 3200 Å. Water vapor and dust in the troposphere absorb more, so that the flux of ultraviolet light at the earth's surface is very small. Nonetheless, enough reaches us to cause a variety of physiologic and pathologic effects. In the former category, we may place the conversion of provitamin D to vitamin D; in the latter, the production of sunburn and tanning.

Vitamin D is produced in the human epidermis from 7-dehydrocholesterol by ultraviolet radiation in the 2900 to 3200 Å band. Since little ultraviolet light reaches the surface of the earth when the sun is less than 20° above the horizon (owing to atmospheric scattering), it is clear that people living in the high north latitudes may be at risk of vitamin D deficiency for a substantial part of each year. This is especially true in industrial urban areas, where air pollution by dust is considerable and where people may have little exposure to sunlight. In these days of vitamin D–supplemented milk, one seldom recalls how serious a problem rickets was and for how long.

Sunburn is produced by ultraviolet light in the band of 2900 to 3200 Å, although large doses of rays longer than 3200 Å do produce erythema. After a latent period of up to several hours following exposure, cutaneous blood vessels dilate, with resultant erythema over the exposed area as well as discomfort and pain. The erythema reaches a peak between 8 and 24 hours following exposure and then gradually fades. If the burn is severe, vesiculation may occur, followed after a variable time by desquamation. A suntan of variable degree replaces the burn. Adaptation of the skin to repeated ultraviolet exposure occurs, manifested by deposition of melanin in the skin, although other adaptive mechanisms may be involved as well.

It should be emphasized that these signs are manifestations of injury to the dermis. Increases in mitotic activity are seen as desquamation takes place, together with marked thickening of the malpighian layer of the epidermis. The relationship between such changes and the eventual development of cancers is not fully understood, although it is clear that repeated sunburn causes degenerative changes in both dermis and epidermis. It has also been shown, both experimentally in animals and by epidemiologic studies in humans, that ultraviolet radiation in the 2800 to 3150 Å band does produce skin cancer.

IONIZING RADIATION

The Nature of Ionizing Radiation. Figure 36-2 shows a dotted line separating ultraviolet from ionizing radiation. There is no clear boundary; we shall see that some of the effects of ionizing radiation differ only in magnitude from those of less energetic forms of radiation. Electromagnetic waves of comparatively low energy can disrupt intramolecular chemical bonds; such disruption is one of the characteristic—and most harmful—effects of waves or particles of higher energy. As with all electromagnetic radiation, the effect of ionizing radiation depends on its absorption within the body. The absorption of ionizing radiation depends in great part on its physical characteristics: whether it is particulate or photon radiation; if particulate, whether it carries a charge; and its energy content.

All radioactive isotopes, or radionuclides, decay at a characteristic rate, which is expressed in terms of the time required for one half of a given quantity to decay. This is the *physical half-life* of the isotope. The decay may involve the emission of a photon, a beta particle, or portions of the nucleus.

It is important to remember that an atom of any element behaves chemically in a characteristic fashion, regardless of whether it is a stable or unstable isotope. The human body has no way to differentiate between isotopes. It turns over each element and compound at a characteristic rate, however; this is the *biologic half-life* of the substance. The *effective half-life* of a radionuclide within the body is a function of how rapidly it decays and of how rapidly it is excreted by the body.

Forms of Ionizing Radiation. An understanding of certain of the physical properties of the various forms of ionizing radiation is a necessary prerequisite to an understanding of the biologic effects of such radiation. The most important forms are as follows:

X-RAYS. These are photons, or quanta, of energy having no mass or charge and traveling at the speed of light. They are produced by transformations of extranuclear orbital electrons or by sudden deceleration of high-speed electrons, as in an x-ray tube. They may have virtually any energy content from very low (a few hundred electron volts) to extremely high. Because they have no mass or charge, their ability to penetrate matter is considerable.

GAMMA RAYS. These, like x-rays, are photons, but they are produced in the process of radioactive decay. Their energy content is a characteristic of the isotope undergoing decay and ranges from low to several million electron volts.

BETA PARTICLES AND HIGH-ENERGY ELECTRONS. Beta particles are energetic electrons carrying either a negative or positive charge. Both are produced by nuclear transformations; negatively charged high-energy electrons can also be produced in accelerating devices. They may have a wide spectrum of energies, although the average energy level of beta particles produced in nuclear transformations is characteristic. Because they are particles, they have momentum; ionization is produced when this momentum is transferred to another particle. Beta particles may also lose energy when decelerated; an x-ray is emitted.

PROTONS. These are nuclear constituents having a positive charge and a mass of one. Because of their charge, they can produce ionization by interacting with other charged particles; they can also produce ionization by transferring momentum to other particles. They are rarely a problem on earth but exist in great numbers in the Van Allen radiation belts surrounding our planet and are produced in enormous numbers during solar flares. They therefore pose a hazard for space travelers and to a lesser extent for persons flying in supersonic transport aircraft at very high altitudes. These aircraft carry warning systems to alert their pilots to the presence of excessive radiation levels.

ALPHA PARTICLES. The alpha particle is identical with the nucleus of the helium atom; it consists of two protons and two neutrons. Because of its large mass and charge, it has enormous ionizing potential but relatively short range in any sort of matter, including air. Alpha particles are produced spontaneously in radioactive decay of heavy elements.

NEUTRONS. These are particles with a mass of one, like protons, but they carry no electrical charge. Their energy is entirely a function of their velocity. Because they carry no charge, they interact with other matter only when they collide with it; ionization occurs indirectly as a result of the energy transfer during such collisions.

It is obvious from the foregoing discussion that the relative effect of these forms of ionizing radiation in biologic tissues will vary considerably. Those forms that have relatively large mass and charge have short ranges in tissues but produce enormous damage within that range; the most penetrating forms of radiation have a much lower likelihood of interacting with tissues. Because of this variation in biologic effect, quantities of radiation are measured in terms that take account only of the number of quanta actually absorbed in the body. The generally accepted radiation dose unit is the *rad* (radiation *a*bsorbed *d*ose). One rad equals 100 ergs of energy absorbed per gram of tissue. The biologic effect of the energy transfer is a function of the type of radiation, its energy content, and the density of the tissue into which it is directed.

Biologic Effects of Ionizing Radiation. The most sensitive structural and chemical component of the cell appears to be the deoxyribonucleic acid molecule. This is not surprising; we have already noted that even thermal radiation may increase the rate of mutations in germinal cells and that ultraviolet radiation's germicidal effectiveness is due to its ability to disrupt the helical structure of DNA.

Although nucleoproteins are at highest risk of alteration from ionizing radiation, lipids and carbohydrates may also be altered by such radiation. At the atomic level, ionizing radiation can result in excitation of an orbital electron or ejection of the electron from its orbit. An ion pair is created when an electron is ejected: an energetic, negatively charged electron and the positively charged residual atom or molecule. These pairs survive only a short time, but they are extremely

reactive and ultimately cause molecular damage by reacting with other cellular components. Because approximately 80 per cent of biologic systems are aqueous, the free radicals formed in water are—OH and—H, in addition to H^+ and OH^- ions. The free radicals react to form H_2, H_2O, and H_2O_2, an active oxidizing agent. It is the last one that is believed to produce physiochemical changes. Organic peroxides may be formed in the same fashion by free-radical action.

Pathologic Physiology of Radiation Injury. The susceptibility of body tissues to injury by ionizing radiation is in general directly proportional to their rate of cell division, or growth rate, and inversely proportional to their degree of differentiation. By this criterion, the hematopoietic system should be highly vulnerable to radiation, the rapidly replaced gastrointestinal mucosal cells should be somewhat less susceptible, and the central nervous system cellular elements should be least sensitive. Within the hematopoietic system, leukocytes and especially lymphocytes are highly susceptible; platelet formation is even more severely affected.

The manifestations of acute radiation injury are predictable. Infection and hemorrhage, particularly in the gastrointestinal tract, are the rule. Platelet deficiencies result in altered coagulation. Multiple tissue and gastrointestinal hemorrhages follow; these phenomena are aggravated by alterations in vascular permeability.

By contrast, although severe exposure and early death may be accompanied by marked central nervous system signs and symptoms, neuronal structural changes are minimal. The predominant changes in central nervous system function are due to altered vascular permeability, resulting in both perivascular and generalized cerebral edema.

Clinical Manifestations of Radiation Injury. The acute syndrome that follows radiation exposure is not unlike other inflammatory or toxic events. The damage depends on the dose of radiation and the period of time over which it is administered. The stages of illness parallel those of viral infections, with a prodrome, a latent period, manifest illness, and finally either death or convalescence and recovery. The periods between the stages are dose-dependent. Cautious predictions as to outcome sometimes can be made within the first 24 to 48 hours.

Since the degree of injury is dependent on the absorbed dose of radiation, a dose-related classification of responses can be described. This may be divided into the following five groups:

GROUP I. Dose, less than 150 rads. Most patients are asymptomatic; a few will have prodomal symptoms but not later signs of illness.

GROUP II. Dose, 200 to 400 rads. Most patients will have a mild form of the acute radiation syndrome with transient prodromal nausea and vomiting and subsequent evidence of hematopoietic alterations (Fig. 36–4). Most will recover; if death occurs it will be due to sequelae of the hematologic depression.

GROUP III. Dose, 400 to 600 rads. The dose that causes 50 per cent mortality in untreated cases is 450 to 500 rads. Persons in group III will exhibit serious effects associated with severe hematopoietic damage and variable degrees of gastrointestinal damage.

GROUP IV. Dose, 600 to 1400 rads. An accelerated version of the acute syndrome is seen, dominated by the effects of gastrointestinal injury. The length of survival depends on the severity of the gastrointestinal damage.

GROUP V. Dose, greater than 2000 rads. The course is fulminating, with severe central nervous system manifestations.

Stages of Illness. As just noted, the course of acute radiation sickness can be divided into the following four stages:

STAGE 1—PRODROMAL STAGE. Regardless of dose, the psychologic concomitants of a known exposure may dominate and obscure the physiopathology of this stage. In general, however, the earlier the onset of symptoms, the higher the likely dose. If no nausea and vomiting occur within the first few hours, the patient has probably received a group I exposure. In groups II and III, these symptoms are usually seen within an hour or so after exposure. In groups IV and V, there is a rapid onset of diarrhea, ataxia, disorientation, coma, and shock.

Prodromal symptoms reach a maximum within 6 to 8 hours. During this time, patients in groups III to V have weakness and fatigue, sweating, and paresthesias. Within 24 to 48 hours, the symptoms subside in groups I and II, become less severe in group III, and progress without a latent period into the manifest illness in group IV and especially group V.

STAGE 2—LATENT PERIOD. In group I patients, the illness usually ends with the prodromal period. In the other groups, the length of the latent period is inversely proportional to dose. Weakness and fatigue may continue through this period.

STAGE 3—MANIFEST ILLNESS. Group II patients may exhibit chills, fever, weight loss, fatigue, and epilation (if the dose was greater than 350 rads). Pharyngitis, upper respiratory infections, melena, hematuria, gingival hemorrhages, and mild purpura reflect the hematopoietic damage. Various combinations of these symptoms may persist for 40 to 50 days, gradually decreasing thereafter.

In group III patients, similar but more severe symptoms and signs appear earlier. Within a month of exposure gastrointestinal damage becomes manifest by severe, bloody diarrhea, abdominal pain, and hematemesis. Hematuria and oliguria may appear. Coma and profound shock may be followed by death in 25 to 40 days.

Group IV patients usually run an abbreviated course and die within 15 to 30 days after exhibiting more severe signs of gastrointestinal damage.

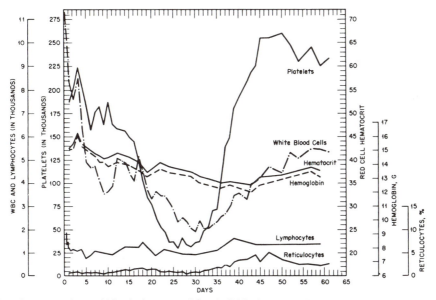

Figure 36–4 Average values of blood elements of five individuals exposed to estimated doses of 200 to 350 rads. (From Saenger, E. L. [ed.]: Medical Aspects of Radiation Accidents: A Handbook for Physicians, Health Physicists and Industrial Hygienists. United States Atomic Energy Commission, 1963.)

Group V patients do not live long enough to manifest hematologic signs. Ataxia, incoherence, disorientation, vomiting, diarrhea, and abdominal cramps occur within 1 or 2 hours after exposure. Although there may be a brief period of mental clarity, the usual course is inexorably downward, regardless of treatment.

It should be noted that this narrative describes the effect of a single dose of ionizing radiation. The effect of fractional doses delivered over a period of time is much less severe.

STAGE 4—RECOVERY. In group II patients, convalescence ordinarily begins between 2 and 3 months after exposure. Clinical recovery usually is apparent within 6 months, although some weakness may persist thereafter. Those patients in groups III and IV who do not die follow a generally similar course, although weakness persists for many months.

Therapeutic Principles. It is obvious that doses in the range above 400 to 500 rads pose severe or insuperable problems. Although measures to replace blood elements are available, there is no way to correct the gastrointestinal defects seen in these groups. Death is probably inevitable after doses of 800 to 1000 rads.

Group I patients may be followed as outpatients. Other patients require hospitalization. Therapy should be directed toward protection against the effects of thrombocytopenia and leukopenia. Hemorrhages may require blood, enriched plasma, or platelet transfusions. Antibiotics, strict antisepsis, and isolation are necessary to protect against infection. Careful maintenance of fluid balance and proper nutrition are essential.

Effects of Surface Irradiation. Irradiation of the skin by low energy x-rays or beta radiation may produce damage restricted to the skin. The effect of such radiation is similar in appearance and course to a thermal burn, although some features of the acute radiation syndrome may appear.

Internal Deposition of Radionuclides. The naturally radioactive elements (uranium, thorium, actinium, plutonium, etc.) decay by emission of alpha particles. Because these particles have such a limited range, they represent only a slight hazard outside the body. Within the body, however, serious damage may be caused because of the intensely ionizing nature of these particles. Inhalation of these substances presents a special risk because even insoluble forms of the elements may be trapped in the lungs. Discussion of this problem is beyond the scope of this chapter, but all cases of suspected inhalation or ingestion of radionuclides should be referred to appropriate specialists immediately for treatment designed to remove as much of the substances as possible prior to their fixation or distribution within the body.

Effects of Local Irradiation. There is suggestive evidence that whole-body irradiation may shorten life span more than local radiation. Local radiation also causes serious effects, however. Such radiation in the range of 600 to 1000 rads to the eye may produce clinically significant cataracts. Elsewhere, degenerative changes in vascular beds may occur, associated with late parenchymal cell destruction. Atrophy of epithelial cells and dermal appendages in the skin is seen, although local areas of hypertrophy may also appear. Progressive fibrosis of the lungs with vascular sclerosis is reported. Arterionephrosclerosis with hypertension may follow local irradiation of the kidneys.

Late Effects of Whole-Body Radiation. The longevity of radiologists in the years prior to 1945 strongly suggests a life-shortening effect from prolonged exposure to relatively small doses of radiation, although this is difficult to establish conclusively. It appears likely, however, that the effects of even small doses of ionizing radiation may be expressed either in the individual (in the form of degenerative lesions or malignancies) or in future generations through the production of inheritable defects. Although germ cells are especially vulnerable to radiation, effects on somatic cells are also possible.

Radiation Carcinogenesis. Among early radiologists, skin cancers were an obvious hazard; the demonstration that leukemia was a late consequence of radiation exposure came much later. Osteosarcomas due to absorption and bone deposition of radium have been well documented, as have been thyroid adenocarcinomas following irradiation of the neck in childhood and lung tumors in uranium miners exposed to radium daughter products.

Whether a threshold dose for carcinogenic effects exists is open to question—a question that cannot, unfortunately, be answered unequivocally. It does seem clear, however, that unlike electromagnetic radiation of longer wavelengths and lower energies, ionizing radiation has no beneficial physiologic effects. For this reason, any preventable exposure to such radiation must be considered from the standpoint of the secondary benefits to be gained compared with the possible costs in terms of later physiopathology.

THE KINETIC ENVIRONMENT

In a previous section, we referred to human mobility as one of the attributes that has made us what we are. Since earliest times, humans have found mobility to be an absolute essential in their attempts to master and control their environment. We cannot synthesize glucose from readily available simpler compounds; we must therefore search out plants that do so. We are puny compared with some of the animal predators (including other humans), so we must be able to flee from them. We reproduce rapidly; crowding and our own desire to know the unknown have led us to explore our entire planet and even to go beyond its confines.

Movement requires work—kinetic energy. In order to understand how we relate to our physical environment, we must understand how we are affected by force fields, either natural or of our own making. That is the purpose of this section. We shall first consider the effects of gravity and its absence, together with the effects of activity and inactivity. The effects of supragravitational force fields will be discussed. Thereafter, vibration and noise will be considered, for they are inevitable concomitants of an industrial society. Finally, we must discuss briefly human responses to combinations of stresses, since environmental stresses are rarely encountered in isolation.

GRAVITY

Humans and all other biologic organisms on earth have evolved under the constant influence of the acceleration of gravity, a force field that pulls us toward the earth's center of mass at roughly 980 cm per sec^2. Each time an individual rises from the supine to the erect position, the column of blood within him is accelerated toward his feet; each time he raises his arms, the action is resisted. When he climbs a hill, he gains potential energy at the cost of an expenditure of roughly five times as much energy, for the human organism works at only about 20 per cent efficiency.

The constant pull of gravity has profound effects on a motile organism, and especially on one that normally extends itself to its full height. The column of blood in the venous reservoir is 150 to 180 cm high; there is, therefore, a gradient in pressure from the top to the bottom of that column of 150 to 180 cm of water, or about 120 mm Hg. Were it not for the valves in our veins, this entire pressure would be exerted on the vessels in our lower legs whenever we assumed an erect position. The heart must supply the brain with blood at adequate perfusion pressures both when the body is supine and the hydrostatic column is horizontal and when it is upright, with a hydrostatic column over 30 cm high.

Humans have learned to cope with this situation, although not without certain consequences. One example is the presence of varicose veins in the lower extremities, a serious and disfiguring problem for many. Stasis ulcers of the skin over the legs are another probably allied problem. More serious for some is postural hypotension, an inability to maintain adequate cardiac output and peripheral resistance in the upright position.

Even in those of us who can cope with sudden changes in position, fairly major physiologic responses are involved. When we assume the recumbent position for any period of time, venous return is improved. The volume receptors in the right atrium sense this, and a water diuresis results.

Over a longer period of time, calcium mobilization and excretion lead to demineralization of bone. The muscles, especially the antigravity muscles, lose strength and mass. The smooth muscle in the walls of blood vessels may also lose tone and the capacity to respond to changes in posture.

All these changes make little difference—as long as we remain supine. If, however, we return to the erect posture, we find ourselves unable to cope with gravitational stress. Bed rest for prolonged periods robs the individual of many of his normal modes of coping with his environment.

WEIGHTLESSNESS

Bed rest is *not* weightlessness, although it is tempting to consider them together. As we began to explore the space above our atmosphere, medical support personnel began to worry about whether the deadaptive changes seen in prolonged recumbency would appear in space flight, in which centrifugal acceleration exactly balances the centripetal acceleration of gravity. It has been found that many of the changes observed are indeed similar, although the data are far from conclusive. Humans have thus far experienced continuous weightlessness for over 7 months. Bone densitometry has suggested that a degree of demineralization occurs; physical deconditioning with diminished exercise tolerance has been observed. Intolerance to upright tilt or lower-body negative pressure has in some cases been profound, although short-lived. Decreases in circulating red cell mass and plasma volume have been noted.

The importance of these and other related findings is still disputed. Some believe that prolonged weightlessness will have profound and dangerous effects on humans; others feel that by 2 weeks of exposure, individuals begin to readapt despite their altered environment. The question is under intense scrutiny by U.S. and Soviet space scientists at this time.

Little research has been done on humans in supragravity force fields, in part because of the very elaborate equipment required. Various investigators have exposed animals, notably fowl, to long periods in strong gravitational fields. They find evidence of adaptation, notably in bone structure, antigravity muscle mass, and postural reflexes.

PHYSICAL ACTIVITY

It has already been noted that prolonged bed rest causes a variety of deadaptive changes in the human organism. The fullest development of heat acclimatization requires both heat and physical work. The importance of physical activity in maintaining the adaptability of the human organism has become a popular topic of discussion; many easily available scientific and popular texts consider this topic in detail. It is necessary, however, that it receive at least brief consideration here as well.

Just as musculoskeletal inactivity causes disuse atrophy and skeletal demineralization, so the performance of musculoskeletal work produces, over a period of time, hypertrophy and increased capillarity of skeletal muscles, optimal mineralization of long bones, and a number of adaptive alterations in the heart and cardiovascular system, including greater cardiac volume and output per stroke, lower resting heart rates, greater work capacity, higher oxygen uptake during work (with consequent sparing of the less efficient anaerobic energy sources), and often an increased sense of well-being.

The induction of these changes requires that the organism be stressed repeatedly by the performance of strenuous physical work. A number of carefully controlled studies indicate that optimal cardiorespiratory fitness can be achieved and maintained better by relatively brief spurts of fairly intense exercise than by much longer periods of less intense exercise. It seems certain, however, that the maintenance of the individual's reserve capacity to deal with physiologic stress requires that stress be experienced on a continuing basis; this truism is nowhere more clear than with respect to a person's capacity to perform muscular work.

PROLONGED ACCELERATION

Aircraft have freedom of motion in all spatial axes. As a result of this freedom, they are capable of accelerations, especially angular, which significantly displace or alter the magnitude of the apparent normal G vector. Detailed consideration of this field, in which much research has been done, is beyond the scope of this review. It will simply be said here that, as an instance, in a 60° banked turn in level flight an acceleration of twice normal gravity (2 G) is imparted to the occupants of an aircraft. The acceleration in this case is parallel to the long axis of the body. Exactly the same acceleration may occur when an airplane pulls out of a dive into level flight or into a climb.

Since the net G vector is the same in both instances, the pilot or occupant may be unable to differentiate those two quite dissimilar situations unless he is provided with gyroscopic instruments to tell him what is occurring. The result is spatial disorientation, a common and dangerous problem in flight. If the natural horizon is not visible, the pilot must use instruments, which are not affected as are his semicircular canals and otoliths by angular and linear accelerations.

With respect to both orientation and cardiovascular physiology, prolonged linear and radial accelerations induce changes that may be adaptive or deadaptive. Several references are provided; standard texts cover these topics in detail.

ABRUPT ACCELERATIONS; IMPACT

Whenever a body acquires momentum, it must dissipate that momentum to return to rest. Since momentum is the product of mass times velocity, the faster we go the more dangerous it becomes to stop abruptly.

Any consideration of the effects of impact on an individual must take into account the rate of onset of the decelerative impulse, the peak magnitude of the deceleration, its duration, the orientation of the person with respect to the force field, and the nature of any protective equipment and of the surrounding environment.

The average magnitude of an impact may be simply estimated in terms of the initial velocity, the final velocity (usually zero), and the distance over which the vehicle or person came to rest. The deceleration thus derived is usually expressed as a ratio, the denominator of which is the acceleration due to gravity. Figure 36–5 shows a variety of deceleration and impact experiences in terms of initial velocity and stopping distance. Body orientation differs in these experiences; the approximate survival limits shown must be interpreted cautiously.

Tolerance limits depend to a considerable extent on the peak acceleration during an impact. Peak transverse accelerations of 100 to 200 G for 0.01 second are tolerated without injury, whereas only 20 to 30 G can be tolerated for 1 second. The duration of an applied acceleration determines whether the body acts as a rigid or a viscoelastic object. During accelerations or decelerations longer than 0.05 to 0.10 second, the internal organs and blood are significantly affected; physiologic adaptations begin to occur.

Tolerance for vertical (longitudinal) impact is substantially less than for transverse (anteroposterior) forces. The outcome of such an impact depends to a considerable extent on whether one's knees are locked or are allowed to flex (thus increasing the distance over which the trunk is decelerated).

Following moderate transverse impacts (15 to 25 G with onset rates from 400 to 1000 G per second), a number of transient physiologic changes are seen in subjects who are free from structural damage. These include hypotension, bradycardia (a vagal effect that is blocked by atropine), transient neurologic changes, changes in blood platelets, psychologic changes, and generalized stress reactions. These effects must be taken into account when one is evaluating the condition of persons involved in automobile accidents.

It should be pointed out here that in automobile crashes, the most serious injuries are usually caused by a secondary impact of occupants with

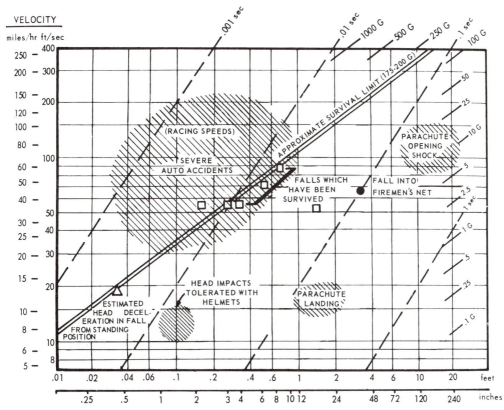

Figure 36–5 This figure brings together a variety of impact and deceleration experiences by plotting the data from a number of sources on the common axes of deceleration distance and velocity. Stopping time and impact force in G units are shown as secondary scales. The data points with hollow squares are for free falls of 50 to 150 ft with survival. The line labeled "approximate survival limit" must be used with caution, since many biophysical factors influence the injury due to deceleration. (From Parker, J. F., and West, V. R. [Eds.]: Bioastronautics Data Book. 2nd ed. Washington, D.C., U. S. Government Printing Office, 1973.)

the steering wheel, an interior structure, the windshield, or (if the occupants are ejected from the vehicle) objects in the vicinity. Adequate restraint systems are now available in new automobiles; the decline in fatalities and in the number and severity of injuries that would result from their universal use would be startling. While automobile manufacturers, prodded by federal standards, have made considerable strides in delethalizing the interiors of vehicles, the simplest way to avoid injury from impacting vehicle parts is not to contact them; there is no substitute for an adequate restraint system in this regard.

VIBRATION

Vibration may be thought of as repeated brief accelerations; these may be sinusoidal or random in character and may be applied to a part of the body (as when vibrating hand tools are used) or to the whole body.

Human responses to vibration depend to a considerable extent on the frequency of the vibra-

tion with respect to the resonant frequencies of various body organs. All studies of whole-body vibration show a sharp decrease in voluntary tolerance at frequencies of 4 to 7 cycles per second owing to resonance of the abdominal organs, as an instance.

G forces during vibration are a function of frequency and amplitude of the applied acceleration. However, the amplitude of the seat, or platform, is usually damped considerably by the body. Head movement, for instance, is usually very much less than seat movement.

Limits of voluntary tolerance for longitudinal vibration in the seated position are from 0.1 to 0.4 G at frequencies of 1 to 40 cycles per second. Minor injury begins to occur at levels of 2 to 5 G, depending on exposure time. Such injuries are the result of mechanical deformation and shear forces on adjacent tissues of differing densities and masses.

A different sort of injury pattern is seen in some workers whose jobs involve prolonged contact with vibrating hand tools. After a variable period of exposure, usually in cold environments, a proportion of these workers will begin to show vascular changes in the hands, with vascular spasm typical of Raynaud's phenomenon. It is not certain whether the changes seen in the arteries are primary or secondary to nerve injury, but considerable thickening of arterial walls has been demonstrated. The disorder is disabling, since once present, it is exacerbated by exposure of the individual or of his hand to cold as well as to vibration.

NOISE

The human ear, like the eye, has an enormous tolerance for cyclic pressure changes that reach the eardrum through the air. The auditory threshold in normal young persons is in the neighborhood of 10^{-4} dynes per cm²; the ear can tolerate sound pressure levels as high as 10^3 dynes per cm². In contemporary society, however, much louder sound

pressure levels are produced by certain machines and by explosives; these sounds and others of lesser magnitude for longer periods of exposure can cause harm. Both acute dysfunction and chronic damage of the very sensitive auditory mechanism result from exposure to high sound pressure levels.

Because of the very wide range of pressures to which the ear can respond, it is conventional to express sound pressure levels (SPLs) in decibels (dB) relative to the threshold of hearing. Figure 36–6 shows the overall SPLs of a variety of common environmental sources of sound.

The frequency spectrum to which the normal ear responds is roughly 30 to 12,000 cycles per second (hertz). Since sounds containing substantial proportions of high-frequency energy are somewhat more injurious than predominantly low-frequency sounds, it is necessary to evaluate the sound environment in terms of its frequency components as well as its overall sound pressure levels.

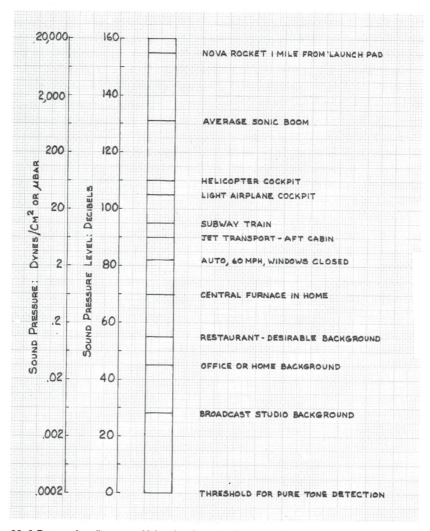

Figure 36–6 Range of auditory sensitivity showing sound pressure levels generated by various sources.

Noise has been defined as "unwanted sound." It has become common practice, therefore, to talk of "noisy environments" and of "the effects of noise." It will be immediately obvious to those who have been exposed to rock-and-roll music in close quarters that one person's sound may be another's noise. However, the damage caused by sound or noise is a function of its energy content, not its information content.

Intense sound (SPL greater than 85 to 95 dB) causes, after a period of exposure, an upward shift in auditory thresholds for pure tones. If sound exposure is terminated or interrupted, this "temporary threshold shift" disappears over a period of a few hours or days, and auditory acuity again becomes normal. The exact physiologic nature of this phenomenon is not known, though it appears to be an end-organ rather than a central response. Regardless of the frequency content of the sound that induces the temporary shift, the shift itself is seen earliest and to the greatest degrees in the range of frequencies between 1500 and 4000 Hz.

If exposures to sound pressure levels of this magnitude are continued over a long time period, a gradual permanent threshold shift occurs. The rate of onset and magnitude of this shift vary considerably, but they are roughly proportional to the intensity of the sound to which persons are exposed. Fairly good normative data are available for continuous noise exposure; the effects of exposure to impulse noise are less well understood.

The permanent threshold shift (which may have a further temporary shift superimposed on it) represents true neural deafness and is irreversible. It results from degeneration of the sensory cells in the organ of Corti. Deafness from noise exposure may be difficult to differentiate from presbycusis, the usual decrease in auditory acuity seen in older people, since both forms cause greater deficits in acuity for tones of high frequencies (4000 to 12,000 Hz). Indeed, some have argued that presbycusis itself is induced by exposure to high sound pressures over a lifetime. (This may be true in part, but it is probably not a full explanation; genetic factors are certainly involved.)

Temporary deafness of a different sort results from obstruction in the external ear canal (water or cerumen), from fluid in the middle ear due to barotitis, or from a ruptured tympanic membrane. Although the human tympanum is very resistant to rupture, an explosive blast or very high pressure differential across the drum may cause traumatic rupture. The lesion is self-limiting, and spontaneous healing ordinarily occurs within a few days. Repeated episodes of serous otitis media, however, may cause thickening of the eardrum, with damping of its motion and loss of elasticity. The threshold shift seen in such cases tends to be roughly uniform across low and high frequencies. A similar picture is seen in otosclerosis. Such hearing losses are characteristic of conductive, as opposed to neural, or perceptive, deafness and are sometimes amenable to medical or surgical treatment.

ULTRASOUND

Mechanical vibrations with frequencies above about 15,000 Hz are not detected by the human ear; such waves therefore are called *ultrasonic*. As frequency increases, propagation through air decreases; extremely high ultrasonic vibrations are readily transmitted only by relatively incompressible (liquid or solid) materials. The energy contained in such waves can, however, be converted to thermal energy in the tissues; this is the basis of continuous output ultrasonic diathermy units. Alternatively, again by proper selection of frequencies and with use of a pulsed wave transmitter and receiver, ultrasound can be used to visualize tissue discontinuities within the body. It is used, for instance, to determine the location of the placenta prior to amniocentesis. The power outputs used in such studies are not hazardous. It has also been suggested that changes in cell membrane permeability can be induced by ultrasound without destruction or denaturation of cell proteins.

COMBINED STRESSES

In this brief review of human responses to the physical environment, most of our discussion has dealt with the effects of single stressors. No such discussion can be complete, however, if it does not emphasize that humans rarely encounter these stressors in isolation. We normally live and work and play in the presence of a great variety of physical, chemical, biologic, and sociocultural stressors, some antagonistic, others additive or synergistic. Indeed, we know from sensory deprivation experiments that too little stress may be at least as damaging to people as too much stress, that individuals function best in a fairly rich environment.

The aluminum foundry worker must perform strenuous work in the face of often severe thermal stress; the mountain climber must exert himself while affected by both hypoxia and cold. Operators of heavy equipment are exposed to high levels of noise and vibration under a wide range of climatic conditions. Each of these persons is working also under the influence of biologic and socioeconomic factors that may or may not impose additional stress upon him.

In dealing with disorders caused by environmental stresses, physicians must keep in mind the pathologic physiology of these disorders if their therapeutic efforts are to be effective. The person who performs muscular work in a hot environment must share his cardiac output between his working muscles, which depend on the blood for oxygen, and his skin, to which heat is carried from the

V—TOXIC PHYSICAL AND CHEMICAL AGENTS

core by blood. These two stresses therefore are additive with respect to their physiologic demands. Their combined effects are multiplied when fluid must be expended for evaporative cooling, reducing the plasma volume.

Many other examples could be cited; the important point is simply that such problems as these are amenable to rational treatment aimed at restoring the body to its normal homeostatic condition or at supporting the patient until he can again adapt to stress. This is the essence of environmental medicine once injury has occurred. The same reasoning, however, based on knowledge of physiology, can as easily be applied to the prevention of such injuries. Herein lie our most stimulating challenges in the field of environmental health.

REFERENCES

Literature concerning this broad area of study is widely spread among journals devoted to medicine, physiology, psychology, and engineering. There are a few publications in which reports relating to a variety of environmental stressors are gathered together. Because of their particular value, they are listed here; individual reports follow in alphabetical order.

Bennett, P. B., and Elliott, D. H.: The Physiology and Medicine of Diving. 3rd ed. Baltimore, Williams and Wilkins Co., 1982.
Calvin, M., and Gazenka, O. (Eds.): Foundations of Space Biology and Medicine. Vol. I: Space as a Habitat. Vol. II: Ecological and Physiological Bases of Space Biology and Medicine. Vol. III: Space Medicine and Biotechnology. Washington, D.C., National Aeronautics and Space Administration, 1975.
Davis, J. C., and Hunt, T. K.: Hyperbaric Oxygen Therapy. Bethesda, Md., Undersea Medical Society, Inc., 1977.
DeHart, R. L. (Ed.): Fundamentals of Aerospace Medicine. Philadelphia, Lea and Febiger Co., 1983.
Dill, D. B. (Ed.): Handbook of Physiology. Section 4, Adaptation to the Environment. Washington, D.C., American Physiological Society, 1964.
Lambertsen, C. J. (Ed.): Proceedings of the Third Symposium on Underwater Physiology. Baltimore, Williams and Wilkins Co., 1967.
Lambertsen, C. J. (Ed.): Proceedings of the Fourth Symposium on Underwater Physiology. New York, Academic Press, 1971.
Lambertsen, C. J., (Ed.): Proceedings of the Fifth Symposium on Underwater Physiology. Bethesda, Md., Federated American Societies for Experimental Biology, 1975.
Leithead, C. S., and Lind, A. R.: Heat Stress and Heat Disorders. Philadelphia, F. A. Davis Co., 1964.
McFarland, A.: Human Factors in Air Transportation. New York, McGraw-Hill Book Co., 1953.
Parker, J. F., Jr., and West, V. R. (Eds.): Bioastronautics Data Book. 2nd ed. NASA SP-3006. Washington, D.C., U.S. Government Printing Office, 1973.
Anonymous: Radiation Induced Cancer. Proceedings Series. Vienna, Austria, International Atomic Energy Agency, 1969.
Bartleson, C. J.: Retinal burns from intense light sources. Am. Industr. Hyg. Assoc. J. 29:415, 1968.
Bass, D. E., Kleeman, R., Quinn, M., et al.: Mechanisms of acclimatization to heat in man. Medicine 34:323, 1955.
Billings, C. E., Brashear, R. E., Bason, R., and Mathews, D. K.: Medical observations during 20 days at 3800 meters. Arch. Environ. Health 18:987, 1969.
Burton, A. C., and Edholm, O. G.: Man in a Cold Environment. London, Edward Arnold, 1955.
Clark, J. M., and Lambertsen, C. J.: Pulmonary oxygen toxicity: A review. Pharmacol. Rev. 23:37, 1971.
Cogan, D. G.: Lesions of the eye from radiant energy. J.A.M.A. 142:145, 1950.
DiGiovanni, C., Jr., and Chambers, R. M.: Physiologic and psychologic aspects of the gravity spectrum. N. Engl. J. Med. 270:35, 88, 134; 1964.
Fenn, W. O.: Possible role of hydrostatic pressure in diving. In Lambertsen, C. J. (Ed.): Underwater Physiology. Baltimore, Williams and Wilkins Co., 1967.
Folk, G. E., Jr.: Introduction to Environmental Physiology: Environmental Extremes and Mammalian Survival. Philadelphia, Lea and Febiger, 1966.

Fox, R. H., Goldsmith, R., Hampton, I. F. G., and Hunt, J. J.: Heat acclimatization by controlled hyperthermia in hot-dry and hot-wet climates. J. Appl. Physiol. 22:39, 1967.
Fox, R. H., Goldsmith, R., Kidd, D. J., and Lewis, H. E.: Acclimatization to heat in man by controlled elevation of body temperature. J. Physiol. 166:530, 1963.
Fryer, D. I.: Subatmospheric Decompression Sickness in Man. Slough, England, Technivision Services, 1969.
Glorig, A., Ward, W. D., and Nixon, J.: Damage risk criteria and noise-induced hearing loss. Arch. Otolaryngol. 74:413, 1961.
Hopps, J. A.: The electric shock hazard in hospitals. Can. Med. Assoc. J. 98:1002, 1968.
Howath, S. M. (Ed.): Cold Injury. New York, Transactions of the Sixth Conference, Josiah Macy, Jr., Foundation, 1960.
International Commission on Radiological Protection: The Evaluation of Risks from Radiation. ICRP Publication No. 8. Oxford, Pergamon Press, 1966.
Kryter, K.D.: The Effects of Noise on Man. New York, Academic Press, 1970.
Largent, E. J., and Ashe, W. F.: Upper limits of thermal stress for workmen. Am. Industr. Hyg. Assoc. J. 19:246, 1958.
Levi, L. (Ed.): Emotional Stress. New York, American Elsevier Publishing Co., 1967.
Lichter, I., Borrie, J., and Miller, W. M.: Radio-frequency hazards with cardiac pacemakers. Br. Med. J. 1:1513, 1965.
Linder, G. S.: Mechanical vibration effects on human beings. Aerospace Med. 33:939, 1962.
Margaria, R.: Exercise at Altitude. New York, Excerpta Medica Foundation, 1967.
Mathews, D. K., Stacy, R. W., and Hoover, G. N.: Physiology of Muscular Activity and Exercise. New York, Ronald Press, 1964.
McCally, M., and Graveline, D. E.: Physiologic aspects of prolonged weightlessness. N. Engl. J. Med. 269:508, 1963.
Menon, N. D.: High-altitude edema. N. Engl. J. Med. 273:66, 1965.
Peyton, M. F. (Ed.): Biological Effects of Microwave Radiation, Vol. I. New York, Plenum Press, 1961.
Roy, S.: Acute mountain sickness in Himalayan terrain. In Hegnauer, A. H. (Ed.): Biomedicine of High Terrestrial Elevations. Washington, D.C., U.S. Army Medical Research and Development Command, January, 1969.
Sacq, Z. M., and Alexander, P. A.: Fundamentals of Radiobiology. Oxford, Pergamon Press, 1961.
Schaefer, K. E., et al.: Pulmonary and circulatory adjustments determining the limits of depth in breathhold diving. Science 162:1020, 1968.
Saenger, E. L. (Ed.): Medical Aspects of Radiation Accidents. A Handbook for Physicians, Health Physicists and Industrial Hygienists. Washington, D.C., U.S. Atomic Energy Commission, 1963.
Sugimoto, T., Schall, S. F., and Wallace, A. G.: Factors determining vulnerability to ventricular fibrillation induced by 60–CPS alternating current. Circ. Res. 21:601, 1967.
Webb, P.: Body heat loss in undersea gaseous environment. Aerospace Med. 41:1283, 1970.
Wood, J. E., and Bass, D. E.: Thermoregulatory and circulatory adjustments during acclimatization to heat in man. J. Clin. Invest. 39:825, 1960.

Chemical Agents and Disease **37**

Edmund B. Flink and Ananda S. Prasad

INTRODUCTION

All biologic processes are dependent on chemical reactions. All living cells contain bundles of innumerable enzymes supported in an orderly arrangement by a chemical skeleton appropriate for the function of an organelle or of the whole cell. For optimal function of all the enzymes in the cells, the physical and chemical architecture must be correct. If one enzyme system is disturbed by a toxic substance, its reaction may be blocked or its equilibrium accelerated or delayed. Such disturbance can cripple or destroy the cell and organism. Many toxic chemicals have profound effects that are grossly evident, but the precise metabolic targets (enzyme or enzyme sequence) may not be known. Adverse effects can be classified in five groups: (1) irritant, caustic, or corrosive (e.g., $HgCl_2$ or "corrosive sublimate" on oral and gastrointestinal mucosa); (2) specific toxicologic reactions (e.g., botulinus toxin on nerve terminals in muscle); (3) mutagenic reactions (e.g., x-ray and radioactive nuclides); (4) carcinogenic reactions (e.g., β-naphthylamine, 1,2 benzanthracene, cresols, butter yellow, methyl cholanthrene, arsenic, and thorium dioxide); and (5) teratogenic reactions (e.g., thalidomide causing phocomelia and alcohol causing the fetal alcohol syndrome).

ROUTE OF ADMINISTRATION OR EXPOSURE

Unique properties of chemicals as well as the anatomic site of exposure determine the reaction to a given chemical. The chemical agent may gain access to the internal milieu by various routes. Most agents must penetrate the cells to do damage; however, they may affect the cell membrane so that its protective action is disrupted. The cell wall has a double-layered lipoprotein structure, with each layer 35 to 50 Å units in thickness. Interaction with the cell membrane depends on both physical and chemical properties, whereas penetration of the cell membrane may be dependent on diffusion (e.g., gases, pinocytosis, or phagocytosis of liquid and particulate matter).

THE PERCUTANEOUS ROUTE

Percutaneous absorption through intact skin depends on the lipid solubility of the chemical. The skin acts as a natural barrier to water-soluble (polar) compounds. This barrier is changed by lipid solvents such as methanol, ethanol, hexane, acetone, or a mixture of chloroform-methanol (2:1), which cause a marked alteration in skin permeability. DDT, carbon tetrachloride, analine, phenol and its derivatives, gasoline, kerosene, tetraethyl lead, steroid hormones, and vitamins D and K can be absorbed through the skin. Petroleum products and especially tetraethyl lead can cause serious chronic toxicity by absorption through the skin. Denuded surfaces such as burns or open wounds bypass the lipid skin barrier and permit absorption of polar compounds, so that an extensive burn can be the portal of entry for drugs applied to the area (e.g., sulfonamides and antibiotics).

THE RESPIRATORY ROUTE

The lungs serve as the route of absorption of many important drugs, such as inhalation anesthetics. For some compounds, such as the two odorless gases, carbon monoxide and nitrous oxide, lethal intoxication occurs only via the lungs. Water soluble chemicals such as NH_3, chlorine, and HCl (gas) can be tolerated in small concentration by the "scrubbing" action of the upper respiratory passages, but in large concentrations these penetrate to cause severe irritation of the lungs with serious or fatal pulmonary edema. Under ordinary urban conditions, air pollution with carbon monoxide, sulfur dioxide, oxides of nitrogen, and fly ash is no real threat to human life. Under abnormal atmospheric conditions, such as has occurred in several well-publicized disasters in Donora, Pennsylvania, and London, England, concentration of pollutants has resulted in many deaths, particularly among the elderly and those with pulmonary or cardiovascular disease.

Pneumoconioses emphasize the specificity and uniqueness of reactions to noxious stimuli. Particulate matter of appropriate size and physical state carried in the air in industrial situations of mining, sand blasting, stone polishing, and cotton milling can cause serious damage to lungs. Particles from 0.5 to 5.0 µ in diameter are capable of reaching alveoli and may be deposited in phagocytes. Reactions vary with both the physical and chemical nature of the particle. Crystalline silicon dioxide is fibrogenic, but amorphous silicates are not. Asbestos fibers are inelastic and produce serious fibrotic changes, but Fiberglas particles of the same size are elastic and deformable and do not cause a parenchymal reaction. Asbestos is also a serious carcinogen in the respiratory tract. Silicosis provides an excellent example of a chronic illness in which the severity depends on time and intensity of exposure. Massive exposure can cause fatal pulmonary insufficiency in a few months, as in the Gaulley Bridge (West Virginia) disaster in 1931, whereas minor exposure over many years will produce some silicotic lung reaction but no pulmonary insufficiency.

THE ORAL ROUTE

Toxic reactions may result from ingestion of appropriate drugs in excessive dose, allergic or hypersensitive responses to accepted dose levels, and the ingestion of chemicals not intended for human consumption, such as accidental ingestion of heavy metals. Foods and beverages may be contaminated with organic mercury compounds, arsenic, cadmium, and lead. Ingestion of lead oxide paint chips (pica) from old houses by young children in urban areas poses one of the more important environmental hazards in our society. In New York City alone, there were 4000 new cases of lead poisoning in 1970 and 1971.

Most ingested chemicals are absorbed by the small intestine, but some, such as alcohol and nitroglycerin, are absorbed also from the mouth and stomach. Slowing of small intestinal motility, particularly after hypnotic drugs (e.g., glutethimide), may result in sequestration and extended absorption with prolonged and fluctuating coma. Many chemicals are fat-soluble and may be stored in fat, permitting cumulative toxicity. This concentration effect can be a source of human intoxication by the ingestion of meat (fat) of animals chronically exposed to DDT, for instance.

Many ingested chemicals are detoxified by the liver. Detoxification begins with oxidation or reduction on the first passage. Certain chemicals are made more toxic by biotransformation. Nevertheless, most chemicals that are completely absorbed are less toxic after an oral dose than those given by the parenteral route in similar doses.

PARENTERAL ROUTE

Toxic reactions can occur following subcutaneous, intramuscular, intravenous, or intraperitoneal administration. Increase in illicit drug use has broadened the opportunities for exposure. Reactions may take many forms. There may be an unexpected sensitivity to an accepted dose or deliberate or accidental overdose. Intravenously administered medication may result in achievement of peak blood levels almost instantaneously. Unless there is an antidote, the only way of ameliorating toxic reactions after parenteral administra-

tion is by elimination of the chemical via renal excretion, hepatic detoxification, or dialysis.

BIOLOGIC COMPLEXITY OF TOXIC REACTIONS

The toxicity of chemical agents is multifaceted. Some agents are tremendously useful therapeutically at appropriate dosage levels but can cause serious toxic and lethal effects with small increases. An excellent example is digitalis and its derivatives. Digitalis affects both the contractility and rhythmicity of the failing heart in a very beneficial way at appropriate doses, but just twice this ideal dose can cause serious and often fatal arrhythmia. Many drugs share this kind of critical dosage consideration. Even glucose can be rendered toxic by causing hyperglycemia, polyuria, dehydration, and ketoacidosis in a totally insulin-deficient person.

This complexity is also illustrated by the importance of dose in relation to time. An example is lead poisoning. A relatively large single dose is tolerated without serious or fatal result, but a much smaller dose repeated over months accumulates and *can* cause serious or fatal intoxication.

Certain toxic chemicals produce reactions that are unique and highly specific. Two examples are cyanide and carbon monoxide. Cyanide poisons heme-containing enzymes, particularly cytochrome A_3, in all cells and causes death quickly by blocking the electron transport system. Carbon monoxide causes tissue anoxia by displacing oxygen from the hemoglobin molecules and also by shifting the oxygen dissociation curve for remaining oxygenated hemoglobin so oxygen is not released normally. Carbon monoxide has an affinity for hemoglobin that is 240 times greater than that of oxygen.

Some chemicals have a high degree of affinity for certain organs such as carbon tetrachloride (CCl_4) and dichloromethane for the liver. Many combinations of chemicals are not only additive but actually synergistic. Moderate doses of CCl_4 inhaled or ingested, particularly by a person also taking alcohol, result in serious renal insufficiency as well as liver damage.

GENETIC FACTORS AND CHEMICAL TOXICITY

Genetically determined serious toxic reactions to usual doses of commonly used drugs (e.g., sulfonamide) or usual servings of a food (e.g., fava bean) are examples of the exquisite sensitivity and specificity of toxic reactions. Four genetically determined sensitivities are illustrated subsequently.

GLUCOSE 6 PHOSPHATE DEHYDROGENASE (G6PD) DEFICIENCY: AN X-LINKED PHENOMENON

Aging red cells are hemolyzed first. G6PD is involved at the beginning of the hexose monophosphate shunt (HMP) and results in an increase in nicotine adenine dinucleotide phosphate (NADP) and consequently in reduced glutathione (GSH) (Fig. 37–1). This sequence helps resist oxidant stresses of fava beans, primaquine, quinine, aspirin, and phenacetin in large doses, the nitrofurans, sulfones, many sulfonamides, para-aminosalicylic acid, probenecid, quinidine, phenylhydrazine, water-soluble analogues of vitamin K, and naphthalene. The severity of the stress varies with the drug and the dose as well as genetic state, whether homozygous or heterozygous. G6PD deficiency occurs in 10 per cent of American blacks and 8 to 20 per cent of West African blacks, but in only 2 per cent of South African Bantus and in virtually no whites other than some of Mediterranean descent who suffer from favism. Eating the bean or inhaling pollen of the broad bean *Vicia fava* causes *favism*—an acute hemolytic anemia due to G6PD deficiency. This occurs in whites only, mostly in Greeks, Italians, Kurdish Jews, and Sardinians. G6PD deficiency may be beneficial in blacks in affording some protection against falciparum malaria.

The unstable hemoglobins Zurich, Shepherd's Bush, and Torino spontaneously form methemoglobin, and hemolysis can be produced by all the drugs listed above under G6PD deficiency. There is a defect in the hemoglobin molecule that resists oxidant stresses poorly.

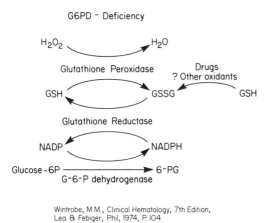

Wintrobe, M.M., Clinical Hematology, 7th Edition, Lea & Febiger, Phil, 1974, P. I04

Figure 37–1 The biochemical interactions of G6PD and glutathione metabolism are shown here. (From Wintrobe, M. M.: Clinical Hematology. 7th ed. Philadelphia, Lea & Febiger, 1974, p. 104.)

ISONIAZID (INH) AND DEFICIENCY OF N-ACETYLTRANSFERASE

Toxicity of INH, a drug of great importance in control of tuberculosis, is related to rate of inactivation by acetylation and excretion. "Rapid inactivators" have an enzyme in the liver that acetylates INH and, therefore, hastens formation of acetyl INH. "Slow inactivators" will form acetyl INH but do so slowly. Toxicity of INH occurs primarily in the slow inactivators. Ability to acetylate is inherited as an autosomal recessive trait. Adjustment of dose and careful surveillance are indicated in patients treated with INH to avoid toxic accumulation.

SUCCINYLCHOLINE SUSCEPTIBILITY

Succinylcholine is a tremendously useful short-acting muscle relaxant employed during anesthesia. Acetylcholinesterase rapidly inactivates the drug. About one in 3000 persons is affected with the trait of acetylcholinesterase deficiency. With failure of inactivation of the muscle relaxant, prolonged apnea results. The setting of anesthesia permits appropriate ventilatory assistance, and the apnea is rarely fatal. Nevertheless, family members should be warned to inform their doctor about this defect so that this drug will not be used during anesthesia for any operation.

MALIGNANT HYPERTHERMIA

Approximately one in 20,000 persons develops malignant hyperthermia (MH) when given certain anesthetic agents. The syndrome is clearly familial, and the pattern fits an autosomal dominant pattern with variable penetrance. The genetic aspects are not clearly established, however. If MH does occur, the person's entire family should be notified, so that the individuals can tell a surgeon who is planning to do surgery. The anesthetics producing MH in susceptible hosts are halothane (Fluothane), methoxyflurane, ketamine hydrochlorate, and the depolarizing agents succinylcholine chloride and decamethonium iodide. Caffeine and halothane act synergistically, but caffeine alone also can cause muscle contracture. Other agents include phencyclidine (chemically related to ketamine), some tranquilizers, tricyclic antidepressants, and monamine oxidase inhibitors. Ketamine can raise the temperature slightly in normal people. Viral infections, lymphomas, emotional upset, and excitement can precipitate MH in susceptible individuals.

A strain of swine has very similar sensitivity, so a great deal of information about the chemical aspects of the syndrome has been elucidated. Studies on porcine and human muscle have led to the theory that control of intracellular ionized calcium levels is abruptly lost and intracellular calcium rises. Aerobic and anaerobic metabolism rise in an attempt to correct these changes. Metabolic and respiratory acidosis result, and a hypermetabolic state ensues with tremendous increase in heat production. There may be generalized increase in permeability of muscle cell membranes. Water, ions, myoglobin, and CPK are lost. A vicious circle results, with temperature rising rapidly as much as 1° C every 5 minutes. Arterial P_{CO_2} greater than 100 torr and a pH less than 7.00 are found. Muscle rigidity, tachycardia, tachypnea, and circulatory instability develop rapidly.

Treatment of MH is a true emergency. Cessation of administration of the anesthetic agent and aggressive attempts to lower body temperature are obviously needed. It has been found that dantrolene is a specific therapeutic drug. It is a lipid soluble hydantoin derivative that acts distal to the end plate in the muscle fiber. It attenuates calcium release and stabilizes calcium metabolism. Specific details of therapy will not be discussed here, but the reader is referred to Gronert's very complete review of the subject.

SUMMARY

The aforementioned genetic variants illustrate the spectacular success of science in defining precise chemical reactions. Obviously, none of these defects (with the possible exception of favism) could have been found if reactions had not occurred to potent and very useful drugs introduced since the 1930's. Undoubtedly, there are many other similar enzyme deficits that are causing adverse reactions. The only way further discoveries can be made is to carry on a careful surveillance with information about family, race, grouping of unusual or unexpected reactions, and so forth. Many reactions now considered to be "idiosyncratic" may well have a genetic basis. Hypersensitivity reactions of allergic nature are dealt with elsewhere in Chapter 5.

ENVIRONMENT

During the past century, the environment has become contaminated by a large number of pollutants as a result of industrial growth. Emissions from chimneys and automobile exhausts pollute the air with sulfur dioxide, oxides of nitrogen, carbon monoxide, chlorides, ammonia, and dust. Sewage from industrial plants has killed aquatic life and made many rivers not fit sources for water for domestic use. Industrial accidents result in massive spills of chemicals, such as carbon tetrachloride, into streams. Transportation of toxic chemicals by truck or train may result in serious

acute local air pollution with lethal or serious concentrations of various gases, such as chlorine. Chemical additives to food represent a threat to all of us. Butter yellow is a classic example that was removed years ago. The U.S. Food and Drug Administration maintains a constant surveillance of such problems.

The home environment poses many serious hazards. Children under 5 years of age are victims of careless storage and failure to seal containers of toxic chemicals, such as caustic soda, liquid drain cleaner, cleaning fluids such as ammonia and carbon tetrachloride, and drugs such as aspirin, acetaminophen, and a whole spectrum of prescription drugs from ferrous sulfate to tricyclic antidepressants. Adults may deliberately take an overdose of any drug. Alcohol is universally available and is the single most important lethal chemical in our society. Its acute effects can cause violent behavior, coma, death, or fatal automobile accidents (50 per cent of fatal automobile accidents are alcohol-related). Its chronic effects result in prolonged serious illnesses and ultimately death. Cigarette smoking causes contamination of one's personal environment by inhaled nicotine, carbon monoxide, and tars, resulting in accelerated atherosclerosis of all arteries, pulmonary insufficiency, and cancer of the respiratory tract. Cigarette smoking is an excellent example of the equation, dose × time = cumulative toxicity.

Important toxic chemical reactions will be discussed in the remainder of the chapter to illustrate the pathophysiology of specific intoxications. The importance of accidental or deliberate poisoning is clearly apparent from the data for 1972 reported to the National Clearinghouse for Poison Information Center. There were 105,018 incidents in children under 5 years of age and a total of 160,824 in all ages. Medicines alone accounted for 47,625 incidents, and of these 8146 were due to ingestion of aspirin in children under 5 years of age. An overwhelming preponderance of accidental ingestion of cleaning and polishing agents, petroleum products, cosmetics, pesticides, turpentine and paints, plants, and miscellaneous agents is recorded in children younger than 5 years. The mortality rate is high. These deaths are preventable.

In the New York Hospital during a 4-year period (1969-1973) the order of frequency of agents involved in severe drug overdose was as follows: alcohol, barbiturates or glutethimide, heroin or methadone, methaqualone, meprobamate, scopolamine, amphetamine, imipramine, lithium, salicylates, phenothiazines, phenytoin, dicumarol, coumadin, tolbutamide, phenformin, and insulin. This order does not apply to the fatality rate.

In the United States, 80 to 90 per cent of chemical-induced deaths in adults involved only four groups of agents: barbiturates and narcotics, carbon monoxide, salicylates, and alcohol. In 1968, in New York City alone, there were 1205 deaths from narcotic abuse. Because of these data, the pathophysiology and possible antidotes for common intoxications will be discussed. Prevention of deaths and injuries of innocent children must have a high priority in medicine. Prevention of accidents by proper labeling and storage also has a high priority.

All favorable and unfavorable chemical reactions are specific, time-related, dose-related from undetectable to toxic and lethal, and often genetically modified or variable, depending on host factors not clearly genetic.

In the clinical setting, it is important to have available an up-to-date detailed data base on all known toxic substances in a retrievable form at the Poison Control Center for the geographic area. For quick reference, the current Physicians' Desk Reference is useful. A different set of rules applies to each chemical agent. It is necessary that each physician know how to have access to the information. A corollary of this is the absolute need to get precise information about the chemical agents taken, the amount, and the route. The label on the bottle of the drug or chemical is the most reliable source of information, so it is vitally important to obtain the container. Because of their overwhelming importance, certain of the toxins (alcohol, aspirin, barbiturates, opiates, carbon monoxide, and acetaminophen) will be discussed in some detail, emphasizing the features of early toxic reaction. Table 37–1 at the end of this chapter gives some basic information about a number of toxic chemicals and naturally occurring poisons.

SALICYLATES

Salicylate intoxication is a leading cause of death in children younger than 5 years. Aspirins or methylsalicylates are ingested because "children's" aspirin tastes like candy or because the odor of methyl salicylate is enticing if these compounds are left in unsafe containers within reach of young children. Infants can be intoxicated by inadvertent therapeutic overdosage because of unfamiliarity with the appropriate dose. Suicide attempts in adolescents or young adults also account for a number of serious or fatal poisonings.

Hyperventilation is the most characteristic manifestation, but delirium, hallucinations, convulsions, coma, and profound shock are also signs of severe intoxication. Chemically, there is, at first, a marked respiratory alkalosis because of stimulation of the respiratory center by salicylates. This changes imperceptibly to metabolic acidosis after a few hours. Arterial blood pH must be determined at regular intervals, since clinical differentiation of respiratory alkalosis and metabolic acidosis is difficult without pH determination. Salicylates act as a general metabolic stimulant capable of uncoupling oxidative phosphorylation with an increase of CO_2 production. There is interference with normal metabolism of carbohydrates and lipids such that ketone bodies and other organic acids accumulate. Toxic levels of salicylate lower brain glucose concentration in the face of normal plasma glucose. Brain edema can occur because of depletion of brain glucose, causing uncal herniation and sudden death. Furthermore, salicylates interfere with normal renal handling of ketones and other metabolic acids. Salicylate excretion is accelerated by alkalinizing the urine by administration of acetazolamide and sodium bicarbonate. Giving sodium bicarbonate alone may not adequately increase the pH of the urine.

The determination of salicylate level is of great importance because a level over 100 mg/dl at zero time (levels can be projected to zero time from a nomogram by Done) is a very serious prognostic sign. Semiquantitative determination of salicylates in the blood can be made by using Phenstix and referring to a color chart with a "small reaction" indicating 25 to 50 mg/dl or a "large reaction" indicating 150 mg/dl or more. Ferric chloride (10 per cent) solution is useful in detecting the presence of salicylate in the urine. $FeCl_3$ reacts with salicylates, resulting in a burgundy red color that is not changed by boiling the urine (acetoacetic acid also gives this color, but acetoacetic acid is volatile and disappears on boiling the urine).

In summary, salicylates have a striking and characteristic effect on metabolism, beginning with respiratory alkalosis and changing to metabolic acidosis. Severe intoxication results in serious cerebral and systemic effects, coma, and death. Treatment includes hydration, induction of vomiting, or intubation and lavage (if seen within 4 hours), potassium administration, monitoring of salicylate level and arterial pH, and alkalinizing urine using acetazolamide and sodium bicarbonate. General supportive measures for circulation and respiration are obviously needed, as in any serious intoxication. Vitamin K is needed to counteract the prothrombin deficiency regularly produced by salicylates. Exchange transfusion for infants, peritoneal dialysis with albumin-containing fluid, or hemodialysis is sometimes needed when the patient is very ill with a very high salicylate level. Prevention should have high priority.

ACETAMINOPHEN

Acetaminophen, or N-acetyl-p-aminophenol (Tylenol, Tempra), has become an important and serious poison in the United States. It has been a serious toxin in England for a number of years. When compared with aspirin, the drug is free of some distressing side effects at modest doses, but in large doses it is toxic to the liver, causing centrilobular necrosis. Renal damage due to tubule necrosis is common in patients surviving more than 2 days.

Acetaminophen is rapidly absorbed from the intestinal tract, and peak plasma concentrations are achieved in 1 to 2 hours. Acetaminophen can cause sudden death before the patient can be admitted to the hospital. Early deaths probably occur from vomiting and aspiration. The concentration in the plasma is the principal predictor of the occurrence of hepatic toxicity. Plasma half-life has been reported to be from 1 to 3 hours in normal subjects to a mean of 4 hours in mild intoxication and a mean of 10 hours in fatal instances. Plasma levels below 150 mg per liter at 4 hours or 50 mg per liter at 12 hours are unlikely to result in severe hepatic toxicity. At 4 hours, a level above 300 mg per liter results in hepatic necrosis. About 80 per cent of a therapeutic dose of acetaminophen is cleared from the blood by biotransformation by microsomal enzymes to a conjugate with glucuronic acid and sulfate. These metabolic products are inactive and excreted. Minor metabolites of acetaminophen are formed by hydroxylation and deacetylation. Production of hydroxylated metabolites involves oxidation by cytochrome P450 and mixed-function oxidases. This minor metabolite is a highly reactive arylating agent. The hydroxylated metabolite is conjugated with hepatic glutathione, further conjugated with cysteine and mercapturic acid, and is excreted in the urine. When a large dose is taken, large amounts of the toxic intermediates accumulate, and hepatic glutathione is depleted. It is important to note that drugs such as phenobarbital induce the cytochrome P450 enzyme system and that consequently there is an acceleration of the formation of hydroxylated intermediates that are active arylating compounds. Glutathione depletion is hastened, with expected toxic consequences. Vital hepatocellular macromolecules bind covalently with these toxic intermediates, causing hepatic necrosis.

A key metabolic feature is depletion of hepatic cellular glutathione, and this has resulted in the suggestion and use of sulfhydryl donors in treatment of patients with plasma levels high enough to indicate moderate to severe hepatic injury. Cysteamine and acetylcysteine have been effective, and one of these agents should be used when plasma levels indicate the probability of hepatic toxicity. Survivors apparently do not have residual liver damage.

Chronic excessive use can cause toxic hepatitis when the drug dose has been in the range of 5 to 8 gm. This dose is just slightly less than the amount that can cause acute intoxication. It is likely that the incidence of liver damage from chronic therapeutic use of large doses will increase.

BARBITURATES, RELATED COMPOUNDS, AND NARCOTICS

Hypnotics and opiates have similar depressive actions on respiratory and circulatory centers and on cerebral function. It is not unusual for a subject to take multiple hypnotic drugs in a suicide attempt. Barbiturates are generally divided into short-acting barbiturates (represented by pentobarbital, secobarbital, and amobarbital) and the long-acting barbiturates (represented by phenobarbital, barbital, and mephobarbital). The long-acting barbiturates are mainly excreted by the kidneys but are also detoxified by the liver. The drug concentration is important for determining prognosis, and it also is important for consideration of hemodialysis in patients with phenobarbital, barbital, or mephobarbital intoxication. Urea- or mannitol-induced diuresis and alkalinization of the urine are helpful in treatment of severe intoxication with both kinds of barbiturates, but particularly the long-acting ones.

Glutethimide intoxication is associated with special problems. Forced diuresis is of little value. Hemodialysis, either aqueous or lipid, does not remove very much drug. Glutethimide is lipid-soluble, and blood levels are not closely correlated with severity of depression. There may be a fluctuating level of consciousness and, particularly, deepening coma, even after starting treatment. Treatment consists of eliminating drug sequestered in the intestine and supporting the respiratory and circulatory systems.

Opiates and synthetic narcotics may cause serious intoxication characterized by coma, severe respiratory slowing or arrest, and shock. Intoxication results from accidental overdose from the use of "street" heroin of uncertain strength or from intentional or suicidal overdose. A competitive inhibitor of narcotics in general, naloxone hydrochloride (Narcan), is very useful therapeutically and diagnostically in an opiate overdose. It should be injected repeatedly as needed, particularly for respiratory depression. It has one undesirable side-effect; namely, it will cause acute withdrawal reaction in an addicted individual. Support of circulation and respiration is, of course, essential.

In all vertebrate studies, the cell membranes of some of the neurons of the central nervous system have synaptosomal receptors. These areas correspond to well-characterized anatomic pathways involved in pain perception. Crude extracts of brain will displace labeled opium derivatives and an opium antagonist like naloxone from synaptosomal preparations. The opiate-like substances are pentapeptides, Leu[5]-enkephalin and Met[5]-enkephalin. The compounds are present in larger molecules derived from an extract of hypothalamus-neurohypophysis, with Met[5]-enkephalin as their N terminal. These latter compounds are called *endorphins*. In synaptosomal opiate-binding assays, α- and γ-endorphins are as active as morphine, and β-endorphin is 5 to 10 times as active. Naloxone can inhibit the action of endorphins. In the intact animal, α-, β-, and γ-endorphins have quite different effects. Naloxone blocks stimulation-produced analgesia and acupuncture analgesia. Endorphins probably will have an enormous impact on future understanding of neurophysiology and neuropharmacology.

The social problems of addiction to heroin and other opium compounds, cocaine, and the sedative and hypnotic drugs are enormous. The effects on the person are shattering. An incidental but very serious effect is the frequent association of systemic bacterial and fungal infections, often with bacterial endocarditis, as a result of "main line" administration. Physical and psychologic dependence is a threat associated with use of any of the aforementioned agents. Withdrawal reactions are similar in many respects, but each group of agents has certain unique and potentially lethal features.

ETHANOL

Ethanol (ethyl alcohol, beverage alcohol) is the most important toxic material in our society today. It accounts for more deaths than any other toxic substance when one considers sudden death from acute overdose, deaths from auto accidents due to drunken driving, and deaths from chronic alcohol-related diseases such as hepatic cirrhosis, chronic brain syndrome, and alcoholic cardiomyopathy.

Ethanol diffuses readily across all biologic membranes except the skin, and so it is absorbed from all parts of the gastrointestinal tract, lungs, urinary bladder, peritoneum, pleura, and from subcutaneous sites. Alcohol distributes uniformly in the total body water by rapidly diffusing across

capillary, cell, and organelle membranes. Alcohols interact with the lipid phase of cell membranes. Very high concentration disrupts the membranes. Ethanol changes membrane permeability to Na^+ and K^+. It depresses the functional activity of nerve cells by a direct effect on the excitable membranes of neuronal tissue. A typical reaction to ethanol ingestion is euphoria and exhilaration, followed by mental slowing and, finally, coma as the alcohol level increases progressively.

Ethanol is converted to acetaldehyde by the enzyme alcohol dehydrogenase; the acetaldehyde is converted to acetate by aldehyde oxidizing enzymes (Fig. 37–2). Alcohol dehydrogenase, 90 per cent of which is located in the cytosol, attaches to a molecule of oxidized coenzyme, nicotine-adenine dinucleotide (NAD). The hydrogen of alcohol is accepted by NAD, which is converted to the reduced form, NADH. This is the rate-limiting step. Accumulation of NADH accounts for some of ethanol's effects on carbohydrate metabolism and on the production of fatty liver. Conversion of NADH or NAD is accomplished by electron transfer along the respiratory chain located in the mitochondria. A large number of alcohols and aldehydes have considerable affinity for alcohol dehydrogenase.

Ethanol has significant effects on the metabolism of carbohydrate. The oxidation of alcohol results in the increase in NADH/NAD in liver cytosol. This increase in NADH/NAD ratio alters the equilibrium between the trioses, dihydroxyacetone phosphate and α-glycerophosphate, favoring the latter. This shift in ratio results in more glycerol and, hence, the formation of hepatic triglycerides. Ethanol inhibits the utilization of galactose metabolism so that galactose is excreted in the urine. When fructose is administered with alcohol, fructose doubles the splanchnic uptake of alcohol and the production of acetate. Alcohol

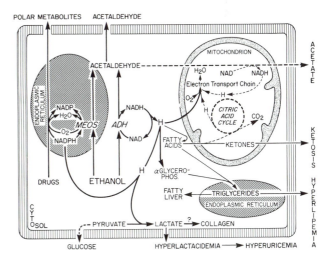

Figure 37–2 Metabolism of ethanol in the hepatocyte and schematic representation of its link to fatty liver, hyperlipemia, hyperuricemia, hyperlactacidemia, and ketosis. Pathways that are decreased by ethanol are represented by dashed lines. ADH, alcohol dehydrogenase; MEOS, microsomal ethanol oxidizing system; NAD, nicotinamide adenine dinucleotide; NADH, nicotinamide adenine dinucleotide, reduced form; NADP, nicotinamide adenine dinuceotide phosphate; NADPH, nicotinamide adenine dinucleotide phosphate, reduced form. (From Lieber, C. M., et al.: Ped. Proc. 34:2061, 1975.)

diverts some fructose to sorbitol via sorbitol dehydrogenase and NADH. This results in a higher proportion of glycerol formation from fructose and more glycerophosphate.

Ethanol can cause hypoglycemia in a fasting subject by slowing down gluconeogenesis. Alanine is the prime regulator of gluconeogenesis. Ethanol lowers circulating levels of alanine and other important glucogenic amino acids and, hence, impairs gluconeogenesis. The high NADH/NAD concentration ratio as a result of oxidation of ethanol to acetate impairs the conversion of glutamic acid to α-ketoglutarate by interfering with the activity of glutamic dehydrogenase. Metabolism of ethanol increases the lactate-pyruvate ratio in the setting of an increased NADH/NAD ratio. In summary, ethanol impairs gluconeogenesis because it preempts mitochondrial cofactors, inhibits enzymes, channels precursors away from gluconeogenic pathways, and blocks uptake of precursors.

The velocity of the reaction of alcohol dehydrogenase (ADH) and ethanol is approximately seven times that for ADH and methanol, and the affinity of ethanol and ADH is twice that of methanol and ADH. For these reasons, ethanol can be given to a person poisoned with methanol, thus preventing the oxidation of methanol to the very toxic products formaldehyde and formic acid. Unchanged methanol can then be excreted by the kidney. Methanol is easily oxidized by catalase, but ethanol is also a good competitive inhibitor of this reaction. Therefore, at this step also, ethanol prevents oxidation of methanol to toxic products so that methanol can be excreted. Similarly, ethylene glycol has a slow velocity of reaction and affinity for ADH compared with ethanol. Ethanol in a large dose competitively inhibits the oxidation of ethylene glycol to the highly toxic oxalic acid and is of considerable practical value in treatment of ethylene glycol poisoning.

Inhibitors of the metabolism of ethanol to acetaldehyde to acetate are useful in treating alcoholism. Disulfiram (Antabuse, tetraethylthiuram disulfide) is converted to diethylthiocarbamate. This compound chelates zinc and the metals of the aldehyde oxidizing system. Disulfiram can inactivate dehydrogenases by formation of disulfide linkages with active sulfhydryl groups of enzymes. The inhibition of alcohol- and aldehyde-metabolizing enzymes causes the disulfiram-alcohol syndrome when the two drugs are taken together. Other compounds, butyraldoxime, sulfonylurea compounds, and metronidazole, produce disulfiram-like reactions.

Catalase found in most animal tissues forms H_2O_2, which reacts with a hydrogen donor. Considerable turnover rates are observed in vitro with methanol, ethanol, and formate. Catalase, however, does not have a major role in normal ethanol metabolism.

Acetate enters the two-carbon pool through acetyl coenzyme A. Two dehydrogenases using NAD as coenzyme, two oxidases producing H_2O_2, and a third group of enzymes, the lyases, are responsible for acetaldehyde oxidation to acetate. Free acetate activation to acetyl coenzyme A is diminished when ethanol is actively being metabolized. Acetate is a central metabolic product and can be oxidized to CO_2 and water or used in the synthesis of fatty acids, steroids, and ketone bodies.

The level of alcohol dehydrogenase is decreased in the livers of animals pretreated with alcohol. The liver shows damage in the form of steatosis. Intolerance to ethanol has been observed in patients with an abnormal liver. A microsomal ethanol oxidizing system (MEOS) of the smooth endoplasmic reticulum has been found by a number of investigators. Chronic ethanol ingestion causes proliferation of the smooth endoplasmic reticulum, which could account for the induction of drug-metabolizing enzymes that results in the increased resistance of alcoholic subjects to the action of sedative drugs. Significant tolerance to ethanol is built up by chronic ingestion of ethanol in persons who do not have overt liver damage.

Ethanol has a direct etiologic role in the pathogenesis of alcoholic fatty liver and cirrhosis. Ethanol fed to normal volunteer men and alcoholic men caused fatty infiltration of the liver in each group, despite a well-balanced standard diet and even massive supplementation with protein and choline. The amount and duration of ethanol intake rather than malnutrition account for fatty liver in adult humans. After ethanol administration, phospholipids are increased in the liver, whereas fatty liver produced by choline deficiency has decreased phospholipids.

Fatty liver induced by moderate amounts of ethanol is reversible and benign. However, a florid kind of fatty metamorphosis called *alcoholic hepatitis* occurs, with extensive cellular degeneration, appearance of alcoholic hyaline of Mallory, hepatic cell necrosis, and inflammatory cells. Ultrastructural cell changes in ordinary fatty liver and alcoholic hepatitis are the same, namely, striking alterations in mitochondria and endoplasmic reticulum and focal cytoplasmic degradation with formation of autophagic vacuoles containing clumps and whorls of osmophilic material. The cisternae and vacuoles of the Golgi apparatus are dilated and filled with osmophilic material, probably lipoprotein particles. The similarity of ultrastructural changes in simple alcoholic fatty liver and in alcoholic hepatitis suggests that the process is a continuum. The pathogenesis of alcoholic cirrhosis clearly is related to fatty metamorphosis, but the exact mechanism is still unclear.

Ethanol intoxication is a phenomenon recognizable by everyone. The blood level of ethanol and, therefore, the dose ingested is related directly to the severity of intoxication. A person unaccustomed to ethanol exhibits intoxication at ethanol levels of 50 to 100 mg/dl, whereas a person who drinks alcohol regularly exhibits intoxication at levels above 150 mg/dl. At 200 mg/dl, most individuals are unmistakably drunk. Intoxication is severe at 350 mg/dl and over. Levels as low as 350 mg/dl have caused death, and levels above 550 mg/dl are usually fatal. By extrapolation of blood levels at time of death to zero time, the levels usually are 500 to 600 mg/dl. This level will kill in a short time or will cause sufficient brain damage to cause death after several hours. The median LD_{50} in terms of blood ethanol has been estimated to be 400 mg/dl. These data emphasize the very serious acute toxic effect of ethanol on the brain.

A very common and serious effect of chronic ethanol abuse is the acute withdrawal reaction manifested as alcoholic hallucinosis and delirium tremens. One of the biochemical phenomena associated with these disturbances is a large increase of free fatty acids in the blood. Another feature is the occurrence of hypomagnesemia and total body magnesium deficit. By careful management, the mortality rate from delirium tremens has been reduced greatly since the 1950s; nevertheless, it is a serious, acute medical emergency.

The most common nervous system lesion is alcoholic neuropathy with all the signs of neuropathy. Thiamine particularly, but also pyridoxine and pantothenic acid, are useful therapeutically, but only if ethanol is stopped.

The mechanism of production of chronic alcoholic encephalopathy is not clear, but certain facts are relevant. Chronic dementia of the Korsakoff type frequently is preceded by acute Wernicke's encephalopathy due to thiamine deficiency. Simple dementia, however, occurs with alcohol-induced brain atrophy. Rare specific localized encephalopathies, such as central pontine myelinolysis, toxic amblyopia, and Marchiafava-Bignami disease, depend on the specific area of the brain affected. Since alcohol causes acute cerebral effects that can be profound and, if repetitive, could have direct degenerative effects on the brain, it is understandable that ethanol can cause chronic encephalopathy. Chronic alcohol dementia accounts for a large number of patients in mental hospitals. Cerebellar degeneration is a common result of alcoholism and may occur with cerebral lesions or may be the only residual lesion.

Ethanol is a direct and frequent cause of gastritis, with serious and sometimes fatal gastric hemorrhage. Ethanol also is the most frequent cause of pancreatitis and all its complications, including a high mortality rate. Ethanol is the usual cause of chronic relapsing pancreatitis.

Alcoholic cardiomyopathy is a serious and often fatal condition caused by continuous high ethanol ingestion. The cause of the cardiomyopathy is not clear, but there is some evidence that acetaldehyde has deleterious effects on both the electrical and mechanical parameters of myocardial function.

Although the relationship between maternal ethanol abuse and undesirable outcomes of pregnancy has been recognized since ancient times, it did not gain scientific validation until this century. Infants and children born to alcoholic mothers exhibit characteristic clinical features. *Fetal alcohol syndrome* refers to these clinical characteristics. Major features of fetal alcohol syndrome are prenatal and postnatal growth retardation, mental deficiency, small head size relative to height, and minor anomalies of the face, eyes, heart, joints, and external genitalia. Mental retardation is the most serious defect. Ocular anomalies include epicanthal folds, convergence defects, ptosis, and palpebral fissures that are below average in length. Minimal diagnostic criteria are physical and mental retardation with associated minor birth defects and a history of chronic maternal alcoholism.

The pathogenesis of the teratogenic effects of ethanol remains unknown. In rats, a deficiency of zinc during crucial stages of gestation is known to be teratogenic. Many enzymes required for DNA synthesis are zinc-dependent, and an adverse effect of zinc deficiency on the activity of deoxythymidine kinase has been reported. Inasmuch as ethanol ingestion may affect zinc balance adversely, one may speculate that the teratogenic effect of alcohol is mediated through zinc enzymes involved in DNA synthesis. Further studies must be carried out in order to understand fully the pathogenic mechanisms of fetal alcohol syndrome so that proper therapeutic measures may be undertaken.

In summary, ethanol is the most serious chemical toxin in modern society because of its widespread use. It causes serious chronic social and physical disturbances that probably exceed the devastation of alcohol-induced death.

CARBON MONOXIDE

Carbon monoxide (CO) is a serious environmental poison. Although CO is used as a highly successful vehicle for suicide, most deaths and morbidity result from accidental poisoning, such as occurs from fires in unventilated rooms, from leaks in smoke ducts, and from destructive fires in buildings. CO is odorless and, therefore, doubly hazardous.

The biochemistry of CO in the body is straightforward, and its toxicity has been known since Claude Bernard reported on it in 1857. J. S. Haldane (1895) was a pioneering investigator of the physiology and toxicology of CO. Hemoglobin has an affinity for CO that is 240 times that for O_2. CO readily displaces O_2 from hemoglobin at partial pressures only 1/240 that of O_2, forming

TABLE 37–1 TOXIC CHEMICALS AND POISONS

Toxin	Special Features of Exposure	Target Tissue of Organ	Enzymes Affected; Physiologic or Pharmacologic Features	Clinical or Pathologic Results	Antidote, Special Form of Treatment, or Prevention
Antimony (Sb^{3+}) Stilbine (SbH$_2$)	Tartar emetic; metallurgy; mining and smelting; rubber manufacture; exposure to nascent H to Sb$_2$O$_3$	CNS; skin; bone	Sulfhydryl group of enzymes	Vomiting; dermatitis; conjunctivitis; acute encephalopathy; acute hemolysis due to stilbene	Administer BAL (British antilewisite, or dimercaprol); avoid generation of stilbene
Arsenic (As^{3+}) As$_2$O$_3$ Arsine (AsH$_3$)	Deliberate (e.g., homicide); Fowler's solution as medicine; industrial exposure nascent H to As$_2$O$_3$	CNS and peripheral nerves; bone marrow; kidney; skin; fingernails	Sulfhydryl groups of many enzymes; carcinogenesis	Shock and death; acute hemolytic anemia; hemoglobinuria; nephropathy; encephalopathy; cardiomyopathy; hyperkeratoses and basal cell cancers (Bowen's disease); Mees' lines; neuropathy	Acute: Administer BAL; initiate hemodialysis for acute renal failure; stop use of Fowler's solution
Cadmium (Cd^{2+})	Industrial waste from battery factories in water supply (Japan); inhalation	Kidney; lungs; bone	Necrosis of respiratory epithelium; renal glucosuria; phosphaturia; hypophosphatemia; low molecular weight proteinuria; interferes with metabolism and utilization of zinc	Pulmonary edema and interstitial pneumonitis; osteomalacia (Itai-Itai, or "ouch-ouch," disease—Japan)	Stop water pollution with cadmium (battery industry); treat osteomalacia, CaNa$_2$ EDTA therapy
Iron ferrous salts	Accidental ingestion in children under 5 years; suicide attempts	CNS; liver; heart	High level of plasma-free iron with transferrin fully saturated	Hypotension; progressive shock; dyspnea; coma	Administer desferoxamine mesylate (Desferal) IV and orally; prevent
Lead (Pb^{2+}) and tetraethyl lead	Pica (eating of paint chips by young children; paint dust in building repair; "moonshine" whiskey; leaded gasoline auto exhaust	CNS; bone marrow; joints; kidneys	Delta amino levulinic acid (ALA) synthetase (probable); ALA dehydratase (Zn dependent); heme synthetase	Encephalopathy; neuropathy of motor nerves; abdominal crises; anemia; nephropathy; hyperuricemia and "Saturnine" gout; possible mental retardation	Give ethylene diamine tetra-acetic acid (CaNa$_2$ EDTA) and penicillamine; eliminate lead in paint and gasoline; maintain appropriate zinc levels (excess dietary zinc is protective against lead toxicity in rats and horses)
Mercury, (Hg^{2+}) mercury bichloride (HgCl$_2$) Calomel (HgCl) (Hg^{1+})	Suicide attempts; industrial use, medicinal use	All tissues; kidney; CNS	Sulfhydryl groups; denaturation of all proteins (corrosive action) and cell death; acute renal tubule cell injury	Corrosion of mucosa and skin; acute renal failure; personality disorder, or "erethism" ("mad as a hatter"); acrodynia (calomel); headache	Administer BAL; initiate hemodialysis; give N-acetyl d.l. penicillamine; eliminate calomel as medication; maintain appropriate levels of dietary selenium (may be protective against toxic effects of methylmercury compounds in rats)

Agent	Source/Remarks	Organs	Properties	Clinical effects	Treatment
Methyl and ethyl mercury	Hg contamination of water, biotransformation by bacteria to organic Hg, then ingestion by fish (tuna and swordfish) (Minamata Bay and Niigata, Japan epidemic)	CNS; fetal intoxication of CNS	Volatile; penetrate mucosa readily; concentrate in CNS	Serious CNS injury (including that found in newborns born to mothers who have ingested alkyl mercury)	Monitor Hg concentration in fish; clean up streams and stop Hg contamination of water; provide N-acetyl d.l. penicillamine
Thallium (Tl$^+$)	Rodent poison; depilatory	CNS; hair follicles; liver; kidney	Degenerative changes in all cells, especially of hair follicles	Alopecia is pathognomonic; encephalopathy with ataxia, choreiform movement, and delirium and coma; central lobular necrosis of liver and renal tubule injury	Administer Prussian blue by mouth as a chelator of Tl in exchange for K$^+$; eliminate use of thallium as domestic rodent poison
Barbiturates, Opiates, Sedatives, and Antidepressants					
Barbiturates; short-acting—amobarbital, pentobarbital, secobarbital; long-acting—phenobarbital, barbital, mephobarbital	Suicide attempts; chronic dependence	CNS	Renal and hepatic elimination of long-acting barbiturates; hepatic detoxification of short-acting barbiturates; physiologic dependence or addiction	Sedation; convulsions; stupor; coma; shock; apnea; death; withdrawal reaction with delirium; intact pupillary reflexes	Support vital functions; induce diuresis and alkalinization of urine; initiate hemodialysis for long-acting barbiturates
Benzodiazepines: diazepam, chlordiazepoxide, flurazepam	Often taken with alcohol or other drugs	CNS	Minor tranquilizer; sedation; physiologic dependence or addiction	Coma, rarely fatal unless other drugs have also been used; withdrawal reaction	Support vital functions
Ethchlorvynol	Storage in fat	CNS	Sedation; physiologic dependence; fat-soluble	Withdrawal reaction; coma; often prolonged because of storage in fat	Support vital functions
Glutethimide (Doriden)	Short-acting like secobarbital	CNS	Sequestered in bowel with fluctuating coma; physiologic dependence; pupillary reflexes lost	Coma, often severe; tends to produce hypotension	Support vital functions
Meprobamate (Equanil)		CNS	Minor tranquilizer; physiologic dependence	Coma; withdrawal seizures common	Support vital functions; treat seizures
Methaqualone (Quaalude)	Abuse common	CNS; blood coagulation	Sedation; rapid physiologic dependence; dangerous dose relatively small	Coma; hallucinations; motor hyperactivity; myoclonus; convulsions; heart failure	Support vital functions; treat seizures
Opium and related compounds	Addiction from therapeutic use and deliberate abuse;	CNS	Narcosis; euphoria; physiologic dependence; endorphins—brain receptors; cocaine—excitement, mania	Special effects on respiratory and circulatory control; altering of pupil reflexes—constricted; stupor; coma; apnea; shock; death	Support vital functions; administer naloxone (Narcan) as often as necessary—opiates
Cocaine	impurity of street drugs and uncertain dose				

Table continued on following page

TABLE 37–1 TOXIC CHEMICALS AND POISONS (*Continued*)

Toxin	Special Features of Exposure	Target Tissue of Organ	Enzymes Affected; Physiologic or Pharmacologic Features	Clinical or Pathologic Results	Antidote, Special Form of Treatment, or Prevention
Tricyclic antidepressants	Often taken with other agents (and prescribed for already depressed patients)	CNS; cardiac conduction	Anticholinergic action	Dry mouth; bladder retention; ileus; blurred vision; sinus tachycardia; agitation; coma	Support vital functions; administer physostigmin salicylate; use activated charcoal as an adsorbent
Solvents and Alcohols					
Carbon tetrachloride	Particularly bad in a person also exposed to alcohols	Liver; kidney	Disruption of lipid membranes	Fatty liver and necrosis; acute tubule necrosis with acute renal failure	Support vital functions; dialysis as needed (peritoneal or hemodialysis); eliminate agent as domestic dry cleaner
Ethanol	Generally available; most widely used toxin	Liver; CNS; all tissues	Alcohol dehydrogenase; physiologic and psychologic dependence	Drunkenness and belligerence; coma and death; hepatic cirrhosis; anemia; acute and chronic brain syndromes	Support vital functions in profound intoxication; prevent alcoholism
Ethylene glycol	Sweet taste; careless storage	Kidney	(1) Oxidase converts it to oxalic acid; (2) Ethanol competes favorably for oxidase, preventing reaction 1.	Calcium oxalate injury to kidney causing acute renal failure and death	Ethanol permits ethylene glycol excretion; initiate hemodialysis or peritoneal dialysis as needed for acute renal failure
Methanol	Careless storage; suicide attempt	Optic nerve; whole body; CNS	(1) Oxidase catalyses it to formaldehyde and formic acid; (2) Ethanol competes favorably for oxidase, preventing reaction 1	Blindness; severe acidosis; death	Initiate dialysis immediately; ethanol competes for methanol oxidation permitting methanol excretion
Miscellaneous Toxins					
Acetylsalicylic acid and salicylates	Careless storage	CNS, respiration center	Stimulate respiration; stimulate metabolism; uncouple oxidative phosphorylation	Respiratory alkalosis; metabolic acidosis; coma and death	Initiate dialysis if severe; provide sodium bicarbonate and acetazolamide to increase excretion of salicylates in alkaline urine; administer glucose
Acetaminophen	Suicidal intent	Liver; kidney; CNS	Hydroxylated intermediate by glutathione under influence of cytochrome P450	Liver necrosis, renal tubule necrosis; toxic metabolites from covalent bonds with macromolecules; depletion glutathione	Administer cysteamine or acetylcysteine (Mucormyst) as sulfhydryl donors
Atropa belladonna	Attractive berries	Many organs (parasympathetic nerves)	Block cholinergic impulses (atropine poisoning)	Dry mouth; wide pupils; tachycardia; delirium; fever; death	Administer pilocarpine; support vital functions

Agent	Source/Occurrence	Site Affected	Mechanism	Effects	Treatment
Datura stramonium (Jimson weed)	Attractive plant	Many organs	Block cholinergic impulse (stramonium poisoning)	Same as those for atropine, belladonna	Administer pilocarpine; support vital functions
Cyanide (CN⁻)	Homicide and suicide; very small dose	Respiratory enzymes (heme-containing) of all cells	Inactivates cytochrome A_3; paralyzes electron transfer	Tissue anoxia and death	Administer Na thiosulfate and Na nitrite → cyanmethemoglobin to neutralize CN⁻
Botulinus toxin (*Clostridium botulinum*)	Contaminated canned food cooked insufficiently or stored in open container	Motor end-plate	Toxin is heat labile; blocks nerve impulse at motor end-plate	Paralysis of skeletal muscle	Administer antitoxin (type-specific); prevent contamination by cooking canned food thoroughly (to boiling)
Cholera toxin (*Vibrio cholerae*)	Epidemic; contaminated water supply	Small intestine mucosa (no inflammation)	Activates adenyl cyclase → cyclic AMP	Massive secretion of salt and water with circulatory collapse and death	Replace H_2O and electrolytes quantitatively
Clostridium perfringens toxin	Contamination of food due to improper refrigeration (toxin is heat labile)	Small intestine mucosa		Massive diarrhea; rarely fatal	Replace losses of H_2O and electrolytes; cook canned or stored food and refrigerate properly
Staphylococcus enterotoxin A, B, C, D	Contamination of food due to improper refrigeration	Probably CNS	Toxin is heat- and trypsin-stable	Abdominal cramping pain; vomiting; diarrhea (variable)	Handle and refrigerate food carefully; replace fluids and electrolytes
Phosphate ester insecticides (parathion, malathion, etc.)	Industrial environments; insecticide sprays and dusting (penetrate skin); careless storage (can result in accidental ingestion)	Parasympathetic nervous system; skeletal muscles; erythrocytes	Produce cholinergic action (powerful anticholinesterases); cause muscle paralysis; decrease RBC cholinesterase	Muscarine effects plus muscle paralysis cause respiratory failure	Administer atropine (2 to 3 mg) and repeat in 5 to 10 min; give pralidoxime chloride – 1 gm IV in 2 min and repeat in 1 hr as needed for adults; prevent problems by careful bathing and handling of clothes, proper equipment, and monitoring of RBC cholinesterase

carbon monoxide hemoglobin (COHG). Furthermore, the O_2 dissociation curve is "shifted to the left," so the oxyhemoglobin present in blood does not dissociate at usual oxygen tensions. Other heme-containing enzymes also react with CO. Generalized tissue anoxia results in a response curve dependent on atmospheric CO. At 0.01 per cent CO, the COHG is 44 per cent; at 0.1 per cent CO, the COHG is 62 per cent. All COHG concentrations above 20 per cent produce cerebral symptoms.

The tissues most easily injured by CO are the brain and myocardium because these tissues have the greatest O_2 consumption. A pre-existing cerebral or myocardial abnormality predisposes the patient to adverse effects of levels not injurious to normals. Late sequelae include late fatal demyelinization, permanent cerebral dysfunction, peripheral neuropathy, and effects on the conduction system of the heart.

Laboratory tests are of obvious diagnostic value, but treatment should be instituted on the basis of history and findings before results are obtained. Arterial blood gases reveal a normal Pa_{CO_2} because the plasma equilibrates with alveolar blood gases, but the blood content of O_2 is seriously decreased.

Treatment is simply administration of 100 per cent oxygen by mask. Two volumes per cent of O_2 are attained by this maneuver. CO excretion is enhanced by O_2 by shifting the equilibrium toward oxyhemoglobin. Brain edema occurs in most severe instances, and dexamethasone treatment is indicated.

Chronic exposure to CO concentrations insufficient to cause clinical (cerebral) symptoms but sufficient to elevate COHG concentrations occurs in our urban society because of the CO output of internal combustion engines and all fossil fuel–using machines. The COHG level in cigarette smokers is directly correlated with the number of cigarettes smoked each day. The COHG can be as high as 5 to 8 per cent in smokers who inhale.

CO may have an etiologic role in atherosclerosis. The deposit of cholesterol in the aorta in rabbits is enhanced by anoxia induced by decreasing partial pressure of O_2 or by slight excess of CO in the atmosphere. Anoxia increases the permeability of artery walls to serum proteins as measured by isotope-labeled protein. It has been postulated that chronic low-grade exposure to CO can result in significant effects on arteries by low-grade hypoxia. Patients who already have coronary artery disease with angina pectoris have such a small margin of safety that an increase in COHG can precipitate ischemic pain. The effects of chronic exposure to increased CO are just now being fully appreciated.

REFERENCES

Arena, J. M.: Salicylates (Poisoning). In Davison's Compleat Pediatrician. Philadelphia, Lea & Febiger, 1969.

Arky, R. A.: Carbohydrate metabolism in alcoholics. In Kissin, B., and Begleiter, H. (Eds.): The Biology of Alcoholism. Vol. I. New York, Plenum Press, 1971, pp. 197–227.

Astrup, P.: Some physiological and pathological effects of moderate carbon monoxide exposure. Br. Med. J. 1:12, 1973.

Beutler, E.: Abnormalities of the hexose monophosphate shunt. Semin. Hematol. 8:311, 1971.

Done, A. K.: Salicylate intoxication. Significance of salicylate in blood cases of acute ingestion. Pediatrics 26:800, 1960.

Dreosti, I. E., and Harley, L. S.: Depressed thymidine kinase activity in zinc deficient rat embryos. Proc. Soc. Exp. Biol. Med. 150:161, 1975.

Flink, E. B.: Mineral metabolism in alcoholism. In Kissin, B., and Begleiter, H. (Eds.): The Biology of Alcoholism. Vol. I. New York, Plenum Press, 1971, pp. 377–396.

Flink, E. B.: Heavy metal poisoning. In Beeson, P., and McDermott, W. (Eds.): Textbook of Medicine. 14th ed. Philadelphia, W. B. Saunders Co., 1975.

French, S. W.: Acute and chronic toxicity of alcohol. In Kissin, B., and Begleiter, H. (Eds.): The Biology of Alcoholism. Vol. I. New York, Plenum Press, 1971, pp. 437–511.

Gleason, M., Gosselin, R., Hodge, H., and Smith, R.: Clinical Toxicology of Commercial Products. 4th ed. Baltimore, Williams & Wilkins Co., 1973.

Goldsmith, J. R., and Landaw, S. A.: Carbon monoxide and human health. Science 162:1352, 1968.

Gronert, G. A.: Malignant hyperthermia. Anesthesiology 53:395, 1980.

Guillemin, R.: Endorphins: brain peptides that act like opiates. N. Engl. J. Med. 296:226, 1977.

Henderson, F., Vietti, T. J. and Brown, E. B.: Desferrioxamine in the treatment of acute toxic reaction to ferrous gluconate. J.A.M.A. 186:1139, 1963.

Henderson, L. W., and Merrill, J. P.: Treatment of barbiturate intoxication. Ann. Int. Med. 64:876, 1966.

Jones, K. L., Smith, D. W., Ulleland, C. N., and Streissguth, A. P.: Pattern of malformation in offspring of chronic alcoholic mothers. Lancet 1:1267, 1973.

Kalant, H.: Effects of biological membranes. In Kissin, B., and Begleiter, H. (Eds.): The Biology of Alcoholism. Vol. I. New York, Plenum Press, 1971, pp. 1–62.

Koch-Weser, J.: Acetaminophen. N. Engl. J. Med. 295:1297, 1976.

Kvenzolok, E. P., Best, L., and Manoguerra, A. S.: Acetaminophen toxicity. Am. J. Hosp. Pharm. 34:391, 1977.

Lieber, C. S., and De Carli, L. M.: Effects of ethanol on lipid, uric acid, intermediary and drug metabolism including pathogenesis of the alcoholic fatty liver. In Kissin, B., and Begleiter, H. (Eds.): The Biology of Alcoholism. Vol. I. New York, Plenum Press, 1971, pp. 264–305.

Loomis, T. A.: Essentials of Toxicology. 2nd ed. Philadelphia, Lea & Febiger, 1974.

Milby, T. H.: Prevention and management of organophosphate poisoning. J.A.M.A. 216:2131, 1971.

Morgan W. K. C., and Seaton, A.: Occupational Lung Diseases. Philadelphia, W. B. Saunders Co., 1975.

Myschetzky, A., and Lassen, N. A.: Forced diuresis in treatment of acute barbiturate poisoning. In Matthew, H. (Ed.): Acute Barbiturate Poisoning. Amsterdam, Excerpta Medica, 1971, pp. 95–204.

Peterson, R. G., and Rumack, B. H.: Treating acute acetaminophen poisoning with acetylcysteine. J.A.M.A. 237:2406, 1977.

Plum, F.: Acute sedative drug poisoning. In Beeson, P., and McDermott, W. (Eds.): Textbook of Medicine. 16th ed. Philadelphia, W. B. Saunders Co., 1982.

Prasad, A. S. (Ed.): Trace Elements in Human Health and Disease. New York, Academic Press, 1976, pp. 1–20, 401–416, 443–476.

Prasad, A. S., and Oberleas, D.: Thymidine kinase activity and incorporation of thymidine into DNA in zinc-deficient tissue. J. Lab. Clin. Med. *83*:634, 1974.

Prescott, L. F., Park, J., Sutherland, G. R., et al.: Cysteamine, methionine, and penicillamine in the treatment of paracetomol poisoning. Lancet 2:109, 1976.

Thurston, J. H., Pollock, P. G., and Warren, S. K.: Reduced brain glucose with normal plasma glucose in salicylate poisoning. J. Clin. Invest. *49*:2139, 1970.

Tobis, J.: Cardiac complications in amitriptyline poisoning: successful treatment with physostigmine. J.A.M.A. *235*:1474, 1976.

Truitt, J. B., Jr., and Walsh, M. J.: The role of acetaldehyde in the action of ethanol. *In* Kissin B., and Begleiter, H. (Eds.): The Biology of Alcoholism. Vol. I. New York, Plenum Press, 1971, pp. 186–187.

Von Wartburg, J. P.: The metabolism of alcohol in normals and alcoholics: enzymes. *In* Kissin, B., and Begleiter, H. (Eds.): The Biology of Alcoholism. Vol. I. New York, Plenum Press, 1971, pp. 63–102.

Wallgren, H.: Effect of ethanol on intracellular respiration and cerebral function. *In* Kissin, B., and Begleiter, H. (Eds.): The Biology of Alcoholism. Vol. I. New York, Plenum Press, 1971, pp. 117–119.

INDEX

Note: Page numbers in *italics* indicate figures; page numbers followed by (t) refer to tables.

Cardiac output, 341(t)
  abnormal states and, 207–208, *208*
  aortic coarctation and, 249
  arterial pressure and, 214–215, 235, *235*
  arterial pulsation and, 226
  autonomic control of, 294
  circulatory filling pressure and, 205–206
  congestive heart failure and, 332–333, 341
  heart and, 204
  hypertension and, 215–216, 343
  in essential hypertension, 251–252
  in postural hypotension, 257, 258(t)
  insufficiency of, 208
  measurement of, Fick method of, 292–293
    indicator dilution method of, 293
    methods of, 206–207, *206*, *207*
    thermodilution technique of, 293
  normal, 293
  peripheral circulation and, 204–207
  peripheral oxygen requirement and, 294
  regulation of, 204–208, 293–294
  renovascular hypertension and, 247
  systemic vascular resistance and, 347
  tachycardia and, 343
  therapeutic control of, 295
  thermoregulation and, 542
  tissue activity and, 203, *203*
  vascular resistance and, 294–295
  venous return and, 205, *206*, *207*
Cardiography, precordial movements and,
    361–362, *362*
Cardiolipin, formation of, 11
Cardiomyopathy, 272, 322
  classification of, 323(t)
  idiopathic, 323–324
  nonobstructive, 324
  obstructive, 323–324
  peripartum, 324
  precordial movements in, 364
  presystolic impulses in, 365
  quadruple rhythm and, 355
  secondary, 325
Cardiopulmonary bypass (CPB), bleeding syn-
    dromes associated with, 753(t)
  hemostasis alterations of, diagnosis of, 753–
    754
    management of, 754
    pathophysiology of, 749–752
    prevention of, 752–753
  platelet counts during, *749*
  vascular defects and, 721
Cardiorespiratory system, pathophysiologic
    changes in, fever and, 542
Cardiovascular disease, congenital, Di-
    George's syndrome and, 154
  erythrocytosis of, 667–668
  hemosiderosis and, 679
Cardiovascular system, allergic disease of,
    517(t)
  arterial pressure and, 235, *235*
  syphilis and, 568
Carditis, rheumatic fever and, 505
Caries, fluoride and, 989, 989(t)
Carotene, 44
Carotid artery, chemoreceptors of, 210
  blood acid-base balance and, 458
  endogenous pyrogen and, 545
Carotid sinus, arterial pressure and, 239

Carpal tunnel syndrome, acromegaly and,
    1003
Cartilage, articular, 490–491, *491*
  degeneration of, 494
  erosion of, 493–494
  joint inflammation and, 497
  fibrillated, erosion of, 494
  trauma to, 496
"Cascade" system, 705
Catabolism, acute infection and, 557
Catalysis, in biologic systems, 26
  macromolecules and, 28
  of enzymes, 41
Catalyst, kinetics of, 26
Cataract, "glass-blower's," 1071
  in galactosemia, 95
  metabolic defect of, 92, 95
  microwave radiation and, 1069
Catecholamine, biosynthesis of, 1029
  blood flow and, 203
  calorigenic activity of, 967
  deficiency of, disorders of, 1030–1031
  degradation of, 1030
  elevation of, congestive heart failure and,
    340
  ileus and, 822
  in chromaffin cells, 117–119
  in endotoxic shock, 533
  in hypersensitivity, 142
  kidney and, 214
  mechanisms of action of, 1029–1030
  myocardial failure and, 339, 339(t)
Catheterization, pulsus alternans and, 227
Cecum, activity in, 857(t)
  inflammatory bowel disease in, 863–864
Cell, chemical composition of, 3
  chemical reactivity in, 27–28
  cycle of, 68, *68*, 105
    interphase in, 68
  division of, kinetics of, 26
  fusion of, in genetic engineering, 49
  informational system of, nucleic acids and,
    28
  metabolism of, iron deficiency and, 677
  normal, vs. malignant, 760–761
  organelles of, 45
  structural properties of, protein and, 28
  surface markers of, 30
Cell division, 26. See also *Meiosis; Mitosis.*
Cell membrane, proteins of, 43
Cellular engineering, 104
Cellulitis, anaerobic, 526
Cellulose, colonic digestion of, 859
Central nervous system, chemical transmis-
    sion in, 143
  chronic viral infections of, 556
  endocrine gland regulation and, 999
  endogenous pyrogens and, 545
  food intake regulation by, 968
  headache and, 546
  ischemic response of, 210
  pain-sensitive structures of, 546
  syphilis and, 568
Central nervous system decompression sick-
    ness, 1063
Centromere, 64, 105
  banding of, 65
Cephalin, 11(t)

Ceramide, 11
Cerebellum, abscess of, 534
  edema of, meningitis and, 572
  hemangioblastoma of, secondary polycy-
    themia due to, 668
Cerebral edema, meningitis and, 572
Cerebrospinal fluid, abnormalities of, menin-
    gitis and, 573, 576
  meningitis and, 572
  respiratory regulation and, 458
Cerebrospinal nerve, abdominal pain and,
    transmission of, 797
Cerebrovascular disease, hypotension and,
    259
Cerebrum, abscess of, 534
  circulation to, postural hypotension and,
    256–257
Cervix, squamous cell carcinoma of, blood
    group antigens and, 162
Chagas' disease, 781
Charcot's joint, 496, 568
Charcot-Leyden crystal, 611
Chediak-Higashi syndrome, 157–158
  platelet function defect in, 723, 726(t)
Chemical(s), ingestion of, 1084
  parenteral administration of, 1084
  percutaneous absorption of, 1083
  respiratory absorption of, 1083–1084
  toxic, 1092–1095(t)
Chemical mediator, cell storage or synthesis
    of, 113–123
Chemoreceptor reflex, 210, 211
  arterial pressure regulation and, 241
Chemotherapy, 603–605, 766
  combination, 767–768
  drug and chemical reactions in, 605
  fibrinolysis and, 754
Chenodeoxycholic acid, 892, 893, 911
  colonic absorption of, 859–860
Chest, lymphatic drainage of, 217
Chest wall, pulsations of, 363
Cheyne-Stokes respiration, acute mountain
    sickness and, 667
Child(ren). See also Infant.
  gamma globulin synthesis in, 153
  innocent murmurs in, 359
  meningitis in, 575
  osteomyelitis in, 580, 581
  poliomyelitis in, 577
  streptococcal infection in, glomerulonephri-
    tis and, 430
  tuberculosis in, meningitis and, 576
Chloramphenicol, aplastic anemia and, 682,
    682(t)
Chloride, colonic absorption of, 859
  in chloridorrhea, 870
  in small intestine, transport of, 840–841
Chloride ion, transport of, kidney and, 408,
    408
Chloride shift, 453
Chloridorrhea, 870
  congenital, 90(t), 91
Chokes, 1063
Cholangiography, endoscopic retrograde, 887
  transhepatic, 886–887
Cholangiopancreatography, endoscopic retro-
    grade (ERCP), 938–939
Cholangitis, sclerosing, 917

Cholecystitis, pathophysiology of, 911–916
  prevalence of, 911
Cholecystokinin, colonic activity and, 856
Cholecystokinin-pancreozymin, 910
  physiologic effects of, 842(t)
  secretion of, 842, 842(t)
Cholelithiasis, hemolytic anemia and, 649
  pathophysiology of, 911–916
  prevalence of, 911
  sickle cell disease and, 671
Cholera, electrolytes in, abnormal fluxes of,
    841
  fluid in, abnormal fluxes of, 841
  pathophysiologic disturbances of, 531
  simple diarrhea and, 861
Cholera enterotoxin, 524(t), 531–532
Choleresis, 910
Cholestasis, 895–896, 895(t)
Cholesterol, 12
  biosynthesis of, coronary heart disease and,
    96, 97
  gallstones of, 896, 912(t), 913–914
  in bile, 892, 892(t), 893
  in red blood cell membrane, 650(t), 651
  metabolism of, 914, 915
  steroid biosynthesis and, 1018
  structure of, 12
  synthesis of, 12, 13
    hypothyroidism and, 1012
    in liver, 896
Cholesterolosis, vs. polypoid lesions, 916
Cholestyramine, bile acid diarrhea and, 863
  mucosal transport defects and, 837
Cholic acid, 911
  synthesis of, 892, 892
Cholinergic receptor, 145
Cholinesterase, serum, 100
Chondrocyte, 489, 491
Christmas disease, 98, 731, 733, 733(t)
Christmas factor, 710(t)
  activation of, 551
Chromaffin cell, 116
  function of, 118–119
Chromatid, 64, 105
Chromatin, 105
  composition of, 84
  female sex, 74–75, 75, 107
  male sex, 74–75, 107
Chromosome, 63–69, 106. See also X chromo-
    some; Y chromosome.
  abnormalities of, 69–71
    classification of, 70(t)
    clinical syndromes and, 53
    Fanconi's anemia and, 683
    human development and, 36
    malignancy and, 760
    numerical, 33, 69, 71–79
    polycythemia vera and, 665
    structural, 69–70, 80–83
  acrocentric, 64, 105
  arm of, 105
  autosome, 105
  balanced translocation of, 105
  banding of, 64–65, 66–68
  break in, 105
    syndromes of, 81–82
  C-band polymorphisms of, 65
  centric fusion of, 80

Free fatty acid. See *Fatty acid, free.*
Friedreich's ataxia, cardiomyopathy and, 324
Frostbite, 1071
Fructose, absorption of, 828, *828*
Fujiwara factor, 710(t)
Functional residual capacity, 438
  airflow resistance and, 441–442
Fundic gland, cells of, gastric secretory products of, 794, *794*
Furosemide, 421

G cell, gastrin in, 792–794
G force, 1079
G vector, 1078
G6P. See *Glucose-6-phosphate.*
G6PD. See *Glucose-6-phosphate dehydrogenase.*
Galactorrhea, hyperprolactinemia and, 1002
Galactose, absorption of, 828, *828*
  congenital malabsorption of, 837–838
Galactosemia, 52, 92, 95
Gallbladder, adenocarcinoma of, 916
  congenital lesions of, 917
  cystic fibrosis and, 961
  disease of, 911–916
    clinical evaluation of, 917
    management of, 918–920
  empyema of, 919
  function of, 910–911
    cholesterol stones and, 914–915
  neoplasms of, 916
  perforation of, 919
  rupture of, 919
  structure of, 910
Gallop rhythm, 355
Gallop sound, 355
  atrial systole and, *356*
Gallstone, bilirubin, formation of, *913*
  bilirubinate, 911–912
  calcium bilirubinate, 912
  cholesterol, 896, 912(t), 913–915
  dissolution of, 915–916, 916(t)
  erythrohepatic protoporphyria and, 700
  pigment, 912–913, 912(t)
  types of, 911–914, 912(t)
Gamma globulin, glomerulonephritis and, 554
  maternal, neonatal hypogammaglobulinemia and, 152–153
  rheumatoid arthritis and, 505
Gamma glutamyl transpeptidase, endoplasmic reticulum injury and, 882
Gamma ray, 1073
Gammopathy, polyclonal, 632
Ganglioneuromatosis, medullary carcinoma and, 1015
Ganglioside, botulinum toxin binding by, 530
  Tay-Sachs disease and, 11
Gangrene, congestive heart failure and, 345
  gas, 526
Gas, diffusion of, in lung, 438
  exchange of, alveolar perfusion and, 449
    dynamic compliance and, 447
  flow of, regulation of, 441
  in large intestine, 860
  transport of, in blood, 451–453
Gas transfer factor, 458
Gaseous environment, 1059–1066

Gastrectomy, Zollinger-Ellison syndrome and, 804
Gastrin, gastric secretion and, 791–793, *792*
  serum, in duodenal ulcer, 802
  Zollinger-Ellison syndrome and, 804
Gastritis, 797–798
  acute, 798–799
  atrophic, 799–800
    gastric carcinoma and, 809
    hypergastrinemia and, 793
  chronic, pernicious anemia and, 687
  chronic superficial, 799–800
  giant hypertrophic, 800
  granulomatous, 801
  hypertrophic glandular, 800
Gastroenteritis, eosinophilic, 800–801
  immunodeficiency syndrome and, 846
  salmonella and, 565
Gastroesophageal reflux, hiatal hernia and, 784
  prevention of, 783–785
  regurgitation and, 784–785
  sphincter pressure and, 783
  strictures and, 780–781
  systemic sclerosis and, 778
Gastrointestinal tract, allergic diseases of, 517(t)
  calcium homeostasis and, 1024
  disease of, primary immunodeficiency syndromes and, 845(t)
  immunoglobulin allergy and, immunodeficiency syndrome and, 846
  lower, bleeding of, simple diverticula and, 864
  lymphoid tissue of, immunologic function of, 844
  mucosa of, esophageal mucosa and, 775–776
  upper, bleeding of, 806
Gaucher's disease, 610
  organomegaly of, 104–105
GBM. See *Glomerular basement membrane.*
Gene, 106
  cloning of, technology of, 50–51, *51*
  frequency of, in population, 60–61
  hemoglobin variants and, 87–88
  insertion of, in genetic engineering, 49–50
  locus of, 106
  mapping of, 82–83, 106
  noncoding sequences of, 46
  of immune response, 128–129
  recombination of, 107
  regulation of, in treatment of heritable disorders, 105
  "sticky" fragments of, 50
  structure of, 30
  trans, in genetics, 107
  transfer of, deficiency disease therapy by, 48
Genetic code, 86
Genetic counseling, 55, 104
Genetic disease. See *Inherited disease.*
Genetic engineering, 49–51
Genetics, 53–112. See also *Inheritance.*
  environment interaction with, 101–102
  glossary of terms in, 105–107
  Hardy-Weinberg law of, 60–63
  Mendelian priciples of, 53–60
  metabolic disorders in, 89–103
  molecular basis of, 83–89

Granulocytopoiesis, ineffective, 606
Granuloma, bone marrow diagnosis of, 586
 immune injury and, 194–195, *195*
Granulomatous disease, chronic (CGD), 598
 in phagocytic disorders, 157
Granulomatous thyroiditis, 1014
Graves' disease, autoimmunity and, 177
 HLA antigen and, 173
Gravity, 1077
Ground substance, 487–489
 proteoglycan in, *488,* 489–490
 synovitis and, 497
Growth, disturbances of, magnetic fields and, *1066*
Growth factor, insulinlike, 1005
Growth failure, pituitary and, 1004–1005
Growth hormone, calorigenic activity of, 967
 function of, 1000
 lipase and, 10
 metabolic regulation by, 22
 obesity and, 972
 secretion of, pituitary tumor and, 1002
Guanethidine, ileus and, 822
Guanidinosuccinic acid, platelet function defect and, 725
Guanosine monophosphate, 21
Guanosine triphosphate, 144
Guanyl nucleotide-binding protein, 144
Guillain-Barré syndrome, vs. diphtheria, 525
Gumma, syphilis and, 568
Gunther's disease, 698

H graft, *885*
Hageman factor, 710(t)
 activation of, *550,* 551
 acute gouty arthritis and, 500
 complement activation and, 713
 deficiency of, 736
 endotoxin activation of, 533
 in synovial fluid, 501
 joint inflammation and, 498
 nephritis and, 430
 plasminogen activation and, 711
Hair, hypopigmentation of, 95
Hallucinosis, alcohol withdrawal and, 1091
Halothane, malignant hyperthermia due to, 1085
Hand-foot syndrome, sickle cell disease and, 671
Hand-Schüller-Christian disease, 609
Haptoglobin, 657
Hardy-Weinberg law, 60–61
Hartnup disease, 90(t), 91, 425
 amino acid transport and, 838
 defective membrane transport in, 90(t), 91
 prevention of, 104
Hashimoto's thyroiditis, 1012, 1014
 Turner's syndrome and, 77
Hassall's corpuscle, 122
Head, squamous cell carcinoma of, blood group antigens and, 162
Headache, fever and, 545–546
Hearing, human range of, heart sounds and, *351*
 loss of, 1081
 sickle cell disease and, 671

Heart. See also *Myocardium.*
 acute failure of, 206–207, *207*
 recovery and, 207
 artificial, 347–348
 as muscle, ventricular hypertrophy of, 337–338
 as pump, ventricular ejection in, 335
 ventricular hypertrophy of, 337–338
 calcium and, 266
 cardiac output and, 204–207
 catheterization of, 295–302
 compliance of, atrial sounds and, 355
 contractile proteins of, 264–268, *265, 267*
 contraction of, 261–291
 actin-myosin linkage in, 279
 excitation-contraction coupling in, 277–287, *280*
 mechanical activation and, 279
 mechanical relaxation in, 282
 mechanism of, 261–291
 mitochondria and, 270
 myosin ATPase activity and, 282
 troponin phosphorylation and, 266
 disease of. See *Cardiovascular disease.*
 ECG and, 368
 electrical impulse and, 371
 excitation of, 277–287
 propagation of, 374
 failure of. See *Congestive heart failure; Heart failure.*
 fiber orientation of, ECG and, 372
 fourth sound of, 355
 hypertrophy of, ECG and, 370
 genetics and, 285
 hyperthyroidism and, 285
 physiologic, 285
 RNA polymerase increase in, 285
 ventricular pressure and, 285
 ischemic disease of. See *Ischemic heart disease.*
 lesions of, ventricular activation and, 377
 murmur of, 357
 performance of, 333–335, 333(t), *334–335*
 left ventricular ejection in, 333
 ventricular contraction patterns in, 333–335, *334, 335*
 precordial movements of, 361–365
 preload state of, congestive heart failure and, 346–347, 346(t)
 protein of, polymerization in, 266
 synthesis mechanisms in, 273–275
 recovery time of, myocardial infarction and, 381–382
 second sound of, fixed splitting of, *355*
 paradoxic splitting of, 352, *354*
 size of, ventricular hypertrophy and, 337
 sounds of, aortic and pulmonary component of, 352, *353, 354*
 subcellular organizational structure of, 261
 superficial membrane system of, 268
 third sound of, 354
 tissue destruction of, ECG and, 381
 valves of, anatomic relationship of, *563*
 disease of. See *Valvular heart disease.*
 heart sounds and, 350
 leakage of, left ventricular ejection and, 333
 ventricle. See *Ventricle.*